The NutriBase

NUTRITION FACTS

DESK REFERENCE

The NutriBase

NUTRITION FACTS

DESK REFERENCE

Avery
a member of Penguin Putnam Inc.
New York

Most Avery books are available at special quantity discounts for bulk purchase for sales promotions, premiums, fund-raising, and educational needs. Special books or book excerpts also can be created to fit specific needs. For details, write Putnam Special Markets, 375 Hudson Street, New York, NY 10014.

a member of
Penguin Putnam Inc.
375 Hudson Street
New York, NY 10014
www.penguinputnam.com

Library of Congress Cataloging-in-Publication Data

The NutriBase nutrition facts desk reference.—2nd ed.
        p.   cm.
      Rev. ed. of: The NutriBase nutrition facts desk reference / Art Ulene.
      ISBN 1-58333-001-1
      1. Food—Composition—Tables.   I. Ulene, Art. NutriBase nutrition facts desk reference.
   II. CyberSoft, Inc.

   TX551 .N75   2001   2001034083
   613.2'8—dc21

Printed in the United States of America
10 9 8 7 6 5 4 3 2 1

CONTENTS

Introduction . . . . *vii*

How to Use This Book . . . . *xvii*

Codes and Abbreviations . . . . *xix*

Table of Measurement Conversions . . . . *xxi*

Part One   **General Nutrient Values** **1**

Calories • Protein • Carbohydrates • Sodium • Fiber • Fat •
Saturated Fat • Cholesterol • Percentage of Calories from Fat

Part Two   **Vitamin and Mineral Values** **665**

Vitamin A • Thiamine • Riboflavin • Niacin • Vitamin B_6 •
Folic Acid • Vitamin B_{12} • Vitamin C • Calcium • Iron •
Magnesium • Potassium • Zinc

Part Three   **Fast-Food/Chain Restaurant Values** **867**

Calories • Protein • Carbohydrates • Sodium • Fiber • Fat •
Saturated Fat • Cholesterol • Percentage of Calories from Fat

INTRODUCTION

For thousands of years, people have recognized the life-sustaining nature of food. But only during the last four or five decades have we begun to understand the many ways in which our choices of foods can affect the quality of our health and the length of our lives. And only during the last five or ten years have we really begun to appreciate how profound the effects of those choices can be.

Now we know that some of the so-called "inevitable" diseases, such as atherosclerosis, osteoporosis, and even cancer are often the consequences of poor nutritional choices. Research has clearly shown the relationship between poor nutritional intake and many of these diseases. The studies prove that a high-fat diet can—and often does—contribute to the development of coronary artery disease; that low fiber intake promotes the development of colon cancer; that folic acid deficiency increases the risk of birth defects; and that inadequate calcium intake fosters the onset of osteoporosis and bone fractures. The list of nutrition-related disorders goes on and on.

There is a hopeful side to this story. Studies have clearly demonstrated the positive effects that good nutritional choices can have on our health. Many cases of cardiovascular disease can be prevented, and even reversed, through dietary changes. The incidence of cancer can be reduced with diets that are low in fat and high in cruciferous vegetables (broccoli and cauliflower, for instance) and through the use of the antioxidant nutrients, such as vitamins C and E. Bone strength can be increased and fracture rates decreased with a diet rich in calcium and vitamin D. Blood cholesterol levels can be reduced with dietary fiber, niacin, and garlic. Blood pressure can be lowered with sodium restriction and calcium and magnesium supplementation. The list of health-promoting nutritional interventions is lengthy and is growing constantly.

THE NEW NUTRITION

Modern research studies are giving rise to a "new" nutrition, one that is both scientifically sound and practical. The new nutrition differs from the old in at least two important ways. First, the old nutrition dealt in generalities, such as the four food groups, and created minimum dietary recommendations designed to prevent deficiency-related disorders. The new nutrition seeks to achieve *optimal* levels of health and creates specific recommendations based on individual differences, such as age, sex, lifestyle, and medical factors. Second, the old nutrition left many nutritional decisions up to the health professionals and food marketers, while the new nutrition puts *you* in control. It empowers you with the information necessary to evaluate confusing and conflicting claims, and it enables you to reject foods that do not meet your nutritional needs and goals.

This book is designed to provide you with that empowering information. It will help you make wiser choices when you buy food and when you dine out. It will help you interpret nutritional stories in the media so you can distinguish useful information from nonsense. It will give you the control you need over your personal nutrition.

Many people refer to books of this sort as "counter" books, because of the nutritional numbers that fill the pages. But this is not a book about counting. This is a book about *control* and *choices*. Use this book to learn more about the foods you should consume—or avoid—so you can meet your particular nutritional needs. Don't be intimidated by the huge number of choices listed or by all the nutritional value numbers that accompany the lists. It is not necessary to memorize these numbers. Instead, just try to familiarize yourself with the foods and food categories that are best suited to your needs. Begin by looking up the foods that you eat most often or in the largest quantities. If these foods are not providing you with the nutrients you need, use the book to find better alternatives that are just as tasty. Once you are familiar with the nutritional content of your most common food choices, gradually look up the remainder of the foods in your diet. You'll be surprised by how easy it is to learn about these foods and to make any necessary changes.

As you take more control over the foods you are eating and put more thought into your choices, keep in mind that good nutrition is just one element of a healthy lifestyle. To achieve maximum benefits from the new nutrition, your life should be filled with physical activity and free of cigarette smoke and other toxic substances. In addition, the stress in your life should be under control. Even the best diet can't overcome the problems caused by smoking, an immoderate use of alcohol, poorly managed stress, or other health-compromising habits.

Finally, be aware that research is constantly adding to our knowledge of nutrition and in the process changing some of our beliefs. As best you can, try to keep up with the new information and, when appropriate, make whatever dietary changes are necessary. But also be skeptical about nutritional news that seems too good to be true. (More often than not, it isn't true.) Be wary of nutritional claims made by people who are trying to sell you something. And be cautious—don't make any drastic changes in your nutritional program without first talking to a health professional who is knowledgeable about nutrition and about your particular medical circumstances. Don't forget: If the right nutritional choices are powerful enough to keep you well, it is only logical that the wrong ones could make you sick.

The following section will explain some of the basics of nutrition. After that, you will learn how to use this book to locate the information you need to improve your diet.

A QUICK LOOK AT THE BASIC NUTRIENTS AND MICRONUTRIENTS

Everyone's diet must contain the four basic nutrients—water, complex carbohydrates, protein, and fats—as well as the micronutrients, which are the vitamins and minerals. These nutrients and micronutrients fuel the body and enable all bodily functions to occur. A proper balance of these essentials is necessary for optimum health.

This book presents the nutrient values of a wide range of foods, both whole and processed. In order to wisely use this information, it is important to have a basic understanding of the function of the nutrients and micronutrients needed by the body.

The Nutrients

Water, complex carbohydrates, protein, and fats are the basic building blocks of a healthy diet. Each works in different ways to fuel the body, build and repair the cells that make up the body, and provide the environment in which the cells live.

Water

The human body is two-thirds water by weight. Indeed, water is an essential nutrient that is involved in every function of the body. It helps transport nutrients and waste products into and out of cells. It is necessary for all digestive, absorptive, circulatory, and excretory functions, and for the utilization of the water-soluble vitamins. And it is needed to maintain proper body temperature.

Most of us are aware of some of the early signs of dehydration: scant or dark urine, thirst, and a dry mouth. If the body continues to be denied adequate water, serious health problems can occur, necessitating hospitalization.

Complex Carbohydrates

Complex carbohydrates provide the body with the energy it needs to function. Signs of an inadequate supply of complex carbohydrates include lack of energy and the breakdown of proteins in tissues.

One type of carbohydrate you may have heard a good deal about is fiber. Referred to in the past as roughage, fiber is actually the part of plant material that our body cannot digest. Yet fiber is known to perform a number of important functions. It promotes feelings of fullness; prevents constipation, hemorrhoids, and other intestinal problems; and is associated with a reduced incidence of colon cancer. In addition, fiber may help lower blood cholesterol levels, reducing the risk of heart disease.

Protein

Protein is essential for growth and development. It provides the body with energy, and is needed for the manufacture of hormones, antibodies, enzymes, and muscle tissues. It also helps maintain the proper acid-alkali balance. Inadequate protein intake can result in stunted growth, diarrhea, vomiting, lack of appetite, and edema, a buildup of fluids in the tissues.

Fats

Much attention has been focused on the need to limit dietary fat intake. Nevertheless, the body does need fats—but the right fats, and in appropriate quantities. Specifically, it needs essential fatty acids, which perform a variety of vital bodily functions. Essential fatty acids carry the fat-soluble vitamins. They are essential for growth and development and for the maintenance of healthy skin, hair, and nails. And they provide the body with energy. A variety of problems can occur if the body fails to receive adequate amounts of essential fatty acids. Signs of deficiency may include retarded growth; skin, hair, and nail disorders; and an impaired metabolism of fats and fat-soluble vitamins.

Most of us are aware that there are several kinds of dietary fat—saturated, polyunsaturated, and monounsaturated—and that some are better than others. To understand the difference between these three types of fats, it is helpful to first learn a little about cholesterol.

Cholesterol is a white, waxy, fatty substance produced by the liver. It is essential to our well-being, as it helps to build cell membranes, to produce hormones, and to manufacture bile acids. The liver is capable of manufacturing all of the cholesterol needed for good health.

The cholesterol manufactured by the liver is carried through the bloodstream by molecules known as low-density lipoproteins, or LDLs. High levels of LDLs in the bloodstream are associated with clogged arteries, high blood pressure, stroke, and heart disease. This is why LDL is sometimes referred to as "bad cholesterol." Fortunately, many people can reduce their LDL levels through proper diet.

High-density lipoproteins, or HDLs, are molecules that carry excess cholesterol from different body tissues back to the liver, where the excess cholesterol is converted into bile acids and then eliminated through the intestines. High levels of HDLs are linked with a decreased risk of cardiovascular disease. This is why HDL is often called "good cholesterol." To a limited extent, HDL levels can be raised through regular exercise.

How are the three types of fats related to cholesterol? Saturated fats—which come from foods of animal origin such as meat, fish, poultry, milk, butter, and cheese, as well as from palm, coconut, and palm kernel oil—have been shown to increase total blood cholesterol levels, especially the undesirable LDL portion. Polyunsaturated fats—found mainly in vegetable oils like corn, sunflower, safflower, and soybean—tend to lower levels of both HDL and LDL. Monounsaturated fats—found mainly in certain vegetable and nut oils, including olive, peanut, and canola—have been shown to reduce total blood cholesterol without lowering levels of the good cholesterol, HDL. Indeed, some monounsaturated fats have been shown to raise HDL levels.

Most experts agree that it is best to limit fat consumption and to choose mostly monounsaturated fats, which increase the levels of HDL while lowering total blood cholesterol. There is, in fact, no biological need for saturated fat!

A Word About Calories

When we talk about foods, we often mention the number of calories a certain food has. Calories are not among the four basic nutrients, nor are they considered micronutrients. What, then, are calories?

A calorie is an energy unit. As already discussed, carbohydrates, protein, and fats provide the body with the energy it needs to function. This energy is measured in calories. There are, for instance, approximately four calories in every gram of protein, four calories in every gram of carbohydrate, and nine calories in every gram of fat. It is no wonder, then, that people who are trying to lose weight are often advised to cut down on fatty foods. On a gram-for-gram basis, fat is more than twice as fattening as carbohydrates or protein.

In addition to having more calories than protein or carbohydrates, dietary fat is metabolized differently. Because dietary fat is similar in chemical composition to body fat, it takes less energy to convert it to body fat. In fact, it takes only 3 percent of the calories in the fat we eat to turn that food into body fat, while it takes at least 25 percent of the calories in the carbohydrates and protein we eat to convert them into body fat. Remember, though, that if you eat more calories than your body needs, regardless of the nutrient source of these calories, the excess will be stored as body fat.

The Micronutrients

Like water, carbohydrates, protein, and fats, vitamins and minerals are essential to life. As such, they are considered nutrients. They are often referred to as micronutrients because they are needed in relatively small amounts compared with the four basic nutrients.

Vitamins

Vitamins are organic compounds, which means that they occur naturally in plants and animals. Generally, vitamins function as coenzymes. Enzymes are the catalysts, or activators, in all of the chemical reactions that are continually taking place in the human body.

As coenzymes, vitamins work with the enzymes and allow all activities that occur within the body to happen quickly and accurately. In addition to this role, some vitamins have other functions. For instance, vitamin D functions as a hormone.

Each vitamin is classified as either water-soluble or fat-soluble, depending on whether fat- or water-based molecules transport that vitamin in the bloodstream. Water-soluble vitamins include all of the B-complex vitamins and vitamin C. These vitamins are either used by the body in a short period of time—two to four days—or excreted. As a result, they must be replenished daily through diet or supplements. Fat-soluble vitamins stay in the body longer, and are stored in the body's fat tissues and in some organs, especially the liver. Vitamins A, D, E, and K are all fat-soluble vitamins.

Each vitamin has specific functions. Even a brief look at the major functions performed by each of these nutrients shows just how important they are to our health.

Vitamin A plays an important role in strengthening the mucous membranes, the immune system, the adrenal glands, and the eyes. Moreover, beta-carotene—a compound that the body converts to vitamin A—is an antioxidant and thus works to neutralize harmful substances known as free radicals. As such, beta-carotene appears to help protect the body against a variety of disorders, including cancer and heart disease. A deficiency of vitamin A can lead to visual problems, including night blindness, an increased susceptibility to infection, impaired growth, and impaired functioning of the reproductive organs.

Thiamine (vitamin B_1) supports the healthy functioning of the heart, muscles, and nerves, and plays a role in the breakdown of carbohydrates. Too little thiamine can result in fatigue, constipation, loss of appetite, memory loss, irritability, and depression. In the most severe cases of thiamine deprivation, a now-rare disease known as beriberi may result.

Riboflavin (vitamin B_2) plays a role in the breakdown and use of carbohydrates, fats, and protein; is involved in cell energy production; supports the production of adrenal hormones; and helps the body utilize other vitamins. Riboflavin deficiency may be signaled by light-sensitivity and other eye problems, loss of appetite, impaired growth, anemia, dry skin, and depression.

Niacin (vitamin B₃) is necessary for the breakdown of carbohydrates and fats, the healthy functioning of the nervous and digestive systems, the production of sex hormones, and the maintenance of healthy skin. Signs of niacin deficiency include fatigue, irritability, depression, confusion, insomnia, blood sugar fluctuations, and arthritis. In the case of severe deficiencies, the now-rare disease known as pellagra may result.

Pantothenic acid (vitamin B₅) is involved in the breakdown and use of carbohydrates and fats, in normal growth and development, in the production of adrenal and sex hormones, and in the body's use of other vitamins. Headaches, nausea, abdominal cramps, fatigue, depression, an increased susceptibility to colds, insomnia, and numbness and tingling in the hands and feet are all possible signs of pantothenic acid deficiency.

Pyridoxine (vitamin B₆) is used in the breakdown of protein, carbohydrates, and fats; in the healthy functioning of the nervous and digestive systems; in the production of red blood cells and antibodies; and in the maintenance of healthy skin. Some of the most common symptoms of pyridoxine deficiency are an impaired immune system, anemia, inflammation of the tongue, weakness, dizziness, nausea and vomiting, and depression.

Cobalamin (vitamin B₁₂) is needed for growth and development, the production of red blood cells, the body's use of folic acid, and healthy nervous system function. Too little of this nutrient can lead to pernicious anemia, a disorder signaled by weakness, weight loss, and pale skin; loss of coordination; tingling in the hands and feet; moodiness; and depression.

Biotin, also a B-complex vitamin, is involved in the metabolism of fatty acids, carbohydrates, and protein; and in the maintenance of healthy skin, hair, sweat glands, nerves, and bone marrow. Biotin deficiency may result in dry and scaly skin, loss of appetite, muscle pain, nausea and vomiting, hair loss, insomnia, and depression.

Folic acid, another B-complex vitamin, is needed for growth, development, and reproduction; in the production of red blood cells; and in the functioning of the nervous system. It also supports the hair and skin. Signs of folic acid deficiency include anemia, digestive problems, and fatigue. In addition, maternal folic acid deficiency has been implicated as a cause of fetal nervous system abnormalities such as spina bifida.

Vitamin C, also known as ascorbic acid, has many functions. It helps maintain normal enzyme function; is important for the healthy growth of teeth, bones, gums, ligaments, and blood vessels; plays an important role in the immune system's response to infection and in healing; and helps in the absorption of iron from the digestive tract. In its role as an antioxidant, this nutrient also protects the body against a variety of disorders, including cancer. Vitamin C deficiency may result in slow wound healing, bleeding gums, recurrent infections, a tendency to bruise easily, and allergies. Severe deficits of vitamin C can result in scurvy, a now-rare disease.

Vitamin D supports bone and tooth formation, muscle function, and thyroid gland function and is necessary for the proper absorption of calcium, phosphorus, magnesium, and zinc. In severe cases, vitamin D deficiency can cause rickets, a disease whose symptoms include loss of appetite, slowed growth, and a softening of the bones.

Vitamin E aids in tissue healing, is essential for normal cell structure, helps maintain normal enzyme function, and is involved in the formation of red blood cells. In its role as an antioxidant, vitamin E protects the lungs against injury from air pollution and helps preserve tissues throughout the body. In addition, several major studies have shown that this nutrient may offer protection from heart disease. Recognized signs of vitamin E deficiency include loss of appetite, difficulty in walking, anemia, nausea, eye problems, and impairment of reproduction function.

Vitamin K is essential for blood clotting and bone formation. A lack of this vitamin is signaled by blood clotting difficulty.

Minerals

Minerals are inorganic elements, which means that they are not produced by plants and animals. Like vitamins, many minerals are needed for proper body function. For instance, minerals are essential in nerve responses and muscle contraction and are needed to maintain proper fluid balance and for the internal processing of nutrients. Some minerals have other functions as well. Calcium and phosphorus, for example, serve as building blocks for bones and teeth.

Depending on the amount in which they are needed in the body, minerals are categorized as either macrominerals or microminerals. The macrominerals, which include calcium, magnesium, phosphorus, potassium, and sodium, are needed in larger amounts than are the microminerals, which include boron, chromium, cobalt, copper, iron, selenium, silicon, and zinc. Each mineral, like each vitamin, performs specific functions in the body.

Calcium plays a role in bone and tooth formation, blood clotting, heart rhythm, nerve-impulse transmission, muscle growth and contraction, and the proper functioning of cell membranes. In addition, calcium contributes to lower blood pressure and may protect against colon cancer. Calcium deficiency can result in muscle cramps, irritability, and insomnia. The most common problem related to long-term calcium deficiency is osteoporosis, a condition in which bones lose their normal density and strength.

Chromium helps to maintain proper blood sugar levels and healthy functioning of the circulatory system. Too little of this mineral can result in blood sugar fluctuations and high cholesterol levels.

Cobalt is involved in the healthy functioning of red blood cells. An inadequate intake of cobalt can result in anemia, weakness, nausea, loss of appetite, and bleeding gums.

Copper plays a role in bone formation, hair and skin color, the healing processes, red blood cell production, and mental and emotional processes. Copper deficiency can show itself as anemia, inflammation, and arthritis.

Iron supports growth and development in children, is needed to produce hemoglobin, and supports a healthy immune system. The most common condition related to inadequate supplies of iron is iron deficiency anemia, a disorder whose symptoms include fatigue, irritability, headaches, shortness of breath, intolerance to cold, and an increased vulnerability to infection.

Magnesium is involved in blood sugar metabolism and energy maintenance, plays a role in the metabolism of calcium and vitamin C, and is used in the structuring of basic genetic material. Too little magnesium can cause depression, fatigue, irritability, muscle weakness or tremors, constipation, nausea, and rapid or irregular heartbeat.

Phosphorus is involved in bone and tooth formation, cell growth and repair, energy maintenance, heart contraction, kidney function, the healthy activity of nerves and muscles, and the body's use of vitamins. Phosphorus deficiency may be indicated by stunted growth, bone malformation and pain, weakness, and loss of appetite.

Potassium is needed for the healthy, steady functioning of the nervous system, and supports the normal functioning of the heart, muscles, kidneys, and blood. Too little potassium can cause muscle weakness, irregular heartbeat, loss of appetite, nausea and vomiting, and irritability.

Selenium is involved in the healthy functioning of cell membranes, may be involved in increasing resistance to cancer, and supports pancreatic function. Also, as an antioxidant, selenium appears to work with vitamin E to prevent injury to cells, and thus may help protect the body from several serious disorders. Poor growth, dry flaky scalp, muscular weakness and discomfort, and skin problems are all possible signs of selenium deficiency.

Silicon is used in bone formation and supports the skin, the major blood vessels, the connective tissue, and the thymus gland. A deficiency of this mineral may cause bone deformities, connective tissue disorders, muscle cramps, irritability, and insomnia.

Sodium helps maintain normal fluid levels in the body, is involved in healthy muscle functioning, and supports the blood and lymphatic systems. Fainting, intolerance to heat, headaches, muscle cramps, and swelling in the extremities may all result from an inadequate intake of sodium. It is important to note, though, that most people get too much sodium in their diets. Nutritionists recommend a maximum intake of about 3,000 milligrams of sodium per day.

Zinc promotes burn and wound healing, supports the immune system, is involved in carbohydrate and protein digestion, and plays a role in reproductive organ growth and development. Possible signs of zinc deficiency include white spots on the fingernails, stretch marks on the skin, hair loss, loss of the sense of smell or taste, joint pain, poor sexual development, menstrual irregularities, slow wound healing, and recurrent infections.

THE FOOD GUIDE PYRAMID

Because the four basic nutrients and the many micronutrients are essential to life and because most of them cannot be made by the body, we must get these nutrients from food or from nutritional supplements. The U.S. Department of Agriculture (USDA) encourages Americans to eat a well-balanced diet, which it illustrates with a diagram known as the Food Guide Pyramid. At the base of the pyramid are breads, cereals, rice, and pasta. Six to eleven servings from this group are recommended daily—more servings than from any other group of foods in the pyramid. The

Fats, Oils & Sweets
USE SPARINGLY

KEY
☐ Fat (naturally occurring and added) ▼ Sugars (added)

These symbols show fats, oils, and added sugars in food.

Milk, Yogurt, & Cheese Group
2-3 SERVINGS

Meats, Poultry, Fish, Dry Beans, Eggs, & Nuts Group
2-3 SERVINGS

Vegetable Group
3-5 SERVINGS

Fruit Group
2-4 SERVINGS

Bread, Cereal, Rice, & Pasta Group
6-11 SERVINGS

Source: U.S. Department of Agriculture &
U.S. Department of Health and Human Services

next level is occupied by vegetables, with three to five daily servings recommended, and by fruit, with two to four servings recommended. Moving upward, the next level is shared by milk, yogurt, and cheese—two to three servings—and meat, poultry, fish, dry beans, eggs, and nuts—two to three servings. Finally, at the peak of the pyramid are fats, oils, and sweets, for which there are no recommended amounts, only a note that they should be consumed sparingly.

To ensure that you have adequate servings of healthful foods, it is a good idea to follow the Food Guide Pyramid and, within each group, to choose foods that are high in the nutrients needed for good health. The remainder of this book shows how each food rates in terms of its nutrient values. To make sure that these foods are still high in nutrients when they reach your table and to help keep your diet low in fat and high in fiber, certain additional guidelines should be followed when selecting foods from each group. These include:

■ When choosing breads, cereals, rice, and pasta, always choose whole-grain, high-fiber, low-fat varieties, preferably without added sugar, coloring, or unnecessary preservatives. Choose brown rice over white rice and whole-grain pastas over pastas made from white flour.

■ Eat your vegetables and fruits fresh and, preferably, raw as often as possible. Water-soluble vitamins such as vitamin C may leach out of foods during normal cooking, be damaged by overprocessing, or be destroyed when foods are overcooked. Even fat-soluble vitamins, which are fairly stable during low-temperature cooking, can be affected by frying. For this reason, it is best to steam or microwave vegetables rather than to boil or fry them. And, unless produce is organically grown, be sure to peel or thoroughly wash it before eating to reduce such unwanted elements as waxes and pesticide residue.

■ Select low-fat and nonfat varieties of milk, yogurt, and cheese. These provide the most nutrients and the least amount of fat. When eating meat, poultry, or fish, choose the leanest cuts available, trim off any excess fat, and bake or broil the foods instead of frying them.

■ Select as few foods as possible from the fats, oils, and sweets category. When you do use fats and oils, choose monounsaturated and polyunsaturated fats instead of saturated ones. Limit your intake of sweets. Choose fresh fruits instead of cakes, cookies, and other high-fat desserts.

FOOD LABELING

Food labels are required to include a "Nutrition Facts" section that identifies how many servings are found in each container and how much of the following components each serving contains:

- Total calories
- Calories from fat
- Total fat
- Saturated fat
- Cholesterol
- Sodium
- Total carbohydrates
- Dietary fiber
- Sugars
- Protein
- Vitamin A
- Vitamin C
- Calcium
- Iron

For the last four nutrients, the amount is expressed only as a percentage of Daily Value—a recommended daily intake based on a 2,000-calorie diet. For most of the other nutrients listed, the amount is expressed both in grams or milligrams and as a percentage of its Daily Value. Reference values are provided to show how much total fat, saturated fat, cholesterol, sodium, total carbohydrates, and dietary fiber should be included in both a 2,000-calorie and a 2,500-calorie diet. All of this information is helpful, but problems remain. Many people—including older people and smaller people—need only 1,200 to 1,800 calories per day, not 2,000 or 2,500. Also, amounts of many nutrients known to be deficient in many people's diets—the B vitamins and magnesium, for instance—are not listed on the label. Also, the Daily Values for vitamins and minerals are based on the *minimum* amounts of these nutrients needed to prevent a deficiency state, not necessarily on the amount that would make for optimal health. Consequently, while they can be helpful for some things, food labels can hardly be considered an adequate source of information about nutrient content.

Then there are the numerous potentially confusing terms you find sprinkled across food labels. What many people do not know is that the U.S. Food and Drug Administration (FDA) has actually standardized some of the terms used on the labels of products it regulates, as well as on processed meat products that are regulated by the USDA. Following are definitions of some of the most frequently used terms:

■ **Free.** This means that the product contains no amount of, or only "physiologically inconsequential" amounts of, one or more of these components: fat, saturated fat, cholesterol, sodium, sugars, and calories. For instance, "calorie-free" means that there are fewer than 5 calories per serving. "Sugar-free" and "fat-free" indicate that there is less than 1/2 of a gram per serving of sugar and fat, respectively.

■ **Low.** This means the food can be eaten frequently without exceeding dietary guidelines for one or more of the following: fat, saturated fat, cholesterol, sodium, and calories. Thus, the following terms are used:

> **Low fat.** 3 grams or less per serving.

> **Low saturated fat.** 1 gram or less per serving.

> **Low sodium.** Less than 140 milligrams per serving.

> **Very low sodium.** Less than 35 milligrams per serving.

> **Low cholesterol.** Less than 20 milligrams per serving.

> **Low calorie.** 40 calories or less per serving.

■ **Lean and extra lean.** The following terms can be used to describe the fat content of meat, poultry, seafood, and game meats:

> **Lean.** Less than 10 grams of fat, less than 4 grams of saturated fat, and less than 95 mil-

ligrams of cholesterol per serving and per 100 grams.

> **Extra lean.** Less than 5 grams of fat, less than 2 grams of saturated fat, and less than 95 milligrams of cholesterol per serving and per 100 grams.

■ **High.** This means that one serving of the food contains 20 percent or more of the recommended daily intake of a particular nutrient.

■ **Good source.** This means that one serving of the food contains 10 to 19 percent of the recommended daily intake of a particular nutrient.

■ **Reduced.** This term denotes a nutritionally altered product that contains 25 percent less of a nutrient or of calories than the regular, or reference, product.

■ **Less.** This denotes a food, whether altered or not, that contains 25 percent less of a nutrient or of calories than the reference food.

■ **Light.** This designates a nutritionally altered product containing one-third fewer calories or half the fat of the reference food, or a low-calorie, low-fat food whose sodium content has been reduced by 50 percent.

■ **More.** This means that one serving of the food, altered or not, contains a nutrient in a quantity that is at least 10 percent of the recommended daily intake more than the reference food.

The following section should provide you with the details you need to better access and understand the data contained in this volume. With this information, and the information that makes up the bulk of this book, you will be equipped to learn more about your unique nutritional needs and the foods you are using to meet those needs. You should enjoy the sense of control this knowledge gives you. More important, you will make better food choices and take a major step toward better health.

HOW TO USE THIS BOOK

This book was designed to provide comprehensive nutritional information on a wide range of foods, both generic and brand name, raw and prepared. The information provided here was gleaned from a number of government agencies, from hundreds of manufacturers, and from food trade associations. This information was compiled and later supplemented through countless hours of follow-up that involved hundreds of additional sources. Because scientific techniques are continually being improved, this book will be continually updated to reflect the most current nutritional data available.

FINDING THE LISTING YOU WANT

This easy-to-use guide is divided into three parts. Part One is an A-to-Z reference to the general nutrients provided by foods. In this section, you will find the amount of calories, protein, carbohydrates, sodium, fiber, fat, saturated fat, and cholesterol, as well as the percentage of calories that come from fat.

Part Two is an A-to-Z reference to the vitamins and minerals provided by foods. This section states the amount of vitamin A, thiamine, riboflavin, niacin, vitamin B_6, folic acid, vitamin B_{12}, vitamin C, calcium, iron, magnesium, potassium, and zinc.

Part Three is an A-to-Z reference to the nutrient values of restaurant-chain foods. In this section, foods are listed alphabetically under the name of the appropriate restaurant, and each food item is accompanied by the amounts of the general nutrients found in that item.

All of the foods in this reference have been listed alphabetically. For instance, if you are looking for the nutrient values of ground beef, you would turn to the *B*'s and look under *Beef.* For convenience, similar foods have sometimes been grouped together in categories such as *Baby Foods, Breads, Candies, Cereals,*

Cheese, Cookies, Pasta, and *Sauces.* Therefore, if the food you are looking for is not listed individually by its own name, you should try looking it up under a logical category.

Always make sure to look in the appropriate part of the book. For instance, if you want to know the amount of a general nutrient, such as fat, look the product up in Part One. If you want to know whether a particular food is high in vitamin A, look in Part Two.

Some foods are known by two or more names. In most cases, the food is listed under just one name and cross-references have been provided to guide you to the proper listing. For instance, chickpeas are also called garbanzo and ceci beans. In this book, you will find the nutrient information under *Chickpeas,* with cross-references under *Ceci* and *Garbanzo.*

If you are unable to find a particular food, look for the entry for a similar food. The nutritional data should be close, if not exact, for any product not listed.

After you locate the listing for the food you are interested in, you may find that abbreviations have been used to provide you with the information you need. Refer to page xix for a key to the abbreviations used throughout this book.

When examining the nutrient values of cooked generic foods, keep in mind that, unless otherwise noted, no additional ingredients have been added during cooking. For processed foods such as cake or pancake mixes, the term "prepared" signifies that the item has been prepared according to the directions on the package, with whatever additional ingredients that requires. Unless otherwise noted, the food values for fish, meats, and poultry are for meat only, and do not include skin or bones.

One feature that sets this book apart from many other nutrition books is the inclusion of the column called "% Fat Calories." Although scientists and nutritionists can use any of several methods to determine the percentage of calories derived from fat, the simplest and most popular is the "4-4-9" method. This technique assumes that 1 gram of protein contains 4 calories, that 1 gram of carbohydrate contains 4 calories, and that 1 gram of fat contains 9 calories. In beverages and foods containing alcohol, it is assumed that each gram of alcohol contains 7 calories. Once you know the total calories and the calories from fat, the calculations used to determine the percentage of calories from fat are, in theory, fairly straightforward and accurate.

When applied to actual published nutrition data, however, several factors make the 4-4-9 method less than ideal. For one thing, many manufacturers consider any nutrient containing fewer than 5 calories to be "nutritionally insignificant." For this reason, the manufacturers round off their published values for protein, carbohydrates, and fats. Sometimes they publish a value of "<1.0 gram" of fat, which means that the fat content might be anywhere from 0.0 grams to 0.99 grams. When a food item contains only a few calories, the "insignificant" rounding of fat values can have significant and misleading consequences.

One consequence of this practice of rounding off values is that when the calorie values for protein, carbohydrates, and fat are added up, they very rarely match the calorie values published by the manufacturer or restaurant. This means that to simply multiply fat grams by 9 will often result in a misleading value for percentage of calories from fat.

To more accurately represent the percentage of calories from fat, we developed a simple method called the compensated 4-4-9 method. Here is how this method was used to calculate the percentage-of-calories-from-fat values that appear in this book.

1. We calculated the total calories from each of the calorie sources by multiplying protein grams by 4, carbohydrate grams by 4, and fat grams by 9. We added these values together to get a "total derived calories" value.

2. We made the assumption that the manufacturer's total calorie value was correct. We then compared our total derived calorie value to the manufacturer's published total calorie value. If our derived value was lower or higher, we adjusted all of the nonzero nutrient values—maintaining the 4-4-9 ratio—to match the manufacturer's total.

3. Using the adjusted nutrient values, we calculated the percentage of calories from fat.

The compensated 4-4-9 method results in percentage-of-calories values for protein, carbohydrates, and fat that both match the manufacturer's calorie figure for each nutrient and add up to 100 percent of the total calories. Using the nutritional information provided by the manufacturers at this time, we feel that this method is the best means of determining accurate values.

CODES AND ABBREVIATIONS

To provide the most comprehensive nutritional information possible, a number of codes and abbreviations have been used throughout this book. A complete translation is given below.

>	greater than		nia	niacin
<	less than		pkg	package
approx	approximately		pot	potassium
cal	calories		prep	prepared according to directions
calc	calcium		prot	protein
carbs	carbohydrates		rib	riboflavin
fl	fluid		sat fat	saturated fat
fol	folic acid		sod	sodium
gm	gram		tbsp	tablespoon
IU	international unit[1]		thi	thiamine
lb	pound		tr	trace
mag	magnesium		(tr)	may contain a trace amount
mcg	microgram(s)		tsp	teaspoon
med	medium-sized		w/	with
mg	milligram(s)		w/o	without
(mq)	may contain a measurable quantity[2]		wt	weight
na	not available		zn	zinc

[1] International units, which are used throughout this book to express vitamin A content, are a measure of fat-soluble vitamin activity. The amounts of all other nutrients are expressed in grams or milligrams, which are units of mass and weight.

[2] The food item may contain a quantity ranging from a trace amount to a substantial amount. This quantity depends upon any one of a number of variables—such as soil condition and mineral content of fertilizer used—that may have affected the food item during growing, processing, and/or preparation.

TABLE OF MEASUREMENT CONVERSIONS

VOLUME MEASUREMENT EQUIVALENTS

Pinch or dash	= less than ⅛ teaspoon		
1 teaspoon	= ⅓ tablespoon		= ⅙ ounce
1 tablespoon	= 3 teaspoons		= ½ fluid ounce
2 tablespoons	= ⅛ cup	= ¹⁄₁₆ pint	= 1 fluid ounce
4 tablespoons	= ¼ cup		= 2 fluid ounces
8 tablespoons	= ½ cup		= 4 fluid ounces
12 tablespoons	= ¾ cup		= 6 fluid ounces
16 tablespoons	= 1 cup	= ½ pint	= 8 fluid ounces
⅛ cup	= 2 tablespoons		= 1 fluid ounce
¼ cup	= 4 tablespoons		= 2 fluid ounces
½ cup	= 8 tablespoons		= 4 fluid ounces
¾ cup	= 12 tablespoons		= 6 fluid ounces
1 cup	= 16 tablespoons	= ½ pint	= 8 fluid ounces
2 cups	= 1 pint	= ½ quart	= 16 fluid ounces
4 cups	= 2 pints	= 1 quart	= 32 fluid ounces
8 cups	= 4 pints	= 2 quarts	= 64 fluid ounces
16 cups	= 8 pints	= 4 quarts / 1 gallon	= 128 fluid ounces
½ pint	= 1 cup		= 8 fluid ounces
1 pint	= 2 cups		= 16 fluid ounces
2 pints	= 4 cups	= 1 quart	= 32 fluid ounces
4 pints	= 8 cups	= 2 quarts	= 64 fluid ounces
8 pints	= 16 cups	= 4 quarts / 1 gallon	= 128 fluid ounces
½ quart	= 2 cups	= 1 pint	= 16 fluid ounces
1 quart	= 4 cups	= 2 pints	= 32 fluid ounces

WEIGHT MEASUREMENT EQUIVALENTS

1 gram	= 0.035 ounce	
100 grams	= 3.57 ounces	
1 ounce		= 28.35 grams
½ pound	= 8 ounces	= 226.8 grams
1 pound	= 16 ounces	= 453.6 grams

The NutriBase

NUTRITION FACTS

DESK REFERENCE

PART ONE

GENERAL NUTRIENT VALUES

Calories • Protein • Carbohydrates • Sodium •
Fiber • Fat • Saturated Fat • Cholesterol •
Percentage of Calories from Fat

A

Food Name	Serving Size	Calories	Prot. gms	Carbs gms	Sod. mgs	Fiber gms	Fat gms	Sat. Fat gms	Chol. mgs	% Fat Cal.
ABALONE, mixed species, raw	3 oz	89	15	5	256	0	0.6	0.1	72	7%
ABALONE MUSHROOM. See MUSHROOM, OYSTER.										
ACEROLA, RAW / Barbados cherry / Puerto Rican cherry / West Indian cherry.										
raw, trimmed	1 medium	2	0	0	0	0	0.0	0.0	0	8%
raw, untrimmed	1 cup	31	0	8	7	1	0.3	0.1	0	8%
ACEROLA JUICE										
....	1 cup	56	1	12	7	1	0.7	0.2	0	11%
....	1 fl oz	7	0	1	1	0	0.1	0.0	0	11%
ACORN										
dried	1 oz	144	2	15	0	na	8.9	1.2	0	52%
raw	1 oz	110	2	12	0	na	6.8	0.9	0	52%
ACORN FLOUR. See under FLOUR.										
ACORN SQUASH. See SQUASH, ACORN.										
ADZUKI BEAN. See BEAN, ADZUKI.										
AGAR. See under SEA VEGETABLE.										
AHI. See under TUNA.										
AKU. See under TUNA.										
ALARIA. See under SEA VEGETABLE.										
ALASKA KING CRAB. See under CRAB.										
ALBACORE. See under TUNA.										
ALE. See BEER, ALE, AND MALT LIQUOR.										
ALCOHOLIC BEVERAGES. See BEER AND ALE; COCKTAIL; COCKTAIL MIX; SHERRY; VERMOUTH; WINE; WINE, COOKING; WINE COOLER; and individual listings.										
ALFALFA SEEDS										
(Arrowhead Mills).......................	1 cup	40	5	4	0	0	1.0	0.0	0	20%
sprouted, raw	1 cup	10	1	1	2	1	0.2	0.0	0	20%
sprouted, raw	1 tbsp	1	0	0	0	0	0.0	0.0	0	20%
ALFALFA TABLETS (Shaklee)	10 tablets	5	0	0	2	0	0.0	0.0	0	0%
ALGAE										
blue-green, Klamath lake algae.	1 gram	3	1	0	3	na	0.0	na	0	10%
spirulina, dried.........................	1 cup	44	9	4	157	1	1.2	0.4	0	22%
ALLIGATOR	1 oz	41	8.3	na	na	na	0.8	0.2	18	18%
ALLSPICE										
ground..................................	1 tbsp	16	0	4	5	1	0.5	0.2	0	28%
ground..................................	1 tsp	5	0	1	1	0	0.2	0.0	0	28%
ground (Durkee)	1 tsp	7	0	0	0	0	0.0	0.0	0	0%
ground (Laurel Leaf)	1 tsp	7	0	0	0	0	0.0	0.0	0	0%
ground (McCormick/Schilling)	1 tsp	6	0	1	1	1	0.0	0.0	0	0%
ground (Spice Islands)	1 tsp	6	0	1	1	0	0.1	0.0	0	14%
ground (Tone's)	1 tsp	5	0	1	2	0	0.2	0.1	0	23%
ALMOND										
ground..................................	1 cup	549	20	19	1	11	48.1	3.7	0	73%
whole kernels, approx 24	1 oz	164	6	6	0	3	14.4	1.1	0	73%
(Beer Nuts)	1 oz	180	5	7	51	0	14.4	0.0	0	73%
(Dole)	1 oz	170	6	12	4	0	14.0	0.0	0	64%
(Fisher)	1 oz	170	3	3	0	0	15.0	1.0	0	85%
natural, chopped (Blue Diamond).........	1 oz	172	6	6	0	4	14.3	1.1	0	73%
natural, sliced (Blue Diamond)	1 oz	172	6	6	0	4	14.3	1.1	0	73%
natural, unsalted (Flanigan Farms)	1 oz	170	6	5	4	na	14.0	na	0	74%
natural, whole (Blue Diamond) natural	1 oz	172	6	6	0	4	14.3	1.1	0	73%
natural, whole or sliced (Azar).	2 oz	340	12	12	6	5	30.0	3.0	0	74%

Food Name	Serving Size	Calories	Prot. gms	Carbs gms	Sod. mgs	Fiber gms	Fat gms	Sat. Fat gms	Chol. mgs	% Fat Cal.
Barbecue (Blue Diamond)	1 oz	167	6	5	243	4	15.0	1.2	0	75%
Blanched										
pieces	1 oz	165	6	6	8	3	14.4	1.1	0	73%
pieces	1 tbsp	53	2	2	3	1	4.6	0.4	0	73%
whole kernels	1 cup	842	32	29	41	15	73.4	5.6	0	73%
(Blue Diamond)	1 oz	175	6	5	2	4	14.5	1.3	0	74%
(Planters)	1 oz	170	6	6	0	0	15.0	2.0	0	74%
slivered (Azar)	2 oz	330	11	10	4	5	29.0	3.0	0	76%
slivered (Blue Diamond)	1 oz	175	6	5	2	4	14.5	1.3	0	74%
whole (Blue Diamond)	1 oz	175	6	5	2	4	14.5	1.3	0	74%
Chili w/lemon (Blue Diamond)	1 oz	172	6	4	245	3	16.0	1.2	0	79%
Dry-roasted										
whole kernels, salted	1 cup	824	30	27	468	16	72.9	5.6	0	74%
whole kernels, salted, approx 22	1 oz	169	6	5	96	3	15.0	1.1	0	74%
whole kernels, unsalted	1 cup	824	30	27	1	16	72.9	5.6	0	74%
whole kernels, unsalted, approx 22	1 oz	169	6	5	0	3	15.0	1.1	0	74%
California, whole (Flanigan Farms)	1/4 cup	170	6	6	0	3	15.0	1.5	0	74%
chopped, unsalted (Flanigan Farms)	1/4 cup	170	6	6	0	3	15.0	1.5	0	74%
(Planters)	1 oz	170	6	6	200	0	15.0	2.0	0	74%
sliced, unsalted (Flanigan Farms)	1/4 cup	170	6	6	0	3	15.0	1.5	0	74%
slivered, unsalted (Flanigan Farms)	1/4 cup	170	6	5	0	3	15.0	1.5	0	75%
unsalted (Blue Diamond)	1 oz	170	6	5	1	3	15.1	1.2	0	75%
w/tamari (Eden Foods)	1 oz	170	8	8	35	4	12.0	1.0	0	63%
Honey-roasted										
unblanched	1 oz	168	5	8	37	4	14.1	1.3	0	70%
whole kernels, unblanched	1 cup	855	26	40	187	20	71.9	6.8	0	70%
(Blue Diamond)	1 oz	170	5	8	37	3	14.2	1.0	0	71%
(Planters)	1 oz	170	5	9	180	0	13.0	1.0	0	68%
Oil-roasted										
whole kernels, salted	1 cup	953	33	28	532	16	86.6	6.6	0	76%
whole kernels, salted, approx 22	1 oz	172	6	5	96	3	15.6	1.2	0	76%
whole kernels, unsalted	1 cup	953	33	28	2	16	86.6	6.6	0	76%
whole kernels, unsalted, approx 22	1 oz	172	6	5	0	3	15.6	1.2	0	76%
Raw										
sliced (Planters)	1 oz	170	6	6	0	0	15.0	2.0	0	74%
slivered (Planters)	1 oz	170	6	6	0	0	15.0	2.0	0	74%
whole (Planters)	1 oz	170	6	6	0	0	15.0	2.0	0	74%
Roasted (Dole)	1 oz	170	6	5	4	0	14.0	0.0	0	74%
Smokehouse (Blue Diamond)	1 oz	173	6	5	169	3	15.8	1.2	0	77%
Unblanched										
sliced	1 cup	549	20	19	1	11	48.1	3.7	0	73%
slivered	1 cup	624	23	21	1	13	54.7	4.2	0	73%
whole	1 cup	821	30	28	1	17	71.9	5.5	0	73%
Yogurt-coated, made w/real fruit juice (Fruit Source)	9 pieces	210	4	19	40	2	14.0	7.0	5	58%
ALMOND BUTTER										
salted	1 cup	1583	38	53	1125	9	147.8	14.0	0	78%
salted	1 tbsp	101	2	3	72	1	9.5	0.9	0	78%
unsalted	1 cup	1583	38	53	28	9	147.8	14.0	0	78%
unsalted	1 tbsp	101	2	3	2	1	9.5	0.9	0	78%
(Hain)										
blanched, toasted	2 tbsp	220	8	3	10	0	19.0	2.0	0	80%
raw, 'Natural'	2 tbsp	190	8	3	5	0	18.0	2.0	0	79%
(Maranatha Natural)										
organic, raw	2 tbsp	190	7	8	5	0	15.0	0.0	0	69%

Food Name	Serving Size	Calories	Prot. gms	Carbs gms	Sod. mgs	Fiber gms	Fat gms	Sat. Fat gms	Chol. mgs	% Fat Cal.
roasted	2 tbsp	190	7	8	5	0	15.0	0.0	0	69%
(Roaster Fresh)										
gourmet	1 oz	184	5	6	4	0	16.0	1.6	0	77%
roasted fresh, creamy, salted	1 oz	184	5	6	4	0	16.0	2.0	0	77%
(Westbrae)										
crunchy, unsalted, 'Natural'	2 tbsp	190	7	7	0	0	17.0	0.0	0	73%
smooth, unsalted, 'Natural'	2 tbsp	190	7	7	0	0	17.0	0.0	0	73%
ALMOND DRINK original flavor (Almond Mylk)	8 fl oz	80	2	8	190	2	4.0	0.0	0	47%
ALMOND MEAL										
partially defatted	4 oz	463	44.8	32.8	8	>2.6c	20.8	2.0	0	38%
partially defatted, salted	4 oz	463	44.8	32.8	846	>2.6c	20.8	2.0	0	38%
ALMOND OIL										
	1 cup	1927	0	0	0	0	218.0	17.9	0	100%
	1 tbsp	120	0	0	0	0	13.6	1.1	0	100%
(Hain)	1 tbsp	120	0	0	0	0	14.0	1.0	0	100%
pure-pressed organic (Spectrum)	1 tbsp	120	0	0	0	0	14.0	1.0	0	100%
sweet (International Collection)	1 tbsp	120	0	0	0	0	14.0	1.0	0	100%
ALMOND PASTE										
	1 oz	130	3	14	3	1	7.9	0.7	0	51%
firmly packed	1 cup	1040	20	109	20	11	63.0	6.0	0	51%
ALOE VERA JUICE										
sodium-free, certified 100% juice (Sunburst)	2 fl oz	5	0	1	3	0	0.0	0.0	0	0%
AMARANTH										
	1 cup	729	28	129	41	30	12.7	3.2	0	15%
(Arrowhead Mills) whole-grain, organic	1/4 cup	170	7	29	0	3	2.0	0.5	0	11%
AMARANTH DISH/ENTRÉE										
(Health Valley) w/vegetables, fat-free, 'Fast Menu'	1 cup	160	8	31	290	9	0.0	0.0	0	0%
AMARANTH FLOUR. See under FLOUR.										
AMARANTH LEAVES										
boiled, drained	1 cup	28	3	5	28	na	0.2	0.1	0	7%
raw	1 cup	6	1	1	6	na	0.1	0.0	0	12%
raw	1 leaf	3	0	1	3	na	0.0	0.0	0	12%
AMARANTH SEED (Arrowhead Mills)	2 oz	200	8	35	1	4	3.0	0.0	0	14%
ANASAZI BEAN. See BEAN, ANASAZI.										
ANCHO PEPPER. See PEPPER, ANCHO.										
ANCHOVY										
Canned										
European, in oil, boneless, drained	1 oz	60	8	0	1040	0	2.8	0.6	24	41%
European, in oil, drained	2 oz	95	13	0	1651	0	4.4	1.0	38	41%
European, in oil, drained	5 medium	42	6	0	734	0	1.9	0.4	17	41%
European, in oil, drained	1 medium	8	1	0	147	0	0.4	0.1	3	41%
flat fillets, in olive oil (Crown Prince)	9 fillets	35	4	0	1050	0	2.5	0.0	15	58%
flat fillets, in olive oil, salt added (Reese)	6 fillets	25	4	0	750	0	1.5	0.0	15	46%
Fresh, European, raw	3 oz	111	17	0	88	0	4.1	1.1	51	33%
ANCHOVY PASTE										
(Reese)	1 tbsp	30	2	0	940	0	2.5	0.5	55	74%
(Roland)	1 tbsp	30	2	0	1140	0	2.5	1.5	24	74%
ANGEL HAIR. See under PASTA; PASTA DISH/ENTRÉE.										
ANGLER FISH. See MONKFISH.										
ANISE, dried (McCormick/Schilling)	1 serving	18	1	2	0	1	0.8	0.0	0	43%
ANISE SEED										
	1 tbsp	23	1	3	1	1	1.1	0.0	0	39%
	1 tsp	7	0	1	0	0	0.3	0.0	0	39%
(Tone's)	1 tsp	7	0	1	2	0	0.3	0.0	0	31%

Food Name	Serving Size	Calories	Prot. gms	Carbs gms	Sod. mgs	Fiber gms	Fat gms	Sat. Fat gms	Chol. mgs	% Fat Cal.
ANTELOPE										
raw	1 oz	32	6	0	14	0	0.6	0.2	27	16%
roasted	3 oz	128	25	0	46	0	2.3	0.8	107	16%
roasted, boneless, yield from 1 lb raw	11.9 oz	510	100	0	184	0	9.1	3.3	428	16%
APPLE										
Canned, sweetened slices, drained	1 cup	137	0	34	6	4	0.9	0.1	0	5%
Dehydrated, sulfured										
low moisture, stewed	1 cup	143	1	38	50	5	0.2	0.0	0	1%
low moisture, uncooked	1 cup	208	1	56	74	7	0.3	0.1	0	1%
rings, uncooked	1 ring	16	0	4	6	1	0.0	0.0	0	1%
stewed	1 cup	145	1	39	51	5	0.2	0.0	0	1%
uncooked	1 cup	209	1	57	75	7	0.3	0.0	0	1%
Fresh										
boiled, peeled, sliced	1 cup	91	0	23	2	4	0.6	0.1	0	6%
microwaved, peeled, sliced	1 cup	95	0	24	2	5	0.7	0.1	0	6%
raw, peeled, quartered or chopped	1 cup	74	0	19	0	3	0.5	0.1	0	5%
raw, peeled, sliced	1 cup	63	0	16	0	2	0.3	0.1	0	5%
raw, peeled, whole, medium, approx 3 per lb	1 apple	73	0	19	0	2	0.4	0.1	0	5%
raw, unpeeled, whole, large, approx 2 per lb	1 apple	125	0	32	0	6	0.8	0.1	0	5%
raw, unpeeled, whole, medium, approx 3 per lb	1 apple	81	0	21	0	4	0.5	0.1	0	5%
raw, unpeeled, whole, small, approx 4 per lb	1 apple	63	0	16	0	3	0.4	0.1	0	5%
Frozen										
unsweetened slices, heated	1 cup	97	1	25	6	4	0.7	0.1	0	6%
unsweetened slices, unheated	1 cup	83	0	21	5	3	0.6	0.1	0	6%
APPLE BUTTER										
(Bama)	2 tsp	25	0	6	5	0	0.0	0.0	0	0%
(Eden Foods)	1 tbsp	25	0	3	0	0	0.0	0.0	na	0%
(Knudsen & Sons) organic	2 tbsp	25	0	6	0	0	0.0	0.0	0	0%
(Lucky Leaf)	4 oz	200	0	49	15	0	1.0	0.0	0	4%
(Musselman's)	4 oz	200	0	49	15	0	1.0	0.0	0	4%
(Smucker's)										
'Autumn Harvest'	1 tsp	12	0	3	0	0	0.0	0.0	0	0%
cider	1 tsp	12	0	3	0	0	0.0	0.0	0	0%
natural	1 tsp	12	0	3	0	0	0.0	0.0	0	0%
'Simply Fruit'	1 tsp	16	0	4	0	0	0.0	0.0	0	0%
spiced	1 tsp	12	0	3	0	0	0.0	0.0	0	0%
(Tap'n Apple)	1 oz	45	1	13	1	1	0.1	0.0	0	2%
(White House)	1 oz	50	0	12	5	0	0.0	0.0	0	0%
APPLE DISH										
escalloped, frozen (Stouffer's)	2/3 cup	182	0	37	71	3	3.0	0.0	0	15%
escalloped, frozen (Stouffer's)	1 oz	31	0	7	1	1	0.5	0.1	0	14%
fried (Luck's)	1/2 cup	130	0	33	0	2	0.0	0.0	0	0%
APPLE JUICE. See also CIDER; CIDER MIX; FRUIT DRINK; FRUIT DRINK MIX; FRUIT JUICE BLEND; FRUIT JUICE DRINK.										
Canned, bottled, or boxed										
w/added vitamin C	1 cup	117	0	29	7	0	0.3	0.0	0	2%
w/added vitamin C	1 fl oz	15	0	4	1	0	0.0	0.0	0	2%
w/o added vitamin C	1 cup	117	0	29	7	0	0.3	0.0	0	2%
w/o added vitamin C	1 fl oz	15	0	4	1	0	0.0	0.0	0	2%
w/o added vitamin C	8.45 fl oz	123	0	31	8	0	0.3	0.1	0	2%
(Flav-R-Pac)	1 cup	120	0	29	15	0	0.0	0.0	0	0%
(Indian Summer)	6 fl oz	90	1	21	10	0	1.0	0.0	0	9%
(J. Hungerford)										
	9.03 fl oz	128	0	32	6	0	0.0	0.0	0	0%
50% juice	9.03 fl oz	119	0	30	8	0	0.0	0.0	0	0%

Food Name	Serving Size	Calories	Prot. gms	Carbs gms	Sod. mgs	Fiber gms	Fat gms	Sat. Fat gms	Chol. mgs	% Fat Cal.
100% juice	9.03 fl oz	112	0	28	17	0	0.0	0.0	0	0%
(Juicy Juice)	6 fl oz	90	0	21	5	0	0.0	0.0	0	0%
(Knudsen)										
clear	8 fl oz	110	0	28	5	na	0.0	0.0	0	0%
Gravenstein	8 fl oz	110	1	28	0	0	0.0	0.0	0	0%
natural	8 fl oz	120	0	30	25	na	0.0	0.0	0	0%
(Kraft) 'Pure 100%'	6 fl oz	80	0	20	5	0	0.0	0.0	0	0%
(Lucky Leaf)										
'Individual Portion Control'	3.8 fl oz	60	0	14	0	0	0.0	0.0	0	0%
100% vitamin-C enriched	6 fl oz	90	0	21	0	0	0.0	0.0	0	0%
(McCain) 100% juice 'Junior'	4.2 fl oz	50	0	13	5	0	0.0	0.0	0	0%
(Mott's)	6 fl oz	88	0	22	13	0	0.0	0.0	0	0%
(Musselman's)										
'Individual Portion Control'	3.8 fl oz	60	0	14	0	0	0.0	0.0	0	0%
100% vitamin-C enriched	6 fl oz	90	0	21	0	0	0.0	0.0	0	0%
(Ocean Spray)	6 fl oz	90	0	23	15	0	0.0	0.0	0	0%
(Red Cheek)										
'Natural'	6 fl oz	97	0	24	16	0	0.0	0.0	0	0%
'100% Pure'	6 fl oz	97	0	24	7	0	0.0	0.0	0	0%
(S&W)										
	8 fl oz	120	0	30	0	0	0.0	0.0	0	0%
'100% Pure Unsweetened'	6 fl oz	85	0	20	5	0	0.0	0.0	0	0%
(S. Martinelli) 'Sparkling'	6 fl oz	100	0	25	5	0	0.0	0.0	0	0%
(Sippin' Pak) 100% pure	8.45 fl oz	110	0	28	25	0	0.0	0.0	0	0%
(Tree Top) 100%										
	8 fl oz	120	0	29	25	0	0.0	0.0	0	0%
(TreeSweet)	6 fl oz	90	0	22	15	0	0.0	0.0	0	0%
(Tropicana)										
100% pure	8 fl oz	116	0	29	17	0	0.0	0.0	0	0%
100% pure	6 fl oz	80	1	20	15	0	1.0	0.0	0	10%
'Pure Premium' 'Orchardstand'	8 fl oz	110	1	27	0	na	0.0	na	na	0%
'Season's Best'	8 fl oz	120	0	29	25	1	0.0	na	na	0%
(Ultra Slim Fast) golden	8 fl oz	153	5	29	167	3	1.0	0.3	7	7%
(Veryfine) '100%'	8 fl oz	107	0	27	10	0	0.0	0.0	0	0%
(Welch's)										
'Orchard Cocktail'	10 fl oz	170	0	42	95	0	0.0	0.0	0	0%
sparkling	6 fl oz	100	0	24	5	0	0.0	0.0	0	0%
(White House)	6 fl oz	87	0	22	5	0	0.0	0.0	0	0%
Chilled or frozen										
concentrate, w/o added vitamin C, prepared	1 cup	112	0	28	17	0	0.2	0.0	0	2%
concentrate, w/o added vitamin C, prepared	1 fl oz	14	0	3	2	0	0.0	0.0	0	2%
concentrate, w/added vitamin C, prepared	1 cup	112	0	28	17	0	0.2	0.0	0	2%
concentrate, w/added vitamin C, prepared	1 fl oz	14	0	3	2	0	0.0	0.0	0	2%
concentrate, w/added vitamin C, undiluted	6-oz can	350	1	87	53	na	0.8	0.1	0	2%
concentrate, w/o added vitamin C, undiluted	6-oz can	350	1	87	53	1	0.8	0.1	0	2%
(A&P) diluted as directed	6 fl oz	90	1	22	0	0	1.0	0.0	0	9%
(Sunkist) diluted as directed	8 fl oz	79	0	19	12	0	0.2	0.0	0	2%
APPLE KIT										
(Concord)										
candy, microwaveable, prepared	1 apple	50	0	14	0	0	0.0	0.0	0	0%
caramel, microwaveable, prepared	1 apple	150	2	27	105	0	3.0	1.5	5	19%
APPLE PIE SPICE. See under SEASONING MIX.										
APPLE SPREAD, no sugar added (Fifty 50)	1 tsp	2	0	1	5	0	0.0	0.0	0	0%
APPLE SYRUP (Knudsen)	1 oz	75	1	15	0	0	1.0	0.0	0	12%

Food Name	Serving Size	Calories	Prot. gms	Carbs gms	Sod. mgs	Fiber gms	Fat gms	Sat. Fat gms	Chol. mgs	% Fat Cal.
APPLE TOPPING (Flav-R-Pac)	2 tbsp	40	0	10	45	0	0.0	0.0	0	0%
APPLESAUCE										
canned, sweetened, w/salt	1 cup	194	0	51	71	3	0.5	0.1	0	2%
canned, sweetened, w/o salt	1 cup	194	0	51	8	3	0.5	0.1	0	2%
canned, sweetened, w/o salt	1 cup	194	0	51	8	3	0.5	0.1	0	2%
canned, unsweetened, w/added vitamin C	1 cup	105	0	28	5	3	0.1	0.0	0	1%
canned, unsweetened w/o added vitamin C	1 cup	105	0	28	5	3	0.1	0.0	0	1%
cinnamon (Tree Top)	1/2 cup	83	0	21	0	1	0.0	0.0	0	0%
cranberry, 'CranFruit' (Ocean Spray)	2 oz	100	0	23	10	0	0.0	0.0	0	0%
original (Tree Top)	1/2 cup	83	0	21	0	1	0.0	0.0	0	0%
unsweetened (Tree Top)	1/2 cup	58	0	15	0	1	0.0	0.0	0	0%
APRICOT										
Canned										
halves, peeled, in extra light syrup, w/liquid	1 cup	121	1	31	5	4	0.2	0.0	0	2%
halves, peeled, in heavy syrup, w/liquid	1 cup	214	1	55	10	4	0.2	0.0	0	1%
halves, unpeeled, in juice, w/liquid	1 cup	117	2	30	10	4	0.1	0.0	0	1%
halves, unpeeled, in light syrup, w/liquid	1 cup	159	1	42	10	4	0.1	0.0	0	1%
halves, unpeeled, in water, w/liquid	1 cup	66	2	16	7	4	0.4	0.0	0	5%
whole, peeled, in heavy syrup, w/o pits, w/liquid	1 cup	236	1	61	32	4	0.1	0.0	0	0%
whole, peeled, in water, w/o pits, w/liquid	1 cup	50	2	12	25	2	0.1	0.0	0	1%
whole, unpeeled, in heavy syrup, w/liquid	1 cup	199	1	52	10	4	0.2	0.0	0	1%
whole, unpeeled, in heavy syrup, w/liquid	1/2 apricot	33	0	9	2	1	0.0	0.0	0	1%
whole, unpeeled, in juice, w/liquid	1/2 apricot	17	0	4	1	1	0.0	0.0	0	1%
whole, unpeeled, in light syrup, w/liquid	1/2 apricot	25	0	7	2	1	0.0	0.0	0	1%
whole, unpeeled, in water, w/liquid	1/2 apricot	10	0	2	1	1	0.1	0.0	0	5%
Dehydrated/sulfured										
halves, stewed	1 cup	213	3	55	8	8	0.4	0.0	0	2%
halves, uncooked	1 cup	309	5	80	13	12	0.6	0.0	0	2%
low-moisture, stewed	1 cup	314	5	81	12	na	0.6	0.0	0	2%
low-moisture, uncooked	1 cup	381	6	99	15	na	0.7	0.1	0	2%
uncooked	1/2 apricot	8	0	2	0	0	0.0	0.0	0	2%
Fresh										
raw, halved	1 cup	74	2	17	2	4	0.6	0.0	0	7%
raw, sliced	1 cup	79	2	18	2	4	0.6	0.0	0	7%
raw, whole	1 med	17	0	4	0	1	0.1	0.0	0	7%
Frozen										
sweetened	1 cup	237	2	61	10	5	0.2	0.0	0	1%
sliced (Flav-R-Pac)	2/3 cup	70	1	18	0	1	0.0	0.0	0	0%
APRICOT KERNEL OIL										
	1 cup	1927	0	0	0	0	218.0	13.7	0	100%
	1 tbsp	120	0	0	0	0	13.6	0.9	0	100%
(Hain)	1 tbsp	120	0	0	0	0	14.0	1.0	0	100%
ARBORIO RICE. See under RICE.										
ARROWHEAD										
boiled, drained	1 medium	9	1	2	2	na	0.0	na	0	1%
powdered (Tone's)	1 tsp	10	0	2	1	0	0.0	0.0	0	0%
raw	1 large	25	1	5	6	na	0.1	na	0	2%
raw	1 medium	12	1	2	3	na	0.0	na	0	2%
ARROWROOT										
raw, whole	1 med root	21	1	4	9	0	0.1	0.0	0	3%
raw, sliced	1 cup	78	5	16	31	2	0.2	0.0	0	3%
ARROWROOT FLOUR. See under FLOUR.										
ARTICHOKE. See also ARTICHOKE, JERUSALEM.										

Food Name	Serving Size	Calories	Prot. gms	Carbs gms	Sod. mgs	Fiber gms	Fat gms	Sat. Fat gms	Chol. mgs	% Fat Cal.
Canned										
globe, bottoms *(Reese)*	2 pieces	35	2	7	260	1	0.0	0.0	0	0%
globe, hearts *(C&W)*	1/2 cup	25	2	4	60	5	0.0	0.0	0	0%
globe, hearts, 5-7 per can *(Reese)*	2 pieces	30	2	6	240	1	0.0	0.0	0	0%
globe, hearts, quartered *(Maria)*	1/2 cup	35	2	6	330	3	0.0	0.0	0	0%
globe, hearts, 10-12 per can *(Reese)*	4 pieces	30	2	6	240	1	0.0	0.0	0	0%
hearts, marinated *(Progresso)*	1/3 cup	160	1	6	290	1	14.0	2.0	0	82%
Fresh										
globe, fresh *(Dole)*	1 large	23	2	5	65	3	0.1	0.0	0	3%
globe or French, boiled, drained	1 medium	60	4	13	114	6	0.2	0.0	0	3%
globe or French, hearts, boiled, drained	1/2 cup	42	3	9	80	5	0.1	0.0	0	3%
globe or French, raw	1 large	76	5	17	152	9	0.2	0.1	0	3%
globe or French, raw	1 medium	60	4	13	120	7	0.2	0.0	0	3%
Frozen										
globe or French, unprepared	9-oz pkg	97	7	20	120	10	1.1	0.3	0	9%
globe or French, w/salt, drained	9-oz pkg	108	7	22	694	11	1.2	0.3	0	9%
globe or French, w/salt, drained	1 cup	76	5	15	486	8	0.8	0.2	0	9%
globe or French, w/salt, drained, 1/3 of 10-oz pkg	1 serving	36	2	7	231	4	0.4	0.1	0	9%
globe or French, w/o salt, drained	1 cup	76	5	15	89	8	0.8	0.2	0	9%
globe or French, w/o salt, drained	9-oz pkg	108	7	22	127	11	1.2	0.3	0	9%
globe or French, w/o salt, drained, 1/3 of 10-oz pkg	1 serving	36	2	7	42	4	0.4	0.1	0	9%
hearts *(Seabrook)*	3 oz	25	3	4	6	1	0.0	0.0	0	0%
hearts, 'Deluxe' *(Birds Eye)*	3 oz	30	2	7	140	0	0.0	0.0	0	0%
ARTICHOKE, JERUSALEM / sunchoke										
raw, sliced	1 cup	114	3	26	6	2	0.0	0.0	0	0%
ARUGULA / rucola / rugula										
raw	1 leaf	1	0	0	1	0	0.0	0.0	0	22%
raw	1/2 cup	3	0	0	3	0	0.1	0.0	0	22%
(Frieda of California)	1 oz	7	1	1	4	0	0.1	0.0	0	12%
ASIAN PEAR / Chinese pear / sand pear										
Fresh										
raw, whole, approx 2.25x2.5-inch diam	1 fruit	51	1	13	0	4	0.3	0.0	0	5%
raw, whole, approx 3-3/8x3-inch diam	1 fruit	116	1	29	0	10	0.6	0.0	0	5%
ASPARAGUS										
Canned										
cuts, green, drained	1 cup	46	5	6	695	4	1.6	0.4	0	29%
cuts, green, w/liquid	1/2 cup	18	2	3	346	1	0.2	0.1	0	10%
cuts, green, 50% less salt, w/liquid *(Green Giant)*	1/2 cup	20	2	3	210	1	0.0	0.0	0	0%
cuts, green *(Stokely)*	1/2 cup	20	2	3	380	0	0.0	0.0	0	0%
cuts, green, w/liquid *(Green Giant)*	1/2 cup	20	2	3	420	1	0.0	0.0	0	0%
cuts, green 'No Salt or Sugar Added' *(Stokely)*	1/2 cup	20	2	3	5	0	0.0	0.0	0	0%
cuts, white, w/liquid *(Green Giant)*	1/2 cup	16	2	3	410	1	0.0	0.0	0	0%
cuts and tips *(Finast)*	1 cup	35	4	6	720	0	0.0	0.0	0	0%
points, green *(S&W)*	1/2 cup	17	4	3	10	0	0.0	0.0	0	0%
spears, drained	1 med spear	3	0	0	52	0	0.1	0.0	0	29%
green, cut *(Green Giant)*	1/2 cup	18	2	3	420	1	0.0	0.0	0	0%
green, cut, 50% less salt *(Green Giant)*	1/2 cup	18	2	3	210	1	0.0	0.0	0	0%
green, cut 'No Salt Added' *(Pathmark)*	1/2 cup	20	3	2	5	0	0.0	0.0	0	0%
green, cut *(Pathmark)*	1/2 cup	20	3	2	450	0	0.0	0.0	0	0%
green, extra large 'LeSueur' *(Green Giant)*	4.5 oz	20	2	3	440	1	0.0	0.0	0	0%
green, extra long *(Green Giant)*	4.5 oz	20	2	3	400	1	0.0	0.0	0	0%
green 'Fancy' *(S&W)*	1/2 cup	18	2	3	320	0	0.0	0.0	0	0%
spears, colossal *(S&W)*	3 pieces	10	1	3	170	1	0.0	0.0	0	0%
white *(Green Giant)*	1/2 cup	16	2	3	410	1	0.0	0.0	0	0%

Food Name	Serving Size	Calories	Prot. gms	Carbs gms	Sod. mgs	Fiber gms	Fat gms	Sat. Fat gms	Chol. mgs	% Fat Cal.
Fresh										
cuts, boiled, drained	1/2 cup	22	2	4	10	1	0.3	0.1	0	11%
cuts, raw	1 cup	31	3	6	3	3	0.3	0.1	0	7%
spears, boiled, drained, whole	4 med spears	14	2	3	7	1	0.2	0.0	0	11%
spears, fresh (Dole)	5 spears	18	2	2	0	2	0.0	0.0	0	0%
spears, raw, extra large, 8.75 to 10-inch long	1 spear	6	1	1	0	1	0.0	0.0	0	7%
spears, raw, large, 7.25 to 8.5-inch long	1 spear	5	0	1	0	0	0.0	0.0	0	7%
spears, raw, medium, 5.25 to 7-inch long	1 spear	4	0	1	0	0	0.0	0.0	0	7%
spears, raw, small, up to 5-inch long	1 spear	3	0	1	0	0	0.0	0.0	0	7%
tips, raw, 2 inches long or less	1 spear tip	1	0	0	0	0	0.0	0.0	0	7%
Frozen										
cuts (Birds Eye)	3.3 oz	25	3	4	5	0	0.0	0.0	0	0%
cuts (Flav-R-Pac)	3/4 cup	20	3	3	5	2	0.0	0.0	0	0%
cuts (Seabrook)	3.3 oz	25	3	4	6	0	0.0	0.0	0	0%
cuts, unprepared	10-oz pkg	68	9	12	23	5	0.7	0.1	0	8%
cuts, w/salt, boiled, drained	10-oz pkg	82	9	14	703	5	1.2	0.3	0	13%
cuts, w/salt, boiled, drained	1 cup	50	5	9	432	3	0.8	0.2	0	13%
cuts, w/o salt, boiled, drained	10-oz pkg	82	9	14	12	5	1.2	0.3	0	13%
cuts, w/o salt, boiled, drained	1 cup	50	5	9	7	3	0.8	0.2	0	13%
cuts and spears (Frosty Acres)	3.3 oz	25	3	4	6	0	0.0	0.0	0	0%
spears (Birds Eye)	3.3 oz	25	3	4	0	0	0.0	0.0	0	0%
spears (Finast)	3.3 oz	25	3	4	5	0	0.0	0.0	0	0%
spears (Frosty Acres)	3.3 oz	25	3	4	4	1	0.0	0.0	0	0%
spears (Seabrook)	3.3 oz	25	3	4	4	1	0.0	0.0	0	0%
spears (Southern)	3.5 oz	27	3	4	20	0	0.2	0.0	0	6%
spears, boiled, drained	4 spears	17	2	3	2	1	0.3	0.1	0	13%
spears, unprepared	4 spears	14	2	2	5	1	0.1	0.0	0	8%

ATLANTIC COD. See under COD.

ATLANTIC MACKEREL. See under MACKEREL.

ATLANTIC OCEAN PERCH. See OCEAN PERCH.

ATLANTIC POLLACK. See POLLACK.

ATLANTIC SALMON. See under SALMON.

AUBERGINE. See EGGPLANT.

AVOCADO

ALL COMMERCIAL VARIETIES

Food Name	Serving Size	Calories	Prot. gms	Carbs gms	Sod. mgs	Fiber gms	Fat gms	Sat. Fat gms	Chol. mgs	% Fat Cal.
Fresh										
raw, cubed	1 cup	242	3	11	15	8	23.0	3.7	0	80%
raw, puréed	1 cup	370	5	17	23	12	35.2	5.6	0	80%
raw, sliced	1 cup	235	3	11	15	7	22.4	3.6	0	80%
raw, whole	1 medium	324	4	15	20	10	30.8	4.9	0	80%
CALIFORNIA										
Fresh										
raw, puréed	1 cup	407	5	16	28	11	39.9	6.0	0	82%
raw, whole, peeled and pitted	1 medium	306	4	12	21	8	30.0	4.5	0	82%
FLORIDA										
Fresh										
raw, puréed	1 cup	258	4	20	12	12	20.4	4.0	0	66%
raw, whole, peeled and pitted	1 medium	340	5	27	15	16	27.0	5.3	0	66%
AVOCADO OIL										
. . . .	1 cup	1927	0	0	0	0	218.0	25.2	na	100%
. . . .	1 tbsp	124	0	0	0	0	14.0	1.6	na	100%
(Hain)	1 tbsp	120	0	0	0	0	14.0	1.0	0	100%
pure-pressed, organic (Spectrum)	1 tbsp	120	0	0	0	0	14.0	2.0	0	100%

AWA / milkfish

Food Name	Serving Size	Calories	Prot. gms	Carbs gms	Sod. mgs	Fiber gms	Fat gms	Sat. Fat gms	Chol. mgs	% Fat Cal.
baked, broiled, grilled, or microwaved...............	3 oz	162	22	0	78	0	7.3	na	57	41%
raw	3 oz	126	17	0	61	0	5.7	1.4	44	41%

B

Food Name	Serving Size	Calories	Prot. gms	Carbs gms	Sod. mgs	Fiber gms	Fat gms	Sat. Fat gms	Chol. mgs	% Fat Cal.
BABASSU OIL. See PALM KERNEL OIL.										
BABY FOOD										
CEREAL										
Barley										
dry..................	1/2 oz	55	2	11	7	1	0.5	0.1	0	8%
dry..................	1 tbsp	9	0	2	1	0	0.1	0.0	0	8%
instant *(Heinz)*..................	3.5 oz	370	9	79	15	0	3.7	0.0	0	9%
instant, prepared w/0.5 oz cereal and 2.4 oz whole milk *(Gerber)*..................	2.9 oz	100	3	14	0	0	4.0	0.0	0	35%
instant, prepared w/2.4 oz formula '1st Foods' *(Gerber)*..................	1/2 oz	110	2	16	0	0	4.0	0.0	0	33%
prepared w/whole milk..................	1 oz	31	1	5	14	na	0.9	na	na	27%
Cereal w/applesauce and bananas, '3rd Foods' *(Gerber)* ...	7 tbsp	82	1	18	3	0	0.6	0.0	0	7%
Cereal w/egg yolks										
junior..................	1 jar	88	3	12	56	2	3.1	1.0	107	30%
strained..................	1 oz	14	1	2	9	0	0.5	0.2	18	31%
w/eggs..................	1 oz	16	1	2	11	na	0.4	0.1	15	23%
Cereal w/egg yolks and bacon, junior..................	1 oz	22	1	2	14	0	1.4	0.5	27	56%
Corn										
instant, dry 'Tropical Foods' *(Gerber)*..................	3.5 oz	390	6	81	55	0	4.6	0.0	0	11%
instant, prepared w/milk 'Tropical Foods' *(Gerber)*	2.4 oz	110	3	15	0	0	4.0	0.0	0	33%
High-protein										
instant, dry..................	1/2 oz	54	5	7	7	1	0.9	0.1	0	14%
instant, dry..................	1 tbsp	9	1	1	1	0	0.1	0.0	0	14%
instant, prepared w/whole milk..................	1 oz	31	2	3	14	na	1.1	na	na	31%
w/apple and orange, instant, dry..................	1/2 oz	53	4	8	15	1	0.9	0.1	0	15%
w/apple and orange, instant, dry..................	1 tbsp	9	1	1	2	0	0.2	0.0	0	15%
w/apple and orange, instant, prepared w/whole milk	1 oz	32	2	4	16	na	1.1	na	na	31%
Mixed										
dry..................	1/2 oz	57	2	11	6	1	0.7	0.1	0	10%
dry..................	1 tbsp	9	0	2	1	0	0.1	0.0	0	10%
prepared w/whole milk..................	1 oz	32	1	5	13	0	1.0	0.5	3	28%
instant, dry *(Earth's Best)*..................	0.5 oz	60	2	11	0	0	0.0	0.0	0	0%
instant, dry, '2nd Foods' *(Gerber)*..................	0.5 oz	60	1	11	0	0	1.0	0.0	0	16%
instant *(Heinz)*..................	3.5 oz	373	13	72	12	0	4.9	0.0	0	12%
instant, prepared w/apple juice, '2nd Foods' *(Gerber)*.....	2.4 oz	90	1	20	0	0	1.0	0.0	0	10%
instant, prepared w/0.5 oz cereal, 2.4 oz formula, 'Stages 2' *(Beech-Nut)*..................	0.5 oz	120	2	17	25	0	4.0	0.0	0	32%
instant, prepared w/0.5 oz cereal, 2.5 oz formula *(Earth's Best)*..................	3 oz	110	3	16	15	0	3.0	0.0	0	26%
instant, prepared w/0.5 oz cereal, 2.4 oz whole milk, 'Stages 2' *(Beech-Nut)*..................	2.9 oz	100	4	14	50	0	3.0	0.0	0	27%
w/apple and bananas, 'Stages 2' *(Beech-Nut)*..........	4.5 oz	90	2	19	0	0	1.0	0.0	0	10%
w/apple and bananas, strained *(Heinz)*................	3.5 oz	70	1	16	3	0	0.3	0.0	0	4%
w/apple 'Stages 2' *(Beech-Nut)*..................	4 oz	70	0	16	0	1	0.0	na	na	0%
w/applesauce and bananas, junior..................	1 oz	24	0	5	10	0	0.1	0.0	0	4%

Food Name	Serving Size	Calories	Prot. gms	Carbs gms	Sod. mgs	Fiber gms	Fat gms	Sat. Fat gms	Chol. mgs	% Fat Cal.
w/applesauce and bananas, strained	1 oz	23	0	5	1	0	0.1	0.0	0	5%
w/applesauce and bananas, '3rd Foods' (Gerber)	7 tbsp	82	1	19	3	0	0.6	0.0	0	6%
w/banana, dry	1/2 oz	59	2	12	18	1	0.7	0.1	0	10%
w/banana, dry	1 tbsp	10	0	2	3	0	0.1	0.0	0	10%
w/bananas, dry, '2nd Foods' (Gerber)	0.5 oz	60	1	11	0	0	1.0	0.0	0	16%
w/fruit and nuts, no sugar added, 1-4 yr, dry (Familia)	1.5 oz	170	4	31	4	0	3.0	0.0	0	16%
w/fruit and nuts, 100% natural, 1-4 yr, dry (Familia)	1.5 oz	170	4	32	1	0	3.0	0.0	0	16%
w/fruit and nuts, 1-4 yr, prepared w/whole milk (Familia)	1.5 oz	270	9	38	77	0	8.0	0.0	0	28%
w/fruit and nuts, 1-4 yr, prepared w/2/3 cup milk (Familia)	1.5 oz	270	9	39	74	0	8.0	0.0	0	27%
Oatmeal										
dry	1/2 oz	60	2	10	5	1	1.2	0.2	0	16%
dry	1 tbsp	10	0	2	1	0	0.2	0.0	0	16%
prepared w/whole milk	1 oz	33	1	4	13	0	1.2	0.6	3	32%
w/apple, 'Stages 2' (Beech-Nut)	4 oz	70	1	16	0	1	0.0	na	na	0%
w/apple and bananas 'Stages 2' (Beech-Nut)	4.5 oz	90	2	17	5	0	1.0	0.0	0	11%
w/apple and bananas, strained (Heinz)	3.5 oz	76	2	16	3	1	0.6	0.0	0	7%
w/apple and cinnamon, instant, '3rd Foods' (Gerber)	1 pkt	90	2	16	50	0	2.0	0.0	0	20%
w/applesauce and bananas, junior	1 oz	21	0	4	9	0	0.2	0.0	0	8%
w/applesauce and bananas, strained	1 oz	21	0	4	1	0	0.2	0.0	0	8%
w/applesauce and bananas, '3rd Foods' (Gerber)	7 tbsp	80	1	17	3	0	0.8	0.0	0	9%
w/bananas, dry	1/2 oz	59	2	11	18	1	0.9	0.2	0	13%
w/bananas, dry	1 tbsp	10	0	2	3	0	0.1	0.0	0	13%
w/bananas, prepared w/whole milk	1 oz	33	1	5	17	na	1.1	na	na	29%
w/bananas, instant '3rd Foods' (Gerber)	1 pkt	90	2	16	50	0	2.0	0.0	0	20%
w/bananas, 100% natural, organic, dry (Healthy Times)	0.5 oz	60	2	12	0	0	0.0	0.0	0	0%
w/bananas, organic, prepared w/2.4 oz formula (Healthy Times)	0.5 oz	100	3	17	15	0	3.0	0.0	0	25%
w/fruit, toddler, instant, dry	0.75 oz	84	2	16	42	2	1.5	0.3	0	16%
w/fruit, toddler, instant, dry	1 tbsp	21	1	4	11	0	0.4	0.1	0	16%
w/honey, dry	1/2 oz	56	2	10	7	na	1.0	na	na	15%
w/honey, dry	1 tbsp	9	0	2	1	na	0.2	na	na	15%
w/honey, prepared w/whole milk	1 oz	33	1	4	14	na	1.1	na	na	31%
Rice										
dry	1/2 oz	59	1	12	5	0	0.7	0.1	0	10%
dry	1 tbsp	10	0	2	1	0	0.1	0.0	0	11%
prepared w/whole milk	1 oz	33	1	5	13	0	1.0	0.7	3	28%
prepared w/formula '1st Foods' (Gerber)	2.4 oz	110	2	16	0	0	4.0	0.0	0	33%
(Heinz)	3.5 oz	376	8	78	12	0	4.1	0.0	0	10%
brown, dry (Earth's Best)	0.5 oz	60	1	12	0	0	0.0	0.0	0	0%
brown, prepared w/0.5 oz cereal, 2.5 oz formula (Earth's Best)	3 oz	110	2	17	15	0	3.0	0.0	0	26%
instant, prepared w/0.5 oz cereal, 2.4 oz whole milk, 'Stages 1' (Beech-Nut) 'Stages 1'	2.9 oz	110	2	17	30	0	3.0	0.0	0	26%
instant, prepared w/0.5 oz cereal, 2.4 oz formula, 'Stages 1' (Beech-Nut)	0.5 oz	120	2	18	20	0	4.0	0.0	0	31%
sprouted (Health Valley)	1 tbsp	60	1	10	5	2	1.0	0.0	0	17%
w/apple, instant, prepared w/0.5 oz cereal, 2.4 oz formula (Beech-Nut)	2.9 oz	120	1	19	20	0	4.0	0.0	0	31%
w/apple, instant, prepared w/0.5 oz cereal, 2.4 oz whole milk (Beech-Nut)	2.9 oz	110	3	17	50	0	3.0	0.0	0	25%
w/apple, 'Stages 2' (Beech-Nut)	4 oz	70	0	16	0	1	0.0	na	na	0%

Food Name	Serving Size	Calories	Prot. gms	Carbs gms	Sod. mgs	Fiber gms	Fat gms	Sat. Fat gms	Chol. mgs	% Fat Cal.
w/apple and bananas, 'Stages 2' (Beech-Nut)	4.5 oz	100	2	24	25	0	0.0	0.0	0	0%
w/apple and bananas, strained (Heinz)	3.5 oz	70	1	16	5	0	0.2	0.0	0	3%
w/applesauce and bananas, '2nd Foods' (Gerber)	7 tbsp	79	1	18	9	0	0.2	0.0	0	2%
w/applesauce and bananas, strained	1 oz	22	0	5	8	0	0.1	0.0	0	4%
w/applesauce and bananas, strained	1 tbsp	13	0	3	4	0	0.1	0.0	0	4%
w/applesauce and bananas, strained, '2nd Foods' (Gerber)	4 oz jar	89	1	19	32	1	0.5	0.1	0	4%
w/applesauce and bananas, strained, 'Strained 2' (Heinz)	4.25 oz jar	95	1	21	34	1	0.5	0.1	0	4%
w/bananas, dry	1 tbsp	10	0	2	2	0	0.1	0.0	0	9%
w/bananas, dry	1/2 oz	61	1	12	14	0	0.6	0.1	0	9%
w/bananas, prepared w/whole milk	1 oz	33	1	5	16	0	1.0	0.6	3	27%
w/bananas, dry, '2nd Foods' (Gerber)	0.5 oz	60	1	11	0	0	1.0	0.0	0	16%
w/bananas, prepared w/0.5 oz cereal, 2.4 oz formula (Beech-Nut)	0.5 oz	120	1	19	20	0	4.0	0.0	0	31%
w/bananas, prepared w/0.5 oz cereal, 2.4 oz whole milk (Beech-Nut)	2.9 oz	100	3	17	50	0	3.0	0.0	0	25%
w/honey, prepared w/whole milk	1 oz	33	1	5	14	na	0.9	na	na	26%
w/mango, dry, 'Tropical Foods' (Gerber)	3.5 oz	386	6	84	20	0	2.6	0.0	0	6%
w/mango, prepared w/milk, 'Tropical Foods' (Gerber)	2.4 oz	100	3	15	0	0	3.0	0.0	0	27%
w/mixed fruit, junior	1 oz	22	0	5	3	0	0.1	0.0	0	2%
w/mixed fruit, junior	1 tbsp	12	0	3	2	0	0.0	0.0	0	2%
w/mixed fruit, junior (Gerber)	6 oz	140	1	31	17	0	1.0	0.0	0	7%
w/mixed fruit, '3rd Foods' (Gerber)	6-oz jar	134	2	31	17	1	0.3	0.1	0	2%
DESSERTS AND SNACKS										
Apple-strawberry dessert, 'Stages 2' (Beech-Nut)	4 oz	100	0	23	0	1	0.0	na	na	0%
Apple-peach-strawberry dessert, 'Stages 2' (Beech-Nut)	4 oz	100	0	22	0	1	0.0	na	na	0%
Banana-pineapple dessert, 'Stages 2' (Beech-Nut)	4 oz	100	0	23	15	0	0.0	0.0	0	0%
Banana-vanilla dessert, (Gerber) 'Tropical Foods'	7 tbsp	85	1	19	11	0	0.9	0.0	0	10%
Cereal snack										
apple-banana, finger snacks, 'Graduates' (Gerber)	3.2 oz	405	8	83	86	0	4.8	0.0	0	11%
apple-cinnamon, finger snacks 'Graduates' (Gerber)	3.2 oz	407	8	83	84	0	5.0	0.0	0	11%
Cookies and crackers										
animal-shaped, baked, chunky (Gerber)	3.5 oz	443	7	75	187	0	13.1	0.0	0	27%
apple, organic, 'Hugga Bears' (Healthy Times)	1 oz	120	2	17	38	0	3.0	0.0	0	26%
arrowroot	1 oz	125	2	20	105	0	4.1	0.9	0	27%
arrowroot	1 cookie	22	0	4	19	0	0.7	0.2	0	27%
arrowroot, baked finger snacks, 'Graduates' (Gerber)	3.5 oz	452	8	70	324	0	15.3	0.0	0	30%
arrowroot, maple, wheat-free (Healthy Times)	1 cookie	120	2	17	38	0	3.0	0.0	0	26%
cinnamon animal cracker, baked 'Graduates' (Gerber)	3.5 oz	449	6	79	369	0	12.3	0.0	0	25%
pretzel	1 oz	113	3	23	76	1	0.6	0.1	0	4%
pretzel, baked, finger snacks, 'Graduates' (Gerber)	3.5 oz	403	11	83	597	0	3.3	0.0	0	7%
strawberry, organic, 'Hugga Bears' (Healthy Times)	1 oz	120	2	17	38	0	3.0	0.0	0	26%
teething biscuit	1 oz	111	3	22	103	0	1.2	0.4	0	9%
teething biscuit	1 biscuit	43	1	8	40	0	0.5	0.2	0	9%
teething, biscuit, baked, chunky, 'Biter Biscuit' (Gerber)	1 biscuit	50	1	9	0	0	1.0	0.0	0	18%
teething toast (Zings!)	1 serving	35	1	5	10	1	1.0	0.5	0	27%
zwieback	1 oz	121	3	21	66	1	2.8	1.1	6	19%
zwieback	1 piece	30	1	5	16	0	0.7	0.3	1	19%
zwieback toast (Gerber)	1 cracker	30	1	5	16	0	0.7	0.3	1	19%
zwieback toast, baked, chunky (Gerber)	3.5 oz	432	13	69	210	0	11.5	0.0	0	24%
Cottage cheese										
w/pineapple, 'Stages 2' (Beech-Nut)	4.5 oz	130	2	26	15	0	1.0	0.0	0	7%

Food Name	Serving Size	Calories	Prot. gms	Carbs gms	Sod. mgs	Fiber gms	Fat gms	Sat. Fat gms	Chol. mgs	% Fat Cal.
w/pineapple 'Stages 3' (Beech-Nut)	6 oz	170	3	36	20	0	2.0	0.0	0	10%
w/pears, 'Stages 2' (Beech-Nut)	4 oz	120	2	24	15	1	1.0	na	na	8%
w/pears, 'Stages 3' (Beech-Nut)	6 oz	180	3	37	20	1	2.0	na	na	10%
Custard/pudding										
banana pudding, 'Stages 2' (Beech-Nut)	4 oz	110	0	26	0	0	0.0	na	na	0%
banana pudding, strained (Heinz)	3.5 oz	74	1	17	9	0	0.5	0.0	0	6%
cherry vanilla pudding, strained	1 oz	19	0	5	5	0	0.1	0.0	3	4%
cherry-vanilla pudding, strained (Gerber)	4.5 oz	90	0	21	12	0	1.0	0.0	3	10%
cherry-vanilla pudding, junior	1 oz	20	0	5	4	0	0.1	0.0	3	3%
custard pudding, junior (Heinz)	3.5 oz	75	2	14	27	0	1.2	0.0	0	14%
custard pudding, strained (Heinz)	3.5 oz	75	2	14	27	0	1.2	0.0	0	14%
orange pudding, strained	1 oz	23	0	5	6	0	0.3	0.2	1	10%
pineapple pudding, junior	1 oz	25	0	6	6	0	0.1	0.0	0	4%
pineapple pudding, junior	1 tbsp	13	0	3	3	0	0.1	0.0	0	4%
pineapple pudding, junior, '3rd Foods' (Gerber)	6-oz jar	148	2	37	37	1	0.7	0.2	0	4%
pineapple pudding, strained	1 oz	23	0	6	5	0	0.1	0.0	0	3%
pineapple pudding, strained	1 tbsp	12	0	3	3	0	0.0	0.0	0	3%
pineapple pudding, strained, '2nd Foods'	4 oz jar	92	1	23	21	1	0.3	0.1	0	3%
tutti frutti pudding, junior (Heinz)	3.5 oz	67	0	16	12	0	0.4	0.0	0	5%
vanilla custard, 'Stages 2' (Beech-Nut)	4 oz	120	2	23	60	0	3.0	0.0	0	21%
vanilla custard, 'Stages 3' (Beech-Nut)	6 oz	180	3	30	80	0	5.0	0.0	0	25%
vanilla custard, '3rd Foods' (Gerber)	6 oz	190	2	32	85	0	6.0	0.0	0	28%
vanilla custard, junior (Gerber)	6 oz	150	3	31	41	0	2.0	0.0	23	12%
vanilla custard, strained (Gerber)	4.5 oz	100	2	22	32	0	1.0	0.0	14	9%
vanilla pudding, junior	1 cup	197	4	40	60	0	2.2	0.7	87	10%
vanilla pudding, junior	1 oz	24	0	5	7	0	0.3	0.1	11	10%
vanilla pudding, junior	1 tbsp	12	0	2	4	0	0.1	0.0	5	10%
vanilla pudding, junior, 'Junior 3' (Heinz)	6 oz jar	146	3	30	44	0	1.7	0.6	65	10%
vanilla pudding, junior, 'Stages 3' (Beech-Nut)	6 oz jar	146	3	30	44	0	1.7	0.6	65	10%
vanilla pudding, junior, '3rd Foods' (Gerber)	6 oz jar	146	3	30	44	0	1.7	0.6	65	10%
vanilla pudding, strained	1 cup	195	4	37	64	0	4.6	2.3	18	21%
vanilla pudding, strained	1 oz	24	0	5	8	0	0.6	0.3	2	21%
vanilla pudding, strained	1 tbsp	12	0	2	4	0	0.3	0.1	1	21%
vanilla pudding, strained, '2nd Foods' (Gerber)	4 oz jar	96	2	18	32	0	2.3	1.1	9	21%
vanilla pudding, strained, 'Stages 2' (Beech-Nut)	4 oz jar	96	2	18	32	0	2.3	1.1	9	21%
vanilla pudding, strained, 'Strained 2' (Heinz)	4 oz jar	96	2	18	32	0	2.3	1.1	9	21%
Dutch apple dessert										
junior	1 oz	22	0	5	1	0	0.0	0.0	0	2%
junior (Heinz)	3.5 oz	69	0	16	5	0	0.4	0.0	0	5%
'Stages 2' (Beech-Nut)	4 oz	100	0	22	10	0	0.0	0.0	0	0%
strained	1 oz	19	0	5	5	0	0.3	0.2	0	11%
strained (Heinz)	3.5 oz	69	0	16	5	0	0.4	0.0	0	5%
'3rd Foods' (Gerber)	7 tbsp	77	0	17	14	0	0.9	0.0	0	11%
Fruit dessert										
junior (Gerber)	6 oz	130	0	30	12	0	1.0	0.0	0	7%
junior (Heinz)	3.5 oz	65	0	16	14	0	0.2	0.0	0	3%
junior, w/o added vitamin C	1 oz	18	0	5	4	0	0.0	0.0	0	0%
junior, w/o added vitamin C	1 tbsp	9	0	3	2	0	0.0	0.0	0	0%
junior, w/o added vitamin C, '3rd Foods' (Gerber)	6-oz jar	107	1	29	22	1	0.0	0.0	0	0%
junior, w/o added vitamin C 'Junior 3' (Heinz)	6-oz jar	107	1	29	22	1	0.0	0.0	0	0%
nonfat, 'Stages 3' (Beech-Nut)	6 oz	120	0	28	0	2	0.0	0.0	0	0%
strained (Gerber)	4.5 oz	100	0	24	13	0	1.0	0.0	0	9%
strained (Heinz)	3.5 oz	66	0	16	11	0	0.2	0.0	0	3%
strained, w/o added vitamin C	1 oz	17	0	5	4	0	0.0	0.0	0	0%

Food Name	Serving Size	Calories	Prot. gms	Carbs gms	Sod. mgs	Fiber gms	Fat gms	Sat. Fat gms	Chol. mgs	% Fat Cal.
strained, w/o added vitamin C.	1 tbsp	9	0	2	2	0	0.0	0.0	0	0%
strained, w/o added vitamin C, '2nd Foods' (Gerber)	4-oz jar	67	0	18	16	1	0.0	0.0	0	0%
strained, w/o added vitamin C, 'Strained 2' (Heinz).	4.25-oz jar	71	0	19	17	1	0.0	0.0	0	0%
'3rd Foods' (Gerber)	7 tbsp	73	0	18	7	0	0.2	0.0	0	2%
Guava dessert										
tropical fruit, 'Stages 2' (Beech-Nut)	4 oz	90	0	22	10	2	0.0	na	na	0%
w/tapioca 'Tropical Foods' (Gerber).	7 tbsp	69	0	17	3	0	0.1	0.0	0	1%
Hawaiian dessert										
Hawaiian delight, '3rd Foods' (Gerber)	7 tbsp	87	1	20	15	0	0.1	0.0	0	1%
Hawaiian delight, junior (Gerber).	6 oz	150	2	33	32	0	1.0	0.0	3	6%
strained (Gerber).	4.5 oz	120	2	25	23	0	1.0	0.0	2	8%
Mango dessert										
tropical fruit dessert, 'Stages 2' (Beech-Nut).	4.5 oz	100	0	25	15	0	0.0	0.0	0	0%
w/tapioca, 'Tropical Foods' (Gerber)	7 tbsp	75	0	18	2	0	0.2	0.0	0	2%
Mango-banana dessert, w/passionfruit,										
'Tropical Foods' (Gerber)	7 tbsp	73	0	18	9	0	0.1	0.0	0	1%
Papaya dessert, w/tapioca, 'Tropical Foods' (Gerber)	7 tbsp	62	0	15	7	0	0.2	0.0	0	3%
Papaya-pineapple dessert, 'Tropical Foods' (Gerber)	7 tbsp	76	0	19	8	0	0.0	0.0	0	0%
Peach cobbler										
junior.	1 oz	19	0	5	3	0	0.0	0.0	0	0%
junior.	1 tbsp	10	0	3	1	0	0.0	0.0	0	0%
junior (Gerber).	6 oz	130	1	30	15	0	1.0	0.0	0	7%
'2nd Foods' (Gerber)	4-oz jar	73	0	20	8	1	0.0	0.0	0	0%
strained	1 oz	18	0	5	2	0	0.0	0.0	0	0%
strained	1 tbsp	10	0	3	1	0	0.0	0.0	0	0%
strained (Gerber).	4.5 oz	100	1	23	9	0	1.0	0.0	0	9%
strained (Heinz).	3.5 oz	72	1	17	6	0	0.3	0.0	0	4%
'Strained 2' (Heinz)	4-oz jar	73	0	20	8	1	0.0	0.0	0	0%
'3rd Foods' (Gerber)	6-oz jar	114	1	31	15	1	0.0	0.0	0	0%
'3rd Foods' (Gerber)	7 tbsp	77	1	18	9	0	0.1	0.0	0	1%
Peach-mango dessert, 'Tropical Foods' (Gerber).	7 tbsp	60	0	17	7	0	0.2	0.0	0	3%
Pineapple-banana dessert, 'Tropical Foods' (Gerber)	7 tbsp	79	0	19	9	0	0.1	0.0	0	1%
Tropical dessert										
island fruit dessert, 'Stages 2' (Beech-Nut).	4 oz	100	0	23	10	0	0.0	na	na	0%
mango dessert, Stages 2' (Beech-Nut).	4 oz	110	0	26	10	1	0.0	na	na	0%
medley, 'Tropical Foods' (Gerber)	7 tbsp	64	0	15	6	0	0.1	0.0	0	1%
papaya dessert, 'Stages 2' (Beech-Nut)	4 oz	100	0	22	10	0	0.0	na	na	0%
w/tapioca, strained (Gerber)	4.5 oz	80	0	20	6	0	0.0	0.0	0	0%
Yogurt										
apple, 'Stages 2' (Beech-Nut)	4 oz	100	1	22	25	0	1.0	0.0	0	9%
apple, 'Breakfast' (Earth's Best)	4.5 oz	100	3	17	20	0	2.0	0.0	0	18%
banana, 'Stages 2' (Beech-Nut)	4 oz	120	1	24	25	0	2.0	0.0	0	15%
banana, strained (Heinz).	3.5 oz	83	1	19	20	0	0.5	0.0	0	5%
blueberry, 'Breakfast' (Earth's Best).	4.5 oz	100	3	16	20	0	2.0	0.0	0	19%
mixed fruit, 'Stages 2' (Beech-Nut)	4 oz	100	1	21	15	1	0.0	na	na	0%
mixed fruit, 'Stages 3' (Beech-Nut)	6 oz	170	1	30	30	1	0.0	na	na	0%
peach, '2nd Foods' (Gerber)	7 tbsp	76	1	17	14	0	0.4	0.0	0	5%
peach, 'Stages 2' (Beech-Nut).	4.5 oz	120	1	25	30	0	2.0	0.0	0	15%
pear, 'Stages 2' (Beech-Nut)	4.5 oz	130	1	29	35	0	2.0	0.0	0	13%
pear, strained (Heinz)	3.5 oz	80	1	18	19	0	0.4	0.0	0	5%
tropical, 'Breakfast' (Earth's Best)	4.5 oz	110	3	19	20	0	2.0	0.0	0	17%
DINNERS AND MAIN DISHES										
Apple and chicken dinner										
'Simple Recipe' '2nd Foods' (Gerber)	4 oz	70	3	12	15	2	1.5	0.0	0	19%

Food Name	Serving Size	Calories	Prot. gms	Carbs gms	Sod. mgs	Fiber gms	Fat gms	Sat. Fat gms	Chol. mgs	% Fat Cal.
'Simple Dinner' 'Stage 2' *(Beech-Nut)*	4 oz	73	2	12	14	2	1.6	0.4	6	19%
strained	1 oz	18	1	3	3	1	0.4	0.1	1	19%
Apple and ham dinner										
'Simple Recipe' '2nd Foods' *(Gerber)*	4 oz	80	3	12	15	2	2.0	0.0	0	22%
strained	1 tbsp	9	0	2	1	0	0.1	0.0	1	13%
Apple and turkey dinner										
'Simple Recipe' '2nd Foods' *(Gerber)*	4 oz	80	3	13	20	0	2.0	0.0	0	22%
strained	1 tbsp	10	0	2	2	0	0.2	0.1	1	18%
Beans and rice dinner, 'Tropical Foods' *(Gerber)*	7 tbsp	52	2	7	8	0	1.5	0.0	0	26%
Beef and rice dinner, toddler	1 oz	23	1	2	101	na	0.8	na	na	31%
Beef and vegetable dinner										
lean meat, junior *(Gerber)*	4.5 oz	100	8	10	29	0	3.0	0.0	12	27%
lean meat, strained *(Gerber)*	4.5 oz	90	7	9	32	0	3.0	0.0	11	30%
'Stage 2' *(Beech-Nut)*	4.5 oz	90	2	10	35	0	4.0	0.0	0	43%
'Stage 3' *(Beech-Nut)*	6 oz	160	6	16	70	0	7.0	0.0	0	42%
Beef dinner										
junior *(Gerber)*	2.5 oz	80	11	1	38	0	4.0	0.0	20	43%
'Stage 1' *(Beech-Nut)*	2.8 oz	90	10	0	40	0	5.0	0.0	0	53%
'Stage 3' *(Beech-Nut)*	6 oz	150	6	14	45	0	8.0	0.0	0	47%
'3rd Foods' *(Gerber)*	7 tbsp	103	15	0	52	0	4.6	0.0	0	40%
Beef lasagna dinner, toddler	1 oz	22	1	3	129	na	0.6	na	na	24%
Beef noodle dinner										
chunky, 'Homestyle' *(Gerber)*	7 tbsp	88	4	10	216	0	3.5	0.0	0	36%
junior	1 oz	16	1	2	5	0	0.5	0.2	2	30%
junior	1 tbsp	9	0	1	3	0	0.3	0.1	1	30%
'Step 3' *(Heinz)*	6 oz	97	4	13	29	2	3.2	1.3	14	30%
strained	1 oz	18	1	2	4	0	0.6	0.3	2	32%
strained	1 tbsp	10	0	1	2	0	0.4	0.1	1	32%
w/egg noodles, '2nd Foods' *(Gerber)*	7 tbsp	62	3	8	10	0	2.0	0.0	0	29%
w/egg noodles, 'Stage 2' *(Beech-Nut)*	4 oz	100	1	8	50	2	6.0	na	na	60%
w/egg noodles, 'Stage 3' *(Beech-Nut)*	6 oz	130	3	13	50	2	6.0	na	na	46%
w/egg noodles, 'Step 2' *(Heinz)*	3.5 oz	49	2	6	15	0	1.8	0.0	0	33%
w/egg noodles, '3rd Foods' *(Gerber)*	6 oz	130	4	18	45	3	1.9	0.0	0	27%
Beef stew										
'Table Time' *(Beech-Nut)*	6 oz	150	10	16	380	0	6.0	0.0	0	34%
toddler	1 oz	14	1	2	98	0	0.3	0.2	4	21%
Broccoli and chicken dinner										
'Simple Recipe' '2nd Foods' *(Gerber)*	4 oz	45	4	3	30	2	2.0	0.5	7	32%
'Step 2' *(Heinz)*	4 oz	47	4	4	21	3	1.7	0.5	7	32%
strained	1 oz	12	1	1	5	1	0.4	0.1	2	32%
Carrot and beef dinner										
'Simple Recipe' '2nd Foods' *(Gerber)*	4 oz	70	4	6	80	2	3.5	0.0	0	38%
strained	1 tbsp	9	1	1	9	0	0.4	0.1	1	38%
Chicken and rice dinner										
'Stage 2' *(Beech-Nut)*	4 oz	80	1	9	70	1	3.0	0.0	0	40%
'Tropical Foods' *(Gerber)*	7 tbsp	48	2	7	14	0	1.3	0.0	0	24%
Chicken and vegetable dinner										
'Stage 2' *(Beech-Nut)*	4.5 oz	90	3	14	65	0	3.0	0.0	0	28%
'Stage 3' *(Beech-Nut)*	6 oz	90	7	13	70	0	2.0	0.0	0	18%
w/broccoli, simple recipe, '2nd Foods' *(Gerber)*	7 tbsp	42	4	3	20	0	1.5	0.0	0	32%
Chicken dinner										
junior *(Gerber)*	2.5 oz	110	11	1	28	0	7.0	0.0	42	57%
'3rd Foods' *(Gerber)*	7 tbsp	132	15	0	39	0	7.9	0.0	0	54%
w/vegetables, lean meat, junior *(Gerber)*	4.5 oz	90	7	10	32	0	3.0	0.0	19	28%

Food Name	Serving Size	Calories	Prot. gms	Carbs gms	Sod. mgs	Fiber gms	Fat gms	Sat. Fat gms	Chol. mgs	% Fat Cal.
w/vegetables, lean meat, strained *(Gerber)*	4.5 oz	90	7	8	31	0	3.0	0.0	18	31%
Chicken noodle dinner										
junior	1 oz	16	1	2	22	0	0.3	0.1	3	19%
junior	1 tbsp	9	0	1	12	0	0.2	0.1	1	19%
'2nd Foods' *(Gerber)*	4 oz	80	3	11	35	2	2.5	0.7	18	28%
'Step 2' *(Heinz)*	4 oz	75	3	10	26	2	2.3	0.7	18	28%
'Step 3' *(Heinz)*	6 oz	94	4	15	133	2	2.0	0.6	15	19%
'Stage 2' *(Beech-Nut)*	4 oz	70	1	7	45	2	4.0	na	na	53%
'Stage 3' *(Beech-Nut)*	6 oz	110	3	14	55	1	4.0	na	na	35%
strained	1 oz	19	1	3	7	1	0.6	0.2	5	28%
strained	1 tbsp	11	0	1	4	0	0.3	0.1	3	28%
'3rd Foods' *(Gerber)*	6 oz	110	4	16	65	4	3.5	0.0	0	29%
w/carrots and peas, chunky *(Gerber)*	7 tbsp	65	4	9	207	0	1.5	0.0	0	21%
Chicken stew										
toddler	1 oz	22	1	2	57	0	1.0	0.3	8	42%
toddler	1 tbsp	12	1	1	32	0	0.6	0.2	5	42%
w/noodles 'Graduates' *(Gerber)*	3.2 oz	69	4	9	308	0	2.0	0.0	0	26%
Green bean and rice dinner *(Earth's Best)*	4.5 oz	70	2	14	0	0	0.0	0.0	0	0%
Green bean and turkey dinner										
'Simple Recipe' '2nd Foods' *(Gerber)*	7 tbsp	55	4	7	11	0	1.5	0.0	0	24%
'Step 2' *(Heinz)*	4 oz	60	4	6	12	3	2.1	0.5	9	31%
strained	1 oz	15	1	2	3	1	0.5	0.1	2	31%
Ham and vegetable dinner										
lean meat, junior *(Gerber)*	4.5 oz	110	8	11	27	0	4.0	0.0	11	32%
lean meat, strained *(Gerber)*	4.5 oz	100	7	10	26	0	4.0	0.0	12	35%
'Stage 2' *(Beech-Nut)*	4.5 oz	80	3	12	30	0	3.0	0.0	0	31%
Lamb and vegetable dinner, 'Stage 2' *(Beech-Nut)*	4.5 oz	90	2	13	40	0	4.0	0.0	0	38%
Macaroni and beef dinner										
in sauce, 'Graduates' *(Gerber)*	3.2 oz	78	5	11	302	0	1.7	0.0	0	19%
'Stage 2' *(Beech-Nut)*	4.5 oz	90	2	13	40	0	4.0	0.0	0	38%
'Stage 3' *(Beech-Nut)*	6 oz	130	3	14	60	2	6.0	0.0	0	44%
Macaroni and cheese										
(Earth's Best)	4.5 oz	100	4	12	10	0	4.0	0.0	0	36%
junior	1 oz	17	1	2	22	0	0.6	0.3	2	29%
strained	1 oz	19	1	3	25	0	0.6	0.4	2	28%
'Table Time' *(Beech-Nut)*	6 oz	200	3	21	320	0	12.0	na	na	53%
Macaroni, tomato, and beef dinner										
junior	1 oz	17	1	3	5	0	0.3	0.1	1	17%
junior	1 tbsp	9	0	2	3	0	0.2	0.1	1	17%
'2nd Foods' *(Gerber)*	4 oz	70	3	11	40	1	1.0	0.5	8	13%
strained	1 oz	17	1	3	11	0	0.4	0.1	2	22%
strained	1 tbsp	10	0	2	6	0	0.2	0.1	1	22%
'Step 2' *(Heinz)*	4 oz	69	3	11	43	1	1.7	0.5	8	22%
'3rd Foods' *(Gerber)*	7 tbsp	60	3	10	12	0	0.9	0.0	0	14%
Pasta dinner										
alphabet pasta w/beef and tomato sauce, chunky *(Gerber)*	7 tbsp	80	4	11	199	0	2.0	0.0	0	22%
(Earth's Best)	4.5 oz	90	3	13	20	0	3.0	0.0	0	30%
pasta w/vegetables *(Gerber)*	4 oz	68	2	9	12	2	2.4	1.4	6	32%
seashells in tomato sauce, 'Table Time' *(Beech-Nut)*	6 oz	150	3	25	170	1	4.0	na	na	24%
Potato and green bean dinner *(Earth's Best)*	4.5 oz	100	4	13	25	0	3.0	0.0	0	28%
Ravioli										
w/beef and sauce, 'Graduates' *(Gerber)*	3.2 oz	97	3	16	322	0	2.0	0.0	0	19%
w/beef and sauce, micro cup, 'Graduates' *(Gerber)*	6 oz	170	6	28	590	0	4.0	0.0	0	21%

Food Name	Serving Size	Calories	Prot. gms	Carbs gms	Sod. mgs	Fiber gms	Fat gms	Sat. Fat gms	Chol. mgs	% Fat Cal.
w/cheese and sauce, 'Graduates' (Gerber)	3.2 oz	99	4	16	297	0	2.2	0.0	0	20%
w/cheese and sauce, micro cup, 'Graduates' (Gerber)	6 oz	170	6	28	510	0	4.0	0.0	0	21%
Rice and beef dinner, w/tomato sauce, chunky (Gerber)	7 tbsp	79	4	12	202	0	1.9	0.0	0	22%
Rice and chicken dinner, saucy, chunky (Gerber)	7 tbsp	67	3	10	222	0	1.5	0.0	0	20%
Rice and lentil dinner (Earth's Best)	4.5 oz	80	3	13	25	0	2.0	0.0	0	22%
Spaghetti										
in tomato sauce w/beef, '3rd Foods' (Gerber)	6 oz	140	5	20	80	2	4.5	0.9	9	28%
rings w/meat sauce, 'Table Time' (Beech-Nut)	6 oz	160	7	20	180	0	6.0	na	na	33%
w/beef, chunky (Gerber)	7 tbsp	85	4	13	223	0	1.9	0.0	0	20%
w/beef, junior (Gerber)	6 oz	120	5	19	41	0	3.0	0.0	7	22%
w/beef, 'Stage 3' (Beech-Nut)	6 oz	130	3	16	70	1	6.0	0.0	0	42%
w/beef, '3rd Foods' (Gerber)	7 tbsp	64	3	11	20	0	1.2	0.0	0	17%
w/meat, junior (Heinz)	3.5 oz	58	2	10	19	0	1.3	0.0	0	20%
w/mini meatballs, 'Graduates' (Gerber)	6 oz	160	7	21	590	0	5.0	0.0	0	29%
w/tomato and meat, junior	1 oz	19	1	3	21	0	0.4	0.2	1	18%
w/tomato and meat, junior	1 tbsp	11	0	2	12	0	0.2	0.1	1	18%
w/tomato and meat, 'Step 3' (Heinz)	6 oz	116	4	19	128	2	2.3	0.9	9	18%
w/tomato and meat, toddler	1 oz	21	2	3	101	na	0.3	na	na	12%
Sweet potato and chicken dinner										
(Earth's Best)	4.5 oz	90	3	13	30	0	2.0	0.0	0	22%
'Stage 2' (Beech-Nut)	4 oz	84	3	12	25	1	2.5	0.6	12	26%
strained	1 tbsp	12	0	2	4	0	0.3	0.1	2	26%
Turkey and barley dinner (Gerber)	4-oz jar	60	3	9	23	2	1.2	0.4	5	19%
Turkey and rice dinner										
junior	1 oz	16	1	3	23	0	0.3	0.1	1	15%
junior	1 tbsp	9	0	2	13	0	0.1	0.0	1	15%
'2nd Foods' (Gerber)	4 oz	60	2	9	30	1	1.5	0.4	6	18%
'Stage 2' (Beech-Nut)	4 oz	70	1	8	50	1	3.0	0.0	0	43%
'Stage 3' (Beech-Nut)	6 oz	100	3	13	60	1	3.0	0.0	0	30%
strained	1 oz	15	1	2	6	0	0.4	0.1	1	21%
strained	1 tbsp	8	0	1	3	0	0.2	0.1	1	21%
w/vegetables, 'Step 2' (Heinz)	4 oz	59	3	9	23	1	1.4	0.4	6	21%
w/vegetables, 'Step 3' (Heinz)	6 oz	95	4	16	136	2	1.6	0.4	7	15%
'3rd Foods' (Gerber)	6 oz	100	4	14	45	2	3.5	0.4	7	31%
Turkey and vegetable dinner										
lean meat, junior (Gerber)	4.5 oz	100	7	10	31	0	4.0	0.0	16	35%
lean meat, strained (Gerber)	4.5 oz	100	7	9	31	0	4.0	0.0	17	36%
Turkey dinner										
junior (Gerber)	2.5 oz	100	10	1	37	0	6.0	0.0	38	55%
supreme, 'Stage 2' (Beech-Nut)	4 oz	90	3	9	45	1	4.0	0.0	0	43%
Turkey stew										
w/rice, 'Graduates' (Gerber)	3.2 oz	59	5	8	298	0	1.0	0.0	0	15%
w/rice, 'Table Time' (Beech-Nut)	6 oz	150	6	14	200	1	7.0	na	na	44%
Vegetable and bacon dinner										
junior	1 oz	20	1	2	13	0	1.1	0.4	1	49%
junior	1 tbsp	11	0	1	7	0	0.6	0.2	0	49%
'Step 2' (Heinz)	4 oz	80	2	10	55	2	3.3	1.2	5	37%
'Step 3' (Heinz)	6 oz	121	3	13	77	2	6.6	2.4	5	49%
'2nd Foods' (Gerber)	4 oz	80	2	10	60	1	3.5	1.2	5	39%
strained	1 oz	20	1	2	14	0	0.8	0.3	1	37%
strained	1 tbsp	11	0	1	8	0	0.5	0.2	1	37%
Vegetable and beef dinner										
chunky (Gerber)	7 tbsp	70	4	9	201	0	2.0	0.0	0	26%
(Earth's Best)	4.5 oz	90	3	11	15	0	3.0	0.0	0	33%

Food Name	Serving Size	Calories	Prot. gms	Carbs gms	Sod. mgs	Fiber gms	Fat gms	Sat. Fat gms	Chol. mgs	% Fat Cal.
junior	1 oz	18	1	3	21	0	0.5	0.2	2	27%
junior	1 tbsp	10	0	1	12	0	0.3	0.1	1	27%
'2nd Foods' (Gerber)	4 oz	70	3	10	35	3	2.5	1.2	7	32%
'Stage 2' (Beech-Nut)	4 oz	80	1	8	45	1	4.0	na	na	50%
'Stage 3' (Beech-Nut)	6 oz	130	3	14	60	2	6.0	na	na	44%
'Step 2' (Heinz)	4 oz	71	3	9	21	2	2.7	1.2	7	35%
'Step 3' (Heinz)	6 oz	105	4	15	128	2	3.1	1.2	14	27%
strained	1 oz	18	1	2	5	1	0.7	0.3	2	35%
strained	1 tbsp	10	0	1	3	0	0.4	0.2	1	35%
'3rd Foods' (Gerber)	6 oz	110	4	15	65	3	3.5	1.2	14	29%
Vegetable and chicken dinner										
junior	1 oz	15	1	2	22	0	0.3	0.1	2	19%
junior	1 tbsp	8	0	1	12	0	0.2	0.0	1	19%
'2nd Foods' (Gerber)	4 oz	70	3	10	35	2	2.0	0.6	12	26%
'Stage 2' (Beech-Nut)	4 oz	80	2	8	40	1	4.0	na	na	47%
'Stage 3' (Beech-Nut)	6 oz	110	4	14	55	1	4.0	na	na	33%
'Step 2' (Heinz)	4-oz jar	67	3	10	27	2	2.0	0.6	12	26%
strained	1 oz	17	1	2	7	1	0.5	0.1	3	26%
strained	1 tbsp	9	0	1	4	0	0.3	0.1	2	26%
'3rd Foods' (Gerber)	6 oz	100	4	15	75	3	3.0	0.5	12	27%
Vegetable and dumpling dinner										
w/beef, 'Step 2' (Heinz)	3.5 oz	49	2	9	15	0	1.3	0.0	0	22%
w/beef, 'Step 3' (Heinz)	3.5 oz	47	2	7	16	0	1.2	0.0	0	23%
Vegetable and ham dinner										
chunky (Gerber)	7 tbsp	70	4	9	200	0	2.3	0.0	0	29%
junior	1 oz	17	1	2	25	0	0.5	0.1	1	28%
junior	1 tbsp	10	0	1	14	0	0.3	0.1	0	28%
'2nd Foods' (Gerber)	4 oz	70	2	10	20	1	2.5	0.9	6	32%
'Stage 2' (Beech-Nut)	4 oz	80	2	9	30	1	3.0	na	na	38%
'Step 2' (Heinz)	4 oz	67	2	9	18	2	2.4	0.9	6	33%
'Step 3' (Heinz)	6 oz	102	3	15	148	2	3.2	0.8	5	28%
strained	1 oz	17	1	2	5	0	0.6	0.2	1	33%
strained	1 tbsp	9	0	1	3	0	0.3	0.1	1	33%
'3rd Foods' (Gerber)	6 oz	120	4	16	55	3	4.0	0.8	5	30%
Vegetable and lamb dinner										
junior	1 oz	14	1	2	4	0	0.5	0.2	1	30%
strained	1 oz	15	1	2	6	0	0.6	0.2	2	34%
strained	1 tbsp	8	0	1	3	0	0.3	0.1	1	34%
'Step 2' (Heinz)	4 oz	59	2	8	23	1	2.3	0.9	7	34%
Vegetable and noodle dinner										
w/chicken, 'Step 2' (Heinz)	3.5 oz	54	2	8	24	0	1.7	0.0	0	28%
w/chicken, 'Step 3' (Heinz)	3.5 oz	57	2	9	21	0	1.8	0.0	0	28%
w/turkey, 'Step 2' (Heinz)	3.5 oz	47	1	7	22	0	1.6	0.0	0	31%
w/turkey, 'Step 3' (Heinz)	3.5 oz	48	1	6	21	0	2.0	0.0	0	37%
Vegetable and turkey dinner										
(Earth's Best)	4.5 oz	60	3	11	15	0	1.0	0.0	0	15%
junior	1 oz	15	0	2	25	0	0.5	0.1	1	30%
junior	1 tbsp	8	0	1	14	0	0.3	0.1	1	30%
strained	1 oz	14	1	2	6	0	0.3	0.1	1	17%
strained	1 tbsp	8	0	1	3	0	0.1	0.0	1	17%
'2nd Foods' (Gerber)	4 oz	60	3	10	30	2	1.0	0.3	5	15%
'3rd Foods' (Gerber)	6 oz	110	4	16	75	3	3.5	0.8	7	29%
toddler	1 oz	23	1	2	95	na	1.0	na	na	38%
Vegetable dinner, 'Summer' (Earth's Best)	4.5 oz	90	3	12	15	0	3.0	0.0	0	31%

Food Name	Serving Size	Calories	Prot. gms	Carbs gms	Sod. mgs	Fiber gms	Fat gms	Sat. Fat gms	Chol. mgs	% Fat Cal.
Vegetable stew										
w/beef, 'Graduates' (Gerber)	6 oz	120	8	15	420	3	2.5	0.0	0	21%
w/beef, 'Table Time' (Beech-Nut)	6 oz	110	4	16	170	1	3.0	na	na	25%
w/chicken, 'Table Time' (Beech-Nut)	6 oz	190	5	23	340	0	8.0	0.0	0	39%
Vegetable and beef dinner										
w/macaroni 'Stage 2' (Beech-Nut)	4 oz	110	2	9	50	1	6.0	na	na	55%
w/dumpling, junior	1 oz	14	1	2	15	na	0.2	na	na	15%
w/dumpling, strained	1 oz	14	1	2	14	na	0.3	na	na	17%
Vegetable, noodle, and chicken dinner										
junior	1 oz	18	0	3	7	0	0.6	na	na	31%
strained	1 oz	18	1	2	6	0	0.7	na	na	35%
Vegetable, noodle, and turkey dinner										
junior	1 oz	15	1	2	5	0	0.4	na	na	26%
strained	1 oz	12	0	2	6	0	0.3	na	na	24%
EGG YOLKS										
(Gerber) '2nd Foods'	7 tbsp	193	10	1	42	0	16.8	0.0	0	78%
FORMULA										
Infant formula, mix										
liquid, w/iron 'Enfamil' (Mead Johnson)	1 fl oz	41	1	4	11	0	2.2	0.9	0	48%
liquid concentrate, low-iron, 'Enfamil' (Mead Johnson)	1 fl oz	41	1	4	11	0	2.2	0.9	0	48%
liquid concentrate, low-iron (Gerber)	1 fl oz	40	1	4	12	0	2.1	0.9	1	48%
liquid concentrate, low-iron, 'Similac' (Ross)	1 fl oz	40	1	4	10	0	2.2	0.8	1	49%
liquid concentrate, low-iron, 'SMA' (Wyeth-Ayerst)	1 fl oz	41	1	4	9	0	2.2	1.0	2	48%
liquid concentrate, w/iron, 'Alsoy' (Carnation)	1 fl oz	41	1	4	17	0	2.3	0.3	0	49%
liquid concentrate, w/iron, 'Enfamil Nutramigen' (Mead Johnson)	1 fl oz	41	1	5	20	0	2.1	0.9	0	45%
liquid concentrate, w/iron, 'Enfamil ProSobee' (Mead Johnson)	1 fl oz	40	1	4	14	0	2.1	0.9	0	48%
liquid concentrate, w/iron, 'Follow-Up' (Carnation)	1 fl oz	41	1	5	16	0	1.7	0.7	1	37%
liquid concentrate, w/iron 'Follow-Up Soy' (Carnation)	1 fl oz	42	1	4	18	0	2.3	0.3	0	48%
liquid concentrate, w/iron (Gerber)	1 fl oz	40	1	4	12	0	2.1	0.9	1	48%
liquid concentrate, w/iron, 'Good Start' (Carnation)	1 fl oz	40	1	4	10	0	2.0	0.9	4	46%
liquid concentrate, w/iron, 'Isomil' (Ross)	1 fl oz	40	1	4	18	0	2.2	0.7	0	49%
liquid concentrate, w/iron, 'Isomil DF' (Ross)	1 fl oz	40	1	4	18	0	2.2	0.9	0	49%
liquid concentrate, w/iron, 'Nursoy' (Wyeth-Ayerst)	1 fl oz	41	1	4	11	0	2.2	1.0	0	48%
liquid concentrate, w/iron, 'Similac with Iron' (Ross)	1 fl oz	40	1	4	10	0	2.2	0.8	1	49%
liquid concentrate, w/iron, 'SMA' (Wyeth-Ayerst)	1 fl oz	41	1	4	9	0	2.2	1.0	3	48%
powder, low-iron, 'Enfamil' (Mead Johnson)	1 scoop	44	1	5	12	0	2.3	1.0	0	48%
powder, low-iron (Gerber)	1 scoop	44	1	5	13	0	2.4	1.0	0	48%
powder, low-iron 'Similac' (Ross)	1 scoop	46	1	5	11	0	2.5	0.9	1	49%
powder, low-iron 'SMA' (Wyeth-Ayerst)	1 scoop	45	1	5	10	0	2.4	1.1	3	47%
powder, soy, w/iron, milk-free, prepared (Gerber)	5 fl oz	100	3	10	47	0	5.3	0.0	0	48%
powder, soy, w/iron, milk-free, prepared 'ProSobee' (Mead Johnson)	5 fl oz	100	3	10	36	0	5.3	0.0	0	48%
powder, soy, w/iron, milk-free (Isomil), prepared	5 fl oz	100	3	10	44	0	5.5	0.0	0	49%
powder, w/iron, 'Alsoy' (Carnation)	1 scoop	22	1	2	9	0	1.2	0.2	0	48%
powder, w/iron, 'Enfamil' (Mead Johnson)	1 scoop	44	1	5	12	0	2.3	1.0	0	48%
powder, w/iron, 'Enfamil Nutramigen' (Mead Johnson)	1 scoop	48	1	5	22	0	2.4	1.0	0	45%
powder, w/iron, 'Follow-Up' (Carnation)	1 scoop	44	1	6	17	0	1.8	0.8	1	37%
powder, w/iron, (Gerber)	1 scoop	44	1	5	13	0	2.4	1.0	0	48%
powder, w/iron, 'Good Start' (Carnation)	1 scoop	45	1	5	10	0	2.3	1.0	4	46%

Food Name	Serving Size	Calories	Prot. gms	Carbs gms	Sod. mgs	Fiber gms	Fat gms	Sat. Fat gms	Chol. mgs	% Fat Cal.
powder, w/iron, 'Isomil' *(Ross)*	1 scoop	45	1	5	20	0	2.5	0.8	0	49%
powder, w/iron, 'Lofenalac' *(Mead Johnson)*	1 scoop	44	1	6	21	0	1.7	0.2	0	35%
powder, w/iron, 'Nursoy' *(Wyeth-Ayerst)*	1 scoop	44	1	5	13	0	2.4	1.1	0	48%
powder, w/iron, 'Portagen' *(Mead Johnson)*	1 scoop	44	2	5	24	0	2.2	1.9	1	44%
powder, w/iron, 'Pregestimil' *(Mead Johnson)*	1 scoop	44	1	4	17	0	2.5	1.5	0	50%
powder, w/iron, prepared, 'Lofenalac' *(Mead Johnson)*	1 fl oz	20	1	3	10	0	0.8	0.1	0	35%
powder, w/iron, prepared 'Portagen' *(Mead Johnson)*	1 fl oz	20	1	2	11	0	1.0	0.8	0	44%
powder, w/iron, prepared 'Enfamil Pregestimil' *(Mead Johnson)*	1 fl oz	20	1	2	8	0	1.1	0.7	0	50%
powder, w/iron, 'ProSobee' *(Mead Johnson)*	1 scoop	44	1	4	16	0	2.3	1.0	0	47%
powder, w/iron, 'SAM' *(Wyeth-Ayerst)*	1 scoop	45	1	5	10	0	2.4	1.1	3	47%
powder, w/iron, 'Similac' *(Ross)*	1 scoop	46	1	5	11	0	2.5	0.9	1	49%
powder, w/iron, 'Soylac' *(Carnation)*	1 scoop	22	1	2	10	0	1.2	0.2	0	48%
Infant formula, ready to use										
low-iron 'Alimentum' *(Ross)*	1 fl oz	20	1	2	9	0	1.1	0.6	0	50%
low-iron, 'Enfamil' *(Mead Johnson)*	1 fl oz	20	0	2	5	0	1.1	0.5	0	47%
low-iron *(Gerber)*	1 fl oz	20	0	2	6	0	1.1	0.5	0	47%
low-iron 'Similac' *(Ross)*	1 fl oz	20	0	2	5	0	1.1	0.4	1	48%
low-iron, 'SMA' *(Wyeth-Ayerst)*	1 fl oz	20	0	2	4	0	1.1	0.5	1	48%
low-iron 'Similac Natural Care' *(Ross)*	1 fl oz	24	1	3	10	0	1.3	0.8	1	49%
w/iron, 'Similac with Iron' *(Ross)*	1 fl oz	24	1	3	10	0	1.3	0.8	1	49%
soy, w/iron, 'Alsoy' *(Carnation)*	1 fl oz	20	1	2	9	0	1.1	0.2	0	48%
soy, w/iron, 'Follow-Up Soy' *(Carnation)*	1 fl oz	20	1	2	9	0	1.1	0.2	0	48%
soy, w/iron, milk-free, 'Enfamil ProSobee' *(Mead Johnson)*	5 fl oz	100	3	10	36	0	5.3	0.0	0	48%
soy, w/iron, milk-free *(Gerber)*	5 fl oz	100	3	10	47	0	5.3	0.0	0	48%
soy, w/iron, milk-free, 'Isomil' *(Ross)*	5 fl oz	100	3	10	44	0	5.4	0.0	0	49%
soy, w/iron, milk-free, 'Nursoy' *(Wyeth-Ayerst)*	5 fl oz	100	3	10	30	0	5.3	0.0	0	48%
soy, w/iron, 'Nursoy' *(Wyeth-Ayerst)*	1 fl oz	20	1	2	5	0	1.1	0.5	0	48%
w/iron, 'Enfamil Nutramigen' *(Mead Johnson)*	1 fl oz	20	1	2	10	0	1.0	0.4	0	45%
w/iron, 'Enfamil with Iron' *(Mead Johnson)*	1 fl oz	20	0	2	5	0	1.1	0.5	0	47%
w/iron, 'Follow-Up' *(Carnation)*	1 fl oz	20	1	3	8	0	0.8	0.4	0	37%
w/iron *(Gerber)*	1 fl oz	20	0	2	6	0	1.1	0.5	0	47%
w/iron, 'Good Start' *(Carnation)*	1 fl oz	20	0	2	5	0	1.0	0.4	2	46%
w/iron, 'Isomil' *(Ross)*	1 fl oz	20	0	2	9	0	1.1	0.4	0	49%
w/iron, 'Isomil DM' *(Ross)*	1 fl oz	20	1	2	9	0	1.1	0.4	0	49%
w/iron, 'Similac' *(Ross)*	1 fl oz	20	0	2	5	0	1.1	0.4	1	48%
w/iron, 'SMA' *(Wyeth-Ayerst)*	1 fl oz	20	0	2	4	0	1.1	0.5	1	48%
Toddler formula, mix										
liquid, prepared, 'Next Step' *(Mead Johnson)*	1 fl oz	20	1	2	7	0	1.1	0.5	0	48%
powder, soy, prepared, 'Next Step Soy' *(Mead Johnson)*	1 fl oz	20	1	2	9	0	0.9	0.4	0	40%
Toddler formula, ready to use										
w/iron *(Pediasure)*	1 fl oz	29	1	3	11	0	1.5	0.4	1	45%
FRUIT										
Apple *(Earth's Best)*	4.5 oz	60	0	14	5	0	1.0	0.0	0	14%
Apple and apricot										
'Stage 2' *(Beech-Nut)*	4 oz	70	0	17	0	1	0.0	na	na	0%
(Earth's Best)	4.5 oz	70	0	15	5	0	1.0	0.0	0	13%
strained *(Heinz)*	3.5 oz	55	0	13	3	0	0.3	0.0	0	5%
Apple and banana										
(Earth's Best)	4.5 oz	80	0	18	15	0	1.0	0.0	0	11%
'2nd Foods' *(Gerber)*	4 oz	60	0	15	0	0	0.0	0.0	0	0%
'Stage 2' *(Beech-Nut)*	4 oz	60	0	14	0	1	0.0	na	na	0%

Food Name	Serving Size	Calories	Prot. gms	Carbs gms	Sod. mgs	Fiber gms	Fat gms	Sat. Fat gms	Chol. mgs	% Fat Cal.
'Stage 3' (Beech-Nut)	6 oz	90	0	21	0	1	0.0	na	na	0%
Apple and blueberry										
(Earth's Best)	4.5 oz	60	0	14	0	0	1.0	0.0	0	14%
junior	1 oz	18	0	5	4	1	0.1	0.0	0	3%
'2nd Foods' (Gerber)	4 oz	60	0	14	1	5	2.0	0.0	0	14%
'Stage 2' (Beech-Nut)	4 oz	70	0	17	0	1	0.0	na	na	0%
strained	1 oz	17	0	5	1	1	0.1	0.0	0	3%
'3rd Foods' (Gerber)	6 oz	80	0	19	2	0	1.0	0.0	0	11%
Apple and cherry, 'Stage 3' (Beech-Nut)	6 oz	110	0	26	0	1	0.0	na	na	0%
Apple and cranberry, w/tapioca, strained (Heinz)	3.5 oz	66	0	16	6	0	0.3	0.0	0	4%
Apple and pear										
'Stage 2' (Beech-Nut)	4 oz	80	0	19	0	1	0.0	na	na	0%
'Step 3' (Heinz)	3.5 oz	57	0	13	1	1	0.2	0.0	0	3%
Apple and plum, (Earth's Best)	4.5 oz	70	0	16	10	0	1.0	0.0	0	12%
Apple and raspberry										
w/sugar, junior..............................	1 oz	16	0	4	1	1	0.1	0.0	0	3%
w/sugar, strained	1 oz	16	0	4	1	1	0.1	0.0	0	3%
Apple and sweet potato, 'Tender Harvest' (Gerber).	4 oz	71	0	17	3	2	0.2	0.0	0	3%
Applesauce										
(Earth's Best)	4.5 oz	52	0	14	3	2	0.3	0.0	0	4%
'1st Foods' (Gerber).	2.5 oz	35	0	9	0	0	0.0	0.0	0	0%
golden delicious, 'Stage 1' (Beech-Nut)	2.5 oz	50	0	11	0	0	0.0	0.0	0	0%
junior (Heinz).	3.5 oz	53	0	12	2	0	0.2	0.0	0	3%
junior	1 oz	10	0	3	1	0	0.0	0.0	0	0%
junior	1 tbsp	6	0	2	0	0	0.0	0.0	0	0%
'2nd Foods' (Gerber)	4 oz	60	0	14	3	0	1.0	0.0	0	14%
'Stage 3' (Beech-Nut)	6 oz	100	0	23	0	2	0.0	0.0	0	0%
'Step 1' (Heinz)	3.5 oz	73	0	18	1	0	0.1	0.0	0	1%
'Step 2' (Heinz)	4 oz	46	0	12	2	2	0.2	0.0	0	4%
'Step 3' (Heinz)	6 oz	63	0	18	3	3	0.0	0.0	0	0%
strained	1 oz	12	0	3	1	0	0.1	0.0	0	4%
strained	1 tbsp	7	0	2	0	0	0.0	0.0	0	4%
'3rd Foods' (Gerber)	6 oz	90	0	20	3	0	1.0	0.0	0	10%
w/apricot	1 oz	13	0	4	1	1	0.1	0.0	0	4%
w/apricot	1 tbsp	8	0	2	0	0	0.0	0.0	0	4%
w/apricot, '2nd Foods' (Gerber)	7 tbsp	53	0	13	1	0	0.2	0.0	0	3%
w/apricot, 'Stage 2' (Beech-Nut)	4.5 oz	80	0	19	0	0	0.0	0.0	0	0%
w/apricot, 'Step 2' (Heinz)	4 oz	51	0	13	3	2	0.2	0.0	0	4%
w/apricot, 'Step 3' (Heinz)	6 oz	80	0	21	5	3	0.3	0.0	0	4%
w/apricot, strained (Earth's Best)	4.5 oz	58	0	15	4	2	0.3	0.0	0	4%
w/apricot, strained..........................	1 oz	13	0	3	1	1	0.1	0.0	0	4%
w/apricot, strained..........................	1 tbsp	7	0	2	0	0	0.0	0.0	0	4%
w/banana, 'Stage 2' (Beech-Nut).	4.5 oz	80	0	18	0	0	0.0	0.0	0	0%
w/banana, 'Stage 3' (Beech-Nut).	6 oz	100	0	25	0	0	0.0	0.0	0	0%
w/banana, strained	1 tbsp	11	0	3	0	0	0.0	0.0	0	1%
w/cherry, 'Stage 2' (Beech-Nut).	4.5 oz	70	0	18	5	0	0.0	0.0	0	0%
w/cherry, 'Stage 3' (Beech-Nut).	6 oz	100	0	24	0	0	0.0	0.0	0	0%
w/cherry, junior	1 oz	16	0	4	0	0	0.0	0.0	0	0%
w/cherry, strained	1 oz	14	0	4	0	0	0.0	0.0	0	0%
w/pineapple, junior	1 oz	11	0	3	1	0	0.0	0.0	0	2%
w/pineapple, strained	1 oz	10	0	3	1	0	0.0	0.0	0	2%
Apricot										
w/pear, 'Stage 3' (Beech-Nut)................	6 oz	120	1	27	0	0	0.0	0.0	0	0%
w/pear and apple, 'Stage 3' (Beech-Nut).	6 oz	130	0	32	0	3	0.0	na	na	0%

Food Name	Serving Size	Calories	Prot. gms	Carbs gms	Sod. mgs	Fiber gms	Fat gms	Sat. Fat gms	Chol. mgs	% Fat Cal.
w/pear and applesauce, 'Stage 2' (Beech-Nut)	4.5 oz	90	0	21	0	0	0.0	0.0	0	0%
w/tapioca, junior	3.5 oz	66	0	16	10	0	0.2	0.0	0	3%
w/tapioca, junior	1 tbsp	9	0	3	1	0	0.0	0.0	0	0%
w/tapioca, '2nd Foods' (Gerber)	4 oz	90	0	20	8	0	1.0	0.0	0	10%
w/tapioca, 'Step 2' (Heinz)	4.25 oz	72	0	20	10	2	0.0	0.0	0	0%
w/tapioca, 'Step 3' (Heinz)	6 oz	107	1	29	10	3	0.0	0.0	0	0%
w/tapioca, strained	3.5 oz	64	0	15	7	0	0.2	0.0	0	3%
w/tapioca, strained	1 tbsp	9	0	2	1	0	0.0	0.0	0	0%
w/tapioca, '3rd Foods' (Gerber)	6 oz	130	1	29	9	0	1.0	0.0	0	7%
Banana										
(Earth's Best)	4.5 oz	100	2	22	60	0	0.0	0.0	0	0%
'1st Foods' (Gerber)	2.5 oz	70	1	17	0	0	0.0	0.0	0	0%
Chiquita, 'Baby's First' (Beech-Nut)	2.5 oz	70	0	16	0	0	0.0	0.0	0	0%
Chiquita, 'Stage 3' (Beech-Nut)	6 oz	160	1	33	0	3	0.0	na	na	0%
'Step 1' (Heinz)	3.5 oz	107	1	25	3	0	0.2	0.0	0	2%
w/pineapple and tapioca, '2nd Foods' (Gerber)	7 tbsp	52	0	12	0	0	0.1	6.0	0	2%
w/pineapple and tapioca, '3rd Foods' (Gerber)	7 tbsp	52	0	12	4	0	0.1	0.0	0	2%
w/tapioca, junior	1 oz	19	0	5	3	0	0.1	0.0	0	3%
w/tapioca, junior	1 tbsp	10	0	3	1	0	0.0	0.0	0	3%
w/tapioca, '2nd Foods' (Gerber)	4 oz	110	1	24	12	0	1.0	0.0	0	8%
w/tapioca, 'Step 2' (Heinz)	3.5 oz	73	0	18	8	0	0.2	0.0	0	2%
w/tapioca, 'Step 3' (Heinz)	3.5 oz	73	0	18	8	0	0.2	0.0	0	2%
w/tapioca, strained	1 oz	16	0	4	3	0	0.0	0.0	0	1%
w/tapioca, strained	1 tbsp	9	0	2	1	0	0.0	0.0	0	1%
w/tapioca, '3rd Foods' (Gerber)	6 oz	140	1	31	15	0	1.0	0.0	0	7%
Banana and apple, strained (Gerber)	4.5 oz	90	0	20	9	0	1.0	0.0	0	10%
Banana and pear, w/applesauce, 'Stage 2' (Beech-Nut)	4.5 oz	100	0	24	0	0	0.0	0.0	0	0%
Banana and pineapple										
'Stage 2' (Beech-Nut)	4.5 oz	110	0	27	15	0	0.0	0.0	0	0%
w/tapioca, junior	1 oz	19	0	5	2	0	0.0	0.0	0	1%
w/tapioca, junior	1 tbsp	10	0	3	1	0	0.0	0.0	0	1%
w/tapioca, '2nd Foods' (Gerber)	4.5 oz	60	1	15	5	0	0.0	0.0	0	0%
w/tapioca, 'Step 2' (Heinz)	3.5 oz	64	0	15	8	0	0.2	0.0	0	3%
w/tapioca, 'Step 3' (Heinz)	6 oz	116	0	31	14	3	0.2	0.1	0	1%
w/tapioca, strained	1 oz	18	0	5	2	0	0.0	0.0	0	0%
w/tapioca, '3rd Foods' (Gerber)	6 oz	90	1	20	7	0	1.0	0.0	0	10%
Guava										
w/tapioca, '2nd Foods' (Gerber)	4 oz	90	0	20	3	0	1.0	0.0	0	10%
w/tapioca, 'Stage 2' (Beech-Nut)	4.5 oz	100	0	24	10	0	0.0	0.0	0	0%
w/tapioca, strained	1 oz	19	0	5	1	1	0.0	na	na	0%
Guava and papaya, w/tapioca, strained	1 oz	18	0	5	1	na	0.0	na	na	1%
Mango										
w/tapioca, '2nd Foods' (Gerber)	4 oz	90	0	21	4	0	1.0	0.0	0	10%
w/tapioca, strained	1 oz	23	0	6	1	0	0.1	0.0	0	2%
w/tapioca, strained	1 tbsp	12	0	3	1	0	0.0	0.0	0	2%
Mango and banana										
w/passionfruit and tapioca, '2nd Foods' (Gerber)	4.5 oz	100	0	25	12	0	0.0	0.0	0	0%
Mixed fruit										
apple, peach, and strawberries 'Stage 2' (Beech-Nut)	4.5 oz	100	0	24	0	0	0.0	0.0	0	0%
apple, pear, and banana 'Stage 2' (Beech-Nut)	4.5 oz	100	0	24	0	0	0.0	0.0	0	0%
Papaya										
'Stage 2' (Beech-Nut)	4.5 oz	100	0	24	15	0	0.0	0.0	0	0%
w/tapioca, '2nd Foods' (Gerber)	4 oz	80	0	19	9	0	1.0	0.0	0	11%
Papaya and applesauce, w/tapioca, strained	1 oz	20	0	5	1	0	0.0	na	na	1%

Food Name	Serving Size	Calories	Prot. gms	Carbs gms	Sod. mgs	Fiber gms	Fat gms	Sat. Fat gms	Chol. mgs	% Fat Cal.
Peach										
'1st Foods' (Gerber)	2.5 oz	30	0	7	0	0	0.0	0.0	0	0%
'2nd Foods' (Gerber)	4 oz	90	1	19	4	0	1.0	0.0	0	10%
'Stage 3' (Beech-Nut)	6 oz	100	0	21	0	4	0.0	0.0	0	0%
'Step 1' (Heinz)	3.5 oz	80	1	18	2	0	0.2	0.0	0	2%
'Step 2' (Heinz)	3.5 oz	68	1	15	7	1	0.3	0.0	0	4%
'Step 3' (Heinz)	3.5 oz	68	1	15	7	1	0.3	0.0	0	4%
'3rd Foods' (Gerber)	6 oz	110	1	25	5	0	1.0	0.0	0	8%
w/banana, 'Stage 2' (Beech-Nut)	4 oz	70	0	15	0	3	0.0	na	na	0%
w/mango and tapioca, '2nd Foods' (Gerber)	4 oz	100	0	24	9	0	1.0	0.0	0	9%
w/oatmeal and banana (Earth's Best)	4.5 oz	70	2	15	5	0	1.0	0.0	0	12%
w/sugar, '1st Foods' (Gerber)	2.5 oz	30	<1	7	0	1	0.0	0.0	0	0%
w/sugar, junior	1 oz	20	0	5	1	0	0.1	0.0	0	2%
w/sugar, junior	1 tbsp	11	0	3	1	0	0.0	0.0	0	2%
w/sugar, '2nd Foods' (Gerber)	4 oz	70	<1	17	10	1	0.0	0.0	0	0%
w/sugar, 'Stage 1' (Beech-Nut)	2.5 oz	50	0	13	4	1	0.1	0.0	0	2%
w/sugar, 'Stage 3' (Beech-Nut)	6 oz	121	1	32	9	3	0.3	0.0	0	2%
w/sugar, 'Step 1' (Heinz)	2.5 oz	50	0	13	4	1	0.1	0.0	0	2%
w/sugar, 'Step 2' (Heinz)	4 oz	80	1	21	7	2	0.2	0.0	0	2%
w/sugar, 'Step 3' (Heinz)	6 oz	121	1	32	9	3	0.3	0.0	0	2%
w/sugar, strained	1 oz	20	0	5	2	0	0.1	0.0	0	2%
w/sugar, strained	1 tbsp	11	0	3	1	0	0.0	0.0	0	2%
w/sugar, '3rd Foods' (Gerber)	6 oz	110	1	26	10	2	0.0	0.0	0	0%
w/yogurt 'Stage 2' (Beech-Nut)	4.5 oz	120	1	25	30	0	2.0	0.0	0	15%
yellow cling, 'Stage 1' (Beech-Nut)	2.5 oz	45	0	10	0	0	0.0	0.0	0	0%
Pear										
Bartlett, 'Stage 1' (Beech-Nut)	2.5 oz	50	0	12	0	0	0.0	0.0	0	0%
Bartlett, 'Stage 3' (Beech-Nut)	6 oz	110	0	27	0	5	0.0	0.0	0	0%
Bartlett, w/applesauce, 'Stage 2' (Beech-Nut)	4 oz	80	0	20	0	0	0.0	0.0	0	0%
(Earth's Best)	4.5 oz	60	0	14	11	0	0.0	0.0	0	0%
'1st Foods' (Gerber)	2.5 oz	40	0	11	2	0	0.0	0.0	0	0%
junior	1 oz	12	0	3	1	1	0.0	0.0	0	2%
junior	1 tbsp	7	0	2	0	1	0.0	0.0	0	2%
'2nd Foods' (Gerber)	4 oz	80	1	16	3	0	1.0	0.0	0	12%
'Step 1' (Heinz)	3.5 oz	76	1	18	3	0	0.2	0.0	0	2%
'Step 2' (Heinz)	3.5 oz	60	0	14	3	0	0.2	0.0	0	3%
'Step 3' (Heinz)	3.5 oz	60	0	14	3	0	0.2	0.0	0	3%
strained	1 oz	12	0	3	1	1	0.1	0.0	0	4%
strained	1 tbsp	7	0	2	0	1	0.0	0.0	0	4%
'3rd Foods' (Gerber)	6 oz	100	1	21	2	0	1.0	0.0	0	9%
Pear and pineapple										
junior	1 oz	12	0	3	0	1	0.1	0.0	0	4%
junior	1 tbsp	7	0	2	0	0	0.0	0.0	0	4%
'2nd Foods' (Gerber)	7 tbsp	55	0	13	1	0	0.2	0.0	0	3%
'Stage 2' (Beech-Nut)	4 oz	46	0	12	5	3	0.1	0.0	0	2%
'Step 2' (Heinz)	4 oz	46	0	12	5	3	0.1	0.0	0	2%
strained	1 oz	12	0	3	1	1	0.0	0.0	0	2%
strained	1 tbsp	7	0	2	1	0	0.0	0.0	0	2%
'3rd Foods' (Gerber)	6 oz	100	1	21	3	0	1.0	0.0	0	9%
Pear and raspberry, (Earth's Best)	4.5 oz	60	0	15	0	0	0.0	0.0	0	0%
Plum										
w/tapioca, junior	1 oz	21	0	6	2	0	0.0	0.0	0	0%
w/tapioca, junior	1 tbsp	11	0	3	1	0	0.0	0.0	0	0%

Food Name	Serving Size	Calories	Prot. gms	Carbs gms	Sod. mgs	Fiber gms	Fat gms	Sat. Fat gms	Chol. mgs	% Fat Cal.
(Gerber) '3rd Foods'	6 oz	120	0	28	10	3	0.0	0.0	0	0%
w/tapioca, '2nd Foods' (Gerber)	4 oz	80	0	19	10	2	0.0	0.0	0	0%
w/tapioca, strained	1 oz	20	0	6	2	0	0.0	0.0	0	0%
w/tapioca, strained	1 tbsp	11	0	3	1	0	0.0	0.0	0	0%
w/tapioca, 'Step 2' (Heinz)	4 oz	80	0	22	7	1	0.0	0.0	0	0%
Prune										
'1st Foods' (Gerber)	2.5 oz	70	1	17	0	0	0.0	0.0	0	0%
w/oatmeal (Earth's Best)	4.5 oz	100	1	24	20	0	0.0	0.0	0	0%
w/pear, 'Stage 2' (Beech-Nut)	4 oz	110	0	24	10	3	0.0	0.0	0	0%
w/tapioca, junior	1 oz	20	0	5	1	1	0.0	0.0	0	1%
w/tapioca, '2nd Foods' (Gerber)	4 oz	100	1	22	5	0	1.0	0.0	0	9%
w/tapioca, 'Step 2' (Heinz)	3.5 oz	90	1	22	8	0	0.2	0.0	0	2%
w/tapioca, strained	1 oz	20	0	5	1	1	0.0	0.0	0	1%
w/tapioca, strained	1 tbsp	11	0	3	1	0	0.0	0.0	0	1%
Tropical fruit, junior	1 oz	17	0	5	2	na	0.0	na	na	0%
JUICE										
Apple										
	1 fl oz	15	0	4	1	0	0.0	0.0	0	2%
beginner, 'Step 1' (Heinz)	4 fl oz	59	0	15	4	0	0.1	0.0	0	2%
(Earth's Best)	4.2 fl oz	62	0	15	4	0	0.1	0.0	0	2%
(Gerber)	4 fl oz	60	<1	14	0	0	0.1	0.0	0	2%
100% juice, 'Junior' (McCain)	4.2 fl oz	50	0	13	5	0	0.0	0.0	0	0%
'Stage 1' (Beech-Nut)	4 fl oz	60	0	15	4	0	0.1	0.0	0	2%
strained, 'Saver Size' (Heinz)	4.2 fl oz	70	0	17	15	0	0.0	0.0	0	0%
Apple-apricot, strained, 'Step 2' (Heinz)	3.5 fl oz	47	0	11	8	0	0.2	0.0	0	4%
Apple-banana										
	1 fl oz	16	0	4	1	0	0.0	0.0	0	2%
(Earth's Best)	4.2 fl oz	60	0	14	2	0	0.0	0.0	0	0%
(Gerber)	4 fl oz	60	<1	15	10	0	0.1	0.0	0	2%
strained, 'Step 2' (Heinz)	3.5 fl oz	52	0	13	6	0	0.2	0.0	0	3%
w/calcium, 'Graduates' (Gerber)	6 fl oz	100	<1	24	20	1	0.0	0.0	0	0%
w/vitamin C, 'Stage 2' (Beech-Nut)	4 fl oz	70	0	16	0	0	0.0	na	na	0%
Apple-cherry										
	1 fl oz	13	0	3	1	0	0.1	0.0	0	4%
'Graduates' (Gerber)	6 fl oz	80	0	21	25	0	0.0	0.0	0	0%
100% juice, 'Junior' (McCain)	4.2 fl oz	50	0	13	5	0	0.0	0.0	0	0%
strained, 'Step 2' (Heinz)	3.5 fl oz	45	0	11	7	0	0.2	0.0	0	4%
w/vitamin C., 'Stage 2' (Beech-Nut)	4 fl oz	70	0	17	10	0	0.0	0.0	0	0%
Apple-cranberry, strained, 'Step 2' (Heinz)	3.5 fl oz	48	0	12	7	0	0.2	0.0	0	4%
Apple-grape										
	1 fl oz	14	0	4	1	0	0.1	0.0	0	4%
(Earth's Best)	4.2 fl oz	60	0	15	4	0	0.3	0.1	0	4%
(Gerber)	4 fl oz	60	<1	15	20	0	0.0	0.1	0	4%
strained, 'Step 2' (Heinz)	4 fl oz	58	0	14	4	0	0.3	0.1	0	4%
w/calcium, 'Graduates' (Gerber)	6 fl oz	98	0	24	8	1	0.2	0.0	0	2%
Apple-peach										
	1 fl oz	13	0	3	0	0	0.0	0.0	0	2%
(Gerber)	3.2 fl oz	47	0	11	5	0	0.1	0.0	0	2%
strained, 'Step 2' (Heinz)	3.5 fl oz	44	0	10	7	0	0.2	0.0	0	4%
Apple-pineapple, strained, 'Step 2' (Heinz)	3.5 fl oz	47	0	11	6	0	0.2	0.0	0	4%
Apple-plum										
	1 fl oz	15	0	4	0	0	0.0	0.0	0	0%
(Gerber)	3.2 fl oz	48	0	12	8	0	0.1	0.0	0	2%

Food Name	Serving Size	Calories	Prot. gms	Carbs gms	Sod. mgs	Fiber gms	Fat gms	Sat. Fat gms	Chol. mgs	% Fat Cal.
Apple-prune										
....	4 fl oz	91	0	23	6	0	0.1	0.0	0	1%
....	1 fl oz	23	0	6	2	0	0.0	0.0	0	1%
strained, 'Step 2' (Heinz)	3.5 oz	50	0	12	7	0	0.2	0.0	0	4%
Apple-white grape, 'Stage 2' (Beech-Nut)	4 fl oz	58	0	14	4	0	0.3	0.1	0	4%
Fruit punch, w/calcium, 'Graduates' (Gerber).	6 fl oz	98	0	24	8	1	0.2	0.0	0	2%
Grape										
'Juice Plus' 'Stage 2' (Beech-Nut)	4 fl oz	100	0	23	10	0	0.0	0.0	0	0%
white (Gerber)........................	4 fl oz	80	0	20	10	0	0.0	0.0	0	1%
white, 'Stage 1' (Beech-Nut)	4 fl oz	100	0	23	10	0	0.0	0.0	0	0%
white, strained, 'Step 2' (Heinz)	3.5 oz	58	0	14	6	0	0.2	0.0	0	3%
Guava, w/mixed fruit, 'Tropical Foods' (Gerber)	3.2 fl oz	58	0	14	6	0	0.1	0.0	0	2%
Mango										
w/mixed fruit, 'Tropical Foods' (Gerber).	3.2 fl oz	59	0	14	5	0	0.1	0.0	0	2%
nectar, w/grape and pear juice, 'Stage 2' (Beech-Nut)	4 fl oz	80	0	19	5	0	0.0	0.0	0	0%
Mixed fruit										
....	1 fl oz	15	0	4	1	0	0.0	0.0	0	2%
....	4 fl oz	59	0	15	5	0	0.1	0.0	0	2%
100% juice, 'Junior' (McCain)	4.2 fl oz	60	0	15	5	0	0.0	0.0	0	0%
strained, 'Step 2' (Heinz)................	3.5 oz	50	0	12	6	0	0.2	0.0	0	4%
Orange										
....	1 fl oz	14	0	3	0	0	0.1	0.0	0	6%
'2nd Foods' (Gerber)...................	4 fl oz	60	<1	13	10	0	0.4	0.0	0	6%
strained, 'Step 2' (Heinz).............	4 fl oz	55	1	13	1	0	0.4	0.0	0	6%
Orange-apple										
....	1 fl oz	13	0	3	1	na	0.1	na	na	4%
strained, 'Step 2' (Heinz).............	3.5 oz	50	0	11	8	0	0.3	0.0	0	5%
Orange-apple-banana										
....	1 fl oz	15	0	4	1	0	0.0	0.0	0	2%
strained, 'Step 2' (Heinz).............	4 fl oz	59	1	14	5	0	0.1	0.0	0	2%
Orange-apricot....................	1 fl oz	14	0	3	2	0	0.0	0.0	0	2%
Orange-banana....................	1 fl oz	16	0	4	1	na	0.0	na	na	2%
Orange-carrot, '3rd Foods' (Gerber).	3.2 fl oz	43	1	10	10	0	0.1	0.0	0	2%
Orange-pineapple	1 fl oz	15	0	4	1	0	0.0	0.0	0	2%
Papaya										
nectar, w/pear and grape juice 'Stage 2' (Beech-Nut).....	4 fl oz	70	0	17	10	0	0.0	0.0	0	0%
Pear										
(Earth's Best)	4.2 fl oz	60	0	15	0	0	0.0	0.0	0	0%
'1st Foods' (Gerber).	3.2 fl oz	46	0	11	1	0	0.1	0.0	0	2%
'Stage 1' (Beech-Nut)	4 fl oz	60	0	15	0	0	0.0	0.0	0	0%
strained, 'Saver Size' (Heinz)	4.2 fl oz	70	0	15	25	0	1.0	0.0	0	13%
strained, 'Step 2' (Heinz)	3.5 oz	49	0	12	9	0	0.2	0.0	0	4%
Pineapple-carrot, '3rd Foods' (Gerber).................	3.2 fl oz	47	0	11	10	0	0.1	0.0	0	2%
Prune-orange.....................	1 fl oz	22	0	5	1	na	0.1	na	na	4%
Tropical blend										
nectar, 'Stage 2' (Beech-Nut)	4 fl oz	90	0	21	10	0	0.0	0.0	0	0%
'Stage 2' (Beech-Nut)	4 fl oz	90	0	19	5	0	0.0	0.0	0	0%
MEAT										
Beef										
and beef gravy, '2nd Foods' (Gerber)	2.5 oz	70	8	3	30	0	3.5	1.8	21	46%
junior....................	1 oz	30	4	0	19	0	1.4	0.7	8	42%
junior....................	1 tbsp	16	2	0	10	0	0.7	0.4	4	42%
junior, 'Step 3' (Heinz)................	2.5 oz	75	10	0	47	0	3.5	1.8	20	42%
strained.....................	1 oz	30	4	0	23	0	1.5	0.7	8	46%

Food Name	Serving Size	Calories	Prot. gms	Carbs gms	Sod. mgs	Fiber gms	Fat gms	Sat. Fat gms	Chol. mgs	% Fat Cal.
strained	1 tbsp	16	2	0	12	0	0.8	0.4	4	46%
strained, 'Step 2' (Heinz)	2.5 oz	76	10	0	58	0	3.8	1.8	21	46%
'3rd Foods' (Gerber)	7 tbsp	103	15	0	52	0	4.6	0.0	0	40%
w/broth, 'Stage 1' (Beech-Nut)	2.5 oz	76	10	0	58	0	3.8	1.8	21	46%
w/broth, strained, 'Step 2' (Heinz)	3.5 oz	123	15	0	53	0	7.2	0.0	0	52%
w/egg yolks (Gerber)	2.5 oz	80	10	0	38	0	4.0	0.0	21	47%
Chicken										
and chicken gravy, '2nd Foods' (Gerber)	2.5 oz	80	8	2	35	0	4.5	1.4	44	51%
junior	1 oz	42	4	0	14	0	2.7	0.7	17	58%
junior	1 tbsp	22	2	0	8	0	1.4	0.4	9	58%
'Stage 1' (Beech-Nut)	2.8 oz	80	10	0	55	0	4.0	0.0	0	47%
strained	1 oz	37	4	0	13	0	2.2	0.6	17	55%
strained	1 tbsp	20	2	0	7	0	1.2	0.3	9	55%
strained, 'Step 2' (Heinz)	2.5 oz	92	10	0	33	0	5.6	1.4	44	55%
'3rd Foods' (Gerber)	7 tbsp	132	15	0	39	0	7.9	0.0	0	54%
w/broth, junior, 'Step 3' (Heinz)	3.5 oz	143	14	1	59	0	9.7	0.0	0	61%
Chicken stick, 'Graduates' (Gerber)	2.5 oz	100	11	1	300	0	5.0	1.5	65	45%
Ham										
and ham gravy, '2nd Foods' (Gerber)	2.5 oz	79	10	0	29	0	4.1	1.4	17	47%
junior	1 oz	35	4	0	19	0	1.9	0.6	8	48%
strained	1 oz	31	4	0	12	0	1.6	0.6	7	47%
strained	1 tbsp	17	2	0	6	0	0.9	0.3	4	47%
'3rd Foods' (Gerber)	7 tbsp	123	15	0	42	0	7.2	0.0	0	53%
w/egg yolks, strained (Gerber)	2.5 oz	90	10	1	30	0	5.0	0.0	17	51%
Lamb										
and lamb gravy, '2nd Foods' (Gerber)	2.5 oz	70	8	2	30	0	3.0	1.6	27	41%
junior	1 oz	32	4	0	21	0	1.5	0.7	11	42%
'Stage 1' (Beech-Nut)	2.8 oz	70	9	0	50	0	3.0	0.0	0	43%
strained	1 oz	29	4	0	18	0	1.3	0.7	11	41%
strained	1 tbsp	15	2	0	9	0	0.7	0.3	6	41%
strained, 'Step 2' (Heinz)	2.5 oz jar	73	10	0	44	0	3.3	1.6	27	41%
w/broth, strained, 'Step 2' (Heinz)	3.5 oz	129	15	0	59	0	7.6	0.0	0	52%
w/egg yolks, strained (Gerber)	2.5 oz	70	10	1	36	0	3.0	0.0	27	38%
Liver, w/broth, strained, 'Step 2' (Heinz)	3.5 oz	100	14	4	49	0	3.2	0.0	0	29%
Meat stick										
'Graduates' (Gerber)	2.5 oz	100	10	1	340	0	7.0	2.5	35	63%
junior	1 stick	18	1	0	55	0	1.5	0.6	7	69%
Pork, strained	1 oz	35	4	0	12	0	2.0	0.7	14	52%
Turkey										
and turkey gravy, '2nd Foods' (Gerber)	2.5 oz	70	7	2	35	0	4.0	1.4	42	46%
'Stage 1' (Beech-Nut)	2.8 oz	100	9	0	50	0	6.0	0.0	0	60%
strained, 'Step 2' (Heinz)	2.5 oz	81	10	0	39	0	4.1	1.4	42	46%
junior	1 oz	37	4	0	20	0	2.0	0.7	15	50%
junior	1 tbsp	19	2	0	11	0	1.1	0.3	8	50%
strained	1 oz	32	4	0	16	0	1.6	0.5	17	46%
strained	1 tbsp	17	2	0	8	0	0.9	0.3	9	46%
'3rd Foods' (Gerber)	7 tbsp	115	15	0	52	0	6.1	0.0	0	48%
w/egg yolks, strained (Gerber)	2.5 oz	100	10	1	38	0	6.0	0.0	42	55%
Turkey stick										
'Graduates' (Gerber)	2.5 oz	100	10	1	300	0	7.0	2.0	60	54%
junior	1 stick	18	1	0	48	0	1.4	0.4	7	68%
Veal										
and veal gravy, '2nd Foods' (Gerber)	2.5 oz	90	8	2	35	0	6.0	1.6	18	60%
junior	1 oz	31	4	0	20	0	1.4	0.7	8	41%

Food Name	Serving Size	Calories	Prot. gms	Carbs gms	Sod. mgs	Fiber gms	Fat gms	Sat. Fat gms	Chol. mgs	% Fat Cal.
'Stage 1' (Beech-Nut)	2.8 oz	60	10	0	50	0	2.0	0.0	0	31%
strained, 'Step 2' (Heinz)	2.5 oz	72	10	0	45	0	3.4	1.6	18	43%
strained	1 oz	29	4	0	18	0	1.4	0.6	7	43%
strained	1 tbsp	15	2	0	10	0	0.7	0.3	4	43%
'3rd Foods' (Gerber)	7 tbsp	108	16	0	56	0	5.0	0.0	0	42%
w/broth, strained, 'Step 2' (Heinz)	3.5 oz	130	15	0	57	1	7.9	0.0	0	54%
w/egg yolks, strained (Gerber)	2.5 oz	80	10	1	38	0	4.0	0.0	18	45%
Veal and beef										
junior (Gerber)	6 oz	110	4	16	31	0	3.0	0.0	7	25%
strained (Gerber)	4.5 oz	90	3	11	17	0	4.0	0.0	5	39%
Veal and ham										
junior (Gerber)	6 oz	120	3	17	24	0	4.0	0.0	7	31%
strained (Gerber) strained	4.5 oz	80	2	11	14	0	3.0	0.0	4	34%
Veal and turkey										
junior (Gerber)	6 oz	100	3	15	24	0	3.0	0.0	19	27%
strained (Gerber)	4.5 oz	70	2	10	17	0	2.0	0.0	12	27%
SOUP										
Chicken										
'Stage 2' (Beech-Nut)	4 oz jar	57	2	8	18	1	1.9	0.3	5	31%
strained	1 oz	14	0	2	5	0	0.5	0.1	1	31%
strained, 'Step 2' (Heinz)	3.5 oz	49	2	7	20	0	1.7	0.0	0	31%
w/stars, 'Table Time' (Beech-Nut)	6 oz	150	7	17	170	1	6.0	0.0	0	36%
Cream of broccoli, '3rd Foods' (Gerber)	3.2 oz	26	1	3	83	0	1.1	0.0	0	38%
Cream of potato, '3rd Foods' (Gerber)	3.2 oz	33	1	5	69	0	0.8	0.0	0	22%
Cream of tomato, '3rd Foods' (Gerber)	3.2 oz	41	1	7	73	0	0.7	0.0	0	15%
Cream of vegetable, '3rd Foods' (Gerber)	3.2 oz	29	1	4	48	0	0.8	0.0	0	24%
VEGETABLES										
Beets										
'2nd Foods' (Gerber)	7 tbsp	39	1	8	91	0	0.2	0.0	0	5%
strained	1 oz	10	0	2	24	1	0.0	0.0	0	2%
strained	1 tbsp	5	0	1	12	0	0.0	0.0	0	2%
strained (Gerber)	4.5 oz	60	1	11	115	0	1.0	0.0	0	16%
strained, 'Step 2' (Heinz)	3.5 oz	40	1	8	34	0	0.2	0.0	0	5%
Carrots										
beginner, 'Step 1' (Heinz)	2.5 oz	19	1	4	26	1	0.1	0.0	0	3%
(Earth's Best)	1 tbsp	4	0	1	5	0	0.0	0.0	0	0%
(Earth's Best)	4.5 oz	40	1	7	70	0	0.0	0.0	0	0%
'1st Foods' (Gerber)	2.5 oz	25	1	5	0	0	0.0	0.0	0	0%
junior	1 oz	9	0	2	14	0	0.1	0.0	0	5%
junior	1 tbsp	4	0	1	7	0	0.0	0.0	0	5%
junior, 'Step 3' (Heinz)	6 oz	54	1	12	83	3	0.3	0.1	0	5%
'2nd Foods' (Gerber)	4 oz	35	1	7	85	2	0.0	0.0	0	0%
'Stage 1' (Beech-Nut)	2.5 oz	25	0	6	80	0	0.0	0.0	0	0%
'Stage 3' (Beech-Nut)	6 oz	70	1	15	170	5	0.0	0.0	0	0%
strained	1 oz	8	0	2	10	0	0.0	0.0	0	3%
strained, 'Step 2' (Heinz)	4 oz	31	1	7	42	2	0.1	0.0	0	3%
'3rd Foods' (Gerber)	6 oz	50	1	11	150	3	0.0	0.0	0	0%
'Vegetable Dices' 'Graduates' (Gerber)	2.5 oz	22	1	4	35	1	0.0	0.0	0	0%
Carrots and parsnips (Earth's Best)	4.5 oz	60	0	14	30	0	0.0	0.0	0	0%
Carrots and peas (Beech-Nut)	4 oz	50	2	10	25	3	0.0	na	na	0%
Corn and butternut squash (Earth's Best)	4.5 oz	90	2	15	0	0	2.0	0.0	0	21%
Corn, creamed										
junior	1 oz	18	0	5	15	1	0.1	0.0	0	5%
junior	1 tbsp	10	0	2	8	0	0.1	0.0	0	5%

Food Name	Serving Size	Calories	Prot. gms	Carbs gms	Sod. mgs	Fiber gms	Fat gms	Sat. Fat gms	Chol. mgs	% Fat Cal.
junior, 'Step 3' *(Heinz)*	6 oz	111	2	28	88	4	0.7	0.1	2	5%
'Stage 2' *(Beech-Nut)*	4 oz	90	1	18	20	2	0.0	0.0	0	0%
'2nd Foods' *(Gerber)*	4 oz	70	2	14	15	0	0.5	0.1	1	6%
strained	1 oz	16	0	4	12	1	0.1	0.0	0	6%
strained	1 tbsp	9	0	2	6	0	0.1	0.0	0	6%
strained, 'Step 2' *(Heinz)*	4 oz	64	2	16	49	2	0.5	0.1	1	6%
Beans, green										
beginner, 'Step 1' *(Heinz)*	2.5 oz	18	1	4	1	1	0.1	0.0	0	3%
creamed, junior	1 oz	9	0	2	3	0	0.1	0.0	0	10%
creamed, junior	1 tbsp	5	0	1	2	0	0.1	0.0	0	10%
creamed, junior *(Gerber)*	6 oz	80	3	16	14	0	1.0	0.0	0	11%
creamed, junior, 'Step 3' *(Heinz)*	6 oz	54	2	12	20	3	0.7	0.1	2	10%
creamed, '3rd Foods' *(Gerber)*	7 tbsp	45	2	9	8	0	0.2	0.0	0	4%
'1st Foods' *(Gerber)*	2.5 oz	25	1	4	1	1	0.0	0.0	0	0%
junior	1 oz	7	0	2	1	1	0.0	0.0	0	3%
junior	1 tbsp	4	0	1	0	0	0.0	0.0	0	3%
'2nd Foods' *(Gerber)*	4 oz	40	1	6	10	1	0.0	0.0	0	0%
'Stage 1' *(Beech-Nut)*	4 oz	35	1	6	0	3	0.0	0.0	0	0%
'Stage 3' *(Beech-Nut)*	6 oz	50	1	10	0	4	0.0	0.0	0	0%
strained	1 oz	7	0	2	1	1	0.0	0.0	0	3%
strained	1 tbsp	4	0	1	0	0	0.0	0.0	0	3%
strained, 'Step 2' *(Heinz)*	3.5 oz	25	1	5	2	1	0.2	0.0	0	7%
'Vegetable Dices' 'Graduates' *(Gerber)*	2.5 oz	21	1	4	23	0	0.1	0.0	0	4%
w/potatoes *(Gerber)*	4 oz	71	2	11	20	2	2.1	1.3	6	27%
w/rice, '3rd Foods' *(Gerber)*	6 oz	70	2	15	20	1	0.0	0.0	0	0%
Garden vegetables										
(Earth's Best)	4.5 oz	70	1	15	15	0	0.0	0.0	0	0%
strained	1 oz	10	1	2	10	0	0.1	0.0	0	5%
'2nd Foods' *(Gerber)*	4 oz	45	2	7	26	2	0.5	0.0	0	10%
'Stage 2' *(Beech-Nut)*	4.5 oz	60	2	11	35	0	0.0	0.0	0	0%
Mixed vegetables										
junior	1 oz	12	0	2	10	0	0.1	0.0	0	8%
junior	1 tbsp	6	0	1	5	0	0.1	0.0	0	8%
'2nd Foods' *(Gerber)*	4 oz	45	1	9	20	2	0.0	0.0	0	0%
'Stage 2' *(Beech-Nut)*	4.5 oz	50	1	12	30	0	0.0	0.0	0	0%
strained	1 oz	12	0	2	4	0	0.1	0.0	0	10%
strained, 'Step 2' *(Heinz)*	3.5 oz	44	1	9	21	0	0.4	0.0	0	8%
'3rd Foods' *(Gerber)*	6 oz	70	2	14	32	0	1.0	0.0	0	12%
'Vegetable Dices' 'Graduates' *(Gerber)*	2.5 oz	35	1	6	55	2	0.0	0.0	0	0%
Peas										
beginner, 'Step 1' *(Heinz)*	2.5 oz	28	2	6	3	1	0.2	0.0	0	6%
creamed, strained	1 oz	15	1	3	4	1	0.5	0.1	1	30%
creamed, strained	1 tbsp	8	0	1	2	0	0.3	0.1	1	30%
creamed, strained, 'Step 2' *(Heinz)*	4 oz	60	2	10	16	2	2.1	0.5	5	30%
'1st Foods' *(Gerber)*	2.5 oz	30	2	6	0	0	0.0	0.0	0	0%
'2nd Foods' *(Gerber)*	4 oz	60	4	10	6	0	1.0	0.0	0	14%
strained	1 oz	11	1	2	1	1	0.1	0.0	0	6%
strained	1 tbsp	6	1	1	1	0	0.0	0.0	0	6%
strained, 'Step 2' *(Heinz)*	4 oz	45	4	9	5	2	0.3	0.1	0	6%
tender, sweet, 'Stage 1' *(Beech-Nut)*	2.5 oz	28	2	6	3	1	0.2	0.0	0	6%
tender, sweet, 'Stage 1' *(Beech-Nut)*	4 oz	45	4	9	5	2	0.3	0.1	0	6%
w/brown rice *(Earth's Best)*	4.5 oz	80	5	16	10	0	0.0	0.0	0	0%
w/rice, '3rd Foods' *(Gerber)*	6 oz	90	5	16	5	0	1.0	0.0	0	10%

Food Name	Serving Size	Calories	Prot. gms	Carbs gms	Sod. mgs	Fiber gms	Fat gms	Sat. Fat gms	Chol. mgs	% Fat Cal.
Potato										
'Graduates' (Gerber)	3.2 oz	38	1	9	6	0	0.1	0.0	0	2%
toddler	1 tbsp	5	0	1	6	0	0.0	0.0	0	2%
Spinach										
creamed, '2nd Foods' (Gerber)	4 oz	50	3	8	55	2	1.0	0.0	0	18%
creamed, strained	1 oz	10	1	2	14	1	0.4	0.2	1	29%
creamed, strained	1 tbsp	6	0	1	7	0	0.2	0.1	1	29%
w/potato (Earth's Best)	4.5 oz	60	2	8	25	0	2.0	0.0	0	31%
Squash										
beginner, 'Step 1' (Heinz)	2.5 oz	17	1	4	1	1	0.1	0.0	0	7%
butternut, 'Stage 1' (Beech-Nut)	2.5 oz	30	0	7	0	0	0.0	0.0	0	0%
'1st Foods' (Gerber)	2.5 oz	25	1	5	0	0	0.0	0.0	0	0%
junior	1 oz	7	0	2	0	1	0.1	0.0	0	7%
junior	1 tbsp	3	0	1	0	0	0.0	0.0	0	7%
'2nd Foods' (Gerber)	4 oz	35	1	7	5	1	0.0	0.0	0	0%
'Stage 1' (Beech-Nut)	4 oz jar	27	1	6	2	2	0.2	0.0	0	7%
strained	1 oz	7	0	2	1	1	0.1	0.0	0	7%
strained (Earth's Best)	4.5 oz	31	1	7	3	3	0.3	0.1	0	7%
strained, 'Step 2' (Heinz)	4 oz	27	1	6	2	2	0.2	0.0	0	7%
'3rd Foods' (Gerber) junior	6 oz	60	1	11	3	0	1.0	0.0	0	16%
w/corn (Gerber)	4 oz	57	2	11	6	2	0.7	0.1	0	11%
winter (Earth's Best)	4.5 oz	50	1	12	10	0	0.0	0.0	0	0%
Sweet potato										
beginner, 'Step 1' (Heinz)	2.5 oz	40	1	9	14	1	0.1	0.0	0	1%
(Earth's Best)	4.5 oz	60	1	12	15	0	1.0	0.0	0	15%
'1st Foods' (Gerber)	2.5 oz	45	1	10	0	0	0.0	0.0	0	0%
junior	1 oz	17	0	4	6	0	0.0	0.0	0	1%
junior	1 tbsp	8	0	2	3	0	0.0	0.0	0	1%
junior, 'Step 3' (Heinz)	6 oz	102	2	24	37	3	0.2	0.0	0	1%
'2nd Foods' (Gerber)	4.5 oz	70	1	16	20	1	0.0	0.0	0	0%
'Stage 1' (Beech-Nut)	2.5 oz	50	0	11	10	0	0.0	0.0	0	0%
'Stage 3' (Beech-Nut)	6 oz	110	1	25	15	1	0.0	0.0	0	0%
strained	1 oz	16	0	4	6	0	0.0	0.0	0	1%
strained (Earth's Best)	1 tbsp	8	0	2	3	0	0.0	0.0	0	1%
strained, 'Step 2' (Heinz)	4 oz	64	1	15	23	2	0.1	0.0	0	1%
'3rd Foods' (Gerber) junior	6 oz	110	1	24	39	0	1.0	0.0	0	8%
WATER, w/fluoride, sodium-free (Beech-Nut)	4 oz	0	0	0	0	0	0.0	0.0	0	0%
BACON										
cured, approx 12 slices per lb, raw	1 slice	211	3	0	277	0	21.9	8.1	25	93%
cured, approx 20 slices per lb, raw	3 slices	378	6	0	496	0	39.1	14.5	46	93%
cured, broiled, pan-fried, or roasted	3 med slices	109	6	0	303	0	9.4	3.3	16	77%
(Hormel)										
'Black Label'	1 oz	142	3	2	192	0	14.0	6.0	18	86%
'Black Label' low-salt	1.76 oz	250	5	2	260	0	25.0	10.0	32	89%
'Black Label' sliced, cooked	2 slices	60	4	0	298	0	5.0	0.0	0	74%
'Range' thick-sliced	1 oz	152	2	2	199	0	16.0	6.0	17	90%
(Hickory Ridge) cured, hickory flavor	2 slices	80	5	0	340	0	6.0	2.5	15	73%
(JM)										
cooked	2 slices	100	4	1	370	0	9.0	0.0	12	80%
'Lower Sodium' cooked	2 slices	100	4	1	260	0	9.0	0.0	0	80%
'Lower Sodium' raw	2 slices	290	5	1	250	0	30.0	0.0	0	92%
raw	2 slices	280	4	1	530	0	29.0	0.0	38	93%
(Jones Dairy Farm) raw	1 slice	165	2	0	187	0	17.0	0.0	25	94%
(Louis Rich) turkey, cooked	1 slice	34	2	0	184	0	2.7	0.7	12	72%

Food Name	Serving Size	Calories	Prot. gms	Carbs gms	Sod. mgs	Fiber gms	Fat gms	Sat. Fat gms	Chol. mgs	% Fat Cal.
(Oscar Mayer)										
....	1 slice	70	4	0	290	0	6.0	2.0	15	77%
approx 0.2-oz slices, cooked...........	1 slice	33	2	0	138	0	2.8	1.2	5	75%
'Center Cut' approx 0.2-oz slices, cooked.......	1 slice	25	2	0	113	0	1.8	0.8	6	66%
'Center Cut' cooked, yield from 1 lb raw........	6 oz	852	69	4	3813	0	62.5	27.5	189	66%
cooked, yield from 16-oz pkg, raw.........	5 oz	784	47	3	3236	0	64.9	25.8	127	74%
lower salt..........................	1 slice	70	5	1	200	0	5.0	2.0	15	65%
thick-cut, cooked....................	1 slice	60	4	0	250	0	5.0	1.5	10	74%
(Range Brand) 'Sliced' cooked...........	2 slices	110	6	0	392	0	9.0	0.0	0	77%
(Red Label) cooked..................	3 slices	110	6	0	0	0	10.0	0.0	0	79%
(West Virginia)										
cured, smoked flavor, cooked..........	2 slices	80	4	0	340	0	7.0	2.5	10	80%
thick-sliced, cooked.................	1 slice	80	3	0	260	0	7.0	2.5	10	84%
BACON, CANADIAN STYLE										
cured, grilled, yield from 6-oz pkg.........	5.9 oz	257	34	2	2149	0	11.7	3.9	81	41%
cured, raw.......................	6 oz	267	35	3	2395	0	11.8	3.8	85	40%
cured, 6 slices per 6 oz, grilled.........	2 slices	86	11	1	719	0	3.9	1.3	27	41%
cured, 6 slices per 6 oz, raw..........	2 slices	89	12	1	799	0	4.0	1.3	28	40%
(Hormel) sliced...................	1 oz	45	6	0	315	0	2.0	0.0	0	43%
(Jones Dairy Farm) unheated.........	1 slice	25	3	0	144	0	1.0	0.0	7	41%
(Light & Lean)....................	2 slices	35	6	0	0	0	1.0	0.0	0	27%
(Oscar Mayer)....................	1 slice	50	8	0	620	0	1.5	1.0	25	30%
BACON BITS										
*(Bac*Os)*										
imitation.........................	2 tsp	25	2	2	90	0	1.0	0.0	0	36%
imitation, bits, cholesterol-free........	1 tbsp	30	3	2	120	0	1.0	0.0	0	31%
(Bac'n Pieces) imitation, chips cholesterol-free..........	1 1/2 tbsp	30	3	2	240	0	1.0	0.0	0	31%
(Hormel)										
....	1 oz	117	12	1	1008	0	7.0	3.0	16	55%
....	1 tbsp	30	3	0	313	0	2.0	0.0	0	60%
50% less fat.......................	1 tsp	30	3	0	250	0	1.5	1.0	5	53%
(Oscar Mayer) real.................	1 tbsp	25	3	0	220	0	1.5	0.5	5	53%
(Schilling) imitation, 'Bac'N Pieces'......	1 tsp	26	2	2	51	0	0.4	0.0	0	18%
(Tone's) imitation.................	1 tsp	7	1	0	59	0	0.3	0.0	0	36%
BACON DISH/ENTRÉE *(Stouffer's)* strata, frozen...	1 oz	52	3	3	125	0	3.5	0.9	31	60%
BACON PIECES (Hormel).................	1 oz	94	12	2	654	0	5.0	2.0	26	45%
BACON SUBSTITUTE										
(Healthy Favorites) turkey, w/pork 'Breakfast Strips'......	11 grams	18	2	0	145	0	1.0	0.3	9	51%
(Heartline)										
Canadian style, vegetarian, nonfat, lite...............	0.5 oz	22	5	1	135	3	0.0	0.0	0	0%
Canadian style, vegetarian, yield from 4 oz cooked.......	2 oz	176	19	9	260	0	7.0	0.0	0	36%
(JM)										
beef, heated......................	2 slices	100	7	1	320	0	7.0	0.0	20	66%
beef, raw.........................	2 slices	200	9	1	430	0	18.0	0.0	53	80%
(Louis Rich) turkey.................	1 slice	30	2	0	190	0	2.5	0.5	10	74%
(Morningstar Farms) vegetarian, 'Breakfast Strips'........	2 strips	56	2	2	220	1	4.4	0.7	0	72%
(Mr. Turkey) turkey, 70% less fat........	1 slice	25	3	0	170	0	2.0	0.5	10	60%
(Sizzlean)										
beef, heated......................	2 strips	70	6	0	480	0	5.0	0.0	0	65%
pork, brown sugar cured, heated.......	2 strips	110	6	2	490	0	9.0	0.0	0	72%
pork, heated......................	2 strips	90	6	0	530	0	8.0	0.0	0	75%
(White Wave SoyFood) vegetarian, 'Healthy'...........	1 oz	27	4	4	310	3	1.0	0.0	0	22%
(Worthington) vegetarian, 'Stripples'........	2 strips	56	2	2	220	1	4.4	0.7	0	72%

Food Name	Serving Size	Calories	Prot. gms	Carbs gms	Sod. mgs	Fiber gms	Fat gms	Sat. Fat gms	Chol. mgs	% Fat Cal.
BAGEL										
BLUEBERRY										
(Earth Grains) 3 oz	1 bagel	245	9	48	210	0	0.0	0.0	0	0%
(Lender's)										
4-inch diam, frozen, 'Bagel Shop'	1 bagel	264	11	53	427	2	1.5	0.3	0	5%
3.13 oz, frozen, 'Big'n Crusty'	1 serving	214	8	46	409	2	0.8	0.2	0	3%
3-inch diam, 'Premium'	1 bagel	209	8	43	409	2	1.3	0.3	0	6%
2.5 oz, frozen	1 bagel	190	7	38	250	0	1.0	0.0	0	5%
(Western Bagel)...............................	1 bagel	240	8	43	410	2	4.0	1.0	0	15%
CINNAMON-RAISIN										
(Earth Grains) 3 oz	1 bagel	245	9	48	210	0	0.0	0.0	0	0%
(Finast) w/cinnamon & honey, 2.5 oz	1 bagel	200	8	40	305	0	1.0	0.0	0	4%
(Lender's) 'Big'n Crusty' 3 1/8 oz	1 bagel	250	8	49	370	0	2.0	0.0	0	7%
(Sara Lee)										
2.5 oz	1 bagel	200	7	39	230	0	2.0	0.0	0	9%
3.1 oz	1 bagel	240	8	48	280	0	2.0	0.0	0	7%
(Thomas')										
....	1 bagel	160	6	36	290	1	1.0	0.0	0	5%
'Deli Style'	1 bagel	170	6	33	230	2	2.0	0.0	0	10%
(Western Bagel).............................	1 bagel	230	8	40	410	4	4.0	1.0	0	16%
EGG										
4.5-inch diam.................................	1 bagel	306	12	58	556	3	2.3	0.5	26	7%
3-inch diam	1 bagel	158	6	30	288	1	1.2	0.2	14	7%
(Lender's)										
'Bakery Style'	1 bagel	210	9	41	450	2	2.0	0.0	5	8%
3.13 oz, frozen, 'Big'n Crusty'	1 bagel	250	9	47	380	0	2.0	0.0	15	7%
2 oz, frozen	1 bagel	160	6	32	340	0	1.0	0.0	0	6%
(Sara Lee)										
3.1 oz, frozen	1 bagel	250	9	48	450	0	2.0	0.0	20	7%
2.5 oz, frozen	1 bagel	200	8	38	360	0	2.0	0.0	15	9%
(Thomas')...................................	1 bagel	170	7	35	280	2	1.5	0.5	15	7%
HONEY RAISIN (Lender's) 2.5 oz	1 bagel	200	8	40	310	0	1.0	0.0	0	4%
HONEY WHEAT (Earth Grains) 3 oz	1 bagel	240	9	45	210	0	0.0	0.0	0	0%
MULTIGRAIN (Thomas')...........................	1 bagel	170	6	35	310	1	1.5	0.5	0	8%
OAT BRAN										
(Lender's) 2.5 oz, frozen	1 bagel	170	7	36	290	3	2.0	0.0	0	9%
(Sara Lee)										
3 oz, frozen	1 bagel	220	9	47	450	0	1.0	0.0	0	4%
2.5 oz, frozen	1 bagel	180	8	38	360	0	1.0	0.0	0	5%
ONION										
4.5-inch diam.................................	1 bagel	303	12	59	587	3	1.8	0.2	0	5%
3-inch diam	1 bagel	157	6	30	304	1	0.9	0.1	0	5%
(Earth Grains) 3 oz bagel.........................	1 bagel	240	9	45	210	0	0.0	0.0	0	0%
(Lender's)										
3.13 oz, frozen, 'Big'n Crusty'	1 bagel	230	9	46	480	0	1.0	0.0	0	4%
2 oz, frozen	1 bagel	160	7	31	290	0	1.0	0.0	0	6%
0.9 oz, frozen, 'Bagelettes'	1 bagel	70	3	14	135	0	1.0	0.0	0	12%
(Sara Lee) 3.1 oz, frozen.........................	1 bagel	230	9	45	560	0	1.0	0.0	0	4%
2.5 oz, frozen	1 bagel	190	7	37	450	0	1.0	0.0	0	5%
(Sprouted Wheat Bagels) w/poppy seeds, organic	1 bagel	250	6	50	320	0	1.0	0.0	0	4%
(Thomas')...................................	1 bagel	170	6	35	300	2	1.5	0.5	0	8%
(Western Bagel)...............................	1 bagel	220	8	39	430	4	4.0	1.0	0	16%
ORGANIC (Bible Bagels)............................	1 bagel	180	11	29	130	4	2.0	0.0	0	10%

Food Name	Serving Size	Calories	Prot. gms	Carbs gms	Sod. mgs	Fiber gms	Fat gms	Sat. Fat gms	Chol. mgs	% Fat Cal.
PLAIN										
4.5-inch diam.	1 bagel	303	12	59	587	3	1.8	0.2	0	5%
4-inch diam	1 bagel	245	9	48	475	2	1.4	0.2	0	5%
3-inch diam	1 bagel	157	6	30	304	1	0.9	0.1	0	5%
2.5-inch diam.	1 bagel	72	3	14	139	1	0.4	0.1	0	5%
(Earth Grains) 3 oz bagel.	1 bagel	240	9	45	210	0	0.0	0.0	0	0%
(Lender's)										
'Bakery Style'	1 bagel	210	8	42	450	2	2.0	0.0	0	8%
soft, 2.5 oz, frozen.	1 bagel	210	7	36	350	0	3.0	0.0	12	14%
3.13 oz, frozen, 'Big'n Crusty'	1 bagel	240	9	47	450	0	1.0	0.0	0	4%
2 oz, frozen	1 bagel	150	6	30	320	0	1.0	0.0	0	6%
0.9 oz, frozen, 'Bagelettes'	1 bagel	70	3	13	170	0	1.0	0.0	0	12%
(Sara Lee)										
3.1 oz, frozen	1 bagel	230	9	46	580	0	1.0	0.0	0	4%
2.5 oz, frozen	1 bagel	190	8	38	460	0	1.0	0.0	0	5%
(Thomas').	1 serving	160	6	35	320	2	1.0	0.5	0	5%
POPPY SEED										
4.5-inch diam.	1 bagel	303	12	59	587	3	1.8	0.2	0	5%
4-inch diam	1 bagel	245	9	48	475	2	1.4	0.2	0	5%
3-inch diam	1 bagel	157	6	30	304	1	0.9	0.1	0	5%
(Lender's) 2 oz, frozen.	1 bagel	160	7	29	370	0	1.0	0.0	0	6%
(Sara Lee)										
3.1 oz, frozen	1 bagel	230	9	46	560	0	1.0	0.0	0	4%
2.5 oz, frozen	1 bagel	190	8	37	450	0	1.0	0.0	0	5%
PUMPERNICKEL *(Lender's)* 2 oz, frozen	1 bagel	160	6	31	330	0	1.0	0.0	0	6%
RAISIN										
(Lender's)										
'Bakery Style'	1 bagel	220	8	44	380	2	2.0	0.0	0	8%
0.9 oz, frozen, 'Bagelettes'	1 bagel	70	2	14	110	0	1.0	0.0	0	12%
RYE *(Lender's)* 2 oz, frozen	1 bagel	150	6	30	310	0	1.0	0.0	0	6%
SESAME SEED										
4.5-inch diam.	1 bagel	303	12	59	587	3	1.8	0.2	0	5%
4-inch diam	1 bagel	245	9	48	475	2	1.4	0.2	0	5%
3-inch diam	1 bagel	157	6	30	304	1	0.9	0.1	0	5%
(Sprouted Wheat Bagels).	1 bagel	250	6	50	320	0	1.0	0.0	0	4%
SPELT *(Rudi's)* organic.	1 bagel	280	11	54	440	0	2.0	0.0	0	6%
WATER *(Western Bagel)*	1 bagel	230	8	41	420	2	4.0	1.0	0	16%
WHEAT *(Lender's)* w/raisin, 2.5 oz	1 bagel	190	6	39	310	0	1.0	0.0	0	5%
WHOLE GRAIN (Natural Ovens)	1 bagel	190	8	36	210	8	2.0	0.0	0	9%
BAGEL CHIPS										
cinnamon raisin *(Original Bagel Crisps)*	1 oz	130	4	20	170	1	4.0	1.0	0	27%
garlic *(Original Bagel Crisps)*	1 oz	130	4	20	190	1	4.0	1.0	0	27%
BAGEL MIX gluten-free *(Gluten Free Pantry)*	1 serving	150	2	36	170	1	0.0	0.0	0	0%
BAKED BEANS, CANNED.										
(B&M)										
red kidney	8 oz	250	15	42	640	11	7.0	0.0	5	22%
yellow eye	8 oz	326	15	50	770	15	7.0	0.0	4	20%
(Beanee Weenee) w/sliced hot dogs	1 cup	30	16	35	1240	8	14.0	4.0	40	38%
(Bearitos)										
black beans, nonfat.	1/2 cup	110	6	22	360	3	0.0	0.0	0	0%
vegetarian, organic, fat-free, original.	1/2 cup	130	6	26	360	3	0.0	0.0	0	0%
(Green Giant)										
barbecue, dry beans in brine	1/2 cup	140	6	28	460	5	0.5	0.0	0	3%
honey bacon, dry beans in brine.	1/2 cup	160	6	34	490	6	0.5	0.0	0	3%

Food Name	Serving Size	Calories	Prot. gms	Carbs gms	Sod. mgs	Fiber gms	Fat gms	Sat. Fat gms	Chol. mgs	% Fat Cal.
(Friends)										
red kidney	8 oz	340	17	57	1060	11	4.0	2.0	4	11%
red kidney, w/pork	8 oz	270	14	55	990	11	4.0	0.0	4	12%
(Green Giant)										
dry beans in brine	1/2 cup	160	6	31	580	7	1.5	1.0	5	8%
w/onion, dry beans in brine	1/2 cup	150	5	28	620	5	1.5	0.5	0	9%
(Health Valley) honey baked, nonfat	1/2 cup	110	7	24	135	7	0.0	0.0	0	0%
(Heinz) vegetarian, in tomato sauce	8 oz	230	13	41	880	11	1.0	0.0	0	4%
(Homestyle) pork and beans, food service product	1/2 cup	157	6	27	621	11	4.8	1.7	2	25%
(Joan of Arc)										
barbecue, dry beans in brine	1/2 cup	140	6	28	460	5	0.5	0.0	0	3%
dry beans in brine	1/2 cup	160	6	31	580	7	1.5	1.0	5	8%
honey bacon, dry beans in brine	1/2 cup	160	6	34	490	6	0.5	0.0	0	3%
w/onion, dry beans in brine	1/2 cup	150	5	28	620	5	1.5	0.5	0	9%
(Luck's)										
October, seasoned w/pork	1/2 cup	140	8	20	340	7	3.0	1.0	3	19%
pork and beans in tomato sauce	1/2 cup	150	6	28	630	6	1.0	0.0	0	6%
(Ranch Style) pork & beans	1/2 cup	140	6	28	740	6	0.5	0.0	5	3%
(S&W) 'Brick Oven'	1/2 cup	160	7	32	620	7	0.5	0.0	0	3%
(Van Camp's)										
nonfat, seasoned w/brown sugar	1/2 cup	130	7	28	430	5	0.0	0.0	0	0%
w/brown sugar and bacon	1/2 cup	140	7	29	520	5	1.0	0.0	0	6%
w/pork, in tomato sauce	1/2 cup	110	6	24	490	6	1.5	0.5	0	10%
w/beef	1 cup	322	17	45	1264	na	9.2	4.5	59	26%
w/franks	1 cup	368	17	40	1114	18	17.0	6.1	16	42%
w/pork	1 cup	268	13	51	1047	14	3.9	1.5	18	13%
w/pork and sweet sauce	1 cup	281	13	53	850	13	3.7	1.4	18	12%
w/pork and tomato sauce	1 cup	248	13	49	1113	12	2.6	1.0	18	9%
w/pork and tomato sauce	1 tbsp	15	1	3	70	1	0.2	0.1	1	9%
BAKER'S YEAST. See under YEAST.										
BAKING CHOCOLATE. See CHOCOLATE, BAKING.										
BAKING MIX										
general purpose, whole wheat, dry *(Insta-Bake)*	1/3 cup	150	4	25	540	3	5.0	1.0	0	28%
BAKING POWDER										
Double-acting										
(Clabber Girl)	1/4 tsp	3	0	1	138	0	0.0	0.0	0	0%
(Rumford)	1/4 tsp	3	0	1	109	0	0.0	0.0	0	0%
sodium aluminum sulfate	1 tsp	2	0	1	488	0	0.0	0.0	0	0%
sodium aluminum sulfate	1/2 tsp	1	0	1	244	0	0.0	0.0	0	0%
straight phosphate	1 tsp	2	0	1	363	0	0.0	0.0	0	0%
straight phosphate	1/2 tsp	1	0	1	182	0	0.0	0.0	0	0%
Low-sodium										
	1 tsp	5	0	2	5	0	0.0	0.0	0	3%
	1/2 tsp	2	0	1	2	0	0.0	0.0	0	3%
(Featherweight)	1 tsp	8	0	2	2	0	0.0	0.0	0	0%
Regular										
(Calumet)	1/4 tsp	0	0	0	100	0	0.0	0.0	0	0%
(Davis)	1 tsp	6	0	2	450	0	0.0	0.0	0	0%
(Tone's)	1 tsp	5	0	1	290	0	0.0	0.0	0	0%
BAKING SODA										
	1 tsp	0	0	0	1259	0	0.0	0.0	0	0%
	1/2 tsp	0	0	0	629	0	0.0	0.0	0	0%
(Arm & Hammer)	1/2 tsp	0	0	0	476	0	0.0	0.0	0	0%
(Tone's)	1 tsp	0	0	0	821	0	0.0	0.0	0	0%

Food Name	Serving Size	Calories	Prot. gms	Carbs gms	Sod. mgs	Fiber gms	Fat gms	Sat. Fat gms	Chol. mgs	% Fat Cal.
BALSAM PEAR / bitter gourd										
Leafy tips										
boiled, drained.	1 cup	20	2	4	8	1	0.1	0.0	0	5%
raw	1/2 cup	7	1	1	3	na	0.2	na	0	19%
raw	1 med leaf	1	0	0	0	na	0.0	na	0	20%
Pods										
boiled, drained, 1/2-inch pieces	1 cup	24	1	5	7	2	0.2	0.0	0	8%
boiled, drained 1/2-inch pieces	1/2 cup	12	1	3	4	1	0.1	0.0	0	8%
raw	1 medium	21	1	5	6	3	0.2	na	0	8%
raw, 1/2-inch pieces	1 cup	16	1	3	5	3	0.2	na	0	8%
BAMBOO SHOOTS										
Canned										
(La Choy)	2 tbsp	3	0	1	0	0	0.1	0.0	0	11%
drained, 1/8-inch slices	1 cup	25	2	4	9	2	0.5	0.1	0	18%
sliced *(China Boy)*	1/2 cup	15	1	3	10	1	0.0	0.0	0	0%
Fresh										
boiled, drained.	1 med shoot	17	2	3	6	1	0.3	0.1	0	15%
boiled, drained, 1/2-inch slices	1 cup	14	2	2	5	1	0.3	0.1	0	15%
raw, 1/2-inch pieces	1/2 cup	21	2	4	3	2	0.2	0.1	0	9%
raw, 1/2-inch slices	1 cup	41	4	8	6	3	0.5	0.1	0	9%
BANANA										
Dehydrated or powdered										
. . . .	1 cup	346	4	88	3	8	1.8	0.7	0	4%
. . . .	1 tbsp	21	0	5	0	0	0.1	0.0	0	4%
Fresh, raw										
mashed	1 cup	207	2	53	2	5	1.1	0.4	0	4%
sliced.	1 cup	138	2	35	2	4	0.7	0.3	0	4%
whole, extra large, 9 inches long and up.	1 banana	140	2	36	2	4	0.7	0.3	0	4%
whole, extra small, up to 6 inches long	1 banana	75	1	19	1	2	0.4	0.1	0	4%
whole, large, 8 to 8 7/8 inches long.	1 banana	125	1	32	1	3	0.7	0.3	0	4%
whole, medium, 7 to 7 7/8 inches long	1 banana	109	1	28	1	3	0.6	0.2	0	4%
whole, small, 6 to 6 7/8 inches long	1 banana	93	1	24	1	2	0.5	0.2	0	4%
BANANA CHIPS										
. . . .	3 oz	441	2	50	5	7	28.6	24.6	0	56%
. . . .	1.5 oz	218	1	25	3	3	14.1	12.2	0	56%
. . . .	1 oz	147	1	17	2	2	9.5	8.2	0	56%
BANANA PEPPER. See PEPPER, BANANA.										
BANANA SQUASH. See SQUASH, BANANA.										
BARBADOS CHERRY. See ACEROLA.										
BARBECUE SPICE. See under SEASONING MIX.										
BARLEY										
. . . .	1 cup	651	23	135	22	32	4.2	0.9	0	5%
pearled, cooked.	1 cup	193	4	44	5	6	0.7	0.1	0	3%
pearled, cooked *(Tone's)*.	1 tsp	8	0	2	1	0	0.1	0.0	0	10%
pearled, quick, raw, 'Scotch Brand' *(Quaker)*	1/3 cup	172	6	36	0	5	0.5	0.0	0	3%
pearled, raw	1 cup	704	20	155	18	31	2.3	0.5	0	3%
pearled, raw *(Arrowhead Mills)*	2 oz	200	5	45	1	7	1.0	0.0	0	4%
BARLEY FLAKES rolled *(Arrowhead Mills)*	1/3 cup	110	4	28	0	5	1.0	0.0	0	7%
BARLEY FLOUR. See under FLOUR.										
BARLEY MALT, natural, organic *(Eden Foods)*.	1/2 tsp	10	0	2	1	0	0.0	0.0	0	0%
BARLEY MALT FLOUR. See under FLOUR.										
BARLEY MIX, organic *(Ener-G Foods)*	1 cup	396	15	85	503	8	1.6	0.0	0	4%
BASELLA. See SPINACH, VINE.										

Food Name	Serving Size	Calories	Prot. gms	Carbs gms	Sod. mgs	Fiber gms	Fat gms	Sat. Fat gms	Chol. mgs	% Fat Cal.
BASIL										
Dried										
(Golden Dipt)	2 grams	8	0	1	36	0	0.0	0.0	0	0%
(McCormick/Schilling)	1 tsp	3	0	0	0	0	0.0	0.0	0	0%
crumbled (Spice Islands)	1 tsp	3	0	1	1	0	0.1	0.0	0	22%
crumbled (Tone's)	1 tsp	4	0	1	1	0	0.1	0.0	0	17%
ground	1 tbsp	11	1	3	2	2	0.2	0.0	0	13%
ground	1 tsp	4	0	1	0	1	0.1	0.0	0	13%
Fresh										
chopped	2 tbsp	1	0	0	0	0	0.0	0.0	0	19%
ground (Durkee)	1 tsp	5	0	0	0	0	0.0	0.0	0	0%
ground (Laurel Leaf)	1 tsp	5	0	0	0	0	0.0	0.0	0	0%
whole leaves	5 med leaves	1	0	0	0	0	0.0	0.0	0	19%
BASMATI RICE. See under RICE.										
BASS, CALICO. See SUNFISH.										
BASS, FRESHWATER										
mixed species, baked, broiled, grilled, or microwaved	3 oz	124	21	0	77	0	4.0	0.9	74	29%
mixed species, raw	3 oz	97	16	0	60	0	3.1	0.7	58	29%
BASS, SEA										
mixed species, baked, broiled, grilled, or microwaved	3 oz	105	20	0	74	0	2.2	0.6	45	19%
mixed species, raw	3 oz	82	16	0	58	0	1.7	0.4	35	19%
BASS, STRIPED										
mixed species, baked, broiled, grilled, or microwaved	3 oz	105	19	0	75	0	2.5	0.6	88	22%
mixed species, raw	3 oz	82	15	0	59	0	2.0	0.4	68	22%
BATTER MIX, ALL PURPOSE										
all-purpose, no MSG, dry mix (Don's Chuck Wagon)	1/4 cup	100	4	20	580	1	0.0	0.0	0	0%
beer, dry mix (Golden Dipt)	1 oz	100	2	22	650	0	0.0	0.0	0	0%
corn dog, dry mix (Golden Dipt)	1 oz	100	3	22	490	0	0.0	0.0	0	0%
fish and chips, no MSG, dry mix (Don's Chuck Wagon)	1/4 cup	100	3	21	740	1	0.0	0.0	0	0%
fish and chips, dry mix (Golden Dipt)	1.25 oz	120	2	27	910	0	0.0	0.0	0	0%
golden mushroom, no MSG, dry mix (Don's Chuck Wagon)	1/4 cup	95	3	21	990	1	0.0	0.0	0	0%
onion ring, no MSG, dry mix (Don's Chuck Wagon)	1/4 cup	100	3	21	690	1	0.0	0.0	0	0%
onion ring, dry mix (Golden Dipt)	1 oz	100	2	22	570	0	0.0	0.0	0	0%
tempura, dry mix (Golden Dipt)	1 oz	100	3	22	130	0	0.0	0.0	0	0%
BAY LEAF										
dried (McCormick/Schilling)	1 tsp	2	0	0	0	0	0.0	0.0	0	0%
dried, crumbled	1 tbsp	6	0	1	0	0	0.2	0.0	0	22%
dried, crumbled	1 tsp	2	0	0	0	0	0.1	0.0	0	22%
dried, crumbled (Durkee)	1 tsp	2	0	0	0	0	0.0	0.0	0	0%
dried, crumbled (Laurel Leaf)	1 tsp	2	0	0	0	0	0.0	0.0	0	0%
dried, crumbled (Spice Islands)	1 tsp	5	0	0	1	0	0.1	0.0	0	36%
dried, crumbled (Tone's)	1 tsp	2	0	1	0	0	0.1	0.1	0	27%
BEAN, ADZUKI										
Canned										
mature seeds, sweetened	1 cup	702	11	163	645	na	0.1	0.0	0	0%
organic, no salt added, very low sodium (Eden Foods)	1/2 cup	80	7	18	10	5	1.0	0.0	0	8%
organic, w/liquid (Eden Foods)	1/2 cup	100	6	17	20	4	1.0	0.0	0	9%
Fresh										
mature seeds, boiled	1 cup	294	17	57	18	17	0.2	0.1	0	1%
mature seeds, raw	1 cup	648	39	124	10	25	1.0	0.4	0	1%
raw (Arrowhead Mills)	2 oz	190	13	35	3	14	1.0	0.0	0	4%
Jarred, organic (Eden Foods)	1/2 cup	90	6	16	35	4	0.0	0.0	0	0%

Food Name	Serving Size	Calories	Prot. gms	Carbs gms	Sod. mgs	Fiber gms	Fat gms	Sat. Fat gms	Chol. mgs	% Fat Cal.
BEAN, ANASAZI, dry *(Arrowhead Mills)*	1/4 cup	150	10	27	0	9	0.5	0.0	0	3%
BEAN, BLACK / black turtle bean										
Canned										
(Green Giant)	1/2 cup	90	7	21	580	6	0.0	0.0	0	0%
(Joan of Arc)	1/2 cup	90	7	21	580	.6	0.0	0.0	0	0%
(Old El Paso)	1/2 cup	100	7	17	400	7	1.0	0.0	0	9%
(Progresso)	1/2 cup	100	7	17	400	7	1.0	0.0	0	9%
(Ranch Style)	1/2 cup	100	6	19	380	5	0.0	0.0	0	0%
(S&W)	1/2 cup	70	5	17	520	6	0.0	0.0	0	0%
'Fiesta' style *(Stokely)*	1/2 cup	100	6	17	600	4	0.5	0.0	0	5%
50% less salt *(S&W)*	1/2 cup	70	5	17	260	6	0.0	0.0	0	0%
'Sun Vista' *(S&W)*	1/2 cup	70	5	20	630	7	1.0	0.0	0	8%
organic, no salt added, very low sodium *(Eden Foods)*	1/2 cup	70	7	17	15	6	1.0	0.0	0	9%
Dry										
mature seeds, boiled	1 cup	227	15	41	2	15	0.9	0.2	0	3%
mature seeds, raw	1 cup	662	42	121	10	29	2.8	0.7	0	3%
mature seeds, raw	1 tbsp	41	3	8	1	2	0.2	0.0	0	3%
raw *(Arrowhead Mills)*	2 oz	190	13	35	9	11	1.0	0.0	0	4%
BEAN, BLACK TURTLE. See BEAN, BLACK.										
BEAN, BROAD. See BEAN, FAVA.										
BEAN, CANNELLINI, CANNED										
(Progresso)	1/2 cup	100	5	18	270	5	0.5	0.0	0	5%
white *(Pathmark)*	1/2 cup	100	6	18	390	0	0.0	0.0	0	0%
BEAN, CRANBERRY / borlotti / Roman bean / rose coco bean										
Canned *(Progresso)*	1/2 cup	110	7	18	420	12	1.0	0.0	0	8%
Dried										
mature seeds, boiled	1 cup	241	17	43	2	18	0.8	0.2	0	3%
mature seeds, canned	1 cup	216	14	39	863	16	0.7	0.2	0	3%
mature seeds, raw	1 cup	653	45	117	12	48	2.4	0.6	0	3%
BEAN, FAVA / broad bean / horse bean / jack bean										
Canned										
(Progresso)	1/2 cup	110	6	20	250	5	0.5	0.0	0	4%
mature seeds	1 cup	182	14	32	1160	9	0.6	0.1	0	3%
Fresh										
immature seeds, raw	1 med bean	6	0	1	4	0	0.0	0.0	0	7%
immature seeds, raw	1 cup	78	6	13	55	5	0.7	0.1	0	7%
mature seeds, boiled	1 cup	187	13	33	9	9	0.7	0.1	0	3%
mature seeds, raw	1 cup	512	39	87	20	38	2.3	0.4	0	4%
mature seeds, raw	1 tbsp	32	2	5	1	2	0.1	0.0	0	4%
raw, in pod	1 cup	111	10	22	32	na	0.9	0.1	0	7%
raw, in pod	1 med pod	5	0	1	2	na	0.0	0.0	0	7%
BEAN, FRENCH / haricots. See also BEAN, GREEN.										
Fresh										
boiled	1 cup	228	12	43	11	17	1.3	0.1	0	5%
raw	1 cup	631	35	118	33	46	3.7	0.4	0	5%
BEAN, GARBANZO. See CHICKPEA.										
BEAN, GOA. See BEAN, WINGED.										
BEAN, GREAT NORTHERN										
Canned										
(A&P)	1 cup	210	14	38	0	0	1.0	0.0	0	4%
(Allens)	1/2 cup	105	5	17	440	0	1.0	0.0	0	9%
(Bush's Best)	1/2 cup	70	5	16	380	5	0.0	0.0	0	0%
(Green Giant)	1/2 cup	80	6	18	290	5	1.0	0.0	0	9%
(Joan of Arc)	1/2 cup	80	6	18	290	5	1.0	0.0	0	9%

Food Name	Serving Size	Calories	Prot. gms	Carbs gms	Sod. mgs	Fiber gms	Fat gms	Sat. Fat gms	Chol. mgs	% Fat Cal.
mature seeds	1 cup	299	19	55	10	13	1.0	0.3	0	3%
mature seeds, no salt added	1 cup	209	15	37	4	12	0.8	0.2	0	3%
organic, w/liquid (Eden Foods)	1/2 cup	110	6	20	15	6	1.0	0.0	0	8%
seasoned, w/pork (Luck's)	1/2 cup	140	7	20	290	6	3.0	1.0	3	20%
'Sun-Vista' (S&W)	1/2 cup	70	6	17	490	6	0.0	0.0	0	0%
w/pork (Allens)	1/2 cup	100	5	19	320	0	1.0	0.0	0	9%
w/pork (Luck's)	7.25 oz	220	12	32	645	13	5.0	0.0	0	20%
Dried										
mature seeds, boiled	1 cup	209	15	37	4	12	0.8	0.2	0	3%
mature seeds, raw	1 cup	620	40	114	26	37	2.1	0.7	0	3%
BEAN, GREEN / string bean / snap bean										
Canned										
(Pathmark)	1/2 cup	20	1	5	350	0	0.0	0.0	0	0%
(Stokely)	1/2 cup	20	1	4	360	0	0.0	0.0	0	0%
almandine (Green Giant)	1/2 cup	45	2	5	300	2	3.0	0.0	0	49%
Blue Lake, cut (Bush's Best)	1/2 cup	20	1	5	360	2	0.0	0.0	0	0%
Blue Lake, cut (Pathmark)	1/2 cup	20	1	4	430	0	0.0	0.0	0	0%
Blue Lake, cut, 'Premium' (S&W)	1/2 cup	20	1	4	385	0	0.0	0.0	0	0%
Blue Lake, French style, (Pathmark)	1/2 cup	20	1	4	430	0	0.0	0.0	0	0%
Blue Lake, French style, 'Premium' (S&W)	1/2 cup	20	1	4	385	0	0.0	0.0	0	0%
cut (A&P)	1/2 cup	20	1	4	350	0	1.0	0.0	0	31%
cut (Allens)	1/2 cup	20	1	4	350	0	1.0	0.0	0	31%
cut (Bush's Best)	1/2 cup	20	1	5	360	2	0.0	0.0	0	0%
cut (Featherweight)	1/2 cup	25	1	5	10	0	0.0	0.0	0	0%
cut (Finast)	1/2 cup	20	1	4	400	0	0.0	0.0	0	0%
cut (Freshlike)	1/2 cup	20	1	4	340	0	0.0	0.0	0	0%
cut (Green Giant)	1/2 cup	16	1	4	300	1	0.0	0.0	0	0%
cut (IGA)	1/2 cup	20	1	5	10	0	0.0	0.0	0	0%
cut (Pathmark)	1/2 cup	20	1	4	430	0	0.0	0.0	0	0%
cut (S&W)	1/2 cup	20	1	4	340	2	0.0	0.0	0	0%
cut (Stokely)	1/2 cup	20	1	4	400	1	0.0	0.0	0	0%
cut (Veg-All)	1/2 cup	20	1	4	340	0	0.0	0.0	0	0%
cut, 'No Frills' (Pathmark)	1 cup	35	2	8	640	0	0.0	0.0	0	0%
cut, 'Pantry Express' (Green Giant)	1/2 cup	12	1	3	20	1	0.0	0.0	0	0%
cut, 'Veri-Green' (Finast)	1/2 cup	20	1	4	320	0	0.0	0.0	0	0%
cut, 50% less salt (Green Giant)	1/2 cup	16	1	4	195	1	0.0	0.0	0	0%
cut, no salt added (Finast)	1/2 cup	20	1	4	10	0	0.0	0.0	0	0%
cut, no salt added (Freshlike)	1/2 cup	20	1	4	5	0	0.0	0.0	0	0%
cut, stringless, w/liquid (S&W)	1/2 cup	20	1	4	3850	0	0.0	0.0	0	0%
cut, water packed, w/o salt (Freshlike)	1/2 cup	20	1	4	5	0	0.0	0.0	0	0%
cut, water packed, w/o sugar or salt (Freshlike)	1/2 cup	20	1	4	5	0	0.0	0.0	0	0%
cut, w/liquid (Del Monte)	1/2 cup	20	1	4	355	0	0.0	0.0	0	0%
cut, w/liquid, no salt added (Del Monte)	1/2 cup	20	1	4	10	0	0.0	0.0	0	0%
dilled (S&W)	1 oz	20	0	5	125	1	0.0	0.0	0	0%
European, slender, whole (Stokely)	1/2 cup	20	1	4	370	1	0.0	0.0	0	0%
50% less salt (Green Giant)	1/2 cup	18	1	4	150	1	0.0	0.0	0	0%
French style (A&P)	1/2 cup	20	1	4	350	0	1.0	0.0	0	31%
French style (Allens)	1/2 cup	20	1	4	350	0	1.0	0.0	0	31%
French style (Bush's Best)	1/2 cup	20	1	5	360	2	0.0	0.0	0	0%
French style (Finast)	1/2 cup	20	1	4	400	0	0.0	0.0	0	0%
French style (Freshlike)	1/2 cup	20	1	4	340	0	0.0	0.0	0	0%
French style (Green Giant)	1/2 cup	16	1	4	390	1	0.0	0.0	0	0%
French style (Stokely)	1/2 cup	20	1	4	400	1	0.0	0.0	0	0%
French style (Veg-All)	1/2 cup	20	1	4	340	0	0.0	0.0	0	0%

Food Name	Serving Size	Calories	Prot. gms	Carbs gms	Sod. mgs	Fiber gms	Fat gms	Sat. Fat gms	Chol. mgs	% Fat Cal.
French style, 'No Frills' (Pathmark)	1 cup	35	2	8	640	0	0.0	0.0	0	0%
French style, cut (TenderSweet)	1/2 cup	20	1	4	400	1	0.0	0.0	0	0%
French style, cut, no salt added (TenderSweet)	1/2 cup	20	1	4	5	0	0.0	0.0	0	0%
French style, no salt added (A&P)	1/2 cup	20	1	4	10	0	1.0	0.0	0	31%
French style, no salt added (Freshlike)	1/2 cup	20	1	4	5	0	0.0	0.0	0	0%
French style, no salt added (Pathmark)	1/2 cup	20	1	5	10	0	0.0	0.0	0	0%
French style, seasoned, w/liquid (Del Monte)	1/2 cup	20	1	4	355	0	0.0	0.0	0	0%
French style, stringless, w/liquid (S&W)	1/2 cup	20	1	4	3850	0	0.0	0.0	0	0%
French style, water packed, no salt added (Freshlike)	1/2 cup	20	1	4	5	0	0.0	0.0	0	0%
Italian, flat, cut (Stokely)	1/2 cup	20	1	4	370	1	0.0	0.0	0	0%
Italian style (Allens)	1/2 cup	18	1	3	260	0	1.0	0.0	0	36%
Italian style, cut (Del Monte)	1/2 cup	25	1	6	355	0	0.0	0.0	0	0%
kitchen-sliced (Green Giant)	1/2 cup	16	1	4	390	1	0.0	0.0	0	0%
kitchen-sliced, 50% less salt (Green Giant)	1/2 cup	20	1	4	200	1	0.0	0.0	0	0%
no salt added (A&P)	1/2 cup	20	1	4	10	0	1.0	0.0	0	31%
no salt added (Pathmark)	1/2 cup	20	1	5	10	0	0.0	0.0	0	0%
no salt added, cut, drained	1 cup	27	2	6	3	3	0.1	0.0	0	4%
no salt added, whole, drained	10 med beans	12	1	3	1	1	0.1	0.0	0	4%
no salt or sugar (Stokely)	1/2 cup	20	1	4	5	0	0.0	0.0	0	0%
regular pack, cut, drained	1 cup	27	2	6	354	3	0.1	0.0	0	4%
regular pack, cut, w/liquid	1/2 cup	18	1	4	311	2	0.1	0.0	0	6%
w/shelly beans, cut (Bush's Best)	1/2 cup	35	3	8	290	4	0.0	0.0	0	0%
whole (A&P)	1/2 cup	20	1	4	350	0	1.0	0.0	0	31%
whole (Bush's Best)	1/2 cup	20	1	5	360	2	0.0	0.0	0	0%
whole (Finast)	1/2 cup	25	1	4	400	0	0.0	0.0	0	0%
whole (Freshlike)	1/2 cup	20	1	4	340	0	0.0	0.0	0	0%
whole (IGA)	1 cup	45	2	8	640	0	0.0	0.0	0	0%
whole (Pathmark)	1/2 cup	20	1	4	430	0	0.0	0.0	0	0%
whole, stringless, w/liquid (S&W)	1/2 cup	20	1	4	3850	0	0.0	0.0	0	0%
whole, w/liquid (Del Monte)	1/2 cup	20	1	4	355	0	0.0	0.0	0	0%
Freeze-Dried (Mountain House) prepared as directed	1/2 cup	35	1	6	0	0	0.0	0.0	0	0%
Fresh										
boiled, drained	1 cup	44	2	10	4	4	0.3	0.1	0	7%
raw, cut	1 cup	34	2	8	7	4	0.1	0.0	0	3%
raw, whole, approx 4-inch long	10 beans	17	1	4	3	2	0.1	0.0	0	3%
Frozen										
(Flav-R-Pac)	2/3 cup	25	1	4	10	2	0.0	0.0	0	0%
cut (A&P)	3 oz	25	1	6	140	0	1.0	0.0	0	24%
cut (Birds Eye)	3 oz	25	1	6	0	2	0.0	0.0	0	0%
cut (Finast)	3 oz	25	1	6	5	0	0.0	0.0	0	0%
cut (Freshlike)	3 oz	25	1	6	5	0	0.0	0.0	0	0%
cut (Frosty Acres)	3 oz	25	1	6	3	1	0.0	0.0	0	0%
cut (Green Giant)	3/4 cup	25	1	5	0	2	0.0	0.0	0	0%
cut (Pictsweet)	2/3 cup	25	1	4	10	2	0.0	0.0	0	0%
cut (Seabrook)	3 oz	25	1	6	3	1	0.0	0.0	0	0%
cut (Veg-All)	3 oz	25	1	6	5	0	0.0	0.0	0	0%
cut, 'Portion Pack' (Birds Eye)	3 oz	25	1	6	0	2	0.0	0.0	0	0%
cut, 'Singles' (Stokely)	3 oz	30	2	6	5	0	1.0	0.0	0	22%
French cut (C&W)	2/3 cup	30	1	5	0	2	0.0	0.0	0	0%
French cut (Flav-R-Pac)	1 cup	25	1	4	10	2	0.0	0.0	0	0%
French style (A&P)	3 oz	25	1	6	0	0	1.0	0.0	0	24%
French style (Birds Eye)	3 oz	25	1	6	0	2	0.0	0.0	0	0%
French style (Finast)	3 oz	25	1	6	5	0	0.0	0.0	0	0%
French style (Freshlike)	3 oz	25	1	6	5	0	0.0	0.0	0	0%

Food Name	Serving Size	Calories	Prot. gms	Carbs gms	Sod. mgs	Fiber gms	Fat gms	Sat. Fat gms	Chol. mgs	% Fat Cal.
French style *(Frosty Acres)*	3 oz	25	1	6	3	1	0.0	0.0	0	0%
French style *(Pictsweet)*	1 cup	25	1	4	10	2	0.0	0.0	0	0%
French style *(Seabrook)*	3 oz	25	1	6	3	1	0.0	0.0	0	0%
French style *(Southern)*	3.5 oz	34	2	.7	20	0	0.1	0.0	0	3%
French style *(Veg-All)*	3 oz	25	1	6	5	0	0.0	0.0	0	0%
French style, w/almonds, 'Combination Vegetable' *(Birds Eye)*	3 oz	50	3	8	340	2	2.0	0.0	0	29%
Italian cut *(C&W)*	3/4 cup	25	1	4	10	2	0.0	0.0	0	0%
Italian cut *(Finast)*	3 oz	30	2	7	5	0	0.0	0.0	0	0%
Italian style *(Birds Eye)*	3 oz	30	2	7	0	3	0.0	0.0	0	0%
Italian style *(Freshlike)*	3 oz	30	2	7	5	0	0.0	0.0	0	0%
Italian style *(Frosty Acres)*	3 oz	30	2	7	3	1	0.0	0.0	0	0%
Italian style *(Seabrook)*	3 oz	30	2	7	3	1	0.0	0.0	0	0%
Italian style *(Veg-All)*	3 oz	30	2	7	5	0	0.0	0.0	0	0%
no salt added, drained	1 cup	38	2	9	12	4	0.2	0.1	0	5%
petite, 'Deluxe' *(Birds Eye)*	2.6 oz	20	1	5	0	2	0.0	0.0	0	0%
petite, whole *(C&W)*	3/4 cup	25	1	4	10	2	0.0	0.0	0	0%
petite, whole *(Flav-R-Pac)*	3/4 cup	25	1	4	10	2	0.0	0.0	0	0%
'Plain Polybag' *(Green Giant)*	1/2 cup	14	1	4	10	1	0.0	0.0	0	0%
whole *(Flav-R-Pac)*	3/4 cup	25	1	4	10	2	0.0	0.0	0	0%
whole *(Freshlike)*	3 oz	25	1	5	5	0	0.0	0.0	0	0%
whole *(Seabrook)*	3 oz	25	1	5	1	1	0.0	0.0	0	0%
whole *(Southern)*	3.5 oz	33	2	7	20	0	0.1	0.0	0	3%
whole *(Veg-All)*	3 oz	25	1	5	5	0	0.0	0.0	0	0%
whole, 'Deluxe' *(Birds Eye)*	3 oz	25	1	5	0	2	0.0	0.0	0	0%
whole 'Farm Fresh' *(Birds Eye)*	4 oz	30	2	7	0	2	0.0	0.0	0	0%
w/almonds 'Harvest Fresh' *(Green Giant)*	2/3 cup	60	2	5	95	2	3.0	0.0	0	49%
w/creamy mushroom 'Garden Gourmet' *(Green Giant)*	1 pkg	220	6	29	860	4	11.0	6.0	25	41%
w/salt, drained	1 cup	38	2	9	331	4	0.2	0.1	0	5%

BEAN, HORSE. See BEAN, FAVA.

BEAN, HYACINTH

Food Name	Serving Size	Calories	Prot. gms	Carbs gms	Sod. mgs	Fiber gms	Fat gms	Sat. Fat gms	Chol. mgs	% Fat Cal.
immature seeds, boiled, drained	1 cup	44	3	8	2	na	0.2	0.1	0	5%
immature seeds, raw	1 cup	37	2	7	2	na	0.2	0.1	0	4%
mature seeds, boiled, drained	1 cup	227	16	40	14	na	1.1	0.2	0	4%
mature seeds, raw	1 cup	722	50	128	44	na	3.5	0.6	0	4%

BEAN, ITALIAN

Food Name	Serving Size	Calories	Prot. gms	Carbs gms	Sod. mgs	Fiber gms	Fat gms	Sat. Fat gms	Chol. mgs	% Fat Cal.
dry beans in brine *(Green Giant)*	1/2 cup	130	5	24	480	5	1.0	0.0	0	7%
dry beans in brine *(Joan of Arc)*	1/2 cup	130	5	24	480	5	1.0	0.0	0	7%

BEAN, JACK. See BEAN, FAVA.

BEAN, KIDNEY

CALIFORNIA RED

Dried

Food Name	Serving Size	Calories	Prot. gms	Carbs gms	Sod. mgs	Fiber gms	Fat gms	Sat. Fat gms	Chol. mgs	% Fat Cal.
mature seeds, boiled	1 cup	219	16	40	7	16	0.2	0.0	0	1%
mature seeds	1 cup	607	45	110	20	46	0.5	0.1	0	1%

DARK RED

Canned

Food Name	Serving Size	Calories	Prot. gms	Carbs gms	Sod. mgs	Fiber gms	Fat gms	Sat. Fat gms	Chol. mgs	% Fat Cal.
(Allens)	1/2 cup	105	5	20	290	0	1.0	0.0	0	8%
(Bush's Best)	1/2 cup	70	6	17	300	6	0.0	0.0	0	0%
(Finast)	1/2 cup	110	6	20	350	0	2.0	0.0	0	15%
(Green Giant)	1/2 cup	90	7	20	330	5	1.0	0.0	0	8%
(Joan of Arc)	1/2 cup	90	7	20	330	5	1.0	0.0	0	8%
(Pathmark)	1/2 cup	110	8	18	370	0	0.0	0.0	0	0%
(Progresso)	1/2 cup	110	7	20	280	8	0.5	0.0	0	4%
(Stokely)	1/2 cup	120	7	21	380	5	0.5	0.0	0	4%

Food Name	Serving Size	Calories	Prot. gms	Carbs gms	Sod. mgs	Fiber gms	Fat gms	Sat. Fat gms	Chol. mgs	% Fat Cal.
(Stokely)	1/2 cup	110	7	20	360	0	1.0	0.0	0	8%
(Van Camp's)	1 cup	182	12	35	830	0	0.5	0.0	0	2%
50% less salt (Green Giant)	1/2 cup	90	7	20	165	5	1.0	0.0	0	8%
50% less salt (Joan of Arc)	1/2 cup	90	7	20	165	5	1.0	0.0	0	8%
50% less salt, 'Lite' (S&W)	1/2 cup	120	7	22	355	0	1.0	0.0	0	7%
'Premium' (S&W)	1/2 cup	120	6	22	596	0	1.0	0.0	0	7%
LIGHT RED										
Canned										
(Allens)	1/2 cup	105	5	2	290	0	1.0	0.0	0	24%
(Bush's Best)	1/2 cup	70	6	17	300	6	0.0	0.0	0	0%
(Finast) light	1/2 cup	110	6	20	350	0	2.0	0.0	0	15%
(Green Giant)	1/2 cup	90	7	20	330	5	1.0	0.0	0	8%
(Joan of Arc)	1/2 cup	90	7	20	330	5	1.0	0.0	0	8%
(Stokely)	1/2 cup	110	7	20	360	0	1.0	0.0	0	8%
(Stokely)	1/2 cup	120	7	21	380	5	0.5	0.0	0	4%
(Van Camp's)	1 cup	184	12	36	650	0	0.5	0.0	0	2%
50% less salt (Green Giant)	1/2 cup	90	7	20	165	5	1.0	0.0	0	8%
50% less salt (Joan of Arc)	1/2 cup	90	7	20	165	5	1.0	0.0	0	8%
RED										
Canned										
(A&P)	1/2 cup	110	7	20	440	0	1.0	0.0	0	8%
(Green Giant)	1/2 cup	90	7	20	250	6	0.0	0.0	0	0%
(Hunt's)	1/2 cup	95	6	20	484	5	0.5	0.0	0	4%
(Joan of Arc)	1/2 cup	90	7	20	250	6	0.0	0.0	0	0%
(Pathmark)	1/2 cup	110	7	20	350	0	0.0	0.0	0	0%
(Pathmark)	1/2 cup	110	8	18	370	0	0.0	0.0	0	0%
(Progresso)	1/2 cup	100	9	21	210	7	1.0	0.0	0	7%
(Stokely)	1/2 cup	110	7	20	360	0	1.0	0.0	0	8%
(Van Camp's)	1 cup	184	12	36	650	0	0.5	0.0	0	2%
50% less salt, 'Lite' (S&W)	1/2 cup	120	7	22	355	0	1.0	0.0	0	7%
mature seeds	1 cup	218	13	40	873	16	0.9	0.1	0	3%
mature seeds	1 tbsp	14	1	2	55	1	0.1	0.0	0	3%
New Orleans style (Van Camp's)	1 cup	178	12	34	940	0	0.6	0.0	0	3%
'Nutradiet' (S&W)	1/2 cup	90	7	16	1	0	1.0	0.0	0	9%
organic, very low-sodium, no salt added (Eden Foods)	1/2 cup	60	8	18	20	10	1.0	0.0	0	8%
'Premium' (S&W)	1/2 cup	120	6	22	596	0	1.0	0.0	0	7%
Dried										
boiled (A&P)	1 cup	230	17	41	5	0	1.0	0.0	0	4%
mature seeds, boiled	1 cup	225	15	40	4	13	0.9	0.1	0	3%
mature seeds, boiled	1 tbsp	14	1	3	0	1	0.1	0.0	0	3%
mature seeds, raw	1 cup	613	43	110	44	46	1.5	0.2	0	2%
mature seeds, raw	1 cup	620	41	113	22	28	1.9	0.3	0	3%
mature seeds, raw	1 tbsp	41	3	7	1	2	0.1	0.0	0	3%
raw (Arrowhead Mills)	2 oz	190	13	35	3	12	1.0	0.0	0	4%
Sprouted, mature seeds	1 cup	53	8	8	11	na	0.9	0.1	0	14%
ROYAL RED										
Dried										
mature seeds, boiled	1 cup	218	17	39	9	16	0.3	0.0	0	1%
mature seeds, raw	1 cup	605	47	107	24	46	0.8	0.1	0	1%
BEAN, LIMA / butterbean										
Canned										
(A&P)	1/2 cup	110	7	20	380	0	1.0	0.0	0	8%
(Featherweight)	1/2 cup	80	5	16	25	0	0.0	0.0	0	0%
(Freshlike)	1/2 cup	80	5	16	320	0	0.0	0.0	0	0%

Food Name	Serving Size	Calories	Prot. gms	Carbs gms	Sod. mgs	Fiber gms	Fat gms	Sat. Fat gms	Chol. mgs	% Fat Cal.
(Green Giant)	1/2 cup	80	6	16	420	4	0.0	0.0	0	0%
(Joan of Arc)	1/2 cup	80	6	16	420	4	0.0	0.0	0	0%
(S&W)	1/2 cup	100	6	19	440	0	1.0	0.0	0	8%
(Stokely)	1/2 cup	80	5	16	390	0	0.0	0.0	0	0%
(Van Camp's)	1 cup	162	11	30	710	0	0.5	0.0	0	3%
(Veg-All)	1/2 cup	80	5	16	320	0	0.0	0.0	0	0%
baby (Bush's Best)	1/2 cup	70	5	16	370	5	0.0	0.0	0	0%
all green (Bush's Best)	1/2 cup	90	4	17	400	4	0.0	0.0	0	0%
baby (C&W)	1/2 cup	90	6	15	80	5	0.5	0.0	0	5%
Fordhook (Stokely)	1/2 cup	80	5	14	300	0	0.0	0.0	0	0%
gem, green and white (Bush's Best)	1/2 cup	80	5	17	300	4	0.0	0.0	0	0%
green (A&P)	1/2 cup	80	5	15	320	0	1.0	0.0	0	10%
giant, seasoned w/pork (Luck's)	1/2 cup	150	8	23	340	5	3.0	1.0	3	18%
green, small, 'Fancy' (S&W)	1/2 cup	80	6	16	390	0	0.0	0.0	0	0%
green, small, w/pork (Luck's)	7.5 oz	220	10	33	640	8	7.0	0.0	0	27%
green, tiny (Allens)	1/2 cup	90	5	15	350	0	1.0	0.0	0	10%
green, w/liquid (Del Monte)	1/2 cup	70	4	14	355	0	0.0	0.0	0	0%
green and white (Allens)	1/2 cup	90	5	15	370	0	1.0	0.0	0	10%
'Harvest Fresh' (Green Giant)	1/2 cup	80	4	15	130	4	0.0	0.0	0	0%
immature seeds, no salt added, w/liquid	1/2 cup	88	5	17	5	4	0.4	0.1	0	3%
immature seeds, regular pack, w/liquid	1/2 cup	88	5	17	312	4	0.4	0.1	0	3%
large (Allens)	1/2 cup	110	5	18	370	0	1.0	0.0	0	9%
large (Bush's Best)	1/2 cup	70	5	16	370	5	0.0	0.0	0	0%
large, mature seeds	1 cup	190	12	36	810	12	0.4	0.1	0	2%
'No Salt or Sugar Added' (Stokely)	1/2 cup	80	5	16	5	0	0.0	0.0	0	0%
seasoned w/pork (Luck's)	1/2 cup	140	6	23	350	5	2.0	1.0	0	13%
speckled (Bush's Best)	1/2 cup	70	5	17	310	5	0.0	0.0	0	0%
speckled, seasoned w/pork (Luck's)	1/2 cup	140	6	22	320	5	3.0	1.0	3	19%
water packed, w/o salt (Freshlike)	1/2 cup	80	5	16	5	0	0.0	0.0	0	0%
w/ham (Dennison's)	7.5 oz	250	14	33	935	9	7.0	0.0	0	25%
w/pork (Luck's)	7.5 oz	230	12	34	720	9	7.0	0.0	0	26%
Dried										
baby, boiled	1 cup	229	15	42	435	14	0.7	0.2	0	3%
baby, boiled (A&P)	1 cup	230	16	40	15	0	1.0	0.0	0	4%
baby, raw	1 cup	677	42	127	26	42	1.9	0.4	0	2%
immature seeds, boiled, drained	1 cup	209	12	40	29	9	0.5	0.1	0	2%
immature seeds, raw	1 cup	176	11	31	12	8	1.3	0.3	0	6%
large, mature seeds, boiled	1 cup	216	15	39	4	13	0.7	0.2	0	3%
large, mature seeds, boiled	1 tbsp	13	1	2	0	1	0.0	0.0	0	3%
mature seeds, raw	1 cup	602	38	113	32	34	1.2	0.3	0	2%
mature seeds, raw	1 tbsp	38	2	7	2	2	0.1	0.0	0	2%
Frozen										
(Flav-R-Pac)	1/2 cup	100	6	20	130	4	0.0	0.0	0	0%
(Green Giant)	1/2 cup	100	6	19	30	5	0.0	0.0	0	0%
(Health Valley)	1/2 cup	94	6	18	26	3	0.0	0.0	0	0%
baby (Birds Eye)	3.3 oz	130	7	24	115	0	0.0	0.0	0	0%
baby (Freshlike)	3.3 oz	130	7	24	100	0	1.0	0.0	0	7%
baby (Frosty Acres)	3.3 oz	130	7	24	125	2	0.0	0.0	0	0%
baby (Seabrook)	3.3 oz	130	7	24	125	2	0.0	0.0	0	0%
baby (Southern)	3.5 oz	135	7	25	125	0	0.5	0.0	0	3%
baby (Veg-All)	3.3 oz	130	7	24	100	0	1.0	0.0	0	7%
baby, butter (Seabrook)	3.3 oz	140	7	26	213	2	1.0	0.0	0	6%
baby, green (A&P)	3.3 oz	130	7	24	130	0	1.0	0.0	0	7%
Fordhook (A&P)	3.3 oz	100	6	19	70	0	1.0	0.0	0	8%

Food Name	Serving Size	Calories	Prot. gms	Carbs gms	Sod. mgs	Fiber gms	Fat gms	Sat. Fat gms	Chol. mgs	% Fat Cal.
Fordhook (Birds Eye)	3.3 oz	100	6	19	100	0	0.0	0.0	0	0%
Fordhook (Flav-R-Pac)	1/2 cup	90	6	17	110	5	0.0	0.0	0	0%
Fordhook (Frosty Acres)	3.3 oz	100	6	19	71	2	0.0	0.0	0	0%
Fordhook (Seabrook)	3.3 oz	100	6	19	71	2	0.0	0.0	0	0%
Fordhook, immature seeds, no salt added, boiled, drained	1/2 cup	85	5	16	45	5	0.3	0.1	0	3%
Fordhook, immature seeds, no salt added, boiled, drained	10-oz pkg	311	19	58	165	18	1.1	0.2	0	3%
Fordhook, immature seeds, unprepared	1/2 cup	85	5	16	46	4	0.3	0.1	0	3%
Fordhook, immature seeds, unprepared	10-oz pkg	301	18	56	165	16	1.0	0.2	0	3%
'Harvest Fresh' (Green Giant)	1/2 cup	80	6	18	170	4	0.0	0.0	0	0%
immature seeds, drained	1/2 cup	95	6	18	239	5	0.3	0.1	0	2%
immature seeds, drained, 10-oz pkg	1 pkg	327	21	60	824	19	0.9	0.2	0	2%
immature seeds, no salt added, drained	1/2 cup	95	6	18	26	5	0.3	0.1	0	2%
immature seeds, no salt added, drained	10-oz pkg	327	21	60	90	19	0.9	0.2	0	2%
speckled (Seabrook)	3.3 oz	120	7	23	19	2	0.0	0.0	0	0%
speckled (Southern)	3.5 oz	135	8	25	30	0	0.4	0.0	0	3%
tiny (Seabrook)	3.3 oz	110	6	21	144	2	1.0	0.0	0	8%
BEAN, MARROW										
regular, boiled	4 oz	158	11.0	28.5	7	7.2	0.4	0.1	0	2%
regular, boiled	1/2 cup	125	8.6	22.5	6	5.7	0.3	0.1	0	2%
regular, raw	1/2 cup	337	23.6	60.9	16	15.4	0.9	0.2	0	2%
regular, raw	1 oz	94	6.6	17.1	5	4.3	0.2	0.1	0	2%
small, boiled	4 oz	161	10.2	29.3	2	5.0	0.7	0.2	0	4%
small, boiled	1/2 cup	127	8.1	23.2	2	3.7	0.6	0.1	0	4%
small, raw	1/2 cup	363	22.8	67.2	13	11.1	1.3	0.3	0	3%
small, raw	1 oz	95	6.0	17.6	3	2.9	0.3	0.1	0	3%
BEAN, MOTH										
mature seeds, boiled	1 cup	207	14	37	18	na	1.0	0.2	0	4%
mature seeds, raw	1 cup	672	45	121	59	na	3.2	0.7	0	4%
BEAN, MUNG										
Canned										
mature seeds, sprouted, drained	1 cup	15	2	3	175	1	0.1	0.0	0	4%
sprouted (La Choy)	2 oz	8	1	1	20	1	0.1	0.0	0	11%
Dried										
mature seeds, boiled	1 cup	212	14	39	4	15	0.8	0.2	0	3%
mature seeds, raw	1 cup	718	49	130	31	34	2.4	0.7	0	3%
mature seeds, raw	1 tbsp	45	3	8	2	2	0.1	0.0	0	3%
Sprouted										
mature seeds, raw	1 cup	31	3	6	6	2	0.2	0.0	0	5%
mature seeds, raw	12-oz pkg	102	10	20	20	6	0.6	0.2	0	5%
mature seeds, stir-fried	1 cup	62	5	13	11	2	0.3	0.0	0	4%
BEAN, MUNGO										
mature seeds, boiled	1 cup	189	14	33	13	12	1.0	0.1	0	4%
mature seeds, raw	1 cup	706	52	122	79	38	3.4	0.2	0	4%
BEAN, NAVY										
Dry										
mature seeds, boiled	1 cup	258	16	48	2	12	1.0	0.3	0	3%
mature seeds raw	1 cup	697	46	126	29	51	2.7	0.7	0	3%
'Michigan #1' cooked (A&P)	1 cup	220	15	40	15	0	1.0	0	0	4%
Canned										
(Allens)	1/2 cup	160	8	24	440	0	1.0	0.1	0	7%
(Bush's Best)	1/2 cup	60	5	17	370	7	0.0	0.0	0	0%
flavored w/bacon (Trappey's)	1/2 cup	130	7	28	430	5	0.0	0.0	0	0%

Food Name	Serving Size	Calories	Prot. gms	Carbs gms	Sod. mgs	Fiber gms	Fat gms	Sat. Fat gms	Chol. mgs	% Fat Cal.
mature seeds	1 cup	296	20	54	1174	13	1.1	0.3	0	3%
organic, no salt added, very low sodium (Eden Foods)	1/2 cup	70	6	18	15	7	1.0	0.0	0	9%
seasoned w/pork (Luck's)	1/2 cup	140	7	19	310	5	4.0	1.0	3	26%
w/ham, 'Homestyle' (Hunt's)	9.03 oz	239	16	38	737	10	2.7	0.9	10	10%
Sprouted, mature seeds, raw	1 cup	70	6	14	14	na	0.7	0.1	0	9%
BEAN, PINK										
mature seeds, boiled	1 cup	252	15	47	3	9	0.8	0.2	0	3%
mature seeds, raw	1 cup	720	44	135	17	27	2.4	0.6	0	3%
BEAN, PINTO										
Dried										
boiled (A&P)	1 cup	230	17	42	5	0	1.0	0.0	0	4%
mature seeds, boiled	1 cup	234	14	44	3	15	0.9	0.2	0	3%
mature seeds, boiled	1 tbsp	15	1	3	0	1	0.1	0.0	0	3%
mature seeds, raw	1 cup	656	40	122	19	47	2.2	0.5	0	3%
mature seeds, raw	1 tbsp	41	3	8	1	3	0.1	0.0	0	3%
raw (Arrowhead Mills)	2 oz	200	13	36	3	11	1.0	0.0	0	4%
raw (Evans)	1 cup	660	43	121	19	0	2.0	0.0	0	3%
Canned										
(Allens)	1/2 cup	105	5	18	480	0	1.0	0.0	0	9%
(Bush's Best)	1/2 cup	60	5	15	350	5	0.0	0.0	0	0%
(Gebhardt)	1/2 cup	92	7	18	505	7	1.2	0.0	0	10%
(Green Giant)	1/2 cup	90	6	20	280	5	1.0	0.0	0	8%
(Joan of Arc)	1/2 cup	90	6	20	280	5	1.0	0.0	0	8%
(Old El Paso)	1/2 cup	100	6	19	320	8	0.0	0.0	0	0%
(Progresso)	1/2 cup	110	7	7	250	7	1.0	0.0	0	14%
(Ranch Style)	1/2 cup	100	6	19	580	5	0.0	0.0	5	0%
baked style, w/pork, 15-oz can (Luck's)	7.5 oz	220	12	30	787	7	6.0	0.0	0	24%
baked style, w/pork, 29 oz can (Luck's)	7.25 oz	220	11	30	520	11	6.0	0.0	0	25%
mature seeds	1 cup	206	12	37	706	11	1.9	0.4	0	8%
organic, no salt added, very low sodium (Eden Foods)	1/2 cup	70	6	17	15	6	1.0	0.0	0	9%
organic, w/liquid (Eden Foods)	1/2 cup	110	6	20	20	6	1.0	0.0	0	8%
picante style (Green Giant)	1/2 cup	100	7	21	580	7	1.0	0.0	0	7%
picante style (Joan of Arc)	1/2 cup	100	7	21	580	7	1.0	0.0	0	7%
seasoned w/pork (Luck's)	1/2 cup	140	7	19	310	6	4.0	1.0	3	26%
'Sun-Vista' (S&W)	1/2 cup	80	3	12	530	3	0.5	0.0	0	7%
w/jalapeño peppers (Ranch Style)	1/2 cup	110	5	21	700	6	0.0	0.0	5	0%
w/onions, seasoned w/pork (Luck's)	1/2 cup	150	7	24	300	6	3.0	1.0	3	18%
Frozen										
(Seabrook)	3.2 oz	160	9	29	0	0	0.0	0.0	0	0%
immature seeds, frozen, no salt added, drained 10-oz pkg	1 pkg	460	26	88	236	24	1.4	0.2	0	2%
immature seeds, unprepared, 10-oz pkg	1 pkg	483	28	92	261	16	1.4	0.2	0	2%
immature seeds, w/salt, drained, 10-oz pkg	1 pkg	460	26	88	906	24	1.4	0.2	0	2%
Jarred, organic, low-sodium (Eden Foods)	1/2 cup	120	7	22	30	6	0.0	0.0	0	0%
BEAN, RED										
Canned										
(A&P)	1/2 cup	120	7	23	400	0	1.0	0.0	0	7%
(Allens)	1/2 cup	115	7	20	350	0	1.0	0.0	0	8%
(Bush's Best)	1/2 cup	70	5	17	350	6	0.0	0.0	0	0%
(Green Giant)	1/2 cup	90	6	19	340	5	1.0	0.0	0	8%
(Joan of Arc)	1/2 cup	90	6	19	340	5	1.0	0.0	0	8%
(Van Camp's)	1 cup	194	11	38	928	0	0.6	0.0	0	3%
small (Hunt's)	4 oz	91	6	18	578	0	0.0	0.0	0	0%
small, baked-style (B&M)	8 oz	223	9	36	725	11	5.0	2.0	5	20%

Food Name	Serving Size	Calories	Prot. gms	Carbs gms	Sod. mgs	Fiber gms	Fat gms	Sat. Fat gms	Chol. mgs	% Fat Cal.
BEAN, ROMAN. See BEAN, CRANBERRY.										
BEAN, ROSE COCO. See BEAN, CRANBERRY.										
BEAN, SHELLY										
Canned										
(Allens)	1/2 cup	35	2	6	395	0	1.0	0.0	0	22%
(Stokely)	1/2 cup	35	2	7	470	0	0.0	0.0	0	0%
w/liquid	1 cup	74	4	15	818	8	0.5	0.1	0	5%
BEAN, SNAP. See BEAN, GREEN; BEAN, WAX.										
BEAN, SOYA. See SOYBEAN.										
BEAN, STRING. See BEAN, GREEN; BEAN, WAX.										
BEAN, WAX / yellow snap bean										
Canned										
(Allens)	1/2 cup	15	1	3	260	0	1.0	0.0	0	36%
(Stokely)	1/2 cup	20	1	4	360	0	0.0	0.0	0	0%
cut (S&W)	1/2 cup	20	1	4	400	1	0.0	0.0	0	0%
cut, 'Premium Golden' (S&W)	1/2 cup	20	1	5	385	0	0.0	0.0	0	0%
cut, water packed, w/o salt (Freshlike)	1/2 cup	18	1	4	5	0	0.0	0.0	0	0%
cut, water packed, w/o sugar or salt (Freshlike)	1/2 cup	18	1	4	5	0	0.0	0.0	0	0%
golden, cut (Del Monte)	1/2 cup	20	0	4	355	0	0.0	0.0	0	0%
golden, French style (Del Monte)	1/2 cup	20	0	4	355	0	0.0	0.0	0	0%
no salt added, cut, drained	1/2 cup	14	1	3	1	1	0.1	0.0	0	4%
no salt added, w/liquid	1/2 cup	18	1	4	17	2	0.1	0.0	0	6%
no salt or sugar (Stokely)	1/2 cup	20	1	4	5	0	0.0	0.0	0	0%
regular pack, cut, drained	1 cup	27	2	6	339	2	0.1	0.0	0	4%
regular pack, whole, drained	10 med beans	12	1	3	156	1	0.1	0.0	0	4%
regular pack, cut, w/liquid	1/2 cup	18	1	4	311	2	0.1	0.0	0	6%
Fresh										
boiled, drained	1 cup	44	2	10	4	4	0.3	0.1	0	7%
raw	1 cup	34	2	8	7	4	0.1	0.0	0	3%
Frozen										
(Flav-R-Pac)	2/3 cup	25	1	4	10	2	0.0	0.0	0	0%
(Frosty Acres)	3 oz	25	2	5	1	1	0.0	0.0	0	0%
cut (Seabrook)	3 oz	25	2	5	1	1	0.0	0.0	0	0%
no salt added, drained	1 cup	38	2	9	12	4	0.2	0.1	0	5%
w/salt, drained	1 cup	38	2	9	331	4	0.2	0.1	0	5%
BEAN, WHITE. See also BEAN, CANNELLINI, CANNED.										
Dried										
mature seeds, boiled	1 cup	249	17	45	11	11	0.6	0.2	0	2%
mature seeds, boiled	1 tbsp	16	1	3	1	1	0.0	0.0	0	2%
mature seeds, raw	1 cup	673	47	122	32	31	1.7	0.4	0	2%
mature seeds, raw	1 tbsp	42	3	8	2	2	0.1	0.0	0	2%
small white, mature seeds, boiled	1 cup	254	16	46	4	19	1.1	0.3	0	4%
small white, mature seeds, raw	1 cup	722	45	134	26	54	2.5	0.7	0	3%
Canned, mature seeds	1 cup	307	19	57	13	13	0.8	0.2	0	2%
BEAN, WINGED / goa bean										
immature seeds, boiled, drained	1 cup	24	3	2	2	na	0.4	0.1	0	15%
immature seeds, raw	1 med pod	8	1	1	1	na	0.1	0.0	0	15%
immature seeds, raw, sliced	1 cup	22	3	2	2	na	0.4	0.1	0	15%
mature seeds, boiled	1 cup	255	16	45	9	18	1.9	0.5	0	6%
mature seeds, boiled	1 cup	253	18	26	22	na	10.0	1.4	0	33%
mature seeds, raw	1 cup	744	54	76	69	na	29.7	4.2	0	33%
BEAN, YARDLONG										
boiled, drained	1 med pod	7	0	1	1	na	0.0	0.0	0	2%
boiled, drained, sliced	1 cup	49	3	10	4	na	0.1	0.0	0	2%

Food Name	Serving Size	Calories	Prot. gms	Carbs gms	Sod. mgs	Fiber gms	Fat gms	Sat. Fat gms	Chol. mgs	% Fat Cal.
boiled, mature seeds...............................	1 cup	202	14	36	9	6	0.8	0.2	0	3%
mature seeds, raw................................	1 cup	579	41	103	28	18	2.2	0.6	0	3%
raw	1 med pod	6	0	1	0	na	0.0	0.0	0	7%
raw, sliced.......................................	1 cup	43	3	8	4	na	0.4	0.1	0	7%
BEAN, YELLOW, dried, mature seeds, raw..............	1 cup	676	43	119	24	49	5.1	1.3	0	6%

BEAN DISH/ENTRÉE. See also BAKED BEANS, CANNED; BEAN SALAD; BEANS, CHILI; BURRITO; CHILI; ENCHILADA.

Food Name	Serving Size	Calories	Prot. gms	Carbs gms	Sod. mgs	Fiber gms	Fat gms	Sat. Fat gms	Chol. mgs	% Fat Cal.
(Amy's Kitchen)										
meatless 'Salisbury steak,' 'Country Dinner'	1 entrée	420	12	63	700	9	16.0	5.0	20	32%
(Banquet) beans and frankfurters, frozen	10 oz	520	17	57	1230	0	25.0	0.0	35	43%
(Bearitos)										
refried beans, low-fat, no salt	1 serving	80	5	14	10	2	2.0	na	0	19%
refried beans, nonfat...........................	1 serving	70	4	14	350	2	0.0	0.0	0	0%
refried beans, organic, canned	1 oz	30	2	5	61	0	0.5	0.0	0	15%
refried beans, organic, no salt, canned.................	1 oz	29	2	5	2	0	0.5	0.0	0	15%
refried beans, spicy, organic, canned	1 oz	31	2	5	56	1	0.6	0.0	0	17%
refried beans, vegetarian, spicy, low-fat, canned	3.2 oz	80	5	14	280	2	2.0	0.0	0	19%
refried beans, w/black beans, low-fat..................	1 serving	80	6	14	320	1	1.0	na	0	10%
refried beans, w/green chilies, nonfat	1/2 cup	40	3	8	245	3	0.0	0.0	0	0%
(Bush's Best) mixed, canned	1/2 cup	70	6	17	410	6	0.0	0.0	0	0%
(Chi-Chi's) refried beans......................	7.5 oz	250	9	29	930	0	11.0	2.0	5	39%
(Del Monte)										
refried beans, canned	1/2 cup	130	6	20	530	0	2.0	0.0	0	15%
refried beans, spicy, canned	1/2 cup	130	6	20	480	0	2.0	0.0	0	15%
(Flav-R-Pac)										
beans Parisian, frozen..........................	1 cup	25	1	4	10	2	0.0	0.0	0	0%
beans Parisian w/buttery sauce, frozen................	1/2 cup	50	2	8	450	2	2.5	0.0	0	36%
beans supreme, frozen	2/3 cup	50	3	9	95	4	0.0	0.0	0	0%
four bean salad, frozen	1/3 cup	70	2	17	370	2	0.5	0.0	0	6%
green beans w/onions and ham, 'Grande Classics'	1/2 cup	40	2	6	460	2	2.0	0.5	5	36%
Oregon bean medley, frozen.......................	2/3 cup	45	3	8	65	3	0.0	0.0	0	0%
(Gebhardt)										
refried beans...............................	1/2 cup	109	6	20	497	6	2.8	1.3	1	19%
refried beans, food service product..................	1/2 cup	109	6	20	497	6	2.8	1.3	1	19%
refried beans, jalapeño	1/2 cup	105	7	19	380	6	3.0	1.4	1	21%
refried beans, nonfat	1/2 cup	92	7	20	480	6	0.5	0.0	0	4%
refried beans, vegetarian	1/2 cup	118	8	21	550	7	2.3	0.3	0	15%
(Green Giant)										
Mexican beans, canned, dry beans in brine	1/2 cup	120	6	21	530	5	1.5	0.0	0	11%
three bean salad, canned	1/2 cup	70	2	16	470	3	0.0	0.0	0	0%
(Health Valley)										
black beans w/garden vegetables, western, 'Fast Menu' ..	7.5 oz	120	13	14	170	15	1.0	0.0	0	8%
(Homestyle)										
beans 'n fixins, food service product..................	1/2 cup	125	2	30	575	8	2.8	1.1	1	16%
country kettle beans, food service product..............	1/2 cup	131	6	26	365	6	2.0	0.6	1	12%
(Hunt's) beans and fixin's, 'Big John's'	1/2 cup	127	7	23	590	6	3.5	1.2	3	21%
(Joan of Arc) Mexican beans, canned, dry beans in brine...	1/2 cup	120	6	21	530	5	1.5	0.0	0	11%
(Kid's Kitchen) beans and wieners, microwave cup........	7.5 oz	310	13	36	750	0	13.0	4.0	45	37%
(Lean Cuisine) three bean chili w/rice	1 entrée	210	8	32	460	7	6.0	2.0	10	25%
(Libby's)										
beans and frankfurters in sauce, micro cup, 'Diner'	7.75 oz	330	15	38	930	4	15.0	6.0	55	39%
(Lipton)										
beans and chicken w/sauce, mix, dry	1/4 pkg	120	6	26	470	0	1.0	0.0	0	7%
beans and chicken w/sauce, mix, prepared	1/2 cup	150	6	26	500	0	4.0	0.0	0	22%
(Little Pancho)										
refried beans, w/green chilies, nonfat, canned	1/2 cup	80	6	15	330	0	0.0	0.0	0	0%

Food Name	Serving Size	Calories	Prot. gms	Carbs gms	Sod. mgs	Fiber gms	Fat gms	Sat. Fat gms	Chol. mgs	% Fat Cal.
(Luck's) pinto and great northern, seasoned w/pork	1/2 cup	130	7	22	370	8	2.0	0.5	3	13%
(Morningstar Farms) 'Spicy Black Bean Burger'	1 patty	110	11	16	470	5	1.0	0.0	0.0	8.2%
(Morton) beans and frankfurters, frozen	10 oz	350	11	46	1490	0	13.0	0.0	30	34%
(Natural Touch)										
'Spicy Black Bean Burger'	1 patty	110	11	15	330	5	1.0	0.0	0	8.2%
'Nine Bean Loaf'	1 slice	160	8	14	350	0	8.0	0.0	0	45%
(Old El Paso)										
refried beans, canned	1/4 cup	55	3	8	200	3	1.0	0.0	1	17%
refried beans, nonfat	1/2 cup	110	6	20	480	6	0.0	0.0	0	0%
refried beans, spicy, canned	1/4 cup	35	1	5	280	2	1.0	0.0	1	27%
refried beans, vegetarian, spicy, canned	1/4 cup	70	6	15	730	5	1.0	0.0	0	10%
refried beans, w/cheese, canned	1/4 cup	36	2	4	280	2	1.0	1.0	2	27%
refried beans, w/green chilies, canned	1/4 cup	49	3	8	252	3	1.0	0.0	0	17%
refried beans, w/sausage, canned	1/2 cup	200	7	14	360	8	13.0	5.0	10	58%
(Rice A Roni) red beans and rice	2.5 oz	158	5	29	675	3	4.0	0.6	0	21%
(Rosarita)										
refried beans	1/2 cup	125	7	22	585	8	2.7	1.2	0	17%
refried beans, nacho cheese	1/2 cup	137	8	24	703	7	3.2	1.9	0	18%
refried beans, no fat	1/2 cup	123	7	28	574	6	0.5	0.0	0	3%
refried beans, original, food service product	1/2 cup	109	6	20	497	6	2.8	1.3	1	19%
refried beans, quick cooking, food service product	1/2 cup	185	11	31	704	10	6.7	1.5	0	27%
refried beans, spicy	1/2 cup	118	7	22	574	6	2.7	1.1	0	17%
refried beans, spicy, food service product	1/2 cup	109	6	20	530	6	2.6	1.3	1	18%
refried beans, vegetarian	1/2 cup	121	7	23	562	6	2.1	0.5	0	13%
refried beans, vegetarian, food service product	1/2 cup	118	8	21	550	6	2.3	0.3	0	15%
refried beans, vegetarian, spicy, canned	4 oz	120	7	19	470	0	2.0	0.0	0	15%
refried beans, vegetarian, w/canola oil	4 oz	100	7	18	480	6	2.0	1.0	0	15%
refried beans, vegetarian, w/soybean oil	4 oz	100	7	18	480	6	2.0	0.5	0	15%
refried beans, w/bacon	1/2 cup	116	8	19	489	8	3.1	1.2	1	21%
refried beans, w/black beans, low-fat	1/2 cup	107	8	23	569	7	0.6	0.0	0	5%
refried beans, w/green chilies	1/2 cup	110	6	20	495	7	2.9	1.8	1	20%
refried beans, w/green chilies, no fat	1/2 cup	101	8	22	565	8	0.1	0.0	0	1%
refried beans, w/onions	1/2 cup	114	6	21	508	6	2.8	1.3	1	19%
salsa refried beans, no fat	1/2 cup	99	6	22	554	8	0.5	0.0	0	3%
(S&W)										
bean salad, deli style, canned	1/2 cup	80	4	20	670	4	0.0	0.0	0	0%
kidney, garbanzo and green beans in vinaigrette, canned	1/2 cup	90	4	17	726	0	1.0	0.0	0	10%
(Santiago)										
refried beans, smooth	1/2 cup	174	7	24	469	10	5.8	2.2	3	29%
refried beans, whole bean style	1/2 cup	174	7	24	469	10	5.8	1.5	0	29%
(Stouffer's) green bean-mushroom casserole	1/2 cup	140	3	13	530	2	8.0	2.0	10	53%
(Swanson) beans and frankfurters frozen	10.5 oz	440	14	53	900	0	19.0	0.0	0	39%
(Weight Watchers) white beans and vegetables Parisian	1 entree	220	13	23	690	13	9.0	3.0	20	36%
BEAN DISH/ENTRÉE MIX										
(Fantastic Foods)										
black beans, instant, prepared	1/3 cup	160	10	29	310	7	1.5	0.0	0	8%
refried beans, instant, prepared	1/3 cup	160	9	29	320	11	1.0	0.0	0	6%
refried beans, instant, prepared w/o added ingredients	1/2 cup	157	10	28	400	0	2.0	0.0	0	11%

BEAN SALAD. See BEAN DISH/ENTRÉE MIX.
BEAN SPROUTS
Canned

(Chun King)	85 grams	5	1	0	15	0	0.0	0.0	0	0%
(La Choy)	1 cup	14	1	1	17	1	0.1	0.0	0	7%

Food Name	Serving Size	Calories	Prot. gms	Carbs gms	Sod. mgs	Fiber gms	Fat gms	Sat. Fat gms	Chol. mgs	% Fat Cal.
(La Choy) food service product	1 cup	12	1	2	20	1	0.1	0.0	0	3%
BEANS, CHILI										
Canned										
(Gebhardt).	1/2 cup	134	7	31	630	7	1.0	0.4	0	6%
(Hunt's).	1/2 cup	87	6	17	597	6	1.0	0.0	0	9%
(S&W)	1/2 cup	110	7	23	580	6	1.0	0.0	1	7%
(Sun Vista).	1/2 cup	110	7	24	360	7	1.0	0.5	0	7%
extra spicy *(Green Giant)*	1/2 cup	100	7	21	580	6	1.0	0.0	0	7%
extra spicy *(Joan of Arc)*	1/2 cup	100	7	21	580	6	1.0	0.0	0	7%
50% less salt *(Green Giant)*	1/2 cup	100	7	21	310	7	1.0	0.0	0	7%
50% less salt *(Joan of Arc)*	1/2 cup	100	7	21	310	7	1.0	0.0	0	7%
hot *(Bush's Best)*.	1/2 cup	70	5	20	420	6	0.0	0.0	0	0%
spiced *(Gebhardt)*	1/2 cup	100	7	19	654	8	1.6	0.6	0	12%
BEANS, REFRIED. See under BEAN DISH/ENTRÉE.										
BEAR										
raw	1 oz	46	6	0	na	0	2.4	na	na	47%
simmered	3 oz	220	28	0	60	0	11.4	3.0	83	47%
simmered, yield from 1 lb raw, boneless.	8 oz	717	90	0	197	0	37.1	9.8	271	47%
BEAVER, RAW										
raw	1 oz	41	7	0	14	0	1.4	na	na	30%
roasted	3 oz	180	30	0	50	0	5.9	1.8	99	30%
roasted, yield from 1 lb raw, boneless.	11 oz	664	109	0	185	0	21.8	6.5	366	30%
BEECHNUT, dried	1 oz	163	2	9	11	na	14.2	1.6	0	73%
BEEF. See also under LUNCHEON MEAT.										
(NOTE: TRIMMED = Lean; separable fat removed after cooking. UNTRIMMED = Separable fat not removed.)										
BRAIN										
pan-fried	3 oz	167	11	0	134	0	13.5	3.2	1696	73%
raw	4 oz	142	11	0	116	0	10.5	2.4	1889	66%
simmered	3 oz	136	9	0	102	0	10.7	2.5	1746	71%
BRISKET										
choice, shredded *(Cripple Creek)*	3 oz	180	18	6	570	0	12.0	6.0	60	53%
choice, sliced *(Cripple Creek)*.	3 oz	120	12	6	540	0	6.0	0.0	60	43%
chopped *(Cripple Creek)*.	3 oz	180	15	6	375	0	12.0	4.5	60	56%
BRISKET, FLAT HALF										
Trimmed										
all grades, 0-inch fat, braised	3 oz	162	27	0	54	0	5.3	1.7	81	29%
all grades, 1/4-inch fat, braised.	3 oz	189	27	0	54	0	8.2	2.7	81	39%
all grades, 1/4-inch fat, raw.	1 oz	42	6	0	21	0	1.8	0.6	17	38%
Untrimmed										
all grades, 0-inch fat, braised	3 oz	183	26	0	53	0	8.0	2.8	81	39%
all grades, 1/8-inch fat, braised.	3 oz	263	23	0	50	0	18.0	6.8	81	62%
all grades, 1/8-inch fat, raw.	4 oz	266	22	0	76	0	19.1	7.4	75	65%
all grades, 1/4-inch fat, braised.	3 oz	309	21	0	48	0	24.2	9.4	81	71%
all grades, 1/4-inch fat, raw	4 oz	328	20	0	70	0	26.7	10.6	79	74%
BRISKET, POINT HALF										
Trimmed										
all grades, 0-inch fat, braised	3 oz	207	24	0	65	0	11.7	4.4	77	51%
all grades, 1/4-inch fat, braised	3 oz	222	24	0	65	0	13.3	5.0	77	54%
all grades, 1/4-inch fat, raw	1 oz	46	6	0	24	0	2.4	0.9	18	47%
Untrimmed										
all grades, 0-inch fat, braised	3 oz	304	20	0	58	0	24.2	9.6	78	72%
all grades, 1/8-inch fat, braised	3 oz	297	21	0	59	0	23.1	9.0	78	70%
all grades, 1/8-inch fat, raw	1 oz	75	5	0	20	0	5.9	2.4	20	71%
all grades, 1/4-inch fat, braised	3 oz	343	19	0	55	0	29.1	11.5	78	77%

Food Name	Serving Size	Calories	Prot. gms	Carbs gms	Sod. mgs	Fiber gms	Fat gms	Sat. Fat gms	Chol. mgs	% Fat Cal.
all grades, 1/4-inch fat, raw	1 oz	94	5	0	18	0	8.2	3.4	22	79%
BRISKET, WHOLE										
Trimmed										
all grades, 0-inch fat, braised,	3 oz	185	25	0	60	0	8.6	3.1	79	42%
all grades, 1/4-inch fat, braised	3 oz	206	25	0	60	0	10.8	3.9	79	48%
all grades, raw	1 oz	44	6	0	22	0	2.1	0.7	18	43%
Untrimmed										
all grades, 0-inch fat, braised	3 oz	247	23	0	55	0	16.6	6.4	79	61%
all grades, 1/8-inch fat, braised	3 oz	281	22	0	54	0	20.8	8.0	79	67%
all grades, 1/8-inch fat, raw	1 oz	71	5	0	20	0	5.4	2.1	19	69%
all grades, 1/4-inch fat, braised	3 oz	327	20	0	52	0	26.8	10.5	80	74%
all grades, 1/4-inch fat, raw	1 oz	88	5	0	18	0	7.5	3.0	21	77%
CHOPPED, canned (Armour)	3 oz	280	11	3	1290	0	24.0	0.0	0	79%
CHUCK, ARM POT ROAST										
Trimmed										
all grades, 0-inch fat, braised	3 oz	179	28	0	56	0	6.5	2.3	86	33%
all grades, 1/4-inch fat, braised	3 oz	184	28	0	56	0	7.1	2.6	86	35%
all grades, 1/4-inch fat, raw	1 oz	37	6	0	19	0	1.2	0.5	17	31%
choice, 0-inch fat, braised	3 oz	186	28	0	56	0	7.4	2.7	86	36%
choice, 1/4-inch fat, braised	3 oz	191	28	0	56	0	7.9	2.9	86	37%
choice, 1/4-inch fat, raw	1 oz	39	6	0	19	0	1.4	0.5	17	34%
prime, 1/2-inch fat, braised	3 oz	222	28	0	56	0	11.4	4.3	86	46%
prime, 1/2-inch fat, raw	1 oz	44	6	0	19	0	2.0	0.8	17	41%
select, 0-inch fat, braised	3 oz	168	28	0	56	0	5.4	1.9	86	29%
select, 1/4-inch fat, braised	3 oz	175	28	0	56	0	6.1	2.2	86	32%
select, 1/4-inch fat, raw	1 oz	35	6	0	19	0	1.0	0.4	17	26%
Untrimmed										
all grades, 0-inch fat, braised	3 oz	238	25	0	53	0	14.5	5.6	85	55%
all grades, 1/8-inch fat, braised	3 oz	263	24	0	52	0	17.6	6.9	85	60%
all grades, 1/8-inch fat, raw	1 oz	69	5	0	17	0	5.2	2.1	19	68%
all grades, 1/4-inch fat, braised	3 oz	282	23	0	51	0	20.2	8.0	84	65%
all grades, 1/4-inch fat, raw	1 oz	69	5	0	17	0	5.2	2.1	19	68%
choice, 1/4-inch fat, braised	3 oz	296	23	0	50	0	21.9	8.6	84	67%
choice, 1/4-inch fat, raw	1 oz	72	5	0	17	0	5.5	2.2	20	69%
prime, 1/2-inch fat, braised	3 oz	332	22	0	49	0	26.3	10.8	84	71%
prime, 1/2-inch fat, raw	1 oz	83	5	0	16	0	6.8	2.9	20	74%
select, 1/8-inch fat, raw	1 oz	62	5	0	17	0	4.4	1.8	19	63%
select, 1/4-inch fat, braised	3 oz	268	24	0	51	0	18.5	7.3	85	62%
select, 1/4-inch fat, raw	1 oz	66	5	0	17	0	4.8	2.0	19	66%
CHUCK, BLADE ROAST										
Trimmed										
all grades, 0-inch fat, braised	3 oz	215	26	0	60	0	11.3	4.4	90	47%
all grades, 1/4-inch fat, braised	3 oz	213	26	0	60	0	11.1	4.3	90	47%
all grades, 1/4-inch fat, raw	1 oz	42	5	0	22	0	2.1	0.8	18	45%
choice, 0-inch fat, braised	3 oz	225	26	0	60	0	12.5	4.8	90	50%
choice, 1/4-inch fat, braised	3 oz	224	26	0	60	0	12.2	4.7	90	49%
choice, 1/4-inch fat, raw	1 oz	45	5	0	22	0	2.4	0.9	18	48%
prime, 1/2-inch fat, braised	3 oz	270	26	0	60	0	17.5	7.1	90	58%
prime, 1/2-inch fat, raw	1 oz	58	5	0	22	0	3.8	1.5	18	60%
select, 0-inch fat, braised	3 oz	202	26	0	60	0	9.9	3.9	90	44%
select, 1/4-inch fat, braised	3 oz	201	26	0	60	0	9.9	3.8	90	44%
select, 1/4-inch fat, raw	1 oz	39	5	0	22	0	1.8	0.7	18	41%
Untrimmed										
all grades, 0-inch fat, braised	3 oz	284	23	0	55	0	20.5	8.2	88	65%

Food Name	Serving Size	Calories	Prot. gms	Carbs gms	Sod. mgs	Fiber gms	Fat gms	Sat. Fat gms	Chol. mgs	% Fat Cal.
all grades, 1/8-inch fat, braised	3 oz	290	23	0	55	0	21.4	8.5	88	66%
all grades, 1/8-inch fat, raw	1 oz	70	5	0	19	0	5.5	2.2	20	71%
all grades, 1/4-inch fat, braised	3 oz	293	23	0	54	0	21.8	8.7	88	67%
all grades, 1/4-inch fat, raw	1 oz	72	5	0	19	0	5.7	2.3	20	71%
choice, 1/8-inch fat, braised	3 oz	305	22	0	54	0	23.2	9.2	88	68%
choice, 1/8-inch fat, raw	1 oz	75	5	0	19	0	6.0	2.4	20	73%
choice, 1/4-inch fat, braised	3 oz	309	22	0	54	0	23.6	9.4	88	69%
choice, 1/4-inch fat, raw	1 oz	77	5	0	19	0	6.3	2.5	20	74%
prime, 1/2-inch fat, braised	3 oz	354	22	0	54	0	29.0	12.1	88	74%
prime, 1/2-inch fat, raw	1 oz	93	5	0	18	0	8.1	3.4	21	79%
select, 1/8-inch fat, braised	3 oz	270	23	0	56	0	19.0	7.6	88	63%
select, 1/8-inch fat, raw	1 oz	65	5	0	20	0	4.9	2.0	20	68%
select, 1/4-inch fat, braised	3 oz	277	23	0	55	0	19.8	7.9	88	65%
select, 1/4-inch fat, raw	1 oz	67	5	0	19	0	5.1	2.1	20	69%
CUBE STEAK, lean cuts, raw *(Lean and Free)*	4 oz	109	24	0	0	0	1.0	0.0	61	9%
FLANK										
Trimmed										
choice, 0-inch fat, broiled	3 oz	176	23	0	71	0	8.6	3.7	57	44%
choice, 0-inch fat, raw	1 oz	44	6	0	21	0	2.1	0.9	14	44%
Untrimmed										
choice, 0-inch fat, braised	3 oz	201	24	0	61	0	11.1	4.7	60	49%
choice, 0-inch fat, broiled	3 oz	192	22	0	69	0	10.7	4.5	58	50%
choice, 0-inch fat, raw	4 oz	203	22	0	80	0	12.0	5.1	59	53%
GROUND										
Extra lean, 17% fat										
baked, medium	3 oz	213	21	0	42	0	13.7	5.4	70	58%
baked, well done	3 oz	233	26	0	54	0	13.6	5.3	91	53%
broiled, medium	3 oz	218	22	0	60	0	13.9	5.5	71	58%
broiled, well done	3 oz	225	24	0	70	0	13.4	5.3	84	54%
pan-fried, medium	3 oz	217	21	0	60	0	14.0	5.5	69	58%
pan-fried, well done	3 oz	224	24	0	69	0	13.6	5.3	79	55%
raw	4 oz	264	21	0	75	0	19.3	7.7	78	66%
raw	1 oz	66	5	0	19	0	4.8	1.9	20	66%
Lean, 21% fat										
baked, medium	3 oz	228	20	0	48	0	15.6	6.1	66	62%
baked, well done	3 oz	248	25	0	60	0	15.6	6.1	84	57%
broiled, medium	3 oz	231	21	0	65	0	15.7	6.2	74	61%
broiled, well done	3 oz	238	24	0	76	0	15.0	5.9	86	57%
lean cuts, raw *(Lean and Free)*	4 oz	161	22	0	0	0	7.5	0.0	67	44%
pan-fried, medium	3 oz	234	21	0	65	0	16.2	6.4	71	63%
pan-fried, well done	3 oz	235	23	0	74	0	15.0	5.9	81	58%
raw	4 oz	298	20	0	78	0	23.4	9.4	85	71%
raw	1 oz	75	5	0	20	0	5.9	2.4	21	71%
Regular, 27% fat										
baked, medium	3 oz	244	20	0	51	0	17.8	7.0	74	66%
baked, well done	3 oz	269	24	0	64	0	18.2	7.2	92	61%
broiled, medium	3 oz	246	20	0	71	0	17.6	6.9	77	65%
broiled, well done	3 oz	248	23	0	79	0	16.5	6.5	86	60%
1/4-pound patties *(Bar-S)*	1 patty	330	18	0	80	0	28.0	11.0	85	78%
1/4-pound patties *(Chuck Wagon)*	1 patty	400	9	5	750	2	35.0	13.0	95	85%
1/4-pound patties *(Manor House)*	1 patty	330	18	0	65	0	28.0	13.0	60	78%
pan-fried, medium	3 oz	260	20	0	71	0	19.2	7.5	76	67%
pan-fried, well done	3 oz	243	23	0	79	0	16.1	6.3	83	60%
raw	4 oz	350	19	0	77	0	30.0	12.2	96	77%

Food Name	Serving Size	Calories	Prot. gms	Carbs gms	Sod. mgs	Fiber gms	Fat gms	Sat. Fat gms	Chol. mgs	% Fat Cal.
raw	1 oz	88	5	0	19	0	7.5	3.1	24	77%
HEART										
raw	4 oz	132	19	3	71	0	4.3	1.3	158	29%
simmered	3 oz	149	24	0	54	0	4.8	1.4	164	29%
KIDNEY										
raw	1 oz	30	5	1	51	0	0.9	0.3	81	26%
simmered	3 oz	122	22	1	114	0	2.9	0.9	329	22%
LIVER										
braised	3 oz	137	21	3	60	0	4.2	1.6	331	27%
pan-fried	3 oz	184	23	7	90	0	6.8	2.3	410	33%
raw	4 oz	162	23	7	82	0	4.4	1.7	400	24%
LOIN, TOP										
Trimmed										
all grades, 0-inch fat, broiled	3 oz	168	24	0	58	0	7.1	2.7	65	38%
all grades, 1/4-inch fat, broiled	3 oz	176	24	0	58	0	8.0	3.1	65	41%
all grades, 1/4-inch fat, raw	1 oz	40	6	0	17	0	1.6	0.6	17	35%
choice, 0-inch fat, broiled	3 oz	178	24	0	58	0	8.2	3.1	65	41%
choice, 1/4-inch fat, broiled	3 oz	182	24	0	58	0	8.6	3.3	65	43%
choice, 1/4-inch fat, raw	1 oz	43	6	0	17	0	1.8	0.7	17	38%
prime, 1/4-inch fat, broiled	3 oz	208	24	0	58	0	11.6	4.6	65	50%
prime, 1/4-inch fat, raw	1 oz	54	6	0	17	0	3.0	1.2	17	51%
prime, 1/2-inch fat, raw	3 oz	208	24	0	58	0	11.6	4.6	65	50%
select, 0-inch fat, broiled	3 oz	156	24	0	58	0	5.9	2.2	65	34%
select, 1/4-inch fat, broiled	3 oz	164	24	0	58	0	6.6	2.5	65	36%
select, 1/4-inch fat, raw	1 oz	38	6	0	17	0	1.3	0.5	17	31%
Untrimmed										
all grades, 0-inch fat, broiled	3 oz	180	24	0	57	0	8.7	3.4	65	44%
all grades, 1/8-inch fat, broiled	3 oz	228	22	0	54	0	14.7	5.8	66	58%
all grades, 1/4-inch fat, broiled	3 oz	244	22	0	54	0	16.8	6.6	67	62%
choice, 0-inch fat, broiled	3 oz	194	24	0	57	0	10.2	4.0	65	48%
choice, 1/8-inch fat, broiled	3 oz	241	22	0	54	0	16.3	6.4	67	61%
choice, 1/4-inch fat, broiled	3 oz	253	22	0	54	0	17.8	7.1	67	64%
prime, 1/8-inch fat, broiled	3 oz	264	22	0	54	0	18.8	7.6	67	64%
prime, 1/4-inch fat, broiled	3 oz	275	22	0	54	0	20.2	8.2	67	67%
prime, 1/2-inch fat, broiled	3 oz	288	21	0	53	0	22.0	9.1	68	69%
select, 0-inch fat, broiled	3 oz	169	24	0	57	0	7.5	2.9	65	40%
select, 1/8-inch fat, broiled	3 oz	215	22	0	55	0	13.2	5.2	66	55%
select, 1/4-inch fat, broiled	3 oz	226	22	0	54	0	14.6	5.8	67	58%
LUNGS										
braised	3 oz	102	17	0	86	0	3.1	1.1	235	28%
raw	4 oz	104	18	0	224	0	2.8	1.0	273	25%
PANCREAS										
braised	3 oz	230	23	0	51	0	14.6	5.0	223	57%
raw	4 oz	266	18	0	76	0	21.0	7.2	232	71%
PORTERHOUSE										
Trimmed										
all grades, 0-inch fat, broiled	3 oz	183	22	0	59	0	9.9	3.4	54	49%
all grades, 1/4-inch fat, broiled	3 oz	180	22	0	59	0	9.3	3.3	56	47%
all grades, 1/4-inch fat, raw	1 oz	45	6	0	16	0	2.1	0.8	16	43%
choice, 0-inch fat, broiled	3 oz	190	22	0	59	0	10.9	3.7	55	52%
choice, 1/4-inch fat, broiled	3 oz	183	22	0	59	0	9.8	3.4	59	48%
choice, 1/4-inch fat, raw	1 oz	45	6	0	16	0	2.3	0.8	17	46%
select, 0-inch fat, broiled	3 oz	165	23	0	59	0	7.5	2.8	49	41%
select, 1/4-inch fat, broiled	3 oz	173	23	0	59	0	8.2	3.1	49	43%

Food Name	Serving Size	Calories	Prot. gms	Carbs gms	Sod. mgs	Fiber gms	Fat gms	Sat. Fat gms	Chol. mgs	% Fat Cal.
select, 1/4-inch fat, raw	1 oz	42	6	0	16	0	1.6	0.6	14	35%
Untrimmed										
all grades, 0-inch fat, broiled	3 oz	237	20	0	55	0	16.7	6.2	57	63%
all grades, 1/8-inch fat, broiled	3 oz	252	20	0	54	0	18.6	7.2	60	66%
all grades, 1/8-inch fat, raw	1 oz	70	5	0	15	0	5.2	2.1	18	68%
all grades, 1/4-inch fat, broiled	3 oz	273	19	0	54	0	21.1	8.2	62	70%
all grades, 1/4-inch fat, raw	1 oz	73	5	0	14	0	5.6	2.3	18	69%
choice, 1/8-inch fat, broiled	3 oz	254	20	0	54	0	18.8	7.2	63	67%
choice, 1/8-inch fat, raw	1 oz	73	5	0	15	0	5.7	2.3	19	70%
choice, 1/4-inch fat, broiled	3 oz	278	19	0	53	0	21.8	8.4	64	71%
choice, 1/4-inch fat, raw	1 oz	73	5	0	15	0	5.7	2.3	19	70%
select, 0-inch fat, broiled	3 oz	227	21	0	55	0	15.3	6.0	54	61%
select, 1/8-inch fat, broiled	3 oz	250	20	0	54	0	18.0	7.1	55	65%
select, 1/8-inch fat, raw	1 oz	63	6	0	15	0	4.2	1.7	16	60%
select, 1/4-inch fat, broiled	3 oz	262	20	0	54	0	19.6	7.7	56	67%
select, 1/4-inch fat, raw	1 oz	63	6	0	15	0	4.2	1.7	16	60%
RIB, LARGE END										
Trimmed										
all grades, ribs 6-9, 0-inch fat, roasted	3 oz	202	23	0	62	0	11.4	4.5	69	51%
all grades, ribs 6-9, 1/4-inch fat, broiled	3 oz	190	21	0	61	0	11.0	4.5	65	52%
all grades, ribs 6-9, 1/4-inch fat, raw	1 oz	47	6	0	19	0	2.6	1.0	17	49%
all grades, ribs 6-9, 1/4-inch fat, roasted	3 oz	201	23	0	62	0	11.2	4.5	69	50%
choice, ribs 6-9, 0-inch fat, roasted	3 oz	215	23	0	62	0	12.8	5.1	69	53%
choice, ribs 6-9, 1/4-inch fat, broiled	3 oz	204	21	0	61	0	12.5	5.1	65	55%
choice, ribs 6-9, 1/4-inch fat, raw	1 oz	50	6	0	19	0	2.9	1.2	17	52%
choice, ribs 6-9, 1/4-inch fat, roasted	3 oz	213	23	0	62	0	12.5	5.0	69	53%
prime, ribs 6-9, 1/4-inch fat, broiled	3 oz	250	21	0	60	0	17.7	7.6	70	64%
prime, ribs 6-9, 1/4-inch fat, raw	1 oz	60	6	0	19	0	4.0	1.7	17	60%
prime, ribs 6-9, 1/4-inch fat, roasted	3 oz	241	23	0	62	0	15.6	6.7	69	58%
prime, ribs 6-9, 1/2-inch fat, broiled	3 oz	250	21	0	60	0	17.7	7.6	70	64%
prime, ribs 6-9, 1/2-inch fat, roasted	3 oz	241	23	0	62	0	15.6	6.7	69	58%
select, ribs 6-9, 0-inch fat, roasted	3 oz	187	23	0	62	0	9.7	3.9	69	47%
select, ribs 6-9, 1/4-inch fat, broiled	3 oz	175	21	0	61	0	9.3	3.8	65	48%
select, ribs 6-9, 1/4-inch fat, raw	1 oz	43	6	0	19	0	2.2	0.9	17	45%
select, ribs 6-9, 1/4-inch fat, roasted	3 oz	187	23	0	62	0	9.7	3.9	69	47%
Untrimmed										
all grades, ribs 6-9, 0-inch fat, roasted	3 oz	300	20	0	55	0	24.0	9.7	72	72%
all grades, ribs 6-9, 1/8-inch fat, broiled	3 oz	287	18	0	54	0	23.1	9.4	68	73%
all grades, ribs 6-9, 1/8-inch fat, raw	1 oz	90	5	0	16	0	7.7	3.2	20	78%
all grades, ribs 6-9, 1/8-inch fat, roasted	3 oz	302	20	0	54	0	24.2	9.8	72	72%
all grades, ribs 6-9, 1/4-inch fat, broiled	3 oz	295	18	0	54	0	24.2	9.8	69	74%
all grades, ribs 6-9, 1/4-inch fat, raw	1 oz	92	5	0	16	0	8.0	3.3	20	79%
all grades, ribs 6-9, 1/4-inch fat, roasted	3 oz	310	19	0	54	0	25.3	10.2	72	74%
choice, ribs 6-9, 0-inch fat, roasted	3 oz	316	19	0	54	0	25.9	10.4	72	74%
choice, ribs 6-9, 1/8-inch fat, broiled	3 oz	315	18	0	54	0	26.5	10.8	69	76%
choice, ribs 6-9, 1/8-inch fat, raw	1 oz	94	5	0	15	0	8.3	3.4	20	79%
choice, ribs 6-9, 1/8-inch fat, roasted	3 oz	334	19	0	54	0	27.8	11.6	72	75%
choice, ribs 6-9, 1/4-inch fat, broiled	3 oz	312	18	0	54	0	26.2	10.6	69	75%
choice, ribs 6-9, 1/4-inch fat, raw	1 oz	98	4	0	15	0	8.7	3.6	21	81%
choice, ribs 6-9, 1/4-inch fat, roasted	3 oz	326	19	0	54	0	27.2	11.0	72	75%
prime, ribs 6-9, 1/8-inch fat, broiled	3 oz	343	18	0	53	0	29.7	12.3	73	78%
prime, ribs 6-9, 1/8-inch fat, raw	1 oz	104	4	0	15	0	9.4	4.0	21	82%
prime, ribs 6-9, 1/4-inch fat, broiled	3 oz	351	17	0	52	0	30.8	12.8	73	79%
prime, ribs 6-9, 1/4-inch fat, raw	1 oz	107	4	0	15	0	9.8	4.1	21	83%

Food Name	Serving Size	Calories	Prot. gms	Carbs gms	Sod. mgs	Fiber gms	Fat gms	Sat. Fat gms	Chol. mgs	% Fat Cal.
prime, ribs 6-9, 1/4-inch fat, roasted	3 oz	342	19	0	54	0	28.8	12.0	72	76%
prime, ribs 6-9, 1/2-inch fat, broiled	3 oz	361	17	0	51	0	32.1	13.6	74	80%
prime, ribs 6-9, 1/2-inch fat, raw	1 oz	109	4	0	15	0	10.0	4.3	21	83%
prime, ribs 6-9, 1/2-inch fat, roasted	3 oz	346	19	0	54	0	29.4	12.5	72	77%
select, ribs 6-9, 1/8-inch fat, broiled	3 oz	275	18	0	54	0	21.9	8.9	68	72%
select, ribs 6-9, 1/8-inch fat, raw	1 oz	84	5	0	16	0	7.0	2.9	20	76%
select, ribs 6-9, 1/8-inch fat, roasted	3 oz	283	20	0	55	0	22.0	8.9	71	70%
select, ribs 6-9, 1/4-inch fat, broiled	3 oz	275	18	0	54	0	21.9	8.9	68	72%
select, ribs 6-9, 1/4-inch fat, raw	1 oz	86	5	0	16	0	7.4	3.0	20	77%
select, ribs 6-9, 1/4-inch fat, roasted	3 oz	289	20	0	55	0	22.7	9.2	72	71%
RIB, SHORTRIB										
Trimmed										
choice, braised	3 oz	251	26	0	49	0	15.4	6.6	79	55%
choice, raw	1 oz	49	5	0	18	0	2.9	1.2	17	53%
Untrimmed										
choice, braised	3 oz	400	18	0	43	0	35.7	15.1	80	80%
choice, raw	1 oz	110	4	0	14	0	10.3	4.5	22	84%
RIB, SMALL END										
Trimmed										
all grades, ribs 10-12, 0-inch fat, broiled	3 oz	181	24	0	59	0	8.8	3.5	68	44%
all grades, ribs 10-12, 1/4-inch fat, broiled	3 oz	188	24	0	59	0	9.5	3.8	68	46%
all grades, ribs 10-12, 1/4-inch fat, raw	1 oz	43	6	0	18	0	2.1	0.8	17	43%
all grades, ribs 10-12, 1/4-inch fat, roasted	3 oz	185	23	0	60	0	9.8	3.9	67	48%
choice, ribs 10-12, 0-inch fat, broiled	3 oz	191	24	0	59	0	9.9	4.0	68	47%
choice, ribs 10-12, 1/4-inch fat, broiled	3 oz	198	24	0	59	0	10.7	4.3	68	49%
choice, ribs 10-12, 1/4-inch fat, raw	1 oz	46	6	0	18	0	2.4	0.9	17	47%
choice, ribs 10-12, 1/4-inch fat, roasted	3 oz	197	23	0	60	0	11.1	4.4	67	51%
prime, ribs 10-12, 1/4-inch fat, broiled	3 oz	221	24	0	59	0	13.2	5.6	68	54%
prime, ribs 10-12, 1/4-inch fat, raw	1 oz	57	6	0	18	0	3.6	1.5	17	57%
prime, ribs 10-12, 1/4-inch fat, roasted	3 oz	258	23	0	64	0	17.9	7.6	68	63%
prime, ribs 10-12, 1/2-inch fat, broiled	3 oz	221	24	0	59	0	13.2	5.6	68	54%
prime, ribs 10-12, 1/2-inch fat, roasted	3 oz	258	23	0	64	0	17.9	7.6	68	63%
select, ribs 10-12, 0-inch fat, broiled	3 oz	168	24	0	59	0	7.4	3.0	68	40%
select, ribs 10-12, 1/4-inch fat, broiled	3 oz	176	24	0	59	0	8.2	3.3	68	42%
select, ribs 10-12, 1/4-inch fat, raw	1 oz	40	6	0	18	0	1.8	0.7	17	39%
select, ribs 10-12, 1/4-inch fat, roasted	3 oz	173	23	0	60	0	8.3	3.3	67	43%
Untrimmed										
all grades, ribs 10-12, 0-inch fat, broiled	3 oz	252	21	0	54	0	17.9	7.3	71	64%
all grades, ribs 10-12, 1/8-inch fat, broiled	3 oz	281	20	0	53	0	21.4	8.7	71	69%
all grades, ribs 10-12, 1/8-inch fat, raw	1 oz	82	5	0	15	0	6.9	2.8	20	75%
all grades, ribs 10-12, 1/8-inch fat, roasted	3 oz	290	19	0	54	0	23.1	9.3	71	72%
all grades, ribs 10-12, 1/4-inch fat, broiled	3 oz	286	20	0	53	0	22.1	8.9	71	70%
all grades, ribs 10-12, 1/4-inch fat, raw	1 oz	84	5	0	15	0	7.1	2.9	20	76%
all grades, ribs 10-12, 1/4-inch fat, roasted	3 oz	295	19	0	54	0	23.8	9.6	71	73%
choice, ribs 10-12, 1/8-inch fat, broiled	3 oz	292	20	0	53	0	22.8	9.2	71	70%
choice, ribs 10-12, 1/8-inch fat, raw	1 oz	86	5	0	15	0	7.3	3.0	20	76%
choice, ribs 10-12, 1/8-inch fat, roasted	3 oz	305	19	0	54	0	24.8	10.0	71	73%
choice, ribs 10-12, 1/4-inch fat, broiled	3 oz	297	20	0	53	0	23.5	9.5	71	71%
choice, ribs 10-12, 1/4-inch fat, raw	1 oz	89	5	0	15	0	7.7	3.1	20	78%
choice, ribs 10-12, 1/4-inch fat, roasted	3 oz	312	19	0	53	0	25.7	10.4	71	74%
prime, ribs 10-12, 1/8-inch fat, broiled	3 oz	301	21	0	54	0	23.7	9.8	71	71%
prime, ribs 10-12, 1/8-inch fat, raw	1 oz	95	5	0	15	0	8.3	3.4	20	79%
prime, ribs 10-12, 1/8-inch fat, roasted	3 oz	349	19	0	55	0	29.9	12.3	71	77%
prime, ribs 10-12, 1/4-inch fat, broiled	3 oz	307	20	0	53	0	24.4	10.1	71	72%

Food Name	Serving Size	Calories	Prot. gms	Carbs gms	Sod. mgs	Fiber gms	Fat gms	Sat. Fat gms	Chol. mgs	% Fat Cal.
prime, ribs 10-12, 1/4-inch fat, raw	1 oz	97	5	0	15	0	8.5	3.5	20	79%
prime, ribs 10-12, 1/4-inch fat, roasted	3 oz	354	19	0	55	0	30.5	12.6	71	78%
prime, ribs 10-12, 1/2-inch fat, broiled.	3 oz	309	20	0	53	0	24.8	10.5	71	72%
prime, ribs 10-12, 1/2-inch fat, raw	1 oz	99	5	0	15	0	8.8	3.8	20	80%
prime, ribs 10-12, 1/2-inch fat, roasted	3 oz	357	19	0	54	0	30.8	13.0	72	78%
select, ribs 10-12, 1/8-inch fat, broiled	3 oz	268	20	0	54	0	20.0	8.1	71	67%
select, ribs 10-12, 1/8-inch fat, raw.	1 oz	78	5	0	15	0	6.4	2.6	20	74%
select, ribs 10-12, 1/8-inch fat, roasted.	3 oz	275	19	0	54	0	21.3	8.5	71	70%
select, ribs 10-12, 1/4-inch fat, broiled	3 oz	273	20	0	53	0	20.6	8.3	71	68%
select, ribs 10-12, 1/4-inch fat, raw	1 oz	81	5	0	15	0	6.7	2.8	20	75%
select, ribs 10-12, 1/4-inch fat, roasted.	3 oz	281	19	0	54	0	22.2	8.9	71	71%
RIB, WHOLE										
Trimmed										
all grades, ribs 6-12, 1/4-inch fat, broiled	3 oz	190	22	0	60	0	10.4	4.2	65	49%
all grades, ribs 6-12, 1/4-inch fat, raw	1 oz	45	6	0	18	0	2.4	0.9	17	47%
all grades, ribs 6-12, 1/4-inch fat, roasted.	3 oz	195	23	0	61	0	10.6	4.2	68	49%
choice, ribs 6-12, 1/4-inch fat, broiled	3 oz	201	22	0	60	0	11.7	4.8	65	53%
choice, ribs 6-12, 1/4-inch fat, raw	1 oz	48	6	0	18	0	2.7	1.1	17	50%
choice, ribs 6-12, 1/4-inch fat, roasted	3 oz	207	23	0	61	0	11.9	4.8	68	52%
prime, ribs 6-12, 1/4-inch fat, broiled.	3 oz	238	22	0	60	0	15.9	6.8	69	60%
prime, ribs 6-12, 1/4-inch fat, raw	1 oz	58	6	0	18	0	3.8	1.6	17	59%
prime, ribs 6-12, 1/4-inch fat, roasted	3 oz	248	23	0	63	0	16.5	7.1	69	60%
prime, ribs 6-12, 1/2-inch fat, broiled.	3 oz	238	22	0	59	0	15.9	6.8	70	60%
prime, ribs 6-12, 1/2-inch fat, roasted	3 oz	248	23	0	63	0	16.5	7.0	69	60%
select, ribs 6-12, 1/4-inch fat, broiled	3 oz	175	22	0	60	0	8.9	3.6	65	46%
select, ribs 6-12, 1/4-inch fat, raw	1 oz	42	6	0	18	0	2.0	0.8	17	43%
select, ribs 6-12, 1/4-inch fat, roasted.	3 oz	181	23	0	61	0	9.1	3.6	68	45%
Untrimmed										
all grades, ribs 6-12, 1/8-inch fat, broiled	3 oz	286	19	0	54	0	22.7	9.2	70	72%
all grades, ribs 6-12, 1/8-inch fat, raw	1 oz	87	5	0	16	0	7.4	3.0	20	77%
all grades, ribs 6-12, 1/8-inch fat, roasted.	3 oz	298	19	0	54	0	23.9	9.6	71	72%
all grades, ribs 6-12, 1/4-inch fat, broiled	3 oz	291	19	0	54	0	23.3	9.5	70	72%
all grades, ribs 6-12, 1/4-inch fat, raw	1 oz	89	5	0	15	0	7.6	3.2	20	78%
all grades, ribs 6-12, 1/4-inch fat, roasted.	3 oz	304	19	0	54	0	24.7	9.9	71	73%
choice, ribs 6-12, 1/8-inch fat, broiled.	3 oz	299	19	0	54	0	24.2	9.8	70	73%
choice, ribs 6-12, 1/8-inch fat, raw	1 oz	91	5	0	15	0	7.9	3.3	20	78%
choice, ribs 6-12, 1/8-inch fat, roasted	3 oz	310	19	0	54	0	25.3	10.2	71	74%
choice, ribs 6-12, 1/4-inch fat, broiled	3 oz	306	19	0	53	0	25.1	10.2	70	74%
choice, ribs 6-12, 1/4-inch fat, raw	1 oz	94	5	0	15	0	8.3	3.4	20	80%
choice, ribs 6-12, 1/4-inch fat, roasted	3 oz	320	19	0	54	0	26.5	10.7	72	75%
prime, ribs 6-12, 1/8-inch fat, broiled.	3 oz	328	19	0	53	0	27.5	11.4	72	76%
prime, ribs 6-12, 1/8-inch fat, raw	1 oz	101	5	0	15	0	9.0	3.7	20	80%
prime, ribs 6-12, 1/8-inch fat, roasted	3 oz	340	19	0	55	0	28.6	11.9	72	76%
prime, ribs 6-12, 1/4-inch fat, broiled.	3 oz	333	18	0	53	0	28.2	11.7	72	76%
prime, ribs 6-12, 1/4-inch fat, raw	1 oz	103	5	0	15	0	9.3	3.9	21	81%
prime, ribs 6-12, 1/4-inch fat, roasted	3 oz	348	19	0	54	0	29.6	12.2	72	77%
prime, ribs 6-12, 1/2-inch fat, broiled.	3 oz	347	18	0	51	0	29.9	12.7	73	78%
prime, ribs 6-12, 1/2-inch fat, raw	1 oz	105	4	0	15	0	9.5	4.1	21	82%
prime, ribs 6-12, 1/2-inch fat, roasted	3 oz	361	18	0	54	0	31.4	13.3	73	78%
select, ribs 6-12, 1/8-inch fat, broiled	3 oz	268	19	0	54	0	20.6	8.3	69	69%
select, ribs 6-12, 1/8-inch fat, raw	1 oz	82	5	0	16	0	6.8	2.8	20	75%
select, ribs 6-12, 1/8-inch fat, roasted.	3 oz	281	20	0	55	0	21.8	8.8	71	70%
select, ribs 6-12, 1/4-inch fat, broiled	3 oz	275	19	0	54	0	21.4	8.7	70	70%
select, ribs 6-12, 1/4-inch fat, raw	1 oz	84	5	0	16	0	7.1	2.9	20	76%

Food Name	Serving Size	Calories	Prot. gms	Carbs gms	Sod. mgs	Fiber gms	Fat gms	Sat. Fat gms	Chol. mgs	% Fat Cal.
select, ribs 6-12, 1/4-inch fat, roasted	3 oz	286	19	0	54	0	22.5	9.1	71	71%
RIB EYE, SMALL END										
Trimmed										
choice, ribs 10-12, 0-inch fat, broiled	3 oz	191	24	0	59	0	9.9	4.0	68	47%
choice, ribs 10-12, 0-inch fat, raw	1 oz	46	6	0	18	0	2.4	0.9	17	47%
lean cuts, raw (Lean and Free)	4 oz	121	25	0	59	0	2.6	0.0	71	19%
Untrimmed										
choice, ribs 10-12, 0-inch fat, broiled	3 oz	261	21	0	54	0	18.9	7.7	71	65%
choice, ribs 10-12, 0-inch fat, raw	1 oz	78	5	0	16	0	6.3	2.6	19	73%
choice, ribs 10-12, 1/8-inch fat, broiled	3 oz	255	21	0	54	0	18.1	7.3	70	64%
choice, ribs 10-12, 1/8-inch fat, raw	1 oz	74	5	0	16	0	5.8	2.4	19	71%
ROLLED, lean cuts, raw (Lean and Free)	4 oz	125	25	0	60	0	2.8	0.0	0	20%
ROUND, BOTTOM										
Trimmed										
all grades, 0-inch fat, braised	3 oz	173	27	0	43	0	6.5	2.2	82	34%
all grades, 0-inch fat, roasted	3 oz	156	24	0	56	0	5.7	1.9	66	33%
all grades, 1/4-inch fat, braised	3 oz	178	27	0	43	0	7.0	2.4	82	35%
all grades, 1/4-inch fat, raw	1 oz	41	6	0	17	0	1.6	0.5	17	35%
all grades, 1/4-inch fat, roasted	3 oz	161	24	0	56	0	6.3	2.1	66	35%
choice, 0-inch fat, braised	3 oz	181	27	0	43	0	7.4	2.5	82	37%
choice, 0-inch fat, roasted	3 oz	164	24	0	56	0	6.6	2.2	66	36%
choice, 1/4-inch fat, braised	3 oz	187	27	0	43	0	8.0	2.7	82	39%
choice, 1/4-inch fat, raw	1 oz	43	6	0	17	0	1.8	0.6	17	38%
choice, 1/4-inch fat, roasted	3 oz	168	24	0	56	0	7.0	2.4	66	38%
prime, 1/2-inch fat, broiled	3 oz	212	27	0	43	0	10.8	3.8	82	46%
prime, 1/2-inch fat, raw	1 oz	45	6	0	17	0	2.1	0.7	17	41%
select, 0-inch fat, braised	3 oz	163	27	0	43	0	5.4	1.8	82	30%
select, 0-inch fat, roasted	3 oz	145	24	0	56	0	4.6	1.5	66	28%
select, 1/4-inch fat, braised	3 oz	167	27	0	43	0	5.8	2.0	82	31%
select, 1/4-inch fat, raw	1 oz	39	6	0	17	0	1.3	0.5	17	31%
select, 1/4-inch fat, roasted	3 oz	152	24	0	56	0	5.3	1.8	66	31%
Untrimmed										
all grades, 0-inch fat, braised	3 oz	181	26	0	43	0	7.5	2.6	82	37%
all grades, 0-inch fat, roasted	3 oz	160	24	0	56	0	6.2	2.1	66	35%
all grades, 1/8-inch fat, braised	3 oz	218	25	0	43	0	12.2	4.5	82	51%
all grades, 1/8-inch fat, raw	1 oz	54	6	0	16	0	3.2	1.2	18	54%
all grades, 1/8-inch fat, roasted	3 oz	195	23	0	54	0	10.6	3.9	67	49%
all grades, 1/4-inch fat, braised	3 oz	234	24	0	43	0	14.4	5.4	82	55%
all grades, 1/4-inch fat, raw	1 oz	59	6	0	16	0	3.8	1.5	18	58%
all grades, 1/4-inch fat, roasted	3 oz	211	23	0	54	0	12.7	4.8	68	54%
choice, 0-inch fat, braised	3 oz	193	26	0	43	0	9.0	3.1	82	42%
choice, 0-inch fat, roasted	3 oz	173	24	0	55	0	7.7	2.7	66	40%
choice, 1/8-inch fat, braised	3 oz	228	25	0	43	0	13.5	5.0	82	53%
choice, 1/8-inch fat, raw	1 oz	57	6	0	16	0	3.5	1.3	18	56%
choice, 1/8-inch fat, roasted	3 oz	205	23	0	54	0	11.8	4.4	67	52%
choice, 1/4-inch fat, braised	3 oz	241	24	0	43	0	15.2	5.7	82	57%
choice, 1/4-inch fat, raw	1 oz	62	6	0	16	0	4.2	1.6	18	61%
choice, 1/4-inch fat, roasted	3 oz	221	22	0	54	0	13.9	5.2	68	57%
prime, 1/2-inch fat, braised	3 oz	252	25	0	43	0	16.2	6.2	82	58%
prime, 1/2-inch fat, raw	1 oz	64	6	0	16	0	4.4	1.8	18	62%
select, 0-inch fat, braised	3 oz	171	26	0	43	0	6.4	2.3	82	34%
select, 0-inch fat, roasted	3 oz	150	24	0	56	0	5.1	1.7	66	31%
select, 1/8-inch fat, braised	3 oz	208	25	0	43	0	11.2	4.2	82	48%
select, 1/8-inch fat, raw	1 oz	51	6	0	16	0	2.9	1.1	18	51%

Food Name	Serving Size	Calories	Prot. gms	Carbs gms	Sod. mgs	Fiber gms	Fat gms	Sat. Fat gms	Chol. mgs	% Fat Cal.
select, 1/8-inch fat, roasted	3 oz	186	23	0	54	0	9.6	3.6	67	47%
select, 1/4-inch fat, braised	3 oz	220	25	0	43	0	12.8	4.8	82	52%
select, 1/4-inch fat, raw	1 oz	55	6	0	16	0	3.4	1.3	18	55%
select, 1/4-inch fat, roasted	3 oz	199	23	0	54	0	11.3	4.3	68	51%
ROUND, EYE OF										
Trimmed										
all grades, 0-inch fat, roasted	3 oz	141	25	0	53	0	4.0	1.4	59	26%
all grades, 1/4-inch fat, raw	1 oz	37	6	0	15	0	1.2	0.4	15	29%
all grades, 1/4-inch fat, roasted	3 oz	143	25	0	53	0	4.2	1.5	59	26%
choice, 0-inch fat, roasted	3 oz	149	25	0	53	0	4.8	1.8	59	29%
choice, 1/4-inch fat, raw	1 oz	39	6	0	15	0	1.4	0.5	15	32%
choice, 1/4-inch fat, roasted	3 oz	149	25	0	53	0	4.8	1.8	59	29%
prime, 1/2-inch fat, raw	1 oz	42	6	0	15	0	1.8	0.6	15	38%
prime, 1/2-inch fat, roasted	3 oz	168	25	0	53	0	7.0	2.7	59	38%
select, 0-inch fat, roasted	3 oz	132	25	0	53	0	3.0	1.1	59	20%
select, 1/4-inch fat, raw	1 oz	35	6	0	15	0	1.0	0.4	15	26%
select, 1/4-inch fat, roasted	3 oz	136	25	0	53	0	3.4	1.2	59	23%
Untrimmed										
all grades, 0-inch fat, roasted	3 oz	145	24	0	53	0	4.6	1.7	59	28%
all grades, 1/8-inch fat, raw	1 oz	47	6	0	14	0	2.4	0.9	16	46%
all grades, 1/8-inch fat, roasted	3 oz	165	24	0	52	0	6.9	2.6	60	38%
all grades, 1/4-inch fat, raw	1 oz	60	6	0	14	0	4.1	1.6	17	61%
all grades, 1/4-inch fat, roasted	3 oz	195	23	0	50	0	10.8	4.2	61	50%
choice, 0-inch fat, roasted	3 oz	153	24	0	53	0	5.4	2.0	59	32%
choice, 1/8-inch fat, raw	1 oz	49	6	0	14	0	2.6	1.0	16	48%
choice, 1/8-inch fat, roasted	3 oz	170	24	0	52	0	7.6	2.9	60	40%
choice, 1/4-inch fat, raw	1 oz	62	6	0	14	0	4.2	1.7	17	61%
choice, 1/4-inch fat, roasted	3 oz	205	23	0	50	0	12.0	4.7	61	53%
select, 1/8-inch fat, raw	1 oz	45	6	0	15	0	2.2	0.8	16	43%
select, 1/8-inch fat, roasted	3 oz	158	24	0	52	0	6.2	2.4	60	36%
select, 1/4-inch fat, raw	1 oz	57	6	0	14	0	3.7	1.5	17	58%
select, 1/4-inch fat, roasted	3 oz	184	23	0	51	0	9.6	3.8	61	47%
prime, 1/2-inch fat, raw	1 oz	63	6	0	14	0	4.3	1.8	17	61%
prime, 1/2-inch fat, roasted	3 oz	213	23	0	50	0	12.7	5.1	61	54%
ROUND, FULL CUT										
Trimmed										
choice, 1/4-inch fat, broiled	3 oz	162	25	0	54	0	6.2	2.2	66	35%
choice, 1/4-inch fat, raw	1 oz	39	6	0	16	0	1.4	0.5	16	32%
select, 1/4-inch fat, broiled	3 oz	146	25	0	54	0	4.4	1.6	66	27%
select, 1/4-inch fat, raw	1 oz	36	6	0	16	0	1.0	0.3	16	25%
Untrimmed										
choice, 1/8-inch fat, broiled	3 oz	200	23	0	53	0	11.0	4.2	67	50%
choice, 1/8-inch fat, raw	1 oz	55	6	0	15	0	3.4	1.3	18	55%
choice, 1/4-inch fat, broiled	3 oz	204	23	0	52	0	11.6	4.4	68	51%
choice, 1/4-inch fat, raw	1 oz	58	6	0	15	0	3.6	1.4	18	57%
select, 1/8-inch fat, broiled	3 oz	185	23	0	53	0	9.4	3.6	67	46%
select, 1/8-inch fat, raw	1 oz	52	6	0	15	0	3.0	1.2	18	52%
select, 1/4-inch fat, broiled	3 oz	190	23	0	53	0	10.0	3.5	47	47%
select, 1/4-inch fat, raw	1 oz	54	6	0	15	0	3.3	1.3	18	55%
ROUND, TOP										
Trimmed										
all grades, 0-inch fat, braised	3 oz	169	31	0	38	0	4.3	1.5	77	23%
all grades, 1/4-inch fat, braised	3 oz	174	31	0	38	0	4.8	1.6	77	25%
all grades, 1/4-inch fat, broiled	3 oz	153	27	0	52	0	4.2	1.4	71	25%

Food Name	Serving Size	Calories	Prot. gms	Carbs gms	Sod. mgs	Fiber gms	Fat gms	Sat. Fat gms	Chol. mgs	% Fat Cal.
all grades, 1/4-inch fat, raw	1 oz	36	6	0	15	0	0.9	0.3	16	23%
choice, 0-inch fat, braised	3 oz	176	31	0	38	0	4.9	1.7	77	25%
choice, 1/4-inch fat, braised	3 oz	181	31	0	38	0	5.5	1.9	77	28%
choice, 1/4-inch fat, broiled	3 oz	161	27	0	52	0	5.0	1.7	71	28%
choice, 1/4-inch fat, pan-fried	3 oz	193	30	0	60	0	7.3	2.1	82	34%
choice, 1/4-inch fat, raw	1 oz	37	6	0	15	0	1.1	0.4	16	27%
lean cuts, raw (Lean Limousin)	4 oz	134	25	0	49	0	4.5	0.0	0	29%
prime, 1/2-inch fat, broiled	3 oz	183	27	0	52	0	7.5	2.6	71	37%
prime, 1/4-inch fat, broiled	3 oz	183	27	0	52	0	7.5	2.6	71	37%
prime, 1/4-inch fat, raw	1 oz	43	6	0	15	0	1.8	0.6	16	37%
select, 0-inch fat, braised	3 oz	162	31	0	38	0	3.4	1.2	77	19%
select, 1/4-inch fat, braised	3 oz	167	31	0	38	0	3.9	1.3	77	21%
select, 1/4-inch fat, broiled	3 oz	144	27	0	52	0	3.1	1.1	71	20%
select, 1/4-inch fat, raw	1 oz	34	6	0	15	0	0.7	0.2	16	19%
Untrimmed										
all grades, 0-inch fat, braised	3 oz	178	30	0	38	0	5.4	1.9	77	27%
all grades, 1/8-inch fat, braised	3 oz	202	29	0	38	0	8.6	3.2	77	38%
all grades, 1/8-inch fat, broiled	3 oz	176	26	0	51	0	7.2	2.7	72	37%
all grades, 1/8-inch fat, raw	1 oz	46	6	0	14	0	2.2	0.9	17	43%
all grades, 1/4-inch fat, braised	3 oz	211	29	0	38	0	9.7	3.7	77	42%
all grades, 1/4-inch fat, broiled	3 oz	184	26	0	51	0	8.2	3.1	72	40%
all grades, 1/4-inch fat, raw	1 oz	50	6	0	14	0	2.7	1.0	17	48%
choice, 0-inch fat, braised	3 oz	184	30	0	38	0	6.0	2.1	77	30%
choice, 1/8-inch fat, braised	3 oz	213	29	0	38	0	9.9	3.7	77	42%
choice, 1/8-inch fat, broiled	3 oz	184	26	0	51	0	8.0	3.0	72	39%
choice, 1/8-inch fat, pan-fried	3 oz	226	28	0	58	0	11.8	3.9	82	47%
choice, 1/8-inch fat, raw	1 oz	48	6	0	14	0	2.4	0.9	17	45%
choice, 1/4-inch fat, braised	3 oz	221	29	0	38	0	10.9	4.1	77	45%
choice, 1/4-inch fat, broiled	3 oz	190	26	0	51	0	9.0	3.3	72	42%
choice, 1/4-inch fat, pan-fried	3 oz	235	28	0	58	0	13.1	4.5	82	50%
choice, 1/4-inch fat, raw	1 oz	51	6	0	14	0	2.8	1.1	17	49%
prime, 1/2-inch fat, broiled	3 oz	201	26	0	51	0	9.9	3.7	72	44%
prime, 1/2-inch fat, raw	1 oz	53	6	0	14	0	3.0	1.2	17	51%
prime, 1/8-inch fat, broiled	3 oz	191	27	0	52	0	8.6	3.1	71	40%
prime, 1/8-inch fat, raw	1 oz	49	6	0	14	0	2.5	0.9	17	45%
prime, 1/4-inch fat, broiled	3 oz	195	26	0	51	0	9.1	3.3	71	42%
prime, 1/4-inch fat, raw	1 oz	51	6	0	14	0	2.7	1.0	17	47%
select, 0-inch fat, braised	3 oz	170	30	0	38	0	4.5	1.6	77	24%
select, 1/8-inch fat, braised	3 oz	191	29	0	38	0	7.3	2.7	77	34%
select, 1/8-inch fat, broiled	3 oz	167	26	0	51	0	6.2	2.3	72	34%
select, 1/8-inch fat, raw	1 oz	44	6	0	14	0	2.0	0.8	17	40%
select, 1/4-inch fat, braised	3 oz	199	29	0	38	0	8.4	3.2	77	38%
select, 1/4-inch fat, broiled	3 oz	175	26	0	51	0	7.2	2.8	72	37%
select, 1/4-inch fat, raw	1 oz	46	6	0	14	0	2.3	0.9	17	44%
ROUND TIP										
Trimmed										
all grades, 0-inch fat, roasted	3 oz	150	24	0	55	0	5.0	1.8	69	30%
all grades, 1/4-inch fat, raw	1 oz	35	6	0	18	0	1.1	0.4	17	28%
all grades, 1/4-inch fat, roasted	3 oz	157	24	0	55	0	5.9	2.0	69	34%
choice, 0-inch fat, roasted	3 oz	153	24	0	55	0	5.4	1.9	69	32%
choice, 1/4-inch fat, raw	1 oz	37	6	0	18	0	1.2	0.4	17	31%
choice, 1/4-inch fat, roasted	3 oz	160	24	0	55	0	6.2	2.2	69	35%
prime, 1/4-inch fat, raw	1 oz	41	6	0	18	0	1.7	0.6	17	38%
prime, 1/2-inch fat, roasted	3 oz	181	24	0	55	0	8.6	3.1	69	43%

Food Name	Serving Size	Calories	Prot. gms	Carbs gms	Sod. mgs	Fiber gms	Fat gms	Sat. Fat gms	Chol. mgs	% Fat Cal.
prime, 1/4-inch fat, roasted	3 oz	181	24	0	55	0	8.6	3.1	69	43%
select, 0-inch fat, roasted	3 oz	145	24	0	55	0	4.5	1.6	69	28%
select, 1/4-inch fat, raw	1 oz	34	6	0	18	0	0.9	0.3	17	24%
select, 1/4-inch fat, roasted	3 oz	153	24	0	55	0	5.4	1.9	69	32%
Untrimmed										
all grades, 0-inch fat, roasted	3 oz	162	24	0	54	0	6.7	2.4	69	37%
all grades, 1/8-inch fat, raw	1 oz	54	6	0	16	0	3.3	1.3	18	56%
all grades, 1/8-inch fat, roasted	3 oz	186	23	0	54	0	9.6	3.6	70	47%
all grades, 1/4-inch fat, raw	1 oz	57	5	0	16	0	3.7	1.5	18	59%
all grades, 1/4-inch fat, roasted	3 oz	199	23	0	54	0	11.3	4.3	70	51%
choice, 0-inch fat, roasted	3 oz	170	24	0	54	0	7.6	2.8	70	40%
choice, 1/8-inch fat, raw	1 oz	56	6	0	16	0	3.6	1.4	18	58%
choice, 1/8-inch fat, roasted	3 oz	194	23	0	54	0	10.5	3.9	70	49%
choice, 1/4-inch fat, raw	1 oz	60	5	0	16	0	4.1	1.6	19	61%
choice, 1/4-inch fat, roasted	3 oz	210	23	0	53	0	12.6	4.8	71	54%
prime, 1/4-inch fat, raw	1 oz	61	6	0	16	0	4.1	1.6	18	61%
prime, 1/4-inch fat, roasted	3 oz	233	22	0	53	0	15.2	5.9	71	59%
prime, 1/2-inch fat, raw	1 oz	63	5	0	16	0	4.6	1.9	19	65%
prime, 1/2-inch fat, roasted	3 oz	241	22	0	52	0	16.3	6.5	71	61%
select, 1/8-inch fat, raw	1 oz	50	6	0	16	0	2.9	1.2	18	53%
select, 1/8-inch fat, roasted	3 oz	179	23	0	54	0	8.7	3.2	70	44%
select, 1/4-inch fat, raw	1 oz	53	6	0	16	0	3.2	1.3	18	55%
select, 1/4-inch fat, roasted	3 oz	191	23	0	54	0	10.3	3.9	70	49%
ROUND STEAK, lean cuts, raw *(Lean and Free)*	4 oz	111	26	0	60	0	1.1	0.0	0	9%
SHANK CROSSCUTS										
Trimmed										
choice, 1/4-inch fat, raw	1 oz	36	6	0	18	0	1.1	0.4	11	27%
choice, 1/4-inch fat, simmered	3 oz	171	29	0	54	0	5.4	1.9	66	29%
Untrimmed										
choice, 1/4-inch fat, raw	3 oz	150	17	0	51	0	8.4	3.2	37	50%
choice, 1/4-inch fat, simmered	3 oz	224	26	0	52	0	12.5	4.8	68	50%
SIRLOIN, TOP										
Trimmed										
all grades, 0-inch fat, broiled	3 oz	162	26	0	56	0	5.8	2.3	76	32%
all grades, 1/4-inch fat, broiled	3 oz	166	26	0	56	0	6.1	2.4	76	33%
all grades, 1/4-inch fat, raw	1 oz	37	6	0	16	0	1.2	0.4	17	31%
choice, 0-inch fat, broiled	3 oz	170	26	0	56	0	6.6	2.6	76	35%
choice, 1/4-inch fat, broiled	3 oz	172	26	0	56	0	6.8	2.6	76	36%
choice, 1/4-inch fat, pan-fried	3 oz	202	28	0	65	0	9.3	3.4	84	42%
choice, 1/4-inch fat, raw	1 oz	39	6	0	16	0	1.4	0.5	17	33%
select, 0-inch fat, broiled	3 oz	153	26	0	56	0	4.8	1.9	76	28%
select, 1/4-inch fat, broiled	3 oz	158	26	0	56	0	5.3	2.0	76	30%
select, 1/4-inch fat, raw	1 oz	35	6	0	16	0	1.0	0.4	17	27%
Untrimmed										
all grades, 0-inch fat, broiled	3 oz	183	25	0	55	0	8.5	3.3	76	42%
all grades, 1/8-inch fat, broiled	3 oz	211	24	0	54	0	12.0	4.8	77	51%
all grades, 1/8-inch fat, raw	1 oz	58	6	0	15	0	3.8	1.5	19	59%
all grades, 1/4-inch fat, broiled	3 oz	219	24	0	54	0	13.1	5.2	77	54%
all grades, 1/4-inch fat, raw	1 oz	62	5	0	15	0	4.3	1.7	19	63%
choice, 0-inch fat, broiled	3 oz	195	25	0	54	0	9.8	3.9	76	46%
choice, 1/8-inch fat, broiled	3 oz	220	24	0	54	0	13.2	5.2	77	54%
choice, 1/8-inch fat, pan-fried	3 oz	266	24	0	60	0	17.9	7.0	83	61%
choice, 1/8-inch fat, raw	1 oz	60	5	0	15	0	4.1	1.6	19	61%
choice, 1/4-inch fat, broiled	3 oz	229	23	0	53	0	14.2	5.7	77	56%

Food Name	Serving Size	Calories	Prot. gms	Carbs gms	Sod. mgs	Fiber gms	Fat gms	Sat. Fat gms	Chol. mgs	% Fat Cal.
choice, 1/4-inch fat, pan-fried	3 oz	277	24	0	60	0	19.4	7.6	83	63%
choice, 1/4-inch fat, raw	1 oz	64	5	0	15	0	4.6	1.8	19	64%
select, 0-inch fat, broiled	3 oz	166	25	0	55	0	6.4	2.5	76	35%
select, 1/8-inch fat, broiled	3 oz	204	24	0	54	0	11.3	4.5	77	50%
select, 1/8-inch fat, raw	1 oz	55	6	0	15	0	3.5	1.4	19	57%
select, 1/4-inch fat, broiled	3 oz	208	24	0	54	0	11.8	4.7	77	51%
select, 1/4-inch fat, raw	1 oz	59	5	0	15	0	3.9	1.6	19	60%
SIRLOIN STEAK, lean cuts, raw *(Lean and Free)*	4 oz	111	24	0	67	0	1.8	0.0	66	14%
SIRLOIN TIP, lean cuts, raw *(Lean and Free)*	4 oz	110	23	0	62	0	1.2	0.0	66	10%
SPLEEN										
braised	3 oz	123	21	0	48	0	3.6	1.2	295	26%
raw	4 oz	119	21	0	96	0	3.4	1.1	297	26%
STRIP LOIN STEAK, lean cuts, raw *(Lean and Free)*	4 oz	113	25	0	61	0	1.8	0.0	67	14%
T-BONE										
Trimmed										
all grades, 0-inch fat, broiled	3 oz	163	22	0	60	0	7.6	2.6	44	42%
all grades, 1/4-inch fat, broiled	3 oz	173	23	0	60	0	8.3	3.0	48	43%
all grades, 1/4-inch fat, raw	1 oz	42	6	0	16	0	1.8	0.7	14	39%
choice, 0-inch fat, broiled	3 oz	168	22	0	60	0	8.2	2.8	44	44%
choice, 1/4-inch fat, broiled	3 oz	174	23	0	60	0	8.5	3.1	50	44%
choice, 1/4-inch fat, raw	1 oz	44	6	0	16	0	2.1	0.8	16	43%
lean cuts, raw *(Lean and Free)*	4 oz	125	26	0	54	0	2.7	0.0	0	19%
select, 0-inch fat, broiled	3 oz	150	22	0	60	0	6.3	2.3	46	38%
select, 1/4-inch fat, broiled	3 oz	168	23	0	60	0	7.6	2.9	43	41%
select, 1/4-inch fat, raw	1 oz	37	6	0	16	0	1.3	0.5	11	31%
Untrimmed										
all grades, 0-inch fat, broiled	3 oz	210	21	0	57	0	13.5	5.1	48	58%
all grades, 1/8-inch fat, broiled	3 oz	238	21	0	56	0	16.5	6.4	53	63%
all grades, 1/8-inch fat, raw	1 oz	62	5	0	15	0	4.3	1.7	16	63%
all grades, 1/4-inch fat, broiled	3 oz	256	20	0	55	0	18.8	7.4	54	66%
all grades, 1/4-inch fat, raw	1 oz	64	5	0	15	0	4.5	1.8	16	64%
choice, 0-inch fat, broiled	3 oz	217	21	0	57	0	14.4	5.3	48	60%
choice, 1/8-inch fat, broiled	3 oz	243	20	0	56	0	17.3	6.7	55	64%
choice, 1/8-inch fat, raw	1 oz	66	5	0	15	0	4.8	1.9	18	65%
choice, 1/4-inch fat, broiled	3 oz	263	20	0	54	0	19.8	7.7	57	68%
choice, 1/4-inch fat, raw	1 oz	67	5	0	15	0	4.9	2.0	18	66%
select, 0-inch fat, broiled	3 oz	194	21	0	58	0	11.6	4.5	49	54%
select, 1/8-inch fat, broiled	3 oz	225	21	0	56	0	14.9	5.9	48	60%
select, 1/8-inch fat, raw	1 oz	54	6	0	16	0	3.4	1.4	13	56%
select, 1/4-inch fat, broiled	3 oz	238	21	0	56	0	16.5	6.5	49	62%
select, 1/4-inch fat, raw	1 oz	56	6	0	15	0	3.5	1.4	13	57%
TENDERLOIN										
Trimmed										
all grades, 0-inch fat, broiled	3 oz	175	24	0	54	0	8.1	3.0	71	42%
all grades, 1/4-inch fat, broiled	3 oz	179	24	0	54	0	8.5	3.2	71	43%
all grades, 1/4-inch fat, raw	1 oz	45	6	0	15	0	2.2	0.8	18	45%
all grades, 1/4-inch fat, roasted	3 oz	189	24	0	52	0	9.8	3.7	71	47%
choice, 0-inch fat, broiled	3 oz	180	24	0	54	0	8.6	3.2	71	43%
choice, 1/4-inch fat, broiled	3 oz	189	24	0	54	0	9.5	3.6	71	46%
choice, 1/4-inch fat, raw	1 oz	47	6	0	15	0	2.4	0.9	18	47%
choice, 1/4-inch fat, roasted	3 oz	196	24	0	61	0	10.6	4.0	71	49%
fillet steak, lean cuts, raw *(Lean and Free)*	4 oz	116	24	0	68	0	2.4	0.0	61	19%
prime, 1/4-inch fat, broiled	3 oz	197	24	0	54	0	10.5	4.1	71	48%
prime, 1/4-inch fat, raw	1 oz	48	6	0	15	0	2.5	1.0	18	47%

Food Name	Serving Size	Calories	Prot. gms	Carbs gms	Sod. mgs	Fiber gms	Fat gms	Sat. Fat gms	Chol. mgs	% Fat Cal.
prime, 1/4-inch fat, roasted	3 oz	217	23	0	50	0	13.0	5.1	73	54%
prime, short loin, 1/2-inch fat, broiled	3 oz	197	24	0	54	0	10.5	4.1	71	48%
prime, short loin, 1/2-inch fat, roasted.	3 oz	217	23	0	50	0	13.0	5.1	73	54%
select, 0-inch fat, broiled	3 oz	170	24	0	54	0	7.5	2.8	71	40%
select, 1/4-inch fat, broiled	3 oz	169	24	0	54	0	7.4	2.8	71	39%
select, 1/4-inch fat, raw	1 oz	43	6	0	15	0	2.0	0.8	18	42%
select, 1/4-inch fat, roasted	3 oz	179	24	0	52	0	8.8	3.3	71	44%
Untrimmed										
all grades, 0-inch fat, broiled	3 oz	200	23	0	53	0	11.2	4.3	72	50%
all grades, 1/8-inch fat, broiled	3 oz	239	22	0	51	0	16.2	6.3	73	61%
all grades, 1/8-inch fat, raw	1 oz	77	5	0	14	0	6.2	2.5	20	72%
all grades, 1/8-inch fat, roasted	3 oz	275	20	0	48	0	20.9	8.3	72	68%
all grades, 1/4-inch fat, broiled	3 oz	247	21	0	50	0	17.2	6.8	73	63%
all grades, 1/4-inch fat, raw	1 oz	80	5	0	14	0	6.5	2.6	20	73%
all grades, 1/4-inch fat, roasted	3 oz	282	20	0	48	0	21.8	8.6	73	70%
choice, 0-inch fat, broiled	3 oz	207	23	0	52	0	12.2	4.7	72	53%
choice, 1/8-inch fat	3 oz	251	22	0	50	0	17.6	6.9	73	63%
choice, 1/8-inch fat, raw	1 oz	79	5	0	14	0	6.3	2.5	20	72%
choice, 1/8-inch fat, roasted	3 oz	281	20	0	55	0	21.6	8.5	72	69%
choice, 1/4-inch fat, broiled	3 oz	258	21	0	50	0	18.6	7.3	73	65%
choice, 1/4-inch fat, raw	1 oz	82	5	0	14	0	6.7	2.7	20	74%
choice, 1/4-inch fat, roasted	3 oz	288	20	0	55	0	22.4	8.9	73	70%
prime, 1/8-inch fat, broiled.	3 oz	262	21	0	50	0	18.9	7.5	73	65%
prime, 1/8-inch fat, raw	1 oz	78	5	0	14	0	6.2	2.5	20	72%
prime, 1/8-inch fat, roasted	3 oz	292	20	0	47	0	22.7	9.0	75	70%
prime, 1/4-inch fat, broiled.	3 oz	269	21	0	50	0	19.9	7.9	73	67%
prime, 1/4-inch fat, raw	1 oz	81	5	0	14	0	6.5	2.7	20	73%
prime, 1/4-inch fat, roasted	3 oz	300	20	0	47	0	23.7	9.5	75	71%
prime, short loin, 1/2-inch fat, broiled	3 oz	270	21	0	50	0	19.9	8.2	73	66%
prime, short loin, 1/2-inch fat, roasted.	3 oz	304	20	0	47	0	24.4	10.0	75	72%
select, 0-inch fat, broiled	3 oz	195	23	0	53	0	10.6	4.1	72	49%
select, 1/8-inch fat, broiled	3 oz	226	22	0	51	0	14.7	5.8	73	59%
select, 1/8-inch fat, raw	1 oz	76	5	0	14	0	6.0	2.4	20	71%
select, 1/8-inch fat, roasted	3 oz	269	20	0	48	0	20.1	8.0	72	68%
select, 1/4-inch fat, broiled	3 oz	230	22	0	51	0	15.2	6.0	73	60%
select, 1/4-inch fat, raw	1 oz	79	5	0	14	0	6.4	2.6	20	73%
select, 1/4-inch fat, roasted	3 oz	275	20	0	48	0	21.0	8.3	73	69%
THYMUS										
braised	3 oz	271	19	0	99	0	21.2	7.3	250	71%
raw.	4 oz	267	14	0	108	0	23.0	7.9	252	78%
TONGUE										
raw	4 oz	253	17	4	78	0	18.2	7.9	98	65%
raw	1 oz	64	4	1	20	0	4.6	2.0	25	65%
simmered	3 oz	241	19	0	51	0	17.6	7.6	91	66%
TRIPE										
canned (Armour).	6 oz	180	33	1	230	0	4.0	0.0	0	21%
raw	4 oz	111	16	0	52	0	4.5	2.3	107	36%
raw	1 oz	28	4	0	13	0	1.1	0.6	27	36%
BEEF, CORNED. See also under HASH.										
Canned										
cured.	1 oz	71	8	0	285	0	4.2	1.8	24	54%
cured, sliced, 0.75-oz slices	1 slice	53	6	0	211	0	3.1	1.3	18	54%
(Dinty Moore)	2 oz	130	15	0	0	0	8.0	0.0	0	55%

Food Name	Serving Size	Calories	Prot. gms	Carbs gms	Sod. mgs	Fiber gms	Fat gms	Sat. Fat gms	Chol. mgs	% Fat Cal.
Fresh										
brisket, cured, cooked	3 oz	213	15	0	964	0	16.1	5.4	83	68%
brisket, cured, raw	1 oz	56	4	0	35	0	4.2	1.3	15	68%
(Eckrich) 'Slender Sliced'	1 oz	40	6	1	270	0	1.0	0.0	0	24%
(Healthy Deli)	1 oz	35	6	1	210	0	1.0	0.0	11	26%
(Healthy Deli) 'St. Paddy's'	1 oz	24	4	1	290	0	0.4	0.0	7	15%
(Hillshire Farm)	1 oz	31	6	1	230	0	0.4	0.0	0	11%
(Oscar Mayer)	0.6 oz	17	3	0	204	0	0.3	0.2	8	16%
BEEF, CORNED, SPREAD, canned *(Hormel)*	0.5 oz	35	2	0	0	0	3.0	0.0	0	77%
BEEF, DRIED, SLICED										
(Armour)	1.1 oz	60	8	2	0	0	2.0	0.0	0	31%
ground and formed, extra lean *(Hormel)*	10 slices	50	8	1	1240	0	1.5	0.5	25	27%
BEEF DINNER/ENTRÉE. See also BEEF, CORNED; BURRITO; CHILI; CHIMICHANGA; HAMBURGER ENTRÉE MIX; MEAT LOAF DINNER/ENTRÉE; RAVIOLI DISH/ENTRÉE; SANDWICH.										
(Armour)										
pepper steak, frozen, 'Classics Lite'	11.25 oz	220	17	29	970	0	4.0	0.0	35	16%
pot roast, Yankee, frozen, 'Classics'	10 oz	310	25	26	670	0	12.0	0.0	85	35%
Salisbury steak, frozen, 'Classics'	11.25 oz	350	22	26	1430	0	17.0	0.0	55	44%
Salisbury steak, frozen, 'Classics Lite'	11.5 oz	300	21	29	1020	0	2.0	0.0	35	8%
Salisbury steak, Parmigiana frozen, 'Classics'	11.5 oz	410	22	32	1120	0	21.0	0.0	60	47%
sirloin, roast, frozen, 'Classics'	10.45 oz	190	19	21	970	0	4.0	0.0	55	18%
sirloin tips, frozen, 'Classics'	10.25 oz	230	22	20	820	0	7.0	0.0	70	27%
stew, canned	8 oz	210	11	16	1200	0	11.0	0.0	0	48%
stew, microwave	7.5 oz	150	10	15	870	0	5.0	0.0	0	31%
Stroganoff, 'Classics Lite'	11.25 oz	250	18	33	510	0	6.0	0.0	55	21%
(Banquet)										
barbecue beef, homestyle 'Healthy Balance'	10.25 oz	270	14	43	680	0	5.0	3.0	25	16%
barbecue beef, sliced, w/sauce, 'Cookin' Bags'	4 oz	100	9	11	0	0	2.0	0.0	0	18%
beef enchilada and tamale entrée	1 entrée	400	10	56	1530	9	15.0	6.0	30	34%
beef entrée, frozen, 'Extra Helping'	16 oz	870	34	50	810	0	61.0	0.0	120	62%
beef entrée, frozen, 'Platters'	10 oz	460	22	20	630	0	34.0	0.0	75	65%
beef pie, frozen	7 oz	510	12	39	870	0	33.0	0.0	25	59%
beef pie, frozen, 'Supreme Microwave'	7 oz	440	14	30	730	0	29.0	0.0	35	60%
beef w/gravy, potatoes, peas in sauce	1 pkg	270	26	19	742	4	10.0	4.3	71	33%
chicken-fried steak	1 entrée	420	15	39	1200	4	23.0	7.0	35	49%
chopped beef entrée, frozen	11 oz	420	21	14	600	0	32.0	0.0	80	67%
creamed, chipped beef, frozen, 'Cook in' Bags'	4 oz	100	7	9	0	0	4.0	0.0	0	36%
meat loaf entrée *(Banquet)*	1 entrée	280	12	23	1020	3	16.0	6.0	60	51%
patty, charbroiled, w/mushroom and onion gravy, frozen	8 oz	300	12	14	0	0	21.0	0.0	0	65%
patty, charbroiled, w/mushroom gravy, frozen	8 oz	290	13	13	0	0	21.0	0.0	0	65%
patty, w/country-style vegetables	1 entrée	310	11	22	1090	3	20.0	8.0	40	58%
patty, Western style	1 entrée	380	14	28	1400	5	23.0	10.0	40	55%
pot roast 'Yankee'	1 entrée	231	14	20	1134	4	10.0	4.0	60	40%
Salisbury steak, frozen	1 entrée	380	12	28	1140	4	24.0	12.0	60	57%
Salisbury steak, frozen	11 oz	500	23	26	600	0	34.0	0.0	80	61%
Salisbury steak, frozen, 'Extra Helping'	18 oz	910	50	49	740	0	60.0	0.0	175	58%
Salisbury steak, w/gravy, frozen, 'Cookin' Bags'	5 oz	190	9	8	0	0	14.0	0.0	0	65%
Salisbury steak, w/gravy, frozen, 'Family Entrées'	8 oz	300	13	12	0	0	22.0	0.0	0	66%
Salisbury steak, w/gravy, potatoes, corn in sauce	1 pkg	398	15	28	na	3	25.0	8.5	51	57%
Salisbury steak, w/gravy, potatoes, corn in sauce, 'Extra Helping'	1 pkg	782	27	47	2195	7	54.1	21.3	131	62%
Salisbury steak, w/mushroom gravy, frozen, 'Extra Helping'	18 oz	890	51	48	685	0	58.0	0.0	169	57%

Food Name	Serving Size	Calories	Prot. gms	Carbs gms	Sod. mgs	Fiber gms	Fat gms	Sat. Fat gms	Chol. mgs	% Fat Cal.
Salisbury steak, charbroiled, frozen, 'Healthy Balance'....	10.5 oz	270	14	34	800	0	8.0	4.0	35	27%
sliced beef entrée..................................	1 entrée	270	26	19	740	4	10.0	4.5	70	33%
sliced beef, w/gravy, frozen, 'Cookin' Bags'.............	4 oz	100	8	5	0	0	5.0	0.0	0	46%
stew, frozen, 'Family Entrees'.......................	7 oz	140	6	18	0	0	5.0	0.0	0	32%
Stroganoff, homestyle, 'Healthy Balance'...............	11.3 oz	360	13	49	710	0	12.0	5.0	30	30%
Stroganoff sauce, w/noodles, 'Family Entrees'..........	7 oz	190	17	18	0	0	6.0	0.0	0	28%
(Budget Gourmet)										
beef Stroganoff.....................................	1 entrée	250	16	30	580	4	7.0	3.5	35	26%
beef Stroganoff, 'Light'..............................	1 entrée	290	20	32	580	3	7.0	4.0	35	23%
beef Stroganoff, frozen, 'Special Selections'...........	1 entrée	260	18	28	500	3	8.0	4.0	35	28%
meatballs w/gravy, 'Light & Healthy'.................	1 dinner	310	22	37	540	5	8.0	3.0	35	23%
Mexicana, frozen...................................	12.8 oz	560	33	56	1290	0	23.0	0.0	50	37%
Oriental, 'Light'....................................	1 entrée	270	16	35	1070	3	8.0	4.0	35	26%
BEEF pepper steak, w/rice...........................	1 entrée	290	18	38	1060	4	8.0	3.0	40	24%
pot roast, Yankee..................................	1 entrée	230	15	30	650	4	5.0	1.5	30	20%
pot roast, Yankee, frozen...........................	11 oz	380	27	22	690	0	21.0	0.0	70	49%
roast beef w/mashed potato and gravy, frozen..........	1 entrée	340	15	33	890	3	17.0	6.0	40	44%
sirloin, roast, frozen................................	9.5 oz	330	13	36	700	0	14.0	0.0	85	39%
sirloin, roast, frozen, 'Supreme'.....................	1 entrée	300	16	32	850	3	13.0	7.0	65	38%
Salisbury steak....................................	1 entrée	240	16	27	550	2	8.0	3.0	40	30%
Salisbury steak, beef sirloin, 'Light'.................	1 entrée	240	21	28	550	2	5.0	2.0	40	19%
Salisbury steak, w/seasoned potatoes................	1 entrée	240	16	30	570	4	6.0	3.5	45	23%
sirloin, in herb sauce, 'Light'.......................	1 entrée	260	19	30	850	5	7.0	4.0	30	24%
sirloin entrée, frozen, 'Light & Healthy'..............	1 dinner	330	23	40	430	5	8.0	3.0	35	22%
sirloin of beef, special recipe.......................	1 entrée	270	19	36	510	5	5.0	2.0	25	17%
sirloin tips, in burgundy sauce, frozen................	11 oz	310	24	28	720	0	11.0	0.0	65	32%
sirloin tips, w/country style vegetables, frozen.........	10 oz	310	16	21	570	0	18.0	0.0	40	52%
sirloin-cheddar melt w/potato wedges, frozen..........	1 entrée	370	17	29	800	3	21.0	10.0	85	51%
stir-fry w/red potato and vegetables, 'Light & Healthy'....	1 dinner	261	18	34	494	7	5.9	2.0	44	20%
(Bryan Foods) puréed beef.........................	1/3 cup	120	12	0	40	0	7.0	3.0	40	57%
(Castleberry Premium)										
stew..	1 pkg	918	42	56	2781	6	58.5	22.0	156	57%
stew..	1 serving	331	15	20	1002	2	21.1	7.9	56	57%
(Chun King)										
teriyaki beef, frozen................................	13 oz	380	22	68	2200	0	2.0	0.0	0	5%
pepper beef Oriental, frozen........................	13 oz	310	17	53	1300	0	3.0	0.0	0	9%
Szechwan beef, frozen.............................	13 oz	340	20	57	1810	0	3.0	0.0	0	8%
(Cripple Creek)										
beef brisket, choice, chopped, w/sauce...............	3 oz	150	15	6	510	0	9.0	2.1	45	49%
(Dining Lite)										
pepper steak, frozen...............................	9 oz	260	18	33	1050	0	6.0	0.0	40	21%
Salisbury steak, frozen.............................	9 oz	200	18	14	1000	0	8.0	0.0	55	36%
teriyaki beef, frozen................................	9 oz	270	20	36	850	0	5.0	0.0	45	17%
(Dinty Moore)										
beef entrée, packaged, 'Micro Meal'.................	1 bowl	260	15	21	1160	3	13.0	6.0	45	45%
meat loaf, w/gravy and mashed potatoes, canned.......	1 bowl	300	18	27	1160	3	13.0	5.0	40	39%
meat loaf w/mashed potatoes and gravy, 'American Classics'...............................	10 oz	262	18	26	0	0	9.0	0.0	0	32%
roasted beef, w/gravy and mashed potatoes, canned.....	1 bowl	240	24	25	860	2	5.0	2.0	35	19%
roasted beef, w/gravy and potatoes, microwave, 'Classics'.....................................	10 oz	260	26	26	910	0	6.0	3.0	45	21%
stew, canned......................................	1 cup	222	11	16	984	3	13.1	5.6	38	53%
stew, microwave bowl..............................	10 oz	260	15	19	1180	0	14.0	6.0	45	48%
stew, microwave cup...............................	7.5 oz	180	11	15	830	0	9.0	1.0	30	44%

Food Name	Serving Size	Calories	Prot. gms	Carbs gms	Sod. mgs	Fiber gms	Fat gms	Sat. Fat gms	Chol. mgs	% Fat Cal.
(Estee) stew, canned	7.5 oz	210	14	15	65	0	11.0	5.0	30	46%
(Featherweight) stew, canned	7.5 oz	160	17	17	400	0	3.0	0.0	35	17%
(Freezer Queen)										
beef patty, charbroiled, frozen	10 oz	300	17	20	1260	0	17.0	0.0	0	51%
beef patty, charbroiled, w/mushroom and onion gravy, frozen	7 oz	200	13	10	960	0	12.0	0.0	0	54%
beef patty, charbroiled, w/mushroom gravy, frozen	7 oz	180	12	9	1050	0	11.0	0.0	0	54%
beef w/peppers in sauce, w/rice, 'Single Serve'	9 oz	260	21	38	810	0	3.0	0.0	0	10%
creamed, chipped beef, frozen, 'Cook-In-Pouch'	5 oz	80	5	11	500	0	2.0	0.0	0	22%
meat loaf, w/tomato sauce, frozen, 'Family Suppers'	7 oz	230	12	15	850	0	13.0	0.0	0	52%
Salisbury steak, frozen	10 oz	380	18	28	1260	0	22.0	0.0	0	52%
Salisbury steak, w/gravy, frozen, 'Cook-In-Pouch'	5 oz	160	9	7	850	0	11.0	0.0	0	61%
Salisbury steak, w/gravy, frozen 'Family Suppers'	7 oz	200	13	9	1110	0	13.0	0.0	0	57%
Salisbury steak, charbroiled, w/vegetable medley, frozen	9 oz	330	22	14	990	0	22.0	0.0	0	58%
sliced beef w/gravy, frozen	10 oz	210	18	18	1010	0	7.0	0.0	0	30%
sliced beef w/gravy, frozen, 'Cook-In-Pouch'	4 oz	60	9	4	500	0	1.0	0.0	0	15%
sliced beef w/gravy, 'Deluxe Family Suppers'	7 oz	130	15	10	870	0	3.0	0.0	0	21%
sliced beef w/mashed potatoes and carrots	1 pkg	207	15	26	648	4	4.8	1.3	31	21%
stew, frozen, 'Family Suppers'	7 oz	150	9	15	820	0	6.0	0.0	0	36%
(Gebhardt)										
beef tamale	1 serving	134	2	9	385	1	10.3	4.8	14	67%
beef tamale, food service product	1 serving	321	3	26	819	3	24.2	10.8	13	66%
(Green Giant)										
burgers, Italian style, frozen	1 burger	140	17	8	370	5	4.5	1.5	0	29%
burgers, original, frozen	1 burger	140	18	8	380	5	4.0	1.5	0	26%
burgers, Southwest style, frozen	1 burger	140	16	9	370	5	4.0	1.5	0	26%
(Healthy Choice)										
barbecue beef, sirloin w/sauce	11 oz	280	17	44	240	0	4.0	2.0	25	13%
beef Bejing, w/broccoli	1 entrée	300	21	45	420	6	4.5	1.5	25	13%
beef Cantonese, w/peppers	1 entrée	280	22	32	480	5	7.0	3.0	55	23%
beef casserole w/macaroni	1 entrée	220	12	34	450	5	4.0	2.0	20	16%
beef dinner w/mesquite, w/barbecue sauce, mashed potato, corn	1 pkg	320	21	38	491	5	9.0	2.9	3	25%
beef macaroni, frozen	1 serving	211	14	33	444	5	2.2	0.7	14	10%
beef patty, charbroiled	1 entrée	280	16	41	550	7	6.0	3.0	25	19%
beef ribs, boneless, w/barbecue sauce, frozen, 11 oz	1 serving	330	28	40	530	0	6.0	2.0	70	17%
beef Stroganoff	1 entrée	310	19	44	440	3	7.0	3.0	60	20%
beef tips, 'Traditional'	1 entrée	260	20	32	390	6	6.0	3.0	40	21%
beef tips Francais	1 entrée	300	20	40	520	4	7.0	2.5	40	21%
meat loaf, 'Traditional'	1 entrée	330	15	52	460	6	7.0	3.5	35	19%
mesquite barbecue beef	1 entrée	320	21	38	490	5	9.0	3.0	55	26%
pepper steak, frozen	9.5 oz	250	18	36	560	0	4.0	2.0	40	14%
pepper steak, Oriental (Healthy Choice)	1 entrée	260	9	34	520	2	5.0	2.5	35	21%
peppercorn steak patty, grilled	1 entrée	220	16	26	470	5	6.0	2.5	30	24%
pot roast 'Yankee'	1 entrée	290	19	38	460	4	7.0	3.0	55	22%
roasted beef, chopped and formed, 'Fresh Trak'	1 slice	30	5	1	240	0	1.0	0.5	10	27%
Salisbury steak, w/mushroom gravy, mashed potato, corn, frozen	1 entrée	326	18	48	466	6	6.9	3.0	49	19%
sirlion tips, traditional, frozen	1 meal	260	20	32	390	6	5.0	2.0	40	18%
(Hereford)										
roasted beef w/gravy, canned, ready-to-serve	2/3 cup	165	23	12	810	0	3.0	1.0	74	16%
(Hormel)										
beef steak, breaded, frozen	4 oz	370	14	13	0	0	30.0	0.0	0	71%

Food Name	Serving Size	Calories	Prot. gms	Carbs gms	Sod. mgs	Fiber gms	Fat gms	Sat. Fat gms	Chol. mgs	% Fat Cal.
beef w/mushrooms, micro cup, 'Health Selections'	7 oz	210	21	25	390	0	3.0	2.0	45	13%
dried beef, sliced, ground and formed, extra lean	10 slices	50	8	1	1240	0	1.5	0.5	25	27%
stew, microwave cup	7.5 oz	230	13	11	1140	0	15.0	5.0	45	58%
(La Choy)										
beef chow mein, bi-pack	1 cup	105	9	15	756	3	1.7	0.8	12	14%
beef chow mein, canned *(LaChoy)*	3/4 cup	40	5	5	960	2	2.0	0.8	16	31%
beef pepper Oriental, bi-pack	1 cup	104	11	11	1065	3	2.7	1.2	22	21%
beef pepper Oriental, frozen, food service product	1 cup	150	8	30	714	2	0.7	0.2	10	4%
beef w/broccoli and rice, frozen, 'Fresh & Lite'	11 oz	260	17	42	1299	5	5.0	0.0	51	16%
pepper beef, canned	3/4 cup	100	7	12	1340	2	4.0	1.6	9	32%
pepper steak	1 serving	175	10	37	4710	7	0.8	0.0	0	4%
pepper steak, frozen	3.81 oz	36	2	7	942	1	0.2	0.0	0	5%
pepper steak, frozen, w/rice and vegetables, 'Fresh & Lite'	10 oz	280	21	33	1082	2	8.0	0.0	36	25%
teriyaki beef, w/rice and vegetables, frozen, 'Fresh & Lite'	10 oz	240	17	40	1198	2	5.0	0.0	57	17%
(Le Menu)										
pepper steak, frozen	11.5 oz	370	26	36	1020	0	13.0	0.0	0	32%
Salisbury steak, frozen	10.5 oz	370	20	28	880	0	20.0	0.0	0	48%
Salisbury steak, frozen, 'Lightstyle'	10 oz	280	18	31	400	0	9.0	0.0	0	29%
sirloin, chopped, frozen	12.25 oz	430	25	28	1010	0	24.0	0.0	0	50%
sirloin tips, frozen	11.5 oz	400	30	29	760	0	18.0	0.0	0	41%
Stroganoff	10 oz	430	26	28	980	0	24.0	0.0	0	50%
(Lean Cuisine)										
beef chop suey, frozen	1 oz	16	2	2	85	0	0.5	0.1	4	27%
beef Oriental	1 entrée	250	14	30	480	4	8.0	3.0	30	29%
beef patty and whipped potatoes, 'Hearty Portions'	1 entrée	370	28	43	790	7	9.0	4.0	50	22%
beef tips barbecue	1 entrée	290	13	47	560	7	6.0	2.0	30	18%
beef w/peppercorns	1 entrée	220	15	23	580	2	7.0	2.0	35	29%
homestyle beef and noodles, 'Hearty Portions'	1 entrée	330	20	46	780	6	7.0	2.5	45	19%
meat loaf	1 entrée	250	18	30	590	4	6.0	3.0	50	22%
meat loaf, w/macaroni and cheese, frozen	9 3/8 oz	280	26	26	540	0	8.0	3.0	55	26%
meat loaf, w/whipped potatoes	1 entrée	250	22	25	570	5	7.0	2.0	45	25%
Oriental beef, w/vegetables and rice, frozen	1 entrée	242	14	36	497	na	4.8	1.8	23	18%
oven roasted beef	1 entrée	260	18	28	590	4	8.0	3.0	50	28%
pot roast	1 entrée	210	13	25	570	6	6.0	2.0	30	26%
pot roast w/whipped potatoes	1 entrée	210	16	21	570	3	7.0	1.5	40	30%
Salisbury steak, w/gravy, frozen, food service product	1 oz	34	3	2	105	0	1.4	0.6	10	38%
Salisbury steak, w/gravy and scalloped potatoes, frozen	9.5 oz	240	23	22	580	0	7.0	2.0	45	26%
Salisbury steak, w/macaroni and cheese, frozen	1 entrée	270	23	27	590	4	8.0	3.5	60	26%
sirloin, peppercorn, frozen, 'Cafe Classics'	1 pkg	210	13	24	480	4	7.0	1.5	25	30%
(Lean Magic)										
mesquite beef patty, flame-broiled	1 piece	138	18	3	218	1	6.4	2.5	42	42%
Salisbury steak, flame broiled	1 piece	148	17	4	400	1	7.2	2.8	41	44%
Salisbury steak, flame broiled, '30'	1 piece	110	15	4	449	1	3.7	1.2	35	30%
(Libby's)										
beef and macaroni, microwave cup, 'Diner'	7.75 oz	230	10	34	670	3	6.0	3.0	20	23%
roasted beef w/gravy	2/3 cup	140	26	2	801	0	3.0	1.5	70	19%
stew, canned, 15 oz package	7.5 oz	160	12	18	870	0	5.0	0.0	0	27%
stew, microwave cup, 'Diner'	7.75 oz	240	12	22	790	0	12.0	6.0	40	44%
stew, hearty, 'Microeasy' prepared	1/4 pkg	370	31	14	800	0	20.0	0.0	0	50%
(Lunch Bucket) stew, hearty, microwave cup	7.5 oz	180	8	13	870	0	11.0	0.0	40	54%
(Lunch Express) beef Oriental	1 entrée	290	12	43	880	4	8.0	1.0	15	25%

Food Name	Serving Size	Calories	Prot. gms	Carbs gms	Sod. mgs	Fiber gms	Fat gms	Sat. Fat gms	Chol. mgs	% Fat Cal.
(Lloyd's) barbecue beef, w/hickory smoked sauce.........	1/2 cup	200	15	21	980	1	7.0	2.5	35	30%
(Marie Callender's)										
meat loaf, w/mashed potatoes and gravy..............	14 oz	540	23	42	1570	6	30.0	12.0	95	51%
pot roast, old fashioned, w/gravy....................	1 cup	260	17	31	790	3	7.0	3.0	45	25%
Salisbury steak, sirloin, w/gravy....................	14 oz	550	30	51	1680	6	25.0	11.0	85	41%
Yankee pot pie...........................	10-oz pie	690	16	57	1390	3	44.0	10.0	25	58%
(Michelinas) Cantonese chow mein, 'Lean n Tasty'........	1 entrée	250	8	42	1340	3	4.5	1.0	5	17%
(Morton)										
Salisbury steak, frozen..........................	10 oz	300	12	23	1420	0	17.0	0.0	40	52%
sliced beef, frozen...........................	10 oz	220	24	20	950	0	5.0	0.0	65	20%
(Mountain House)										
beef w/rice and onions, freeze-dried, prepared.........	1 cup	330	11	42	265	0	12.0	0.0	0	34%
stew, freeze-dried, prepared......................	1 cup	260	16	26	75	0	9.0	0.0	0	33%
Stroganoff, freeze-dried, prepared.................	1 cup	270	10	26	118	0	13.0	0.0	0	45%
(Myers)										
beef pie, frozen...............................	3.5 oz	123	7	10	343	0	6.0	0.0	0	44%
creamed, chipped beef, frozen....................	3.5 oz	136	9	7	863	0	8.0	0.0	0	53%
Stroganoff...................................	3.5 oz	112	8	7	346	0	6.0	0.0	0	47%
(Nalley's)										
stew, canned, 'Big Chunk'......................	7.5 oz	200	10	24	790	0	7.0	0.0	0	32%
stew, canned, 'Homestyle'.......................	8 oz	180	11	22	810	0	5.0	0.0	0	25%
(Nestlé)										
stew, 'Chef-Mate'.............................	1 pkg	2305	181	228	14285	39	74.0	27.3	394	29%
stew, 'Chef-Mate'.............................	1 cup	192	15	19	1187	3	6.1	2.3	33	29%
(Pathmark) stew, canned, 'No Frills'...................	8 oz	190	10	25	625	0	4.0	0.0	0	20%
(Pierre)										
beef and onion patty, breaded, flame-broiled, frozen, 'Two-Fers'...............	1 piece	96	6	1	129	0	7.8	3.1	18	73%
beef and onion patty, flame-broiled, frozen, product 3879....	1 piece	161	16	2	317	1	9.8	3.9	42	54%
beef and onion patty, flame-broiled, frozen, product 9675....	1 piece	177	15	2	265	1	11.7	4.7	43	60%
beef and onion patty, flame-broiled, frozen, product 9680....	1 piece	473	28	4	636	2	38.4	15.4	90	73%
beef finger, country-fried, frozen, product 3714.........	1 piece	79	4	3	114	0	5.5	1.5	11	63%
beef finger, country-fried, frozen, product 3813.........	1 piece	82	4	4	126	0	5.5	1.4	10	60%
beef finger, country-fried, frozen, product 3814.........	1 piece	100	5	4	121	0	7.0	1.9	15	63%
beef nugget, country-fried, frozen, product 1910........	1 piece	54	2	2	54	0	4.0	1.2	8	66%
beef nugget, country-fried, frozen, product 1935........	1 piece	49	2	2	71	0	3.4	0.9	5	63%
beef nugget, country-fried, frozen, product 3711........	1 piece	47	3	2	76	0	3.1	0.9	8	59%
beef nugget, country-fried, frozen, product 3811........	1 piece	51	3	2	74	0	3.1	1.0	9	55%
beef patty, country-fried, frozen, product 1840..........	1 piece	356	18	16	519	2	24.8	6.5	42	63%
beef patty, country-fried, frozen, product 1845..........	1 piece	292	15	14	427	1	20.3	5.4	31	63%
beef patty, country-fried, frozen, product 3712..........	1 piece	306	17	16	364	1	20.1	5.6	41	59%
beef patty, country-fried, frozen, product 3713..........	1 piece	360	18	17	401	1	24.6	6.5	46	62%
beef patty, country-fried, frozen, product 3812..........	1 piece	304	17	15	479	1	19.9	5.1	38	59%
beef patty, deluxe, flame-broiled, frozen, product 9100.....	1 piece	216	16	2	323	1	15.9	6.4	47	66%
beef patty, deluxe, flame-broiled, frozen, product 9110.....	1 piece	160	12	1	239	1	11.8	4.7	35	66%
beef patty, flame-broiled, frozen, product 3771..........	1 piece	153	16	2	248	1	8.9	3.6	41	53%
beef patty, flame-broiled, frozen, product 3774..........	1 piece	211	23	2	367	1	12.3	4.9	57	53%
beef patty, flame-broiled, frozen, product 3781..........	1 piece	154	17	2	250	1	9.0	3.6	41	53%
beef patty, flame-broiled, frozen, product 3871..........	1 piece	158	16	2	291	1	9.5	3.8	41	54%

Food Name	Serving Size	Calories	Prot. gms	Carbs gms	Sod. mgs	Fiber gms	Fat gms	Sat. Fat gms	Chol. mgs	% Fat Cal.
beef patty, flame-broiled, frozen, product 3874	1 piece	218	22	2	401	1	13.1	5.2	57	54%
beef patty, flame-broiled, frozen, product 3881	1 piece	158	16	2	293	1	9.6	3.8	42	55%
beef patty, flame-broiled, frozen, product 9220	1 piece	186	11	2	313	1	15.1	6.1	31	73%
beef patty, flame-broiled, frozen, product 9230	1 piece	229	13	2	386	2	18.6	7.5	38	73%
beef patty, jalapeño, flame-broiled, product 3778	1 piece	154	16	2	340	1	9.0	3.6	41	53%
beef patty, jalapeño, flame-broiled, frozen, product 3878	1 piece	159	16	2	335	1	9.6	3.8	41	54%
beef patty, less fat, flame-broiled, product 3772	1 piece	143	16	2	298	1	7.9	3.1	36	49%
beef patty, mesquite, deluxe, flame-broiled, frozen, product 9103	1 piece	216	15	2	277	1	16.3	6.5	42	68%
beef patty, mesquite, flame-broiled, frozen, product 3870	1 piece	158	16	2	246	1	9.5	3.8	41	54%
beef patty, mesquite, flame-broiled, frozen, product 3880	1 piece	159	16	2	247	1	9.6	3.8	42	54%
beef patty, mesquite, flame-broiled, product 3770	1 piece	153	16	2	248	1	8.9	3.5	41	53%
beef patty, mesquite, flame-broiled, product 3780	1 piece	154	17	2	250	1	9.0	3.6	41	53%
beef patty w/onions, flame-broiled, product 3779	1 piece	153	16	2	315	1	8.8	3.5	41	52%
beef steak, country-fried, frozen, product 3710	1 piece	315	17	14	494	0	21.0	6.9	59	60%
beef steak, country-fried, frozen, product 1610	1 piece	356	17	14	377	0	25.6	7.9	52	65%
beef steak, country-fried, frozen, product 3810	1 piece	343	21	16	498	0	21.1	6.8	64	55%
beef steak, flame-broiled, frozen, product 9010	1 piece	249	18	0	285	0	18.9	7.6	64	69%
beef steak, flame-broiled, frozen, product 9017	1 piece	237	18	1	360	0	17.4	6.9	64	66%
beef steak, flame-broiled, frozen, product 9503	1 piece	177	16	1	309	0	12.0	4.8	52	61%
beef steak, flame-broiled, product 3760	1 piece	164	16	1	259	0	10.2	4.1	47	56%
beef steak, flame-broiled, product 3765	1 piece	164	16	1	259	0	10.2	4.1	47	56%
beef steak, flame-broiled, product 3860	1 piece	189	17	1	261	0	12.8	5.1	56	61%
beef steak, mesquite, flame-broiled, frozen, product 3863	1 piece	194	17	1	297	0	13.1	5.2	57	61%
beef steak, mesquite, flame-broiled, product 3763	1 piece	169	17	1	295	0	10.5	4.2	48	56%
flame-broiled, frozen, 'Two-Fers' product 9684	1 piece	98	6	1	130	0	7.8	3.1	19	72%
meat loaf, flame-broiled, product 3724	1 piece	162	16	4	363	1	9.1	3.6	41	51%
meat loaf, flame-broiled, product 3725	1 piece	152	16	4	360	1	8.2	3.2	36	48%
meat loaf, flame-broiled, frozen, product 3824	1 piece	170	16	4	364	1	10.1	4.0	44	53%
mesquite beef patty, flame-broiled, less fat, product 3773	1 piece	145	16	3	231	1	7.9	3.1	36	49%
New York strip, flame-broiled, frozen, product 3877	1 piece	164	16	2	340	1	10.2	4.0	44	56%
New York strip, flame-broiled, product 3777	1 piece	159	17	2	345	0	9.5	3.8	44	54%
Salisbury steak, flame-broiled, frozen, product 3820	1 piece	161	16	3	500	1	9.8	3.9	42	55%
Salisbury steak, flame-broiled, frozen, product 9600	1 piece	186	16	2	553	1	12.4	4.9	45	60%
Salisbury steak, flame-broiled, less fat	1 piece	147	16	3	512	1	8.2	3.2	36	50%
Salisbury steak, flame-broiled, product 3720	1 piece	157	16	2	503	0	9.3	3.7	42	53%
(Pillsbury) casserole, frozen, 'Microwave Classic'	1 pkg	430	16	34	1100	0	25.0	0.0	0	53%
(Rib-B-Q)										
beef and onion patty, flame-broiled, frozen, 'Lean Magic'	1 piece	138	17	2	313	1	6.7	2.6	42	44%
beef and turkey barbecue, flame-broiled, frozen, product 9126, 'Lean Magic 30'	1 piece	116	14	8	560	1	3.1	1.0	29	24%
beef and turkey patty, flame-broiled, w/tangy glaze, 'Lean Magic 30'	1 piece	120	17	7	541	1	3.1	1.1	35	23%
beef and turkey patty, flame-broiled, w/teriyaki sauce, 'Lean Magic 30'	1 piece	28	4	2	127	0	0.7	0.2	8	23%
beef barbecue, flame-broiled, frozen, product 3732, 'Lean Magic 30'	1 piece	139	15	4	398	1	7.3	2.9	33	47%
beef patty, flame-broiled, 'Lean Magic'	1 piece	136	18	2	280	1	6.5	2.5	42	43%

Food Name	Serving Size	Calories	Prot. gms	Carbs gms	Sod. mgs	Fiber gms	Fat gms	Sat. Fat gms	Chol. mgs	% Fat Cal.
beef rib barbecue, flame-broiled, frozen, product 3733	1 piece	154	16	3	403	1	8.6	3.4	39	50%
beef rib barbecue, flame-broiled, frozen, product 3833	1 piece	175	16	3	405	1	10.7	4.2	47	55%
beef rib barbecue, flame-broiled, frozen, product 4150	1 piece	204	12	3	387	1	15.9	6.4	35	70%
beef rib barbecue, flame-broiled, frozen, product 3832, 'Lean Magic'	1 piece	156	15	3	400	1	9.0	3.6	39	52%
(Rice A Roni)										
beef and mushroom rice dish, prepared	2.5 oz	164	4	29	714	1	3.4	0.6	0	19%
(Right Course)										
Dijon beef, w/pasta and vegetables, frozen	9.5 oz	290	20	31	580	0	9.0	2.0	40	28%
fiesta, w/corn pasta	8 7/8 oz	270	18	33	590	0	7.0	2.0	30	24%
pot roast, homestyle, frozen	9.25 oz	220	17	22	550	0	7.0	2.0	35	29%
ragout, w/rice pilaf, frozen	10 oz	300	19	38	550	0	8.0	2.0	50	24%
(Steak-Umm) sandwich steak	2 oz	180	9	0	50	0	16.0	0.0	0	80%
(Stouffer's)										
beef pie	1 entrée	450	19	36	1140	3	26.0	9.0	65	52%
beef pot pie	1 pie	415	11	41	740	2	23.0	9.0	25	50%
beef stew, frozen, food service product	1 oz	23	2	2	103	0	1.0	0.3	5	39%
beef Stroganoff, frozen, food service product	1 oz	41	3	1	116	0	2.7	1.0	10	59%
beef Stroganoff w/noodles	1 entrée	390	23	30	1100	2	20.0	7.0	85	46%
creamed chipped beef entrée	1 entrée	160	10	6	690	1	11.0	3.0	40	61%
creamed chipped beef, frozen	1 pkg	435	25	18	1546	na	29.5	12.5	109	61%
creamed chipped beef, frozen	1 serving	175	10	7	621	na	11.9	5.0	44	61%
creamed chipped beef, frozen, food service product	1 oz	40	2	1	156	0	2.8	0.6	9	65%
homestyle beef w/noodles, gravy, vegetable	8 3/8 oz	230	16	26	720	0	7.0	0.0	0	27%
meat loaf, w/whipped potatoes, 'Homestyle'	1 entrée	390	20	24	910	3	24.0	8.0	80	55%
pepper steak, beef w/rice, frozen	10.5 oz	310	20	35	700	0	10.0	0.0	0	29%
Salisbury steak, w/gravy, macaroni and cheese, frozen	9 5/8 oz	350	25	23	1130	0	17.0	0.0	0	44%
Salisbury steak w/gravy, macaroni and cheese, 'Homestyle'	1 pkg	386	23	26	1015	na	21.2	8.0	63	49%
steak w/green pepper *(Stouffer's)*	1 entrée	330	17	45	650	3	9.0	3.0	35	25%
(Swanson)										
barbecue beef w/sauce	11 oz	460	30	51	860	0	17.0	0.0	0	32%
beef enchilada entrée	1 entrée	500	21	68	1220	11	16.0	6.0	25	29%
beef entrée, frozen	11.25 oz	310	26	38	770	0	6.0	0.0	0	17%
beef pot pie, 'Hungry Man'	1 pie	660	24	70	1590	6	31.0	13.0	50	43%
beef w/gravy	1 entrée	370	19	40	700	6	15.0	6.0	40	36%
chopped beef steak, frozen, 'Hungry Man'	16.75 oz	640	35	41	1600	0	37.0	0.0	0	52%
chopped sirloin w/gravy	1 entrée	380	19	37	730	5	14.0	6.0	40	36%
meat loaf	1 entrée	380	19	37	730	5	14.0	6.0	35	36%
Salisbury steak	1 entrée	340	16	35	920	6	15.0	6.0	30	40%
Salisbury steak, frozen, 'Homestyle Recipe'	10 oz	320	21	22	980	0	16.0	0.0	0	46%
Salisbury steak, in gravy, w/mashed potatoes, frozen	1 entrée	330	17	24	1040	3	18.0	10.0	30	50%
Salisbury steak, frozen, 'Hungry Man'	1 entrée	610	34	46	1620	10	33.0	17.0	80	48%
sirloin, chopped, frozen	10.75 oz	340	20	28	790	0	16.0	0.0	0	43%
sirloin tips, in burgundy sauce, frozen, 'Homestyle Recipe'	7 oz	160	12	16	550	0	5.0	0.0	0	29%
sirloin tips, w/noodles and beef gravy, frozen	1 entrée	290	16	34	530	5	11.0	5.0	50	33%
sliced beef, frozen, 'Hungry Man'	15.25 oz	450	37	49	1060	0	12.0	0.0	0	24%
(Top Shelf)										
beef and potatoes, microwave bowl	1 serving	254	29	22	1211	0	6.0	0.0	88	21%
beef entrée, packaged	10 oz	320	25	22	910	0	15.0	7.0	70	42%

Food Name	Serving Size	Calories	Prot. gms	Carbs gms	Sod. mgs	Fiber gms	Fat gms	Sat. Fat gms	Chol. mgs	% Fat Cal.
beef ribs, boneless, packaged, microwave bowl.........	1 serving	440	28	29	550	0	24.0	0.0	90	49%
beef sukiyaki, packaged, microwave bowl.............	1 serving	330	24	36	1700	0	10.0	0.0	45	27%
Oriental beef entrée, packaged, microwave bowl	1 serving	290	25	25	1700	0	10.0	0.0	45	31%
roasted beef, tender, frozen	10 oz	240	28	19	880	0	6.0	2.0	60	22%
roasted beef, tender, packaged, microwave bowl	1 serving	240	27	18	980	0	7.0	0.0	65	26%
Stroganoff, microwave bowl	1 serving	320	29	24	1250	0	12.0	0.0	48	34%
(Tyson)										
champignon, frozen, 'Gourmet Selection'	10.5 oz	370	27	31	830	0	15.0	0.0	0	37%
pepper steak, beef, frozen, 'Gourmet Selection'	11.25 oz	330	20	38	1130	0	11.0	0.0	0	30%
pot roast w/potatoes, 'Homestyle'	1 entrée	270	19	25	640	4	10.0	3.0	40	34%
Salisbury steak, supreme, frozen, 'Gourmet Selection'....	10 oz	430	16	34	810	0	26.0	0.0	0	54%
short ribs in gravy, frozen :......................	9 oz	350	30	12	900	0	20.0	0.0	0	52%
short ribs, frozen, 'Gourmet Selection'	11 oz	470	25	38	950	0	24.0	0.0	0	46%
stir-fry, w/rice, Oriental vegetables, frozen	1 pkg	867	52	142	3167	na	10.0	na	na	10%
stir-fry, w/rice, Oriental vegetables, frozen	1 serving	433	26	71	1584	na	5.0	na	na	10%
(Ultra Slim Fast)										
beef w/mushroom gravy, frozen	10.5 oz	290	19	44	830	0	5.0	0.0	35	15%
meat loaf, beef, w/tomato sauce, frozen	10.5 oz	340	19	52	780	0	9.0	0.0	35	22%
pepper steak, beef, w/parsley rice, frozen.............	12 oz	270	22	36	690	0	4.0	0.0	45	13%
(Weight Watchers)										
beef Cantonese, w/rice, frozen, 'Stir Fry'.............	9 oz	200	14	27	530	0	4.0	1.0	15	18%
beef Romanoff, supreme, w/pasta and vegetables, frozen	9 oz	230	12	29	540	0	7.0	3.0	20	28%
beef stir-fry, frozen, 'Jade Garden'	9 oz	150	13	17	490	0	3.0	2.0	20	18%
London broil, frozen, 'Ultimate 200'..................	7.5 oz	110	17	4	320	0	3.0	1.0	25	24%
London broil, in mushroom sauce, frozen..............	7.37 oz	140	18	9	510	0	3.0	1.0	40	20%
pepper steak	1 entrée	240	18	33	690	4	4.5	1.5	35	17%
Salisbury steak, grilled, w/gravy	1 entrée	260	19	24	620	3	10.0	5.0	40	34%
sirloin tips, frozen, 'Ultimate 200'..................	7.5 oz	200	20	20	560	0	6.0	3.0	30	25%
stew, chunky, microwave cup	7.5 oz	120	14	14	450	0	2.0	1.0	20	14%
(Wolf Brand) stew, canned........................	1 cup	179	10	18	1043	1	7.5	0.0	0	38%
(Yu Sing)										
beef and pepper Oriental, w/rice....................	1 container	230	8	38	820	2	5.0	2.0	10	20%
BEEF DINNER/ENTRÉE MIX. See also HAMBURGER ENTRÉE MIX.										
(Hamburger Helper) meat loaf mix, prepared	1 slice	270	24	11	580	0	14.0	6.0	110	47%
(Lipton)										
meat loaf mix, homestyle, mix only, 'Microeasy'	1/4 pkg	90	4	15	630	0	1.0	0.0	0	11%
meat loaf mix, homestyle, prepared w/ground beef, 'Microeasy'................................	1/4 pkg	390	31	15	700	0	22.0	0.0	0	52%
BEEF JERKY										
chopped and formed.............................	1 oz	116	9	3	627	1	7.3	3.1	14	56%
cured, dried	1 oz	47	8	0	984	0	1.1	0.5	12	21%
(Eagle)										
kippered beefsteak	0.8 oz	50	10	1	550	0	0.5	0.5	20	9%
kippered beefsteak, hot...........................	0.8 oz	50	9	2	560	0	0.5	0.5	20	9%
kippered turkey steak	0.8 oz	60	9	2	580	0	1.5	0.5	20	23%
(Frito-Lay's)										
....	0.21-oz piece	25	3	1	200	0	1.0	0.0	10	36%
'Tender'	0.7 oz	120	5	2	370	0	10.0	0.0	25	76%
(Hickory Farms)	1 oz	100	16	4	1360	0	3.0	0.0	73	25%
(Hormel) 'Lumberjack'	1 oz	101	5	0	304	0	9.0	0.0	0	80%
(Pemmican)										
'Arrowhead'	0.7 -oz piece	70	8	2	580	0	3.0	0.0	0	40%
'Steakers'	0.14-oz piece	40	5	2	160	0	1.0	0.0	0	24%

Food Name	Serving Size	Calories	Prot. gms	Carbs gms	Sod. mgs	Fiber gms	Fat gms	Sat. Fat gms	Chol. mgs	% Fat Cal.
jalapeño..............................	0.25 oz	25	3	1	220	0	1.0	0.0	0	36%
natural................................	0.25 oz	25	3	1	220	0	1.0	0.0	0	36%
peppered...........................	0.25 oz	25	3	1	220	0	1.0	0.0	0	36%
Tabasco............................	0.25 oz	25	3	1	220	0	1.0	0.0	0	36%
'Tender Brave'....................	1 oz	80	14	2	830	0	2.0	0.0	0	22%
'Tender Chief'.....................	1 oz	80	14	2	830	0	2.0	0.0	0	22%
'Tender Tomahawk'..............	0.25 oz	20	3	1	210	0	1.0	0.0	0	36%
'Tender Trail'......................	1 oz	80	14	2	830	0	2.0	0.0	0	22%
'Tender Tribe'.....................	1 oz	80	14	2	830	0	2.0	0.0	0	22%
teriyaki..............................	0.25 oz	20	3	1	200	0	1.0	0.0	0	36%
(Rustlers Roundup).............	5 servings	20	2	1	115	1	1.5	0.5	5	57%
(Slim Jim)										
'Big Jerk'...........................	0.25-oz piece	25	3	1	220	0	1.0	0.0	0	36%
'Giant Jerk'........................	0.63-oz piece	60	7	2	510	0	2.0	0.0	0	33%
	0.14-oz piece	20	2	1	120	0	1.0	0.0	0	43%
regular, 'Super Jerk'...........	0.31-oz piece	30	4	1	250	0	1.0	0.0	0	31%
Tabasco 'Super Jerk'...........	0.31-oz piece	30	4	1	250	0	1.0	0.0	0	31%
(Tumen)										
hot pepperoni style............	1/2 oz	50	5	2	125	1	2.0	0.0	0	39%
smoked ham style..............	1/2 oz	50	5	2	125	1	2.0	0.0	0	39%
spicy Italian style..............	1/2 oz	50	5	2	125	1	2.0	0.0	0	39%

BEEF SEASONING. See under HAMBURGER ENTRÉE MIX; MARINADE; MARINADE MIX; SEASONING MIX.

BEEF STEW. See under BEEF DINNER/ENTRÉE.

BEEF SPREAD

Food Name	Serving Size	Calories	Prot. gms	Carbs gms	Sod. mgs	Fiber gms	Fat gms	Sat. Fat gms	Chol. mgs	% Fat Cal.
(Hormel) roast beef, canned	0.5 oz	31	2	0	0	0	2.0	0.0	0	69%
(Underwood)										
roast beef, canned	2 1/8 oz	140	9	1	360	0	11.0	5.0	45	71%
roast beef, canned, 'Light'........	2 1/8 oz	90	9	2	210	0	6.0	2.0	30	55%
roast beef, canned, mesquite smoked	2 1/8 oz	126	9	1	300	0	11.0	5.0	45	71%

BEEF STICK

Food Name	Serving Size	Calories	Prot. gms	Carbs gms	Sod. mgs	Fiber gms	Fat gms	Sat. Fat gms	Chol. mgs	% Fat Cal.
(Eagle).............................	1 oz	110	7	1	480	0	9.0	5.0	20	72%
(Eagle) pepperoni sausage	1.25 oz	150	10	3	740	0	11.0	5.0	25	66%

BEEF SUBSTITUTE

Food Name	Serving Size	Calories	Prot. gms	Carbs gms	Sod. mgs	Fiber gms	Fat gms	Sat. Fat gms	Chol. mgs	% Fat Cal.
(Heartline)										
lite, vegetarian, 'Beef Fillet Style'	0.5 oz	22	5	1	135	3	0.0	0.0	0	0%
lite, vegetarian, 'Ground Beef Style'	0.5 oz	22	2	1	135	3	0.0	0.0	0	0%
vegetarian, 'Beef Fillet Style'	2 oz	176	19	9	480	0	7.0	0.0	0	36%
vegetarian, 'Ground Beef Style'	2 oz	176	19	9	480	0	7.0	0.0	0	36%
vegetarian, 'Teriyaki Beef Style'	2 oz	176	19	9	450	0	7.0	0.0	0	36%
(Morningstar Farms)										
ground beef substitute, vegetarian, 'Burger Style Recipe Crumbles'.................	2/3 cup	80	10	4	210	2	2.5	0.0	0	28.1%
ground beef substitute, vegetarian, 'Ground Meatless'....	1/2 cup	60	10	4	260	2	0.0	0.0	0	0%
(Worthington)										
beef style, vegetarian, meatless	1 slice	113	9	4	624	3	6.8	1.3	0	54%
corned beef style, vegetarian, roll, frozen.............	2.5 oz	150	12	9	660	0	7.0	1.0	0	43%
corned beef style, vegetarian, frozen, approx 2-oz slices	4 slices	120	9	8	740	0	6.0	1.0	0	44%
ground beef style, vegetarian, 'Burger Crumbles'........	1 pkg	3809	365	109	7855	83	213.1	53.7	0	50%
ground beef style, vegetarian, 'Burger Crumbles'........	1 cup	231	22	7	476	5	12.9	3.3	0	50%
ground beef style, vegetarian, 'Burger Crumbles'........	1 serving	116	11	3	238	3	6.5	1.6	0	50%
roll, vegetarian, frozen, approx 2.5-oz slices...........	4 slices	130	12	7	750	0	6.0	0.0	0	42%
smoked, roll, frozen, approx. 2-oz slices	3 slices	120	10	7	790	0	6.0	0.0	0	44%
steak style, 'Stakelets'.................	1 serving	144	12	6	484	2	8.0	1.4	2	50%

Food Name	Serving Size	Calories	Prot. gms	Carbs gms	Sod. mgs	Fiber gms	Fat gms	Sat. Fat gms	Chol. mgs	% Fat Cal.
(White Wave)										
roast beef style, vegetarian, sandwich sliced	1 slice	90	14	8	270	1	0.0	0.0	0	0%
BEEF SUBSTITUTE DINNER/ENTRÉE										
(Amy's Kitchen)										
burger, vegetarian, 'California'	1 serving	100	4	17	290	3	3.0	0.0	0	24%
burger, vegetarian, organic, frozen	2.5-oz burger	173	6	22	181	1	4.0	0.0	0	24%
Salisbury steak, meatless, 'Country Dinner'	1 entrée	420	12	63	700	9	16.0	5.0	20	32%
(Boca Burger)										
burger, vegetarian, frozen, 'Chef Max's Favorite'	1 burger	110	14	9	296	4	0.0	0.0	0	0%
burger, vegetarian, original, frozen	1 burger	84	12	9	227	5	0.0	0.0	0	0%
(Fantastic Foods)										
burger, tofu, vegetarian, prepared w/o cooking fat	3.4-oz burger	133	11	14	320	0	5.0	0.0	0	31%
(Gardenburger)										
burger, vegetarian, original	2.5 oz	130	8	18	290	5	2.9	1.0	11	20%
burger, vegetarian, soy-free	2.5 oz	140	8	21	180	5	2.5	0.5	0	16%
burger, Greek, classic, vegetarian, 'Gourmet'	2.5 oz	121	6	17	306	2	2.9	1.4	8	22%
hamburger style, vegetarian, low-fat	2.5 oz	115	16	7	381	3	2.6	0.8	4	20%
veggie medley patty, vegetarian	2.5 oz	100	6	17	280	3	0.7	0.1	0	6%
zesty bean patty, vegetarian	2.5 oz	120	7	19	290	5	2.5	1.0	10	18%
(Green Giant)										
burger, vegetable protein, vegetarian, original, 'Harvest Burger'	1 pkg	552	72	28	1654	23	16.7	4.1	0	27%
burger, vegetable protein, vegetarian, original, 'Harvest Burger'	1 patty	137	18	7	411	6	4.1	1.0	0	27%
burger, vegetarian, all-vegetable, Southwestern style, 'Harvest Burger'	1 patty	140	16	9	370	5	4.0	1.5	0	26%
(Heartline) burger, vegetarian, meatless	4 oz	176	19	9	480	5	7.0	0.0	0	36%
(Ken & Robert's)										
burger, vegetarian.	1 serving	130	5	26	260	3	1.0	0.0	0	7%
burger, vegetarian, frozen, 2.5 oz, 'Truly Amazing'	1 patty	110	5	19	390	0	2.0	0.0	0	16%
(Legume)										
stew, beef style	1 cup	150	10	29	450	5	0.0	0.0	0	0%
tamale, beef style, vegetarian, low-fat	3 tamales	220	10	40	350	3	2.5	0.0	0	10%
(Loma Linda)										
burger, vegetarian, dry mix, 'Patty Mix'	1/3 cup	90	14	7	480	5	1.0	0.0	0	10.0%
dinner loaf, dry mix, 'Savory Dinner Loaf'	1/3 cup	90	14	7	560	5	1.5	0.0	0	15.0%
(Love Natural Foods)										
burger, vegetarian, prepared, 'Loveburger'	4-oz burger	245	17	20	224	8	11.0	0.0	0	40%
(Morningstar Farms)										
burger, vegetarian, 'Better'N Burgers'	1 patty	80	13	8	360	3	0.0	0.0	0	0%
burger, vegetarian, 'Grillers'	1 patty	140	15	5	260	2	6.0	1.0	0	38.5%
burger, vegetarian, 'Hard Rock Café All-Natural Veggie Burgers'	1 patty	170	6	18	340	3	8.0	1.0	0	42.3%
burger, vegetarian, 'Harvest Burgers' Italian style	1 patty	140	17	8	370	5	4.5	1.5	0	28.9%
burger, vegetarian, 'Harvest Burgers' original flavor	1 patty	140	18	8	370	5	4.0	1.5	0	25.7%
burger, vegetarian, 'Harvest Burgers' Southwestern style. .	1 patty	140	16	9	370	5	4.0	1.5	0	25.7%
burger, vegetarian, 'Harvest Burgers' recipe crumbles	1/2 cup	70	12	5	200	3	0.0	0.0	0	0%
burger, vegetarian, frozen, 'Oven Roasted Veggie Burgers'	1 patty	120	14	40	400	2	8.0	3.5	10	60%
burger, vegetarian, 'Quarter Prime'	1 patty	140	24	6	370	3	2.0	0.0	0	12.8%
burger, vegetarian, and cheese, 'Stuffed Sandwiches'	1 sandwich	290	14	10	400	2	8.0	3.5	10	24.8%
(Natural Touch)										
burger, vegetarian, 'Hard Rock Cafe All Natural Veggie Burgers'	1 patty	170	6	18	340	3	8.0	1.0	0	42.3%
burger, vegetarian, 'Vegan Burger'	1 patty	70	11	6	370	3	0.0	0.0	0	0%

Food Name	Serving Size	Calories	Prot. gms	Carbs gms	Sod. mgs	Fiber gms	Fat gms	Sat. Fat gms	Chol. mgs	% Fat Cal.
'Loaf Mix' dry mix	4 tbsp	100	14	10	700	7	0.5	0.0	0	4.5%
'Stroganoff Mix' dry mix	4 tbsp	90	5	10	610	3	3.5	2.0	10	35.0%
(Naturally Tofu) burger, vegetarian, meatless	4 oz	165	20	25	52	9	2.0	0.5	0	9%
(Nature's Burger)										
burger, vegetarian, prepared w/o cooking fat, 'Original'	3-oz burger	152	7	21	228	0	4.0	0.0	0	24%
burger, barbecue, vegetarian, prepared w/o cooking fat	3-oz burger	117	4	24	423	0	0.8	0.0	0	6%
burger, pizza, vegetarian, prepared w/o cooking fat	3-oz burger	121	5	24	406	0	1.0	0.0	0	7%
(Tempeh) burger, soy and rice, vegetarian, frozen	2 2/3 oz	140	12	13	0	5	5.0	0.5	0	31%
(White Wave)										
burger, vegetarian, 'Veggielife'	1 serving	130	6	20	250	3	3.5	0.0	0	23%
tempeh burger, vegetarian	1 serving	110	12	10	270	6	2.5	0.0	0	20%
(Worthington)										
burger, vegetarian, 'FriPats'	1 patty	132	15	4	323	4	6.3	0.9	2	43%
burger, vegetarian, 'Vegetarian Burger'	1/4 cup	60	9	2	270	1	2.0	0.0	0	30%
'Meatless Corned Beef' 72-oz roll	3/8-inch slice	130	9	4	510	2	9.0	1.0	0	62.3%
'Meatless Corned Beef' 8-oz carton	4 slices	140	10	5	520	2	9.0	1.0	0	57.9%
'Meatless Smoked Beef'	6 slices	120	11	6	730	3	6.0	1.0	0	45.0%
pie, vegetarian, frozen	8 oz	360	9	44	1940	0	16.0	0.0	0	40%
stew, vegetarian, 'Country Stew'	1 cup	210	13	20	830	5	9.0	1.0	0	38.6%
roast, vegetarian, 'Dinner Roast'	3/4-inch slice	180	12	5	580	3	12.0	1.5	<5	60.0%
sliced, vegetarian, 'Savory Slices'	3 slices	150	10	6	540	3	9.0	3.5	0	54.0%
steak, vegetarian, 'Prime Stakes'	1 piece	136	9	4	445	4	9.3	1.4	2	61%
steak, vegetarian, 'Stakelets'	1 piece	140	12	6	480	2	8.0	1.0	0	51.4%
steak, vegetarian, 'Vegetable Steaks'	2 slices	80	15	3	300	3	1.5	0.5	0	16.9%
BEEF SUBSTITUTE DINNER/ENTRÉE MIX										
(Fantastic Foods)										
Stroganoff, creamy, 'Tofu Classics' mix only	1/2 cup	190	10	35	660	3	5.0	3.0	5	20%
(Loma Linda) vegetarian 'Vita-Burger Chunks'	1/4 cup	75	10	6	353	4	1.1	0.3	0	13%
(Tofu Classics)										
Stroganoff, creamy, vegetarian, prepared w/tofu	1/2 cup	94	7	11	264	0	3.0	0.0	0	27%
Stroganoff, creamy, vegetarian, prepared w/tofu, 2 tbsp salted butter	1/2 cup	127	7	11	310	0	7.0	0.0	0	47%
BEEF SUBSTITUTE JERKY										
original flavor, meatless (Pemmican)	1 pkg	420	17	59	90	9	13.0	2.0	0	28%
vegetarian, 'Spicy Italian Style' (Cajun Jerky)	0.5 oz	50	5	2	125	1	2.0	0.0	0	39%
vegetable protein, 'Jerquee' (Stonewall's)	0.5 oz	50	5	2	125	1	2.0	0.0	0	39%
BEEF TALLOW										
	1 cup	1849	0	0	0	0	205.0	102.1	223	100%
	1 tbsp	115	0	0	0	0	12.8	6.4	14	100%
BEEFALO										
composite of cuts, raw	1 oz	41	7	0	22	0	1.4	0.6	12	30%
composite of cuts, roasted	3 oz	160	26	0	70	0	5.4	2.3	49	30%
BEER AND ALE										
ALE										
(McSorley's)	12 fl oz	166	2	15	6	0	0.0	0.0	0	0%
(Tiger Head)	12 fl oz	166	2	15	6	0	0.0	0.0	0	0%
BEER										
	12 fl oz	146	1	13	18	1	0.0	0.0	0	0%
light	12 fl oz	99	1	5	11	0	0.0	0.0	0	0%
(Anheuser Marzen)	12 fl oz	168	2	15	12	0	0.0	0.0	0	0%
(Beck's)	12 fl oz	148	2	10	14	0	0.0	0.0	0	0%
(Budweiser)										
	12 fl oz	144	1	11	12	0	0.0	0.0	0	0%
light, 'Bud Light'	12 fl oz	110	1	7	12	0	0.0	0.0	0	0%

Food Name	Serving Size	Calories	Prot. gms	Carbs gms	Sod. mgs	Fiber gms	Fat gms	Sat. Fat gms	Chol. mgs	% Fat Cal.
(Busch)	12 fl oz	144	1	12	12	0	0.0	0.0	0	0%
(Carlsberg)										
. . . .	12 fl oz	149	1	12	12	0	0.0	0.0	0	0%
light	12 fl oz	110	1	7	12	0	0.0	0.0	0	0%
(Coors)										
. . . .	12 fl oz	137	1	12	1	0	0.0	0.0	0	0%
'Coors Dry'	12 fl oz	119	0	6	1	0	0.0	0.0	0	0%
'Extra Gold'	12 fl oz	151	1	13	1	0	0.0	0.0	0	0%
light, 'Coors Light'	12 fl oz	103	1	5	1	0	0.0	0.0	0	0%
3.2%										
. . . .	12 fl oz	119	1	10	1	0	0.0	0.0	0	0%
3.2%, 'Coors Dry'	12 fl oz	101	1	5	1	0	0.0	0.0	0	0%
3.2%, 'Extra Gold'	12 fl oz	121	1	10	1	0	0.0	0.0	0	0%
3.2, light, 'Coors Light'	12 fl oz	98	1	5	1	0	0.0	0.0	0	0%
(Cutter) nonalcoholic	12 fl oz	76	1	20	1	0	0.0	0.0	0	0%
(Dribeck's)	12 fl oz	94	1	7	14	0	0.0	0.0	0	0%
(Kaliber) nonalcoholic	12 fl oz	71	1	11	3	0	0.0	0.0	0	0%
(Keystone)										
. . . .	12 fl oz	121	1	7	1	0	0.0	0.0	0	0%
'Keystone Dry'	12 fl oz	121	1	6	1	0	0.0	0.0	0	0%
light, 'Keystone Light'	12 fl oz	100	1	4	1	0	0.0	0.0	0	0%
3.2%	12 fl oz	104	1	6	1	0	0.0	0.0	0	0%
3.2%, light, 'Keystone Light'	12 fl oz	99	0	5	1	0	0.0	0.0	0	0%
(Killian's)										
. . . .	12 fl oz	161	1	15	1	0	0.0	0.0	0	0%
3.2%	12 fl oz	128	1	11	1	0	0.0	0.0	0	0%
(Knickerbocker)	12 fl oz	140	1	12	9	0	0.0	0.0	0	0%
(LA) light alcohol	12 fl oz	114	1	16	12	0	0.0	0.0	0	0%
(Lite)										
. . . .	12 fl oz	96	1	3	6	0	0.0	0.0	0	0%
'Genuine Draft'	12 fl oz	98	1	4	6	0	0.0	0.0	0	0%
(Lowenbrau)										
'Dark Special'	12 fl oz	158	1	14	7	0	0.0	0.0	0	0%
'Special'	12 fl oz	158	1	14	7	0	0.0	0.0	0	0%
(Meister Brau)										
. . . .	12 fl oz	141	1	13	6	0	0.0	0.0	0	0%
light	12 fl oz	98	1	4	6	0	0.0	0.0	0	0%
(Michelob)										
. . . .	12 fl oz	156	2	14	12	0	0.0	0.0	0	0%
'Classic Dark'	12 fl oz	158	2	14	12	0	0.0	0.0	0	0%
'Dry'	12 fl oz	133	1	8	12	0	0.0	0.0	0	0%
light	12 fl oz	134	1	12	12	0	0.0	0.0	0	0%
(Miller)										
'Genuine Draft'	12 fl oz	147	1	13	7	0	0.0	0.0	0	0%
'High-Life'	12 fl oz	147	1	13	7	0	0.0	0.0	0	0%
'Magnum'	12 fl oz	162	1	10	8	0	0.0	0.0	0	0%
(Milwaukee)										
'Milwaukee's Best'	12 fl oz	133	1	11	6	0	0.0	0.0	0	0%
'Milwaukee's Best Light'	12 fl oz	98	1	4	6	0	0.0	0.0	0	0%
(Natural Light) light	12 fl oz	110	1	7	12	0	0.0	0.0	0	0%
(O'Doul's) nonalcoholic	12 fl oz	70	1	15	0	0	0.0	0.0	0	0%
(Prior) 'Double Dark'	12 fl oz	171	1	15	10	0	0.0	0.0	0	0%
(Rheingold)										
. . . .	12 fl oz	148	1	13	9	0	0.0	0.0	0	0%

Food Name	Serving Size	Calories	Prot. gms	Carbs gms	Sod. mgs	Fiber gms	Fat gms	Sat. Fat gms	Chol. mgs	% Fat Cal.
light	12 fl oz	96	1	3	7	0	0.0	0.0	0	0%
(Rolling Rock)										
light	12 fl oz	104	0	8	1	0	0.0	0.0	0	0%
'Premium'	12 fl oz	145	0	10	1	0	0.0	0.0	0	0%
(Schmidt's)										
. . . .	12 fl oz	148	1	13	9	0	0.0	0.0	0	0%
'Classic'	12 fl oz	144	1	13	10	0	0.0	0.0	0	0%
light	12 fl oz	96	1	3	7	0	0.0	0.0	0	0%
(Sharp's) nonalcoholic	12 fl oz	86	1	10	5	0	0.0	0.0	0	0%
BEET										
Fresh										
boiled, drained, whole, approx 2-inch diam.	2 med beets	44	2	10	77	2	0.2	0.0	0	3%
boiled, drained, sliced	1/2 cup	37	1	8	65	2	0.2	0.0	0	3%
raw, sliced	1 cup	58	2	13	106	4	0.2	0.0	0	3%
raw, whole, approx 2-inch diam.	1 med beet	35	1	8	64	2	0.1	0.0	0	3%
Canned										
cut (Stokely)	1/2 cup	40	1	8	300	0	0.0	0.0	0	0%
diced (S&W)	1/2 cup	40	1	9	270	0	0.0	0.0	0	0%
diced (Stokely)	1/2 cup	35	1	7	300	0	0.0	0.0	0	0%
diced, drained	1 cup	49	1	11	305	3	0.2	0.0	0	4%
Harvard (Green Giant)	1/3 cup	60	1	15	270	2	0.0	0.0	0	0%
Harvard (Stokely)	1/2 cup	70	1	18	135	0	0.0	0.0	0	0%
Harvard, sliced, w/liquid	1 cup	180	2	45	399	6	0.1	0.0	0	1%
no salt, 'No Salt or Sugar Added' (Stokely)	1/2 cup	40	1	8	40	0	0.0	0.0	0	0%
no salt, w/liquid	1 cup	69	2	16	52	3	0.2	0.0	0	2%
pickled (Freshlike)	1/2 cup	40	1	9	650	0	0.0	0.0	0	0%
pickled (Stokely)	1/2 cup	100	1	25	400	0	0.0	0.0	0	0%
pickled (Veg-All)	1/2 cup	100	1	25	650	0	0.0	0.0	0	0%
pickled, crinkle sliced, w/liquid (Del Monte)	1/2 cup	80	1	19	375	0	0.0	0.0	0	0%
pickled, sliced, w/liquid	1 cup	148	2	37	599	6	0.2	0.0	0	1%
pickled, sliced, w/red wine vinegar, 'Party' (S&W)	1 oz	15	0	4	50	1	0.0	0.0	0	0%
pickled, sliced, w/red wine vinegar, regular (S&W)	1/2 cup	70	1	16	215	0	0.0	0.0	0	0%
pickled, whole (S&W)	1 oz	15	0	4	50	1	0.0	0.0	0	0%
pickled, whole, extra small (S&W)	1/2 cup	70	1	16	215	0	0.0	0.0	0	0%
regular pack, w/liquid	1 cup	69	2	16	620	3	0.2	0.0	0	2%
shredded, drained	1 cup	60	2	14	378	3	0.3	0.0	0	4%
sliced (A&P)	1/2 cup	40	1	9	300	0	1.0	0.0	0	18%
sliced (Featherweight)	1/2 cup	45	1	10	55	0	0.0	0.0	0	0%
sliced (Finast)	1/2 cup	40	1	9	390	0	0.0	0.0	0	0%
sliced (Green Giant)	1/2 cup	35	1	8	260	2	0.0	0.0	0	0%
sliced (Pathmark)	1/2 cup	45	1	10	330	0	0.0	0.0	0	0%
sliced (Stokely)	1/2 cup	40	1	8	300	0	0.0	0.0	0	0%
sliced, no salt added (A&P)	1/2 cup	35	1	8	50	0	1.0	0.0	0	20%
sliced, no salt added (Finast)	1/2 cup	40	1	9	40	0	0.0	0.0	0	0%
sliced, no salt added (Green Giant)	1/2 cup	35	1	8	60	2	0.0	0.0	0	0%
sliced, no salt added (Pathmark)	1/2 cup	35	1	7	35	0	0.0	0.0	0	0%
sliced, 'Nutradiet' (S&W)	1/2 cup	35	1	9	40	0	0.0	0.0	0	0%
sliced, drained	1 cup	53	2	12	330	3	0.2	0.0	0	4%
sliced, drained	1 slice	2	0	1	16	0	0.0	0.0	0	4%
sliced, small (Freshlike)	1/2 cup	40	1	9	260	0	0.0	0.0	0	0%
sliced, small, tender, 'Premium' (S&W)	1/2 cup	40	1	9	270	0	0.0	0.0	0	0%
sliced, water packed, w/o salt (Freshlike)	1/2 cup	40	1	9	50	0	0.0	0.0	0	0%
sliced, water packed, w/o sugar or salt (Freshlike)	1/2 cup	40	1	9	50	0	0.0	0.0	0	0%
sliced, w/liquid, no salt added (Del Monte)	1/2 cup	35	1	8	100	0	0.0	0.0	0	0%

Food Name	Serving Size	Calories	Prot. gms	Carbs gms	Sod. mgs	Fiber gms	Fat gms	Sat. Fat gms	Chol. mgs	% Fat Cal.
whole (A&P)	1/2 cup	40	1	9	300	0	1.0	0.0	0	18%
whole (Green Giant)	1/2 cup	35	1	8	260	2	0.0	0.0	0	0%
whole (IGA)	1/2 cup	40	1	9	275	0	0.0	0.0	0	0%
whole (Stokely)	1/2 cup	40	1	8	300	0	0.0	0.0	0	0%
whole, baby, 'LeSueur' (Green Giant)	1/2 cup	35	1	8	260	2	0.0	0.0	0	0%
whole, drained	1 beet	7	0	2	47	0	0.0	0.0	0	4%
whole, drained	1 cup	51	1	12	316	3	0.2	0.0	0	4%
whole, small (Freshlike)	1/2 cup	40	1	9	260	0	0.0	0.0	0	0%
Jarred										
pickled (Stokely)	1/2 cup	90	1	22	280	0	0.0	0.0	0	0%
pickled, sliced (Stokely)	1 oz	25	0	6	100	0	0.0	0.0	0	0%
pickled, whole (Stokely)	1 oz	25	0	6	100	0	0.0	0.0	0	0%
BEET GREENS										
boiled, drained, 1-inch pieces	1 cup	39	4	8	347	4	0.3	0.0	0	6%
boiled, drained, 1-inch pieces	1/2 cup	19	2	4	174	2	0.1	0.0	0	6%
raw	1 cup	7	1	2	76	1	0.0	0.0	0	3%
raw	1 med leaf	6	1	1	64	1	0.0	0.0	0	3%
raw, 1-inch pieces	1/2 cup	4	0	1	38	1	0.0	0.0	0	3%
BEET ROOT JUICE (Biotta) bottled	6 fl oz	75	2	16	128	0	0.1	0.0	0	1%
BELL PEPPER. See PEPPER, BELL.										
BELLYFISH. See MONKFISH.										
BERRIES. See also individual listings.										
mixed, Oregon, frozen (Flav-R-Pac)	4.9 oz	70	1	16	20	6	0.0	0.0	0	0%
BISCOTTI										
chocolate chip, gluten-free (Ener-G Foods)	1 serving	122	1	17	136	0	5.1	1.3	0	39%
orange walnut, gluten-free (Gluten Free Pantry)	1 serving	110	1	22	25	1	2.5	0.0	0	20%
plain, gluten-free (Ener-G Foods)	1 serving	81	1	11	96	0	3.3	0.7	0	38%
BISCUIT										
dough, mixed-grain	1 oz	75	2	13	190	na	1.6	0.4	0	19%
dough, mixed-grain, baked, 2.25-inch diam	1 biscuit	116	3	21	295	na	2.5	0.6	0	19%
dough, plain or buttermilk	1 oz	90	2	12	314	0	3.8	1.0	0	37%
dough, plain or buttermilk, baked	1 oz	98	2	13	341	0	4.2	1.1	0	38%
dough, plain or buttermilk, baked, 2.25-inch diam	1 biscuit	93	2	13	325	0	4.0	1.0	0	38%
dough, plain or buttermilk, less fat	1 oz	73	2	13	354	0	1.3	0.3	0	15%
dough, plain or buttermilk, less fat, baked	1 oz	85	2	16	411	1	1.5	0.4	0	16%
dough, plain or buttermilk, less fat, baked, 2.25-inch diam	1 biscuit	63	2	12	305	0	1.1	0.3	0	16%
(Awrey's)										
2-inch square	1 oz	80	2	12	260	0	3.0	1.0	0	33%
3-inch square	2 oz	160	4	23	520	1	5.0	1.0	0	29%
(Bridgford) frozen	2 oz	180	4	28	632	0	6.0	0.0	1	30%
(Ballard)										
light, oven-ready, 'Extra Lights'	1 piece	50	1	10	180	0	0.0	0.0	0	0%
(Big Country)										
butter	1 biscuit	100	2	13	300	0	4.0	1.0	0	38%
'Butter Tastin"	1 piece	100	2	14	320	0	4.0	1.0	0	36%
buttermilk	1 biscuit	100	2	14	300	0	4.0	1.0	0	36%
Southern style	1 biscuit	100	2	14	300	0	4.0	1.0	0	36%
(1869 Brand)										
baking powder	1 biscuit	100	2	12	300	0	5.0	1.5	0	45%
'Butter Tastin"	1 piece	100	2	12	300	0	5.0	1.0	0	45%
buttermilk	1 biscuit	100	2	12	300	0	5.0	1.5	0	45%
(Good 'N Buttery)										
fluffy	1 biscuit	90	1	11	270	0	5.0	1.0	0	48%

Food Name	Serving Size	Calories	Prot. gms	Carbs gms	Sod. mgs	Fiber gms	Fat gms	Sat. Fat gms	Chol. mgs	% Fat Cal.
(Hungry Jack)										
buttermilk, 'Extra Rich'	1 piece	50	1	9	180	0	1.0	1.0	0	18%
flaky	2 biscuits	170	3	23	600	1	7.0	1.5	0	38%
flaky, 'Honey Tastin''	2 biscuits	180	3	25	580	1	7.0	1.5	0	36%
flaky, Southern style	1 biscuit	80	2	12	300	0	4.0	1.0	0	39%
fluffy	2 biscuits	180	3	23	570	1	8.0	2.0	0	41%
(Lite Fluff) buttermilk, ready to bake, Texas style	1 biscuit	90	2	16	250	0	2.5	0.5	0	24%
(Mrs. Wright's)										
butter-flavored, ready to bake, 'Jumbos'	1 biscuit	180	4	24	360	2	9.0	2.5	0	42%
butter-flavored, ready to bake, Texas style	1 biscuit	100	2	15	260	1	3.0	1.0	0	28%
buttermilk, ready to bake, 'Jumbos'	1 biscuit	180	4	23	360	2	9.0	2.5	0	43%
buttermilk, ready to bake, Texas style	1 biscuit	90	2	16	250	0	2.5	0.5	0	24%
(Pillsbury)										
'Big Premium Heat 'n Eat'	2 biscuits	280	5	32	610	0	15.0	3.0	0	48%
butter, 'Grands'	1 biscuit	200	4	23	580	1	10.0	2.5	0	45%
buttermilk, 'Grands'	1 biscuit	200	4	23	570	1	10.0	3.0	0	45%
buttermilk, 'Heat 'n Eat'	2 biscuits	170	4	27	530	0	5.0	1.0	0	27%
buttermilk, light, 'Extra Lights'	3 biscuits	150	4	29	490	1	2.0	0.0	0	12%
cinnamon-raisin	1 biscuit	200	4	28	580	1	8.0	2.0	0	36%
flaky, 'Grands'	1 biscuit	190	4	23	530	0	8.0	2.0	0	40%
home style, 'Grands'	1 biscuit	190	4	24	600	1	9.0	2.5	0	42%
Southern style 'Grands'	1 biscuit	200	4	23	580	1	10.0	2.5	0	45%
w/cinnamon and raisin, 'Grands'	1 biscuit	190	3	27	540	0	7.0	2.0	0	34%
(Roman Meal)										
	2 biscuits	180	4	32	456	1	3.8	0.9	0	19%
oat bran, w/honey and nuts	1 biscuit	131	2	20	278	1	4.7	1.2	0	32%
white, 'Premium'	1 biscuit	127	2	19	308	0	4.7	1.2	0	33%
(Stilwell) buttermilk, 3-inch diam	1 biscuit	210	4	30	370	0	9.0	2.5	0	37%
(Wonder)	1 piece	80	2	14	140	1	1.0	0.0	0	12%
BISCUIT, TOASTER										
(Northridge) English muffin	1 muffin	80	2	16	135	0	1.0	0.0	0	11%
(Oroweat) 'Australian'	1 biscuit	180	6	30	440	1	5.0	1.0	0	24%
(Oroweat) w/cinnamon and raisin	1 biscuit	200	5	34	410	1	5.0	1.0	0	22%
BISCUIT DOUGH										
buttermilk, artificial flavor, refrigerated *(Pillsbury)*	1 serving	154	5	30	547	na	1.4	0.3	na	8%
BISCUIT MIX										
plain or buttermilk, dry mix	1 cup	548	10	81	1633	3	19.7	5.1	3	32%
plain or buttermilk, dry mix	1 oz	121	2	18	362	1	4.4	1.1	1	32%
plain or buttermilk, prepared	1 oz	95	2	14	271	1	3.4	0.8	1	33%
plain or buttermilk, prepared, 3-inch diam	1 biscuit	191	4	28	544	1	6.9	1.6	2	33%
(Arrowhead Mills)	2 oz	100	4	19	96	0	1.0	0.0	0	9%
(Bisquick)	1/2 cup	240	4	37	700	0	8.0	2.0	0	31%
(Bisquick)	1/3 cup	170	3	25	481	1	6.0	1.5	0	33%
(Gold Medal)	1/3 cup	170	3	26	470	1	6.0	2.0	0	32%
(Health Valley) buttermilk, 'Biscuit & Pancake Mix'	1 oz	100	4	20	170	3	1.0	0.0	0	9%
(Kentucky Kernel) all natural, dry mix	1/4 cup	171	3	28	659	1	5.0	1.0	0	27%
(Krusteaz)										
prepared, 2-inch diam	1 biscuit	90	2	14	260	0	3.0	0.7	1	30%
w/cinnamon and raisin, glazed, prepared, 3-inch diam	1 biscuit	200	2	39	150	1	4.0	0.0	0	18%
(Martha White)										
'BixMix' prepared w/2% milk	1 biscuit	90	2	15	240	0	2.0	0.0	2	21%
buttermilk, dry mix	1 serving	171	3	26	504	na	5.9	1.1	na	31%
(Robin Hood) 'Pouch Mix' 0.7 oz mix prepared w/skim milk	1/8 mix	90	2	14	270	0	3.0	1.0	0	30%

Food Name	Serving Size	Calories	Prot. gms	Carbs gms	Sod. mgs	Fiber gms	Fat gms	Sat. Fat gms	Chol. mgs	% Fat Cal.
(Tone's) buttermilk	1 tsp	1	0	0	1	0	0.0	0.0	0	0%
BISON / American buffalo										
raw	1 oz	31	6	0	15	0	0.5	0.2	18	15%
ribeye, trimmed to 0-inch fat, raw	1 oz	33	6	0	14	na	0.7	0.3	18	19%
ribeye, trimmed to 0-inch fat, raw	4 oz	131	25	0	54	na	2.7	1.0	70	19%
roasted	3 oz	122	24	0	48	0	2.1	0.8	70	15%
roasted, boneless, yield from 1 lb raw	11.9 oz	486	97	0	194	0	8.2	3.1	279	15%
shoulder, trimmed to 0-inch fat	4 oz	123	24	0	67	na	2.4	0.8	75	17%
shoulder, trimmed to 0-inch fat, raw	1 oz	31	6	0	17	na	0.6	0.2	19	17%
top round, trimmed to 0-inch fat, raw.	1 oz	31	6	0	14	na	0.5	0.2	19	13%
top round, trimmed to 0-inch fat, raw.	4 oz	124	25	0	58	na	1.8	0.7	75	13%
BITTER GOURD. See BALSAM PEAR.										
BITTER LEMON. See under SOFT DRINKS AND MIXERS.										
BLACK BEAN. See BEAN, BLACK.										
BLACK CHERRY JUICE										
(Knudsen)	8 fl oz	180	2	43	40	na	0.0	0.0	0	0%
(Smucker's) 'Naturally 100%'	8 fl oz	130	0	31	10	0	0.0	0.0	0	0%
BLACK CURRANT. See under CURRANT.										
BLACK PEPPER. See under PEPPER, GROUND.										
BLACK TURTLE BEAN. See BEAN, BLACK.										
BLACKBERRIES										
Canned, in heavy syrup, w/liquid	1 cup	236	3	59	8	9	0.4	0.0	0	1%
Fresh, raw	1 cup	75	1	18	0	8	0.6	0.0	0	6%
Frozen										
Marion *(Flav-R-Pac)*	1 cup	80	2	19	5	7	0.0	0.0	0	0%
unsweetened	18-oz pkg	326	6	80	5	26	2.2	0.1	0	6%
unsweetened	1 cup	97	2	24	2	8	0.6	0.0	0	6%
BLACKBERRY SYRUP. See under SYRUP.										
BLACK-EYED PEAS / cowpeas										
Canned										
(Allens)	1/2 cup	100	7	18	370	0	1.0	0.0	0	8%
Crowder, 'Fresh' *(Allens)*	1/2 cup	80	5	15	370	0	1.0	0.0	0	10%
Crowder, frozen *(Seabrook)*	3 oz	130	8	23	0	1	1.0	0.0	0	7%
Crowder, seasoned w/pork, canned *(Luck's)*	1/2 cup	120	6	18	280	4	3.0	1.0	3	22%
Crowder, Southern, mature seeds, boiled, drained	1 cup	200	13	36	7	11	0.9	0.2	0	4%
Crowder, Southern, mature seeds, w/pork	1 cup	199	7	40	840	8	3.8	1.5	17	17%
immature seeds, drained.	1 cup	160	5	34	7	8	0.6	0.2	0	3%
mature *(A&P)*	7.5 oz	120	7	20	410	0	1.0	0.0	0	8%
mature *(Allens)*	1/2 cup	105	5	18	300	0	1.0	0.0	0	9%
mature *(Green Giant)*	1/2 cup	90	7	18	300	4	1.0	0.0	0	8%
mature *(Joan of Arc)*	1/2 cup	90	7	18	300	4	1.0	0.0	0	8%
packed from fresh shelled *(Bush's Best)*	1/2 cup	70	5	16	350	3	0.0	0.0	0	0%
packed from soaked dry *(Bush's Best)*	1/2 cup	70	5	16	350	3	0.0	0.0	0	0%
seasoned w/bacon *(Bush's Best)*	1/2 cup	90	7	16	420	3	1.0	0.0	0	9%
seasoned w/pork *(Luck's)*	1/2 cup	130	6	18	280	3	3.0	1.0	3	22%
'Sun-Vista' *(S&W)*	1/2 cup	70	6	15	550	4	0.0	0.0	0	0%
w/jalapeño peppers *(Ranch Style)*	1/2 cup	110	6	19	660	4	0.5	0.0	5	4%
w/snaps *(Allens)*	1/2 cup	100	5	20	370	0	1.0	0.0	0	8%
Dried										
Catjang, mature seeds, boiled, drained	1 cup	200	14	35	32	6	1.2	0.3	0	5%
Catjang, mature seeds, uncooked	1 cup	573	40	100	97	18	3.5	0.9	0	5%
Crowder, Southern, mature seeds, uncooked.	1 cup	561	39	100	27	18	2.1	0.6	0	3%
Crowder, Southern, mature seeds, uncooked.	1 tbsp	35	2	6	2	1	0.1	0.0	0	3%
immature seeds, uncooked.	1 cup	131	4	27	6	7	0.5	0.1	0	3%

Food Name	Serving Size	Calories	Prot. gms	Carbs gms	Sod. mgs	Fiber gms	Fat gms	Sat. Fat gms	Chol. mgs	% Fat Cal.
mature, boiled (A&P)	1 cup	230	15	41	15	0	1.0	0.0	0	4%
Fresh										
leafy tips, boiled, drained, chopped	1 cup	12	2	1	3	na	0.1	0.0	0	4%
leafy tips, raw, chopped	1 cup	10	1	2	3	na	0.1	0.0	0	7%
leafy tips, raw, whole	1 med leaf	1	0	0	0	na	0.0	0.0	0	8%
young pods w/seeds, boiled, drained	1 cup	32	2	7	3	na	0.3	0.1	0	7%
young pods w/seeds, raw, chopped	1 cup	41	3	9	4	na	0.3	0.1	0	6%
young pods w/seeds, raw, whole	1 med pod	5	0	1	0	na	0.0	0.0	0	6%
Frozen										
(Flav-R-Pac)	1/2 cup	110	7	21	10	4	1.0	0.0	0	7%
(Freshlike)	3.3 oz	130	9	23	5	0	1.0	0.0	0	7%
(Frosty Acres)	3.3 oz	130	9	23	6	1	1.0	0.0	0	7%
(Pictsweet)	1/2 cup	110	7	21	10	4	1.0	0.0	0	7%
(Seabrook)	3.3 oz	130	9	23	6	1	1.0	0.0	0	7%
(Southern)	3.5 oz	136	9	24	20	0	0.7	0.0	0	5%
(Veg-All)	3.3 oz	130	9	23	5	0	1.0	0.0	0	7%
immature seeds, drained	1 cup	224	14	40	9	11	1.1	0.3	0	4%
immature seeds, unprepared	10-oz pkg	395	26	71	17	14	2.0	0.5	0	4%
immature seeds, unprepared	1 cup	222	14	40	10	8	1.1	0.3	0	4%
BLINTZ										
apple, kosher (Empire Kosher)	2 blintzes	220	6	36	260	5	5.5	1.5	5	23%
blueberry (Golden)	1 crepe	90	2	18	150	0	1.0	0.0	10	10%
blueberry, kosher (Empire Kosher)	2 blintzes	190	4	36	260	2	4.0	1.0	10	18%
cheese, kosher (Empire Kosher)	2 blintzes	200	11	29	310	3	6.0	2.0	20	25%
cheese, low-fat (Golden)	1 crepe	80	6	13	135	0	2.0	0.5	13	19%
cherry (Golden)	1 crepe	95	3	18	145	0	1.0	0.0	5	10%
cherry, kosher (Empire Kosher)	2 blintzes	200	5	38	280	3	4.0	1.0	10	17%
potato, kosher (Empire Kosher)	2 blintzes	190	6	32	530	3	6.0	1.5	10	26%
BLUE CRAB. See under CRAB.										
BLUEBERRIES										
Canned, in heavy syrup, w/liquid	1 cup	225	2	56	8	4	0.8	0.1	0	3%
Fresh										
raw	1 pint	225	3	57	24	11	1.5	0.1	0	6%
raw	50 berries	38	0	10	4	2	0.3	0.0	0	6%
Frozen										
sweetened	10-oz pkg	230	1	62	3	6	0.4	0.0	0	1%
sweetened, thawed	1 cup	186	1	50	2	5	0.3	0.0	0	1%
unsweetened	20-oz pkg	289	2	69	6	15	3.6	0.3	0	11%
unsweetened, unthawed	1 cup	79	1	19	2	4	1.0	0.1	0	11%
(Flav-R-Pac)	1 cup	70	1	16	10	4	0.0	0.0	0	0%
BLUEBERRY JUICE. See also FRUIT DRINK, FRUIT DRINK MIX; FRUIT JUICE BLEND.										
mountain blueberry, organic (Mountain Sun)	8 fl oz	108	0	27	0	0	0.0	0.0	0	0%
BLUEBERRY TOPPING (Flav-R-Pac)	2 tbsp	40	0	10	5	1	0.0	0.0	0	0%
BLUEFIN TUNA. See under TUNA.										
BLUEFISH										
baked, broiled, grilled, or microwaved	3 oz	135	22	0	65	0	4.6	1.0	65	31%
raw	3 oz	105	17	0	51	0	3.6	0.8	50	31%
BOAR, WILD										
raw	1 oz	35	6	0	na	0	0.9	0.3	na	25%
roasted	3 oz	136	24	0	51	0	3.7	1.1	65	25%
roasted, boneless, yield from 1 lb raw	11.9 oz	544	96	0	204	0	14.9	4.4	262	25%
BOBWHITE. See QUAIL.										
BOK CHOY / Chinese cabbage / napa cabbage / pak-choi / pe-tsai										
boiled, drained	1 leaf	2	0	0	1	0	0.0	0.0	0	10%

Food Name	Serving Size	Calories	Prot. gms	Carbs gms	Sod. mgs	Fiber gms	Fat gms	Sat. Fat gms	Chol. mgs	% Fat Cal.
boiled, drained, shredded	1 cup	20	3	3	58	3	0.3	0.0	0	11%
fresh, shredded *(Dole)*	1/2 cup	5	1	1	23	0	0.1	0.0	0	10%
raw	1 head	109	13	18	546	8	1.7	0.2	0	13%
raw	1 leaf	2	0	0	9	0	0.0	0.0	0	13%
raw, shredded	1 cup	12	1	2	7	2	0.2	0.0	0	10%
BORAGE, raw, 1-inch pieces	1 cup	19	2	3	71	na	0.6	0.2	0	28%
BORECOLE. See KALE.										
BORLOTTI. See BEAN, CRANBERRY.										
BOYSENBERRIES										
Canned, in heavy syrup	1 cup	225	3	57	8	7	0.3	0.0	0	1%
Frozen										
(Flav-R-Pac)	1 cup	59	2	20	18	7	0.0	0.0	0	0%
unsweetened	10-oz pkg	142	3	35	3	11	0.7	0.0	0	4%
unsweetened	1 cup	66	1	16	1	5	0.3	0.0	0	4%
BOYSENBERRY JUICE (Smucker's) 'Naturally 100%'	8 fl oz	120	0	30	10	0	0.0	0.0	0	0%
BRAMBLE. See RASPBERRY.										
BRATWURST. See under SAUSAGE.										
BRAZIL NUT / paranut										
dried, unblanched, approx 6-8 kernels	1 oz	186	4	4	1	2	18.8	4.6	0	84%
dried, unblanched, shelled, approx 32 kernels	1 cup	918	20	18	3	8	92.7	22.6	0	84%
BREAD										
ALFALFA SPROUT										
(Vermont Bread Company)										
. . . .	1 slice	80	2	15	115	2	1.0	0.0	0	12%
'Sandwich'	1 slice	90	3	17	130	2	1.5	0.0	0	14%
APPLE WALNUT *(Arnold)*	1 slice	64	2	13	103	1	1.3	0.0	1	17%
APPLE HONEY *(Brownberry)* wheat	1 slice	69	2	11	148	2	1.9	0.0	0	24%
AUSTRIAN *(Du Jour)* brown and serve	1 oz	70	3	13	140	1	1.0	0.0	0	12%
BARBECUE *(Colombo Brand)* 'BBQ Loaf'	2 oz	139	8	24	318	0	1.6	0.0	0	10%
BRAN										
(Brownberry)										
'Bran'nola'	1 slice	85	4	18	137	3	1.4	0.0	0	13%
whole, 'Natural'	1 slice	58	2	12	167	2	1.4	0.0	0	18%
w/raisins	1 slice	61	2	12	108	2	1.3	0.0	0	17%
(Earth Grains) 'Gold'N Bran'	1 oz	70	3	12	150	0	1.0	0.0	0	13%
(Oroweat) original, natural, 'Bran'nola'	1 slice	100	4	19	160	2	1.0	0.0	0	9%
(Pepperidge Farm) honey, 1.5-lb loaf	1 slice	90	3	18	160	1	1.0	0.0	0	10%
BROWN										
canned	1 slice	88	2	19	284	2	0.7	0.1	0	6%
canned	1 oz	55	1	12	179	1	0.4	0.1	0	6%
(B&M)										
plain, 1/2-inch slice	1 slice	92	2	21	345	2	0.0	0.0	0	0%
w/raisins, 1/2-inch slice *(B&M)*	1 slice	94	2	22	320	2	0.0	0.0	0	0%
(Friends)										
plain, 1/2-inch slice	1 slice	92	2	21	345	2	0.0	0.0	0	0%
w/raisins, 1/2-inch slice *(Friends)*	1 slice	94	2	22	320	2	0.0	0.0	0	0%
(S&W) canned, 'New England'	2 slices	76	2	17	172	0	0.0	0.0	0	0%
BROWN RICE										
(Ener-G Foods)										
gluten free	1 slice	122	1	20	25	1	4.3	0.2	1	32%
gluten free, yeast-free	1 slice	154	1	25	282	3	3.5	0.3	0	23%
(Mystic Lake Dairy) wheat gluten-free	1 slice	155	2	22	0	0	6.0	0.0	0	36%

Food Name	Serving Size	Calories	Prot. gms	Carbs gms	Sod. mgs	Fiber gms	Fat gms	Sat. Fat gms	Chol. mgs	% Fat Cal.
BUTTERMILK										
(Grant's Farm)	1 slice	70	3	12	190	0	1.0	0.0	0	13%
(Oroweat)	1 slice	100	4	20	210	1	1.0	0.0	0	9%
CINNAMON RAISIN										
(Arizona Original Homestyle) 100% stone ground	1 slice	116	4	23	130	2	0.0	0.0	0	0%
(Arnold)	1 slice	67	2	13	86	1	1.4	0.0	2	17%
(Pepperidge Farm)	1 slice	90	2	16	100	2	2.0	0.0	0	20%
CINNAMON OATMEAL (Oatmeal Goodness)	1 slice	90	4	15	140	1	2.0	0.0	0	19%
CINNAMON SWIRL (Pepperidge Farm)	1 slice	90	2	15	110	2	3.0	0.0	0	28%
DARK (Hollywood)	1 slice	70	3	13	160	1	1.0	0.0	0	12%
DATE										
(Dromedary) date nut roll	1/2-inch slice	80	1	13	160	0	2.0	0.0	0	24%
(Thomas') date nut loaf	1 oz	80	1	15	160	1	2.5	0.0	5	26%
EGG										
5x3x1/2-inch slices	1 slice	115	4	19	197	1	2.4	0.6	20	19%
(Ener-G Foods) gluten-free	1 slice	176	3	23	83	1	6.8	0.7	7	38%
FLAXSEED (Natural Ovens) 'Flax 'N Honey'	1 slice	70	3	15	70	3	0.5	0.0	0	6%
FRENCH										
large slices, approx 5 x 2-1/2 x 1 inch	1 slice	96	3	18	213	1	1.1	0.2	0	10%
medium slices, approx 4-3/4 x 4 x 1/2 inch	1 slice	69	2	13	152	1	0.8	0.2	0	10%
small slices, approx 2-1/2 x 2 x 1/2 inch	1 slice	41	1	8	91	0	0.5	0.1	0	10%
(Colombo Brand)										
extra sour	2 oz	150	8	27	311	0	1.3	0.0	0	8%
sweet, 'French Stick'	2 oz	154	7	27	331	0	1.9	0.0	0	11%
(DiCarlo) 'Parisian'	1 slice	70	3	13	180	1	1.0	0.0	0	12%
(Du Jour) brown and serve	1 oz	70	3	13	140	1	1.0	0.0	0	12%
(Farm Hearth) twin loaves	1 oz	80	3	15	160	0	1.0	0.0	0	11%
(Monterey Baking) high-fiber, low-calorie	1 slice	48	2	10	98	3	0.1	na	0	2%
(Pepperidge Farm)										
enriched	1 slice	130	4	25	280	1	1.5	1.0	0	10%
enriched, twin loaves	1 slice	130	4	26	270	1	1.5	0.5	0	10%
'Hearth'	1 oz	75	3	14	160	1	1.0	0.0	0	12%
(Pillsbury)	1 slice	150	6	28	370	1	1.0	0.0	0	6%
GARLIC										
(Campione) frozen	1 serving	101	2	12	154	1	4.7	0.8	na	42%
(Cole's) mini-loaf, ready-to-serve	1.8 oz	180	4	21	290	1	8.0	2.0	2	42%
(Colombo Brand)	2 oz	185	6	17	331	0	10.1	0.0	0	49%
(Mamma Bella)										
frozen	2 slices	150	3	16	240	1	8.0	2.0	0	49%
sliced	2 slices	160	3	16	260	1	9.0	2.5	5	52%
(Marie Callender's) original	1 piece	190	4	25	290	2	8.0	2.0	0	38%
(Pepperidge Farm)										
crusty, Italian	1 serving	186	4	21	200	na	9.6	2.4	5	46%
heat and serve	1.7 oz	170	4	19	240	3	9.0	2.5	20	47%
HAWAIIAN (King's Hawaiian Bread)	2 oz	180	6	30	160	2	4.0	1.0	20	20%
HEALTH (Brownberry) 'Health Nut'	1 slice	71	2	12	158	3	2.6	0.0	0	28%
HONEY WHEAT BERRY (Arnold)	1 slice	77	3	17	143	2	1.2	0.0	0	12%
HONEY BRAN (Pepperidge Farm)	1 slice	90	3	18	160	1	1.0	0.0	0	10%
HONEY NUT (Roman Meal) w/rice bran	1 slice	71	3	13	127	1	1.6	0.0	0	19%
INDIAN FRY										
Navajo, 10.5-inch diam	1 serving	526	11	85	1112	3	15.2	3.7	0	26%
Navajo, 5-inch diam	1 serving	296	6	48	626	2	8.6	2.1	0	26%
ITALIAN										
large slices, approx 4-1/2 x 3-1/4 x 3/4 inch	1 slice	81	3	15	175	1	1.1	0.3	0	11%

Food Name	Serving Size	Calories	Prot. gms	Carbs gms	Sod. mgs	Fiber gms	Fat gms	Sat. Fat gms	Chol. mgs	% Fat Cal.
medium slices	1 slice	54	2	10	117	1	0.7	0.2	0	11%
small slices, approx 3-1/4 x 2-1/2 x 1/2 inch	1 slice	27	1	5	58	0	0.3	0.1	0	11%
(Arnold)										
'Francisco International'	1 slice	72	3	14	190	1	1.1	0.0	0	13%
'Francisco International' sliced thick	1 slice	66	2	14	111	1	0.8	0.0	0	10%
light, 'Bakery'.	1 slice	45	2	10	90	2	0.5	0.0	0	8%
(Brownberry) 'Light'	1 slice	44	2	10	89	2	0.5	0.0	0	8%
(Monk's) 'Hi-Fibre'	1 slice	70	3	13	80	1	1.0	0.0	0	12%
(Monterey Baking) twist	1 slice	71	2	15	148	0	0.2	0.1	0	3%
(Pepperidge Farm)										
enriched, brown and serve	1 slice	130	4	24	260	1	2.0	1.0	0	14%
'Hearth'	1 oz	80	2	14	150	0	1.0	0.0	0	12%
(Wonder) 'Family'	1 slice	70	2	13	160	1	1.0	0.0	0	13%
LIGHT (Hollywood)	1 slice	70	3	13	150	1	1.0	0.0	0	12%
MILLET, 'Sunny Millet' (Natural Ovens)	1 slice	50	3	15	80	7	0.0	0.0	0	0%
MIXED GRAIN										
7-grain, w/whole grain, large slices	1 slice	80	3	15	156	2	1.2	0.3	0	13%
7-grain, w/whole-grain, medium slices	1 slice	65	3	12	127	2	1.0	0.2	0	13%
(Arizona Original Homestyle) 9-grain, 100%										
stone-ground	1 slice	94	4	23	102	2	0.0	0.0	0	0%
(Arnold) bran, nutty, 'Bran'nola'	1 slice	85	4	17	144	3	1.6	0.0	0	14%
(Aunt Hattie's) 7-grain	1 slice	100	4	17	200	0	2.0	0.0	0	18%
(Beefsteak) multigrain	1 slice	70	3	11	130	2	1.0	0.0	0	14%
(BreadMill Bakery) 5-grain, organic	1 slice	122	6	23	298	0	1.0	0.0	0	7%
(Brownberry) bran, 'Bran'nola Nutty Grains'	1 slice	85	4	17	144	3	1.6	0.0	0	14%
(Colonial) w/honey, 'Family Recipe'	1 slice	70	3	14	180	0	1.0	0.0	0	12%
(Earth Grains) 12-grain	1 oz	70	3	13	140	0	1.0	0.0	0	12%
(Food for Life) multigrain, w/wheat, rice, and almond,										
gluten-free	1 slice	120	5	22	5	0	2.5	0.0	0	17%
(Grant's Farm)										
7-grain	1 slice	60	3	13	140	0	1.0	0.0	0	12%
7-grain, 'Light'	1 slice	40	2	9	115	0	1.0	0.0	0	17%
w/honey	1 slice	70	3	13	170	0	1.0	0.0	0	12%
(Healthy Choice)										
multigrain.	1 slice	60	3	12	120	2	0.5	0.0	0	7%
7-grain	1 slice	80	4	18	170	3	1.0	0.0	0	9%
(Home Pride) 7-grain	1 slice	70	3	12	140	1	1.0	0.0	0	13%
(Kilpatrick's) w/honey, 'Family Recipe'	1 slice	70	3	14	180	0	1.0	0.0	0	12%
(Monterey Baking)										
9-grain.	1 slice	111	4	23	220	1	0.4	0.1	0	3%
9-grain, low salt	1 slice	111	4	23	50	1	0.4	0.1	0	3%
(Natural Ovens)										
7-grain.	1 slice	70	3	15	70	3	0.5	0.0	0	6%
whole wheat, flax, millet, and soy, 'Stay Trim'	1 slice	50	2	15	90	7	0.0	0.0	0	0%
(Oroweat)										
9-grain, 'Light'	1 slice	40	2	10	135	2	0.0	0.0	0	0%
12-grain.	1 slice	110	5	20	210	1	2.0	0.0	0	15%
(Pepperidge Farm)										
multigrain, granola, w/oat and honey	1 slice	60	2	12	105	2	2.0	0.0	0	24%
7-grain, 'Hearty Slice'	2 slices	180	5	36	340	2	2.0	0.0	0	10%
(Rainbo) w/honey, 'Family Recipe'	1 slice	70	3	14	180	0	1.0	0.0	0	12%
(Roman Meal)										
multigrain, 'Round Top'	1 slice	67	3	13	140	1	0.8	0.0	0	10%
multigrain, sliced, sandwich thin	1 slice	55	2	11	114	1	0.7	0.0	0	11%

Food Name	Serving Size	Calories	Prot. gms	Carbs gms	Sod. mgs	Fiber gms	Fat gms	Sat. Fat gms	Chol. mgs	% Fat Cal.
multigrain, 'Sun Grain'	1 slice	68	3	12	140	2	1.4	0.0	0	17%
(Rudi's) 'Ancient Grain Bread'	1 slice	85	3	14	215	0	2.0	0.0	0	21%
(Vermont Bread Company) 'Soft 10'	1 piece	90	3	16	130	2	2.0	0.0	0	19%
(Weight Watchers) multigrain	1 slice	40	2	9	100	0	1.0	0.0	0	17%
NUT (Oroweat) 'Health Nut'	1 slice	110	4	20	200	2	2.0	0.0	0	16%
OAT										
(Colonial) split top, 'Family Recipe'	1 slice	70	3	13	140	0	1.0	0.0	0	12%
(Earth Grains) w/honey and nuts	1 oz	80	3	14	85	0	2.0	0.0	0	21%
(Kilpatrick's) split top, 'Family Recipe'	1 slice	70	3	13	140	0	1.0	0.0	0	12%
(Oroweat) light, 'Country Oat'	1 slice	40	2	10	135	2	0.0	0.0	0	0%
(Pepperidge Farm)										
hearty, crunchy	1 slice	100	4	17	180	2	2.0	0.0	0	18%
honey granola	1 slice	60	2	12	105	2	2.0	0.0	0	24%
(Rainbo) split top 'Family Recipe'	1 slice	70	3	13	140	0	1.0	0.0	0	12%
OAT BRAN										
	1 slice	71	3	12	122	1	1.3	0.2	0	16%
lower calorie	1 slice	46	2	9	81	3	0.7	0.1	0	14%
(Awrey's)	1 slice	50	2	10	130	1	0.0	0.0	0	0%
(BreadMill Bakery)										
organic, 'Light'	1 slice	113	4	22	229	0	1.0	0.0	0	8%
w/honey, whole wheat, organic	1 slice	121	5	23	315	0	1.0	0.0	0	7%
(Earth Grains) w/honey	1 oz	80	3	13	105	0	1.0	0.0	0	12%
(Grant's Farm)	1 slice	70	3	14	140	0	1.0	0.0	0	12%
(Monterey Baking)										
	1 slice	100	3	18	160	3	1.5	0.0	0	14%
low-salt	1 slice	99	4	16	50	3	4.1	0.7	0	32%
(Oatmeal Goodness) 'Light'	1 slice	40	2	6	90	0	1.0	0.0	0	22%
(Oroweat) natural, 'Bran'nola Country'	2 slices	230	8	39	390	3	4.0	1.0	0	16%
(Roman Meal)										
'Split-Top'	1 slice	68	3	13	140	1	0.9	0.0	0	11%
w/honey	1 slice	71	3	13	130	1	1.2	0.0	0	15%
w/honey and nut	1 slice	72	3	12	130	1	1.6	0.0	0	19%
(Vermont Bread Company)										
w/oatmeal, low-sodium	1 slice	70	2	14	120	2	1.0	0.0	0	12%
w/oatmeal, 'Sandwich Bread'	1 slice	100	3	18	120	2	1.5	0.0	0	14%
(Weight Watchers)	1 slice	40	1	10	100	0	1.0	0.0	0	17%
OATMEAL										
	1 slice	73	2	13	162	1	1.2	0.2	0	14%
lower calorie	1 slice	48	2	10	89	na	0.8	0.1	0	14%
(Arnold) light, 'Bakery'	1 slice	44	2	10	98	2	0.6	0.0	0	10%
(Grant's Farm) w/toasted almonds	1 slice	80	3	14	135	0	1.0	0.0	0	12%
(Hearty Grains) twists	1 serving	80	2	15	120	1	2.0	0.0	0	21%
(Oatmeal Goodness)										
cinnamon	1 slice	90	4	15	140	1	2.0	0.0	0	19%
w/bran	1 slice	90	4	15	140	1	2.0	0.0	0	19%
w/sunflower seeds	1 slice	90	4	15	140	1	2.0	0.0	0	19%
	1 slice	90	3	17	200	1	1.0	0.2	0	10%
'Light Style'	1 slice	45	2	9	95	1	0.0	0.0	0	0%
1.5 lb. loaf	1 slice	90	3	17	200	1	1.0	0.0	0	10%
'Very Thin'	1 slice	40	1	8	80	0	1.0	0.0	0	20%
OATNUT (Oroweat)	1 slice	100	3	18	200	1	2.0	0.0	0	18%
ORANGE RAISIN (Brownberry)	1 slice	67	2	13	83	1	1.2	0.0	0	15%
PITA										
white, large, 6.5-inch diam	1 pita	165	5	33	322	1	0.7	0.1	0	4%

Food Name	Serving Size	Calories	Prot. gms	Carbs gms	Sod. mgs	Fiber gms	Fat gms	Sat. Fat gms	Chol. mgs	% Fat Cal.
white, small, 4-inch diam.	1 pita	77	3	16	150	1	0.3	0.0	0	4%
whole wheat, large, 6.5-inch diam.	1 pita	170	6	35	340	5	1.7	0.3	0	8%
whole wheat, small, 4-inch diam.	1 pita	74	3	15	149	2	0.7	0.1	0	8%
(Kangaroo) w/onion, nonfat, sliced, no oils	1 pita	75	4	15	160	0	0.0	0.0	0	0%
(Sahara)										
oat bran	1/2 piece	66	2	15	163	2	0.3	0.0	0	4%
100% whole wheat	1 pita	130	7	28	310	5	1.0	0.0	0	6%
original	1 pita	150	6	31	290	1	1.0	0.0	0	6%
sourdough	1 pita	150	5	33	320	2	0.5	0.0	0	3%
white	1/2 piece	79	3	16	147	0	0.5	0.0	0	6%
white, mini	1 slice	79	3	16	147	0	0.5	0.0	0	6%
whole wheat	1 piece	150	6	28	320	1	2.0	0.0	0	12%
(Vermont Bread Company)	1/2 pita	80	3	16	90	3	0.5	0.0	0	6%
POTATO *(Ener-G Foods)* gluten-free	1 slice	170	3	24	77	1	5.4	0.5	0	31%
PROTEIN, w/gluten	1 slice	47	2	8	104	1	0.4	0.1	0	8%
PUMPERNICKEL										
regular slices	1 slice	65	2	12	174	2	0.8	0.1	0	11%
snack size	1 slice	18	1	3	47	0	0.2	0.0	0	11%
thick slices, approx 5x4x3/8 inch	1 slice	80	3	15	215	2	1.0	0.1	0	11%
thin slices	1 slice	50	2	10	134	1	0.6	0.1	0	11%
(Arnold)	1 slice	70	3	15	198	1	0.9	0.0	0	10%
(Pepperidge Farm)										
'Family'	1 slice	80	3	15	230	2	1.0	0.0	0	11%
small, 'Party'	4 slices	60	2	12	160	1	1.0	0.0	0	14%
RAISIN										
large slices	1 slice	88	3	17	125	1	1.4	0.3	0	14%
medium slices	1 slice	71	2	14	101	1	1.1	0.3	0	14%
thin slices	1 slice	63	2	12	90	1	1.0	0.2	0	14%
(BreadMill Bakery) whole wheat, organic	1 slice	120	5	24	327	0	1.0	0.0	0	7%
(Brownberry)										
bran	1 slice	61	2	12	108	2	1.3	0.0	0	17%
cinnamon	1 slice	66	1	13	107	1	1.3	0.0	0	17%
walnut	1 slice	68	2	11	96	2	2.7	0.0	0	31%
(Ener-G Foods)										
gluten-free, egg-free	1 slice	116	1	20	139	1	2.7	0.3	0	22%
gluten-free, w/egg	1 slice	154	3	32	56	2	1.5	0.2	0	9%
(Monk's) cinnamon	1 slice	70	3	10	85	0	2.0	0.0	0	26%
(Northridge) walnut, royal	1 slice	90	2	16	90	0	2.0	0.0	0	20%
(Pepperidge Farm)										
cinnamon swirl	1 slice	90	2	16	100	1	2.0	0.0	0	20%
(Pillsbury) oatmeal, 'Hearty Grain'	1 serving	90	2	16	210	1	2.0	0.0	0	20%
(Vermont Bread Company)										
cinnamon, low-fat, low-sodium	1 slice	80	3	17	115	2	0.5	0.0	0	5%
RICE										
(Ener-G Foods)										
gluten-free, 'Papa's Loaf'	1 slice	144	1	19	98	3	5.9	0.5	0	40%
white rice, yeast free, gluten-free	1 slice	147	1	24	272	3	3.1	0.2	0	22%
(French Meadow)										
sourdough, whole grain, yeast-free, organic	1.35 oz	84	4	17	180	3	1.0	0.0	0	10%
RICE BRAN										
	1 slice	66	2	12	119	1	1.2	0.2	0	16%
(Monk's) golden	1 slice	70	3	14	80	2	1.0	0.0	0	12%
(Roman Meal)										
	1 slice	70	3	12	132	1	1.5	0.0	0	18%

Food Name	Serving Size	Calories	Prot. gms	Carbs gms	Sod. mgs	Fiber gms	Fat gms	Sat. Fat gms	Chol. mgs	% Fat Cal.
w/honey and nuts	1 slice	71	3	13	127	1	1.6	0.0	0	19%
RICE STARCH *(Med Diet)* low-protein	1 slice	155	0	29	25	6	4.0	1.1	0	24%
RYE										
lower calorie, medium slices	1 slice	47	2	9	93	3	0.7	0.1	0	12%
lower calorie, thick slices	1 slice	65	3	13	130	4	0.9	0.1	0	12%
lower calorie, thin slices	1 slice	41	2	8	81	2	0.6	0.1	0	12%
regular, medium slices	1 slice	83	3	15	211	2	1.1	0.2	0	11%
regular, snack size	1 slice	18	1	3	46	0	0.2	0.1	0	11%
regular, thin slices	1 slice	52	2	10	132	1	0.7	0.1	0	11%
(Arnold) w/dill	1 slice	71	3	14	187	1	1.0	0.0	0	12%
(Beefsteak)										
'Hearty'	1 slice	70	3	13	180	1	1.0	0.0	0	12%
'Mild'	1 slice	70	3	13	180	1	1.0	0.0	0	12%
'Soft'	1 slice	70	3	13	170	1	1.0	0.0	0	12%
w/onion	1 slice	70	3	12	170	1	1.0	0.0	0	13%
w/wheat berries	1 slice	70	3	13	160	1	1.0	0.0	0	12%
(Braun's) 'Old Allegheny'	1 slice	70	3	13	160	1	1.0	0.0	0	12%
(Brownberry)										
seedless, natural, sliced thin	1 slice	45	2	10	118	1	0.6	0.0	0	11%
w/caraway, 'Natural'	1 slice	73	3	15	185	1	0.8	0.0	0	9%
(Earth Grains) sliced very thin, 'Light'	1 oz	70	3	14	230	0	1.0	0.0	0	12%
(Food for Life) white, 100% wheat-free, no preservatives	2 slices	217	4	42	257	0	4.0	0.0	0	16%
(Grant's Farm) cracked rye, w/honey	1 slice	70	3	13	190	0	1.0	0.0	0	12%
(Levy's)										
Jewish, seeded	1 slice	76	3	16	181	1	0.9	0.0	0	10%
Jewish, seedless	1 slice	75	3	16	178	1	0.8	0.0	0	9%
(Mrs. Wright's) Jewish, w/seeds	2 slices	110	3	20	320	1	1.5	0.0	0	13%
(Natural Ovens) mild	1 slice	70	3	13	70	4	0.5	0.0	0	7%
(Oroweat) hearty, 'Light'	1 slice	40	2	10	135	2	0.0	0.0	0	0%
(Pepperidge Farm)										
Dijon	1 slice	50	2	9	170	1	1.0	0.0	0	17%
Dijon, 'Hearty'	1 slice	70	3	15	260	2	1.0	0.0	0	11%
seedless, 'Family'	1 slice	80	3	16	210	2	1.0	0.0	0	11%
small, 'Party'	4 slices	60	2	12	250	1	1.0	0.0	0	14%
w/seeds, 'Family'	1 slice	80	3	16	220	2	1.0	0.0	0	11%
(Vermont Bread Company)										
	1 slice	70	2	14	115	2	1.0	0.0	0	12%
'Black Russian'	1 slice (1/2")	110	3	23	120	3	0.0	0.0	0	0%
'Sandwich'	1 slice	100	3	18	120	3	1.5	0.0	0	14%
(Weight Watchers)	1 slice	40	2	10	100	0	1.0	0.0	0	16%
(Wonder)	1 slice	70	2	13	150	1	1.0	0.0	0	13%
SOURDOUGH										
(Boudin)	2 slices	130	5	27	297	0	1.0	0.0	0	7%
(DiCarlo)	1 slice	70	3	12	140	1	1.0	0.0	0	13%
(Earth Grains) 'Light'	1 slice	40	2	9	115	0	1.0	0.2	0	17%
(French Meadow) yeast-free, organic	2 oz	132	7	29	0	0	0.9	0.0	0	5%
(Monterey Baking)	1 slice	75	3	16	152	1	0.2	0.0	0	2%
(Rainbo) 'Light'	1 slice	40	2	9	110	2	1.0	0.0	0	17%
SPELT *(French Meadow)* sprouted, yeast-free, organic	1.5 oz	93	5	18	160	4	0.0	0.0	0	0%
SPLIT TOP *(Healthy Choice)*	1 slice	60	3	12	120	2	0.5	0.0	0	7%
SUNFLOWER										
(BreadMill Bakery) w/whole wheat, organic	1 slice	129	6	21	287	0	2.0	0.0	0	14%
(Monk's) w/bran	1 slice	70	3	12	80	2	1.0	0.0	0	13%
SUNFLOWER SESAME *(Vermont Bread Company)*	1 slice	70	3	14	120	2	1.0	0.0	0	12%

Food Name	Serving Size	Calories	Prot. gms	Carbs gms	Sod. mgs	Fiber gms	Fat gms	Sat. Fat gms	Chol. mgs	% Fat Cal.
SWEET (Vermont Bread Company)	1 slice	70	3	15	120	2	0.0	0.0	0	0%
TAPIOCA										
(Ener-G Foods)										
gluten free	1 slice	141	1	19	175	4	6.0	0.4	0	41%
gluten free, thin sliced	1 slice	88	0	12	109	2	3.7	0.3	0	41%
THREE SEED (Monterey Baking)	1 slice	100	4	16	220	na	2.5	na	0	22%
VIENNA										
(Pepperidge Farm)										
'Light Style'	1 slice	45	2	10	100	1	0.0	0.0	0	0%
sliced thick, 'Hearth'	1 slice	70	2	13	125	0	1.0	0.0	0	13%
WHEAT										
(Arizona Original Homestyle)										
w/honey, 100% stone ground	1 slice	110	5	23	380	2	0.0	0.0	0	0%
(Arnold)										
'Brick Oven'	1 slice	57	2	11	104	2	1.5	0.0	0	21%
light, golden, 'Bakery'	1 slice	44	2	10	86	2	0.5	0.0	0	9%
(Aunt Hattie's)										
buttertop	1 slice	70	3	13	140	0	1.0	0.0	5	12%
w/buttermilk	1 slice	70	3	12	130	0	1.0	0.0	0	13%
(Beefsteak)										
light, 'Hearty'	1 slice	70	3	11	160	1	1.0	0.0	0	14%
'Soft'	1 slice	70	3	12	160	2	1.0	0.0	0	13%
(BreadMill Bakery)										
w/oat bran and honey, all-natural, organic	1 slice	120	5	23	400	1	1.0	0.0	0	7%
w/sunflower, all natural, organic	1 slice	130	6	1	380	2	2.0	0.0	0	39%
(Brownberry)										
	1 slice	74	3	13	127	1	1.8	0.0	0	20%
'Hearth'	1 oz	70	3	14	150	2	1.4	0.0	0	16%
'Natural'	1 slice	80	3	17	183	2	1.3	0.0	0	13%
w/apple and honey	1 slice	69	2	11	148	2	1.9	0.0	0	24%
(Colonial)										
'Family Recipe'	1 slice	70	3	14	150	0	1.0	0.0	0	12%
honey buttered, split top	1 slice	70	3	14	140	0	1.0	0.0	0	12%
stone ground, 'Family Recipe'	1 slice	70	3	14	150	0	1.0	0.0	0	12%
(Country Grain)	1 slice	70	3	12	160	1	1.0	0.0	0	13%
(Earth Grains)										
cracked wheat	1 oz	70	2	12	180	0	1.0	0.0	0	14%
'Light 35'	1 oz	35	2	8	100	0	1.0	0.0	0	18%
sliced very thin	1 oz	70	2	13	150	0	1.0	0.0	0	13%
(Fresh and Natural)	1 slice	70	3	13	140	2	1.0	0.0	0	12%
(Grant's Farm)										
'Light'	1 slice	40	2	9	115	0	1.0	0.0	0	17%
stone ground	1 slice	60	3	12	150	0	1.0	0.0	0	13%
(Healthy Choice) honey wheat	1 slice	60	3	12	120	2	0.5	0.0	0	7%
(Hearty Grains) cracked wheat, w/honey, twists	1 serving	80	2	14	120	1	2.0	0.0	0	22%
(Home Pride)										
butter top wheat	1 slice	80	2	14	190	1	1.0	0.0	0	12%
stone ground	1 slice	70	3	12	140	2	1.0	0.0	0	13%
(Kamut) stone-ground, yeast-free, organic, frozen	1 slice	120	7	23	140	4	0.0	0.0	0	0%
(Kilpatrick's)										
'Family Recipe'	1 slice	70	3	14	150	0	1.0	0.0	0	12%
stone ground, 'Family Recipe'	1 slice	70	3	14	150	0	1.0	0.0	0	12%
(Mrs. Wright's)										
	2 slices	100	4	18	240	2	1.5	0.0	0	13%

Food Name	Serving Size	Calories	Prot. gms	Carbs gms	Sod. mgs	Fiber gms	Fat gms	Sat. Fat gms	Chol. mgs	% Fat Cal.
crushed wheat, sliced, round top	1 slice	70	2	15	160	1	0.5	0.0	0	6%
crushed wheat, sliced, sandwich thin	1 slice	60	2	12	130	1	0.5	0.0	0	7%
dark wheat, 'Bran'nola'	1 slice	83	4	18	166	3	1.0	0.0	0	9%
(Natural Ovens) cracked wheat	1 slice	80	4	16	70	3	0.5	0.0	0	5%
(Oatmeal Goodness)										
w/oatmeal	1 slice	90	4	15	140	1	2.0	0.0	0	19%
w/oatmeal, 'Light'	1 slice	40	2	6	90	0	1.0	0.0	0	22%
(Pepperidge Farm)										
cracked wheat	1 slice	70	2	13	140	1	1.0	0.0	0	13%
'Light Style'	1 slice	45	2	9	90	1	0.0	0.0	0	0%
1.5-lb loaf	1 slice	90	3	18	190	2	2.0	0.0	0	18%
sprouted	1 slice	70	3	11	100	2	2.0	0.0	0	24%
2-lb loaf, 'Family'	1 slice	70	2	13	130	2	1.0	0.0	0	13%
w/sesame, 'Hearty'	2 slices	190	7	36	340	3	3.0	1.0	0	14%
(Pipin' Hot) thick sliced	1 slice	70	2	12	170	0	2.0	0.0	0	24%
(Rainbo)										
'Family Recipe'	1 slice	70	3	14	150	0	1.0	0.0	0	12%
honey buttered, split top	1 slice	70	3	14	140	0	1.0	0.0	0	12%
'Light'	1 slice	40	2	9	100	2	1.0	0.0	0	17%
stone ground, 'Family Recipe'	1 slice	70	3	14	150	0	1.0	0.0	0	12%
(Vermont Bread Company)										
low-sodium	1 slice	80	2	15	115	2	1.0	0.0	0	12%
sodium-free	1 slice	90	3	15	0	2	2.0	0.0	0	20%
sprouted	1 slice	70	3	15	115	2	0.5	0.0	0	6%
(Weight Watchers)	1 slice	40	2	9	100	0	1.0	0.0	0	17%
(Wonder)										
nonfat, 'Light'	1 slice	40	3	7	120	0	1.0	0.0	0	18%
sliced	1 slice	80	2	14	160	0	1.0	0.0	0	12%
sliced, 'Family'	1 slice	80	2	13	160	1	1.0	0.0	0	13%
WHEAT BERRY										
(Arizona Original Homestyle) cracked, stone-ground	1 slice	93	4	23	135	2	0.0	0.0	0	0%
(Arnold) w/honey	1 slice	77	3	17	143	2	1.2	0.0	0	12%
(Earth Grains) w/honey	1 oz	70	3	12	160	0	1.0	0.0	0	13%
(Grant's Farm)	1 slice	70	3	13	150	0	1.0	0.0	0	12%
(Healthy Choice)	1 slice	80	4	18	170	3	1.0	0.0	0	9%
(Oroweat) w/honey	1 slice	90	3	17	180	2	1.0	0.0	0	10%
WHEAT BRAN (Grant's Farm) w/honey	1 slice	70	3	14	120	0	1.0	0.0	0	12%
WHEAT GERM	1 slice	73	3	14	155	1	0.8	0.2	0	10%
WHITE										
medium slices	1 slice	67	2	12	135	1	0.9	0.1	0	12%
medium slices, crust removed	1 slice	32	1	6	65	0	0.4	0.1	0	12%
thick slices	1 slice	80	2	15	161	1	1.1	0.2	0	12%
thin slices	1 slice	53	2	10	108	0	0.7	0.1	0	12%
very thin slices	1 slice	40	1	7	81	0	0.5	0.1	0	12%
(Arnold)										
'Brick Oven'	1 slice	61	2	11	134	1	1.2	0.0	0	17%
'Country White'	1 slice	98	3	19	204	1	1.8	0.0	0	16%
extra fiber, 'Brick Oven'	1 slice	55	2	12	93	2	0.8	0.0	0	11%
'Light Premium'	1 slice	42	2	10	89	2	0.5	0.0	0	9%
(Aunt Hattie's)										
buttertop, 'Homestyle'	1 slice	70	3	13	140	0	1.0	0.0	0	12%
w/buttermilk, 'Homestyle'	1 slice	80	3	13	140	0	1.0	0.0	0	12%
(Beefsteak) 'Robust'	1 slice	70	3	13	140	1	1.0	0.0	0	12%

Food Name	Serving Size	Calories	Prot. gms	Carbs gms	Sod. mgs	Fiber gms	Fat gms	Sat. Fat gms	Chol. mgs	% Fat Cal.
(Brownberry)										
'Light Premium'	1 slice	42	2	10	89	2	0.5	0.0	0	9%
'Natural'	1 slice	59	2	11	136	1	1.1	0.0	0	16%
(Colonial) honey buttered, split top	1 slice	80	3	14	140	0	1.0	0.0	0	12%
(Earth Grains)										
'Light 35'	1 oz	35	2	8	105	0	1.0	0.0	0	18%
very thin sliced	1 oz	80	2	14	160	0	1.0	0.0	0	12%
(Grant's Farm) 'Light'	1 slice	40	2	9	115	0	1.0	0.0	0	17%
(Holsum)										
enriched, 'Country Style'	1 slice	70	2	14	135	0	1.0	0.0	0	12%
thin sliced	1 slice	70	2	14	160	0	1.0	0.0	0	12%
(Kilpatrick's) honey buttered, split top	1 slice	80	3	14	140	0	1.0	0.0	0	12%
(Monk's)	1 slice	60	3	10	95	0	1.0	0.0	0	15%
(Mrs. Wright's)										
enriched	2 slices	100	3	20	190	1	1.0	0.0	0	9%
sliced, Sandwich style, 'Winners'	1 slice	70	3	13	160	2	1.0	0.0	0	12%
(Northridge) 'Old Fashioned'	1 slice	70	2	13	125	0	1.0	0.0	0	13%
(Pepperidge Farm)										
'Hearty Country'	2 slices	190	7	38	340	2	2.0	1.0	0	9%
sliced, sandwich style	2 slices	130	4	24	260	0	2.0	0.0	0	14%
thin sliced, 1-lb loaf	1 slice	80	2	14	130	0	2.0	0.0	0	22%
'Toasting'	1 slice	90	3	17	200	1	1.0	0.0	0	10%
2-lb loaf, 'Large Family'	1 slice	70	2	13	150	0	1.0	0.0	0	13%
very thin sliced	1 slice	40	1	8	80	0	0.0	0.0	0	0%
(Pipin' Hot) loaf, thick sliced	1 slice	70	2	12	170	0	2.0	0.0	0	24%
(Rainbo)										
honey buttered, split top	1 slice	80	3	14	140	0	1.0	0.0	0	12%
'Light'	1 slice	40	2	9	100	2	1.0	0.0	0	17%
thin sliced, special recipe, 'Iron Kids'	1 slice	60	3	13	140	2	1.0	0.0	0	12%
(Vermont Bread Company)										
'Old Fashioned Sandwich'	1 slice	70	2	14	100	1	1.0	0.0	0	12%
'Soft'	1 piece	80	2	15	115	1	1.0	0.0	0	12%
(Weight Watchers)	1 slice	40	2	10	100	0	1.0	0.0	0	16%
(Wonder)										
'High-Fiber'	1 slice	40	2	6	80	3	0.0	0.0	0	0%
'Light'	1 slice	40	3	7	110	2	0.0	0.0	0	0%
sliced	1 slice	70	2	14	150	0	1.0	0.0	0	12%
sliced thin	1 slice	50	2	10	120	1	1.0	0.0	0	16%
w/buttermilk	1 slice	70	2	13	160	1	1.0	0.0	0	13%
WHOLE GRAIN										
(Healthy Choice)	1 slice	80	4	18	170	3	1.0	0.0	0	9%
(Natural Ovens)	1 slice	70	4	13	70	5	0.5	0.0	0	6%
WHOLE WHEAT										
	1 slice	69	3	13	148	2	1.2	0.3	0	15%
(Arnold) 100%, stone ground	1 slice	48	2	10	97	2	0.7	0.0	0	11%
(Aunt Hattie's)	1 slice	90	4	14	170	0	2.0	0.0	0	20%
(BreadMill Bakery)										
w/orange, organic	1 slice	130	5	24	420	1	1.0	0.0	0	7%
w/poppyseed, organic	1 slice	120	6	22	340	1	1.0	0.0	0	7%
w/raisin, organic	1 slice	120	5	24	410	1	1.0	0.0	0	7%
(Daily)	1 piece	140	6	26	0	0	0.0	0.0	0	0%
(Earth Grains)	1 oz	70	3	11	150	0	1.0	0.0	0	14%
(Monk's) 100% stone ground	1 slice	70	3	13	110	0	1.0	0.0	0	12%

Food Name	Serving Size	Calories	Prot. gms	Carbs gms	Sod. mgs	Fiber gms	Fat gms	Sat. Fat gms	Chol. mgs	% Fat Cal.
(Northridge) 100%										
....	1 slice	60	3	11	120	2	1.0	0.0	0	14%
(Oroweat) 100% stone ground..........	1 slice	60	3	11	125	2	1.0	0.0	0	14%
(Pepperidge Farm)										
thin sliced, 1-lb loaf..........	1 slice	60	2	12	110	2	1.0	0.0	0	14%
very thin sliced	1 slice	35	2	7	75	0	0.0	0.0	0	0%
(Vermont Bread Company)										
'Sandwich'..........	1 slice	90	3	18	120	3	1.0	0.0	0	10%
'Soft Whole Wheat'	1 piece	80	3	15	110	2	1.0	0.0	0	11%
sourdough..........	1 slice	80	3	16	120	3	0.5	0.0	0	6%
(Wonder)										
'High-Fiber'	1 slice	40	2	6	80	3	0.0	0.0	0	0%
'Light'..........	1 slice	40	3	7	120	2	0.0	0.0	0	0%
100%..........	1 slice	70	3	12	160	2	1.0	0.0	0	13%
'Soft 100%'	1 slice	70	4	10	140	2	1.0	0.0	0	14%
BREAD, QUICK										
cornbread *(Ballard)*..........	1 piece	130	4	23	520	2	2.5	1.0	25	17%
cornbread *(Marie Callender's)*..........	1 piece	150	2	27	310	2	3.0	1.0	5	19%
raisin loaf, fat-free, cholesterol-free *(Entenmann's)*......	1 slice	140	2	33	150	1	0.0	0.0	0	0%
BREAD, QUICK, MIX										
APPLE CINNAMON										
(Pillsbury)										
mix only..........	1/12 pkg	140	2	30	160	0	1.0	0.0	0	7%
prepared w/1/4 cup oil, 1/4 cup egg substitute	1/12 loaf	190	2	31	170	0	6.0	1.0	0	29%
prepared w/water, 1/4 cup oil, 1 egg..........	1/12 loaf	180	2	31	170	0	6.0	1.0	20	29%
BANANA										
(Keebler) individual, 'Elfin Loaf' prepared w/margarine	1 loaf	186	2	31	172	1	6.0	1.3	25	29%
(Krusteaz) w/nuts, prepared	3/4-inch slice	190	3	33	300	2	6.0	0.0	3	27%
(Pillsbury)										
mix only..........	1/12 pkg	120	2	27	190	0	1.0	0.0	0	7%
prepared, regular recipe	1/12 loaf	170	3	27	220	0	6.0	0.0	0	31%
prepared w/water, 3 tbsp oil, 1/2 cup egg substitute......	1/12 loaf	170	3	27	210	0	6.0	1.0	0	31%
prepared w/water, 3 tbsp oil, 2 eggs..........	1/12 loaf	170	3	27	200	0	5.0	1.0	35	27%
BLUEBERRY										
(Pillsbury)										
mix only..........	1/12 pkg	130	2	29	160	0	1.0	0.0	0	7%
nut, prepared..........	1/12 loaf	150	2	26	150	0	4.0	0.0	0	24%
prepared, regular recipe	1/12 loaf	150	2	26	150	0	4.0	0.0	0	24%
prepared w/water, 1/4 cup oil, 1 egg..........	1/12 loaf	180	2	30	160	0	6.0	1.0	20	30%
prepared w/water, 1/4 cup oil, 1/4 cup egg substitute.....	1/12 loaf	180	2	30	170	0	6.0	1.0	0	30%
CHERRY *(Pillsbury)* prepared, regular recipe	1/12 loaf	180	3	29	150	0	5.0	0.0	0	26%
CORNBREAD										
(Aunt Jemima) 'Easy'..........	1/3 cup	150	2	26	450	1	4.0	1.0	0	24%
(Ballard)										
mix only..........	1/16 pkg	120	2	24	560	0	2.0	1.0	0	15%
prepared	1 serving	110	2	21	500	1	1.5	0.0	0	13%
(Dromedary)										
mix only..........	3 tbsp	100	2	19	280	0	2.0	0.0	0	18%
prepared, 2x2-inch pieces..........	1 piece	130	3	20	480	0	3.0	0.0	0	23%
(Gluten Free Pantry) gluten-free, prepared	1 serving	130	3	29	290	2	0.0	0.0	0	0%
(Gold Medal)										
white, 'Pouch Mix' prepared w/egg, whole milk..........	1/6 pan	150	4	22	490	0	5.0	0.0	0	30%
yellow, 'Pouch Mix' prepared w/egg, whole milk	1/6 pan	150	4	23	500	0	5.0	0.0	0	29%

Food Name	Serving Size	Calories	Prot. gms	Carbs gms	Sod. mgs	Fiber gms	Fat gms	Sat. Fat gms	Chol. mgs	% Fat Cal.
(Hodgson Mill)										
Mexican, w/jalapeño, mix only.	1/4 cup	100	4	21	310	1	1.0	0.0	0	8%
and muffin mix, whole-grain cornmeal	1/4 cup	130	4	28	240	3	1.0	0.0	0	7%
(Kentucky Kernel) sweet, all-natural, mix only	1/4 cup	120	2	24	310	0	2.0	0.0	0	15%
(Krusteaz)										
Southern, prepared, 2 x 2-inch pieces	1 piece	140	3	27	450	0	3.0	0.0	8	18%
w/honey, prepared.	1/16 loaf	120	2	21	230	0	3.0	0.0	17	23%
(Martha White)										
'Cotton Pickin' prepared w/water.	1/6 pan	110	2	21	360	0	2.0	0.0	0	16%
'Cotton Pickin' prepared	1/4 pan	170	3	31	540	0	3.0	0.0	2	17%
Mexican, prepared w/2% milk.	1/6 pan	140	2	24	410	0	4.0	0.0	25	26%
w/buttermilk, prepared w/water.	1/6 pan	110	2	21	360	0	2.0	0.0	0	16%
yellow, 'Light Crust' prepared.	2 oz	140	4	21	400	0	4.0	0.0	26	26%
yellow, prepared w/water.	1/6 pan	130	2	27	310	0	2.0	0.0	0	13%
(Pillsbury)										
prepared	1/18 pkg	130	4	23	520	1	2.5	1.0	25	17%
twists, prepared.	1 serving	130	3	17	320	0	6.0	1.5	0	40%
(Robin Hood)										
white, 'Pouch Mix' prepared w/egg, whole milk	1/6 pan	150	4	22	490	0	5.0	0.0	0	30%
yellow, 'Pouch Mix' prepared w/egg, whole milk	1/6 pan	150	4	23	500	0	5.0	0.0	0	29%
CRANBERRY										
(Pillsbury)										
mix only.	1/12 pkg	140	2	30	150	0	1.0	0.0	0	7%
prepared w/water, 2 tbsp oil, 1 egg.	1/12 loaf	160	2	30	150	0	4.0	1.0	20	22%
prepared w/water, 2 tbsp oil 1/4 cup egg substitute	1/12 loaf	170	3	30	160	0	4.0	1.0	0	21%
CRANBERRY-ORANGE										
(Gluten Free Pantry) gluten-free, prepared	1 serving	150	1	35	150	1	0.0	0.0	0	0%
DATE NUT										
(Dromedary)										
mix only.	1/12 pkg	166	2	26	242	0	7.0	0.0	0	36%
prepared	1/12 loaf	183	2	26	248	0	8.0	0.0	0	39%
(Pillsbury)										
mix only.	1/12 pkg	140	2	31	140	0	1.0	0.0	0	6%
prepared.	1/12 loaf	180	3	32	160	1	4.0	1.0	20	20%
prepared w/water, 1 tbsp oil, 1/4 cup egg substitute	1/12 loaf	160	2	32	150	0	3.0	1.0	0	17%
IRISH SODA *(Gluten Free Pantry)* gluten-free.	1 serving	130	3	28	270	1	1.0	0.0	5	7%
NUT										
(Pillsbury)										
mix only.	1/12 pkg	150	3	27	180	0	3.0	1.0	0	18%
prepared w/water, 2 tbsp oil, 1 egg.	1/12 loaf	170	3	27	190	0	6.0	1.0	20	31%
prepared w/water, 2 tbsp oil, 1/4 cup egg substitute	1/12 loaf	170	3	28	190	0	6.0	1.0	0	30%
OATMEAL-RAISIN										
(Pillsbury)										
mix only.	1/12 pkg	140	3	30	170	0	2.0	0.0	0	12%
prepared w/water, 1/4 cup oil, 1 egg.	1/12 loaf	190	3	30	180	0	7.0	1.0	20	32%
prepared w/1/4 cup oil, 1/4 cup egg substitute	1/12 loaf	190	3	30	180	0	7.0	1.0	0	32%
PUMPKIN										
(Pillsbury)										
mix only.	1/12 pkg	130	2	26	190	1	1.5	0.0	0	11%
prepared.	1/12 loaf	170	3	27	200	1	6.0	1.0	35	31%
BREAD CRUMBS										
Italian, dry, grated *(Tone's)*.	1 tsp	8	0	2	15	0	0.1	0.1	1	11%
Italian or plain, whole wheat, organic *(Jaclyn's)*	14 grams	28	4	13	5	0	1.0	0.0	0	12%
Italian style *(Devonsheer)*.	1 oz	104	4	21	408	1	1.3	0.0	0	11%

Food Name	Serving Size	Calories	Prot. gms	Carbs gms	Sod. mgs	Fiber gms	Fat gms	Sat. Fat gms	Chol. mgs	% Fat Cal.
Italian style *(Progresso)*	1/4 cup	110	4	20	430	1	1.5	0.0	0	12%
Italian style *(Progresso)*	2 tbsp	60	2	11	240	0	1.0	0.0	0	15%
Italian style, whole wheat *(Jaclyn's)*	0.5 oz	28	4	13	5	0	1.0	0.0	0	12%
plain *(Contadina)*	1/3 cup	100	3	19	701	1	1.5	0.4	0	13%
plain *(Devonsheer)*	1 oz	108	4	22	272	1	1.4	0.0	0	11%
plain *(Progresso)*	1/4 cup	100	4	19	210	1	1.5	0.0	0	13%
plain *(Progresso)*	2 tbsp	60	2	11	110	0	1.0	0.0	0	15%
plain, dry, grated	1 cup	427	14	78	931	3	5.8	1.3	0	12%
plain, dry, grated	1 oz	112	4	21	244	1	1.5	0.3	0	12%
plain, dry, grated *(Tone's)*	1 tsp	8	0	2	15	0	0.1	0.1	1	11%
seasoned, dry, grated	1 cup	440	17	84	3180	5	3.1	0.9	1	6%
seasoned, dry, grated	1 oz	104	4	20	751	1	0.7	0.2	0	6%

BREAD DOUGH

Food Name	Serving Size	Calories	Prot. gms	Carbs gms	Sod. mgs	Fiber gms	Fat gms	Sat. Fat gms	Chol. mgs	% Fat Cal.
cracked wheat, unbleached, high-protein, frozen *(Rhodes)*	1 oz	75	3	15	0	0	1.0	0.0	0	11%
French, crusty, refrigerated, prepared, 1-inch slice *(Pillsbury)*	1 slice	60	2	11	120	0	1.0	0.0	0	15%
raisin, unbleached flour, no preservatives, frozen, prepared *(Rhodes)*	1 slice	70	2	13	0	0	1.0	0.0	0	13%
refrigerated *(Roman Meal)*	1 oz	85	2	13	199	1	2.8	0.9	0	30%
wheat, refrigerated, prepared, thick sliced *(Pipin' Hot)*	1 slice	70	0	12	170	0	2.0	0.0	0	27%
white, enriched, frozen *(Bridgford)*	2 oz	150	5	28	325	0	2.0	0.0	0	12%
white, frozen *(Bridgford)*	1 oz	76	3	14	156	0	1.2	0.0	0	14%
white, frozen *(Rhodes)*	1 slice	139	5	26	280	2	2.3	0.0	0	14%
white, frozen *(Rich's)*	2 slices	120	4	23	300	0	1.0	0.0	0	8%
white, refrigerated, prepared, 1-inch slice *(Pipin' Hot)*	1 slice	70	3	12	170	0	2.0	0.0	0	23%
w/honey, frozen *(Bridgford)*	2 oz	150	6	27	304	0	2.0	0.0	0	12%
w/honey, unbleached high-protein flour, frozen *(Rhodes)*	1 slice	125	6	23	219	3	2.0	0.0	0	13%
w/walnuts and honey, frozen *(Bridgford)*	1 oz	76	3	14	152	0	0.9	0.0	0	11%

BREAD MIX

Food Name	Serving Size	Calories	Prot. gms	Carbs gms	Sod. mgs	Fiber gms	Fat gms	Sat. Fat gms	Chol. mgs	% Fat Cal.
caraway rye, mix only *(Hodgson Mill)*	1/4 cup	120	5	22	190	3	2.0	1.0	0	14%
caraway rye, gluten-free *(Gluten Free Pantry)*	1 serving	110	4	23	170	1	0.0	0.0	0	0%
cracked wheat, for bread machines *(Pillsbury)*	1/12 pkg	130	4	25	260	2	2.0	0.0	0	13%
European cheese and herb, low-fat, cholesterol-free, mix only *(Hodgson Mill)*	1/4 cup	130	5	21	250	1	2.0	0.0	0	15%
French, country, gluten-free, prepared *(Gluten Free Pantry)*	1 slice	110	1	25	115	1	0.0	0.0	0	0%
Italian, frozen *(Rhodes)*	1 slice	130	5	23	280	1	2.0	0.0	0	14%
9-grain, low-fat, mix only *(Hodgson Mill)*	1/4 cup	130	5	22	150	2	2.0	0.0	0	14%
oatmeal, w/raisin, mix only *(Pillsbury)*	1/12 pkg	140	3	30	170	0	2.0	0.0	0	12%
oatmeal, w/raisin, prepared w/water, 1/4 cup oil, 1 egg *(Pillsbury)*	1/12 pkg	190	3	30	180	0	7.0	1.0	20	32%
oatmeal, w/raisin, prepared w/water, 1/4 cup oil, 1/4 cup egg substitute *(Pillsbury)*	1/12 pkg	190	3	30	180	0	7.0	1.0	0	32%
potato, fat free, cholesterol free, mix only *(Hodgson Mill)*	1/4 cup	120	5	23	170	1	0.0	0.0	0	0%
sandwich, gluten-free, 'Favorite' *(Gluten Free Pantry)*	1 slice	110	3	24	170	1	0.0	0.0	0	0%
tapioca, gluten-free *(Gluten Free Pantry)*	1 serving	110	2	25	115	1	0.0	0.0	0	0%
white, crusty, for bread machines *(Pillsbury)*	1/8 pkg	130	4	25	250	1	2.0	0.0	0	13%
white, unbleached flour, mix only *(Hodgson Mill)*	1/4 cup	120	5	22	170	3	2.0	1.0	0	14%
whole grain, stone ground, w/honey, mix only *(Hodgson Mill)*	1/4 cup	120	5	22	160	3	2.0	1.0	0	14%

Food Name	Serving Size	Calories	Prot. gms	Carbs gms	Sod. mgs	Fiber gms	Fat gms	Sat. Fat gms	Chol. mgs	% Fat Cal.
whole wheat, low-fat, cholesterol free, mix only										
(Hodgson Mill)	1/4 cup	120	5	22	160	3	2.0	na	na	14%
whole wheat, 100% all natural, stone ground										
(Bob's Red Mill)	1.5 oz	152	7	28	245	2	2.0	0.5	0	11%
BREAD PUDDING										
w/apples, frozen, food service product (Stouffer's)	1 oz	42	2	5	77	1	1.6	0.4	30	34%
BREADFRUIT										
Fresh, raw, whole, small fruit	1/4 fruit	99	1	26	2	5	0.2	0.0	0	2%
Frozen, unthawed	1 cup	227	2	60	4	11	0.5	0.1	0	2%
BREADFRUIT SEEDS										
boiled	1 oz	48	2	9	7	1	0.7	0.2	0	11%
raw	1 oz	54	2	8	7	1	1.6	0.4	0	25%
roasted	1 oz	59	2	11	8	2	0.8	0.2	0	11%
BREADNUT TREE SEEDS / Jamaican breadnut										
dried	1 cup	587	14	127	85	24	2.7	0.7	0	4%
dried	1 oz	104	2	23	15	4	0.5	0.1	0	4%
raw, 8–14 seeds	1 oz	62	2	13	9	na	0.3	0.1	0	4%
BREADSTICK										
garlic, frozen (Cole's)	1.9 oz	170	4	27	290	1	5.0	1.0	1	27%
garlic, Italian style (Barbara's Bakery)	1 oz	120	4	18	170	0	3.0	0.0	0	23%
garlic and sesame (Angonoa's)	7 pieces	120	4	19	120	1	3.0	0.5	0	23%
onion (Stella D'oro)	1 piece	40	1	6	0	0	1.3	0.0	0	29%
pizza (Fattorie & Pandea)	3 pieces	59	2	10	100	0	1.0	0.0	0	16%
pizza (Stella D'oro)	1 piece	43	1	7	0	0	1.2	0.0	0	25%
plain (Angonoa's)	6 pieces	120	4	20	280	1	2.5	0.5	0	19%
plain (Stella D'oro)	1 piece	41	1	7	0	0	1.2	0.0	0	26%
plain, 4.25-inch length	1 breadstick	21	1	3	33	0	0.5	0.1	0	20%
plain, 7-5/8 x 5/8 inch	1 breadstick	41	1	7	66	0	0.9	0.1	0	20%
plain, 9-1/4 x 3/8 inch	1 breadstick	25	1	4	39	0	0.6	0.1	0	20%
plain, dietetic (Stella D'oro)	1 piece	46	1	7	10	0	1.4	0.0	0	27%
plain, regular (Barbara's Bakery)	1 oz	120	4	18	170	0	3.0	0.0	0	23%
sesame, dietetic (Stella D'oro)	1 piece	49	1	6	10	0	2.1	0.0	0	39%
soft (Pillsbury)	1 serving	110	3	18	290	1	2.5	0.5	0	21%
sesame (Fattorie & Pandea)	3 pieces	65	2	10	100	0	2.0	0.0	0	27%
sesame (Stella D'oro)	1 piece	51	1	6	0	0	2.2	0.0	0	39%
sesame, Italian style (Barbara's Bakery)	1 oz	120	4	18	170	0	3.0	0.0	0	23%
soft, refrigerated ready-to-bake (Mrs. Wright's)	1 stick	100	3	17	300	1	2.5	1.0	0	22%
soft, refrigerated (Roman Meal)	1 piece	117	3	17	274	1	3.9	1.2	0	30%
wheat (Stella D'oro)	1 piece	42	1	6	0	0	1.4	0.0	0	30%
whole wheat, w/sesame (Angonoa's)	5 pieces	130	4	19	220	3	4.0	0.5	0	28%
whole wheat (Fattorie & Pandea)	3 pieces	57	2	10	100	0	1.0	0.0	0	16%
BREAKFAST BAR										
(Carnation)										
chocolate chip	1 bar	200	6	20	180	1	11.0	4.2	1	49%
chocolate crunch	1 bar	190	6	20	150	1	10.0	3.9	1	46%
peanut butter chocolate chip	1 bar	200	6	20	170	1	11.0	3.0	1	49%
peanut butter crunch	1 bar	190	6	20	180	1	10.0	2.8	1	46%
BREAKFAST BURRITO. See under BURRITO.										
BREAKFAST DRINK MIX										
(Carnation)										
regular, prepared w/8 fl oz 2% milk	9 oz	250	12	39	220	na	5.0	na	na	18%
sugarless, prepared w/8 fl oz 2% milk	9 oz	190	12	24	220	na	5.0	na	na	24%
(Ovaltine) traditional flavor, 'Classic'	4 tbsp	80	2	17	65	0	0.0	0.0	0	0%

Food Name	Serving Size	Calories	Prot. gms	Carbs gms	Sod. mgs	Fiber gms	Fat gms	Sat. Fat gms	Chol. mgs	% Fat Cal.
(Pillsbury)										
chocolate, variety pack, dry mix, 'Instant Breakfast'	1/10 pkg	130	6	25	135	0	0.0	0.0	0	0%
BREAKFAST SANDWICH										
(Great Starts)										
egg, beefsteak, and cheese	4.9 oz	360	17	27	730	0	20.0	0.0	0	51%
egg, Canadian bacon, cheese	5.2 oz	420	16	37	1845	0	22.0	0.0	0	48%
muffin w/egg, Canadian style bacon, cheese	1 pkg	290	14	25	750	2	15.0	6.0	95	46%
muffin w/egg, sausage, cheese	1 pkg	490	18	36	1110	3	30.0	12.0	145	56%
sausage, egg, and cheese biscuit	1 entree	460	16	37	1060	3	28.0	11.0	115	54%
(Jimmy Dean)										
biscuit w/egg, bacon, cheese	1 biscuit	300	11	28	890	2	16.0	6.0	95	48%
biscuit w/egg, ham, cheese	1 biscuit	240	13	26	720	1	10.0	3.0	100	37%
biscuit w/egg, sausage, cheese	1 biscuit	390	14	28	1040	2	27.0	10.0	115	59%
biscuit w/sausage, frozen	1 pkg	385	10	23	881	1	28.2	8.6	31	66%
biscuit w/sausage, frozen	1 sandwich	192	5	12	441	1	14.1	4.3	16	66%
biscuit w/sausage, frozen	1 serving	385	10	23	881	1	28.2	8.6	31	66%
biscuit w/sausage, microwavable	2 sandwiches	310	9	23	850	1	20.0	7.0	30	58%
sausage, refrigerated, microwave	1 sandwich	160	5	10	360	0	11.0	0.0	0	62%
(La Choy) ham, egg, and cheese breakfast roll, food										
service product	1 serving	237	10	22	463	2	12.6	3.6	91	47%
(Morningstar Farms)										
vegetarian, 'Breakfast Sandwich' w/muffin, patty,										
cheese, and Scramblers	1 sandwich	280	28	35	1000	5	3.0	0.5	10	9.6%
vegetarian, Scramblers patty sandwich	1 serving	300	18	29	590	na	12.0	na	na	36%
(Owens)										
sausage, biscuit, refrigerated, 'Border Breakfasts'	2 oz	210	6	14	400	0	14.0	0.0	0	61%
sausage, egg, and cheese, biscuit, refrigerated,										
'Border Breakfasts'	2.5 oz	250	8	15	500	0	15.0	0.0	0	59%
sausage, smoked, biscuit, refrigerated,										
'Border Breakfasts'	2 oz	200	4	15	786	0	6.0	0.0	0	42%
(Red Baron)										
bacon scramble, 'Sunrise Singles'	1 unit	420	16	34	830	2	24.0	9.0	65	52%
(Pierre)										
ham and cheese, wrapped, product 1295, 'Ham n Go'	1 piece	236	11	26	677	1	10.6	3.5	26	40%
ham, wrapped, product 1293, 'Ham-n-Go'	1 piece	223	11	26	660	1	8.9	2.3	26	36%
wrapped, 'Link-N-Dog' 'Dine'n w/Pierre'	1 piece	203	11	20	364	2	9.1	3.3	22	40%
wrapped, 'Saus-A-Rage' 'Dine'n w/Pierre'	1 piece	263	11	26	495	2	13.2	4.2	22	45%
(Quick Meal)										
sausage, biscuit	3.7 oz	350	10	29	870	0	22.0	0.0	40	56%
sausage, w/cheese, biscuit	4.3 oz	420	13	31	1060	0	27.0	10.0	60	58%
sausage, w/egg and cheese, muffin	5.1 oz	76	3	5	143	0	4.0	0.0	26	53%
sausage, w/egg, biscuit	4.5 oz	350	11	30	780	0	21.0	0.0	110	54%
(Red Baron)										
ham scramble, 'Sunrise Singles'	1 unit	370	15	34	770	2	19.0	7.0	65	47%
(Sunny Fresh)										
biscuit w/ham and cheese, pre-cooked, frozen	1 pkg	29206	1470	3028	87040	14	1165.4	316.2	13736	36%
biscuit w/ham and cheese, pre-cooked, frozen	1 serving	243	12	25	725	0	9.7	2.6	114	36%
egg and cheese biscuit, pre-cooked, frozen	1 pkg	26910	1187	2957	67751	0	1066.9	282.8	13336	36%
egg and cheese biscuit, pre-cooked, frozen	1 serving	224	10	25	565	0	8.9	2.4	111	36%
egg and cheese pocket sandwich, pre-cooked, frozen,										
'Breakfast Stuff-Its'	1 pkg	17605	814	1760	27862	115	913.9	366.7	11176	47%
egg and cheese pocket sandwich, pre-cooked, frozen,										
'Breakfast Stuff-Its'	1 serving	147	7	15	232	1	7.6	3.1	93	47%
(Red Baron) sausage scramble 'Sunrise Singles'	1 unit	380	15	34	730	2	21.0	8.0	65	49%

Food Name	Serving Size	Calories	Prot. gms	Carbs gms	Sod. mgs	Fiber gms	Fat gms	Sat. Fat gms	Chol. mgs	% Fat Cal.
(Swanson) egg, sausage & cheese 'Great Starts'	5.5 oz	460	18	35	1310	0	28.0	0.0	0	54%
(Weight Watchers) sausage, biscuit.	1 biscuit	230	11	20	660	2	11.0	3.5	25	44%

BREAKFAST STRIPS. See under BACON SUBSTITUTE.
BREWER'S YEAST. See under YEAST.
BROAD BEAN. See BEAN, FAVA.
BROCCOLI
Fresh

Food Name	Serving Size	Calories	Prot. gms	Carbs gms	Sod. mgs	Fiber gms	Fat gms	Sat. Fat gms	Chol. mgs	% Fat Cal.
boiled, drained, chopped............................	1/2 cup	22	2	4	20	2	0.3	0.0	0	10%
boiled, drained, spears, large, 11-12 inches long	1 spear	78	8	14	73	8	1.0	0.2	0	10%
boiled, drained, spears, medium, 7.5 - 8 inches long	1 spear	50	5	9	47	5	0.6	0.1	0	10%
boiled, drained, spears, small, 5 inches long	1 spear	39	4	7	36	4	0.5	0.1	0	10%
raw, bunch..	1 medium	170	18	32	164	18	2.1	0.3	0	10%
raw, chopped.....................................	1 cup	25	3	5	24	3	0.3	0.0	0	10%
raw, chopped or diced.,..........................	1/2 cup	12	1	2	12	1	0.2	0.0	0	10%
raw, florets......................................	1 cup	20	2	4	19	na	0.2	0.0	0	10%
raw, florets......................................	1 medium	3	0	1	3	na	0.0	0.0	0	11%
raw, spears, medium (Dole)	1 spear	40	5	4	75	5	1.0	0.0	0	20%
raw, spears, medium, 7.5-8 inches long	1 spear	42	5	8	41	5	0.5	0.1	0	10%
raw, spears, small, 5 inches long	1 spear	9	1	2	8	1	0.1	0.0	0	11%

Frozen

Food Name	Serving Size	Calories	Prot. gms	Carbs gms	Sod. mgs	Fiber gms	Fat gms	Sat. Fat gms	Chol. mgs	% Fat Cal.
(Flav-R-Pac)..........................	1 cup	25	2	4	20	2	0.0	0.0	0	0%
(Health Valley).......................	1/2 cup	26	3	5	24	3	0.0	0.0	0	0%
chopped (A&P).......................	3.3 oz	25	3	5	25	0	1.0	0.0	0	22%
chopped (Birds Eye)..................	3.3 oz	25	3	5	15	3	0.0	0.0	0	0%
chopped (Finast).....................	3.3 oz	25	3	5	20	3	0.0	0.0	0	0%
chopped (Flav-R-Pac).................	3/4 cup	30	2	5	5	3	0.0	0.0	0	0%
chopped (Frosty Acres)...............	3.3 oz	25	3	5	18	1	0.0	0.0	0	0%
chopped (Seabrook)..................	3.3 oz	25	3	5	18	1	0.0	0.0	0	0%
chopped (Southern)	3.5 oz	28	3	4	25	0	0.3	0.0	0	8%
chopped, drained	1 cup	52	6	10	478	6	0.2	0.0	0	4%
chopped, no salt added, drained......	1 cup	52	6	10	44	6	0.2	0.0	0	4%
chopped, 'Plain Polybag' (Green Giant)	3/4 cup	25	2	4	25	2	0.0	0.0	0	0%
chopped, unprepared	1 cup	41	4	7	37	5	0.5	0.1	0	9%
chopped, unprepared	10-oz pkg	74	8	14	68	9	0.8	0.1	0	9%
cuts (A&P)...........................	3.3 oz	25	3	5	25	0	1.0	0.0	0	22%
cuts (Birds Eye)......................	3.2 oz	25	3	5	25	3	0.0	0.0	0	0%
cuts (Flav-R-Pac)	1 cup	25	2	4	20	2	0.0	0.0	0	0%
cuts (Frosty Acres)	3.3 oz	25	3	5	50	1	0.0	0.0	0	0%
cuts (Pictsweet).....................	1 cup	25	2	4	20	2	0.0	0.0	0	0%
cuts (Seabrook).....................	3.3 oz	25	3	5	50	1	0.0	0.0	0	0%
cuts, 'Plain Polybag' (Green Giant)	1/2 cup	18	2	5	25	4	0.0	0.0	0	0%
cuts, 'Portion Pack' (Birds Eye)	3 oz	20	3	4	20	2	0.0	0.0	0	0%
cuts, 'Singles' (Stokely)	3 oz	25	3	5	15	0	1.0	0.0	0	22%
drained	1/2 cup	26	3	5	239	3	0.1	0.0	0	3%
drained	10-oz pkg	70	8	13	650	8	0.3	0.0	0	3%
florets (C&W)........................	3.3 oz	25	3	5	20	0	0.0	0.0	0	0%
florets (Frosty Acres).................	3.3 oz	30	3	5	14	1	0.0	0.0	0	0%
florets, 'Deluxe' (Birds Eye)..........	3.3 oz	25	3	5	20	3	0.0	0.0	0	0%
florets, 'Select Polybag' (Green Giant)	1 1/3 cup	25	2	4	25	2	0.0	0.0	0	0%
Normandy (Flav-R-Pac)	3/4 cup	25	2	4	30	2	0.0	0.0	0	0%
Normandy, w/buttery sauce (Flav-R-Pac)............	1/2 cup	45	2	7	490	3	2.5	0.0	0	38%
spears (A&P)........................	3.3 oz	25	3	5	20	0	1.0	0.0	0	22%
spears (Birds Eye)....................	3.3 oz	25	3	5	20	3	0.0	0.0	0	0%
spears (Frosty Acres)	3.3 oz	25	3	5	20	1	0.0	0.0	0	0%

Food Name	Serving Size	Calories	Prot. gms	Carbs gms	Sod. mgs	Fiber gms	Fat gms	Sat. Fat gms	Chol. mgs	% Fat Cal.
spears *(Seabrook)*.	3.3 oz	25	3	5	20	1	0.0	0.0	0	0%
spears *(Southern)*.	3.5 oz	30	3	5	30	0	0.2	0.0	0	5%
spears and florets, 'Deluxe' *(Birds Eye)*.	3.3 oz	25	3	5	20	3	0.0	0.0	0	0%
spears, 'Select Polybag' *(Green Giant)*.	3 oz	25	2	4	25	2	0.0	0.0	0	0%
spears, baby *(Seabrook)*.	3.3 oz	30	3	5	14	1	0.0	0.0	0	0%
spears, baby, 'Deluxe' *(Birds Eye)*.	3.3 oz	30	3	5	15	3	0.0	0.0	0	0%
spears, mini, *(Green Giant)*.	1/5 pkg	18	2	5	25	3	0.0	0.0	0	0%
spears, no salt added, drained	10-oz pkg	70	8	13	60	8	0.3	0.0	0	3%
spears, no salt added, drained	1/2 cup	26	3	5	22	3	0.1	0.0	0	3%
spears, whole, 'Farm Fresh' *(Birds Eye)*	4 oz	30	4	6	25	3	0.0	0.0	0	0%
unprepared	2-lb pkg	263	28	49	154	27	3.1	0.5	0	10%
unprepared	10-oz pkg	82	9	15	48	9	1.0	0.1	0	10%
BROCCOLI, CHINESE, cooked	1 cup	19	1	3	6	2	0.6	0.1	0	27%
BROCCOLI DISH/ENTRÉE										
(A&P) w/cauliflower, frozen	3.2 oz	25	2	4	20	0	1.0	0.0	0	27%
(Amy's Kitchen)										
pie, w/cheddar cheese, organic	8-oz pie	390	10	46	500	3	18.0	0.0	0	42%
pot pie	1 serving	430	11	46	630	4	22.0	10.0	45	46%
(Birds Eye)										
stir-fry, 'Farm Fresh Mixtures'	1 cup	30	2	5	30	2	0.0	0.0	0	0%
w/baby carrots and water chestnuts, 'Farm Fresh'	4 oz	45	2	10	35	3	0.0	0.0	0	0%
(Flav-R-Pac) cheddar broccoli Normandy, frozen,										
'Grande Classics'	1/2 cup	45	3	6	210	2	2.0	1.0	5	33%
(Frosty Acres) w/cauliflower, 'Swiss Mix'	3 oz	25	2	5	36	1	0.0	0.0	0	0%
(Green Giant)										
'Broccoli Fanfare' 'Valley Combinations'	1/2 cup	80	3	14	340	3	2.0	0.0	0	21%
in cheese flavored sauce	1 pkg	188	6	25	1344	na	7.0	1.3	na	33%
in cheese flavored sauce	1 cup	113	4	15	806	na	4.2	0.8	na	33%
in cheese flavored sauce	1 serving	75	3	10	538	na	2.8	0.5	na	33%
w/cauliflower, 'Valley Combinations'	1/2 cup	60	2	9	340	3	2.0	0.0	0	29%
w/red peppers, 'Select'	1/2 cup	25	2	4	15	2	0.0	0.0	0	0%
(Nancy's) broccoli-cheddar quiche, frozen, microwave,										
'French Baked'	1 quiche	490	17	33	750	2	33.0	16.0	165	60%
(Pepperidge Farm) w/cheese, in pastry, frozen	1 piece	230	5	18	380	0	16.0	0.0	0	61%
(Stokely)										
w/cauliflower 'Singles'	3 oz	20	2	4	15	0	1.0	0.0	0	27%
w/whole baby carrots, and water chestnuts, 'Singles'	3 oz	30	2	6	22	0	1.0	0.0	0	22%
(Stouffer's)										
and cheese soufflé, frozen, food service product	1 oz	35	2	2	129	0	2.1	0.9	32	54%
au gratin, frozen, food service product	1 oz	27	1	3	105	0	1.3	0.5	3	43%
BROCCOLI DISH/ENTRÉE MIX										
(Pasta Roni) and mushroom noodles entrée, 'Tenderthin'	1 serving	260	7	28	644	1	13.6	2.8	3	47%
(Rice A Roni)										
and cheese rice, 'Fast Cook'	2.5 oz	169	4	23	412	1	6.8	1.4	3	36%
au gratin	2.5 oz	209	4	27	500	1	9.6	2.3	3	41%
au gratin, w/rice, 1/3 less sodium	2.5 oz	181	4	28	333	1	6.2	1.4	3	31%
BROTH. See under SOUP.										
BROWN RICE. See under RICE.										
BROWNIE. See under CAKE, SNACK.										
BRUSSELS SPROUTS										
Fresh										
boiled, drained	1/2 cup	30	2	7	16	2	0.4	0.1	0	11%
boiled, drained, whole	1 medium	8	1	2	4	1	0.1	0.0	0	11%
raw	1 cup	38	3	8	22	3	0.3	0.1	0	6%

Food Name	Serving Size	Calories	Prot. gms	Carbs gms	Sod. mgs	Fiber gms	Fat gms	Sat. Fat gms	Chol. mgs	% Fat Cal.
raw	1 medium	8	1	2	5	1	0.1	0.0	0	6%
raw (Dole)	1/2 cup	19	1	4	11	2	0.1	0.0	0	4%
Frozen										
(A&P)	3.3 oz	35	3	7	15	0	1.0	0.0	0	18%
(Birds Eye)	3.3 oz	35	3	7	15	3	0.0	0.0	0	0%
(Flav-R-Pac)	6 medium	35	3	5	25	3	0.0	0.0	0	0%
(Frosty Acres)	3.3 oz	35	3	7	12	1	0.0	0.0	0	0%
(Pictsweet)	85 grams	35	3	5	25	3	0.0	0.0	0	0%
(Seabrook)	3.3 oz	35	3	7	12	1	0.0	0.0	0	0%
(Southern)	3.5 oz	37	3	8	20	0	0.0	0.0	0	0%
baby (Seabrook)	3.3 oz	40	4	7	5	1	0.0	0.0	0	0%
no salt, drained	1 cup	65	6	13	36	6	0.6	0.1	0	8%
petite (C&W)	3.2 oz	30	3	5	25	3	0.0	0.0	0	0%
'Plain Polybag' (Green Giant)	1/2 cup	25	2	6	10	2	0.0	0.0	0	0%
'Singles' (Stokely)	3 oz	35	4	7	10	0	0.0	0.0	0	0%
unprepared	2-lb pkg	372	34	71	91	34	3.7	0.8	0	8%
unprepared	10-oz pkg	116	11	22	28	11	1.2	0.2	0	8%
w/salt, drained	1 cup	65	6	13	401	6	0.6	0.1	0	8%
BUBBLE GUM. See under CANDY.										
BUCKWHEAT	1 cup	583	23	122	2	17	5.8	1.3	0	8%
BUCKWHEAT FLOUR. See under FLOUR.										
BUCKWHEAT GROATS, ROASTED / kasha										
cooked	1 cup	155	6	33	7	5	1.0	0.2	0	6%
dry	1 cup	567	19	123	18	17	4.4	1.0	0	7%
(Wolff's Kasha)	3/4 cup	150	4	35	2	4	0.0	0.0	0	0%
BUFFALO. See BISON.										
BULGUR. See also CEREAL, HOT.										
cooked	1 cup	151	6	34	9	8	0.4	0.1	0	2%
cooked	1 tbsp	7	0	2	0	0	0.0	0.0	0	2%
dry	1 cup	479	17	106	24	26	1.9	0.3	0	3%
BULGUR DISH/ENTRÉE MIX										
(Casbah)										
pilaf mix, dry	1 oz	100	3	21	270	2	0.0	0.0	0	0%
tabbouleh, seasoned, prepared	2/3 cup	120	6	24	410	1	0.5	0.0	0	4%
(Fantastic Foods) tabbouleh, seasoned	1/4 cup	120	4	26	450	6	0.5	0.0	0	4%
BULLOCK'S HEART. See CUSTARD APPLE.										
BUN. See also BISCUIT; BUN, FRANKFURTER; BUN, HAMBURGER; BUN, SWEET; CROISSANT; ENGLISH MUFFIN; ROLL.										
hoagie, deli (Wonder)	1 serving	260	8	49	500	2	3.5	0.5	0	12%
'Sof-Buns' (Holsum)	1 bun	120	3	23	190	0	2.0	0.0	0	15%
spelt, yeast-free, organic (French Meadow)	1 bun	160	9	33	155	5	1.4	0.0	0	7%
w/sesame seeds, 'Big BBQ Buns' (Holsum)	1 bun	200	5	38	320	0	3.0	0.0	0	14%
BUN, FRANKFURTER										
	1 oz	81	2	14	159	1	1.4	0.3	0	16%
(Arnold)										
	1 bun	100	3	20	162	1	1.8	0.0	0	15%
'New England Style'	1 bun	108	4	21	178	1	2.0	0.0	0	15%
oat bran	1 bun	110	4	20	210	1	2.0	0.0	0	16%
(Aunt Hattie's) potato	1 bun	150	5	23	260	0	4.0	0.0	0	24%
(Country Grain)	1 bun	100	4	18	230	1	1.0	0.0	0	9%
(Mrs. Wright's)										
crushed wheat	1 bun	110	4	20	230	1	1.5	0.0	0	12%
enriched	1 bun	100	3	19	190	1	1.5	0.0	0	13%
(Pepperidge Farm)										
	1 bun	140	5	24	270	1	3.0	1.0	0	19%

Food Name	Serving Size	Calories	Prot. gms	Carbs gms	Sod. mgs	Fiber gms	Fat gms	Sat. Fat gms	Chol. mgs	% Fat Cal.
Dijon	1 bun	160	5	23	230	2	5.0	1.0	0	29%
(Roman Meal)										
'Original'	1 bun	104	4	20	210	2	1.9	0.0	0	15%
whole-grain	1 bun	120	4	19	210	0	3.0	0.0	0	23%
(Wonder)										
	1 bun	110	3	21	220	0	1.5	0.0	0	12%
footlong Coney	1 bun	220	7	42	430	1	3.0	0.5	0	12%
'Light'	1 bun	80	5	13	210	4	1.0	0.0	0	11%
BUN, HAMBURGER										
	1 oz	81	2	14	159	1	1.4	0.3	0	16%
(Arnold)	1 bun	115	4	22	223	2	2.2	0.0	0	16%
(Aunt Hattie's) potato	1 bun	150	5	23	260	0	4.0	0.0	0	24%
(Mrs. Wright's)										
crushed wheat	1 bun	110	3	21	240	1	1.5	0.0	0	12%
enriched	1 bun	110	3	21	190	1	1.5	0.0	0	12%
enriched, w/sesame	1 bun	110	4	21	190	1	1.5	0.0	0	12%
(Pepperidge Farm)	1 bun	130	5	22	240	1	2.0	1.0	0	14%
(Roman Meal)										
'Original'	1 bun	113	5	21	228	2	1.9	0.0	0	14%
whole grain	1 bun	130	4	20	230	0	3.0	0.0	0	22%
(Wonder)										
	1 bun	110	3	21	220	0	1.5	0.0	0	12%
4-inch diam (Wonder)	1 bun	110	3	21	220	1	1.5	0.0	0	12%
'Light'	1 bun	80	5	13	210	4	1.0	0.0	0	11%
BUN, SWEET. See also PASTRY; ROLL, SWEET.										
(Aunt Fanny's)										
honey	3 oz	360	4	42	150	0	30.0	0.0	10	59%
honey, apple bear	4 oz	460	6	50	220	0	26.0	0.0	5	51%
honey, applesauce-filled	1 bun	330	6	43	300	4	17.0	4.0	0	44%
honey, banana creme filled	1 bun	350	5	32	290	2	18.0	4.0	0	52%
honey, birdie, jelly-filled	4 oz	450	6	53	210	0	24.0	0.0	5	48%
honey, bogie, creme-filled	4 oz	460	6	49	200	0	27.0	0.0	10	52%
honey, chocolate creme filled	1 bun	350	5	32	290	2	18.0	4.0	0	52%
honey, iced	1 bun	350	5	32	290	2	18.0	4.0	0	52%
honey, lemon bear	4 oz	440	5	52	200	0	23.0	0.0	5	48%
honey, raspberry-filled	1 bun	350	5	45	290	2	17.0	5.0	0	43%
honey, regular	1 bun	360	5	41	300	2	20.0	5.0	0	49%
honey, snow bear	4 oz	480	6	60	220	0	24.0	0.0	5	45%
honey, vanilla creme filled	1 bun	350	5	32	290	2	18.0	4.0	0	52%
(Break Cake)										
apple honey, multi pak, 1.5 oz	1 bun	170	2	20	90	0	10.0	2.7	0	51%
honey, 3 oz	1 bun	420	4	38	160	0	28.0	7.8	0	60%
honey, multi pak, 2.75 oz	1 bun	380	3	34	150	0	24.0	7.2	0	59%
(Entenmann's)										
blueberry cheese, nonfat, no cholesterol	1 serving	140	4	31	150	1	0.0	0.0	0	0%
cheese-topped	1 bun	240	5	29	240	0	12.0	0.0	0	44%
cinnamon	1 bun	230	4	31	200	0	10.0	0.0	0	39%
pineapple cheese, nonfat, no cholesterol	1 serving	140	4	30	150	1	0.0	0.0	0	0%
raspberry cheese, nonfat, no cholesterol	1 serving	160	4	36	135	1	0.0	0.0	0	0%
(Hostess)										
honey glazed, 'Breakfast Bake Shop'	1 piece	360	5	38	230	1	21.0	10.0	15	52%
honey iced, 'Breakfast Bake Shop'	1 piece	430	5	55	240	2	22.0	10.0	20	45%
(Morton) honey, microwave	1 bun	250	3	35	160	2	10.0	2.5	0	37%
(Pepperidge Farm) cinnamon, frozen, '2/pkg.'	1 piece	280	4	34	190	0	14.0	0.0	0	45%

Food Name	Serving Size	Calories	Prot. gms	Carbs gms	Sod. mgs	Fiber gms	Fat gms	Sat. Fat gms	Chol. mgs	% Fat Cal.
(Rich's)										
cinnamon, frozen, 2.5 oz, *'Ever Fresh'*	1 bun	293	4	38	0	0	14.6	0.0	0	44%
honey, frozen, mini, *'Ever Fresh'*	1.36 oz	133	2	18	0	0	6.6	0.0	0	43%
(Tastykake)										
honey glazed	3.25 oz	362	6	42	219	4	20.4	4.3	2	49%
honey iced	3.25 oz	348	5	50	254	2	14.9	3.3	2	38%
(Weight Watchers)										
cheese bun, frozen, 'Microwave'	1/2 pkg	180	5	32	5	0	4.0	1.0	210	20%
BURBOT										
baked, broiled, grilled, or microwaved	3 oz	98	21	0	105	0	0.9	0.2	65	8%
raw	3 oz	77	16	0	82	0	0.7	0.1	51	8%
BURDOCK ROOT / gobo										
boiled, drained, sliced, 1-inch pieces	1 cup	110	3	26	5	2	0.2	0.0	0	1%
boiled, drained, whole	1 med root	146	3	35	7	3	0.2	0.0	0	1%
raw, sliced, 1-inch pieces	1 cup	85	2	20	6	4	0.2	0.0	0	2%
raw, whole	1 med root	112	2	27	8	5	0.2	0.0	0	2%
BURGER. See under BEEF DINNER/ENTRÉE; BEEF SUBSTITUTE DINNER/ENTRÉE; and individual ground meat listings.										
BURGUNDY. See under WINE.										
BURRITO										
(Amy's Kitchen)										
bean and cheese burrito	1 burrito	280	10	43	460	6	8.0	2.5	10	25%
bean and rice burrito	1 burrito	250	9	44	450	6	5.0	0.2	0	18%
bean burrito, w/rice and cheese, organic, frozen, 6 oz	1 burrito	280	10	43	460	6	8.0	2.5	10	25%
breakfast burrito	1 serving	230	9	38	480	5	5.0	0.5	0	19%
(Don Miguel)										
beef, cheese & green chili	1 burrito	390	20	53	910	3	11.0	4.0	40	25%
chicken, cheese, no beans	1 burrito	410	18	52	950	3	14.0	4.0	45	31%
(Great Starts)										
breakfast burrito, hot and spicy	1 pkg	220	9	30	490	3	7.0	3.0	55	29%
breakfast burrito, w/cheese and chili peppers, 'Original'	1 pkg	200	8	25	510	2	8.0	3.0	60	35%
breakfast burrito, w/eggs, bacon, cheese	1 pkg	250	10	27	540	0	11.0	4.0	90	40%
breakfast, burrito, w/eggs, ham, cheese	1 pkg	210	9	29	350	0	6.0	2.0	60	26%
breakfast, burrito, w/eggs, pepperoni, cheese w/pizza sauce	1 pkg	240	9	28	410	0	9.0	3.0	60	35%
(Healthy Choice)										
beef and bean, 'Quick Meals'	5.2 oz	270	12	42	520	0	7.0	3.0	15	23%
chicken con queso, frozen, 'Quick Meals'	5.4 oz	280	15	40	500	0	8.0	2.0	20	25%
chicken con queso entrée	1 entrée	350	14	60	590	6	6.0	2.5	35	15%
(Homestyle Kitchens) black bean, organic, frozen	1 burrito	190	8	36	240	7	1.5	0.0	0	7%
(Hormel)										
beef, frozen	1 piece	205	9	31	780	0	8.0	0.0	0	31%
cheese, frozen	1 piece	210	9	32	792	0	5.0	0.0	0	22%
chicken and rice, frozen	1 piece	200	9	32	594	0	4.0	0.0	0	18%
chili, hot, frozen	1 piece	240	9	33	619	0	8.0	0.0	0	30%
(Las Campanas)										
bean and cheese, no lard	1 burrito	272	10	42	480	6	7.0	3.0	3	23%
beef and bean, frozen	1 pkg	2964	87	382	5791	8	120.8	41.8	125	37%
beef and bean, frozen	1 serving	296	9	38	579	1	12.1	4.2	13	37%
beef and bean, no lard	1 burrito	304	10	39	504	5	12.0	5.0	12	36%
(Maria's)										
bean and cheese, jalapeño	1 burrito	360	12	54	620	8	11.0	3.5	10	27%
beef and bean	1 burrito	420	13	49	660	5	19.0	6.0	25	41%

Food Name	Serving Size	Calories	Prot. gms	Carbs gms	Sod. mgs	Fiber gms	Fat gms	Sat. Fat gms	Chol. mgs	% Fat Cal.
(Marquez Pimera)										
beef, green chili, and cheese, 'Primera'	1 burrito	330	14	43	950	2	11.0	4.0	30	30%
beef, green chili, and Monterey Jack cheese, frozen	1 pkg	324	15	40	768	na	11.6	3.8	27	32%
(Old El Paso)										
bean and cheese, frozen	1 burrito	330	14	45	740	0	11.0	0.0	0	30%
beef and bean, frozen, 'Festive Dinners'	11 oz	470	23	72	1180	0	9.0	0.0	0	18%
beef and bean, hot, frozen	1 burrito	310	12	41	710	0	11.0	0.0	0	32%
beef and bean, medium, frozen	1 burrito	330	13	41	630	0	13.0	5.0	29	35%
beef and bean, mild, frozen	1 burrito	320	13	42	500	0	11.0	0.0	0	31%
packaged, prepared, w/filling	1 burrito	299	11	36	430	4	13.0	4.0	23	38%
(Patio)										
beef and bean, frozen	5 oz	370	11	43	830	0	16.0	0.0	0	40%
beef and bean, frozen, 'Britos'	3.63 oz	250	6	33	340	0	10.0	0.0	15	37%
beef and bean, green chili, frozen	5 oz	330	12	43	770	0	12.0	0.0	0	33%
beef and bean, nacho, frozen, 'Britos'	3.63 oz	270	9	30	420	0	13.0	0.0	25	43%
beef and bean, red chili, frozen	5 oz	340	11	44	810	0	13.0	0.0	0	35%
beef and bean, w/green chili, mild	1 pkg	325	10	44	879	4	11.9	4.0	20	33%
beef and bean, w/green chili, mild	1 serving	325	10	44	879	4	11.9	4.0	20	33%
chicken, spicy, frozen, 'Britos'	3.63 oz	250	6	33	330	0	10.0	0.0	25	37%
frozen	12 oz	517	18	74	1643	0	16.0	0.0	0	28%
green chili, frozen, 'Britos'	3.63 oz	250	6	33	420	0	10.0	0.0	15	37%
nacho cheese, frozen, 'Britos'	3.63 oz	250	7	32	330	0	10.0	0.0	20	37%
red chili, frozen, 'Britos'	3.63 oz	240	6	31	370	0	10.0	0.0	15	38%
red hot, frozen, 'Britos'	5 oz	360	12	43	800	0	15.0	0.0	0	38%
(Ruiz)										
beefsteak fajita, 'Supreme'	1 burrito	290	11	42	240	1	9.0	2.0	5	28%
chicken fajita, 'Supreme'	1 burrito	260	12	50	500	10	1.0	1.0	5	4%
BURRITO FILLING										
beans *(Del Monte)*	1/2 cup	110	6	20	900	0	1.0	0.0	0	8%
'Manwich' *(Hunt's)*	1/4 cup	25	1	6	559	4	0.2	0.0	0	7%
BURRITO SEASONING. See under SEASONING MIX.										
BUSH NUT. See MACADAMIA NUT.										
BUTTER										
light, salted, stick *(Land O'Lakes)* stick	1 tbsp	50	0	0	70	0	6.0	4.0	20	100%
light, salted, whipped *(Land O'Lakes)* whipped	1 tbsp	35	0	0	45	0	4.0	2.5	10	100%
light, unsalted, stick *(Land O'Lakes)*	1 tbsp	50	0	0	5	0	6.0	4.0	15	100%
lightly salted *(Darigold)*	1 tsp	25	0	0	25	0	3.0	1.7	7	100%
lightly salted *(Hotel Bar)*	1 tsp	35	0	0	35	0	4.0	0.0	0	100%
lightly salted *(Kellers)*	1 tsp	35	0	0	35	0	4.0	0.0	0	100%
lightly salted, stick *(Breakstone's)*	1 tbsp	100	0	0	90	0	11.0	7.0	35	100%
lightly salted, whipped *(Breakstone's)*	1 tbsp	70	0	0	65	0	7.0	4.0	20	100%
lightly salted, whipped *(Breakstone's)*	1 tbsp	70	0	0	65	0	7.0	4.0	20	100%
'Quarters' *(Darigold)*	1 tsp	35	0	0	2	0	4.0	2.5	11	100%
salted	1 cup	1628	2	0	1875	0	184.1	114.6	497	99%
salted	1 pat	36	0	0	41	0	4.1	2.5	11	99%
salted	1 stick	813	1	0	937	0	92.0	57.3	248	99%
salted	1 tbsp	102	0	0	117	0	11.5	7.2	31	99%
salted *(Hotel Bar)*	1 tsp	35	0	0	35	0	4.0	0.0	0	100%
salted *(Kellers)*	1 tsp	35	0	0	35	0	4.0	0.0	0	100%
salted, 'Quarters' *(Darigold)*	1 tsp	35	0	0	40	0	4.0	2.5	11	100%
salted, stick *(Land O'Lakes)*	1 tbsp	100	0	0	85	0	11.0	7.0	30	100%
salted, whipped *(Land O'Lakes)*	1 tsp	25	0	0	25	0	3.0	0.0	5	100%
salted, whipped	1 cup	1082	1	0	1248	0	122.5	76.2	331	99%
salted, whipped	1 pat	27	0	0	31	0	3.1	1.9	8	99%

Food Name	Serving Size	Calories	Prot. gms	Carbs gms	Sod. mgs	Fiber gms	Fat gms	Sat. Fat gms	Chol. mgs	% Fat Cal.
salted, whipped	1 stick	542	1	0	625	0	61.3	38.2	165	99%
salted, whipped	1 tbsp	67	0	0	78	0	7.6	4.7	21	99%
unsalted	1 pat	36	0	0	1	0	4.1	2.5	11	99%
unsalted	1 cup	1628	2	0	25	0	184.1	114.6	497	99%
unsalted	1 stick	813	1	0	12	0	92.0	57.3	248	99%
unsalted	1 tbsp	102	0	0	2	0	11.5	7.2	31	99%
unsalted (Land O'Lakes)	1 tsp	35	0	0	0	0	4.0	0.0	10	100%
unsalted, sweet, stick (Breakstone's)	1 tbsp	100	0	0	0	0	11.0	7.0	35	100%
unsalted, sweet, whipped (Breakstone's)	1 tbsp	70	0	0	0	0	7.0	4.0	20	100%
unsalted, whipped (Darigold)	1 tsp	25	0	0	2	0	3.0	1.6	7	100%
unsalted, whipped (Land O'Lakes)	1 tsp	25	0	0	0	0	3.0	0.0	5	100%
whipped (Breakstone's)	1 tbsp	70	0	0	0	0	7.0	0.0	0	100%
whipped (Darigold)	1 tsp	25	0	0	2	0	3.0	1.6	7	100%
whipped (Land O'Lakes)	1 tsp	25	0	0	0	0	3.0	0.0	5	100%
BUTTER ALTERNATIVE										
(Canola Harvest) canola oil spread	1 tbsp	100	0	0	110	0	11.0	1.0	0	100%
(Fleischmann's) corn oil spread, 60% oil, 'Light'	1 tbsp	80	0	0	70	0	8.0	1.0	0	100%
(I Can't Believe It's Not Butter!)										
buttermilk, no salt	1 tbsp	90	0	0	0	0	10.0	2.0	0	100%
buttermilk, stick	1 tbsp	90	0	0	95	0	10.0	2.0	0	100%
cream, buttermilk, squeezable	1 tbsp	90	0	0	90	0	10.0	2.0	0	100%
light spread, 40% vegetable oil, stick	1 tbsp	50	0	0	90	0	6.0	1.0	0	100%
soft, 70% vegetable oil	1 tbsp	90	0	0	95	0	10.0	2.0	0	100%
whipped	1 tbsp	60	0	0	70	0	7.0	1.5	0	100%
(Land O'Lakes)										
stick, no salt	1 tbsp	90	na	na	0	0	10.0	2.0	0	100%
tub	1 tbsp	80	na	na	70	0	8.0	2.0	0	100%
w/sweet cream, salted, stick	1 tbsp	90	na	na	95	0	10.0	2.0	0	100%
(Mazola) corn oil spread, 40% corn oil, light	1 tbsp	50	0	0	100	0	6.0	1.0	0	100%
(Spectrum Naturals) canola oil spread, 100% dairy-free, nonhydrogenated	1 tbsp	94	0	0	84	0	11.0	7.0	0	100%
BUTTER FLAVORING										
(Butter Buds) fat-free, sprinkles	1 tsp	5	0	2	120	na	0.0	na	0	0%
(Fry's)	1/2 tsp	4	0	0	70	0	0.0	0.0	0	0%
(Molly McButter) fat-free, natural butter flavor, sprinkles	1 tsp	5	0	1	180	na	0.0	0.0	0	0%
(Schilling) naturally flavored, 'Best 'O Butter'	1/2 tsp	4	1	1	65	0	1.0	0.0	0	53%
BUTTER OIL										
anhydrous	1 cup	1796	1	0	3	0	203.9	126.9	525	100%
anhydrous	1 tbsp	112	0	0	0	0	12.7	7.9	33	100%
BUTTERBEAN. See BEAN, LIMA.										
BUTTERBUR / fuki										
Canned										
chopped	1 cup	4	0	0	5	na	0.2	na	0	36%
stalks, whole	3 medium	1	0	0	2	na	0.1	na	0	37%
Fresh										
raw, chopped	1 cup	13	0	3	7	na	0.0	na	0	2%
raw, petioles, whole	1 medium	1	0	0	0	na	0.0	na	0	2%
BUTTERFISH										
baked, broiled, grilled, or microwaved	3 oz	159	19	0	97	0	8.7	na	71	50%
raw	3 oz	124	15	0	76	0	6.8	2.9	55	50%
BUTTERHEAD LETTUCE. See under LETTUCE.										
BUTTERMILK										
cultured (A&P)	1 cup	90	8	12	260	0	1.0	0.0	0	10%
cultured (Crowley)	1 cup	110	9	12	390	0	4.0	0.0	15	30%

Food Name	Serving Size	Calories	Prot. gms	Carbs gms	Sod. mgs	Fiber gms	Fat gms	Sat. Fat gms	Chol. mgs	% Fat Cal.
cultured, low-fat..............................	1 quart	396	32	47	1028	0	8.6	5.4	34	19%
cultured, low-fat..............................	1 cup	99	8	12	257	0	2.2	1.3	9	19%
cultured, low-fat..............................	1 fl oz	12	1	1	32	0	0.3	0.2	1	19%
cultured, 1.5%, 'Golden Churn' (Borden)..............	1 cup	120	8	11	250	0	4.0	0.0	0	32%
cultured, 1.5%, 'Unsalted' (Friendship)...............	1 cup	120	9	12	125	0	4.0	0.0	14	30%
cultured, 2%, (Knudsen)........................	1 cup	120	8	12	140	0	5.0	0.0	0	36%
cultured, 'Unsalted' (Crowley)...................	1 cup	110	9	12	130	0	4.0	0.0	15	30%
cultured, 'Unsalted' (Friendship)................	1 cup	120	9	12	125	0	4.0	0.0	14	30%
dry..	1 cup	464	41	59	621	0	6.9	4.3	83	13%
dry..	1 tbsp	25	2	3	34	0	0.4	0.2	5	13%
dry, blend, cultured (Saco Foods)...............	3.5 tbsp	79	8	11	168	0	0.7	0.0	0	8%
BUTTERNUT										
dried	1 cup	734	30	14	1	6	68.4	1.6	0	78%
dried	1 oz	174	7	3	0	1	16.2	0.4	0	78%
dried	1 nutmeat	18	1	0	0	0	1.7	0.0	0	78%
BUTTERNUT SQUASH. See under SQUASH.										
BUTTERSCOTCH. See under CANDY.										
BUTTERSCOTCH TOPPING										
(Kraft)	1 tbsp	60	0	13	70	0	1.0	0.0	0	15%
(Smucker's)...................................	2 tbsp	140	0	33	75	0	1.0	0.0	0	6%
BUTTON MUSHROOM. See MUSHROOM, WHITE.										

C

Food Name	Serving Size	Calories	Prot. gms	Carbs gms	Sod. mgs	Fiber gms	Fat gms	Sat. Fat gms	Chol. mgs	% Fat Cal.
CABBAGE, COMMON										
boiled, drained, shredded	1/2 cup	17	1	3	6	2	0.3	0.0	0	16%
boiled, drained, whole, medium, approx										
5.75-inch diam	1 head	278	13	56	101	29	5.4	0.7	0	16%
raw, chopped................................	1 cup	22	1	5	16	2	0.2	0.0	0	9%
raw, leaf, large leaf	1 leaf	8	0	2	6	1	0.1	0.0	0	9%
raw, leaf, medium leaf......................	1 leaf	6	0	1	4	1	0.1	0.0	0	9%
raw, leaf, small leaf	1 leaf	4	0	1	3	0	0.0	0.0	0	9%
raw, shredded	1 cup	18	1	4	13	2	0.2	0.0	0	9%
raw, whole, large, approx 7-inch diam............	1 head	312	18	68	225	29	3.4	0.4	0	9%
raw, whole, medium head, approx 5.75-inch diam	1 head	227	13	49	163	21	2.5	0.3	0	9%
raw, whole, small head, approx 4.5-inch diam	1 head	179	10	39	129	16	1.9	0.2	0	9%
CABBAGE, DANISH										
raw, shredded	1/2 cup	8	0	2	6	1	0.1	0.0	0	6%
raw, whole, medium........................	1 head	218	11	49	163	21	1.6	0.2	0	6%
CABBAGE, NAPA. See BOK CHOY.										
CABBAGE, RED										
Canned or jarred										
sweet and sour (Green Giant)................	1/2 cup	90	1	21	640	2	0.0	0.0	0	0%
sweet and sour (S&W)	2 tbsp	15	0	3	160	0	0.0	0.0	0	0%
Fresh										
boiled, drained, leaf........................	1 leaf	5	0	1	2	0	0.0	0.0	0	8%
boiled, drained, shredded	1/2 cup	16	1	3	6	2	0.1	0.0	0	8%
raw, chopped................................	1 cup	24	1	5	10	2	0.2	0.0	0	8%
raw, leaf, medium	1 leaf	6	0	1	3	0	0.1	0.0	0	8%
raw, shredded	1 cup	19	1	4	8	1	0.2	0.0	0	8%
raw, whole, large, approx 5.5-inch diam	1 head	306	16	69	125	23	2.9	0.4	0	8%

Food Name	Serving Size	Calories	Prot. gms	Carbs gms	Sod. mgs	Fiber gms	Fat gms	Sat. Fat gms	Chol. mgs	% Fat Cal.
raw, whole, medium, approx 5-inch diam	1 head	227	12	51	92	17	2.2	0.3	0	8%
raw, whole, small, approx 4-inch diam	1 head	153	8	35	62	11	1.5	0.2	0	8%
CABBAGE, SAVOY										
boiled, drained, shredded	1 cup	35	3	8	35	4	0.1	0.0	0	3%
raw, shredded	1 cup	19	1	4	20	2	0.1	0.0	0	3%
CABBAGE, SKUNK / swamp cabbage / water convolvulus										
boiled, drained, chopped	1 cup	20	2	4	120	2	0.2	0.0	0	10%
raw, chopped	1 cup	11	1	2	63	1	0.1	na	0	9%
raw, medium shoot	1 shoot	2	0	0	15	0	0.0	na	0	9%
CABBAGE DISH/ENTRÉE										
(Lean Cuisine)										
stuffed cabbage, w/whipped potatoes	1 entrée	220	11	27	460	5	7.0	1.5	25	29%
stuffed cabbage w/meat and tomato sauce, potato	1 pkg	199	12	26	412	6	5.6	1.7	24	26%
(Efficienc)										
stuffed cabbage roll entrée, food service product	1 serving	168	11	17	1026	na	6.0	na	na	33%
(Stouffer's)										
stuffed cabbage, w/o sauce, frozen, food service product	1 oz	36	2	3	136	1	1.9	0.7	6	48%
stuffed cabbage, w/sauce, frozen, food service product	1 oz	27	1	3	128	0	1.2	0.3	3	41%
CABBAGE TURNIP. See KOHLRABI.										
CAJUN SEASONING. See under MARINADE MIX; SEASONING MIX; SEASONING AND COATING MIX.										
CAKE. See also BREAD, QUICK; CAKE, SNACK; CAKE MIX.										
(Awrey's)										
'Best Wishes' 6-inch diam	1/4 cake	150	1	18	170	0	9.0	3.0	25	52%
'Four-in-One Occasion'	1.3 oz	150	1	18	170	0	8.0	2.0	25	49%
BANANA										
(Entenmann's)										
crunch, fat-free, cholesterol-free	1 slice	140	2	33	150	2	0.0	0.0	0	0%
loaf, fat-free, cholesterol-free	1 slice	150	2	34	190	1	0.0	0.0	0	0%
(Sara Lee) single layer, iced	1/8 cake	170	1	28	160	0	6.0	0.0	0	32%
BLACK FOREST										
(Awrey's) torte	1/14 cake	350	3	38	330	1	21.0	7.0	50	54%
(Sara Lee) two-layer, frozen	1/8 cake	190	2	28	100	0	8.0	0.0	0	38%
BLUEBERRY										
(Entenmann's) crunch, fat-free, cholesterol-free	1 slice	140	2	32	200	2	0.0	0.0	0	0%
BOSTON CREAM PIE										
(Pepperidge Farm)	1 slice	260	3	42	120	1	9.0	2.5	45	31%
(Weight Watchers) frozen, approx 1/2 pkg	3 oz	160	3	34	260	0	4.0	1.0	5	20%
CARAMEL FUDGE *(Weight Watchers)* à la mode	1 serving	160	4	29	180	0	3.0	1.0	5	17%
CARROT										
(Awrey's) cream cheese iced, three-layer	1/12 cake	390	5	44	310	1	23.0	5.0	45	51%
(Entenmann's) fat-free, cholesterol-free	1 slice	170	3	40	230	1	0.0	0.0	0	0%
(Pepperidge Farm)										
cream cheese iced, frozen, 'Old Fashioned'	1.5 oz	150	1	19	160	0	9.0	3.0	15	50%
'Deluxe'	1 slice	310	2	39	320	1	16.0	4.0	40	47%
(Sara Lee) single layer, iced, frozen	1/8 cake	250	3	30	240	0	13.0	0.0	25	47%
(Stilwell) frozen, 'Oregon Farms'	1/6 cake	280	4	38	370	3	15.0	2.5	30	45%
(Weight Watchers) frozen, 1/2 pkg	3 oz	170	4	27	280	0	5.0	1.0	5	27%
CHEESECAKE										
(Sara Lee)										
cream strawberry, frozen	1/6 cake	222	4	34	171	0	8.0	0.0	0	32%
cream, cherry, frozen	1/6 cake	243	4	35	184	0	8.0	0.0	0	32%
cream, plain, frozen	1/6 cake	230	5	27	153	0	11.0	0.0	0	44%
French, frozen, 'Classics'	1/8 cake	250	4	23	120	0	16.0	0.0	20	57%

Food Name	Serving Size	Calories	Prot. gms	Carbs gms	Sod. mgs	Fiber gms	Fat gms	Sat. Fat gms	Chol. mgs	% Fat Cal.
strawberry, French, frozen, 'Classics'	1/8 cake	240	3	28	125	0	13.0	0.0	20	49%
(Tofutti) nondairy, frozen, 'Better than Cheesecake'	1/10 cake	160	2	16	110	0	10.0	0.0	0	56%
(Weight Watchers)										
brownie	1 serving	200	9	33	220	4	6.0	2.0	5	24%
frozen	3.9 oz	210	10	29	230	0	7.0	2.0	20	29%
New York style	1 serving	150	6	21	140	0	5.0	2.0	10	29%
strawberry, frozen, 'Sweet Celebrations'	3.9 oz	180	7	28	210	0	4.0	2.0	20	20%
triple chocolate	1 serving	200	7	32	200	1	5.0	2.5	10	22%
triple chocolate, frozen, 'Sweet Celebrations'	1 cake	190	8	30	220	0	4.0	2.0	5	19%
CHERRY (Weight Watchers) cherries and cream, frozen	3 oz	190	3	32	200	0	6.0	1.0	5	28%
CHOCOLATE										
(Awrey's)										
double chocolate torte	1/14 cake	340	3	51	300	2	15.0	4.0	35	38%
double chocolate, three-layer	1/12 cake	310	3	48	290	2	14.0	4.0	35	38%
double chocolate, two-layer	1/12 cake	250	3	38	260	1	11.0	3.0	35	38%
German, iced, 2x2-inch piece	1 piece	160	2	19	150	0	9.0	3.0	20	49%
German chocolate, three-layer	1/12 cake	350	3	46	300	1	18.0	6.0	40	45%
'Happy Birthday'	1.4 oz	150	1	18	150	1	8.0	3.0	25	49%
milk chocolate, yellow, two-layer	1/12 cake	290	3	33	320	0	17.0	5.0	50	52%
white iced, two-layer	1/12 cake	270	3	34	290	1	15.0	5.0	40	48%
(Entenmann's)										
crunch, fat-free, cholesterol-free	1 slice	130	2	32	170	2	0.0	0.0	0	0%
devil's food, fudge iced	1.2 oz	130	2	19	120	0	5.0	0.0	0	35%
fudge iced, fat-free, cholesterol-free	1 slice	210	3	51	270	2	0.0	0.0	0	0%
loaf, fat-free, cholesterol-free	1 slice	130	3	30	250	1	0.0	0.0	0	0%
(Pepperidge Farm)										
chocolate mousse	1 slice	250	2	35	120	2	10.0	3.0	25	38%
devil's food, layer	1 slice	290	2	40	220	2	14.0	5.0	35	43%
frozen, 'Supreme'	2 7/8 oz	300	3	37	140	0	16.0	7.0	25	47%
fudge layer cake	1 slice	300	2	38	230	2	16.0	5.0	35	47%
fudge stripe layer cake	1 slice	290	2	38	150	2	14.0	3.0	35	44%
German chocolate, layer	1 slice	300	2	37	280	2	16.0	4.0	35	48%
(Sara Lee)										
chocolate mousse, frozen, 'Classics'	1/8 cake	260	3	23	100	0	17.0	0.0	20	60%
double chocolate, three layer, frozen	1/8 cake	220	3	26	130	0	11.0	0.0	20	46%
frozen, 'Free & Light'	1/8 cake	110	2	26	140	0	0.0	0.0	0	0%
(Stilwell) bar cake, frozen	1/6 cake	260	3	43	410	2	9.0	2.0	40	31%
(Weight Watchers)										
devil's food, 'Sweet Rewards'	1 serving	160	2	36	370	1	1.5	0.5	0	8%
double fudge	1 serving	190	4	36	200	2	4.5	1.0	0	20%
frozen	2.5 oz	180	5	31	250	0	5.0	1.0	5	24%
German chocolate, frozen	2.5 oz	200	4	31	220	0	7.0	1.0	5	31%
CHOCOLATE VANILLA ROLL										
(Ener-G Foods) gluten-free	2 oz	168	0	28	59	0	4.0	1.1	102	24%
CINNAMON (Pillsbury) swirl, refrigerated	1/8 pkg	180	2	22	170	0	9.0	2.0	0	46%
CINNAMON APPLE										
(Entenmann's) twist, fat-free, cholesterol-free	1 slice	150	3	35	110	1	0.0	0.0	0	0%
COCONUT										
(Pepperidge Farm) layer	1 slice	300	2	41	200	1	14.0	4.0	40	42%
(Awrey's) yellow, three-layer	1/12 cake	350	3	40	340	0	21.0	7.0	50	52%
COFFEECAKE										
(Awrey's)										
caramel nut	1/12 cake	140	2	15	150	0	8.0	2.0	5	51%
'Long John'	1/12 cake	160	2	19	130	0	8.0	2.0	10	46%

Food Name	Serving Size	Calories	Prot. gms	Carbs gms	Sod. mgs	Fiber gms	Fat gms	Sat. Fat gms	Chol. mgs	% Fat Cal.
(Entenmann's)										
cheese....	1.6 oz	150	3	20	140	0	7.0	0.0	0	41%
cinnamon apple, fat-free, cholesterol-free.	1 slice	130	2	29	110	2	0.0	0.0	0	0%
crumb	1.3 oz	160	3	21	160	0	7.0	0.0	0	40%
crumb, cheese-filled	1.4 oz	130	3	18	140	0	6.0	0.0	0	39%
(Pillsbury)										
cinnamon swirl, w/icing	1 serving	230	3	29	240	0	11.0	2.0	0	44%
pecan crumb, w/icing	1 serving	230	3	29	240	0	12.0	2.0	0	46%
(Sara Lee)										
cheese, all butter, frozen	1/8 cake	210	4	25	220	0	11.0	0.0	0	46%
pecan, all butter, frozen	1/8 cake	160	3	19	180	0	8.0	0.0	0	45%
streusel, all butter, frozen	1/8 cake	160	3	20	160	0	7.0	0.0	0	41%
CRUMB										
(Entenmann's)										
apple spice, fat-free, cholesterol-free	1 slice	138	2	32	148	2	0.0	0.0	0	0%
French, all butter	1.6 oz	180	2	26	220	0	8.0	0.0	0	39%
golden, French, fat-free, cholesterol-free	1 slice	140	2	35	150	2	0.0	0.0	0	0%
FRUIT *(Ener-G Foods)* loaf, gluten-free	1 slice	118	3	22	130	7	2.2	0.4	13	17%
FUNNEL *(Funnel Cake Factory)* 5-inch	1 serving	270	4	31	230	1	14.0	3.0	30	47%
GOLDEN										
(Entenmann's)										
fudge iced, fat-free, cholesterol-free	1 slice	220	3	52	200	2	0.0	0.0	0	0%
thick fudge	1.2 oz	130	2	20	120	0	6.0	0.0	0	38%
(Pepperidge Farm) layer	1 slice	290	3	38	230	1	14.0	3.0	50	43%
LEMON										
(Awrey's)										
three-layer	1/12 cake	320	2	38	310	0	19.0	5.0	45	52%
yellow, two-layer	1/12 cake	290	2	33	310	0	17.0	5.0	45	52%
(Pepperidge Farm)										
lemon coconut, frozen, 'Supreme'	3 oz	280	3	38	220	0	13.0	6.0	30	42%
lemon cream, frozen, 'Supreme'	1 5/8 oz	170	2	21	120	0	9.0	3.0	20	47%
LOUISIANA CRUNCH										
(Entenmann's)										
	1.7 oz	180	2	27	180	0	8.0	0.0	0	38%
fat-free, cholesterol-free	1 slice	220	3	51	220	1	0.0	0.0	0	0%
MARBLE *(Entenmann's)* loaf, fat-free, cholesterol-free	1 slice	130	2	29	190	1	0.0	0.0	0	0%
NEAPOLITAN *(Awrey's)* torte	1/14 cake	380	3	43	370	0	22.0	7.0	55	52%
ORANGE *(Awrey's)* three-layer	1/12 cake	320	2	40	320	0	17.0	4.0	35	48%
PEANUT BUTTER *(Awrey's)* torte	1/14 cake	380	7	44	340	1	22.0	5.0	40	49%
PECAN STREUSEL *(Pillsbury)* refrigerated	1/8 pkg	180	2	21	170	0	9.0	2.0	0	47%
PINEAPPLE										
(Entenmann's) crunch	1 oz slice	70	1	16	85	0	0.0	0.0	0	0%
(Pepperidge Farm) pineapple cream, frozen, 'Supreme'	2 oz	190	2	28	130	0	7.0	2.0	20	34%
PISTACHIO *(Awrey's)* torte	1/12 cake	370	3	41	370	1	22.0	7.0	35	53%
POUND										
(Awrey's) golden	1/14 loaf	130	2	19	150	0	5.0	1.0	20	35%
(Ener-G Foods) gluten-free	1 serving	236	4	32	576	3	9.9	2.4	9	38%
(Entenmann's)										
all butter, loaf	1 oz	110	2	15	150	0	5.0	0.0	0	40%
sour cream, loaf	1 oz	120	1	14	90	0	7.0	0.0	0	51%
(Pepperidge Farm) frozen, 'Old Fashioned Cholesterol-Free'	1 oz	110	1	13	85	0	6.0	1.0	0	49%
(Sara Lee)										
all butter, frozen, 'Family Size Original'	1/15 cake	130	2	14	85	0	7.0	0.0	0	50%
all butter, frozen, 'Original'	1/10 cake	130	2	14	85	0	7.0	0.0	0	50%

Food Name	Serving Size	Calories	Prot. gms	Carbs gms	Sod. mgs	Fiber gms	Fat gms	Sat. Fat gms	Chol. mgs	% Fat Cal.
all butter, frozen, 1.6 oz.	1 piece	200	2	23	190	0	11.0	0.0	0	50%
frozen, 'Free & Light'	1/10 cake	70	1	17	105	0	0.0	0.0	0	0%
RASPBERRY										
(Awrey's) nut	1/16 cake	310	3	39	220	0	16.0	3.0	30	46%
(Entenmann's) twist, fat-free, cholesterol-free	1 slice	140	3	33	125	2	0.0	0.0	0	0%
(Great Cakes) bar, all natural	3 oz	175	7	35	4	16	2.0	0.0	0	10%
SHORTCAKE (Sara Lee) strawberry, frozen	1/8 cake	190	2	26	90	0	8.0	0.0	0	39%
SPONGE (Awrey's) 2x2-inch piece	1 piece	80	1	11	125	0	3.0	1.0	15	36%
STRAWBERRY										
(Awrey's) strawberry supreme torte	1/14 cake	270	3	38	310	1	12.0	3.0	45	40%
(Pepperidge Farm)										
strawberry cream, frozen, 'Supreme'	2 oz	190	1	30	120	0	7.0	3.0	20	34%
strawberry stripe, layer	1 slice	310	2	47	150	1	13.0	4.0	65	37%
VANILLA (Pepperidge Farm) layer	1 slice	290	2	41	190	1	13.0	2.5	45	40%
WALNUT (Awrey's) torte	1/14 cake	320	2	38	290	0	19.0	4.0	30	52%
YELLOW (Awrey's) white iced, 2x2-inch piece	1 piece	150	1	18	180	0	9.0	3.0	25	52%
CAKE, SNACK										
(Awrey's) 'Best Wishes, Miniature'	3 oz	320	5	33	280	0	22.0	9.0	0	57%
(Break Cake)										
filled twins, 3 oz.	2 cakes	310	2	53	260	0	10.0	2.7	15	29%
filled twins, multi-pak, 1.5 oz.	1 cake	150	1	26	130	0	5.0	1.3	5	29%
(Drake's)										
cream filled, 'Sunny Doodle'	1 piece	100	1	16	100	0	3.0	1.0	10	28%
cream filled, 'Ring Ding'	1 piece	100	1	16	110	0	4.0	1.0	0	35%
'Funny Bone'	1.25 oz	150	3	18	110	0	8.0	2.0	0	46%
'Zoinks'	1.25 oz	130	1	20	130	0	5.0	1.0	10	35%
(Erewhon) 'Poppets'	1 oz	110	2	24	10	1	1.0	0.0	0	8%
(Hostess)										
dessert cup	1 piece	90	2	18	170	0	2.0	1.0	15	18%
'Lil' Angels'	1 piece	90	1	14	95	0	2.0	0.0	2	23%
'Snowballs'	1 serving	180	1	31	190	1	5.0	2.5	5	26%
'Suzy Q's'	1 serving	230	2	35	270	1	9.0	4.0	10	35%
'Tiger Tail'	1 piece	240	4	38	290	1	8.0	4.0	25	30%
'Twinkie'	1 serving	150	1	25	200	0	5.0	2.0	20	30%
(Little Debbie)										
'Be My Valentine'	2.5 oz	330	2	44	125	0	17.0	0.0	1	45%
'Caravella'	1.2 oz	200	2	26	95	0	9.0	0.0	1	42%
Christmas tree	1 cake	190	1	26	100	0	10.0	2.0	0	45%
dessert cup	0.79 oz	80	1	4	170	0	1.0	0.0	1	31%
'Doodle Dandies'	2.5 oz	320	2	44	140	0	16.0	0.0	1	44%
'Easter Bunny'	2.5 oz	320	2	45	135	0	15.0	0.0	1	42%
'Tiger Cake'	1 cake	310	2	44	190	1	15.0	3.5	0	42%
(Sunbelt) bar, baked	1.31 oz	130	1	28	130	0	2.0	0.0	1	13%
(Tastykake) 'Tasty Twist'	1 piece	18	0	3	0	0	0.6	0.0	0	31%
ANGEL FOOD (Break Cake)	1 oz	70	1	16	100	0	0.0	0.0	0	0%
APPLE										
(Aunt Fanny's) applesauce	2.5 oz	234	3	40	230	0	7.0	0.0	0	27%
(Awrey's) apple streusel	1 piece	160	2	18	120	0	9.0	1.0	15	50%
(Erewhon) 'Apple Stroodles'	1 oz	90	3	23	15	3	0.0	0.0	0	0%
(Hostess) 'Light'	1 piece	130	2	29	150	1	1.0	1.0	0	7%
(Little Debbie)										
'Apple Delight'	1.25 oz	140	2	24	95	0	4.0	0.0	1	26%
apple spice, 2.2 oz	1 piece	270	2	41	180	0	11.0	0.0	1	37%

Food Name	Serving Size	Calories	Prot. gms	Carbs gms	Sod. mgs	Fiber gms	Fat gms	Sat. Fat gms	Chol. mgs	% Fat Cal.
(Pepperidge Farm)										
apple spice, frozen, 'Dessert Lights' 4.25 oz	1 piece	170	2	37	105	0	2.0	0.0	10	10%
(Sara Lee) frozen, apple crisp 'Lights' 3 oz	1 piece	150	1	31	130	0	2.0	0.0	5	12%
(Weight Watchers) apple raisin bar	1 bar	70	1	14	60	2	2.0	0.5	0	23%
BANANA										
(Awrey's) iced	1 piece	140	1	17	120	0	8.0	2.0	20	50%
(Break Cake) banana marshmallow pie	1 pie	150	1	25	80	0	5.0	1.4	0	30%
(Hostess) 'Suzy Q's'	1 piece	240	2	4	200	0	9.0	0.0	20	78%
(Little Debbie) banana slices	3 oz	340	3	54	260	0	12.0	0.0	1	32%
(Tastykake) 'Creamie'	1.5 oz	185	2	25	91	1	7.1	1.6	8	38%
BLACK FOREST *(Sara Lee)* frozen, 3.6 oz, 'Lights'	1 piece	170	3	34	85	0	5.0	0.0	10	23%
BOSTON CREAM *(Pepperidge Farm)* frozen, 'Hyannis'	1 piece	230	4	34	125	2	10.0	4.0	70	37%
BROWN RICE TREAT										
(Glenny's)										
98% fat-free, 100% natural	1 pkg	120	1	28	25	1	3.0	0.0	0	19%
caramel, 100% natural	1.25 oz	120	1	29	70	1	0.0	0.0	0	0%
chocolate, 100% natural	1.25 oz	120	1	28	10	2	0.0	0.0	0	0%
BROWNIE										
(Auburn Farms)										
butterscotch, nonfat, 'Jammers'	1 serving	100	2	22	90	2	0.0	0.0	0	0%
cappuccino fudge, nonfat, 'Jammers'	1 serving	90	2	22	90	2	0.0	0.0	0	0%
chocolate fudge, nonfat, 'Jammers'	1 serving	90	2	22	95	2	0.0	0.0	0	0%
butterscotch, nonfat, 'Jammers'	1 brownie	100	2	22	65	2	0.0	0.0	0	0%
cappuccino fudge, nonfat, 'Jammers'	1 brownie	100	2	22	90	2	0.0	0.0	0	0%
chocolate fudge, nonfat, 'Jammers'	1 brownie	90	2	22	95	2	0.0	0.0	0	0%
raspberry fudge, nonfat, 'Jammers'	1 brownie	90	2	22	95	2	0.0	0.0	0	0%
whole wheat fudge	1 serving	90	2	22	35	2	0.0	0.0	0	0%
(Awrey's)										
Dutch chocolate, 'Cake'	1/16 cake	340	3	40	260	1	20.0	4.0	35	51%
fudge nut, iced, 'Sheet Cake' 2.5 oz	1 brownie	300	3	36	210	1	17.0	3.0	40	50%
fudge nut, 'Sheet Cake' 1.25 oz	1 brownie	150	2	16	115	1	9.0	1.0	25	53%
(Break Cake)										
chocolate nut, mini, 0.5 oz	1 brownie	70	1	9	60	0	4.0	0.6	0	47%
fudge, 2.8 oz	1 brownie	370	4	47	260	0	18.0	4.1	35	44%
(Ener-G Foods) gluten free	1 serving	108	2	16	178	2	4.1	1.0	10	34%
(Entenmann's) fudge, cholesterol-free	1 piece	110	2	27	140	1	0.0	0.0	0	0%
(Frito-Lay's) fudge nut, 3 oz	1 brownie	360	3	56	225	0	14.0	0.0	8	35%
(Health Valley) fudge brownie bar, nonfat	1 bar	110	3	26	30	4	0.0	0.0	0	0%
(Hostess) fudge, chocolate iced, lowfat, 'Lights'	1 brownie	140	2	29	95	1	2.6	0.5	10	16%
(Little Debbie)										
fudge	1 brownie	270	2	39	170	1	13.0	2.5	15	42%
low-fat	1 serving	190	3	39	200	1	3.0	0.0	0	14%
twin wrapped	1 pkg	247	3	39	190	1	9.9	2.6	10	35%
(Nestlé)										
chocolate chip, frozen, 'Toll House Ready to Bake'	1.4 oz	150	2	19	60	0	7.0	0.0	0	43%
(Pepperidge Farm) hot fudge, 'Newport'	1 ramekin	400	4	50	160	0	20.0	10.0	80	45%
(Tastykake) fudge walnut, 3 oz	1 brownie	335	4	53	222	5	14.2	3.3	22	36%
(Weight Watchers)										
brownie à la mode	1 serving	190	5	34	170	2	4.0	1.5	5	19%
chocolate, frosted	1 serving	100	2	22	135	3	2.5	1.0	0	19%
chocolate, frozen, 'Sweet Celebrations'	1/3 pkg	100	3	16	150	0	3.0	1.0	5	26%
mint frosted 'Sweet Celebrations'	1.23 oz	100	2	18	130	0	2.0	1.0	5	18%
peanut butter fudge	1 serving	110	2	21	140	3	2.5	0.5	0	20%
Swiss mocha fudge, 'Sweet Celebrations'	1.23 oz	90	2	18	140	0	2.0	1.0	5	18%

Food Name	Serving Size	Calories	Prot. gms	Carbs gms	Sod. mgs	Fiber gms	Fat gms	Sat. Fat gms	Chol. mgs	% Fat Cal.
BUTTERSCOTCH *(Tastykake)* 'Krimpets'	1 oz	103	1	19	83	0	2.6	1.2	22	22%
CARAMEL *(Little Debbie)* peanut filled, chocolate coated	1 piece	230	3	28	120	0	12.0	0.0	1	47%
CARROT										
(Break Cake)										
multi pak, 1.2 oz	1 cake	120	1	20	115	0	4.0	0.7	5	30%
3.5 oz	2 cakes	370	3	64	380	0	12.0	2.2	20	29%
(Pepperidge Farm) frozen 'Classic' 2.5 oz	1 piece	260	2	32	280	0	16.0	6.0	50	51%
(Sara Lee)										
frozen, 1.8 oz, 'Deluxe'	1 piece	180	3	26	200	0	7.0	0.0	0	35%
frozen, 2.5 oz, 'Lights'	1 piece	170	4	30	75	0	4.0	0.0	5	21%
CHEESECAKE										
(Pepperidge Farm) strawberry, frozen, 'Manhattan'	1 piece	300	6	49	250	0	9.0	5.0	150	27%
(Sara Lee)										
classic, 2 oz	1 piece	200	4	16	150	0	14.0	0.0	0	61%
French, frozen, 3.2 oz, 'Lights'	1 piece	150	5	24	90	0	4.0	0.0	15	24%
French, strawberry, frozen, 3.5 oz, 'Lights'	1 piece	150	3	29	65	0	2.0	0.0	5	12%
(Weight Watchers)										
brownie, 'Sweet Celebrations'	3.5 oz	200	9	34	260	0	5.0	1.0	10	21%
strawberry, 'Sweet Celebrations'	3.9 oz	180	7	28	210	0	4.0	2.0	20	20%
CHERRY *(Pepperidge Farm)* frozen, supreme, 3.25 oz, 'Dessert Lights'	1 piece	170	0	38	35	0	2.0	0.0	80	11%
CHOCOLATE										
(Aunt Fanny's)										
chocolate fudge	2.5 oz	222	4	39	402	0	6.0	0.0	0	24%
fingers, devil's food	3 oz	288	4	49	438	0	9.0	0.0	0	28%
(Awrey's) one piece	0.8 oz	70	1	11	110	0	3.0	1.0	15	36%
(Break Cake)										
chocolate marshmallow pie	1 pie	150	1	24	70	0	5.0	1.4	0	31%
chocolate marshmallow pie, double-decker	1 pie	360	3	61	170	0	11.0	3.2	0	28%
devil's food marshmallow pie	1 pie	140	1	25	85	0	4.0	1.4	0	26%
rounds, multi pak, 1.3 oz	1 cake	160	1	24	125	0	7.0	1.7	0	39%
rounds, 3.25 oz	2 cakes	390	3	58	300	0	16.0	4.0	0	37%
(Drake's)										
Swiss chocolate roll, cream filled	1.4 oz	170	2	22	140	0	8.0	2.0	15	43%
chocolate mint, cream filled 'Ring Ding'	1.5 oz	190	2	22	115	0	11.0	3.0	0	51%
chocolate roll, cream filled, 'Yodel'	1.1 oz	150	2	16	65	0	9.0	2.0	5	53%
cream filled, 'Devil Dog'	1.5 oz	160	2	24	135	0	6.0	1.0	0	34%
cream filled, 'Ring Ding'	1.5 oz	180	2	23	115	0	10.0	3.0	0	47%
(Hostess)										
'Choco Bliss'	1 piece	200	2	29	210	1	9.0	4.0	5	40%
'Chocodiles'	1 serving	240	2	33	180	1	11.0	8.0	20	41%
'Chocolicious'	1 serving	190	1	30	210	1	7.0	2.5	10	34%
creme filled, 'Ding Dongs'	1 serving	368	3	45	241	2	19.4	10.9	14	47%
vanilla pudding filled, 'Light'	1 piece	130	2	28	180	1	1.0	1.0	0	7%
(Little Debbie)										
	2.5 oz	320	2	45	135	0	14.0	0.0	1	40%
'Be My Valentine'	1 cake	270	2	39	160	1	13.0	3.0	0	42%
'Choco-Cake'	2.17 oz	270	2	37	220	0	13.0	0.0	1	43%
'Choco-Jel'	1.16 oz	150	1	21	80	0	7.0	0.0	1	42%
chocolate fudge, crispy	2.1 oz	260	2	48	90	0	7.0	0.0	1	24%
chocolate fudge, round	2.75 oz	330	3	55	180	0	12.0	0.0	1	32%
chocolate slices	3 oz	320	3	56	280	0	9.0	0.0	1	26%
chocolate twins	2.2 oz	240	2	41	200	0	7.0	0.0	1	27%

Food Name	Serving Size	Calories	Prot. gms	Carbs gms	Sod. mgs	Fiber gms	Fat gms	Sat. Fat gms	Chol. mgs	% Fat Cal.
(Pepperidge Farm)										
chocolate fudge, frozen, 1.6 oz cake.	1 piece	190	2	24	125	0	10.0	0.0	0	46%
double chocolate, frozen, 2.25 oz, 'Classic'	1 piece	250	2	31	180	0	13.0	4.0	35	47%
double chocolate, frozen, 2.5 oz, 'Lights'	1 piece	150	4	23	85	0	5.0	0.0	10	29%
German chocolate, frozen, 2.25 oz, 'Classic'	1 piece	250	2	29	230	0	13.0	4.0	45	49%
mousse, frozen, 1.5 oz, 'Dessert Lights'	1 piece	190	3	25	260	0	9.0	3.0	5	42%
mousse, frozen, 3 oz serving	1 piece	180	5	20	125	0	9.0	0.0	15	45%
mousse, frozen, 3 oz, 'Lights'	1 piece	170	4	20	60	0	8.0	0.0	10	43%
(Snackwell's)										
devil's food cookie cake, nonfat.	1 cookie	50	1	13	25	1	0.0	0.0	0	0%
double fudge cookie cake, nonfat	1 serving	50	1	12	70	1	0.0	0.0	0	0%
frosted fudge cake.	1 cake	180	1	25	130	1	10.0	2.0	5	46%
(Tastykake)										
cream filled, 'Krimpets'	1 piece	124	1	20	113	0	4.3	0.0	6	31%
'Creamie'	1.5 oz	168	2	24	126	1	7.6	2.0	12	40%
'Juniors'	3.3 oz	341	4	57	223	4	12.3	3.4	60	31%
'Kandy Kakes'	0.7 oz	78	1	13	35	1	3.1	2.3	0	34%
CHOCOLATE CHIP *(Little Debbie)*.	1 cake	290	2	42	210	1	14.0	3.5	0	42%
CINNAMON *(Aunt Fanny's)* twirl.	1 oz	110	1	16	85	0	4.0	1.0	0	33%
COCONUT										
(Little Debbie)										
coconut creme cake	1 cake	210	1	30	140	0	10.0	3.0	0	42%
coconut crunch	2 oz	320	2	35	80	0	19.0	0.0	2	54%
(Pepperidge Farm) frozen, 2.25 oz, 'Classic'	1 piece	230	2	31	160	0	11.0	4.0	20	43%
(Tastykake) 'Juniors'	3.3 oz	296	4	60	304	4	6.0	3.0	49	17%
COFFEECAKE										
(Drake's)										
cinnamon crumb	1.33 oz	150	2	22	110	0	6.0	1.0	10	36%
'Jr.'	1.1 oz	140	2	18	90	0	6.0	1.0	10	40%
'Small'	2 oz	220	3	33	160	0	9.0	2.0	15	36%
(Hostess Snack Cake)	1 serving	130	1	19	110	0	5.0	2.0	10	36%
(Little Debbie)										
. . . .	2.1 oz	250	3	39	210	0	9.0	0.0	1	33%
apple streusel	1 cake	230	2	39	190	1	7.0	1.5	10	28%
(Sara Lee)										
apple cinnamon, individually wrapped	1 piece	290	4	40	270	0	13.0	0.0	0	40%
butter streusel, individually wrapped.	1 piece	230	4	27	270	0	12.0	0.0	0	47%
pecan, individually wrapped	1 piece	280	5	30	270	0	16.0	0.0	0	51%
(Tastykake)										
cream filled, 'Koffee Kake'	1 oz	110	1	18	81	0	4.0	0.9	16	32%
'Koffee Kake Juniors'	2.5 oz	261	3	44	212	1	8.5	2.1	410	29%
(Weight Watchers) cinnamon streusel, 'Microwave'	1/2 pkg	190	3	28	250	0	7.0	1.0	5	34%
CRUMB *(Hostess)*	1 serving	90	1	19	100	0	0.5	0.0	0	5%
CUPCAKE										
(Aunt Fanny's) orange	3 oz	334	3	54	363	0	12.0	0.0	0	32%
(Break Cake)										
chocolate, 3.5 oz	2 cupcakes	350	3	64	350	0	9.0	3.5	0	23%
chocolate, multi-pak, 1.3 oz	1 cupcake	130	1	24	135	0	4.0	1.3	0	26%
white, 1.3 oz	1 cupcake	130	1	24	115	0	3.0	1.2	0	21%
(Hostess)										
chocolate.	1 cupcake	180	2	30	290	1	6.0	3.0	5	30%
chocolate, creme-filled, 'Light'	1 cupcake	120	2	25	160	0	2.0	0.0	0	14%
orange.	1 serving	160	1	27	160	0	5.0	2.0	10	29%

Food Name	Serving Size	Calories	Prot. gms	Carbs gms	Sod. mgs	Fiber gms	Fat gms	Sat. Fat gms	Chol. mgs	% Fat Cal.
(Tastykake)										
butter cream, cream filled, 1.1 oz	1 cupcake	118	1	20	120	1	4.2	1.5	6	31%
chocolate, 'Royale'	1 cupcake	171	2	28	130	2	6.6	1.8	7	33%
chocolate, cream filled, 1.1 oz.	1 cupcake	118	1	19	119	1	4.2	1.3	4	31%
chocolate, cream filled, 1.1 oz, 'Tastylite'	1 cupcake	100	1	22	116	1	1.3	0.5	0	11%
'Kreme Kup'	0.9 oz	86	1	15	113	1	2.8	1.0	4	28%
vanilla, cream filled, 'Tastylite'	1 cupcake	100	1	21	121	1	1.5	0.6	0	13%
FRUIT *(Hostess)* 'Fruit Loaf'	1 piece	400	4	77	520	0	9.0	0.0	7	20%
GOLDEN *(Hostess)* creme-filled, 'Twinkies'	1 piece	150	2	27	200	1	5.0	2.0	20	28%
JELLY										
(Little Debbie) jelly roll	2.2 oz	250	1	43	160	0	9.0	0.0	1	32%
(Tastykake) 'Krimpets'	1 oz	85	1	19	82	1	1.0	0.7	21	10%
LEMON										
(Little Debbie) lemon stix	1.5 oz	220	2	29	55	0	10.0	0.0	1	42%
(Pepperidge Farm) frozen, supreme 'Dessert Lights'	1 piece	170	4	26	100	0	5.0	1.0	50	27%
(Sara Lee) frozen, lemon cream 'Lights'	1 piece	180	3	29	60	0	6.0	0.0	10	30%
(Tastykake) 'Juniors'.	3.3 oz	306	3	64	255	0	4.0	0.0	0	12%
ORANGE *(Tastykake)* 'Juniors'	3.3 oz	337	3	61	236	1	9.2	2.6	5	24%
PEANUT BUTTER										
(Little Debbie) wafer, 'Peanut Butter Naturals'	1.25 oz	170	5	19	90	0	10.0	0.0	1	48%
(Tastykake) 'Kandy Kakes'	0.7 oz	87	2	11	38	1	4.2	2.4	5	42%
PECAN										
(Aunt Fanny's) twirls.	2 twirls	210	2	33	160	2	8.0	1.5	5	34%
(Little Debbie) twins . . . , ...	2 oz	220	3	34	170	0	10.0	0.0	1	38%
(Tastykake) twirls	1 oz	109	1	17	74	0	4.9	0.0	0	38%
POUND										
(Aunt Fanny's)	2.5 oz	260	3	41	253	0	9.0	0.0	0	32%
(Drake's) approx. 1.1 oz.	1/10 cake	110	2	16	70	0	5.0	1.0	25	38%
(Sara Lee) frozen, all butter, 1.6 oz	1 piece	200	2	23	190	0	11.0	0.0	0	50%
PUDDING *(Hostess)*.	1 piece	170	2	32	200	0	4.0	0.0	8	21%
RASPBERRY										
(Aunt Fanny's) fingers	3 oz	303	3	53	337	0	9.0	0.0	0	27%
(Little Debbie) raspberry angel cake	1 cake	120	2	28	100	1	1.5	0.0	0	10%
(Pepperidge Farm) vanilla swirl, frozen, 'Dessert Lights'	1 piece	160	4	25	140	0	5.0	1.0	15	28%
SHORTCAKE										
(Pepperidge Farm) strawberry, frozen, 'Dessert Lights'	1 piece	170	2	30	50	1	5.0	1.0	70	26%
(Weight Watchers) strawberry à la mode	1 serving	170	3	33	150	0	2.0	1.0	5	11%
SPICE										
(Aunt Fanny's) fingers	3 oz	290	3	49	433	0	9.0	0.0	0	28%
(Little Debbie)	1 cake	300	2	44	230	0	14.0	3.5	10	41%
STRAWBERRY *(Hostess)* 'Twinkies Fruit N Creme'.	1.75 oz	160	2	32	210	1	3.0	0.0	20	17%
VANILLA										
(Aunt Fanny's) fingers	3 oz	250	3	50	380	0	9.0	2.0	25	28%
(Little Debbie)	2.6 oz	330	2	46	135	0	16.0	0.0	1	43%
(Pepperidge Farm) fudge swirl, frozen, 'Classic'	1 piece	250	2	33	160	0	11.0	4.0	35	41%
(Tastykake)										
cream filled 'Krimpets'	1.1 oz	116	1	19	77	1	4.1	1.4	19	31%
'Creamie'	1.5 oz	184	1	25	117	1	9.0	2.2	26	44%
YELLOW *(Awrey's)* one piece	0.9 oz	80	1	12	135	0	3.0	1.0	20	34%
CAKE, SNACK, MIX										
APPLE										
(Pillsbury)										
apple streusel bar, deluxe, mix only	1/24 pkg	130	1	22	40	1	4.5	1.0	0	31%
apple streusel bar, deluxe, prepared.	1/24 pkg	150	1	23	55	1	6.0	1.5	0	36%

Food Name	Serving Size	Calories	Prot. gms	Carbs gms	Sod. mgs	Fiber gms	Fat gms	Sat. Fat gms	Chol. mgs	% Fat Cal.
BROWNIE										
regular, mix only	1 oz	123	1	22	86	na	4.2	0.7	0	30%
regular, mix only	21.5-oz pkg	2647	24	467	1848	na	90.9	15.4	0	30%
(Betty Crocker)										
caramel, 'Supreme' prepared	1 brownie	110	1	21	110	0	2.0	0.0	0	17%
caramel, 'Supreme' prepared w/1/4 cup oil, 1 egg	1 brownie	120	1	21	115	0	4.0	0.0	10	29%
chocolate chip, 'Supreme' prepared	1 brownie	110	1	20	85	0	3.0	0.0	0	24%
chocoplate chip, 'Supreme' prepared w/1/4 cup oil, 1 egg	1 brownie	130	1	20	90	0	5.0	0.0	10	35%
frosted, 'Supreme' prepared	1 brownie	140	1	26	100	0	3.0	0.0	0	20%
frosted, 'Supreme' prepared w/1/4 cup oil, 1 egg	1 brownie	160	1	26	105	0	6.0	0.0	10	33%
German chocolate, prepared w/oil, margarine, egg, 2% milk	1 brownie	160	1	24	120	0	7.0	0.0	10	39%
original, 'Supreme' prepared w/1/4 cup oil, 2 eggs	1 brownie	140	1	22	95	0	5.0	0.0	20	33%
party, 'Supreme' prepared	1 brownie	140	1	26	100	0	3.0	0.0	0	20%
party, 'Supreme' prepared w/1/4 cup oil, 1 egg	1 brownie	160	1	26	105	0	6.0	0.0	10	33%
peanut butter candies 'Supreme' mix only	1/24 pkg	120	2	21	80	0	3.0	0.0	0	23%
peanut butter candies 'Supreme' prepared	1/24 pkg	140	2	21	85	0	5.0	0.0	0	33%
(Duncan Hines)										
blonde, prepared	1 piece	160	2	22	100	0	8.0	1.5	10	43%
'Dark 'n Fudgy' prepared	1 piece	170	2	25	110	1	8.0	1.5	15	40%
double fudge, 'Brownies Plus' mix only	1 brownie	120	1	22	100	0	3.0	0.0	0	23%
double fudge, 'Brownies Plus' prepared	1 brownie	150	2	22	105	0	6.0	0.0	0	36%
double fudge, prepared	1 piece	170	2	29	130	1	7.0	1.5	20	34%
fudge, chewy, prepared	1 piece	160	2	25	120	1	7.0	1.5	10	37%
fudge, prepared	1 brownie	130	1	18	90	0	5.0	0.0	0	37%
fudge, mix only	1 brownie	100	1	18	85	0	18.0	2.0	0	68%
'Gourmet Turtle' mix only	1 brownie	160	2	27	120	0	5.0	0.0	0	28%
'Gourmet Turtle' prepared	1 brownie	200	2	27	125	0	9.0	0.0	0	41%
milk chocolate, 'Brownies Plus' prepared	1 brownie	160	1	20	95	0	8.0	0.0	0	46%
milk chocolate, 'Brownies Plus' mix only	1 brownie	120	1	20	90	0	4.0	0.0	0	30%
milk chocolate chunk, prepared	1 piece	170	2	26	120	1	7.0	1.0	20	36%
Mississippi mud, prepared	1 piece	160	1	26	100	0	6.0	1.0	10	33%
peanut butter, 'Brownies Plus'	1 brownie	150	3	16	105	0	8.0	0.0	0	49%
peanut butter, 'Brownies Plus' mix only	1 brownie	120	3	16	100	0	5.0	0.0	0	37%
peanut butter, prepared	1 piece	160	2	23	120	1	8.0	1.5	10	42%
w/walnuts, 'Brownies Plus'	1 brownie	150	1	19	90	0	7.0	0.0	0	44%
w/walnuts 'Brownies Plus' mix only	1 brownie	120	1	19	85	0	4.0	0.0	0	31%
turtle, prepared	1 piece	160	2	26	110	1	6.0	1.5	10	33%
walnut, prepared	1 piece	170	2	24	105	0	8.0	1.5	10	41%
(Estee) prepared, 2-inch square	1 brownie	50	1	11	0	0	2.0	1.0	0	27%
(Finast)										
fudge, 'Ultra Moist'	1/16 pkg	130	2	20	120	0	5.0	0.0	0	34%
w/walnuts, 'Ultra Moist'	11/16 pkg	130	1	19	110	0	6.0	0.0	0	40%
(General Mills)										
caramel 'Supreme' prepared	1 brownie	110	1	21	110	0	2.0	0.0	0	17%
caramel 'Supreme' prepared w/1/4 cup oil, 1 egg	1 brownie	120	1	21	115	0	4.0	0.0	10	29%
chocolate chip, 'Supreme' prepared	1 brownie	110	1	20	85	0	3.0	0.0	0	24%
chocolate chip, 'Supreme' prepared w/1/4 cup oil, 1 egg	1 brownie	130	1	20	90	0	5.0	0.0	10	35%
frosted, 'Supreme' prepared	1 brownie	140	1	26	100	0	3.0	0.0	0	20%
frosted, 'Supreme' prepared w/1/4 cup oil, 1 egg	1 brownie	160	1	26	105	0	6.0	0.0	10	33%
fudge, 'Family Size' prepared as directed	1 brownie	110	1	22	95	0	2.0	0.0	0	16%
fudge, 'Family Size' prepared w/1/4 cup oil, 1 egg	1 brownie	140	1	22	100	0	5.0	0.0	10	33%

Food Name	Serving Size	Calories	Prot. gms	Carbs gms	Sod. mgs	Fiber gms	Fat gms	Sat. Fat gms	Chol. mgs	% Fat Cal.
fudge, 'Light' prepared	1 brownie	100	1	21	90	0	1.0	0.0	0	9%
fudge, 'Regular Size' prepared	1 brownie	110	1	23	100	0	2.0	0.0	0	16%
fudge, 'Regular Size' prepared w/1/4 cup oil, 1 egg	1 brownie	150	1	23	105	0	6.0	0.0	15	36%
German chocolate, 'Supreme' prepared	1 brownie	130	1	24	105	0	3.0	0.0	0	21%
German chocolate, prepared w/oil, margarine, egg, 2% milk	1 brownie	160	1	24	120	0	7.0	0.0	10	39%
original, 'Supreme' prepared	1 brownie	120	1	22	90	0	3.0	0.0	0	23%
original, 'Supreme' prepared w/1/4 cup oil, 2 eggs	1 brownie	140	1	22	95	0	5.0	0.0	20	33%
party, 'Supreme' prepared	1 brownie	140	1	26	100	0	3.0	0.0	0	20%
party, 'Supreme' prepared w/1/4 cup oil, 1 egg	1 brownie	160	1	26	105	0	6.0	0.0	10	33%
walnut, 'Supreme' prepared	1 brownie	110	1	18	85	0	4.0	0.0	0	32%
walnut, 'Supreme' prepared w/1/4 cup oil, 1 egg	1 brownie	130	1	18	85	0	6.0	0.0	10	42%
(Gluten Free Pantry) chocolate truffle, gluten-free	1 serving	150	1	30	65	2	2.5	1.5	0	15%
(Gold Medal)										
fudge, prepared	1 brownie	120	2	24	100	1	2.0	1.0	0	15%
fudge, 'Pouch Mix'	1/16 pkg	100	1	16	85	0	4.0	0.0	0	35%
(Great Additions)										
double chocolate, mix only	1/24 pkg	110	1	19	70	0	3.0	1.0	0	25%
double chocolate, prepared w/1/3 cup oil, 1egg, 2-inch square	1 brownie	140	1	19	75	0	6.0	2.0	10	40%
double chocolate, prepared w/1/3 cup oil, 2 egg whites, 2-inch square	1 brownie	130	1	19	75	0	6.0	2.0	0	40%
frosted, 'Funfetti Frosted' mix only	1/24 pkg	100	1	18	80	0	2.0	1.0	0	19%
frosted, 'Funfetti' prepared w/1/3 cup oil, 1 egg, 2-inch square	1 brownie	160	1	23	100	0	7.0	1.0	10	40%
frosted, 'Funfetti' prepared w/1/3 cup oil, 1 egg white, 2-inch square	1 brownie	150	1	23	100	0	6.0	1.0	0	36%
walnut, mix only	1/24 pkg	110	1	16	70	0	4.0	1.0	0	35%
walnut, prepared w/water, 1/3c oil 2 egg whites, 2-inch square	1 brownie	130	2	16	75	0	7.0	1.0	0	47%
walnut, prepared w/water, 1/3 cup oil 1 egg, 2-inch square	1 brownie	140	2	16	70	0	8.0	1.0	10	50%
(Krusteaz) fudge, prepared	1.5 oz mix	190	1	28	135	0	8.0	0.0	19	38%
(Lovin' Lites)										
fudge, mix only	1/24 pkg	100	1	19	80	0	2.0	1.0	0	18%
fudge, prepared w/water, 1 egg	1/24 pkg	100	1	19	80	0	2.0	1.0	10	18%
fudge, prepared w/water, 2 egg whites	1/24 pkg	100	1	19	85	0	2.0	1.0	0	18%
(Martha White) mix only	1 serving	114	1	23	138	na	1.8	0.4	na	14%
(MicroRave)										
frosted	1 brownie	180	2	27	130	0	7.0	0.0	0	35%
'Singles' prepared	1 brownie	250	4	39	230	0	9.0	0.0	0	32%
walnut, 1.1 oz	1 brownie	160	2	21	95	0	7.0	2.0	0	41%
w/hot fudge topping, 'Singles'	1 brownie	340	5	54	270	0	12.0	0.0	0	31%
(Mixed Company) organic, chewy	1/4 cup	150	3	31	10	1	2.0	0.0	0	12%
(Pillsbury)										
caramel fudge chunk, prepared, 2-inch square	1 brownie	170	2	25	105	0	7.0	0.0	0	37%
chocolate chip, deluxe, mix only	1/20 pkg	140	1	28	110	1	3.0	0.5	0	19%
chocolate chip, deluxe, prepared	1/20 pkg	180	2	28	110	1	7.0	1.5	10	34%
cream cheese swirl, mix only	1/20 pkg	140	1	22	90	1	5.0	2.0	5	33%
cream cheese swirl, prepared	1/20 pkg	180	2	22	95	1	9.0	2.5	25	46%
double fudge, 2-inch square	1 brownie	160	2	24	105	0	6.0	0.0	0	34%
fudge, deluxe 'Lovin' Bites'	1 piece	160	2	29	125	0	3.5	1.0	15	20%
fudge, 15-oz pkg, mix only	1/16 pkg	110	1	21	90	0	2.0	1.0	0	17%
fudge, 15-oz, prep	1/16 pkg	150	1	22	95	1	6.0	0.5	15	37%

Food Name	Serving Size	Calories	Prot. gms	Carbs gms	Sod. mgs	Fiber gms	Fat gms	Sat. Fat gms	Chol. mgs	% Fat Cal.
fudge, mix only	1/9 pkg	130	2	25	110	0	3.0	1.0	0	20%
fudge, prepared	1 brownie	190	2	25	105	0	9.0	0.0	0	43%
fudge, prepared w/1/4 cup oil	1/9 pkg	190	2	25	110	0	9.0	2.0	0	43%
fudge, prepared w/1/2 cup oil, 2 egg whites, 2-inch square	1 brownie	150	1	20	90	0	7.0	1.0	0	43%
fudge, prepared w/water, 1/4 cup oil, 1 egg, 2-inch square	1 brownie	140	2	21	95	0	6.0	1.0	15	37%
fudge, prepared w/water, 1/4 cup oil, 1 egg white, 2-inch square	1 brownie	140	1	21	95	0	6.0	1.0	0	38%
fudge, 21.5-oz pkg, mix only	1/24 pkg	100	1	20	85	0	2.0	1.0	0	18%
fudge, 21.5-oz, prepared	1/20 pkg	180	2	25	105	1	8.0	1.5	10	40%
fudge, w/fudge frosting, 'Microwave Mix'	1/9 pkg	50	0	7	30	0	2.0	1.0	0	39%
fudge, w/fudge frosting, mix only	1/9 pkg	130	2	25	110	0	3.0	1.0	0	20%
fudge, w/fudge frosting, prepared w/1/4 cup oil, frosting	1/9 pkg	240	2	32	140	0	11.0	3.0	0	42%
fudge deluxe, 'Family Size' 2-inch square	1 brownie	150	1	20	95	0	7.0	0.0	0	43%
fudge deluxe, 2-inch square	1 brownie	150	2	21	100	0	6.0	0.0	0	37%
fudge deluxe, w/walnuts, 2-inch square	1 brownie	150	2	19	90	0	8.0	0.0	0	46%
fudge swirl cookie bar, deluxe, mix only	1/20 pkg	150	1	25	105	1	5.0	1.0	0	30%
fudge swirl cookie bar, deluxe, prepared	1/20 pkg	180	1	25	110	1	8.0	1.5	10	41%
hot fudge, mix	1/24 pkg	130	1	24	100	1	3.5	1.5	0	24%
hot fudge, prepared	1/24 pkg	160	1	24	100	1	7.0	2.0	10	39%
rocky road, fudge, 2-inch square	1 brownie	170	2	24	95	0	8.0	0.0	0	41%
walnut, mix only	1/18 pkg	140	2	22	90	1	5.0	1.0	0	32%
walnut, prepared	1/18 pkg	180	2	22	90	1	9.0	1.5	10	46%
traditional, mix only	1 serving	132	1	23	88	na	3.6	0.8	na	25%
triple fudge, chunky, 2-inch square	1 brownie	170	2	25	105	0	7.0	0.0	0	37%
(Robin Hood) fudge, 'Pouch Mix'	1/16 pkg	100	1	16	85	0	4.0	0.0	0	35%
(Weight Watchers) fudge, low-fat, 'Sweet Rewards'	1 serving	130	2	27	115	1	2.5	1.0	0	16%
CHEESECAKE										
(Pillsbury)										
lemon, bar, mix only	1/24 pkg	170	1	20	45	0	9.0	3.0	10	49%
lemon, bar, prepared	1/24 pkg	180	2	20	50	0	10.0	3.5	25	51%
CHOCOLATE										
(Pillsbury)										
Oreo bar, deluxe, mix only	1/24 pkg	130	1	22	125	1	4.0	1.0	0	28%
Oreo bar, deluxe, prepared	1/24 pkg	150	1	22	130	1	6.0	1.5	10	37%
CUPCAKE										
(Funfetti)										
chocolate, microwave, mix only	1/9 pkg	100	1	14	160	0	4.0	1.0	10	38%
chocolate, microwave, w/chocolate fudge frosting, prepared	1/9 pkg	160	1	24	190	0	7.0	2.0	10	39%
yellow, microwave, mix only	1/9 pkg	110	1	17	135	0	5.0	1.0	10	38%
yellow, microwave, w/vanilla frosting, prepared	1/9 pkg	180	1	28	160	0	7.0	2.0	10	35%
GINGERBREAD										
(Betty Crocker)										
'Classic' cholesterol-free recipe, prepared	1/9 pkg	210	3	35	330	0	6.0	0.0	0	26%
'Classic' prepared w/1 egg	1/9 pkg	220	3	35	330	0	7.0	0.0	30	29%
(Dromedary) mix only	3 tbsp	100	1	19	190	0	2.0	0.0	0	18%
(Hodgson Mill) whole wheat, mix only	1/4 cup	110	2	24	260	2	0.0	0.0	0	0%
(Pillsbury)										
	1 serving	220	3	40	340	1	5.0	1.5	0	21%
prepared, 3-inch square	1 piece	190	2	36	310	0	4.0	0.0	0	19%
prepared w/water	1/9 pkg	180	2	32	300	0	5.0	1.0	0	25%

Food Name	Serving Size	Calories	Prot. gms	Carbs gms	Sod. mgs	Fiber gms	Fat gms	Sat. Fat gms	Chol. mgs	% Fat Cal.
(Sweet 'n Low) w/'Sweet 'n Low' mix only	1/6 cake	150	2	30	30	1	3.0	1.0	0	17%
NUT										
(Pillsbury)										
Nutter Butter bar, deluxe, mix only	1/18 pkg	150	2	26	140	0	4.0	0.5	0	24%
Nutter Butter bar, deluxe, prepared	1/18 pkg	180	3	26	170	0	7.0	1.5	15	35%
CAKE DECORATION. See also under FROSTING.										
candies, rainbow mix *(Dec-a-Cake)*	1 tsp	15	0	3	5	0	0.5	0.0	0	27%
candies, sugar crystals *(Dec-a-Cake)*	1 tsp	15	0	3	0	0	0.0	0.0	0	0%
CAKE MIX										
ANGEL FOOD										
(Betty Crocker)										
confetti, 'SuperMoist'	1/12 cake	150	3	34	320	0	0.0	0.0	0	0%
one-step white, SuperMoist' prepared	1/12 cake	140	3	32	320	0	0.0	0.0	0	0%
'Traditional' mix only	1/12 mix	130	3	30	170	0	0.0	0.0	0	0%
'Traditional' 'Supermoist' prepared	1/12 cake	130	3	30	150	0	0.0	0.0	0	0%
(Duncan Hines)										
mix only	1/12 mix	140	3	30	130	0	0.0	0.0	0	0%
prepared	1/12 cake	130	3	30	320	0	0.0	0.0	0	0%
(General Mills)										
chocolate, mix only	1/12 mix	150	3	34	300	0	0.0	0.0	0	0%
confetti, mix only	1/12 mix	150	3	34	300	0	0.0	0.0	0	0%
lemon custard, mix only	1/12 mix	150	3	34	300	0	0.0	0.0	0	0%
lemon pudding, mix only	1/12 mix	150	3	34	300	0	0.0	0.0	0	0%
strawberry, mix only	1/12 mix	150	3	35	260	0	0.0	0.0	0	0%
white, one-step, mix only	1/12 mix	150	3	34	300	0	0.0	0.0	0	0%
(Gluten Free Pantry) gluten-free	1 serving	140	4	32	90	0	0.0	0.0	0	0%
(Lovin' Loaf)										
mix only	1/8 pkg	90	2	20	210	0	0.0	0.0	0	0%
prepared w/water	1/8 pkg	90	2	20	210	0	0.0	0.0	0	0%
(Pillsbury)										
'Moist Supreme' mix only	1/12 pkg	140	3	31	330	0	0.0	0.0	0	0%
prepared	1/12 cake	150	3	34	360	0	0.0	0.0	0	0%
APPLE										
(Betty Crocker)										
apple cinnamon, 'SuperMoist' prepared	1/12 cake	250	3	36	280	0	10.0	2.0	55	37%
apple cinnamon, 'SuperMoist' prepared, cholesterol-free recipe	1/12 cake	210	3	36	280	0	6.0	2.0	0	26%
(Gold Medal) applesauce raisin, mix only	1/9 mix	140	1	28	160	0	3.0	0.0	0	19%
(MicroRave)										
apple streusel, prepared	1/12 cake	240	2	33	190	0	11.0	3.0	45	41%
apple streusel, prepared w/cholesterol-free egg product	1/12 cake	210	2	33	200	0	8.0	2.0	0	34%
(Robin Hood) applesauce raisin, mix only	1/9 mix	140	1	28	160	0	3.0	0.0	0	19%
BANANA										
(Duncan Hines)										
'Banana Supreme' prepared	1/12 cake	250	3	36	270	0	11.0	2.0	45	39%
cholesterol-free recipe, prepared	1/12 cake	250	3	36	285	0	10.0	2.0	0	37%
mix only	1/12 pkg	190	2	36	280	0	4.0	11.0	0	19%
(Gold Medal) banana walnut, mix only	1/9 mix	150	1	27	200	0	4.0	0.0	0	24%
(Pillsbury)										
microwave, mix only	1/9 pkg	110	1	17	140	0	5.0	1.0	10	38%
'Moist Supreme' mix only	1/12 pkg	180	2	35	260	0	4.0	1.5	0	20%
'Moist Supreme' prepared	1/12 pkg	260	3	36	280	0	11.0	2.5	55	39%
'Pillsbury Plus' prepared	1/12 cake	260	3	36	280	0	11.0	2.5	55	39%

Food Name	Serving Size	Calories	Prot. gms	Carbs gms	Sod. mgs	Fiber gms	Fat gms	Sat. Fat gms	Chol. mgs	% Fat Cal.
'Pillsbury Plus' prepared w/water, 1/3 cup oil, 3 eggs	1/12 pkg	250	3	35	280	0	11.0	3.0	55	39%
'Pillsbury Plus' prepared w/water, 3 egg whites, 2 tbsp flour	1/12 pkg	190	3	36	280	0	4.0	1.0	0	19%
w/vanilla frosting, microwave, 'Snack' prepared	1/9 pkg	170	1	26	160	0	7.0	2.0	10	37%
(Robin Hood) banana walnut, mix only	1/9 mix	150	1	27	200	0	4.0	0.0	0	24%
(Sweet 'n Low) mix only	1/6 cake	150	2	30	30	1	3.0	1.0	0	17%
BLACK FOREST										
(Duncan Hines) mousse,'Tiarra'	1/12 cake	260	3	33	270	0	13.0	0.0	0	45%
(Pillsbury)										
cherry 'Bundt Ring Cake' mix only	1/16 pkg	200	2	40	310	0	4.0	1.0	0	18%
cherry, 'Bundt' prepared	1/16 cake	240	3	38	310	0	8.0	0.0	0	31%
cherry, prepared w/1/2 cup oil, 3 egg whites	1/16 pkg	270	3	41	320	0	12.0	2.0	40	38%
cherry, prepared w/1/2 cup oil, 4 egg whites	1/16 pkg	260	3	41	320	0	11.0	2.0	0	36%
BLUEBERRY										
(Streusel Swirl)										
streusel, mix only	1/16 pkg	210	2	39	190	0	5.0	1.0	0	22%
streusel, prepared w/1/3 cup oil, 3 eggs	1/16 pkg	260	3	39	200	0	11.0	2.0	40	37%
streusel, prepared w/1/3 cup oil, 4 egg whites	1/16 pkg	250	3	39	200	0	10.0	2.0	0	35%
BOSTON CREAM										
(Betty Crocker)										
'Classic' mix only	1/8 pkg	230	1	48	370	0	4.0	0.0	0	16%
'Classic' prepared w/egg, 2% milk	1/8 pkg	270	4	50	390	0	6.0	0.0	30	20%
(Pillsbury)										
'Bundt' prepared	1/16 cake	270	3	43	310	0	10.0	0.0	0	33%
chocolate éclair, 'Bundt Ring' mix only	1/16 pkg	210	1	42	280	0	4.0	1.0	0	17%
chocolate éclair, prepared w/1/2 cup oil, 4 egg whites	1/16 cake	250	2	42	300	0	9.0	2.0	0	32%
chocolate éclair, prepared w/1/3 cup oil, 3 eggs	1/16 pkg	260	3	42	290	0	10.0	2.0	40	33%
BUTTER BRICKLE										
(Betty Crocker)										
'SuperMoist' prepared	1/12 cake	250	3	38	280	0	10.0	2.0	55	35%
'SuperMoist' prepared w/cholesterol-free egg product	1/12 cake	220	3	38	280	0	6.0	2.0	0	25%
BUTTER PECAN										
(Betty Crocker)										
'SuperMoist' mix only	1/12 mix	180	1	35	300	0	4.0	0.0	0	20%
'SuperMoist' prepared w/3 eggs, 1/3 cup oil	1/12 cake	250	3	35	320	0	11.0	0.0	55	39%
'SuperMoist' prepared w/oil, cholesterol-free egg product	1/12 cake	220	3	35	320	0	7.0	0.0	0	29%
CARAMEL (Duncan Hines) prepared	1/12 cake	250	3	36	270	0	11.0	2.0	45	39%
CARROT										
(Betty Crocker)										
'SuperMoist' mix only	1/12 mix	180	1	36	280	0	3.0	0.0	0	15%
'Supermoist' prepared	1/12 cake	200	2	42	320	0	3.0	1.0	0	13%
'SuperMoist' prepared w/1/3 cup oil, 3 eggs	1/12 cake	250	3	36	300	0	10.0	0.0	55	37%
'SuperMoist' prepared w/1/3 cup oil, egg substitute	1/12 cake	210	3	36	300	0	6.0	0.0	0	26%
(Dromedary) prepared	1/12 cake	232	3	23	292	0	15.0	0.0	0	56%
(Estee) prepared	1/10 cake	100	1	18	65	0	2.0	1.0	0	19%
(Pillsbury)										
carrot 'n spice, 'Pillsbury Plus' prepared	1/12 cake	260	3	36	330	0	11.0	0.0	0	39%
microwave, mix only	1/9 pkg	110	1	17	170	0	5.0	1.0	10	38%
'Moist Supreme' mix only	1/12 pkg	180	2	35	280	1	4.0	1.5	0	20%
'Moist Supreme' prepared	1/12 pkg	260	3	35	290	1	12.0	2.5	55	42%
'Pillsbury Plus' prepared w/1/3 cup oil, 3 eggs	1/12 pkg	260	3	34	300	0	12.0	3.0	55	42%
'Pillsbury Plus' prepared w/water, 3 egg whites, 2 tbsp flour	1/12 pkg	190	3	35	300	0	5.0	1.0	0	23%

Food Name	Serving Size	Calories	Prot. gms	Carbs gms	Sod. mgs	Fiber gms	Fat gms	Sat. Fat gms	Chol. mgs	% Fat Cal.
'Quick Bread Mix' mix only	1/12 pkg	110	2	22	150	1	1.0	0.0	0	9%
'Quick Bread Mix' prepared	1/12 pkg	140	2	22	150	1	5.0	1.0	25	32%
w/cream cheese frosting, microwave, prepared	1/9 pkg	170	1	25	200	0	7.0	2.0	10	38%
CHEESECAKE										
(Jell-O)										
lemon, no bake, mix only	1 pkg	170	4	31	300	0	3.0	0.0	0	16%
lemon, no bake, prepared, 8-inch cake	1/8 cake	270	5	36	400	0	13.0	0.0	25	42%
New York style, no bake, mix only	1 pkg	180	4	33	320	0	3.0	0.0	0	15%
New York style, no bake, prepared, 8-inch cake	1/8 cake	280	6	38	420	0	12.0	0.0	30	38%
strawberry, no bake, prepared	1/12 cake	340	5	52	400	1	12.0	4.5	5	32%
(Royal)										
lite, 'No-Bake'	1/8 cake	210	5	23	380	0	10.0	0.0	0	45%
real, 'No-Bake'	1/8 cake	280	5	31	370	0	9.0	0.0	0	36%
CHERRY										
(Betty Crocker)										
cherry chip, 'SuperMoist' mix only	1/12 mix	180	2	37	250	0	3.0	0.0	0	15%
cherry chip, 'SuperMoist' prepared w/3 egg whites	1/12 mix	190	3	37	270	0	3.0	0.0	0	14%
(Duncan Hines)										
cherries and cream 'Tiarra'	1/12 cake	250	4	34	265	0	11.0	0.0	0	39%
cherry vanilla, prepared	1/12 cake	250	3	36	270	0	11.0	2.0	45	39%
CHOCOLATE										
(Betty Crocker)										
butter recipe, 'SuperMoist' mix only	1/12 mix	190	2	35	300	0	5.0	0.0	0	23%
butter recipe, 'SuperMoist' prepared w/1/2 cup butter, 3 eggs	1/12 mix	280	4	35	400	0	14.0	0.0	75	45%
chocolate chocolate chip, 'SuperMoist' prepared w/1/3 cup oil, 3 eggs	1/12 mix	260	3	34	400	0	12.0	0.0	55	42%
chocolate chocolate chip, 'SuperMoist' mix only	1/12 mix	190	2	34	380	0	5.0	0.0	0	24%
chocolate fudge, 'SuperMoist' mix only	1/12 mix	180	2	35	430	0	4.0	0.0	0	20%
chocolate fudge, 'SuperMoist' prepared w/1/3 cup oil, 3 eggs	1/12 mix	260	3	35	450	0	12.0	0.0	55	42%
chocolate pudding, 'Classic Dessert' mix only	1/6 pkg	220	2	44	240	0	4.0	0.0	0	16%
chocolate pudding, 'Classic Dessert' prepared w/1 egg	1/6 pkg	230	3	44	250	0	5.0	0.0	35	19%
devil's food 'SuperMoist' 'Light' cholesterol-free recipe, prepared	1/12 mix	180	3	36	370	0	3.0	0.0	0	15%
devil's food 'SuperMoist' 'Light' mix only	1/12 mix	180	2	36	330	0	3.0	0.0	0	15%
devil's food 'SuperMoist' 'Light' prepared w/3 eggs	1/12 mix	200	4	36	340	0	4.0	0.0	55	18%
devil's food, 'SuperMoist' mix only	1/12 mix	190	2	35	410	0	5.0	0.0	0	23%
devil's food, 'SuperMoist' prepared w/1/3 cup oil, 3 eggs	1/12 mix	260	4	35	430	0	12.0	0.0	55	41%
devil's food, 'SuperMoist' prepared w/oil, cholesterol-free egg product	1/12 mix	220	3	35	430	0	7.0	0.0	0	29%
fudge marble, 'SuperMoist' mix only	1/12 mix	180	1	36	270	0	4.0	0.0	0	20%
fudge marble, 'SuperMoist' prepared w/1/3 cup oil, 3 eggs	1/12 mix	260	3	36	290	0	11.0	0.0	55	39%
fudge marble, 'SuperMoist' prepared w/oil, cholesterol-free egg substitute	1/12 mix	220	3	36	290	0	7.0	0.0	0	29%
German chocolate, 'SuperMoist' cholesterol-free recipe, prepared	1/12 mix	220	3	35	420	0	8.0	0.0	0	32%
German chocolate, 'SuperMoist' mix only	1/12 mix	180	2	35	400	0	4.0	0.0	0	20%
German chocolate, 'SuperMoist' prepared w/1/3 cup oil, 3 eggs	1/12 mix	260	3	35	420	0	12.0	0.0	55	42%
milk chocolate, 'SuperMoist' cholesterol-free recipe, prepared	1/12 mix	210	3	34	340	0	7.0	0.0	0	30%

Food Name	Serving Size	Calories	Prot. gms	Carbs gms	Sod. mgs	Fiber gms	Fat gms	Sat. Fat gms	Chol. mgs	% Fat Cal.
milk chocolate, 'SuperMoist' mix only	1/12 mix	190	2	34	320	0	5.0	0.0	0	24%
milk chocolate, 'SuperMoist' prepared w/1/3 cup oil, 3 eggs.	1/12 mix	260	4	34	340	0	12.0	0.0	55	42%
sour cream, 'SuperMoist' mix only.	1/12 mix	180	2	35	410	0	4.0	0.0	0	20%
sour cream, 'SuperMoist' prepared w/egg substitute	1/12 mix	220	3	35	430	0	8.0	0.0	0	32%
sour cream, 'SuperMoist' prepared w/1/3 cup oil, 3 eggs.	1/12 mix	260	3	35	430	0	12.0	0.0	55	42%
(Duncan Hines)										
chocolate mousse, Amaretto, 'Tiarra' prepared.	1/12 cake	270	3	29	230	0	16.0	0.0	0	53%
chocolate mousse, 'Tiarra' prepared	1/12 cake	270	3	29	235	0	16.0	0.0	0	53%
dark Dutch fudge, prepared	1/12 cake	280	4	33	470	0	15.0	4.0	65	48%
dark Dutch fudge, cholesterol-free recipe, prepared.	1/12 cake	270	4	33	380	0	14.0	2.0	0	46%
dark Dutch fudge, mix only	1/12 cake	190	2	33	455	0	5.0	2.0	0	24%
devil's food, cholesterol-free recipe, prepared.	1/12 cake	270	4	33	380	0	14.0	2.0	0	46%
devil's food, mix only	1/12 pkg	190	2	33	360	0	5.0	2.0	0	24%
devil's food, prepared	1/12 cake	280	4	33	375	0	15.0	2.0	65	48%
fudge, butter recipe, mix only . . . . ─	1/12 cake	190	2	34	240	0	4.0	2.0	0	20%
fudge, butter recipe, prepared.	1/12 cake	320	3	40	300	2	17.0	8.0	80	47%
fudge, butter recipe, prepared w/stick margarine	1/12 cake	270	3	34	350	0	13.0	4.0	65	44%
fudge marble, cholesterol-free recipe, prepared	1/12 cake	250	3	36	285	0	10.0	2.0	0	37%
fudge marble, mix only	1/12 cake	190	2	36	280	0	4.0	11.0	0	19%
fudge marble, prepared.	1/12 cake	260	3	36	295	0	11.0	3.0	65	39%
Swiss chocolate, cholesterol-free recipe, prepared	1/12 cake	270	4	33	380	0	14.0	2.0	0	46%
Swiss chocolate, mix only.	1/12 pkg	190	2	33	360	0	5.0	2.0	0	24%
Swiss chocolate, prepared	1/12 cake	280	4	33	375	0	15.0	4.0	65	48%
(Estee) prepared	1/10 cake	100	1	18	100	0	2.0	1.0	0	19%
(Finast) devil's food, 'Ultra Moist' prepared	1/12 cake	250	3	33	360	0	11.0	0.0	0	41%
(Gold Medal) mix, chocolate chip fudge, mix only	1/9 mix	150	2	25	210	0	5.0	0.0	0	29%
(Krusteaz) devil's food, 8-inch double cake, prepared.	1/12 cake	190	4	37	330	0	2.0	0.0	25	10%
(MicroRave)										
chocolate fudge, w/vanilla frosting, prepared	1/6 cake	310	3	40	300	0	15.0	4.0	35	44%
devil's food, 'Lovin' Lites' mix only	1/12 pkg	160	3	32	370	0	2.0	1.0	0	11%
devil's food, 'Lovin' Lites' prepared w/water, 2 eggs	1/12 pkg	170	4	32	380	0	3.0	1.0	35	16%
devil's food, 'Lovin' Lites' prepared w/water, 3 egg whites	1/12 pkg	160	4	32	380	0	2.0	1.0	0	11%
devil's food, microwave, 'Singles' mix only.	1 cake	250	5	35	450	0	10.0	0.0	50	36%
devil's food, w/chocolate frosting, microwave, mix only	1/6 pkg	210	2	35	240	0	7.0	0.0	0	30%
devil's food, w/chocolate frosting, microwave, prepared.	1/6 pkg	310	3	36	250	0	17.0	0.0	35	50%
devil's food, w/chocolate frosting, microwave, prepared w/egg substitute	1/6 pkg	240	3	36	250	0	9.0	0.0	0	34%
devil's food, w/chocolate frosting, microwave, 'Singles' prepared.	1 cake	450	5	65	520	0	19.0	0.0	50	38%
German chocolate, w/frosting, microwave, mix only	1/6 pkg	230	2	37	240	0	8.0	0.0	0	32%
German chocolate, w/frosting, microwave, prepared	1/6 pkg	320	3	37	350	0	18.0	0.0	35	50%
(Pillsbury)										
butter recipe, 'Moist Supreme' mix only.	1/12 pkg	180	2	33	330	1	4.0	1.5	0	20%
butter recipe, 'Moist Supreme' mix only.	1/12 pkg	270	4	33	420	1	13.0	7.0	75	44%
butter recipe, 'Pillsbury Plus' mix only	1/12 pkg	170	2	32	330	0	4.0	1.0	0	21%
butter recipe, 'Pillsbury Plus' prepared	1/12 pkg	270	4	33	430	2	13.0	7.0	75	44%
butter recipe, 'Pillsbury Plus' prepared w/1/2 cup margarine,4 egg whites	1/12 cake	240	3	32	420	0	12.0	1.0	0	44%
caramel nut, 'Bundt Ring Cake' mix.	1/16 pkg	180	2	28	200	1	7.0	2.0	0	34%

Food Name	Serving Size	Calories	Prot. gms	Carbs gms	Sod. mgs	Fiber gms	Fat gms	Sat. Fat gms	Chol. mgs	% Fat Cal.
caramel nut, 'Bundt Ring Cake' prepared	1/16 cake	290	3	28	210	1	18.0	3.5	40	57%
caramel, 'Bundt Ring Cake' mix only	1/16 pkg	220	2	43	350	0	5.0	1.0	5	20%
caramel, prepared w/1/3 cup oil, 4 egg whites	1/16 cake	280	3	43	370	0	12.0	2.0	5	37%
caramel, prepared w/water, 1/2 cup oil, 3 eggs	1/16 cake	290	3	43	370	0	13.0	2.0	45	39%
chocolate macaroon, prepared w/1/2c oil, 4 egg whites	1/16 cake	270	3	37	340	0	14.0	4.0	0	44%
chocolate macaroon, 'Bundt Ring Cake' mix only	1/16 pkg	210	2	37	330	0	7.0	3.0	0	29%
chocolate macaroon, prepared w/1/2 cup oil, 3 eggs	1/16 cake	280	3	37	340	0	14.0	4.0	40	44%
chocolate mousse, 'Bundt Ring Cake' mix only	1/16 pkg	180	2	37	300	0	4.0	1.0	0	19%
chocolate mousse, prepared w/1/2 cup oil, 3 eggs	1/16 cake	260	3	37	310	0	12.0	2.0	40	40%
chocolate mousse, prepared w/1/2 cup oil, 4 egg whites	1/16 cake	250	3	37	320	0	11.0	2.0	0	38%
dark chocolate, 'Moist Supreme' mix only	1/12 pkg	180	2	34	320	1	4.0	1.5	0	20%
dark chocolate, 'Moist Supreme' prepared	1/12 cake	250	3	34	340	1	11.0	2.5	55	40%
dark chocolate, 'Pillsbury Plus' prepared w/3 egg whites, 2 tbsp flour	1/12 cake	180	3	33	340	0	5.0	2.0	0	24%
dark chocolate, 'Pillsbury Plus' prepared w/water, 1/3 cup oil, 3 eggs	1/12 cake	250	3	32	340	0	12.0	3.0	55	44%
devil's food, 'Lovin Lites' prepared	1/10 cake	230	4	41	420	2	5.0	2.0	45	20%
devil's food, 'Lovin' Lites' mix only	1/10 pkg	210	2	41	410	2	4.5	1.5	0	19%
devil's food, 'Moist Supreme' mix only	1/12 pkg	180	2	33	330	1	4.0	1.5	0	20%
devil's food, 'Moist Supreme' prepared	1/12 cake	270	4	33	340	1	14.0	3.0	55	46%
devil's food, 'Pillsbury Plus' prepared w/water, 3 egg whites, 2 tbsp flour	1/12 cake	180	3	33	340	0	4.0	1.0	0	20%
double hot fudge, bundt, prepared	1/12 cake	280	3	32	220	1	16.0	5.0	40	51%
double supreme, microwave, prepared	1/8 cake	330	3	39	340	0	19.0	0.0	0	50%
fudge, 'Tunnel of Fudge' mix only	1/16 pkg	210	2	42	330	0	4.0	1.0	0	17%
fudge, 'Tunnel of Fudge' prepared w/3/4c oil, 4 egg whites	1/16 pkg	300	3	42	340	0	15.0	3.0	0	43%
fudge, 'Tunnel of Fudge' prepared w/3/4 cup oil, 3 eggs	1/16 cake	310	3	42	340	0	16.0	3.0	40	44%
fudge swirl, 'Moist Supreme' mix only	1/12 pkg	200	2	37	280	1	4.5	1.5	0	21%
fudge swirl, 'Moist Supreme' prepared	1/12 cake	250	3	37	290	1	10.0	2.0	55	36%
fudge swirl, 'Pillsbury Plus' prepared w/1/3 cup oil, 3 eggs	1/12 cake	270	3	36	300	0	12.0	3.0	55	41%
fudge swirl, 'Pillsbury Plus' prepared w/water, 3 egg whites, 2 tbsp flour	1/12 cake	200	3	37	290	0	5.0	2.0	0	22%
German chocolate, 'Moist Supreme' mix only	1/12 pkg	180	2	34	270	1	4.0	1.5	0	20%
German chocolate, 'Moist Supreme' prepared	1/12 cake	250	3	34	280	1	11.0	2.5	35	40%
German chocolate, 'Pillsbury Plus' prepared w/1/3 cup oil, 3 eggs	1/12 cake	250	3	34	280	0	11.0	3.0	55	40%
German chocolate, 'Pillsbury Plus' prepared w/3 egg whites, 2 tbsp flour	1/12 cake	180	3	34	280	0	4.0	1.0	0	20%
microwave, mix only	1/9 pkg	110	1	16	180	0	5.0	2.0	10	40%
microwave, prepared	1/8 cake	210	2	23	260	0	13.0	0.0	0	54%
'Pillsbury Plus' prepared	1/12 cake	260	3	34	330	1	12.0	3.0	55	42%
'Pillsbury Plus' prepared w/1/2 cup butter, 3 eggs	1/12 pkg	250	4	32	420	0	13.0	6.0	75	45%
w/chocolate frosting, microwave, prepared	1/8 cake	300	2	35	310	0	17.0	0.0	0	51%
w/chocolate fudge frosting, prepared	1/9 pkg	160	2	24	210	0	7.0	2.0	10	38%
w/vanilla frosting, microwave, prepared	1/8 cake	300	2	36	300	0	17.0	0.0	0	50%
(Robin Hood) mix, chocolate chip fudge, mix only	1/9 mix	150	2	25	210	0	5.0	0.0	0	29%
(Sweet 'n Low) low-fat, low-sodium, low-cholesterol, microwave, prepared	1/10 cake	90	2	16	40	1	2.0	0.0	5	20%
mix only	1/6 cake	150	2	30	30	1	3.0	1.0	0	17%

Food Name	Serving Size	Calories	Prot. gms	Carbs gms	Sod. mgs	Fiber gms	Fat gms	Sat. Fat gms	Chol. mgs	% Fat Cal.
CHOCOLATE CHIP										
(Betty Crocker)										
'SuperMoist' mix only	1/12 mix	180	2	35	280	0	4.0	0.0	0	20%
'SuperMoist' prepared w/oil, cholesterol-free egg substitute	1/12 mix	220	3	35	300	0	8.0	0.0	0	32%
'SuperMoist' prepared w/1/2 cup oil, 3 eggs	1/12 mix	290	3	35	300	0	15.0	0.0	55	47%
(Gold Medal) golden, mix only	1/9 mix	140	1	26	190	0	4.0	0.0	0	25%
(Pillsbury)										
'Moist Supreme' mix only	1/12 pkg	190	2	35	270	1	5.0	2.0	0	23%
'Moist Supreme' prepared	1/12 cake	240	3	35	280	1	10.0	3.0	35	37%
'Pillsbury Plus' prepared w/1/4 cup oil, 2 eggs	1/12 cake	240	3	34	280	0	10.0	3.0	35	38%
'Pillsbury Plus' w/2 egg whites, 2 tbsp flour	1/12 cake	190	3	35	280	0	5.0	2.0	0	23%
(Robin Hood) golden, mix only	1/9 mix	140	1	26	190	0	4.0	0.0	0	25%
CINNAMON										
(MicroRave)										
pecan, microwave	1/6 cake	290	3	39	210	0	13.0	3.0	45	41%
pecan, microwave, prepared w/cholesterol-free egg product	1/6 cake	240	3	39	220	0	8.0	2.0	0	30%
(Pillsbury)										
streusel, microwave, 'Streusel Swirl' prepared	1/8 cake	240	2	33	180	0	11.0	0.0	0	41%
streusel, 'Streusel Swirl' mix only	1/16 pkg	210	2	38	210	0	5.0	1.5	0	22%
streusel, 'Streusel Swirl' prepared	1/16 cake	260	3	38	200	0	11.0	0.0	0	38%
streusel, 'Streusel Swirl' prepared w/1/3 cup oil, 4 egg whites	1/16 pkg	250	2	38	200	0	10.0	2.0	0	36%
streusel, 'Streusel Swirl' prepared w/water, 1/3 cup oil, 3 eggs	1/16 pkg	260	3	38	200	0	11.0	2.0	40	38%
COFFEECAKE										
(Aunt Jemima) 'easy'	1/3 cup	170	2	30	240	1	5.0	1.0	0	26%
(Pillsbury) apple cinnamon	1/8 cake	240	3	40	150	0	7.0	0.0	0	27%
FRUIT										
(Duncan Hines) tropical fruit, prepared	1/12 cake	250	3	36	270	0	11.0	2.0	45	39%
GOLDEN										
(Betty Crocker) vanilla, 'Supermoist' prepared	1/12 cake	170	1	35	270	0	3.0	1.0	0	16%
(Duncan Hines)										
golden, butter recipe, mix only	1/12 pkg	190	2	36	160	0	4.0	2.0	0	19%
golden, butter recipe, prepared	1/12 cake	320	3	42	190	2	16.0	7.0	80	44%
golden, butter recipe, prepared w/stick margarine	1/12 cake	270	3	36	270	0	13.0	4.0	65	43%
KEY LIME *(Duncan Hines)* prepared	1/12 cake	250	3	36	270	0	11.0	2.0	45	39%
LEMON										
(Betty Crocker)										
'SuperMoist' mix only	1/12 mix	180	1	36	260	0	4.0	0.0	0	20%
'SuperMoist' prepared w/1/3 cup oil, 3 eggs	1/12 mix	260	3	37	280	0	11.0	0.0	55	38%
'SuperMoist' prepared w/3 tbsp oil, egg substitute	1/12 mix	220	3	37	280	0	7.0	0.0	0	28%
lemon chiffon, 'Classic Dessert' mix only	1/12 pkg	190	3	36	190	0	4.0	0.0	0	19%
lemon chiffon, 'Classic Dessert' w/2 eggs	1/12 pkg	200	4	36	200	0	5.0	0.0	35	22%
lemon pudding, 'Classic Dessert' mix only	1/6 pkg	220	1	45	260	0	4.0	0.0	0	16%
lemon pudding, 'Classic Dessert' prepared w/1 egg	1/6 pkg	230	2	45	270	0	5.0	0.0	35	19%
(Duncan Hines)										
lemon supreme	1/12 cake	260	3	36	295	0	11.0	3.0	65	39%
lemon supreme, cholesterol-free recipe, prepared	1/12 cake	250	3	36	285	0	10.0	2.0	0	37%
lemon supreme, mix only	1/12 cake	190	2	36	280	0	4.0	11.0	0	19%
(Estee)	1/10 cake	100	1	18	68	0	2.0	1.0	0	19%
(MicroRave) w/lemon frosting	1/6 cake	300	2	37	250	0	16.0	4.0	45	48%

Food Name	Serving Size	Calories	Prot. gms	Carbs gms	Sod. mgs	Fiber gms	Fat gms	Sat. Fat gms	Chol. mgs	% Fat Cal.
(Pillsbury)										
'Moist Supreme' mix only	1/10 pkg	210	2	42	330	1	4.0	1.5	0	17%
'Moist Supreme' prepared	1/10 pkg	300	4	42	350	1	13.0	3.0	65	39%
'Pillsbury Plus' prepared w/1/3 cup oil, 3 eggs	1/12 pkg	240	3	34	280	0	10.0	2.0	55	38%
'Pillsbury Plus' prepared w/water, 3 egg whites, 2 tbsp flour	1/12 pkg	180	3	35	280	0	3.0	1.0	0	15%
'Pillsbury Plus' prepared	1/12 cake	310	4	43	340	1	13.0	3.0	65	38%
Bundt, 'Tunnel of Lemon' mix only	1/16 pkg	210	1	44	270	0	4.0	1.0	0	17%
Bundt, 'Tunnel of Lemon' prepared	1/16 cake	270	2	45	300	0	9.0	0.0	0	30%
Bundt, 'Tunnel of Lemon' prepared w/1/3 cup oil, 3 eggs	1/16 pkg	270	2	44	280	0	9.0	2.0	40	31%
Bundt, 'Tunnel of Lemon' prepared w/1/3 cup oil, 4 egg whites	1/16 pkg	260	2	44	280	0	8.0	2.0	0	28%
double supreme, microwave, prepared	1/8 cake	300	2	40	210	0	15.0	0.0	0	45%
microwave, prepared	1/8 cake	220	2	23	180	0	13.0	0.0	0	54%
w/lemon frosting, microwave, prepared	1/8 cake	300	2	37	220	0	17.0	0.0	0	50%
(Streusel Swirl)										
lemon supreme, mix only	1/16 pkg	200	2	37	290	0	6.0	1.0	0	26%
lemon supreme, prepared	1/16 cake	270	3	39	340	0	11.0	0.0	0	37%
lemon supreme, prepared w/water, 1/3 cup oil, 3 eggs	1/16 pkg	260	3	37	300	0	11.0	2.0	40	38%
lemon supreme, prepared w/water, 1/3c oil, 4 egg whites	1/16 pkg	250	3	37	300	0	10.0	2.0	0	36%
(Sweet 'N Low) mix only	1/6 cake	150	2	30	30	1	3.0	1.0	0	17%
ORANGE										
(Duncan Hines)										
orange supreme, cholesterol-free recipe, prepared	1/12 cake	250	3	36	285	0	10.0	2.0	0	37%
orange supreme, mix only	1/12 cake	190	2	36	280	0	4.0	11.0	0	19%
orange supreme, prepared	1/12 cake	260	3	36	295	0	11.0	3.0	65	39%
PEACH *(Duncan Hines)* prepared	1/12 cake	250	3	36	270	0	11.0	2.0	45	39%
PINEAPPLE										
(Betty Crocker)										
upside down, prepared w/egg substitute	1/9 cake	270	2	43	240	0	10.0	0.0	0	33%
upside down, prepared w/eggs, margarine	1/9 cake	270	2	43	240	0	10.0	0.0	25	33%
supreme, cholesterol-free recipe, prepared	1/12 cake	250	3	36	285	0	10.0	2.0	0	37%
supreme, mix only	1/12 cake	190	2	36	280	0	4.0	11.0	0	19%
supreme, prepared	1/12 cake	260	3	36	295	0	11.0	3.0	65	39%
(Pillsbury)										
crème, Bundt, mix only	1/16 pkg	200	1	42	270	0	3.0	1.0	0	14%
crème, Bundt, prepared	1/16 cake	260	2	41	300	0	9.0	0.0	0	32%
crème, prepared w/water, 1/2 cup oil, 4 egg whites	1/16 pkg	270	2	42	280	0	10.0	2.0	0	34%
crème, prepared w/water, 1/3 cup oil, 3 eggs	1/16 pkg	280	2	42	280	0	11.0	2.0	40	36%
POUND										
(Betty Crocker) golden 'Classic Dessert' mix only	1/12 pkg	190	1	28	150	0	8.0	0.0	0	38%
(Dromedary)										
mix only	5 tbsp	130	1	20	140	0	5.0	0.0	0	35%
prepared	1 slice (1/2")	150	2	21	160	0	6.0	0.0	0	37%
(Estee) prepared	1/8 cake	120	2	23	85	0	2.5	1.0	0	19%
(Martha White) prepared	1/10 cake	120	2	19	110	0	4.0	0.0	20	30%
RAINBOW CHIP										
(Betty Crocker)										
party cake, 'SuperMoist' mix only	1/12 mix	180	2	35	300	0	4.0	0.0	0	20%
party cake, 'Supermoist' prepared	1/12 cake	220	2	41	340	0	5.0	2.5	0	21%
party cake, 'SuperMoist' prepared w/1/3 cup oil, 3 eggs	1/12 cake	250	3	35	320	0	11.0	0.0	55	39%
RASPBERRY *(Duncan Hines)* prepared	1/12 cake	250	3	36	270	0	11.0	2.0	45	39%

Food Name	Serving Size	Calories	Prot. gms	Carbs gms	Sod. mgs	Fiber gms	Fat gms	Sat. Fat gms	Chol. mgs	% Fat Cal.
SPICE										
(Betty Crocker)										
'SuperMoist' mix only	1/12 mix	180	1	36	300	0	4.0	0.0	0	20%
'SuperMoist' prepared w/1/3 cup oil, 3 eggs	1/12 cake	260	3	36	320	0	11.0	0.0	55	39%
'SuperMoist' prepared w/3 tbsp oil, cholesterol-free egg product	1/12 cake	220	3	36	320	0	7.0	0.0	0	29%
(Duncan Hines)										
cholesterol-free recipe, prepared	1/12 cake	250	3	36	285	0	10.0	2.0	0	37%
mix only	1/12 cake	190	2	36	280	0	4.0	11.0	0	19%
prepared	1/12 cake	260	3	36	295	0	11.0	3.0	65	39%
(Estee)	1/8 cake	120	1	23	80	0	3.0	1.0	0	22%
(Gluten Free Pantry) gluten-free	1 serving	110	1	26	170	0	0.0	0.0	0	0%
STRAWBERRY										
(Duncan Hines)										
supreme, mix only	1/12 pkge	190	2	36	280	0	4.0	11.0	0	19%
supreme, prepared	1/12 cake	260	3	36	295	0	11.0	3.0	65	39%
supreme, prepared, cholesterol-free recipe	1/12 cake	250	3	36	285	0	10.0	2.0	0	37%
(Pillsbury)										
'Moist Supreme' mix only	1/12 pkg	180	1	36	280	1	4.0	1.5	0	20%
'Moist Supreme' prepared	1/12 cake	260	3	36	300	1	11.0	2.5	55	39%
cream cheese, 'Bundt Ring Cake' mix only	1/16 pkg	190	1	34	180	0	5.0	2.5	5	24%
cream cheese, 'Bundt RingCake' prepared	1/16 cake	300	3	34	200	0	17.0	4.5	60	51%
'Pillsbury Plus' prepared	1/12 cake	260	3	36	310	0	11.0	2.5	55	39%
'Pillsbury Plus' prepared w/1/3 cup oil & 3 eggs	1/12 pkg	190	3	36	310	0	4.0	1.0	0	19%
SWIRL										
(Betty Crocker)										
party cake, 'SuperMoist' mix only	1/12 mix	190	2	36	270	0	4.0	0.0	0	19%
party cake, 'SuperMoist' prepared, cholesterol-free recipe,	1/12 cake	220	3	36	290	0	7.0	0.0	0	29%
party cake, 'SuperMoist' prepared w/1/3 cup oil, 3 eggs	1/12 cake	260	3	36	280	0	11.0	0.0	55	39%
(Pillsbury)										
white and fudge, 'Moist Supreme' mix only	1/12 pkg	200	2	37	280	1	4.5	1.5	0	21%
white and fudge, 'Moist Supreme' prepared	1/12 pkg	250	3	37	290	1	10.0	2.5	35	36%
white and fudge, 'Pillsbury Plus' mix only	1/12 pkg	190	2	36	280	0	4.0	1.0	0	19%
white and fudge, 'Pillsbury Plus' prepared	1/12 pkg	250	3	36	290	0	10.0	2.0	35	37%
white and fudge, 'Pillsbury Plus' prepared, cholesterol-free recipe	1/12 pkg	200	3	37	290	0	4.0	1.0	0	18%
VANILLA										
(Betty Crocker)										
golden, 'SuperMoist' mix only	1/12 mix	180	1	36	250	0	4.0	0.0	0	20%
golden, 'SuperMoist' prepared w/1/2 cup oil, 3 eggs	1/12 mix	280	3	36	270	0	14.0	0.0	55	45%
golden, 'SuperMoist' prepared w/oil, egg substitute	1/12 mix	220	3	36	270	0	7.0	0.0	0	29%
(Duncan Hines)										
French, mix only	1/12 cake	190	2	36	280	0	4.0	11.0	0	19%
French, prepared	1/12 cake	260	3	36	295	0	11.0	3.0	65	39%
French, prepared, cholesterol-free recipe	1/12 cake	250	3	36	285	0	10.0	2.0	0	37%
(MicroRave) golden	1/6 cake	320	2	40	230	0	17.0	5.0	35	48%
(Pillsbury)										
French, 'Moist Supreme' mix only	1/10 pkg	220	2	42	330	1	5.0	1.5	0	20%
French, 'Moist Supreme' prepared	1/10 pkg	300	3	42	350	1	13.0	3.0	45	39%
French, 'Pillsbury Plus' mix only	1/10 pkg	230	2	41	340	1	6.0	2.0	0	24%
French, 'Pillsbury Plus' prepared	1/10 pkg	320	4	41	360	1	15.0	3.5	65	43%
sunshine, 'Moist Supreme' mix only	1/12 pkg	190	1	34	280	1	5.0	1.5	0	24%
sunshine, 'Moist Supreme' prepared	1/12 cake	260	3	34	300	1	12.0	3.0	55	42%

Food Name	Serving Size	Calories	Prot. gms	Carbs gms	Sod. mgs	Fiber gms	Fat gms	Sat. Fat gms	Chol. mgs	% Fat Cal.
sunshine, 'Pillsbury Plus' prepared w/3 egg white, 2 tbsp flour	1/12 pkg	190	3	35	300	0	5.0	2.0	0	23%
WHITE										
(Betty Crocker)										
'Light' prepared	1/12 mix	180	1	37	320	0	3.0	0.0	0	15%
'Light' mix only	1/12 mix	180	2	34	300	0	4.0	0.0	0	20%
'Light' prepared w/3 egg whites	1/12 mix	180	2	37	330	0	3.0	0.0	0	15%
sour cream, 'SuperMoist' mix only	1/12 mix	180	2	36	280	0	3.0	0.0	0	15%
sour cream, 'SuperMoist' prepared	1/12 cake	210	2	41	370	0	4.5	1.5	0	19%
sour cream, 'SuperMoist' prepared w/3 egg whites	1/12 mix	180	3	36	290	0	3.0	0.0	0	15%
'SuperMoist' prepared w/1/3 cup oil, 3 eggs	1/12 mix	230	2	34	320	0	10.0	0.0	0	38%
(Duncan Hines)										
cholesterol-free recipe, prepared	1/12 cake	240	3	36	270	0	10.0	2.0	0	37%
mix only	1/12 cake	190	2	36	250	0	4.0	2.0	0	19%
prepared	1/12 cake	240	2	35	220	0	10.0	2.0	0	38%
(Estee)	1/10 cake	100	1	18	68	0	2.0	1.0	0	19%
(Krusteaz) prepared, 8-inch double cake	1/12 cake	190	3	37	280	0	3.0	0.0	2	14%
(Lovin' Loaf)										
mix only	1/12 pkg	170	2	35	300	0	2.0	1.0	0	11%
prepared w/water, 2 eggs	1/12 cake	180	3	35	310	0	3.0	1.0	35	15%
prepared w/water, 3 egg whites	1/12 cake	170	3	35	310	0	2.0	1.0	0	11%
(Pillsbury)										
'Lovin Lites' mix only	1/10 pkg	210	2	42	340	1	4.0	1.5	0	17%
'Lovin Lites' prepared	1/10 cake	230	3	42	350	1	5.0	1.5	45	20%
'Moist Supreme' mix only	1/10 pkg	220	2	41	330	1	5.0	1.5	0	21%
'Moist Supreme' prepared	1/10 cake	280	3	41	350	1	11.0	2.5	0	36%
'Pillsbury Plus' mix only	1/12 pkg	170	2	35	300	0	2.0	1.0	0	11%
'Pillsbury Plus' prepared w/water, egg whites	1/12 cake	170	3	35	310	0	2.0	1.0	0	11%
'Pillsbury Plus' prepared w/water, eggs	1/12 cake	180	3	35	310	0	3.0	1.0	35	15%
'Pillsbury Plus' prepared w/1/4 cup oil, 3 egg whites	1/12 cake	220	3	34	290	0	9.0	2.0	0	35%
'Pillsbury Plus' prepared w/water, 3 egg whites, 2 tbsp flour	1/12 cake	190	3	35	290	0	4.0	1.0	0	19%
(Sweet 'n Low) lowfat, mix only	1/6 pkg	140	2	30	30	1	3.0	1.0	0	17%
(Weight Watchers) low-fat, 'Sweet Rewards'	1 serving	170	2	36	300	0	2.0	0.5	0	11%
YELLOW										
(Betty Crocker)										
'Supermoist' 'Light' prepared	1/12 cake	180	1	37	290	0	3.0	0.0	0	15%
'Supermoist' 'Light' prepared w/3 eggs	1/12 cake	200	3	37	310	0	4.0	0.0	55	18%
'Supermoist' 'Light' prepared w/egg substitute	1/12 cake	190	3	37	330	0	3.0	0.0	0	14%
'Supermoist' mix only	1/12 mix	180	1	36	280	0	4.0	0.0	0	20%
'Supermoist' prepared w/1/3 cup oil, 3 eggs	1/12 cake	260	3	36	300	0	11.0	0.0	55	39%
'Supermoist' prepared w/3 tbsp oil, egg substitute	1/12 cake	220	3	36	300	0	7.0	0.0	0	29%
(Duncan Hines)										
cholesterol-free recipe, prepared	1/12 cake	250	3	36	285	0	10.0	2.0	0	37%
mix only	1/12 pkg	190	2	36	280	0	4.0	11.0	0	19%
prepared	1/12 cake	260	3	36	295	0	11.0	3.0	65	39%
(Finast) 'Ultra Moist' prepared	1/12 cake	240	3	34	280	0	10.0	0.0	0	38%
(Krusteaz) prepared, 8-inch double cake	1/12 cake	200	3	36	330	1	5.0	1.3	0	22%
(Lovin' Loaf)										
prepared w/water, 2 eggs	1/12 pkg	180	3	35	300	0	3.0	1.0	35	15%
prepared w/water, 3 egg whites	1/12 pkg	170	3	35	310	0	2.0	1.0	0	11%
(MicroRave)										
microwave, 'Singles' prepared	1 cake	260	3	36	450	0	11.0	0.0	50	39%
w/chocolate frosting, microwave, mix only	1/6 pkg	210	1	36	210	0	7.0	0.0	0	30%

Food Name	Serving Size	Calories	Prot. gms	Carbs gms	Sod. mgs	Fiber gms	Fat gms	Sat. Fat gms	Chol. mgs	% Fat Cal.
w/chocolate frosting, microwave, 'Singles' prepared	1 cake	460	4	65	510	0	20.0	0.0	50	39%
w/chocolate frosting, microwave, prepared w/1 tbsp oil, egg substitute	1/6 pkg	230	2	36	230	0	9.0	0.0	0	35%
yellow, w/chocolate frosting, microwave, prepared w/1/4 cup oil, 1 egg	1/6 pkg	300	2	36	220	0	17.0	0.0	35	50%
(Pillsbury)										
butter recipe, 'Moist Supreme' mix only	1/12 pkg	170	1	35	270	0	3.0	1.0	0	16%
butter recipe, 'Pillsbury Plus' prepared	1/12 cake	260	3	36	370	0	12.0	6.0	75	41%
butter recipe, 'Pillsbury Plus' prepared w/1/2 cup butter, 3 eggs	1/12 cake	260	3	35	370	0	12.0	5.0	75	42%
butter recipe, 'Pillsbury Plus' prepared w/1/2 cup margarine, 4 egg whites	1/12 cake	250	3	35	360	0	11.0	1.0	0	39%
butter recipe, 'SuperMoist' mix only	1/12 mix	170	1	37	250	0	2.0	0.0	0	11%
butter recipe, 'SuperMoist' prepared w/1/2 cup butter, 3 eggs	1/12 mix	260	3	37	340	0	11.0	0.0	75	38%
'Lovin' Lites' mix only	1/10 pkg	220	2	43	370	1	4.0	1.5	0	17%
'Lovin' Lites' prepared	1/10 cake	230	3	43	380	1	5.0	1.5	45	20%
microwave, prepared	1/8 cake	220	2	23	170	0	13.0	0.0	0	54%
'Moist Supreme' mix only	1/12 pkg	180	2	35	280	1	4.0	1.5	0	20%
'Moist Supreme' prepared	1/12 cake	240	3	35	290	1	10.0	2.5	55	37%
'Pillsbury Plus' prepared w/1/3 cup oil, 3 eggs	1/12 cake	260	3	34	300	0	12.0	3.0	55	42%
'Pillsbury Plus' prepared w/water, 3 egg whites, 2 tbsp flour	1/12 cake	190	3	35	300	0	5.0	2.0	0	23%
w/chocolate frosting, microwave, prepared	1/8 cake	300	2	36	220	0	17.0	0.0	0	50%
(Sweet 'n Low)										
low-fat, low-sodium, low-cholesterol, microwave, prepared	1/10 cake	90	2	16	40	1	2.0	0.0	5	20%
mix only	1/6 pkg	150	2	30	30	1	3.0	1.0	0	17%
(Weight Watchers) less fat 'Sweet Rewards'	1 serving	160	2	37	280	0	1.0	0.5	0	5%

CALABASH GOURD. See GOURD, BOTTLE.

CALAMARI. See SQUID.

CALICO BASS. See SUNFISH.

CALZONE. See under SANDWICH.

CANADIAN BACON. See BACON, CANADIAN STYLE.

CANARY TREE. See PILI NUT.

CANDY. See also CANDY COATING.

Food Name	Serving Size	Calories	Prot. gms	Carbs gms	Sod. mgs	Fiber gms	Fat gms	Sat. Fat gms	Chol. mgs	% Fat Cal.
(Boyer) 'Smoothie'	1.6 oz	250	5	24	0	0	15.0	0.0	0	54%
(Brach's) 'Bridge Mix'	1 oz	140	2	17	30	0	7.0	0.0	0	45%
(Estee) 'Estee-ets'	5 pieces	35	1	4	10	0	2.0	1.0	1	47%
(Nestlé) 'Butterfinger' round 'BBs'	10 pieces	125	3	17	51	1	4.9	2.7	0	35%
(Russell Stover) 'Home Fashioned Favorites'	1.4 oz	170	1	27	60	1	7.0	4.5	5	36%
ALMOND										
(Brach's) candy-coated, 'Jordan Almonds'	1 oz	120	2	23	0	0	2.0	0.0	0	15%
(Estee) chocolate covered	2 squares	60	1	5	10	0	4.5	2.0	2	65%
(Featherweight) chocolate covered	1 section	90	1	6	20	0	7.0	0.0	0	69%
(Hershey's) chocolate covered, solitaires, 'Hershey's Golden Collection' 2.8-oz pieces	1 piece	444	9	37	44	3	28.9	11.9	10	59%
(M&M Mars) candy-coated, 'M&M's'	1 oz	150	2	17	30	0	8.0	0.0	0	49%
(Russell Stover) 'Almond Delights'	1.4 oz	210	3	22	55	1	12.0	5.0	10	52%
BUTTERSCOTCH *(Russell Stover)* squares	1.4 oz	180	1	29	65	1	6.5	5.0	5	33%
CANDY BAR										
(Barat)										
chocolate tofu, w/almonds	1 oz	170	3	13	10	0	11.0	0.0	0	61%
chocolate tofu, w/almonds and raisins	1 oz	160	3	14	10	0	11.0	0.0	0	59%

Food Name	Serving Size	Calories	Prot. gms	Carbs gms	Sod. mgs	Fiber gms	Fat gms	Sat. Fat gms	Chol. mgs	% Fat Cal.
chocolate tofu truffle, w/pralines	1 oz	170	4	12	10	0	11.0	0.0	0	61%
(Cadbury)										
chocolate, w/crisps and honey	1 oz	150	2	18	40	0	7.0	0.0	0	44%
chocolate, w/fruit and nuts	1 oz	150	2	17	40	0	8.0	0.0	0	49%
chocolate, w/roasted almonds	1 oz	150	3	15	40	0	9.0	0.0	0	53%
'Dairy Milk'	1 oz	150	2	17	45	0	8.0	0.0	0	49%
(Carafection)										
'Almond Crunch' date sweetened carob	1 oz	139	2	17	26	0	7.0	0.0	0	45%
'Cashew Coconut Crunch' carob	1 oz	139	2	17	26	0	7.0	0.0	0	45%
'Crispy Crunch' date sweetened carob	1 oz	139	2	17	26	0	7.0	0.0	0	45%
'Mint Honey Graham' carob coated	1 oz	139	2	17	26	0	7.0	0.0	0	45%
'Mint' date sweetened carob	1 oz	139	2	17	26	0	7.0	0.0	0	45%
'Original Honey Graham' carob coated	1 oz	139	2	17	26	0	7.0	0.0	0	45%
'Peanut Crunch' date sweetened, carob	1 oz	139	2	17	26	0	7.0	0.0	0	45%
plain, date sweetened, carob	1 oz	139	2	17	26	0	7.0	0.0	0	45%
(Caroby) carob	4 sections	150	4	13	55	0	9.0	0.0	0	54%
(Cocofection) original	1 oz	155	2	15	23	0	10.0	0.0	0	57%
(Estee)										
chocolate, coconut	2 squares	60	1	5	15	0	4.0	2.5	5	60%
chocolate, dark, deluxe	2 squares	50	1	6	0	0	3.0	2.0	0	49%
chocolate, fruit and nut	2 squares	60	1	5	10	0	4.5	2.0	2	65%
chocolate, milk	2 squares	60	1	5	15	0	4.0	2.5	5	60%
crunch	2 squares	45	1	4	10	0	3.0	2.0	2	57%
mint	2 squares	50	1	6	0	0	3.0	2.0	0	49%
(Fantastic Foods) 'Halvah'	1.5 oz	232	8	17	0	0	10.0	0.0	0	47%
(Fifty 50)										
chocolate, milk, extra thick, w/o sugar	1 section	80	1	6	25	0	6.0	0.0	0	66%
chocolate, milk, mini	4 pieces	90	2	6	20	0	6.0	0.0	0	63%
chocolate, w/almonds, extra thick, w/o sugar	1 section	90	2	6	20	0	6.0	0.0	0	63%
crunch, chocolate, extra thick, w/o sugar	1 section	70	1	6	20	0	5.0	0.0	0	62%
fruit and nut, chocolate, extra thick, w/o sugar	1 section	80	1	6	20	0	5.0	0.0	0	62%
(Ghirardelli)										
chocolate, dark, 'Premier Bar'	1 bar	428	4	51	5	5	28.6	17.1	0	54%
chocolate, dark, w/almonds, 'Premier Bar'	1 bar	442	6	45	6	6	31.6	14.5	0	58%
chocolate, dark, w/raspberries, 'Premier Bar'	1 bar	423	4	52	4	5	27.6	16.4	0	53%
(Heath) 'Soft'n Crunchy Bar' 2 pieces	1.19 oz serving	190	1	19	85	0	12.0	0.0	0	57%
(Hershey's)										
'Almond Joy' 1.7-oz bar	1 bar	229	2	29	72	2	13.1	8.5	2	52%
'Almond Joy' snack size, 0.7 oz	1 bar	93	1	12	29	1	5.4	3.5	1	52%
'Caramello' 5-oz bar	1 bar	673	9	90	195	2	30.8	19.9	38	41%
'Caramello' 1.6-oz bar	1 bar	213	3	29	62	1	9.8	6.3	12	41%
chocolate, 'Hershey's Milk Chocolate Bar'	1.55 oz	240	4	25	40	0	14.0	0.0	10	52%
chocolate, snack size, 0.7-oz bar	1 bar	91	1	11	28	1	4.8	3.9	0	47%
chocolate, w/almonds, 'Hershey's Milk Chocolate Bar w/Almonds'	1.45 oz	230	5	20	55	0	14.0	0.0	10	56%
chocolate almond, 'Golden Collection'	2.8 oz	448	10	36	52	4	29.7	12.8	12	60%
'Cookies 'N' Mint'	1 bar	220	3	26	75	0	12.0	0.0	0	48%
'5th Avenue' 2-oz bar	1 bar	280	5	38	94	1	12.1	4.5	3	39%
'5th Avenue' snack size, 0.6 oz	1 bar	79	1	11	26	0	3.4	1.3	1	39%
'Kit Kat' 3.375-oz bar	1 bar	493	7	61	72	2	24.5	15.6	6	45%
'Kit Kat' 2.8-oz bar	1 bar	401	6	50	59	1	19.9	12.7	5	45%
'Kit Kat' 1.62-oz bar	1 bar	236	3	29	35	1	11.7	7.5	3	45%
'Kit Kat' 1.5-oz bar	1 bar	216	3	27	32	1	10.7	6.8	3	45%
'Kit Kat' mini, 0.35-oz bar	1 bar	51	1	6	8	0	2.5	1.6	1	45%

Food Name	Serving Size	Calories	Prot. gms	Carbs gms	Sod. mgs	Fiber gms	Fat gms	Sat. Fat gms	Chol. mgs	% Fat Cal.
'Krackel' 7-oz pkg	1 pkg	982	12	114	255	4	53.1	33.5	35	49%
'Krackel' 2.2-oz bar	1 bar	329	4	38	86	1	17.8	11.2	12	49%
'Krackel' 1.5-oz bar	1 bar	218	3	25	57	1	11.8	7.4	8	49%
'Mounds' 1.9-oz bar.	1 bar	253	2	31	79	3	13.3	10.8	1	47%
'Mr. Goodbar' 2.6-oz bar	1 bar	398	8	38	109	3	25.5	10.9	6	58%
'Mr. Goodbar' 1.75-oz bar	1 bar	267	5	25	73	2	17.1	7.3	4	58%
'Skor' 1.4-oz bar	1 bar	217	2	23	108	1	13.3	8.5	20	55%
'Special Dark' extra large, 8 oz	1 bar	1253	11	138	16	11	73.5	46.1	2	53%
'Special Dark' large, 4-oz bar	1 bar	624	6	68	8	6	36.6	22.9	1	53%
'Special Dark' 2.8-oz bar.	1 bar	436	4	48	6	4	25.6	16.0	1	53%
'Special Dark' 2.2-oz bar	1 bar	342	3	38	4	3	20.1	12.6	1	53%
'Special Dark' 1.45-oz bar.	1 bar	226	2	25	3	2	13.3	8.3	0	53%
'Symphony' 1.5-oz bar.	1 bar	232	3	24	39	1	13.8	na	9	53%
'Symphony' 2.4-oz bar.	1 bar	371	5	39	62	1	22.0	na	15	53%
'Whatchamacallit' 1.7-oz bar	1 bar	214	4	29	99	1	9.3	4.5	5	39%
(M&M Mars)										
'Bounty' milk chocolate	1 oz	140	1	17	30	0	7.0	0.0	0	47%
'Dove' dark chocolate	1 bar	200	2	22	0	2	12.0	7.0	5	53%
'Dove' dark chocolate, miniatures	4 pieces	130	1	14	0	0	8.0	0.0	0	55%
'Dove' milk chocolate.	1 bar	200	2	22	25	1	12.0	7.0	5	53%
'Dove' milk chocolate, miniatures	4 pieces	130	1	14	20	0	8.0	0.0	0	55%
'Mars' almond, 1.76-oz bar	1 bar	234	4	31	85	1	11.5	3.6	9	42%
'Milky Way' 2.15-oz bar	1 bar	258	3	44	146	1	9.8	4.8	9	33%
'Milky Way' 2.1-oz bar	1 bar	254	3	43	144	1	9.7	4.7	8	33%
'Milky Way' 2.05-oz bar	1 bar	245	3	42	139	1	9.3	4.5	8	33%
'Milky Way' 1.9-oz bar	1 bar	228	2	39	130	1	8.7	4.2	8	33%
'Milky Way' 0.8-oz bar	1 bar	97	1	16	55	0	3.7	1.8	3	33%
'Milky Way' fun size	1 bar	76	1	13	43	0	2.9	1.4	3	33%
'Munch'	1.42 oz	220	6	19	110	0	14.0	0.0	0	56%
'Snickers' king size, 4-oz bar.	1 bar	541	9	67	301	3	27.8	10.2	15	46%
'Snickers' 2-oz bar.	1 bar	273	5	34	152	1	14.0	5.1	7	46%
'Snickers' fun size	1 bar	72	1	9	40	0	3.7	1.3	2	46%
'3 Musketeers' 2.13-oz bar	1 bar	250	2	46	116	1	7.7	3.9	7	27%
'3 Musketeers' 1.813-oz bar	1 bar	212	2	39	99	1	6.6	3.3	6	27%
'3 Musketeers' 0.8-oz bar	1 bar	96	1	18	45	0	3.0	1.5	3	27%
'3 Musketeers' fun size	1 bar	69	1	13	32	0	2.1	1.1	2	27%
'Twix' 11-oz pkg.	1 pkg	1557	14	205	602	3	76.1	27.8	16	44%
'Twix' 3.35-oz bar.	4 bars	474	4	62	183	1	23.2	8.5	5	44%
'Twix' 2.06-oz bar.	2 bars	289	3	38	112	1	14.1	5.2	3	44%
'Twix' 2-oz pkg.	1 pkg	284	3	37	110	1	13.9	5.1	3	44%
'Twix' peanut, 9.43-oz pkg.	1 pkg	1415	27	141	726	9	85.9	30.4	13	55%
'Twix' peanut, 2.06-oz pkg.	1 pkg	307	6	31	158	2	18.7	6.6	3	55%
'Twix' peanut, 1.89-oz pkg.	1 pkg	286	5	28	147	2	17.4	6.2	3	55%
'Twix' peanut, 1.77-oz pkg.	1 pkg	265	5	26	136	2	16.1	5.7	3	55%
(Natures Warehouse)										
'A-Ok' fruit juice sweetened.	1 oz	130	3	17	32	0	6.2	0.0	0	41%
'My O My' fruit juice sweetened.	1 oz	103	2	21	42	0	1.4	0.0	0	12%
'No How' peanut butter, fruit juice sweetened	1 oz	140	6	11	48	0	10.0	0.0	0	57%
'Non Stop' fruit juice sweetened	1 oz	122	2	18	48	0	5.0	0.0	0	36%
'Nut Wit' carob caramel and peanuts.	1 oz	135	3	17	32	0	6.3	0.0	0	42%
(Necco) 'Sky Bar'	1.5 oz	196	2	32	57	0	7.1	0.0	0	32%
(Nestlé)										
'100 Grand' 1.5-oz bar.	1 bar	200	2	30	89	1	7.8	4.8	8	35%
'100 Grand' miniature	1 bar	98	1	15	43	0	3.8	2.3	4	35%

Food Name	Serving Size	Calories	Prot. gms	Carbs gms	Sod. mgs	Fiber gms	Fat gms	Sat. Fat gms	Chol. mgs	% Fat Cal.
'Aero' regular size	1 bar	210	0	20	20	0	12.0	0.0	0	57%
'Aero' bite size	2 bars	85	0	10	0	0	5.0	0.0	10	53%
'Baby Ruth' 2.28-oz bar	1 bar	313	5	42	147	2	13.8	8.0	3	40%
'Baby Ruth' 2.1-oz bar	1 bar	289	4	39	136	2	12.7	7.4	2	40%
'Baby Ruth' 1.2-oz bar	1 bar	164	3	22	77	1	7.2	4.2	1	40%
'Baby Ruth' miniature	1 bar	101	2	14	47	1	4.4	2.6	1	40%
'Baby Ruth' fun size	1 bar	67	1	9	32	0	3.0	1.7	1	40%
'Butterfinger' king size	1 bar	518	13	71	214	3	20.2	11.2	1	35%
'Butterfinger' 2.16-oz bar	1 bar	293	8	40	121	1	11.4	6.3	1	35%
'Butterfinger' 1.6-oz bar	1 bar	216	6	30	89	1	8.4	4.7	0	35%
'Butterfinger' fun size	1 bar	101	3	14	42	1	3.9	2.2	0	35%
'Butterfinger' bite size	1 bar	34	1	5	14	0	1.3	0.7	0	35%
'Chunky' 1.4-oz bar	1 bar	198	4	23	21	2	11.7	9.3	4	51%
'Chunky' 1.25-oz bar	1 bar	173	3	20	19	2	10.2	8.1	4	51%
'Crunch' 1.55-oz bar	1 bar	230	3	29	59	1	11.6	6.7	6	45%
'Crunch' 1.4-oz bar	1 bar	209	2	26	53	1	10.5	6.1	5	45%
'Crunch' miniature	1 bar	52	1	7	13	0	2.6	1.5	1	45%
'Oh Henry!' 2-oz bar	1 bar	246	6	37	135	2	9.6	3.8	5	34%
(Pay Day) 'Pay Day'	1.85 oz	250	9	28	200	0	12.0	0.0	0	42%
(Russell Stover)										
French chocolate	1 bar	200	3	20	30	1	13.0	8.0	10	56%
mint, French chocolate	1 bar	230	3	20	25	2	15.5	9.5	10	60%
peanut butter	1 bar	290	7	22	130	3	19.0	6.0	5	60%
(Weight Watchers)										
caramel nut	1 bar	130	2	14	25	0	8.0	3.5	5	53%
English toffee crunch	1 bar	120	2	12	25	0	7.0	3.5	5	53%
(Yogafection)										
'Brazil Nut Crunch'	1 oz	180	2	17	70	0	10.0	9.0	5	54%
'Cashew Nut Crunch'	1 oz	180	2	17	70	0	10.0	9.0	5	54%
CARAMEL										
(Allen Wertz)										
	1 piece	37	0	6	2	0	2.0	0.0	1	43%
nougat swirl	1 piece	32	0	6	2	0	1.0	0.0	1	27%
(Brach's) chocolate, 'Milk Maid'	1 oz	110	1	20	55	0	3.0	0.0	0	24%
(Estee)										
chocolate	2 pieces	50	1	9	25	0	2.0	1.0	0	31%
vanilla	2 pieces	50	1	9	25	0	2.0	1.0	0	31%
(Featherweight)	1 piece	30	0	5	10	0	1.0	0.0	0	31%
(Hershey's)										
in milk chocolate, 1.91-oz pkg 'Rolo'	1 pkg	218	3	28	93	0	10.6	6.5	10	44%
in milk chocolate, 1.74-oz roll 'Rolo'	1 roll	202	2	26	86	0	9.8	6.0	9	44%
in milk chocolate, 0.2-oz pieces 'Rolo'	1 piece	12	0	2	5	0	0.6	0.4	1	44%
(Kraft)	1 piece	30	0	6	25	0	1.0	0.0	0	27%
(Pom Poms) chocolate coated	1 oz	100	1	15	70	0	3.0	0.0	0	30%
(Russell Stover)										
butter cream, squares	1.4 oz	170	1	26	95	1	7.5	5.5	10	38%
marshmallow, milk chocolate, soft-chewy, squares	1.4 oz	190	2	25	85	5	10.0	5.0	0	45%
CHERRY										
(Brach's)										
chocolate cream	1 oz	110	1	21	20	0	2.0	0.0	0	17%
dark chocolate coated	1 oz	110	1	22	20	0	2.0	0.0	0	16%
milk chocolate covered, 'Villa'	1 oz	110	1	22	20	0	2.0	0.0	0	16%
(Russell Stover)										
'Cherry Cordials'	1.4 oz	170	1	25	25	2	7.5	4.5	5	39%

Food Name	Serving Size	Calories	Prot. gms	Carbs gms	Sod. mgs	Fiber gms	Fat gms	Sat. Fat gms	Chol. mgs	% Fat Cal.
squares	1.4 oz	160	1	28	40	1	5.5	4.5	0	30%
CHOCOLATE										
(Allen Wertz) assortment, 'Gourmet'	11.9 grams	55	1	9	13	0	2.0	0.0	1	31%
(Barat)										
tofu, 'Passionettes'	1 piece	70	1	6	5	0	5.0	0.0	0	62%
tofu pastilles 'Bits'	0.75 oz	120	2	11	10	0	8.0	0.0	0	58%
(Brach's)										
assorted, wrapped	1 oz	110	0	24	20	0	2.0	0.0	0	16%
'Jots'	1 oz	130	1	21	30	0	5.0	0.0	0	34%
milk, 'Stars'	1 oz	150	2	17	30	0	8.0	0.0	0	49%
milk chocolate coated, 'Malted Milk Balls'	1 oz	130	1	21	40	0	5.0	0.0	0	34%
(Callard and Bowser) cream	1 oz	120	0	22	0	0	3.7	0.0	0	27%
(Cocofection) trail mix, premium	1 oz	130	4	13	14	0	9.0	0.0	0	54%
(Featherweight)										
crunch	1 section	80	1	7	20	0	6.0	0.0	0	63%
milk	1 section	80	1	7	20	0	6.0	0.0	0	63%
(Great Cakes) amaretto, confection, 'Buffalo Ball'	1 ball	105	3	27	15	6	3.5	0.0	0	21%
(Hershey's)										
milk, 'Kisses'	6 pieces	150	2	16	25	0	9.0	0.0	5	53%
milk, creamy, w/almonds and toffee chips.	0.75 oz	280	5	26	50	0	17.0	0.0	0	55%
w/almonds, 'Kisses w/Almonds'	6 pieces	160	3	14	25	0	10.0	0.0	0	57%
(M&M Mars)										
'M&M's' mini, 5-oz pkg.	1 pkg	707	7	95	97	4	33.1	20.5	21	42%
'M&Ms' plain	1 cup	1023	9	148	127	5	44.0	27.2	29	39%
'M&Ms' plain	10 pieces	34	0	5	4	0	1.5	0.9	1	39%
'M&Ms' plain, 1.69-oz pkg	1 pkg	236	2	34	29	1	10.1	6.3	7	39%
'M&Ms' plain, 1.48-oz box	1 box	207	2	30	26	1	8.9	5.5	6	39%
(Nabisco) milk, 'Stars' approx 13 pieces	1 oz	160	2	19	35	0	8.0	0.0	0	46%
(Russell Stover)										
dark and milk mix, 'The Gift Box'	1.4 oz	180	2	26	45	0	8.5	4.5	5	41%
milk, assortment	1.4 oz	190	2	27	50	0	8.5	5.0	5	40%
(Saco Foods)										
'Choc'Oh's'	1.5 oz	111	1	14	14	0	6.6	2.4	0	50%
chunks.	3.5 oz	466	4	67	26	0	26.4	14.9	0	45%
(Spangler)										
coated, creme center	1 piece	80	1	15	40	0	2.0	0.0	0	22%
coated, creme center caramel, w/nuts	1 piece	100	2	11	30	0	6.0	0.0	0	51%
coated, creme center cherry, w/nuts	1 piece	110	2	12	20	0	5.0	0.0	0	45%
coated, creme center fudge, w/nuts	1 piece	140	2	17	25	0	6.0	0.0	0	42%
coated, creme center fudge, w/pecans	1 piece	140	1	18	40	0	7.0	0.0	0	45%
coated, creme center maple, w/nuts	1 piece	110	2	12	15	0	5.0	0.0	0	45%
coated, creme center vanilla, w/nuts	1 piece	110	2	13	20	0	5.0	0.0	0	43%
(Tootsie Roll) chewy roll.	1 oz	112	0	23	6	0	2.5	0.6	0	20%
(Whoppers) milk chocolate coated, malted milk balls	1 oz	136	1	20	0	0	6.0	0.0	0	39%
COCONUT										
(Brach's) Neapolitan	1 oz	120	1	24	40	0	2.0	0.0	0	15%
(Sunbelt) chocolate coated 'Macaroo'	2 oz	288	3	33	75	0	16.0	0.0	1	50%
COFFEE										
(Allen Wertz)										
'Coffee Time'	1 piece	20	0	4	2	0	1.0	0.0	1	36%
'Coffee Time' assorted.	1 piece	28	0	5	2	0	1.0	0.0	1	31%
'Coffee Time' decaffeinated.	1 piece	20	0	4	2	0	1.0	0.0	1	36%
(Brach's).	1 oz	120	0	25	35	0	2.0	0.0	0	15%

Food Name	Serving Size	Calories	Prot. gms	Carbs gms	Sod. mgs	Fiber gms	Fat gms	Sat. Fat gms	Chol. mgs	% Fat Cal.
FRUIT										
(Bonkers!) chews, all flavors	1 piece	20	0	5	0	0	0.0	0.0	0	0%
(Featherweight)										
berry patch	1 piece	12	0	3	0	0	0.0	0.0	0	0%
drops, all flavors	0.33 oz	30	0	8	15	0	0.0	0.0	0	0%
orchard	1 piece	12	0	3	0	0	0.0	0.0	0	0%
tropical blend	1 piece	12	0	3	0	0	0.0	0.0	0	0%
(Glenny's)										
black cherry, 'Drops'	1 drop	6	1	1	1	0	1.0	0.0	0	53%
lemon, twist of, 'Drops'	1 drop	6	1	1	1	0	1.0	0.0	0	53%
mandarin orange, 'Drops'	1 drop	6	1	1	1	0	1.0	0.0	0	53%
mixed fruit, 'Drops'	1 drop	6	1	1	1	0	1.0	0.0	0	53%
(Hershey's) 'Jujyfruits'	11 pieces	100	1	25	0	0	1.0	0.0	0	8%
(M&M Mars)										
'Skittles' original, bite size	1 cup	830	0	186	33	0	9.0	1.8	0	10%
'Skittles' original, bite size, 4-oz pkg	1 pkg	458	0	102	18	0	4.9	1.0	0	10%
'Skittles' original, bite size, 2.3-oz pkg.	1 pkg	263	0	59	10	0	2.8	0.6	0	10%
'Skittles' original, bite size, 2.17-oz pkg.	1 pkg	251	0	56	10	0	2.7	0.5	0	10%
'Skittles' original, bite size, 2-oz pkg	1 pkg	231	0	52	9	0	2.5	0.5	0	10%
'Skittles' original, bite size	10 pieces	43	0	10	2	0	0.5	0.1	0	10%
chews, 'Starburst'	1 piece	20	0	4	3	0	0.4	0.1	0	18%
chews, 'Starburst' 2.07-oz pkg.	1 pkg	234	0	50	33	0	4.9	0.7	0	18%
chews, 'Starburst' fun size	1 pkg	166	0	35	24	0	3.5	0.5	0	18%
(Rascals) chews, all flavors	1 piece	4	0	1	0	0	0.0	0.0	0	0%
(SweeTARTS) chewy	1 oz	113	0	25	0	0	1.0	0.0	0	8%
FUDGE										
(Kraft) 'Fudgies'	1 piece	35	0	6	25	0	1.0	0.0	0	27%
(Woodys)										
cheese, w/walnuts	1 oz	120	2	18	25	0	4.0	2.0	5	31%
chocolate, w/walnuts	1 oz	120	2	18	25	0	4.0	2.0	5	31%
maple walnut	1 oz	120	1	19	25	0	4.0	1.0	5	31%
mint, w/walnuts	1 oz	120	2	18	25	0	4.0	2.0	5	31%
GUM										
(Beech-Nut)										
candy-coated, 'Beechies'	1 piece	6	0	2	0	0	0.0	0.0	0	0%
cinnamon	1 piece	10	0	2	0	0	0.0	0.0	0	0%
fruit	1 piece	10	0	2	0	0	0.0	0.0	0	0%
peppermint	1 piece	10	0	2	0	0	0.0	0.0	0	0%
spearmint	1 piece	10	0	2	0	0	0.0	0.0	0	0%
(Brach's) balls, 'Gumdinger' all flavors,	1 oz	110	0	24	5	0	2.0	0.0	0	16%
(Bubble Yum)										
bananaberry split	1 piece	25	0	7	0	0	0.0	0.0	0	0%
checkermint	1 piece	25	0	7	0	0	0.0	0.0	0	0%
cherry	1 piece	25	0	7	0	0	0.0	0.0	0	0%
fruit	1 piece	25	0	7	0	0	0.0	0.0	0	0%
fruit, sugarless	1 piece	20	0	5	0	0	0.0	0.0	0	0%
grape	1 piece	25	0	7	0	0	0.0	0.0	0	0%
grape, sugarless	1 piece	20	0	5	0	0	0.0	0.0	0	0%
Hawaiian punch	1 piece	25	0	7	0	0	0.0	0.0	0	0%
lime, luscious	1 piece	25	0	7	0	0	0.0	0.0	0	0%
peppermint, sugarless	1 piece	20	0	5	0	0	0.0	0.0	0	0%
strawberry stripe	1 piece	25	0	7	0	0	0.0	0.0	0	0%
strawberry, sugarless	1 piece	20	0	5	0	0	0.0	0.0	0	0%
3-flavor, grape, cherry, and fruit	1 piece	25	0	7	0	0	0.0	0.0	0	0%

Food Name	Serving Size	Calories	Prot. gms	Carbs gms	Sod. mgs	Fiber gms	Fat gms	Sat. Fat gms	Chol. mgs	% Fat Cal.
watermelon, wet 'n wild	1 piece	25	0	7	0	0	0.0	0.0	0	0%
(Bubblicious)										
original	1 piece	25	0	6	0	0	0.0	0.0	0	0%
sugarless	1 piece	5	0	1	0	0	0.0	0.0	0	0%
(Care Free)										
bubble, fruit, sugarless	1 piece	10	0	2	0	0	0.0	0.0	0	0%
bubble, wild cherry, sugarless	1 piece	10	0	2	0	0	0.0	0.0	0	0%
bubble, wintergreen, sugarless	1 piece	10	0	2	0	0	0.0	0.0	0	0%
cinnamon, sugarless	1 piece	8	0	2	0	0	0.0	0.0	0	0%
peppermint, sugarless	1 piece	8	0	2	0	0	0.0	0.0	0	0%
spearmint, sugarless	1 piece	8	0	2	0	0	0.0	0.0	0	0%
(Chewels) all flavors	1 piece	8	0	2	0	0	0.0	0.0	0	0%
(Chiclets)										
	10 pieces	55	0	15	1	0	0.0	0.0	0	1%
candy-coated	1 piece	6	0	2	0	0	0.0	0.0	0	0%
candy-coated, 'Tiny'	1 pkg	8	0	0	0	0	0.0	0.0	0	0%
(Clorets) stick, all flavors	1 piece	9	0	2	0	0	0.0	0.0	0	0%
(Dentyne)										
all flavors	1 piece	6	0	2	0	0	0.0	0.0	0	0%
all flavors, sugarless	1 piece	5	0	1	0	0	0.0	0.0	0	0%
(Extra)										
bubble, classic	1 piece	6	0	0	0	0	0.0	0.0	0	0%
bubble, original	1 piece	7	0	0	0	0	0.0	0.0	0	0%
cinnamon	1 stick	8	0	0	0	0	0.0	0.0	0	0%
peppermint	1 stick	8	0	0	0	0	0.0	0.0	0	0%
spearmint	1 stick	8	0	0	0	0	0.0	0.0	0	0%
winter fresh	1 stick	8	0	0	0	0	0.0	0.0	0	0%
(Freedent)										
cinnamon	1 stick	10	0	2	0	0	0.0	0.0	0	0%
peppermint	1 stick	10	0	2	0	0	0.0	0.0	0	0%
spearmint	1 stick	10	0	2	0	0	0.0	0.0	0	0%
(Freshen-Up) all flavors	1 piece	13	0	3	0	0	0.0	0.0	0	0%
(Fruit Stripe)										
bubble, cherry	1 piece	8	0	2	0	0	0.0	0.0	0	0%
bubble, fruit	1 piece	8	0	2	0	0	0.0	0.0	0	0%
bubble, grape	1 piece	8	0	2	0	0	0.0	0.0	0	0%
bubble, lemon	1 piece	8	0	2	0	0	0.0	0.0	0	0%
cherry	1 piece	10	0	2	0	0	0.0	0.0	0	0%
lemon	1 piece	10	0	2	0	0	0.0	0.0	0	0%
lime	1 piece	10	0	2	0	0	0.0	0.0	0	0%
orange	1 piece	10	0	2	0	0	0.0	0.0	0	0%
(Hubba Bubba)										
all flavors except cola and grape	1 piece	23	0	6	0	0	0.0	0.0	0	0%
cola	1 piece	23	0	5	0	0	0.0	0.0	0	0%
grape, sugar-free	1 piece	13	0	0	0	0	0.0	0.0	0	0%
original, sugar-free	1 piece	14	0	0	0	0	0.0	0.0	0	0%
(Wrigley's)										
	1 serving	10	0	2	0	0	0.0	0.0	0	0%
'Big Red'	1 piece	10	0	2	0	0	0.0	0.0	0	0%
'Doublemint'	1 piece	10	0	2	0	0	0.0	0.0	0	0%
'Juicy Fruit'	1 piece	10	0	2	0	0	0.0	0.0	0	0%
'Spearmint'	1 piece	10	0	2	0	0	0.0	0.0	0	0%
GUMDROP										
1-inch diam	1 gumdrop	45	0	11	5	0	0.0	0.0	0	0%

Food Name	Serving Size	Calories	Prot. gms	Carbs gms	Sod. mgs	Fiber gms	Fat gms	Sat. Fat gms	Chol. mgs	% Fat Cal.
3/4-inch diam.	1 gumdrop	16	0	4	2	0	0.0	0.0	0	0%
(Estee)	4 pieces	25	0	6	0	0	0.0	0.0	0	0%
HARD CANDY										
(Brach's)										
butterscotch, 'Disks'	1 oz	110	0	27	220	0	0.0	0.0	0	0%
cinnamon, 'Disks'	1 oz	110	0	27	15	0	0.0	0.0	0	0%
cinnamon, 'Imperials'	1 oz	110	0	27	5	0	0.0	0.0	0	0%
'Cut Rock'	1 oz	110	0	27	10	0	0.0	0.0	0	0%
filled, assorted	1 oz	110	0	27	15	0	0.0	0.0	0	0%
lemon drops	1 oz	110	0	27	5	0	0.0	0.0	0	0%
raspberry filled	1 oz	110	0	27	15	0	0.0	0.0	0	0%
ribbon, crimp	1 oz	110	0	27	15	0	0.0	0.0	0	0%
'Royals'	1 oz	100	1	20	60	0	2.0	0.0	0	18%
'Spicettes'	1 oz	100	0	26	15	0	0.0	0.0	0	0%
sour balls	1 oz	110	0	27	15	0	0.0	0.0	0	0%
(Breath Savers)										
mint-cinnamon	1 piece	8	0	2	0	0	0.0	0.0	0	0%
mint-cinnamon, cores	1 piece	2	0	1	0	0	0.0	0.0	0	0%
peppermint	1 piece	8	0	2	0	0	0.0	0.0	0	0%
peppermint, cores	1 piece	2	0	1	0	0	0.0	0.0	0	0%
spearmint	1 piece	8	0	2	0	0	0.0	0.0	0	0%
spearmint, cores	1 piece	2	0	1	0	0	0.0	0.0	0	0%
wintergreen	1 piece	8	0	2	0	0	0.0	0.0	0	0%
wintergreen, cores	1 piece	2	0	1	0	0	0.0	0.0	0	0%
(Callard and Bowser) butterscotch	1 oz	115	0	25	0	0	1.9	0.0	0	15%
(Ce De) 'Smarties'	1 roll	25	0	6	0	0	0.0	0.0	0	0%
(Certs)										
mini, sugar-free	1 piece	1	0	0	0	0	0.0	0.0	0	0%
mints, sugar-free	1 piece	6	0	2	0	0	0.0	0.0	0	0%
(Clorets)										
clear mint	1 piece	8	0	2	0	0	0.0	0.0	0	0%
pressed mints	1 piece	6	0	2	0	0	0.0	0.0	0	0%
(Estee)	2 pieces	25	0	6	0	0	0.0	0.0	0	0%
(Featherweight)										
butterscotch	1 piece	25	0	6	25	0	0.0	0.0	0	0%
tropical blend, 'Sweet Pretenders'	1 piece	12	0	3	0	0	0.0	0.0	0	0%
(Fruit Juicers)										
mixed berries	1 piece	8	0	2	0	0	0.0	0.0	0	0%
citrus fruits	1 piece	8	0	2	0	0	0.0	0.0	0	0%
fruit punch	1 piece	8	0	2	0	0	0.0	0.0	0	0%
grape	1 piece	8	0	2	0	0	0.0	0.0	0	0%
strawberry	1 piece	8	0	2	0	0	0.0	0.0	0	0%
(Glenny's)										
fruit	1 piece	19	1	4	1	0	1.0	0.0	0	31%
peppermint	1 piece	19	1	4	1	0	1.0	0.0	0	31%
(Jolly Joes)	1 piece	9	0	2	1	0	0.0	0.0	0	0%
(Jolly Rancher)										
apple	1 piece	23	0	6	5	0	0.0	0.0	0	0%
butterscotch	1 piece	25	0	6	37	0	1.0	0.0	0	27%
cherry	1 piece	23	0	6	3	0	0.0	0.0	0	0%
fire cinnamon	1 piece	23	0	6	5	0	0.0	0.0	0	0%
fruit punch	1 piece	23	0	6	5	0	0.0	0.0	0	0%
grape	1 piece	23	0	6	5	0	0.0	0.0	0	0%
lemon	1 piece	23	0	6	5	0	0.0	0.0	0	0%

Food Name	Serving Size	Calories	Prot. gms	Carbs gms	Sod. mgs	Fiber gms	Fat gms	Sat. Fat gms	Chol. mgs	% Fat Cal.
orange	1 piece	23	0	6	4	0	0.0	0.0	0	0%
peach	1 piece	23	0	6	3	0	0.0	0.0	0	0%
peppermint	1 piece	23	0	6	3	0	0.0	0.0	0	0%
pink lemonade	1 piece	23	0	6	5	0	0.0	0.0	0	0%
raspberry	1 piece	23	0	6	5	0	0.0	0.0	0	0%
strawberry	1 piece	23	0	6	3	0	0.0	0.0	0	0%
watermelon	1 piece	23	0	6	5	0	0.0	0.0	0	0%
(Jurassic Park)										
jawbreakers, tropical flavors										
jawbreakers, wild cherry, 'Raptor Bites'	13 pieces	60	0	15	0	0	0.0	0.0	0	0%
(Life Savers)										
butter creme mint	1 piece	8	0	2	5	0	0.0	0.0	0	0%
butter rum	1 piece	8	0	2	10	0	0.0	0.0	0	0%
butter rum, 'Holes'	1 piece	2	0	1	0	0	0.0	0.0	0	0%
butterscotch	1 piece	8	0	2	10	0	0.0	0.0	0	0%
'Cin-O-Mon'	1 piece	8	0	2	0	0	0.0	0.0	0	0%
'Cryst-O-Mint'	1 piece	8	0	2	0	0	0.0	0.0	0	0%
fancy fruits	1 piece	8	0	2	0	0	0.0	0.0	0	0%
five flavor	1 piece	8	0	2	0	0	0.0	0.0	0	0%
five flavor, 'Holes'	1 piece	2	0	1	0	0	0.0	0.0	0	0%
'Pep-O-Mint'	1 piece	8	0	2	0	0	0.0	0.0	0	0%
'Pep-O-Mint,' 'Holes'	1 piece	2	0	1	0	0	0.0	0.0	0	0%
root beer flavor	1 piece	8	0	2	0	0	0.0	0.0	0	0%
'Spear-O-Mint'	1 piece	8	0	2	0	0	0.0	0.0	0	0%
sunshine fruits	1 piece	8	0	2	0	0	0.0	0.0	0	0%
sunshine fruits, 'Holes'	1 piece	2	0	1	0	0	0.0	0.0	0	0%
tangerine, 'Holes'	1 piece	2	0	1	0	0	0.0	0.0	0	0%
tropical fruits	1 piece	8	0	2	0	0	0.0	0.0	0	0%
wild cherry	1 piece	8	0	2	0	0	0.0	0.0	0	0%
'Wint-O-Green'	1 piece	8	0	2	0	0	0.0	0.0	0	0%
'Wint-O-Green,' 'Holes'	1 piece	2	0	1	0	0	0.0	0.0	0	0%
(Mike and Ike)	1 piece	9	0	2	1	0	0.0	0.0	0	0%
(Russell Stover) mixed, sugar-free	3 pieces	70	0	18	5	0	0.0	0.0	0	0%
'Spitters'	13 pieces	60	0	15	0	0	0.0	0.0	0	0%
(Spree) fruit	1 oz	110	0	26	0	0	0.0	0.0	0	0%
(SweeTARTS) fruit	1 oz	110	0	26	0	0	0.0	0.0	0	0%
(Sunmark) jawbreakers, 'Willy Wonka's Everlasting Gobstoppers'	6 pieces	59	0	15	1	na	0.0	na	na	0%
HOLIDAY										
(Brach's) holiday mints	1 oz	110	0	26	0	0	1.0	0.0	0	8%
Christmas										
(Brach's)										
bell, chocolate, in foil	1 oz	150	2	17	25	0	8.0	0.0	0	49%
candy cane	1 oz	110	0	27	10	0	0.0	0.0	0	0%
chocolate, assorted	1 oz	110	0	23	25	0	2.0	0.0	0	16%
jellies	1 oz	100	0	24	10	0	0.0	0.0	0	0%
jellies, snowbase	1 oz	100	0	24	5	0	0.0	0.0	0	0%
'Jots'	1 oz	130	1	21	30	0	5.0	0.0	0	34%
mint 'Pearls'	1 oz	110	0	25	5	0	1.0	0.0	0	8%
mint 'Starlight'	1 oz	110	0	27	15	0	0.0	0.0	0	0%
nougat	1 oz	110	0	24	20	0	2.0	0.0	0	16%
ornaments	1 oz	150	2	17	50	0	8.0	0.0	0	49%
'Perkys'	1 oz	90	0	23	20	0	0.0	0.0	0	0%
Santa, chocolate, in foil	1 oz	140	2	18	40	0	7.0	0.0	0	44%

Food Name	Serving Size	Calories	Prot. gms	Carbs gms	Sod. mgs	Fiber gms	Fat gms	Sat. Fat gms	Chol. mgs	% Fat Cal.
Santa, marshmallow	1 oz	120	1	23	35	0	3.0	0.0	0	22%
(Just Born)										
snowman, marshmallow, large	1 piece	111	1	27	8	0	0.1	0.0	0	1%
snowman, marshmallow, small	1 piece	37	0	9	3	0	0.1	0.0	0	2%
tree, marshmallow, large	1 piece	111	1	27	8	0	0.1	0.0	0	1%
tree, marshmallow, small	1 piece	37	0	9	3	0	0.1	0.0	0	2%
(Spangler) candy cane	1 piece	60	1	14	0	0	1.0	0.0	0	13%
Easter										
(Brach's)										
assorted, 'Chicks and Rabbits'	1 oz	100	0	26	10	0	0.0	0.0	0	0%
assorted, 'Easter Fun'	1 oz	100	0	26	10	0	0.0	0.0	0	0%
corn	1 oz	100	0	26	66	0	0.0	0.0	0	0%
eggs, 'Hide'n Seek'	1 oz	110	0	27	5	0	0.0	0.0	0	0%
eggs, chocolate malted milk	1 oz	130	1	21	40	0	5.0	0.0	0	34%
eggs, chocolate, in foil	1 oz	150	2	17	25	0	8.0	0.0	0	49%
eggs, creme, chocolate coated buttercream	1 oz	120	1	22	50	0	3.0	0.0	0	23%
eggs, creme, chocolate coated cherry	1 oz	110	1	23	20	0	2.0	0.0	0	16%
eggs, creme, chocolate coated coconut	1 oz	110	0	22	40	0	3.0	0.0	0	23%
eggs, creme, chocolate coated fruit and nut	1 oz	110	0	23	35	0	2.0	0.0	0	16%
eggs, creme, chocolate coated maple	1 oz	110	0	23	30	0	2.0	0.0	0	16%
eggs, creme, chocolate coated vanilla	1 oz	110	0	23	25	0	2.0	0.0	0	16%
eggs, jelly	1 oz	100	0	24	15	0	0.0	0.0	0	0%
eggs, jelly, 'Tiny'	1 oz	100	0	26	10	0	0.0	0.0	0	0%
eggs, jelly, speckled	1 oz	110	0	27	40	0	0.0	0.0	0	0%
eggs, jelly, spiced	1 oz	90	0	22	10	0	0.0	0.0	0	0%
eggs, marshmallow	1 oz	100	0	25	5	0	0.0	0.0	0	0%
eggs, pastel 'Fiesta'	1 oz	120	1	23	25	0	3.0	0.0	0	22%
lollipop, pastels, 'Easter'	1 lollipop	40	0	10	0	0	0.0	0.0	0	0%
mint, 'Starlight'	1 oz	110	0	27	15	0	0.0	0.0	0	0%
nougats	1 oz	100	0	24	25	0	1.0	0.0	0	9%
rabbits, jel, 'Jube'	1 oz	100	0	24	15	0	0.0	0.0	0	0%
rabbits, marshmallow	1 oz	120	1	22	55	0	3.0	0.0	0	23%
'Robin's Eggs'	1 oz	140	1	20	30	0	6.0	0.0	0	39%
(Cadbury)										
eggs, creme	1.37 oz	190	2	26	0	0	8.0	0.0	0	39%
eggs, creme, mini	1 oz	140	2	20	0	0	7.0	0.0	0	42%
(Just Born) peeps, marshmallow	1 piece	27	0	7	2	0	0.1	0.0	0	3%
Halloween										
(Brach's)										
corn, Indian	1 oz	100	0	26	75	0	0.0	0.0	0	0%
corn, three color	1 oz	100	0	26	95	0	0.0	0.0	0	0%
jelly beans	1 oz	100	0	26	15	0	0.0	0.0	0	0%
lollipops 'Picture Pops'	1 oz	110	0	27	10	0	0.0	0.0	0	0%
'Mellowcremes'	1 oz	100	0	26	40	0	0.0	0.0	0	0%
pumpkin heads, crazy	1 oz	100	0	24	15	0	1.0	0.0	0	9%
pumpkins	1 oz	100	0	26	65	0	0.0	0.0	0	0%
'Scary Cats'	1 oz	100	0	26	85	0	0.0	0.0	0	0%
'Trick or Treat Party Pack'	1 oz	110	0	27	20	0	0.0	0.0	0	0%
witches' teeth	1 oz	100	0	26	75	0	0.0	0.0	0	0%
(Just Born)										
cats, marshmallow	1 piece	28	0	7	2	0	0.1	0.0	0	3%
pumpkins, marshmallow, large	1 piece	111	1	27	8	0	0.1	0.0	0	1%
pumpkins, marshmallow, small	1 piece	14	0	3	1	0	0.1	0.0	0	6%

Food Name	Serving Size	Calories	Prot. gms	Carbs gms	Sod. mgs	Fiber gms	Fat gms	Sat. Fat gms	Chol. mgs	% Fat Cal.
Valentine's Day										
(Brach's)										
chocolate, 'I Luv U'	1 oz	150	2	17	25	0	8.0	0.0	0	49%
'Heart Box' 1/2-lb box	1 oz	110	1	23	35	0	2.0	0.0	0	16%
hearts	1 oz	110	1	23	30	0	2.0	0.0	0	16%
hearts, cherry jel 'Jube'	1 oz	100	0	26	20	0	0.0	0.0	0	0%
hearts, cinnamon 'Imperial'	1 oz	110	0	27	5	0	0.0	0.0	0	0%
hearts, 'Conversation' large	1 oz	110	0	27	5	0	0.0	0.0	0	0%
hearts, 'Conversation' small	1 oz	110	0	27	0	0	0.0	0.0	0	0%
hearts, fruity	1 oz	100	0	24	5	0	0.0	0.0	0	0%
hearts, jelly, red	1 oz	100	0	24	10	0	0.0	0.0	0	0%
hearts, 'Sassy Hearts'	1 oz	100	0	25	0	0	0.0	0.0	0	0%
kisses, nougat	1 oz	110	0	24	15	0	2.0	0.0	0	16%
'Love'	1 oz	150	2	17	25	0	8.0	0.0	0	49%
'Mellowcremes'	1 oz	100	0	26	75	0	0.0	0.0	0	0%
'Valentine Heart' 1/3-lb box	1 oz	110	1	23	25	0	2.0	0.0	0	16%
'Valentine Heart' 1-lb box	1 oz	110	1	23	30	0	2.0	0.0	0	16%
JELLIED AND GUMMED										
jellybeans, large	10 pieces	104	0	26	7	0	0.1	0.0	0	1%
jellybeans, small	10 pieces	40	0	10	3	0	0.1	0.0	0	1%
(Brach's)										
cinnamon bears	1 oz	80	0	21	10	0	0.0	0.0	0	0%
'Fruit Bunch'	1 oz	100	0	24	10	0	0.0	0.0	0	0%
gummi bears	1 oz	100	2	22	15	0	0.0	0.0	0	0%
gummi worms	1 oz	100	2	22	15	0	0.0	0.0	0	0%
jelly beans	1 oz	100	0	26	5	0	0.0	0.0	0	0%
jelly nougat	1 oz	100	0	24	35	0	1.0	0.0	0	9%
'Jels' sour cherry	1 oz	100	0	26	10	0	0.0	0.0	0	0%
'Jube'	1 oz	100	0	24	10	0	0.0	0.0	0	0%
jube jels	1 oz	100	0	24	10	0	0.0	0.0	0	0%
mint, assorted	1 oz	100	0	26	0	0	0.0	0.0	0	0%
'Rainbow Bears'	1 oz	100	0	24	10	0	0.0	0.0	0	0%
'Spearmint Leaves'	1 oz	100	0	24	5	0	0.0	0.0	0	0%
spicettes	1 oz	100	0	26	15	0	0.0	0.0	0	0%
(Callard and Bowser) juicy	1 oz	90	0	23	0	0	0.0	0.0	0	0%
(Estee)										
gummi bears	4 pieces	20	1	4	0	0	0.0	0.0	0	0%
ring, 1.25-inch diam.	1 piece	39	0	10	4	0	0.0	0.0	0	0%
(Hershey's)										
gummi bears, 'Amazin Fruit' 12 pieces	1 oz	90	2	21	20	0	1.0	0.0	0	9%
gummi bears, tropical, 'Amazin Fruit'	1 oz	90	2	21	20	0	1.0	0.0	0	9%
(Hot Tamales) cinnamon, hot	1 piece	9	0	2	1	0	0.0	0.0	0	0%
(Jurassic Park) gummi dinosaurs, tropical	15 pieces	140	3	31	0	0	0.0	0.0	0	0%
(Just Born)										
eggs, 'Petite'	1 piece	4	0	1	1	0	0.0	0.0	0	0%
'Teenee Beanee Gourmet'	1 piece	4	0	1	1	0	0.0	0.0	0	0%
(Life Savers) 'Gummi Savers'	1 piece	12	0	3	0	0	0.0	0.0	0	0%
(Rodda) eggs	1 piece	7	0	2	1	0	0.0	0.0	0	0%
LEMON *(Russell Stover)* squares	1.4 oz	160	1	27	35	2	5.5	4.5	0	31%
LICORICE										
(Brach's)										
'Red Laces'	1 oz	100	2	22	10	0	0.0	0.0	0	0%
'Twin Twists'	1 oz	100	2	22	10	0	0.0	0.0	0	0%
'Twists'	1 oz	100	2	22	50	0	1.0	0.0	0	9%

Food Name	Serving Size	Calories	Prot. gms	Carbs gms	Sod. mgs	Fiber gms	Fat gms	Sat. Fat gms	Chol. mgs	% Fat Cal.
(Good and Fruity) candy-coated	1 oz	106	1	26	8	0	0.1	0.0	0	1%
(Hershey's)										
cherry bits, 'Twizzlers'	5 oz pkg	474	5	110	351	2	2.3	0.6	0	4%
cherry bits, 'Twizzlers' 4-oz bag	22 pieces	139	1	31	85	1	1.0	0.2	0	6%
strawberry bits, 'Twizzlers' 2.5-oz pkg	1 pkg	237	2	55	175	1	1.1	0.3	0	4%
LOLLIPOP										
(Brach's) all flavors, 'Pops'	1 oz	110	0	27	10	0	0.0	0.0	0	0%
(Estee) all flavors	1 lollipop	30	0	7	0	0	0.0	0.0	0	0%
(Fruit Juicers)										
black raspberry	1 lollipop	40	0	10	0	0	0.0	0.0	0	0%
fruit punch	1 lollipop	40	0	10	0	0	0.0	0.0	0	0%
pineapple	1 lollipop	40	0	10	0	0	0.0	0.0	0	0%
strawberry	1 lollipop	40	0	10	0	0	0.0	0.0	0	0%
(Glenny's)										
fruit	1 lollipop	21	1	5	1	0	1.0	0.0	0	27%
Vit-C	1 lollipop	35	1	8	1	0	1.0	0.0	0	20%
(Life Savers)										
assorted	1 lollipop	45	0	11	10	0	0.0	0.0	0	0%
swirled	1 lollipop	45	0	11	10	0	0.0	0.0	0	0%
(Sorbee) assorted fruit flavors	1 lollipop	22	0	5	0	0	0.0	0.0	0	0%
(Spangler)										
all flavors, 'Dum Dums'	1 lollipop	25	1	6	0	0	1.0	0.0	0	24%
all flavors, 'Saf-T-Pops'	1 lollipop	45	1	11	0	0	1.0	0.0	0	16%
bubble gum center, all flavors	1 lollipop	57	1	14	5	0	1.0	0.0	0	13%
(Tootsie Pop)										
all flavors except chocolate	1 oz	111	0	26	1	0	0.6	0.1	0	5%
chocolate	1 oz	110	0	26	2	0	0.6	0.2	0	5%
MARSHMALLOW										
(Boyer) 'Mallow Cup'	2 pieces	224	2	30	0	0	11.0	0.0	0	44%
(Brach's) 'Perkys Circus Peanuts'	1 oz	100	0	26	10	0	0.0	0.0	0	0%
(Campfire) large	2 pieces	40	0	10	10	0	0.0	0.0	0	0%
(FunMallows)										
	1 piece	30	0	7	15	0	0.0	0.0	0	0%
miniature	10 pieces	18	0	5	5	0	0.0	0.0	0	0%
(Just Born) coconut, toasted	1 piece	30	0	6	6	1	0.6	0.0	0	17%
(Spangler) 'Circus Peanuts'	4 pieces	110	1	26	5	0	1.0	0.0	0	8%
MINT										
(Andes) chocolate mint thins, 'Creme de Menthe'	6 pieces	150	2	16	20	0	9.0	0.0	0	53%
(Barat)										
chocolate tofu, 'Bits'	0.75 oz	120	2	11	15	0	8.0	0.0	0	58%
chocolate tofu, after dinner	1 piece	40	1	4	0	0	2.0	0.0	0	47%
(Brach's)										
'Kentucky Mints'	1 oz	110	0	27	0	0	0.0	0.0	0	0%
chocolate covered, thin	1 oz	110	0	24	10	0	2.0	0.0	0	16%
'Coolers/Starlight'	1 oz	110	0	27	15	0	0.0	0.0	0	0%
creme, chocolate covered, regular	1 oz	110	0	24	10	0	2.0	0.0	0	16%
'Creme de Menthe'	1 oz	150	2	16	20	0	9.0	0.0	0	53%
'Dessert Mints' assorted	1 oz	110	0	27	0	0	0.0	0.0	0	0%
'Jots/Pearls'	1 oz	120	0	25	10	0	2.0	0.0	0	15%
parfait	1 oz	150	2	16	35	0	9.0	0.0	0	53%
peppermint, 'Star Brites'	3 pieces	59	0	15	6	na	0.0	na	na	0%
peppermint kisses	1 oz	100	0	24	25	0	1.0	0.0	0	9%
straws, filled	1 oz	110	0	26	10	0	1.0	0.0	0	8%

Food Name	Serving Size	Calories	Prot. gms	Carbs gms	Sod. mgs	Fiber gms	Fat gms	Sat. Fat gms	Chol. mgs	% Fat Cal.
(Featherweight)										
'Cool Blue'	1 piece	25	0	6	0	0	0.0	0.0	0	0%
peppermint swirls	1 piece	20	0	5	0	0	0.0	0.0	0	0%
(Glenny's) gentle, 'Drops'	1 piece	6	1	1	1	0	1.0	0.0	0	53%
(Hershey's)										
'Peppermnt Pattie' large, 1.5 oz.	1 piece	165	1	34	10	1	3.0	1.8	0	16%
'Peppermint Pattie' 0.6 oz	1 patty	67	0	14	4	0	1.2	0.7	0	16%
'Peppermint Pattie' 0.5 oz	1 patty	55	0	11	3	0	1.0	0.6	0	16%
(Kraft)										
butter	1 piece	8	0	2	0	0	0.0	0.0	0	0%
party	1 piece	8	0	2	0	0	0.0	0.0	0	0%
(Mint) 'Meltaway'	1 piece	50	0	5	10	0	3.0	0.0	0	57%
(Nestlé)										
'After Eight'	5 pieces	147	1	31	5	1	5.6	3.4	0	32%
'After Eight'	1 piece	29	0	6	1	0	1.1	0.7	0	32%
(Rowntree) dark chocolate, wafer thin, 'After Eight'	1 piece	35	0	6	0	0	1.0	0.0	0	27%
(Russell Stover) squares	1.4 oz	160	1	28	35	1	5.0	4.0	0	28%
(Saco Foods) 'Mint'Oh's'	1.5 oz	111	1	14	14	0	6.6	2.4	0	50%
(Spangler) dark chocolate coated	1 piece	80	1	14	25	0	2.0	0.0	0	23%
(Velamints)										
all flavors except cocoamint	1 piece	7	0	2	0	0	0.0	0.0	0	0%
cocoamint	1 piece	7	5	2	0	0	0.3	0.0	0	10%
NONPAREILS										
(Brach's) dark chocolate	1 oz	140	1	20	20	0	6.0	0.0	0	39%
(Nestlé) 'Sno-Caps'	1 oz	140	1	21	0	0	6.0	0.0	0	38%
ORANGE										
(Brach's)										
'Orangettes'	1 oz	100	0	24	20	0	0.0	0.0	0	0%
sticks, chocolate coated	1 oz	110	1	23	25	0	2.0	0.0	0	16%
PEANUT										
(Barat) chocolate tofu, dipped, 'Bits'	1 oz	120	4	8	15	0	8.0	0.0	0	60%
(Brach's)										
caramel cluster	1 oz	150	4	15	50	0	8.0	0.0	0	49%
chocolate covered 'Small'	1 oz	140	4	15	40	0	7.0	0.0	0	45%
filled	1 oz	110	1	25	20	0	1.0	0.0	0	8%
French, burnt	1 oz	130	4	18	5	0	5.0	0.0	0	34%
'Jots'	1 oz	140	3	18	25	0	6.0	0.0	0	39%
milk chocolate coated	1 oz	150	3	15	30	0	9.0	0.0	0	53%
milk chocolate, 'Peanut Clusters'	1 oz	150	3	15	25	0	9.0	0.0	0	53%
'Nut Goodies'	1 oz	130	2	21	10	0	4.0	0.0	0	28%
parfait	1 oz	160	3	14	60	0	10.0	0.0	0	57%
(Cocofection) enrobed in chocolate	1 oz	140	5	10	12	0	12.0	0.0	0	64%
(Estee)										
candy-coated	10 pieces	70	2	8	10	0	4.0	1.0	0	47%
chocolate-covered	2 squares	60	1	5	10	0	4.5	2.0	2	65%
(M&M Mars)										
chocolate, candy-coated, 'M&Ms'	1 cup	877	16	103	82	6	44.6	17.6	15	46%
chocolate, candy-coated, 'M&Ms' 1.74-oz pkg	1 pkg	253	5	30	24	2	12.9	5.1	4	46%
chocolate, candy-coated, 'M&Ms' 1.67-oz pkg	1 pkg	243	4	28	23	2	12.3	4.9	4	46%
chocolate, candy-coated, 'M&Ms' fun size pkg	1 pkg	108	2	13	10	1	5.5	2.2	2	46%
chocolate, candy-coated, 'M&Ms'	10 pieces	103	2	12	10	1	5.2	2.1	2	46%
(Nabisco) chocolate covered, approx 14 pieces	1 oz	160	4	14	15	0	9.0	0.0	0	53%
(Nestlé)										
chocolate-covered, 'Goobers' 7-oz pkg	1 pkg	1016	27	96	81	12	66.3	24.2	18	56%

Food Name	Serving Size	Calories	Prot. gms	Carbs gms	Sod. mgs	Fiber gms	Fat gms	Sat. Fat gms	Chol. mgs	% Fat Cal.
chocolate-covered, 'Goobers'	1/4 cup	210	6	20	17	3	13.7	5.0	4	56%
chocolate-covered, 'Goobers' 1.375-oz pkg	1 pkg	200	5	19	16	2	13.1	4.8	4	56%
chocolate-covered, 'Goobers'	10 pieces	51	1	5	4	1	3.4	1.2	1	56%
(Russell Stover) 'Peanut Delights'	1.4 oz	210	4	22	130	1	12.0	5.0	10	51%
PEANUT BRITTLE										
(Estee)	0.5 oz	60	1	10	20	0	2.0	1.0	0	29%
(Kraft)	1 oz	130	3	20	135	0	5.0	1.0	0	33%
(Sophie Mae)	1.4 oz	170	4	30	130	1	5.0	1.0	0	25%
PEANUT BUTTER										
(Boyer)										
cup	1.6 oz	250	5	23	0	0	15.0	0.0	0	55%
cup, 0.5 oz.	1 piece	75	3	12	0	0	7.5	0.0	0	54%
(Brach's) kisses	1 oz	110	1	22	135	0	2.0	0.0	0	16%
(Estee) cup	1 piece	40	1	3	20	0	3.0	2.5	1	63%
(Hershey's)										
'Reese's Crunchy Peanut Butter Cup'	1.8 oz	280	7	24	130	0	18.0	0.0	5	57%
'Reese's Peanut Butter Cup' individual, 0.6 oz	1 piece	92	2	9	54	1	5.3	1.9	1	52%
'Reese's Peanut Butter Cup' miniature	5 pieces	211	4	21	124	1	12.2	4.3	2	52%
'Reese's Peanut Butter Cup' miniature	1 piece	38	1	4	22	0	2.2	0.8	0	52%
'Reese's Peanut Butter Cup' 2-pack, 1.6 oz	1 pkg	243	5	25	143	1	14.1	5.0	2	52%
'Reese's Pieces'	1/4 cup	231	6	29	69	1	9.9	8.5	1	39%
'Reese's Pieces'	1.6-oz pkg	226	6	28	68	1	9.7	8.3	1	39%
'Reese's Pieces'	50 pieces	191	5	24	57	1	8.2	7.1	1	39%
'Reese's Pieces'	10 pieces	39	1	5	12	0	1.7	1.4	0	39%
(M&M Mars)										
chocolate-covered, 'Kudos'	1.3 oz	200	4	19	80	0	12.0	0.0	0	54%
chocolate-covered cookie, 'PB Max'	1 piece	240	5	20	150	0	15.0	0.0	0	57%
PECAN										
(Russell Stover)										
'Pecan Crowns'	1.4 oz	200	2	19	60	1	13.0	4.0	5	58%
'Pecan Delights'	1.4 oz	220	2	19	55	1	14.5	5.5	5	61%
(Demet's)										
turtles	6-oz pkg	825	11	99	160	4	47.3	18.4	37	49%
turtles	1 piece	82	1	10	16	0	4.7	1.8	4	49%
POWDER CANDY										
(Lik-m-aid Fun Dip)	1 oz	110	0	26	0	0	0.0	0.0	0	0%
(Pixy Stix)	1 oz	100	0	26	0	0	0.0	0.0	0	0%
RAISIN										
(Barat) chocolate tofu, 'Bits'	1 oz	120	1	14	10	0	7.0	0.0	0	51%
(Brach's) chocolate-coated	1 oz	130	1	20	30	0	5.0	0.0	0	35%
(Cocofection) enrobed in chocolate	1 oz	120	1	20	14	0	5.0	0.0	0	35%
(Estee) chocolate-coated	8 pieces	30	1	5	5	0	1.0	1.0	0	27%
(Fruit Source) yogurt-coated, made w/real fruit juice	9 pieces	170	3	27	35	1	7.0	5.0	0	34%
(Harmony) chocolate-coated	44 pieces	160	2	29	15	1	5.0	2.5	5	27%
(Nabisco) chocolate-coated, approx 29 pieces	1 oz	130	1	21	15	0	5.0	0.0	1	34%
(Nestlé)										
chocolate-covered, 'Raisinets'	1.58-oz pkg	185	2	32	16	2	7.2	3.3	2	34%
chocolate-covered, 'Raisinets'	10 pieces	41	0	7	4	1	1.6	0.7	0	34%
TAFFY										
(Brach's)										
(Beich's)										
all flavors, 'Salt Water Taffy'	1 oz	100	0	24	30	0	1.0	0.0	0	9%
apple flavor chews, 'Laffy Taffy'	2 pieces	110	0	26	55	0	1.0	0.0	0	8%
banana flavor chews, 'Laffy Taffy'	2 pieces	120	0	26	55	0	1.0	0.0	0	8%

Food Name	Serving Size	Calories	Prot. gms	Carbs gms	Sod. mgs	Fiber gms	Fat gms	Sat. Fat gms	Chol. mgs	% Fat Cal.
cherry flavor chews, 'Laffy Taffy'	2 pieces	110	0	26	55	0	1.0	0.0	0	8%
grape flavor chews, 'Laffy Taffy'	2 pieces	110	0	26	60	0	1.0	0.0	0	8%
passion punch flavor, 'Laffy Taffy'	2 pieces	120	0	26	50	0	1.0	0.0	0	8%
strawberry flavor chews, 'Laffy Taffy'	2 pieces	110	0	26	55	0	1.0	0.0	0	8%
watermelon flavor chews, 'Laffy Taffy'	2 pieces	110	0	26	55	0	1.0	0.0	0	8%
TOFFEE										
(Brach's)	1 oz	110	1	23	80	0	2.0	0.0	0	16%
(Callard and Bowser)	1 oz	135	1	19	0	0	6.5	0.0	0	43%
(Flavor House) peanut butter	1 oz	150	4	17	90	0	7.0	0.0	0	43%
(Heath)										
'Bits O'Brickle'	3 oz	448	1	50	472	0	28.0	0.0	0	55%
English, 'Bits O'Heath'	3.5 oz	520	3	62	390	0	31.0	0.0	0	52%
English, 'Heath Bar'	2 pieces	180	1	20	130	0	11.0	0.0	0	54%
CANDY COATING										
bars, butterscotch, confectioner's coating	1 oz	153	1	19	25	0	8.2	6.8	0	49%
bars, white, confectioner's coating	3 oz	458	5	50	77	0	27.3	16.5	18	52%
chips, butterscotch, confectioner's coating	1 cup	916	4	114	151	0	49.4	41.0	0	49%
chip, white, confectioner's coating	1 cup	916	10	101	153	0	54.6	33.0	36	52%
CANNELLINI BEAN. See BEAN, CANNELLINI.										
CANOLA OIL										
	1 cup	1927	0	0	0	0	218.0	15.5	0	100%
	1 tbsp	124	0	0	0	0	14.0	1.0	0	100%
(Hain)	1 tbsp	120	0	0	0	0	14.0	1.0	0	100%
(Kroger)	1 tbsp	122	0	0	0	0	13.6	1.0	0	100%
(Smart Beat)	1 tbsp	117	0	0	0	0	13.6	1.0	0	100%
(Wesson)	1 tbsp	122	0	0	0	0	13.6	1.0	0	100%
(Westbrae Naturals)	1 tbsp	100	0	0	90	0	11.0	0.5	5	100%
cholesterol-free, no sodium (Country Pure)	1 tbsp	120	0	0	0	0	14.0	0.0	0	100%
'Food Service' (Wesson)	1 tbsp	122	0	0	0	0	13.6	1.0	0	100%
'Heart Beat' (Nucoa)	1 tbsp	120	0	0	0	0	14.0	1.0	0	100%
100% pure pressed (Loriva')	1 tbsp	120	0	0	0	0	14.0	1.0	0	100%
pure pressed, organic, lowest in saturated fat (Spectrum Naturals)	1 tbsp	120	0	0	0	0	14.0	1.0	0	100%
CANTALOUPE. See MELON, CANTALOUPE.										
CAPERS										
canned, drained	1 tbsp	2	0	0	255	0	0.1	0.0	0	31%
canned, drained (Progresso)	1 tsp	0	0	0	105	0	0.0	0.0	0	0%
canned, non-pareilles (Reese)	1 tsp	0	0	0	105	0	0.0	0.0	0	0%
CAPPUCCINO. See under COFFEE, FLAVORED.										
CARAMBOLA. See STAR FRUIT.										
CARAMEL. See under CANDY.										
CARAMEL TOPPING										
(Kraft)	2 tbsp	120	2	28	90	0	0.0	0.0	0	0%
(Mrs. Richardson's)										
	2 tbsp	130	1	28	90	0	2.0	0.0	5	13%
nonfat	2 tbsp	130	1	31	55	0	0.0	0.0	0	0%
(Smucker's)										
hot	2 tbsp	150	1	28	75	0	4.0	0.0	0	24%
'Special Recipe'	2 tbsp	160	1	33	40	0	3.0	0.0	0	17%
CARAWAY SEED										
	1 tbsp	22	1	3	1	3	1.0	0.0	0	37%
	1 tsp	7	0	1	0	1	0.3	0.0	0	37%
(Spice Islands)	1 tsp	8	0	1	1	0	0.4	0.0	0	43%
(Tone's)	1 tsp	7	0	1	1	1	0.3	0.1	0	31%

Food Name	Serving Size	Calories	Prot. gms	Carbs gms	Sod. mgs	Fiber gms	Fat gms	Sat. Fat gms	Chol. mgs	% Fat Cal.
dried *(McCormick/Schilling)*	1 tsp	14	1	1	0	1	0.8	0.0	0	47%
whole seeds *(Durkee)*	1 tsp	9	0	0	0	0	0.0	0.0	0	0%
whole seeds *(Laurel Leaf)* whole seeds	1 tsp	9	0	0	0	0	0.0	0.0	0	0%
CARDAMOM										
ground	1 tbsp	18	1	4	1	2	0.4	0.0	0	18%
ground	1 tsp	6	0	1	0	1	0.1	0.0	0	18%
ground *(Tone's)*	1 tsp	6	0	1	1	0	0.1	0.1	0	13%
ground, fresh *(Durkee)*	1 tsp	7	0	0	0	0	0.0	0.0	0	0%
ground, fresh *(Laurel Leaf)*	1 tsp	7	0	0	0	0	0.0	0.0	0	0%
whole *(McCormick/Schilling)*	1 tsp	7	0	2	0	1	0.0	0.0	0	0%
whole *(Spice Islands)*	1 tsp	6	0	1	0	0	0.1	0.0	0	13%
CARDONI. See CARDOON.										
CARDOON / cardoni										
boiled, drained	4 oz	25	0.9	6.0	200	2.1	0.1	<.1	0	3%
raw, shredded	1 cup	36	1.0	9.0	303	3.0	0.2	0.0	0	4%
CARIBOU										
raw	1 oz	36	6	0	16	0	1.0	0.4	24	24%
roasted	3 oz	142	25	0	51	0	3.8	1.4	93	24%
CARISSA / Natal plum										
Fresh										
raw, sliced	1 cup	93	1	20	5	na	1.9	na	0	18%
raw, whole, peeled and seeded	1 fruit	12	0	3	1	na	0.3	na	0	18%
CAROB CHIPS, unsweetened *(Sunspire)*	1 oz	133	4	15	123	0	6.0	6.0	2	42%
CAROB FLAVOR DRINK										
mix, powder	1 tbsp	45	0	11	12	1	0.0	0.0	0	0%
mix, powder, prepared w/milk	8 fl oz	195	8	23	133	1	8.2	5.1	33	38%
CAROB FLOUR. See under FLOUR.										
CARP										
baked, broiled, grilled, or microwaved	3 oz	138	19	0	54	0	6.1	1.2	71	40%
raw	3 oz	108	15	0	42	0	4.8	0.9	56	40%
CARROT										
Canned										
(A&P)	1/2 cup	30	1	6	300	0	1.0	0.0	0	24%
(Stokely)	1/2 cup	35	1	7	300	0	0.0	0.0	0	0%
baby, petite, whole *(Stokely)*	4.5 oz	30	0	5	390	2	0.0	0.0	0	0%
baby, whole *(Allens)*	1/2 cup	30	1	6	240	0	1.0	0.0	0	24%
baby, whole, 'LeSueur' *(Green Giant)*	1/2 cup	35	1	8	410	3	0.0	0.0	0	0%
crinkle sliced *(Freshlike)*	1/2 cup	30	1	6	300	0	0.0	0.0	0	0%
crinkle sliced *(Stokely)*	1/2 cup	35	1	7	300	na	0.0	0.0	na	0%
crinkle sliced *(Veg-All)*	1/2 cup	30	1	6	300	0	0.0	0.0	0	0%
diced *(Allens)*	1/2 cup	30	1	5	190	0	1.0	0.0	0	27%
diced, 'Fancy' *(S&W)*	1/2 cup	30	1	7	240	0	0.0	0.0	0	0%
diced, w/liquid *(Del Monte)*	1/2 cup	30	0	7	265	0	0.0	0.0	0	0%
mashed, no salt added, drained	1 cup	57	1	13	96	3	0.4	0.1	0	6%
no salt added *(A&P)*	1/2 cup	25	1	6	40	0	1.0	0.0	0	24%
no salt or sugar added *(Stokely)*	1/2 cup	35	1	7	35	0	0.0	0.0	0	0%
regular pack, mashed, drained	1 cup	57	1	13	552	3	0.4	0.1	0	6%
regular pack, sliced, drained	1 cup	37	1	8	353	2	0.3	0.1	0	6%
regular pack, sliced, drained	1 slice	1	0	0	7	0	0.0	0.0	0	6%
regular pack, sliced, w/liquid	1/2 cup	28	1	7	295	2	0.2	0.0	0	5%
sliced *(Featherweight)*	1/2 cup	30	1	6	30	0	0.0	0.0	0	0%
sliced *(Finast)*	1/2 cup	35	1	8	370	0	0.0	0.0	0	0%
sliced *(Green Giant)*	1/2 cup	25	1	6	380	2	0.0	0.0	0	0%
sliced *(IGA)*	1/2 cup	30	1	6	300	0	0.0	0.0	0	0%

Food Name	Serving Size	Calories	Prot. gms	Carbs gms	Sod. mgs	Fiber gms	Fat gms	Sat. Fat gms	Chol. mgs	% Fat Cal.
sliced (Pathmark)	1/2 cup	35	1	7	310	0	0.0	0.0	0	0%
sliced, no salt added, drained	1 cup	37	1	8	61	2	0.3	0.1	0	6%
sliced, no salt added, drained	1 slice	1	0	0	1	0	0.0	0.0	0	6%
sliced, no salt added, w/liquid	1/2 cup	28	1	7	42	2	0.2	0.0	0	5%
sliced, large (Allens)	1/2 cup	30	1	7	250	0	1.0	0.0	0	22%
sliced, medium (Allens)	1/2 cup	30	1	7	250	0	1.0	0.0	0	22%
sliced, Nutradiet (S&W)	1/2 cup	30	0	7	50	0	0.0	0.0	0	0%
sliced, small (Allens)	1/2 cup	30	1	7	250	0	1.0	0.0	0	22%
sliced no salt added (Finast)	1/2 cup	35	1	8	30	0	0.0	0.0	0	0%
sliced no salt added (Pathmark)	1/2 cup	35	1	8	35	0	0.0	0.0	0	0%
sliced, water packed, no salt (Freshlike)	1/2 cup	30	1	6	40	0	0.0	0.0	0	0%
Fresh										
baby, raw, large	1 carrot	6	0	1	5	0	0.1	0.0	0	12%
baby, raw, medium	1 carrot	4	0	1	4	0	0.1	0.0	0	12%
boiled, drained, sliced	1/2 cup	35	1	8	51	3	0.1	0.0	0	3%
boiled, drained, whole, medium	1 carrot	21	1	5	30	2	0.1	0.0	0	3%
raw, chopped	1 cup	55	1	13	45	4	0.2	0.0	0	4%
raw, cut, 3-inch strips	1 strip	3	0	1	2	0	0.0	0.0	0	4%
raw, cut, strips or slices	1 cup	52	1	12	43	4	0.2	0.0	0	4%
raw, grated	1 cup	47	1	11	39	3	0.2	0.0	0	4%
raw, shredded	1/2 cup	24	0.6	5.6	19	1.7	0.1	0.0	0	4%
raw, whole, medium (Dole)	1 carrot	40	1.0	8.0	40	1.0	1.0	na	na	20%
raw, whole, large, 7.25–8.5-inch long	1 carrot	31	1	7	25	2	0.1	0.0	0	4%
raw, whole, small, 5.5-inch long	1 carrot	22	1	5	18	2	0.1	0.0	0	4%
Frozen										
(A&P)	3.3 oz	40	1	9	45	0	1.0	0.0	0	18%
(Seabrook)	3.3 oz	40	1	9	44	1	0.0	0.0	0	0%
baby, cut, 'Select Polybag' (Green Giant)	3/4 cup	30	1	7	40	3	0.0	0.0	0	0%
baby, whole (C&W)	2/3 cup	35	1	7	60	3	0.0	0.0	0	0%
baby, whole (Flav-R-Pac)	2/3 cup	35	1	6	45	2	0.0	0.0	0	0%
baby, whole, 'Deluxe' (Birds Eye)	3.3 oz	40	1	9	45	2	0.0	0.0	0	0%
baby, whole, 'Harvest Fresh' (Green Giant)	1/2 cup	18	1	5	75	2	0.0	0.0	0	0%
baby, whole, 'Select' (Green Giant)	1/2 cup	20	1	7	35	2	0.0	0.0	0	0%
baby, whole, 'Singles' (Stokely)	3 oz	35	1	8	50	0	0.0	0.0	0	0%
Parisienne, 'Deluxe' (Birds Eye)	2.6 oz	30	1	7	35	2	0.0	0.0	0	0%
sliced (Birds Eye)	3.2 oz	35	1	8	40	1	0.0	0.0	0	0%
sliced (Flav-R-Pac)	2/3 cup	35	1	6	45	2	0.0	0.0	0	0%
sliced (Frosty Acres)	3.3 oz	40	1	9	44	1	0.0	0.0	0	0%
sliced, drained	1 cup	53	2	12	431	5	0.2	0.0	0	3%
sliced, no salt, drained	1 cup	53	2	12	86	5	0.2	0.0	0	3%
sliced, unprepared	10-oz pkg	111	3	26	168	9	0.6	0.1	0	5%
sliced, unprepared	1/2 cup	25	1	6	38	2	0.1	0.0	0	4%
small, round, European style, 'Parisienne' (C&W)	2/3 cup	40	0	10	50	3	0.0	0.0	0	0%
whole (Southern)	3.5 oz	42	1	9	60	0	0.2	0.0	0	4%
CARROT CHIPS										
(Hain)										
	1 oz	150	2	16	160	0	9.0	0.0	0	53%
barbecue	1 oz	140	2	16	160	0	8.0	0.0	0	50%
no salt added	1 oz	150	2	16	30	0	7.0	0.0	0	47%
CARROT DISH										
(Birds Eye)										
w/sweet peas, pearl onions, 'Deluxe'	3.3 oz	50	2	10	60	2	0.0	0.0	0	0%
(Flav-R-Pac)										
baby, orange glazed, 'Grande Classics'	1/2 cup	60	1	14	85	3	1.5	0.0	0	18%

Food Name	Serving Size	Calories	Prot. gms	Carbs gms	Sod. mgs	Fiber gms	Fat gms	Sat. Fat gms	Chol. mgs	% Fat Cal.
baby, whole, w/buttery sauce	1/2 cup	45	1	9	420	3	2.0	0.0	0	31%
shoestring, frozen	1 cup	35	1	6	45	2	0.0	0.0	0	0%
CARROT JUICE										
Canned or bottled										
	1 cup	94	2	22	68	2	0.4	0.1	0	3%
	1 fl oz	12	0	3	9	0	0.0	0.0	0	3%
(Biotta)	6 fl oz	51	2	11	158	0	0.1	0.0	0	2%
(Hain)	6 fl oz	80	1	17	170	0	0.0	0.0	0	0%
(Hollywood)	6 fl oz	80	1	17	170	2	0.0	0.0	0	0%
CASABA MELON. See MELON, CASABA.										
CASHEW / heart nut										
(Beer Nuts)	1 oz	170	5	8	65	0	13.0	0.0	0	69%
(Frito-Lay's)	1 oz	170	4	9	115	0	14.0	0.0	0	71%
halves (Fisher)	1 oz	160	5	8	0	0	13.0	3.0	0	69%
halves, lightly salted (Eagle)	1 oz	180	5	8	65	1	14.0	3.0	0	71%
lightly salted (Eagle)	1 oz	190	5	8	65	1	14.0	3.0	0	71%
pieces (Fisher)	1 oz	170	5	8	135	0	14.0	3.0	0	71%
salted, whole (Guy's)	1 oz	170	5	5	140	0	14.0	0.0	0	76%
salted (Pathmark)	1 oz	170	4	9	150	0	13.0	0.0	0	69%
salted, 'No Frills' (Pathmark)	1 oz	170	5	8	220	0	13.0	3.0	0	69%
salted (Planters)	1 oz	160	5	9	230	0	13.0	3.0	0	68%
unsalted, natural (Flanigan Farms)	1/4 cup	160	4	9	0	2	13.0	2.5	0	69%
whole (Fisher)	1 oz	160	5	8	100	0	13.0	3.0	0	69%
Dry roasted										
halves and whole, salted	1 cup	786	21	45	877	4	63.5	12.5	0	68%
halves and whole, unsalted	1 cup	786	21	45	22	4	63.5	12.5	0	68%
lightly salted (Planters)	1 oz	160	5	9	0	0	13.0	2.0	0	68%
salted	1 oz	163	4	9	181	1	13.1	2.6	0	68%
unsalted	1 oz	163	4	9	5	1	13.1	2.6	0	68%
unsalted	1 tbsp	49	1	3	1	0	4.0	0.8	0	68%
unsalted (Planters)	1 oz	160	5	9	0	0	13.0	3.0	0	68%
Honey roasted										
(Eagle)	1 oz	180	4	9	130	1	14.0	3.0	0	71%
(Planters)	1 oz	170	4	11	170	0	12.0	2.0	0	64%
halves (Eagle)	1 oz	180	4	9	130	1	14.0	3.0	0	71%
halves (Fisher)	1 oz	150	4	7	0	0	13.0	3.0	0	73%
whole (Fisher)	1 oz	150	4	7	90	0	13.0	3.0	0	73%
w/peanuts (Planters)	1 oz	170	5	9	170	0	12.0	2.0	0	66%
Oil roasted										
halves, salted (Fisher)	1/4 cup	170	5	8	160	1	15.0	2.5	0	72%
halves, salted (Planters)	1 oz	170	5	8	135	0	14.0	3.0	0	71%
halves, salted (Planters)	1 oz	170	5	8	135	0	14.0	3.0	0	71%
halves, unsalted (Planters)	1 oz	170	5	8	0	0	14.0	3.0	0	71%
halves and whole, salted	1 cup	749	21	37	814	5	62.7	12.4	0	70%
halves and whole, unsalted	1 cup	749	21	37	22	5	62.7	12.4	0	70%
lightly salted (Planters)	1 oz	160	5	8	80	0	14.0	3.0	0	71%
salted (Flavor House)	1 oz	180	7	3	125	0	16.0	0.0	0	78%
salted (Pathmark)	1 oz	170	5	8	150	0	14.0	0.0	0	71%
salted, approx 18 kernels	1 oz	163	5	8	177	1	13.7	2.7	0	70%
salted, 'Fancy' (Planters)	1 oz	170	5	8	135	0	14.0	3.0	0	71%
salted, 'No Frills' (Pathmark)	1 oz	170	5	8	150	0	14.0	0.0	0	71%
unsalted, approx 18 kernels	1 oz	163	5	8	5	1	13.7	2.7	0	70%
w/almonds (Fisher)	1 oz	170	5	6	95	0	15.0	2.0	0	75%
whole (Fisher)	1/4 cup	170	5	8	130	1	15.0	2.5	0	72%

Food Name	Serving Size	Calories	Prot. gms	Carbs gms	Sod. mgs	Fiber gms	Fat gms	Sat. Fat gms	Chol. mgs	% Fat Cal.
CASHEW BUTTER										
creamy, roasted fresh, no salt added *(Roaster Fresh)*	1 oz	165	4	9	4	0	14.0	3.0	0	71%
gourmet *(Roaster Fresh)*............................	1 oz	165	4	9	4	0	14.0	2.9	0	71%
peanut date *(Maranatha Natural)*	2 tbsp	190	8	8	8	0	14.0	0.0	0	66%
peanut date, 'Natural' *(Westbrae)*	2 tbsp	200	6	8	2	0	15.0	0.0	0	71%
raw *(Hain)*	2 tbsp	190	6	8	0	0	15.0	3.0	0	71%
raw, 'Natural' *(Westbrae)*.........................	2 tbsp	300	6	8	0	0	28.0	0.0	0	82%
raw, unsalted *(Hain)*	2 tbsp	210	5	8	10	0	19.0	3.0	0	77%
roasted *(Maranatha Natural)*.......................	2 tbsp	190	6	10	5	0	14.0	0.0	0	66%
roasted, 'Natural' *(Westbrae)*.....................	2 tbsp	190	6	8	0	0	17.0	0.0	0	73%
roasted, organic *(Maranatha Natural)*	2 tbsp	210	8	8	9	6	16.0	2.0	0	69%
salted...	1 oz	166	5	8	174	1	14.0	2.8	0	70%
salted...	1 tbsp	94	3	4	98	0	7.9	1.6	0	70%
toasted *(Hain)*	2 tbsp	210	7	7	15	0	17.0	3.0	0	73%
unsalted...	1 oz	166	5	8	4	1	14.0	2.8	0	70%
unsalted...	1 tbsp	94	3	4	2	0	7.9	1.6	0	70%
unsalted, 'Fancy' *(Planters)*	1 oz	170	5	8	0	0	14.0	2.0	0	71%
CASSAVA / manioc / yuca										
raw, chopped or sliced	1 cup	330	3	78	29	4	0.6	0.2	0	1%
raw, whole......................................	1 root	653	6	155	57	7	1.1	0.3	0	1%
CATFISH, CHANNEL										
Fresh										
breaded, fried	3 oz	195	15	7	238	1	11.3	2.8	69	53%
farmed, baked, broiled, grilled, or microwaved	3 oz	129	16	0	68	0	6.8	1.5	54	48%
farmed, raw.....................................	3 oz	115	13	0	45	0	6.5	1.5	40	51%
wild, baked, broiled, grilled, or microwaved...........	3 oz	89	16	0	43	0	2.4	0.6	61	24%
wild, raw.......................................	3 oz	81	14	0	37	0	2.4	0.6	49	27%
Frozen, fillets *(Delta Pride)*	4 oz	132	18	5	1	0	4.9	0.0	62	33%
CATFISH, OCEAN. See WOLF FISH.										
CATSUP / ketchup										
....	1 cup	250	4	65	2846	3	0.9	0.1	0	3%
....	1 tbsp	16	0	4	178	0	0.1	0.0	0	3%
....	1 pkt	6	0	2	71	0	0.0	0.0	0	3%
low-salt...	1 cup	250	4	65	48	3	0.9	0.1	0	3%
low-salt...	1 tbsp	16	0	4	3	0	0.1	0.0	0	3%
low-salt...	1 pkt	6	0	2	1	0	0.0	0.0	0	3%
(Del Monte)										
....	1/4 cup	60	1	16	675	0	0.0	0.0	0	0%
....	1 tbsp	15	0	4	190	0	0.0	0.0	0	0%
'No Salt Added'	1/4 cup	60	1	16	25	0	0.0	0.0	0	0%
(Estee)...	1 tbsp	6	0	0	20	0	0.0	0.0	0	0%
(Featherweight)	1 tbsp	6	0	1	5	0	0.0	0.0	0	0%
(Hain)										
'Natural'..	1 tbsp	16	0	4	155	0	0.0	0.0	0	0%
'Natural No Salt Added'............................	1 tbsp	16	0	4	5	0	0.0	0.0	0	0%
(Healthy Choice)	0.5 oz	9	0	2	97	0	0.1	0.0	0	9%
(Heinz)										
hot...	1 tbsp	16	0	4	195	0	0.0	0.0	0	0%
light	1 tbsp	10	0	3	95	0	0.0	0.0	0	0%
regular...	1 tbsp	16	0	4	213	0	0.0	0.0	0	0%
w/onions	1 tbsp	19	5	0	289	0	0.0	0.0	0	0%
(Hunt's)										
....	1 tbsp	16	0	4	158	0	0.1	0.0	0	5%
bulk packaged, food service product.................	1 tbsp	16	0	4	197	0	0.1	0.0	0	4%

Food Name	Serving Size	Calories	Prot. gms	Carbs gms	Sod. mgs	Fiber gms	Fat gms	Sat. Fat gms	Chol. mgs	% Fat Cal.
no salt added.	1 tbsp	16	0	3	6	0	0.1	0.0	0	7%
packets, food service product	1 pkt	10	0	2	96	0	0.1	0.0	0	4%
(Life) 'All Natural'	1 tbsp	17	0	4	10	0	0.0	0.0	0	0%
(Millina's Finest)										
organic	1 oz	17	1	4	143	0	0.1	0.0	0	5%
organic, fruit juice sweetened	1 tbsp	25	0	6	143	0	0.0	0.0	0	0%
(Smucker's)	1 tsp	8	0	2	45	0	0.0	0.0	0	0%
(Snider's)	1 tbsp	16	0	4	158	0	0.1	0.0	0	5%
(Stokely)	1 tbsp	20	0	5	190	0	0.0	0.0	0	0%
(Weight Watchers)	2 tsp	8	0	2	110	0	0.0	0.0	0	0%
(Westbrae)										
fruit sweetened	1 tbsp	12	0	2	110	0	0.0	0.0	0	0%
fruit sweetened, no salt	1 tbsp	12	0	2	10	0	0.0	0.0	0	0%
unsweetened	1 tbsp	5	0	1	60	0	0.0	0.0	0	0%
unsweetened 'Unketchup'	1 tbsp	8	0	1	105	0	0.0	0.0	0	0%
CAULIFLOWER										
Canned or jarred										
pickled, 'Hot & Spicy' *(Vlasic)*	1 oz	4	0	1	435	0	0.0	0.0	0	0%
sweet *(Vlasic)*	1 oz	35	0	9	225	0	0.0	0.0	0	0%
Fresh										
green, cooked	1/5 head	29	3	6	21	3	0.3	0.0	0	8%
green, raw, chopped	1 cup	20	2	4	15	2	0.2	0.0	0	8%
green, raw, florets	1 floret	8	1	2	6	1	0.1	0.0	0	8%
green, raw, whole, large, approx 6-7-inch diam.	1 head	158	15	31	118	16	1.5	0.2	0	8%
green, raw, whole, medium, approx 5-6-inch diam	1 head	134	13	26	99	14	1.3	0.2	0	8%
green, raw, whole, small, approx 4-inch diam	1 head	101	10	20	75	10	1.0	0.2	0	8%
white, boiled, drained, florets	3 florets	12	1	2	8	1	0.2	0.0	0	16%
white, boiled, drained, 1-inch pieces	1/2 cup	14	1	3	9	2	0.3	0.0	0	16%
white, raw, chopped.	1 cup	25	2	5	30	3	0.2	0.0	0	7%
white, raw, florets.	1 floret	3	0	1	4	0	0.0	0.0	0	7%
white, raw, whole, large, approx 6-7-inch diam	1 head	210	17	44	252	21	1.8	0.3	0	7%
white, raw, whole, medium, approx 5-6-inch diam.	1 head	144	11	30	173	14	1.2	0.2	0	7%
white, raw, whole, small, approx 4-inch diam	1 head	66	5	14	80	7	0.6	0.1	0	7%
Frozen										
(A&P).	3.3 oz	25	2	5	20	0	1.0	0.0	0	24%
(Birds Eye)	3.3 oz	25	2	5	20	2	0.0	0.0	0	0%
(Finast)	3.3 oz	25	2	5	15	0	0.0	0.0	0	0%
(Flav-R-Pac)	4 pieces	20	2	3	25	2	0.0	0.0	0	0%
(Frosty Acres)	3.3 oz	25	2	5	16	1	0.0	0.0	0	0%
(Kohl's)	3 oz	20	2	4	15	0	1.0	0.0	0	27%
(Seabrook)	3.3 oz	25	2	5	16	1	0.0	0.0	0	0%
(Southern)	3.5 oz	26	2	5	30	0	0.2	0.0	0	6%
cuts *(Green Giant)*.	1/2 cup	12	1	3	25	1	0.0	0.0	0	0%
cuts, no salt, drained, 1-inch pieces	1 cup	34	3	7	32	5	0.4	0.1	0	10%
cuts, unprepared, 1-inch pieces	1/2 cup	16	1	3	16	2	0.2	0.0	0	9%
cuts, w/salt, drained, 1-inch pieces.	1 cup	34	3	7	457	5	0.4	0.1	0	10%
florets, 'Plain Polybag' *(Green Giant)*	1/2 cup	12	1	3	25	2	0.0	0.0	0	0%
'Singles' *(Stokely)*	3 oz	20	2	4	20	0	0.0	0.0	0	0%
unprepared	10-oz pkg	68	6	13	68	7	0.8	0.1	0	9%
CAULIFLOWER DISH										
(Green Giant) w/cheese flavored sauce	1/2 cup	60	2	8	510	2	2.5	0.5	3	36%
CAVATELLI. See under PASTA DISH/ENTRÉE.										
CAVIAR										
black or red, granular	1 oz	71	7	1	425	0	5.1	1.2	167	64%
black or red, granular	1 tbsp	40	4	1	240	0	2.9	0.7	94	64%

Food Name	Serving Size	Calories	Prot. gms	Carbs gms	Sod. mgs	Fiber gms	Fat gms	Sat. Fat gms	Chol. mgs	% Fat Cal.
CAYENNE. See under PEPPER, GROUND.										
CECI. See CHICKPEA.										
CELERIAC										
boiled, drained, chopped.	1 cup	42	1	9	95	2	0.3	na	0	6%
raw, chopped.	1 cup	66	2	14	156	3	0.5	0.1	0	6%
CELERY										
boiled, drained, diced	1 cup	27	1	6	137	2	0.2	0.1	0	7%
boiled, drained, whole.	2 stalks	14	1	3	68	1	0.1	0.0	0	7%
raw, cut, approx 4-inch strips.	1 cup	20	1	5	108	2	0.2	0.0	0	7%
raw, cut, approx 4-inch strips.	1 strip	1	0	0	3	0	0.0	0.0	0	8%
raw, diced	1 cup	19	1	4	104	2	0.2	0.0	0	7%
raw, diced	1 tbsp	1	0	0	7	0	0.0	0.0	0	8%
raw, whole, large, 11–12 inches long	1 stalk	10	0	2	56	1	0.1	0.0	0	7%
raw, whole, medium, 7.5 –8 inches long	1 stalk	6	0	1	35	1	0.1	0.0	0	7%
raw, whole, small, approx 5 inches long	1 stalk	3	0	1	15	0	0.0	0.0	0	7%
CELERY FLAKES (Tone's).	1 tsp	9	0	1	4	0	0.5	0.1	0	46%
CELERY ROOT JUICE, bottled (Biotta)	6 fl oz	67	3	13	195	0	0.2	0.0	0	3%
CELERY SALT (Tone's)	1 tsp	6	0	1	1584	0	0.4	0.1	0	50%
CELERY SEED										
. . . .	1 tbsp	25	1	3	10	1	1.6	0.1	0	54%
. . . .	1 tsp	8	0	1	3	0	0.5	0.0	0	54%
(McCormick/Schilling)	1 tsp	7	0	1	3	1	0.4	0.0	0	43%
(Spice Islands)	1 tsp	11	0	1	4	0	0.5	0.1	0	43%
(Tone's)	1 tsp	9	0	1	4	0	0.5	0.1	0	46%
whole seeds (Durkee).	1 tsp	9	0	0	0	0	0.0	0.0	0	0%
whole seeds (Laurel Leaf).	1 tsp	9	0	0	0	0	0.0	0.0	0	0%
CELLOPHANE NOODLES. See under NOODLE.										
CELTUCE, fresh, raw	1 med leaf	1	0	0	1	0	0.0	na	0	14%
CEREAL, HOT										
(Krusteaz)										
'Ala'	1/4 cup	150	4	33	0	7	0.0	0.0	0	0%
'Zoom'	1/3 cup	120	5	24	0	4	0.0	0.0	0	0%
(Malt-O-Meal)										
'Maple Brown Sugar' 30% formulation, prepared,										
w/2% milk	1 oz	160	7	28	60	1	3.0	0.0	10	16%
'Maple Brown Sugar' 30% formulation, unprepared	1 oz	100	3	22	0	1	0.0	0.0	0	0%
(Quaker) plus fiber, prepared w/1/2 cup nonfat milk	1/2 cup	170	10	27	66	6	2.5	0.5	0	13%
BARLEY										
(Erewhon) organic	1 oz	110	3	22	0	1	1.0	0.0	0	8%
(Quaker) Scotch, quick	1/3 cup	170	5	37	0	5	1.0	0.0	0	5%
BRAN										
(Breadshop) oat, rice, corn, 'Triple Bran' unprepared	1 oz	100	6	15	5	6	2.0	0.0	0	18%
(H-O Brand) 'Super Bran' unprepared	1/3 cup	110	4	18	0	8	2.0	0.0	0	17%
BULGUR										
(Arrowhead Mills).	2 oz	200	6	43	0	5	1.0	0.0	0	4%
(Hodgson Mill) w/soy grits, unprepared	1/4 cup	120	6	24	0	1	1.0	0.0	0	7%
CORN GRITS. See GRITS.										
FARINA										
(H-O Brand) instant, unprepared	1 pkt	110	3	22	235	3	0.0	0.0	0	0%
(Krusteaz)	1 oz	100	3	22	1	1	0.0	0.0	0	0%
(Pillsbury)										
unprepared	1/12 pkg	80	3	18	0	0	0.0	0.0	0	0%
prepared w/water, 1/8 tsp salt.	2/3 cup	80	3	18	270	0	0.0	0.0	0	0%
(Quaker).	1/4 cup	154	5	33	1	1	0.4	0.1	0	2%

Food Name	Serving Size	Calories	Prot. gms	Carbs gms	Sod. mgs	Fiber gms	Fat gms	Sat. Fat gms	Chol. mgs	% Fat Cal.
GRANOLA										
(Breadshop)										
almond raisin, nectarsweet	1 oz	120	4	18	2	3	4.0	0.0	0	30%
'Blueberry 'N Cream' nectarsweet	1 oz	115	4	19	2	3	3.0	0.0	0	23%
'California Orange Crunch' honeysweet	1 oz	130	4	18	1	2	5.0	0.0	0	34%
'Cinnapple Spice' honeysweet	1 oz	125	3	19	2	2	4.5	0.5	0	32%
'Crunchy Oat Bran' nectarsweet	1 oz	120	3	18	2	3	5.0	0.5	0	35%
'Golden Maple Nut' honeysweet	1 oz	130	4	17	2	2	5.0	0.8	0	35%
'Golden Maple Nut'	1/2 cup	230	6	32	0	4	9.5	1.5	0	36%
'Gone Nuts!' nectarsweet	1 oz	125	4	17	2	3	5.0	0.5	0	35%
honey apple blueberry, honeysweet	1 oz	125	4	18	1	3	5.0	0.5	0	34%
'Honey Gone Nuts!' honeysweet	1 oz	130	4	18	2	3	5.5	0.5	0	37%
'New England Supernatural'	1/2 cup	220	5	31	0	3	9.0	1.0	0	36%
orange almond	1/2 cup	240	7	35	0	5	8.5	1.0	0	31%
orange almond, nectarsweet	1 oz	120	4	18	2	3	4.0	0.5	0	30%
'Oregon Blueberry Crunch' honeysweet	1 oz	125	4	18	2	3	5.0	0.8	0	34%
'Peaches 'N Cream' nectarsweet	1 oz	115	4	19	2	3	3.0	0.5	0	23%
raspberries and cream, w/organic oats	1/2 cup	220	6	34	0	4	7.5	1.0	0	30%
'Raspberry 'N Cream' nectarsweet	1 oz	115	4	19	2	3	3.0	0.5	0	23%
'Strawberry 'N Cream' nectarsweet	1 oz	110	3	16	5	3	4.0	0.0	0	32%
'Supernatural New England' honeysweet	1 oz	130	3	18	2	2	5.0	0.5	0	35%
'Supernatural' honeysweet	1 oz	100	4	18	2	4	5.0	0.8	0	35%
(Ener-G Foods) gluten-free	1 cup	436	9	47	178	7	26.8	5.6	0	52%
(Erewhon)										
apple, spiced	1 oz	130	3	17	55	0	6.0	0.0	0	40%
honey almond	1 oz	130	3	17	65	0	6.0	0.0	0	40%
maple	1 oz	130	3	17	55	0	5.0	0.0	0	36%
'Sunflower Crunch'	1 oz	130	3	18	60	0	4.0	0.0	0	30%
w/bran, '#9'	1 oz	130	3	17	10	4	6.0	0.0	0	40%
w/dates and nuts	1 oz	130	3	17	45	0	6.0	0.0	0	40%
(Golden Temple)										
apple cinnamon, low-fat	1/2 cup	190	6	39	5	4	2.0	0.0	0	9%
blueberry	1 oz	132	4	19	6	2	5.0	1.0	0	33%
blueberry, coconut-free	1 oz	131	4	19	3	2	4.5	0.5	0	31%
blueberry, wild	1/2 cup	230	6	33	5	4	9.0	2.0	0	34%
cashew almond	1 oz	129	4	19	3	4	3.5	0.5	0	26%
cinnamon apple raisin	1 oz	125	3	20	3	2	3.5	0.5	0	26%
coconut almond	1 oz	145	4	18	3	2	3.5	0.5	0	26%
fruit and nut	1 oz	129	3	19	26	2	4.5	0.5	0	32%
golden	1 oz	138	4	19	25	2	6.0	1.0	0	37%
Hawaiian	1 oz	126	4	19	3	2	4.0	1.0	0	28%
high-protein	1 oz	124	4	19	6	2	3.5	0.5	0	26%
honey almond	1 oz	130	4	20	25	3	3.5	0.5	0	25%
honey blueberry apple	1 oz	128	4	20	2	2	3.5	0.5	0	25%
'Lite & Crunchy'	1/2 cup	220	6	33	5	4	8.0	1.0	0	32%
maple almond	1 oz	129	4	20	25	2	3.5	0.5	0	25%
'Natural Delite'	1 oz	128	3	20	26	2	3.5	0.5	0	26%
oat bran, w/berries	1 oz	120	4	20	3	3	3.5	0.5	0	25%
oat bran, w/raisins and almonds	1 oz	119	3	19	3	3	3.5	0.5	0	26%
orange almond	1 oz	133	4	19	25	2	4.0	1.0	0	28%
'Rainforest Granola'	1/2 cup	240	7	33	0	4	10.0	2.0	0	36%
raisin apricot date	1 oz	127	3	20	25	2	3.5	0.5	0	26%
'Super Nutty'	1 oz	135	4	19	25	3	5.0	1.0	0	33%
'Super Nutty'	1/2 cup	230	6	33	45	4	9.0	2.0	0	34%

Food Name	Serving Size	Calories	Prot. gms	Carbs gms	Sod. mgs	Fiber gms	Fat gms	Sat. Fat gms	Chol. mgs	% Fat Cal.
'Sweet Home Farm' low-fat	1 oz	110	3	22	65	2	2.0	0.5	0	15%
(Health Valley)										
date and almond, nonfat	1 oz	90	2	21	20	3	0.0	0.0	0	0%
raisin cinnamon, nonfat	1 oz	90	2	21	20	3	0.0	0.0	0	0%
raspberry, nonfat	1 oz	140	2	35	5	3	0.0	0.0	0	0%
tropical fruit, nonfat	1 oz	90	2	21	20	3	0.0	0.0	0	0%
(Stone-Buhr) apple, no preservatives, no added sugar	1/3 cup	130	5	31	0	5	1.0	0.0	0	6%
GRITS. See GRITS.										
MULTIGRAIN										
(Arrowhead Mills)										
four grain, unprepared	1 oz	94	4	18	1	7	1.0	0.0	0	9%
seven grain, unprepared	1 oz	100	4	17	1	4	1.0	0.0	0	10%
(Pritikin) hearty, microwave, prepared	1 pkt	190	9	38	65	0	2.0	0.0	0	9%
(Quaker)										
unprepared	1/2 cup	133	5	29	1	5	1.0	0.2	0	7%
prepared w/1/2 cup nonfat milk	1/2 cup	170	9	30	65	5	1.5	0.5	0	8%
(Roman Meal)										
oats, wheat, and other grains, prepared w/water	1 cup	170	7	34	540	8	1.9	0.2	0	9%
oats, wheat, and other grains, prepared w/water	3/4 cup	128	5	26	405	6	1.4	0.1	0	9%
oats, wheat, and other grains, unprepared	1 cup	340	15	69	20	na	4.0	na	0	10%
oats, wheat, and other grains, unprepared	1/4 cup	85	4	17	5	na	1.0	na	0	10%
wheat w/other grains, plain, prepared w/water	1 cup	147	7	33	198	8	1.0	0.1	0	5%
wheat w/other grains, plain, prepared w/water	3/4 cup	110	5	25	148	6	0.7	0.1	0	5%
wheat w/other grains, unprepared	1 cup	299	13	67	6	17	2.0	0.3	0	6%
wheat w/other grains, unprepared	1/3 cup	100	4	22	2	6	0.7	0.1	0	6%
wheat w/other grains, unprepared	1 tbsp	19	1	4	0	1	0.1	0.0	0	6%
w/apple cinnamon, prepared	2/3 cup	112	4	24	14	6	2.8	0.0	1	19%
OAT BRAN										
(Arrowhead Mills) unprepared	1 oz	110	6	17	1	5	1.0	0.0	0	9%
(Breadshop)										
'Oat Bran Muesli' unprepared	1 oz	100	4	20	5	3	2.0	0.0	0	16%
100% pure 'Oat Bran' unprepared	1 oz	100	6	17	5	4	2.0	0.0	0	16%
(Erewhon) w/toasted wheat germ *(Erewhon)*	1 oz	115	5	18	15	3	2.0	0.0	0	16%
(Health Valley)										
apple/cinnamon, 'Natural' unprepared	1/4 cup	100	3	19	10	4	1.0	0.0	0	9%
raisin, nonfat	1 oz	100	3	19	10	4	1.0	na	0	9%
(Hodgson Mill) low-fat, cholesterol-free, unprepared	1/4 cup	120	6	23	3	6	3.0	1.0	0	19%
(Malt-O-Meal)										
'Plus 40% Oat Bran' prepared, w/1/2 cup nonfat milk	1.3 oz	170	10	31	65	3	2.0	0.0	0	10%
'Plus 40% Oat Bran' prepared, w/1/2 cup 2% milk	1.3 oz	190	10	31	65	3	4.0	0.0	10	18%
'Plus 40% Oat Bran' unprepared	1.3 oz	130	6	25	0	3	2.0	0.0	0	13%
(Mother's)										
prepared w/o salt	2/3 cup	92	6	17	1	4	2.0	0.2	0	17%
prepared w/1/2 cup whole milk, w/o salt	1 oz	180	10	22	60	1	7.0	0.0	15	33%
unprepared	1/3 cup	92	6	17	1	4	2.1	0.2	0	17%
(Quaker) 'Mother's' unprepared	1/2 cup	146	7	25	2	6	3.2	0.6	0	20%
(3-Minute Brand)										
'Quick' unprepared	1 oz	100	5	18	0	3	2.0	0.0	0	16%
'Regular' unprepared	1 oz	90	6	17	0	4	2.0	0.0	0	16%
(Wholesome 'N Hearty)										
apple cinnamon, unprepared	1 pkt	130	3	30	160	5	2.0	0.0	0	12%
honey, unprepared	1 pkt	110	3	26	160	5	2.0	0.0	0	13%
regular, unprepared	1 oz	100	4	18	0	5	2.0	0.0	0	17%

Food Name	Serving Size	Calories	Prot. gms	Carbs gms	Sod. mgs	Fiber gms	Fat gms	Sat. Fat gms	Chol. mgs	% Fat Cal.
OATMEAL AND OATS										
(Arrowhead Mills)										
apple, date, and almond, unprepared	1 oz	130	5	23	3	4	3.0	0.0	0	19%
apple spice, unprepared	1 oz	130	5	23	1	3	2.0	0.0	0	14%
cinnamon, raisin, almond, unprepared	1 oz	140	6	23	3	4	3.0	0.0	0	19%
instant, unprepared	1 oz	100	6	18	0	4	2.0	0.0	0	16%
(Erewhon)										
apple cinnamon, instant	1.25 oz	145	4	25	100	0	3.0	0.0	0	19%
apple cinnamon, 100% natural, instant	1 pkt	130	5	24	100	3	2.0	0.5	0	13%
apple raisin, instant	1.3 oz	150	4	27	100	0	3.0	0.0	0	18%
apple raisin, 100% natural, instant	1 pkt	150	4	27	100	0	3.0	0.0	0	18%
maple spice, instant	1.2 oz	140	4	24	100	0	3.0	0.0	0	19%
maple spice, 100% natural, instant	1 pkt	130	2	25	100	3	2.0	0.5	0	14%
w/oat bran, instant	1.25 oz	125	6	23	0	4	3.0	0.0	0	19%
w/raisins, dates, and walnuts, instant	1.2 oz	130	3	24	60	3	3.0	0.0	0	20%
(General Mills)										
apple and cinnamon, instant, unprepared	1.5 oz	150	4	32	105	3	2.0	0.0	0	11%
cinnamon raisin, unprepared	1.8 oz	170	4	38	130	3	2.0	0.0	0	10%
(H-O Brand)										
apple and bran w/fiber, instant, unprepared	1 pkt	130	3	26	140	3	2.0	0.0	0	13%
apple and cinnamon, instant, unprepared	1 pkt	130	3	26	220	3	2.0	0.0	0	13%
'Gourmet' unprepared	1/3 cup	100	5	18	0	3	2.0	0.0	0	16%
instant, unprepared	1 pkt	110	4	18	230	3	2.0	0.0	0	17%
instant, unprepared	1/2 cup	130	5	22	5	3	2.0	0.0	0	14%
maple brown sugar, unprepared	1 pkt	160	4	32	285	3	2.0	0.0	0	11%
'Quick' unprepared	1/2 cup	130	5	23	5	3	2.0	0.0	0	14%
raisin and bran, w/fiber, instant, unprepared	1 pkt	150	4	32	140	3	2.0	0.0	0	11%
raisins and spice, instant, unprepared	1 pkt	150	4	32	240	3	2.0	0.0	0	11%
sweet'n mellow, instant, unprepared	1 pkt	150	5	30	270	3	2.0	0.0	0	11%
w/fiber, instant, unprepared	1 pkt	110	5	18	140	3	2.0	0.0	0	16%
w/fiber, instant, unprepared	1/3 cup	100	5	15	5	3	2.0	0.0	0	18%
(Maypo)										
maple flavored, 'Vermont Style' unprepared	1 oz	105	4	20	0	2	1.0	0.0	0	9%
'Maypo' prepared w/water, salt	1 cup	170	6	32	259	6	2.4	0.4	0	12%
'Maypo' prepared w/water, salt	3/4 cup	128	4	24	194	4	1.8	0.3	0	12%
'Maypo' prepared w/water, no salt added	1 cup	170	6	32	10	6	2.4	0.4	0	12%
'Maypo' prepared w/water, no salt added	3/4 cup	128	4	24	7	4	1.8	0.3	0	12%
'Maypo' prepared w/water, no salt added	1 tbsp	11	0	2	1	0	0.1	0.0	0	12%
'Maypo' '30 Second' unprepared	1 oz	100	4	19	0	2	1.0	0.0	0	9%
'Maypo' unprepared	1 cup	362	12	68	18	10	5.0	na	0	12%
'Maypo' unprepared	1/2 cup	181	6	34	9	5	2.5	na	0	12%
(Mother's)										
instant, prepared w/1/2 cup whole milk	1 oz	190	9	24	60	0	6.0	0.0	15	29%
instant, unprepared	1 oz	110	5	18	0	0	2.0	0.0	0	16%
(Oatmeal Swirlers)										
cherry, unprepared	1.7 oz	150	3	33	130	2	2.0	0.0	0	11%
cinnamon spice, unprepared	1.6 oz	160	3	35	100	2	2.0	0.0	0	11%
maple brown sugar, unprepared	1.6 oz	160	3	35	100	2	2.0	0.0	0	11%
milk chocolate, unprepared	1.7 oz	170	3	37	100	2	2.0	0.0	0	10%
apple and cinnamon, instant, unprepared	1.7 oz	160	3	34	120	2	2.0	0.0	0	11%
strawberry, unprepared	1.6 oz	150	3	32	120	2	2.0	0.0	0	11%
(Quaker)										
apple spice, microwave, 'Quick 'n Hearty'	1 pkt	166	4	35	306	3	2.0	0.4	0	11%
apples and cinnamon, instant, unprepared	1 pkt	130	4	26	105	3	1.5	0.5	0	10%

Food Name	Serving Size	Calories	Prot. gms	Carbs gms	Sod. mgs	Fiber gms	Fat gms	Sat. Fat gms	Chol. mgs	% Fat Cal.
apples and spice, instant, 'Extra' unprepared	1 pkt	133	4	27	191	3	1.9	0.3	0	12%
brown sugar cinnamon, microwave, 'Quick 'n Hearty'	1 pkt	155	4	31	255	3	2.2	0.4	0	13%
cinnamon and spice, instant, unprepared	1 pkt	164	5	35	322	3	2.1	0.4	0	11%
cinnamon double raisin, microwave, 'Quick 'n Hearty'	1 pkt	169	4	35	275	3	2.2	0.4	0	12%
cinnamon graham, instant, 'Kids' Choice' unprepared.	1 pkt	140	4	29	170	3	2.0	0.0	0	12%
cinnamon graham cookie, instant, 'Kids Choice'	1 pkt	190	8	35	230	3	2.0	0.0	0	9%
cinnamon toast, instant, unprepared.	1 pkt	130	3	27	160	2	2.0	0.0	0	13%
'Cinnamagic' instant, unprepared	1 pkt	144	4	30	165	3	2.0	0.4	0	12%
'Extra' unprepared.	1 pkt	95	4	18	219	3	2.0	0.2	0	17%
fruit punch flavor, instant, 'Power Rangers' unprepared.	1 pkt	149	4	31	165	3	2.0	0.4	0	12%
fruit and cream, instant, unprepared.	1 pkt	135	3	26	169	2	2.5	0.5	0	17%
fruit and cream blueberry, instant, unprepared	1 pkt	130	3	27	140	2	2.5	0.5	0	16%
honey bran, microwave, 'Quick 'n Hearty'	1 pkt	151	4	31	253	3	2.1	0.4	0	13%
honey nut, instant, unprepared	1 pkt	130	3	25	210	2	3.0	0.5	0	19%
instant, unprepared	1 pkt	94	4	18	270	3	2.0	0.3	0	17%
low-salt, instant, unprepared	1 pkt	103	4	19	78	3	2.0	0.4	0	17%
maple and brown sugar, instant, prepared w/water	1 pkt	153	4	31	234	3	1.8	0.4	0	10%
maple and brown sugar, instant, 'Kids' Choice' unprepared.	1 pkt	140	4	31	240	3	2.0	0.0	0	11%
maple and brown sugar, instant, unprepared	1 pkt	152	5	32	320	3	2.1	0.4	0	12%
'Old Fashioned' prepared	2/3 cup	99	4	19	1	3	2.0	0.3	0	16%
'Old Fashioned' unprepared	1/3 cup	99	4	19	1	3	2.0	0.3	0	16%
peaches and cream, instant, unprepared	1 pkt	129	3	26	179	2	2.2	0.9	0	14%
plus fiber, instant, unprepared.	1/2 cup	130	6	21	0	6	2.5	0.5	0	17%
'Quick' prepared	2/3 cup	99	4	19	1	3	2.0	0.3	0	16%
'Quick' unprepared	1/3 cup	99	4	19	1	3	2.0	0.3	0	16%
radical raspberry, instant, 'Kids' Choice' unprepared.	1 pkt	150	4	28	170	3	3.0	0.0	0	17%
raisin bran, plus fiber, instant, unprepared	1 pkt	190	9	34	125	6	2.0	0.5	0	9%
raisins and cinnamon, instant, 'Extra' unprepared.	1 pkt	129	4	27	119	3	1.9	0.3	0	12%
raisins and spice, instant, unprepared	1 pkt	149	4	32	266	3	2.0	0.3	0	11%
raisins, dates, and walnuts, instant, unprepared.	1 pkt	141	4	25	216	2	3.8	0.4	0	23%
regular flavor, instant.	1 pkt	94	4	18	270	3	2.0	0.3	0	17%
regular flavor, microwave, 'Quick 'n Hearty'.	1 pkt	106	4	19	153	2	2.1	0.4	0	18%
strawberries and cream, instant, unprepared	1 pkt	129	3	27	204	2	2.0	1.1	0	13%
strawberries and stuff, instant, 'Kids' Choice' unprepared.	1 pkt	140	4	30	170	3	2.0	0.0	0	12%
unprepared	1/3 cup	99	4	19	1	3	2.0	0.3	0	16%
w/apples and cinnamon, instant, prepared w/water	1 pkt	125	3	26	121	3	1.4	0.3	0	10%
w/apples and cinnamon, instant, unprepared	1 pkt	128	3	27	121	3	1.5	0.3	0	10%
(Ralston)										
prepared w/water, salt	1 cup	134	6	28	476	6	0.8	0.1	0	5%
prepared w/water, salt	3/4 cup	101	4	21	357	5	0.6	0.1	0	5%
(3-Minute Brand)										
'Old Fashioned' unprepared	1 oz	100	5	18	0	3	2.0	0.0	0	16%
'Quick' unprepared	1 oz	100	5	18	0	3	2.0	0.0	0	16%
raisin, unprepared	1 oz	100	5	18	0	3	2.0	0.0	0	16%
raisin, w/oat bran, unprepared	1 oz	100	4	18	0	3	2.0	0.0	0	17%
(Total)										
instant, unprepared.	1.2 oz	110	4	22	220	3	2.0	0.0	0	15%
maple brown sugar, unprepared	1.6 oz	160	4	34	150	3	2.0	0.0	0	11%
'Quick' unprepared	1 oz	90	4	18	0	3	2.0	0.0	0	17%
(Under Cover Bears) plain, instant, prepared w/water.	1 pkt	71	3	12	195	2	1.2	0.2	0	14%

Food Name	Serving Size	Calories	Prot. gms	Carbs gms	Sod. mgs	Fiber gms	Fat gms	Sat. Fat gms	Chol. mgs	% Fat Cal.
RICE										
(Arrowhead Mills)										
brown, 'Rise and Shine' unprepared	1.5 oz	160	3	35	1	2	1.0	0.0	0	6%
(Cream of Rice)										
cream of, prepared w/water, no salt	1 cup	127	2	28	2	0	0.2	0.1	0	2%
cream of, prepared w/water, no salt	3/4 cup	95	2	21	2	0	0.2	0.0	0	2%
cream of, prepared w/water, no salt	1 tbsp	8	0	2	0	0	0.0	0.0	0	2%
cream of, prepared w/water, salt.	1 cup	127	2	28	422	0	0.2	0.0	0	2%
cream of, prepared w/water, salt.	3/4 cup	95	2	21	317	0	0.2	0.0	0	2%
cream of, unprepared	1 cup	640	11	143	10	1	0.9	0.2	0	1%
cream of, unprepared	1 tbsp	38	1	8	1	0	0.1	0.0	0	1%
(Erewhon)										
brown, cream of, organic.	1 oz	110	3	23	20	0	1.0	0.0	0	8%
(Lundberg Family)										
almond-date, 'Hot'n Creamy' prepared	1 oz	110	2	24	25	0	1.0	0.0	0	8%
organic, 'Hot'n Creamy' prepared	1 oz	110	3	23	20	0	1.0	0.0	0	8%
RYE										
(Breadshop) 'Rye Date Muesli' unprepared	1 oz	100	3	19	5	4	2.0	0.0	0	17%
(Roman Meal) cream of, unprepared.	1/3 cup	110	4	27	0	5	1.0	0.0	0	7%
WHEAT										
(Ancient Harvest) whole-grain, steam rolled	1/3 cup	105	3	23	5	3	1.0	0.0	0	8%
(Arrowhead Mills)										
'Bear Mush' unprepared	1 oz	100	3	21	1	1	0.0	0.0	0	0%
cracked wheat, unprepared.	2 oz	180	7	40	1	2	1.0	0.0	0	5%
(Cream of Wheat)										
cream of, apple, banana and maple flavored, instant,										
'Mix 'N Eat' prepared	1 pkt	132	2	29	242	0	0.5	0.1	0	3%
cream of, apple, banana and maple flavored, instant,										
'Mix 'N Eat' unprepared	1 pkt	132	2	29	241	1	0.4	na	0	2%
cream of, apple and cinnamon, 'Mix'n Eat' unprepared. . . .	1 oz	130	2	29	250	1	0.0	0.0	0	0%
cream of, brown sugar cinnamon, 'Mix'n Eat'										
unprepared.	1 oz	130	2	29	230	1	0.0	0.0	0	0%
cream of, instant, prepared w/water, no salt	1 cup	121	4	26	1	1	0.2	0.0	0	1%
cream of, instant, prepared w/water, no salt	3/4 cup	116	3	24	5	2	0.4	0.1	0	3%
cream of, instant, prepared w/water, salt.	1 serving	96	3	20	160	1	0.2	0.0	0	2%
cream of, instant, prepared w/water, salt.	1 cup	154	4	32	364	3	0.5	0.1	0	3%
cream of, instant, prepared w/water, salt.	3/4 cup	116	3	24	273	2	0.4	0.1	0	3%
cream of, instant, prepared w/water, salt.	1 tbsp	10	0	2	0	0	0.0	0.0	0	3%
cream of, instant, unprepared	1 cup	651	19	134	27	6	2.5	0.4	0	3%
cream of, instant, unprepared	1 tbsp	42	1	9	2	0	0.2	0.0	0	3%
cream of, maple brown sugar, 'Mix'n Eat' unprepared.	1 oz	130	2	29	180	1	0.0	0.0	0	0%
cream of, original, 'Mix'n Eat' unprepared	1 oz	100	3	21	170	1	0.0	0.0	0	0%
cream of, plain, instant, 'Mix 'N Eat' prepared	1 pkt	102	3	21	241	0	0.3	0.0	0	2%
cream of, plain, instant, 'Mix 'N Eat' unprepared	1 pkt	102	3	21	241	1	0.3	0.1	0	3%
cream of, quick, prepared w/water	1 cup	129	4	27	139	1	0.5	0.1	0	3%
cream of, quick, prepared w/water	3/4 cup	97	3	20	104	1	0.4	0.1	0	3%
cream of, quick, prepared w/water	1 tbsp	8	0	2	9	0	0.0	0.0	0	3%
cream of, quick, prepared w/water, salt.	1 cup	129	4	27	464	1	0.5	0.1	0	3%
cream of, quick, prepared w/water, salt.	3/4 cup	97	3	20	347	1	0.4	0.1	0	3%
cream of, quick, unprepared	1 cup	635	18	132	688	5	2.3	0.4	0	3%
cream of, quick, unprepared	1 tbsp	40	1	8	43	0	0.1	0.0	0	3%
cream of, regular, prepared w/water, no salt.	1 cup	133	4	28	3	2	0.5	0.1	0	3%
cream of, regular, prepared w/water, no salt.	3/4 cup	100	3	21	2	1	0.4	0.1	0	3%
cream of, regular, prepared w/water, no salt.	1 tbsp	8	0	2	0	0	0.0	0.0	0	3%

Food Name	Serving Size	Calories	Prot. gms	Carbs gms	Sod. mgs	Fiber gms	Fat gms	Sat. Fat gms	Chol. mgs	% Fat Cal.
cream of, regular, prepared w/water, salt	1 cup	133	4	28	336	2	0.5	0.1	0	3%
cream of, regular, prepared w/water, salt	3/4 cup	100	3	21	252	1	0.4	0.1	0	3%
cream of, regular, unprepared	1 cup	640	18	132	12	7	2.6	0.4	0	3%
cream of, regular, unprepared	1 tbsp	39	1	8	1	0	0.2	0.0	0	3%
(General Mills)										
'Wheat Hearts' prepared, w/3/4 cup nonfat milk	3/4 cup	170	10	29	95	1	1.0	0.0	0	5%
'Wheat Hearts' unprepared	1 oz	110	4	21	0	0	1.0	0.0	0	8%
(Wheat Hearts) unprepared	1 oz	110	4	21	0	0	1.0	0.0	0	8%
(H-O Brand) wheat farina, cream of, unprepared	3 tbsp	120	3	26	0	3	0.0	0.0	0	0%
(Hodgson Mill) cracked, coarse milled, unprepared.	1/4 cup	110	4	26	0	8	1.0	0.0	0	7%
(Malt-O-Meal)										
and barley, chocolate, prepared, w/1/2 cup 2% milk	1 oz	160	7	28	60	1	3.0	0.0	10	16%
and barley, chocolate, unprepared	1 cup	607	17	128	17	na	1.5	na	0	2%
and barley, chocolate, unprepared	1 oz	100	3	22	0	1	0.0	0.0	0	0%
and barley, plain or chocolate, prepared w/water	1 cup	122	4	26	2	1	0.2	0.1	0	2%
and barley, plain or chocolate, prepared w/water	3/4 cup	92	3	19	2	1	0.2	0.1	0	2%
and barley, plain or chocolate, prepared w/water	1 tbsp	8	0	2	0	0	0.0	0.0	0	2%
and barley, plain or chocolate, prepared w/water, salt	1 cup	122	4	26	324	1	0.2	0.0	0	2%
and barley, plain or chocolate, prepared w/water, salt	3/4 cup	92	3	19	243	1	0.2	0.0	0	2%
and barley, plain, unprepared	1 cup	607	17	128	12	na	1.5	na	0	2%
and barley, plain, unprepared	1 tbsp	38	1	8	1	na	0.1	na	0	2%
(Maltex)										
and barley, unprepared	1 oz	105	3	21	0	3	1.0	0.0	0	9%
'Maltex' prepared w/water, no salt	1 cup	179	6	40	10	3	1.0	0.2	0	5%
'Maltex' prepared w/water, no salt	3/4 cup	135	4	30	7	2	0.7	0.1	0	5%
'Maltex' prepared w/water, no salt	1 tbsp	11	0	2	1	0	0.1	0.0	0	5%
'Maltex' prepared w/water, salt	1 cup	179	6	40	189	3	1.0	0.2	0	5%
'Maltex' prepared w/water, salt	3/4 cup	135	4	30	142	2	0.7	0.1	0	5%
'Maltex' unprepared	1 cup	532	17	117	26	6	3.2	0.5	0	5%
'Maltex' unprepared	1/4 cup	134	4	29	6	2	0.8	0.1	0	5%
(Mother's)										
whole wheat, prepared, w/1/2 cup whole milk.	1 oz	180	8	26	60	1	5.0	0.0	0	25%
whole wheat, unprepared	1/3 cup	92	3	21	1	2	0.6	0.1	0	5%
(Nabisco)										
cream of, apple cinnamon, prepared	1 serving	114	2	25	202	1	0.3	0.1	0	3%
cream of, apple cinnamon, unprepered	1 oz	108	2	24	192	1	0.3	0.1	0	3%
cream of, enriched w/iron, quick, prepared	1 cup	78	3	16	59	1	0.3	0.1	0	3%
cream of, enriched w/iron, quick, unprepared	1 cup	629	21	127	474	8	2.1	0.4	0	3%
cream of, enriched w/iron, unprepared	1 oz	105	3	21	233	1	0.4	0.1	0	4%
(Ralston)										
100% wheat, prepared	1/2 cup	160	5	31	0	5	1.0	0.2	0	6%
'Ralston' prepared w/water, no salt	1 cup	134	6	28	5	6	0.8	0.1	0	5%
'Ralston' prepared w/water, no salt	3/4 cup	101	4	21	4	5	0.6	0.1	0	5%
'Ralston' prepared w/water, no salt	1 tbsp	8	0	2	0	0	0.0	0.0	0	5%
'Ralston' unprepared	1 cup	402	17	85	13	16	2.5	na	0	5%
'Ralston' unprepared	1/4 cup	102	4	22	3	4	0.6	na	0	5%
(Roman Meal)										
w/dates, raisins, almonds, unprepared	1/3 cup	140	4	26	0	3	3.0	0.0	0	18%
w/honey, coconut, almond.	1/3 cup	150	5	21	5	3	6.0	0.0	0	34%
w/rye, bran, flax, unprepared	1/3 cup	116	5	25	5	5	1.7	0.0	0	11%
(Wheatena)										
wheat, unprepared	1 oz	100	3	21	0	4	1.0	0.0	0	9%
'Wheatena' prepared w/water, no salt	1 cup	136	5	29	5	7	1.2	0.2	0	7%
'Wheatena' prepared w/water, no salt	3/4 cup	102	4	21	4	5	0.9	0.1	0	7%

Food Name	Serving Size	Calories	Prot. gms	Carbs gms	Sod. mgs	Fiber gms	Fat gms	Sat. Fat gms	Chol. mgs	% Fat Cal.
'Wheatena' prepared w/water, salt	1 cup	136	5	29	578	7	1.2	0.2	0	7%
'Wheatena' prepared w/water, salt	3/4 cup	102	4	21	433	5	0.9	0.2	0	7%
'Wheatena' unprepared	1 cup	503	18	107	18	18	4.1	0.6	0	7%
'Wheatena' unprepared	1/4 cup	125	5	26	5	4	1.0	0.1	0	7%

CEREAL, READY-TO-EAT
(Arrowhead Mills)

Food Name	Serving Size	Calories	Prot. gms	Carbs gms	Sod. mgs	Fiber gms	Fat gms	Sat. Fat gms	Chol. mgs	% Fat Cal.
bran flakes	1 oz	100	5	21	100	4	1.0	0.0	0	8%
buckwheat groats, brown	2 oz	190	7	41	1	7	1.0	0.0	0	4%
buckwheat groats, white	2 oz	190	7	41	1	7	1.0	0.0	0	4%
corn flakes	1 oz	100	2	25	100	2	0.0	0.0	0	0%
corn flakes, organic	1 cup	130	3	30	65	2	0.0	0.0	0	0%
'Maple Corns'	1 oz	100	3	23	75	3	1.0	0.0	0	8%
'Maple Corns' organic	1 cup	190	5	43	140	6	3.0	0.5	0	12%
multigrain, organic	1 cup	140	3	29	130	3	1.5	0.0	0	10%
'Nature-O's' organic	1 cup	130	5	24	5	3	2.0	0.5	0	13%
oat bran flakes	1 oz	100	5	19	100	3	2.0	0.0	0	16%
oat flakes	2 oz	220	10	39	1	8	4.0	0.0	0	16%
oat groats	2 oz	220	8	38	1	6	4.0	0.0	0	16%
puffed corn	0.5 oz	50	3	11	1	3	0.0	0.0	0	0%
puffed rice	0.5 oz	50	1	12	1	3	0.0	0.0	0	0%
puffed wheat	0.5 oz	50	2	11	1	6	0.0	0.0	0	0%
wheat flakes	2 oz	210	8	42	1	7	1.0	0.0	0	4%

(Barbara's Bakery)

Food Name	Serving Size	Calories	Prot. gms	Carbs gms	Sod. mgs	Fiber gms	Fat gms	Sat. Fat gms	Chol. mgs	% Fat Cal.
raisin bran	1 oz	170	3	36	80	0	1.0	0.0	0	5%
'Shredded Spoonfuls' natural, 97% fat-free	3/4 cup	120	5	23	200	4	1.5	0.0	0	11%
'Shredded Wheat'	2 biscuits	140	4	31	0	5	1.0	0.0	0	6%

(Breadshop)

Food Name	Serving Size	Calories	Prot. gms	Carbs gms	Sod. mgs	Fiber gms	Fat gms	Sat. Fat gms	Chol. mgs	% Fat Cal.
'Almond Raisin' nectarsweet premium	1 oz	120	4	18	2	3	4.0	0.0	0	30%
'Blueberry 'N Cream' nectarsweet gourmet	1 oz	115	4	19	2	3	3.0	0.0	0	23%
'California Orange Crunch' honeysweet premium	1 oz	130	4	18	1	2	5.0	0.0	0	34%
'Cinnapple Spice' honeysweet premium	1 oz	125	3	19	2	2	4.5	0.5	0	32%
'Crunchy Oat Bran' nectarsweet gourmet	1 oz	120	3	18	2	3	5.0	0.5	0	35%
'Golden Maple Nut' honeysweet premium	1 oz	130	4	17	2	2	5.0	0.8	0	35%
'Gone Nuts!' nectarsweet premium	1 oz	125	4	17	2	3	5.0	0.5	0	35%
'Honey Apple Blueberry' honeysweet premium	1 oz	125	4	18	1	3	5.0	0.5	0	34%
'Honey Gone Nuts!' honeysweet premium	1 oz	130	4	18	2	3	5.5	0.5	0	37%
'Orange Almond' nectarsweet premium	1 oz	120	4	18	2	3	4.0	0.5	0	30%
'Oregon Blueberry Crunch' honeysweet gourmet	1 oz	125	4	18	2	3	5.0	0.8	0	34%
'Peaches 'N Cream' nectarsweet gourmet	1 oz	115	4	19	2	3	3.0	0.5	0	23%
'Raspberry 'N Cream' nectarsweet gourmet	1 oz	115	4	19	2	3	3.0	0.5	0	23%
'Strawberry 'N Cream' nectarsweet gourmet	1 oz	110	3	16	5	3	4.0	0.0	0	32%
'Supernatural' honeysweet gourmet	1 oz	100	4	18	2	4	5.0	0.8	0	35%
'Supernatural New England' honeysweet gourmet	1 oz	130	3	18	2	2	5.0	0.5	0	35%
(Eden Foods) 'Puffed Rice' five-flavor	30 puffs	110	3	24	160	2	0.0	0.0	0	0%

(Erewhon)

Food Name	Serving Size	Calories	Prot. gms	Carbs gms	Sod. mgs	Fiber gms	Fat gms	Sat. Fat gms	Chol. mgs	% Fat Cal.
'Aztec' natural, nonfat	1 cup	110	2	26	70	1	0.0	0.0	0	0%
'Banana-O's' organic, natural	3/4 cup	110	2	26	15	2	0.0	0.0	0	8%
'Brown Rice' crispy	1 oz	110	2	24	185	4	1.0	0.0	0	8%
brown rice, crispy, low-sodium	1 oz	110	2	24	5	4	1.0	0.0	0	8%
brown rice, crispy, nonfat	1 cup	110	2	25	180	1	0.0	0.0	0	0%
corn flakes, natural, no sweeteners	3/4 cup	100	2	22	50	1	1.0	0.0	0	9%
'Crisp Rice' brown, natural	1 cup	110	2	25	180	1	0.0	0.0	0	0%
'Fruit 'N Wheat'	1 oz	100	2	21	75	3	1.0	0.0	0	9%
'Galaxy Grahams' natural, organic	3/4 cup	100	3	23	60	2	0.5	0.0	0	4%

Food Name	Serving Size	Calories	Prot. gms	Carbs gms	Sod. mgs	Fiber gms	Fat gms	Sat. Fat gms	Chol. mgs	% Fat Cal.
kamut flakes	3/4 cup	90	4	18	60	0	0.0	0.0	0	0%
'Poppets' natural, organic	1 cup	120	2	25	10	0	1.0	0.0	0	8%
raisin bran	1 oz	100	3	22	80	3	0.0	0.0	0	0%
raisin bran, high-fiber, low-fat, low-sodium	1 cup	170	5	40	100	6	1.0	0.0	0	5%
'Raisin Grahams' natural, nonfat, low-sodium	3/4 cup	100	4	23	55	3	0.0	0.0	0	0%
'Right Start'	1 oz	90	3	24	80	5	0.0	0.0	0	0%
'Right Start w/Raisins'	1 oz	90	3	22	80	5	0.0	0.0	0	0%
'Wheat Flakes'	1 oz	110	3	22	75	4	0.0	0.0	0	0%
'Super O's'	1 oz	110	3	24	5	4	0.0	0.0	0	0%
(General Mills)										
'Addam's Family'	1 oz	110	1	25	65	0	1.0	0.0	0	8%
'Basic 4'	1 cup	201	4	42	323	3	2.8	0.4	0	13%
'Batman Returns'	1 oz	110	1	26	190	0	0.0	0.0	0	0%
'Berry Berry Kix'	3/4 cup	120	1	26	185	0	1.2	0.2	0	9%
'Body Buddies'	1 cup	115	2	26	288	1	0.9	0.2	0	7%
'Boo Berry'	1 cup	116	1	27	214	0	0.5	0.1	0	4%
'Bunuelitos'	1 oz	120	1	25	120	0	2.0	0.0	0	15%
'Cheerios'	1 cup	110	3	23	284	3	1.8	0.4	0	15%
'Cheerios' apple cinnamon	3/4 cup	118	2	25	150	2	1.6	0.3	0	12%
'Cheerios' apple cinnamon, breakfast pack	1-oz box	120	2	24	200	2	2.0	0.0	0	15%
'Cheerios' honey nut	1 cup	115	3	24	259	2	1.2	0.2	0	10%
'Cheerios' multigrain	1 cup	112	3	24	254	2	1.1	0.2	0	9%
'Cheerios Plus' multigrain	1 cup	108	3	24	201	3	1.1	0.2	0	9%
'Cheerios-To-Go' apple cinnamon	1 pouch	110	2	22	180	2	2.0	0.0	0	16%
'Cheerios-To-Go' honey nut	1 pouch	110	3	23	250	2	1.0	0.0	0	8%
'Cheerios-To-Go'	1 pouch	80	3	15	220	2	2.0	0.0	0	20%
'Chex' corn	1 cup	113	2	26	289	1	0.4	0.1	0	3%
'Chex' honey nut	3/4 cup	117	2	26	224	0	0.7	0.1	0	5%
'Chex' multi-bran	1 cup	165	4	41	325	6	1.2	0.2	0	7%
'Chex' rice	1.25 cup	117	2	27	291	0	0.2	0.0	0	1%
'Chex' wheat	1 cup	104	3	24	269	3	0.7	0.1	0	6%
'Cinnamon Streusel' Betty Crocker	3/4 cup	120	2	25	167	1	1.3	0.3	0	10%
'Cinnamon Toast Crunch'	3/4 cup	124	2	24	210	2	3.0	0.5	0	22%
'Cocoa Puffs'	1 cup	119	1	27	181	0	0.9	0.2	0	7%
'Cookie-Crisp'	1 cup	120	2	26	207	0	1.1	0.6	0	8%
'Corn Flakes'	1 cup	98	2	22	239	0	0.1	na	0	1%
'Count Chocula'	1 cup	117	1	26	209	0	0.9	0.2	0	7%
'Country Corn Flakes'	1 cup	114	2	26	284	0	0.5	0.1	0	4%
'Crispy Wheats 'N Raisins'	1 cup	191	4	44	285	3	0.8	0.2	0	4%
'Crunchy Bran'	3/4 cup	90	2	23	253	5	0.9	0.2	0	9%
'Dutch Apple' Betty Crocker	1 cup	219	4	46	309	2	2.0	0.4	0	8%
'Fiber One'	1/2 cup	62	3	24	143	14	0.8	0.1	0	12%
'Fingos' cinnamon	1 oz	110	1	22	170	2	3.0	0.0	0	23%
'Fingos' honey toasted oat	1 oz	110	2	21	210	2	3.0	0.0	0	23%
'40% Bran Flakes'	1 cup	159	6	39	456	7	0.7	na	0	4%
'Frankenberry'	1 cup	117	1	27	209	0	0.5	0.1	0	4%
'Golden Grahams'	3/4 cup	116	2	26	275	1	1.1	0.2	0	8%
'Hidden Treasures' fruit juice added	3/4 cup	120	1	25	140	0	2.0	0.0	0	15%
'Honey Almond Delight'	1 oz	110	2	23	200	1	2.0	0.0	0	15%
'Honey Frosted Wheaties'	3/4 cup	110	2	26	211	2	0.3	0.1	0	2%
'Honey Nut Clusters'	1 cup	213	5	43	239	4	3.5	0.4	0	15%
'Kaboom'	1.25 cup	118	3	24	275	2	1.1	0.2	0	9%
'Kix'	1 1/3 cup	114	2	26	263	1	0.6	0.2	0	5%
'Lucky Charms'	1 cup	116	2	25	203	1	1.1	0.2	0	8%

Food Name	Serving Size	Calories	Prot. gms	Carbs gms	Sod. mgs	Fiber gms	Fat gms	Sat. Fat gms	Chol. mgs	% Fat Cal.
'Muesli' apple almond	1.45 oz	150	4	31	140	3	2.0	0.0	0	11%
'Muesli' banana walnut	1.45 oz	150	4	30	150	3	3.0	0.0	0	17%
'Muesli' cranberry walnut	1.45 oz	150	4	30	95	3	3.0	0.0	0	17%
'Muesli' date almond	1.45 oz	140	4	32	95	3	2.0	0.0	0	11%
'Muesli' peach pecan	1.45 oz	150	4	30	150	3	3.0	0.0	0	17%
'Muesli' raspberry almond	1.45 oz	150	4	30	140	3	3.0	0.0	0	17%
'Nature Valley Granola' cinnamon and raisin	3/4 cup	235	5	38	88	3	7.7	1.0	0	29%
'Nature Valley Granola' fruit, low-fat	2/3 cup	212	5	44	205	3	3.0	0.4	0	13%
'Nature Valley Granola' fruit and nut	2/3 cup	253	6	34	77	3	11.2	1.9	0	40%
'Nature Valley Granola' fruit and nut	1/3 cup	130	2	19	45	1	5.0	0.0	0	35%
'Nature Valley Granola' toasted oats	3/4 cup	248	6	36	89	4	9.7	1.3	0	35%
'Nature Valley Granola' toasted oats	1/3 cup	130	2	20	50	1	5.0	0.0	0	34%
'Oatmeal Crisp w/Almonds'	1 cup	219	6	42	250	4	4.6	0.6	0	19%
'Oatmeal Crisp w/Apples'	1 cup	205	4	46	282	4	1.8	0.4	0	8%
'Oatmeal Raisin Crisp'	1 cup	204	4	44	224	4	2.4	0.4	0	11%
'Raisin Bran'	1 cup	178	4	46	486	8	0.3	0.0	0	1%
'Raisin Bran'	1-1/3 oz box	120	3	31	328	5	0.2	0.0	0	1%
'Raisin Nut Bran'	1 cup	209	5	41	246	5	4.4	0.7	0	19%
'Reese's Peanut Butter Puffs'	3/4 cup	129	3	23	177	0	3.2	0.6	0	22%
'Ripple Crisp'	1 oz	110	1	24	280	1	1.0	0.0	0	8%
'Ripple Crisp' honey bran	1 oz	100	2	24	210	3	1.0	0.0	0	8%
'S'Mores Grahams'	3/4 cup	117	2	26	212	1	1.2	0.2	0	9%
'Sprinkle Spangles' corn puffs w/sprinkles	1 oz	110	1	25	130	0	1.0	0.0	0	8%
'Sugar Frosted Flakes'	1 cup	149	2	34	247	1	0.5	0.3	0	3%
'Sun Crunchers'	1 cup	216	5	44	380	2	3.2	0.3	0	13%
'Sunflakes' multigrain	1 oz	100	2	24	240	0	1.0	0.0	0	8%
'Team Cheerios'	1 cup	113	2	25	224	2	1.1	0.2	na	9%
'Teenage Mutant Ninja Turtles'	1 oz	110	1	26	190	0	0.0	0.0	0	0%
'Total'	3/4 cup	105	3	24	199	3	0.7	0.2	0	6%
'Total Corn Flakes'	1 1/3 cup	112	2	26	203	1	0.5	0.2	0	4%
'Total Raisin Bran'	1 cup	178	4	43	240	5	1.0	0.2	0	5%
'Triples'	1 cup	116	2	25	191	1	1.0	0.3	0	8%
'Trix'	1 cup	122	1	26	197	1	1.7	0.4	0	13%
'Urkel-O's'	1 oz	110	1	25	160	0	1.0	0.0	0	8%
'Wheaties'	1 cup	110	3	24	222	2	0.9	0.2	0	8%
'Wheaties' honey gold'	3/4 cup	100	2	25	200	1	1.0	0.0	0	8%
(Glenny's)										
'Maple Frosted Corn' mini puffs	1 oz	109	4	20	50	0	0.5	0.0	0	4%
'Oat Mini Puffs'	1 oz	108	5	22	30	0	0.5	0.0	0	4%
'Oat Mini Puffs' no salt, no sugar	1 oz	108	5	22	7	0	0.5	0.0	0	4%
'Rice Mini Puffs'	1 oz	109	4	20	30	0	0.5	0.0	0	4%
(Golden Temple)										
'Almond Raisin' low-fat	1 oz	110	2	22	57	2	1.5	0.5	0	12%
'Apple Cinnamon' low-fat	1 oz	110	2	22	59	2	1.5	0.5	0	12%
'Cashew Almond Granola'	1 oz	129	4	19	3	4	3.5	0.5	0	26%
'Cinnamon & Spice Crunch' psyllium and chia seed	1 oz	132	3	20	26	2	4.5	0.5	0	31%
'Cinnamon Granola' apple and raisin	1 oz	125	3	20	3	2	3.5	0.5	0	26%
'Coconut Almond Granola'	1 oz	145	4	18	26	3	7.0	2.0	0	42%
'Fruit 'N Nut Granola'	1 oz	129	3	19	26	2	4.5	0.5	0	32%
'Golden Granola'	1 oz	138	4	19	25	2	6.0	1.0	0	37%
'Hawaiian Granola'	1 oz	126	4	19	3	2	4.0	1.0	0	28%
'Hazelnut Boysenberry' organic oats	1 oz	135	4	19	2	3	5.5	0.5	0	35%
'High-Protein Granola'	1 oz	124	4	19	6	2	3.5	0.5	0	26%
'Honey Almond Granola'	1 oz	130	4	20	25	3	3.5	0.5	0	25%

Food Name	Serving Size	Calories	Prot. gms	Carbs gms	Sod. mgs	Fiber gms	Fat gms	Sat. Fat gms	Chol. mgs	% Fat Cal.
'Honey Blueberry Granola' apple	1 oz	128	4	20	2	2	3.5	0.5	0	25%
'Lite 'N Crunchy Granola'	1 oz	129	4	19	9	2	4.5	0.5	0	31%
'Lite Muesli'	1 oz	102	3	20	60	2	1.0	0.0	0	9%
'Maple Almond Granola'	1 oz	129	4	20	25	2	3.5	0.5	0	25%
'Natural Blueberry Granola'	1 oz	132	4	19	3	2	5.0	1.0	0	33%
'Natural Blueberry Granola' coconut-free	1 oz	131	4	19	3	2	4.5	0.5	0	31%
'Natural Delite Granola'	1 oz	128	3	20	26	2	3.5	0.5	0	26%
'Natural Foods' almond and raisin, lowfat	1 oz	110	3	22	3	2	1.0	0.0	0	8%
'Natural Foods' apple and cinnamon, lowfat	1 oz	110	3	22	3	2	1.0	0.0	0	8%
'Natural Foods' strawberry and raspberry, lowfat	1 oz	111	3	22	3	2	1.0	0.0	0	8%
'Oat Bran Almond'	1 oz	120	4	20	3	3	3.5	0.5	0	25%
'Oat Bran Apple'	1 oz	112	4	19	3	3	3.5	0.5	0	26%
'Oat Bran Granola' berries	1 oz	120	4	20	3	3	3.5	0.5	0	25%
'Oat Bran Granola' raisins and almonds	1 oz	119	3	19	3	3	3.5	0.5	0	26%
'Oat Bran Muesli' dates and almonds	1 oz	108	3	21	79	2	1.5	0.0	0	12%
'Oat Bran Muesli' raisins and hazelnut	1 oz	102	3	20	59	3	1.5	0.0	0	13%
'Oat Bran Oregonberry'	1 oz	116	4	20	3	3	3.5	0.5	0	25%
'100% Natural Almond'	1 oz	123	3	18	15	2	4.0	1.0	0	30%
'100% Natural Apple/Cinnamon'	1 oz	120	3	18	14	2	4.0	1.0	0	30%
'100% Natural Oat Bran'	1 oz	70	5	19	1	5	2.5	0.5	0	19%
'100% Natural Raisin/Almond'	1 oz	120	3	19	7	2	4.0	1.0	0	29%
'Orange Almond Granola'	1 oz	133	4	19	25	2	4.0	1.0	0	28%
'Raisin Granola' apricot and dates	1 oz	127	3	20	25	2	3.5	0.5	0	26%
'Six-Grain Crisp' fruit and flaxseed	1 oz	118	3	20	73	2	3.5	0.5	0	26%
'Super Nutty Granola'	1 oz	135	4	19	25	3	5.0	1.0	0	33%
'Sweet Home Farm Almond'	1 oz	123	3	18	14	2	4.0	1.0	0	30%
'Sweet Home Farm Granola' lowfat	1 oz	110	3	22	65	2	2.0	0.5	0	15%
'Sweet Home Farm Muesli' crunchy, lowfat	1 oz	105	3	21	98	2	2.0	0.5	0	16%
'Sweet Home Farm Raisin'	1 oz	120	3	19	13	2	4.0	1.0	0	29%
'Swiss Style Muesli'	1 oz	105	3	19	15	3	1.5	0.0	0	13%
'35% Fruit Muesli'	1 oz	97	3	19	16	3	1.0	0.0	0	9%
(Health Valley)										
'Almond Flavor O's' fat-free	1 oz	90	3	19	5	5	0.0	0.0	0	0%
granola, date and almond flavor, nonfat	1 oz	90	2	21	20	3	0.0	0.0	0	0%
granola, raisin cinnamon, nonfat	1 oz	90	2	21	20	3	0.0	0.0	0	0%
granola, tropical fruit, nonfat	1 oz	90	2	21	20	3	0.0	0.0	0	0%
'High-Fiber O's, nonfat'	1 oz	90	3	19	5	5	0.0	0.0	0	0%
'100% Organic Blue Corn Flakes'	1 oz	90	3	19	10	3	1.0	0.0	0	9%
'Organic Amaranth Flakes'	1 oz	90	3	20	10	3	0.0	0.0	0	0%
'Sprouts 7' bananas and Hawaiian fruit, nonfat	1 oz	90	3	16	0	4	0.0	0.0	0	0%
'Sprouts 7' raisins, nonfat	1 oz	90	4	16	0	5	0.0	0.0	0	0%
(Heartland)										
'Heartland Natural' plain	1 cup	499	12	79	293	7	17.7	4.5	0	31%
'Heartland Natural, plain	1 oz	123	3	19	72	2	4.4	1.1	0	31%
'Heartland Natural' w/coconut	1 cup	463	11	71	213	7	17.1	6.2	0	32%
'Heartland Natural' w/coconut	1 oz	125	3	19	58	2	4.6	1.7	0	32%
'Heartland Natural' w/raisins	1 cup	468	11	76	226	6	15.6	4.0	0	29%
(Honeybran)										
'Honeybran'	1 cup	119	3	29	202	4	0.7	0.3	0	5%
'Honeybran'	1 oz	97	2	23	164	3	0.6	0.2	0	5%
(Kashi)										
'Multigrain' medley	1 oz	100	4	20	50	2	1.0	0.0	0	9%
'Puffed' honey, no refined sugars, no added oils	2 oz	120	3	25	6	2	1.0	0.0	0	7%
'Puffed' sodium-free	2 oz	70	3	19	0	2	1.0	0.0	0	9%

Food Name	Serving Size	Calories	Prot. gms	Carbs gms	Sod. mgs	Fiber gms	Fat gms	Sat. Fat gms	Chol. mgs	% Fat Cal.
(Kellogg's)										
'All-Bran'	1/2 cup	79	4	23	61	10	0.9	0.2	0	11%
'All-Bran Bran Buds'	1/3 cup	83	3	24	200	12	0.7	0.1	0	8%
'All-Bran' w/extra fiber	1/2 cup	53	4	23	127	15	0.9	0.2	0	16%
'Apple Jacks'	1 cup	116	1	27	134	1	0.4	0.1	0	3%
'Apple Raisin Crisp'	1 cup	185	3	47	373	4	0.5	0.1	0	2%
'Bran Flakes'	3/4 cup	95	3	23	226	5	0.6	0.1	0	6%
'Cinnamon Mini Buns'	3/4 cup	115	1	27	208	1	0.6	0.1	0	5%
'Cocoa Frosted Flakes'	3/4 cup	120	1	28	208	0	0.5	0.4	0	4%
'Cocoa Krispies'	3/4 cup	120	2	27	210	0	0.8	0.6	0	6%
'Common Sense Oat Bran Flakes'	3/4 cup	109	4	23	270	4	1.2	0.4	0	10%
'Corn Flakes'	1 cup	102	2	24	298	1	0.2	0.1	0	2%
'Corn Pops'	1 cup	118	1	28	123	0	0.2	0.1	0	1%
'Cracklin' Oat Bran'	3/4 cup	225	5	40	195	7	7.0	2.9	0	28%
'Crispix'	1 cup	108	2	25	240	1	0.3	0.1	0	2%
'Double Dip Crunch'	3/4 cup	115	1	27	176	0	0.1	0.0	0	1%
'Fiberwise'	1 oz	90	3	23	140	5	1.0	0.0	0	8%
'Froot Loops'	1 cup	117	1	26	141	1	0.9	0.4	0	7%
'Frosted Bran'	3/4 cup	101	2	25	206	3	0.3	0.0	0	3%
'Frosted Flakes'	3/4 cup	119	1	28	200	1	0.2	0.1	0	1%
'Frosted Krispies'	3/4 cup	113	1	27	219	0	0.2	0.1	0	2%
'Frosted Mini-Wheats' bite size	1 cup	187	5	45	2	6	0.9	0.2	0	5%
'Frosted Mini-Wheats' regular	1 cup	173	5	42	2	5	0.8	0.2	0	4%
'Fruity Marshmallow Krispies'	3/4 cup	113	1	27	179	0	0.1	0.0	0	1%
granola, w/o raisins, low-fat	1/2 cup	213	5	44	135	3	3.2	0.5	0	14%
granola, w/raisins, low-fat	2/3 cup	202	5	44	124	3	2.8	0.9	0	12%
'Healthy Choice Almond Crunch with Raisins'	1 cup	198	5	43	215	5	2.6	0.4	0	12%
'Healthy Choice Multigrain' clusters w/raisins and almonds	1 1/4 cup	200	4	44	240	4	2.0	0.0	0	9%
'Healthy Choice Multigrain' flakes w/brown sugar	1 cup	110	3	26	210	3	0.0	0.0	0	0%
'Healthy Choice Multigrain' flakes	1 cup	104	3	25	174	3	0.4	0.0	0	3%
'Healthy Choice Multigrain' squares w/honey	1 1/4 cup	190	5	45	0	6	1.0	0.0	0	4%
'Healthy Choice Toasted Brown Sugar Squares'	1.25 cup	189	5	45	2	5	1.0	0.2	0	5%
'Honey Crunch Corn Flakes'	3/4 cup	115	2	26	216	1	0.9	0.1	0	7%
'Just Right' fruit and nut	1 cup	193	4	44	266	3	1.6	0.3	0	7%
'Just Right' w/crunchy nuggets	1 cup	204	4	46	338	3	1.5	0.1	0	7%
'Kenmei Rice Bran'	3/4 cup	110	2	24	230	1	1.0	0.0	0	8%
'Mini-Wheats' apple cinnamon	3/4 cup	182	4	44	20	5	1.0	0.2	0	5%
'Mini-Wheats' blueberry	3/4 cup	182	4	44	20	5	1.0	0.2	0	5%
'Mini-Wheats' raisin	3/4 cup	187	4	43	3	5	1.5	0.2	0	7%
'Mini-Wheats' strawberry	1 cup	187	4	43	17	5	1.3	0.2	0	6%
'Mueslix' apple and orange crunch	3/4 cup	211	5	41	270	5	5.0	1.0	0	21%
'Mueslix' raisin and almond crunch, w/dates	2/3 cup	200	4	40	160	4	3.2	0.4	0	15%
'Nut & Honey Crunch'	1.25 cup	223	4	46	370	1	2.5	0.5	0	10%
'Nutri-Grain Raisin Bran'	1 cup	130	4	31	200	5	1.0	0.0	0	6%
'Nutri-Grain Wheat'	3/4 cup	101	3	24	221	4	1.0	0.1	0	9%
'Oatbake Honey Bran'	1/3 cup	110	2	21	190	3	3.0	1.0	0	23%
'Oatbake Raisin Nut'	1 oz	110	2	21	190	3	3.0	1.0	0	23%
'Pop Tarts Crunch' cinnamon, brown sugar, frosted	3/4 cup	120	1	26	160	1	1.0	0.0	0	8%
'Pop-Tarts Crunch' strawberry, frosted	3/4 cup	118	1	27	114	0	0.8	0.3	0	6%
'Product 19'	1 cup	110	3	25	216	1	0.4	0.0	0	3%
'Raisin Bran'	1 cup	186	6	47	354	8	1.5	0.0	0	7%
'Razzle Dazzle Rice Krispies'	3/4 cup	108	1	25	166	0	0.3	0.1	0	2%
'Rice Krispies'	1.25 cup	124	2	29	354	0	0.4	0.1	0	3%

Food Name	Serving Size	Calories	Prot. gms	Carbs gms	Sod. mgs	Fiber gms	Fat gms	Sat. Fat gms	Chol. mgs	% Fat Cal.
'Rice Krispies' apple cinnamon	3/4 cup	112	2	27	223	0	0.1	0.0	0	1%
'Rice Krispies Treats'	3/4 cup	120	1	26	190	0	1.6	0.4	0	12%
'Smacks'	3/4 cup	103	2	24	51	1	0.5	0.3	0	5%
'Smart Start'	1 cup	183	3	43	313	2	0.7	0.1	0	3%
'Special K'	1 cup	115	6	22	250	1	0.3	0.0	0	2%
'Temptations' French vanilla almond	3/4 cup	119	2	25	207	1	1.6	1.1	0	12%
'Temptations' honey roasted pecan	1 cup	122	2	24	248	1	2.3	0.5	0	17%
'Whole Grain Shredded Wheat'	1 oz	90	3	23	0	4	0.0	0.0	0	0%
(Kolln) 'Oat Bran Crunch'	1 oz	100	5	20	0	0	2.0	0.0	0	15%
(Krusteaz)										
'Corn Flakes'	1 oz	110	2	24	280	1	1.0	0.0	0	8%
'Crisp Rice'	1 oz	110	2	25	270	1	0.0	0.0	0	0%
'Fruit Whirls'	1 oz	110	1	25	120	1	1.0	0.0	0	8%
'Honey Nut O's'	1 oz	110	3	23	190	2	1.0	0.0	0	8%
'Raisin Bran'	3/4 cup	120	3	30	210	4	1.0	0.0	0	6%
'Sugar Frosted Flakes'	1 oz	110	1	26	230	1	0.0	0.0	0	0%
'Toasted Oats'	1 oz	110	4	22	290	2	1.0	0.0	0	8%
(Lundberg Family) 'Crunchies' brown rice	1 cup	171	3	38	7	0	0.8	0.0	0	4%
(Malt-O-Meal)										
'Apple & Cinnamon Toasted Oat'	1 oz	110	2	22	180	1	2.0	0.0	0	16%
'Berry Colossal Crunch'	3/4 cup	120	1	26	220	1	1.7	0.4	0	13%
'Bran Flakes'	1 oz	90	3	23	210	5	1.0	0.0	0	8%
'Colossal Crunch'	3/4 cup	120	1	26	230	1	1.7	0.4	0	13%
'Corn Bursts'	1 cup	118	1	29	122	0	0.1	0.1	0	1%
'Corn Flakes'	1 oz	110	2	25	290	1	0.0	0.0	0	0%
'Crisp 'N' Crackling Rice'	1 oz	110	2	25	240	0	0.0	0.0	0	0%
'Crispy Rice'	1 cup	125	2	29	320	0	0.4	0.1	0	3%
'Fruit & Frosted O's' multigrain	1 oz	110	2	25	120	1	1.0	0.0	0	8%
'Honey & Nut Toasted Oat'	1 oz	110	3	23	190	2	1.0	0.0	0	8%
'Marshmallow Mateys'	1 cup	115	2	25	211	1	1.0	0.2	0	8%
'Puffed Rice'	0.5 oz	50	1	12	0	0	0.0	0.0	0	0%
'Puffed Wheat'	0.5 oz	50	2	10	0	1	0.0	0.0	0	0%
'Raisin Bran Flakes'	1.4 oz	130	3	30	200	5	2.0	0.0	0	12%
'Sugar Frosted Flakes'	1 oz	110	1	26	170	1	0.0	0.0	0	0%
'Sugar Puffs'	1 oz	110	2	25	25	0	0.0	0.0	0	0%
'Sweetened Puffed Wheat'	1 oz	110	2	25	25	1	0.0	0.0	0	0%
'Toasted Oats'	1 oz	110	4	20	240	2	2.0	0.0	0	16%
'Toasty O's'	1 cup	112	3	22	284	3	1.8	0.4	0	15%
'Tootie Fruities'	1 cup	125	2	28	149	1	1.0	0.3	0	7%
(Nabisco)										
'Fruit Wheats' apple	1 oz	90	2	23	15	3	0.0	0.0	0	0%
'Team Flakes'	1 oz	110	2	24	180	0	1.0	0.0	0	8%
(Nature Valley) See under General Mills.										
(Nature's Path) 'Heritage O's'	1 cup	165	5	34	140	5	1.0	0.0	0	5%
(Perky's) 'Rice' nutty	1/2 cup	210	4	47	110	2	1.5	0.0	0	6%
(Post)										
'Alpha-Bits' w/marshmallows	1 cup	115	2	25	206	0	1.0	0.2	0	7%
'Banana Nut Crunch'	1 cup	249	5	44	253	4	6.1	0.8	0	22%
'Blueberry Morning'	1.25 cup	211	4	43	266	2	2.5	0.3	0	11%
'Bran Flakes'	3/4 cup	96	3	24	220	5	0.7	0.1	0	6%
'C.W. Post Hearty Granola'	1 oz	130	2	21	80	0	4.0	0.0	0	28%
'Cocoa Pebbles'	3/4 cup	115	1	25	157	0	1.2	1.1	0	10%
'Dino Pebbles'	1 oz	110	1	25	150	0	1.0	0.0	0	8%
'Frosted Alpha-Bits'	1 cup	130	3	27	212	1	1.3	0.3	0	9%

Food Name	Serving Size	Calories	Prot. gms	Carbs gms	Sod. mgs	Fiber gms	Fat gms	Sat. Fat gms	Chol. mgs	% Fat Cal.
'Frosted Shredded Wheat' bite size	1 cup	183	4	44	10	5	1.0	0.2	0	5%
'Fruit & Fibre' tropical fruit	1.25 oz	120	3	27	170	5	3.0	0.0	0	18%
'Fruit & Fibre' w/dates, raisins and walnuts	1 cup	212	4	42	280	5	3.1	0.4	0	13%
'Fruity Pebbles'	3/4 cup	108	1	24	158	0	1.1	0.2	0	9%
'Golden Crisp'	3/4 cup	107	1	25	41	0	0.4	0.1	0	3%
'Grape-Nuts'	1/2 cup	208	6	47	354	5	1.1	0.2	0	5%
'Grape-Nuts Flakes'	3/4 cup	106	3	24	140	3	0.8	0.2	0	7%
'Great Grains' crunchy pecan	2/3 cup	216	5	38	214	4	6.3	0.7	0	26%
'Great Grains' double pecan	1 oz	120	3	20	60	3	3.0	0.0	0	23%
'Great Grains' raisin, date, and pecan	2/3 cup	204	4	40	156	4	4.5	0.6	0	20%
'Honey Bunches Of Oats'	3/4 cup	118	2	25	193	1	1.6	0.2	0	13%
'Honey Bunches Of Oats' w/almonds	3/4 cup	126	2	24	187	1	2.6	0.3	0	19%
'Honeycomb'	1 1/3 cup	115	2	26	215	1	0.6	0.2	0	5%
'Oat Flakes'	1 oz	110	4	21	130	2	1.0	0.0	0	8%
'100% Bran'	1/3 cup	83	4	23	121	8	0.6	0.1	0	7%
'Oreo O's'	3/4 cup	112	1	22	128	1	2.4	0.4	0	19%
'Raisin Bran'	1 cup	187	5	46	360	8	1.1	0.2	0	5%
'Raisin Grape-Nuts'	1 oz	100	3	23	140	2	0.0	0.0	0	0%
'Shredded Wheat' original	2 biscuits	156	5	38	3	5	0.6	0.1	0	3%
'Shredded Wheat' spoon size	1 cup	167	5	41	3	6	0.5	0.1	0	3%
'Shredded Wheat N Bran' original	1.25 cup	197	7	47	3	8	0.8	0.1	0	4%
'Smurf-Magic Berries'	1 oz	120	2	26	60	0	1.0	0.0	0	7%
'Toasties' corn flakes	1 cup	101	2	24	266	1	0.0	0.0	0	0%
'Waffle Crisp'	1 cup	129	2	24	130	1	2.9	0.4	0	21%
(Quaker)										
'Apple Zaps'	3/4 cup	118	1	27	132	1	1.0	0.3	0	8%
'Cap'n Crunch'	3/4 cup	107	1	23	208	1	1.4	0.4	0	11%
'Cap'n Crunch's Crunchberries'	3/4 cup	104	1	22	190	1	1.3	0.3	0	11%
'Cap'n Crunch's Peanut Butter Crunch'	3/4 cup	112	2	22	204	1	2.3	0.5	0	19%
'Cinnamon Life'	1 cup	190	4	40	220	3	1.7	0.3	0	8%
'Cinnamon Oatmeal Squares'	1 cup	232	8	47	266	5	2.6	0.5	0	10%
'Cocoa Blasts'	1 cup	129	1	29	133	1	1.2	0.4	0	8%
'Corn Blasts'	1 cup	133	1	28	240	1	1.9	0.5	0	13%
'Frosted Flakers'	3/4 cup	117	1	28	281	1	0.2	0.0	0	2%
'Fruitangy Oh!s'	1 cup	122	2	27	152	1	1.1	0.3	0	8%
'Honey Graham Oh!'	3/4 cup	112	1	23	178	1	1.9	0.6	0	15%
'King Vitaman'	1.25 cup	120	2	26	260	1	1.1	0.3	0	8%
'Kretschmer Honey Crunch Wheat Germ'	1 2/3 tbsp	52	4	8	2	1	1.1	0.2	0	19%
'Marshmallow Safari'	3/4 cup	119	2	25	192	1	1.5	0.4	0	11%
'Oat Bran'	1.25 cup	213	9	41	205	6	2.9	0.5	0	12%
'Oat Life, Plain'	3/4 cup	121	3	25	174	2	1.3	0.2	0	9%
'Oatmeal Squares'	1 cup	216	7	43	263	4	2.6	0.5	0	11%
'100% Natural,' oats, honey, and raisins	1/2 cup	218	5	36	11	4	7.3	3.2	1	30%
'100% Natural,' oats and honey'	1/2 cup	213	5	33	13	4	7.9	3.5	0	33%
'100% Natural,' whole grain w/raisins, lowfat	1/2 cup	195	4	40	129	3	2.7	0.8	1	12%
'Puffed Rice'	1 cup	54	1	12	1	0	0.1	0.0	0	2%
'Puffed Wheat'	1.25 cup	55	2	11	1	1	0.3	0.1	0	5%
'Quisp'	1 cup	109	1	23	194	1	1.5	0.4	0	12%
'Sun Country Granola' w/almonds'	1/2 cup	266	7	38	19	3	10.3	1.3	0	35%
'Sun Country Granola' w/raisins and dates	1/2 cup	135	3	22	8	2	4.2	0.6	0	28%
'Toasted Oatmeal' honey nut	1 cup	191	5	39	166	3	2.7	0.5	0	13%
'Toasted Oatmeal' original	1 oz	100	3	22	160	2	1.0	0.2	0	8%
(Rainforest Flake)										
flakes w/cashews, Brazil nuts, and raisins	4 oz	230	7	35	40	5	8.0	1.0	0	30%

Food Name	Serving Size	Calories	Prot. gms	Carbs gms	Sod. mgs	Fiber gms	Fat gms	Sat. Fat gms	Chol. mgs	% Fat Cal.
'Honey Nut Clusters' lowfat	4 oz	210	4	45	200	4	1.5	0.0	0	6%
(Ralston Purina) See under *(General Mills)*.										
(Rice Krinkles)										
'Frosted Rice Krinkles'	1 cup	173	2	41	284	0	0.1	0.0	0	0%
'Frosted Rice Krinkles' single serving box	0.75 oz	82	1	19	134	0	0.0	0.0	0	0%
(Stone-Buhr)										
'Cereal Mates' 4-grain	1/3 cup	140	6	31	0	5	1.5	0.0	0	8%
'Cereal Mates' 7-grain	1/3 cup	140	6	31	0	7	2.0	0.0	0	11%
(Sunbelt)										
granola, banana almond	1 oz	130	3	20	25	0	4.0	0.0	2	28%
granola, fruit and nut	1 oz	120	3	19	20	0	5.0	0.0	0	34%
(US Mills) 'Uncle Sam'	1 oz	110	4	20	65	7	1.0	0.0	0	9%
(Wonder)										
'Apple Cinnamon Corn Flakes'	1 oz	110	2	25	200	0	0.0	0.0	0	0%
'Crunch Graham Oat Rings'	1 oz	110	2	24	125	0	1.0	0.0	0	8%
'Honey Nut Crispy Rice'	1 oz	110	2	25	205	0	1.0	0.0	0	8%
CEREAL BAR. See GRANOLA/CEREAL BAR.										
CEREAL GRAIN BEVERAGE. See COFFEE SUBSTITUTE.										
CEREAL SNACK. See also GRANOLA/CEREAL BAR.										
(Barbara's Bakery)										
chocolate chip, 'Grrr-nola Treat'	1 serving	80	1	15	5	1	2.0	0.0	0	22%
peanut butter and jelly, 'Grrr-nola Treat'	1 serving	80	1	14	5	1	3.0	0.0	0	31%
(General Mills)										
'Cheerios-to-Go' apple cinnamon	1 pouch	110	2	22	180	2	2.0	0.0	0	16%
'Cheerios-to-Go' honey nut	1 pouch	110	3	23	250	2	1.0	0.0	0	8%
'Cheerios-to-Go' plain	1 pouch	80	3	15	220	2	2.0	0.0	0	20%
'Fingos' cinnamon	1 oz	110	1	22	170	2	3.0	0.0	0	23%
'Fingos' honey toasted oat	1 oz	110	2	21	210	2	3.0	0.0	0	23%
(Natural Nectar)										
granola, almond butter crunch 'Nectar Nuggets'	1 cup	120	3	11	30	5	7.0	0.0	0	53%
granola, almond cappuccino crunch 'Nectar Nuggets'	1 cup	110	2	14	30	5	5.0	0.0	0	41%
granola, coconut almond crunch, 'Nectar Nuggets'	1 cup	110	2	15	20	4	5.0	0.0	0	40%
granola, peanut butter crunch, 'Nectar Nuggets'	1 cup	120	4	11	30	5	7.0	0.0	0	51%
(Nature Valley)										
granola, apple-cinnamon, 'Granola Bites'	1 pouch	170	3	25	100	2	7.0	0.0	0	36%
granola, honey nut, 'Granola Bites'	1 pkg	170	3	24	120	2	8.0	1.0	0	40%
granola, variety pack, 'Granola Bites'	1 pkg	170	3	24	120	2	8.0	1.0	0	40%
(Nature's Choice)										
granola, chocolate chip, 'Grrr-Nola Treats'	0.75 oz	80	1	15	5	0	2.0	0.0	0	22%
granola, cinnamon toast, 'Grrr-Nola Treats'	0.75 oz	80	1	15	5	0	2.0	0.0	0	22%
granola, peanut butter and jelly, 'Grrr-Nola Treats'	0.75 oz	80	1	14	5	0	3.0	0.0	0	31%
granola, tutti-frutti, 'Grrr-Nola Treats'	0.75 oz	75	1	15	5	0	2.0	0.0	0	22%
CHARD. See SWISS CHARD.										
CHAYOTE										
Fresh										
boiled, drained, chopped, 1-inch pieces	1 cup	38	1	8	2	4	0.8	0.1	0	17%
raw, chopped, 1-inch pieces	1 cup	25	1	6	3	2	0.2	0.0	0	6%
raw, whole, 5.75-inches	1 chayote	39	2	9	4	3	0.3	0.1	0	6%
CHEDDARWURST. See under SAUSAGE, CHEESE.										
CHEESE. See also CHEESE FOOD; CHEESE PRODUCT; CHEESE SPREAD; CHEESE SUBSTITUTE.										
AMERICAN										
pasteurized, process	1 oz	106	6	0	184	0	8.9	5.6	27	73%
pasteurized process, w/disodium phosphate added	1 oz	106	6	0	406	0	8.9	5.6	27	73%

Food Name	Serving Size	Calories	Prot. gms	Carbs gms	Sod. mgs	Fiber gms	Fat gms	Sat. Fat gms	Chol. mgs	% Fat Cal.
(Borden)										
processed, 'Light'	1-1/3 slices	70	6	1	420	0	4.0	0.0	15	56%
processed, 'Loaf'	1 oz	110	6	1	40	0	9.0	0.0	0	74%
processed, nonfat, low-cholesterol	1 oz	40	6	4	380	0	0.0	0.0	5	0%
processed, 'Slices'	1 oz	110	6	1	40	0	9.0	0.0	0	74%
processed, slices, 'Premium'	1 oz	110	6	1	460	0	9.0	0.0	0	74%
(Dorman's)										
processed	1 oz	110	6	1	440	0	9.0	0.0	0	74%
processed, low-sodium, 'Loaf'	1 oz	110	6	1	140	0	9.0	0.0	0	74%
(Healthy Choice)										
white, singles	1 slice	40	5	2	200	0	1.0	0.5	5	24%
yellow, singles	1 slice	40	5	2	200	0	1.0	0.5	5	24%
(Healthy Favorites) processed	2/3 oz	45	4	2	260	0	2.0	1.0	10	43%
(Hoffman's) processed	1 oz	110	6	1	400	0	9.0	0.0	0	74%
(Kraft)										
processed, 'Deluxe Loaf'	1 oz	110	6	1	430	0	9.0	5.0	25	74%
processed, 'Deluxe Slices'	1 oz	110	6	1	450	0	9.0	5.0	25	74%
(Land O'Lakes)										
processed	1 oz	110	6	1	405	0	9.0	6.0	25	74%
processed, sharp	1 oz	100	6	1	360	0	9.0	6.0	30	74%
(Old English)										
processed, sharp, 'Loaf'	1 oz	110	6	1	400	0	9.0	5.0	30	74%
processed, sharp, 'Slices'	1 oz	110	6	1	440	0	9.0	5.0	30	74%
(Sargento) hot pepper, pasteurized process	1 oz	106	6	0	406	0	8.9	0.0	27	75%
(Smart Beat) fat-free	1 slice	25	4	3	180	0	0.0	0.0	0	0%
(Weight Watchers) low-fat	1 slice	30	5	2	151	0	0.0	0.0	0	0%
ASIAGO *(Frigo)* natural, wheel	1 oz	110	7	1	400	0	9.0	0.0		72%
BABYBEL										
(Laughing Cow)										
natural	1 oz	91	7	0	227	0	7.0	0.0	22	69%
natural, mini	3/4 oz	74	5	0	170	0	6.0	0.0	18	74%
BEL PAESE										
(Bel Paese)										
'Domestic Traditional'	1 oz	101	6	1	145	0	8.0	0.0	20	73%
'Imported'	1 oz	90	6	0	196	0	7.4	0.0	22	74%
'Lite'	1 oz	76	7	1	155	0	5.0	0.0	16	58%
primavera, 'Lite'	1 oz	68	6	2	165	0	4.0	0.0	14	53%
BLUE										
	1 oz	100	6	1	396	0	8.1	5.3	21	72%
(Dorman's)										
natural, 'Castello 70%'	1 oz	134	4	0	286	0	12.3	9.0	29	88%
natural, 'Danablu 50%'	1 oz	100	6	0	200	0	8.2	5.0	23	73%
natural, 'Danablu 60%'	1 oz	108	5	0	200	0	9.7	6.9	31	81%
natural, 'Saga 70%'	1 oz	134	4	0	286	0	12.3	9.0	29	88%
(Frigo) natural	1 oz	100	6	1	400	0	8.0	0.0	0	72%
(Hickory Farms) natural, 'Domestic'	1 oz	101	6	1	396	0	8.3	0.0	21	73%
(Kraft) natural	1 oz	100	6	1	330	0	9.0	5.0	30	74%
(Sargento)										
crumbled	1/4 cup	100	6	1	380	0	8.0	5.0	20	72%
natural	1 oz	100	6	1	400	0	8.0	0.0	21	72%
BONBEL										
(Laughing Cow)										
mini	3/4 oz	74	5	0	170	0	6.0	0.0	18	74%
natural	1 oz	100	6	0	227	0	8.0	0.0	24	75%

Food Name	Serving Size	Calories	Prot. gms	Carbs gms	Sod. mgs	Fiber gms	Fat gms	Sat. Fat gms	Chol. mgs	% Fat Cal.
BONBINO *(Laughing Cow)* natural	1 oz	103	7	0	227	0	9.0	0.0	27	74%
BRICK										
	1 oz	105	7	1	159	0	8.4	5.3	27	70%
(Dorman's) natural	1 oz	110	7	1	180	0	8.0	0.0	0	69%
(Kraft) natural	1 oz	110	7	0	180	0	9.0	5.0	30	74%
(Land O'Lakes) natural	1 oz	110	7	1	160	0	8.0	5.0	25	69%
BRIE										
	1 oz	95	6	0	178	0	7.8	4.9	28	73%
(Dorman's) natural	1 oz	81	5	0	229	0	6.6	4.0	20	73%
(Sargento) natural	1 oz	100	6	0	180	0	8.0	0.0	28	75%
BURGER *(Sargento)* natural	1 oz	110	6	1	410	0	9.0	0.0	27	76%
BUTTERNIP *(Hickory Farms)* natural	1 oz	110	5	1	82	0	9.4	0.0	25	77%
CAJUN *(Sargento)*	1 oz	110	7	0	165	0	9.0	0.0	28	74%
CALJACK *(Churny)*	1 oz	100	6	1	0	0	8.0	0.0	0	72%
CAMEMBERT										
	1 cup	737	49	1	2071	0	59.7	37.5	177	71%
(Dorman's)										
'45%'	1 oz	82	6	0	226	0	6.3	3.9	17	69%
'50%'	1 oz	89	6	0	285	0	7.3	4.4	23	74%
(Hickory Farms)	1 oz	90	6	0	239	0	7.0	0.0	26	72%
(Sargento)	1 oz	90	6	0	240	0	7.0	0.0	20	72%
CHEDDAR										
	1 oz	114	7	0	176	0	9.4	6.0	30	72%
low-fat	1 oz	49	7	1	174	0	2.0	1.2	6	36%
low-salt	1 oz	113	7	1	6	0	9.2	5.9	28	72%
(Alpine Lace)										
'Cheddar Flavored'	1 oz	100	7	1	95	0	8.0	5.0	25	69%
milk, natural, shredded, 'Ched-R-Lo'	1 oz	80	7	1	95	0	5.0	0.0	20	58%
(Alta Dena)										
mild, natural	1 oz	110	7	1	200	0	9.0	0.0	0	72%
sharp, natural	1 oz	110	7	1	200	0	9.0	0.0	0	72%
(Axelrod)										
extra sharp	1 oz	110	7	1	200	0	9.0	0.0	30	72%
sharp	1 oz	110	7	1	200	0	9.0	0.0	30	72%
(Boar's Head) sharp sliced	1 oz	110	7	1	100	0	9.0	0.0	18	72%
(Darigold)	1 oz	110	7	1	170	0	9.0	5.9	29	72%
(Dorman's)										
	1 oz	110	7	1	200	0	9.0	0.0	0	72%
'Chedda-Delite'	1 oz	90	7	1	100	0	7.0	0.0	0	66%
cheddar Jack, low-salt	1 oz	80	8	1	140	0	5.0	3.0	19	56%
less fat, 'Low Sodium'	1 oz	80	8	1	100	0	5.0	3.4	20	56%
low-salt, low-fat	1 oz	80	8	1	140	0	5.0	3.0	20	56%
w/Monterey Jack, 'Chedda-Jack'	1 oz	90	7	1	100	0	7.0	0.0	0	66%
(Featherweight) 'Low Sodium'	1 oz	110	7	1	5	0	9.0	0.0	0	72%
(Frigo)										
	1 oz	110	7	1	200	0	9.0	0.0	0	72%
low-fat	1 oz	20	3	1	20	0	1.0	0.0	5	36%
(Golden Balance)										
mild, natural, shredded 'Natural Shreds'	1 oz	90	8	1	150	0	6.0	3.0	20	60%
sharp, natural, shredded 'Natural Shreds'	1 oz	90	8	1	130	0	6.0	3.0	20	60%
(Healthy Choice)										
low-fat, 'Fancy Shreds'	1/4 cup	50	8	1	220	1	1.5	1.0	3	27%
mild, natural, 'Fancy Shreds'	1 oz	70	8	0	220	0	4.0	2.0	15	53%

Food Name	Serving Size	Calories	Prot. gms	Carbs gms	Sod. mgs	Fiber gms	Fat gms	Sat. Fat gms	Chol. mgs	% Fat Cal.
(Hickory Farms)										
....	1 oz	110	7	1	176	0	9.0	0.0	30	72%
raw milk, 'Light Choice Low Sodium'.	1 oz	114	6	0	100	0	8.0	0.0	30	75%
(Hoffman's) super sharp, processed	1 oz	110	6	2	390	0	8.0	0.0	0	69%
(Kraft)										
mild, natural.	1 oz	110	7	1	180	0	9.0	6.0	30	73%
mild, natural, low-fat, made w/2% milk	1 oz	90	7	1	240	0	6.0	4.0	20	64%
mild, natural, shredded 'Light Naturals'.	1 oz	80	8	1	220	0	5.0	3.0	20	56%
sharp, less fat, 'Light Naturals'	1 oz	80	9	1	220	0	5.0	3.0	20	53%
sharp, low-fat, natural, made w/2% milk	1 oz	90	7	1	240	0	6.0	4.0	20	64%
sharp, natural, made w/2% milk, 'Cracker Barrel'	1 oz	90	7	1	240	0	6.0	4.0	20	64%
sharp, white, light, 'Cracker Barrel'	1 oz	80	9	1	220	0	5.0	3.0	20	53%
(Land O'Lakes)										
natural	1 oz	110	7	1	175	0	9.0	6.0	30	72%
natural, 'Chedarella'	1 oz	100	7	1	180	0	8.0	5.0	25	69%
(Laughing Cow)										
. . . .	1 oz	110	7	0	227	0	9.0	0.0	28	74%
'Reduced Mini'.	3/4 oz	45	6	0	170	0	2.5	0.0	8	48%
(Sargento)										
. . . .	1 oz	110	7	0	176	0	9.0	0.0	30	73%
mild, fancy, shredded, 'Preferred Light'	1/4 cup	70	8	1	200	0	4.5	3.0	10	54%
mild, light, 'Mootown Snackers'	1 piece	60	7	1	170	0	4.0	2.5	10	55%
mild, shredded, 'Classic Supreme'	1/4 cup	110	6	1	160	0	9.0	6.0	30	74%
mild or sharp, 'Mootown Snackers'	1 piece	100	5	1	130	0	8.0	5.0	25	75%
'New York'	1 oz	110	7	0	180	0	9.0	0.0	30	73%
sliced.	1 slice	110	6	1	160	0	9.0	6.0	30	74%
(Smart Beat) sharp, nonfat	1 slice	25	4	3	230	0	0.0	0.0	0	0%
(Stilwell) cheddar, frozen 'Bumpers'.	1 piece	60	1	6	230	1	3.0	1.5	5	49%
(Weight Watchers)										
mild, 'Natural'.	1 oz	80	8	1	150	0	5.0	3.0	15	56%
mild, shredded, 'Natural'	1 oz	80	8	1	150	0	5.0	3.0	15	56%
sharp, 'Natural'	1 oz	80	8	1	150	0	5.0	3.0	15	56%
CHESHIRE.	1 oz	110	7	1	198	0	8.7	5.5	29	69%
CHUTTER *(Hickory Farms)* 'Cold Pack'	1 oz	87	6	3	213	0	5.8	0.0	46	60%
COLBY										
. . . .	1 oz	112	7	1	171	0	9.1	5.7	27	72%
low-fat	1 oz	49	7	1	174	0	2.0	1.2	6	36%
low-salt	1 oz	113	7	1	6	0	9.2	5.9	28	72%
(Alpine Lace) 'Colby-Lo'.	1 oz	80	7	1	85	0	5.0	4.0	20	58%
(Dorman's)	1 oz	110	7	1	190	0	9.0	0.0	0	72%
(Hickory Farms)										
'Light Choice Low Sodium'	1 oz	100	8	1	4	0	6.0	0.0	20	60%
'Longhorn'	1 oz	112	7	1	171	0	8.6	0.0	27	72%
low-fat, calcium-enriched 'Light Choice'	1 oz	100	7	1	180	0	8.0	0.0	0	69%
(Kraft)										
. . . .	1 oz	110	7	1	180	0	9.0	5.0	30	72%
made w/2% milk, natural.	1 oz	80	7	0	220	0	6.0	4.0	20	66%
w/Monterey Jack, less fat, 'Light Naturals'.	1 oz	80	8	1	220	0	5.0	3.0	20	56%
w/Monterey Jack, natural, shredded, 'Light Naturals'	1 oz	80	8	1	220	0	5.0	3.0	20	56%
(Land O'Lakes) natural	1 oz	110	7	1	170	0	9.0	6.0	25	72%
(Sargento)										
. . . .	1 oz	110	7	1	170	0	9.0	0.0	27	72%
Jack.	1 oz	110	7	1	160	0	9.0	0.0	27	73%
Jack, 'Mootown Snackers'.	1 piece	90	5	1	160	0	8.0	5.0	20	77%

Food Name	Serving Size	Calories	Prot. gms	Carbs gms	Sod. mgs	Fiber gms	Fat gms	Sat. Fat gms	Chol. mgs	% Fat Cal.
Jack, shredded, 'Fancy Supreme'	1/4 cup	110	6	1	190	0	9.0	6.0	25	76%
sliced.	1 slice	110	6	0	190	0	9.0	6.0	30	77%
(Weight Watchers) 'Natural'	1 oz	80	8	1	130	0	5.0	2.0	15	56%
COTTAGE CHEESE										
creamed, not packed.	1 cup	217	26	6	850	0	9.5	6.0	31	38%
dry, large or small curd, not packed	1 cup	123	25	3	19	0	0.6	0.4	10	4%
nonfat, dry, large or small curd	4 oz	96	20	2	14	0	0.5	0.3	8	4%
(Bison)										
chive, creamed	1/2 cup	120	14	4	420	0	5.0	0.0	20	38%
creamed, low-fat, 1% milk fat	1/2 cup	90	14	4	350	0	2.0	0.0	5	20%
creamed, 4% milk fat.	1/2 cup	120	14	4	420	0	5.0	0.0	20	38%
garden salad, creamed	1/2 cup	110	12	4	420	0	4.0	0.0	15	36%
w/pineapple, creamed.	1/2 cup	140	10	18	340	0	4.0	0.0	15	24%
(Borden)										
creamed, 4% milk fat.	1/2 cup	120	14	4	400	0	5.0	0.0	0	38%
creamed, 4% milk fat, unsalted.	1/2 cup	120	14	4	40	0	5.0	0.0	0	38%
dry curd, unsalted	1/2 cup	80	18	3	20	0	1.0	0.0	0	10%
(Breakstone's)										
creamed	4 oz	110	13	3	370	0	5.0	3.0	25	41%
creamed, low-fat, 2% milk fat	4 oz	100	14	4	510	0	2.0	1.0	15	20%
dry curd, nonfat, unsalted	4 oz	90	16	6	65	0	0.0	0.0	10	0%
(Carnation)										
large curd, 4% milk fat.	1/2 cup	115	14	4	440	0	5.0	0.0	0	38%
low-fat, 1.5% milk fat, 'Slender'	1/2 cup	90	14	4	440	0	2.0	0.0	0	20%
small curd, 4% milk fat	1/2 cup	115	14	4	440	0	5.0	0.0	0	38%
w/pineapple, 4% milk fat,.	1/2 cup	130	10	12	430	0	5.0	0.0	0	34%
(Crowley)										
calcium-fortified, creamed, low-fat, 1% milk fat.	1/2 cup	90	14	4	390	0	1.0	0.0	5	11%
creamed, 4% milk fat.	1/2 cup	120	14	4	390	0	5.0	0.0	15	38%
creamed, low-fat, 1% milk fat	1/2 cup	90	14	4	390	0	1.0	0.0	5	11%
no salt added, creamed, low-fat, 1% milk fat.	1/2 cup	90	14	4	50	0	1.0	0.0	5	11%
w/peaches, creamed, 4% milk fat	1/2 cup	140	10	17	340	0	3.0	0.0	10	20%
w/pineapple, creamed, 4% milk fat	1/2 cup	140	11	15	330	0	4.0	0.0	15	26%
w/pineapple, creamed, low-fat, 1% milk fat.	1/2 cup	110	11	15	330	0	1.0	0.0	5	8%
(Darigold)										
creamed, 4% milk fat.	4 oz	120	14	4	510	0	4.2	3.2	17	34%
dry curd, unsalted	4 oz	80	18	3	15	0	1.0	0.4	10	10%
'Trim' creamed, low-fat, 2% milk fat	4 oz	100	14	4	510	0	3.2	2.0	17	29%
(Friendship)										
'California Style' creamed, 4% milk fat	1/2 cup	120	14	4	380	0	5.0	0.0	17	38%
creamed, low-fat, 1% milk fat	1/2 cup	90	14	4	350	0	1.0	0.0	5	11%
lactose-reduced, creamed, low-fat, 1% milk fat.	1/2 cup	90	14	4	350	0	1.0	0.0	5	11%
no salt added, creamed, low-fat, 1% milk fat.	1/2 cup	90	14	4	31	0	1.0	0.0	5	11%
pot style, large curd, creamed, low-fat, 2% milk fat.	1/2 cup	100	14	4	405	0	2.0	0.0	9	20%
w/pineapple, creamed, 4% milk fat	1/2 cup	140	11	15	300	0	4.0	0.0	17	26%
w/pineapple, creamed, low-fat, 1% milk fat	1/2 cup	110	11	15	300	0	1.0	0.0	5	8%
(Knudsen)										
creamed, 4% milk fat.	4 oz	120	14	4	340	0	5.0	3.0	20	38%
low-fat, 2% milk fat	4 oz	100	14	4	370	0	2.0	1.0	15	20%
nonfat	1/2 cup	80	14	4	380	0	0.0	0.0	0	0%
nonfat	4 oz	70	15	3	420	0	0.0	0.0	5	0%
small curd, creamed, 4% milk fat	4 oz	120	14	4	370	0	5.0	3.0	20	38%
w/fruit cocktail low-fat, 2% milk fat.	4 oz	130	11	16	330	0	2.0	2.0	10	14%
w/mandarin orange, low-fat, 2% milk fat	4 oz	110	11	11	320	0	2.0	2.0	10	17%

Food Name	Serving Size	Calories	Prot. gms	Carbs gms	Sod. mgs	Fiber gms	Fat gms	Sat. Fat gms	Chol. mgs	% Fat Cal.
w/peach, low-fat, 2% milk fat.	6 oz	170	16	19	270	0	2.0	2.0	15	11%
w/pear, low-fat, 2% milk fat	4 oz	110	11	12	320	0	2.0	2.0	10	16%
w/pineapple, creamed, 4% milk fat	4 oz	140	10	14	260	0	5.0	3.0	25	32%
w/pineapple, low-fat, 2% milk fat.	6 oz	170	16	18	300	0	2.0	2.0	15	12%
w/spiced apple, low-fat, 2% milk fat	6 oz	180	16	20	280	0	2.0	2.0	15	11%
w/strawberry, low-fat, 2% milk fat	6 oz	170	16	19	320	0	2.0	2.0	15	11%
(Light n' Lively)										
garden salad, low-fat, 1% milk fat	4 oz	80	18	5	350	0	2.0	1.0	10	16%
low-fat, 1% milk fat	4 oz	80	14	4	370	0	2.0	1.0	10	20%
nonfat	4 oz	90	14	7	400	0	0.0	0.0	10	0%
w/peach and pineapple, low-fat.	4 oz	100	11	12	320	0	1.0	1.0	10	9%
(Lite-Line) creamed, low-fat 1.5% milk fat	1/2 cup	90	14	4	400	0	2.0	0.0	0	20%
(Lucerne)										
no added salt.	1/2 cup	80	14	4	40	0	1.0	0.5	5	11%
nonfat	1/2 cup	70	14	4	420	0	0.0	0.0	0	0%
(Sealtest) low-fat, 2% milk fat.	4 oz	100	14	4	340	0	2.0	1.0	15	20%
(Weight Watchers)										
creamed, low-fat, 1% milk fat	1/2 cup	90	14	4	460	0	1.0	0.0	0	11%
creamed, low-fat, 2% milk fat	1/2 cup	100	14	4	460	0	2.0	0.0	0	20%
CREAM CHEESE										
	1 cup	810	18	6	686	0	80.9	51.0	255	88%
	3-oz pkg	297	6	2	251	0	29.6	18.7	93	88%
	1 oz	99	2	1	84	0	9.9	6.2	31	88%
	1 tbsp	51	1	0	43	0	5.1	3.2	16	88%
whipped.	1 tbsp	35	1	0	30	0	3.5	2.2	11	88%
(Alta Dena) pasteurized	1 oz	100	2	2	110	0	10.0	0.0	0	85%
(Crowley)	1 oz	110	2	1	100	0	9.0	0.0	30	87%
(Darigold)	1 oz	99	2	1	84	0	9.9	6.2	31	88%
(Dorman's)										
'65%'	1 oz	90	3	1	200	0	8.4	5.1	26	84%
'70%'	1 oz	102	3	1	200	0	9.9	6.1	30	87%
(Friendship) soft	1 oz	103	2	1	70	0	10.0	0.0	31	91%
(Healthy Choice) plain, nonfat	2 tbsp	25	4	2	200	1	0.0	0.0	0	0%
(Healthy Favorites)	1 oz	60	3	2	110	0	5.0	2.0	15	69%
(Philadelphia Brand)										
	1 oz	100	2	1	90	0	10.0	6.0	30	88%
brick.	1 oz	100	2	1	90	0	10.0	6.0	30	90%
light, soft	2 tbsp	70	3	2	150	0	5.0	3.5	15	69%
nonfat, 'Free'	1 oz	25	4	1	170	0	0.0	0.0	5	0%
pasteurized process, 'Light'	1 oz	60	3	2	160	0	5.0	3.0	10	69%
soft	2 tbsp	100	2	1	100	0	10.0	7.0	30	88%
strawberry, soft	2 tbsp	110	1	5	100	0	9.0	6.0	25	77%
whipped.	2 tbsp	70	1	1	85	0	7.0	4.5	25	91%
w/chives	1 oz	90	2	1	125	0	9.0	5.0	30	87%
w/chives, brick.	1 oz	90	2	1	135	0	9.0	6.0	25	89%
w/chives, whipped.	2 tbsp	70	1	1	130	0	6.0	4.0	20	90%
w/chives and onion, soft	2 tbsp	110	1	2	135	0	10.0	7.0	30	88%
w/herb and garlic, soft	1 oz	100	1	2	160	0	9.0	5.0	25	87%
w/olive and pimiento, nonfat	1 oz	90	2	2	160	0	8.0	0.0	0	82%
w/olive and pimiento, soft	1 oz	90	2	2	160	0	8.0	5.0	25	82%
w/onion, whipped	1 oz	90	2	2	170	0	8.0	5.0	25	82%
w/pimiento.	1 oz	90	2	1	150	0	9.0	5.0	30	87%
w/pineapple, soft	2 tbsp	100	1	4	100	0	9.0	6.0	25	80%
w/salmon, soft	2 tbsp	100	2	1	200	0	9.0	6.0	30	87%

Food Name	Serving Size	Calories	Prot. gms	Carbs gms	Sod. mgs	Fiber gms	Fat gms	Sat. Fat gms	Chol. mgs	% Fat Cal.
w/smoked salmon, whipped	2 tbsp	70	2	1	140	0	6.0	4.0	20	82%
(Stilwell) frozen, 'Bumpers'	1 piece	60	2	5	210	0	3.0	2.0	5	49%
(Temp-Tee) whipped	1 oz	100	2	1	85	0	10.0	6.0	30	88%
CREMA DANIA (Dorman's) 'Crema Dania 70%'	1 oz	134	4	0	286	0	12.3	9.0	29	88%
DANBO										
(Dorman's)										
45%										
	1 oz	98	7	0	200	0	7.5	4.6	23	69%
20%										
	1 oz	62	9	0	200	0	2.8	1.7	9	41%
EDAM										
	1 oz	101	7	0	274	0	7.9	5.0	25	69%
(Dorman's)										
	1 oz	100	7	1	200	0	8.0	0.0	0	69%
45%										
	1 oz	91	7	0	200	0	7.0	4.3	21	69%
(Hickory Farms) 'Domestic'	1 oz	100	6	1	182	0	8.4	0.0	24	73%
(Kaukauna)	1 oz	100	7	1	275	0	8.0	0.0	25	69%
(Kraft)	1 oz	90	8	0	310	0	7.0	4.0	20	66%
(Land O'Lakes) natural	1 oz	100	7	1	275	0	8.0	5.0	25	69%
(Laughing Cow)	1 oz	100	6	0	227	0	8.0	0.0	26	75%
(May-Bud)	1 oz	100	7	0	275	0	8.0	0.0	0	72%
(Sargento)	1 oz	100	7	0	270	0	8.0	0.0	25	71%
FARMER										
(Friendship)										
	1/2 cup	160	16	4	356	0	12.0	0.0	40	57%
'No Salt Added'	1/2 cup	160	16	4	8	0	12.0	0.0	40	57%
(Hickory Farms)										
	1 oz	90	6	1	210	0	7.0	0.0	20	69%
'Light Choice'	1 oz	90	6	1	150	0	7.0	0.0	20	69%
(Kaukauna)	1 oz	100	7	1	0	0	8.0	0.0	25	69%
(May-Bud)	1 oz	90	6	1	210	0	7.0	0.0	20	69%
(Sargento)	1 oz	100	7	1	130	0	8.0	0.0	26	69%
FETA										
	1 oz	75	4	1	316	0	6.0	4.2	25	71%
(Churny) 'Natural'	1 oz	75	5	1	316	0	6.5	4.2	25	71%
(Dorman's) 45%										
	1 oz	91	6	0	0	0	7.3	0.0	0	72%
(Sargento)	1 oz	80	4	1	320	0	6.0	0.0	25	73%
FONTINA										
	1 oz	110	7	0	227	0	8.8	5.4	33	70%
(Sargento)	1 oz	110	7	0	0	0	9.0	0.0	33	73%
GJETOST										
	1 oz	132	3	12	170	0	8.4	5.4	27	56%
(Sargento)	1 oz	130	3	12	170	0	8.0	0.0	0	55%
GOAT										
hard	1 oz	128	9	1	98	0	10.1	7.0	30	69%
semisoft	1 oz	103	6	1	146	0	8.5	5.9	22	72%
soft	1 oz	76	5	0	104	0	6.0	4.1	13	69%
GOUDA										
	1 oz	101	7	1	232	0	7.8	5.0	32	68%
(Dorman's)	1 oz	100	7	1	210	0	8.0	0.0	0	69%
(Kaukauna)										
	1 oz	100	7	1	230	0	8.0	0.0	30	69%

Food Name	Serving Size	Calories	Prot. gms	Carbs gms	Sod. mgs	Fiber gms	Fat gms	Sat. Fat gms	Chol. mgs	% Fat Cal.
w/caraway seed........................	1 oz	100	7	1	230	0	8.0	0.0	30	69%
w/hickory smoke flavor	1 oz	100	7	1	230	0	8.0	0.0	25	69%
(Kraft).................................	1 oz	110	7	0	200	0	9.0	5.0	30	74%
(Land O'Lakes) natural	1 oz	100	7	1	230	0	8.0	5.0	30	69%
(Laughing Cow)										
....	1 oz	110	7	0	227	0	9.0	0.0	28	74%
mini	3/4 oz	80	5	0	170	0	6.4	0.0	21	73%
(May-Bud)	1 oz	100	7	1	230	0	8.0	0.0	0	69%
(Sargento)	1 oz	100	7	1	230	0	8.0	0.0	32	69%
GRUYERE	1 oz	117	8	0	95	0	9.2	5.4	31	69%
HAVARTI										
(Casino).............................	1 oz	120	6	0	140	0	11.0	7.0	35	80%
(Dorman's)										
45%										
....	1 oz	91	7	0	200	0	7.0	4.3	21	69%
60%										
....	1 oz	118	5	0	200	0	10.6	6.5	31	81%
(Hickory Farms) 'Danish Special'......	1 oz	117	5	0	198	0	10.5	0.0	31	81%
(Sargento)	1 oz	120	5	0	200	0	11.0	0.0	31	82%
HORSERADISH (Kaukauna) hearty, cold pack 'Cup'........	1 oz	100	6	3	250	0	7.0	0.0	25	64%
HOT PEPPER (Hickory Farms)	1 oz	106	6	1	406	0	8.9	0.0	27	75%
ITALIAN STYLE										
(Sargento)										
grated	1 oz	110	8	1	105	0	8.0	0.0	26	67%
6-cheese blend, 'Recipe Blend'.......	1/4 cup	90	7	0	180	0	7.0	4.0	20	69%
JACK. See MONTEREY JACK.										
JARLSBERG										
(Hickory Farms)	1 oz	100	7	1	130	0	7.0	0.0	16	66%
(Norseland)	1 oz	97	7	1	135	0	7.0	4.2	18	66%
(Sargento) sliced	1 slice	120	9	1	160	0	9.0	5.0	20	67%
LIMBURGER										
....	1 cup	438	27	1	1072	0	36.5	22.4	121	73%
(Mohawk Valley) natural 'Little Gem' ...	1 oz	90	6	0	250	0	8.0	5.0	25	75%
(Sargento)	1 oz	90	6	0	230	0	8.0	0.0	26	75%
MASCARPONE (Galbani) 'Imported'	1 oz	128	2	1	17	0	13.1	0.0	39	92%
MEXICAN STYLE										
(Healthy Choice) fancy shreds........	1/4 cup	50	8	1	220	1	1.5	1.0	3	27%
(Sargento) 4-cheese blend, 'Recipe Blend'	1/4 cup	110	6	1	200	0	9.0	6.0	25	76%
(Velveeta) mild, pasteurized process, shredded	1/4 cup	120	8	3	520	0	9.0	6.0	30	65%
MONTEREY JACK										
....	1 oz	106	7	0	152	0	8.6	5.4	25	71%
(Alpine Lace)										
'Monti-Jack-Lo'	1 oz	80	7	1	75	0	5.0	4.0	15	58%
natural, milk cheese 'Monti-Jack-Lo' ...	1 oz	80	7	1	75	0	5.0	3.0	15	58%
(Alta Dena)										
natural.............................	1 oz	100	7	1	180	0	8.0	0.0	0	69%
natural, w/jalapeño peppers	1 oz	100	7	1	180	0	8.0	0.0	0	69%
(Axelrod)										
....	1 oz	100	6	1	150	0	8.0	0.0	30	72%
w/jalapeño pepper....................	1 oz	100	6	1	220	0	8.0	0.0	30	72%
(Darigold)............................	1 oz	110	7	1	150	0	8.0	0.0	25	69%
(Dorman's)										
....	1 oz	100	6	1	180	0	8.0	0.0	0	72%
less fat, 'Low Sodium'	1 oz	80	8	1	90	0	5.0	3.1	18	56%

Food Name	Serving Size	Calories	Prot. gms	Carbs gms	Sod. mgs	Fiber gms	Fat gms	Sat. Fat gms	Chol. mgs	% Fat Cal.
low-salt	1 oz	80	8	1	140	0	5.0	2.6	18	56%
'Slim Jack'	1 oz	90	6	1	90	0	7.0	0.0	0	69%
(Hickory Farms) 'Light Choice Low Sodium'	1 oz	110	6	0	100	0	8.0	0.0	30	75%
(Kaukauna)	1 oz	110	7	1	150	0	9.0	0.0	25	72%
(Kraft)										
	1 oz	110	6	0	190	0	9.0	5.0	30	77%
natural, low-fat, made w/2% milk	1 oz	80	7	1	240	0	6.0	4.0	20	64%
natural, w/jalapeño peppers	1 oz	110	7	1	190	0	9.0	6.0	30	73%
w/caraway	1 oz	100	7	1	180	0	8.0	5.0	30	69%
w/peppers, less fat, 'Light Naturals'	1 oz	80	8	1	220	0	5.0	3.0	20	56%
(Land O'Lakes)										
natural	1 oz	110	7	1	150	0	9.0	5.0	20	72%
natural, hot pepper	1 oz	110	7	1	150	0	9.0	5.0	20	72%
processed, 'Jalapeño Jack'	1 oz	90	5	1	430	0	8.0	5.0	20	75%
(May-Bud)	1 oz	110	7	0	150	0	9.0	0.0	0	74%
(Sargento)										
	1 oz	110	7	0	150	0	9.0	0.0	25	74%
shredded	1/4 cup	100	6	0	190	0	9.0	5.0	30	77%
sliced	1 slice	100	6	0	190	0	9.0	5.0	30	77%
(Weight Watchers) 'Natural'	1 oz	80	8	1	120	0	5.0	2.0	15	56%
MOZZARELLA										
part skim	1 oz	72	7	1	132	0	4.5	2.9	16	55%
part skim, low-moisture	1 oz	79	8	1	150	0	4.9	3.1	15	54%
part skim, low-moisture, diced	1 cup	370	36	4	697	0	22.6	14.4	71	54%
part skim, low moisture, shredded	1 cup	316	31	4	596	0	19.3	12.3	61	54%
whole milk	1 oz	80	6	1	106	0	6.1	3.7	22	67%
whole milk, low moisture	1 oz	90	6	1	118	0	7.0	4.4	25	68%
whole milk, low-moisture, shredded	1 cup	315	22	2	418	0	24.2	14.7	88	67%
(Alpine Lace)										
natural, shredded	1 oz	70	7	1	75	0	5.0	0.0	15	58%
natural, sliced	1 oz	70	7	1	75	0	5.0	3.0	15	58%
part skim, low-moisture	1 oz	70	7	1	75	0	5.0	3.0	15	58%
(Crowley)										
part skim	1 oz	70	8	1	240	0	4.0	0.0	15	50%
whole milk	1 oz	90	5	1	240	0	7.0	0.0	25	72%
(Dorman's)										
	1 oz	90	7	1	190	0	6.0	0.0	0	63%
less fat, 'Low Sodium'	1 oz	80	9	1	90	0	4.0	2.5	17	47%
low-salt	1 oz	80	9	1	140	0	4.0	2.7	15	47%
part skim, low-moisture, 'Low Sodium'	1 oz	80	8	1	90	0	5.0	2.6	15	56%
(Frigo)										
part skim, low-moisture	1 oz	80	7	1	190	0	5.0	0.0	10	58%
part skim, low-moisture, less fat	1 oz	60	8	1	150	0	3.0	2.0	10	43%
whole milk, low-moisture	1 oz	90	6	1	190	0	7.0	4.0	15	69%
(Healthy Choice)										
ball	1 oz	45	10	1	200	1	0.0	0.0	0	0%
fat-free, shredded	1 oz	40	9	1	200	0	0.0	0.0	5	0%
low-fat, fancy, shredded	1/4 cup	50	8	1	220	0	1.5	1.0	3	27%
natural, fat-free, chunk	1 oz	40	9	1	200	0	0.0	0.0	5	0%
string	1 oz	50	8	1	220	0	1.5	1.0	3	27%
(Hickory Farms)										
	1 oz	72	7	1	132	0	4.5	0.0	16	57%
low-salt, 'Light Choice Low Sodium'	1 oz	80	8	1	90	0	5.0	0.0	15	56%

Food Name	Serving Size	Calories	Prot. gms	Carbs gms	Sod. mgs	Fiber gms	Fat gms	Sat. Fat gms	Chol. mgs	% Fat Cal.
(Kraft)										
....	1 oz	90	6	1	190	0	7.0	4.0	20	69%
less fat, 'Light Naturals'	1 oz	80	8	1	200	0	4.0	3.0	15	50%
natural, low-fat, made w/2% milk....................	1/3 cup	80	9	1	210	0	5.0	3.0	15	54%
part skim, low-moisture....................	1 oz	80	8	1	200	0	5.0	3.0	15	56%
part skim, w/jalapeño pepper	1 oz	80	8	1	230	0	5.0	3.0	20	56%
(Land O'Lakes) natural, low moisture, part skim	1 oz	80	8	1	150	0	5.0	3.0	15	56%
(Polly-O)										
fresh 'Fior di Latte'....................	1 oz	80	5	1	20	0	6.0	0.0	20	69%
grated	1 oz	130	11	1	530	0	10.0	0.0	25	65%
'Lite'....................	1 oz	70	7	1	200	0	4.0	0.0	15	53%
part skim....................	1 oz	80	6	1	280	0	5.0	0.0	15	62%
whole milk....................	1 oz	90	5	1	280	0	6.0	0.0	20	69%
(Sargento)										
light, sliced, 'Preferred Light'	1 slice	90	11	0	230	0	5.0	3.0	15	51%
part skim, low-moisture....................	1 oz	80	8	1	150	0	5.0	3.0	15	56%
shredded, 'Classic Supreme'....................	1/4 cup	80	7	1	150	0	6.0	3.5	15	63%
shredded, 'Preferred Light'....................	1/4 cup	70	8	1	140	0	3.0	2.0	10	44%
sliced....................	1 slice	130	11	2	230	0	9.0	6.0	25	61%
whole milk....................	1 oz	90	6	1	120	0	7.0	0.0	25	69%
(Weight Watchers)										
'Natural'....................	1 oz	70	8	1	150	0	4.0	2.0	15	50%
shredded, 'Natural'	1 oz	80	8	1	150	0	4.0	2.0	15	50%
MUENSTER										
....	1 oz	104	7	0	178	0	8.5	5.4	27	72%
(Alpine Lace)										
....	1 oz	100	7	1	85	0	8.0	5.0	30	69%
low-salt, natural, sliced 'Low Sodium'	1 oz	100	7	1	85	0	9.0	6.0	25	72%
(Dorman's)										
....	1 oz	110	7	0	190	0	9.0	0.0	0	74%
50%										
....	1 oz	100	6	0	200	0	8.2	5.0	24	73%
less fat, 'Low Sodium'	1 oz	80	8	0	140	0	5.0	3.1	18	58%
low-salt....................	1 oz	80	8	0	140	0	5.0	2.7	18	58%
low-salt, 'Low Sodium'....................	1 oz	110	7	0	95	0	9.0	0.0	0	74%
(Hickory Farms)										
....	1 oz	100	7	0	180	0	8.5	0.0	25	73%
low-salt, 'Light Choice Low Sodium'	1 oz	110	7	0	95	0	9.0	0.0	27	74%
(Kaukauna)	1 oz	110	7	1	180	0	9.0	0.0	25	72%
(Land O'Lakes) natural	1 oz	100	7	1	180	0	9.0	5.0	25	72%
(Sargento) sliced	1 slice	100	6	1	200	0	9.0	6.0	25	76%
NACHO *(Sargento)* shredded, 'Fancy Supreme'	1/4 cup	110	6	1	240	0	9.0	5.0	25	74%
NEUFCHATEL CHEESE										
....	3-oz pkg	221	8	2	339	0	19.9	12.6	65	79%
....	1 oz	74	3	1	113	0	6.6	4.2	22	79%
(Hickory Farms)										
chocolate....................	1 oz	110	2	8	90	0	8.0	0.0	33	64%
date nut, rum....................	1 oz	100	2	4	80	0	8.0	0.0	31	75%
orange....................	1 oz	100	2	4	75	0	8.0	0.0	45	75%
peach	1 oz	90	2	3	85	0	8.0	0.0	39	78%
pineapple....................	1 oz	90	2	2	60	0	8.0	0.0	33	82%
strawberry	1 oz	90	2	3	70	0	8.0	0.0	32	78%
(Kaukauna)										
garlic and herbs....................	1 oz	80	3	1	150	0	7.0	0.0	25	80%

Food Name	Serving Size	Calories	Prot. gms	Carbs gms	Sod. mgs	Fiber gms	Fat gms	Sat. Fat gms	Chol. mgs	% Fat Cal.
vegetable, garden	1 oz	80	3	1	200	0	7.0	0.0	25	80%
(Philadelphia Brand)										
	1 oz	70	3	1	120	0	6.0	4.0	20	79%
'Light'	1 oz	80	3	1	115	0	7.0	4.0	25	80%
NEW HOLLAND										
(Hickory Farms) w/herbs, 'Light Choice'	1 oz	90	7	1	100	0	8.0	0.0	27	69%
PARMESAN										
grated	1 cup	456	42	4	1862	0	30.0	19.1	79	58%
grated	1 oz	129	12	1	528	0	8.5	5.4	22	58%
grated	1 tbsp	23	2	0	93	0	1.5	1.0	4	58%
hard	1 oz	111	10	1	454	0	7.3	4.7	19	58%
shredded	1 tbsp	21	2	0	85	0	1.4	0.9	4	58%
(Churny) 'Natural'	1 oz	110	10	1	455	0	7.0	4.0	20	59%
(Frigo)										
fresh, grated	1 oz	110	10	1	350	0	7.0	0.0	0	59%
grated	1 oz	130	12	1	510	0	9.0	0.0	0	61%
wheel	1 oz	110	10	1	350	0	7.0	0.0	0	59%
w/Romano cheese, grated	1 oz	130	12	1	510	0	9.0	0.0	0	61%
(Hickory Farms)	1 oz	110	10	1	350	0	7.0	0.0	0	59%
(Kraft)										
	1 oz	100	9	1	290	0	7.0	4.0	20	61%
grated	1 oz	130	12	1	430	0	9.0	5.0	30	61%
(Polly-O) grated	1 oz	130	11	1	530	0	9.0	0.0	20	63%
(Progresso) grated	1 tbsp	23	2	1	95	0	2.0	1.0	4	60%
(Sargento)										
fresh	1 oz	110	10	1	450	0	7.0	0.0	19	59%
grated	1 oz	130	12	2	530	0	9.0	0.0	22	59%
shredded, 'Fancy Supreme'	1/4 cup	110	9	1	300	0	7.0	5.0	25	61%
w/Romano, grated	1 oz	110	10	1	400	0	7.0	0.0	24	59%
w/Romano, shredded, 'Fancy Supreme'	1/4 cup	110	9	1	340	0	7.0	5.0	25	61%
PARMESANO REGGIANO *(Galbani)* 'Imported'	1 oz	105	10	1	188	0	7.1	0.0	21	59%
PIZZA										
(Frigo)										
low-fat, shredded	1 oz	65	9	1	150	0	3.0	0.0	10	40%
shredded	1 oz	90	6	1	190	0	7.0	0.0	20	69%
(Healthy Choice) low-fat, fancy, shredded	1/4 cup	50	8	1	220	1	1.5	1.0	5	27%
(Precious) mozzarella cheddar, natural, shredded	1 oz	95	7	1	180	0	7.0	0.0	0	66%
(Sargento)										
double cheese, shredded, 'Fancy Supreme'	1/4 cup	90	7	1	150	0	6.0	4.5	20	63%
shredded, 'Classic Supreme'	1/4 cup	90	7	0	210	0	6.0	4.0	20	66%
PORT DU SALUT	1 oz	100	7	0	151	0	8.0	4.7	35	71%
PORT WINE *(Hickory Farms)* natural	1 oz	97	6	2	262	0	6.9	0.0	18	66%
POT *(Sargento)*	1 oz	25	5	1	1	0	0.2	0.0	0	7%
PROVOLONE										
	1 oz	100	7	1	248	0	7.5	4.8	20	67%
(Alpine Lace) 'Provo-Lo'	1 oz	70	7	1	85	0	5.0	5.0	15	58%
(Dorman's)										
	1 oz	90	7	1	290	0	7.0	0.0	0	66%
low-salt	1 oz	80	9	1	140	0	4.0	3.0	17	47%
(Frigo)										
	1 oz	100	7	1	230	0	7.0	0.0	0	66%
smoked	1 oz	100	7	1	230	0	7.0	0.0	0	66%
(Hickory Farms) low-salt, 'Light Choice Low Sodium'	1 oz	90	7	1	140	0	7.0	0.0	20	66%
(Kraft)	1 oz	100	7	1	260	0	7.0	4.0	25	66%

Food Name	Serving Size	Calories	Prot. gms	Carbs gms	Sod. mgs	Fiber gms	Fat gms	Sat. Fat gms	Chol. mgs	% Fat Cal.
(Land O'Lakes) natural	1 oz	100	7	1	250	0	8.0	5.0	20	69%
(Sargento) sliced	1 slice	100	7	0	190	0	8.0	5.0	25	72%
PUB *(Hickory Farms)*	1 oz	94	6	2	237	0	6.9	0.0	18	66%
QUESO ANEJO										
Mexican	1 oz	106	6	1	321	0	8.5	5.4	30	71%
Mexican, crumbled	1 cup	492	28	6	1493	0	39.6	25.1	139	71%
QUESO ASEDERO										
Mexican	1 oz	101	6	1	186	0	8.0	5.1	30	70%
Mexican, diced	1 cup	470	30	4	865	0	37.3	23.7	139	70%
Mexican, shredded	1 cup	402	26	3	740	0	31.9	20.3	119	70%
QUESO BLANCO *(Sargento)*	1 oz	100	7	0	180	0	9.0	0.0	27	74%
QUESO CHIHUAHUA										
Mexican	1 oz	106	6	2	175	0	8.4	5.3	30	70%
Mexican, diced	1 cup	494	28	7	814	0	39.2	24.9	139	70%
Mexican, shredded	1 cup	423	24	6	697	0	33.5	21.3	119	70%
QUESO DE PAPA *(Sargento)*	1 oz	110	7	0	180	0	9.0	0.0	30	73%
QUESO DE TACO *(Hickory Farms)*	1 oz	106	6	1	450	0	8.9	0.0	27	75%
RICOTTA										
part skim	1 cup	340	28	13	307	0	19.5	12.1	76	50%
part skim	1 oz	39	3	1	35	0	2.2	1.4	9	50%
whole milk	1 cup	428	28	7	207	0	31.9	20.4	124	66%
(Breakstone's) whole milk	4 oz	200	12	6	95	0	15.0	8.0	55	65%
(Crowley)										
part skim	2 oz	80	7	3	50	0	4.0	0.0	15	47%
whole milk	2 oz	100	6	3	50	0	7.0	0.0	25	64%
(Frigo)										
low-fat	1/4 cup	64	9	3	98	0	1.9	1.2	11	26%
nonfat	1/4 cup	48	8	2	122	0	0.4	0.3	6	8%
nonfat, 'Truly Lite'	1 oz	20	4	2	15	0	0.0	0.0	3	0%
part skim	1 oz	45	3	1	100	0	3.0	0.0	10	63%
whole milk	1 oz	50	3	1	100	0	4.0	0.0	15	69%
(Gardenia) low-fat	1/4 cup	65	8	2	159	0	2.8	1.7	14	39%
(Polly-O)										
light, 'Lite'	2 oz	80	7	3	65	0	4.0	0.0	15	47%
part skim	2 oz	90	7	2	45	0	6.0	0.0	20	60%
whole milk	2 oz	100	7	2	45	0	7.0	0.0	20	64%
(Precious) low-fat, natural	1 oz	40	3	2	20	0	2.0	1.0	10	47%
(Sargento)										
	1 oz	40	3	1	25	0	3.0	0.0	13	63%
light	1/4 cup	60	5	3	55	0	2.5	1.5	15	41%
old fashioned	1/4 cup	90	7	3	75	0	6.0	4.0	25	57%
part skim	1/4 cup	80	7	2	75	0	5.0	3.0	20	56%
ROMANO										
	1 oz	110	9	1	340	0	7.6	4.9	29	61%
(Frigo)										
grated	1 oz	130	12	1	510	0	9.0	0.0	0	61%
wedge	1 oz	110	9	1	350	0	8.0	0.0	0	64%
(Kraft) grated	1 oz	130	11	1	350	0	9.0	6.0	30	63%
(Hickory Farms) loaf	1 oz	110	9	1	350	0	8.0	0.0	0	64%
(Kraft) 'Natural'	1 oz	100	8	1	250	0	7.0	4.0	20	64%
(Polly-O) grated	1 oz	130	11	1	530	0	10.0	0.0	30	65%
(Progresso) grated	1 tbsp	23	2	1	70	0	2.0	1.0	6	60%
(Sargento)	1 oz	110	9	1	340	0	8.0	0.0	29	64%
ROQUEFORT	1 oz	105	6	1	513	0	8.7	5.5	26	73%

Food Name	Serving Size	Calories	Prot. gms	Carbs gms	Sod. mgs	Fiber gms	Fat gms	Sat. Fat gms	Chol. mgs	% Fat Cal.
SMOKED										
(Hickory Farms) 'Light Choice Smoky Lyte'	1 oz	80	7	1	449	0	6.0	0.0	5	63%
(Hoffman's) sharp, processed	1 oz	110	6	1	440	0	9.0	0.0	0	74%
(Sargento) 'Smokestick'	1 oz	100	7	1	390	0	7.0	0.0	24	66%
SOY. See under CHEESE SUBSTITUTE.										
STRING										
(Frigo)	1 oz	80	7	1	190	0	5.0	0.0	0	58%
(Kraft) low moisture	1 oz	80	8	1	230	0	5.0	3.0	20	56%
(Polly-O)	1 oz slice	90	7	2	200	0	6.0	0.0	15	60%
(Sargento)										
	1 oz	80	8	1	150	0	5.0	0.0	15	56%
light , 'Mootown Snackers'	1 piece	60	7	1	200	0	3.0	2.0	10	47%
smoked	1 oz	80	8	1	150	0	5.0	0.0	15	56%
SWISS										
	1 oz	107	8	1	74	0	7.8	5.0	26	64%
diced	1 cup	496	38	4	343	0	36.2	23.5	121	64%
pasteurized process, w/disodium phosphate added	1 oz	95	7	1	388	0	7.1	4.5	24	66%
shredded	1 cup	406	31	4	281	0	29.6	19.2	99	64%
(Alpine Lace)										
light, 'Swiss-Lo'	1 oz	100	8	1	35	0	7.0	4.0	20	64%
natural, milk, sliced, 'Swiss-Lo'	1 oz	90	8	1	35	0	6.0	4.0	20	60%
(Boar's Head)										
'Domestic'	1 oz	110	7	1	75	0	8.0	0.0	25	69%
no salt added	1 oz	100	8	1	12	0	8.0	0.0	26	67%
(Borden)										
processed	1 oz	100	7	1	380	0	8.0	0.0	0	69%
processed, fat-free, low cholesterol	1 oz	40	6	4	0	0	0.0	0.0	5	0%
(Casino)	1 oz	110	8	1	35	0	8.0	5.0	30	67%
(Dorman's)										
	1 oz	100	8	0	80	0	8.0	0.0	0	69%
less fat	1 oz	90	10	0	80	0	5.0	2.8	17	53%
low-fat, low-sodium	1 oz	90	10	0	60	0	5.0	3.0	17	53%
no salt added	1 oz	100	8	0	8	0	8.0	0.0	0	69%
no salt added, 'Deli Light'	1 oz	100	8	0	8	0	8.0	5.0	26	69%
smoked	1 oz	100	7	1	390	0	7.0	0.0	0	66%
(Healthy Favorites) less fat, natural, sliced	1 oz	80	9	1	70	0	4.0	2.0	15	47%
(Hickory Farms)										
creamy, 'Cold Pack'	1 oz	92	6	3	237	0	7.2	0.0	24	67%
'Domestic'	1 oz	110	8	1	75	0	7.8	0.0	25	66%
light, 'Light Choice Lorraine'	1 oz	100	8	0	35	0	7.8	0.0	25	69%
low-salt, 'Light Choice Low Sodium'	1 oz	100	8	0	8	0	8.0	0.0	26	69%
(Hoffman's) w/cheddar, smoky	1 oz	110	7	1	410	0	8.0	0.0	0	69%
(Kraft)										
	1 oz	110	8	1	40	0	8.0	5.0	25	67%
aged	1 oz	110	8	1	45	0	8.0	5.0	25	67%
light, 'Light Naturals'	1 oz	90	10	1	45	0	5.0	3.0	20	51%
low-salt, '75% Very Low Sodium'	1 oz	110	8	1	10	0	8.0	5.0	25	67%
natural, baby, 'Cracker Barrel'	1 oz	110	7	0	65	0	9.0	5.0	25	74%
natural, less fat, 'Light Naturals'	1 oz	90	10	1	70	0	5.0	3.0	20	51%
processed, 'Deluxe'	1 oz	90	7	1	420	0	7.0	4.0	25	66%
processed, 'Light'	1 oz	70	6	2	350	0	3.0	2.0	15	46%
(Land O'Lakes) natural	1 oz	110	8	1	75	0	8.0	5.0	25	67%
(Sargento)										
'Finland'	1 oz	110	8	1	75	0	8.0	0.0	26	67%

Food Name	Serving Size	Calories	Prot. gms	Carbs gms	Sod. mgs	Fiber gms	Fat gms	Sat. Fat gms	Chol. mgs	% Fat Cal.
light, thin sliced, 'Preferred Light'	1 slice	80	9	1	50	0	4.0	2.5	15	49%
mild, wafer thin sliced	1 slice	110	8	0	40	0	9.0	5.0	25	72%
shredded, 'Fancy Supreme'	1/4 cup	110	8	0	40	0	8.0	5.0	30	69%
sliced	1 slice	80	6	0	30	0	6.0	4.0	20	69%
(Weight Watchers)										
'Natural'	1 oz	90	9	1	50	0	5.0	3.0	15	53%
nonfat	1 slice	30	5	2	281	0	0.0	0.0	0	0%
TACO										
(Frigo) shredded	1 oz	110	7	1	200	0	9.0	0.0	0	72%
(Kraft) shredded	1 oz	110	7	1	190	0	9.0	5.0	30	72%
(Sargento)										
	1 oz	110	7	1	160	0	9.0	0.0	27	73%
shredded, 'Classic Supreme'	1/4 cup	110	6	1	220	0	9.0	6.0	25	74%
shredded, 'Preferred Light'	1/4 cup	70	8	1	240	0	4.5	2.5	15	54%
TALEGGIO (Tal-Fino) natural, 'Brand Imported'	1 oz	89	5	0	176	0	7.4	0.0	0	75%
TILSIT										
	1 oz	96	7	1	213	0	7.4	4.8	29	67%
(Sargento)	1 oz	100	7	1	210	0	7.0	0.0	29	66%
TYBO										
(Dorman's) 45%	1 oz	98	7	0	200	0	7.5	4.7	23	69%
(Sargento) red wax	1 oz	100	7	0	200	0	7.0	0.0	23	68%
VERMONT (Churny)	1 oz	110	7	1	180	0	9.0	5.0	30	72%
CHEESE-BALL										
cheddar, sharp, w/almonds (Kaukauna)	1 oz	100	6	3	250	0	7.0	0.0	25	64%
cheddar, w/almonds and bacon (Kaukauna)	1 oz	100	6	3	250	0	7.0	0.0	25	64%
green onion flavor, w/almonds (Kaukauna)	1 oz	100	6	3	250	0	7.0	0.0	25	64%
Port wine, w/almonds (Kaukauna)	1 oz	100	6	3	250	0	7.0	0.0	25	64%
CHEESE DISH/ENTRÉE										
(Snow's) Welsh rarebit, canned	1/2 cup	170	9	10	460	0	11.0	0.0	0	57%
(Stouffer's)										
Swiss cheese strata, frozen, food service product	4 oz	176	8	10	376	1	11.2	4.4	119	58%
Welsh rarebit	1/4 cup	120	5	5	280	0	9.0	4.0	20	67%
CHEESE FLAVORED SEASONING										
(Molly McButter)	1/2 tsp	4	0	1	61	0	0.1	na	0	29%
CHEESE FLAVORED SNACK										
(Barbara's Bakery)										
cheese flavored puffs, tangy triple cheese, 'Pinta Puffs'	1 oz	70	2	10	100	0	2.0	0.0	5	27%
cheese puff bakes (Barbara's Bakery)	1 1/2 cup	160	2	13	190	0	11.0	2.0	0	62%
(Bearitos)										
cheddar flavored puffs, light	1 oz	120	2	20	150	na	4.0	1.0	0	29%
cheddar flavored puffs, original	1 oz	160	2	14	260	na	10.0	2.0	4	58%
(Cheetos)										
cheddar valley	1 oz	160	2	16	240	1	9.0	0.0	0	53%
cheese flavored puffs	1 oz	160	2	15	370	1	10.0	2.5	0	57%
cheese flavored puffs, balls	1 oz	150	2	15	300	1	10.0	3.0	0	57%
cheese flavored puffs, crunchy	1 oz	160	2	15	290	1	10.0	2.5	0	57%
cheese flavored puffs, curls	1 oz	150	2	15	290	1	10.0	3.0	0	57%
cheese flavored puffs, flamin' hot	1 oz	160	2	15	240	1	10.0	2.0	0	57%
cheese flavored puffs, jumbo	1 oz	160	2	13	350	0	10.0	2.5	0	60%
light, approx 38 pieces	1 oz	140	2	19	280	1	6.0	0.0	0	39%
paws, approx 16 pieces	1 oz	160	1	15	310	1	10.0	0.0	0	58%
(Eagle)										
cheese crunch, 'Cheegles'	1 cup	160	2	15	240	0	10.0	2.0	0	57%
cheese flavored balls, 'Cheegles'	2 1/2 cups	160	2	15	260	0	10.0	2.0	0	57%

Food Name	Serving Size	Calories	Prot. gms	Carbs gms	Sod. mgs	Fiber gms	Fat gms	Sat. Fat gms	Chol. mgs	% Fat Cal.
cheese flavored balls, less fat, 'Cheegles'	2 1/2 cups	150	2	18	200	0	6.0	1.5	0	40%
'Shamu Shapes'	1 cup	160	2	15	260	0	10.0	2.0	0	57%
(Flavor Tree)										
cheese flavored sticks, cheddar	1/4 cup	129	3	12	335	0	8.1	0.0	0	56%
(Health Valley)										
cheese flavored puffs, baked, w/organic corn,										
'Cheddar Lite'	0.25 oz	40	1	4	35	0	2.0	0.0	0	47%
cheese flavored puffs, nonfat	1 cup	73	2	15	173	1	0.0	0.0	0	0%
cheese flavored puffs, w/chili, nonfat	1 oz	100	3	21	75	0	0.0	0.0	0	0%
(Keebler)										
zesty cheddar, 'RC Ricers'	1 oz	140	2	17	200	0	8.0	2.0	0	49%
(Planters)										
cheese flavored balls, 'Cheez Balls'	1 oz	160	2	14	270	0	11.0	2.0	5	61%
cheese flavored balls, nacho, 'Cheez Balls'	1 oz	160	2	15	290	0	10.0	2.0	5	57%
cheese flavored curls, 'Cheez Curls'	1 oz	160	2	14	290	0	11.0	2.0	5	61%
cheese flavored curls, nacho, 'Cheez Curls'	1 oz	160	2	15	290	0	10.0	2.0	5	57%
(Ralston)										
cheddar snacks, 'Stop & Shop'	18 crackers	150	2	20	240	2	7.0	1.0	na	42%
(Weight Watchers)										
cheese curls	1 serving	70	1	10	85	0	2.5	1.0	0	34%
(Wise)										
cheese flavored puffs, baked, 'Cheez Doodles'	1 oz	150	2	16	360	0	9.0	0.0	0	53%
cheese flavored spirals, nacho cheese	1 oz	160	2	16	190	0	10.0	0.0	0	56%
'Cheez Waffies'	1 oz	140	3	14	420	0	8.0	0.0	0	51%
cheese flavored twists, nacho cheese, crispy	1 oz	160	2	16	190	0	10.0	0.0	0	56%
fried, crunchy, 'Cheez Doodles'	1 oz	160	2	16	230	0	10.0	0.0	0	56%
CHEESE FOOD. See also CHEESE PRODUCT.										
(Kraft)										
nonfat, processed, singles, 'Free'	1 oz	45	6	4	430	0	0.0	0.0	5	0%
pasteurized process, shredded, 'Velveeta'	1/4 cup	130	8	3	500	0	9.0	6.0	30	65%
shredded, 'Velveeta'	1 oz	100	6	3	410	0	7.0	4.0	20	64%
(Land O'Lakes)										
processed	1 oz	90	5	2	350	0	6.0	4.0	20	66%
processed, slices	3/4 oz	70	4	2	260	0	5.0	3.0	15	65%
(Nippy)	1 oz	90	5	2	380	0	7.0	4.0	20	69%
AMERICAN										
(Borden)										
processed, sharp, 'Singles'	1 oz	90	5	2	470	0	7.0	0.0	0	69%
processed, 'Singles'	1 oz	90	5	3	350	0	7.0	0.0	0	66%
processed, 'Slices'	1 oz	100	6	2	420	0	7.0	0.0	0	66%
(Darigold) processed	1 oz	80	5	2	381	0	6.0	3.8	16	66%
(Hoffman's) processed, colored	1 oz	100	5	3	490	0	7.0	0.0	0	66%
(Kraft)										
processed, grated	1 oz	130	8	8	740	0	7.0	4.0	25	50%
processed, 'Light'	1 oz	70	6	2	420	0	4.0	3.0	15	53%
processed, 'Singles'	1 oz	90	5	2	390	0	7.0	4.0	25	69%
processed, white, 'Singles'	1 oz	90	5	2	400	0	7.0	4.0	20	69%
(Land O'Lakes) processed, w/Swiss cheese	1 oz	100	7	1	400	0	8.0	5.0	25	69%
BACON										
(Hoffman's) 'Chees'N Bacon'	1 oz	90	6	3	540	0	6.0	0.0	0	60%
(Kraft)										
'Chees'N Bacon'	1 oz	90	6	2	400	0	7.0	4.0	25	66%
'Cracker Barrel'	1 oz	90	5	3	280	0	7.0	4.0	20	66%
CARAWAY *(Hoffman's)* 'Swisson Rye'	1 oz	90	6	2	400	0	7.0	0.0	0	66%

Food Name	Serving Size	Calories	Prot. gms	Carbs gms	Sod. mgs	Fiber gms	Fat gms	Sat. Fat gms	Chol. mgs	% Fat Cal.
CHEDDAR										
(Alpine Lace) nonfat	1 oz	45	8	2	280	0	0.0	0.0	0	0%
(Kaukauna)										
extra sharp, cold pack, 'Cup'	1 oz	100	6	3	250	0	7.0	0.0	25	64%
nacho, processed, cold pack 'Cup'	1 oz	100	6	3	250	0	7.0	0.0	25	64%
sharp, 'Lite'	1 oz	70	5	5	230	0	4.0	0.0	15	47%
sharp, cold pack, 'Cup'	1 oz	100	6	3	250	0	7.0	0.0	25	64%
sharp, cup, 'Lite 50'	1 oz	70	5	5	190	0	3.0	2.0	15	40%
smoky, 'Lite'	1 oz	70	5	5	230	0	4.0	0.0	15	47%
w/bacon and horseradish, cold pack, 'Cup'	1 oz	100	6	3	250	0	7.0	0.0	25	64%
(Kraft)										
extra sharp, processed, 'Cracker Barrel'	1 oz	90	5	3	240	0	7.0	4.0	20	66%
sharp, processed, 'Cracker Barrel'	1 oz	100	4	4	230	0	7.0	4.0	20	66%
sharp, 'Singles'	1 oz	100	6	1	400	0	8.0	5.0	25	72%
(Land O'Lakes)										
extra sharp, processed	1 oz	100	6	1	370	0	9.0	6.0	30	74%
'La Chedda'	1 oz	90	6	2	335	0	7.0	4.0	20	66%
processed, w/bacon	1 oz	110	6	1	350	0	9.0	5.0	25	74%
(Wispride) sharp, cold pack	1 oz	100	5	2	210	0	7.0	0.0	25	69%
GARLIC (Kraft) pasteurized process	1 oz	90	5	2	370	0	7.0	4.5	20	69%
ITALIAN HERB (Land O'Lakes) processed	1 oz	90	6	2	430	0	7.0	4.0	20	66%
JALAPEÑO										
(Hoffman's)	1 oz	90	5	2	580	0	7.0	0.0	0	69%
(Kraft)										
pasteurized process	1 oz	90	5	2	370	0	7.0	5.0	20	69%
'Singles'	1 oz	90	5	2	450	0	7.0	4.0	25	69%
(Land O'Lakes)										
	1 oz	90	6	2	360	0	7.0	4.0	20	66%
processed	1 oz	90	6	2	400	0	7.0	4.0	20	66%
MEXICAN										
(Kraft)										
hot, pasteurized process, shredded, 'Velveeta'	1/4 cup	130	8	3	540	0	9.0	6.0	30	65%
hot, shredded, 'Velveeta'	1 oz	100	6	3	430	0	7.0	4.0	25	64%
mild, shredded, 'Velveeta'	1 oz	100	6	3	420	0	7.0	4.0	25	64%
ONION										
(Hoffman's) 'Chees'N Onion'	1 oz	100	5	3	490	0	7.0	0.0	0	66%
(Land O'Lakes) processed	1 oz	90	6	2	330	0	7.0	4.0	15	66%
PEPPERONI (Land O'Lakes) processed	1 oz	90	6	1	395	0	7.0	4.0	20	69%
PIMIENTO										
(Kraft)										
'Singles'	1 oz	90	5	2	390	0	7.0	4.0	25	69%
processed, 'Deluxe'	1 oz	100	6	1	440	0	8.0	5.0	25	72%
PORT WINE										
(Kaukauna)										
cold pack, 'Cup'	1 oz	100	6	3	250	0	7.0	0.0	25	64%
cup, 'Lite 50'	1 oz	70	5	5	190	0	3.0	2.0	15	40%
(Wispride) cold pack	1 oz	100	5	3	210	0	7.0	0.0	25	66%
SALAMI										
(Hoffman's) 'Chees'N Salami'	1 oz	90	5	3	560	0	6.0	0.0	0	63%
(Land O'Lakes) processed	1 oz	90	6	2	410	0	7.0	4.0	20	66%
SMOKY (Kaukauna) cold pack 'Cup'	1 oz	100	6	3	250	0	7.0	0.0	25	64%
SWISS										
(Borden) processed, slices 'Singles'	1 oz	100	6	2	420	0	7.0	0.0	0	66%

Food Name	Serving Size	Calories	Prot. gms	Carbs gms	Sod. mgs	Fiber gms	Fat gms	Sat. Fat gms	Chol. mgs	% Fat Cal.
(Kaukauna)										
almond, cup, 'Lite 50'	1 oz	70	5	5	180	0	3.0	2.0	15	40%
country, cold pack 'Cup'	1 oz	100	6	3	250	0	7.0	0.0	25	64%
country, 'Lite'	1 oz	70	6	5	200	0	4.0	0.0	15	45%
(Kraft)										
fat-free, singles, 'Free'	1 oz	45	6	4	390	0	0.0	0.0	5	0%
singles	1 oz	90	6	2	440	0	7.0	4.0	25	66%
(Velveeta)	1 oz	100	6	3	410	0	7.0	4.0	20	64%
CHEESE-LOG										
CHEDDAR										
(Kraft)										
sharp, w/almonds, 'Cracker Barrel'	1 oz	90	5	4	410	0	6.0	3.0	15	60%
smoky, w/almonds, 'Cracker Barrel'	1 oz	90	5	4	410	0	6.0	3.0	15	60%
(Kaukauna)										
white, sharp, w/green onion	1 oz	100	6	3	250	0	7.0	0.0	25	64%
white, sharp hickory smoke	1 oz	100	6	3	250	0	7.0	0.0	25	64%
(Sargento)										
Port wine	1 oz	100	6	3	250	0	7.0	0.0	18	64%
sharp	1 oz	100	6	3	250	0	7.0	0.0	18	64%
SWISS										
(Kaukauna) w/almonds	1 oz	100	6	3	250	0	7.0	0.0	25	64%
(Sargento) w/almonds	1 oz	90	6	2	350	0	7.0	0.0	21	66%
CHEESE NUGGET, mozzarella, breaded, frozen,										
'Cheese Hot Bites' *(Banquet)*	2.63 oz	240	14	16	530	0	13.0	0.0	0	49%
CHEESE NUT										
(Kraft)										
cheddar, sharp, 'Cracker Barrel'	1 oz	100	5	4	250	0	7.0	3.0	20	64%
Port wine, 'Cracker Barrel'	1 oz	90	5	4	260	0	6.0	3.0	15	60%
(Kaukauna) sharp, w/bell and jalapeno peppers	1 oz	100	6	3	250	0	7.0	0.0	25	64%
CHEESE PRODUCT										
(Borden) 'Singles' processed, slices, fat-free	1 oz	40	6	4	380	0	0.0	0.0	5	0%
(Kraft)										
'Cheez Whiz' light, pasteurized process	2 tbsp	75	6	6	597	0	3.3	2.2	12	40%
'Cheez Whiz' pasteurized process	2 tbsp	91	4	3	541	0	6.9	4.3	25	68%
'Velveeta' less fat, pasteurized process	1 oz	62	5	3	444	0	3.0	2.0	12	43%
(Lite-Line) slices, processed, fat-free	1 slice	25	4	3	250	0	0.0	0.0	5	0%
(Lunch Wagon) sandwich slices, processed	1 oz	90	5	2	370	0	7.0	2.0	5	69%
AMERICAN FLAVOR										
(Alpine Lace) processed	1 oz	90	6	2	200	0	7.0	4.0	20	66%
(Borden) processed, 'Light'	1 oz	70	6	1	420	0	5.0	0.0	0	62%
(Harvest Moon) processed	1 oz	70	6	2	420	0	4.0	2.0	15	53%
(Kraft)										
pasteurized process	1 slice	31	5	2	273	0	0.2	0.1	3	6%
processed, 'Light Singles'	1 oz	70	6	2	420	0	4.0	3.0	15	53%
white, processed, 'Light Singles'	1 oz	70	6	2	410	0	4.0	2.0	15	53%
(Light n' Lively) white, processed, 'Singles'	1 oz	70	6	2	410	0	4.0	2.0	15	53%
(Lite-Line)										
processed	1 oz	50	7	1	410	0	2.0	0.0	0	36%
processed, reduced sodium	1 oz	70	6	2	90	0	4.0	0.0	0	53%
processed, 'Sodium Lite'	1 oz	70	6	2	200	0	4.0	0.0	0	53%
CHEDDAR FLAVOR										
(Kraft)										
sharp, processed, 'Free'	1 oz	45	6	4	390	0	0.0	0.0	5	0%
sharp, processed, 'Light'	1 oz	70	6	2	380	0	4.0	2.0	15	53%

Food Name	Serving Size	Calories	Prot. gms	Carbs gms	Sod. mgs	Fiber gms	Fat gms	Sat. Fat gms	Chol. mgs	% Fat Cal.
sharp, processed, 'Singles'	1 oz	100	6	1	400	0	8.0	0.0	25	72%
(Light n' Lively) sharp, processed, 'Singles'	1 oz	70	6	2	380	0	4.0	2.0	15	53%
(Lite-Line)										
mild, processed	1 oz	50	7	1	380	0	2.0	0.0	0	36%
sharp, processed	1 oz	50	7	1	440	0	2.0	0.0	0	36%
sharp, processed, slices	1 slice	35	4	1	300	0	2.0	0.0	5	47%
(Spreadery)										
medium, processed	1 oz	70	5	3	250	0	4.0	2.0	15	53%
sharp, processed	1 oz	70	5	3	240	0	4.0	2.0	15	53%
Vermont white, processed	1 oz	70	5	3	230	0	4.0	2.0	15	53%
CREAM CHEESE FLAVOR										
(Philadelphia Brand) processed, 'Light'	1 oz	60	3	2	160	0	5.0	3.0	10	69%
MEXICAN FLAVOR										
(Spreadery) mild, w/jalapeños, processed	1 oz	70	5	3	260	0	4.0	3.0	15	53%
MOZZARELLA FLAVOR										
(Alpine Lace) nonfat	1 oz	45	8	2	280	0	0.0	0.0	0	0%
(Lite-Line) processed	1 oz	50	7	1	340	0	2.0	0.0	0	36%
MUENSTER FLAVOR (Lite-Line) processed	1 oz	50	7	1	450	0	2.0	0.0	0	36%
NACHO FLAVOR (Spreadery) processed	1 oz	70	5	3	240	0	4.0	2.0	15	53%
NEUFCHATEL										
(Spreadery)										
French onion, processed	1 oz	70	2	2	135	0	6.0	4.0	20	77%
garden vegetable, processed	1 oz	70	2	2	220	0	6.0	3.0	20	77%
garlic and herb, processed	1 oz	70	2	1	140	0	6.0	4.0	20	82%
ranch, classic, processed	1 oz	70	2	1	190	0	7.0	4.0	20	84%
strawberry, processed	1 oz	70	2	1	270	0	5.0	3.0	15	79%
PORT WINE FLAVOR (Spreadery) processed	1 oz	70	5	3	250	0	4.0	2.0	15	53%
SWISS FLAVOR										
(Kraft) processed, slices, 'Free Singles'	1 oz	45	6	4	390	0	0.0	0.0	5	0%
(Light n' Lively) processed, 'Singles'	1 oz	70	6	2	350	0	3.0	2.0	15	46%
(Lite-Line) processed	1 oz	50	7	1	380	0	2.0	0.0	0	36%
CHEESE SPREAD										
(Kraft)										
'Velveeta'	1 oz	80	5	3	430	0	6.0	4.0	20	63%
'Velveeta' pasteurized process	1 oz	85	5	3	420	0	6.2	4.0	22	65%
'Velveeta' slices	1 oz	90	5	3	400	0	6.0	4.0	20	63%
(Land O'Lakes) processed, 'Golden Velvet'	1 oz	80	5	2	380	0	6.0	4.0	15	66%
(Laughing Cow) 'Cheezbits'	1/6 oz	13	1	0	55	0	1.0	0.0	3	71%
(Micro Melt)	1 oz	80	4	2	380	0	6.0	0.0	15	69%
AMERICAN										
(Easy Cheese) pasteurized process	2 tbsp	100	6	2	400	0	7.0	4.0	25	66%
(Kraft) processed	1 oz	80	4	2	470	0	6.0	3.0	15	69%
(Nabisco) 'Easy Cheese American'	1 oz	80	4	2	350	0	6.0	0.0	0	69%
(Sargento)										
sharp, processed, 'Cracker Snacks'	1 oz	110	6	1	410	0	9.0	0.0	27	76%
w/pimento, processed, 'Cracker Snacks'	1 oz	110	6	1	410	0	9.0	0.0	27	76%
BACON										
(Kraft)	1 oz	80	5	1	560	0	7.0	4.0	20	72%
(Squeez-A-Snak)	1 oz	80	5	1	500	0	7.0	4.0	20	72%
BLUE (Roka)	1 oz	70	3	2	270	0	6.0	4.0	20	73%
BRICK 'Cracker Snacks' (Sargento)	1 oz	100	6	1	430	0	9.0	0.0	25	74%
CHEDDAR										
(Kraft)										
extra sharp, 'Cracker Barrel'	2 tbsp	80	3	1	180	0	8.0	5.0	20	84%

Food Name	Serving Size	Calories	Prot. gms	Carbs gms	Sod. mgs	Fiber gms	Fat gms	Sat. Fat gms	Chol. mgs	% Fat Cal.
sharp, and cream cheese, 'Cracker Barrel'	2 tbsp	80	3	1	180	0	8.0	5.0	20	84%
(Nabisco)										
'Easy Cheese Cheddar'	1 oz	80	4	2	370	0	6.0	0.0	0	69%
'Easy Cheese Cheddar 'n Bacon'	1 oz	80	4	2	350	0	6.0	0.0	0	69%
'Easy Cheese Sharp Cheddar'	1 oz	80	4	2	320	0	6.0	0.0	0	69%
(Old English) sharp	1 oz	80	5	1	480	0	7.0	4.0	20	72%
(Squeez-A-Snak) sharp	1 oz	80	5	1	440	0	7.0	4.0	20	72%
(Weight Watchers) sharp, 'Cup'	1 oz	70	4	7	190	0	3.0	2.0	10	38%
GARLIC *(Squeez-A-Snak)*	1 oz	80	5	1	430	0	7.0	4.0	20	72%
HICKORY SMOKE *(Squeez-A-Snak)*	1 oz	80	5	1	440	0	7.0	4.0	20	72%
JALAPEÑO										
(Kraft)										
	1 oz	70	2	3	95	0	5.0	3.0	15	69%
loaf	1 oz	80	5	2	470	0	6.0	4.0	20	66%
(Squeez-A-Snak)	1 oz	80	5	1	510	0	6.0	4.0	20	69%
LIMBURGER *(Mohawk Valley)*	1 oz	70	4	0	420	0	6.0	3.0	20	77%
MEXICAN *(Velveeta)* mild	1 oz	80	5	3	440	0	6.0	3.0	20	63%
NACHO *(Nabisco)* 'Easy Cheese Nacho'	1 oz	80	4	2	340	0	6.0	0.0	0	69%
OLIVE *(Kraft)* olives and pimiento	1 oz	60	2	2	160	0	5.0	3.0	15	74%
PIMIENTO										
(Kraft)	1 oz	70	2	3	120	0	5.0	3.0	15	69%
'Velveeta' *(Kraft)*	1 oz	80	5	3	400	0	6.0	3.0	20	63%
PINEAPPLE *(Kraft)*	1 oz	70	2	4	15	0	5.0	3.0	75	65%
PORT WINE 'Cup' *(Weight Watchers)*	1 oz	70	4	7	190	0	3.0	2.0	10	38%
GARLIC										
(Alouette) and spices	1 oz	95	2	2	165	0	9.0	0.0	31	84%
(Rondel) w/herbs, soft, 'Lite'	1 oz	70	3	2	170	0	6.0	3.0	15	73%
HERB										
(Alouette) and garlic, soft, 'Light'	1 oz	60	3	2	130	0	4.5	0.0	15	67%
(Rondel) soft, 'Fines Herbes'	1 oz	90	3	2	170	0	8.0	0.0	0	78%
HORSERADISH *(Alouette)* and chive	1 oz	85	2	1	130	0	8.0	0.0	28	86%
LIMBURGER *(Mohawk Valley)*	1 oz	70	4	0	420	0	6.0	3.0	20	77%
MEXICAN										
(Kraft)										
hot, 'Velveeta'	1 oz	80	5	3	520	0	6.0	3.0	20	63%
mild, 'Velveeta'	1 oz	80	5	3	440	0	6.0	3.0	20	63%
ONION *(Alouette)* French	1 oz	95	2	2	205	0	9.0	0.0	31	84%
PIMENTO										
(Kraft)										
	1 oz	70	2	3	120	0	5.0	3.0	15	69%
'Velveeta'	1 oz	80	5	3	400	0	6.0	3.0	20	63%
PINEAPPLE *(Kraft)*	1 oz	70	2	4	75	0	5.0	3.0	15	65%
PORT WINE *(Weight Watchers)* 'Cup'	1 oz	70	4	7	190	0	3.0	2.0	10	38%
SALMON *(Alouette)*	1 oz	70	2	2	140	0	6.0	0.0	20	77%
SPINACH *(Alouette)* creamy	1 oz	90	2	2	125	0	8.0	0.0	0	82%
SWISS *(Sargento)* 'Cracker Snacks'	1 oz	100	7	1	390	0	7.0	0.0	24	66%
VEGETABLE										
(Alouette) spring, soft, 'Light'	1 oz	60	3	1	120	0	4.5	0.0	15	72%
(Rondel) garden, soft	1 oz	90	3	3	160	0	8.0	0.0	0	75%
CHEESE STICK										
CHEDDAR										
(Farm Rich) breaded, frozen	3 oz	300	11	19	740	0	21.0	0.0	0	61%
(Flavor Tree) snack	1/4 cup	129	3	12	335	0	8.1	0.0	0	56%
(Stilwell) battered, frozen	1 piece	80	4	8	40	1	4.0	2.0	10	43%

Food Name	Serving Size	Calories	Prot. gms	Carbs gms	Sod. mgs	Fiber gms	Fat gms	Sat. Fat gms	Chol. mgs	% Fat Cal.
PEPPER										
(Farm Rich) hot, breaded, frozen	3 oz	260	8	20	700	0	17.0	0.0	0	58%
(Stilwell) jalapeño, breaded, frozen	1 piece	70	4	8	220	1	3.0	2.0	10	36%
MOZZARELLA										
(Farm Rich) breaded, frozen	3 oz	240	10	19	570	0	13.0	0.0	0	50%
(Frigo) string, natural, 'Truly Lite'	0.83 oz	50	8	1	116	0	2.0	2.0	7	33%
(Stilwell)										
baby, battered, frozen	3 pieces	80	4	8	350	1	4.0	2.0	10	43%
battered, frozen	1 piece	80	4	7	180	1	5.0	2.5	10	51%
premium, battered, frozen	1 piece	100	5	9	180	0	5.0	3.0	15	45%
PROVOLONE										
(Farm Rich) provolone, breaded, frozen	3 oz	270	10	22	820	0	16.0	0.0	0	53%
CHEESE SUBSTITUTE. See also CHEESE FOOD; CHEESE PRODUCT.										
(Cheeztwin)	1 oz	90	5	3	400	0	6.0	0.0	0	63%
(Fisher) 'Sandwich-Mate'	1 oz	90	5	3	400	0	6.0	0.0	0	63%
(Lite-Line) low-cholesterol	1 oz	90	5	2	430	0	7.0	0.0	0	69%
(Nucoa) 'Heart Beat'	1 1/2 slices	50	7	2	280	0	2.0	1.0	0	33%
AMERICAN STYLE										
(Delicia)										
	1 oz	80	6	1	300	0	6.0	0.0	3	66%
hickory smoked	1 oz	80	6	0	470	0	6.0	0.0	1	69%
w/caraway	1 oz	80	6	1	275	0	6.0	0.0	3	66%
w/hot pepper	1 oz	80	6	1	300	0	6.0	0.0	3	66%
w/salami	1 oz	80	6	1	370	0	6.0	0.0	3	66%
(Formagg) lactose-free, singles	3/4 oz	70	5	1	280	0	5.0	1.0	0	65%
(Golden Image)	1 oz	90	7	2	360	0	6.0	2.0	5	60%
CHEDDAR STYLE										
(Fisher) shredded, 'Ched-O-Mate'	1 oz	90	6	1	330	0	7.0	0.0	0	69%
(Formagg) fancy, shredded	1 oz	70	7	1	70	0	5.0	1.0	0	58%
(Frigo)	1 oz	90	5	1	280	0	7.0	1.0	0	72%
(Golden Image) mild	1 oz	110	7	0	190	0	9.0	2.0	5	74%
(Nu Tofu)										
	1 oz	70	6	1	190	0	4.0	0.5	0	56%
low salt	1 oz	70	7	1	75	0	4.0	0.5	0	53%
nonfat	1 oz	40	7	2	240	0	0.0	0.0	0	0%
(Rella Good)										
California style, 'AlmondRella'	1 oz	50	7	1	170	0	1.4	0.2	0	28%
California style, 'Zero-Fat Rella'	1 oz	45	8	3	170	0	0.0	0.0	0	0%
mild, 'TofuRella'	1 oz	80	8	1	170	0	5.0	0.8	0	56%
mild, slices, 'TofuRella'	0.75-oz slice	60	5	1	280	0	4.0	0.6	0	60%
(Sargento)										
	1 oz	90	7	1	350	0	6.0	0.0	2	63%
shredded, 'Fancy Supreme'	1/4 cup	90	5	2	420	0	7.0	1.5	0	69%
(Savoldi)	1 oz	90	6	1	400	0	6.0	1.0	0	66%
(Soya Kaas)	1 oz	79	6	2	250	0	5.4	0.0	0	61%
COLBY STYLE										
(Golden Image)	1 oz	110	7	1	190	0	9.0	2.0	5	72%
(Delicia) Longhorn style	1 oz	80	6	1	550	0	6.0	0.0	3	66%
(Dorman's) 'LoChol'	1 oz	90	7	1	140	0	6.0	1.1	1	63%
CREAM CHEESE STYLE										
(Soya Kaas)	1 oz	90	2	0	60	0	9.4	0.0	0	90%
(Tofutti) 'Better Than Cheese'	1 tbsp	40	1	1	68	na	4.0	1.0	0	90%
(Weight Watchers)	1 oz	35	3	1	40	0	2.0	0.0	0	53%

Food Name	Serving Size	Calories	Prot. gms	Carbs gms	Sod. mgs	Fiber gms	Fat gms	Sat. Fat gms	Chol. mgs	% Fat Cal.
GARLIC HERB										
(Rella Good)										
'AlmondRella'	1 oz	60	5	3	250	1	3.0	0.5	0	46%
'TofuRella'	1 oz	80	5	2	290	0	5.0	1.0	0	62%
ITALIAN STYLE										
(Rella Good) 'VeganRella'	1 oz	60	1	7	130	1	3.0	0.0	0	46%
(Weight Watchers) Italian topping, grated, nonfat	1 tbsp	20	2	2	60	0	0.0	0.0	0	0%
JACK										
(Nu Tofu)										
. . . .	1 oz	70	6	2	210	0	4.0	0.5	0	53%
nonfat	1 oz	40	7	2	240	0	0.0	0.0	0	0%
(Rella Good) 'TofuRella'	1 oz	80	5	2	290	0	5.0	1.0	0	62%
JALAPEÑO										
(Rella Good)										
jack, 'Zero-FatRella'	1 oz	45	8	3	170	0	0.0	0.0	0	0%
'TofuRella'	1 oz	80	5	2	290	0	5.0	1.0	0	62%
'Zero-FatRella'	1 oz	40	7	3	250	0	0.0	0.0	0	0%
(Soya Kaas) 'Jalapeño Mexi Kaas'	1 oz	77	7	0	160	0	5.3	0.0	0	63%
MEXICAN *(Rella Good)* 'VeganRella'	1 oz	60	1	7	130	1	3.0	0.0	0	46%
MOZZARELLA STYLE										
(Fisher) shredded, 'Pizza-Mate'	1 oz	90	6	1	310	0	7.0	0.0	0	69%
(Frigo)	1 oz	90	6	1	240	0	7.0	1.0	0	69%
(Nu Tofu)										
. . . .	1 oz	70	6	2	190	0	4.0	0.5	0	53%
low sodium	1 oz	70	6	2	80	0	4.0	0.5	0	53%
nonfat	1 oz	40	7	2	220	0	0.0	0.0	0	0%
(Rella Good)										
'AlmondRella'	1 oz	60	5	3	250	1	3.0	0.5	0	46%
slices	0.75-oz slice	60	5	1	280	0	4.0	0.6	0	60%
'TofuRella'	1 oz	80	5	2	290	0	5.0	1.0	0	62%
'Zero-Fat Rella'	1 oz	40	7	3	250	0	0.0	0.0	0	0%
(Sargento)										
. . . .	1 oz	80	7	1	310	0	6.0	0.0	2	63%
'Classic Supreme'	1/4 cup	80	6	1	320	0	6.0	1.0	0	68%
(Savoldi)	1 oz	80	6	1	360	0	6.0	1.0	0	66%
(Soya Kaas)	1 oz	78	7	2	155	0	5.6	0.0	0	60%
MUENSTER STYLE 'LoChol' *(Dorman's)*	1 oz	100	7	1	140	0	7.0	1.1	1	66%
PARMESAN STYLE *(Soyco)* grated	1 tbsp	23	3	1	120	0	0.8	0.0	0	31%
SWISS STYLE										
(Dorman's) 'LoChol'	1 oz	100	7	1	140	0	7.0	1.1	1	66%
(Formagg) lactose-free, singles	3/4 oz	70	5	1	280	0	5.0	1.0	0	65%
CHEESE TOPPING *(Tone's)* cheddar, w/bacon	1 tsp	10	1	1	81	0	1.0	0.5	1	65%
CHERIMOYA. See CUSTARD APPLE.										
CHERRY										
SOUR										
Canned										
red, in extra heavy syrup, w/liquid	1 cup	298	2	76	18	2	0.2	0.1	0	1%
red, in heavy syrup, w/liquid	1 cup	233	2	60	18	3	0.3	0.1	0	1%
red, in light syrup, w/liquid	1 cup	189	2	49	18	2	0.3	0.1	0	1%
red, in water, w/liquid	1 cup	88	2	22	17	3	0.2	0.1	0	2%
Fresh										
red, raw	1 cup	52	1	13	3	2	0.3	0.1	0	5%
red, raw, pitted	1 cup	78	2	19	5	2	0.5	0.1	0	5%

Food Name	Serving Size	Calories	Prot. gms	Carbs gms	Sod. mgs	Fiber gms	Fat gms	Sat. Fat gms	Chol. mgs	% Fat Cal.
Frozen										
red, unsweetened	18-oz pkg	235	5	56	5	8	2.2	0.5	0	8%
red, unsweetened, unthawed	1 cup	71	1	17	2	2	0.7	0.2	0	8%
SWEET										
Canned										
pitted, in extra heavy syrup w/liquid	1 cup	266	2	68	8	4	0.4	0.1	0	1%
pitted, in heavy syrup, w/liquid	1 cup	210	2	54	8	4	0.4	0.1	0	2%
pitted, in juice, w/liquid	1 cup	135	2	35	8	4	0.1	0.0	0	0%
pitted, in light syrup, w/liquid	1 cup	169	2	44	8	4	0.4	0.1	0	2%
pitted, in water, w/liquid	1 cup	114	2	29	2	4	0.3	0.1	0	2%
Fresh										
raw	1 cup	84	1	19	0	3	1.1	0.3	0	11%
raw, medium	1 cherry	5	0	1	0	0	0.1	0.0	0	11%
raw, pitted	1 cup	104	2	24	0	3	1.4	0.3	0	11%
Frozen										
	10-oz pkg	253	3	64	3	6	0.4	0.1	0	1%
thawed	1 cup	231	3	58	3	5	0.3	0.1	0	1%
CHERRY JUICE. See also BLACK CHERRY JUICE; FRUIT DRINK; FRUIT JUICE DRINK; FRUIT DRINK MIX.										
Canned, bottled, or boxed										
(Dole) blend 'Pure & Light Mountain Cherry'	6 fl oz	87	0	22	8	0	0.1	0.0	0	1%
(Juicy Juice)	6 fl oz	90	0	22	5	0	0.0	0.0	0	0%
(Knudsen & Sons) tart	8 fl oz	125	1	30	0	0	0.0	0.0	0	0%
(Mountain Sun) organic, 'Mountain Cherry'	8 fl oz	109	0	27	0	0	0.0	0.0	0	0%
(Santa Cruz Natural) organic, 'Cruz'	8 fl oz	125	1	29	0	0	1.0	0.0	0	7%
(Welch's) 'Orchard'	6 fl oz	180	0	45	10	0	0.0	0.0	0	0%
Frozen										
(Welch's) concentrate, 'Welchade'	2 fl oz	130	0	31	15	0	0.0	0.0	0	0%
CHERRY PEPPER. See PEPPER, CHERRY.										
CHERRY, SURINAM. See PITANGA.										
CHERVIL										
dried	1 tbsp	4	0	1	2	0	0.1	0.0	0	14%
dried	1 tsp	1	0	0	0	0	0.0	0.0	0	14%
dried *(McCormick/Schilling)*	1 tsp	2	0	0	1	0	0.0	0.0	0	0%
dried *(Tone's)*	1 tsp	1	0	0	2	0	0.1	0.0	0	36%
CHESTNUT, CHINESE										
boiled or steamed	1 oz	43	0.8	9.6	1	>0.3 c	0.2	0.0	0	4%
dried	1 oz	103	1.9	22.6	1	>0.8 c	0.5	0.1	0	4%
raw	1 oz	64	1.2	13.9	1	>0.5 c	0.3	0.1	0	4%
raw, in shell	1 lb	852	16.0	187.0	13	>6.2 c	4.2	0.6	0	4%
roasted	1 oz	68	1.3	14.9	1	>0.5 c	0.3	0.1	0	4%
CHESTNUT, EUROPEAN / Italian chestnut / sweet chestnut										
boiled or steamed, shelled	1 oz	37	0.8	7.9	8	>.2 c	0.4	0.1	0	9%
dried, in shell	1 lb	1357	23.2	280.5	135	>19.8 c	16.1	3.0	0	11%
dried, shelled, peeled	1 oz	105	1.4	22.3	11	>1.4 c	1.1	02	0	10%
dried, shelled, unpeeled	1 oz	106	1.8	22.0	11	3.3	1.3	0.2	0	11%
raw, in shell	1 lb	714	8.1	152.8	9	33.3	7.6	1.4	0	10%
raw, shelled, peeled	1 oz	56	0.5	12.5	1	>.3 c	0.4	0.1	0	7%
raw, shelled, unpeeled	1 cup	309	3.5	66.0	4	11.7	3.3	0.6	0	10%
raw, shelled, unpeeled	1 oz	60	0.7	12.9	1	2.3	0.6	0.1	0	9%
roasted, in shell	1 lb	700	9.1	151.3	6	33.4	6.3	1.2	0	8%
roasted, in shell	1 cup	350	4.5	75.7	3	18.4	3.2	0.6	0	8%
roasted, in shell	1 oz	70	0.9	15.0	1	3.7	0.6	0.1	0	8%
roasted, shelled	1 oz	70	0.9	15.0	1	3.3	0.6	0.1	0	8%
roasted, shelled, approx 17 nuts	1 cup	350	4.3	75.7	3	16.7	3.2	0.6	0	8%

Food Name	Serving Size	Calories	Prot. gms	Carbs gms	Sod. mgs	Fiber gms	Fat gms	Sat. Fat gms	Chol. mgs	% Fat Cal.
CHESTNUT, ITALIAN. See CHESTNUT, EUROPEAN.										
CHESTNUT, JAPANESE										
boiled or steamed	1 oz	16	0.2	3.6	1	>.1 c	0.1	0.0	0	6%
dried, in shell	1 lb	1078	15.7	243.7	101	>6.8 c	3.7	0.5	0	3%
dried, shelled	1 oz	102	1.5	23.1	10	>.6 c	0.4	0.1	0	4%
dried, shelled	1 cup	558	8.1	126.2	53	>3.5 c	1.9	0.3	0	3%
raw, in shell	1 lb	462	6.7	104.5	43	>2.9 c	1.6	0.2	0	3%
raw, shelled	1 oz	44	0.6	9.9	4	>.3 c	0.2	0.0	0	4%
roasted	1 oz	57	0.8	12.8	5	>.3 c	0.2	0.0	0	3%
CHESTNUT, SWEET. See CHESTNUT, EUROPEAN.										
CHESTNUT FLOUR. See under FLOUR.										
CHEWING GUM. See under CANDY, GUM.										
CHIA SEEDS, dried	1 oz	134	4.7	13.6	11	>7.2 c	7.4	3.0	0	48%
CHICKEN										
AVERAGE OF ALL PARTS										
Fresh										
capon, meat and skin, raw	1 lb	1056	84.8	0.0	208	0	76.8	22.4	336	67%
capon, meat and skin, raw	1 oz	66	5.3	0.0	13	0	4.8	1.4	21	67%
capon, meat and skin, roasted	4 oz	260	32.8	0.0	56	0	13.2	3.7	98	48%
roaster, meat and skin, raw	1 lb	976	78.4	0.0	304	0	72.0	20.8	336	67%
roaster, meat and skin, raw	1 oz	61	4.9	0.0	19	0	4.5	1.3	21	67%
roaster, meat and skin, roasted	4 oz	253	27.2	0.0	83	0	15.2	4.2	86	56%
stewing, meat and skin, raw	1 oz	73	5.0	0.0	20	0	5.8	1.6	20	72%
stewing, meat and skin, stewed	4 oz	323	30.5	0.0	83	0	21.4	5.8	90	61%
BACK										
Fresh										
broiler/fryer, meat and skin, flour-coated, fried	4 oz	375	31.5	7.4	102	>.1 c	23.5	6.4	101	58%
broiler/fryer, meat and skin, raw	1 oz	90	4.0	0.0	18	0	8.1	2.4	22	82%
broiler/fryer, meat and skin, roasted	4 oz	340	29.4	0.0	99	0	23.8	6.6	100	65%
broiler/fryer, meat and skin, stewed	4 oz	293	25.2	0.0	73	0	20.6	5.7	88	65%
broiler/fryer, meat only, raw	1 lb	624	88.0	0.0	400	0	28.8	8.0	400	41%
broiler/fryer, meat only, raw	1 oz	39	5.5	0.0	23	0	1.7	0.4	23	41%
broiler/fryer, meat only, roasted	4 oz	271	32.0	0.0	109	0	14.9	4.1	102	51%
broiler/fryer, meat only, stewed	4 oz	237	28.7	0.0	76	0	12.7	3.4	96	50%
BREAST										
Canned										
chunk *(Hormel)*	6.75 oz	350	41	0	855	0	20.0	0.0	0	52%
Fresh										
broiler/fryer, meat and skin, batter-dipped, fried	4 oz	295	28.2	10.2	312	0.4	15.0	4.0	96	47%
broiler/fryer, meat and skin, flour-coated, fried	4 oz	252	36.1	1.9	86	>.1 c	10.1	2.8	101	37%
broiler/fryer, meat and skin, raw	1 lb	784	94.4	0.0	288	0	41.6	12.8	288	50%
broiler/fryer, meat and skin, raw	1 oz	49	5.9	0.0	18	0	2.6	0.8	18	50%
broiler/fryer, meat and skin, roasted	4 oz	223	33.8	0.0	81	0	8.8	2.5	95	37%
broiler/fryer, meat and skin, stewed	4 oz	209	31.1	0.0	70	0	8.4	2.4	85	38%
broiler/fryer, meat only, raw	1 lb	496	104.0	0.0	288	0	6.4	1.6	256	12%
broiler/fryer, meat only, raw	1 oz	31	6.5	0.0	18	0	0.4	0.1	16	12%
broiler/fryer, meat only, roasted	4 oz	187	35.2	0.0	84	0	4.0	1.1	96	20%
broiler/fryer, meat only, stewed	4 oz	171	32.9	0.0	71	0	3.4	1.0	87	19%
Frozen or refrigerated										
Breast										
baked, 'Classic' *(Carving Board)*	1 slice	40	9	1	530	0	0.5	0.0	25	10%
boneless, barbecue marinated, frozen *(Tyson)*	3.75 oz	120	22	5	400	0	3.0	0.0	0	20%
boneless, butter garlic marinated *(Tyson)*	3.75 oz	160	21	3	320	0	7.0	0.0	0	40%
boneless, Italian marinated, frozen *(Tyson)*	3.75 oz	130	22	6	320	0	2.0	0.0	0	14%

Food Name	Serving Size	Calories	Prot. gms	Carbs gms	Sod. mgs	Fiber gms	Fat gms	Sat. Fat gms	Chol. mgs	% Fat Cal.
boneless, teriyaki marinated, frozen *(Tyson)*	3.75 oz	130	22	6	290	0	2.0	0.0	0	14%
broiler/fryer, baked *(Tyson)*	3 oz	116	24	0	63	0	1.5	0.0	72	12%
fillet, barbecue, boneless, frozen *(Tyson)*	3 oz	110	14	6	310	0	3.0	0.0	35	25%
fillet, boneless, grilled *(Tyson)*	2.75 oz	100	15	4	410	0	3.0	0.0	45	26%
fillet, boneless, skinless, raw *(Delightful Farms)*	1 med breast	140	29	0	85	0	1.5	0.0	75	10%
fillet, lemon-pepper breast, boneless, frozen *(Tyson)*	2.75 oz	100	14	4	380	0	3.0	0.0	40	27%
grilled *(Carving Board)*	1 slice	40	9	1	530	0	0.5	0.0	25	10%
half, roasted, w/skin *(Tyson)*	1 med piece	250	34	1	670	0	13.0	4.0	110	46%
hickory smoked, nonfat *(Tyson)*	1 slice	35	7	1	450	0	0.0	0.0	0	0%
honey flavor, nonfat *(Tyson)*	1 slice	35	7	2	450	0	0.0	0.0	0	0%
mesquite flavor, roasted, nonfat *(Tyson)*	1 slice	35	7	1	440	0	0.0	0.0	0	0%
peppered, roasted, nonfat *(Tyson)*	1 slice	35	7	1	480	0	0.0	0.0	0	0%
roasted, nonfat *(Tyson)*	1 slice	35	7	1	460	0	0.0	0.0	0	0%
split, skinless, raw *(Hudson)*	1 med breast	140	29	0	85	0	1.5	0.0	75	10%
split, w/skin, raw *(Hudson)*	1 med breast	270	33	0	100	0	14.0	4.0	100	49%
w/rib meat, boneless, skinless, raw *(Hudson)*	1 med breast	140	29	0	85	0	1.5	0.0	75	10%
CHUNK										
Canned										
(Featherweight)	3 oz	90	16	0	60	0	3.0	0.0	65	30%
(Swanson)	1 cup	360	64	8	800	0	12.0	4.0	140	27%
DARK MEAT										
Canned, chunk *(Hormel)*	6.75 oz	327	42	0	933	0	18.0	0.0	0	49%
Fresh										
broiler/fryer, meat and skin, batter-dipped, fried	4 oz	338	24.8	10.6	335	>.1 c	21.1	5.6	101	57%
broiler/fryer, meat and skin, flour-coated, fried	4 oz	323	30.9	4.6	101	>.1 c	19.2	5.2	104	55%
broiler/fryer, meat and skin, raw	1 oz	67	4.7	0.0	21	0	5.2	1.5	23	71%
broiler/fryer, meat and skin, roasted	4 oz	287	29.4	0.0	99	0	17.9	5.0	103	58%
broiler/fryer, meat and skin, stewed	4 oz	264	26.6	0.0	79	0	16.6	4.6	93	58%
broiler/fryer, meat only, fried, chopped or diced	1 cup	335	40.6	3.6	136	0	16.3	4.4	134	45%
broiler/fryer, meat only, raw	1 oz	35	6.0	0.0	24	0	1.2	0.3	23	32%
broiler/fryer, meat only, roasted	1 cup	287	38.3	0.0	130	0	13.6	3.7	130	44%
broiler/fryer, meat only, roasted	4 oz	232	31.0	0.0	105	0	11.0	3.0	105	44%
broiler/fryer, meat only, roasted, chopped or diced	1 cup	286	38.3	0.0	130	0	13.6	3.7	130	44%
broiler/fryer, meat only, stewed	1 cup	269	36.4	0.0	104	0	12.6	3.4	123	44%
broiler/fryer, meat only, stewed	4 oz	218	29.4	0.0	84	0	10.2	2.8	100	44%
broiler/fryer, meat only, stewed, chopped or diced	1 cup	269	36.4	0.0	104	0	12.6	3.4	123	44%
roaster, meat only, raw	1 oz	32	5.3	0.0	27	0	1.0	0.3	20	30%
roaster, meat only, roasted	4 oz	202	26.4	0.0	108	0	9.9	2.8	85	46%
stewing, meat only, raw	1 oz	45	5.6	0.0	29	0	2.3	0.6	22	48%
stewing, meat only, stewed	1 cup	361	39.4	0.0	133	0	21.4	5.7	133	55%
stewing, meat only, stewed	4 oz	293	31.9	0.0	108	0	17.3	4.6	108	55%
DRUMSTICK										
Fresh										
broiler/fryer, meat and skin, batter-dipped, fried	4 oz	304	24.9	9.4	305	>.1 c	17.9	4.7	98	54%
broiler/fryer, meat and skin, flour-coated, fried	4 oz	278	30.6	1.8	101	>.1 c	15.6	4.2	102	52%
broiler/fryer, meat and skin, raw	1 lb	736	88.0	0.0	384	0	40.0	11.2	368	51%
broiler/fryer, meat and skin, raw	1 oz	46	5.5	0.0	24	0	2.5	0.7	23	51%
broiler/fryer, meat and skin, roasted	4 oz	245	30.7	0.0	102	0	12.6	3.5	103	48%
broiler/fryer, meat and skin, stewed	4 oz	231	28.7	0.0	86	0	12.1	3.3	94	49%
broiler/fryer, meat only, raw	1 lb	544	92.8	0.0	400	0	16.0	3.2	352	28%
broiler/fryer, meat only, raw	1 oz	34	5.8	0.0	25	0	1.0	0.2	22	28%
broiler/fryer, meat only, roasted	4 oz	195	32.1	0.0	108	0	6.4	1.7	105	31%
broiler/fryer, meat only, stewed	4 oz	192	31.2	0.0	91	0	6.5	1.7	100	32%

Food Name	Serving Size	Calories	Prot. gms	Carbs gms	Sod. mgs	Fiber gms	Fat gms	Sat. Fat gms	Chol. mgs	% Fat Cal.
DRUMSTICK AND WING										
Frozen										
drumette and wing portions, raw (Delightful Farms)	4 sections	150	13	0	310	0	10.0	3.0	70	63%
GIBLETS										
Fresh										
all classes, fried	1 cup	402	47.2	6.3	164	0	19.5	5.5	647	45%
all classes, simmered	1 cup	228	37.5	1.4	84	0	6.9	2.2	570	29%
broiler/fryer, fried, chopped or diced	1 cup	402	47	6	164	0	19.5	5.5	647	44%
broiler/fryer, raw	2.6 oz	93	13	1	58	0	3.4	1.0	197	33%
broiler/fryer, simmered, chopped or diced	1 cup	228	37	1	84	0	6.9	2.2	570	27%
capon, raw	1 lb	592	83.2	6.4	352	0	24.0	8.0	1328	38%
capon, raw	1 oz	37	5.2	0.4	22	0	1.5	0.5	83	38%
capon, simmered	1 cup	238	38.3	1.1	80	0	7.8	2.6	629	31%
capon, simmered	4 oz	186	29.9	0.9	62	0	6.1	20.0	492	31%
roaster, simmered	1 Cup	239	38.8	1.3	87	0	7.6	2.4	518	30%
stewing, raw	1 lb	560	81.6	8.0	352	0	20.8	6.4	1184	34%
stewing, raw	1 oz	35	5.1	0.5	22	0	1.3	0.4	74	34%
stewing, simmered	1 cup	281	37.3	0.2	81	0	13.5	3.9	515	45%
GIZZARD										
Fresh										
all classes, simmered	1 cup	222	39.4	1.6	97	0	5.3	1.5	281	23%
broiler-fryer, raw, approx 1.3 oz.	1 medium	44	6.7	0.2	28	0	1.6	0.4	48	34%
broiler-fryer, simmered, approx .8 oz	1 medium	34	6.0	0.3	15	0	0.8	0.2	43	22%
roaster, raw	1 medium	44	7	0	28	0	1.6	0.4	48	32%
roaster, simmered	1 medium	11	2	0	5	0	0.3	0.1	14	22%
roaster, simmered, chopped or diced	1 cup	222	39	2	97	0	5.3	1.5	281	22%
HEART										
Fresh										
all classes, simmered	1 cup	268	38.3	0.2	70	0	11.5	3.3	351	40%
broiler-fryer, raw, 1 heart	2 oz	9	1.0	<.1	5	0	0.6	0.2	8	55%
broiler-fryer, simmered	4 oz	210	29.9	0.1	54	0	9.0	2.6	275	40%
roaster, raw	1 medium	9	1	0	5	0	0.6	0.2	8	55%
roaster, simmered, chopped or diced	1 cup	268	38	0	70	0	11.5	3.3	351	39%
LEG										
Fresh										
broiler/fryer, meat and skin, batter-dipped, fried	4 oz	310	24.7	9.9	316	>.1 c	18.3	4.9	102	54%
broiler/fryer, meat and skin, flour-coated, fried	4 oz	285	30.1	2.8	99	>.1 c	16.2	4.4	105	53%
broiler/fryer, meat and skin, raw	1 lb	848	81.6	0.0	352	0	54.4	16.0	384	60%
broiler/fryer, meat and skin, raw	1 oz	53	5.1	0.0	22	0	3.4	1.0	24	60%
broiler/fryer, stewed	4 oz	249	27.4	0.0	83	0	14.7	4.0	95	55%
broiler/fryer, meat only, raw	1 lb	544	91.2	0.0	384	0	17.6	4.8	368	30%
broiler/fryer, meat only, raw	1 oz	34	5.7	0.0	24	0	1.1	0.3	23	30%
broiler/fryer, meat only, roasted	4 oz	217	30.7	0.0	103	0	9.6	2.6	107	41%
broiler/fryer, meat only, stewed	4 oz	210	29.8	0.0	88	0	9.1	2.5	101	41%
Frozen or refrigerated										
broiler/fryer, baked (Tyson)	3 oz	131	23	0	81	0	3.8	0.0	79	27%
raw (Delightful Farms)	1 med drumstick	200	24	0	105	0	11.0	3.0	100	51%
w/skin (Hudson)	2 med drumsticks	230	27	0	115	0	12.0	3.0	115	50%
LIGHT MEAT										
Fresh										
broiler/fryer, meat and skin, batter-dipped, fried	4 oz	312	26.6	10.7	324	>.1 c	17.4	4.7	94	51%
broiler/fryer, meat and skin, flour-coated, fried	4 oz	279	34.5	2.1	87	>.1 c	13.7	3.8	99	46%
broiler/fryer, meat and skin, raw	1 oz	53	5.7	0.0	18	0	3.1	0.9	19	55%
broiler/fryer, meat and skin, roasted	4 oz	252	32.9	0.0	85	0	12.3	3.5	95	46%

Food Name	Serving Size	Calories	Prot. gms	Carbs gms	Sod. mgs	Fiber gms	Fat gms	Sat. Fat gms	Chol. mgs	% Fat Cal.
broiler/fryer, meat and skin, stewed	4 oz	228	29.6	0.0	71	0	11.3	3.2	84	46%
broiler/fryer, meat only, fried	8 oz	269	46.0	0.6	113	0	7.8	2.1	126	27%
broiler/fryer, meat only, raw	1 oz	32	6.6	0.0	19	0	0.5	0.1	16	15%
broiler/fryer, meat only, roasted	1 cup	242	43.3	0.0	108	'0	6.3	1.8	119	25%
broiler/fryer, meat only, roasted	4 oz	196	35.1	0.0	87	0	5.1	1.4	96	25%
broiler/fryer, meat only, roasted, chopped or diced	1 cup	242	43.3	0.0	108	0	6.3	1.8	118	25%
broiler/fryer, meat only, stewed, chopped or diced	1 cup	223	40.4	0.0	91	0	5.6	1.6	107	24%
broiler/fryer, meat only, stewed	4 oz	180	32.7	0.0	74	0	4.5	1.3	87	24%
roaster, meat only, raw	1 oz	31	6.3	0.0	14	0	0.5	0.1	16	15%
roaster, meat only, roasted	4 oz	174	30.8	0.0	58	0	4.6	1.2	85	25%
roaster, meat only, roasted, chopped or diced	1 cup	214	38.0	0.0	71	0	5.7	1.5	105	25%
stewing, meat only, raw	1 oz	39	6.5	0.0	15	0	1.2	0.3	13	29%
stewing, meat only, stewed	1 cup	298	46.3	0.0	81	0	11.2	2.8	98	35%
stewing, meat only, stewed	4 oz	242	37.5	0.0	66	0	9.0	2.2	79	35%
LIVER										
Fresh										
all classes, simmered	1 cup	220	34.1	1.2	71	0	7.6	2.6	883	33%
broiler-fryer, chopped, simmered	1 cup	219	34.1	1.2	71	0	7.6	2.6	883	33%
broiler-fryer, raw, approx 1.1 oz.	1 liver	40	5.8	1.1	25	0	1.2	0.4	140	28%
broiler-fryer, simmered	4 oz	178	27.6	1.0	58	0	6.2	2.1	716	33%
NECK										
Fresh										
broiler/fryer, meat and skin, batter-dipped, fried	4 oz	374	22.5	9.9	313	>.1 c	26.7	7.1	103	65%
broiler/fryer, meat and skin, flour-coated, fried	4 oz	376	27.2	4.8	93	>.1 c	26.8	7.2	107	65%
broiler/fryer, meat and skin, raw	1 lb	1344	64.0	0.0	288	0	118.4	33.6	448	81%
broiler/fryer, meat and skin, raw	1 oz	84	4.0	0.0	18	0	7.4	2.1	28	81%
broiler/fryer, meat and skin, simmered	4 oz	280	22.2	0.0	59	0	20.5	5.7	79	68%
broiler/fryer, meat only, raw	1 lb	704	80.0	0.0	368	0	40.0	9.6	384	53%
broiler/fryer, meat only, raw	1 oz	44	5.0	0.0	23	0	2.5	0.6	24	53%
broiler/fryer, meat only, simmered	4 oz	203	27.9	0.0	73	0	9.3	2.4	90	43%
SKIN										
Fresh										
broiler/fryer, batter-dipped, fried	1 oz	112	2.9	6.6	165	>.1 c	8.2	2.2	21	66%
broiler/fryer, roasted	1 oz	129	5.8	0.0	18	0	11.5	3.2	24	82%
broiler/fryer, stewed	1 oz	103	4.3	0.0	16	0	9.4	2.6	18	83%
THIGH										
Fresh										
broiler/fryer, meat and skin, batter-dipped, fried	4 oz	314	24.5	10.3	327	>.1 c	18.7	5.0	105	55%
broiler/fryer, meat and skin, flour-coated, fried	4 oz	297	30.3	3.6	100	>.1 c	17.0	4.6	110	53%
broiler/fryer, meat and skin, raw	1 lb	960	78.4	0.0	352	0	68.8	19.2	384	66%
broiler/fryer, meat and skin, raw	1 oz	60	4.9	0.0	22	0	4.3	1.2	24	66%
broiler/fryer, meat and skin, roasted	4 oz	280	28.4	0.0	95	0	17.6	4.9	105	58%
broiler/fryer, meat and skin, stewed	4 oz	263	26.4	0.0	81	0	16.7	4.7	95	59%
broiler/fryer, meat only, raw	1 lb	544	89.6	0.0	384	0	17.6	4.8	384	31%
broiler/fryer, meat only, raw	1 oz	34	5.6	0.0	24	0	1.1	0.3	24	31%
broiler/fryer, meat only, roasted	4 oz	237	29.4	0.0	100	0	12.3	3.4	108	49%
broiler/fryer, meat only, stewed	4 oz	221	28.4	0.0	85	0	11.1	3.1	102	47%
Frozen or refrigerated										
boneless, skinless, raw (Hudson)	1 med thigh	100	16	0	70	0	3.0	1.0	70	30%
broiler/fryer, baked (Tyson)	3 oz	152	21	0	75	0	6.7	0.0	81	42%
roasted, w/skin (Tyson)	1 med piece	270	22	1	490	0	19.0	6.0	140	65%
w/skin, raw (Hudson)	1 med thigh	230	19	0	85	0	17.0	5.0	90	67%
THIGH AND DRUMSTICK										
Frozen, 'Plump and Juicy' (Swanson)	3.25 oz	290	15	17	610	0	18.0	0.0	0	56%

Food Name	Serving Size	Calories	Prot. gms	Carbs gms	Sod. mgs	Fiber gms	Fat gms	Sat. Fat gms	Chol. mgs	% Fat Cal.
WHITE AND DARK MEAT										
Canned										
(Swanson)	2.5 oz	100	16	0	240	0	4.0	0.0	40	36%
chunk (Hormel)	6.75 oz	340	39	0	857	0	20.0	0.0	0	54%
chunk, unsalted (Hormel)	6.75 oz	330	42	0	75	0	18.0	0.0	0	49%
cooked, in water, 96% fat-free (Valley Fresh)	2 oz	80	15	0	130	0	2.0	0.5	50	23%
puréed (Bryan foods)	1/3 cup	120	12	0	45	0	7.0	2.0	45	57%
WHITE MEAT										
Canned										
(Swanson)	2.5 oz	100	15	0	235	0	4.0	0.0	35	38%
chunk, cooked, in water, 98% fat-free (Valley Fresh)	2 oz	70	15	0	130	0	1.0	0.0	25	13%
chunk, premium (Swanson)	3 oz	80	16	1	340	1	1.0	0.5	40	12%
WHOLE										
Frozen or refrigerated										
barbecue (Empire Kosher)	5 oz	280	31	1	460	0	17.0	4.5	110	54%
broiler/fryer, baked (Tyson)	3 oz	134	23	0	73	0	4.1	0.0	76	29%
roasted, w/skin (Tyson)	3 oz	180	19	1	300	0	12.0	3.0	100	57%
WING										
Fresh										
broiler/fryer, meat and skin, batter-dipped, fried	4 oz	367	22.5	12.4	363	>.1 c	24.7	6.6	90	61%
broiler/fryer, meat and skin, flour-coated, fried	4 oz	364	29.6	2.7	87	>.1 c	25.1	6.9	92	64%
broiler/fryer, meat and skin, raw	1 lb	1008	83.2	0.0	336	0	72.0	20.8	352	66%
broiler/fryer, meat and skin, raw	1 oz	63	5.2	0.0	21	0	4.5	1.3	22	66%
broiler/fryer, meat and skin, roasted	4 oz	329	30.5	0.0	93	0	22.1	6.2	95	62%
broiler/fryer, meat and skin, stewed	4 oz	282	25.8	0.0	76	0	19.1	5.3	79	63%
broiler/fryer, meat only, raw	1 lb	576	99.2	0.0	368	0	16.0	4.8	256	27%
broiler/fryer, meat only, raw	1 oz	36	6.2	0.0	23	0	1.0	0.3	16	27%
broiler/fryer, meat only, roasted	4 oz	230	34.5	0.0	104	0	9.2	2.6	96	38%
broiler/fryer, meat only, stewed	4 oz	205	30.8	0.0	83	0	8.1	2.3	84	37%
Frozen or refrigerated										
w/skin (Hudson)	3 med wings	280	23	0	90	0	20.0	6.0	95	66%
broiler/fryer, baked (Tyson)	3 oz	147	23	0	78	0	5.6	0.0	72	35%

CHICKEN DINNER/ENTRÉE. See also BURRITO; CHICKEN; CHICKEN DINNER/ENTRÉE MIX; CHILI; CHIMICHANGA; ENCHILADA; FAJITA; LUNCH COMBINATION, PACKAGED; RAVIOLI DISH/ENTRÉE; SANDWICH; TORTELLINI DISH/ENTRÉE.

Food Name	Serving Size	Calories	Prot. gms	Carbs gms	Sod. mgs	Fiber gms	Fat gms	Sat. Fat gms	Chol. mgs	% Fat Cal.
(Armour)										
à la king, frozen, 'Classics Lite'	11.25 oz	290	19	38	630	0	7.0	0.0	55	22%
Burgundy, frozen, 'Classics Lite'	10 oz	210	23	25	780	0	2.0	0.0	45	9%
glazed, frozen, 'Classics'	10.75 oz	300	15	24	960	0	16.0	0.0	60	48%
Marsala, frozen, 'Classics Lite'	10.5 oz	250	20	27	930	0	7.0	0.0	80	25%
mesquite, frozen, 'Classics'	9.5 oz	370	15	42	660	0	16.0	0.0	55	39%
Oriental, 'Classics Lite'	10 oz	180	18	24	660	0	1.0	0.0	35	5%
parmigiana, frozen, 'Classics'	11.5 oz	370	22	27	1060	0	19.0	0.0	75	47%
sweet and sour, frozen, 'Classics Lite'	11 oz	240	18	39	820	0	2.0	0.0	35	7%
w/noodles, frozen, 'Classics'	11 oz	230	19	23	660	0	7.0	0.0	50	27%
w/wine and mushroom sauce, frozen, 'Classics'	10.75 oz	280	22	24	900	0	11.0	0.0	50	35%
(Banquet)										
à la king, frozen, 'Cookin' Bags'	4 oz	110	8	9	0	0	5.0	0.0	0	40%
and dumplings, w/gravy	1 entrée	270	13	35	780	3	9.0	3.0	40	30%
breast patty, fried, w/biscuit, frozen, 'Southern'	4 oz	320	12	37	980	0	14.0	0.0	0	39%
chow mein, w/egg roll	1 entrée	210	9	28	850	3	7.0	2.0	30	30%
drumsticks, frozen, 'Drumsnackers' 'Platters'	7 oz	430	20	49	690	0	19.0	0.0	0	38%
fingers, barbecue	1 entrée	340	13	36	800	3	16.0	4.0	60	42%
fried, 'Original'	1 entrée	470	21	35	1500	2	27.0	9.0	90	52%
fried, white meat	1 entrée	480	18	40	1100	3	28.0	11.0	100	52%

Food Name	Serving Size	Calories	Prot. gms	Carbs gms	Sod. mgs	Fiber gms	Fat gms	Sat. Fat gms	Chol. mgs	% Fat Cal.
fried, white meat, frozen, 'Extra Helping'	16 oz	570	20	70	1470	0	28.0	0.0	0	41%
fried, white meat, hot 'n spicy, frozen, 'Platter'	9 oz	430	38	21	0	0	22.0	0.0	105	46%
fried, w/mashed potatoes and corn, seasoned sauce	1 entrée	470	21	35	1500	2	27.0	9.3	89	52%
grilled	1 entrée	330	16	37	1210	3	13.0	3.0	50	36%
hot 'n spicy, frozen, 'Snack'n'	3.75 oz	140	6	8	480	0	9.0	0.0	0	59%
nugget meal, frozen	1 meal	410	18	38	650	4	21.0	5.0	45	46%
nuggets, fried	1 entrée	430	14	42	650	4	23.0	8.0	50	48%
nuggets, hot'n spicy, w/barbecue sauce	4.5 oz	360	20	23	820	0	21.0	0.0	0	52%
nuggets, sweet and sour, 'Extra Helping'	10 oz	650	28	64	0	0	34.0	0.0	0	45%
nuggets, sweet and sour, w/sauce, 'Microwave'	4.5 oz	360	20	22	770	0	21.0	0.0	0	53%
nuggets, w/BBQ sauce, 'Extra Helping'	10 oz	640	29	56	1390	0	36.0	0.0	0	49%
nuggets, w/BBQ sauce, frozen, 'Southern'	4.5 oz	370	19	20	930	0	23.0	0.0	0	57%
Oriental, w/egg rolls	1 entrée	260	10	36	790	3	9.0	2.5	40	31%
parmigiana	1 entrée	320	10	29	900	3	18.0	4.5	50	51%
patty, frozen, 'Platters'	7.5 oz	380	15	34	760	0	21.0	0.0	0	49%
pie, frozen	7 oz	550	15	39	860	0	36.0	0.0	35	60%
pie, frozen, 'Supreme Microwave'	7 oz	430	15	30	740	0	28.0	0.0	40	58%
pot pie, frozen	1 serving	382	10	36	948	1	22.0	8.9	40	52%
primavera, w/vegetable, frozen, 'Cookin' Bags'	4 oz	100	6	14	0	0	2.0	0.0	0	18%
primavera, w/vegetable, frozen, 'Family Entrees'	7 oz	140	9	18	0	0	3.0	0.0	0	20%
Southern fried	1 entrée	560	26	40	1540	3	33.0	8.0	100	53%
sweet and sour, frozen, 'Cookin' Bags'	4 oz	130	5	22	0	0	2.0	0.0	0	14%
w/dumplings, frozen	10 oz	430	17	34	940	0	24.0	0.0	45	51%
(Barber Foods)										
cordon bleu, w/cheese and ham, frozen	1 pkg	697	52	30	1527	na	41.5	11.5	163	54%
cordon bleu, w/cheese and ham, frozen	1 serving	344	26	15	754	na	20.5	5.7	81	54%
w/broccoli and cheese stuffing, frozen	1 pkg	527	42	12	1054	na	34.7	8.9	126	59%
w/broccoli and cheese stuffing, frozen	1 serving	260	21	6	521	na	17.1	4.4	62	59%
(Budget Gourmet)										
and egg noodles, w/broccoli, frozen	10 oz	450	23	31	1110	0	26.0	0.0	130	52%
au gratin, 'Light'	1 entrée	250	18	26	820	3	8.0	5.0	45	29%
breast, herbed, frozen, 'Special Selections'	1 entrée	300	25	34	620	5	8.0	3.0	65	23%
breast, honey mustard	1 entrée	310	19	45	620	3	6.0	1.5	35	17%
breast, honey mustard, 'Light & Healthy'	1 dinner	310	20	46	540	6	6.0	1.5	50	17%
breast, orange glazed	1 entrée	280	11	51	790	2	3.0	1.0	30	10%
breast, orange glazed, 'Light'	1 entrée	300	15	56	920	1	2.0	1.0	30	6%
cacciatore, frozen	11 oz	300	20	27	810	0	13.0	0.0	60	38%
French, light, w/vegetables, potato, sauce	1 serving	179	23	9	864	6	5.6	1.4	26	28%
French recipe, 'Light'	1 entrée	200	13	19	950	4	8.0	3.0	30	36%
frozen, w/egg noodles, frozen	1 entrée	410	21	30	930	3	23.0	12.0	110	50%
herbed, w/fettuccini	1 entrée	260	19	29	640	4	8.0	3.0	80	27%
Italian style, frozen, 'Special Selections'	1 entrée	280	10	44	660	3	7.0	2.0	25	23%
Mandarin, w/vegetables, frozen, 'Special Selections'	1 entrée	250	16	37	850	4	5.0	1.0	45	18%
Marsala, frozen	10 oz	250	15	37	660	0	5.0	0.0	65	18%
Mexican, frozen	12.8 oz	510	23	70	1210	0	15.0	0.0	40	27%
Oriental, w/vegetables	1 entrée	290	11	43	730	3	8.0	2.5	25	25%
Oriental, w/vegetables, 'Light & Healthy'	9 oz	280	19	44	690	0	6.0	1.0	20	18%
Oriental, w/vegetables and rice, frozen, 'Special Selections'	1 entrée	290	11	42	720	4	9.0	1.5	15	28%
roasted, frozen	11.2 oz	280	19	34	1110	0	7.0	0.0	40	23%
roasted, w/herb gravy	1 entrée	260	14	34	610	4	8.0	3.5	45	27%
sweet and sour, w/rice	10 oz	350	18	53	640	0	7.0	0.0	40	18%
Szechuan, spicy, w/vegetable, frozen, 'Special Selections'	1 entrée	300	14	41	710	5	9.0	1.5	10	27%

Food Name	Serving Size	Calories	Prot. gms	Carbs gms	Sod. mgs	Fiber gms	Fat gms	Sat. Fat gms	Chol. mgs	% Fat Cal.
teriyaki, frozen	12 oz	360	20	44	610	0	12.0	0.0	55	30%
teriyaki, w/Oriental style vegetables, frozen, 'Light and Healthy'	1 entrée	317	19	52	675	4	3.7	0.6	25	11%
w/fettuccini	1 entrée	380	20	33	810	3	19.0	10.0	85	45%
w/rigatoni, broccoli 'Special Selections'	1 entrée	310	17	46	670	5	6.0	2.5	15	18%
white meat, w/Chinese style vegetables, rice	1 entrée	250	8	39	640	3	7.0	2.5	15	25%
white meat, w/Italian style vegetables, rice	1 entrée	250	8	39	540	2	7.0	2.5	25	25%
(Celentano)										
breaded, w/pasta marinara w/cheese	10 oz tray	390	19	36	1040	8	19.0	4.0	50	44%
parmigiana, frozen	9 oz	330	32	15	560	0	20.0	0.0	0	49%
primavera, frozen	11.5 oz	270	25	18	580	0	10.0	0.0	0	34%
(Chicken By George)										
Cajun, boneless, skinless	1 med breast	120	20	2	650	0	4.0	1.0	55	29%
Cajun, packaged	5 oz	180	25	4	890	0	8.0	1.0	80	38%
Caribbean grill, packaged	5 oz	200	25	10	610	0	6.0	0.0	80	28%
Italian bleu cheese, packaged	5 oz	180	26	2	890	0	8.0	0.0	85	39%
lemon herb, boneless, skinless, raw	1 med breast	120	19	3	800	0	3.0	1.0	50	23%
lemon herb, packaged	5 oz	170	24	6	870	0	6.0	1.0	70	31%
lemon oregano, packaged	5 oz	160	26	4	580	0	4.0	1.0	75	23%
mesquite barbecue, packaged	5 oz	170	25	6	790	0	6.0	1.0	70	30%
mustard dill, packaged	5 oz	180	26	3	640	0	7.0	0.0	80	35%
roasted, packaged	5 oz	150	26	2	710	0	4.0	0.0	70	24%
teriyaki, breast, boneless, skinless, raw	1 med breast	130	20	6	650	0	3.0	1.0	50	21%
tomato herb, w/basil, packaged,	5 oz	190	25	7	800	0	7.0	0.0	80	33%
(Chun King)										
chow mein, frozen	13 oz	370	25	53	1560	0	6.0	0.0	0	15%
imperial, frozen	13 oz	300	17	54	1540	0	1.0	0.0	0	3%
sweet and sour, w/vegetables, fruit, and sauce, canned	1 pkg	802	28	154	2739	na	8.6	na	111	10%
sweet and sour, w/vegetables, fruit, and sauce, canned	1 serving	165	6	32	564	na	1.8	na	23	10%
walnut, crunchy, frozen	13 oz	310	16	49	1700	0	5.0	0.0	0	15%
(Contadina) parmigiana, frozen, food service product	1 oz	43	2	3	130	0	2.3	0.6	7	48%
(Country Pride) primavera, sticks, frozen	3 oz	240	10	16	400	0	15.0	0.0	0	56%
(Dining Lite)										
à la king, frozen	9 oz	240	14	30	780	0	7.0	0.0	40	26%
and noodles, frozen	9 oz	240	17	28	570	0	7.0	0.0	50	26%
chow mein, frozen	9 oz	180	10	31	650	0	2.0	0.0	30	10%
glazed, frozen	9 oz	220	17	30	680	0	4.0	0.0	45	16%
(Dinty Moore)										
and dumplings, microwave cup	1 cup	100	6	12	940	1	3.0	1.0	35	27%
stew, microwave cup	7.5 oz	260	11	15	850	0	18.0	4.0	80	61%
w/dumplings, microwave cup	7.5 oz	166	12	17	683	0	5.0	0.0	19	28%
w/gravy and mashed potatoes, packaged	1 bowl	220	22	24	1180	2	4.0	1.5	25	16%
w/noodles, 'Micro Meal'	1 bowl	260	21	26	1150	2	8.0	4.0	80	28%
(Empire Kosher)										
breast, battered and breaded, fried, kosher	3 oz	170	21	3	440	1	8.0	2.0	45	43%
cutlets, battered and breaded, fried, kosher	1 med cutlet	200	18	11	320	2	9.0	1.5	25	41%
nuggets, battered and breaded, fried, kosher	5 nuggets	200	13	9	650	1	13.0	2.5	30	57%
nuggets, kosher	5 nuggets	180	13	12	370	1	9.0	1.5	15	45%
pie, kosher	1 pie	440	23	41	960	11	21.0	5.0	30	42%
(Featherweight)										
stew, w/wild rice, canned	7.5 oz	140	10	23	400	0	1.0	0.0	20	6%
w/dumplings, canned	7.5 oz	160	12	18	115	0	5.0	0.0	0	27%
(Freezer Queen)										
à la king, frozen, 'Cook-In-Pouch'	4 oz	70	9	6	460	0	1.0	0.0	0	13%

Food Name	Serving Size	Calories	Prot. gms	Carbs gms	Sod. mgs	Fiber gms	Fat gms	Sat. Fat gms	Chol. mgs	% Fat Cal.
à la king, w/rice, frozen, 'Single Serve'	9 oz	270	20	37	520	0	5.0	0.0	0	16%
cacciatore, frozen, 'Single Serve'	9 oz	270	20	33	710	0	6.0	0.0	0	20%
croquettes, breaded, 'Family Suppers'	7 oz	240	12	20	1000	0	12.0	0.0	0	46%
nuggets, frozen, 'Deluxe Family Suppers'	3 oz	270	14	15	770	0	17.0	0.0	0	57%
nuggets, platter, frozen	6 oz	410	14	36	950	0	23.0	0.0	0	51%
patty, frozen, 'Platter'	7.5 oz	360	17	33	1160	0	17.0	0.0	0	43%
primavera, sliced, w/gravy, 'Cook-In-Pouch'	5 oz	80	7	6	820	0	3.0	0.0	0	34%
sweet and sour, w/rice, frozen, 'Single Serve'	9 oz	300	20	48	700	0	4.0	0.0	0	12%
(Green Giant) and broccoli, frozen, 'Entrées'	9.5 oz	340	23	28	890	0	15.0	0.0	0	40%
(Healthy Choice)										
à l'orange, frozen	9 oz	260	23	38	340	0	2.0	1.0	40	7%
and broccoli, 'Hearty Handfuls'	1 entrée	320	17	51	580	5	5.0	1.5	20	14%
and mushrooms, 'Hearty Handfuls'	1 entrée	310	17	49	590	4	5.0	1.5	20	15%
broccoli Alfredo	1 entrée	300	25	34	530	2	7.0	3.0	50	21%
cacciatore	1 entrée	340	21	52	590	6	5.0	2.0	20	13%
cacciatore, in sauce, w/vegetables	1 serving	266	22	36	552	5	4.0	1.0	32	13%
Cantonese	1 entrée	280	22	34	480	2	6.0	3.0	50	19%
chow mein, lowfat, low-cholesterol, frozen	9 oz	240	20	29	530	0	5.0	2.0	45	19%
country breaded	1 entrée	350	16	51	480	5	9.0	2.0	45	23%
country glazed	1 entrée	230	17	30	480	3	4.0	1.5	45	16%
country herb	1 entrée	320	18	44	540	3	8.0	3.0	45	23%
Dijon	1 entrée	270	23	33	470	6	5.0	2.0	40	17%
divan, w/pasta, frozen	11.5 oz	300	25	41	520	0	4.0	2.0	50	12%
entrée	1 entrée	250	17	31	470	3	6.0	2.0	50	22%
Francesca	1 entrée	330	23	46	600	4	6.0	2.5	30	16%
garlic, 'Hearty Handfuls'	1 entrée	330	20	53	600	6	5.0	1.5	25	13%
glazed, frozen	8.5 oz	220	21	27	510	0	3.0	1.0	45	12%
grilled, Sonoma	1 entrée	230	18	30	530	5	4.0	0.5	15	16%
grilled, Southwestern	1 entrée	260	21	30	450	4	6.0	3.0	40	21%
grilled, w/mashed potatoes	1 entrée	170	18	18	600	3	3.5	1.5	40	18%
herb roasted, frozen	11 oz	380	26	56	470	0	7.0	3.0	60	16%
honey mustard	1 entrée	290	21	38	520	1	6.0	2.5	40	19%
Mandarin	1 entrée	280	20	44	520	4	2.5	0.0	35	8%
Marsala, w/vegetables	1 entrée	240	20	32	440	3	4.0	2.0	30	15%
mesquite barbecue	1 entrée	310	18	48	480	6	5.0	2.0	55	15%
mesquite barbecue, w/rice, vegetable, apple raisin cobbler	1 serving	310	18	48	483	6	5.0	2.0	54	14%
Mexican, low-fat, low-cholesterol, frozen	12.5 oz	340	25	51	550	0	5.0	2.0	60	13%
Milano, garlic	1 entrée	260	18	34	510	3	6.0	2.5	35	21%
Oriental, frozen	11.25 oz	200	19	32	440	0	1.0	1.0	35	4%
parmigiana	1 entrée	330	19	46	490	3	8.0	3.0	40	22%
picante	1 entrée	250	18	30	550	4	7.0	3.0	45	25%
roasted	1 entrée	230	20	25	480	6	5.0	2.5	45	20%
roasted, frozen	1 serving	290	25	39	430	0	4.0	2.0	50	12%
'Salsa Chicken Dinner' frozen	1 serving	240	20	36	450	0	2.0	1.0	50	7%
sesame	1 entrée	250	16	38	600	2	4.0	1.0	35	14%
Shanghai, sesame	1 entrée	360	19	54	600	4	7.0	2.0	20	18%
stir-fry, w/vermicelli, frozen, 'Extra Portion'	12 oz	300	23	42	550	0	5.0	1.0	30	15%
sweet and sour	1 entrée	360	20	53	360	5	7.0	3.0	45	18%
sweet and sour, frozen	11.5 oz	280	20	52	320	0	2.0	1.0	35	6%
teriyaki	1 entrée	270	17	37	600	3	6.0	3.0	45	20%
teriyaki, w/rice, vegetable, apple cherry compote	1 serving	268	17	37	602	3	5.6	3.0	44	19%
(Heinz) stew, w/dumplings, canned	7.5 oz	210	9	22	850	0	9.0	0.0	0	40%
(Hormel) loaf, canned	2 oz	130	7	0	608	0	10.0	0.0	0	76%

Food Name	Serving Size	Calories	Prot. gms	Carbs gms	Sod. mgs	Fiber gms	Fat gms	Sat. Fat gms	Chol. mgs	% Fat Cal.
(Hot Bites)										
breast tenders, boneless.	2.25 oz	150	11	12	280	0	6.0	0.0	0	37%
breast tenders, boneless, 'Microwave'.	4 oz	260	19	24	560	0	10.0	0.0	0	34%
drumsticks, frozen, 'Drumsnackers'.	2.63 oz	220	10	13	530	0	15.0	0.0	0	59%
nuggets, fried, frozen, 'Southern'	2.63 oz	220	10	13	530	0	14.0	0.0	0	58%
nuggets, frozen.	2.63 oz	210	11	11	550	0	14.0	0.0	0	59%
nuggets, hot'n spicy, frozen.	2.63 oz	250	10	10	380	0	19.0	0.0	0	68%
nuggets, w/cheddar, frozen.	2.63 oz	250	11	11	560	0	18.0	0.0	0	65%
sticks, primavera, frozen.	2.63 oz	220	10	11	350	0	15.0	0.0	0	62%
(Kid Cuisine)										
fried, frozen 'Mega Meal'.	10.8 oz	720	34	53	1400	0	41.0	0.0	0	51%
fried, frozen.	7.25 oz	420	15	41	1050	0	22.0	0.0	0	47%
fried, white meat, w/potato, corn, chocolate pudding, frozen.	1 meal	440	19	48	710	6	20.0	6.0	65	40%
nuggets, frozen.	6.25 oz	400	11	46	610	0	19.0	0.0	60	43%
nuggets, frozen, 'Mega Meal'.	8.4 oz	470	21	51	1010	0	20.0	0.0	0	38%
nuggets, w/macaroni and cheese, corn, pudding, 'Cosmic'.	1 serving	524	18	53	974	3	26.7	6.6	49	46%
nuggets, w/macaroni, corn, chocolate pudding.	1 meal	360	14	46	500	6	13.0	3.0	30	33%
(La Choy)										
almond, w/rice, vegetable, 'Fresh and Lite'.	9.75 oz	270	14	40	1092	3	8.0	0.0	42	25%
chow mein, canned.	1 cup	80	8	6	1352	3	3.5	1.0	9	37%
chow mein, canned, 'Bi-Pack'.	3/4 cup	80	7	8	980	1	3.0	0.0	18	31%
chow mein, canned, food service product.	1 cup	91	5	11	865	2	3.6	0.9	9	33%
chow mein, frozen, food service product.	1 cup	133	8	19	857	1	3.1	1.2	5	21%
imperial, w/rice, frozen, 'Fresh and Lite'.	11 oz	260	13	45	1269	3	6.0	0.0	46	19%
Oriental, canned, 'Bi-Pack'.	3/4 cup	240	9	47	1400	1	2.0	0.0	0	7%
Oriental, spicy, frozen, 'Fresh and Lite'.	9.75 oz	270	11	52	560	4	4.0	0.0	42	13%
Oriental, w/noodles, canned, 'Bi-Pack'.	9 oz	160	11	23	1163	4	3.8	1.0	13	20%
sweet and sour, canned.	3/4 cup	240	8	47	1420	1	2.0	0.5	19	8%
sweet and sour, canned, 'Dinner Classics'.	1/4 pkg	120	1	29	840	1	1.0	0.0	0	7%
sweet and sour, packaged, 'Dinner Classics'.	3/4 cup	310	32	30	860	1	6.0	1.1	50	18%
sweet and sour, w/noodles, frozen.	1 cup	256	7	49	697	9	3.1	1.3	10	11%
sweet and sour, w/rice, vegetables, frozen 'Fresh & Lite'.	10 oz	260	13	50	601	4	3.0	0.0	53	10%
Szechwan, spicy, bi-pack.	1 cup	98	8	11	857	1	2.6	1.0	19	23%
(Le Menu)										
à la king, w/seasoned rice, frozen, 'LightStyle'.	8.25 oz	240	19	29	670	0	5.0	1.0	30	19%
breast, glazed, frozen, 'LightStyle'.	10 oz	230	25	25	430	0	3.0	0.0	55	12%
breast, roasted, w/herbs, rice, and vegetable.	7.75 oz	260	22	29	500	0	6.0	2.0	45	21%
cordon bleu, frozen.	11 oz	460	23	47	850	0	20.0	0.0	0	39%
Dijon, w/pasta and vegetables, 'LightStyle'.	8.5 oz	240	22	21	500	0	7.0	2.0	40	27%
herb roasted, frozen, 'LightStyle'.	10 oz	240	27	18	400	0	7.0	0.0	70	26%
in wine sauce, frozen.	10 oz	280	26	27	680	0	7.0	0.0	0	23%
Kiev, frozen.	8 oz	530	20	24	780	0	39.0	0.0	0	67%
Oriental, à la king, frozen.	10.25 oz	330	23	29	830	0	13.0	0.0	0	36%
parmigiana, frozen.	11.75 oz	410	26	31	1030	0	20.0	0.0	0	44%
sweet and sour, frozen.	11.25 oz	400	19	41	1020	0	18.0	0.0	0	40%
sweet and sour, frozen, 'LightStyle'.	10 oz	250	18	29	530	0	7.0	0.0	2	25%
(Lean Cuisine)										
'Fiesta' frozen.	8.5 oz	240	19	30	560	0	5.0	2.0	40	19%
à l'orange.	1 entrée	260	19	40	260	1	2.5	0.5	40	9%
à l'orange, in sauce, w/broccoli and rice.	1 serving	268	24	39	360	na	1.8	0.4	46	6%
and vegetables, w/vermicelli.	1 pkg	252	19	32	582	5	5.6	1.0	24	20%

Food Name	Serving Size	Calories	Prot. gms	Carbs gms	Sod. mgs	Fiber gms	Fat gms	Sat. Fat gms	Chol. mgs	% Fat Cal.
and vegetables, w/vermicelli, frozen	11.75 oz	240	18	30	500	0	5.0	1.0	30	19%
baked	1 entrée	230	18	31	520	5	4.0	1.5	35	16%
baked, w/whipped potatoes	1 entrée	250	19	30	590	2	6.0	0.5	30	22%
barbecue, w/rice pilaf, frozen	8.75 oz	260	20	32	500	0	6.0	1.0	50	21%
barbecue, w/sauce, 'Hearty Portions'	1 entrée	380	23	58	790	7	6.0	1.5	45	14%
breaded, baked, w/potato and vegetable, frozen	8 oz	200	17	21	480	0	5.0	2.0	35	23%
cacciatore, w/vermicelli, frozen	10 7/8 oz	280	22	31	570	0	7.0	2.0	45	23%
Calypso, frozen, 'Café Classics'	1 pkg	280	15	42	590	3	6.0	2.0	40	19%
carbonara	1 entrée	280	18	33	580	2	8.0	2.0	30	26%
chow mein	1 entrée	220	12	33	560	3	5.0	1.0	35	20%
chow mein, w/rice, frozen	9 oz	240	14	34	530	0	5.0	1.0	30	19%
classica, frozen, food service product	1 oz	23	2	2	85	0	0.8	0.2	5	31%
fiesta, w/rice and vegetables	1 entrée	260	19	35	550	3	5.0	0.5	40	17%
Florentine, 'Hearty Portions'	1 entrée	420	23	61	720	5	9.0	3.0	60	19%
glazed	1 entrée	240	22	25	480	0	6.0	1.0	55	22%
glazed, frozen, food service product	1 oz	26	3	1	101	0	1.1	0.2	9	39%
glazed, w/vegetable rice, frozen	8.5 oz	250	21	24	590	0	7.0	2.0	50	26%
grilled, and penne pasta, 'Hearty Portions'	1 entrée	380	25	52	750	7	8.0	2.5	45	19%
grilled, w/salsa, frozen, 'Café Classics'	1 pkg	240	15	32	550	4	6.0	1.5	40	22%
herb roasted	1 entrée	210	13	27	540	3	5.0	1.0	40	22%
herb roasted, 'Café Classics'	1 entrée	210	17	25	430	4	5.0	1.0	40	21%
honey mustard, 'Café Classics'	1 entrée	270	16	39	580	3	5.0	2.0	35	17%
honey mustard, frozen	7.5 oz	230	18	30	540	1	4.0	1.0	40	16%
honey roasted	1 entrée	290	14	46	590	5	6.0	2.0	25	18%
in peanut sauce	1 entrée	290	23	35	550	4	6.0	1.0	30	19%
Italienne, frozen, food service product	1 oz	20	2	1	122	0	0.9	0.2	7	40%
medallions, w/creamy cheese sauce	1 entrée	260	16	31	590	4	8.0	3.0	50	28%
Marsala, w/vegetables, frozen	8-1/8 oz	180	22	13	430	0	4.0	1.0	55	20%
Mediterranean, frozen, 'Café Classics'	1 pkg	260	19	36	580	4	4.0	1.0	35	14%
Mexicali style, frozen, food service product	1 oz	20	2	2	48	1	0.7	0.2	6	32%
Oriental	1 entrée	250	19	30	530	4	6.0	1.5	35	22%
Oriental, glazed, 'Hearty Portions'	1 entrée	410	19	69	790	4	6.0	1.0	50	13%
Oriental, w/vermicelli, frozen	9 oz	280	22	31	480	0	7.0	2.0	35	23%
parmesan	1 entrée	220	18	27	560	4	5.0	1.5	50	20%
parmesan, 'Café Classics'	1 entrée	240	20	25	580	4	7.0	2.5	50	26%
piccata	1 entrée	270	13	41	530	2	6.0	2.0	25	20%
picatta, frozen, 'Café Classics'	1 pkg	290	15	45	540	1	6.0	1.5	30	18%
pie	1 entrée	320	18	39	590	3	10.0	2.5	35	28%
pie, 100% white meat, frozen	1 pkg	310	23	32	590	0	10.0	2.0	40	29%
primavera, frozen, food service product	1 oz	16	1	1	82	0	0.7	0.1	5	39%
roasted, w/herbs, frozen, 'Café Classics'	1 pkg	210	17	25	430	4	5.0	1.0	40	21%
roasted, w/mushrooms, 'Hearty Portions'	1 entrée	380	21	57	790	4	7.0	1.0	35	17%
sweet and sour, frozen, food service product	1 oz	22	2	3	40	0	0.5	0.1	4	20%
sweet and sour, w/rice, frozen	9 oz	280	17	39	490	0	6.0	1.0	50	19%
tenderloins, in herb sauce, frozen	9.5 oz	240	29	19	490	0	5.0	2.0	60	19%
tenderloins, in peanut sauce, frozen	9 oz	290	23	33	530	0	7.0	2.0	45	22%
w/bow tie pasta, frozen, 'Café Classics'	1 pkg	270	19	34	550	5	6.0	1.5	60	20%
w/rice and vegetables	1 entrée	240	22	24	460	2	6.0	1.0	60	23%
(Libby's)										
chow mein, microwave cup	7.75 oz	130	5	19	830	2	4.0	1.0	10	27%
w/pasta spirals, microwave cup, 'Diner'	7.75 oz	120	8	16	910	2	3.0	1.0	15	22%
(Lloyds) breast fillet, roasted, barbecue, w/sauce	1 fillet	140	16	12	930	1	3.0	1.0	60	19%
(Luck's)										
and dumplings, microwave bowl	1 serving	150	16	21	1400	1	1.0	0.0	35	6%

Food Name	Serving Size	Calories	Prot. gms	Carbs gms	Sod. mgs	Fiber gms	Fat gms	Sat. Fat gms	Chol. mgs	% Fat Cal.
and rice, microwaveable bowl	1 serving	140	14	19	1180	1	1.0	0.0	30	6%
Brunswick stew, microwave bowl.	1 serving	130	9	23	910	3	0.0	0.0	0	0%
thighs and wings, w/dumplings, in sauce	1 cup	340	24	23	810	2	20.0	4.0	140	49%
w/dumplings, canned	7.25 oz	240	16	18	605	0	11.0	0.0	0	42%
(Lunch Bucket)										
w/beans and rice, micro cup, 'Light'n Healthy'	7.5 oz	170	7	28	600	0	3.0	0.0	10	16%
w/dumplings, microwave lunch cup.	7.5 oz	140	4	25	880	0	2.0	0.0	0	13%
(Lunch Express)										
Alfredo.	1 entrée	373	19	33	588	4	18.5	7.0	57	45%
chow mein.	1 entrée	260	13	43	940	3	4.0	1.0	30	14%
Mandarin.	1 entrée	270	12	41	520	2	6.0	1.0	30	20%
Oriental	1 entrée	370	11	55	910	3	12.0	1.5	28	29%
stir-fry, w/rice and vegetables, frozen	1 entrée	270	12	40	632	6	7.4	0.9	26	25%
w/vegetables and rice	1 entrée	340	15	45	750	2	11.0	3.0	30	29%
(Manor House) fried, assorted pieces	3 oz	270	14	13	620	1	18.0	5.0	65	60%
(Marie Callender's)										
and noodles	13 oz	520	21	42	1320	5	30.0	11.0	65	52%
and noodles, escalloped, frozen	1 pkg	629	21	61	1597	na	33.6	11.5	na	48%
and noodles, escalloped, frozen	1 cup	397	13	38	1007	na	21.2	7.3	na	48%
and noodles, escalloped, frozen	1 serving	292	10	28	742	na	15.6	5.4	na	48%
chicken and dumplings	1 cup	250	13	22	1030	3	12.0	5.0	80	44%
cordon bleu	13 oz	590	33	58	1920	7	25.0	8.0	55	38%
country fried, w/gravy	16 oz	620	24	63	2300	6	30.0	9.0	75	44%
grilled, in mushroom sauce	14 oz	480	33	54	1030	7	15.0	6.0	65	28%
grilled, w/rice pilaf	11.7 oz	360	20	38	1070	6	14.0	4.0	40	35%
herb roasted, w/mashed potatoes.	14 oz	670	43	32	2100	7	31.0	15.0	205	48%
Marsala	14 oz	450	33	42	1260	6	17.0	7.0	70	34%
parmigiana, breaded	16 oz	620	31	63	730	9	27.0	8.0	50	39%
pot pie	1 pie	600	14	53	1070	4	37.0	9.0	15	55%
pot pie, au gratin	1 pie	690	19	50	1300	4	46.0	13.0	30	60%
pot pie, frozen	1 pkg	999	25	88	2078	na	61.1	25.2	28	55%
pot pie, frozen	1 serving	501	12	44	1041	na	30.6	12.6	14	55%
pot pie, w/broccoli	1 pie	670	16	54	1000	4	43.0	12.0	25	58%
sweet and sour	14 oz	530	25	86	700	1	9.0	2.0	35	15%
(Michelinas)										
primavera, w/spirals, 'Lean 'n' Tasty'	1 entrée	250	13	32	860	2	7.0	3.5	35	26%
teriyaki, w/rice 'Lean 'n' Tasty'	1 entrée	290	9	65	1140	2	3.0	0.5	15	8%
(Mrs. Paterson's) pie, hand held pie, frozen, 'Aussie Pie'. . . .	1 serving	434	15	40	799	na	24.0	7.2	48	50%
(Mountain House) stew, freeze-dried, prepared.	1 cup	230	9	30	209	0	8.0	0.0	0	32%
(Myers)										
à la king, frozen.	3.5 oz	137	9	6	357	0	9.0	0.0	0	57%
and noodles, frozen.	3.5 oz	136	8	9	399	0	8.0	0.0	0	51%
creamed, frozen	3.5 oz	151	12	5	372	0	10.0	0.0	0	57%
croquettes, frozen	3.5 oz	168	16	10	364	0	7.0	0.0	0	38%
frozen, à la gratin, frozen.	3.5 oz	129	9	9	276	0	7.0	0.0	0	47%
pie, frozen	3.5 oz	129	7	10	253	0	7.0	0.0	0	48%
(Pierre)										
barbecue, frozen, 'Chix-B-Q' product 9845	1 piece	137	14	6	418	1	5.8	1.6	36	38%
breaded, frozen, 'Two-Fers' product 1870	1 piece	92	5	4	194	0	6.5	1.2	12	64%
breast, breaded, frozen, cooked, product 1881	1 piece	95	5	3	193	0	6.6	1.3	14	63%
breast patty, fillet-shaped, flame-broiled, 'Caboose' product 9863	1 piece	121	15	3	320	1	5.4	1.5	35	40%
breast patty, fillet-shaped, flame-broiled, product 9820. . . .	1 piece	157	21	4	473	1	6.0	1.7	49	35%
breast patty, fillet-shaped, flame-broiled, product 9916. . . .	1 piece	152	19	4	417	1	6.3	1.8	47	37%

Food Name	Serving Size	Calories	Prot. gms	Carbs gms	Sod. mgs	Fiber gms	Fat gms	Sat. Fat gms	Chol. mgs	% Fat Cal.
breast patty, mesquite, fillet-shaped, flame-broiled, product 9816	1 piece	149	18	1	382	1	7.4	2.1	45	45%
nuggets, breaded, frozen, product 3800	1 piece	47	2	2	99	0	3.3	0.7	6	64%
patty, breaded, frozen, product 1915	1 piece	185	9	7	390	1	13.1	2.5	25	64%
patty, cutlet-shaped, flame-broiled, frozen, product 9835	1 piece	145	18	4	379	1	6.2	1.8	47	39%
patty, cutlet-shaped, honey mustard, flame-broiled, frozen, product 9852	1 piece	167	18	8	611	1	7.1	1.9	47	38%
patty, cutlet-shaped, mesquite, flame-broiled, frozen, product 9805	1 piece	138	18	1	337	1	6.3	1.8	47	41%
patty, cutlet-shaped, rotisserie style, flame-broiled, frozen, product 9878	1 piece	133	19	2	297	1	5.7	1.6	45	38%
patty, cutlet-shaped, teriyaki sauce, flame-broiled, frozen, product 9829	1 piece	165	18	7	576	1	6.7	1.9	47	37%
patty, fillet-shaped, flame-broiled, frozen, product 9840	1 piece	123	14	3	325	1	5.8	1.6	37	43%
(Pilgrim's Pride)										
Cajun style, frozen	3 oz	241	13	9	480	0	17.0	0.0	51	64%
primavera, frozen	3 oz	183	14	8	640	0	10.4	0.0	21	51%
(Pillsbury)										
casserole, frozen, 'Microwave Classic'	1 pkg	400	21	30	890	0	22.0	0.0	0	49%
w/cheese, casserole, 'Microwave Classic'	1 pkg	480	21	33	940	0	29.0	0.0	0	55%
(Redi-Serve) nuggets, white meat, breaded and cooked	6 nibblers	270	14	17	610	2	16.0	4.0	35	54%
(Rice A Roni)										
w/mushrooms, rice	2.5 oz	203	5	29	835	1	7.9	1.4	0	34%
w/vegetable rice	2.5 oz	164	3	29	830	1	4.0	0.6	0	21%
(Right Course)										
primavera, sesame, frozen	10 oz	320	25	34	590	0	9.0	2.0	50	26%
tenderloins, barbecue, w/sauce, frozen	8.75 oz	270	20	35	590	0	6.0	1.0	40	20%
tenderloins, in peanut sauce, frozen	9.25 oz	330	27	32	570	0	10.0	2.0	50	28%
(Shanghai) stir-fry, frozen	10.3 oz	190	22	19	1220	0	3.0	0.0	30	14%
(Shelton's)										
pie, white flour	1 serving	230	15	18	370	1	10.0	5.0	55	41%
pie, whole wheat	1 serving	230	16	18	370	3	10.0	5.0	55	40%
(Smart Ones)										
à l'orange, frozen	8 oz	190	12	34	530	0	1.0	1.0	15	5%
chow mein	1 entrée	200	12	34	490	3	2.0	0.5	25	9%
chow mein, frozen	9 oz	170	14	27	470	0	1.0	1.0	20	5%
fiesta	1 entrée	220	12	38	480	5	2.0	0.5	25	8%
Francais, w/garlic vegetables, frozen	8.5 oz	150	15	18	400	0	1.0	1.0	5	6%
grilled, glazed, w/sauce, frozen	8 oz	130	12	17	540	0	1.0	1.0	20	7%
honey mustard	1 entrée	200	13	33	340	6	2.0	0.5	30	9%
honey mustard, w/sauce, frozen	7.5 oz	140	11	20	220	0	1.0	1.0	10	7%
Marsala	1 entrée	150	10	22	500	6	2.0	0.5	25	12%
Mexican, w/Spanish rice, frozen, 'Fiesta'	8 oz	210	14	37	390	0	1.0	1.0	20	4%
Mexican style, w/rice, frozen, 'Monterey'	1 pkg	410	23	35	700	4	20.0	9.0	75	44%
Mirabella	1 entrée	170	11	26	470	6	2.0	0.5	20	11%
picatta	1 entrée	190	10	34	460	3	2.0	0.5	25	9%
Szechwan style, spicy, w/vegetables	1 entrée	220	11	39	730	3	2.0	0.5	10	8%
(Stouffer's)										
à la king	1 entrée	320	15	43	750	3	10.0	3.0	55	28%
à la king, w/rice, frozen	9.5-oz pkg	270	18	38	800	0	5.0	0.0	0	17%
and dumplings, frozen, food service product	1 oz	39	2	3	109	0	2.3	0.5	9	52%
and noodles, escalloped	1 entrée	450	17	32	1170	1	28.0	6.0	50	56%

Food Name	Serving Size	Calories	Prot. gms	Carbs gms	Sod. mgs	Fiber gms	Fat gms	Sat. Fat gms	Chol. mgs	% Fat Cal.
and noodles, escalloped, frozen	1 entrée	365	17	4	1211	na	31.4	6.6	76	77%
and noodles, escalloped, frozen, food service product	1 oz	42	2	3	122	0	2.5	1.0	11	54%
and noodles, 'Homestyle'	1 entrée	300	20	25	950	3	13.0	3.0	90	39%
and vegetables, w/cream sauce, frozen	1 oz	31	1	2	113	0	2.0	0.5	9	58%
baked, w/mashed potatoes, 'Homestyle'	1 entrée	270	22	19	750	2	12.0	3.0	75	40%
chow mein, w/rice, frozen	10 3/4 oz pkg	250	13	39	720	0	5.0	0.0	0	18%
creamed	1 entrée	280	17	8	720	0	20.0	7.0	80	64%
creamed, frozen, food service product	1 oz	46	2	1	108	0	3.7	1.4	11	72%
divan, frozen	8-oz pkg	220	24	11	610	0	10.0	0.0	0	39%
fried, w/mashed potatoes, 'Homestyle'	1 entrée	330	18	29	780	3	16.0	4.0	55	43%
grilled, homestyle, w/BBQ sauce, frozen	7 5/8 oz	210	23	14	550	0	7.0	0.0	0	30%
Monterey, w/Mexican rice, homestyle, food service product	1 entrée	410	23	35	700	4	20.0	9.0	75	44%
noodle, homestyle, frozen, food service product	1 oz	31	2	2	120	0	1.6	0.3	6	47%
parmigiana, w/pasta Alfredo, homestyle, frozen	9 7/8 oz	360	31	24	990	0	15.0	0.0	0	38%
parmigiana, w/spaghetti, 'Homestyle'	1 entrée	320	27	30	890	4	10.0	2.0	75	28%
pie, frozen	1 entrée	572	23	37	942	3	37.1	10.7	76	58%
tenders, breaded, w/potatoes, homestyle	8 3/8 oz	430	20	46	950	0	18.0	0.0	0	38%
w/dumplings, in broth, frozen, food service product	1 oz	26	2	2	103	0	1.1	0.3	11	38%
(Swanson)										
à la king, canned	1 cup	320	15	17	1080	0	22.0	8.0	60	61%
à la king, canned	5.25 oz	190	10	9	690	0	12.0	0.0	0	59%
and dumplings, canned	1 cup	260	13	22	1120	0	13.0	5.0	65	46%
boneless, 'Hungry Man'	1 entrée	630	26	80	1680	9	22.0	6.0	55	32%
cacciatore, frozen, 'Homestyle Recipe'	10.95 oz	260	15	33	1030	0	8.0	0.0	0	27%
fried, barbecue flavored, frozen	10 oz	540	25	61	1160	0	22.0	0.0	0	37%
fried, dark meat	1 entrée	580	24	54	1430	5	30.0	10.0	105	46%
fried, dark meat, 'Hungry Man'	1 entrée	780	33	74	1700	8	39.0	12.0	105	45%
fried, mostly white meat, 'Hungry Man'	1 entrée	800	35	79	2380	6	39.0	11.0	85	43%
fried, white meat	1 entrée	630	26	62	1700	5	31.0	8.0	55	44%
grilled, white meat, w/garlic sauce, almonds	10 oz	310	17	39	630	0	9.0	0.0	30	27%
nibbles, frozen, 'Homestyle Recipe'	4.25 oz	340	10	29	730	0	20.0	0.0	0	54%
nibbles, 'Plump and Juicy'	3.25 oz	300	12	19	690	0	19.0	0.0	0	58%
nuggets, 'Plump and Juicy'	3 oz	230	13	14	360	0	14.0	0.0	0	54%
nuggets, fried	1 entrée	590	20	71	990	5	25.0	7.0	35	38%
nuggets, frozen	8.75 oz	470	19	47	650	0	23.0	0.0	0	44%
parmigiana, frozen, 'Budget'	10 oz	300	7	35	780	0	15.0	0.0	0	45%
pie, frozen, 'Homestyle Recipe'	8 oz	410	15	41	1030	0	21.0	0.0	0	46%
pot pie	1 pie	410	10	43	780	2	22.0	9.0	25	48%
pot pie, 'Hungry Man'	1 pie	650	19	64	1500	3	35.0	14.0	65	49%
stew, canned	1 cup	180	11	17	1110	2	8.0	3.0	35	39%
(Sweet Sue)										
and dumplings, canned	1 pkg	620	43	65	2683	7	21.1	5.1	102	31%
chicken and dumplings, canned	1 serving	218	15	23	946	3	7.4	1.8	36	31%
(Swift)										
cordon bleu, frozen, 'International'	6 oz	360	30	23	1010	0	17.0	0.0	0	42%
Kiev, frozen, 'International'	6 oz	420	27	22	1030	0	24.0	0.0	0	52%
(Top Shelf)										
à la king, packaged	10 oz	360	18	49	890	0	10.0	4.0	37	25%
Acapulco, packaged	1 serving	390	28	41	1320	0	13.0	0.0	55	30%
cacciatore, packaged	10 oz	210	21	25	810	0	3.0	0.0	50	13%
glazed, packaged	10 oz	170	19	19	780	0	2.0	1.0	35	11%
sweet and sour, packaged	1 serving	270	24	41	280	0	1.0	0.0	60	3%
w/Spanish rice, packaged	10 oz	400	27	38	810	0	15.0	7.0	75	34%

Food Name	Serving Size	Calories	Prot. gms	Carbs gms	Sod. mgs	Fiber gms	Fat gms	Sat. Fat gms	Chol. mgs	% Fat Cal.
(Tyson)										
à l'orange, 'Gourmet Selection' frozen	9.5 oz	300	21	36	670	0	8.0	0.0	0	24%
barbecue, frozen	12.5 oz	400	27	56	600	0	8.0	0.0	50	18%
barbecue, glazed, frozen, 'Yosemite Sam'	7.38 oz	230	12	28	510	0	8.0	0.0	45	31%
barbecue, w/potato and vegetable medley	1 entrée	560	19	73	1190	9	21.0	5.0	30	34%
blackened, w/Spanish rice and corn	1 entrée	260	17	36	480	4	5.0	1.0	30	18%
breast patty, breaded	1 piece	80	10	9	430	1	0.0	0.0	0	0%
breast patty, breaded, Southern fried	1 entrée	180	11	8	360	0	12.0	2.5	30	59%
chunks, frozen, 'Chick'n Chunks'	2.6 oz	220	10	11	500	0	15.0	0.0	35	62%
chunks, frozen, 'Looney Tunes Bugs Bunny'	7.7 oz	290	17	31	480	0	11.0	0.0	28	34%
chunks, Southern fried 'Chick'n Chunks'	2.6 oz	220	10	11	540	0	15.0	0.0	35	62%
cordon bleu, wholesale club item, 'Mini Cordon Bleu'	1 piece	90	8	5	210	0	4.0	0.0	17	41%
cordon bleu, wholesale club item, frozen	7 oz	480	40	28	1030	0	22.0	0.0	0	42%
divan, w/candied carrots and pasta	1 entrée	370	20	38	530	2	15.0	4.0	50	37%
drummettes, frozen, ' Tazmanian Devil'	8 oz	310	14	31	480	0	14.0	0.0	40	41%
drumsticks, roasted, w/skin	3 med pieces	330	40	1	870	0	18.0	5.0	225	50%
Francais, frozen, 'Gourmet Selection'	9.5 oz	280	19	20	1130	0	14.0	0.0	0	45%
fried, w/mashed potatoes, gravy, corn	1 entrée	360	16	30	5	4	15.0	3.0	4	42%
glazed, w/sauce 'Gourmet Selections'	9.25 oz	240	22	29	930	0	4.0	0.0	44	15%
grilled, w/corn O'Brien and ranch beans	1 entrée	230	19	30	590	7	4.0	1.0	30	16%
grilled, w/Italian style w/pasta and vegetable medley	1 entrée	190	21	19	440	3	3.5	1.5	30	16%
'Herb Chicken Meal' frozen	13.75 oz	340	32	43	550	0	4.0	0.0	50	11%
honey Dijon, w/pasta and peas	1 entrée	340	20	49	900	6	7.0	1.5	25	19%
'Honey Mustard Chicken Meal' frozen	13.75 oz	390	31	52	520	0	6.0	0.0	50	14%
honey roasted, frozen, 'Gourmet Selections'	9 oz	220	26	23	500	0	4.0	0.0	48	16%
Italian, grilled, 'Gourmet Selections'	9 oz	210	28	19	420	0	3.0	0.0	40	13%
'Italian Style Chicken Meal' frozen	13.75 oz	310	30	38	600	0	4.0	0.0	50	12%
Kiev, w/rice pilaf, broccoli, carrots	1 entrée	440	18	36	900	2	25.0	11.0	85	51%
'Looney Tunes Road Runner' frozen	6.7 oz	300	8	42	490	0	11.0	0.0	24	33%
marinara, frozen	13.75 oz	340	31	37	590	0	7.0	0.0	45	19%
Marsala, w/carrots and red potatoes	1 entrée	180	15	19	520	4	5.0	1.5	30	25%
mesquite breast tenders, boneless, frozen	2.75 oz	110	17	4	420	0	3.0	0.0	45	24%
mesquite, w/barbecue sauce, corn, potato	1 entrée	321	18	45	793	4	7.8	2.6	26	22%
mesquite, w/corn, pea, and au gratin	1 entrée	320	18	44	780	4	8.0	2.0	25	23%
'Mesquite Chicken Meal' frozen	13.25 oz	330	34	38	600	0	5.0	0.0	45	14%
nuggets, frozen, 'Microwave'	3.5 oz	220	10	11	0	0	15.0	0.0	0	62%
Oriental, breast strips, boneless, frozen	2.75 oz	110	14	6	250	0	3.0	0.0	40	25%
Oriental, frozen, 'Gourmet Selection'	10.25 oz	270	20	32	1140	0	7.0	0.0	0	23%
parmigiana, frozen, 'Gourmet Selection'	11.25 oz	380	19	37	1100	0	17.0	0.0	0	41%
picatta, w/broccoli and parslied potatoes	1 entrée	190	17	18	500	5	6.0	2.0	35	28%
pie, premium, frozen	9 oz	390	16	36	1065	0	20.0	0.0	43	46%
pie, white meat, premium, frozen	9 oz	400	22	33	783	0	20.0	0.0	56	45%
primavera	1 entrée	350	25	48	610	5	6.0	2.5	30	16%
roasted, frozen, 'Gourmet Selections'	9 oz	200	21	21	430	0	2.0	0.0	42	10%
roasted, w/garlic sauce, pasta, vegetable	1 entrée	214	17	22	467	4	6.7	1.3	28	28%
'Salsa Chicken Meal' frozen	13.75 oz	370	34	52	470	0	6.0	0.0	45	14%
sesame, frozen, 'Healthy Portions'	13.5 oz	390	27	58	410	0	5.0	1.0	45	12%
stir-fry, w/vegetable, frozen, wholesale club item	3.5 oz	130	11	13	710	0	5.0	0.0	45	32%
supreme, frozen, 'Gourmet Selections'	9 oz	230	21	23	480	0	6.0	0.0	51	23%
sweet and sour, frozen, 'Gourmet Selection'	11 oz	420	22	50	850	0	15.0	0.0	0	32%
tabasco barbecue	1 entrée	260	13	37	610	5	7.0	1.5	25	24%
tenders, frozen 'Microwave'	3.5 oz	230	16	19	0	0	11.0	0.0	0	41%
w/cheddar, boneless, 'Chick'n Cheddar'	2.6 oz	220	11	11	310	0	15.0	0.0	40	61%
wholesale club item, 'Classic Colonial'	3.5 oz	180	13	11	190	0	9.0	0.0	40	46%

Food Name	Serving Size	Calories	Prot. gms	Carbs gms	Sod. mgs	Fiber gms	Fat gms	Sat. Fat gms	Chol. mgs	% Fat Cal.
wings, hot, wholesale club item, frozen 'Wings of Fire'	3.5 oz	220	26	2	390	0	12.0	0.0	105	49%
wings, teriyaki style	4 pieces	190	21	2	210	2	12.0	3.0	120	54%
(Ultra Slim Fast)										
and vegetables	12 oz	290	24	45	850	0	3.0	0.0	30	9%
chow mein	12 oz	320	25	43	580	0	6.0	0.0	60	17%
in mushroom sauce	12 oz	280	25	30	830	0	6.0	0.0	55	20%
mesquite	12 oz	350	29	61	300	0	1.0	0.0	65	2%
sweet and sour, frozen	12 oz	330	20	57	340	0	2.0	0.0	45	6%
(Weaver)										
'Honey Batter Tenders' frozen	3 oz	220	13	14	500	0	12.0	0.0	0	50%
'Italian Rondolet' frozen	2.6 oz	190	11	11	560	0	11.0	0.0	0	53%
'Original Rondolet' frozen	3 oz	190	13	13	610	0	10.0	0.0	0	46%
'Premium Tenders' frozen	3 oz	170	12	11	500	0	9.0	0.0	0	47%
assorted pieces, frozen, 'Crispy Dutch Frye'	3.6 oz	290	16	16	550	0	18.0	0.0	0	56%
breast, frozen 'Crispy Dutch Frye'	4.5 oz	350	22	17	520	0	22.0	0.0	0	56%
crispy, light, skinless, frozen	2.9 oz	170	14	9	320	0	9.0	0.0	0	47%
croquettes, frozen	2 pieces	280	14	22	780	0	16.0	0.0	0	50%
frozen, 'Cheese Rondolet'	2.6 oz	190	11	12	520	0	11.0	0.0	0	52%
mini drums, herb and spice, frozen	3 oz	200	13	13	320	0	11.0	0.0	0	49%
mini-drums, crispy, frozen	3 oz	210	13	13	480	0	12.0	0.0	0	51%
(Weight Watchers)										
barbecue glazed	1 entrée	230	20	33	440	4	2.5	0.5	30	10%
barbecue, glazed, w/vegetables, frozen, 'Ultimate 200'	7 oz	200	19	22	450	0	6.0	3.0	30	25%
barbecue, w/sauce, mixed vegetables, frozen, 'Ultimate 200'	1 serving	217	19	26	405	na	4.4	1.0	48	18%
cordon bleu	1 entrée	230	15	31	650	2	4.5	1.5	20	18%
cordon bleu, w/vegetables, frozen, 'Ultimate 200'	7.7 oz	170	19	15	560	0	5.0	1.0	40	25%
divan, w/baked potato, frozen	11.25 oz	280	17	38	480	0	7.0	2.0	30	22%
glazed	1 entrée	240	18	29	550	4	6.0	1.0	20	22%
grilled, glazed, frozen, 'Ultimate 200'	7.5 oz	150	15	17	520	0	2.0	1.0	20	12%
grilled, w/Spanish rice, frozen, 'Suiza'	8.6 oz	220	21	18	590	0	7.0	2.0	60	29%
Hunan, w/vegetables, frozen, 'Stir Fry'	9 oz	160	15	21	430	0	2.0	1.0	15	11%
imperial, frozen, 'Ultimate 200'	8.5 oz	200	18	25	430	0	3.0	1.0	25	14%
Kiev, w/vegetables, rice, frozen, 'Ultimate 200'	7 oz	190	14	22	470	0	5.0	2.0	15	24%
orange glazed, w/rice, frozen, 'Stir Fry'	9 oz	170	14	25	360	0	2.0	1.0	10	10%
parmigiana	1 entrée	310	21	39	500	4	7.0	2.0	30	21%
patty, Southern baked, w/vegetables, frozen, 'Ultimate 200'	6.3 oz	170	17	10	520	0	7.0	2.0	45	37%
Polynesian, frozen, 'Stir Fry'	9 oz	190	12	34	240	0	1.0	1.0	20	5%
sesame, w/lo mein noodles, frozen, 'Stir Fry'	9 oz	200	19	23	420	0	4.0	2.0	10	18%
teriyaki, frozen, 'Ultimate 200'	7.6 oz	150	21	7	590	0	4.0	1.0	50	24%
teriyaki, w/spring vegetables, frozen, 'Stir Fry'	9 oz	140	13	16	470	0	3.0	2.0	20	19%
w/Spanish rice, frozen 'TexMex'	8.3 oz	250	18	33	590	0	5.0	2.0	35	18%
(Wonderbites)										
barbecue, flame-broiled, frozen, 'Dippers'	1 piece	41	4	2	127	0	1.7	0.5	12	36%
breast, flame-broiled, frozen, 'Dippers'	1 piece	35	4	1	91	0	1.5	0.4	11	38%
Buffalo flavored, flame-broiled, frozen, 'Dippers'	1 piece	33	4	1	199	0	1.5	0.4	11	40%
chili salsa, breaded, frozen, 'Dippers'	1 piece	69	4	3	121	0	4.8	0.9	8	63%
flame-broiled, frozen, 'Dippers'	1 piece	35	4	1	92	0	1.5	0.4	11	39%
honey mustard, flame-broiled, frozen, 'Dippers'	1 piece	40	4	2	151	0	1.6	0.4	12	37%
Italian, flame-broiled, frozen, 'Dippers'	1 piece	33	4	0	124	0	1.4	0.4	11	40%
rotisserie style, flame-broiled, frozen, 'Dippers' product 9896	1 piece	34	5	0	75	0	1.4	0.4	11	38%
teriyaki, flame broiled, frozen, 'Dippers' product 3727	1 piece	45	4	2	128	0	2.3	0.9	11	47%

Food Name	Serving Size	Calories	Prot. gms	Carbs gms	Sod. mgs	Fiber gms	Fat gms	Sat. Fat gms	Chol. mgs	% Fat Cal.
teriyaki, flame broiled, frozen, 'Dippers' product 3827.....	1 piece	45	4	2	127	0	2.4	0.9	10	48%
teriyaki, flame broiled, frozen, 'Dippers' product 9879.....	1 piece	41	4	2	142	0	1.7	0.5	12	37%
(Yu Sing)										
lo mein, frozen..........................	1 container	230	13	35	950	3	5.0	2.0	15	19%
sweet and sour, w/rice........................	1 container	300	12	50	480	2	6.0	2.5	20	18%
w/almonds, w/rice, frozen....................	1 container	250	12	33	770	3	8.0	2.0	20	29%
CHICKEN DINNER/ENTRÉE MIX										
(Chicken Helper)										
cheesy broccoli, 'Skillet' dry....	1/5 pkg	160	4	32	700	0	2.0	0.0	5	11%
cheesy broccoli, 'Skillet' prepared........	7 oz	310	24	34	790	0	9.0	0.0	65	26%
stir-fry, 'Skillet' mix only..............	1/5 pkg	170	4	36	800	0	1.0	0.0	0	5%
stir-fry, 'Skillet' prepared.............	7 oz	370	25	36	950	0	14.0	0.0	145	34%
creamy, 'Skillet' mix only.............	1/5 pkg	170	6	26	720	0	5.0	0.0	40	26%
creamy, 'Skillet' prepared.........	8.25 oz	330	26	29	820	0	13.0	0.0	100	35%
fettuccini Alfredo, 'Skillet' mix only...	1/5 pkg	160	6	25	690	0	4.0	0.0	10	23%
fettuccini Alfredo, 'Skillet' prepared.........	7.5 oz	320	26	27	780	0	12.0	0.0	70	34%
creamy mushroom, 'Skillet' mix only.........	1/5 pkg	170	5	28	720	0	4.0	0.0	30	21%
creamy mushroom, 'Skillet' prepared..........	8 oz	320	25	31	810	0	11.0	0.0	90	31%
(Lipton)										
barbecue, 'Microeasy' mix only............	1/4 pkg	110	2	24	980	0	1.0	0.0	0	8%
barbecue, 'Microeasy' prepared.............	1/4 pkg	220	16	24	1020	0	6.0	0.0	0	25%
country style, 'Microeasy' mix only...........	1/4 pkg	80	3	15	840	0	1.0	0.0	0	11%
country style, 'Microeasy' prepared...........	1/4 pkg	190	18	15	880	0	6.0	0.0	0	29%
(Skillet Chicken Helper) stir-fried.............	1/4 cup	140	4	30	690	1	0.5	0.0	0	3%
CHICKEN FAT										
....	1 cup	1846	0.0	0.0	0	0	204.6	61.1	174	100%
....	1 oz	178	1.1	0.0	9	0	19.3	5.7	16	98%
....	1 tbsp	115	0.0	0.0	0	0	12.8	3.8	11	100%
kosher, retail rendered *(Empire Kosher)*..............	1 tbsp	120	0	1	0	0	13.0	4.0	0	97%
CHICKEN SALAD SPREAD										
(Libby's) 'Spreadables'..........................	1 pkg	329	11	23	1062	na	21.3	4.4	59	58%
(Libby's) 'Spreadables'..........................	1/3 cup	140	7	7	340	2	9.0	1.5	25	59%
(Libby's) 'Spreadables'..........................	1 serving	171	6	12	552	na	11.1	2.3	31	58%
CHICKEN SPREAD										
(Hormel) canned..........................	0.5 oz	30	2	0	0	0	2.0	0.0	0	69%
(Underwood) canned, chunky.....................	2 1/8 oz	150	10	2	440	0	9.0	3.0	40	63%
(Underwood) canned, 'Light'....................	2 1/8 oz	80	11	2	330	0	3.0	1.0	30	34%
(Underwood) canned, smoky.....................	2 1/8 oz	150	10	10	290	0	8.0	2.0	40	47%
CHICKEN SUBSTITUTE										
(Heartline)										
vegetarian, 'Chicken Fillet Style'..................	2 oz	176	19	9	260	0	7.0	0.0	0	36%
vegetarian, lite, 'Chicken Fillet Style'..................	0.5 oz	22	5	1	135	3	0.0	0.0	0	0%
(Morningstar Farms)										
nuggets, vegetarian, 'Chik Nuggets'..................	4 nuggets	160	13	17	670	5	4.0	0.5	0	22.5%
nuggets, vegetarian, homestyle, frozen,										
'Country Crisps'..........................	3 oz	250	8	18	480	0	16.0	0.0	0	58%
nuggets, vegetarian, zesty, frozen, 'Country Crisps'......	3 oz	280	9	17	740	0	19.0	3.0	0	62%
patty, vegetarian, 'Chik Patty'..................	1 patty	177	7	15	536	2	9.8	1.3	1	50%
patty, vegetarian, frozen, 'Country Crisps'..............	2.5 oz	220	8	13	620	0	15.0	2.0	0	62%
vegetarian, 'Meatless Chicken'..................	1 patty	170	8	13	590	0	10.0	2.0	0	52%
(Worthington)										
chicken style, vegetarian....................	1 slice	86	10	1	374	1	4.6	0.8	1	48%
diced, vegetarian, 'Diced Chik'..................	1/4 cup drained	40	7	1	270	1	0.0	0.0	0	0%
diced, vegetarian, frozen, 5-lb pkg 'Meatless Chicken'....	1/4 cup	50	10	2	400	1	0.0	0.0	0	0%

Food Name	Serving Size	Calories	Prot. gms	Carbs gms	Sod. mgs	Fiber gms	Fat gms	Sat. Fat gms	Chol. mgs	% Fat Cal.
nuggets, vegetarian, 'Chik Stiks'	1 serving	111	9	3	355	2	7.3	1.2	1	59%
pie, vegetarian, frozen	8 oz	380	7	43	1200	0	20.0	3.0	0	47%
roll, vegetarian, 4-lb pkg, 'Meatless Chicken'	3/8-inch slice	80	9	1	360	<1	4.5	1.0	0	50.6%
roll, vegetarian, frozen, 'Meatless Chicken'	2.5 oz	150	11	4	570	0	10.0	1.0	0	60%
sliced, vegetarian, 'Chic-Ketts'	2 3/8-inch slices	120	13	2	390	2	7.0	1.0	0	52.5%
sliced, vegetarian, 'Sliced Chik'	3 slices	70	14	2	430	2	0.5	0.0	0	6.4%
slices, vegetarian, 8-oz pkg, 'Meatless Chicken'	2 slices	80	9	1	370	1	4.5	1.0	0	50.6%
slices, vegetarian, frozen, 'Meatless Chicken' 2 oz	2 slices	130	9	3	460	0	9.0	1.0	0	63%
vegetarian, 'Chic-Ketts'	1 slice	121	13	2	390	2	6.5	1.0	0	49%
vegetarian, diced, canned drained	1/4 cup	90	4	2	330	0	8.0	0.0	0	75%
vegetarian, diced, frozen, 'Meatless Chicken'	1/2 cup	190	13	5	680	0	13.0	2.0	0	62%
vegetarian, frozen, 'Crispy Chik'	3 oz	280	10	17	500	0	19.0	0.0	0	61%
vegetarian, sliced, canned, drained, 2.1 oz.	2 slices	90	4	2	330	0	8.0	0.0	0	75%

CHICKEN SUBSTITUTE DINNER/ENTRÉE

(Loma Linda)

croquette, loaf, or patty, vegetarian, dry mix, 'Chicken Supreme'	1/3 cup	90	15	6	720	4	1.0	0.0	0	10.0%
fried chicken style, vegetarian, 'Fried Chik'n with Gravy'	2 pieces	160	12	4	440	2	10.0	1.5	0	56.2%
nuggets, vegetarian, 'Meatless Chik-Nuggets'	5 pieces	240	12	13	710	5	16.0	2.5	0	60.0%

(Morningstar Farms)

wings, vegetarian, 'Meat-Free Buffalo Wings'	5 nuggets	200	13	16	730	3	9.0	1.5	0	40.5%

(Worthington)

croquettes, vegetarian, 'Golden Croquettes'	4 pieces	210	14	14	600	3	10.0	1.5	0	42.9%
drumsticks, vegetarian, 'Chik Stiks'	1 piece	110	9	3	360	2	7.0	1.0	0	57.2%
fried chicken style, vegetarian, 'FriChik'	2 pieces	120	10	1	430	1	8.0	1.0	0	60.0%
fried chicken style, vegetarian, low-fat, 'Low Fat FriChik'	2 pieces	80	18	21	870	11	1.0	0.0	0	11.3%
patties, vegetarian, lightly breaded, seasoned, 'Crispy Chik Patties'	1 pattie	150	8	15	600	2	6.0	1.0	0	36.0%

CHICKEN SEASONING. See under SEASONING MIX.

CHICKEN SEASONING AND COATING MIX. See under SEASONING AND COATING MIX.

CHICKPEA / ceci / garbanzo

Canned

	1 cup	286	12	54	718	11	2.7	0.3	0	8%
(A&P)	1/2 cup	100	6	17	270	0	1.0	0.0	0	9%
(Allens)	1/2 cup	110	5	18	320	0	1.0	0.0	0	9%
(Bush's Best)	1/2 cup	80	5	21	350	6	0.0	0.0	0	0%
(Finast)	8 oz	210	10	35	250	0	3.0	0.0	0	13%
(Green Giant)	1/2 cup	90	6	18	320	5	2.0	0.0	0	16%
(Old El Paso)	1/2 cup	190	5	16	250	0	1.0	0.0	0	10%
(Progresso)	1/2 cup	110	9	22	200	6	1.0	0.0	0	7%
'Nutradiet' *(S&W)*	1/2 cup	100	5	19	5	0	1.0	0.0	0	9%
dry beans in brine *(Green Giant)*	1/2 cup	110	6	18	380	5	1.5	0.0	0	12%
50% less salt *(Green Giant)*	1/2 cup	90	6	18	160	5	2.0	0.0	0	16%
50% less salt *(Joan of Arc)*	1/2 cup	90	6	18	160	5	2.0	0.0	0	16%
large 'Lite 50% Less Salt' *(S&W)*	1/2 cup	110	6	21	295	0	1.0	0.0	0	8%
organic, no salt added *(Eden Foods)*	1/2 cup	90	6	17	10	4	1.0	0.0	0	9%
organic, w/liquid *(Eden Foods)*	1/2 cup	110	6	17	15	4	2.0	0.0	0	16%

Fresh

mature seed, boiled	1 cup	269	15	45	11	12	4.2	0.4	0	13%
mature seed, raw	1 cup	728	39	121	48	35	12.1	1.3	0	14%
mature seed, raw	1 tbsp	46	2	8	3	2	0.8	0.1	0	14%
raw *(Arrowhead Mills)*	2 oz	200	12	35	9	7	3.0	0.0	0	13%

Food Name	Serving Size	Calories	Prot. gms	Carbs gms	Sod. mgs	Fiber gms	Fat gms	Sat. Fat gms	Chol. mgs	% Fat Cal.
Jarred, organically grown *(Eden Foods)*	1/2 cup	110	7	20	95	4	1.0	0.0	0	8%
CHICKPEA FLOUR. See under FLOUR.										
CHICORY										
trimmed	1 oz	7	0.5	1.3	13	(mq)	0.1	<.1	0	11%
trimmed, chopped	1/2 cup	21	1.5	4.2	41	3.6	0.3	0.1	0	11%
untrimmed	1 lb	87	6.3	17.5	167	(mq)	1.1	0.3	0	9%
CHICORY, WITLOOF										
raw	1/2 cup	8	0.4	1.8	1	1.4	0.0	0.0	0	0%
raw, medium, approx 2.1 oz	1 head	9	0.5	2.1	1	1.6	0.1	0.0	0	8%
trimmed	1 oz	4	0.3	0.9	2	(mq)	<.1	tr	0	<16%
untrimmed	1 lb	61	4.0	12.9	28	(mq)	0.4	0.1	0	5%
CHICORY ROOT										
raw, medium, approx 2.6 oz	1 root	44	0.8	10.5	30	>1.2 c	0.1	0.0	0	2%
raw, 1-inch pieces	1/2 cup	33	0.6	7.9	23	>.9 c	0.1	0.0	0	3%
trimmed	1 oz	21	0.4	5.0	14	>.6 c	0.1	<.1	0	4%
untrimmed	1 lb	272	5.2	65.1	186	>7.3 c	0.7	0.2	0	2%
CHILE PEPPER. See PEPPER, CHILI.										
CHILI										
(Armour)										
hot, w/beans, canned	7.5 oz	390	13	27	1080	0	26.0	0.0	0	59%
w/beans, canned	7.5 oz	390	13	27	1080	0	26.0	0.0	0	59%
w/beans, canned, 'Premium Lite'	7.5 oz	260	16	27	1110	0	10.0	0.0	0	34%
w/beans, microwave	7.5 oz	300	16	26	1120	0	14.0	0.0	0	43%
w/o beans, canned	7.5 oz	390	13	14	1150	0	31.0	0.0	0	72%
(Bearitos)										
black bean, low-fat, 'Premium'	1 cup	150	9	20	550	5	1.0	0.0	0	7%
original, lowfat, 'Premium'	1 cup	190	10	36	550	6	1.0	0.0	0	5%
spicy, lowfat, 'Premium'	1 cup	190	10	36	550	5	1.0	0.0	0	5%
(Chef Boyardee)										
beef, w/beans, canned	7.5 oz	330	15	30	1005	0	17.0	0.0	0	46%
'Chili Mac' canned	7.5 oz	230	8	26	1410	0	11.0	0.0	0	42%
(Chili Bowl) homestyle	1 cup	680	24	12	1210	8	59.0	26.0	10	79%
(Cimmaron)										
beef, w/beans, canned	7.5 oz	230	17	21	0	0	9.0	0.0	35	35%
chicken, w/beans, canned	7.5 oz	180	12	22	970	0	5.0	0.0	60	25%
(Dennison's)										
chunky, w/beans, canned	7.5 oz	310	16	28	780	10	14.0	0.0	0	42%
hot, w/beans, 15-oz can	7.5 oz	310	16	26	910	7	16.0	0.0	0	46%
w/beans, 15-oz can	7.5 oz	310	16	27	875	8	15.0	0.0	0	44%
'Cook-Off' w/beans, canned	7.5 oz	340	17	25	915	8	19.0	0.0	0	50%
w/o beans, 15-oz can	7.5 oz	300	17	15	1380	0	19.0	0.0	0	57%
(El Rio)										
con carne, w/o beans, canned	1 pkg	497	25	26	1322	6	32.7	12.2	81	59%
con carne, w/o beans, canned	1 serving	305	15	16	812	4	20.1	7.5	50	59%
(Estee) w/beans, canned	7.5 oz	370	16	27	125	0	20.0	10.0	60	51%
(Featherweight) w/beans, canned	7.5 oz	280	19	29	440	0	10.0	0.0	30	32%
(Gebhardt)										
hot, w/beans, canned	1 cup	470	16	47	1000	6	27.0	9.8	65	49%
hot, w/beans, canned	4 oz	189	7	9	497	2	14.2	0.2	17	66%
longhorn, w/beans	1 cup	450	18	32	1089	8	31.4	14.5	33	58%
plain	1 cup	412	20	15	1324	7	30.4	13.5	40	66%
plain, w/o beans	1 cup	530	21	20	990	1	41.0	16.0	150	69%
vegetarian, canned	4 oz	219	10	7	555	0	17.1	0.0	0	70%
w/beans	1 cup	322	15	32	673	15	14.9	5.7	29	42%

Food Name	Serving Size	Calories	Prot. gms	Carbs gms	Sod. mgs	Fiber gms	Fat gms	Sat. Fat gms	Chol. mgs	% Fat Cal.
(Hain)										
w/chicken, canned	7.5 oz	130	11	19	1030	0	2.0	0.0	40	13%
spicy Tempeh, vegetarian, canned	7.5 oz	160	7	24	1350	0	4.0	0.0	0	23%
vegetarian, spicy, canned	7.5 oz	160	7	29	1060	0	1.0	0.0	0	6%
vegetarian, spicy, canned, 'Reduced Sodium'	7.5 oz	170	7	31	200	0	1.0	0.0	0	6%
(Health Valley)										
three-bean, vegetarian, mild, fat-free	5 oz	90	10	12	180	9	0.0	0.0	0	0%
w/beans, vegetarian, mild, canned, 'No Salt Added'	4 oz	130	8	16	25	8	3.0	0.0	0	22%
w/beans, vegetarian, spicy, canned, 'No Salt Added'	4 oz	130	8	16	25	8	3.0	0.0	0	22%
w/black beans, vegetarian, mild, fat-free	5 oz	140	11	23	290	12	0.0	0.0	0	0%
w/black beans, vegetarian, spicy, canned	5 oz	70	7	9	180	8	0.0	0.0	0	0%
w/lentils, vegetarian, mild, 'No Salt Added'	4 oz	130	8	16	50	8	3.0	0.0	0	22%
w/lentils, vegetarian, mild, canned	4 oz	130	8	16	200	8	3.0	0.0	0	22%
(Heinz)										
'Chili Con Carne' canned	7.75 oz	350	15	27	1000	0	21.0	0.0	0	53%
'Chili Mac' canned	7.5 oz	250	10	26	860	0	12.0	0.0	0	43%
hot, w/beans, canned	7.75 oz	330	15	30	1140	0	16.0	0.0	0	44%
(Hormel)										
'Chili Mac' microwave	7.5 oz	192	10	18	977	0	9.0	4.0	22	42%
chunky, w/beans, canned	7.5 oz	290	15	25	780	0	14.0	0.0	50	44%
hot, w/beans, 15-oz can	7.5 oz	310	16	24	1121	0	16.0	0.0	0	47%
hot, w/beans, microwave	7.38 oz	250	15	24	977	0	11.0	4.0	49	39%
hot, w/o beans, 15-oz can	7.5 oz	370	17	12	985	0	28.0	0.0	0	68%
microwave	1 cup	220	15	27	1050	6	6.0	2.5	30	24%
turkey, w/beans, canned	1 cup	203	19	26	1198	6	2.8	0.7	35	12%
vegetarian, w/beans, canned	1 cup	205	12	38	778	10	0.7	0.1	0	3%
w/beans, canned	1 cup	240	17	34	1163	8	4.4	1.8	25	16%
w/beans, 15-oz can	7.5 oz	310	17	23	1127	0	17.0	0.0	0	49%
w/beans, 40-oz can	8 oz	320	17	25	1135	0	17.0	0.0	0	48%
w/beans, microwave	7.5 oz	250	15	23	980	0	11.0	0.0	65	39%
w/o beans, canned	10.5 oz	540	24	19	1384	0	41.0	0.0	0	68%
w/o beans, canned	1 cup	194	17	18	970	3	6.6	2.2	35	31%
w/o beans, 15-oz can	7.5 oz	370	17	12	1012	0	28.0	0.0	0	68%
w/o beans, microwave	7.38 oz	290	18	15	830	0	17.0	8.0	60	54%
(Just Rite)										
hot, w/beans, hot, canned	4 oz	195	11	16	495	1	10.0	3.5	33	45%
vegetarian, w/beans, canned	4.55 oz	190	9	15	616	6	13.3	6.3	18	55%
w/beans, canned	4 oz	200	10	16	500	1	11.0	4.0	33	49%
w/o beans, canned	4 oz	180	13	9	515	1	11.0	3.7	41	53%
(Lean Cuisine) 3-bean, frozen, food service product	1/2 cup	80	4	12	340	4	2.0	0.4	0	22%
(Legume) chicken style, vegetarian	1 cup	160	10	29	460	7	1.0	0.0	0	5%
(Libby's)										
w/beans, 15-oz can	7.5 oz	270	13	25	810	0	13.0	0.0	0	43%
w/beans, microwave, 'Diner'	7.75 oz	280	15	29	820	4	12.0	6.0	40	38%
w/o beans, canned	7.5 oz	390	18	11	800	0	30.0	0.0	0	70%
(Luck's) hot, w/pinto beans	1/2 cup	120	6	20	310	6	1.0	0.0	0	8%
(Lunch Bucket) w/beans, microwave	7.5 oz	300	16	26	1120	0	14.0	0.0	45	43%
(Marie Callender's) w/cornbread	1 cup	350	14	45	1380	5	13.0	6.0	30	33%
(Michelinas) black bean, 'Lean 'n' Tasty'	1 entree	400	13	77	480	10	5.0	1.0	0	11%
(Mountain House)										
w/beans, freeze-dried, prepared	1 cup	390	20	38	153	0	16.0	0.0	0	38%
w/beef, freeze-dried, prepared	1 cup	250	12	31	115	0	8.0	0.0	0	30%
(Nalley's)										
chunky, w/o beans, canned, 'Big Chunk'	7.5 oz	270	17	14	810	0	16.0	0.0	0	54%

Food Name	Serving Size	Calories	Prot. gms	Carbs gms	Sod. mgs	Fiber gms	Fat gms	Sat. Fat gms	Chol. mgs	% Fat Cal.
con carne, w/beans, canned	1 serving	281	40	12	1231	13	8.0	2.8	26	26%
hot jalapeño, w/beans, canned	7.5 oz	260	14	29	920	0	10.0	0.0	0	34%
hot, w/beans, canned	7.5 oz	280	17	30	810	0	10.0	0.0	0	32%
w/beans	7.5 oz	260	17	27	880	0	9.0	0.0	0	32%
w/beans, canned, 'Thick'	7.5 oz	260	16	29	840	0	9.0	0.0	0	31%
(Natural Touch)										
vegetarian, 'Low Fat Vegetarian Chili'	1 cup	170	18	21	870	11	1.0	0.0	0	5.3%
vegetarian, spicy, canned	2/3 cup	230	12	19	890	0	12.0	1.0	0	47%
(Nestlé)										
spicy, w/beans, canned, 'Chef Mate'	1 cup	423	17	33	1485	4	24.7	10.7	56	53%
w/beans, canned 'Chef Mate'	1 cup	412	18	29	1171	11	25.0	10.9	56	55%
w/o beans, canned, 'Chef Mate'	1 cup	430	19	18	1588	3	31.6	14.4	85	66%
(Norpac) w/beans, vegetarian, lowfat. 'Soup Supreme'	1 cup	130	7	27	1150	8	1.0	0.0	0	6%
(Old El Paso)	1 serving	249	18	22	588	10	10.3	2.1	36	37%
(Open Range)										
vegetarian, plain, canned	4.41 oz	176	9	9	608	3	12.8	5.7	24	61%
vegetarian, w/beans, canned	4.5 oz	136	9	13	645	5	8.0	3.7	13	46%
w/beans, food service product	1 cup	281	17	25	1291	10	16.0	7.3	26	46%
w/o beans, food service product	1 cup	353	18	19	1216	6	25.6	7.3	48	61%
(Right Course) vegetarian, frozen	9.75 oz	280	9	45	590	0	7.0	1.0	0	23%
(Shelton's)										
chicken, mild or spicy	1 cup	210	21	26	970	7	3.0	1.0	45	13%
turkey, mild or spicy	1 cup	210	19	26	990	4	4.0	2.0	45	17%
(Stagg)										
chicken, w/beans, canned	7.5 oz	200	14	21	0	0	6.0	0.0	0	28%
chicken, w/beans, canned, 'Ranch House'	7.5 oz	210	17	26	0	0	5.0	0.0	0	21%
country, w/beans, canned	7.5 oz	270	14	25	0	0	12.0	0.0	0	41%
w/beans, canned, 'Chunkero'	1 cup	330	19	28	880	16	15.0	5.0	40	42%
w/beans, canned, 'Classic'	1 cup	324	17	29	825	7	16.3	6.7	42	45%
w/beans, canned, 'Country'	1 cup	319	15	29	1131	6	15.8	6.8	40	45%
w/beans, canned, 'Dynamite'	1 cup	333	18	31	862	8	15.4	5.7	44	41%
w/beans, canned, 'Laredo'	7.5 oz	260	15	22	0	0	12.0	0.0	0	42%
w/beans, canned, 'Ranchhouse'	1 cup	284	19	32	813	9	8.9	2.6	47	28%
w/beans, canned, 'Silverado'	1 cup	227	18	33	865	8	2.8	1.0	40	11%
w/o beans, canned, 'Steak House'	7.5 oz	300	16	17	0	0	19.0	0.0	0	56%
(Stouffer's)										
con carne, w/beans, frozen	8.75 oz	280	20	28	910	0	10.0	0.0	0	32%
con carne, w/beans, frozen, food service product	4 oz	128	8	12	376	4	4.8	2.0	23	34%
w/beans	1 entrée	270	15	29	1130	8	10.0	4.0	35	34%
(Swanson) con carne, frozen, 'Homestyle Recipe'	8.25 oz	270	20	26	740	0	10.0	0.0	0	33%
(Top Shelf) con carne suprema, packaged	1 serving	320	24	30	1140	0	12.0	0.0	65	33%
(Tyson) chicken, frozen, wholesale club item	3.5 oz	105	8	11	420	0	3.0	0.0	0	26%
(Van Camp's)										
w/beans, canned	1 cup	352	15	21	1215	2	23.2	0.0	0	59%
w/franks, w/o beans, canned, 'ChileeWeenee'	1 cup	309	14	28	1057	2	15.7	0.0	0	46%
w/o beans, canned	1 cup	412	15	12	1499	2	33.5	0.0	0	73%
(Wolf Brand)										
extra spicy, w/beans, canned	7.75 oz	324	14	21	926	2	20.6	0.0	0	57%
extra spicy, w/o beans, canned	7.5 oz	363	19	15	962	2	24.9	0.0	0	62%
w/beans, canned	8 oz	345	15	22	1013	2	22.0	0.0	0	57%
w/o beans, canned	8 oz	387	21	16	1042	2	26.6	0.0	0	62%
w/o beans, canned, 'Chili-Mac'	7.75 oz	317	12	23	854	1	19.9	0.0	0	57%
(Worthington)										
vegetarian, 'Chili'	1 cup	290	19	21	1130	9	15.0	2.5	0	46.5%

Food Name	Serving Size	Calories	Prot. gms	Carbs gms	Sod. mgs	Fiber gms	Fat gms	Sat. Fat gms	Chol. mgs	% Fat Cal.
vegetarian, 'Low Fat Chili'	1 cup	170	18	21	870	11	1.0	0.0	0	5.3%

CHILI BEANS. See BEANS, CHILI, CANNED.

CHILI MIX

(Gebhardt) 'Chili Quik' mix only	1.5 oz pkt	82	3	17	2784	3	1.1	0.1	0	11%
(Mountain House)										
w/beans, freeze-dried, prepared.	1 cup	390	20	38	153	0	16.0	0.0	0	38%
w/beef, freeze-dried, 'Chili Mac' prepared.	1 cup	250	12	31	115	0	8.0	0.0	0	30%
(Old El Paso)										
'Chili con Carne' prepared.	1 cup	162	19	8	510	2	7.0	0.0	47	37%
w/beans, prepared	1 cup	217	15	17	480	6	10.0	0.0	32	41%

CHILI PEPPER. See PEPPER, CHILI. See also under PEPPER, GROUND.

CHILI POWDER. See under SEASONING MIX.

CHILI SEASONING. See under SEASONING MIX.

CHIMICHANGA

(Banquet)	1 entree	500	13	56	1180	9	24.0	8.0	20	44%
(Fiesta Cafe) beef and bean, frozen	1 serving	422	24	56	804	6	11.6	2.2	36	25%
(Marquez) shredded beef 'Primera'	1 chimichanga	380	13	42	890	2	17.0	5.0	30	41%
(Old El Paso)										
bean and cheese, frozen.	1 pkg	380	12	40	610	0	19.0	0.0	20	45%
beef, frozen.	1 piece	370	12	34	470	0	21.0	0.0	0	51%
beef and cheese, frozen, 'Festive Dinners'	11 oz	510	22	53	1400	0	23.0	0.0	0	41%
beef and pork, frozen	1 pkg	340	13	35	700	0	16.0	0.0	0	43%
beef, frozen, 'Festive Dinners'.	11 oz	540	23	65	1200	0	21.0	0.0	0	35%
chicken, frozen	1 piece	360	13	33	470	0	20.0	0.0	0	49%

CHINESE APPLE. See POMEGRANATE.

CHINESE BROCCOLI. See BROCCOLI, CHINESE.

CHINESE CABBAGE. See BOK CHOY.

CHINESE DATE

dried	1 oz	81	1.0	20.1	3	>.9 c	0.3	(tr)	0	3%
raw, seeded.	1 oz	22	0.3	5.7	1	>.4 c	0.1	(tr)	0	4%
raw, w/seeds	1 lb	331	5.1	85.3	11	>5.9 c	0.8	na	0	2%

CHINESE FUNGUS / Jew's ear / pepeao

approx 0.2 oz	1 piece	2	0.0	0.4	0	0	(tr)	(tr)	0	0%
dried	1 cup	72	1	19	17	na	0.1	na	0	1%
sliced.	1/2 cup	13	0.2	3.3	5	0	(tr)	(tr)	0	0%
trimmed.	1 oz	7	0.1	1.9	3	0	na	(tr)	0	0%
untrimmed.	1 lb	111	2.1	30.0	41	0	0.2	(tr)	0	1%

CHINESE GOOSEBERRY. See KIWI FRUIT.

CHINESE JUJUBE. See JUJUBE, CHINESE.

CHINESE NOODLE. See under NOODLE.

CHINESE PARSLEY. See CORIANDER LEAF; CORIANDER SEED.

CHINESE PARSLEY LEAF. See CORIANDER LEAF.

CHINESE PARSLEY SEED. See CORIANDER SEED.

CHINESE PEA PODS. See PEAS, SNOW.

CHINESE PEAR. See ASIAN PEAR.

CHINESE RADISH. See DAIKON.

CHINESE WATERMELON. See GOURD, WHITE.

CHINESE YAM. See JICAMA.

CHIVES

Fresh

raw	1 oz	7	0.8	1.1	2	0.9	0.2	<.1	0	19%
raw, chopped.	1 tbsp	1	0.1	0.1	0	0.1	0.0	0.0	0	0%
raw, chopped.	1 tsp	0	0.0	0.0	0	na	0.0	0.0	0	0%
Dried (McCormick/Schilling)	1 tsp	1	0	0	0	0	0.0	0.0	0	0%

Food Name	Serving Size	Calories	Prot. gms	Carbs gms	Sod. mgs	Fiber gms	Fat gms	Sat. Fat gms	Chol. mgs	% Fat Cal.
Freeze-dried										
. . . .	1/4 cup	2	0.2	0.5	1	>.1 c	0.0	0.0	0	0%
. . . .	1 tbsp	1	0.0	0.1	0	tr	0.0	0.0	0	0%
(McCormick/Schilling)	1 tsp	1	0	0	0	0	0.0	0.0	0	0%
(Tone's)	1 tsp	1	0	0	0	0	0.0	0.0	0	0%
CHOCOLATE. See CHOCOLATE, BAKING. See also under CANDY.										
CHOCOLATE, BAKING										
Bars										
bittersweet *(Ghirardelli)*	1 bar	551	7	63	8	9	39.3	23.6	0	56%
dark, dark *(Ghirardelli)*	1 bar	570	5	68	6	6	38.0	22.7	0	54%
semisweet *(Baker's)*	1/2 bar	70	1	8	0	1	4.5	2.5	0	53%
semisweet *(Ghirardelli)*	1 bar	555	6	66	7	8	38.1	22.9	9	54%
semisweet *(Nestlé)*	1 oz	160	2	16	0	0	9.0	0.0	0	53%
semisweet, 'Premium' *(Hershey's)*	1 oz	140	1	16	0	0	8.0	0.0	0	51%
unsweetened *(Baker's)*	1/2 bar	70	2	4	0	2	7.0	4.5	0	72%
unsweetened *(Ghirardelli)*	1 serving	571	14	33	16	17	59.9	36.5	0	74%
unsweetened *(Hershey's)*	1 oz	190	4	7	5	0	16.0	0.0	0	77%
unsweetened *(Nestlé)*	1 oz	180	4	9	0	0	14.0	0.0	0	71%
unsweetened, 'Premium' *(Hershey's)*	1 oz	190	4	7	5	0	16.0	0.0	0	77%
white *(Baker's)*	1/2 bar	80	1	8	15	0	4.5	3.0	3	53%
white, classic *(Ghirardelli)*	1 bar	627	6	66	111	0	39.5	23.6	13	56%
white, 'Premier' *(Nestlé)*	1 oz	150	2	18	15	0	9.0	0.0	0	50%
Chips										
less fat *(Hershey's)*	1 tbsp	60	1	10	0	0	3.5	3.5	0	43%
milk chocolate *(Baker's)*	1/2 oz	70	1	9	10	0	4.0	2.0	0	47%
milk chocolate *(Hershey's)*	1/4 cup	220	2	27	55	0	12.0	0.0	10	48%
milk chocolate *(Hershey's)*	1 oz	150	2	27	55	0	12.0	0.0	10	48%
milk chocolate *(Hershey's)*	1 tbsp	79	1	9	16	0	4.2	2.7	2	47%
chips, milk chocolate, 'Big Chips' *(Baker's)*	1/4 cup	240	3	30	40	0	13.0	0.0	10	47%
milk chocolate, 'Mini Baking Bits' *(M&M Mars)*	1 oz	142	2	20	20	0	6.6	4.2	4	42%
mint chocolate *(Hershey's)*	1.5 oz	230	2	28	1	0	12.0	0.0	0	47%
semisweet *(Baker's)*	1/2 oz	60	1	9	0	1	3.5	2.0	0	44%
semisweet *(Hershey's)*	1.5 oz	220	2	27	0	0	12.0	0.0	0	48%
semisweet, 'Big Chips' *(Baker's)*	1/4 cup	220	2	31	0	0	13.0	0.0	0	47%
semisweet, mini, approx 1/4 cup *(Hershey's)*	1.5 oz	220	2	26	5	0	12.0	0.0	0	49%
semisweet, 'Mini Baking Bits' *(M&M Mars)*	1 oz	146	2	18	0	2	7.4	4.4	0	46%
white *(Hershey's)*	1.5 oz	240	3	25	65	0	14.0	0.0	0	53%
Chunks										
milk chocolate *(Hershey's)*	12 pieces	160	2	16	25	0	9.0	0.0	10	53%
semisweet *(Hershey's)*	1 oz	140	1	15	0	0	8.0	0.0	0	53%
semisweet *(Saco Foods)*	12-oz bag	466	4	67	26	0	26.5	14.9	0	46%
white, 'Premier Treasures' *(Nestlé)*	1 oz	160	2	15	25	0	10.0	0.0	0	57%
Liquid, unsweetened, premelted, 'Choco Bake' *(Nestlé)* . . .	1 oz	190	4	7	0	0	16.0	0.0	0	77%
Shreds *(Tone's)*	1 tsp	21	0	2	1	0	1.4	0.8	0	58%
Squares, Mexican	1 square	85	1	15	1	1	3.1	1.7	0	31%
CHOCOLATE FLAVORED DRINK. See also CHOCOLATE MILK.										
(Frostee) canned	8 fl oz	200	2	30	160	0	8.0	0.0	0	36%
(Yoo-Hoo)	9 fl oz	140	3	27	130	0	1.0	0.0	0	7%
CHOCOLATE FLAVORED DRINK MIX										
(Butterfinger) Butterfinger flavored, w/vitamins A										
and D prepared w/2% milk	8 fl oz	200	8	30	120	1	5.0	3.0	20	23%
(Hershey's)										
'Hershey's Genuine' prepared	8 fl oz	150	5	28	85	0	2.0	0.0	0	12%
'Hershey's Chocolate Milk Mix' mix only	3 heaping tsp	90	1	22	40	0	1.0	0.0	0	9%

Food Name	Serving Size	Calories	Prot. gms	Carbs gms	Sod. mgs	Fiber gms	Fat gms	Sat. Fat gms	Chol. mgs	% Fat Cal.
(Nestlé)										
chocolate raspberry truffle, prepared....	8 fl oz	180	15	23	280	6	2.0	0.0	0	11%
classic chocolate chip, prepared.	8 fl oz	180	15	24	300	6	2.0	0.0	0	10%
classic chocolate chip, mix only	1.13 oz	90	7	12	170	6	2.0	0.0	0	19%
creamy milk chocolate, prepared.	8 fl oz	180	15	24	280	6	2.0	0.0	0	10%
creamy milk chocolate, mix only	1.13 oz	90	7	12	150	6	2.0	0.0	0	19%
dark chocolate fudge, mix only	1.13 oz	90	7	11	150	6	2.0	0.0	0	20%
'Quik' prepared w/1 cup skim milk.	8 fl oz	170	9	31	150	0	1.0	0.0	0	5%
'Quik' prepared w/1 cup whole milk.	8 fl oz	230	9	31	150	0	9.0	0.0	0	34%
sugar-free, 'Quik' prepared w/1 cup 2% milk.	8 fl oz	140	9	15	150	0	5.0	0.0	0	32%
sugar-free, 'Quik' dry, mix only	1 heaping tsp	18	1	3	35	0	1.0	0.0	0	36%
(Swiss Miss) 'Chocolate Milk Maker'	0.67 oz	73	1	17	55	0	0.3	0.2	0	4%
(Weight Watchers) chocolate fudge shake mix	1 serving	80	6	12	140	2	1.0	0.0	0	11%
CHOCOLATE MILK										
1% fat	1 quart	630	32	104	607	5	10.0	6.2	29	14%
1% fat	1 cup	158	8	26	152	1	2.5	1.5	7	14%
2% fat	1 quart	715	32	104	602	5	20.0	12.4	68	25%
2% fat	1 cup	179	8	26	151	1	5.0	3.1	17	25%
2% fat	1 fl oz	22	1	3	19	0	0.6	0.4	2	25%
2% fat, vitamin A and D enriched *(Lucerne)*	1 cup	200	8	29	200	0	5.0	3.0	25	23%
2% low-fat *(Darigold)*	1 cup	190	8	28	210	0	5.0	3.1	17	24%
2% low-fat *(Hershey's)*	1 cup	190	8	29	130	0	5.0	0.0	20	23%
2% low-fat, 'Dutch Brand' *(Borden)*	1 cup	180	8	25	180	0	5.0	0.0	0	25%
3.5% fat *(Hershey's)*	1 cup	210	7	28	120	0	8.0	0.0	0	34%
whole	1 quart	834	32	103	596	8	33.9	21.0	122	36%
whole	1 cup	208	8	26	149	2	8.5	5.3	31	36%
whole	1 fl oz	26	1	3	19	0	1.1	0.7	4	36%
whole, ready to drink, 'Quik' *(Nestlé)*	1 cup	230	7	31	120	0	9.0	5.0	30	35%
whole, vitamin D added *(Meadow Gold)*	1 cup	210	8	25	240	0	8.0	0.0	0	35%
CHOCOLATE TOPPING. See also DESSERT TOPPING; FUDGE TOPPING.										
(Kraft)	2 tbsp	110	2	26	30	1	0.0	0.0	0	0%
(Mrs. Richardson's)										
fudge, dark	2 tbsp	130	1	19	55	0	6.0	0.0	0	40%
fudge, dark, microwaveable	2 tbsp	130	1	19	55	0	6.0	0.0	0	40%
(Nestlé)										
milk, w/almonds, 'Candytops'	1.25 oz	230	2	14	15	0	18.0	0.0	0	72%
milk, w/crisps, 'Crunch Candytops'	2 tbsp	220	2	16	40	0	17.0	0.0	0	68%
white, w/almonds, 'Candytops'	1.25 oz	230	3	12	20	0	19.0	0.0	0	74%
(Smucker's)										
dark, 'Special Recipe'	2 tbsp	130	1	31	45	0	1.0	0.0	0	7%
fudge, 'Magic Shell'	2 tbsp	190	1	16	50	0	15.0	0.0	0	67%
fudge, milk, Swiss	2 tbsp	140	3	31	70	0	1.0	0.0	0	6%
'Magic Shell'	2 tbsp	190	1	16	25	0	15.0	0.0	0	67%
nut, 'Magic Shell'	2 tbsp	200	2	25	40	0	16.0	0.0	0	57%
CHOP SUEY SEASONING. See under SEASONING MIX.										
CHORIZO. See under SAUSAGE.										
CHOW MEIN SEASONING. See under SEASONING MIX.										
CHRYSANTEMUM LEAVES										
raw, whole	1 leaf	4	1	1	21	1	0.1	na	0	20%
raw, chopped	1 cup	12	2	2	60	2	0.3	na	0	20%
CHRYSANTHEMUM GARLAND										
boiled, drained, 1-inch pieces	1 cup	20	2	4	53	2	0.1	0.0	0	4%
raw, 1-inch pieces	1 cup	5	0	1	13	1	0.0	na	0	7%
raw, whole, approx 8.75-inch long	1 stem	3	0	1	7	0	0.0	na	0	7%

Food Name	Serving Size	Calories	Prot. gms	Carbs gms	Sod. mgs	Fiber gms	Fat gms	Sat. Fat gms	Chol. mgs	% Fat Cal.
CHUB / cisco										
raw	3 oz	83	16	0	47	0	1.6	0.4	43	18%
smoked	3 oz	150	14	0	409	0	10.1	1.5	27	61%
smoked	1 oz	50	5	0	136	0	3.4	0.5	9	61%
CHURRO. See under PASTRY.										
CIDER										
APPLE										
(Alpine) spiced	8 fl oz	80	0	21	20	0	0.0	0.0	0	0%
(Indian Summer) canned or bottled	6 fl oz	80	1	20	10	0	1.0	0.0	0	10%
(Knudsen) and spice	8 fl oz	110	1	28	0	0	0.0	0.0	0	0%
(Krusteaz) spiced	8 fl oz	16	0	4	30	0	0.0	0.0	0	0%
(Lucky Leaf)										
canned or bottled	6 fl oz	90	0	21	0	0	0.0	0.0	0	0%
sparkling, canned or bottled	6 fl oz	80	0	18	45	0	0.0	0.0	0	0%
(Musselman's) canned or bottled	6 fl oz	90	0	21	0	0	0.0	0.0	0	0%
(Tree Top) canned or frozen, prepared	6 fl oz	90	0	22	10	0	0.0	0.0	0	0%
APPLE CHERRY (Indian Summer)	6 fl oz	100	1	25	10	0	1.0	0.0	0	8%
APPLE CINNAMON (Indian Summer) canned or bottled	6 fl oz	90	1	21	10	0	1.0	0.0	0	9%
APPLE CRANBERRY (Indian Summer)	6 fl oz	100	1	24	10	0	1.0	0.0	0	8%
CHERRY										
(Knudsen)										
	8 fl oz	100	1	24	0	0	0.0	0.0	0	0%
blend	8 fl oz	130	0	33	35	na	0.0	0.0	0	0%
CIDER MIX										
APPLE										
spiced, instant (Alpine)	1 pouch	80	0	19	20	0	0.0	0.0	0	0%
spiced, instant, sugar-free (Alpine)	1 pouch	15	0	4	25	0	0.0	0.0	0	0%
(Swiss Miss)	0.78 oz	84	0	20	58	1	0.3	0.0	0	3%
CILANTRO LEAF										
dried (McCormick/Schilling)	1 tsp	2	0	0	4	0	0.0	0.0	0	0%
dried (Tone's)	1 tsp	2	0	0	1	0	0.1	0.0	0	36%
raw, chopped	1 cup	11	1	2	25	1	0.2	0.0	0	17%
raw, minced	1 tsp	0	0	0	1	0	0.0	0.0	0	17%
CILANTRO SEED (Spice Islands)	1 tsp	6	0	1	1	0	0.3	0.1	0	40%
CINNAMON										
ground	1 tbsp	18	0	5	2	4	0.2	0.0	0	10%
ground	1 tsp	6	0	2	1	1	0.1	0.0	0	10%
ground (McCormick/Schilling)	1 tsp	6	0	1	0	1	0.0	0.0	0	0%
ground (Spice Islands)	1 tsp	6	0	1	1	0	0.1	0.0	0	13%
ground (Tone's)	1 tsp	6	0	2	1	1	0.1	0.1	0	11%
ground, fresh (Durkee)	1 tsp	8	0	0	0	0	0.0	0.0	0	0%
ground, fresh (Laurel Leaf)	1 tsp	8	0	0	0	0	0.0	0.0	0	0%
CISCO, RAW. See CHUB.										
CITRONELLA. See LEMONGRASS.										
CLAM										
Canned										
baby (S&W)	1/4 cup	50	8	2	260	0	1.5	0.5	40	25%
baby, smoked (S&W)	2 oz	130	9	2	220	0	10.0	2.0	20	67%
baby, smoked, in cottonseed oil (Crown Prince)	1/3 cup	90	10	2	330	2	5.0	1.5	43	48%
chopped (Gorton's)	1/2 can	70	12	4	640	0	1.0	0.0	0	12%
chopped (Progresso)	1/2 cup	70	12	2	140	0	1.0	0.0	31	14%
chopped (S&W)	1/4 cup	20	4	1	360	0	0.0	0.0	0	0%
chopped, w/liquid (Doxsee)	6.5 oz	100	14	8	1160	0	1.0	0.0	0	9%
chopped, w/liquid (Orleans)	6.5 oz	100	14	8	1160	0	1.0	0.0	0	9%

Food Name	Serving Size	Calories	Prot. gms	Carbs gms	Sod. mgs	Fiber gms	Fat gms	Sat. Fat gms	Chol. mgs	% Fat Cal.
minced (Gorton's)	1/2 can	70	12	4	640	0	1.0	0.0	0	12%
minced (Progresso)	1/2 cup	70	12	2	140	0	1.0	0.0	31	14%
minced (S&W)	1/4 cup	20	8	1	360	0	0.0	0.0	0	0%
minced, in clam juice (Gorton's)	1/4 cup	20	4	1	360	0	0.0	0.0	10	0%
minced, w/liquid (Doxsee)	6.5 oz	100	14	8	1160	0	1.0	0.0	0	9%
minced, w/liquid (Orleans)	6.5 oz	100	14	8	1160	0	1.0	0.0	0	9%
mixed species, drained	1 cup	237	41	8	179	0	3.1	0.3	107	12%
mixed species, drained	3 oz	126	22	4	95	0	1.7	0.2	57	12%
Fresh										
mixed species, boiled or steamed	3 oz	126	22	4	95	0	1.7	0.2	57	12%
mixed species, boiled or steamed, small	20 clams	281	49	10	213	0	3.7	0.4	127	12%
mixed species, breaded, fried	3 oz	172	12	9	309	na	9.5	2.3	52	49%
mixed species, breaded, fried, small	20 clams	380	27	19	684	na	21.0	5.0	115	49%
mixed species, raw	3 oz	63	11	2	48	0	0.8	0.1	29	12%
mixed species, raw, large	9 clams	133	23	5	101	0	1.7	0.2	61	12%
mixed species, raw, large	1 clam	15	3	1	11	0	0.2	0.0	7	12%
mixed species, raw, medium	1 clam	11	2	0	8	0	0.1	0.0	5	12%
mixed species, raw, small	1 clam	7	1	0	5	0	0.1	0.0	3	12%
CLAM DISH/ENTRÉE										
(Gorton's) 'Crunchy Clam Strips' microwave,										
5.8-oz pkg.	1/2 pkg	270	8	20	350	0	17.0	0.0	20	58%
(Matlaw's) stuffed, New England style	2 clams	180	8	21	730	3	8.0	1.0	0	38%
CLAM JUICE										
(Doxsee)	3 fl oz	4	1	0	110	0	0.0	0.0	0	0%
(S&W)	9.6 fl oz	0	8	0	740	0	0.0	0.0	0	0%
(Snow's)	3 fl oz	4	1	0	110	0	0.0	0.0	0	0%
all natural (Reese)	1 tbsp	0	1	0	100	0	0.0	0.0	0	0%
CLAM-TOMATO JUICE										
canned	5.5-oz can	80	1	18	601	0	0.3	0.1	0	4%
canned	1 fl oz	14	0	3	109	0	0.1	0.0	0	4%
CLARIFIED BUTTER. See GHEE.										
CLOUD EAR FUNGUS										
dried	1 cup	80	3	20	10	20	0.2	na	0	2%
dried, whole	1 medium	13	0	3	2	3	0.0	na	0	2%
CLOVES										
ground	1 tbsp	21	0	4	16	2	1.3	0.4	0	52%
ground	1 tsp	7	0	1	5	1	0.4	0.1	0	52%
ground (McCormick/Schilling)	1 tsp	5	0	1	4	0	0.3	0.0	0	38%
ground (Spice Islands)	1 tsp	7	0	1	4	0	0.2	0.0	0	26%
ground (Tone's)	1 tsp	7	0	1	5	0	0.4	0.1	0	38%
ground, fresh (Durkee)	1 tsp	9	0	0	0	0	0.0	0.0	0	0%
ground, fresh (Laurel Leaf)	1 tsp	9	0	0	0	0	0.0	0.0	0	0%
COATING MIX. See SEASONING AND COATING MIX.										
COBBLER										
Fresh										
(Awrey's)										
apple, deep dish	1/8 cobbler	320	2	48	300	1	14.0	3.0	0	39%
blueberry, deep dish	1/8 pie	310	2	45	360	2	14.0	3.0	0	40%
Frozen										
(Pet-Ritz)										
apple, 4.33-oz pkg.	1/6 pkg	290	1	50	0	0	9.0	0.0	0	28%
blackberry, 4.33-oz pkg	1/6 pkg	250	2	39	0	0	10.0	0.0	0	35%
blueberry, 4.33-oz pkg.	1/6 pkg	370	3	50	0	0	12.0	0.0	0	34%
cherry, 4.33-oz pkg	1/6 pkg	280	2	46	0	0	10.0	0.0	0	32%

Food Name	Serving Size	Calories	Prot. gms	Carbs gms	Sod. mgs	Fiber gms	Fat gms	Sat. Fat gms	Chol. mgs	% Fat Cal.
peach, 4.33-oz pkg	1/6 pkg	260	2	46	0	0	10.0	0.0	0	32%
strawberry, 4.33-oz pkg	1/6 pkg	290	1	50	0	0	9.0	0.0	0	28%
(Stilwell)										
apple, 'Deli'	1/8 cobbler	240	2	39	370	3	9.0	4.0	0	33%
apple, light, 'Deli Lite'	1/8 cobbler	140	3	22	300	2	4.5	1.0	0	29%
apple, 'Thrifty House'	1/22 cobbler	290	4	45	190	2	11.0	3.5	0	34%
apricot	1/8 cobbler	240	3	39	230	3	9.0	4.0	0	33%
berry, 'Festival of Berry'	1/8 cobbler	250	3	42	250	3	9.0	4.0	0	31%
berry, light, 'Festival of Berry-Lite'	1/8 cobbler	140	3	22	140	2	4.5	1.0	0	29%
blackberry, 'Deli'	1/8 cobbler	250	3	39	230	4	9.0	4.0	0	33%
blackberry, light, 'Deli Lite'	1/8 cobbler	150	3	24	150	2	4.5	1.0	0	27%
blackberry, 'Thrifty House'	1/22 cobbler	320	3	46	105	2	14.0	3.5	0	39%
blueberry	1/18 cobbler	270	3	42	250	4	10.0	5.0	0	33%
cherry, 'Deli'	1/8 cobbler	250	3	39	280	3	9.0	4.0	0	33%
cherry, light, 'Deli Lite'	1/8 cobbler	150	3	24	170	1	4.5	1.0	0	27%
cherry, 'Thrifty House'	1/22 cobbler	330	3	47	125	2	14.0	3.5	0	39%
peach, 'Deli'	1/8 cobbler	240	3	38	250	3	9.0	4.0	0	33%
peach, light, 'Deli Lite'	1/8 cobbler	140	3	22	150	1	4.5	1.0	0	29%
peach, 'Thrifty House'	1/22 cobbler	300	4	43	170	0	12.0	3.0	0	36%
pecan	1/6 cobbler	440	5	66	310	3	17.0	3.5	50	35%
strawberry	1/8 cobbler	260	3	41	200	3	9.0	4.0	0	32%

COBNUT. See HAZELNUT.

COCA-COLA. See under SOFT DRINKS AND MIXERS.

COCKTAIL. See also COCKTAIL MIX; LIQUEUR; SHERRY; VERMOUTH; WINE.

DAIQUIRI

Food Name	Serving Size	Calories	Prot. gms	Carbs gms	Sod. mgs	Fiber gms	Fat gms	Sat. Fat gms	Chol. mgs	% Fat Cal.
canned	6.8 fl oz	259	0	32	83	0	0.0	0.0	0	0%
canned	1 fl oz	38	0	5	12	0	0.0	0.0	0	0%

PIÑA COLADA

| canned | 6.8 fl oz | 526 | 1 | 61 | 158 | 0 | 16.9 | 14.6 | 0 | 27% |
| canned | 1 fl oz | 77 | 0 | 9 | 23 | 0 | 2.5 | 2.1 | 0 | 27% |

TEQUILA SUNRISE

canned	6.8 fl oz	232	1	24	120	0	0.2	0.0	0	1%
canned	1 fl oz	34	0	4	18	0	0.0	0.0	0	1%
TOM COLLINS	1 fl oz	16	0.0	0.4	5	0	0.0	0.0	0	0%

WHISKEY SOUR

| canned | 6.8 fl oz | 249 | 0 | 28 | 92 | 0 | 0.0 | 0.0 | 0 | 0% |
| canned | 1 fl oz | 37 | 0 | 4 | 14 | 0 | 0.0 | 0.0 | 0 | 0% |

COCKTAIL MIX

BLOODY MARY

(Holland House) bottled 'Smooth 'N' Spicy'	1 fl oz	3	0	1	329	0	0.0	0.0	0	0%
(Mr. & Mrs. T)										
bottled	4.5 fl oz	20	1	4	670	0	0.0	0.0	0	0%
bottled, rich and spicy	4.5 fl oz	30	1	6	500	0	0.0	0.0	0	0%
(V8)	8 fl oz	49	2	9	1256	1	0.0	0.0	0	0%

DAIQUIRI

(Bacardi)										
banana, frozen, prepared w/rum	7 fl oz	210	0	35	0	0	1.0	0.0	0	6%
banana, frozen, prepared w/water	7 fl oz	150	0	35	0	0	1.0	0.0	0	6%
lime, shelf-stable, prepared w/rum	7 fl oz	210	0	33	10	0	0.0	0.0	0	0%
lime, shelf-stable, prepared w/water	7 fl oz	130	0	33	10	0	0.0	0.0	0	0%
peach, frozen, prepared w/rum	7 fl oz	200	0	33	5	0	0.0	0.0	0	0%
peach, frozen, prepared w/water	7 fl oz	130	0	33	5	0	0.0	0.0	0	0%
strawberry, frozen, prepared w/rum	7 fl oz	200	0	34	0	0	0.0	0.0	0	0%
strawberry, frozen, prepared w/water	7 fl oz	140	0	34	0	0	0.0	0.0	0	0%

Food Name	Serving Size	Calories	Prot. gms	Carbs gms	Sod. mgs	Fiber gms	Fat gms	Sat. Fat gms	Chol. mgs	% Fat Cal.
strawberry, shelf-stable, prepared w/rum	7 fl oz	200	0	31	15	0	0.0	0.0	0	0%
strawberry, shelf-stable, prepared w/water	7 fl oz	130	0	31	15	0	0.0	0.0	0	0%
(Holland House)										
bottled	1 fl oz	36	0	9	111	0	0.0	0.0	0	0%
instant, dry	0.56 oz	65	0	16	21	0	0.0	0.0	0	0%
prepared w/liquor	3.5 fl oz	177	0	18	50	0	0.0	0.0	0	0%
raspberry, bottled	1 fl oz	30	0	7	4	0	0.0	0.0	0	0%
strawberry, bottled	1 fl oz	31	0	7	3	0	0.0	0.0	0	0%
GRENADINE SYRUP *(Roses)*	1 fl oz	65	0	16	27	0	0.0	0.0	0	0%
MAI TAI										
(Holland House)										
bottled	1 fl oz	32	0	8	60	0	0.0	0.0	0	0%
instant, dry	0.56 oz	64	0	16	4	0	0.0	0.0	0	0%
MANHATTAN *(Holland House)* bottled	1 fl oz	28	0	7	5	0	0.0	0.0	0	0%
MARGARITA										
(Bacardi)										
frozen, prepared w/rum	7 fl oz	160	0	24	5	0	0.0	0.0	0	0%
frozen, prepared w/water	7 fl oz	90	0	24	0	0	0.0	0.0	0	0%
shelf stable, prepared w/rum	7 fl oz	210	0	33	10	0	0.0	0.0	0	0%
shelf stable, prepared w/water	7 fl oz	130	0	33	10	0	0.0	0.0	0	0%
(Holland House)										
bottled	1 fl oz	27	0	6	92	0	0.0	0.0	0	0%
instant, dry	0.5 oz	57	0	14	4	0	0.0	0.0	0	0%
strawberry, bottled	1 fl oz	31	0	7	3	0	0.0	0.0	0	0%
strawberry, instant, dry	0.56 oz	66	0	16	1	0	0.0	0.0	0	0%
(Mr. & Mrs. T)										
bottled	3 fl oz	80	1	20	35	0	1.0	0.0	0	10%
strawberry, bottled	3.5 fl oz	100	1	24	10	0	1.0	0.0	0	8%
OLD-FASHIONED DRINK *(Holland House)* bottled	1 fl oz	33	0	8	6	0	0.0	0.0	0	0%
PIÑA COLADA										
(Bacardi)										
frozen, prepared w/rum	7 fl oz	260	1	37	25	0	6.0	0.0	0	26%
frozen, prepared w/water	7 fl oz	200	1	37	25	0	6.0	0.0	0	26%
shelf-stable, prepared w/rum	7 fl oz	240	0	36	20	0	2.0	0.0	0	11%
shelf-stable, prepared w/water	7 fl oz	170	0	36	20	0	2.0	0.0	0	11%
(Holland House)										
bottled	1 fl oz	33	0	8	4	0	0.0	0.0	0	0%
instant, dry	0.56 oz	82	0	12	1	0	3.0	0.0	0	36%
(Mr. & Mrs. T) bottled	4 fl oz	150	1	39	120	0	1.0	0.0	0	5%
RUM RUNNER										
(Bacardi)										
shelf-stable, prepared w/rum	7 fl oz	210	0	33	15	0	0.0	0.0	0	0%
shelf-stable, prepared w/water	7 fl oz	140	0	33	15	0	0.0	0.0	0	0%
STRAWBERRY COLADA										
(Bacardi)										
shelf-stable, prepared w/rum	7 fl oz	230	0	34	15	0	1.0	0.0	0	6%
shelf-stable, prepared w/water	7 fl oz	150	0	34	15	0	1.0	0.0	0	6%
SWEET AND SOUR DRINK										
(Holland House) liquid	1 fl oz	34	0	8	107	0	0.0	0.0	0	0%
(Mr. & Mrs. T) bottled	3 fl oz	70	1	17	45	0	1.0	0.0	0	11%
TOM COLLINS										
(Holland House)										
bottled	1 fl oz	47	0	11	96	0	0.0	0.0	0	0%
instant, dry	0.56 oz	65	0	16	14	0	0.0	0.0	0	0%

Food Name	Serving Size	Calories	Prot. gms	Carbs gms	Sod. mgs	Fiber gms	Fat gms	Sat. Fat gms	Chol. mgs	% Fat Cal.
WHISKEY SOUR										
bottled	1 fl oz	26	0	7	32	0	0.0	0.0	0	1%
bottled, w/added potassium and sodium	1 fl oz	27	0	7	11	0	0.0	0.0	0	1%
instant, dry	1 pkt	64	0	16	46	0	0.0	0.0	0	0%
(Bar-Tender's) powder, prepared w/whiskey	3.5 fl oz	177	0	18	50	0	0.0	0.0	0	0%
(Holland House)										
bottled	1 fl oz	37	0	9	105	0	0.0	0.0	0	0%
instant, dry	0.56 oz	64	0	16	16	0	0.0	0.0	0	0%
COCKTAIL ONIONS. See under ONION.										
COCOA										
baking, 'Premium' (Saco Foods)	1 tbsp	15	2	4	51	0	0.9	0.5	0	28%
100% (Nestlé)	1 oz	80	7	5	5	10	5.0	0.0	0	48%
powder (Bensdorp)	1 oz	130	6	8	5	0	7.0	0.0	1	53%
powder (Nestlé)	1.5 oz	180	11	21	6	0	6.0	0.0	0	30%
unsweetened, European style (Hershey's)	1 cup	332	20	45	42	25	8.0	5.0	0	22%
unsweetened, European style (Hershey's)	1 tbsp	19	1	3	2	1	0.5	0.3	0	22%
unsweetened, powder	1 cup	197	17	47	18	29	11.8	6.9	0	50%
unsweetened, powder	1 tbsp	12	1	3	1	2	0.7	0.4	0	50%
unsweetened, processed w/alkali, powder	1 cup	191	16	47	16	26	11.3	6.7	0	49%
unsweetened, processed w/alkali, powder	1 tbsp	12	1	3	1	2	0.7	0.4	0	49%
COCOA, HOT, MIX										
(Alba '66)										
milk chocolate flavor, mix only	0.68 oz	60	6	10	160	0	0.0	0.0	0	0%
milk chocolate flavor, w/marshmallows, mix only	0.68 oz	60	6	10	160	0	0.0	0.0	0	0%
w/aspartame, mix only	1 pkt	61	5	11	214	0	0.6	0.3	2	8%
(Carnation)										
chocolate fudge flavor, mix only	1 pkt	110	1	24	135	0	1.3	1.1	1	10%
mocha flavor, 'Sugar-free' mix only	1 pkt	50	3	9	140	0	0.3	0.2	2	5%
rich, mix only	1 pkt	112	1	24	102	1	1.1	0.3	2	9%
'70-Calorie' mix only	1 pkt	70	3	16	135	0	0.3	0.2	1	3%
sugarless, mix only	1 pkt	55	4	8	142	1	0.4	0.2	3	7%
w/marshmallows, mix only	1 pkt	112	1	24	96	1	1.0	0.4	2	8%
(Featherweight)										
mix only	0.44 oz	50	2	8	110	0	1.0	0.0	0	18%
(Finast)										
regular, prepared	6 fl oz	110	2	24	150	0	1.0	0.0	0	8%
w/mini marshmallows, prepared	6 fl oz	110	2	24	150	0	1.0	0.0	0	8%
(Hills Bros)										
regular, mix only	2 tbsp	110	3	23	55	0	1.0	0.0	0	8%
'Sugar-free' mix only	3 tbsp	60	2	9	145	0	2.0	0.0	0	29%
(Land O'Lakes)										
chocolate and mint 'Cocoa Classics' mix only	1 pkt	160	4	24	160	0	5.0	0.0	0	29%
chocolate and raspberry, 'Cocoa Classics' mix only	1 pkt	160	4	25	160	0	5.0	0.0	0	28%
chocolate cinnamon, mix only	1.25 oz pkt	160	4	25	180	0	5.0	4.5	0	28%
chocolate mint, mix only	1.25-oz pkt	160	4	25	180	0	5.0	4.5	0	28%
chocolate raspberry, mix only	1.25-oz pkt	160	4	25	180	0	5.0	4.5	0	28%
chocolate supreme, 'Cocoa Classics' mix only	1.25-oz pkt	160	4	25	160	0	5.0	0.0	0	28%
(Pathmark)										
chocolate flavor, mix only	1 oz	110	2	24	110	0	1.0	0.0	0	8%
w/mini marshmallows, mix only	1 oz	110	2	24	140	0	1.0	0.0	0	8%
(Saco Foods)										
milk chocolate flavor, mix only	1 oz	110	2	24	150	0	1.0	0.0	0	8%
sugar-free, sweetened w/NutraSweet, mix only	1 pkt	50	3	9	150	0	1.0	0.0	0	16%

Food Name	Serving Size	Calories	Prot. gms	Carbs gms	Sod. mgs	Fiber gms	Fat gms	Sat. Fat gms	Chol. mgs	% Fat Cal.
(Swiss Miss)										
Amaretto creme flavor, mix only	1.25 oz	150	2	29	220	0	3.0	0.0	0	18%
Bavarian chocolate, mix only	1 oz	110	1	20	170	0	3.0	1.3	2	24%
chocolate Bavarian mint, mix only	1.23 oz	142	2	28	231	2	2.3	69.0	1	15%
chocolate flavor, mix only	1 oz	110	1	24	125	0	1.0	0.0	0	8%
chocolate flavor, 'Sugar-free' mix only	0.5 oz	50	2	9	130	0	1.0	0.2	1	17%
chocolate praline and crème, mix only	1.23 oz	142	3	29	223	2	2.3	0.7	1	14%
diet, mix only	0.26 oz	20	2	3	180	0	1.0	0.0	1	31%
double rich chocolate flavor, mix only	1 oz	110	2	24	125	0	1.0	0.0	0	8%
fat-free, mix only	1 serving	50	3	9	197	1	0.3	0.0	2	5%
light, mix only	0.75 oz	74	1	17	197	2	0.5	0.2	0	5%
'Marshmallow Lovers' 'Hot Cocoa Mix' mix only	1.2 oz	132	2	24	167	1	1.5	0.3	2	12%
milk chocolate, 'Hot Cocoa Mix' mix only	1.2 oz	133	2	29	169	1	1.5	0.3	2	10%
milk chocolate, sugar-free, mix only	1 serving	49	2	10	179	1	0.2	0.1	0	3%
milk chocolate, w/ marshmallows, 'Hot Cocoa Mix' mix only	1.2 oz	132	2	29	181	1	1.5	0.5	1	10%
milk chocolate flavor, mix only	1-oz pkt	110	1	20	170	0	3.0	1.3	1	24%
sugar free, mix only	1 serving	51	1	11	159	1	0.6	0.2	1	10%
vending machine product, 'Hot Cocoa Mix'	1.34 oz	146	2	32	185	1	1.7	0.3	2	10%
w/aspartame, w/added calcium or phosphorus, w/o added salt or vitamin A, mix only	1 pkt	48	4	9	98	0	0.5	0.3	1	8%
w/aspartame, w/added salt and vitamin A, w/o added calcium or phosphorus, mix only	1 pkt	48	4	9	168	0	0.5	0.3	1	8%
w/mini marshmallows, 'Sugar-Free' mix only	0.5-oz pkt	50	3	9	120	0	1.0	0.0	0	16%
(Weight Watchers) rich milk flavor, w/marshmallows, mix only	1 pkt	60	6	10	160	0	0.0	0.0	0	0%
COCOA BUTTER OIL										
	1 cup	1927	0	0	0	0	218.0	130.1	0	100%
	1 tbsp	120	0	0	0	0	13.6	8.1	0	100%
COCONUT										
Dried										
meat, creamed	1 oz	194	2	6	10	na	19.6	17.4	0	85%
meat, sweetened, flaked, canned	1 cup	341	3	32	15	3	24.4	21.6	0	60%
meat, sweetened, flaked, canned	4 oz	505	4	47	23	5	36.1	32.0	0	60%
meat, sweetened, flaked, packaged	1 cup	351	2	35	189	3	23.8	21.1	0	57%
meat, sweetened, flaked, packaged	1 oz	134	1	13	73	1	9.1	8.1	0	57%
meat, sweetened, flaked, packaged, 'Snowflake' *(Finast)*	1 oz	137	1	12	1	0	9.0	0.0	0	61%
meat, sweetened, shredded	1 cup	466	3	44	244	4	33.0	29.3	0	59%
meat, sweetened, shredded	7-oz pkg	997	6	95	521	9	70.6	62.6	0	59%
meat, sweetened, shredded, 'Angel Flake' *(Baker's)*	2 tbsp	70	1	6	45	1	5.0	5.0	0	62%
meat, sweetened, shredded, canned, 'Angel Flake' *(Baker's)*	2 tbsp	70	1	6	0	1	6.0	5.0	0	66%
meat, sweetened, shredded, premium *(Baker's)*	2 tbsp	70	1	6	45	1	5.0	5.0	0	62%
meat, sweetened, toasted	1 oz	168	2	13	10	na	13.3	11.8	0	66%
meat, sweetened, toasted, flaked, packaged *(Baker's)*	1/3 cup	200	2	17	85	0	17.0	0.0	0	67%
meat, unsweetened	1 oz	187	2	7	10	5	18.3	16.2	0	82%
Fresh										
mature kernel, in shell	1 lb	834	7.9	35.9	47	21.2	79.0	70.0	0	80%
mature kernel, shelled	1 oz	100	0.9	4.3	6	2.6	9.5	8.4	0	80%
mature kernel, shelled, grated, packed	1 cup	460	4.3	19.8	26	11.7	43.5	38.6	0	80%
meat, raw, shredded	1 cup	283	2.7	12.2	16	7.2	26.8	23.8	0	80%
meat, raw, 2x2x1/2-inch pieces	1 piece	159	1	7	9	4	15.1	13.4	0	79%
meat, raw, whole, medium	1 coconut	1405	13	60	79	36	133.0	117.9	0	79%

Food Name	Serving Size	Calories	Prot. gms	Carbs gms	Sod. mgs	Fiber gms	Fat gms	Sat. Fat gms	Chol. mgs	% Fat Cal.
COCONUT CREAM										
Canned										
liquid expressed from grated meat	1 cup	568	8	25	148	7	52.5	46.5	0	77%
liquid expressed from grated meat	1 tbsp	36	1	2	10	0	3.4	3.0	0	77%
sweetened *(Coco Lopez)*	2 tbsp	120	0	20	10	0	5.0	0.0	0	36%
Fresh										
liquid expressed from grated meat, raw	1 cup	792	9	16	10	5	83.2	73.8	0	88%
liquid expressed from grated meat, raw	1 tbsp	50	1	1	1	0	5.2	4.6	0	88%
COCONUT MILK										
Canned										
liquid expressed from grated meat and water	1 cup	445	5	6	29	na	48.2	42.7	0	91%
liquid expressed from grated meat and water	1 tbsp	30	0	0	2	na	3.2	2.8	0	91%
Fresh										
liquid expressed from grated meat and water, raw	1 cup	552	5	13	36	5	57.2	50.7	0	87%
liquid expressed from grated meat and water, raw	1 tbsp	35	0	1	2	0	3.6	3.2	0	87%
Frozen										
liquid expressed from grated meat and water	1 cup	485	4	13	29	na	49.9	44.3	0	86%
liquid expressed from grated meat and water	1 tbsp	30	0	1	2	na	3.1	2.8	0	86%
COCONUT OIL										
	1 cup	1879	0	0	0	0	218.0	188.6	0	100%
	1 tbsp	117	0	0	0	0	13.6	11.8	0	100%
(Hain)	1 tbsp	120	0	0	0	0	14.0	12.0	0	100%
COCONUT WATER										
liquid from coconuts	1 cup	46	2	9	252	3	0.5	0.4	0	9%
liquid from coconuts	1 tbsp	3	0	1	16	0	0.0	0.0	0	9%
COD										
Frozen										
(Booth) fillet, 'Individually Wrapped'	4 oz	90	20	0	80	0	1.0	0.0	0	10%
(Finast) fillet, skinless	4 oz	80	18	0	200	0	1.0	0.0	0	11%
(SeaPak) fillet	4 oz	90	20	0	135	0	1.0	0.0	0	10%
(Van de Kamp's) fillet, light	1 piece	250	17	20	510	0	11.0	2.0	35	40%
(Van de Kamp's) fillet, natural	4 oz	90	20	0	90	0	1.0	0.0	25	10%
ALASKAN / sablefish / skil										
Fresh										
baked, broiled, grilled, or microwaved	3 oz	213	15	0	61	0	16.7	3.5	54	71%
raw	3 oz	166	11	0	48	0	13.0	2.7	42	71%
smoked	3 oz	218	15	0	626	0	17.1	3.6	54	71%
ATLANTIC										
Canned, w/liquid	3 oz	89	19	0	185	0	0.7	0.1	47	7%
Dried/salted										
	1 oz	82	18	0	1992	0	0.7	0.1	43	7%
	3 oz	247	53	0	5973	0	2.0	0.4	129	7%
Fresh										
baked, broiled, grilled, or microwaved	3 oz	89	19	0	66	0	0.7	0.1	47	7%
raw	3 oz	70	15	0	46	0	0.6	0.1	37	7%
PACIFIC										
baked, broiled, grilled, or microwaved	3 oz	89	20	0	77	0	0.7	0.1	40	7%
raw	3 oz	70	15	0	60	0	0.5	0.1	31	7%
COD DISH/ENTRÉE										
(Gorton's) cod cakes, canned	4 oz	100	8	16	640	0	0.5	0.0	15	4%
(Booth)										
fillet, au gratin, frozen	9.5 oz	280	27	18	1160	0	11.0	0.0	0	35%
fillet, Florentine, frozen	9.5 oz	244	20	29	880	0	6.0	0.0	0	22%
fillet, w/lemon butter sauce and rice, frozen	9.5 oz	567	22	27	1330	0	38.0	0.0	0	64%

Food Name	Serving Size	Calories	Prot. gms	Carbs gms	Sod. mgs	Fiber gms	Fat gms	Sat. Fat gms	Chol. mgs	% Fat Cal.
fillet, w/mushroom sauce and rice, frozen.............	9.5 oz	280	27	19	1010	0	11.0	0.0	0	35%

COD LIVER OIL. See under FISH OIL.

COFFEE

Brewed

decaffeinated, prepared w/tap water..................	6 fl oz	4	0	1	4	0	0.0	0.0	0	0%
regular, prepared w/distilled water	6 fl oz	4	0	1	2	0	0.0	0.0	0	0%
regular, prepared w/tap water.......................	6 fl oz	4	0	1	4	0	0.0	0.0	0	0%

Instant

regular, powder, mix only	1 rounded tsp	4	0	1	1	0	0.0	0.0	0	2%
regular, powder, mix only	1 tsp	2	0	0	0	0	0.0	0.0	0	2%
regular, powder, prepared	6 fl oz	4	0	1	5	0	0.0	0.0	0	0%
w/chicory, powder, prepared	6 fl oz	7	0	1	11	0	0.0	0.0	0	0%
(Brim) decaffeinated mix only	1 tsp	4	1	1	0	0	0.0	0.0	0	0%
(Kava) regular, powder, mix only	1 tsp	2	0	1	5	0	0.0	0.0	0	0%
(Nescafé)										
decaffeinated, 'Decaf' prepared......................	8 fl oz	4	1	1	0	0	1.0	0.0	0	53%
regular, prepared.................................	8 fl oz	4	1	1	0	0	1.0	0.0	0	53%
regular, 'Brava' prepared	8 fl oz	4	1	1	0	0	1.0	0.0	0	53%
regular, 'Classic' prepared.........................	8 fl oz	4	1	1	0	0	1.0	0.0	0	53%
regular, 'Silka' prepared...........................	8 fl oz	4	1	1	0	0	1.0	0.0	0	53%
w/chicory, 'Mountain Blend' prepared	8 fl oz	6	1	1	0	0	1.0	0.0	0	53%
(Sanka)										
decaffeinated, mix only	1 tsp	4	1	1	0	0	0.0	0.0	0	0%
decaffeinated, prepared	8 fl oz	3	0	1	0	0	0.0	0.0	0	0%
(Sunrise) w/chicory, prepared	8 fl oz	6	1	1	0	0	1.0	0.0	0	53%
(Taster's Choice)										
dark roast, decaffeinated, freeze-dried, 'Maragor' prepared...	8 fl oz	4	1	1	0	0	1.0	0.0	0	53%
dark roast, freeze-dried, 'Maragor' prepared...........	8 fl oz	4	1	1	0	0	1.0	0.0	0	53%
decaffeinated, freeze-dried, 'Original' prepared	8 fl oz	4	1	1	0	0	1.0	0.0	0	53%
regular, freeze-dried, 'Colombian Select' prepared.......	8 fl oz	4	1	1	0	0	1.0	0.0	0	53%
regular, freeze-dried, 'Original' prepared..............	8 fl oz	4	1	1	0	0	1.0	0.0	0	53%
(Yuban) regular, mix only	1 tsp	4	1	1	0	0	0.0	0.0	0	0%

FLAVORED

Instant

(General Foods)										
Belgian café, 'International Coffees' mix only	1-1/3 tbsp	70	1	12	65	0	2.0	0.5	0	26%
café Amaretto, mix only............................	1-1/3 tbsp	60	1	8	105	0	3.5	0.5	0	48%
café Francais, 'International Coffees' mix only	1-1/3 tbsp	60	1	7	25	0	3.5	1.0	0	51%
café Francais, 'International Coffees' prepared..........	6 fl oz	62	1	7	93	0	3.5	0.8	0	50%
café Francais, sugar-free, 'International Coffees' prepared...	6 fl oz	35	0	3	30	0	2.0	0.0	0	60%
café Vienna, 'International Coffees' mix only............	1-1/3 tbsp	70	1	11	110	0	2.5	0.5	0	33%
café Vienna, sugar-free, 'International Coffees' mix only	1-1/3 tbsp	30	1	3	75	0	1.5	0.5	0	49%
cappuccino, Italian, mix only	1-1/3 tbsp	50	1	10	50	0	1.5	0.5	0	24%
cappuccino, sugar-free, mix only.....................	1-1/3 tbsp	30	1	3	75	0	1.5	0.5	0	49%
double Dutch chocolate, 'International Coffees, prepared...	6 fl oz	50	0	8	15	0	2.0	0.0	0	36%
Dutch chocolate mint, 'International Coffees' prepared....	6 fl oz	50	0	8	80	0	2.0	0.0	0	36%
French vanilla, sugarless, 'International Coffees' mix only	1 1/3 tbsp	35	1	4	55	0	2.0	0.5	0	50%
French vanilla, sugarless, 'International Coffees' prepared...	8 fl oz	25	0	5	65	0	0.0	0.0	0	0%

Food Name	Serving Size	Calories	Prot. gms	Carbs gms	Sod. mgs	Fiber gms	Fat gms	Sat. Fat gms	Chol. mgs	% Fat Cal.
Irish crème café, 'International Coffees' prepared........	6 fl oz	50	0	8	15	0	2.0	0.0	0	36%
Kahlua café, mix only	1 1/3 tbsp	60	1	10	55	0	2.0	0.5	0	30%
Suisse mocha, 'International Coffees' mix only..........	1 1/3 tbsp	60	1	8	50	0	2.5	0.5	0	40%
Suisse mocha, decaffeinated, 'International Coffees' mix only......................................	1 1/3 tbsp	60	1	8	40	0	3.0	0.5	0	44%
Suisse mocha, decaffeinated, sugar-free, 'International Coffees' mix only	1 1/3 tbsp	30	1	4	35	0	1.5	0.5	0	43%
Suisse mocha, sugar-free, 'International Coffees' mix only .....'............	1 1/3 tbsp	30	1	4	30	0	2.0	0.5	0	50%
Suisse mocha, sugar-free, 'International Coffees' prepared.........................	8 fl oz	25	0	5	35	1	0.0	0.0	0	0%
Viennese chocolate, 'International Coffees' mix only	1 1/3 tbsp	60	1	10	30	0	2.0	1.0	0	30%
(Hills Bros)										
café Vienna, 'Cafe Coffees' prepared	6 fl oz	60	1	9	35	0	2.0	0.0	0	31%
Capri orange, 'Cafe Coffees' prepared	6 fl oz	60	1	9	30	0	2.0	0.0	0	31%
Swiss mocha, 'Cafe Coffees' prepared	6 fl oz	60	1	8	10	0	2.0	0.0	0	33%
Swiss mocha, sugarless, 'Cafe Coffees' prepared	6 fl oz	40	1	5	25	0	2.0	0.0	0	43%
(Maxwell House)										
'Cinnamon Hot Cappuccino' prepared	6 fl oz	60	2	11	100	0	1.0	0.0	0	15%
'Coffee Hot Cappuccino' prepared	6 fl oz	60	1	12	110	0	1.0	0.0	0	15%
'Mocha Hot Cappuccino' prepared	6 fl oz	70	2	12	80	0	2.0	0.0	0	24%
(MJB)										
mocha, banana nut, sugar-free, prepared..............	6 fl oz	39	1	5	60	0	1.8	0.0	0	42%
mocha, cherry, prepared..........................	6 fl oz	53	1	10	17	0	1.4	0.0	0	24%
mocha, fudge, sugar-free, prepared	6 fl oz	39	1	5	88	0	1.8	0.0	0	42%
mocha, mint, prepared	6 fl oz	53	0	10	16	0	1.3	0.0	0	22%
mocha, mint, sugar-free, prepared	6 fl oz	37	1	6	43	0	1.3	0.0	0	32%
mocha, prepared................................	6 fl oz	52	1	10	54	0	1.3	0.0	0	22%
mocha, vanilla, sugar-free, prepared.................	6 fl oz	39	1	5	50	0	1.7	0.0	0	39%
(Superior) cappuccino, mix only.....................	1 serving	90	1	13	75	0	3.0	2.5	0	33%
Ready to drink										
(Cappio)										
cappuccino, cinnamon, iced	8 fl oz	130	2	25	70	0	3.0	0.0	15	20%
cappuccino, ooffee flavored, iced	8 fl oz	120	2	23	75	0	3.0	0.0	15	21%
cappuccino, mocha, iced.........................	8 fl oz	130	2	25	65	0	2.0	0.0	15	14%
cappuccino, vanilla, iced.........................	8 fl oz	130	2	25	65	0	2.0	0.0	15	14%
COFFEE SUBSTITUTE										
cereal grain beverage, mix only....................	1 tsp	8	0	2	2	0	0.1	0.0	0	9%
cereal grain beverage, prepared w/milk	6 fl oz	120	6	10	91	0	6.1	3.8	24	46%
cereal grain beverage, prepared w/water	6 fl oz	9	0	2	7	0	0.0	0.0	0	0%
(Cafix)										
all natural, 100% caffeine-free......................	1.5 grams	6	0	1	3	0	0.0	0.0	0	0%
(Inka)										
grain beverage, caffeine-free, instant, 'Naturalis' mix only (Inka)	1 tsp	0	1	1	3	0	1.0	0.0	0	0%
(Kaffree Roma)										
cereal grain beverage, coffee flavor, prepared	8 fl oz	6	0	1	0	0	0.0	0.0	0	0%
(Pero)										
cereal grain beverage, caffeine-free, mix only..........	1 serving	4	1	1	2	0	0.0	0.0	0	0%
cereal grain beverage, caffeine-free, prepared	5 fl oz	4	1	1	2	0	0.0	0.0	0	0%
(Pionier)										
cereal grain beverage, coffee flavor, mix only	1 serving	6	0	1	0	0	0.0	0.0	0	0%
(Postum)										
cereal grain beverage, coffee flavor, 'Instant' prepared	6 fl oz	12	0	3	0	0	0.0	0.0	0	0%

Food Name	Serving Size	Calories	Prot. gms	Carbs gms	Sod. mgs	Fiber gms	Fat gms	Sat. Fat gms	Chol. mgs	% Fat Cal.
COLE. See KALE.										
COLESLAW										
fresh	1/2 cup	41	1	7	14	1	1.6	0.2	5	34%
fresh	1 tbsp	6	0	1	2	0	0.2	0.0	1	34%
COLESLAW DRESSING. See under SALAD DRESSING.										
COLEWORT. See KALE.										
COLLARDS										
Canned										
chopped (Allens)	1/2 cup	20	2	2	15	0	1.0	0.0	0	36%
chopped, greens (Bush's Best)	1/2 cup	30	2	5	320	0	0.0	0.0	0	0%
seasoned w/pork (Luck's)	1 cup	60	2	5	290	2	3.0	1.0	3	49%
Fresh										
boiled, drained, chopped	1 cup	49	4	9	17	5	0.7	0.1	0	12%
raw, chopped	1 cup	11	1	2	7	1	0.2	0.0	0	12%
Frozen										
chopped (Flav-R-Pac)	1/2 cup	30	2	2	20	2	0.0	0.0	0	0%
chopped (Seabrook)	3.3 oz	25	3	4	45	1	0.0	0.0	0	0%
chopped (Southern)	3.5 oz	30	3	5	60	0	0.4	0.0	0	11%
chopped, unprepared	3-lb pkg	449	37	88	653	49	5.0	0.7	0	9%
chopped, unprepared	10-oz pkg	94	8	18	136	10	1.1	0.1	0	9%
no salt added, chopped, drained	1 cup	61	5	12	85	5	0.7	0.1	0	10%
COLLINS MIXER. See under SOFT DRINKS AND MIXERS.										
COLORADO PINYON. See PINE NUT.										
COOKIE										
(Archway)										
'Aunt Bea's Pound Cake' 'Home Style'	1 serving	105	1	16	83	0	4.1	1.0	15	35%
hermits, 'Home Style'	1 serving	95	1	17	147	1	2.7	0.7	5	26%
'Select Assortment'	1 piece	50	1	7	40	0	2.0	0.0	5	36%
windmill, old fashioned, 'Home Style'	1 serving	91	1	14	93	1	3.5	0.7	0	34%
(Break Cake)										
'Hermit'	1 cookie	230	3	38	280	0	7.0	1.5	10	28%
'Striper Wafer'	1 wafer	190	2	23	80	0	10.0	3.2	0	47%
(Carr's) 'Hob-Nobs'	1 piece	72	1	10	78	0	3.2	0.0	0	40%
(Featherweight) double	1 piece	45	1	6	0	0	2.0	0.0	0	39%
(Frookie) 'Trolls'	11 cookies	60	1	10	65	0	2.0	0.0	0	29%
(Glenny's) 'Nookie'	1.5 oz	180	3	18	24	0	12.0	0.0	0	56%
(Lu)										
'Crokine'	2 cookies	35	1	7	70	0	0.0	0.0	0	0%
'Little Schoolboy'	1 cookie	70	1	8	35	0	4.0	0.0	0	50%
'Marie Lu'	1 cookie	50	1	8	45	0	2.0	0.0	0	33%
'Marie Lu' mini	5 cookies	50	1	8	45	0	2.0	0.0	0	33%
'Pims'	2 cookies	95	1	18	25	0	2.0	0.0	0	19%
wafer, creme filled	3 cookies	110	1	11	50	0	7.0	0.0	0	57%
(Made'em Myself) ready-to-decorate	0.25 oz piece	45	0	7	35	0	2.0	0.0	0	39%
(Mother's)										
dinosaur, original, mini	7 cookies	60	1	9	40	0	1.0	0.0	0	18%
wafer, checkerboard	5 cookies	85	1	13	15	0	4.0	0.0	0	39%
(Nabisco) wafer, striped, 'Cookies, 'N Fudge'	1 piece	70	1	8	25	0	4.0	1.0	0	50%
(Oven Lovin')										
candy	1 cookie	70	0	10	40	0	3.0	1.0	0	40%
w/Reese's Pieces	1 cookie	70	1	9	50	0	3.0	0.0	5	40%
(Stella D'oro)										
'Angel Bars'	1 piece	76	1	7	0	0	4.7	0.0	0	56%
'Angel Wings'	1 piece	74	1	7	0	0	4.7	0.0	0	57%

Food Name	Serving Size	Calories	Prot. gms	Carbs gms	Sod. mgs	Fiber gms	Fat gms	Sat. Fat gms	Chol. mgs	% Fat Cal.
'Angelica Goodies'	1 piece	106	2	16	0	0	4.0	0.0	0	34%
'Como Delight'	1 piece	145	2	18	0	0	7.2	0.0	0	45%
'Holiday Trinkets'	1 piece	38	1	5	0	0	1.9	0.0	0	45%
'Hostess' assorted	1 piece	42	1	6	0	0	2.0	0.0	0	43%
'Lady Stella' assorted	1 piece	42	1	6	0	0	2.0	0.0	0	42%
'Love Cookies'	1 piece	106	1	13	0	0	5.2	0.0	0	44%
'Royal Nuggets'	1 piece	2	0	0	0	0	0.1	0.0	0	53%
ALMOND										
(Ener-G Foods)										
amaretti, gluten-free	1 serving	141	4	14	36	2	4.7	0.4	0	37%
butter, gluten-free	2 cookies	119	2	13	85	1	6.1	1.0	3	48%
French, gluten-free	1 serving	104	2	17	31	1	3.6	0.3	0	30%
macaroon, gluten-free	1 serving	109	2	16	13	1	4.1	0.8	5	34%
(Mother's) shortbread	2 cookies	120	1	13	50	0	7.0	0.0	0	53%
(Natures Warehouse) butter	2 cookies	122	2	19	41	0	4.1	0.0	0	30%
(Stella D'oro)										
'Breakfast Treats'	1 cookie	101	2	15	0	0	3.6	0.0	0	32%
'Chinese Dessert'	1 cookie	169	2	20	0	0	8.9	0.0	0	48%
toast, 'Mandel'	1 piece	58	1	10	0	0	1.4	0.0	0	22%
AMARANTH										
(Hansa) whole grain, biscuit, organic	1 cookie	120	3	22	50	3	3.0	1.5	5	21%
(Health Valley)	1 cookie	90	2	12	30	2	3.0	0.0	0	33%
ANIMAL CRACKERS										
(Barbara's Bakery) vanilla	1 oz	145	2	18	85	0	7.0	0.0	0	44%
(Barnum's)	12 cookies	141	2	23	160	1	4.0	0.5	0	26%
(Finast)	5 cookies	120	2	22	110	0	3.0	0.0	0	22%
(Frookie) cinnamon, 'Animal Frackers'	6 cookies	60	1	9	45	0	2.0	0.0	0	31%
(Glenny's) peanut butter, 'Noah 'N Friends Animal Cookies'	0.5 oz	65	1	9	35	0	3.0	0.0	0	40%
(Grandma's) candied	5 cookies	140	1	20	80	0	6.0	0.0	0	39%
(Keebler)	5 cookies	70	1	11	75	0	2.0	1.0	0	27%
(Mother's) circus animals	4 cookies	110	1	14	40	0	6.0	0.0	0	47%
(Ralston)	12 cookies	130	2	22	80	1	3.0	1.0	1	22%
(Sunshine)	14 cookies	140	2	24	125	1	4.0	1.0	0	26%
ANISE										
(Biscotti Thins) fat- and cholesterol-free, low-sodium	5 cookies	80	1	20	25	0	0.0	0.0	0	0%
(Stella D'oro)										
'Anisette Sponge'	1 piece	51	1	10	0	0	0.8	0.0	0	14%
'Anisette Toast'	1 piece	46	1	9	0	0	0.6	0.0	0	12%
'Anisette Toast Jumbo'	1 piece	109	2	23	0	0	1.0	0.0	0	8%
APPLE										
(Archway) cinnamon 'Home Style'	1 serving	106	1	17	132	0	3.7	0.9	0	31%
(Bakery Wagon)										
oatmeal, filled	1 cookie	90	1	14	115	0	4.0	0.0	2	38%
w/cinnamon	1 cookie	100	1	17	100	0	3.0	0.0	2	27%
w/walnuts and raisins	1 cookie	100	2	17	110	0	3.0	0.0	2	26%
(Estee) w/cinnamon, 'Snack Crisps'	0.66 oz	80	1	15	75	0	2.0	1.0	0	22%
(Frookie)										
'Fruitins'	1 cookie	60	1	12	25	0	1.0	0.0	0	15%
w/spice, nonfat	1 cookie	50	1	11	80	1	0.0	0.0	0	0%
(Great Cakes)	4.5 oz	260	10	40	20	21	6.0	0.0	0	21%
(Health Valley)										
raspberry, nonfat	2 cookies	67	1	16	33	2	0.0	0.0	0	0%
spice, nonfat	1 serving	33	1	8	17	1	0.0	0.0	0	0%

Food Name	Serving Size	Calories	Prot. gms	Carbs gms	Sod. mgs	Fiber gms	Fat gms	Sat. Fat gms	Chol. mgs	% Fat Cal.
w/cinnamon, nonfat 'Mini Fruit Centers'	3 cookies	75	2	17	60	3	0.0	0.0	0	0%
w/raisin, nonfat, 'Fruit Chunks'	3 cookies	85	2	19	80	3	0.0	0.0	0	0%
(Healthy Times) organic, 'Hugga Bears'	1 oz	120	2	17	38	0	3.0	0.0	0	26%
(Nabisco) nonfat, 'Newton's'	2 cookies	100	1	24	60	1	0.0	0.0	0	0%
(Natures Warehouse) cinnamon	1 bar	54	1	10	10	0	1.0	0.0	0	18%
(Stella D'oro)										
bar, Dutch	1 piece	112	1	19	0	0	3.3	0.0	0	27%
pastry, dietetic	1 piece	86	1	13	10	0	3.3	0.0	0	35%
(Sunshine) low-fat, 'Golden Fruit'	1 serving	70	1	15	60	1	1.0	0.0	0	12%
(Weight Watchers) fruit-filled	1 cookie	80	1	21	35	0	1.0	0.0	0	9%
APPLE RAISIN										
(Archway)										
'Apple n' Raisin'	1 piece	120	2	20	169	1	3.0	0.0	10	23%
filled, 'Home Style'	1 serving	100	1	16	80	0	3.5	1.4	7	31%
gourmet, 'Home Style'	1 serving	111	1	17	121	1	4.2	0.9	5	34%
(Health Valley)										
almond, 'Fancy Fruit Chunks'	2 pieces	90	2	14	45	2	4.0	0.0	0	36%
apple, nonfat, 'Fruit Chunks'	3 cookies	85	2	19	80	3	0.0	0.0	0	0%
delight, nonfat	1 serving	33	1	8	17	1	0.0	0.0	0	0%
nonfat, 'Fruit Centers'	1 cookie	80	2	17	80	2	0.0	0.0	0	0%
nonfat, jumbo	1 serving	80	2	19	35	3	0.0	0.0	0	0%
(Pepperidge Farm) raspberry, 'Zurich'	1 piece	60	1	10	30	0	2.0	1.0	0	29%
ARROWROOT (Nabisco) 'National Arrowroot'	1 oz	130	2	21	85	0	4.0	1.0	10	28%
BANANA										
(Break Cake) creme	1 cookie	240	2	37	200	0	9.0	2.2	5	34%
(Frookie) nonfat	1 cookie	45	1	10	90	1	0.0	0.0	0	0%
(Health Valley) spice, nonfat	2 cookies	67	1	16	33	2	0.0	0.0	0	0%
(Natures Warehouse)										
all natural, nonfat	1 cookie	75	1	17	69	0	0.4	0.0	0	5%
wheat-free, nonfat	1 cookie	80	1	19	65	1	0.0	0.0	0	0%
BLUEBERRY (Great Cakes)	4.5 oz	260	10	40	20	21	6.0	0.0	0	21%
BRAN (Archway) w/raisin	1 piece	100	2	18	95	1	3.0	0.0	5	25%
BROWNIE										
(Break Cake) creme	1 cookie	240	2	38	150	0	8.0	1.8	5	31%
(Eagle) chocolate fudge, 'Gourmet'	1 cookie	330	5	42	120	3	16.0	5.0	15	43%
(Pepperidge Farm)										
chocolate nut, 'Old Fashioned'	2 pieces	110	1	11	45	0	7.0	2.0	5	57%
cream sandwich, 'Capri'	1 piece	80	0	10	45	0	5.0	1.0	0	53%
BUTTER										
(Barbara's Bakery) pecan, bites, 'Small Indulgences'	1 oz	140	2	16	95	0	8.0	0.0	20	50%
(Delicious) frosted, made w/Land O'Lakes butter	1 cookie	88	1	11	44	0	5.0	1.0	10	48%
(Fifty 50)										
fructose-sweetened	4 cookies	160	2	20	65	1	8.0	6.0	25	45%
fructose-sweetened, low-sodium	1 cookie	40	1	5	20	0	2.0	0.0	5	43%
(Hansa) biscuit, whole-grain, organic	1 cookie	130	3	24	75	3	3.5	2.0	10	23%
(Keebler)										
chocolate coated, 'Baby Bear'	3 pieces	70	1	10	55	0	2.0	1.0	0	29%
chocolate coated, 'E.L. Fudge'	2 pieces	80	1	10	40	0	4.0	1.0	5	45%
(Lu) 'Petit Beurre'	1 cookie	40	1	7	45	0	1.0	0.0	0	22%
(Mother's)	5 cookies	140	2	20	130	0	6.0	0.0	0	38%
CARAMEL										
(Barbara's Bakery) apple minis, nonfat	6 cookies	110	2	24	125	1	0.0	0.0	0	0%
(FFV) patties	2 pieces	150	1	20	125	0	7.0	0.0	0	43%
(Little Debbie) bar	1 bar	160	1	22	85	0	8.0	1.5	0	44%

Food Name	Serving Size	Calories	Prot. gms	Carbs gms	Sod. mgs	Fiber gms	Fat gms	Sat. Fat gms	Chol. mgs	% Fat Cal.
(Natures Warehouse)										
crisp, all natural, nonfat	1 cookie	80	1	19	55	2	0.0	0.0	0	0%
wheat-free, crisp, nonfat	1 cookie	80	1	19	55	2	0.0	0.0	0	0%
(Snackwell's) 'Caramel Delights'	1 serving	69	1	13	33	0	2.0	0.5	0	26%
CAROB										
(Great Cakes) w/cherry	4.5 oz	280	10	40	20	21	8.0	0.0	0	26%
(Heaven Scent) fudge, wheat-free	1 cookie	70	2	15	55	1	1.0	0.0	0	12%
(Jennies) macaroon, gluten- and lactose-free	1 cookie	310	2	41	20	6	15.0	14.0	0	44%
(Natures Warehouse) fudge	2 cookies	116	1	21	78	0	3.1	0.0	0	24%
(Westbrae) 'Rice Malt Snap'	1 oz	140	2	18	70	0	7.0	0.0	0	44%
CARROT										
(Archway) cake, gourmet, 'Home Style'	1 serving	120	1	18	176	1	5.0	1.5	4	37%
(Pepperidge Farm) w/walnut, lowfat, soft, 'Wholesome Choice'	1 cookie	60	1	11	45	0	1.0	1.0	0	16%
CHERRY										
(Archway) filled, 'Home Style'	1 serving	100	1	16	83	0	3.5	1.4	7	31%
(Natures Warehouse)										
all natural, nonfat	1 cookie	72	1	17	69	0	0.4	0.0	0	5%
wheat-free, nonfat	1 cookie	80	1	18	60	1	0.5	0.0	0	6%
CHOCOLATE										
(Archway)										
devil's food, nonfat, 'Home Style'	1 serving	68	1	16	79	1	0.2	0.1	0	2%
mud pie, 'Home Style'	1 serving	107	1	15	103	1	4.9	2.1	5	41%
(Auburn Farms)										
chewy, nonfat	2 cookies	80	2	19	65	2	0.5	0.0	0	5%
w/mint, nonfat	2 cookies	90	1	20	95	2	0.0	0.0	0	0%
(Barbara's Bakery)										
double chocolate, minis, nonfat	6 cookies	100	2	23	135	1	0.0	0.0	0	0%
w/raspberry, 'Cookies & Creme'	2 cookies	120	2	18	80	0	5.0	0.0	15	36%
(Betty Crocker) w/peanut butter creme, 'Dunkaroos'	1 tray	140	3	15	140	0	8.0	0.0	0	50%
(Biscotti Thins) fat- and cholesterol-free, low sodium	5 cookies	80	1	20	25	0	0.0	0.0	0	0%
(Break Cake) wafer	4 wafers	200	2	30	95	0	9.0	3.8	0	39%
(Cookietree) fudge, nonfat	1 cookie	120	2	27	180	1	0.0	0.0	0	0%
(Delicious) wafer	1 wafer	34	1	2	5	0	2.0	0.0	0	60%
(Drake's)	2 pieces	130	2	19	85	0	5.0	1.0	0	35%
(Ener-G Foods)										
nut, gluten-free	1 serving	102	2	12	7	1	4.5	0.4	0	42%
walnut, gluten-free	1 serving	109	1	11	107	1	6.8	2.0	5	56%
(Estee) 'Snack Crisps'	0.66 oz	80	1	15	65	0	2.0	1.0	0	22%
(FFV) devil's food, 'Trolley Cakes' 2 oz serving	2 pieces	120	2	25	80	0	2.0	0.0	0	14%
(Frookie)										
'Animal Frackers'	6 cookies	60	1	9	70	0	2.0	0.0	0	31%
'Funky Monkeys'	8 cookies	60	1	10	60	0	2.0	0.0	0	29%
(Grandma's) cookie bits	1 oz	140	2	19	180	0	6.0	0.0	0	39%
(Health Valley) fudge, nonfat	2 cookies	70	2	17	20	3	0.0	0.0	0	0%
(Heaven Scent) wheat-free	1 cookie	71	2	15	54	1	1.0	0.0	0	12%
(Keebler) devil's food, fat free, 'Elfin Delights'	1 serving	70	1	14	110	0	0.0	0.0	0	0%
(Lu)										
'Chocolatiers'	2 cookies	85	1	10	10	0	4.0	0.0	0	45%
dipped, 'Chocolatiers'	2 cookies	105	1	12	15	0	6.0	0.0	0	51%
(M&M Mars) fudge, and crunchy, 'Twix'	1 bar	100	1	11	35	0	6.0	0.0	0	53%
(Nabisco)										
'Pure Chocolate Middles'	0.5 oz piece	80	1	9	35	0	5.0	2.0	5	53%
cake, 'Mallomars'	1 piece	60	1	8	20	0	3.0	1.0	0	43%

Food Name	Serving Size	Calories	Prot. gms	Carbs gms	Sod. mgs	Fiber gms	Fat gms	Sat. Fat gms	Chol. mgs	% Fat Cal.
devil's food, cakes	1 piece	70	1	15	40	0	1.0	1.0	0	12%
w/peanut butter, 'Ideal Bars'	0.5 oz piece	90	1	10	80	0	5.0	2.0	0	51%
(Snackwell's) devil's food	1 serving	49	1	12	28	0	0.2	0.1	0	3%
(Stella D'oro)										
'Castelets'	1 piece	64	1	9	0	0	2.8	0.0	0	39%
'Margherite'	1 piece	72	1	10	0	0	3.1	0.0	0	39%
(Tastykake) 'Soft, 'n Chewy'	1.4 oz	171	2	26	111	1	7.0	2.1	3	36%
(Weight Watchers)	3 cookies	80	1	13	70	0	3.0	0.0	0	33%
CHOCOLATE CHIP										
(Almost Home)	0.5 oz piece	60	1	8	45	0	3.0	1.0	2	43%
(Archway)										
	1 piece	50	1	7	40	0	3.0	0.0	5	46%
and toffee, gourmet, 'Home Style'	1 serving	131	1	18	124	1	6.1	1.8	6	42%
drop, 'Home Style'	1 serving	101	1	15	78	0	3.7	1.1	14	33%
ice box, 'Home Style'	1 serving	117	1	15	59	0	5.7	1.8	8	44%
no sugar, 'Home Style'	1 serving	108	1	16	64	0	5.3	1.5	0	45%
rocky road, gourmet, 'Home Style'	1 serving	127	2	18	71	1	5.9	1.5	11	42%
rocky road, sugarless, 'Home Style'	1 serving	101	1	15	66	1	4.9	1.2	0	44%
(Barbara's Bakery) crisp, 'Small Indulgences'	1 oz	140	2	18	105	0	7.0	0.0	15	44%
(Break Cake)	5 cookies	140	2	20	115	0	6.0	1.4	5	38%
(Drake's)	2 pieces	140	1	18	110	0	6.0	2.0	0	42%
(Duncan Hines) milk chocolate	2 pieces	110	1	15	85	0	5.0	2.0	0	41%
(Eagle)										
	1 cookie	190	2	26	170	1	8.0	2.5	15	39%
peanut butter, 'Gourmet'	1 cookie	360	7	39	110	4	20.0	6.0	15	49%
(Ener-G Foods) potato, gluten-free	1 serving	91	1	12	34	0	3.9	1.1	4	40%
(Entenmann's)	3 cookies	140	1	19	85	0	7.0	0.0	0	44%
(Estee)	3 cookies	110	1	13	20	0	5.0	2.0	0	45%
(Featherweight)	1 piece	45	1	6	0	0	2.0	0.0	0	39%
(Fifty 50) fructose sweetened	1 cookie	35	1	4	10	0	2.0	0.0	0	47%
(Finast)	1 oz	90	1	18	60	0	7.0	0.0	0	45%
(Frookie)										
Mandarin	1 cookie	45	1	7	35	0	2.0	0.5	0	38%
mint	1 cookie	45	1	7	35	0	2.0	0.5	0	38%
(Grandma's)										
'Big Cookies'	1 serving	200	2	28	125	1	9.0	3.0	15	40%
'Rich'N Chewy'	3 cookies	140	1	20	80	0	6.0	0.0	5	39%
(Keebler)										
bakery crisp, 'Chips Deluxe'	1 cookie	60	1	7	45	0	3.0	1.0	0	46%
chewy, 'Elfin Delights'	1 cookie	65	1	11	55	0	2.0	1.0	0	27%
'Chips Deluxe'	1 piece	80	1	10	75	0	4.0	1.0	5	45%
'Coconut Chocolate Drop'	1 cookie	80	1	10	60	0	5.0	2.0	0	51%
food service product, 'Old Fashioned'	1 serving	80	1	10	60	0	4.0	1.0	0	45%
less fat, 'Chips Deluxe'	1 serving	70	1	11	70	0	3.0	1.0	0	36%
rainbow chips 'Chips Deluxe'	1 piece	80	1	11	45	0	3.0	1.0	5	36%
regular, enriched, 'Rich, 'n Chips'	1 large	67	1	9	44	0	3.2	1.0	0	41%
'Soft Batch'	1 serving	80	1	10	70	1	3.5	1.0	0	43%
(Mother's)										
	1 cookie	70	1	10	55	0	3.0	0.0	0	38%
angel	2 cookies	120	1	14	45	0	8.0	0.0	0	55%
(Nabisco)										
'Chips Ahoy'	1 cookie	68	1	9	45	0	3.2	1.1	0	41%
chunky, 'Chips Ahoy!'	0.5 oz piece	90	1	10	65	0	5.0	2.0	10	51%
chunky, 'Chips Ahoy!'	1 serving	80	1	11	60	1	4.0	3.0	10	43%

Food Name	Serving Size	Calories	Prot. gms	Carbs gms	Sod. mgs	Fiber gms	Fat gms	Sat. Fat gms	Chol. mgs	% Fat Cal.
mini, 'Chips Ahoy!'	0.5 oz	70	1	9	50	0	3.0	1.0	0	40%
mini, 'Chips Ahoy!'	1 cookie	11	0	1	7	0	0.5	0.2	0	41%
pecan, 'Selections' 'Chips Ahoy!'	0.5 oz piece	100	1	10	65	0	6.0	2.0	10	55%
'Rockers' 'Chips Ahoy!'	1 cookie	60	1	8	40	0	3.0	1.0	0	43%
walnut, 'Selections' 'Chips Ahoy!'	0.5 oz piece	100	1	9	70	0	6.0	2.0	5	57%
walnut, w/white fudge chunks 'Chips Ahoy!'	1 cookie	90	1	11	75	0	5.0	2.0	5	48%
(Oven Lovin')	1 cookie	70	0	9	50	0	3.0	0.0	5	43%
(Pepperidge Farm)										
'Family Request'	2 cookies	90	1	15	55	0	5.0	1.0	5	41%
'Old Fashioned'	2 pieces	100	1	12	45	0	5.0	2.0	5	46%
w/pecan, regular, enriched	1 cookie	58	1	8	38	0	2.7	0.9	0	41%
(Pillsbury)	1 serving	130	1	17	85	1	6.0	1.5	3	43%
(Snackwell's) less fat	13 cookies	130	2	22	170	1	3.5	1.5	0	25%
(Soft Batch)	1 piece	80	1	10	70	0	4.0	1.0	0	45%
(Tastykake)										
bar	1 piece	193	3	28	97	1	8.4	1.5	4	38%
'Soft 'n Chewy'	1.4 oz	174	2	26	168	1	7.3	2.1	10	37%
CHOCOLATE CHOCOLATE CHIP										
(Lady J.) 100% natural	1 cookie	120	2	15	85	1	7.0	1.0	0	48%
(Natures Warehouse)	2 cookies	130	3	16	69	0	6.1	0.0	0	42%
(Pillsbury) 'Pillsbury's Best'	1 cookie	70	1	9	35	0	3.0	1.0	0	40%
CINNAMON										
(Archway) honey hearts, nonfat, 'Home Style'	1 serving	106	1	25	123	0	0.2	0.1	0	2%
(Biscotti Thins) fat- and cholesterol-free, low sodium	5 cookies	80	1	20	25	0	0.0	0.0	0	0%
(Natures Warehouse) w/nuts	2 cookies	113	1	19	71	0	3.6	0.0	0	29%
COCOA										
(Archway) Dutch, 'Home Style'	1 serving	98	1	17	87	1	3.3	0.8	3	30%
(Barbara's Bakery) mocha, minis, nonfat	6 cookies	100	2	23	125	1	0.0	0.0	0	0%
(Westbrae)										
'Rice Malt Snap'	1 oz	140	2	17	70	0	7.0	0.0	0	45%
w/cocoa chip, 'Rice Malt Snap'	1 oz	130	2	18	60	0	7.0	0.0	0	44%
COCONUT										
(Archway) macaroon, 'Home Style'	1 serving	106	1	12	38	1	6.1	5.4	0	52%
(Break Cake) macaroon	2 cookies	270	2	34	160	0	14.0	12.5	0	47%
(Drake's)	2 pieces	130	2	20	95	0	5.0	2.0	0	34%
(Estee)	3 cookies	110	1	14	15	0	5.0	1.0	0	43%
(Fifty 50) fructose-sweetened	4 cookies	160	2	18	0	1	10.0	3.0	0	53%
(Glenny's) w/almonds and raisins, 'Nookie Bar'	1.15 oz	138	2	18	0	0	3.0	0.0	0	25%
(Jennies) macaroon, gluten- and lactose-free	1 cookie	270	2	34	20	5	14.0	13.0	0	47%
(Mother's)										
'Cocadas'	4 cookies	120	2	17	150	0	6.0	0.0	0	42%
macaroon	1 cookie	80	1	8	40	0	5.0	0.0	0	56%
(Mrs. Denson's) macaroon, quinoa	2 cookies	150	2	14	25	2	12.0	7.0	0	63%
(Pepperidge Farm) chocolate-filled, 'Tahiti'	1 piece	90	0	9	25	0	6.0	2.0	5	60%
(Stella D'oro)										
dietetic	1 piece	52	1	7	10	0	2.4	0.0	0	42%
macaroon	1 piece	60	1	7	0	0	3.4	0.0	0	51%
COFFEE-FLAVORED										
(Barbara's Bakery) cake crunch, 'Small Indulgences'	1 oz	130	2	18	140	0	6.0	0.0	20	40%
(Pepperidge Farm) chocolate, praline-filled, 'Cappuccino'	1 piece	50	0	6	20	0	3.0	1.0	5	53%
CRANBERRY										
(Frookie) orange, nonfat	1 cookie	45	1	10	75	1	0.0	0.0	0	0%
(Nabisco) nonfat, 'Newton's'	2 cookies	100	1	23	95	1	0.0	0.0	0	0%

Food Name	Serving Size	Calories	Prot. gms	Carbs gms	Sod. mgs	Fiber gms	Fat gms	Sat. Fat gms	Chol. mgs	% Fat Cal.
(Pepperidge Farm) honey, soft, 'Wholesome Choice'	1 cookie	60	1	11	50	0	2.0	1.0	0	27%
(Sunshine) low-fat, 'Golden Fruit'	1 serving	70	1	15	60	1	1.0	0.0	0	12%
CREAM										
(Break Cake)										
'Chips & Creme'	1 cookie	140	1	21	130	0	6.0	1.3	2	38%
devil's food creme	1 cookie	130	1	20	120	0	5.0	1.0	0	35%
w/raisins	1 cookie	140	1	22	120	0	5.0	1.0	2	33%
(Delicious) mini	1 wafer	24	1	3	2	0	1.0	0.0	0	36%
(Eagle)										
lemon	6 sandwiches	260	3	37	190	0	11.0	2.5	0	38%
vanilla	6 sandwiches	260	3	37	170	0	11.0	2.5	0	38%
DATE										
(Ener-G Foods) gluten-free	1 serving	76	1	13	75	1	2.3	0.6	3	27%
(Health Valley)										
almond, 'Fruit Jumbos'	1 cookie	70	2	10	30	1	3.0	0.0	0	36%
delight	1 serving	33	1	8	17	1	0.0	0.0	0	0%
granola, nonfat	2 cookies	67	1	16	33	2	0.0	0.0	0	0%
w/pecan, 'Fancy Fruit Chunks'	2 pieces	90	2	15	45	2	4.0	0.0	0	35%
(Lady J.)										
w/almond, 100% natural	1 cookie	120	2	14	75	2	6.0	0.5	0	46%
w/pecan, 100% natural	1 cookie	110	1	16	90	2	5.0	1.0	0	40%
(Pepperidge Farm) w/pecan, 'Kitchen Hearth'	2 pieces	110	1	15	40	0	5.0	2.0	10	41%
EGG BISCUIT										
(Estee) 'Original Sandwich'	1 cookie	45	1	6	5	0	2.0	1.0	0	39%
(FFV)										
'Kreem Pilot Bread'	1 piece	60	1	9	60	0	2.0	0.0	0	31%
'Royal Dainty' 7 oz serving	2 pieces	120	1	14	90	0	6.0	0.0	0	47%
'T.C. Rounds' 1 oz serving	2 pieces	160	1	20	65	0	8.0	0.0	0	46%
'Tango' 1.2 oz serving	2 pieces	160	1	26	50	0	5.0	0.0	0	29%
(Stella D'oro)										
'Anginetti'	1 piece	31	1	5	0	0	1.0	0.0	0	29%
dietetic	1 piece	43	2	7	10	0	1.1	0.0	0	23%
dietetic, 'Kitchen'	1 piece	8	0	1	10	0	0.5	0.0	0	56%
'Jumbo'	1 piece	47	1	9	0	0	0.7	0.0	0	13%
'Roman'	1 piece	137	3	20	0	0	5.0	0.0	0	33%
sugared	1 piece	75	2	14	0	0	1.4	0.0	0	17%
FIG										
(Estee) bar	2 cookies	90	1	21	60	0	1.0	0.0	0	9%
(FFV)										
w/vanilla, bar	1 piece	70	1	12	55	0	1.0	1.0	0	15%
whole wheat, bar	1 piece	70	1	11	50	0	2.0	1.0	0	27%
(Figaroo) bar	1 cookie	150	2	30	151	2	3.1	0.5	0	18%
(Frookie)										
'Fruitins'	1 cookie	60	1	12	25	0	1.0	0.0	0	15%
nonfat, 'Fruitins'	2 cookies	90	1	21	75	1	0.0	0.0	0	0%
(Keebler) bar	1 piece	60	1	11	70	0	2.0	1.0	0	27%
(Little Debbie) snack squares, 'Figaroos'	1 cookie	150	1	31	110	1	3.5	1.0	0	20%
(Mother's)										
bar	2 cookies	110	1	23	85	0	2.0	0.0	0	16%
whole wheat	2 cookies	120	2	25	105	0	2.0	0.0	0	14%
(Nabisco)										
'Newton's'	2 cookies	110	1	20	120	1	2.5	1.0	0	21%
nonfat, 'Newton's'	2 cookies	100	1	22	125	2	0.0	0.0	0	0%

Food Name	Serving Size	Calories	Prot. gms	Carbs gms	Sod. mgs	Fiber gms	Fat gms	Sat. Fat gms	Chol. mgs	% Fat Cal.
(Natures Warehouse)										
fruit juice sweetened	1 bar	70	1	12	20	1	1.5	0.0	1	21%
wheat-free, bar	1 oz	98	1	19	18	.0	2.0	0.0	0	18%
wheat-free, fruit juice sweetened	1 bar	54	1	10	10	0	1.0	0.0	0	18%
whole wheat, bar	1 oz	98	1	19	18	0	2.0	0.0	0	18%
w/apple and cinnamon, bar, wheat-free	1 oz	98	1	19	18	0	2.0	0.0	0	18%
w/raspberry, bar, wheat-free	1 oz	98	1	19	18	0	2.0	0.0	0	18%
(Stella D'oro) pastry, dietetic	1 piece	89	1	13	10	0	3.7	0.0	0	37%
(Weight Watchers) filled	1 serving	70	1	16	50	0	0.0	0.0	0	0%
FORTUNE										
(La Choy) food service product	1 serving	112	2	26	11	1	0.2	0.1	0	2%
(Umeya)	30 grams	110	4	24	90	1	0.0	0.0	0	0%
FRUIT										
(Archway) and honey, bar, 'Home Style'	1 serving	103	1	18	107	0	3.3	0.8	6	29%
(Bakery Wagon) honey, bar	1 cookie	100	1	16	70	0	3.0	0.0	2	28%
(Barbara's Bakery) w/nuts	1 oz	140	2	18	55	0	6.0	0.0	0	40%
(Hansa) whole grain, organic, biscuit, 'Fruit, 'n Nut'	1 cookie	120	2	20	45	1	3.5	1.5	5	26%
(Health Valley)										
'Fruit & Fitness'	5 pieces	200	4	40	249	4	6.0	0.0	0	23%
Hawaiian, nonfat	1 serving	33	1	8	17	1	0.0	0.0	0	0%
tropical, 'Fancy Fruit Chunks'	2 pieces	80	2	13	45	2	3.0	0.0	0	31%
tropical, 'Fruit Jumbos'	1 piece	70	1	10	26	2	2.0	0.0	0	29%
tropical, nonfat, 'Fruit Centers'	1 cookie	80	2	17	80	2	0.0	0.0	0	0%
(Nabisco) chewy, nonfat, "Newton's"	2 cookies	100	1	22	115	1	0.0	0.0	0	0%
(Stella D'oro) slices	1 piece	60	1	9	0	0	2.2	0.0	0	34%
FUDGE										
(Almost Home) w/chocolate chips	0.5 oz piece	70	1	9	50	0	3.0	1.0	2	40%
(Eagle) w/chocolate chips	1 cookie	260	3	36	120	3	11.0	4.0	20	39%
(Estee)	1 cookie	30	1	4	0	0	1.0	1.0	0	31%
(Grandma's)										
'Big Cookies'	2 pieces	350	4	54	380	0	13.0	0.0	5	34%
w/chocolate chips, 'Big Cookies'	1 serving	190	2	28	80	1	7.0	2.5	10	34%
(Mother's) wafer, 'Flaky Flix'	2 cookies	130	1	14	30	0	9.0	0.0	0	57%
(Nabisco)										
middles	0.5 oz piece	80	1	9	35	0	5.0	2.0	5	53%
mini bites, 'Little Fudgies' 'Chips Ahoy!'	1 oz	230	3	27	105	0	12.0	4.0	0	47%
snaps	4 pieces	70	1	11	75	0	2.0	1.0	2	27%
wafer, 'Famous Wafers'	5 pieces	70	1	11	110	0	2.0	1.0	2	27%
w/caramel and peanuts, 'Heyday Bars'	0.75 oz	110	2	13	40	1	6.0	2.0	0	47%
(Stella D'oro) 'Swiss'	1 piece	68	1	9	0	0	3.4	0.0	0	45%
(Tastykake) bar	1.8 oz	205	2	35	155	1	6.8	2.1	6	29%
GINGER										
(Archway)										
snap, 54 per package	1 piece	35	0	6	30	0	1.0	0.0	0	27%
snap, 80 per package	1 piece	25	1	4	20	0	1.0	0.0	0	31%
snap, iced, 'Home Style'	1 serving	172	1	26	132	0	7.0	2.1	0	37%
snap, less fat, 'Home Style'	1 serving	136	1	25	141	0	3.6	0.9	0	24%
(Break Cake) snap	5 cookies	130	2	20	110	0	5.0	1.2	0	34%
(Delicious) snap	0.5 oz	64	1	11	78	0	1.7	0.0	1	24%
(Eagle) 'Gourmet'	1 cookie	240	4	49	180	0	3.5	1.0	20	13%
(Ener-G Foods) gluten-free	1 serving	75	1	12	134	1	2.7	0.6	3	32%
(FFV) boys	1.25 oz pkg	150	2	26	210	0	5.0	1.0	0	29%
(Frookie) spice	1 cookie	45	1	7	35	0	2.0	0.5	0	38%
(Little Debbie)	1 cookie	90	1	15	60	0	3.0	1.0	5	30%

Food Name	Serving Size	Calories	Prot. gms	Carbs gms	Sod. mgs	Fiber gms	Fat gms	Sat. Fat gms	Chol. mgs	% Fat Cal.
(Sunshine) snap................................	5 pieces	100	1	16	120	0	3.0	1.0	0	28%
(Westbrae) 'Rice Malt Snap'........................	1 oz	130	2	20	140	0	5.0	0.0	0	34%
GRAHAM										
(Betty Crocker)										
cinnamon, w/vanilla frosting, 'Dunkaroos'............	1 serving	130	1	21	60	0	4.5	1.5	0	32%
w/chocolate frosting, 'Dunkaroos'....................	1 tray	130	1	19	70	0	5.0	0.0	0	36%
w/vanilla frosting, 'Dunkaroos'......................	1 tray	130	1	21	60	0	5.0	0.0	0	34%
(Carafection)										
honey, carob coated, 'Original'....................	1 oz	139	2	17	26	0	7.0	0.0	0	45%
mint honey, carob coated........................	1 oz	139	2	17	26	0	7.0	0.0	0	45%
(Carr's) wheat and honey, 'Home Wheat Graham'........	1 piece	74	1	11	1	0	3.3	0.0	0	38%
(Delicious)										
w/cinnamon....................................	0.5 oz	60	1	11	50	0	2.0	0.5	0	27%
w/honey.......................................	0.5 oz	60	1	11	50	0	2.0	0.3	0	27%
(Eagle) peanut butter.............................	6 sandwiches	250	4	36	200	1	10.0	2.5	0	36%
(Health Valley)										
amaranth, nonfat...............................	8 pieces	100	4	23	30	3	0.0	0.0	0	0%
honey, 'Fancy'.................................	7 pieces	130	3	21	89	4	5.0	0.0	0	32%
oat bran, nonfat...............................	1 serving	13	1	3	4	0	0.0	0.0	0	0%
(Honey Grahams) honey........................	4 pieces	70	1	12	85	0	2.0	1.0	0	26%
(Keebler)										
....	4 crackers	70	1	12	85	0	2.0	1.0	0	26%
chocolate, 'Selects'..........................	4 cookies	60	1	9	55	0	3.0	1.0	0	40%
chocolate, 'Selects'..........................	4 crackers	60	1	9	55	0	3.0	1.0	0	40%
chocolate, 'Thin Bits'........................	12 pieces	70	1	9	75	0	3.0	1.0	0	40%
cinnamon, 'Alpha Grahams'....................	6 pieces	70	1	10	55	0	2.0	1.0	0	29%
cinnamon, 'Cinnamon Crisp'....................	4 pieces	70	1	11	85	0	2.0	1.0	0	27%
cinnamon, fudge covered, 'Deluxe'..............	2 pieces	90	1	11	60	0	4.0	1.0	0	43%
cinnamon, 'Thin Bits'........................	12 pieces	70	1	10	50	0	3.0	1.0	0	38%
honey nut, 'Selects'.........................	4 cookies	60	1	9	70	0	3.0	1.0	0	40%
(Mi-Del) 100% whole wheat......................	1 cracker	60	1	12	110	1	1.5	0.0	0	21%
(Mother's)										
cinnamon, dinosaurs...........................	1 cookie	80	1	12	50	0	3.0	0.0	0	34%
cinnamon, dinosaurs, mini's...................	7 cookies	70	1	9	40	0	2.0	0.0	0	31%
dinosaurs, original...........................	1 cookie	70	1	12	50	0	2.0	0.0	0	26%
(Nabisco)										
....	1 serving	119	2	21	185	1	2.8	0.4	0	21%
....	2 pieces	60	1	11	90	1	1.0	0.0	0	16%
apple cinnamon, 'Honey Maid Graham Bites'..........	11 crackers	60	1	11	80	0	2.0	1.0	0	27%
brown sugar, 'Honey Maid Graham Bites'..............	11 crackers	60	1	11	80	0	2.0	1.0	0	27%
'Bugs Bunny'....................................	0.5 oz	60	1	11	70	0	2.0	0.0	0	27%
chocolate......................................	11 pieces	60	1	10	90	0	2.0	1.0	0	29%
chocolate, 'Bugs Bunny'.........................	0.5 oz	60	1	10	80	0	2.0	2.0	0	29%
chocolate, w/vanilla creme, 'Bearwichs' 'Teddy Grahams'..	4 pieces	70	1	10	60	0	3.0	1.0	0	38%
'Chocolate Grahams'............................	0.5 oz piece	150	3	17	80	0	7.0	0.0	0	44%
cinnamon, 'Bearwichs' 'Teddy Grahams'............	0.5 oz	70	1	10	60	0	3.0	1.0	0	38%
cinnamon, 'Bugs Bunny'.........................	0.5 oz	60	1	11	80	0	2.0	2.0	0	27%
cinnamon, 'Honey Maid'.........................	2 pieces	60	1	12	85	0	1.0	1.0	0	15%
cinnamon, w/fudge, 'Cookies'N Fudge'.............	1 piece	45	1	6	35	0	2.0	1.0	0	39%
honey, 'Honey Maid'............................	2 pieces	60	1	11	90	0	1.0	1.0	0	16%
honey vanilla..................................	11 pieces	60	1	10	75	0	2.0	1.0	0	29%
oat bran, w/honey, 'Graham Bites' 'Honey Maid'........	0.5 oz	60	1	11	55	0	2.0	1.0	0	27%
vanilla and honey, 'Bearwichs' 'Teddy Grahams'.........	4 pieces	70	1	10	65	0	3.0	1.0	0	38%

Food Name	Serving Size	Calories	Prot. gms	Carbs gms	Sod. mgs	Fiber gms	Fat gms	Sat. Fat gms	Chol. mgs	% Fat Cal.
(Pepperidge Farm)										
cinnamon, 'Goldfish'	1 oz	130	2	19	130	0	7.0	2.0	10	43%
'Goldfish'	1 oz	140	2	18	140	0	7.0	2.0	10	44%
honey hazelnut, 'Old Fashioned'	2 pieces	110	1	15	75	0	6.0	2.0	0	46%
(Regal)	2 crackers	140	1	19	120	0	7.0	0.0	0	44%
(Rokeach)	8 crackers	120	2	21	0	0	3.0	0.0	0	23%
(Sunshine)										
cinnamon	1 piece	70	1	11	95	0	3.0	1.0	0	36%
'Grahamy Bears'	9 crackers	130	2	21	160	0	5.0	1.0	0	33%
GRANOLA										
(Health Valley) 'Healthy'	3 cookies	75	2	17	60	3	0.0	0.0	0	0%
(Incredibites)										
w/chocolate filling	1 pouch	170	2	24	150	0	7.0	1.0	0	38%
w/peanut butter	1 pouch	170	2	23	160	0	8.0	1.0	0	42%
w/vanilla creme	1 pouch	170	2	24	180	0	7.0	1.0	0	38%
HONEY										
(Health Valley)										
w/cinnamon, crisp, 'Honey Jumbos'	1 piece	70	1	10	35	3	2.0	0.0	0	29%
w/oat bran, fancy, 'Honey Jumbos'	1 piece	70	1	10	22	2	2.0	0.0	0	29%
w/peanut butter, crisp, 'Honey Jumbos'	1 piece	70	2	10	24	2	2.0	0.0	0	27%
JELLY *(Delicious)* jelly top	0.8 oz	112	2	14	34	0	5.3	0.0	1	43%
LEMON										
(Archway)										
drop, 'Home Style'	1 serving	93	1	15	95	0	3.3	0.8	9	32%
frosty, 'Home Style'	1 serving	112	1	17	95	0	4.4	1.5	0	36%
nuggets, nonfat, 'Home Style'	1 serving	115	1	27	117	0	0.2	0.1	0	2%
snap, 'Home Style'	1 serving	152	2	20	117	0	7.3	1.7	7	43%
(Cookietree) poppyseed, nonfat	1 cookie	130	2	28	150	1	0.0	0.0	0	0%
(Estee)										
	3 cookies	100	1	14	15	0	5.0	1.0	0	43%
'Snack Crisps'	0.66 oz	80	1	15	75	0	2.0	1.0	0	22%
(Featherweight)	1 piece	45	1	6	0	0	2.0	0.0	0	39%
(Westbrae) 'Rice Malt Snap'	1 oz	130	2	20	70	0	6.0	0.0	0	38%
MACADAMIA										
(Eagle) w/coconut, 'Gourmet Cookie'	1 cookie	330	5	42	230	3	16.0	5.0	20	43%
(Pepperidge Farm) 'Special Collection'	1 piece	70	1	8	35	0	4.0	1.0	5	50%
MARSHMALLOW										
(Nabisco)										
cake, chocolate-coated, 'Mallomars'	0.5-oz piece	60	1	9	20	0	3.0	1.0	0	40%
cake, chocolate-coated, 'Pinwheels'	1 piece	130	1	20	35	0	5.0	3.0	0	35%
(Suddenly S'Mores) fudge graham	0.75-oz piece	100	1	15	90	0	4.0	2.0	0	36%
MINT										
(Girl Scout) thin	4 cookies	160	1	20	140	2	9.0	6.0	0	49%
(Little Debbie) creme, wafers	1 wafer	150	1	18	40	1	9.0	1.5	0	52%
(Snackwell's) creme	1 serving	108	1	19	72	1	3.6	0.9	0	30%
(Soft Batch)	1 piece	80	1	10	70	0	4.0	1.0	0	45%
MOLASSES										
(Archway)										
	1 piece	100	1	18	155	2	2.0	0.0	10	19%
dark, 'Home Style'	1 serving	115	1	20	154	0	3.4	0.8	0	27%
iced, 'Home Style'	1 serving	114	1	20	130	0	3.6	1.1	0	28%
old fashioned, 'Home Style'	1 serving	105	1	18	138	0	3.0	0.7	8	25%
3.5-4-inch diam	1 cookie	138	2	24	147	0	4.1	1.0	0	26%
(Bakery Wagon) iced	1 cookie	100	1	17	120	0	4.0	0.0	5	33%

Food Name	Serving Size	Calories	Prot. gms	Carbs gms	Sod. mgs	Fiber gms	Fat gms	Sat. Fat gms	Chol. mgs	% Fat Cal.
(Little Debbie)	1 cookie	86	1	15	92	0	2.6	0.6	0	26%
(Nabisco) 'Pantry'	0.5 oz piece	80	1	13	75	0	3.0	1.0	0	33%
MUESLI (Carr's)	1 piece	84	1	11	30	0	4.1	0.0	0	44%
OAT BRAN										
(Awrey's) w/raisins	1 piece	100	1	14	115	1	4.0	1.0	0	38%
(Frookie) muffin cookie	1 cookie	45	1	7	35	0	2.0	0.5	0	38%
(Health Valley)										
animal cookies	7 pieces	110	3	20	50	3	4.0	0.0	0	28%
w/fruit and nuts	2 pieces	110	3	17	70	3	4.0	0.0	0	31%
w/fruit, 'Oat Bran Fruit Jumbos'	1 piece	70	1	10	22	2	2.0	0.0	0	29%
w/raisins, 'Fancy Fruit Chunks'	2 pieces	90	2	15	95	2	3.0	0.0	0	28%
(Natures Warehouse)										
w/chocolate chips	2 cookies	139	4	17	55	0	6.0	0.0	0	40%
wheat-free	2 cookies	129	2	16	54	0	6.2	0.0	0	43%
OATMEAL										
(Almost Home) w/raisins	0.5 oz piece	70	1	10	40	1	3.0	1.0	2	38%
(Archway)										
	1 piece	110	2	19	90	1	3.0	0.0	5	24%
apple-filled	1 piece	90	1	18	115	1	1.0	0.0	5	11%
apple-filled, 'Home Style'	1 serving	99	1	16	103	1	3.2	0.7	2	29%
date-filled	1 piece	100	1	18	105	1	2.0	0.0	5	19%
date-filled, 'Home Style'	1 serving	99	1	17	98	1	3.1	0.7	3	28%
golden, gourmet, 'Ruth's 'Home Style'	1 serving	122	2	18	107	1	5.0	1.0	4	37%
'Home Style'	1 serving	106	2	17	87	1	3.8	0.9	3	32%
iced	1 piece	140	2	22	107	2	5.0	0.0	5	32%
pecan, gourmet, 'Home Style'	1 serving	134	2	16	103	1	6.8	2.4	5	46%
raisin, 'Home Style'	1 serving	107	1	17	98	1	3.5	0.8	3	30%
raisin, nonfat, 'Home Style'	1 serving	106	1	24	165	1	0.5	0.1	0	4%
raspberry, nonfat, 'Home Style'	1 serving	109	1	25	166	1	0.5	0.1	0	4%
'Ruth's Golden'	1 piece	120	2	20	122	1	4.0	0.0	5	29%
sugar-free, 'Home Style'	1 serving	106	1	16	74	0	5.0	1.2	0	43%
w/raisins	1 piece	50	1	7	20	0	2.0	0.0	0	36%
(Auburn Farms) raisin, nonfat, 'Jammers'	2 cookies	80	2	19	70	2	0.5	0.0	0	5%
(Bakers Bonus)	0.5 oz piece	80	1	12	65	0	3.0	1.0	0	34%
(Bakery Wagon)										
date-filled	1 cookie	90	1	15	100	0	3.0	0.0	2	30%
soft	1 cookie	100	2	15	105	0	5.0	0.0	2	40%
w/chocolate chunks	1 cookie	100	2	17	80	0	3.0	0.0	2	26%
w/walnuts and raisins	1 cookie	100	2	16	80	0	4.0	0.0	2	33%
(Barbara's Bakery)										
raisin, minis, nonfat	6 cookies	110	2	24	105	2	0.0	0.0	0	0%
w/raisins	1 oz	100	2	19	50	0	2.0	0.0	0	18%
(Break Cake)										
	5 cookies	140	1	20	60	0	6.0	1.2	0	39%
w/creme	1 cookie	140	1	21	140	0	5.0	1.0	2	34%
(Cookietree) raisin, nonfat	1 cookie	120	2	27	110	1	0.0	0.0	0	0%
(Drake's)	2 pieces	120	2	19	50	0	4.0	1.0	0	30%
(Duncan Hines) w/raisins	2 pieces	110	1	15	85	0	5.0	2.0	0	41%
(Eagle)										
creme pie	1 cookie	310	4	46	340	2	12.0	3.0	5	35%
fudge stripe, creme pie	1 cookie	310	3	47	180	2	12.0	4.0	5	35%
'Gourmet Oatmeal Raisin Cookie'	1 cookie	330	5	40	190	4	17.0	4.0	10	46%
iced	1 cookie	170	2	28	110	1	5.0	1.0	0	27%
w/raisins	3 cookies	100	2	14	15	0	4.0	1.0	0	36%

Food Name	Serving Size	Calories	Prot. gms	Carbs gms	Sod. mgs	Fiber gms	Fat gms	Sat. Fat gms	Chol. mgs	% Fat Cal.
(Fifty 50) hearty, fructose sweetened..................	1 cookie	35	1	5	15	0	1.0	0.0	0	27%
(Frookie)										
7-grain..	1 cookie	45	1	7	35	0	2.0	0.5	0	38%
w/raisins	1 cookie	45	1	7	35	0	2.0	0.5	0	38%
w/raisins, nonfat	1 cookie	50	1	11	75	1	0.0	0.0	0	0%
(Glenny's) wheat-free, 'Noah, 'N Friends Animal'	0.5 oz	65	1	10	20	0	2.0	0.0	0	29%
(Grandma's)										
raisin, 'Big Cookies'............................	1 serving	180	2	30	240	1	6.0	1.5	3	30%
w/apple and spice, 'Big Cookies'...............	2 pieces	330	5	51	570	0	12.0	0.0	10	33%
(Health Valley)										
raisin, nonfat	1 serving	33	1	8	17	1	0.0	0.0	0	0%
w/raisins and cinnamon, nonfat, 'Fruit Chunks'	3 cookies	85	2	19	80	3	0.0	0.0	0	0%
w/raisins, nonfat	3 cookies	80	2	18	80	3	0.0	0.0	0	0%
(Keebler)										
caramel, oatmeal, w/apple, 'Elfin Delights'	1 cookie	65	1	12	55	0	2.0	1.0	0	26%
food service product, 'Old Fashioned'	1 serving	80	1	10	75	0	3.5	1.0	0	42%
raisin, 'Soft Batch'	1 serving	70	1	10	65	1	3.0	1.0	0	39%
w/caramel and apple, 50% less fat, 'Elfin Delights'	1 cookie	70	1	13	80	1	1.5	1.0	0	19%
(Little Debbie)	2.75 oz	340	5	52	440	0	12.0	0.0	2	32%
(Magic Middles) chocolate-filled	1 piece	80	1	8	30	0	5.0	1.0	0	56%
(Mother's)										
....	1 cookie	60	1	8	80	0	3.0	0.0	0	43%
iced	1 cookie	70	1	10	70	0	3.0	0.0	0	38%
w/chocolate chips	1 cookie	70	1	10	85	0	3.0	0.0	0	38%
w/walnuts and chocolate chips	1 cookie	70	1	9	60	0	3.0	0.0	0	40%
(Nabisco) w/chocolate chips, 'Selections' 'Chips Ahoy!'.....	0.5 oz piece	90	1	10	60	0	5.0	2.0	5	51%
(Natures Warehouse) w/raisins	2 cookies	135	2	17	44	0	6.4	0.0	0	43%
(Pepperidge Farm)										
'Family Request'	2 cookies	90	1	13	70	0	4.0	1.0	10	39%
w/chocolate chunks, 'Dakota'	1 piece	110	1	15	70	1	6.0	2.0	5	46%
(Raisin Ruckus)										
w/chocolate-covered raisins	1 cookie	70	1	11	70	0	3.0	1.0	0	36%
w/raisins, chewy	1 cookie	70	1	10	45	0	3.0	1.0	0	38%
(Snackwell's) oatmeal w/raisins, less fat	2 cookies	110	2	20	135	1	2.5	0.0	0	20%
(Weight Watchers) spice	3 cookies	80	1	13	75	0	2.0	0.0	0	24%
(Westbrae) 'Rice Malt Snap'	1 oz	130	2	19	130	0	5.0	0.0	0	35%
ORANGE										
(Archway) frosty, 'Home Style'	1 serving	113	1	17	94	0	4.6	1.4	0	37%
(Biscotti Thins) fat and cholesterol free, low sodium	5 cookies	80	1	20	25	0	0.0	0.0	0	0%
(Ener-G Foods) almond, gluten-free	1 cookie	74	2	9	39	1	3.7	0.4	0	44%
(Health Valley) pineapple, nonfat, 'Mini Fruit Centers'	3 cookies	75	2	17	60	3	0.0	0.0	0	0%
(Lady J.) pineapple, 100% natural....................	1 cookie	100	2	16	175	2	4.0	0.5	0	33%
PEACH										
(FFV)										
apricot, whole wheat, bar	1 piece	70	1	11	50	0	2.0	1.0	0	27%
apricot, w/vanilla, bar	1 piece	70	1	14	50	0	1.0	1.0	0	13%
(Great Cakes)	4.5 oz	260	10	40	20	21	6.0	0.0	0	21%
(Health Valley) apricot, nonfat	2 cookies	70	2	19	25	2	0.0	0.0	0	0%
(Stella D'oro)										
apricot, pastry.................................	1 piece	93	1	14	0	0	3.8	0.0	0	37%
apricot, pastry, dietetic	1 piece	87	1	12	10	0	3.7	0.0	0	38%
PEANUT										
(Archway) jumble, 'Home Style'	1 serving	116	2	13	77	1	6.2	1.6	4	48%
(Cookietree) crunchy, nonfat	1 cookie	130	3	28	100	1	0.0	0.0	0	0%

Food Name	Serving Size	Calories	Prot. gms	Carbs gms	Sod. mgs	Fiber gms	Fat gms	Sat. Fat gms	Chol. mgs	% Fat Cal.
(Health Valley) chunky, 'Fancy Peanut Chunks'	2 pieces	100	2	14	585	2	3.0	0.0	0	30%
(Nabisco) creme, 'Nutter Butter Patties'	0.5 oz	80	2	8	45	0	4.0	1.0	0	47%
PEANUT BUTTER										
(Archway)										
gourmet, old fashioned, 'Home Style'	1 serving	117	2	14	118	1	5.9	1.3	9	45%
'Home Style'	1 serving	101	2	12	85	1	5.1	1.1	8	46%
(Auburn Farms) nonfat, natural, 'P'nutty crisp'	2 cookies	90	1	19	90	2	0.0	0.0	0	0%
(Bakery Wagon) w/oatmeal	1 cookie	110	3	12	150	0	7.0	0.0	2	51%
(Break Cake)										
	1 cookie	140	2	18	110	0	7.0	1.4	0	44%
wafer, w/peanut butter	1 wafer	180	2	24	75	0	9.0	2.7	0	44%
(Delicious) made w/Skippy peanut butter	1 cookie	80	2	7	65	1	5.0	1.0	0	56%
(Eagle) bar	1 bar	170	2	19	75	1	10.0	3.0	0	52%
(Ener-G Foods) gluten-free	1 serving	94	2	11	108	1	4.6	0.8	0	43%
(Featherweight)	1 piece	40	1	5	10	0	2.0	0.0	0	43%
(Fiber Classic)	1 serving	220	3	36	320	7	9.0	2.2	0	34%
(Fifty 50) fructose-sweetened	1 cookie	40	1	5	10	0	2.0	0.0	0	43%
(Grandma's)										
'Big Cookies'	1 serving	200	4	24	200	1	10.0	2.5	10	45%
cookie bits	1 oz	140	3	19	125	0	6.0	0.0	0	38%
(Keebler) food service product, 'Old Fashioned'	1 serving	80	1	9	80	0	4.5	1.0	0	50%
(Little Debbie)										
bar	1 bar	270	4	32	190	1	15.0	3.0	0	48%
wafer, w/peanut butter, chocolate covered	1 serving	312	5	31	127	na	18.7	3.6	na	54%
(Natures Warehouse)										
	2 cookies	128	4	18	29	0	6.1	0.0	0	39%
w/chocolate chips	2 cookies	139	4	14	50	0	8.5	0.0	0	52%
(Pepperidge Farm) w/chocolate chunks, 'Cheyenne'	1 piece	110	2	13	80	1	6.0	2.0	5	47%
(Planters) crispy, 'P.B. Crisps'	1 oz	140	3	17	125	0	7.0	2.0	0	44%
(Soft Batch)										
w/chocolate chips	1 piece	80	1	9	55	0	5.0	1.0	0	53%
w/nuts	1 piece	80	1	9	60	0	4.0	1.0	0	47%
PECAN										
(Archway)										
crunch	1 piece	60	1	8	45	0	3.0	0.0	5	43%
iced, 'Home Style'	1 serving	120	1	15	75	0	6.3	1.4	6	47%
(FFV) praline	1 piece	40	1	10	40	0	2.0	1.0	5	29%
(Keebler)										
shortbread, less fat, 'Sandies'	1 serving	70	1	10	50	0	3.0	0.5	0	38%
shortbread, rich, 'Sandies'	1 serving	80	1	9	75	1	5.0	1.0	3	54%
(Pepperidge Farm)										
chunk, 'Chesapeake'	1 piece	120	1	14	60	1	7.0	2.0	5	51%
chunk, 'Special Collection'	1 piece	70	0	8	25	0	4.0	1.0	10	53%
PRUNE (Stella D'oro) pastry, dietetic	1 piece	95	1	15	10	2	3.4	0.0	0	32%
RAISIN										
(Almost Home)	0.5 oz piece	70	1	10	40	0	3.0	1.0	2	38%
(Archway)	1 piece	100	2	18	107	1	3.0	0.0	5	25%
(Entenmann's) nonfat	2 pieces	80	1	17	120	0	0.0	0.0	0	0%
(Featherweight)	1 piece	45	1	6	0	0	2.0	0.0	0	39%
(Grandma's) soft, 'Big Cookies'	2 pieces	320	3	54	280	0	10.0	0.0	10	28%
(Health Valley)										
jumbo, nonfat	1 serving	80	2	19	35	3	0.0	0.0	0	0%
w/nuts, 'Fruit Jumbos'	1 piece	70	2	10	35	1	3.0	0.0	0	36%
(Keebler) iced, bar	1 piece	80	1	11	85	0	4.0	1.0	0	43%

Food Name	Serving Size	Calories	Prot. gms	Carbs gms	Sod. mgs	Fiber gms	Fat gms	Sat. Fat gms	Chol. mgs	% Fat Cal.
(Mother's) iced	1 cookie	80	1	11	45	0	4.0	0.0	0	43%
(Pepperidge Farm)										
'Old Fashioned'	2 pieces	110	1	15	115	0	5.0	2.0	10	41%
'Santa Fe'	1 piece	100	1	16	70	1	4.0	1.0	5	35%
w/bran, 'Kitchen Hearth'	2 pieces	110	1	13	55	0	5.0	2.0	5	45%
(Soft Batch)	1 piece	70	1	10	65	0	3.0	1.0	0	38%
(Stella D'oro) 'Golden Bars'	1 piece	109	2	16	0	0	4.3	0.0	0	35%
(Sunshine)										
. . . .	2 pieces	110	1	16	125	0	5.0	1.0	0	40%
'Golden Fruit'	1 serving	80	1	15	50	1	1.5	0.5	0	17%
(Tastykake)										
bar	1.8 oz	212	3	32	255	1	8.3	2.2	17	35%
'Soft'n Chewy'	1.4 oz	161	3	27	158	1	5.4	1.0	3	29%
(Weight Watchers) w/spice	3 cookies	80	1	13	75	0	2.0	0.0	0	24%
RASPBERRY										
(Archway) filled, 'Home Style'	1 serving	101	1	16	84	0	3.5	1.4	7	31%
(Bakery Wagon) filled	1 cookie	90	1	16	125	0	3.0	0.0	2	28%
(Frookie) nonfat, 'Fruitins'	2 cookies	90	1	21	75	1	0.0	0.0	0	0%
(Great Cakes)	4.5 oz	260	10	40	20	21	6.0	0.0	0	21%
(Health Valley)										
center, nonfat	1 serving	70	2	18	20	2	0.0	0.0	0	0%
jumbo, nonfat	1 serving	80	2	19	35	3	0.0	0.0	0	0%
(Nabisco) nonfat, 'Newton's'	2 cookies	100	1	23	115	1	0.0	0.0	0	0%
(Natural Nectar) swirl, 'Incredible Edible Novelties'	1 cookie	220	4	33	115	0	8.0	0.0	20	33%
(Natures Warehouse)										
all natural, nonfat	1 cookie	80	2	19	60	1	0.0	0.0	0	0%
wheat-free, nonfat	1 cookie	80	2	19	60	1	0.0	0.0	0	0%
(Pepperidge Farm)										
filled, 'Chantilly'	1 piece	80	1	14	35	0	2.0	1.0	5	23%
filled, w/chocolate, 'Chantilly'	1 piece	90	1	14	35	0	3.0	1.0	5	31%
tart, lowfat, 'Wholesome Choice'	1 cookie	60	1	11	35	0	1.0	1.0	0	16%
(Weight Watchers) filled	1 serving	70	1	16	45	0	0.0	0.0	0	0%
SANDWICH										
(Break Cake) apple	1 cookie	90	1	15	70	0	3.0	0.5	5	30%
(Delicious) peanut butter, w/jelly, 'Skippy & Welchs'	1 cookie	120	2	15	90	1	6.0	1.5	0	44%
(Ener-G Foods) lemon, gluten-free	1 serving	194	0	30	55	2	8.2	2.2	0	38%
(Estee)										
chocolate	1 cookie	50	1	7	15	0	2.0	1.0	0	36%
original	2 cookies	110	1	17	25	0	4.0	1.0	0	33%
vanilla	2 cookies	110	1	17	20	0	4.0	1.0	0	33%
w/peanut butter	1 cookie	50	1	5	35	0	3.0	1.0	0	53%
(FFV)										
mint	2 pieces	160	2	22	50	0	7.0	0.0	0	40%
w/peanut butter	2 pieces	170	2	21	110	0	8.0	0.0	0	44%
(Frookie)										
chocolate, 'Frookwich'	1 cookie	50	1	7	30	0	2.0	0.0	0	36%
chocolate, w/vanilla filling, 'Frookwich'	1 cookie	50	1	7	30	0	2.0	0.0	0	36%
lemon, 'Frookwich'	1 cookie	50	1	7	30	0	2.0	0.0	0	36%
vanilla, 'Frookwich'	1 cookie	50	1	7	30	0	2.0	0.0	0	36%
w/peanut butter, 'Frookwich'	1 cookie	50	1	7	30	0	2.0	0.0	0	36%
(Great Cakes) peanut butter, w/jelly	4.5 oz	280	10	40	20	21	8.0	0.0	0	26%
(Keebler)										
butter flavor, w/fudge creme, 'E.L. Fudge'	3 cookies	170	2	24	105	1	8.0	2.0	5	41%
chocolate, 'E.L. Fudge'	1 cookie	70	1	9	50	0	3.0	1.0	0	40%

Food Name	Serving Size	Calories	Prot. gms	Carbs gms	Sod. mgs	Fiber gms	Fat gms	Sat. Fat gms	Chol. mgs	% Fat Cal.
chocolate, w/chocolate filling, 'E.L. Fudge'	1 cookie	60	1	8	35	0	3.0	1.0	5	43%
chocolate, w/fudge creme, 'Elfin Delights'	1 cookie	55	1	10	50	0	2.0	1.0	0	29%
chocolate, w/fudge creme, 50% less fat, 'Elfin Delights'	3 cookies	150	2	27	135	1	3.5	1.0	0	21%
chocolate, w/peanut butter, 'E.L. Fudge'	1 cookie	50	1	7	50	0	3.0	1.0	0	46%
chocolate, w/vanilla creme, 'E.L. Fudge'	3 cookies	170	2	23	125	1	8.0	2.0	0	42%
chocolate, w/vanilla creme, 50% less fat, 'Elfin Delights'	3 cookies	150	2	26	170	1	3.5	1.0	0	22%
chocolate-filled sandwich creme, 50% less fat, 'Elfin Delights'	3 cookies	150	1	27	125	1	3.5	1.0	0	22%
fudge 'E.L. Fudge'	3 cookies	160	2	23	100	1	7.0	2.0	0	39%
fudge, food service product	1 serving	80	1	12	70	0	3.5	1.0	0	38%
less fat, 'Elfin Delights'	2 cookies	110	1	19	100	1	2.5	0.5	0	22%
praline cream, 'Sandies'	1 cookie	80	1	9	35	0	6.0	1.5	0	57%
vanilla, French, 'Classic Collection'	1 serving	80	1	12	65	0	3.5	1.0	0	38%
vanilla, French, food service product	1 serving	80	1	12	85	0	3.5	1.0	0	38%
(Little Debbie) chocolate	1.8 oz	250	3	35	260	0	12.0	0.0	1	42%
(Mother's)										
duplex	2 cookies	105	1	15	70	0	5.0	0.0	0	41%
English tea	1 cookie	100	1	14	60	0	4.0	0.0	0	38%
fudge, double	2 cookies	100	2	15	75	0	4.0	0.0	0	35%
taffy	1 cookie	100	1	12	60	0	6.0	0.0	0	51%
w/peanut butter, 'Gaucho'	1 cookie	90	1	12	75	0	5.0	0.0	0	46%
(Nabisco)										
chocolate, w/creme filling, 'Big Stuf Oreo'	0.25-oz piece	200	2	27	220	1	9.0	3.0	5	41%
chocolate, w/creme filling, 'Oreo'	1 oz	140	1	20	170	0	6.0	0.0	0	39%
peanut butter, 'Nutter Butter'	0.5-oz piece	70	1	9	50	0	3.0	1.0	0	40%
vanilla, w/creme, 'Cameo'	0.5-oz piece	70	1	10	50	0	3.0	0.0	0	38%
vanilla, w/vanilla creme, 'Cameo'	0.5-oz piece	70	1	10	50	0	3.0	1.0	0	38%
vanilla, w/vanilla creme, 'Cookie Break'	1 piece	50	1	7	35	0	2.0	0.0	0	36%
vanilla, w/vanilla creme, 'Giggles'	2 cookies	60	1	8	20	0	3.0	1.0	2	43%
(Pepperidge Farm)										
butter, chocolate filled, 'Brussels'	2 cookies	110	1	13	65	0	5.0	2.0	0	45%
butter, chocolate filled, 'Double Chocolate Milano'	2 cookies	150	2	18	45	0	8.0	3.0	10	47%
butter, chocolate filled, 'Hazelnut Milano'	2 cookies	130	2	15	30	0	8.0	2.0	5	51%
butter, chocolate filled, 'Lido'	1 cookie	90	1	10	30	0	5.0	1.0	5	51%
butter, chocolate filled, 'Milano'	2 cookies	120	1	15	45	0	6.0	2.0	5	46%
butter, chocolate filled, 'Orleans'	2 cookies	120	1	14	40	0	8.0	2.0	0	55%
butter, chocolate mint filled, 'Brussels Mint'	2 cookies	130	1	17	40	0	7.0	2.0	0	47%
butter, chocolate mint filled, 'Mint Milano'	2 cookies	150	1	17	60	0	7.0	2.0	5	47%
butter, chocolate orange filled, 'Orange Milano'	2 cookies	150	1	17	60	0	7.0	2.0	5	47%
(Pitter Patter) peanut butter, cream filled	1 cookie	90	2	12	115	0	4.0	1.0	0	39%
(Tastykake) shortbread, w/vanilla creme	0.4 oz	55	1	6	31	0	3.0	0.7	0	49%
SESAME										
(Glenny's) bite size, 'Nookie'	0.5 oz	60	1	6	8	0	4.0	0.0	0	56%
(Stella D'oro)										
dietetic, 'Regina'	1 piece	41	1	5	10	0	2.0	0.0	0	43%
'Regina'	1 piece	48	1	6	0	0	2.2	0.0	0	41%
SHORTBREAD										
(Archway) sugarless, 'Home Style'	1 serving	107	1	16	47	0	5.4	1.3	0	45%
(Break Cake)	5 cookies	140	1	19	70	0	6.0	1.1	5	40%
(Ener-G Foods) lemon, gluten-free	1 serving	110	0	16	18	4	5.0	1.2	0	41%
(FFV) country style	1 piece	70	1	9	45	0	4.0	1.0	5	47%

Food Name	Serving Size	Calories	Prot. gms	Carbs gms	Sod. mgs	Fiber gms	Fat gms	Sat. Fat gms	Chol. mgs	% Fat Cal.
(Keebler)										
fudge-covered, 'Toffee Toppers'	2 cookies	60	1	10	50	0	4.0	3.0	0	45%
pecan, bite size, 'Sandies'	4 cookies	90	1	9	50	0	5.0	1.0	5	53%
pecan, 'Sandies'	1 piece	80	1	9	75	0	5.0	1.0	5	53%
toffee, "Sandies"	2 cookies	130	1	16	90	1	7.0	2.0	1	48%
w/toffee pieces, 'Sandies'	1 cookie	70	1	8	45	0	4.0	1.0	0	50%
(Magic Middles) w/chocolate center	1 piece	80	1	9	25	0	5.0	1.0	5	53%
(Mother's) striped	2 cookies	100	1	14	55	0	5.0	0.0	0	43%
(Nabisco)										
fudge-striped, 'Cookies 'n Fudge'	0.5 oz piece	60	1	7	50	0	3.0	1.0	0	46%
pecan, supreme, low-cholesterol	1 cookie	80	1	9	45	0	5.0	1.0	2	53%
(Pepperidge Farm) pecan, 'Old Fashioned'	1 piece	70	1	7	15	0	5.0	2.0	0	58%
SPICE										
(Stella D'oro) drops, 'Pfeffernusse'	1 piece	35	1	7	0	0	0.8	0.0	0	20%
(Westbrae) 5-spice wafer	4 1/2 wafers	40	1	8	30	0	0.0	0.0	0	0%
STRAWBERRY										
(Archway) filled, 'Home Style'	1 serving	100	1	16	84	0	3.5	1.4	7	31%
(Health Valley) nonfat, 'Mini Fruit Centers'	3 cookies	75	2	17	60	3	0.0	0.0	0	0%
(Healthy Times) organic, 'Hugga Bears'	1 oz	120	2	17	38	0	3.0	0.0	0	26%
(Little Debbie) fruits	1 cookie	130	1	33	105	1	0.0	0.0	0	0%
(Nabisco) nonfat, 'Newton's'	2 cookies	100	1	23	115	1	0.0	0.0	0	0%
(Natural Nectar) swirl, 'Incredible Edible Novelties'	1 cookie	220	4	33	115	0	8.0	0.0	20	33%
(Suddenly S'Mores)	0.75-oz piece	100	1	15	90	0	4.0	2.0	0	36%
SUGAR										
(Almost Home) 'Old Fashioned'	0.5 oz piece	70	1	10	80	0	3.0	1.0	2	38%
(Archway)										
'Home Style'	1 serving	98	1	17	162	0	3.1	0.8	5	28%
nonfat, 'Home Style'	1 serving	71	1	17	80	0	0.2	0.1	0	2%
(Cookietree) butter, 'Thaw & Serve'	1 cookie	120	2	18	120	0	4.5	1.0	10	34%
(Ener-G Foods) crisp, gluten-free	1 serving	93	3	14	218	2	3.1	0.8	2	30%
(Keebler) food service product, 'Old Fashioned'	1 serving	80	1	10	45	0	4.0	1.0	0	45%
(Mother's)	1 cookie	70	1	8	35	0	4.0	0.0	0	50%
(Pepperidge Farm) cinnamon, 'Family Request'	2 cookies	80	1	12	40	0	4.0	1.0	15	41%
SUGAR WAFER										
(Break Cake) strawberry	4 wafers	220	1	28	100	0	11.0	3.1	0	46%
(Delicious)										
chocolate, w/strawberry creme	1 wafer	35	1	3	4	0	2.0	0.0	0	53%
lemon	1 wafer	35	1	4	3	0	2.0	0.0	0	47%
strawberry	1 wafer	35	1	4	3	0	2.0	0.0	0	47%
vanilla w/strawberry	1 wafer	35	1	4	3	0	2.0	0.0	0	47%
(Estee)										
chocolate, w/chocolate creme	4 wafers	90	1	11	0	0	5.0	1.0	0	48%
strawberry	3 wafers	100	1	14	0	0	5.0	1.0	0	43%
vanilla	3 wafers	100	1	14	0	0	5.0	1.0	0	43%
w/vanilla creme	4 wafers	90	1	12	0	0	4.0	1.0	0	41%
(Featherweight)										
chocolate, w/chocolate creme	1 piece	20	0	3	0	0	1.0	0.0	0	43%
peanut butter	1 piece	25	1	3	0	0	1.0	0.0	0	36%
w/strawberry cream	1 piece	20	0	3	0	0	1.0	0.0	0	43%
w/vanilla creme	1 piece	20	0	3	0	0	1.0	0.0	0	43%
(Fifty 50)										
chocolate, cream filled, sugarless	1 wafer	35	1	4	10	0	2.0	0.0	0	47%
w/vanilla creme filled, sugarless	1 wafer	35	1	4	5	0	2.0	0.0	0	47%
(Tastykake) vanilla	10 pieces	34	0	4	11	0	1.9	0.5	0	49%

Food Name	Serving Size	Calories	Prot. gms	Carbs gms	Sod. mgs	Fiber gms	Fat gms	Sat. Fat gms	Chol. mgs	% Fat Cal.
TEA BISCUIT (Nabisco) 'Social Tea'	0.5 oz	60	1	11	60	0	2.0	0.0	5	27%
TOFFEE										
(Delicious) w/Heath English toffee	1 cookie	90	1	10	45	1	5.0	1.0	8	51%
(Nabisco) Heath chunk, 'Selections' 'Chips Ahoy!'	1 piece	90	1	5	85	0	5.0	2.0	5	65%
(Pepperidge Farm) 'Old Fashioned'	2 pieces	100	1	12	75	0	5.0	2.0	5	46%
TOFU (Health Valley) 'The Great Tofu Cookie'	2 pieces	90	2	16	29	1	3.0	0.0	0	27%
VANILLA										
(Archway) wafer	1 piece	30	0	6	30	0	1.0	0.0	0	27%
(Biscotti Thins) fat- and cholesterol-free, low sodium	5 cookies	80	1	20	25	0	0.0	0.0	0	0%
(Break Cake) wafer	4 wafers	220	1	28	105	0	11.0	3.7	0	46%
(Delicious) wafer	1 wafer	35	1	4	3	0	2.0	0.0	0	47%
(Estee)	3 cookies	100	1	14	15	0	5.0	1.0	0	43%
(Featherweight)	1 piece	45	1	6	0	0	2.0	0.0	0	39%
(FFV) wafer	8 cookies	130	1	19	100	0	5.0	1.0	5	36%
(Fiber Classic) 'Original'	1 serving	210	3	37	280	0	8.0	2.2	0	31%
(Frookie) 'Funky Monkeys'	8 cookies	60	1	10	60	0	2.0	0.0	0	29%
(Glenny's) 'Noah, 'N Friends Animal Cookies'	0.5 oz	65	1	10	35	0	2.0	0.0	0	29%
(Keebler)										
wafer, 'Keebler Golden'	1 serving	147	2	22	120	na	6.0	1.1	na	37%
wafer, golden, 30% less fat	8 wafers	130	2	25	140	1	3.5	0.5	0	23%
(Mother's) wafer, 'Flaky Flix'	2 cookies	115	1	18	25	0	5.0	0.0	0	37%
(Nabisco)										
wafer, 'Nilla Wafers'	3 1/2 cookies	60	1	11	45	0	2.0	1.0	5	27%
wafer, w/cinnamon, 'Nilla Wafers'	3 1/2 cookies	60	1	11	45	0	2.0	1.0	5	27%
(Pepperidge Farm)										
chocolate nut coated, 'Geneva'	2 pieces	130	1	14	50	0	6.0	2.0	0	47%
chocolate-coated, 'Orleans'	3 pieces	90	0	11	30	0	6.0	2.0	0	55%
chocolate-laced, 'Pirouettes'	2 pieces	70	1	8	20	0	4.0	1.0	5	50%
'Goldfish'	1 oz	140	2	19	50	0	7.0	2.0	15	43%
'Pirouettes'	2 pieces	70	0	9	35	0	4.0	1.0	5	50%
(Stella D'oro)										
'Castelets'	1 piece	72	1	10	0	0	3.1	0.0	0	39%
'Margherite'	1 piece	72	1	11	0	0	2.8	0.0	0	35%
VANILLA CHIP (Mrs. Denson's) macaroon	2 cookies	150	2	14	30	2	11.0	6.0	0	61%
WALNUT										
(Archway) black, ice box, 'Home Style'	1 serving	119	1	15	77	0	6.2	1.4	10	46%
(Mother's) w/fudge	1 cookie	70	1	8	50	0	4.0	0.0	0	50%
(Soft Batch)	1 piece	80	1	10	70	0	4.0	1.0	0	45%
WHOLE WHEAT (Lu) w/cinnamon, 'Marie Lu'	1 cookie	45	1	8	55	0	1.0	0.0	0	20%
COOKIE CRUMB TOPPING										
(Nabisco) 'Oreo Crunchies'	1 serving	52	1	8	58	0	2.4	0.5	na	41%
COOKIE CRUMBS										
graham cracker (Sunshine)	3 tbsp	80	2	13	150	1	2.0	0.5	0	23%
graham cracker, food service product (Keebler)	1 cup	550	8	81	480	3	23.0	5.0	0	37%
'Nilla' (Nabisco)	2 tbsp	70	1	13	55	1	2.5	0.5	3	29%
'Oreo' (Nabisco)	2 tbsp	80	1	13	140	1	3.0	0.5	0	33%
COOKIE DOUGH										
(Pillsbury)										
dinosaurs, ready to bake, prepared	2 cookies	120	2	17	95	1	5.0	1.5	5	37%
holiday, ready to bake, prepared	2 cookies	130	1	16	105	0	7.0	2.0	5	48%
teddy bears, ready to bake, prepared	2 cookies	120	1	18	105	0	5.0	1.0	5	37%
CANDY (Pillsbury) ready to bake	1 oz	130	1	18	80	1	6.0	2.0	5	42%
CHOCOLATE CHIP										
(Mrs. Goodcookie) gourmet, ready to bake, prepared	2 cookies	120	1	15	80	0	6.0	2.0	0	46%

Food Name	Serving Size	Calories	Prot. gms	Carbs gms	Sod. mgs	Fiber gms	Fat gms	Sat. Fat gms	Chol. mgs	% Fat Cal.
(Nestlé) ready to bake	2 tbsp	150	2	23	120	1	6.0	2.0	10	35%
(Pillsbury)										
. . . . .	1 serving	127	1	18	88	1	5.7	1.8	na	40%
ready to bake, prepared	1 cookie	70	1	9	55	0	3.0	1.0	5	40%
(Toll House)										
double chips	1.2 oz	150	2	19	60	0	7.0	0.0	0	43%
ready to bake	1.2 oz	150	1	20	115	0	7.0	0.0	0	43%
w/nuts, ready to bake	1.2 oz	160	2	19	90	0	8.0	0.0	0	46%
CHOCOLATE CHOCOLATE CHIP *(Nestlé)*	2 tbsp	150	2	21	110	2	6.0	2.0	10	37%
OATMEAL										
(Nestlé) w/Raisinets	2 tbsp	150	2	22	120	2	6.0	2.0	10	36%
(Pillsbury)										
w/chocolate chips, ready to bake	1 oz	120	1	16	95	1	6.0	1.5	5	44%
w/raisins, prepared	1 cookie	60	1	9	55	0	3.0	1.0	0	40%
(Toll House) w/raisins, ready to bake	1.2 oz	130	2	21	55	0	5.0	0.0	0	33%
PEANUT BUTTER *(Pillsbury)* prepared	1 cookie	70	1	9	75	0	3.0	1.0	5	40%
COOKIE MIX										
(Krusteaz) 'Deluxe' prepared	1 cookie	120	1	16	126	0	5.0	0.0	11	40%
CHOCOLATE CHIP										
(Big Batch) prepared	2 cookies	120	1	16	100	0	6.0	0.0	0	44%
(Duncan Hines) prepared	2 cookies	130	1	20	85	0	5.0	0.0	0	35%
(Estee) prepared	2 cookies	90	1	13	80	0	4.0	1.0	0	39%
(Finast) prepared	2 cookies	110	1	16	290	0	5.0	0.0	0	40%
(Gluten-Free Pantry) gluten-free, prepared	1 serving	60	1	12	50	0	1.0	0.5	0	15%
(Pillsbury)										
bar, 'Chips Ahoy' mix only	1/18 pkg	140	1	26	100	1	4.0	1.5	0	25%
bar, 'Chips Ahoy' prepared	1/18 pkg	180	2	26	125	1	7.0	2.0	10	36%
(Sweet 'n Low) low-fat, w/'Sweet 'n Low, prepared	4 cookies	120	2	22	30	0	2.5	0.5	0	19%
DATE *(Betty Crocker)* bar, prepared	1 serving	150	1	23	90	1	6.0	2.0	0	36%
OATMEAL *(Duncan Hines)* w/raisins, prepared	2 cookies	130	2	18	70	0	6.0	0.0	0	40%
PEANUT BUTTER *(Duncan Hines)* prepared	2 cookies	140	3	15	120	0	7.0	0.0	0	47%
SUGAR										
(Duncan Hines) golden, prepared	2 cookies	130	1	17	70	0	6.0	0.0	0	43%
(Gluten-free Pantry) gluten-free, prepared	1 serving	130	1	31	130	0	0.0	0.0	0	0%
COOKING OIL. See individual listings.										
COOKING SPRAY										
(Canola Harvest) Canola, nonstick	0.25 grams	0	0	0	0	0	0.0	0.0	0	0%
(I Can't Believe It's Not Butter)	1 spray	0	0	0	0	0	0.0	0.0	0	0%
(Mazola)										
corn oil	2.5-sec spray	6	0	0	0	0	1.0	0.1	0	100%
corn oil	1 tsp	2	0	0	0	0	0.2	0.0	0	100%
(Pam)										
. . . . .	1 serving	0	0	0	0	0	0.0	0.0	0	0%
butter-flavored	1 serving	0	0	0	0	0	0.0	0.0	0	0%
olive oil	1 serving	0	0	0	0	0	0.0	0.0	0	0%
(Town House) Canola oil	0.25 grams	0	0	0	0	0	0.0	0.0	0	0%
(Weight Watchers)										
. . . . .	1-sec spray	2	0	0	0	0	1.0	0.0	0	100%
butter flavor, 'Buttery Spray'	1 spray	2	0	0	0	0	1.0	0.0	0	100%
Canola oil	0.33 grams	2	0	0	0	0	1.0	0.0	0	100%
(Wesson)										
. . . . .	0.25 grams	2	0	0	0	0	0.3	0.0	0	100%
lite	0.27 grams	1	0	0	0	0	1.0	0.0	0	100%

COOKING WINE. See WINE, COOKING.

Food Name	Serving Size	Calories	Prot. gms	Carbs gms	Sod. mgs	Fiber gms	Fat gms	Sat. Fat gms	Chol. mgs	% Fat Cal.
CORIANDER LEAF / Chinese parsley leaf										
dried	1 tbsp	5	0	1	4	0	0.1	0.0	0	14%
dried	1 tsp	2	0	0	1	0	0.0	0.0	0	15%
dried *(Tone's)*	1 tsp	2	0	0	1	0	0.1	0.0	0	36%
fresh, raw, chopped	1/4 cup	1	0	0	1	0	0.0	0.0	0	25%
fresh, raw, whole, med plants	9 plants	4	0	1	6	0	0.1	0.0	0	25%
CORIANDER SEED / Chinese parsley seed										
round *(McCormick/Schilling)*	1 tsp	7	0	1	0	1	0.4	0.0	0	43%
whole	1 tbsp	15	1	3	2	2	0.9	0.1	0	50%
whole	1 tsp	5	0	1	1	1	0.3	0.0	0	50%
whole *(Durkee)* whole seeds	1 tsp	8	0	0	0	0	0.0	0.0	0	0%
whole *(Laurel Leaf)* whole seeds	1 tsp	8	0	0	0	0	0.0	0.0	0	0%
whole *(McCormick/Schilling)*	1 tsp	12	0	2	1	2	0.4	0.0	0	31%
whole *(Spice Islands)*	1 tsp	6	0	1	1	0	0.3	0.1	0	40%
CORN. See also CORN DISH/ENTRÉE.										
Canned										
(Del Monte)	1/2 cup	90	3	22	355	0	1.0	0.0	0	8%
'Crisp 'N Sweet' *(Freshlike)*	1/2 cup	80	2	18	5	0	1.0	0.0	0	10%
'Crisp 'N Sweet' *(Stokely)*	1/2 cup	80	2	13	240	2	1.5	0.0	0	18%
'Delicorn' *(Green Giant)*	1/2 cup	80	2	19	350	2	1.0	0.0	0	10%
50% less sodium, 'Niblets' *(Green Giant)*	1/3 cup	60	2	14	115	1	0.0	0.0	0	0%
in brine, w/liquid *(Green Giant)*	1/2 cup	70	2	18	350	2	0.0	0.0	0	0%
kernels, extra sweet, 'Niblets' *(Green Giant)*	1/3 cup	50	2	10	200	2	0.5	0.0	0	9%
kernels, 'Niblets' *(Green Giant)*	1/2 cup	80	2	20	310	2	0.0	0.0	0	0%
kernels, w/liquid *(A&P)*	1/2 cup	80	2	20	350	0	1.0	0.0	0	9%
kernels, w/liquid *(Featherweight)*	1/2 cup	80	2	16	10	0	1.0	0.0	0	11%
kernels, w/liquid *(Finast)*	1/2 cup	90	2	20	390	0	1.0	0.0	0	9%
kernels, w/liquid *(Green Giant)*	1/2 cup	80	2	18	280	3	0.0	0.0	0	0%
kernels, w/liquid, 50% less salt, no sugar *(Green Giant)*	1/2 cup	50	2	11	140	2	1.0	0.0	0	15%
kernels, w/liquid, 'No Frills' *(Pathmark)*	1 cup	160	5	38	550	0	1.0	0.0	0	5%
kernels, w/liquid, 'No Salt Added' *(A&P)*	1/2 cup	80	2	18	10	0	1.0	0.0	0	10%
kernels, w/liquid, 'No Salt Added' *(Finast)*	1/2 cup	80	3	19	10	0	1.0	0.0	0	9%
kernels, w/liquid, 'No Salt Added' *(Pathmark)*	1/2 cup	70	2	16	10	0	1.0	0.0	0	11%
kernels, w/liquid, 'Nutradiet' *(S&W)*	1/2 cup	80	2	15	0	0	1.0	0.0	0	12%
no salt or sugar added, 'Niblets' *(Green Giant)*	1/2 cup	80	2	18	0	2	1.0	0.0	0	10%
sweet *(TenderSweet)*	1/2 cup	100	2	20	340	1	1.0	0.0	0	9%
sweet, select *(Green Giant)*	1/2 cup	60	2	15	280	3	1.0	0.0	0	12%
vacuum pack, w/liquid, 'No Salt Added' *(Del Monte)*	1/2 cup	90	3	22	10	0	1.0	0.0	0	8%
Dried, approx 4 oz prepared *(John Cope's)*	1 oz	101	3	21	0	0	1.2	0.0	0	10%
Freeze-Dried, prepared *(Mountain House)*	1/2 cup	90	2	18	1	0	1.0	0.0	0	10%
Frozen										
(Health Valley)	1/2 cup	76	2	17	4	2	0.0	0.0	0	0%
kernels *(Finast)*	3.3 oz	80	3	20	5	0	1.0	0.0	0	9%
kernels, cut *(Frosty Acres)*	3.3 oz	80	3	20	3	1	1.0	0.0	0	9%
kernels, cut *(Seabrook)*	3.3 oz	80	3	20	3	1	1.0	0.0	0	9%
kernels, cut *(Southern)*	3.5 oz	98	3	21	20	0	0.7	0.0	0	6%
kernels, cut, petite, 'Deluxe' *(Birds Eye)*	2.6 oz	70	2	16	0	2	1.0	0.0	0	11%
kernels, cut, 'Portion Pack' *(Birds Eye)*	3 oz	70	3	18	0	2	1.0	0.0	0	10%
kernels, cut, 'Portion Pack' *(Birds Eye)*	3 oz	70	3	18	0	2	1.0	0.0	0	10%
kernels, cut, 'Singles' *(Stokely)*	3 oz	75	3	18	5	0	1.0	0.0	0	10%
kernels, cut, whole *(Flav-R-Pac)*	2/3 cup	80	3	19	10	1	1.0	0.0	0	9%
on the cob, half ears, 'Sweet Select' *(Green Giant)*	2 half-ears	90	3	19	10	2	2.0	0.0	0	17%
kernels, harvest fresh, 'Niblets' *(Green Giant)*	1/2 cup	80	2	17	40	2	1.0	0.0	0	11%

Food Name	Serving Size	Calories	Prot. gms	Carbs gms	Sod. mgs	Fiber gms	Fat gms	Sat. Fat gms	Chol. mgs	% Fat Cal.
kernels, 'Niblets' (Green Giant)	1/2 cup	90	2	19	5	2	1.0	0.0	0	10%
kernels, plain polybag, 'Nibblers' (Green Giant)	1 ear	70	2	14	5	1	0.5	0.0	0	7%
kernels, plain polybag, 'Niblets' (Green Giant)	1/2 cup	90	2	19	5	2	1.0	0.0	0	10%
kernels, supersweet, 'Niblets' (Green Giant)	1/2 cup	60	2	13	5	2	1.0	0.0	0	13%
kernels, 'Sweet' (Birds Eye)	3.3 oz	80	3	20	0	2	1.0	0.0	0	9%
kernels, 'Tender Sweet Deluxe' (Birds Eye)	3.3 oz	80	3	20	0	2	1.0	0.0	0	9%
on the cob (A&P)	1 ear	120	4	28	0	0	1.0	0.0	0	7%
on the cob (Birds Eye)	1 ear	120	4	29	0	0	1.0	0.0	0	6%
on the cob (Frosty Acres)	1 ear	120	4	29	0	0	1.0	0.0	0	6%
on the cob (Ore-Ida)	1 ear	180	5	39	40	0	2.0	0.0	0	9%
on the cob, baby, 'Deluxe' (Birds Eye)	2.6 oz	25	2	4	10	2	0.0	0.0	0	0%
on the cob, 'Big Ears' (Birds Eye)	1 ear	160	5	37	0	0	1.0	0.0	0	5%
on the cob, 'Cob Treats' (A&P)	2 ears	130	5	28	5	0	1.0	0.0	0	6%
on the cob, 5-inch ear (Seabrook)	1 ear	120	4	29	4	1	1.0	0.0	0	6%
on the cob, 5-inch ear (Southern)	1 ear	140	5	30	0	0	1.0	0.0	0	6%
on the cob, 'Little Ears' (Birds Eye)	2 ears	130	4	30	0	0	1.0	0.0	0	6%
on the cob, miniature, 'Mini-Gold' (Ore-Ida)	2 ears	180	5	39	40	0	2.0	0.0	0	9%
on the cob, mini-cob (Superior Pride)	1 ear	80	3	18	10	1	1.0	0.0	0	10%
on the cob, mini-cob (Trader Joe's)	1/2 cup	90	3	20	230	2	0.5	0.0	0	5%
on the cob, 'Niblet Ears' (Green Giant)	1 ear	120	4	27	10	2	1.0	0.0	0	7%
on the cob, 'One Serving' (Green Giant)	2 half-ears	120	4	26	10	2	1.0	1.0	0	7%
on the cob, 'Plain Polybag' (Green Giant)	1 ear	120	4	22	0	3	2.0	0.0	0	15%
on the cob, 6-ear pkg, 'Nibblers' (Green Giant)	2 ears	120	4	27	10	2	1.0	0.0	0	7%
on the cob, supersweet, 'Nibblers' (Green Giant)	2 ears	90	3	19	10	2	2.0	0.0	0	17%
on the cob, supersweet, 'Niblet Ears' (Green Giant)	1 ear	90	3	19	10	2	2.0	0.0	0	17%
on the cob, sweet, no salt added, mini-cob (TenderSweet)	1/2 cup	80	2	19	5	0	1.0	0.0	0	10%
on the cob, sweet, unprepared, med ears	1 ear	123	4	29	6	4	1.0	0.1	0	7%
on the cob, 'Sweet Select' (Green Giant)	1 ear	90	3	19	10	2	2.0	0.0	0	17%
sweet (Birds Eye)	3.3 oz	80	3	20	0	2	1.0	0.0	0	9%
sweet, petite, 'Early Harvest' (C&W)	2/3 cup	80	3	19	10	1	1.0	0.0	0	9%
sweet, select, 'Plain Polybag' (Green Giant)	1/2 cup	60	2	13	5	2	1.0	0.0	0	13%
sweet, tender, 'Deluxe' (Birds Eye)	3.3 oz	80	3	20	0	2	1.0	0.0	0	9%
GOLD AND WHITE, canned (Stokely)	1/2 cup	60	2	10	250	2	1.5	0.0	0	22%
GOLDEN										
Canned										
(Pathmark)	1/2 cup	90	2	19	330	0	1.0	0.0	0	10%
(Stokely)	1/2 cup	90	2	20	300	0	0.0	0.0	0	0%
50% less salt (Green Giant)	1/2 cup	70	2	16	175	2	1.0	0.0	0	11%
kernels (Veg-All)	1/2 cup	80	2	19	320	0	1.0	0.0	0	10%
kernels, sweet (Green Giant)	1/2 cup	70	2	18	360	2	0.0	0.0	0	0%
kernels, sweet, 50% less salt (Green Giant)	1/2 cup	70	2	16	180	2	1.0	0.0	0	11%
kernels, vacuum packed (Freshlike)	1/2 cup	100	3	22	260	0	1.0	0.0	0	8%
kernels, vacuum packed (Veg-All)	1/2 cup	100	3	22	260	0	1.0	0.0	0	8%
kernels, water pack, w/o salt (Freshlike)	1/2 cup	80	2	19	5	0	1.0	0.0	0	10%
kernels, water pack, w/o sugar, salt (Freshlike)	1/2 cup	80	2	19	5	0	1.0	0.0	0	10%
no salt added (Del Monte)	1/2 cup	80	2	18	10	0	1.0	0.0	0	10%
no salt or sugar added (Green Giant)	1/2 cup	80	3	18	0	2	1.0	0.0	0	10%
no salt or sugar added (Stokely)	1/2 cup	80	2	16	5	0	0.0	0.0	0	0%
'Pantry Express' (Green Giant)	1/2 cup	80	2	18	210	1	1.0	0.0	0	10%
vacuum-packed (Green Giant)	1/2 cup	80	2	20	330	2	0.0	0.0	0	0%
vacuum-packed (Stokely)	1/2 cup	90	3	22	300	0	0.0	0.0	0	0%
w/liquid (Del Monte)	1/2 cup	70	2	17	355	0	1.0	0.0	0	11%

Food Name	Serving Size	Calories	Prot. gms	Carbs gms	Sod. mgs	Fiber gms	Fat gms	Sat. Fat gms	Chol. mgs	% Fat Cal.
WHITE										
Canned										
(Green Giant)	1/2 cup	80	2	20	310	2	0.0	0.0	0	0%
(Stokely)	1/2 cup	90	3	21	290	0	0.0	0.0	0	0%
kernels, sweet, drained	1 cup	133	4	30	530	3	1.6	0.3	0	10%
kernels, sweet, no salt, vacuum pack	1/2 cup	83	3	20	3	2	0.5	0.1	0	5%
kernels, sweet, no salt, w/liquid	1/2 cup	82	2	20	15	1	0.6	0.1	0	7%
kernels, sweet, w/liquid	1/2 cup	82	2	20	273	2	0.6	0.1	0	7%
sweet, vacuum packed	1/2 cup	83	3	20	286	2	0.5	0.1	0	5%
vacuum-packed (A&P)	1/2 cup	100	2	25	300	0	1.0	0.0	0	8%
vacuum-packed (Finast)	4 oz	90	5	20	150	0	1.0	0.0	0	8%
vacuum-packed (Green Giant)	1/2 cup	80	2	20	290	2	0.0	0.0	0	0%
vacuum-packed (Pathmark)	1/2 cup	120	3	25	350	0	1.0	0.0	0	7%
vacuum-packed, 'Niblets' (Green Giant)	1/2 cup	80	3	16	280	2	1.0	0.0	0	11%
w/liquid (Del Monte)	1/2 cup	70	2	16	355	0	0.0	0.0	0	0%
young, tender ,'Premium' (S&W)	1/2 cup	90	2	20	295	0	1.0	0.0	0	9%
Fresh										
kernels, sweet, boiled, drained	1/2 cup	76	3	18	3	2	0.6	0.1	0	7%
kernels, sweet, raw	1 cup	132	5	29	23	4	1.8	0.3	0	11%
on the cob, sweet, large ears, 7.75 to 9 inches	1 ear	123	5	27	21	4	1.7	0.3	0	11%
on the cob, sweet, med ears, 6.75 to 7.5 inches	1 ear	83	3	19	13	2	1.0	0.2	0	10%
on the cob, sweet, small ears, 5.5 to 6.5 inches	1 ear	63	2	14	11	2	0.9	0.1	0	11%
Frozen										
(Green Giant)	1/2 cup	90	2	19	5	2	1.0	0.0	0	10%
(Seabrook)	3.3 oz	80	3	19	3	1	1.0	0.0	0	9%
kernels, sweet, boiled, drained	1/2 cup	66	2	16	4	2	0.4	0.1	0	5%
kernels, sweet, boiled, drained	10-oz pkg	227	8	56	14	7	1.2	0.2	0	5%
kernels, sweet, unprepared	1/2 cup	72	2	17	2	2	0.6	0.1	0	7%
kernels, sweet, unprepared	10-oz pkg	250	9	59	9	7	2.2	0.3	0	7%
on the cob, sweet, unprepared, med ears	1 ear	123	4	29	6	4	1.0	0.1	0	7%
petite, 'Early Harvest' (C&W)	2/3 cup	80	3	19	10	1	1.0	0.0	0	9%
shoepeg, 'Harvest Fresh' (Green Giant)	1/2 cup	90	3	19	60	2	1.0	0.0	0	9%
shoepeg, 'Select' (Green Giant)	1/2 cup	90	2	19	5	2	1.0	0.0	0	10%
YELLOW										
Canned										
kernels, sweet, drained	12-oz can	171	6	39	452	4	2.1	0.3	0	10%
kernels, sweet, drained	1 cup	133	4	30	351	3	1.6	0.3	0	10%
kernels, sweet, regular pack, w/liquid	1/2 cup	82	2	20	273	2	0.6	0.1	0	7%
sweet, no salt, vacuum-packed	1/2 cup	83	3	20	3	2	0.5	0.1	0	5%
sweet, no salt, w/liquid	1/2 cup	82	2	20	15	2	0.6	0.1	0	7%
Fresh										
baby, sweet, whole, boiled, drained	1 ear	9	0	2	1	0	0.1	0.0	0	10%
kernels, sweet, boiled, drained	1/2 cup	76	3	18	3	2	0.6	0.1	0	7%
kernels, sweet, raw	1 cup	132	5	29	23	4	1.8	0.3	0	11%
on the cob, large ears, 7.75 to 9 inches	1 ear	123	5	27	21	4	1.7	0.3	0	11%
on the cob, medium ears, 6.75 to 7.5 inches	1 ear	77	3	17	14	2	1.1	0.2	0	11%
on the cob, small ears, 5.5 to 6.5 inches	1 ear	63	2	14	11	2	0.9	0.1	0	11%
Frozen										
kernels, sweet, boiled, drained	10-oz pkg	227	8	56	14	7	1.2	0.2	0	5%
kernels, sweet, unprepared	10-oz pkg	250	9	59	9	7	2.2	0.3	0	7%
kernels, sweet, unprepared	1/2 cup	72	2	17	2	2	0.6	0.1	0	7%
CORN, CREAMED. See under CORN DISH/ENTRÉE.										
CORN BRAN, crude	1 cup	170	6	65	5	65	0.7	0.1	0	3%

Food Name	Serving Size	Calories	Prot. gms	Carbs gms	Sod. mgs	Fiber gms	Fat gms	Sat. Fat gms	Chol. mgs	% Fat Cal.
CORN CAKE										
apple cinnamon flavor *(Roman Meal)*	1 cake	49	1	11	5	0	1.0	0.0	0	16%
caramel flavor, nonfat *(Roman Meal)*	1 cake	50	1	11	5	0	0.0	0.0	0	0%
caramel flavored *(Quaker)*	1 serving	50	1	12	30	0	0.0	0.0	0	0%
cheddar flavor *(Roman Meal)*	1 cake	43	1	9	14	0	1.0	0.0	0	18%
natural butter flavor, nonfat *(Roman Meal)*	1 cake	40	1	8	35	0	0.0	0.0	0	0%
popcorn, butter flavor *(Chico-San)*	1 cake	40	1	8	45	0	0.0	0.0	0	0%
popcorn, caramel *(Chico-San)*	1 cake	50	1	10	55	0	0.0	0.0	0	0%
popcorn, lightly salted *(Chico-San)*	1 cake	40	1	8	45	0	0.0	0.0	0	0%
popcorn, white cheddar cheese *(Chico-San)*	1 cake	50	1	9	65	0	1.0	0.0	0	18%
popped, butter flavor *(Quaker)*	1 cake	35	1	7	55	0	0.0	0.0	0	0%
white cheddar, mild *(Quaker)*	1 serving	40	1	8	100	0	0.0	0.0	0	0%
white cheddar flavor, nonfat *(Roman Meal)*	1 cake	45	1	9	15	0	0.0	0.0	0	0%
CORN CHIPS AND SNACKS. See also TORTILLA CHIPS.										
(Arrowhead Mills)										
chips, blue corn, 'Corn Curls'	1 oz	120	3	22	54	4	2.0	0.0	0	15%
chips, blue corn, unsalted, 'Corn Curls'	1 oz	120	3	22	1	4	2.0	0.0	0	15%
chips, yellow, 'Corn Chips'	0.75 oz	90	2	18	31	3	1.0	0.0	0	10%
chips, yellow, w/cheese, 'Corn Chips'	0.75 oz	90	2	15	30	3	2.0	0.0	0	21%
(Azteca) chips, 'Unsalted'	1 oz	140	2	18	110	0	7.0	0.0	0	44%
(Bachman)										
chips	1 oz	160	2	15	160	0	10.0	0.0	0	57%
chips, barbecue	1 oz	150	1	17	230	0	9.0	0.0	0	53%
(Barbara's Bakery)										
chips, blue corn	15 chips	140	3	16	40	1	7.0	0.5	0	45%
chips, blue corn, no salt added	15 chips	140	3	16	0	1	7.0	0.5	0	45%
chips, chipotle chili, 'Potilla'	1 oz	140	2	18	180	0	8.0	0.0	0	47%
chips, 'Potilla'	1 oz	140	2	18	120	0	8.0	0.0	0	47%
chips, salsa, 'Pinta Puffs'	1 oz	70	2	10	130	0	2.0	0.0	0	27%
(Corn Snackers)										
chips	0.5-oz pkg	60	1	10	190	0	2.0	0.0	0	29%
chips, nacho cheese	0.5-oz pkg	60	1	10	240	0	2.0	0.0	0	29%
(Cornuts)										
nuggets, toasted, barbecue	1 oz	124	3	20	277	2	4.1	0.7	0	29%
nuggets, toasted, chili picante	1 oz	120	2	22	260	2	4.0	0.0	0	27%
nuggets, toasted, nacho	1 oz	124	3	20	180	2	4.0	0.7	1	28%
nuggets, toasted, plain	1 oz	124	2	21	156	2	4.0	0.7	0	28%
nuggets, toasted, ranch	1 oz	120	2	20	190	2	4.0	0.0	0	29%
nuggets, toasted, unsalted	1 oz	120	2	19	30	3	4.0	0.0	0	30%
(Dipsy Doodles) chips, rippled, 'Rippled Corn Chips'	1 oz	160	2	15	180	0	10.0	0.0	0	57%
(Doritos)										
chips, 'Nacho Cheesier'	1 oz	140	2	17	360	1	7.0	1.5	3	45%
chips, '3-D's'	1 oz	140	2	18	350	1	6.0	1.5	3	40%
(Featherweight)										
chips, 'Low-Salt'	1 oz	170	2	15	3	0	11.0	0.0	0	59%
puffs, cheese, low-salt 'Cheese Curls'	1 oz	150	2	16	81	0	9.0	0.0	0	53%
(Fritos)										
chips, 'Bar-B-Q'	34 pieces	150	2	16	320	0	9.0	0.0	0	53%
chips, barbecue, 'Rowdy Rustlers'	34 chips	150	2	17	300	1	9.0	0.0	0	52%
chips, chili cheese flavor	34 chips	160	2	15	300	1	10.0	0.0	0	57%
chips, 'Dip Size'	13 pieces	150	2	17	210	0	9.0	0.0	0	52%
chips, nacho cheese, 'Non-Stop'	34 chips	150	2	16	220	1	9.0	0.0	1	53%
chips, original	34 pieces	150	1	16	230	0	9.0	0.0	0	54%
chips, 'Wild 'N Mild'	32 chips	160	2	16	240	1	9.0	0.0	0	53%

Food Name	Serving Size	Calories	Prot. gms	Carbs gms	Sod. mgs	Fiber gms	Fat gms	Sat. Fat gms	Chol. mgs	% Fat Cal.
nuggets, toasted	1.38 oz	170	3	29	265	0	5.0	0.0	0	26%
(Harry's)										
chips, bean 'Garden Vegetable Chips'	1 oz	144	3	17	1	2	7.0	1.2	0	44%
chips, bean, mild, 'Garden Vegetable Chips'	1 oz	144	3	17	74	2	7.0	1.2	0	44%
chips, bean, wild, 'Garden Vegetable Chips'	1 oz	141	3	18	51	3	6.0	0.8	0	39%
chips, beet-garlic, 'Garden Vegetable Chips'	1 oz	134	2	20	43	2	5.0	0.8	0	34%
chips, bell pepper, 'Garden Vegetable Chips'	1 oz	140	2	19	40	2	6.0	0.7	0	39%
chips, blue corn, garlic 'Garden Vegetable Chips'	1 oz	129	3	21	28	3	4.0	0.5	0	28%
chips, carrot caraway 'Garden Vegetable Chips'	1 ez	131	2	20	31	2	4.0	0.6	0	29%
chips, vegetable, 'Garden Vegetable Chips'	1 oz	141	2	18	40	3	7.0	0.7	0	44%
(Health Valley)										
chips	1 oz	160	1	13	90	1	11.0	0.0	0	64%
chips, 'No Salt Added'	1 oz	160	1	13	1	1	11.0	0.0	0	64%
puffs, caramel, nonfat, orignal	1 cup	110	2	24	60	2	0.0	0.0	0	0%
puffs, caramel corn, peanut flavor	1 oz	100	3	21	65	0	0.0	0.0	0	0%
puffs, cheddar cheese	1 oz	160	3	15	120	1	10.0	0.0	2	56%
(Jax)										
puffs, cheese 'Crunchy'	1 oz	160	2	14	250	0	11.0	0.0	0	61%
puffs, cheese, 'Baked'	1 oz	140	2	17	290	0	7.0	0.0	0	45%
(Maine Coast)										
chips, corn-dulse-kelp-onion-garlic, organic	1 oz	146	2	17	65	4	6.6	0.0	0	43%
(Peddlers)										
chips, bean 'Offbeat Originals'	1 oz	144	3	17	1	2	7.0	1.2	0	44%
chips, bean, mild, 'Offbeat Originals'	1 oz	144	3	17	74	2	7.0	1.2	0	44%
chips, bean, wild, 'Offbeat Originals'	1 oz	141	3	18	51	3	6.0	0.8	0	39%
chips, beet-garlic 'Offbeat Originals'	1 oz	134	2	20	43	2	5.0	0.8	0	34%
chips, bell pepper 'Offbeat Originals'	1 oz	140	2	19	40	2	6.0	0.7	0	39%
chips, blue corn, garlic 'Offbeat Originals'	1 oz	129	3	21	28	3	4.0	0.5	0	28%
chips, carrot caraway 'Offbeat Originals'	1 oz	131	2	20	31	2	4.0	0.6	0	29%
chips, vegetable, 'Offbeat Originals'	1 oz	141	2	18	40	3	7.0	0.7	0	44%
(Planters) chips	1 oz	160	2	15	160	0	10.0	2.0	0	57%
(Skinny Snacks)										
chips, barbecue	1 cup	60	1	12	140	1	1.0	0.8	0	15%
chips, nacho flavor	1 cup	60	1	12	105	1	1.0	0.8	0	15%
chips, no salt	1 cup	60	1	12	0	1	1.0	0.8	0	15%
chips, salted	1 cup	60	1	12	58	1	1.0	0.8	0	15%
chips, sour cream and onion	1 cup	65	1	12	70	1	1.0	0.8	0	15%
(Snyder's)										
chips	1 oz	160	2	14	150	0	11.0	2.0	0	61%
(Tio Sancho) nachos	0.5 oz	70	4	1	282	0	5.7	0.0	0	73%
(Ultra Slim Fast) curls, cheese, 'Great Tasting'	1 oz	110	2	20	360	3	3.0	0.0	0	23%
(Wise)										
corn chips	1 oz	160	2	15	180	0	10.0	0.0	0	57%
chips, ridged	1 oz	160	2	15	180	0	10.0	0.0	0	57%
crunchies	1 oz	160	2	15	180	0	10.0	0.0	0	57%
puffs, cheese, fried, 'Cheez Doodles Corn Puffs'	1 oz	160	2	15	220	0	10.0	0.0	0	57%
puffs, cheese, baked, 'Cheez Doodles Corn Puffs'	1 oz	150	2	17	360	0	8.0	0.0	0	49%
spirals	1 oz	160	2	15	125	0	10.0	0.0	0	57%
twists	1 oz	160	2	15	125	0	10.0	0.0	0	57%
CORN DISH/ENTRÉE										
(A&P)										
cream style, canned	1/2 cup	100	2	25	330	0	1.0	0.0	0	8%
kernels, cream style, frozen	3.3 oz	80	3	18	0	0	1.0	0.0	0	10%

Food Name	Serving Size	Calories	Prot. gms	Carbs gms	Sod. mgs	Fiber gms	Fat gms	Sat. Fat gms	Chol. mgs	% Fat Cal.
(Del Monte)										
cream style, no salt added, canned	1/2 cup	90	2	20	10	2	1.0	0.0	0	9%
golden, cream style, canned	1/2 cup	80	2	18	355	0	1.0	0.0	0	10%
golden, cream style, no salt added, canned	1/2 cup	80	2	20	10	0	1.0	0.0	0	9%
(Diamond A) sweet, cream style, canned	1 cup	245	5	50	650	0	1.0	0.0	0	4%
(Finast) cream style, canned	1/2 cup	105	2	25	350	0	1.0	0.0	0	8%
(Flav-R-Pac)										
cream style, frozen	1/2 cup	130	3	24	380	2	3.0	0.5	0	20%
w/buttery sauce, frozen	1/2 cup	130	3	24	420	2	3.0	0.5	0	20%
(Freshlike)										
and peppers, vacuum packed	1/2 cup	90	3	23	300	0	1.0	0.0	0	8%
golden, cream style, canned	1/2 cup	110	2	25	290	0	1.0	0.0	0	8%
golden, cream style, no salt added, canned	1/2 cup	110	2	25	15	0	1.0	0.0	0	8%
(Green Giant)										
cream style, canned	1/2 cup	100	2	24	390	2	1.0	0.0	0	8%
cream style, canned	1/2 cup	110	2	23	330	2	1.0	0.0	0	8%
w/peppers, canned, 'Mexicorn'	1/2 cup	80	2	19	450	2	1.0	0.0	0	10%
(IGA) golden, sweet, cream style, canned	1/2 cup	70	2	16	10	0	1.0	0.0	0	11%
(Pathmark)										
cream style, canned, 'No Frills'	1 cup	210	5	51	700	0	1.0	0.0	0	4%
golden, cream style, canned	1/2 cup	100	2	25	350	0	1.0	0.0	0	8%
(S&W)										
cream style, canned	1/2 cup	100	2	24	340	1	1.0	0.0	0	8%
cream style, canned, 'Nutradiet'	1/2 cup	100	3	21	0	0	1.0	0.0	0	9%
cream style, no starch added, canned, 'Premium Homestyle'	1/2 cup	120	3	24	285	0	1.0	0.0	0	8%
cream style, starch added, canned, 'Premium Homestyle'	1/2 cup	105	2	25	435	0	1.0	0.0	0	8%
(Stokely)										
gold and white, cream style, canned	1/2 cup	100	2	23	380	0	0.0	0.0	0	0%
gold and white, w/red peppers, canned	1/2 cup	60	2	10	250	2	1.5	0.0	0	22%
white, cream style, canned	1/2 cup	100	2	21	400	1	1.0	0.0	0	9%
(Stouffer's)										
pudding, frozen, food service product	1 oz	38	1	5	126	0	1.7	0.3	15	41%
soufflé	1/2 cup	170	5	21	490	1	7.0	2.0	65	38%
(Veg-All)										
golden, cream style, canned	1/2 cup	110	2	25	290	0	1.0	0.0	0	8%
w/peppers, vacuum packed	1/2 cup	90	3	23	300	0	1.0	0.0	0	8%
CORN DOG. See under FRANKFURTER.										
CORN FLOUR. See under FLOUR. See also CORNMEAL.										
CORN OIL										
(Hain)	1 tbsp	120	0	0	0	0	14.0	2.0	0	100%
(Kroger)	1 tbsp	122	0	0	0	0	13.6	1.9	0	100%
(Mazola)	1 tbsp	120	0	0	0	0	14.0	2.0	0	100%
(Wesson)	1 tbsp	122	0	0	0	0	13.6	1.8	0	100%
'No Frills' *(Pathmark)*	1 tbsp	130	0	0	0	0	14.0	2.0	0	100%
pure pressed, organic *(Spectrum)*	1 tbsp	120	0	0	0	0	14.0	1.5	0	100%
CORN SYRUP										
dark	1 cup	925	0	251	508	0	0.0	0.0	0	0%
dark	1 tbsp	56	0	15	31	0	0.0	0.0	0	0%
dark *(Karo)*	1 tbsp	60	0	15	40	0	0.0	0.0	0	0%
high-fructose	1 cup	871	0	236	6	0	0.0	0.0	0	0%
high-fructose	1 tbsp	53	0	14	0	0	0.0	0.0	0	0%
light	1 cup	925	0	251	397	0	0.0	0.0	0	0%

Food Name	Serving Size	Calories	Prot. gms	Carbs gms	Sod. mgs	Fiber gms	Fat gms	Sat. Fat gms	Chol. mgs	% Fat Cal.
light	1 tbsp	56	0	15	24	0	0.0	0.0	0	0%
light *(Karo)*	1 tbsp	60	0	15	30	0	0.0	0.0	0	0%
table blend, w/sugar	1 cup	1008	0	265	224	0	0.0	0.0	0	0%
table blend, w/sugar	1 tbsp	64	0	17	14	0	0.0	0.0	0	0%
CORNBREAD. See under BREAD, QUICK.										
CORNBREAD MIX. See under BREAD, QUICK, MIX.										
CORNED BEEF. See BEEF, CORNED.										
CORNED BEEF HASH. See under HASH.										
CORNISH GAME HEN										
meat and skin, raw	1/2 medium	336	29	0	102	0	23.6	6.5	170	63%
meat and skin, roasted	1/2 medium	335	29	0	83	0	23.5	6.5	169	63%
meat only, raw	1/2 medium	139	24	0	82	0	4.0	1.0	109	26%
meat only, roasted	1/2 medium	147	26	0	69	0	4.3	1.1	117	26%
(Tyson)										
meat and skin, frozen	3.5 oz	250	27	1	80	0	15.0	0.0	155	55%
meat only, frozen	3.5 oz	240	28	0	70	0	14.0	0.0	75	53%
CORNISH GAME HEN DINNER/ENTRÉE										
(Tyson) w/wild rice, wholesale club item	3.5 oz	190	19	6	125	0	11.0	0.0	85	50%
CORNMEAL										
organic, stone ground, gluten free *(Hodgson Mill)*	1/4 cup	100	3	22	0	3	1.0	0.0	0	8%
whole-grain, high-lysine *(Arrowhead Mills)*	2 oz	210	4	43	1	7	2.0	0.0	0	9%
whole-grain, stone-ground *(Hodgson Mill)*	1/4 cup	100	3	22	0	3	1.0	0.0	0	8%
BLUE										
(Arrowhead Mills)	1/4 cup	120	3	27	0	3	1.0	0.0	0	7%
whole-grain *(Arrowhead Mills)*	2 oz	210	6	41	1	6	3.0	0.0	0	13%
WHITE										
Regular										
(Albers)	1 oz	100	2	22	0	2	1.0	0.0	0	9%
bolted *(Aunt Jemima)*	1/6 cup	99	2	21	337	0	0.7	0.0	0	6%
enriched *(Aunt Jemima)*	3 tbsp	102	2	22	1	1	0.5	0.0	0	4%
enriched, degermed	1 cup	505	12	107	4	10	2.3	0.3	0	4%
unenriched, degermed	1 cup	505	12	107	4	10	2.3	0.3	0	4%
whole-grain	1 cup	442	10	94	43	9	4.4	0.6	0	8%
whole-grain, stone-ground *(Hodgson Mill)* . . .	1/4 cup	100	3	22	0	3	1.0	0.0	0	8%
Self-rising										
(Aunt Jemima)	1/6 cup	98	2	21	381	0	0.5	0.0	0	5%
bolted, plain, enriched	1 cup	407	10	86	1521	8	4.1	0.6	0	9%
bolted, w/wheat flour added, enriched	1 cup	592	14	125	2242	11	4.8	0.7	0	7%
buttermilk *(Aunt Jemima)*	3 tbsp	101	3	20	439	0	1.1	0.0	0	10%
enriched, degermed	1 cup	490	12	103	1860	10	2.4	0.3	0	4%
YELLOW										
Regular										
(Albers)	1 oz	100	2	22	0	2	1.0	0.0	0	9%
bolted *(Tone's)*	1 tsp	9	0	2	0	0	0.1	0.1	0	10%
degermed, unenriched	1 cup	505	12	107	4	10	2.3	0.3	0	4%
enriched *(Aunt Jemima)*	3 tbsp	102	2	22	1	1	0.5	0.0	0	4%
enriched, degermed	1 cup	505	12	107	4	10	2.3	0.3	0	4%
whole-grain	1 cup	442	10	94	43	9	4.4	0.6	0	8%
whole-grain *(Arrowhead Mills)*	2 oz	210	4	43	1	7	2.0	0.0	0	9%
Self-rising										
(Aunt Jemima)	3 tbsp	100	2	21	490	0	1.0	0.0	0	9%
bolted, plain, enriched	1 cup	407	10	86	1521	8	4.1	0.6	0	9%
bolted, w/wheat flour added, enriched	1 cup	592	14	125	2242	11	4.8	0.7	0	7%

Food Name	Serving Size	Calories	Prot. gms	Carbs gms	Sod. mgs	Fiber gms	Fat gms	Sat. Fat gms	Chol. mgs	% Fat Cal.
enriched, degermed	1 cup	490	12	103	1860	10	2.4	0.3	0	4%
whole-grain *(Hodgson Mill)*	1/4 cup	90	3	21	260	3	1.0	0.0	0	9%
CORNSTARCH										
	1 cup	488	0	117	12	1	0.1	0.0	0	0%
(Argo)	1 tbsp	30	0	7	0	0	0.0	0.0	0	0%
(Cream)	1 tbsp	29	0	7	0	0	0.0	0.0	0	0%
(Kingsford)	1 tbsp	30	0	7	0	0	0.0	0.0	0	0%
(Tone's)	1 tsp	10	0	2	0	0	0.1	0.0	0	9%
100% pure *(Hodgson Mill)*	2 tsp	35	0	9	0	0	0.0	0.0	0	0%
COTTAGE CHEESE. See under CHEESE.										
COTTONSEED FLOUR. See under FLOUR.										
COTTONSEED KERNELS										
roasted	1 cup	754	49	33	37	8	54.1	14.5	0	60%
roasted	1 tbsp	51	3	2	3	1	3.6	1.0	0	60%
COTTONSEED MEAL, partially defatted	1 oz	104	14	11	10	na	1.4	0.3	0	11%
COTTONSEED OIL										
	1 cup	1927	0	0	0	0	218.0	56.5	0	100%
	1 tbsp	120	0	0	0	0	13.6	3.5	0	100%
(Wesson)	1 tbsp	122	0	0	0	0	13.6	3.2	0	100%
w/ sesame oil, seasoned, 'Mongolian Fire Oil'										
(House of Tsang)	1 tsp	45	0	0	0	0	5.0	1.0	0	100%
COUSCOUS										
cooked	1 cup	176	6	36	8	2	0.3	0.0	0	1%
savory, prepared *(Fantastic Foods)*	2/3 cup	160	6	33	300	3	0.7	0.0	0	4%
uncooked	1 cup	591	20	123	26	7	0.8	0.2	0	1%
uncooked	1 oz	96	3	20	4	1	0.1	0.0	0	1%
uncooked *(Near East)*	1.25 oz	120	4	26	5	0	0.0	0.0	0	0%
uncooked 'Elegant Grains' *(Fantastic Foods)*	1/4 cup	210	7	43	5	3	0.0	0.0	0	0%
whole wheat, prepared w/2 tbsp salted butter										
(Fantastic Foods)	1/2 cup	111	4	20	23	0	2.0	0.0	0	16%
whole wheat, uncooked, 'Elegant Grains'										
(Fantastic Foods)	1/4 cup	210	8	45	0	7	1.0	0.0	0	4%
COUSCOUS DISH/ENTRÉE										
pilaf, cooked *(Casbah)*	3/4 cup	220	8	40	480	1	0.5	0.0	0	2%
pilaf, savory, prepared w/2 tbsp salted butter										
(Quick Pilaf)	1/2 cup	124	4	19	254	0	3.0	0.0	0	23%
pilaf, savory, prepared w/o additional ingredients										
(Quick Pilaf)	1/2 cup	94	4	19	215	0	0.0	0.0	0	0%
pilaf, uncooked *(Casbah)*	28 grams	100	4	20	280	1	0.0	0.0	0	0%
w/lentils, cooked *(Fantastic Foods)*	1 serving	220	12	47	140	9	1.0	0.0	0	4%
w/lentils, uncooked *(Fantastic Foods)*	2.3 oz	220	12	47	140	9	1.0	0.0	0	4%
CRAB										
ALASKA KING										
boiled, poached, or steamed	1 med leg	130	26	0	1436	0	2.1	0.2	71	14%
boiled, poached, or steamed	3 oz	82	16	0	911	0	1.3	0.1	45	14%
raw	1 med leg	144	31	0	1438	0	1.0	0.2	72	6%
raw	3 oz	71	16	0	711	0	0.5	0.1	36	6%
BLUE										
Canned										
	1 cup	134	28	0	450	0	1.7	0.3	120	11%
	3 oz	84	17	0	283	0	1.0	0.2	76	11%
	1 oz	28	6	0	94	0	0.3	0.1	25	11%
drained	6.5-oz can	124	26	0	416	0	1.5	0.3	111	11%

Food Name	Serving Size	Calories	Prot. gms	Carbs gms	Sod. mgs	Fiber gms	Fat gms	Sat. Fat gms	Chol. mgs	% Fat Cal.
Fresh										
boiled, poached, or steamed	3 oz	87	17	0	237	0	1.5	0.2	85	16%
boiled, poached, or steamed, flakes and pieces	1 cup	120	24	0	329	0	2.1	0.3	118	16%
boiled, poached, or steamed, pieces	1 cup	138	27	0	377	0	2.4	0.3	135	16%
boiled, poached, or steamed, w/o shell	1 oz	29	6	0	79	0	0.5	0.1	28	16%
raw	1 med crab	18	4	0	62	0	0.2	0.0	16	11%
raw	3 oz	74	15	0	249	0	0.9	0.2	66	11%
DUNGENESS										
Canned (*S&W*)	1/3 cup	80	18	0	310	0	1.0	0.0	60	11%
Fresh										
boiled, poached, or steamed	1 med crab	140	28	1	480	0	1.6	0.2	97	10%
boiled, poached, or steamed	3 oz	94	19	1	321	0	1.1	0.1	65	10%
raw	1 med crab	140	28	1	481	0	1.6	0.2	96	10%
raw	3 oz	73	15	1	251	0	0.8	0.1	50	10%
MIXED SPECIES										
15% leg meat, canned (*Crown Prince*)	1/2 can	50	12	1	300	0	0.0	0.0	75	0%
white meat, canned (*Crown Prince*)	1/2 can	50	12	0	340	0	0.0	0.0	70	0%
QUEEN										
boiled, poached, or steamed	3 oz	98	20	0	587	0	1.3	0.2	60	12%
raw	3 oz	77	16	0	458	0	1.0	0.1	47	12%
SNOW										
frozen (*Wakefield*)	3 oz	60	13	0	270	0	1.0	0.0	0	15%
raw, Opilio, clusters (*Peter Pan Seafoods*)	3.5 oz	91	21	0	539	0	1.2	0.0	55	12%
raw, Opilio, scored, 'Snap 'n' Eat' (*Peter Pan Seafoods*)	3.5 oz	91	21	0	539	0	1.2	0.0	55	12%
SOFTSHELL										
boiled	4 oz	116	22.9	0.0	316	0	2.0	0.3	113	16%
boiled, approx 4.75 oz	1 cup	138	27.3	0.0	376	0	2.4	0.3	135	17%
poached	4 oz	116	22.9	0.0	316	0	2.0	0.3	113	16%
poached, approx 4.75 oz	1 cup	138	27.3	0.0	376	0	2.4	0.3	135	17%
raw	1 lb	395	81.9	0.2	1329	0	4.9	1.0	355	12%
raw	1 oz	25	5.1	<.1	83	0	0.3	0.1	22	12%
raw, approx 0.7 oz	1 crab	18	3.8	<.1	62	0	0.2	<.1	16	10%
steamed	4 oz	116	22.9	0.0	316	0	2.0	0.3	113	16%
steamed, approx 4.75 oz	1 cup	138	27.3	0.0	376	0	2.4	0.3	135	17%
CRAB ENTRÉE/DINNER (*Wakefield*) w/shrimp, frozen	3 oz	60	13	0	210	0	1.0	0.0	0	15%
CRAB SUBSTITUTE										
Alaska King style, made from surimi	3 oz	87	10	9	715	0	1.1	0.2	17	12%
made from surimi	1 oz	28	4	2	41	0	0.3	0.1	9	8%
made from surimi	3 oz	84	13	6	122	0	0.8	0.2	26	8%
(*Icicle Brand*)	3.5 oz	99	12	11	900	0	0.1	0.0	10	1%
(*Peter Pan Seafoods*)										
leg style, made from surimi and 10% crab, 'Classic Seablends'	3.5 oz	85	10	0	890	0	0.4	0.0	31	8%
leg style, made from surimi, 'Standard Seablends'	3.5 oz	88	9	0	845	0	0.4	0.0	34	9%
salad style made from surimi and 10% crab, 'Classic Seablends Combo'	3.5 oz	85	10	0	890	0	0.4	0.0	31	8%
salad style, made from surimi 'Standard Seablends Combo'	3.5 oz	88	9	0	845	0	0.4	0.0	34	9%
(*Trader Joe's*) made from surimi	1/2 cup	80	6	14	670	0	1.0	0.0	15	10%
CRABAPPLE, raw, sliced	1 cup	84	0	22	1	na	0.3	0.1	0	3%
CRACKER										
(*Adrienne's*)										
lahvosh, 'Classic Island'	7 crackers	140	4	21	290	1	4.0	1.5	25	26%

Food Name	Serving Size	Calories	Prot. gms	Carbs gms	Sod. mgs	Fiber gms	Fat gms	Sat. Fat gms	Chol. mgs	% Fat Cal.
lahvosh, onion	4 crackers	66	2	10	120	0	1.9	0.5	10	26%
lahvosh, 10-grain	4 crackers	59	2	10	120	0	1.6	0.3	0	23%
(Ak-Mak) wheat, 100% stone ground, w/sesame	5 crackers	116	5	19	214	4	2.3	0.5	0	18%
(American Classic)										
butter flavor	4 crackers	70	1	9	140	0	3.0	1.0	2	40%
cracked wheat	4 crackers	70	1	8	140	0	4.0	1.0	0	50%
golden, w/sesame	4 crackers	70	1	9	120	0	3.0	1.0	0	40%
onion, minced	4 crackers	70	1	10	120	0	3.0	1.0	0	38%
toasted poppy	4 crackers	70	1	9	140	0	3.0	1.0	0	40%
(Auburn Farms)										
onion, 7-grain, nonfat, bite size	0.5 oz	60	2	12	105	1	0.0	0.0	0	0%
7-grain, bite size	1 oz	120	2	24	220	2	0.0	0.0	0	0%
vegetable, 7-grain, nonfat, bite size	1 oz	120	4	24	210	2	0.0	0.0	0	0%
(Barbara's Bakery)										
'Wheatines' less salt	1 serving	50	1	10	110	1	1.5	0.0	0	23%
'Wheatines' unsalted tops	0.5 oz	60	2	9	45	0	2.0	0.0	0	29%
'Wheatines' sesame, less salt	1 serving	50	1	10	110	1	1.5	0.0	0	23%
'Wheatines,' w/pepper	1 serving	50	1	10	110	1	1.5	1.0	0	23%
'Wheatine' bits	0.5 oz	60	2	9	132	0	2.0	0.0	0	29%
(Breton)										
low-sodium	3 crackers	70	2	8	30	0	3.0	1.5	0	40%
sesame	3 crackers	80	2	9	120	0	3.5	2.0	0	42%
(Cabaret)	3 crackers	70	1	9	160	0	3.5	1.5	0	44%
(Carr's)										
'Monterey' savory wheat	3 crackers	70	<1	9	95	1	2.5	0.0	0	36%
'Monterey' hearty wheat	3 crackers	60	1	9	100	<1	2.0	0.0	0	33%
'Monterey' sesame and onion	3 crackers	70	<1	9	110	<1	3.0	0.0	0	36%
'Monterey' roasted vegetable	3 crackers	60	<1	10	160	<1	2.0	0.0	0	33%
'Table Water'	5 crackers	70	1	13	100	<1	1.5	0.0	0	21%
'Table Water' w/toasted sesame seeds	5 crackers	70	1	13	95	<1	1.5	0.0	0	21%
'Table Water' w/cracked pepper	5 crackers	70	1	13	100	<1	1.5	0.0	0	21%
'Table Water' w/roasted garlic and herbs	5 crackers	70	1	13	140	<1	1.5	0.0	0	21%
(Cheddar Wedges) cheese flavor, bite size	31 pieces	70	1	9	150	0	3.0	1.0	0	40%
(Cheez-It)										
cheese flavor	12 crackers	70	2	7	135	0	4.0	1.0	2	50%
hot and spicy	12 crackers	70	1	8	160	0	4.0	1.0	2	50%
low-salt	12 crackers	70	2	7	65	0	4.0	1.0	2	50%
party mix	1/2 cup	140	4	19	270	1	5.0	1.0	0	33%
white cheddar	12 crackers	76	1	9	160	0	4.0	1.0	2	47%
(Club Partners) garlic bread flavor	4 crackers	60	1	10	140	0	2.0	0.5	0	29%
(Crackups)										
cheddar	0.5 oz	70	1	10	100	0	3.0	0.0	0	38%
salsa	0.5 oz	70	1	9	100	0	3.0	0.0	0	40%
(Crisp & Light)										
'Crackerbread'	1 slice	17	1	3	25	0	1.0	0.0	0	36%
'Crackerbread' salt-free	1 slice	17	1	3	1	0	1.0	0.0	0	36%
(Dandy) soup and oyster, 5 oz serving	20 crackers	60	1	10	220	0	2.0	1.0	0	29%
(Dar-Vida)										
crispbread, regular	1 cracker	20	1	4	40	0	1.0	0.0	0	31%
crispbread, sesame	1 cracker	22	1	4	40	0	1.0	0.0	0	31%
sesame, 'Crispbread'	1 cracker	22	1	4	40	0	1.0	0.0	0	31%
(Delicious)										
bacon flavor	0.5 oz	70	1	10	190	0	3.0	0.0	0	38%
bite size	0.5 oz	70	1	9	135	0	3.0	0.5	1	40%

Food Name	Serving Size	Calories	Prot. gms	Carbs gms	Sod. mgs	Fiber gms	Fat gms	Sat. Fat gms	Chol. mgs	% Fat Cal.
cheese flavor, 'Big'.	25 crackers	140	3	19	220	1	6.0	1.0	5	38%
'Crackerdiles'.	0.5 oz	70	1	9	135	0	3.0	0.5	1	40%
garden vegetable.	0.5 oz	70	1	10	220	0	3.0	0.0	0	38%
garlic 'Discos'	0.5 oz	78	1	6	184	0	5.0	0.0	0	62%
low-sodium, bite size.	0.5 oz	70	1	9	55	0	3.0	1.0	0	40%
nacho cheese.	0.5 oz	89	1	8	150	0	5.0	0.0	0	56%
onion, 'Discos'.	0.5 oz	76	1	7	156	0	5.0	0.0	0	58%
pumpernickel.	0.5 oz	70	1	9	160	0	3.0	0.0	0	40%
'Regency'.	0.5 oz	70	1	9	100	0	3.0	0.5	0	40%
'Snackers'.	0.5 oz	70	1	9	90	0	3.0	1.0	0	40%
sour cream, w/onion, 'Discos'.	0.5 oz	79	1	6	162	0	5.0	0.0	0	62%
sourdough.	0.5 oz	70	1	9	160	0	3.0	0.0	0	40%
'Wheat On'.	0.5 oz	68	1	8	86	0	3.0	0.5	0	43%
wheat wafer, w/sesame.	0.5 oz	80	1	9	170	0	4.0	0.0	0	47%
'Wheatstone'.	0.5 oz	70	2	9	180	0	3.0	0.0	0	38%
(Devonsheer)										
Melba toast, honey bran.	1 cracker	16	1	3	25	0	0.4	0.1	0	18%
Melba toast, honey bran, 'Rounds'.	0.5 oz	52	2	10	98	1	0.9	0.0	0	14%
Melba toast, plain.	1 cracker	16	1	3	30	0	0.4	0.1	0	18%
Melba toast, plain, 'Rounds'.	0.5 oz	53	2	11	111	1	0.6	0.0	0	9%
Melba toast, plain, 'Unsalted'.	1 cracker	16	1	3	5	0	0.4	0.1	0	18%
Melba toast, plain, 'Unsalted Rounds'.	0.5 oz	52	2	11	5	1	0.6	0.0	0	10%
Melba toast, rye.	1 cracker	16	1	3	30	0	0.4	0.1	0	18%
Melba toast, rye, 'Rounds'.	0.5 oz	53	2	11	130	1	0.6	0.0	0	10%
Melba toast, rye, 'Unsalted'.	1 cracker	16	1	3	5	0	0.4	0.1	0	18%
Melba toast, sesame.	1 cracker	16	1	3	25	0	0.5	0.1	0	22%
Melba toast, sesame, 'Rounds'.	0.5 oz	57	2	9	131	1	1.8	0.0	0	26%
Melba toast, w/onion, 'Rounds'.	0.5 oz	51	2	11	120	1	0.6	0.0	0	10%
Melba toast, w/vegetable.	1 cracker	16	1	3	25	0	0.4	0.1	0	18%
Melba toast, whole wheat.	1 cracker	16	1	3	30	0	0.4	0.1	0	18%
Melba toast, whole wheat, unsalted.	1 cracker	16	1	3	5	0	0.4	0.1	0	18%
(Distinctive)										
cracked wheat.	3 crackers	100	2	14	180	1	4.0	1.0	0	36%
'English Water Biscuit'.	4 crackers	70	2	13	100	0	1.0	0.0	0	13%
sesame.	4 crackers	80	2	12	140	2	4.0	1.0	0	39%
thins.	4 crackers	70	1	10	115	0	3.0	1.0	5	38%
toasted wheat.	4 crackers	80	2	12	140	0	3.0	1.0	0	33%
wheat.	4 crackers	100	2	13	140	1	5.0	1.0	0	43%
(Eagle)										
'Cheese on Cheese'.	6 crackers	210	3	24	390	1	11.0	3.0	5	48%
peanut butter and cheese sandwich.	6 crackers	230	6	25	320	1	12.0	2.0	0	47%
peanut butter on toast.	6 crackers	210	5	23	430	1	10.0	2.5	0	45%
wheat, w/cheddar cheese.	6 crackers	200	4	24	400	1	10.0	3.0	5	45%
(Eden Foods)										
nori maki.	15 crackers	110	3	24	160	2	0.0	0.0	0	0%
rice, brown.	5 crackers	120	3	22	230	2	2.0	0.0	0	15%
(Escort) butter flavor.	3 crackers	70	1	9	115	0	4.0	1.0	0	47%
(Estee)										
Melba toast, wheat, '6-calorie'.	1 cracker	6	1	1	5	0	1.0	1.0	0	53%
Melba toast, wheat, 'Snax'.	1 oz	100	4	22	15	0	1.0	1.0	0	8%
saltine, unsalted.	4 crackers	60	1	9	0	0	2.0	1.0	0	31%
ranch flavor 'Snack Crisps'.	0.66 oz	80	2	13	135	0	2.0	1.0	0	23%
(Euphrates)										
wheat.	1 cracker	19	0	3	32	0	0.8	0.2	0	38%

Food Name	Serving Size	Calories	Prot. gms	Carbs gms	Sod. mgs	Fiber gms	Fat gms	Sat. Fat gms	Chol. mgs	% Fat Cal.
wheat, low-salt	1 cracker	19	0	3	11	0	0.8	0.2	0	38%
(Featherweight) low-salt	2 pieces	30	0	5	1	0	1.0	0.0	0	31%
(FFV)										
'Schooners'	0.5 oz	60	1	10	130	0	2.0	1.0	0	29%
sesame, 'Crisp'	1 cracker	60	1	10	120	0	2.0	1.0	0	29%
soda, 'Ocean Crisps'	1 cracker	60	1	10	120	0	2.0	1.0	0	29%
stoned wheat	4 crackers	60	1	10	170	0	2.0	1.0	0	29%
wafer, w/sesame, 'Crisp'	4 crackers	60	2	9	140	0	2.0	1.0	0	29%
wheat, 'Crispy Wafer'	6 crackers	70	1	9	80	0	3.0	0.0	0	40%
(FiberRich) bran	1 cracker	18	1	6	10	3	1.0	0.0	0	24%
(Finast)										
snack	12 crackers	70	1	9	135	0	3.0	0.0	0	40%
wheat, 'Snacks'	7 crackers	70	1	9	85	0	3.0	0.0	0	40%
(Finn Crisp)										
crispbread, dark	2 crackers	38	1	9	130	2	1.0	0.0	0	18%
crispbread, light, 'Hi-Fiber'	1 cracker	35	1	8	60	0	1.0	0.0	0	20%
crispbread, regular	2 crackers	38	1	9	130	2	1.0	0.0	0	18%
crispbread, rye, original, 'Hi-Fiber'	1 cracker	40	1	10	95	0	0.0	0.0	0	0%
crispbread, w/caraway	2 slices	38	1	9	130	2	1.0	0.0	0	18%
(Flavor Tree)										
sesame chips	1/4 cup	163	3	11	380	0	9.2	0.0	0	60%
sesame sticks	1/4 cup	133	3	11	358	0	9.1	0.0	0	60%
sesame sticks, no salt	1/4 cup	131	3	13	7	0	8.1	0.0	0	52%
(Frito-Lay's)										
cheddar	0.5 oz	70	1	8	150	0	4.0	0.0	0	50%
cheese-filled	1.5 oz	210	4	24	470	0	10.0	0.0	5	45%
Italian, zesty	0.5 oz	70	1	9	115	0	3.0	0.0	0	40%
peanut butter, bar	1.75 oz	270	2	30	65	0	16.0	0.0	0	53%
peanut butter filled	6 crackers	210	6	24	450	0	10.0	0.0	0	43%
(Frookie)										
garlic, w/herbs, nonfat, 'Gourmet'	4 crackers	35	1	7	120	0	0.0	0.0	0	0%
pepper, nonfat, 'Gourmet'	4 crackers	35	1	7	40	0	0.0	0.0	0	0%
water, nonfat, 'Gourmet'	4 crackers	35	1	7	60	0	0.0	0.0	0	0%
whole wheat, nonfat, 'Gourmet'	4 crackers	35	1	7	60	0	0.0	0.0	0	0%
(Garden Crisps) vegetables	15 crackers	130	2	22	290	1	3.5	0.5	0	25%
(Grand Union) cheese flavor, 'Big'	25 crackers	140	3	19	220	1	6.0	1.0	5	38%
(Hain)										
cheese flavor	1 oz	130	3	17	180	0	6.0	0.0	0	40%
onion flavor	1 oz	130	3	17	160	0	6.0	0.0	0	40%
onion flavor, no salt added	1 oz	130	3	17	5	0	6.0	0.0	0	40%
'Rich'	1 oz	130	3	18	160	0	5.0	0.0	0	35%
'Rich' no salt added	1 oz	130	3	18	15	0	5.0	0.0	0	35%
rye	1 oz	120	3	19	200	0	4.0	0.0	0	29%
rye, no salt added	1 oz	120	3	19	10	0	4.0	0.0	0	29%
sesame	1 oz	140	3	16	210	0	7.0	0.0	0	45%
sesame, no salt added	1 oz	140	3	16	5	0	7.0	0.0	0	45%
sour cream, w/chive	1 oz	130	3	15	150	0	6.0	0.0	0	43%
sour cream, w/chive, no salt added	1 oz	130	3	15	25	0	6.0	0.0	0	43%
sourdough	0.5 oz	65	2	9	100	0	3.0	0.0	0	38%
sourdough, low-salt	1 oz	130	3	18	10	0	5.0	0.0	0	35%
vegetable, no salt added	1 oz	130	3	18	10	0	5.0	0.0	0	46%
(Health Valley)										
cheese, organic, nonfat	0.5 oz	40	1	9	80	2	0.0	0.0	0	0%
cheese, whole wheat, nonfat	5 crackers	50	2	11	80	2	0.0	0.0	0	0%

Food Name	Serving Size	Calories	Prot. gms	Carbs gms	Sod. mgs	Fiber gms	Fat gms	Sat. Fat gms	Chol. mgs	% Fat Cal.
herb, organic, nonfat	0.5 oz	40	1	9	80	2	0.0	0.0	0	0%
onion, organic, nonfat	0.5 oz	40	1	9	80	2	0.0	0.0	0	0%
rice bran	7 crackers	130	4	19	64	2	4.0	0.0	0	28%
7-grain, stoned wheat	13 crackers	120	3	17	125	3	5.0	0.0	0	36%
7-grain, stoned wheat, no salt added	13 crackers	120	3	17	20	3	5.0	0.0	0	36%
7-grain, w/vegetable, organic	0.5 oz	40	1	9	80	2	0.0	0.0	0	0%
stoned wheat	13 crackers	120	3	17	85	4	6.0	0.0	0	40%
stoned wheat, no salt added	13 crackers	120	3	17	10	4	6.0	0.0	0	40%
stoned wheat, w/herbs, no salt added	13 crackers	120	3	17	30	4	6.0	0.0	0	40%
stoned wheat, w/sesame	13 crackers	130	3	16	150	3	6.0	0.0	0	42%
stoned wheat, w/sessame, no salt added	13 crackers	130	3	17	20	3	6.0	0.0	0	40%
whole wheat, nonfat	5 crackers	50	2	11	80	2	0.0	0.0	0	0%
whole wheat, w/herbs, nonfat	5 crackers	50	2	11	80	2	0.0	0.0	0	0%
whole wheat, w/onions, nonfat	5 crackers	50	2	11	80	2	0.0	0.0	0	0%
whole wheat, w/vegetables, nonfat	5 crackers	50	2	11	80	2	0.0	0.0	0	0%
(Kraft)										
'Handi-Snacks' bacon flavor, w/cheese	1 pkg	130	4	8	410	0	9.0	4.0	20	63%
'Handi-Snacks' peanut butter and cheese sandwich	1 pkg	190	6	11	180	0	14.0	4.0	0	65%
(Hickory Farms)										
cracked wheat wafers	8 crackers	100	2	17	290	0	3.0	0.0	0	26%
'Old Fashioned' *(Hickory Farms)*	10 pieces	90	2	16	170	0	3.0	0.0	0	27%
'Rounds O' Rye' barbecue flavor	1 oz	153	3	13	60	0	10.6	0.0	0	60%
'Rounds O' Rye' garlic	1 oz	147	3	15	126	0	8.9	0.0	0	54%
'Rounds O' Rye' natural	1 oz	156	3	12	93	0	10.9	0.0	0	62%
'Rounds O'Rye' sour cream	1 oz	155	3	13	130	0	10.7	0.0	0	61%
rye wafers	8 crackers	90	2	17	250	0	2.0	0.0	0	19%
rye wafers, salt-free	8 crackers	90	2	18	0	0	1.0	0.0	0	10%
stoned wheat wafers, salt-free	8 crackers	100	2	18	0	0	2.0	0.0	0	18%
'Wheat Mill Wafers' salt-free	4 crackers	50	1	9	0	0	1.0	0.0	0	18%
(Kavli)										
Norwegian crispbread, thick	1 slice	35	1	8	31	2	0.3	0.0	0	7%
Norwegian crispbread, thin	2 slices	40	1	8	32	6	0.3	0.0	0	7%
(Keebler)										
cheese, sandwich, w/peanut butter	2 crackers	70	2	9	150	0	3.0	1.0	0	38%
'Club' low-salt	4 crackers	60	1	9	75	0	3.0	1.0	0	40%
'Hi Ho'	5 crackers	70	1	10	140	1	2.5	0.5	0	34%
'Krispy' saltine	5 crackers	60	1	11	210	0	1.0	1.0	0	16%
'Krispy' saltine, mild cheddar	5 crackers	60	2	10	180	0	2.0	1.0	2	27%
'Krispy' saltine, unsalted tops	5 crackers	60	1	11	120	0	1.0	1.0	0	16%
peanut butter and toast sandwich	2 crackers	70	2	9	120	0	3.0	1.0	0	38%
sesame breadstix, food service product	2 pieces	26	1	4	47	0	0.8	0.1	0	30%
'Toasteds' bacon flavor	4 crackers	60	1	8	125	0	3.0	1.0	0	43%
'Toasteds' buttercrisp	4 crackers	60	1	8	125	0	3.0	1.0	0	43%
'Toasteds' cheddar, juniors	8 pieces	80	1	8	95	0	4.0	1.0	5	50%
'Toasteds' onion flavor	4 crackers	60	1	9	140	0	3.0	1.0	0	40%
'Toasteds' rye	4 crackers	60	1	8	140	0	3.0	1.0	0	43%
'Toasteds' sesame	4 crackers	60	1	8	130	0	3.0	1.0	0	43%
'Town House'	4 crackers	70	1	8	120	0	4.0	1.0	0	50%
'Town House' 50% less fat	5 crackers	70	1	11	180	1	2.0	0.5	0	27%
'Town House' food service product	2 crackers	35	0	4	60	0	2.0	0.5	0	50%
'Town House' low-salt	4 crackers	70	1	8	60	0	4.0	1.0	0	50%
'Town House' sandwich, cheddar	1 cracker	70	1	6	105	0	4.0	1.0	5	56%
'Waldorf' no salt, food service product	2 crackers	30	1	5	1	0	1.0	0.2	0	28%
wheat, sandwich, w/American cheese	1 cracker	70	1	7	85	0	4.0	1.0	5	53%

Food Name	Serving Size	Calories	Prot. gms	Carbs gms	Sod. mgs	Fiber gms	Fat gms	Sat. Fat gms	Chol. mgs	% Fat Cal.
wheats, whole grain, food service product	2 crackers	35	1	5	50	0	1.5	0.3	0	37%
'Wheatables'	12 crackers	70	1	9	140	0	3.0	1.0	0	40%
'Wheatables' low-salt	1 cracker	5	0	1	3	0	0.2	0.1	0	38%
'Wheatables' reduced-fat	29 crackers	130	3	21	320	1	3.5	1.0	0	25%
'Zesta' saltine	5 crackers	60	1	10	190	0	2.0	1.0	0	29%
'Zesta' saltine, 50% less salt	5 crackers	60	1	11	95	1	2.0	0.5	0	27%
'Zesta' saltine, food service product	2 crackers	25	1	4	80	0	1.0	0.1	0	33%
'Zesta' saltine, low-salt	5 crackers	60	1	10	95	0	2.0	1.0	0	29%
'Zesta' saltine, nonfat	5 crackers	50	1	11	90	1	0.0	0.0	0	0%
'Zesta' saltine, unsalted tops	5 crackers	60	1	10	85	0	2.0	1.0	0	29%
'Zesta' saltine, unsalted tops, food service product	2 crackers	25	1	4	35	0	1.0	0.2	0	33%
'Zesta' saltine, wheat	5 crackers	60	1	10	190	0	2.0	1.0	0	29%
(Lite 'N Krispy)										
rice sticks	6 sticks	40	1	8	150	1	0.5	0.0	0	11%
rice sticks, no salt	6 sticks	40	1	8	0	1	0.5	0.0	0	11%
(Little Debbie) wheat, w/cheddar cheese	1 serving	140	3	15	230	0	8.0	2.0	3	50%
(M&M Mars)										
'Combos' cheese flavor	1.8 oz	240	5	34	580	0	10.0	0.0	0	37%
'Combos' peanut butter	1.8 oz	240	6	30	360	0	10.0	0.0	0	38%
(Manischewitz)										
'Tam Tams'	10 crackers	147	2	17	171	0	8.0	6.0	0	49%
'Tam Tams' no salt	10 crackers	138	2	18	10	0	7.0	5.0	0	44%
'Garlic Tams'	10 crackers	153	2	19	165	0	8.0	6.0	0	46%
matzo, American	1 matzo	115	3	22	168	0	1.9	0.4	0	14%
matzo, board, 'Daily Unsalted'	1 oz	110	3	24	1	0	0.3	0.0	0	2%
matzo, board, 'Passover'	1.1 oz	129	3	27	5	0	0.4	0.0	0	3%
matzo, board, thin	0.9 oz	100	3	21	0	0	0.3	0.0	0	3%
matzo, dietetic, thin	0.8 oz	91	3	19	1	0	0.4	0.0	0	4%
matzo, egg and onion, board	1 oz	112	3	23	180	0	1.0	0.2	15	8%
matzo, egg, board, 'Passover'	1.2 oz	132	4	27	5	0	2.0	0.0	25	13%
matzo, egg, miniature, 'Passover'	10 crackers	108	3	20	10	0	2.0	0.0	20	16%
matzo, miniature	10 crackers	90	2	20	10	0	1.0	0.0	0	9%
matzo, tea, thin	1 matzo	100	3	22	3	0	0.3	0.1	0	3%
matzo, whole wheat, w/bran, board	1 oz	110	4	21	1	1	0.6	0.0	0	5%
'Onion Tams'	10 crackers	150	2	18	157	0	8.0	6.0	0	47%
'Wheat Tams'	10 crackers	150	2	18	180	0	8.0	6.0	0	47%
(McCrakens)										
cheddar, tangy	1 oz	140	2	18	170	0	8.0	0.0	0	47%
country butter flavor	1 oz	140	2	18	170	0	8.0	0.0	0	47%
sour cream w/chive flavor	1 oz	140	2	18	170	0	8.0	0.0	0	47%
wheat, toasted	1 oz	140	2	18	170	0	8.0	0.0	0	47%
(Meal Mates)										
bread wafer, w/sesame	3 crackers	70	1	9	160	0	3.0	1.0	0	40%
crispbread, w/sesame	3 crackers	70	1	9	160	0	3.0	1.0	0	40%
(Musso's) garlic toast, w/cheese	3 pieces	70	2	11	180	1	2.5	0.5	0	30%
(Nabisco)										
bacon-flavored	15 crackers	160	3	19	460	0	8.0	1.5	0	45%
'Bran Thins' *(Nabisco)*	7 crackers	60	1	9	70	0	3.0	1.0	0	40%
cheese, sandwich, w/peanut butter	4 pieces	130	3	15	320	0	7.0	1.0	0	47%
'Cheese Nips'	13 pieces	70	1	9	130	0	3.0	1.0	0	40%
'Chicken in a Biskit'	7 pieces	80	1	8	130	0	5.0	1.0	0	56%
'Crown Pilot'	1 cracker	70	1	13	85	1	1.5	0.0	0	19%
'Harvest Crisps' oat	6 crackers	60	1	10	135	0	2.0	1.0	0	29%
'Harvest Crisps' rice	6 crackers	60	1	11	135	1	2.0	0.0	0	27%

Food Name	Serving Size	Calories	Prot. gms	Carbs gms	Sod. mgs	Fiber gms	Fat gms	Sat. Fat gms	Chol. mgs	% Fat Cal.
'Harvest Wheat'	4 crackers	60	1	8	95	0	3.0	1.0	0	43%
'Harvest Wheat' low-salt	1 cracker	14	0	2	8	0	0.6	0.2	0	38%
'Oat Thins'	18 crackers	140	3	20	190	2	6.0	1.0	0	37%
'Oysterettes' soup and oyster	18 crackers	60	1	10	140	0	1.0	1.0	0	17%
'Premium' saltine, low salt	5 crackers	60	1	10	35	1	1.0	0.0	0	17%
'Premium' saltine, multigrain	5 crackers	60	1	10	150	1	1.5	0.0	0	23%
'Premium' saltine, original	5 crackers	59	2	10	178	0	1.4	0.3	0	22%
'Premium' saltine, unsalted tops	5 crackers	60	1	10	135	1	1.5	0.0	0	23%
'Premium' saltine, wheat	4 crackers	60	1	10	130	1	2.0	0.0	0	29%
'Ritz'	4 crackers	70	1	9	140	0	4.0	1.0	0	47%
'Ritz' low-salt	5 crackers	80	1	10	35	1	4.0	0.5	0	45%
'Ritz' wheat	1 cracker	14	0	2	24	0	0.6	0.2	0	38%
'Ritz' wheat, low salt	1 cracker	14	0	2	8	0	0.6	0.2	0	38%
'Ritz' whole wheat	5 crackers	70	1	9	135	0	3.0	1.0	0	40%
'Ritz Bits' cheese flavor	22 pieces	70	1	8	130	0	4.0	0.0	0	50%
'Ritz Bits Sandwiches' w/peanut butter	12 crackers	80	2	8	80	0	4.0	0.0	0	47%
'Ritz Bits Sandwiches' w/cheese	6 crackers	80	1	7	135	0	5.0	1.0	0	58%
'Royal Lunch' milk biscuit	1 cracker	60	1	10	80	1	2.0	0.0	0	29%
'Royal Lunch' soda	0.5 oz	60	1	17	125	0	3.0	1.0	0	27%
Swiss cheese, 'Naturally Flavored'	7 crackers	70	1	9	170	0	3.0	1.0	0	40%
'Toast Sandwich' w/peanut butter	4 pieces	130	3	15	300	0	7.0	1.0	0	47%
'Triscuit' wheat	10 bits	44	1	7	66	1	1.7	0.3	0	34%
'Triscuit' wheat, low-salt	3 crackers	60	1	10	35	0	2.0	1.0	0	29%
'Triscuit Bits'	15 pieces	60	1	10	85	0	3.0	0.0	0	38%
'Triscuit Bits' wheat	8 crackers	60	1	10	75	0	2.0	1.0	0	29%
'Twigs' cheese	1 cracker	10	0	1	20	0	0.5	0.2	0	44%
'Uneeda Biscuits' no salt tops	2 crackers	60	1	10	100	0	2.0	0.0	0	29%
'Waverly Wafer'	4 crackers	70	1	10	160	0	3.0	1.0	0	38%
'Waverly Wafer' low-salt	4 crackers	70	1	10	80	0	3.0	1.0	0	38%
'Wheat Thins'	16 crackers	140	2	19	170	2	6.0	1.0	0	39%
'Wheat Thins'	7 crackers	70	1	9	170	0	4.0	1.0	0	47%
'Wheat Thins' less fat	18 crackers	120	2	21	220	2	4.0	0.5	0	28%
'Wheat Thins' low-salt	1 cracker	14	0	2	8	0	0.6	0.2	0	38%
'Wheat Thins' multigrain	17 crackers	130	2	21	291	2	4.0	0.5	0	28%
'Wheatsworth'	1 cracker	14	0	2	24	0	0.6	0.2	0	38%
'Wheatsworth' low-salt	1 cracker	14	0	2	8	0	0.6	0.2	0	38%
(Nature's Path)										
unleavened bread, carrot raisin, flourless, sprouted, organic	2 oz	130	5	22	5	0	1.0	1.0	0	8%
unleavened bread, millet-rice, flourless, sprouted, organic	2 oz	140	5	23	0	0	1.0	0.0	0	7%
unleavened bread, rye, w/carrot and raisin, organic	1 slice	120	3	26	0	6	0.0	0.0	0	0%
unleavened bread, salt-free, organic, 'Sun Seed'	1 slice	160	6	29	3	7	2.0	0.0	0	11%
unleavened bread, w/apple and spice, organic	1 slice	130	5	9	6	5	0.0	0.0	0	0%
unleavened bread, w/fruit and nuts, organic	1 slice	140	6	27	7	6	0.0	0.0	0	0%
unleavened bread, whole rye, flourless, sprouted, organic	2 oz	140	5	23	0	0	1.0	0.0	0	7%
unleavened bread, whole wheat, flourless, sprouted, organic	2 oz	140	5	23	0	0	1.0	0.0	0	7%
(North Castles) soda, 'English'	1 cracker	10	0	3	14	0	0.0	0.0	0	0%
(Old London)										
Melba toast, bacon, 'Rounds'	0.5 oz	53	2	10	126	1	1.0	0.0	0	16%
Melba toast, garlic, 'Rounds'	0.5 oz	56	2	10	132	1	1.2	0.0	0	18%
Melba toast, pumpernickel	0.5 oz	54	2	11	156	1	0.6	0.0	0	10%

Food Name	Serving Size	Calories	Prot. gms	Carbs gms	Sod. mgs	Fiber gms	Fat gms	Sat. Fat gms	Chol. mgs	% Fat Cal.
Melba toast, rye.	0.5 oz	52	2	11	132	1	0.7	0.0	0	11%
Melba toast, rye, 'Rounds'.	0.5 oz	52	2	11	132	1	0.7	0.0	0	11%
Melba toast, sesame.	0.5 oz	55	2	9	148	1	1.8	0.0	0	27%
Melba toast, sesame, 'Rounds'.	0.5 oz	56	2	9	149	1	1.8	0.0	0	27%
Melba toast, sesame, unsalted.	0.5 oz	55	2	9	5	1	1.8	0.0	0	27%
Melba toast, wheat.	0.5 oz	51	2	11	121	1	0.7	0.0	0	11%
Melba toast, white.	0.5 oz	51	2	10	111	1	0.6	0.0	0	10%
Melba toast, white, 'Rounds'.	0.5 oz	48	2	10	111	1	0.6	0.0	0	10%
Melba toast, white, unsalted.	0.5 oz	51	2	11	4	1	0.6	0.0	0	10%
Melba toast, whole grain.	0.5 oz	52	2	10	116	1	0.9	0.0	0	14%
Melba toast, whole grain, 'Rounds'.	0.5 oz	54	2	10	102	1	1.2	0.0	0	18%
Melba toast, whole grain, unsalted.	0.5 oz	53	2	10	4	1	1.0	0.0	0	16%
(Orchard Crisps)										
apple cinnamon.	0.5 oz	60	1	11	40	0	2.0	1.0	0	27%
banana walnut *(Orchard Crisps)*.	0.5 oz	60	1	11	40	0	2.0	1.0	0	27%
(OTC) soup and oyster.	1 cracker	25	1	4	65	0	1.0	1.0	0	31%
(Pacific Grain)										
barbecue, baked, 94% fat-free.	30 grams	120	2	25	140	1	1.5	0.0	0	11%
potato, 100% natural, baked, 94% fat-free.	30 grams	120	2	26	150	1	0.5	0.0	0	4%
potato, au gratin flavored, baked, 94% nonfat.	1 oz	120	2	24	140	1	2.0	0.0	0	15%
sour cream, w/chive, baked, 94% fat-free.	30 grams	120	2	24	140	1	2.0	0.0	0	15%
(Pepperidge Farm)										
'Flutters'.	0.75 oz	100	2	15	150	0	4.0	1.0	5	35%
'Flutters' garden herb.	0.75 oz	100	2	14	190	0	4.0	1.0	0	36%
'Flutters' golden, w/sesame.	0.75 oz	110	2	13	150	0	5.0	1.0	0	43%
'Flutters' toasted wheat.	0.75 oz	110	2	13	170	0	5.0	1.0	0	43%
'Goldfish' cheddar.	1 oz	120	4	19	230	1	4.0	1.0	5	28%
'Goldfish' cheddar, original.	1 oz	130	3	18	190	1	5.0	1.0	0	35%
'Goldfish' Parmesan cheese.	1 oz	120	4	19	330	1	4.0	1.0	5	28%
'Goldfish' pizza.	1 oz	130	4	19	220	1	5.0	1.0	5	33%
'Goldfish Snack' honey nut, w/roasted cashews and almonds.	1/2 cup	180	5	20	330	2	9.0	1.5	25	45%
'Goldfish Snack' w/roasted peanuts.	1/2 cup	170	5	21	360	2	8.0	1.5	5	41%
'Goldfish Thins' cheddar.	4 crackers	50	1	8	160	0	2.0	0.0	0	33%
'Guppies' cheddar.	12 pieces	40	1	5	95	0	2.0	0.0	0	43%
'Snack Sticks'.	8 crackers	130	4	19	400	1	5.0	2.0	0	33%
'Snack Sticks' pumpernickel.	8 crackers	140	3	20	330	1	6.0	1.0	0	37%
'Snack Sticks' sesame.	8 crackers	140	4	19	280	1	5.0	1.0	0	33%
(Premier Japan)										
rice, sembei, 'Fire & Spice'.	4 crackers	50	1	10	150	1	1.0	0.0	0	17%
rice sembei, w/sesame, wheat-free, lowfat.	4 crackers	60	1	10	260	1	1.0	0.0	0	17%
(Ralston)										
'Oat Bran Krisps'.	0.5 oz	60	1	9	140	3	3.0	0.0	0	40%
'Oat Krisp'.	0.5 oz	50	1	7	140	3	2.0	0.0	0	36%
vegetable.	17 crackers	150	2	19	270	1	7.0	1.0	na	43%
vegetable, less fat.	21 crackers	120	2	23	280	1	3.0	0.0	0	21%
wheat, w/sesame, 'Jacquet'.	8 crackers	140	2	18	150	1	6.0	1.5	na	40%
(Red Oval Farms)										
stoned wheat, w/toasted sesame, mini.	19 crackers	140	4	21	440	2	4.0	0.5	0	26%
(Rokeach)										
cheese flavor.	1 oz	140	3	16	0	0	8.0	0.0	0	49%
saltine.	10 pieces	120	2	20	0	0	3.0	0.0	0	23%
snack.	9 crackers	130	2	19	0	0	5.0	0.0	0	35%

Food Name	Serving Size	Calories	Prot. gms	Carbs gms	Sod. mgs	Fiber gms	Fat gms	Sat. Fat gms	Chol. mgs	% Fat Cal.
(Roman Meal)										
wheat, w/onion, baked	6 crackers	70	1	9	120	1	3.0	1.0	0	40%
wheat, w/sesame, baked	6 crackers	70	1	9	120	0	3.0	1.0	0	40%
whole wheat, baked	6 crackers	70	2	9	105	0	3.0	1.0	0	38%
whole wheat, rye and bran, baked	6 crackers	70	1	9	140	0	3.0	1.0	0	40%
(RyKrisp)										
'Rykrisp Twindividuals' 2 triple pieces	0.5 oz	45	1	11	105	3	1.0	0.0	0	16%
crispbread, original	2 crackers	60	2	8	75	4	0.0	0.0	0	0%
crispbread, rye, triple cracker	1 wafer	92	2	21	66	4	0.3	0.0	0	3%
crispbread, rye, w/sesame, 2 triple pieces	0.5 oz	50	1	10	105	3	2.0	0.0	0	29%
crispbread, seasoned	2 crackers	60	1	10	90	3	1.5	0.0	0	23%
crispbread, sesame	2 crackers	60	2	11	80	3	1.5	0.0	0	21%
(Ryvita)										
crispbread, dark rye	1 cracker	26	1	6	35	1	1.0	0.0	0	25%
crispbread, high-fiber, 'Crisp Bread'	1 cracker	23	1	4	10	2	1.0	0.0	0	31%
crispbread, high-fiber, 'Snackbread'	1 cracker	14	1	3	25	1	1.0	0.0	0	38%
crispbread, light	1 cracker	26	1	6	20	1	1.0	0.0	0	25%
crispbread, rye, light	1 cracker	26	1	6	20	1	1.0	0.0	0	25%
crispbread, rye, dark	1 cracker	26	1	6	35	1	1.0	0.0	0	25%
crispbread, rye, w/sesame	1 cracker	31	1	5	10	1	1.0	0.0	0	27%
wheat, 'Original Snackbread'	1 cracker	20	1	4	20	0	1.0	0.0	0	33%
(Snackwell's)										
cheese, zesty	1 serving	129	2	23	315	1	3.0	0.7	1	21%
cracked pepper	7 crackers	61	1	10	117	0	1.6	0.3	0	23%
French onion	1 serving	128	2	23	275	1	3.0	0.5	1	21%
golden, reduced fat	6 crackers	60	1	11	140	0	1.0	0.0	0	16%
Italian ranch	1 serving	128	2	23	311	1	3.0	0.6	1	21%
salsa, snack	1 serving	128	2	23	321	1	3.0	0.5	1	21%
wheat	1 serving	62	1	12	150	1	1.5	na	na	22%
wheat, nonfat	5 crackers	60	2	12	170	1	0.0	0.0	0	0%
wheat thins, baked	1 serving	136	2	20	168	1	5.8	0.9	0	38%
(Spicer's)										
diet, natural, for weight control	1 oz	100	4	11	65	9	4.0	0.0	0	38%
w/onion, for weight control	1 oz	100	4	12	150	6	4.0	0.0	0	36%
wheat, barbecue, for weight control	1 oz	100	5	12	75	9	5.0	0.0	0	40%
(Stop & Shop) cheese flavor, 'Big'	25 crackers	140	3	19	220	1	6.0	1.0	5	38%
(Sunshine)										
heart shaped	1 cracker	9	0	1	6	0	0.4	0.1	0	38%
soup and oyster	16 crackers	60	1	11	190	0	1.0	1.0	0	16%
wheat	8 crackers	70	1	9	170	0	4.0	1.0	0	47%
wheat, heart shaped	1 cracker	9	0	1	16	0	0.4	0.1	0	38%
(Valley Bakery)	8 crackers	110	3	21	140	1	1.0	0.0	0	9%
'Janet Saghatelian's Hearts'	8 crackers	110	3	21	140	1	1.0	0.0	0	9%
lahvosh, 5-inch rounds	1.2 oz	140	5	26	180	1	1.5	0.0	0	10%
lahvosh, 5-inch wheat rounds	1.2 oz	130	5	26	180	2	1.5	0.0	0	10%
lahvosh, hearts	1 oz	110	4	21	140	1	1.0	0.0	0	8%
lahvosh, 'Sweet-heart Crispies'	1 oz	120	3	22	130	1	2.5	1.0	0	18%
lahvosh, 3-inch rounds	1 oz	110	4	21	140	1	1.0	0.0	0	8%
lahvosh, 3-inch wheat rounds	1 oz	110	4	20	140	2	1.0	0.0	0	9%
lahvosh, 2-inch rounds	1 oz	110	4	21	140	1	1.0	0.0	0	8%
rounds, hors d'oeurvre size	1 cracker	28	1	6	41	0	0.3	0.0	0	10%
rounds, snack size	2 crackers	130	4	26	170	1	1.0	0.0	0	7%
w/sesame seed, original, Armenian	1 slice	190	6	37	250	1	2.0	0.0	0	9%
(Vivant) vegetable	3 crackers	70	1	9	125	0	3.0	1.5	0	40%

Food Name	Serving Size	Calories	Prot. gms	Carbs gms	Sod. mgs	Fiber gms	Fat gms	Sat. Fat gms	Chol. mgs	% Fat Cal.
(Wasa)										
crispbread, 'Extra Crisp'	1 cracker	25	1	5	40	0	0.0	0.0	0	0%
crispbread, cinnamon toast	1 slice	60	2	11	65	1	1.0	0.0	0	15%
crispbread, corn, original, gluten- and wheat-free	1 slice	40	1	7	90	0	1.0	0.0	0	23%
crispbread, light, 'Crisp 'N Light'	1 cracker	25	1	5	40	1	0.0	0.0	0	0%
crispbread, multigrain, original	1 slice	45	2	8	85	2	0.0	0.0	0	0%
crispbread, rye	1 crispbread	37	1	8	26	2	0.1	0.0	0	3%
crispbread, rye, fiber	1 slice	30	1	4	60	2	1.0	0.0	0	31%
crispbread, rye, golden	1 cracker	35	1	7	55	1	0.0	0.0	0	0%
crispbread, rye, hearty	1 slice	45	1	9	40	2	0.0	0.0	0	0%
crispbread, rye, light	1 slice	25	1	5	40	1	0.0	0.0	0	0%
crispbread, rye, organic, salt-free	1 slice	25	1	7	50	1	0.0	0.0	0	0%
crispbread, rye, original	1 slice	30	1	7	0	2	0.0	0.0	0	0%
crispbread, sesame, savory	1 cracker	30	2	4	40	2	1.0	0.0	0	27%
crispbread, sourdough rye, light, 'Crisp 'N Light'	3 pieces	60	2	12	120	1	0.0	0.0	0	0%
crispbread, sourdough rye, original	1 slice	35	1	7	55	1	0.0	0.0	0	0%
crispbread, sourdough, crisp	3 pieces	50	2	11	100	2	0.0	0.0	0	0%
crispbread, wheat, light, 'Crisp 'N Light'	2 crackers	50	2	10	100	1	0.0	0.0	0	0%
crispbread, wheat, toasted, original	1 slice	50	2	8	85	1	1.5	0.0	0	25%
crispbread, wheat, w/sesame	1 cracker	50	2	8	65	1	2.0	0.0	0	31%
crispbread, whole wheat	1 slice	30	2	4	40	2	1.0	0.0	0	27%
crispbread, whole wheat, original	1 slice	50	2	11	55	1	0.5	0.0	0	8%
(Weight Watchers)										
crispbread, garlic flavor	2 crackers	30	1	7	55	0	0.0	0.0	0	0%
crispbread, harvest rice	2 crackers	30	1	7	55	0	0.0	0.0	0	0%
(Westbrae)										
no salt, wafer	4-1/2 wafers	40	1	8	0	0	0.0	0.0	0	0%
onion garlic, wafer	4-1/2 wafers	40	1	8	50	0	0.0	0.0	0	0%
tamari, wafer	4-1/2 wafers	40	1	8	60	0	0.0	0.0	0	0%
w/sesame, wafer	4-1/2 wafers	40	1	8	60	0	0.0	0.0	0	0%
(Wheat Krisp) wheat	0.5 oz	50	2	11	220	0	1.0	0.0	0	15%
(Zings)										
cracker chips, cheddar, baked	0.5 oz	70	1	9	140	0	3.0	1.0	2	40%
cracker chips, ranch flavor, baked	0.5 oz	70	1	9	140	0	3.0	1.0	2	40%
CRACKER CRUMBS										
'Ritz' *(Nabisco)*	1/3 cup	140	2	17	270	1	7.0	1.0	0	45%
'Premium' *(Nabisco)*	1/4 cup	100	3	23	0	1	0.0	0.0	0	0%
CRACKER MEAL										
	1 cup	440	11	93	32	3	2.0	0.3	0	4%
	1 oz	109	3	23	8	1	0.5	0.1	0	4%
(Golden Dipt)	1 oz	100	3	22	0	0	0.0	0.0	0	0%
(Nabisco)	1/4 cup	110	3	24	10	1	0.0	0.0	0	0%
extra fine, food service product *(Keebler)*	4 tbsp	130	3	23	0	1	0.0	0.0	0	0%
matzo *(Manischewitz)*	1/2 cup	243	6	54	7	2	0.3	0.0	0	1%
matzo, 'Daily' *(Manischewitz)*	1 cup	514	13	109	3	1	1.4	0.0	0	3%
matzo, 'Farfel' *(Manischewitz)*	1 cup	280	7	60	2	0	0.8	0.0	0	3%
CRANBERRY										
Fresh										
raw, chopped	1 cup	54	0	14	1	5	0.2	0.0	0	3%
raw, whole	1 cup	47	0	12	1	4	0.2	0.0	0	3%
CRANBERRY BEAN. See BEAN, CRANBERRY.										
CRANBERRY JUICE										
(J. Hungerford) 100% juice	9.03 fl oz	133	0	33	19	0	0.0	0.0	0	0%

Food Name	Serving Size	Calories	Prot. gms	Carbs gms	Sod. mgs	Fiber gms	Fat gms	Sat. Fat gms	Chol. mgs	% Fat Cal.
(Knudsen)										
....	8 fl oz	60	0	14	25	na	0.0	0.0	0	0%
'Just Cranberry'.................................	8 fl oz	40	1	10	0	0	0.0	0.0	0	0%
'Yankee'..	8 fl oz	120	0	30	25	na	0.0	0.0	0	0%
(Lucky Leaf)..................................	6 fl oz	110	0	26	10	0	0.0	0.0	0	0%
(Ocean Spray) 'Crantastic'....................	6 fl oz	100	0	26	15	0	0.0	0.0	0	0%
(Santa Cruz Natural) organic, 'Sparkling'......	8 fl oz	90	1	22	0	0	1.0	0.0	0	9%
CRANBERRY JUICE COCKTAIL. See under FRUIT JUICE DRINK.										
CRANBERRY SAUCE										
Canned										
(A&P).	2 oz	100	1	25	15	0	1.0	0.0	0	8%
(Knudsen)	1 oz	30	1	8	0	0	1.0	0.0	0	20%
jellied *(Finast)*	2 oz	90	0	22	10	0	0.0	0.0	0	0%
jellied *(Ocean Spray)*.	2 oz	80	0	22	10	0	0.0	0.0	0	0%
jellied *(Pathmark)*	2 oz	90	0	22	10	0	0.0	0.0	0	0%
jellied *(S&W)*	1/4 cup	100	0	26	15	1	0.0	0.0	0	0%
jellied, 'Old Fashioned' *(S&W)*	1/2 cup	90	0	22	20	0	0.0	0.0	0	0%
sweetened, 1/2-inch slices	1 slice	86	0	22	17	1	0.1	0.0	0	1%
sweetened.	1 cup	418	1	108	80	3	0.4	0.0	0	1%
whole berry *(Finast)*	2 oz	90	0	22	10	0	0.0	0.0	0	0%
whole berry *(Ocean Spray)*.	2 oz	80	0	21	10	0	0.0	0.0	0	0%
whole berry *(S&W)*	1/4 cup	100	0	26	15	1	0.0	0.0	0	0%
whole berry, 'Old Fashioned' *(S&W)*	1/2 cup	90	0	22	20	0	0.0	0.0	0	0%
CRAPPIE. See SUNFISH.										
CRAYFISH										
mixed species, farmed, cooked....................	3 oz	74	15	0	82	0	1.1	0.2	116	13%
mixed species, farmed, raw.......................	3 oz	61	13	0	53	0	0.8	0.1	91	12%
mixed species, wild, cooked	3 oz	70	14	0	80	0	1.0	0.2	113	13%
mixed species, wild, raw.........................	3 oz	65	14	0	49	0	0.8	0.1	97	11%
CRAYFISH DINNER/ENTRÉE										
(Cajun Cookin') crayfish etouffee, frozen................	12 oz	390	23	51	1110	0	10.0	0.0	0	23%
CREAM										
half and half.	1 cup	315	7	10	98	0	27.8	17.3	89	78%
half and half.	1 fl oz	39	1	1	12	0	3.5	2.2	11	78%
half and half.	1 tbsp	20	0	1	6	0	1.7	1.1	6	78%
half and half *(Crowley)*	1 fl oz	35	1	1	10	0	3.0	0.0	15	77%
half and half *(Darigold)*.	8 fl oz	310	8	11	120	0	27.0	17.3	89	76%
half and half *(Knudsen)*........................	4 fl oz	150	4	5	60	0	13.0	0.0	0	76%
half and half *(Rockview)*	2 tbsp	35	1	0	15	0	3.0	2.0	15	87%
Hawaiian macadamia flavored *(International Delight)*......	1 tbsp	30	0	7	5	0	0.0	0.0	0	0%
heavy, whipping.................................	8 fl oz	821	5	7	89	0	88.1	54.8	326	94%
heavy, whipping.................................	1 fl oz	103	1	1	11	0	11.0	6.9	41	94%
heavy, whipping.................................	1 tbsp	52	0	0	6	0	5.5	3.5	21	94%
heavy, whipping *(Crowley)*......................	1 oz	110	1	1	10	0	11.0	0.0	40	93%
heavy, whipping *(Darigold)*	1 cup	790	6	8	90	0	81.0	50.8	290	93%
heavy, whipping, 'Classic' *(Darigold)*	1 cup	858	5	7	77	0	90.0	23.7	334	94%
heavy, whipping, ultra-pasteurized *(Darigold)*...........	1 cup	790	6	8	90	0	81.0	50.8	290	93%
light	1 cup	469	6	9	95	0	46.3	28.8	159	87%
light	1 fl oz	59	1	1	12	0	5.8	3.6	20	87%
light	1 tbsp	29	0	1	6	0	2.9	1.8	10	87%
light, whipping	1 cup	699	5	7	82	0	73.9	46.2	265	93%
light, whipping	1 tbsp	44	0	0	5	0	4.6	2.9	17	93%
CREAM CHEESE. See under CHEESE.										

Food Name	Serving Size	Calories	Prot. gms	Carbs gms	Sod. mgs	Fiber gms	Fat gms	Sat. Fat gms	Chol. mgs	% Fat Cal.
CREAM OF TARTAR										
....	1 tsp	8	0	2	2	0	0.0	0.0	0	0%
....	1/2 tsp	4	0	1	1	0	0.0	0.0	0	0%
(Tone's)	1 tsp	2	0	1	0	0	0.0	0.0	0	0%
CREAM SUBSTITUTE										
Liquid										
(Carnation)										
butter rum flavored, nondairy, nonfat............	1 tbsp	25	0	6	20	0	0.0	0.0	0	0%
French vanilla flavored, nondairy, nonfat............	1 tbsp	25	0	6	20	0	0.0	0.0	0	0%
Irish cream flavored, nondairy, nonfat............	1 tbsp	25	0	6	20	0	0.0	0.0	0	0%
(Coffee-Mate)										
....	1 tbsp	16	0	2	5	0	1.0	0.3	0	53%
French vanilla flavored, nondairy	1 tbsp	40	0	5	5	0	2.0	0.0	0	47%
mocha almond flavored, nondairy............	2 tsp	60	0	9	20	0	3.0	3.0	0	43%
nondairy, 'Amaretto'....................	1 tbsp	40	0	5	5	0	2.0	0.0	0	47%
nondairy, 'Cinnamon Creme'............	1 tbsp	40	0	5	5	0	2.0	0.0	0	47%
nondairy, 'Hazelnut'....................	1 tbsp	40	0	5	5	0	2.0	0.0	0	47%
nondairy, 'Irish Creme'............	1 tbsp	40	0	5	5	0	2.0	0.0	0	47%
nondairy, fat-free....................	1 tbsp	10	0	2	0	0	0.0	0.0	0	0%
nondairy, light....................	1 tbsp	10	0	1	5	0	0.5	0.0	0	53%
(Crowley) nondairy....................	0.5 fl oz	16	1	1	5	0	1.0	0.0	5	53%
(Finast) nondairy, frozen....................	0.5 fl oz	20	0	2	10	0	2.0	1.0	0	69%
(International Delight)										
Amaretto flavored, nondairy............	1 tbsp	45	0	7	5	0	1.5	0.0	0	33%
Hawaiian macadamia flavored, dairy	1 tbsp	30	0	7	5	0	0.0	0.0	0	0%
Irish cream flavored, nondairy............	1 tbsp	45	0	7	5	0	1.5	0.0	0	33%
(Lucerne) nondairy, 100% milk-free............	0.5 fl oz	16	1	1	5	0	2.0	0.0	0	69%
(Mocha Mix)										
nondairy....................	1 tbsp	20	0	1	5	0	1.5	0.0	0	77%
nondairy, lite....................	1 tbsp	10	0	1	0	0	1.0	0.0	0	69%
(Rich's)										
nondairy, frozen, 'Coffee Rich'............	0.5 fl oz	20	0	2	10	0	2.0	1.0	0	69%
nondairy, frozen, 'Farm Rich'............	0.5 fl oz	20	0	1	5	0	2.0	0.0	0	82%
nondairy, frozen, 'Poly Rich'............	0.5 fl oz	20	0	2	5	0	1.0	1.0	0	53%
(Saco Foods) nondairy, 'Kwik Kream'............	1 tbsp	10	0	2	0	0	1.0	0.0	0	53%
(Westbrae) nondairy............	1 tbsp	10	1	2	10	0	1.0	0.0	0	43%
(WestSoy) nondairy, lite, all natural............	1 tbsp	10	1	2	10	0	1.0	0.0	0	43%
Powder										
(Coffee-Mate)										
nondairy....................	1 tsp	10	1	1	5	0	1.0	0.7	0	53%
nondairy, 'Amaretto'....................	2 tsp	60	0	9	15	0	3.0	3.0	0	43%
nondairy, 'Hazelnut'....................	2 tsp	60	0	0	15	0	3.0	3.0	0	100%
nondairy, 'Irish Creme'....................	2 tsp	60	0	9	15	0	3.0	3.0	0	43%
nondairy, light....................	1 tsp	10	0	2	0	0	0.0	0.0	0	0%
nondairy, nonfat....................	1 tsp	10	0	2	0	0	0.0	0.0	0	0%
(Cremora) nondairy....................	1 tsp	10	0	1	5	0	1.0	0.0	0	69%
(Diehl) nondairy....................	1 tsp	10	0	1	0	0	1.0	0.0	0	69%
(IGA) nondairy....................	1 tsp	10	0	2	5	0	1.0	0.0	0	53%
(Pathmark) nondairy, 'No Frills'............	1 tsp	10	0	1	5	0	0.0	0.0	0	0%
CREAM TOPPING										
(Birds Eye)										
chocolate, nondairy, frozen, 'Cool Whip'............	1 tbsp	12	0	1	0	0	1.0	0.0	0	69%
extra creamy, nondairy, frozen, 'Cool Whip Dairy Recipe'....................	1 tbsp	14	0	1	0	0	1.0	0.0	0	69%

Food Name	Serving Size	Calories	Prot. gms	Carbs gms	Sod. mgs	Fiber gms	Fat gms	Sat. Fat gms	Chol. mgs	% Fat Cal.
nondairy, frozen, 'Cool Whip Lite'	1 tbsp	8	0	1	0	0	1.0	0.0	0	69%
nondairy, frozen, 'Cool Whip'	1 tbsp	12	0	1	0	0	1.0	0.0	0	69%
(Crowley)										
whipped, pressurized can	1 tbsp	20	1	1	10	0	1.0	0.0	5	53%
whipping, heavy	1 oz	110	1	1	10	0	11.0	0.0	40	93%
(Darigold)										
whipping, heavy	1 cup	790	6	8	90	0	81.0	50.8	290	93%
whipping, heavy, 'Classic'	1 cup	858	5	7	77	0	90.0	23.7	334	94%
whipping, heavy, ultra-pasteurized	1 cup	790	6	8	90	0	81.0	50.8	290	93%
(Estee) nondairy, prewhipped	1 tbsp	4	1	1	0	0	1.0	1.0	0	53%
(Kraft)										
frozen, whipped, 'Real Cream'	1/4 cup	30	0	2	5	0	2.0	2.0	10	69%
nondairy, frozen, 'Whipped Topping'	1/4 cup	35	0	2	10	0	3.0	3.0	0	77%
(La Creme) frozen, whipped	1 tbsp	16	0	1	5	0	1.0	0.0	1	69%
(Pet) nondairy, frozen, 'Whip'	1 tbsp	14	0	1	0	0	1.0	0.0	0	69%
(Rich's)										
nondairy, pressurized can, 'Richwhip'	0.25 oz	20	0	1	5	0	2.0	0.0	0	82%
nondairy, prewhipped, 'Richwhip'	1 tbsp	12	0	1	0	0	1.0	0.0	0	69%
(Saco Foods)										
chocolate, dark, 'Dolci Frutta Con Cioccolatta'	1 serving	111	1	14	14	0	6.6	2.4	0	50%
white, 'Dolci Frutta Crema Bianca'	1 serving	112	1	12	14	0	6.0	2.1	0	51%
CREAM TOPPING MIX										
(D-Zerta) prepared	1 tbsp	8	0	0	5	0	1.0	0.0	0	100%
(Dream Whip)										
mix only	1 tbsp	6	0	1	0	0	0.0	0.0	0	0%
prepared w/whole milk	1 tbsp	10	0	1	0	0	0.0	0.0	0	0%
(Featherweight) prepared	1 tbsp	4	0	0	5	0	0.0	0.0	0	0%
(Rich's) mix only, 'Richwhip'	0.25 oz	20	0	1	10	0	2.0	0.0	0	82%
CREOLE SEASONING. See under SEASONING MIX.										
CREPE MIX *(Krusteaz)* prepared, 7-inch diam	2 crepes	80	2	14	110	0	1.0	0.0	0	12%
CRIMINI MUSHROOM. See MUSHROOM, CRIMINI.										
CROAKER, ATLANTIC										
breaded, fried	3 oz	188	15	6	296	0	10.8	3.0	71	52%
raw	3 oz	88	15	0	48	0	2.7	0.9	52	28%
CROISSANT										
(Awrey's)										
butter	1 oz	100	2	10	90	0	6.0	3.0	15	53%
margarine	1.25 oz	120	2	13	180	0	7.0	2.0	5	51%
wheat	2.5 oz	240	4	24	390	1	14.0	3.0	5	53%
(Pepperidge Farm)										
butter, petite, frozen	1 piece	140	3	13	160	0	7.0	0.0	0	50%
'Sandwich Quartet'	1 croissant	170	4	22	250	0	7.0	0.0	0	38%
(Sara Lee) butter, petite, frozen	1 croissant	120	3	13	160	0	6.0	0.0	0	46%
CROOKNECK SQUASH. See SQUASH, CROOKNECK. Also see under SQUASH, SUMMER.										
CROUTONS										
(Brownberry)										
Caesar salad flavored	0.5 oz	62	2	8	165	1	2.6	0.0	1	37%
cheddar cheese flavored	0.5 oz	63	2	8	155	0	2.8	0.0	3	38%
onion and garlic flavored	0.5 oz	60	2	9	190	0	2.2	0.0	1	32%
seasoned	1/2 oz	59	2	9	155	1	2.2	0.0	1	33%
toasted	0.5 oz	56	2	10	145	0	1.4	0.0	0	22%
(Ener-G Foods)										
Italian, gluten free	1 cup	241	4	31	305	4	12.5	1.7	4	45%
onion and garlic, gluten free	1 cup	147	2	37	267	4	0.4	0.1	0	2%

Food Name	Serving Size	Calories	Prot. gms	Carbs gms	Sod. mgs	Fiber gms	Fat gms	Sat. Fat gms	Chol. mgs	% Fat Cal.
plain, gluten free	1 cup	125	1	17	135	3	7.0	0.5	0	48%
(Fresh Gourmet)										
Caesar flavor	4 croutons	30	1	4	85	0	1.0	0.0	0	31%
cheese and garlic flavor, homestyle	4 croutons	30	1	4	100	0	1.0	0.0	0	31%
herb seasoned	4 croutons	30	1	5	90	0	1.0	0.0	0	27%
(Hidden Valley Ranch)										
Parmesan, Italian style, 'Salad Crispins'	1 serving	30	1	5	80	na	0.9	0.1	na	27%
(Just Off Melrose)										
cheese and garlic	3 croutons	25	1	3	30	0	1.5	1.0	5	46%
garlic	3 croutons	30	0	3	25	0	2.0	0.0	0	60%
sun-dried tomato and basil	3 croutons	30	0	3	25	0	2.0	0.0	0	60%
(Other Fine Foods) whole grain, all natural	1 oz	110	3	15	115	0	4.0	0.5	0	33%
(Pepperidge Farm)										
cheddar and romano	9 croutons	30	1	4	95	0	1.0	0.0	0	31%
cheese and garlic	9 croutons	35	1	4	80	0	1.5	0.0	0	40%
onion and garlic	9 pieces	30	1	5	80	0	1.0	0.0	0	27%
seasoned	9 croutons	35	1	4	85	0	1.5	0.0	0	40%
seasoned, classic style	1 serving	33	1	4	97	na	1.3	0.3	na	36%
sour cream and chive	0.5 oz	70	2	9	170	0	3.0	1.0	0	38%
(Reese) Caesar salad flavored	0.5 oz	60	2	9	130	0	2.0	0.0	0	29%
(Rothbury Farms)										
onion flavor poppy toast, nonfat	9 grams	35	1	7	135	0	0.0	0.0	0	0%
seasoned, French style, nonfat	7 grams	25	1	5	105	0	0.0	0.0	0	0%
seasoned, nonfat	7 grams	25	1	5	105	0	0.0	0.0	0	0%

CROWDER PEA. See under BLACK-EYED PEAS.

CRUMPET

(Wolferman's)										
blueberry, low-fat, cholesterol-free	1 crumpet	90	3	21	250	1	1.0	0.0	0	9%
brown sugar-cinnamon, lowfat	1 crumpet	110	3	21	220	2	2.0	0.0	0	16%
raspberry, low-fat, cholesterol-free	1 crumpet	90	3	20	260	1	1.0	0.0	0	9%

CUCUMBER

Fresh										
peeled, raw, chopped	1 cup	16	1	3	3	1	0.2	0.1	0	11%
peeled, raw, sliced	1 cup	14	1	3	2	1	0.2	0.1	0	11%
peeled, raw, sticks, 4-inches	1 stick	1	0	0	0	0	0.0	0.0	0	11%
peeled, raw, whole, large, 8.25 inches	1 cucumber	34	2	7	6	2	0.4	0.1	0	11%
peeled, raw, whole, small 6-3/8 inches	1 cucumber	19	1	4	3	1	0.3	0.1	0	11%
w/peel, raw, whole, large, 8.25 inches	1 cucumber	39	2	8	6	2	0.4	0.1	0	8%
w/peel, raw, sliced	1/2 cup	7	0	1	1	0	0.1	0.0	0	8%

CUMIN SEED

ground *(McCormick/Schilling)*	1 tsp	11	0	1	5	1	0.4	0.0	0	43%
whole	1 tbsp	22	1	3	10	1	1.3	0.1	0	50%
whole	1 tsp	8	0	1	4	0	0.5	0.0	0	50%
whole *(Durkee)*	1 tsp	10	0	0	0	0	0.0	0.0	0	0%
whole *(Laurel Leaf)*	1 tsp	10	0	0	0	0	0.0	0.0	0	0%
whole *(McCormick/Schilling)*	1 tsp	16	1	2	7	1	0.8	0.0	0	43%
whole *(Spice Islands)*	1 tsp	7	0	1	3	0	0.4	0.0	0	47%
whole *(Tone's)*	1 tsp	7	0	1	3	0	0.4	0.0	0	41%

CUPU ASSU OIL

	1 cup	1927	0	0	0	0	218.0	116.0	0	98%
	1 tbsp	120	0	0	0	0	13.6	7.2	0	98%

CURRANT

BLACK / European currant, raw	1 cup	71	2	17	2	na	0.5	0.0	0	5%
RED OR WHITE, raw	1 cup	63	2	15	1	5	0.2	0.0	0	3%

Food Name	Serving Size	Calories	Prot. gms	Carbs gms	Sod. mgs	Fiber gms	Fat gms	Sat. Fat gms	Chol. mgs	% Fat Cal.
ZANTE										
dried	1 cup	408	6	107	12	10	0.4	0.0	0	1%
dried *(Sun-Maid)*	1/4 cup	130	1	31	10	3	0.0	0.0	0	0%
dried *(S&W)*..........................	1/4 cup	130	1	31	10	2	0.0	0.0	0	0%
CURRY POWDER. See under SEASONING MIX.										
CUSK / torsk / tusk										
baked, broiled, grilled, or microwaved................	3 oz	95	21	0	34	0	0.7	na	45	7%
raw	3 oz	74	16	0	26	0	0.6	0.1	35	7%
CUSTARD APPLE / bullock's heart / cherimoya										
Fresh, raw, skin and seeds removed	1 fruit	514	7	131	na	13	2.2	na	0	4%
CUTTLEFISH										
mixed species, cooked	3 oz	134	28	1	632	0	1.2	0.2	190	8%
mixed species, raw	3 oz	67	14	1	316	0	0.6	0.1	95	8%

D

Food Name	Serving Size	Calories	Prot. gms	Carbs gms	Sod. mgs	Fiber gms	Fat gms	Sat. Fat gms	Chol. mgs	% Fat Cal.
DAIKON / Chinese radish / Oriental radish										
boiled, drained..........................	4 oz	19	0.8	3.9	15	>.6 c	0.3	0.1	0	13%
boiled, drained, sliced	1 cup	25	1	5	19	2	0.4	0.1	0	12%
boiled, drained, sliced	1/2 cup	13	0.5	2.5	10	1.2	0.2	0.1	0	13%
dried	1 cup	314	9	74	322	na	0.8	0.3	0	2%
dried	1/2 cup	157	4.6	36.8	161	>4.9 c	0.4	0.1	0	2%
dried	1 oz	77	2.2	18.0	79	>2.4 c	0.2	0.1	0	2%
raw, trimmed	1 oz	5	0.2	1.2	6	>.2 c	<.1	tr	0	<14%
raw, trimmed *(Frieda's)*	1 lb	86	4.1	19.1	(mq)	(mq)	0.5	(mq)	0	5%
raw, trimmed *(Frieda's)*	1 oz	5	0.3	1.2	(mq)	(mq)	<.1	tr	0	<13%
raw, trimmed, sliced	1/2 cup	8	0.3	1.8	9	0.7	<.1	<.1	0	<10%
raw, untrimmed	1 lb	65	2.2	14.7	75	>2.3 c	0.4	0.1	0	5%
raw, whole, approx 7 inches long, 2 1/4 inch diam	1 daikon	62	2.0	13.9	71	5.4	0.3	0.1	0	4%
DAIQUIRI. See under COCKTAIL; COCKTAIL MIX.										
DANDELION GREENS										
boiled, drained, chopped.........................	1 cup	35	2	7	46	3	0.6	0.2	0	15%
raw, chopped.........................	1 cup	25	1	5	42	2	0.4	0.1	0	13%
DANISH CABBAGE. See CABBAGE, DANISH.										
DANISH PASTRY. See under PASTRY; PASTRY, TOASTER.										
DASHEEN										
cooked...........................	4 oz	161	0.6	39.2	11	>1.0 c	0.1	<.1	0	1%
cooked, sliced.........................	1/2 cup	94	0.3	22.8	10	>.6 c	0.1	<.1	0	1%
raw, sliced..........................	1/2 cup	56	0.8	13.8	6	>.4 c	0.1	<.1	0	2%
raw, trimmed	1 oz	30	0.4	7.5	3	>.2 c	0.1	<.1	0	3%
raw, untrimmed	1 lb	419	5.9	103.2	43	>3.1 c	0.8	0.2	0	2%
DASHEEN LEAF										
raw	1/2 cup	6	0.7	0.9	1	>.3 c	0.1	<.1	0	12%
raw, trimmed	1 oz	12	1.4	1.9	1	>.6 c	0.2	<.1	0	12%
raw, untrimmed	1 lb	115	13.5	18.3	8	>5.5 c	2.0	0.4	0	12%
steamed	1/2 cup	18	2.0	3.0	2	>.4 c	0.3	0.1	0	12%
steamed	4 oz	27	3.1	4.6	2	>.6 c	0.5	0.1	0	13%
DASHEEN SHOOTS										
cooked...........................	4 oz	16	0.8	3.6	2	>.6 c	0.1	<.1	0	5%
cooked, sliced	1/2 cup	10	0.5	2.2	1	>.4 c	0.1	<.1	0	8%
raw, sliced...........................	1/2 cup	5	0.4	1.0	<1	>.3 c	<.1	tr	0	<14%

Food Name	Serving Size	Calories	Prot. gms	Carbs gms	Sod. mgs	Fiber gms	Fat gms	Sat. Fat gms	Chol. mgs	% Fat Cal.
raw, trimmed	1 oz	3	0.3	0.7	<1	>.2 c	<.1	tr	0	<18%
raw, untrimmed	1 lb	45	3.7	9.3	4	>2.3 c	0.4	0.1	0	7%
DATE										
Domestic, natural and dry										
	1 lb	1123	8.0	300.1	10	20.8	1.8	na	0	1%
chopped	1/2 cup	245	1.8	65.4	3	4.5	0.4	na	0	1%
pitted	1 oz	78	0.6	20.8	1	1.4	0.1	na	0	1%
pitted (Dole)	1/2 cup	280	5.0	62.0	0	(mq)	0.0	0.0	0	0%
pitted, whole, approx 10 dates	2.9 oz	228	1.6	61.0	2	4.2	0.4	na	0	1%
Imported, pitted										
(Amport Foods)										
chopped	1.5 oz	135	0.0	36.0	0	5	0.0	na	0	0%
whole	1.5 oz	135	0.0	36.0	0	5	0.0	na	0	0%
(Bordo)										
	2 oz	204	1.2	47.2	5	>1.5 c	1.2	na	0	5%
diced	2 oz	203	1.0	47.5	5	>1.2 c	1.1	na	0	5%
(Dromedary)										
chopped	1/4 cup	130	1.0	31.0	0	(mq)	0.0	0.0	0	0%
whole, approx 5 dates	1 oz	100	1.0	23.0	0	(mq)	0.0	0.0	0	0%
DATE, INDIAN. See TAMARIND.										
DEER										
raw	1 lb	544	104.1	0.0	231	na	11.0	4.3	386	19%
raw	1 oz	34	6.4	0.0	14	na	0.7	0.3	24	20%
roasted	3 oz	134	25.7	0.0	46	na	2.7	1.1	95	19%
DESSERT TOPPING										
(Nestlé)										
'Butterfinger'	1 cup	835	22	114	345	4	32.5	18.0	2	35%
'Butterfinger'	2 tbsp	120	3	16	50	1	4.7	2.6	0	35%
'Crunch'	2 tbsp	125	1	16	32	1	6.3	3.6	3	45%
crunchy, 'Buncha Crunch'	1 serving	103	1	13	46	0	5.1	2.4	3	44%
crunchy, 'Buncha Crunch'	2 lb pkg	4671	52	598	2095	15	230.7	108.3	127	44%
crunchy, 'Buncha Crunch'	2 tbsp	103	1	13	46	0	5.1	2.4	3	44%
'Rainbow Morsel'	1 pkt	68	1	10	0	1	2.7	1.6	0	36%
'Rainbow Morsel'	1 serving	68	1	10	0	1	2.7	1.6	0	36%
'Rainbow Morsel'	3 lb pkg	6628	57	1008	41	75	263.8	157.9	27	36%
(Snack Pack)										
chocolate fudge	3.88 oz	166	2	25	148	0	6.3	2.0	0	34%
chocolate, w/dinosaurs	3.84 oz	163	2	26	167	0	5.8	1.4	0	32%
milk chocolate sprinkles	3.88 oz	178	2	28	156	0	6.3	1.7	1	32%
vanilla chocolate sprinkles	3.88 oz	166	2	26	132	0	6.1	1.7	0	33%
DIET BAR. See under SPORTS AND DIET/NUTRITION BARS.										
DIET DRINK. See under SPORTS AND DIET/NUTRITION DRINKS.										
DILL SEASONING. See under SEASONING MIX.										
DILL SEED										
whole	1 tbsp	20	1	4	1	1	1.0	0.0	0	40%
whole	1 tsp	6	0	1	0	0	0.3	0.0	0	40%
whole (Durkee)	1 tsp	9	0	0	0	0	0.0	0.0	0	0%
whole (Laurel Leaf)	1 tsp	9	0	0	0	0	0.0	0.0	0	0%
whole (McCormick/Schilling)	1 tsp	13	0	2	1	2	0.4	0.0	0	31%
whole (Spice Islands)	1 tsp	9	0	1	1	0	0.4	0.0	0	38%
whole (Tone's)	1 tsp	6	0	1	2	0	0.3	0.1	0	31%
DILL WEED										
dried	1 tbsp	8	1	2	6	0	0.1	0.0	0	14%
dried	1 tsp	3	0	1	2	0	0.0	0.0	0	15%

Food Name	Serving Size	Calories	Prot. gms	Carbs gms	Sod. mgs	Fiber gms	Fat gms	Sat. Fat gms	Chol. mgs	% Fat Cal.
dried *(McCormick/Schilling)*	1 tsp	4	0	0	10	0	0.0	0.0	0	0%
dried *(Tone's)*...................................	1 tsp	3	0	1	2	0	0.1	0.0	0	22%
fresh, sprigs...............................	1 cup sprigs	4	0	1	5	0	0.1	0.0	0	22%
fresh, sprigs...............................	5 med sprigs	0	0	0	1	0	0.0	0.0	0	21%
DINNER ROLL. See under ROLL.										
DIP										
ACAPULCO *(Ortega)* nonfat	1 oz	8	0	2	0	0	0.0	0.0	0	0%
AVOCADO										
(Kraft).................................	2 tbsp	60	1	4	240	0	4.0	3.0	0	64%
(Rod's Dips)............................	2 tbsp	110	1	2	210	0	11.0	3.0	5	89%
BACON AND HORSERADISH										
(Breakstone's)	2 tbsp	70	1	2	270	0	6.0	3.0	15	82%
(Kraft)										
	2 tbsp	60	1	3	220	0	5.0	3.0	0	74%
'Premium'	2 tbsp	50	1	2	270	0	5.0	3.0	15	79%
(Sealtest)	2 tbsp	70	1	2	270	0	6.0	3.0	15	82%
BACON AND ONION										
(Breakstone's) 'Gourmet'	2 tbsp	70	1	2	210	0	6.0	3.0	15	82%
(Kraft) 'Premium'	2 tbsp	60	1	2	170	0	5.0	3.0	15	79%
BEAN										
(Bearitos)										
black bean, vegetarian, organic, fat-free	1 oz	24	2	4	135	0	0.0	0.0	0	0%
vegetarian, organic, fat-free	1 oz	25	1	5	135	0	0.0	0.0	0	0%
(Chi-Chi's) 'Fiesta'	1 oz	30	1	4	126	0	1.0	0.0	3	31%
(Eagle)										
black bean......................................	2 tbsp	35	2	5	220	1	1.0	0.0	0	24%
mild	2 tbsp	40	2	5	160	2	1.5	0.0	0	33%
(Frito-Lay's)										
	2 tbsp	40	2	6	140	0	1.0	0.5	0	22%
hot.......................................	2 tbsp	40	2	5	170	1	1.0	0.0	0	24%
(Garden of Eden)										
Baja black bean, organic.....................	2 tbsp	25	2	5	80	1	0.0	0.0	0	0%
chipotle red bean, organic.......................	2 tbsp	25	1	5	90	2	0.0	0.0	0	0%
(Guiltless Gourmet)										
barbecue, mild, nonfat...........................	2 tbsp	23	1	4	100	2	0.0	0.0	0	0%
barbecue, spicy, nonfat...........................	2 tbsp	35	2	6	125	1	0.0	0.0	0	0%
black bean, barbecue, nonfat	2 tbsp	35	2	6	125	1	0.0	0.0	0	0%
black bean, spicy, nonfat........................	2 tbsp	30	2	5	100	1	0.0	0.0	0	0%
mild, nonfat......................................	2 tbsp	23	1	4	100	2	0.0	0.0	0	0%
pinto bean, barbecue, mild	2 tbsp	27	2	5	100	2	0.0	0.0	0	0%
pinto bean, barbecue, spicy	2 tbsp	40	2	7	110	2	0.0	0.0	0	0%
pinto bean, mild............................	2 tbsp	27	2	5	100	2	0.0	0.0	0	0%
pinto bean, spicy, nonfat	2 tbsp	35	2	6	100	2	0.0	0.0	0	0%
(Hain)										
hot......................................	4 tbsp	70	4	10	250	0	1.0	0.0	5	14%
Mexican......................................	4 tbsp	60	4	9	260	0	1.0	0.0	5	15%
w/onion	4 tbsp	70	4	10	270	0	1.0	0.0	5	14%
(Mi Ranchito)										
low-fat......................................	2 tbsp	30	2	8	100	0	1.0	1.0	0	18%
spicy, low-fat	2 tbsp	27	2	7	105	0	1.0	0.0	0	20%
(Old El Paso) black bean	2 tbsp	20	1	4	150	1	0.0	0.0	0	0%
(Tostitos) black, medium, nonfat	2 tbsp	30	2	6	210	2	0.0	0.0	0	0%
BLUE CHEESE										
(Kraft) 'Premium'	2 tbsp	50	1	2	210	0	4.0	2.0	10	75%

Food Name	Serving Size	Calories	Prot. gms	Carbs gms	Sod. mgs	Fiber gms	Fat gms	Sat. Fat gms	Chol. mgs	% Fat Cal.
(Litehouse)										
and dressing, refrigerated, 'Lite'	1 tbsp	33	1	1	86	0	3.0	0.0	0	77%
and dressing, refrigerated, 'Original'	1 tbsp	77	1	0	82	0	8.0	0.0	0	95%
country, and dressing, refrigerated	1 tbsp	76	1	0	84	0	8.0	0.0	0	95%
CAESAR *(Litehouse)* and dressing, refrigerated	1 tbsp	57	0	0	84	0	6.0	0.0	0	100%
CHEESE										
(Chi-Chi's) 'Fiesta'	1 oz	41	1	3	296	0	3.0	1.0	9	63%
(Frito-Lay's) cheddar, mild	2 tbsp	60	1	3	330	0	4.0	1.5	5	69%
(Kraft) nacho, 'Premium'	2 tbsp	55	2	2	200	0	4.0	2.0	10	69%
(Guiltless Gourmet)										
queso, mild	2 tbsp	20	1	5	150	0	0.0	0.0	0	0%
queso, spicy	2 tbsp	20	1	5	150	0	0.0	0.0	0	0%
CHEESE AND SALSA										
(Eagle) medium	2 tbsp	40	1	3	300	0	3.0	1.0	5	63%
(Old El Paso) mild or medium	2 tbsp	40	1	3	300	0	3.0	1.0	3	66%
CHILI *(La Victoria)*	1 tbsp	6	1	1	90	0	1.0	0.0	0	53%
CLAM										
(Breakstone's)										
	2 tbsp	50	1	2	220	0	4.0	3.0	15	75%
'Gourmet Chesapeake'	2 tbsp	50	1	2	200	0	4.0	3.0	20	75%
(Kraft)	2 tbsp	60	1	3	250	0	4.0	3.0	0	69%
(Sealtest)	2 tbsp	50	1	2	220	0	4.0	3.0	15	75%
CUCUMBER *(Kraft)* creamy, 'Premium'	2 tbsp	50	1	2	130	0	4.0	3.0	10	75%
CUCUMBER AND ONION										
(Breakstone's)	2 tbsp	50	1	2	160	0	4.0	3.0	15	75%
(Sealtest)	2 tbsp	50	1	2	160	0	4.0	3.0	15	75%
DILL *(Nasoya)* creamy, 'Vegi-Dip'	1 oz	60	2	4	100	0	4.0	0.0	0	60%
GARLIC										
(Life) and dressing, w/tofu, 'All Natural'	1 tbsp	70	1	1	75	0	7.1	0.0	0	87%
(Nasoya) and herb, 'Vegi-Dip'	1 oz	50	2	6	100	0	2.0	0.0	0	36%
GREEN ONION, *(Kraft)*	2 tbsp	60	1	4	190	0	4.0	3.0	0	64%
GUACAMOLE										
(Kraft)	2 tbsp	50	1	3	210	0	4.0	2.0	0	69%
(Lucerne)	2 tbsp	80	1	1	170	0	8.0	1.5	5	90%
(Rod's Dips)	2 tbsp	80	1	1	170	0	8.0	1.5	5	90%
HONEY MUSTARD *(Litehouse)* and dressing, refrigerated	1 tbsp	67	0	2	55	0	7.0	0.0	0	89%
ITALIAN *(Litehouse)* creamy, and dressing, refrigerated	1 tbsp	60	0	0	76	0	6.0	0.0	0	100%
JALAPEÑO										
(Breakstone's) cheddar, 'Gourmet'	2 tbsp	70	2	2	90	0	6.0	3.0	15	77%
(Frito-Lay's)										
and cheddar cheese	2 tbsp	50	1	4	300	0	4.0	1.0	5	64%
bean	1 oz	30	1	4	115	0	1.0	0.0	0	31%
(Hain) bean, medium	4 tbsp	70	4	10	150	0	1.0	0.0	5	14%
(Kraft)	2 tbsp	60	1	3	260	0	4.0	3.0	0	69%
(Old El Paso) bean, nonfat	1 tbsp	14	1	2	53	1	0.0	0.0	0	0%
(Price's) nacho	1 oz	80	3	2	0	0	7.1	0.0	0	78%
(Wise) bean, nonfat	2 tbsp	25	1	5	100	0	0.0	0.0	0	0%
MUSHROOM *(Breakstone's)* and herb, 'Gourmet'	2 tbsp	50	1	2	150	0	4.0	3.0	10	75%
NACHO *(Guiltless Gourmet)* spicy, nonfat	2 tbsp	25	1	5	150	0	0.0	0.0	0	0%
ONION										
(Bison) French	1 oz	60	1	2	180	0	5.0	0.0	20	79%
(Breakstone's)										
French	2 tbsp	50	1	2	140	0	5.0	3.0	15	79%
toasted, 'Gourmet'	2 tbsp	50	1	2	170	0	5.0	3.0	10	79%
(Frito-Lay's) French	2 tbsp	60	1	4	230	0	5.0	3.0	15	69%

Food Name	Serving Size	Calories	Prot. gms	Carbs gms	Sod. mgs	Fiber gms	Fat gms	Sat. Fat gms	Chol. mgs	% Fat Cal.
(Heluva Good) French, real sour cream	2 tbsp	50	1	2	160	0	5.0	3.0	20	79%
(Kraft)										
creamy, 'Premium'	2 tbsp	45	1	2	160	0	4.0	2.0	10	75%
French	2 tbsp	60	1	4	230	0	4.0	3.0	0	64%
French, 'Premium'	2 tbsp	45	1	2	150	0	4.0	2.0	10	75%
(Lucerne) French	2 tbsp	70	1	2	160	0	6.0	3.0	5	82%
(Nasoya) French, 'Vegi-Dip'	1 oz	50	2	4	100	0	3.0	0.0	0	53%
(Rod's Dips)										
French	2 tbsp	70	1	2	160	0	6.0	3.0	5	82%
French, nonfat	2 tbsp	25	2	3	40	0	0.0	0.0	0	0%
French, w/bacon	2 tbsp	70	1	2	180	0	6.0	2.5	5	82%
(Sealtest) French	2 tbsp	50	1	2	140	0	5.0	3.0	15	79%
PEPPERCORN *(Litehouse)* and dressing, refrigerated	1 tbsp	67	0	0	66	0	7.0	0.0	0	100%
PICANTE										
(Frito-Lay's) nonfat	1 oz	10	0	3	160	0	0.0	0.0	0	0%
(Tostitos) medium	1 tbsp	8	0	2	125	1	0.0	0.0	0	0%
(Wise) nonfat	2 tbsp	12	0	3	130	0	0.0	0.0	0	0%
POPPYSEED *(Litehouse)* and dressing, refrigerated	1 tbsp	65	0	3	83	0	6.0	0.0	0	82%
RANCH										
(Heluva Good) real sour cream	2 tbsp	60	1	2	180	0	5.0	3.0	20	79%
(Litehouse)										
and dressing, refrigerated	1 tbsp	59	0	1	67	0	6.0	0.0	0	93%
and dressing, refrigerated, 'Lite'	1 tbsp	35	1	1	80	0	3.0	0.0	0	77%
country, and dressing, refrigerated	1 tbsp	61	0	1	75	0	7.0	0.0	0	94%
jalapeño, and dressing, refrigerated	1 tbsp	60	0	1	80	0	6.0	0.0	0	93%
refrigerated, 'Veggie Dip'	1 tbsp	60	0	1	68	0	7.0	0.0	0	94%
(Lucerne)	2 tbsp	110	1	2	160	0	11.0	2.0	10	89%
(Rod's Dips)										
nonfat	2 tbsp	25	2	3	40	0	0.0	0.0	0	0%
w/bacon	2 tbsp	110	1	2	180	0	11.0	2.0	5	89%
SALSA										
(Eagle)										
medium	2 tbsp	10	3	2	250	1	0.0	0.0	0	0%
mild	2 tbsp	10	3	2	250	1	0.0	0.0	0	0%
(Pace)										
medium, 'Chunky'	2 tbsp	4	1	1	102	0	1.0	0.0	0	53%
mild, 'Chunky'	2 tbsp	4	1	1	101	0	1.0	0.0	0	53%
SOUR CREAM AND CHIVES										
(Litehouse) vinaigrette, and dressing, refrigerated	1 tbsp	63	0	1	72	0	7.0	0.0	0	94%
TACO										
(Hain) and sauce	4 tbsp	25	1	5	350	0	1.0	0.0	5	27%
(Wise) nonfat	2 tbsp	12	0	3	115	0	0.0	0.0	0	0%
THOUSAND ISLAND										
(Litehouse) and dressing, refrigerated	1 tbsp	65	0	1	99	0	7.0	0.0	0	94%
VEGETABLE *(Marzetti)* and dressing	1 tbsp	88	0	1	120	0	10.0	0.0	2	96%
DIP MIX										
onion and chive *(Knorr)*	1/20 pkg	5	0	1	110	0	0.0	0.0	0	0%
sour cream *(Durkee)*	2 tsp	25	1	4	200	0	0.5	0.0	0	18%
nacho cheese, 'Microwave Snacks' *(Tio Sancho)*	3.5 oz	247	15	2	995	0	20.0	0.0	0	73%
DISHCLOTH GOURD. See GOURD, DISHCLOTH.										
DOCK										
Fresh										
boiled, drained, chopped	3.5 oz	20	1.8	2.9	3	>.7c	0.6	na	0	22%
boiled, drained, chopped	4 oz	23	2.1	3.3	3	>.8 c	0.7	(tr)	0	23%
raw, chopped	1 cup	29	3	4	5	4	0.9	na	0	27%

Food Name	Serving Size	Calories	Prot. gms	Carbs gms	Sod. mgs	Fiber gms	Fat gms	Sat. Fat gms	Chol. mgs	% Fat Cal.
raw, chopped	1/2 cup	15	1.3	2.1	3	1.94	0.5	na	0	25%
raw, trimmed	1 oz	6	0.6	0.9	1	>.2 c	0.2	(tr)	0	23%
raw, untrimmed	1 lb	70	6.4	10.2	13	>2.5 c	2.2	na	0	23%

DOLPHIN FISH. See MAHI MAHI.

DOUGHNUT

(Awrey's)

Food Name	Serving Size	Calories	Prot. gms	Carbs gms	Sod. mgs	Fiber gms	Fat gms	Sat. Fat gms	Chol. mgs	% Fat Cal.
crunch	1 doughnut	600	7	65	730	2	34.0	8.0	40	52%
plain.	1 doughnut	490	6	48	650	1	30.0	7.0	35	56%
sugared	1 doughnut	610	7	68	735	2	35.0	8.0	40	51%
(Break Cake)										
chocolate, gem	1 doughnut	70	1	7	60	0	4.0	1.0	5	53%
chocolate, 1 oz	1 doughnut	130	1	14	115	0	8.0	2.0	5	55%
cinnamon, gem	1 doughnut	60	1	8	70	0	3.0	0.8	5	43%
cinnamon, 1 oz	1 doughnut	120	1	15	130	0	6.0	1.6	5	46%
dunkin stix, 3 oz	2 stix	420	3	43	320	0	27.0	0.0	0	57%
powdered sugar, gem	1 doughnut	60	1	8	70	0	3.0	0.7	5	43%
powdered sugar, 1 oz	1 doughnut	120	1	16	135	0	5.0	1.4	5	40%
(Ener-G Foods) pumpkin, gluten-free	1 serving	128	0	18	7	na	5.9	na	na	42%
(Entenmann's)										
crumb-topped	1 doughnut	260	3	34	220	0	12.0	0.0	0	42%
devil's food crumb	1 doughnut	250	3	34	200	0	12.0	0.0	0	42%
frosted, rich	1 doughnut	280	3	27	210	0	18.0	0.0	0	57%
(Hostess)										
cinnamon, 'Breakfast Bake Shop Donette Gems'	1 doughnut	60	1	7	70	0	3.0	2.0	5	46%
cinnamon, 'Breakfast Bake Shop Family Pack'	1 doughnut	120	2	14	140	1	6.0	3.0	5	46%
cinnamon, 'Breakfast Bake Shop Pantry'	1 doughnut	190	3	24	240	1	10.0	5.0	10	45%
cinnamon, apple-filled, mini.	1 doughnut	70	1	10	70	0	3.0	1.0	5	38%
crumb, 'Breakfast Bake Shop'	1 doughnut	160	1	16	140	1	10.0	5.0	10	57%
frosted, 'Breakfast Bake Shop Donette Gems'	1 doughnut	80	1	8	70	0	5.0	3.0	5	56%
frosted, 'Breakfast Bake Shop' 1.5 oz	1 doughnut	190	2	20	180	1	12.0	7.0	5	55%
frosted, 'O's'.	1 doughnut	260	3	32	240	2	14.0	9.0	5	47%
glazed, 'Breakfast Bake Shop Old Fashioned'	1 doughnut	250	3	33	230	1	12.0	5.0	15	43%
glazed, whirl, 'Breakfast Bake Shop'.	1 doughnut	190	3	27	230	1	7.0	3.0	5	34%
honey wheat, 'Breakfast Bake Shop'.	1 doughnut	250	3	32	280	1	12.0	6.0	25	44%
'Krunch'.	1 doughnut	110	1	16	130	0	4.0	0.0	4	35%
plain, 'Breakfast Bake Shop Donette Gems'	1 doughnut	60	1	6	80	0	3.0	2.0	5	49%
plain, 'Breakfast Bake Shop Family Pack'	1 doughnut	120	2	13	160	1	6.0	3.0	5	47%
plain, 'Breakfast Bake Shop Old Fashioned'	1 doughnut	170	3	21	230	1	9.0	4.0	10	46%
plain, 'Breakfast Bake Shop Pantry'	1 doughnut	190	3	21	270	1	11.0	5.0	10	51%
plain, 'O's'.	1 doughnut	230	3	34	230	1	10.0	4.0	5	38%
powdered sugar, 'Breakfast Bake Shop Pantry'	1 doughnut	190	2	24	230	1	10.0	5.0	10	46%
powdered sugar, mini	1 doughnut	60	1	7	70	0	3.0	2.0	5	46%
strawberry-filled, frosted, mini.	1 doughnut	80	1	10	70	1	4.0	3.0	5	45%
strawberry-filled, powdered sugar, mini.	1 doughnut	70	1	10	70	0	3.0	1.0	5	38%
(Rich's)										
glazed, frozen, 1.2 oz, 'Ever Fresh'	1 doughnut	141	2	17	0	0	7.0	0.0	0	45%
jelly, frozen, 2.17 oz, 'Ever Fresh'	1 doughnut	213	4	26	0	0	9.5	0.0	0	42%
(Tastykake)										
cinnamon, mini	1 doughnut	48	1	6	54	0	2.4	0.6	4	43%
cinnamon, 1.6 oz	1 doughnut	179	3	25	211	1	8.2	2.1	11	41%
frosted, rich, mini	1 doughnut	61	1	8	59	1	3.2	1.9	4	46%
frosted, rich, 2 oz	1 doughnut	258	4	28	196	3	16.0	7.6	9	53%
honey wheat, mini	1 doughnut	40	1	7	48	0	1.2	0.3	3	26%
honey wheat, mini.	1 doughnut	40	1	7	48	0	1.2	0.3	3	26%
honey wheat, 2 oz.	1 doughnut	209	2	33	190	1	7.5	0.0	15	32%

Food Name	Serving Size	Calories	Prot. gms	Carbs gms	Sod. mgs	Fiber gms	Fat gms	Sat. Fat gms	Chol. mgs	% Fat Cal.
orange glazed, 2 oz.	1 doughnut	219	3	32	178	1	9.1	2.5	10	37%
plain, 1.6 oz.	1 doughnut	185	3	22	171	1	10.1	2.5	12	48%
powdered sugar, mini	1 doughnut	42	1	7	71	0	1.3	0.3	4	28%
powdered sugar, 1.6 oz.	1 doughnut	188	3	24	221	1	8.6	2.2	10	42%
DOUGHNUT HOLES (Ener-G Foods) gluten free	1 serving	17	1	2	69	0	0.6	0.2	4	31%
DRAGON'S EYE. See LONGAN.										
DREAM WHIP. See under TOPPING.										
DRESSING. See SALAD DRESSING; STUFFING.										
DRUM, FRESHWATER										
Fresh										
baked, broiled, grilled, or microwaved	3 oz	130	19	0	82	0	5.4	1.2	70	37%
raw	3 oz	101	15	0	64	0	4.2	1.0	54	37%
DUCK										
AVERAGE OF ALL PARTS										
Domestic										
meat and skin, cooked	10 oz	1159	33	0	181	0	112.9	37.9	218	88%
meat and skin, roasted, chopped or diced	1 cup	472	27	0	83	0	39.7	13.5	118	76%
meat only, raw	4.8 oz	181	25	0	101	0	8.2	3.2	105	41%
meat only, roasted, chopped or diced	1 cup	281	33	0	91	0	15.7	5.8	125	50%
Wild, meat and skin, raw	8.3 oz	504	42	0	134	0	36.3	12.0	191	65%
BREAST										
Domestic										
meat and skin, roasted	3 oz	172	21	0	71	na	9.2	2.5	116	48%
meat only, broiled	3 oz	119	23	0	89	na	2.1	0.5	122	16%
meat only, broiled, chopped or diced	1 cup	244	48	0	183	na	4.3	1.0	249	16%
Wild, meat only, raw	3 oz	102	16	0	47	0	3.5	1.1	64	31%
LEG										
Domestic										
meat and skin, braised, chopped or diced	1 cup	310	51	0	188	na	10.4	2.3	183	30%
meat and skin, roasted	3 oz	184	23	0	94	na	9.7	2.5	97	47%
meat only, braised	3 oz	151	25	0	92	na	5.1	1.1	89	30%
LIVER, domestic, raw	1 oz	39	5.3	1.0	(mq)	0	1.3	0.4	146	32%
DUCK FAT										
	1 cup	1846	0	0	0	0	204.6	68.1	205	98%
	1 tbsp	115	0	0	0	0	12.8	4.3	13	98%
DULSE. See under SEA VEGETABLE.										
DUMPLING										
(Creamette) egg noodle, w/pasteurized eggs	2 oz	220	8	40	20	0	3.0	0.0	70	12%
(Stilwell) apple dumpling, w/3tbsp sauce	1 dumpling	390	4	59	240	3	15.0	3.0	0	35%
DUNGENESS CRAB. See under CRAB.										
DURIAN										
raw or frozen, chopped or diced	1 cup	357	4	66	2	9	13.0	na	0	30%
raw or frozen, whole	1 medium	885	9	163	6	23	32.1	na	0	30%

E

Food Name	Serving Size	Calories	Prot. gms	Carbs gms	Sod. mgs	Fiber gms	Fat gms	Sat. Fat gms	Chol. mgs	% Fat Cal.
ÉCLAIR. See under PASTRY.										
EEL										
mixed species, baked, broiled, grilled, or microwaved	3 oz	201	20	0	55	0	12.7	2.6	137	57%
mixed species, baked, broiled, grilled, or microwaved, 1-inch cubes	1 piece	40	4	0	11	0	2.5	0.5	27	57%

Food Name	Serving Size	Calories	Prot. gms	Carbs gms	Sod. mgs	Fiber gms	Fat gms	Sat. Fat gms	Chol. mgs	% Fat Cal.
mixed species, raw	3 oz	156	16	0	43	0	9.9	2.0	107	57%
EGG										
CHICKEN										
Dried										
white, flakes, glucose-reduced	1/2 lb	797	175	9	2624	0	0.1	0.0	0	0%
white, powdered, 100% egg whites *(Nutra/Balance)*	1 tbsp	30	6	1	96	0	0.0	0.0	0	0%
white, stabilized, glucose-reduced, flakes	1 oz	100	21.8	1.2	328	0	<.1	0.0	0	<1%
white, stabilized, glucose-reduced, powder	1 cup	402	88.2	4.8	1325	0	<.1	0.0	0	<1%
white, stabilized, glucose-reduced, powder	1 oz	107	23.4	1.3	351	0	<.1	0.0	0	<1%
whole	1 tbsp	30	2	0	26	0	2.0	0.6	86	62%
whole, powder, glucose-reduced	1 tbsp	53	12	1	173	0	0.0	0.0	0	0%
whole, powder, glucose-reduced, sifted	1 cup	402	88	5	1325	0	0.0	0.0	0	0%
whole, sifted	1 cup	505	40	4	445	0	34.8	10.8	1458	62%
whole, stabilized, glucose-reduced	1 tbsp	31	2	0	27	0	2.2	0.7	101	64%
whole, stabilized, glucose-reduced, sifted	1 cup	523	41	2	466	0	37.4	11.2	1714	64%
yolk, powdered	1 tbsp	27	1	0	5	0	2.2	0.7	93	76%
yolk, powdered, sifted	1 cup	446	23	2	90	0	37.4	11.5	1564	76%
Fresh										
white, raw	1 cup	122	25.6	2.5	399	0	0.0	na	na	0%
white, raw	1 oz	14	3.0	0.3	46	0	0.0	0.0	0	0%
white, raw, large	1 white	17	3.5	0.3	55	0	0.0	na	na	0%
whole, cooked, omelet	1 tbsp	23	2	0	41	0	1.7	0.5	53	68%
whole, cooked, omelet-style, large	1 egg	93	6	1	165	0	7.0	1.9	214	68%
whole, fried, large	1 egg	92	6	1	162	0	6.9	1.9	211	68%
whole, hard-boiled	1 tbsp	13	1	0	11	0	0.9	0.3	36	62%
whole, hard-boiled, chopped	1 cup	211	17	2	169	0	14.4	4.4	577	62%
whole, hard-boiled, large	1 egg	78	6	1	62	0	5.3	1.6	212	62%
whole, poached, large	1 egg	75	6	1	140	0	5.0	1.5	212	60%
whole, raw	1 cup	362	30	3	306	0	24.3	7.5	1033	61%
whole, raw, brown, grade AA *(Lucerne)*	1 egg	70	6	1	65	0	4.5	1.5	215	59%
whole, raw, extra large	1 egg	86	7	1	73	0	5.8	1.8	247	61%
whole, raw, extra large, grade AA *(Lucerne)*	1 egg	80	7	1	70	0	5.0	1.5	240	58%
whole, raw, jumbo	1 egg	97	8	1	82	0	6.5	2.0	276	61%
whole, raw, jumbo, grade A *(Lucerne)*	1 egg	90	8	1	80	0	5.0	2.0	270	56%
whole, raw, large	1 egg	75	6	1	63	0	5.0	1.6	213	61%
whole, raw, medium	1 egg	66	5	1	55	0	4.4	1.4	187	61%
whole, raw, medium, grade AA *(Lucerne)*	1 egg	70	6	1	55	0	4.0	1.5	190	58%
whole, raw, small	1 egg	55	5	0	47	0	3.7	1.1	157	61%
whole, scrambled	1 cup	365	24	5	616	0	26.9	8.1	774	66%
whole, scrambled	1 tbsp	23	2	0	38	0	1.7	0.5	48	66%
whole, scrambled, large	1 egg	101	7	1	171	0	7.4	2.2	215	66%
yolk, raw	1 cup	870	41	4	104	0	75.0	23.2	3113	78%
yolk, raw, large	1 yolk	59	3	0	7	0	5.1	1.6	213	78%
Frozen										
diced *(Sunny Fresh)*	1 serving	80	6	1	125	0	5.0	2.0	215	62%
liquid, 'Country Gold' *(Sunny Fresh)*	1/2 cup	130	12	2	310	0	9.0	3.0	315	59%
whole	1/2 lb	688	35	3	152	0	58.1	17.8	2440	76%
whole, raw, sugared	1/2 lb	697	31	25	152	0	51.6	15.8	2177	67%
Pickled *(Penrose)* approx 2 oz	1 egg	80	8	1	230	0	5.0	0.0	0	56%
DUCK										
whole, fresh, raw	1 large	130	9.0	1.0	102	0	9.6	2.6	619	68%
whole, fresh, raw	1 oz	52	3.6	0.4	41	0	3.9	1.0	251	69%
GOOSE										
whole, fresh, raw	1 large	267	20.0	1.9	199	0	19.1	5.2	1227	66%

Food Name	Serving Size	Calories	Prot. gms	Carbs gms	Sod. mgs	Fiber gms	Fat gms	Sat. Fat gms	Chol. mgs	% Fat Cal.
whole, fresh, raw	1 oz	52	3.9	0.4	na	0	3.8	1.0	(mq)	67%
QUAIL										
whole, fresh, raw	1 oz	45	3.7	0.1	na	0	3.1	1.0	239	65%
whole, fresh, raw	1 large	14	1.2	0.0	13	0	1.0	0.3	76	65%
TURKEY										
whole, fresh, raw	1 large	135	10.8	0.9	120	0	9.4	2.9	737	64%
whole, fresh, raw	1 oz	48	3.9	0.3	na	0	3.4	1.0	265	65%
EGG DISH/MEAL										
(Aunt Jemima)										
scrambled, w/cheddar cheese and fried potatoes	5.9 oz	250	11	22	910	0	13.0	0.0	0	47%
scrambled, w/sausages and hash browns, frozen	5.7 oz	290	12	14	810	0	20.0	0.0	0	63%
scrambled, w/sausages and pancakes, frozen	5.2 oz	270	13	21	880	0	14.0	0.0	0	48%
(Downyflake)										
scrambled, w/ham and hash browns, frozen	6.25 oz	360	13	17	730	0	26.0	0.0	0	66%
scrambled, w/ham and pecan twirl, frozen	6.25 oz	470	15	40	670	0	28.0	0.0	0	53%
scrambled, w/hash browns and sausage link	6.25 oz	420	12	17	790	0	34.0	0.0	0	73%
scrambled, w/sausages and pecan twirl, frozen	6.25 oz	510	16	39	710	0	33.0	0.0	0	57%
(Great Starts) scrambled, w/home fried potatoes	1 pkg	200	7	15	390	2	12.0	8.0	190	55%
(Healthy Choice)										
omelet, turkey sausage, on English muffin, frozen	1 serving	210	16	30	470	0	4.0	2.0	20	16%
omelet, Western style, on English muffin, frozen	1 serving	200	16	29	480	0	3.0	2.0	15	13%
(Mountain House)										
omelet, cheese, freeze-dried, prepared	1/2 pkg	180	13	8	207	0	9.0	0.0	0	49%
w/bacon, freeze-dried, prepared	1/2 pkg	170	12	7	165	0	10.0	0.0	0	54%
w/bacon, precooked, , freeze-dried, prepared	1/2 pkg	180	12	3	0	0	12.0	0.0	0	64%
w/butter, freeze-dried, prepared	1/2 pkg	160	11	8	174	0	8.0	0.0	0	49%
(Sunny Fresh)										
scrambled, precooked	2 oz	90	7	2	180	0	5.0	2.0	215	56%
scrambled, squares	1 serving	60	5	1	50	0	3.5	1.0	145	57%
(Swanson)										
omelet w/cheese sauce, w/ham, 'Great Starts'	7 oz	390	19	15	1220	0	29.0	0.0	0	66%
scrambled, w/bacon and home fries	5.6 oz	340	11	16	690	0	26.0	0.0	0	68%
scrambled, w/cheese and cinnamon pancakes	3.4 oz	290	7	14	380	0	23.0	0.0	0	71%
scrambled, w/sausages and hash browns, frozen	6.5 oz	430	13	19	760	0	34.0	0.0	0	71%
w/mini oat bran muffins, reduced cholesterol	4.75 oz	250	10	27	400	0	12.0	0.0	0	42%
(Weight Watchers)										
ham and cheese omelet, 'Handy'	1 serving	220	13	30	440	2	5.0	2.5	30	21%
omelet sandwich, 'Classic'	1 sandwich	220	15	26	410	2	5.0	2.5	20	22%
omelet sandwich, 'Garden'	3.60 oz	210	9	28	480	0	6.0	2.0	15	27%
EGG DISH/MEAL MIX										
(LaChoy)										
egg foo yung, w/3 oz sauce, 'Dinner Classics' prepared	2 patties	170	8	20	1390	1	7.0	2.2	275	36%
egg foo yung, packaged, 'Dinner Classics'	1/4 pkg	85	3	19	1250	1	1.0	0.0	0	9%
EGG ROLL										
(Chun King)										
chicken, mini	6 egg rolls	210	6	25	650	2	9.0	2.5	15	40%
pork and shrimp, mini	6 egg rolls	210	6	27	540	2	9.0	2.5	15	38%
shrimp, mini	6 egg rolls	190	5	28	730	2	6.0	1.5	10	29%
(La Choy)										
pork, spicy, frozen, food service product	1 roll	196	6	23	537	2	9.4	2.2	5	42%
shrimp, frozen, food service product	1 roll	187	6	26	400	2	7.1	1.3	4	34%
vegetable, food service product	1 roll	174	4	28	456	2	5.1	0.9	2	26%
(Worthington) vegetarian	1 serving	181	6	20	384	2	8.5	1.7	1	42%
EGG ROLL WRAPPER										

Food Name	Serving Size	Calories	Prot. gms	Carbs gms	Sod. mgs	Fiber gms	Fat gms	Sat. Fat gms	Chol. mgs	% Fat Cal.
(Azumaya) square	2 wraps	130	4	26	200	1	0.0	0.0	5	0%
(Azumaya) wonton	5 wraps	100	3	21	160	0	0.0	0.0	5	0%
(Nasoya)	1 piece	23	1	5	19	0	0.0	0.0	0	0%
EGG SUBSTITUTE										
(Best of Egg) 99% egg white product	1/4 cup	30	6	1	100	na	0.0	0.0	0	0%
(Ener-G Foods) egg-free, gluten-free	1 1/2 tsp	15	0	4	7	0	0.0	0.0	0	0%
(Fantastic Foods) dry, 'Tofu Scrambler'	2 1/2 tbsp	60	3	12	480	3	0.5	0.0	0	7%
(Featherweight)	2 eggs	120	9	2	250	0	8.0	0.0	15	62%
(Fleischmann's)										
cheese omelet mix, 'Egg Beaters'	1/2 cup	110	14	2	480	0	5.0	2.0	5	41%
'Egg Beaters'	1/4 cup	30	6	1	100	0	0.0	0.0	0	0%
vegetable omelet mix, 'Egg Beaters'	1/2 cup	50	7	5	170	0	0.0	0.0	0	0%
(Healthy Choice) 'Cholesterol-Free Egg Product'	1/4 cup	30	5	1	90	0	1.0	0.0	0	27%
(Morningstar Farms)										
vegetarian, 'Better 'N Eggs'	1/4 cup	23	5	0	90	0	0.3	0.1	2	12%
vegetarian, 'Scramblers'	1/4 cup	37	6	2	97	0	0.4	na	2	10%
(Nu Laid) nonfat, cholesterol-free	1/4 cup	30	6	1	100	0	0.0	0.0	0	0%
(Second Nature)										
cholesterol-free, real egg product	1/4 cup	60	6	3	110	0	2.0	0.0	0	33%
nonfat, real egg product	1/4 cup	40	6	3	115	0	0.0	0.0	0	0%
(Tofu Scrambler)										
mix, prepared w/tofu	1/2 cup	98	11	7	252	0	5.0	0.0	0	38%
mix, prepared w/tofu, 3 tbsp salt	1/2 cup	158	11	7	335	0	12.0	0.0	0	60%
(Tofutti)										
frozen, 'Egg Watchers'	2 oz	50	7	2	100	0	2.0	0.0	0	33%
nonfat, 'Egg Watchers'	1/4 cup	30	6	1	80	0	0.0	0.0	0	0%
(Wonder Slim)										
for cooking, baking, and salad dressing	1/4 cup	45	0	9	10	1	1.0	0.0	0	20%
nonfat, no animal or dairy products	1/4 cup	35	1	8	10	1	0.0	0.0	0	0%
EGG SUBSTITUTE DISH/MEAL										
(Morningstar Farms)										
frozen, w/hash browns and links 'Scramblers'	7 oz	360	16	22	660	0	23.0	0.0	0	58%
frozen, w/pancakes and links 'Scramblers'	6.8 oz	380	18	33	900	0	19.0	0.0	0	46%
EGG WHITE STABILIZER (Tone's)	1 tsp	12	0	3	1	0	0.0	0.0	0	0%
EGGNOG										
Canned										
(Borden) nonalcoholic	1/2 cup	160	3	16	80	0	9.0	0.0	0	52%
Refrigerated										
(Crowley) nonalcoholic	6 fl oz	270	6	34	200	0	13.0	0.0	100	42%
(Darigold) nonalcoholic	8 fl oz	350	6	43	120	0	17.0	0.0	0	44%
(Darigold) nonalcoholic 'Classic'	8 fl oz	390	10	48	170	0	17.0	0.0	0	40%
(Lucerne)	1/2 cup	170	5	19	75	0	9.0	5.0	75	46%
EGGPLANT / aubergine										
Fresh										
boiled, drained, cubed	1 cup	28	1	7	3	2	0.2	0.0	0	7%
raw, cubed	1 cup	21	1	5	2	2	0.1	0.0	0	6%
raw, whole, approx 1.25 lb, peeled	1 eggplant	119	5	28	14	11	0.8	0.2	0	6%
raw, whole, approx 1.25 lb, unpeeled	1 eggplant	142	6	33	16	14	1.0	0.2	0	6%
Frozen										
cutlets (Celentano)	3/4 cup	330	7	23	170	7	23.0	4.0	45	63%
cutlets, breaded (Bernardi)	1/2 cup	180	3	17	220	2	11.0	2.0	0	55%
rollettes (Celentano)	11 oz	320	14	36	210	0	14.0	0.0	0	39%
rollettes, 'Great Choice' (Celentano)	10-oz tray	330	11	39	660	7	15.0	4.0	55	40%
rollettes, 'Selects' (Celentano)	10-oz tray	360	11	27	490	6	23.0	4.5	45	58%

Food Name	Serving Size	Calories	Prot. gms	Carbs gms	Sod. mgs	Fiber gms	Fat gms	Sat. Fat gms	Chol. mgs	% Fat Cal.
EGGPLANT DISH/ENTRÉE										
(Celentano) Parmigiana	10 oz tray	420	14	30	800	23	27.0	9.0	45	58%
(Progresso) appetizer, canned, 'Caponata'	2 tbsp	30	0	2	130	2	2.0	0.0	0	69%
ELDERBERRY										
Fresh										
raw	1 lb	329	3.0	83.5	na	>31.8 c	2.3	na	0	6%
raw	1 oz	21	0.2	5.2	na	>2.0 c	0.1	(tr)	0	4%
raw	1 cup	106	1.0	26.7	na	>10.1 c	0.7	na	0	5%
ELK										
raw	1 lb	504	104.1	0.0	263	na	6.6	2.4	249	13%
raw	1 oz	31	6.4	0.0	16	na	0.4	0.2	15	12%
roasted	3 oz	124	25.7	0.0	52	na	1.6	0.6	62	12%
roasted	4 oz	166	34.2	0.0	69	0	2.2	0.8	83	13%
roasted, diced, approx 4.9 oz	1 cup	204	42.3	0.0	85	0	2.7	1.0	102	13%
ENCHILADA/ENCHILADA ENTRÉE										
(Amy's Kitchen)										
black bean and vegetable	1 serving	130	4	20	390	2	4.0	0.0	0	27%
cheese.	1 serving	210	11	16	390	2	9.0	2.5	20	43%
(Banquet)										
. . . .	1 entrée	360	10	55	1390	9	11.0	5.0	20	28%
chicken	1 entrée	350	12	54	1580	9	10.0	3.0	25	25%
beef, frozen	12 oz	500	19	72	1810	0	15.0	0.0	0	27%
beef, w/chili and gravy, 'Family Entrées'	7 oz	270	10	28	0	0	13.0	0.0	0	43%
cheese.	1 entrée	360	12	56	1500	8	10.0	4.0	20	25%
cheese, frozen.	12 oz	550	22	71	2170	0	19.0	0.0	0	31%
(Gebhardt)										
. . . .	2 enchiladas	310	5	20	460	2	24.0	9.0	58	68%
. . . .	5.71 oz	258	4	20	687	3	19.1	8.9	25	63%
beef.	1 serving	129	2	10	344	2	9.6	4.5	13	63%
(Healthy Choice)										
beef, frozen, 13.4 oz	1 serving	370	15	66	450	0	5.0	2.0	30	12%
chicken, frozen, 9.5 oz	1 serving	310	14	44	480	0	9.0	3.0	35	26%
chicken, frozen, 13.4 oz	1 serving	340	14	61	470	0	5.0	2.0	30	13%
chicken, suprema	1 entrée	300	13	46	560	4	7.0	3.0	40	21%
chicken, suprema, w/green sauce, rice, corn,										
apple raspberry	1 serving	298	13	46	563	4	6.7	3.1	38	20%
chicken, Suiza.	1 entrée	280	14	43	440	5	4.0	3.0	40	14%
(Hormel)										
beef, frozen	1 piece	140	6	17	573	0	5.0	0.0	0	33%
cheese, frozen.	1 piece	151	6	18	676	0	6.0	0.0	0	36%
(Le Menu) chicken, frozen, 'Light Style'	8 oz	280	21	32	530	0	8.0	0.0	35	25%
(Legume) w/organic tofu, vegetarian	1 serving	270	14	36	390	10	8.0	na	0	26%
(Lean Cuisine)										
beef and bean, frozen.	9.25 oz	240	15	32	480	0	6.0	3.0	45	22%
chicken enchilada Suiza	1 entrée	280	11	48	520	3	5.0	1.5	25	16%
chicken enchilada Suiza, w/sour cream sauce, rice	1 serving	298	11	52	538	4	4.8	1.5	20	15%
(Legume) vegetable, w/tofu and sauce, frozen	11 oz	270	14	36	390	10	8.0	3.0	0	26%
(Old El Paso)										
beef, frozen	1 pkg	210	8	16	720	0	13.0	0.0	10	55%
beef, frozen, 'Festive Dinners'	11 oz	390	24	56	1200	0	8.0	0.0	0	18%
cheese, frozen.	1 pkg	250	10	24	830	0	12.0	0.0	0	44%
cheese, frozen, 'Festive Dinners'	11 oz	590	24	51	1200	0	31.0	0.0	0	48%
chicken, frozen	1 pkg	220	8	20	740	0	12.0	0.0	0	49%

Food Name	Serving Size	Calories	Prot. gms	Carbs gms	Sod. mgs	Fiber gms	Fat gms	Sat. Fat gms	Chol. mgs	% Fat Cal.
chicken, frozen, 'Festive Dinners'	11 oz	460	21	54	770	0	18.0	0.0	0	35%
chicken, w/sour cream sauce, frozen	1 pkg	280	10	18	520	0	19.0	0.0	0	60%
(Patio)										
beef, frozen	13.25 oz	520	16	59	1810	0	24.0	0.0	40	42%
cheese, frozen	12.25 oz	380	14	59	2010	0	10.0	0.0	20	24%
(Soypreme) tofu, organic, all-natural, frozen	11 oz	370	21	45	490	0	11.0	0.0	0	27%
(Stouffer's)										
cheese, frozen, 1 pkg	9.75 oz	490	23	33	550	0	29.0	0.0	0	54%
cheese, w/Mexican rice	1 entrée	370	12	48	890	5	14.0	5.0	25	34%
chicken, frozen, 1 pkg.	10 oz	490	21	31	860	0	31.0	0.0	0	57%
chicken enchanadas, frozen, food service product	1 oz	46	2	4	105	0	2.7	1.0	10	52%
chicken enchilada, w/Mexican rice, Monterey Jack sauce	1 serving	376	12	48	1002	5	14.7	3.4	25	35%
chicken enchiladas, w/Mexican rice	1 entrée	370	16	45	970	3	14.0	3.5	30	34%
(Tio Sancho) 'Dinner Kit'	1 shell	80	1	11	2	1	3.5	0.0	0	39%
(Ultimate 200) beef, Ranchero, frozen	9.12 oz	190	18	18	500	0	5.0	2.0	20	24%
(Van de Kamp's)										
beef, frozen, 'Mexican Dinner'	1/2 pkg	200	8	27	740	0	7.0	0.0	0	31%
beef, frozen, 'Mexican Entrées Family Pack'	1/4 pkg	150	7	19	530	0	5.0	0.0	0	30%
beef, frozen, 'Mexican Entrées'	1 pkg	270	11	30	1040	0	12.0	0.0	0	40%
beef, shredded, frozen, 'Mexican Entrées'	1 pkg	360	20	40	1010	0	14.0	0.0	0	34%
cheese, frozen, 'Mexican Dinner'	1/2 pkg	220	8	26	620	0	9.0	0.0	0	37%
cheese, frozen, 'Mexican Entrées'	1 pkg	300	11	31	980	0	15.0	0.0	0	45%
cheese, frozen, 'Mexican Entrées Family Pack'	1/4 pkg	200	7	19	460	0	10.0	0.0	0	46%
chicken, frozen, 'Mexican Entrées'	1 pkg	260	13	27	1010	0	11.0	0.0	0	38%
ranchero, frozen, 'Mexican Entrées'	1/2 pkg	260	11	26	630	0	12.0	0.0	0	42%
Suiza, frozen, 'Mexican Entrées'	1 pkg	230	12	23	390	0	10.0	0.0	0	39%
(Weight Watchers)										
chicken, nacho Grande, frozen 'Mexican Style'	9 oz	280	14	38	590	0	8.0	3.0	20	26%
chicken, Suiza, frozen	9 oz	230	16	25	530	0	7.0	2.0	40	28%
chicken enchiladas, nacho grande	1 entrée	290	15	42	560	4	8.0	2.5	20	24%
chicken enchiladas Suiza	1 entrée	270	14	33	540	4	9.0	4.5	40	30%
chicken enchilada Suiza, w/sour cream sauce and cheese	1 serving	283	16	33	518	4	9.7	3.7	64	31%

ENCHILADA SEASONING. See under SEASONING MIX.

ENDIVE

Food Name	Serving Size	Calories	Prot. gms	Carbs gms	Sod. mgs	Fiber gms	Fat gms	Sat. Fat gms	Chol. mgs	% Fat Cal.
raw, chopped	1/2 cup	4	0	1	6	1	0.1	0.0	0	10%
raw, whole, approx 1.3 lb.	1 head	87	6	17	113	16	1.0	0.2	0	10%

ENERGY BAR. See under SPORTS AND DIET/NUTRITION BARS.

ENGLISH MUFFIN

Food Name	Serving Size	Calories	Prot. gms	Carbs gms	Sod. mgs	Fiber gms	Fat gms	Sat. Fat gms	Chol. mgs	% Fat Cal.
(Earth Grains)										
oat bran, 12-oz pkg.	1 muffin	120	5	24	410	2	1.0	0.4	0	7%
plain, 12 oz pkg.	1 muffin	120	5	25	390	1	1.0	0.2	0	7%
sourdough, 12-oz pkg.	1 muffin	120	5	25	390	1	1.0	0.2	0	7%
w/raisins, 14-oz pkg	1 muffin	160	5	33	300	1	2.0	0.3	0	11%
w/raisins, 15-oz pkg, 'Sun Maid'	1 muffin	160	5	34	180	2	1.0	0.4	0	5%
wheat berry, 14-oz pkg.	1 muffin	140	6	28	470	2	1.0	0.4	0	6%
whole wheat, 14-oz pkg.	1 muffin	130	6	26	420	4	1.0	0.4	0	7%
whole wheat, 15-oz pkg.	1 muffin	140	6	28	450	4	2.0	0.4	0	12%
(Ener-G Foods) gluten-free	1 serving	203	4	37	1067	14	3.9	0.6	0	17%
(Hi Fiber)										
multigrain	1 muffin	120	4	23	240	4	1.0	0.0	0	8%
plain	1 muffin	110	5	21	280	5	1.0	0.0	0	8%
w/cinnamon and raisins	1 muffin	110	4	21	275	5	1.0	0.0	0	8%

Food Name	Serving Size	Calories	Prot. gms	Carbs gms	Sod. mgs	Fiber gms	Fat gms	Sat. Fat gms	Chol. mgs	% Fat Cal.
(Oatmeal Goodness)										
oatmeal, w/cinnamon and raisins	1 muffin	140	5	26	160	2	2.0	0.0	0	13%
oatmeal, w/honey	1 muffin	140	5	26	160	2	2.0	0.0	0	13%
(Organic Grains)										
7-grain, sprouted, organic	1 muffin	140	10	29	150	3	2.0	0.0	0	10%
w/cinnamon and raisins, organic	1 muffin	170	8	33	165	3	1.0	0.0	0	5%
(Oroweat)										
extra crisp	1 muffin	130	4	26	260	0	1.0	0.0	0	7%
'Health Nut'	1 muffin	170	6	29	220	1	4.0	0.0	0	20%
sourdough	1 muffin	140	4	27	370	0	1.0	0.0	0	7%
(Pepperidge Farm)										
plain	1 muffin	140	5	27	220	0	1.0	0.0	0	7%
sourdough	1 muffin	135	4	27	260	0	1.0	0.0	0	7%
w/cinnamon and apple	1 muffin	140	4	27	210	0	1.0	0.0	0	7%
w/cinnamon and raisins	1 muffin	150	4	29	200	0	2.0	0.0	0	12%
w/cinnamon chips	1 muffin	160	4	28	180	0	3.0	0.0	0	17%
(Roman Meal)										
honey nut, w/oat bran, refrigerated	1/2 muffin	81	3	15	114	1	1.3	0.2	0	15%
'Original'	1 muffin	146	6	29	350	3	1.8	0.0	0	10%
plain, refrigerated	1/2 muffin	71	2	14	88	1	0.5	0.1	0	6%
(Thomas')										
honey wheat	1 serving	110	5	24	190	3	1.0	0.0	0	7%
oat bran	1 serving	120	4	26	210	2	1.0	0.5	0	7%
plain	1 muffin	130	4	25	206	0	1.3	0.0	0	9%
plain, sandwich size	1 serving	190	7	38	280	2	2.0	0.0	0	9%
raisin	1 serving	140	4	31	170	1	1.0	0.1	0	6%
rye	1 muffin	120	5	27	210	3	1.0	0.0	0	7%
sourdough	1 serving	120	4	25	190	1	1.0	0.0	0	7%
sourdough, sandwich size	1 muffin	200	7	41	310	2	2.0	0.0	0	9%
w/onion, sandwich size	1 muffin	180	6	40	270	2	1.5	0.0	0	7%
wheat, sandwich size	1 serving	180	8	39	280	4	1.5	0.0	0	7%
(Wonder) plain	1 serving	130	4	25	290	1	1.0	0.0	0	7%

ENOKI. See MUSHROOM, ENOKI.

ENSURE. See under MEDICAL NUTRITIONALS.

EPAZOTE

Food Name	Serving Size	Calories	Prot. gms	Carbs gms	Sod. mgs	Fiber gms	Fat gms	Sat. Fat gms	Chol. mgs	% Fat Cal.
fresh, raw, whole sprigs	1 medium	1	0	0	1	0	0.0	na	0	13%
fresh, raw, chopped	1 tbsp	0	0	0	0	0	0.0	na	0	13%
EPPAW, raw	1 cup	150	5	32	12	na	1.8	na	0	10%

EUROPEAN CHESTNUT. See CHESTNUT, EUROPEAN.

EUROPEAN CURRANT. See under CURRANT.

F

Food Name	Serving Size	Calories	Prot. gms	Carbs gms	Sod. mgs	Fiber gms	Fat gms	Sat. Fat gms	Chol. mgs	% Fat Cal.
FAJITA/FAJITA ENTRÉE										
(Healthy Choice)										
beef, frozen	7 oz	210	19	26	250	0	4.0	2.0	35	17%
chicken, fiesta	1 entrée	260	21	36	410	4	4.0	1.0	30	14%
chicken, frozen	7 oz	200	17	25	310	0	3.0	1.0	35	14%
(Wonderbites)										
beef, flame-broiled, 'Dippers'	1 piece	33	4	1	86	0	1.5	0.6	9	41%
beef, flame-broiled, frozen, product 9971	1 piece	51	4	1	106	0	3.6	1.4	11	64%

FIG 261

Food Name	Serving Size	Calories	Prot. gms	Carbs gms	Sod. mgs	Fiber gms	Fat gms	Sat. Fat gms	Chol. mgs	% Fat Cal.
(Chicken By George) refrigerated	5 oz	170	28	2	370	0	6.0	0.0	85	31%
FAJITA MIX										
(Hudson) beef, meal kit, prepared	1 fajita	220	11	22	560	1	9.0	5.0	35	38%
(Tyson)										
chicken, kit, frozen	1 pkg	915	57	123	2472	na	23.2	5.9	91	23%
chicken, kit, frozen	1 serving	129	8	17	350	na	3.3	0.8	13	23%
kit	4 oz	80	7	2	240	0	2.0	0.0	0	33%
kit, wholesale club item	3.5 oz	160	10	18	420	0	5.0	0.0	30	29%
FAJITA SEASONING. See under SEASONING MIX.										
FALAFEL MIX										
(Casbah) mix only	1.5 oz	160	6	20	530	2	3.0	0.0	0	21%
(Fantastic Foods) prepared	1/2 cup	250	15	42	610	11	4.0	0.5	0	14%
FARINA. See under CEREAL, HOT.										
FAT SUBSTITUTE										
(Wonder Slim) for cooking, baking, and salad dressing	1/4 cup	45	0	9	10	1	1.0	0.0	0	20%
(Rokeach) 'Neutral Nyafat'	1 tbsp	99	0	0	0	0	11.0	0.0	0	100%
FATHEAD. See SHEEPSHEAD.										
FAVA BEAN. See BEAN, FAVA.										
FEIJOA										
raw, puréed	1 cup	119	3	26	7	na	1.9	na	0	13%
raw, whole, trimmed	1 medium	25	1	5	2	na	0.4	na	0	13%
FENNEL / finnochio										
fresh, raw *(Frieda of California)*	1 oz	4	0	1	26	0	0.1	0.0	0	18%
fresh, raw, sliced	1 cup	27	1	6	45	3	0.2	na	0	5%
fresh, raw, whole, bulb	1 medium	73	3	17	122	7	0.5	na	0	5%
FENNEL SEED										
whole	1 tbsp	20	1	3	5	2	0.9	0.0	0	36%
whole	1 tsp	7	0	1	2	1	0.3	0.0	0	36%
whole *(Durkee)*	1 tsp	7	0	0	0	0	0.0	0.0	0	0%
whole *(Laurel Leaf)*	1 tsp	7	0	0	0	0	0.0	0.0	0	0%
whole *(McCormick/Schilling)*	1 tsp	14	1	2	4	1	0.8	0.0	0	43%
whole *(Spice Islands)*	1 tsp	8	0	1	2	0	0.2	0.0	0	23%
whole *(Tone"s)*	1 tsp	7	0	1	2	0	0.3	0.1	0	33%
FENUGREEK SEED										
whole	1 tbsp	36	3	6	7	3	0.7	0.2	0	17%
whole	1 tsp	12	1	2	2	1	0.2	0.1	0	17%
FETTUCCINE. See under PASTA.										
FETTUCCINE DISH/ENTRÉE. See under PASTA DISH/ENTRÉE.										
FIELD PEAS. See PEAS, FIELD.										
FIG										
Canned										
in extra heavy syrup, w//liquid	1 cup	279	1	73	3	na	0.3	0.1	0	1%
in heavy syrup, w/liquid	1 cup	228	1	59	3	6	0.3	0.1	0	1%
in heavy syrup, w/liquid	1 medium	25	0	6	0	1	0.0	0.0	0	1%
in light syrup, w/liquid	1 cup	174	1	45	3	5	0.3	0.1	0	1%
in light syrup, w/liquid	1 medium	19	0	5	0	1	0.0	0.0	0	1%
in water, w/liquid	1 cup	131	1	35	2	5	0.2	0.1	0	2%
in water, w/liquids	1 medium	14	0	4	0	1	0.0	0.0	0	2%
Dried										
raw, chopped	1 cup	507	6	130	22	24	2.3	0.5	0	4%
raw, whole	1 medium	48	1	12	2	2	0.2	0.0	0	4%
stewed	1 cup	280	3	71	13	13	1.3	0.3	0	4%
Fresh										
raw, large, approx 2.5-inch diam.	1 fig	47	0	12	1	2	0.2	0.0	0	3%

Food Name	Serving Size	Calories	Prot. gms	Carbs gms	Sod. mgs	Fiber gms	Fat gms	Sat. Fat gms	Chol. mgs	% Fat Cal.
raw, medium, approx 2.25-inch diam	1 fig	37	0	10	1	2	0.1	0.0	0	3%
raw, small, approx 1.5-inch diam.....................	1 fig	30	0	8	0	1	0.1	0.0	0	3%
FILBERT. See HAZELNUT.										
FILBERT BUTTER (Maranatha Natural)										
roasted	2 tbsp	180	5	6	5	0	16.0	0.0	0	77%
FILO DOUGH. See PHYLLO DOUGH.										
FINNIAN HADDIE. See under HADDOCK.										
FINNOCHIO. See FENNEL.										
FIREWEED LEAVES										
raw, chopped.....................................	1 cup	24	1	4	8	2	0.6	na	0	22%
raw, whole	1 med plant	23	1	4	7	2	0.6	na	0	22%
FISH. See individual listings.										
FISH AND CHIPS. See under FISH DINNER/ENTRÉE.										
FISH DINNER/ENTRÉE										
(Banquet)										
fillet	1 entrée	290	11	33	820	4	13.0	3.5	30	40%
frozen, 'Platters'.................................	8.75 oz	450	31	33	0	0	22.0	0.0	95	44%
(Fisher Boy)										
batter-dipped, crispy, frozen	1 fillet	170	7	15	310	0	9.0	2.0	20	48%
batter-dipped, crunchy, 'Portions'	1 portion	110	6	10	450	0	6.0	1.0	5	46%
sticks, crunchy, frozen...........................	5 sticks	230	12	19	530	2	11.0	3.0	15	44%
(Gorton's)										
breaded, garlic and herb, frozen....................	2 fillets	250	10	20	720	0	14.0	4.0	25	51%
breaded, hot and spicy, frozen	2 fillets	270	10	19	630	0	17.0	5.0	30	57%
in herb sauce, frozen............................	1 pkg	190	26	3	450	0	8.0	5.0	90	38%
sticks, mini, breaded, frozen	9 sticks	190	8	14	390	0	11.0	3.0	20	53%
(Healthy Choice) lemon pepper	1 entrée	320	14	50	480	5	7.0	2.0	30	20%
(Kid Cuisine) nuggets, frozen....................	7 oz	320	13	33	750	0	15.0	0.0	45	42%
(Lean Cuisine)										
baked	1 entrée	270	17	36	540	3	6.0	2.0	45	20%
fillet, divan, frozen.............................	10 3/8 oz	210	27	13	490	0	5.0	2.0	65	22%
fillet, Florentine, frozen	9 5/8 oz	220	26	13	590	0	7.0	3.0	65	29%
(Morton) frozen	9.75 oz	370	18	46	910	0	13.0	0.0	65	31%
(Mrs. Paul's)										
Dijon, frozen, 'Light'.............................	8.75 oz	200	21	17	650	0	5.0	2.0	60	23%
fillet, Florentine, frozen, 'Light'...................	8 oz	220	25	10	820	0	8.0	4.0	95	34%
Mornay, frozen, 'Light'	9 oz	230	24	12	670	0	10.0	4.0	80	38%
(Stouffer's) fillet, w/macaroni and cheese, 'Homestyle'	1 entrée	430	24	37	930	2	21.0	5.0	70	44%
(Swanson)										
fish 'n chips, battered and fried	1 entrée	490	19	59	1030	5	20.0	4.0	45	37%
w/fries, frozen, 'Home Style Recipe'	6.5 oz	340	11	37	670	0	16.0	0.0	0	43%
(Tyson) sticks, , frozen 'Looney Tunes Sylvester'	7.5 oz	290	13	36	510	0	11.0	0.0	17	34%
(Van de Kamp's)										
breaded, baked, 97% fat-free, frozen, 'Crisp and Healthy'	2 fillets	150	12	18	420	0	3.0	1.0	25	18%
fillet, baked, breaded, frozen, microwaveable	2 fillets	150	12	18	420	0	3.0	1.0	25	18%
fillet, battered, frozen............................	1 serving	180	8	12	340	0	11.0	1.5	20	55%
fillet, breaded.................................	2 pieces	280	11	18	280	0	18.0	3.0	35	58%
fillet, breaded, baked, frozen, 'Crisp and Healthy'	2 pieces	150	12	18	350	0	3.0	1.0	25	18%
fillet, breaded, frozen, 'Snack Pack'.................	2 pieces	220	8	13	280	0	10.0	2.0	20	52%
fillet, crispy, frozen, microwave	1 piece	140	6	9	210	0	9.0	2.0	15	57%
fillet, large, crispy, frozen, microwave	1 piece	290	12	21	640	0	17.0	3.0	25	54%
nuggets, battered, frozen	4 pieces	130	5	8	310	0	9.0	1.0	10	61%
sticks, battered, frozen	4 pieces	160	8	12	380	0	9.0	2.0	20	50%

Food Name	Serving Size	Calories	Prot. gms	Carbs gms	Sod. mgs	Fiber gms	Fat gms	Sat. Fat gms	Chol. mgs	% Fat Cal.
sticks, breaded, baked, frozen, 'Crisp and Healthy'	4 pieces	120	9	17	330	0	2.0	1.0	15	15%
sticks, breaded, frozen 'snack Pack'	4 pieces	170	8	13	270	0	10.0	2.0	20	52%
sticks, breaded, frozen 'Value Pack'	4 pieces	170	8	13	270	0	10.0	2.0	20	52%
sticks, breaded, frozen	4 pieces	200	9	15	290	0	12.0	2.0	20	53%
sticks, crispy, frozen, microwave	3 pieces	130	7	11	280	0	7.0	1.0	15	47%
sticks, mini, breaded, frozen, 'Crisp and Healthy'	10 sticks	180	8	14	280	0	10.0	2.0	20	51%
(Wakefield)										
gems, fancy style, frozen	4 oz	80	11	11	0	0	1.0	0.0	0	9%
gems, salad style, frozen	3 oz	70	10	8	0	0	1.0	0.0	0	11%
(Weight Watchers) oven-baked, w/vegetable medley,										
frozen, 'Ultimate 200'	6.64 oz	120	16	10	390	0	2.0	1.0	0	15%
FISH BATTER SEASONING MIX. See under SEASONING AND COATING MIX.										
FISH OIL										
COD LIVER										
	1 cup	1966	0.0	0.0	0	0	218.0	49.3	1243	100%
	1 tbsp	123	0.0	0.0	0	0	13.6	3.1	78	100%
(Hain)										
cherry	1 tbsp	120	0	0	0	0	14.0	0.0	75	100%
mint	1 tbsp	120	0	0	0	0	14.0	0.0	85	100%
regular	1 tbsp	120	0	0	0	0	14.0	0.0	85	100%
HERRING										
	1 cup	1966	0	0	0	0	218.0	46.4	1670	100%
	1 tbsp	123	0	0	0	0	13.6	2.9	104	100%
MENHADEN										
	1 cup	1966	0	0	0	0	218.0	66.3	1136	100%
	1 tbsp	123	0	0	0	0	13.6	4.1	71	100%
fully hydrogenated	1 cup	1849	0	0	0	0	205.0	196.0	1025	100%
fully hydrogenated	1 tbsp	113	0	0	0	0	12.5	11.9	63	100%
SALMON										
	1 cup	1966	0	0	0	0	218.0	43.3	1057	100%
	1 tbsp	123	0	0	0	0	13.6	2.7	66	100%
SARDINE										
	1 cup	1966	0	0	0	0	218.0	65.2	1548	100%
sardine	1 tbsp	123	0	0	0	0	13.6	4.1	97	100%
FISH PASTE CAKE										
Japanese, block, steamed, 'Kamoboko'	4 oz	111	13.6	11.0	1134	na	1.0	(mq)	(mq)	8%
Japanese, stick, grilled, 'Chikuwa'	4 oz	143	13.8	15.3	1134	na	2.4	(mq)	(mq)	16%
FISH SEASONING. See under SEASONING MIX; SEASONING AND COATING MIX.										
FISH STICKS. See under FISH DINNER/ENTRÉE.										
FISH SUBSTITUTE DINNER/ENTRÉE										
(Worthington) vegetarian, 'Fillets'	2 pieces	180	16	8	750	4	10.0	2.0	0	50.0%
(Loma Linda) vegetarian, 'Ocean Platter' dry mix	1/3 cup	90	14	8	450	4	1.0	0.0	0	10.0%
FIVE-SPICE SEASONING. See under SEASONING MIX.										
FLAN MIX. See under PUDDING MIX.										
FLATFISH. See FLOUNDER; HALIBUT; SOLE.										
FLAX OIL										
organic *(Spectrum Naturals)*	1 tbsp	120	0.0	0.0	0	(tr)	14.0	1.0	(tr)	100%
organic, cinnamon flavored *(Spectrum Naturals)*	1 tbsp	120	0.0	0.0	0	(tr)	14.0	1.0	(tr)	100%
FLAXSEED										
	1 cup	763	30	53	53	43	52.7	5.0	0	58%
	1 tbsp	59	2	4	4	3	4.1	0.4	0	58%
(Arrowhead Mills)	1 oz	140	5	11	1	6	10.0	0.0	0	58%
FLORIDA POMPANO. See POMPANO, FLORIDA.										

Food Name	Serving Size	Calories	Prot. gms	Carbs gms	Sod. mgs	Fiber gms	Fat gms	Sat. Fat gms	Chol. mgs	% Fat Cal.
FLOUNDER										
Fresh										
baked, broiled, grilled, or microwaved...............	3 oz	99	20.5	0.0	89	0	1.3	0.3	58	13%
raw	3 oz	77	16.0	0.0	69	0	1.0	0.2	41	12%
Frozen										
(Finast)	4 oz	90	19	0	150	0	1.0	0.0	0	11%
(SeaPak)...........	4 oz	90	20	0	120	0	1.0	0.0	0	10%
Atlantic (Booth)	4 oz	90	19	0	180	0	1.0	0.0	0	11%
fillet (Van de Kamp"s)	1 serving	110	22	0	105	0	2.0	0.0	45	17%
fillet, 'Light' (Van de Kamp's)	1 piece	260	18	21	480	0	12.0	2.0	45	41%
'Natural' (Van de Kamp's)	4 oz	100	22	0	100	0	2.0	0.0	35	17%
FLOUNDER DINNER/ENTRÉE										
(Gorton's) stuffed, 'Microwave Entrees'	1 pkg	350	25	21	850	0	18.0	7.0	120	47%
FLOUR. See also individual listings.										
ACORN, full-fat...........	1 oz	142	2	15	0	na	8.6	1.1	0	50%
AMARANTH (Arrowhead Mills)	1/4 cup	110	4	19	0	2	1.5	0.0	0	13%
ARROWROOT...........	1 cup	457	0	113	3	4	0.1	0.0	0	0%
BARLEY										
....	1 cup	511	16	110	6	15	2.4	0.5	0	4%
(Arrowhead Mills)...........	2 oz	200	7	35	1	7	1.0	0.0	0	5%
(Arrowhead Mills)...........	1.4 cup	75	3	19	0	3	0.5	0.0	0	5%
BARLEY MALT...........	1 cup	585	17	127	18	12	3.0	0.6	0	4%
BUCKWHEAT										
100% stone ground (Hodgson Mill)...........	1/3 cup	160	7	33	10	2	1.0	0.0	0	5%
whole-grain (Arrowhead Mills)...........	2 oz	190	7	41	0	7	1.0	0.0	0	4%
whole-groat...........	1 cup	402	15	85	13	12	3.7	0.8	0	8%
CAROB										
....	1 cup	229	5	92	36	41	0.7	0.1	0	3%
....	1 tbsp	18	0	7	3	3	0.1	0.0	0	3%
CHESTNUT...........	100 gm	362	6.1	76.2	11	>2.0 c	3.7	0.0	0	9%
CHICKPEA										
(Arrowhead Mills)	2 oz	200	12	35	9	7	3.0	0.0	0	13%
besan	1 cup	339	21	53	59	10	6.2	0.6	0	15%
CORN. See also CORNMEAL.										
masa, enriched...........	1 cup	416	11	87	6	11	4.3	0.6	0	9%
masa harina, enriched (Quaker)...........	1/4 cup	110	3	25	0	2	1.0	0.0	0	7%
masa harina de maiz (Quaker)...........	1/3 cup	137	4	27	5	3	1.5	0.0	0	10%
masa trigo (Quaker)	1/3 cup	149	4	25	794	1	4.0	0.0	0	24%
white, masa harina (Tone's)	1 tsp	8	0	2	1	0	0.1	0.1	0	11%
white, whole grain	1 cup	422	8	90	6	11	4.5	0.6	0	9%
yellow, degermed, unenriched	1 cup	473	7	104	1	2	1.8	0.2	0	3%
yellow, enriched...........	1 cup	416	11	87	6	na	4.3	0.6	0	9%
yellow, whole grain	1 cup	422	8	90	6	16	4.5	0.6	0	9%
COTTONSEED										
low-fat...........	1 oz	94	14	10	10	na	0.4	0.1	0	4%
partially defatted	1 cup	337	39	38	33	3	5.8	1.5	0	14%
partially defatted	1 tbsp	18	2	2	2	0	0.3	0.1	0	14%
GARBANZO (Arrowhead Mills) toasted	1/4 cup	90	5	15	0	3	1.0	0.0	0	10%
GRAHAM										
(Hodgson Mill) whole wheat, organic	1/4 cup	100	3	22	0	3	1.0	0.0	na	8%
(Hodgson Mill) whole grain, stone ground, organic.......	1/4 cup	100	3	22	0	3	1.0	0.0	0	8%
KAMUT (Arrowhead Mills)	1/4 cup	110	4	25	0	4	0.5	0.0	0	4%
MILLET (Arrowhead Mills)	1/4 cup	110	4	26	0	2	1.0	0.0	0	7%
MUSTARD (McCormick/Schilling) ground	1 tsp	12	1	0	0	0	0.8	0.0	0	60%

Food Name	Serving Size	Calories	Prot. gms	Carbs gms	Sod. mgs	Fiber gms	Fat gms	Sat. Fat gms	Chol. mgs	% Fat Cal.
OAT										
(Arrowhead Mills)	1/3 cup	120	5	20	0	4	2.0	0.0	0	15%
blend (Gold Medal)	1 cup	390	14	81	0	4	3.0	0.0	0	7%
OAT BRAN										
blend, all natural (Hodgson Mill)	1/4 cup	110	3	24	3	3	1.0	0.0	0	8%
all-natural (Hodgson Mill)	1/4 cup	110	3	23	4	3	2.0	1.0	na	15%
organic, wheat-free (Hodgson Mill)	1/4 cup	110	3	24	120	3	1.0	0.0	0	8%
PEANUT										
defatted	1 cup	196	31	21	108	9	0.3	0.0	0	1%
defatted	1 oz	93	15	10	51	4	0.2	0.0	0	1%
low-fat	1 cup	257	20	19	1	9	13.1	1.8	0	43%
low-fat	1 oz	121	10	9	0	4	6.2	0.9	0	43%
POTATO										
	1 cup	571	11	133	88	9	0.5	0.1	0	1%
gluten-free (Ener-G Foods)	1 cup	527	14	136	58	10	1.4	0.4	0	2%
QUINOA										
whole-grain, gluten-free (Ancient Harvest)	1/4 cup	132	4	24	10	5	2.0	0.0	0	14%
whole-grain, gluten-free (Quinoa)	1/4 cup	132	4	24	10	5	2.0	0.0	0	14%
RICE										
(Featherweight)	1 cup	500	11	113	7	0	1.0	0.0	0	2%
brown	1 cup	574	11	121	13	7	4.4	0.9	0	6%
brown (Arrowhead Mills)	2 oz	200	4	44	3	3	1.0	0.0	0	4%
brown, whole-grain, stone ground (Hodgson Mill)	1/4 cup	110	3	23	0	1	1.0	0.0	0	8%
sweet, gluten-free (Ener-G Foods)	1 cup	406	8	91	18	0	1.1	0.0	0	3%
white	1 cup	578	9	127	0	4	2.2	0.6	0	3%
RICE STARCH										
gluten-free (Ener-G Foods)	1 cup	263	0	69	0	0	0.0	0.0	0	0%
RYE										
(Krusteaz)	1 cup	351	11	73	1	3	2.0	1.0	0	5%
'Bohemian Style' (Pillsbury)	1/4 cup	100	3	22	0	2	0.0	0.0	0	0%
medium (Pillsbury)	1/4 cup	100	3	22	0	2	0.0	0.0	0	0%
stone-ground (Robin Hood)	1 cup	360	13	86	10	13	2.0	0.0	0	4%
dark	1 cup	415	18	88	1	29	3.4	0.4	0	7%
light	1 cup	374	9	82	2	15	1.4	0.1	0	3%
medium	1 cup	361	10	79	3	15	1.8	0.2	0	4%
organic (Hodgson Mill)	1/4 cup	90	3	22	0	5	1.0	0.0	0	8%
whole-grain (Arrowhead Mills)	2 oz	190	9	39	1	8	1.0	0.0	0	4%
whole-grain, stone-ground (Hodgson Mill)	1/4 cup	90	3	22	0	5	1.0	0.0	0	8%
SESAME										
high-fat	1 oz	149	9	8	12	na	10.5	1.5	0	59%
low-fat	1 oz	94	14	10	11	na	0.5	0.1	0	4%
partially defatted	1 oz	108	11	10	12	na	3.4	0.5	0	26%
SOY										
(Arrowhead Mills)	2 oz	250	20	18	1	8	11.0	0.0	0	39%
defatted	1 tbsp	20	3	2	1	1	0.1	0.0	0	3%
defatted, stirred	1 cup	329	47	38	20	18	1.2	0.1	0	3%
full-fat	1 tbsp	23	2	2	1	0	1.1	0.2	0	40%
full-fat, roasted, stirred	1 cup	366	29	30	11	8	17.3	2.5	0	40%
full-fat, stirred	1 cup	375	30	29	10	8	18.6	2.7	0	41%
gluten-free (Hodgson Mill)	1/4 cup	80	15	9	10	na	0.0	0.0	0	0%
gluten-free, organic (Hodgson Mill)	1/4 cup	110	9	9	0	4	5.0	1.0	0	38%
low-fat	1 tbsp	20	3	2	1	1	0.4	0.1	0	15%
low-fat, stirred	1 cup	327	41	33	16	9	5.9	0.9	0	15%
organic (Hodgson Mill)	1/4 cup	110	9	9	0	4	5.0	1.0	na	38%

Food Name	Serving Size	Calories	Prot. gms	Carbs gms	Sod. mgs	Fiber gms	Fat gms	Sat. Fat gms	Chol. mgs	% Fat Cal.
SPELT										
(Arrowhead Mills)	1/4 cup	100	4	24	0	5	0.5	0.0	0	4%
wheat-free, oragnic, raw (Hodgson Mill)	1/4 cup	115	4	22	0	2	1.0	0.0	0	8%
SUNFLOWER SEED										
partially defatted	1 cup	209	31	23	2	3	1.0	0.1	0	4%
partially defatted	1 tbsp	13	2	1	0	0	0.1	0.0	0	4%
TAPIOCA, cassava flour, gluten-free (Ener-G Foods)	1 cup	313	0	100	4	0	0.0	0.0	0	0%
TEFF, whole-grain (Arrowhead Mills)	2 oz	200	7	41	6	8	1.0	0.0	0	4%
TRITICALE, whole-grain	1 cup	439	17	95	3	19	2.4	0.4	0	4%
WHEAT										
Semolina										
golden, and extra fancy durum (Hodgson Mill)	1/4 cup	110	4	22	0	2	1.0	0.0	0	8%
pasta flour, unbleached (Bob's Red Mill)	1/4 cup	150	5	31	0	0	0.5	0.0	0	3%
White										
all-purpose (Ballard)	1 cup	400	11	87	0	2	1.0	0.0	0	2%
all-purpose (Ceresota)	4 oz	390	13	83	0	0	1.0	0.0	0	2%
all-purpose (Gold Medal)	1 cup	400	11	87	0	0	1.0	0.0	0	2%
all-purpose (Heckers)	4 oz	390	13	83	0	0	1.0	0.0	0	2%
all-purpose (Red Band)	1 cup	390	10	85	0	0	1.0	0.0	0	2%
all-purpose (Robin Hood)	1 cup	400	13	85	0	0	1.0	0.0	0	2%
all-purpose (White Deer)	1 cup	400	11	87	0	0	1.0	0.0	0	2%
all-purpose, bleached (Pillsbury)	1/4 cup	100	3	23	0	1	0.0	0.0	0	0%
all-purpose, bleached, 'Pillsbury's Best' (Pillsbury)	1 cup	400	11	87	0	2	1.0	0.0	0	2%
all-purpose, unbleached (Gold Medal)	1 cup	400	11	87	0	0	1.0	0.0	0	2%
all-purpose, unbleached (Hodgson Mill)	1/4 cup	100	3	23	0	1	0.0	0.0	0	0%
all-purpose, unbleached (Pillsbury)	1/4 cup	100	3	21	0	1	0.0	0.0	0	0%
all-purpose, unbleached (Robin Hood)	1 cup	400	13	85	0	0	1.0	0.0	0	2%
all-purpose, unbleached, 'Pillsbury's Best' (Pillsbury)	1 cup	400	12	86	0	3	1.0	0.0	0	2%
bread (Hodgson Mill)	1/4 cup	100	4	22	0	1	0.0	0.0	0	0%
bread (Pillsbury)	1/4 cup	100	4	22	0	1	0.0	0.0	0	0%
bread, 'Better for Bread' (Gold Medal)	1 cup	400	14	83	0	0	1.0	0.0	0	2%
bread, high-protein, high-gluten (Hodgson Mill)	1/4 cup	100	4	22	5	1	0.0	0.0	0	0%
bread, 'Pillsbury's Best' (Pillsbury)	1 cup	400	14	83	0	0	2.0	0.0	0	4%
bread, enriched	1 cup	495	16	99	3	3	2.3	0.3	0	4%
cake, enriched	1 cup	496	11	107	3	2	1.2	0.2	0	2%
'Drifted Snow (Red Band)	1 cup	400	11	87	0	0	1.0	0.0	0	2%
enriched bleached	1 cup	455	13	95	3	3	1.2	0.2	0	2%
enriched, unbleached	1 cup	455	13	95	3	3	1.2	0.2	0	2%
'La Pina' (Red Band)	1 cup	400	10	87	0	0	1.0	0.0	0	2%
organic, unbleached, (Hodgson Mill)	1/4 cup	100	3	23	0	1	0.0	0.0	0	0%
self-rising (Ballard)	1 cup	380	9	84	1290	0	1.0	0.0	0	2%
self-rising (Gold Medal)	1 cup	380	10	83	1520	0	1.0	0.0	0	2%
self-rising (Red Band)	1 cup	380	9	83	1520	0	1.0	0.0	0	2%
self-rising, bleached (Pillsbury)	1/4 cup	100	3	22	360	1	0.0	0.0	0	0%
self-rising, bleached, 'Pillsbury's Best' (Pillsbury)	1 cup	380	9	84	1290	2	1.0	0.0	0	2%
self-rising, enriched (Aunt Jemima)	1/4 cup	109	3	24	368	0	0.3	0.0	0	2%
self-rising, unbleached, 'Pillsbury's Best' (Pillsbury)	1 cup	380	9	84	1290	2	1.0	0.0	0	2%
self-rising, unbleached (Pillsbury)	1/4 cup	100	2	22	360	1	0.0	0.0	0	0%
shake and blend (Pillsbury)	1/4 cup	100	3	23	0	1	0.0	0.0	0	0%
'Softasilk' (Red Band)	1/4 cup	100	2	23	0	0	0.0	0.0	0	0%
tortilla, enriched	1 cup	450	11	75	751	na	11.8	4.6	0	22%
unbleached (Arrowhead Mills)	2 oz	200	7	53	1	0	1.0	0.0	0	4%
unbleached (Gold Medal)	1 cup	400	11	87	0	0	1.0	0.0	0	2%
unbleached (Robin Hood)	1 cup	400	13	85	0	0	1.0	0.0	0	2%

Food Name	Serving Size	Calories	Prot. gms	Carbs gms	Sod. mgs	Fiber gms	Fat gms	Sat. Fat gms	Chol. mgs	% Fat Cal.
unbleached (Stone-Buhr)	1 cup	400	11	87	5	0	1.0	0.0	0	2%
unenriched	1 cup	455	13	95	3	3	1.2	0.2	0	2%
'Wondra' (Red Band)	1 cup	400	11	87	0	0	1.0	0.0	0	2%
White and whole wheat										
50/50 blend (Hodgson Mill)	1/4 cup	100	4	21	0	2	1.0	0.0	0	8%
whole grain, blend (Gold Medal)	1 cup	380	14	84	0	8	2.0	0.0	0	4%
whole wheat blend (Gold Medal)	1 cup	380	14	84	0	8	2.0	0.0	0	4%
Whole wheat										
	1 cup	407	16	87	6	15	2.2	0.4	0	5%
(Gold Medal)	1 cup	350	16	78	0	10	2.0	0.0	0	5%
(Krusteaz)	1 cup	450	17	90	5	15	2.0	1.0	0	4%
(Pillsbury)	1/4 cup	120	5	22	0	4	1.0	0.0	0	8%
100% hard white wheat (Hodgson Mill)	1/4 cup	100	4	21	0	3	1.0	0.0	0	8%
pastry, organic (Hodgson Mill)	1/4 cup	110	3	22	0	3	1.0	0.0	0	8%
pastry, stone-ground (Hodgson Mill)	1/4 cup	110	3	22	0	3	1.0	na	na	8%
pastry, whole-grain (Arrowhead Mills)	2 oz	180	6	41	1	7	1.0	0.0	0	5%
whole-grain, stone-ground (Arrowhead Mills)	2 oz	200	8	40	1	7	1.0	0.0	0	4%
whole-grain (Ceresota)	4 oz	400	15	80	0	0	2.0	0.0	0	5%
whole-grain (Gold Medal)	1 cup	350	16	78	0	10	2.0	0.0	0	5%
whole-grain (Heckers)	4 oz	400	15	80	0	0	2.0	0.0	0	5%
whole-grain, 'Pillsbury's Best' (Pillsbury)	1 cup	400	15	80	10	0	2.0	0.0	0	5%
WHEAT AND RYE										
'Bohemian Style' (Pillsbury)	1 cup	400	11	86	0	0	1.0	0.0	0	2%
'Pillsbury's Best' (Pillsbury)	1 cup	400	12	83	0	9	2.0	0.0	0	5%
FRANKFURTER										
(Armour)										
beef, 25% less sodium	1 frank	180	7	2	470	0	16.0	6.0	30	80%
jumbo, 25% less sodium	1 frank	160	7	2	470	0	14.0	4.0	50	78%
(Ball Park)										
beef, pork, and chicken, 'Lite'	1 frank	140	7	1	0	0	12.0	0.0	0	77%
light	1 serving	110	7	4	730	0	8.0	2.0	20	62%
mini-franks on a bun	1 pkg	180	6	15	450	1	10.0	3.0	25	52%
nonfat	1 serving	40	6	4	560	0	0.0	0.0	0	0%
(Boar's Head)										
beef	1 oz	80	4	1	0	0	7.0	0.0	15	76%
pork and beef	1 oz	80	4	1	250	0	7.0	0.0	15	76%
(Butcher Boy Meats) turkey	1 serving	134	8	3	651	0	10.2	3.3	58	68%
(Butterball)										
nonfat	1 frank	45	6	4	480	0	0.0	0.0	0	0%
turkey	1 frank	140	7	2	610	0	11.0	0.0	0	73%
(Eckrich)										
beef, 'Bunsize'	1 frank	190	6	2	520	0	17.0	0.0	0	83%
beef, 1 lb pkg.	1 frank	150	5	2	400	0	14.0	0.0	0	82%
'Bun Size'	1 frank	190	6	2	500	0	17.0	0.0	0	83%
cheesefurter	1 frank	180	7	2	530	0	16.0	0.0	0	80%
'Jumbo Lean Supreme'	1 frank	140	7	2	490	0	12.0	0.0	0	75%
1-lb pkg	1 frank	160	5	2	420	0	14.0	0.0	0	82%
(Empire Kosher)										
chicken, kosher	1 frank	100	21	46	820	0	23.0	5.0	25	44%
turkey, kosher	1 frank	90	0	1	410	0	6.0	1.5	35	93%
(Health Valley)										
chicken, 'Weiners'	1 frank	96	5	1	90	0	8.0	0.0	49	75%
turkey, 'Weiners'	1 frank	96	5	1	112	0	8.0	0.0	35	75%

Food Name	Serving Size	Calories	Prot. gms	Carbs gms	Sod. mgs	Fiber gms	Fat gms	Sat. Fat gms	Chol. mgs	% Fat Cal.
(Healthy Choice)										
beef, w/natural smoke flavor, low-fat	1 frank	60	7	5	430	0	1.5	1.0	15	22%
turkey, pork, and beef, lowfat, bun size	1 frank	60	6	6	430	0	1.5	0.5	20	22%
(Healthy Favorites)										
turkey and beef, 97% fat-free	1 frank	60	9	2	570	0	1.5	0.5	25	23%
w/turkey	2 oz	57	9	2	572	0	1.6	0.6	24	25%
(Hebrew National) beef	1 frank	149	6	1	497	0	14.0	0.0	15	82%
(Hillshire Farm)										
beef, bun size	1 serving	180	6	2	530	0	16.0	6.0	40	82%
cheesefurter, 'Bun Size Wieners'	2 oz	180	7	2	530	0	16.0	0.0	0	80%
hot, 'Hot Franks'	2 oz	190	8	2	530	0	16.0	0.0	0	78%
(Hormel)										
batter-wrapped, frozen, 'Corn Dogs'	1 piece	220	7	21	656	0	12.0	0.0	0	49%
batter-wrapped, frozen, 'Tater Dogs'	1 piece	210	6	15	170	0	14.0	0.0	0	60%
beef, 1-lb pkg	1 frank	140	5	1	463	0	13.0	0.0	0	83%
beef, 12-oz pkg	1 frank	100	4	1	362	0	10.0	0.0	0	82%
beef, smoked, 'Wranglers'	1 frank	170	7	2	619	0	15.0	0.0	0	79%
chili, 'Frank 'n Stuff'	1 frank	165	7	2	517	0	15.0	0.0	0	79%
'Light & Lean 97'	1.6 oz	45	6	2	390	0	1.0	2.0	15	22%
meat, 1-lb pkg	1 frank	140	5	1	486	0	13.0	0.0	0	83%
meat, 12-oz pkg	1 frank	110	4	1	378	0	10.0	0.0	0	82%
'Mexicali Dogs'	5 oz	400	14	41	952	0	21.0	0.0	0	46%
smoked, 'Range Brand Wranglers'	1 frank	170	7	1	600	0	16.0	0.0	0	82%
smoked, w/cheese 'Wranglers'	1 frank	180	8	1	546	0	16.0	0.0	0	80%
'Wrangler'	1 frank	162	7	1	557	na	14.4	5.9	38	80%
(Hygrade) chicken, 'Grillmaster'	1 frank	130	7	3	0	0	11.0	0.0	0	71%
(JM)										
10 per lb	1 frank	140	5	1	490	0	13.0	0.0	22	83%
beef	1 frank	100	4	1	350	0	9.0	0.0	20	80%
beef, 'Jumbo'	1 frank	180	6	2	600	0	16.0	0.0	33	82%
beef, 10 per lb	1 frank	140	5	1	480	0	13.0	0.0	26	83%
cheesefurter, 'Cheese Franks'	1.6 oz	140	5	2	540	0	13.0	0.0	0	81%
'German Brand'	1 frank	160	7	1	620	0	14.0	0.0	0	80%
'Jumbo'	1 frank	190	6	2	620	0	17.0	0.0	27	83%
1 frank	1.2 oz	110	4	1	370	0	10.0	0.0	16	82%
w/cheese, 'German Brand' 1 frank	2 oz	160	8	2	620	0	14.0	0.0	37	76%
(Kahn's)										
beef	1 frank	140	5	2	500	0	13.0	0.0	0	81%
beef, 'Bun Size Franks'	1 frank	190	6	3	560	0	17.0	0.0	0	81%
beef, 'Jumbo'	1 frank	190	6	3	560	0	18.0	0.0	0	82%
beef, smoked, 'Bun Size Beef Smokey'	1 frank	190	7	2	530	0	17.0	0.0	0	81%
beef, w/cheddar cheddar, 'Beef n' Cheddar'	1 frank	180	7	2	640	0	16.0	0.0	0	80%
'Bun Size Frank'	1 frank	190	6	2	560	0	17.0	0.0	0	83%
'Cheese Wiener'	1 frank	150	6	1	490	0	13.0	0.0	0	81%
'Jumbo'	1 frank	190	6	2	560	0	17.0	0.0	0	83%
smoked, 'Big Red Smokey'	1 frank	170	8	2	550	0	14.0	0.0	0	76%
smoked, 'Bun Size Smokey'	1 frank	180	8	2	550	0	15.0	0.0	0	77%
'Wieners'	1 frank	140	5	1	500	0	13.0	0.0	0	83%
(King Kold) beef	2 oz	173	9	1	815	0	16.3	0.0	0	79%
(Loma Linda)										
vegetarian, canned, 'Big Franks'	1 pkg	1315	135	17	2489	17	78.7	9.0	0	54%
vegetarian, canned, 'Big Franks'	1 link	118	12	2	224	2	7.1	0.8	0	54%
(Longacre)										
chicken	1 oz	63	4	1	230	0	5.0	0.0	30	69%

Food Name	Serving Size	Calories	Prot. gms	Carbs gms	Sod. mgs	Fiber gms	Fat gms	Sat. Fat gms	Chol. mgs	% Fat Cal.
turkey	1 oz	66	4	0	260	0	6.0	0.0	30	77%
(Louis Rich)										
cheese	1 frank	90	5	2	420	0	7.0	2.5	40	69%
turkey	1 frank	101	6	1	505	0	8.2	2.7	42	73%
turkey, w/cheese	1 frank	109	6	1	523	0	8.9	2.9	44	73%
turkey and chicken	1 frank	85	5	2	511	0	6.1	1.7	41	65%
turkey and chicken, bun size	1 frank	110	7	3	630	0	8.0	2.5	50	64%
turkey and chicken, w/cheese	1 frank	90	6	2	482	0	6.5	2.3	42	65%
(Morningstar Farms)										
corn dog, vegetarian, 'Meat-Free Corn Dogs'	1 corn dog	150	7	22	500	3	4.0	0.5	0	24.0%
corn dog, vegetarian, 'Meat-Free Mini Corn Dogs'	1 corn dog	150	11	21	580	1	4.5	0.5	0	24.0%
hot dog, vegetarian, 'Veggie Dogs'	1 frank	80	11	6	580	1	0.5	0.0	0	5.6%
vegetarian, 'Deli Franks'	1 serving	109	10	3	524	3	6.5	1.0	2	54%
(Mr. Turkey)										
turkey, 10 per lb.	1 frank	106	6	1	440	0	8.9	0.0	31	76%
turkey, w/cheese	1 frank	109	6	1	526	0	9.1	0.0	29	75%
(Natural Touch) vegetarian	1 frank	99	10	2	471	2	5.5	0.9	1	50%
(OHSE)										
beef	1 oz	85	3	1	280	0	8.0	0.0	0	82%
chicken, beef, and pork	1 oz	85	3	1	260	0	8.0	0.0	0	82%
'Wieners'	1 oz	90	3	1	300	0	8.0	0.0	0	82%
(Oscar Mayer)										
bacon and cheddar cheese, 'Hot Dogs'	1 frank	137	6	1	501	0	12.0	5.0	29	79%
beef, deli-style, 'Big & Juicy'	1 frank	230	9	1	680	0	22.0	10.0	50	83%
beef, 'Franks'	1 frank	181	6	1	583	0	16.7	7.0	35	83%
beef, 'Light Franks'	1 frank	131	7	1	594	0	11.1	4.6	23	76%
beef, original, 'Big & Juicy'	1 frank	240	9	1	700	0	22.0	9.0	45	83%
beef, quarter pound, 'Big & Juicy'	1 frank	350	13	2	1050	0	33.0	13.0	65	83%
beef, w/cheddar, 'Franks'	1 frank	163	8	1	655	0	14.3	6.4	36	79%
beef, w/garlic, 'Big & Juicy'	2.7 oz	239	9	0	652	0	22.5	9.4	51	85%
fat free	1 frank	35	6	2	490	0	0.0	0.0	0	0%
light	1 frank	110	6	2	620	0	8.0	3.5	30	69%
pork and turkey	1 frank	150	5	1	450	0	13.0	5.0	30	83%
pork, turkey, and beef, light	1 frank	111	7	2	591	0	8.5	3.0	35	69%
turkey, w/cheese	1 frank	143	5	1	514	0	12.9	4.5	33	81%
wiener, hot and spicy, 'Big & Juicy'	1 wiener	220	10	1	750	0	20.0	8.0	45	80%
wiener, original, 'Big & Juicy'	1 wiener	240	9	1	690	0	22.0	9.0	45	83%
wiener, smokie link, 'Big & Juicy'	1 wiener	220	10	1	770	0	19.0	7.0	50	80%
(Pilgrim's Pride)										
1-lb pkg	1 frank	118	8	1	456	0	8.8	0.0	31	69%
12-oz pkg	1 frank	88	6	1	342	0	6.6	0.0	24	69%
(Quick Meal) w/chili and cheese	4.5 oz	340	14	25	540	0	20.0	8.0	80	54%
(Smart Dog) vegetarian, fat-free, 'Lightlife'	1.5 oz	40	8	1	290	0	0.0	0.0	0	0%
(State Fair) beef, batter-wrapped, on a stick, 'Corn Dogs'	2.67 oz	210	6	24	0	0	10.0	0.0	0	43%
(Tyson)										
chicken	1 frank	115	6	1	700	0	10.0	0.0	0	76%
chicken, batter-wrapped, 'Corn Dogs'	3.5 oz	280	9	28	70	0	14.0	0.0	75	46%
w/cheese	1 frank	145	7	1	680	0	11.0	0.0	0	76%
(White Wave SoyFood) vegetarian, 'Healthy'	1.5 oz	120	7	5	340	0	8.0	1.0	0	60%
(Worthington) vegetarian, 'Leanies'	1 serving	106	7	2	425	1	7.8	1.3	1	66%

FRENCH ARTICHOKE. See under ARTICHOKE.
FRENCH BEAN. See BEAN, FRENCH.
FRENCH TOAST

Food Name	Serving Size	Calories	Prot. gms	Carbs gms	Sod. mgs	Fiber gms	Fat gms	Sat. Fat gms	Chol. mgs	% Fat Cal.
(Aunt Jemima)										
cinnamon, frozen	1 slice	240	10	35	330	2	7.0	2.0	90	26%

Food Name	Serving Size	Calories	Prot. gms	Carbs gms	Sod. mgs	Fiber gms	Fat gms	Sat. Fat gms	Chol. mgs	% Fat Cal.
homestyle, frozen	1 slice	240	10	35	310	2	7.0	2.0	95	26%
original, frozen	3 oz	166	7	27	554	1	4.4	1.0	46	23%
sticks, and syrup, frozen, 'Homestyle'	5.2 oz	400	7	48	640	0	20.0	0.0	0	45%
wedges, and sausages, frozen, 'Homestyle'	5.3 oz	360	13	40	780	0	17.0	0.0	0	42%
(Downyflake)										
frozen	1 slice	130	4	22	270	0	3.0	1.0	25	21%
frozen, 'Extra Thick'	1 slice	150	5	11	340	0	9.0	0.0	0	56%
Texas style, w/sausage, frozen	4.25 oz	400	10	37	550	0	24.0	0.0	0	53%
(Farm Rich)										
sticks, apple cinnamon	3 oz	310	6	39	300	0	15.0	0.0	0	43%
sticks, blueberry	3 oz	310	6	37	280	0	14.0	0.0	0	42%
sticks, original	3 oz	300	5	37	280	0	15.0	0.0	0	45%
(French Toast Boat) cinnamon	1 piece	224	5	28	267	1	11.1	1.8	4	45%
(Krusteaz)										
cinnamon swirl, w/sausage, frozen	1 pkg	415	13	38	502	2	23.2	7.3	98	50%
cinnamon swirl, frozen	2 slices	270	10	46	370	0	5.0	0.0	120	17%
regular, frozen	2 slices	250	11	38	380	0	6.0	1.3	120	22%
(Morningstar Farms)										
vegetarian, cinnamon swirl, w/patties, frozen	6.5 oz	380	24	37	1220	4	15.0	0.0	0	36%
(Pierre) cinnamon, wedge, product 1847	1 piece	118	2	16	163	1	5.1	0.9	32	39%
(Stilwell) sticks, frozen, 'Qwik-Krisp'	5 pieces	400	6	46	370	1	21.0	5.0	40	48%
(Sunny Fresh)										
bagel, w/maple syrup, frozen	1 pkg	15196	1120	1678	22623	0	426.4	100.3	10263	25%
bagel, w/maple syrup, frozen	1 serving	190	14	21	283	0	5.3	1.3	128	25%
cinnamon swirl, frozen	1 serving	190	6	26	220	1	7.0	2.0	75	33%
(Swanson)										
cinnamon swirl, w/sausage, frozen, 'Great Starts'	5.5 oz	390	12	37	530	0	21.0	0.0	0	49%
mini, w/sausage, frozen, 'Great Starts'	2.5 oz	190	6	22	320	0	9.0	0.0	0	42%
oatmeal, w/lite links, frozen, 'Great Starts'	4.65 oz	310	13	35	500	0	13.0	0.0	0	38%
sticks, w/syrup, 'Great Starts'	1 pkg	320	7	50	260	2	10.0	5.0	25	28%
w/sausage, 'Great Starts'	1 pkg	410	13	33	580	3	26.0	9.0	110	56%
w/sausage, frozen, 'Great Starts'	1 entree	410	13	33	580	3	26.0	9.0	110	56%

FRESHWATER BASS. See BASS, FRESHWATER.

FRIED RICE SEASONING. See under SEASONING MIX.

FRITTER

Food Name	Serving Size	Calories	Prot. gms	Carbs gms	Sod. mgs	Fiber gms	Fat gms	Sat. Fat gms	Chol. mgs	% Fat Cal.
corn, frozen *(Mrs. Paul's)*	2 pieces	240	5	35	560	0	9.0	0.0	10	34%
apple, frozen *(Mrs. Paul's)*	2 pieces	240	4	35	500	0	9.0	0.0	5	34%

FROG

Food Name	Serving Size	Calories	Prot. gms	Carbs gms	Sod. mgs	Fiber gms	Fat gms	Sat. Fat gms	Chol. mgs	% Fat Cal.
legs, raw	3.5 oz	73	16.4	0.0	58	0	0.3	0.0	50	4%
legs, raw	1 oz	21	4.6	0.0	(mq)	0	<1.0	(mq)	(mq)	<33%

FROGFISH. See MONKFISH.

FROSTING

(Betty Crocker)

Food Name	Serving Size	Calories	Prot. gms	Carbs gms	Sod. mgs	Fiber gms	Fat gms	Sat. Fat gms	Chol. mgs	% Fat Cal.
Amaretto almond, 'Creamy Deluxe'	1/12 can	160	0	27	50	0	6.0	2.0	0	33%
butter pecan 'Creamy Deluxe'	1/12 tub	170	0	26	50	0	7.0	0.0	0	38%
chocolate, light, 'Creamy Deluxe'	1/12 tub	130	1	28	60	0	2.0	0.0	0	13%
chocolate, w/dinosaurs, 'Creamy Deluxe Party'	1/12 tub	160	1	24	60	0	7.0	0.0	0	39%
chocolate, w/red gel 'Creamy Deluxe Party'	1/12 tub	160	1	24	50	0	7.0	0.0	0	39%
chocolate, w/turbo racers, 'Creamy Deluxe Party'	1/12 tub	160	1	24	50	0	7.0	0.0	0	39%
chocolate chip, 'Creamy Deluxe'	1/12 tub	170	1	27	30	0	7.0	0.0	0	36%
chocolate chip, 'Creamy Deluxe Party'	1/12 can	160	1	24	60	0	7.0	2.0	0	39%
chocolate coconut almond, 'Creamy Deluxe'	1/12 can	160	1	21	55	0	8.0	3.0	0	45%
double chocolate chip, 'Creamy Deluxe'	1/12 can	170	1	24	60	0	8.0	3.0	0	42%
Dutch fudge, dark, 'Creamy Deluxe'	1/12 tub	160	1	22	70	0	7.0	0.0	0	41%

Food Name	Serving Size	Calories	Prot. gms	Carbs gms	Sod. mgs	Fiber gms	Fat gms	Sat. Fat gms	Chol. mgs	% Fat Cal.
milk chocolate 'Creamy Deluxe Light'	1/12 tub	140	1	29	60	0	2.0	0.0	0	13%
rocky road, 'Creamy Deluxe'	1/12 can	150	1	20	50	0	8.0	2.0	0	46%
vanilla, 'Creamy Deluxe Light'	1/12 tub	140	0	30	30	0	2.0	0.0	0	13%
vanilla, w/blue gel, 'Creamy Deluxe Party'	1/12 tub	160	0	27	30	0	6.0	0.0	0	33%
vanilla, w/teddy bears, 'Creamy Deluxe Party'	1/12 tub	160	0	27	25	0	6.0	0.0	0	33%
(Duncan Hines)										
chocolate	1/12 can	160	0	24	90	0	7.0	0.0	0	40%
cream cheese	1/12 can	160	0	24	120	0	8.0	2.0	0	43%
cream cheese, 'Homestyle'	1/12 can	160	0	26	75	0	6.0	2.0	0	34%
dark chocolate 'Homestyle'	1/12 can	160	0	25	75	0	6.0	2.0	0	35%
Dutch fudge	1/12 can	160	0	24	95	0	7.0	2.0	0	40%
lemon	1/24 tub	60	0	9	30	0	3.0	1.0	0	43%
milk chocolate	1/12 can	160	0	24	85	0	7.0	2.0	0	40%
milk chocolate, 'Homestyle'	1/12 can	160	0	25	75	0	6.0	2.0	0	35%
vanilla	1/12 can	160	0	24	80	0	7.0	2.0	0	40%
vanilla, 'Homestyle'	1/12 can	160	0	26	75	0	6.0	2.0	0	34%
wild cherry	1 tbsp	140	0	22	60	0	5.0	1.5	0	34%
(Finast) milk	1/12 can	160	0	25	105	0	6.0	0.0	0	35%
(Pathmark)										
chocolate, creamy	1/12 can	160	0	25	95	0	6.0	0.0	0	35%
fudge, creamy	1/12 can	160	0	25	100	0	7.0	0.0	0	39%
white, creamy	1/12 can	160	0	25	95	0	6.0	0.0	0	35%
(Pillsbury)										
butter fudge, 'Frosting Supreme'	1/12 pkg	140	1	22	50	0	6.0	2.0	0	37%
candy, creamy, 'Creamy Supreme'	2 tbsp	150	0	22	95	0	7.0	2.0	0	42%
candy, creamy, 'Frosting Supreme'	2 tbsp	150	0	22	95	0	7.0	2.0	0	42%
caramel pecan, 'Frosting Supreme'	1/12 pkg	150	0	20	70	0	8.0	2.0	0	47%
chocolate, 'Creamy Supreme'	2 tbsp	140	0	21	80	0	6.0	1.5	0	39%
chocolate, 'Frost It Hot'	1/8 cake	50	0	12	50	0	0.0	0.0	0	0%
chocolate, 'Frosting Supreme'	2 tbsp	140	0	21	75	0	6.0	1.5	0	39%
chocolate, 'Funfetti, Creamy Supreme'	2 tbsp	140	0	22	80	0	6.0	1.5	0	38%
chocolate, dark, 'Creamy Supreme'	2 tbsp	130	0	20	45	0	6.0	1.5	0	40%
chocolate, dark, 'Frosting Supreme'	2 tbsp	130	0	20	45	0	7.0	1.5	0	44%
chocolate, double Dutch, 'Frosting Supreme'	1/12 can	140	1	22	45	0	6.0	0.0	0	37%
chocolate chip, 'Frosting Supreme'	1/12 can	150	0	27	70	0	5.0	0.0	0	29%
chocolate fudge, 'Funfetti' 'Frosting Supreme'	1/12 pkg	140	0	23	80	0	6.0	2.0	0	37%
chocolate fudge, 'Frosting Supreme'	1/12 pkg	150	0	22	85	0	6.0	2.0	0	38%
chocolate fudge, 'Lovin Lites'	1/12 pkg	130	1	28	95	1	2.0	1.0	0	13%
chocolate fudge, lowfat, 'Creamy Supreme'	2 tbsp	140	0	26	85	0	3.5	1.0	0	23%
coconut almond, 'Frosting Supreme'	1/12 can	150	1	17	60	0	9.0	0.0	0	53%
coconut pecan, 'Frosting Supreme'	1/12 can	160	0	17	60	0	10.0	0.0	0	57%
cream cheese, 'Frosting Supreme'	1/12 can	160	0	26	115	0	6.0	0.0	0	34%
decorator, all flavors except chocolate	1 tbsp	70	0	12	0	0	2.0	0.0	0	27%
decorator, chocolate	1 tbsp	60	0	11	0	0	2.0	0.0	0	29%
fudge, 'Frosting Supreme'	1/12 can	150	1	24	80	0	6.0	0.0	0	35%
lemon, 'Frosting Supreme'	1/12 can	160	0	26	80	0	6.0	0.0	0	34%
milk, 'Frosting Supreme'	1/12 can	150	0	23	60	0	6.0	0.0	0	37%
milk chocolate, 'Creamy Supreme'	2 tbsp	140	0	21	60	1	6.0	1.5	0	39%
milk chocolate, 'Frosting Supreme'	1/12 pkg	150	0	23	65	0	6.0	2.0	0	37%
milk chocolate, 'Lovin' Lites'	2 tbsp	130	0	25	85	1	3.0	1.0	0	21%
milk chocolate, w/fudge glaze, 'Creamy Supreme'	2 tbsp	140	0	22	75	1	6.0	1.5	0	38%
milk chocolate, w/fudge swirl, 'Frosting Supreme'	1/12 pkg	150	0	23	65	0	6.0	2.0	0	37%
mint, 'Frosting Supreme'	1/12 can	150	1	24	80	0	7.0	0.0	0	39%
mocha, 'Frosting Supreme'	1/12 can	150	1	24	60	0	6.0	0.0	0	35%

Food Name	Serving Size	Calories	Prot. gms	Carbs gms	Sod. mgs	Fiber gms	Fat gms	Sat. Fat gms	Chol. mgs	% Fat Cal.
Oreo, 'Frosting Supreme'	2 tbsp	150	0	23	75	0	6.0	1.5	0	37%
sour cream vanilla, 'Frosting Supreme'	1/12 can	160	0	27	80	0	6.0	0.0	0	33%
strawberry, 'Frosting Supreme'	1/12 can	160	0	26	75	0	6.0	0.0	0	34%
vanilla	1/8 cake	120	0	19	60	0	5.0	0.0	0	37%
vanilla, 'Creamy Supreme'	2 tbsp	150	0	23	70	0	6.0	1.5	0	37%
vanilla, 'Frosting Supreme'	1/12 can	160	0	26	75	0	6.0	0.0	0	34%
vanilla, 'Funfetti'	2 tbsp	150	0	25	75	0	6.0	1.5	0	35%
vanilla, 'Funfetti Pink'	2 tbsp	150	0	24	70	0	6.0	1.5	0	36%
vanilla, 'Lovin Lites'	1/12 pkg	130	0	29	70	0	2.0	1.0	0	13%
vanilla, French, 'Creamy Supreme'	2 tbsp	150	0	25	80	0	6.0	1.5	0	35%
vanilla, French, 'Frosting Supreme'	2 tbsp	160	0	26	75	0	6.0	1.5	0	34%
vanilla, pink and white, 'Frosting Supreme'	1/12 can	150	0	24	70	0	6.0	0.0	0	36%
vanilla, w/fudge glaze, 'Creamy Supreme'	2 tbsp	150	0	25	75	0	6.0	1.5	0	35%
vanilla, w/fudge swirl, 'Frosting Supreme'	1/12 pkg	150	0	25	75	0	6.0	2.0	0	35%
white, fluffy	1/12 can	60	0	15	65	0	0.0	0.0	0	0%
white, fluffy, 'Frost It Hot'	1/8 cake	50	0	12	50	0	0.0	0.0	0	0%
(Weight Watchers)										
chocolate, less fat, 'Sweet Rewards'	2 tbsp	120	1	24	55	0	2.5	1.0	0	19%
milk chocolate, less fat, 'Sweet Rewards'	2 tbsp	120	0	24	60	0	2.5	1.0	0	19%
vanilla, 'less fat, Sweet Rewards'	2 tbsp	120	0	26	65	0	2.0	0.5	0	15%
FROSTING MIX										
(Betty Crocker)										
cherry, creamy, prepared w/margarine	1/12 pkg	180	0	31	100	0	6.0	3.0	0	30%
chocolate fudge, creamy, prepared w/1/4 cup butter	1/12 mix	180	1	30	70	0	6.0	0.0	10	30%
chocolate fudge, creamy, prepared w/1/4 cup margarine	1/12 mix	180	1	30	70	0	6.0	0.0	0	30%
chocolate fudge, sour cream, creamy, prepared w/margarine	1/12 pkg	180	1	30	75	0	6.0	2.0	0	30%
coconut pecan, creamy, mix only	1/12 mix	110	1	19	5	0	4.0	0.0	0	31%
coconut pecan, creamy, prepared w/butter, 2% milk	1/12 mix	150	1	19	50	0	8.0	0.0	10	47%
coconut pecan, creamy, prepared w/margarine, skim milk	1/12 mix	150	1	19	50	0	8.0	0.0	0	47%
milk chocolate, creamy, prepared w/margarine	1/12 pkg	170	1	29	40	0	5.0	1.0	0	27%
rainbow chip, creamy, prepared w/margarine	1/12 pkg	190	1	32	50	0	7.0	2.0	0	32%
vanilla, creamy, mix only	1/12 mix	150	0	32	5	0	2.0	0.0	0	12%
vanilla, creamy, prepared w/1/4 cup butter	1/12 mix	170	0	32	50	0	5.0	0.0	10	26%
vanilla, creamy, prepared w/1/4 cup margarine	1/12 mix	170	0	32	50	0	5.0	0.0	0	26%
white, sour cream, creamy, prepared w/margarine	1/12 pkg	170	0	31	100	0	5.0	1.0	0	27%
(Sweet 'n Low)										
chocolate fudge, low sodium w/'Sweet 'N Low'	3 tbsp	140	2	16	30	0	8.0	3.0	0	50%
white, low-sodium w/Sweet 'N Low	3 tbsp	120	2	16	30	0	8.0	3.0	0	50%
FRUCTOSE										
(Estee)	1 tsp	16	0	4	0	0	0.0	0.0	0	0%
(Featherweight)	1 tsp	12	0	3	0	0	0.0	0.0	0	0%
crystalline, pure *(Esculent)*	1 tsp	15	0	4	0	0	0.0	0.0	0	0%
crystalline, pure *(Fifty 50)*	1 tsp	15	0	4	0	0	0.0	0.0	0	0%
crystalline, pure *(Healthy Edge)*	1 tsp	15	0	4	0	0	0.0	0.0	0	0%
liquid *(Sweet Lite)*	1 tsp	20	0	6	0	0	0.0	0.0	0	0%
packet *(Estee)*	1 pkt	12	0	3	0	0	0.0	0.0	0	0%
FRUIT, MIXED										
(Flav-R-Pac)										
frozen	2/3 cup	60	1	14	0	2	0.0	0.0	0	0%
melons, mixed, frozen	3/4 cup	40	1	10	16	1	0.0	0.0	0	0%
w/pineapple, frozen	2/3 cup	60	1	15	0	2	0.0	0.0	0	0%

Food Name	Serving Size	Calories	Prot. gms	Carbs gms	Sod. mgs	Fiber gms	Fat gms	Sat. Fat gms	Chol. mgs	% Fat Cal.
FRUIT AND NUT MIX										
(Eden Foods)	1 oz	160	7	10	0	3	10.0	1.5	0	57%
(Estee)	14 pieces	70	2	6	15	0	5.0	2.0	0	58%
(Fisher)										
'California Style'	1/4 cup	140	2	16	20	2	8.0	3.0	0	50%
classic	1/4 cup	150	5	11	70	2	11.0	1.5	0	61%
(Planters)										
'Caribbean Crunch'	1 oz	150	3	14	130	0	10.0	3.0	0	57%
'Fruit 'n Nut'	1 oz	150	5	13	90	0	9.0	2.0	0	53%
FRUIT BAR. See also FRUIT BAR, FROZEN.										
APPLE										
(Health Valley)										
nonfat	1 bar	140	3	35	0	3	0.0	0.0	0	0%
nonfat, 'Bakes'	1 bar	70	2	18	30	2	0.0	0.0	0	0%
APPLE RAISIN (Weight Watchers)	1 bar	70	1	14	60	2	2.0	0.5	0	23%
APRICOT, nonfat (Health Valley)	1 bar	140	3	35	5	4	0.0	0.0	0	0%
BLUEBERRY, nonfat (Parnasa)	1 bar	120	1	28	20	0	0.0	0.0	0	0%
CRANBERRY, natural (Hearty Balance)	1 bar	150	4	30	60	3	0.5	0.5	0	3%
DATE										
(Health Valley)										
	1 bar	140	3	34	5	3	0.0	0.0	0	0%
nonfat, 'Bakes'	1 bar	70	2	18	30	2	0.0	0.0	0	0%
RAISIN										
(Health Valley)										
nonfat	1 bar	140	2	35	5	3	0.0	0.0	0	0%
nonfat, 'Bakes'	1 bar	70	2	18	30	2	0.0	0.0	0	0%
RASPBERRY (Parnasa) nonfat	1 bar	120	1	29	15	1	0.0	0.0	0	0%
FRUIT BAR, FROZEN										
(Dole)										
blueberry and cream, 'Fruit & Cream'	1 bar	90	1	19	20	0	1.4	0.0	5	13%
cherry, 'Fresh Lites'	1 bar	25	1	6	6	0	1.0	0.0	0	24%
chocolate, banana, and cream, 'Fruit & Cream'	1 bar	175	2	22	20	0	9.0	0.0	0	46%
chocolate, strawberry, and cream, 'Fruit & Cream'	1 bar	140	2	23	20	0	8.0	0.0	0	42%
grape, nonfat, no sugar added	1 bar	25	0	6	5	0	0.0	0.0	0	0%
grape, 'SunTops'	1 bar	40	1	9	5	0	1.0	0.0	0	18%
lemon, 'Fresh Lites'	1 bar	25	1	6	16	0	1.0	0.0	0	24%
lemonade, 'SunTops'	1 bar	40	1	9	5	0	1.0	0.0	0	18%
orange, tropical, 'SunTops'	1 bar	40	1	9	5	0	1.0	0.0	0	18%
peach and cream, 'Fruit & Cream'	1 bar	90	1	19	19	0	1.4	0.0	5	13%
piña colada, 'Fruit 'n Juice'	1 bar	90	1	16	2	0	3.0	0.0	0	28%
pineapple, 'Fruit & Juice'	1 bar	70	0	17	4	0	0.1	0.0	0	1%
pineapple-orange, 'Fresh Lites'	1 bar	25	1	6	7	0	1.0	0.0	0	24%
punch, 'SunTops'	1 bar	40	1	9	5	0	1.0	0.0	0	18%
raspberry, 'Fresh Lites'	1 bar	25	1	6	6	0	1.0	0.0	0	24%
raspberry, 'Fruit & Juice'	1 bar	70	0	16	14	0	0.1	0.0	0	1%
raspberry, nonfat, no sugar added	1 bar	25	0	6	5	0	0.0	0.0	0	0%
raspberry and cream, 'Fruit & Cream'	1 bar	90	1	20	23	0	1.4	0.0	5	13%
strawberry, 'Fruit n' Juice'	1 bar	70	0	16	6	0	0.1	0.0	0	1%
strawberry, nonfat, no sugar added	1 bar	25	0	6	5	0	0.0	0.0	0	0%
strawberry and cream, 'Fruit & Cream'	1 bar	90	1	19	22	0	1.4	0.0	5	13%
(Fruit a Freeze)										
banana, all natural	1 bar	99	2	16	28	1	4.0	3.0	10	33%
strawberry, all-natural	1 bar	100	1	18	35	0	3.0	2.0	10	26%
(Minute Maid) all flavors, nonfat, 'Fruit Juicee'	1 bar	60	0	14	0	0	0.0	0.0	0	0%

Food Name	Serving Size	Calories	Prot. gms	Carbs gms	Sod. mgs	Fiber gms	Fat gms	Sat. Fat gms	Chol. mgs	% Fat Cal.
(Natural Nectar)										
lemony lime, juice snack, all natural, nonfat	1 bar	70	1	17	10	0	0.0	0.0	0	0%
strawberry nectar, juice snack	1 bar	70	1	16	55	0	1.0	0.0	0	12%
'Tropical Delight' juice snack, all-natural, nonfat	1 bar	70	1	16	10	0	0.0	0.0	0	0%
(Sunkist)										
coconut	1 bar	170	3	15	70	0	10.0	0.0	0	56%
lemonade, nonfat	1 bar	90	0	24	5	0	0.0	0.0	0	0%
orange, nonfat, 'Juice Bar'	1 bar	100	0	25	0	0	0.0	0.0	0	0%
strawberry and cream	1 bar	90	0	19	30	0	1.0	0.0	0	11%
wildberry, nonfat	1 bar	140	0	33	15	0	0.0	0.0	0	0%
FRUIT COCKTAIL *(Hunt's)*	1/2 cup	90	0	23	15	1	0.0	0.0	0	0%
FRUIT DESSERT MIX										
apple-cinnamon, w/Nutrasweet *(Sans Sucre de Paris)*	1/4 cup	60	0	14	10	1	0.0	0.0	0	0%
pina colada, w/Nutrasweet *(Sans Sucre de Paris)*	1/4 cup	70	0	12	10	1	1.5	1.0	0	22%
FRUIT DRINK. See also CIDER; FRUIT DRINK MIX; FRUIT JUICE BLEND; FRUIT JUICE DRINK.										
(A&P)										
cranberry apple	6 fl oz	130	1	32	1	0	0.0	0.0	0	0%
grape	6 fl oz	100	1	25	0	0	1.0	0.0	0	8%
lemonade, frozen, prepared	8 fl oz	110	1	28	0	0	1.0	0.0	0	7%
lemonade, pink, frozen, prepared	8 fl oz	110	1	28	0	0	1.0	0.0	0	7%
raspberry, w/cranberry	6 fl oz	110	1	27	0	0	1.0	0.0	0	7%
(Awake) orange, frozen concentrate, prepared	6 fl oz	80	0	20	10	0	0.0	0.0	0	0%
(Bama)										
fruit punch	8.45 fl oz	130	0	32	15	0	0.0	0.0	0	0%
grape	8.45 fl oz	120	0	29	25	0	0.0	0.0	0	0%
orange	8.45 fl oz	120	0	29	60	0	0.0	0.0	0	0%
(Bel-Air) lemonade, pink, concentrate, prepared	6 fl oz	110	0	27	0	0	0.0	0.0	0	0%
(Bright & Early)										
'Bright & Early Fruit Punch' prepared	6 fl oz	90	0	22	5	0	0.0	0.0	0	0%
grape, 'Bright & Early Grape'	6 fl oz	100	0	24	0	0	0.0	0.0	0	0%
orange, 'Bright & Early Orange'	6 fl oz	90	0	21	20	0	0.0	0.0	0	0%
pineapple, 'Bright & Early Pineapple'	6 fl oz	90	0	23	0	0	0.0	0.0	0	0%
(Castle Crest)										
fruit punch, artificially flavored	8 fl oz	120	0	31	15	0	0.0	0.0	0	0%
grape flavored	8 fl oz	120	0	31	15	0	0.0	0.0	0	0%
lemonade drink, artificially flavored	8 fl oz	120	0	31	15	0	0.0	0.0	0	0%
(Crowley)										
fruit punch	8 fl oz	130	0	32	15	0	0.0	0.0	0	0%
grape	8 fl oz	130	0	32	15	0	0.0	0.0	0	0%
lemon	8 fl oz	130	0	32	15	0	0.0	0.0	0	0%
orange	8 fl oz	130	0	32	15	0	0.0	0.0	0	0%
(Del Monte)										
pineapple, w/grapefruit	6 fl oz	90	0	24	50	0	0.0	0.0	0	0%
pineapple, w/pink grapefruit	6 fl oz	90	0	24	50	0	0.0	0.0	0	0%
pineapple-orange	6 fl oz	90	0	24	20	0	0.0	0.0	0	0%
(Finast)										
cranberry grape	6 fl oz	103	0	26	5	0	0.0	0.0	0	0%
raspberry, w/cranberry	6 fl oz	110	0	27	10	0	0.0	0.0	0	0%
(Five Alive)										
berry citrus drink	6 fl oz	90	0	22	5	0	0.0	0.0	0	0%
tropical citrus	6 fl oz	90	0	21	0	0	0.0	0.0	0	0%
(Flav-R-Pac) lemonade	8 fl oz	110	0	27	0	0	0.0	0.0	0	0%
(Frostee) strawberry-flavored	8 fl oz	180	2	27	150	0	7.0	0.0	0	35%
(Fruit Corners) soda pop snacks 'Soda Licious'	1 pouch	100	1	22	20	0	1.0	0.0	0	9%

Food Name	Serving Size	Calories	Prot. gms	Carbs gms	Sod. mgs	Fiber gms	Fat gms	Sat. Fat gms	Chol. mgs	% Fat Cal.
(Hawaiian Punch)										
fruit punch, red, 'Fruit Juicy Lite'	6 fl oz	60	0	15	30	0	0.0	0.0	0	0%
fruit punch, red, 'Fruit Juicy'	6 fl oz	90	0	22	20	0	0.0	0.0	0	0%
fruit punch, tropical	6 fl oz	90	0	22	30	0	0.0	0.0	0	0%
fruit punch, tropical, wild fruit	6 fl oz	90	0	23	35	0	0.0	0.0	0	0%
fruit punch cocktail, island fruit	6 fl oz	90	0	22	30	0	0.0	0.0	0	0%
orange	6 fl oz	100	0	24	20	0	0.0	0.0	0	0%
'Very Berry'	6 fl oz	90	0	22	30	0	0.0	0.0	0	0%
(Hi-C)										
'Boppin' Berry'	6 fl oz	90	0	23	25	0	0.0	0.0	0	0%
'Candy Apple Cooler'	6 fl oz	94	0	23	17	0	0.1	0.0	0	1%
cherry, aseptic box	6 fl oz	100	0	24	25	0	0.0	0.0	0	0%
'Double Fruit Cooler'	6 fl oz	93	0	23	18	0	0.1	0.0	0	1%
'Ecto Cooler'	6 fl oz	95	0	23	17	0	0.1	0.0	0	1%
'Fruity Bubble Gum'	6 fl oz	90	0	22	20	0	0.0	0.0	0	0%
grape	6 fl oz	90	0	23	25	0	0.0	0.0	0	0%
'Hula Cooler'	6 fl oz	97	0	24	17	0	0.1	0.0	0	1%
'Hula Punch'	6 fl oz	87	0	21	17	0	0.1	0.0	0	1%
'Jammin' Apple Drink' aseptic box	6 fl oz	90	0	23	20	0	0.0	0.0	0	0%
lemonade	8.45 fl oz	109	0	27	73	0	0.1	0.0	0	1%
orange	6 fl oz	95	0	23	17	0	0.1	0.0	0	1%
peach	6 fl oz	100	0	24	20	0	0.0	0.0	0	0%
'Stompin' Banana Berry'	6 fl oz	90	0	22	25	0	0.0	0.0	0	0%
wild berry	6 fl oz	92	0	23	17	0	0.1	0.0	0	1%
(J. Hungerford)										
fruit punch, 20% plus juice	9.03 fl oz	43	0	11	32	0	0.0	0.0	0	0%
grape, 20% plus juice	9.03 fl oz	41	0	11	31	0	0.0	0.0	0	0%
lemon, 20% plus juice	9.03 fl oz	41	0	11	38	0	0.0	0.0	0	0%
lemonade, pink, 20% plus juice	9.03 fl oz	41	0	11	39	0	0.0	0.0	0	0%
orange, 20% plus juice	9.03 fl oz	41	0	11	23	0	0.0	0.0	0	0%
punch juice	9.03 fl oz	133	0	33	2	0	0.0	0.0	0	0%
(Juicy Juice)										
fruit punch	6 fl oz	100	1	23	10	0	0.0	0.0	0	0%
tropical	6 fl oz	100	1	24	5	0	0.0	0.0	0	0%
(Kern's)										
apple-strawberry nectar, canned or bottled	6 fl oz	110	0	26	0	0	0.0	0.0	0	0%
apricot-mango nectar	11.5 fl oz	220	1	53	10	0	0.0	0.0	0	0%
apricot nectar, canned or bottled	6 fl oz	110	1	27	0	0	0.0	0.0	0	0%
apricot-pineapple nectar	11.5 fl oz	220	1	53	5	2	0.0	0.0	0	0%
banana-pineapple nectar	11.5 fl oz	220	1	52	5	0	0.0	0.0	0	0%
coconut-pineapple nectar, can or bottle	6 fl oz	140	1	26	25	0	4.0	0.0	0	25%
(Knudsen)										
apricot nectar	8 fl oz	105	1	24	0	0	0.0	0.0	0	0%
blueberry nectar	8 fl oz	135	1	34	0	0	0.0	0.0	0	0%
boysenberry nectar	8 fl oz	110	1	33	0	0	0.0	0.0	0	0%
calamansi punch, 'Rain Forest'	8 fl oz	115	1	27	0	0	0.0	0.0	0	0%
cherry lemonade	8 fl oz	120	0	29	35	na	0.0	0.0	0	0%
coconut nectar	8 fl oz	140	1	26	55	na	5.0	na	na	29%
guanabana punch, 'Rain Forest'	8 fl oz	125	1	29	0	0	0.0	0.0	0	0%
hibiscus cooler	8 fl oz	95	1	24	0	0	0.0	0.0	0	0%
lime cactus cooler blend *(Knudsen)*	8 fl oz	120	0	29	35	na	0.0	0.0	0	0%
lemonade, 'Natural'	8 fl oz	100	1	26	0	0	0.0	0.0	0	0%
lime, tropical	8 fl oz	130	1	32	0	0	0.0	0.0	0	0%
papaya, concentrate	1.5 fl oz	90	1	22	37	0	0.0	0.0	0	0%

Food Name	Serving Size	Calories	Prot. gms	Carbs gms	Sod. mgs	Fiber gms	Fat gms	Sat. Fat gms	Chol. mgs	% Fat Cal.
passionfruit, tropical	8 fl oz	80	1	20	0	0	0.0	0.0	0	0%
rainforest punch, cupu assu	8 fl oz	110	1	25	0	0	0.0	0.0	0	0%
rainforest punch, fruit juice sweetened	8 fl oz	120	1	29	20	0	0.0	0.0	0	0%
raspberry float	8 fl oz	130	2	31	0	0	0.0	0.0	0	0%
raspberry lemonade	8 fl oz	110	1	28	0	0	0.0	0.0	0	0%
strawberry lemonade	8 fl oz	90	1	21	0	0	0.0	0.0	0	0%
tropical punch	8 fl oz	120	0	29	20	na	0.0	0.0	0	0%
(Kool-Aid)										
cherry, 'Koolers'	8.45 fl oz	140	0	38	10	0	0.0	0.0	0	0%
grape, 'Koolers'	8.45 fl oz	140	0	35	10	0	0.0	0.0	0	0%
grape-berry, 'Kool-Aid Splash'	1 serving	116	0	31	35	0	0.0	0.0	0	0%
'Great Bluedini' 'Koolers'	8.45 fl oz	110	0	29	10	0	0.0	0.0	0	0%
mountain berry punch, 'Koolers'	8.45 fl oz	140	0	37	10	0	0.0	0.0	0	0%
rainbow punch, 'Koolers'	8.45 fl oz	130	0	36	10	0	0.0	0.0	0	0%
'Rock-A-Dile Red' 'Koolers'	8.45 fl oz	130	0	34	10	0	0.0	0.0	0	0%
tropical punch, 'Koolers'	8.45 fl oz	130	0	35	10	0	0.0	0.0	0	0%
tropical, 'Kool-Aid Burst'	1 serving	90	0	24	29	0	0.0	0.0	0	0%
(Lemonade Chillers) 'Key Lime'	8 fl oz	110	0	26	0	0	0.0	0.0	0	0%
(Libby's)										
apricot nectar	5.5 fl oz	105	0	25	5	0	0.0	0.0	0	0%
banana nectar	8 fl oz	132	0	33	24	0	0.0	0.0	0	0%
banana nectar	6 fl oz	110	0	26	15	0	0.0	0.0	0	0%
(Minute Maid)										
apple punch, prepared	6 fl oz	90	0	23	20	0	0.0	0.0	0	0%
berry punch	6 fl oz	90	0	23	20	0	0.0	0.0	0	0%
berry punch, frozen concentrate, prepared	6 fl oz	90	0	23	0	0	0.0	0.0	0	0%
cranberry lemonade	6 fl oz	90	0	23	20	0	0.0	0.0	0	0%
cranberry lemonade, frozen, concentrate, prepared	6 fl oz	90	0	22	0	0	0.0	0.0	0	0%
lemonade, country style	6 fl oz	80	0	21	20	0	0.0	0.0	0	0%
lemonade, country style, frozen concentrate, prepared	6 fl oz	90	0	22	0	0	0.0	0.0	0	0%
lemonade, pink	6 fl oz	80	0	21	20	0	0.0	0.0	0	0%
lemonade, pink, frozen concentrate, prepared	6 fl oz	90	0	22	0	0	0.0	0.0	0	0%
limeade, frozen concentrate, prepared	6 fl oz	70	0	19	0	0	0.0	0.0	0	0%
orange punch	6 fl oz	80	0	20	20	0	0.0	0.0	0	0%
raspberry lemonade	6 fl oz	90	0	23	20	0	0.0	0.0	0	0%
raspberry lemonade, frozen concentrate, prepared	6 fl oz	90	0	22	0	0	0.0	0.0	0	0%
tropical punch	6 fl oz	90	0	22	20	0	0.0	0.0	0	0%
(Mott's)										
apple cranberry	10 fl oz	176	0	44	3	0	0.0	0.0	0	0%
apple raspberry drink	10 fl oz	158	0	40	17	0	0.0	0.0	0	0%
punch	9.5 fl oz	161	0	40	4	0	0.0	0.0	0	0%
grape-apple	10 fl oz	167	0	42	1	0	0.0	0.0	0	0%
(Mountain Sun)										
cherry lemonade, organic	8 fl oz	101	0	25	0	0	0.0	0.0	0	0%
lemonade, organic	8 fl oz	110	0	27	0	0	0.0	0.0	0	0%
(Natural Choice)										
apple cranberry, 5% juice, vitamin C added	1 cup	120	0	30	20	0	0.0	0.0	0	0%
(Nestlé) strawberry-flavored, ready to drink, 'Quik'	1 cup	230	7	31	100	0	9.0	5.0	30	35%
(Ocean Spray)										
'Cran-Apple'	6 fl oz	120	0	31	15	0	0.0	0.0	0	0%
'Cran-Apple Low-calorie'	6 fl oz	35	0	9	15	0	0.0	0.0	0	0%
cranberry, citrus 'Refreshers'	6 fl oz	100	0	26	15	0	0.0	0.0	0	0%
'Cran-Grape'	6 fl oz	120	0	31	15	0	0.0	0.0	0	0%
'Cranicot'	6 fl oz	120	0	29	15	0	0.0	0.0	0	0%

Food Name	Serving Size	Calories	Prot. gms	Carbs gms	Sod. mgs	Fiber gms	Fat gms	Sat. Fat gms	Chol. mgs	% Fat Cal.
'Cran-Blueberry'	6 fl oz	120	0	31	10	0	0.0	0.0	0	0%
'Cran-Raspberry' low-calorie	6 fl oz	40	0	9	15	0	0.0	0.0	0	0%
'Cran-Raspberry'	6 fl oz	110	0	27	15	0	0.0	0.0	0	0%
'Cran-Strawberry'	6 fl oz	110	0	27	15	0	0.0	0.0	0	0%
guava-passionfruit, Hawaiian, 'Mauna La'i'	6 fl oz	100	0	25	10	0	0.0	0.0	0	0%
lemonade drink, w/cranberry juice	8 fl oz	110	0	26	35	0	0.0	0.0	0	0%
orangecranberry, 'Refreshers'	6 fl oz	100	0	26	15	0	0.0	0.0	0	0%
peach, citrus, 'Refreshers'	6 fl oz	90	0	23	15	0	0.0	0.0	0	0%
(Orange Julius)										
piña colada flavored	16 fl oz	300	2	71	15	0	1.0	0.0	0	3%
raspberry cream supreme	16 fl oz	510	4	76	40	0	23.0	0.0	0	39%
strawberry, regular	16 fl oz	340	1	82	15	0	1.0	0.0	0	3%
tropical cream supreme	16 fl oz	510	5	67	40	0	25.0	0.0	95	44%
(Orlando Sun)										
pineapple-orange-banana	8 fl oz	110	1	29	0	0	0.0	0.0	0	0%
strawberry-guava	8 fl oz	110	1	29	0	0	0.0	0.0	0	0%
(P&Q) cranberry apple	6 fl oz	130	1	32	1	0	0.0	0.0	0	0%
(Pathmark)										
cranberry-apple	6 fl oz	130	0	32	10	0	0.0	0.0	0	0%
cranberry-grape	6 fl oz	103	0	26	5	0	0.0	0.0	0	0%
fruit punch	6 fl oz	90	0	22	0	0	0.0	0.0	0	0%
grape	6 fl oz	90	0	22	0	0	0.0	0.0	0	0%
guava-passionfruit, Hawaiian, 'Hawaii'	6 fl oz	100	0	25	10	0	0.0	0.0	0	0%
orange, 'No Frills Sodium-free'	6 fl oz	80	0	22	0	0	0.0	0.0	0	0%
pineapple, w/grapefruit	6 fl oz	80	0	21	0	0	0.0	0.0	0	0%
raspberry, w/cranberry	6 fl oz	110	0	27	10	0	0.0	0.0	0	0%
raspberry, w/cranberry, 'Sodium-free'	6 fl oz	110	0	27	0	0	0.0	0.0	0	0%
(Red Cheek) apple punch drink	6 fl oz	113	0	28	7	0	0.0	0.0	0	0%
(S&W)										
apricot nectar, canned or bottled	8 fl oz	140	1	35	15	1	0.0	0.0	0	0%
apricot nectar, canned or bottled	5.5 fl oz	100	1	24	10	1	0.0	0.0	0	0%
apricot-pineapple nectar	4 fl oz	35	0	12	20	0	0.0	0.0	0	0%
(Santa Cruz Natural)										
apricot nectar, certified organic	8 fl oz	150	1	38	25	0	0.0	0.0	0	0%
berry nectar, organic	8 fl oz	90	1	22	0	0	1.0	0.0	0	9%
cherry lemonade, dark, sweet, organic	8 fl oz	60	1	20	0	0	1.0	0.0	0	10%
cranberry guava nectar, certified organic	8 fl oz	110	1	24	25	0	0.0	0.0	0	0%
lemonade, certified organic	8 fl oz	120	1	29	35	0	0.0	0.0	0	0%
lemonade, organic	8 fl oz	60	1	21	0	0	1.0	0.0	0	9%
lemonade, organic, 'Sparkling'	8 fl oz	85	1	20	0	0	1.0	0.0	0	10%
limeade, organic, 'Sparkling'	8 fl oz	60	1	23	0	0	1.0	0.0	0	9%
orangeade, organic	8 fl oz	90	1	22	0	0	1.0	0.0	0	9%
orangeade, organic, 'Sparkling'	8 fl oz	90	1	24	0	0	1.0	0.0	0	8%
organic, 'Kauai Punch'	8 fl oz	120	1	28	0	0	1.0	0.0	0	7%
raspberry lemonade, organic	8 fl oz	60	1	20	0	0	1.0	0.0	0	10%
raspberry lemonade, organic, 'Sparkling'	8 fl oz	85	1	20	0	0	1.0	0.0	0	10%
red raspberry, organic, 'Cruz'	8 fl oz	120	1	28	0	0	1.0	0.0	0	7%
strawberry lemonade, organic	8 fl oz	60	1	20	0	0	1.0	0.0	0	10%
tropical punch, organic	8 fl oz	110	1	26	0	0	1.0	0.0	0	8%
(Shasta) lemonade	12 fl oz	146	0	39	106	0	0.0	0.0	0	0%
(Squeezit)										
'Berry B. Wild'	6.75 fl oz	120	0	29	5	0	0.0	0.0	0	0%
'Chucklin' Cherry'	1 serving	110	0	28	0	0	0.0	0.0	0	0%
'Grumpy Grape'	1 serving	110	0	28	0	0	0.0	0.0	0	0%

Food Name	Serving Size	Calories	Prot. gms	Carbs gms	Sod. mgs	Fiber gms	Fat gms	Sat. Fat gms	Chol. mgs	% Fat Cal.
'Mean Green Puncher'	6.75 fl oz	100	0	25	5	0	0.0	0.0	0	0%
orange fruit, 'Smarty Arty'	1 serving	110	0	27	45	0	0.0	0.0	0	0%
'Rockin Red Puncher'	6.75 fl oz	110	0	28	5	0	0.0	0.0	0	0%
'Silly Billy Strawberry'	6.75 fl oz	90	0	23	5	0	0.0	0.0	0	0%
strawberry	1 serving	110	0	29	0	0	0.0	0.0	0	0%
(Sunkist)										
lemonade	8 fl oz	141	0	36	0	0	0.0	0.0	0	0%
lemonade, frozen, prepared	8 fl oz	92	0	24	1	0	0.0	0.0	0	0%
(Sunny Delight) orange, 'California Style'	8 fl oz	130	0	31	130	0	0.0	0.0	0	0%
(Tang)										
berry blend drink, 'Fruit Box'	8.45 fl oz	140	0	36	10	0	0.0	0.0	0	0%
orange, tropical, 'Fruit Box'	8.45 fl oz	150	0	37	10	0	0.0	0.0	0	0%
strawberry-flavored	8.45 fl oz	120	0	32	10	0	0.0	0.0	0	0%
(10-K)										
apple	8 fl oz	60	0	15	55	0	0.0	0.0	0	0%
fruit punch	8 fl oz	60	0	15	55	0	0.0	0.0	0	0%
grape, 'Clear'	8 fl oz	60	0	15	55	0	0.0	0.0	0	0%
lemonade, pink	8 fl oz	60	0	15	55	0	0.0	0.0	0	0%
lemon-lime	8 fl oz	60	0	15	55	0	0.0	0.0	0	0%
orange	8 fl oz	60	0	15	55	0	0.0	0.0	0	0%
strawberry	8 fl oz	60	0	15	55	0	0.0	0.0	0	0%
(Thick & Easy)										
apple, honey consistency	1/2 cup	70	0	17	30	0	0.0	0.0	0	0%
cranberry, honey consistency	1/2 cup	70	0	17	20	0	0.0	0.0	0	0%
cranberry, nectar consistency	1/2 cup	60	0	15	20	0	0.0	0.0	0	0%
orange, honey consistency	1/2 cup	60	0	16	25	0	0.0	0.0	0	0%
orange, nectar consistency	1/2 cup	60	0	15	25	0	0.0	0.0	0	0%
(Tree Top) fruit punch, 100%	8 fl oz	119	0	30	24	0	0.0	0.0	0	0%
(Tropicana)										
apple, 'Single Serve'	10 fl oz	175	0	43	3	0	0.0	0.0	0	0%
berry, 'Berries & Berries'	6 fl oz	90	1	23	20	0	1.0	0.0	0	9%
cranberry raspberry, w/strawberry	8 fl oz	120	0	31	5	na	0.0	0.0	0	0%
cranberry raspberry, w/strawberry, light	8 fl oz	45	0	11	10	na	0.0	0.0	0	0%
fruit punch, 'Single Serve'	10 fl oz	148	0	37	3	0	0.0	0.0	0	0%
grape	6 fl oz	90	1	22	10	0	1.0	0.0	0	9%
lemonade, 'Single Serve'	8 fl oz	120	0	30	3	0	0.0	0.0	0	0%
orange, 'Single Serve'	10 fl oz	132	0	33	3	0	0.0	0.0	0	0%
pineapple, w/grapefruit	6 fl oz	100	1	24	10	0	1.0	0.0	0	8%
(Veryfine)										
fruit punch, '100% Juice Punch'	8 fl oz	122	1	30	10	0	0.0	0.0	0	0%
grape	8 fl oz	130	0	34	10	0	0.0	0.0	0	0%
guava-strawberry, 'Refresher'	8 fl oz	120	0	30	25	0	0.0	0.0	0	0%
lemonade	8 fl oz	120	0	30	25	0	0.0	0.0	0	0%
lemon-lime	8 fl oz	120	0	30	10	0	0.0	0.0	0	0%
orange	8 fl oz	130	1	33	70	0	0.0	0.0	0	0%
papaya punch	8 fl oz	120	1	30	10	0	0.0	0.0	0	0%
pineapple-orange	8 fl oz	130	0	32	10	0	0.0	0.0	0	0%
(Welch's)										
cranberry-apple cocktail, frozen, prepared	6 fl oz	120	0	30	0	0	0.0	0.0	0	0%
cranberry-grape cocktail, frozen, prepared	6 fl oz	110	0	27	0	0	0.0	0.0	0	0%
fruit punch cocktail, 'Orchard Fruit Harvest Punch'	10 fl oz	180	0	45	0	0	0.0	0.0	0	0%
raspberry cocktail, 'Orchard' *(Welch's)*	10 fl oz	160	0	40	10	0	0.0	0.0	0	0%
(Wyler's)										
fruit punch, tropical, 'Fruit Slush'	4 fl oz	157	0	39	10	0	0.0	0.0	0	0%

Food Name	Serving Size	Calories	Prot. gms	Carbs gms	Sod. mgs	Fiber gms	Fat gms	Sat. Fat gms	Chol. mgs	% Fat Cal.
'Fruit Tea Punch'	12 fl oz	118	0	30	1	0	0.0	0.0	0	0%
grape, 'Fruit Slush'	4 fl oz	157	0	39	10	0	0.0	0.0	0	0%
lemonade	6 fl oz	64	0	17	33	0	0.0	0.0	0	0%
lemonade, pink, 'Fruit Slush'	4 fl oz	157	0	39	10	0	0.0	0.0	0	0%
orange, 'Fruit Slush'	4 fl oz	157	0	39	10	0	0.0	0.0	0	0%
FRUIT DRINK MIX										
(Continental Mills) apple flavored, instant, powdered	1 pouch	83	0	21	0	na	0.0	na	na	0%
(Country Time)										
lemonade, pink, sugar-free, w/vitamin C, mix only	1/8 cap/tub	5	0	2	0	na	0.0	na	na	4%
lemonade, w/vitamin C, mix only	1/8 cap/tub	64	0	18	13	na	0.2	na	na	3%
lemonade drink, pink, prepared	8 fl oz	80	0	20	20	0	0.0	0.0	0	0%
lemonade drink, pink, sugar-free, prepared	8 fl oz	4	0	0	0	0	0.0	0.0	0	0%
lemonade drink, pink, sugar-sweetened, prepared	8 fl oz	80	0	20	20	0	0.0	0.0	0	0%
lemonade drink, pink, w/NutraSweet, prepared	8 fl oz	4	0	0	0	0	0.0	0.0	0	0%
lemonade drink, prepared	8 fl oz	80	0	20	20	0	0.0	0.0	0	0%
lemonade punch, prepared	8 fl oz	80	0	20	15	0	0.0	0.0	0	0%
lemonade punch, sugar-sweetened, prepared	8 fl oz	80	0	20	15	0	0.0	0.0	0	0%
(Crystal Light)										
berry blend, sugar-free, prepared	8 fl oz	4	0	0	0	0	0.0	0.0	0	0%
cherry, cranberry, low-calorie, sugarless	1/8 pkt	5	0	0	0	0	0.0	0.0	0	0%
fruit punch, sugar-free, prepared	8 fl oz	4	0	0	0	0	0.0	0.0	0	0%
lemonade drink, low-calorie, prepared	8 fl oz	5	0	0	20	0	0.0	0.0	0	0%
lemonade drink, mix only	1 serving	5	0	0	0	0	0.0	0.0	0	0%
lemonade drink, sugar-free, prepared	8 fl oz	4	0	0	0	0	0.0	0.0	0	0%
lemonade drink, w/NutraSweet, prepared	8 fl oz	4	0	0	0	0	0.0	0.0	0	0%
lemon-lime, mix only	1 serving	5	0	0	0	0	0.0	0.0	0	0%
lemon-lime, sugar-free, prepared	8 fl oz	4	0	0	0	0	0.0	0.0	0	0%
(Finast)										
cherry, prepared	8 fl oz	80	0	21	15	0	0.0	0.0	0	0%
grape, prepared	8 fl oz	80	0	21	15	0	0.0	0.0	0	0%
lemonade drink, prepared	8 fl oz	80	0	20	15	0	0.0	0.0	0	0%
orange, breakfast, prepared	8 fl oz	80	0	20	15	0	0.0	0.0	0	0%
(Kool-Aid)										
berry blend, sugar-free, w/NutraSweet, mix, prepared	8 fl oz	4	0	0	5	0	0.0	0.0	0	0%
berry blue, mix, prepared w/sugar	8 fl oz	100	0	25	0	0	0.0	0.0	0	0%
berry blue, mix, sugar-sweetened, prepared	8 fl oz	80	0	21	5	0	0.0	0.0	0	0%
berry blue, mix, unsweetened, prepared	8 fl oz	2	0	0	0	0	0.0	0.0	0	0%
black cherry, prepared w/sugar	8 fl oz	100	0	25	0	0	0.0	0.0	0	0%
black cherry, unsweetened, prepared	8 fl oz	2	0	0	0	0	0.0	0.0	0	0%
cherry, sugar-free, prepared	8 fl oz	4	0	0	0	0	0.0	0.0	0	0%
cherry, sugar-sweetened, prepared	8 fl oz	80	0	20	0	0	0.0	0.0	0	0%
cherry, unsweetened, prepared	8 fl oz	2	0	0	0	0	0.0	0.0	0	0%
cherry, w/aspartame and vitamin C, sugarless	1/8 envelope	3	0	1	5	na	0.0	na	na	1%
grape, sugar-free, prepared	8 fl oz	4	0	0	0	0	0.0	0.0	0	0%
grape, sugar-sweetened	8 fl oz	80	0	20	25	0	0.0	0.0	0	0%
grape, unsweetened	8 fl oz	2	0	0	0	0	0.0	0.0	0	0%
'Great Bluedini' prepared w/sugar	8 fl oz	100	0	25	0	0	0.0	0.0	0	0%
'Great Bluedini' sugar-free, prepared	8 fl oz	4	0	0	0	0	0.0	0.0	0	0%
'Great Bluedini' unsweetened, prepared	8 fl oz	2	0	0	0	0	0.0	0.0	0	0%
'Incrediberry' sugar-free, mix only	1/8 envelope	5	0	0	0	0	0.0	0.0	0	0%
lemonade drink, pink, prepared w/sugar	8 fl oz	100	0	25	0	0	0.0	0.0	0	0%
lemonade drink, pink, unsweetened, prepared	8 fl oz	2	0	0	0	0	0.0	0.0	0	0%
lemonade drink, w/NutraSweet, prepared	8 fl oz	4	0	0	0	0	0.0	0.0	0	0%
lemonade drink, sugar-sweetened, prepared	8 fl oz	80	0	20	0	0	0.0	0.0	0	0%

Food Name	Serving Size	Calories	Prot. gms	Carbs gms	Sod. mgs	Fiber gms	Fat gms	Sat. Fat gms	Chol. mgs	% Fat Cal.
lemon-lime, prepared w/sugar	8 fl oz	100	0	25	0	0	0.0	0.0	0	0%
lemon-lime, unsweetened, prepared	8 fl oz	2	0	0	0	0	0.0	0.0	0	0%
mountain berry punch, prepared w/sugar	8 fl oz	100	0	25	15	0	0.0	0.0	0	0%
mountain berry punch, sugar-free, prepared	8 fl oz	4	0	0	35	0	0.0	0.0	0	0%
mountain berry punch, sugar-sweetened, prepared	8 fl oz	80	0	20	15	0	0.0	0.0	0	0%
mountain berry punch, unsweetened, prepared	8 fl oz	2	0	0	15	0	0.0	0.0	0	0%
orange, prepared w/sugar	8 fl oz	100	0	25	0	0	0.0	0.0	0	0%
orange, sugar-free, prepared	8 fl oz	4	0	0	0	0	0.0	0.0	0	0%
orange, sugar-sweetened, prepared	8 fl oz	80	0	20	0	0	0.0	0.0	0	0%
orange, unsweetened, prepared	8 fl oz	2	0	0	0	0	0.0	0.0	0	0%
'Purplesaurus Rex' prepared w/sugar	8 fl oz	100	0	25	5	0	0.0	0.0	0	0%
'Purplesaurus Rex' sugar-free, prepared	8 fl oz	4	0	0	5	0	0.0	0.0	0	0%
'Purplesaurus Rex' unsweetened, prepared	8 fl oz	2	0	0	5	0	0.0	0.0	0	0%
rainbow punch, prepared w/sugar	8 fl oz	100	0	25	0	0	0.0	0.0	0	0%
rainbow punch, sugar-sweetened, prepared	8 fl oz	80	0	21	20	0	0.0	0.0	0	0%
rainbow punch, unsweetened, prepared	8 fl oz	2	0	0	0	0	0.0	0.0	0	0%
raspberry punch, prepared w/sugar	8 fl oz	100	0	25	25	0	0.0	0.0	0	0%
raspberry punch, sugar-sweetened, prepared	8 fl oz	80	0	20	25	0	0.0	0.0	0	0%
raspberry punch, unsweetened, prepared	8 fl oz	2	0	0	25	0	0.0	0.0	0	0%
'Rock-A-Dile Red' prepared w/sugar	8 fl oz	100	0	25	0	0	0.0	0.0	0	0%
'Rock-A-Dile Red' sugar-free, prepared	8 fl oz	4	0	0	0	0	0.0	0.0	0	0%
'Rock-A-Dile Red' unsweetened, prepared	8 fl oz	2	0	0	0	0	0.0	0.0	0	0%
'Sharkleberry Fin' prepared w/sugar	8 fl oz	100	0	25	0	0	0.0	0.0	0	0%
'Sharkleberry Fin' sugar-free, prepared	8 fl oz	4	0	0	0	0	0.0	0.0	0	0%
'Sharkleberry Fin' sugar-sweetened, prepared	8 fl oz	80	0	21	0	0	0.0	0.0	0	0%
'Sharkleberry Fin' unsweetened, prepared	8 fl oz	2	0	0	0	0	0.0	0.0	0	0%
strawberry punch, prepared w/sugar	8 fl oz	100	0	25	25	0	0.0	0.0	0	0%
strawberry punch, sugar-sweetened, prepared	8 fl oz	80	0	20	0	0	0.0	0.0	0	0%
strawberry punch, unsweetened, prepared	8 fl oz	2	0	0	25	0	0.0	0.0	0	0%
strawberry-flavored, prepared	8 fl oz	100	0	25	25	0	0.0	0.0	0	0%
strawberry-flavored, presweetened, prepared	8 fl oz	80	0	20	0	0	0.0	0.0	0	0%
'Surfin' Berry' prepared w/sugar	8 fl oz	100	0	25	25	0	0.0	0.0	0	0%
'Surfin' Berry' sugar-free, prepared	8 fl oz	4	0	0	10	0	0.0	0.0	0	0%
'Surfin' Berry' unsweetened, prepared	8 fl oz	2	0	0	25	0	0.0	0.0	0	0%
tropical punch, sugar-sweetened, mix only	1 serving	64	0	16	2	0	0.0	0.0	0	0%
tropical punch, sugar-sweetened, prepared	8 fl oz	80	0	21	0	0	0.0	0.0	0	0%
tropical punch, unsweetened, mix only	1 serving	1	0	0	15	0	0.0	0.0	0	0%
tropical punch, unsweetened, prepared	8 fl oz	2	0	0	0	0	0.0	0.0	0	0%
(Kroger)										
lemonade drink, light, diet, 15% vitamin C, mix only	1/8 pkt	5	0	1	0	0	0.0	0.0	0	0%
lemonade drink, sugar, 10% vitamin C, no preservatives, mix only	1 1/2 tbsp	65	0	16	40	0	0.0	0.0	0	0%
lemon-lime, light, diet, 15% vitamin C	1/8 pkt	6	0	2	0	0	0.0	0.0	0	0%
(Minute Maid)										
grape punch, chilled	6 fl oz	90	0	23	20	0	0.0	0.0	0	0%
grape punch, frozen concentrate, prepared	6 fl oz	90	0	23	0	0	0.0	0.0	0	0%
(Nestlé)										
strawberry-flavored, 'Quik' mix only	0.75 oz	80	0	21	0	0	0.0	0.0	0	0%
strawberry-flavored, 'Quik' prepared w/skim milk	8 fl oz	160	8	32	125	0	0.0	0.0	0	0%
strawberry-flavored, 'Quik' prepared wwhole milk	8 fl oz	220	8	32	120	0	8.0	0.0	0	31%
(Pathmark)										
cherry, 'No Frills' prepared	8 fl oz	90	0	22	65	0	0.0	0.0	0	0%
fruit punch, 'No Frills' prepared	8 fl oz	90	0	22	85	0	0.0	0.0	0	0%
grape, 'No Frills Sodium-free' prepared	6 fl oz	80	0	22	0	0	0.0	0.0	0	0%

Food Name	Serving Size	Calories	Prot. gms	Carbs gms	Sod. mgs	Fiber gms	Fat gms	Sat. Fat gms	Chol. mgs	% Fat Cal.
grape, 'No Frills' prepared	8 fl oz	90	0	22	20	0	0.0	0.0	0	0%
lemon, 'No Frills' prepared	8 fl oz	90	0	20	55	0	0.0	0.0	0	0%
orange, breakfast, 'No Frills' prepared	4 fl oz	60	0	15	0	0	0.0	0.0	0	0%
mango flavor, prepared	6 fl oz	80	0	20	0	0	0.0	0.0	0	0%
(Tang)										
orange, mix only	2 tbsp	100	0	24	0	0	0.0	0.0	0	0%
orange, prepared	8 fl oz	90	0	23	0	0	0.0	0.0	0	0%
orange, sugar-free, 'Breakfast Beverage Crystals'										
prepared	6 fl oz	6	0	1	0	0	0.0	0.0	0	0%
orange, sugar-free, prepared	6 fl oz	6	0	1	0	0	0.0	0.0	0	0%
orange-flavored, mix only	2 tbsp	92	0	25	2	0	0.0	0.0	0	0%
orange-flavored, prepared	8 fl oz	92	0	25	2	0	0.0	0.0	0	0%
orange-flavored, sugarless, prepared	8 fl oz	5	0	2	2	0	0.0	0.0	0	0%
orange, 'Breakfast Beverage Crystals' prepared	6 fl oz	90	0	22	0	0	0.0	0.0	0	0%
(Welch's) grape, frozen concentrate, 'Welchade'	2 fl oz	130	0	31	10	0	0.0	0.0	0	0%
(Wyler's)										
cherry, 'Fruit Slush' prepared	4 fl oz	157	0	39	10	0	0.0	0.0	0	0%
fruit punch, tropical, 'Crystals' prepared	8 fl oz	85	0	21	18	0	0.1	0.0	0	1%
lemonade drink, 'Crystals' prepared	8 fl oz	92	0	20	44	0	1.5	0.0	0	15%
strawberry-flavored, 'Crystals' prepared	8 fl oz	85	0	21	43	0	0.3	0.0	0	3%
FRUIT JUICE BLEND. See also CIDER; FRUIT DRINK; FRUIT JUICE DRINK.										
AMBROSIA *(Knudsen)*	8 fl oz	110	1	27	0	0	0.0	0.0	0	0%
APPLE APRICOT *(Knudsen)*	8 fl oz	120	0	30	35	na	0.0	0.0	0	0%
APPLE BANANA *(Knudsen)*	8 fl oz	120	0	30	25	na	0.0	0.0	0	0%
APPLE BLACKBERRY										
(Knudsen)	8 fl oz	100	1	24	0	0	0.0	0.0	0	0%
organic *(Santa Cruz Natural)*	8 fl oz	120	1	29	0	0	1.0	0.0	0	7%
APPLE BOYSENBERRY										
organic *(Santa Cruz Natural)*	8 fl oz	120	1	29	0	0	1.0	0.0	0	7%
(Knudsen)	8 fl oz	120	0	30	25	na	0.0	0.0	0	0%
APPLE CARROT 100% pure juice *(Vruit)*	8.45 fl oz	120	1	28	60	na	0.0	na	na	0%
APPLE CHERRY										
'Breakfast Cocktail' *(Musselman's)*	6 fl oz	100	1	26	5	0	0.0	0.0	0	0%
'Naturally 100%' *(Red Cheek)*	6 fl oz	113	0	28	11	0	0.0	0.0	0	0%
100% juice 'Junior' *(McCain)*	4.2 fl oz	50	0	13	5	0	0.0	0.0	0	0%
APPLE CITRUS, canned or frozen *(Tree Top)*	6 fl oz	90	1	22	10	0	0.0	0.0	0	0%
APPLE CRANBERRY										
(Apple & Eve)	6 fl oz	80	0	19	5	0	0.0	0.0	0	0%
(Knudsen)	8 fl oz	120	0	30	25	na	0.0	0.0	0	0%
(Lucky Leaf)	6 fl oz	130	0	32	10	0	0.0	0.0	0	0%
(Mott's)	6 fl oz	83	0	24	17	0	0.0	0.0	0	0%
(Santa Cruz Natural) organic	8 fl oz	115	1	28	0	0	1.0	0.0	0	7%
(Smucker's) 'Naturally 100%'	8 fl oz	120	0	32	10	0	0.0	0.0	0	0%
(Tree Top) canned or frozen	6 fl oz	100	0	25	10	0	0.0	0.0	0	0%
(Veryfine) cocktail	8 fl oz	130	0	33	10	0	0.0	0.0	0	0%
APPLE CRANBERRY RASPBERRY *(Ultra Slim Fast)*	8 fl oz	153	5	32	167	3	1.0	0.3	7	6%
APPLE GRAPE CHERRY										
(Welch's) frozen, 'Orchard Cocktail'	6 fl oz	90	0	22	10	0	0.0	0.0	0	0%
(Welch's) 'Orchard Cocktails-In-A-Box'	8.45 fl oz	150	0	38	20	0	0.0	0.0	0	0%
APPLE GRAPE										
(Juicy Juice)	6 fl oz	90	0	22	10	0	0.0	0.0	0	0%
(Mott's)	6 fl oz	86	0	23	17	0	0.0	0.0	0	0%
(Musselman's) 'Breakfast Cocktail'	6 fl oz	110	0	28	5	0	0.0	0.0	0	0%
(Red Cheek)	6 fl oz	109	0	27	9	0	0.0	0.0	0	0%

Food Name	Serving Size	Calories	Prot. gms	Carbs gms	Sod. mgs	Fiber gms	Fat gms	Sat. Fat gms	Chol. mgs	% Fat Cal.
(Tree Top) 100%	8 fl oz	130	0	32	30	0	0.0	0.0	0	0%
(Welch's) 'Orchard Cocktail'	6 fl oz	110	0	27	20	0	0.0	0.0	0	0%
APPLE GRAPE RASPBERRY										
(Welch's) 'Orchard Cocktail' frozen, prepared	6 fl oz	90	0	22	10	0	0.0	0.0	0	0%
(Welch's) 'Orchard Cocktails-In-A-Box'	8.45 fl oz	140	0	35	20	0	0.0	0.0	0	0%
APPLE ORANGE PINEAPPLE										
(Welch's) 'Orchard Tropical Cocktails'	6 fl oz	100	0	25	20	0	0.0	0.0	0	0%
APPLE PEACH *(Knudsen)*	8 fl oz	120	0	30	25	na	0.0	0.0	0	0%
APPLE PEAR *(Tree Top)* 100%	8 fl oz	120	0	29	25	0	0.0	0.0	0	0%
APPLE RASPBERRY										
(Knudsen)	8 fl oz	120	0	30	25	na	0.0	0.0	0	0%
(Mott's)	6 fl oz	83	0	22	48	0	0.0	0.0	0	0%
(Red Cheek)	6 fl oz	113	0	28	8	0	0.0	0.0	0	0%
(Santa Cruz Natural) organic	8 fl oz	120	1	29	0	0	1.0	0.0	0	7%
(Tree Top) 100%	8 fl oz	116	0	28	22	0	0.0	0.0	0	0%
(Veryfine) cocktail	8 fl oz	110	0	27	15	0	0.0	0.0	0	0%
APPLE STRAWBERRY										
(Knudsen)	8 fl oz	120	0	30	25	na	0.0	0.0	0	0%
(Santa Cruz Natural) organic	8 fl oz	120	1	29	0	0	1.0	0.0	0	7%
APPLE WHITE GRAPE										
(Welch's) cocktail, frozen 'No Sugar Added'	6 fl oz	40	0	10	5	0	0.0	0.0	0	0%
BERRY										
(Juicy Juice) bottled.	6 fl oz	90	1	22	10	0	0.0	0.0	0	0%
CRANBERRY BLUEBERRY										
(Knudsen)	8 fl oz	115	1	36	0	0	0.0	0.0	0	0%
CRANBERRY RASPBERRY										
(Knudsen)	8 fl oz	140	0	36	35	na	0.0	0.0	0	0%
(Welch's) light, frozen, prepared	6 fl oz	40	0	10	0	0	0.0	0.0	0	0%
GRAPE *(Juicy Juice)* juice blend	6 fl oz	100	0	25	5	0	0.0	0.0	0	0%
GUAVA CRANBERRY										
(Santa Cruz Natural) organic 'Cruz'	8 fl oz	130	1	30	0	0	1.0	0.0	0	7%
HIBISCUS CRANBERRY *(Knudsen)*	8 fl oz	120	0	30	35	na	0.0	0.0	0	0%
LEMON GINGER *(Santa Cruz Natural)* organic 'Cruz'.	8 fl oz	125	1	29	0	0	1.0	0.0	0	7%
MANGO PEACH *(Knudsen)*	8 fl oz	120	0	30	50	na	0.0	0.0	0	0%
ORANGE *(Minute Maid)* blend, 'Juices To Go'	6 fl oz	90	1	22	20	0	0.0	0.0	0	0%
ORANGE APRICOT *(Musselman's)* 'Breakfast Cocktail'	6 fl oz	90	0	21	20	0	0.0	0.0	0	0%
ORANGE BANANA *(Smucker's)* 'Naturally 100%'	8 fl oz	120	0	30	10	0	0.0	0.0	0	0%
ORANGE CRANBERRY *(Santa Cruz Natural)*										
organic 'Cruz'	8 fl oz	125	1	29	0	0	1.0	0.0	0	7%
ORANGE GRAPEFRUIT										
(Kraft) chilled, 'Pure 100%'	6 fl oz	80	1	19	0	0	0.0	0.0	0	0%
(Tropicana) ruby red, 'Pure Premium'	8 fl oz	120	1	28	0	1	0.0	na	na	0%
ORANGE KIWI PASSIONFRUIT										
(Tropicana) 100% pure	6 fl oz	80	1	17	35	0	1.0	0.0	0	11%
(Tropicana) 'Pure Premium'.	8 fl oz	100	1	26	15	1	0.0	na	na	0%
ORANGE MANGO										
(Knudsen)	8 fl oz	120	0	30	50	na	0.0	0.0	0	0%
(Tropicana) 'Twister'.	6 fl oz	90	1	21	45	0	1.0	0.0	0	9%
ORANGE PASSIONFRUIT *(Tropicana)* 'Twister'	6 fl oz	80	1	19	35	0	1.0	0.0	0	10%
ORANGE PEACH *(Tropicana Twister)*	8 fl oz	120	0	31	20	na	0.0	0.0	0	0%
ORANGE PEACH MANGO										
(Tropicana) 100% pure	6 fl oz	80	1	19	20	0	1.0	0.0	0	10%
(Tropicana) 'Pure Premium'	8 fl oz	110	1	28	15	1	0.0	na	na	0%

Food Name	Serving Size	Calories	Prot. gms	Carbs gms	Sod. mgs	Fiber gms	Fat gms	Sat. Fat gms	Chol. mgs	% Fat Cal.
ORANGE PINEAPPLE										
(Kraft) 'Pure 100%'	6 fl oz	80	1	19	0	0	0.0	0.0	0	0%
(Musselman's) 'Breakfast Cocktail'	6 fl oz	90	1	23	15	0	0.0	0.0	0	0%
(Tropicana) 100% pure	6 fl oz	80	1	19	15	0	1.0	0.0	0	10%
(Tropicana) 'Pure Premium'	8 fl oz	110	1	27	15	1	0.0	na	na	0%
(Ultra Slim Fast)	8 fl oz	153	5	33	181	3	1.0	0.3	7	6%
ORANGE STRAWBERRY BANANA										
(Tropicana) 100% pure	6 fl oz	80	1	18	25	0	1.0	0.0	0	11%
(Ultra Slim Fast)	8 fl oz	153	5	33	167	3	1.0	0.3	7	6%
PAPAYA LIME (Knudsen)	8 fl oz	115	1	29	0	0	0.0	0.0	0	0%
PASSIONFRUIT RASPBERRY (Knudsen)	8 fl oz	130	1	32	0	0	0.0	0.0	0	0%
PINEAPPLE COCONUT (Knudsen)	8 fl oz	130	0	32	50	na	0.0	0.0	0	0%
PINEAPPLE GRAPEFRUIT										
(Dole) frozen, prepared	6 fl oz	90	1	22	10	0	0.0	0.0	0	0%
(Dole) w/pink grapefruit	6 fl oz	101	0	25	0	0	0.1	0.0	0	1%
PINEAPPLE ORANGE										
(Dole)	6 fl oz	90	0	22	10	0	0.0	0.0	0	0%
(Dole) w/banana	6 fl oz	100	0	23	10	0	0.0	0.0	0	0%
(Dole) w/guava	6 fl oz	100	1	21	10	0	0.0	0.0	0	0%
(Minute Maid)	6 fl oz	90	1	23	0	0	0.0	0.0	0	0%
PINEAPPLE PASSIONFRUIT (Dole) w/banana	6 fl oz	100	1	21	10	0	0.0	0.0	0	0%
RASPBERRY										
(Apple & Eve) w/cranberry	6 fl oz	90	0	21	10	0	0.0	0.0	0	0%
(Dole) blend, 'Pure & Light Country Raspberry'	6 fl oz	87	0	24	15	0	0.2	0.0	0	2%
(Knudsen) blend, 'Razzleberry'	8 fl oz	90	1	21	0	0	0.0	0.0	0	0%
RASPBERRY PEACH (Knudsen)	8 fl oz	120	0	31	25	na	0.0	0.0	0	0%
STRAWBERRY BANANA (Knudsen)	8 fl oz	120	0	30	25	na	0.0	0.0	0	0%
STRAWBERRY GUAVA (Knudsen)	8 fl oz	105	1	26	0	0	0.0	0.0	0	0%
TOMATO-BEEF COCKTAIL (Beefamato)	6 fl oz	80	1	19	240	0	0.0	0.0	0	0%
TOMATO-CHILE COCKTAIL (Snap-E-Tom)	6 fl oz	40	2	8	500	1	0.0	0.0	0	0%
TOMATO-CLAM COCKTAIL (Clamato)	6 fl oz	96	1	23	815	0	0.0	0.0	0	0%
FRUIT JUICE DRINK										
(A&P)										
cranberry juice cocktail, bottled	6 fl oz	100	1	26	0	0	1.0	0.0	0	8%
(Capri Sun)										
fruit punch	1 serving	100	0	26	20	0	0.0	0.0	0	0%
'Pacific Cooler'	1 serving	100	0	26	20	0	0.0	0.0	0	0%
Maui punch	1 serving	100	0	27	20	0	0.0	0.0	0	0%
wild cherry	1 serving	110	0	30	20	0	0.0	0.0	0	0%
(Citrus Hill)										
grapefruit, 'Plus Calcium'	6 fl oz	70	1	19	10	0	1.0	0.0	0	10%
orange, 'Lite Premium'	6 fl oz	60	1	14	10	0	1.0	0.0	0	13%
(Clinical Resource)										
orange	8 fl oz	180	9	36	70	na	0.0	0.0	0	0%
peach	8 fl oz	180	9	36	70	na	0.0	0.0	0	0%
wild berry	8 fl oz	180	9	36	70	na	0.0	0.0	0	0%
(Del Monte) apricot nectar	6 fl oz	100	1	26	10	0	0.0	0.0	0	0%
(Hi-C)										
cherry	8.45 fl oz	141	0	35	24	0	0.1	0.0	0	1%
grape	6 fl oz	96	0	24	17	0	0.1	0.0	0	1%
(IGA) pink grapefruit	6 fl oz	80	0	20	15	0	0.0	0.0	0	0%
(J. Hungerford)										
cranberry juice cocktail	9.03 fl oz	141	1	36	0	0	0.0	0.0	0	0%
cranberry juice cocktail, 50% juice	9.03 fl oz	134	0	35	7	0	0.1	0.0	0	1%

Food Name	Serving Size	Calories	Prot. gms	Carbs gms	Sod. mgs	Fiber gms	Fat gms	Sat. Fat gms	Chol. mgs	% Fat Cal.
fruit punch, 50% juice	9.03 fl oz	107	0	27	7	0	0.0	0.0	0	0%
fruit punch, 100% juice	9.03 fl oz	116	1	30	11	0	0.0	0.0	0	0%
grape, 50% juice	9.03 fl oz	135	0	34	0	0	0.0	0.0	0	0%
grapefruit, 50% juice	9.03 fl oz	109	1	27	0	0	0.0	0.0	0	0%
pineapple, 50% juice	9.03 fl oz	123	0	31	0	0	0.0	0.0	0	0%
(Kern's)										
guava nectar	11.5 fl oz	216	0	55	7	0	0.0	0.0	0	0%
mango nectar	11.5 fl oz	216	0	52	7	52	0.0	0.0	0	0%
mango-orange nectar	8 fl oz	140	0	35	10	0	0.0	0.0	0	0%
orange-banana nectar	6 fl oz	110	1	25	0	0	0.0	0.0	0	0%
orange-guava nectar	8 fl oz	150	0	36	10	0	0.0	0.0	0	0%
papaya nectar	11.5 fl oz	210	1	51	10	0	0.0	0.0	0	0%
peach nectar	11.5 fl oz	210	1	52	5	0	0.0	0.0	0	0%
peach-passionfruit nectar	11.5 fl oz	220	1	53	5	2	0.0	0.0	0	0%
pear nectar	11.5 fl oz	220	0	54	5	3	0.0	0.0	0	0%
pineapple-orange-passionfruit nectar	8 fl oz	146	2	33	7	0	0.0	0.0	0	0%
strawberry nectar	6 fl oz	110	0	28	0	0	0.0	0.0	0	0%
strawberry-banana nectar	8 fl oz	150	0	36	5	0	0.0	0.0	0	0%
tropical nectar	11.5 fl oz	210	3	48	10	0	0.0	0.0	0	0%
(Knudsen)										
breakfast juice, natural	8 fl oz	110	1	27	35	na	0.0	0.0	0	0%
breakfast juice, natural, concentrate, prepared	8 fl oz	110	1	27	35	na	0.0	0.0	0	0%
kiwi nectar	8 fl oz	60	1	14	0	0	0.0	0.0	0	0%
orange juice float	8 fl oz	140	1	33	60	na	0.0	0.0	0	0%
papaya nectar	8 fl oz	130	0	34	35	na	0.0	0.0	0	0%
peach nectar	8 fl oz	120	0	30	25	na	0.0	0.0	0	0%
pineapple juice float	8 fl oz	130	2	31	0	0	0.0	0.0	0	0%
raspberry nectar, concentrate, prepared	8 fl oz	120	0	30	25	na	0.0	0.0	0	0%
red raspberry nectar	8 fl oz	120	1	30	0	0	0.0	0.0	0	0%
strawberry juice float	8 fl oz	130	2	32	0	0	0.0	0.0	0	0%
strawberry nectar	8 fl oz	120	0	30	25	na	0.0	0.0	0	0%
(Kool-Aid) orange, 'Koolers'	8.45 fl oz	110	0	30	10	0	0.0	0.0	0	0%
(Libby's)										
guanabana nectar	8 fl oz	147	0	35	17	0	0.0	0.0	0	0%
guava nectar	8 fl oz	153	0	38	7	0	0.0	0.0	0	0%
mango nectar	6 fl oz	110	0	26	0	0	0.0	0.0	0	0%
papaya nectar	6 fl oz	110	0	28	10	0	0.0	0.0	0	0%
peach nectar	6 fl oz	100	0	24	5	0	0.0	0.0	0	0%
pineapple nectar	6 fl oz	110	0	27	30	0	0.0	0.0	0	0%
strawberry nectar	6 fl oz	110	0	27	0	0	0.0	0.0	0	0%
(Minute Maid) pink grapefruit, 'Juices To Go'	6 fl oz	80	0	20	20	0	0.0	0.0	0	0%
(Mott's) orange	10 fl oz	144	1	35	6	0	0.0	0.0	0	0%
(Musselman's) w/grapefruit juice, 'Breakfast Cocktail'	6 fl oz	90	1	22	20	0	0.0	0.0	0	0%
(Ocean Spray)										
cranberry juice cocktail, bottled	6 fl oz	110	0	26	10	0	0.0	0.0	0	0%
cranberry juice cocktail, bottled, 'Low-calorie'	6 fl oz	40	0	9	15	0	0.0	0.0	0	0%
cranberry juice drink, citrus, 'Refreshers'	6 fl oz	100	0	26	15	0	0.0	0.0	0	0%
orange juice cocktail	6 fl oz	100	0	25	15	0	0.0	0.0	0	0%
pineapple cocktail, w/grapefruit juice	6 fl oz	110	0	26	5	0	0.0	0.0	0	0%
pink grapefruit	6 fl oz	80	0	20	15	0	0.0	0.0	0	0%
(Orange Julius) orange	16 fl oz	265	1	66	15	0	1.0	0.0	0	3%
(P&Q) cranberry juice cocktail, bottled	6 fl oz	100	1	24	0	0	1.0	0.0	0	8%
(Pathmark)										
cranberry juice cocktail, bottled, 'No Frills'	6 fl oz	100	0	26	10	0	0.0	0.0	0	0%
pink grapefruit	6 fl oz	80	0	20	15	0	0.0	0.0	0	0%

Food Name	Serving Size	Calories	Prot. gms	Carbs gms	Sod. mgs	Fiber gms	Fat gms	Sat. Fat gms	Chol. mgs	% Fat Cal.
(Santa Cruz Natural)										
papaya nectar, certified organic	8 fl oz	110	1	28	35	0	0.0	0.0	0	0%
red raspberry nectar, certified organic	8 fl oz	100	1	26	35	0	0.0	0.0	0	0%
strawberry-guava nectar, certified organic	8 fl oz	100	1	24	25	0	0.0	0.0	0	0%
(Snapple)										
'Apple Crisp' *(Snapple)*	10 fl oz	140	0	36	30	0	0.0	0.0	0	0%
'Cranberry Royale'	10 fl oz	150	0	37	25	0	0.0	0.0	0	0%
'Passion Supreme'	10 fl oz	160	0	39	20	0	0.0	0.0	0	0%
(Sunkist)										
cranberry juice cocktail, bottled	6 fl oz	110	0	28	8	0	0.1	0.0	0	1%
cranberry juice cocktail, frozen, prepared	6 fl oz	110	0	28	0	0	0.1	0.0	0	1%
grape, frozen, prepared	6 fl oz	69	0	17	3	0	0.1	0.0	0	1%
(Tang)										
cherry, 'Fruit Box'	8.45 fl oz	130	0	34	10	0	0.0	0.0	0	0%
grape, 'Fruit Box'	8.45 fl oz	130	0	34	10	0	0.0	0.0	0	0%
mixed fruit, 'Fruit Box'	8.45 fl oz	140	0	36	10	0	0.0	0.0	0	0%
orange, 'Fruit Box'	8.45 fl oz	130	0	32	10	0	0.0	0.0	0	0%
strawberry, 'Fruit Box'	8.45 fl oz	120	0	32	10	0	0.0	0.0	0	0%
(TreeSweet) pink grapefruit 'Lite'	6 fl oz	40	1	10	15	0	0.0	0.0	0	0%
(Tropic Isle) fruit punch, vitamin-enriched	6 fl oz	90	0	22	5	0	0.0	0.0	0	0%
(Tropicana)										
apple raspberry blackberry drink, 'Twister'	8 fl oz	130	0	31	20	na	0.0	0.0	0	0%
cranberry juice drink, 'Season's Best' 'Medley'	10 fl oz	140	1	35	30	1	0.0	na	na	0%
cranberry juice drink, 'Season's Best' 'Medley'	8 fl oz	120	1	29	20	1	0.0	na	na	0%
'Cranberry Orchard Juice Sparkler'	8 fl oz	120	0	30	20	0	0.0	0.0	0	0%
grapefruit, 'Juice Sparkler'	8 fl oz	110	0	26	50	0	0.0	0.0	0	0%
pink grapefruit, 'Twister'	8 fl oz	110	0	28	1	0	0.0	0.0	0	0%
grapefruit, ruby red w/cranberry, 'Twister'	8 fl oz	120	0	30	20	na	0.0	na	na	0%
Mandarin orange-papaya, 'Twister'	6 fl oz	90	1	21	30	0	1.0	0.0	0	9%
orange-cranberry, 'Twister'	8 fl oz	130	0	32	45	na	0.0	0.0	0	0%
orange-cranberry, light, 'Twister'	8 fl oz	30	0	7	20	na	0.0	0.0	0	0%
orange-raspberry, 'Twister'	6 fl oz	80	1	20	30	0	1.0	0.0	0	10%
orange-raspberry, light, 'Twister'	8 fl oz	35	0	9	20	na	0.0	0.0	0	0%
orange-strawberry-banana, 'Twister'	8 fl oz	130	0	32	45	na	0.0	0.0	0	0%
orange-strawberry-banana, light, 'Twister'	8 fl oz	35	1	9	20	na	0.0	0.0	0	0%
orange-strawberry-guava, 'Twister'	8 fl oz	120	0	29	20	na	0.0	0.0	0	0%
pineapple, w/grapefruit juice, 'Twister'	8 fl oz	125	0	32	2	0	0.0	0.0	0	0%
pineapple-grapefruit, 'Twister'	8 fl oz	120	0	29	20	na	0.0	0.0	0	0%
pineapple-grapefruit, light, 'Twister'	8 fl oz	35	0	9	20	na	0.0	0.0	0	0%
'Season's Best' 'Medley'	8 fl oz	130	1	32	25	1	0.0	na	na	0%
wild berry, 'Juice Sparkler'	8 fl oz	110	0	27	15	0	0.0	0.0	0	0%
(Veryfine)										
apple cherry berry	8 fl oz	130	0	33	25	0	0.0	0.0	0	0%
cranberry juice cocktail, bottled	8 fl oz	160	1	40	10	0	0.0	0.0	0	0%
'Passionfruit Refresher' w/orange, tropical	8 fl oz	110	1	26	25	0	0.0	0.0	0	0%
pink grapefruit	8 fl oz	120	1	29	15	0	0.0	0.0	0	0%
(Welch's)										
cranberry juice cocktail, frozen, diluted as directed	6 fl oz	100	0	26	0	0	0.0	0.0	0	0%
cranberry juice cocktail, no sugar added, frozen, prepared	6 fl oz	40	0	10	5	0	0.0	0.0	0	0%
cranberry juice cocktail, w/raspberry, frozen, prepared	6 fl oz	110	0	28	0	0	0.0	0.0	0	0%
cranberry juice cocktail, w/blueberry, frozen, prepared	6 fl oz	110	0	27	0	0	0.0	0.0	0	0%
cranberry juice cocktail, lite, frozen, prepared	6 fl oz	40	0	10	20	0	0.0	0.0	0	0%
grape juice cocktail, no sugar added, frozen concentrate, prepared	6 fl oz	40	0	10	5	0	0.0	0.0	0	0%

Food Name	Serving Size	Calories	Prot. gms	Carbs gms	Sod. mgs	Fiber gms	Fat gms	Sat. Fat gms	Chol. mgs	% Fat Cal.
grape juice cocktail, 'Orchard Cocktails-In-A-Box'	8.45 fl oz	150	0	38	20	0	0.0	0.0	0	0%
grape juice cocktail, 'Orchard'	6 fl oz	110	0	27	20	0	0.0	0.0	0	0%
orange juice cocktail, 'Orchard'	10 fl oz	150	0	37	0	0	0.0	0.0	0	0%
'Orchard Harvest Blend Cocktails-In-A-Box'	8.45 fl oz	150	0	38	20	0	0.0	0.0	0	0%
'Orchard Harvest Blend' frozen, prepared	6 fl oz	110	0	27	10	0	0.0	0.0	0	0%
passionfruit cocktail, 'Orchard Tropical Cocktails-In-A-Box'	8.45 fl oz	140	0	34	20	0	0.0	0.0	0	0%
passionfruit cocktail, 'Orchard Tropicals' frozen, prepared	6 fl oz	100	0	25	20	0	0.0	0.0	0	0%
pineapple cocktail, w/banana, 'Orchard Tropicals'	6 fl oz	100	0	24	20	0	0.0	0.0	0	0%
pineapple cocktail, w/banana, 'Orchard Tropicals'	8.45 fl oz	140	0	34	20	0	0.0	0.0	0	0%
(Wyler's)										
grapefruit, 'Fruit Slush'	4 fl oz	157	0	39	10	0	0.0	0.0	0	0%
strawberry, 'Fruit Slush'	4 fl oz	157	0	39	10	0	0.0	0.0	0	0%
FRUIT ROLL. See FRUIT SNACK.										
FRUIT SNACK										
(Betty Crocker)										
all flavors, 'Berry Bears'	1 pouch	100	1	22	20	0	1.0	0.0	0	9%
all flavors, 'Fruit Roll-Ups Peel-Outs'	1 roll	50	1	12	40	0	1.0	0.0	0	15%
assorted flavors, 'Bugs Bunny & Friends'	1 pouch	90	1	21	30	0	1.0	0.0	0	9%
assorted flavors, 'Tasmanian Devil'	1 pouch	90	1	21	30	0	1.0	0.0	0	9%
berry fruit roll-up, w/vitamin C	2 rolls	104	0	24	89	na	1.0	0.3	na	8%
blueberry, 'Wild Blue' 'Garfield & Friends'	1 roll	50	1	12	20	0	1.0	0.0	0	15%
cherry, 'Fruit by the Foot'	1 roll	80	1	17	45	0	2.0	0.0	0	20%
cherry, 'Fruit Roll-Ups'	0.5 oz roll	50	1	12	40	0	1.0	0.0	0	15%
crazy colors, 'Fruit Roll-Ups'	0.5 oz roll	50	1	12	40	0	1.0	0.0	0	15%
grape, 'Fruit by the Foot'	1 roll	80	1	17	45	0	2.0	0.0	0	20%
grape, 'Fruit Roll-Ups'	0.5 oz roll	50	1	12	40	0	1.0	0.0	0	15%
grape, 'Gushin Grape Gushers'	1 pouch	90	1	21	45	0	1.0	0.0	0	9%
raspberry, 'Fruit Roll-Ups'	0.5 oz roll	50	1	12	40	0	1.0	0.0	0	15%
strawberry, 'Fruit by the Foot'	1 roll	80	1	17	45	0	2.0	0.0	0	20%
strawberry, 'Fruit Roll-Ups'	0.5-oz roll	50	1	12	40	0	1.0	0.0	0	15%
strawberry, 'Gushers'	1 pouch	90	1	21	45	0	1.0	0.0	0	9%
wild cherry, 'Gushers'	1 pouch	90	1	21	40	0	1.0	0.0	0	9%
(Farley)										
assorted flavors, 'Dinosaurs'	1 oz	90	1	22	0	0	1.0	0.0	0	9%
assorted flavors, 'Teenage Mutant Ninja Turtles'	1 oz	90	1	22	0	0	1.0	0.0	0	9%
assorted flavors, 'Trolls'	1 oz	90	1	22	0	0	1.0	0.0	0	9%
w/vitamins A, C, and E	1 pouch	89	1	21	9	na	0.0	na	na	0%
(Flavor Tree)										
apple roll	1 piece	75	0	19	17	0	0.0	0.0	0	0%
apricot roll	1 piece	76	0	18	17	0	0.5	0.0	0	6%
assorted flavors, 'Fruit Circus Fruit Bears'	1.05 oz	117	0	25	12	0	1.6	0.0	0	12%
cherry roll	1 piece	75	0	18	18	0	0.1	0.0	0	1%
grape roll	1 piece	76	0	19	13	0	0.1	0.0	0	1%
raspberry roll	1 piece	75	0	18	20	0	0.1	0.0	0	1%
strawberry roll	1 piece	74	0	18	11	0	0.1	0.0	0	1%
(Fruit Parade)										
assorted flavors, 'Chip 'N Dale Rescue Rangers'	1 pouch	100	0	22	10	0	1.0	0.0	0	9%
assorted flavors, 'Darkwing Duck'	1 pouch	100	0	22	10	0	1.0	0.0	0	9%
assorted flavors, 'Tale Spin'	1 pouch	100	0	22	10	0	1.0	0.0	0	9%
(Rokeach) compote	4 oz	120	1	31	4	0	1.0	0.0	0	7%
(Stretch Island)										
'Berry Blackberry' 100% fruit	1 oz	90	0	24	0	2	0.0	0.0	0	0%
'Chunky Cherry' 100% fruit	1 oz	90	0	24	0	2	0.0	0.0	0	0%

Food Name	Serving Size	Calories	Prot. gms	Carbs gms	Sod. mgs	Fiber gms	Fat gms	Sat. Fat gms	Chol. mgs	% Fat Cal.
'Great Grape' 100% fruit	1 oz	90	0	24	0	2	0.0	0.0	0	0%
'Rave Raspberry' 100% fruit	1 oz	90	0	24	0	2	0.0	0.0	0	0%
apple, 100% fruit, 'Snappy Apple'	1 oz	90	0	25	0	2	0.0	0.0	0	0%
apricot, 'Tangy Apricot' 100% fruit	1 oz	90	1	23	0	2	0.0	0.0	0	0%
(Sunkist)										
assorted flavors, 'Fun Fruits Fantastic Fruit'	1 pouch	100	0	22	10	0	1.4	0.0	0	13%
assorted flavors, all shapes, 'Fun Fruits'	1 pouch	100	0	22	10	0	1.4	0.0	0	13%
berry, 'Fun Fruits Berry Bunch'	1 pouch	100	0	22	10	0	1.4	0.0	0	13%
cherry, 'Fun Fruits'	1 pouch	100	0	22	10	0	1.4	0.0	0	13%
grape, 'Fun Fruits'	1 pouch	100	0	22	10	0	1.4	0.0	0	13%
orange, 'Fun Fruits'	1 pouch	100	0	22	10	0	1.4	0.0	0	13%
strawberry roll, w/vitamins A, C, and E	1 roll	72	0	17	23	2	0.2	na	na	3%
strawberry, 'Fun Fruits'	1 pouch	100	0	22	10	0	1.4	0.0	0	13%
strawberry, yogurt-coated, 'Creme Supremes'	1 pouch	114	0	20	19	0	3.6	0.0	0	29%
(Sun-Maid) raisin, muscat, seeded	1/2 cup	270	2	67	25	0	1.0	0.0	0	3%
(Weight Watchers)										
apple	1 pouch	50	1	13	75	0	1.0	0.0	0	14%
apple chips	0.75 oz	70	0	19	110	0	0.0	0.0	0	0%
cinnamon flavor	1 pouch	50	1	13	75	0	1.0	0.0	0	14%
peach	0.5 oz	50	1	13	75	0	1.0	0.0	0	14%
strawberry	1 pouch	50	1	13	75	0	1.0	0.0	0	14%

FRUIT SPREAD. See also JAM AND PRESERVES.

Food Name	Serving Size	Calories	Prot. gms	Carbs gms	Sod. mgs	Fiber gms	Fat gms	Sat. Fat gms	Chol. mgs	% Fat Cal.
(Fifty 50)										
apple, no sugar added	1 tsp	2	0	1	5	0	0.0	0.0	0	0%
grape, no sugar added	1 tsp	2	0	1	5	0	0.0	0.0	0	0%
grape spread, no sugar added, contains phenylalanine	1 tbsp	10	0	3	10	0	0.0	0.0	0	0%
orange marmalade, no sugar added	1 tsp	2	0	1	5	0	0.0	0.0	0	0%
raspberry, no sugar added	1 tsp	2	0	1	5	0	0.0	0.0	0	0%
strawberry, no sugar added	1 tsp	2	0	1	5	0	0.0	0.0	0	0%
(Knott's Berry Farm)										
apricot-pineapple	1 tsp	16	0	4	0	0	0.0	0.0	0	0%
apricot-pineapple, 'Light'	1 tsp	8	0	2	0	0	0.0	0.0	0	0%
apricot-pineapple, portion pack	0.5 oz	35	0	9	0	0	0.0	0.0	0	0%
blackberry	1 tsp	16	0	4	0	0	0.0	0.0	0	0%
blackberry, 'Light'	1 tsp	8	0	2	0	0	0.0	0.0	0	0%
blackberry, portion pack	0.5 oz	35	0	9	0	0	0.0	0.0	0	0%
boysenberry	1 tsp	16	0	4	0	0	0.0	0.0	0	0%
boysenberry, 'Light'	1 tsp	8	0	2	0	0	0.0	0.0	0	0%
boysenberry, portion pack	0.5 oz	35	0	9	0	0	0.0	0.0	0	0%
orange marmalade	1 tsp	16	0	4	0	0	0.0	0.0	0	0%
orange marmalade, 'Light'	1 tsp	8	0	2	0	0	0.0	0.0	0	0%
orange marmalade, portion pack	0.5 oz	35	0	9	0	0	0.0	0.0	0	0%
red raspberry	1 tsp	16	0	4	0	0	0.0	0.0	0	0%
red raspberry, 'Light'	1 tsp	8	0	2	0	0	0.0	0.0	0	0%
red raspberry, portion pack	0.5 oz	35	0	9	0	0	0.0	0.0	0	0%
strawberry, 'Light'	1 tsp	8	0	2	0	0	0.0	0.0	0	0%
(Knudsen)										
calamansi, 'Tropical Rainforest'	2 tsp	35	0	8	0	0	0.0	0.0	0	0%
guanabana, 'Tropical Rainforest'	2 tsp	35	0	8	0	0	0.0	0.0	0	0%
(Polaner)										
apricot, 'All Fruit Spreadable Fruit'	1 tsp	14	0	4	0	0	0.0	0.0	0	0%
black cherry, 'All Fruit Spreadable Fruit'	1 tsp	14	0	4	0	0	0.0	0.0	0	0%
blueberry, 'All Fruit Spreadable Fruit'	1 tsp	14	0	4	0	0	0.0	0.0	0	0%
grape, 'All Fruit Spreadable Fruit'	1 tsp	14	0	4	0	0	0.0	0.0	0	0%
orange, 'All Fruit Spreadable Fruit'	1 tsp	14	0	4	0	0	0.0	0.0	0	0%

Food Name	Serving Size	Calories	Prot. gms	Carbs gms	Sod. mgs	Fiber gms	Fat gms	Sat. Fat gms	Chol. mgs	% Fat Cal.
raspberry, seedless, 'All Fruit Spreadable Fruit'	1 tsp	14	0	4	0	0	0.0	0.0	0	0%
strawberry, 'All Fruit Spreadable Fruit'	1 tsp	14	0	4	0	0	0.0	0.0	0	0%
(Smucker's)										
all flavors, 'Homestyle'	1 tsp	15	0	3	0	0	0.0	0.0	0	0%
all flavors, 'Slenderella'	1 tsp	7	0	2	0	0	0.0	0.0	0	0%
apricot, low-sugar	1 tsp	8	0	2	10	0	0.0	0.0	0	0%
apricot, 'Simply Fruit'	1 tsp	16	0	4	0	0	0.0	0.0	0	0%
black raspberry, 'Simply Fruit'	1 tsp	16	0	4	0	0	0.0	0.0	0	0%
blackberry, low-sugar	1 tsp	8	0	2	10	0	0.0	0.0	0	0%
blackberry, 'Simply Fruit'	1 tsp	16	0	4	0	0	0.0	0.0	0	0%
blueberry, 'Simply Fruit'	1 tsp	16	0	4	0	0	0.0	0.0	0	0%
boysenberry, low-sugar	1 tsp	8	0	2	10	0	0.0	0.0	0	0%
concord grape, low-sugar	1 tsp	8	0	2	0	0	0.0	0.0	0	0%
grape, 'Imitation'	1 tsp	2	0	1	2	0	0.0	0.0	0	0%
grape, 'Simply Fruit'	1 tsp	16	0	4	0	0	0.0	0.0	0	0%
orange marmalade, low-sugar	1 tsp	8	0	2	10	0	0.0	0.0	0	0%
orange marmalade, 'Simply Fruit'	1 tsp	16	0	4	0	0	0.0	0.0	0	0%
peach, 'Simply Fruit'	1 tsp	16	0	4	0	0	0.0	0.0	0	0%
red raspberry, low-sugar	1 tsp	8	0	2	0	0	0.0	0.0	0	0%
red raspberry, 'Simply Fruit'	1 tsp	16	0	4	0	0	0.0	0.0	0	0%
strawberry, 'Imitation'	1 tsp	2	0	1	2	0	0.0	0.0	0	0%
strawberry, low-sugar	1 tsp	8	0	2	0	0	0.0	0.0	0	0%
strawberry, 'Simply Fruit'	1 tsp	16	0	4	0	0	0.0	0.0	0	0%
(Weight Watchers)										
grape	1 tsp	8	0	2	0	0	0.0	0.0	0	0%
raspberry	1 tsp	8	0	2	0	0	0.0	0.0	0	0%
strawberry	1 tsp	8	0	2	0	0	0.0	0.0	0	0%
FRUIT TOPPING, pourable, 'Fruit 'n Maple'										
(Knudsen)	1 oz	105	0	26	0	0	0.0	0.0	0	0%
FUDGE. See under CANDY.										
FUDGE TOPPING. See also CHOCOLATE TOPPING.										
(Kraft) hot	2 tbsp	140	1	24	100	1	4.5	2.0	0	29%
(Mrs. Richardson's)										
caramel, microwavable	2 tbsp	130	1	28	90	0	2.0	0.0	5	13%
hot	2 tbsp	140	1	20	75	0	7.0	0.0	0	43%
hot, microwaveable	2 tbsp	140	1	20	75	0	7.0	0.0	0	43%
(Smucker's)										
	2 tbsp	130	1	31	50	0	1.0	0.0	0	7%
hot	2 tbsp	110	1	18	55	0	4.0	0.0	0	32%
hot, 'Light'	2 tbsp	70	2	19	35	0	0.0	0.0	0	0%
hot, 'Special Recipe'	2 tbsp	150	2	23	60	0	5.0	0.0	0	31%
'Magic Shell'	2 tbsp	190	1	16	50	0	15.0	0.0	0	67%
FUKI. See BUTTERBUR.										

G

Food Name	Serving Size	Calories	Prot. gms	Carbs gms	Sod. mgs	Fiber gms	Fat gms	Sat. Fat gms	Chol. mgs	% Fat Cal.
GARBANZO BEAN. See CHICKPEA.										
GARDEN CRESS										
boiled, drained	1 cup	31	3	5	11	1	0.8	0.0	0	22%
boiled, drained	1/2 cup	16	1	3	5	0	0.4	0.0	0	22%
raw	1 cup	16	1	3	7	1	0.3	0.0	0	18%

Food Name	Serving Size	Calories	Prot. gms	Carbs gms	Sod. mgs	Fiber gms	Fat gms	Sat. Fat gms	Chol. mgs	% Fat Cal.
GARLIC AND HERB SEASONING. See under SEASONING MIX.										
GARLIC										
Fresh										
raw, chopped	1 cup	203	9	45	23	3	0.7	0.1	0	3%
raw, chopped	1 tsp	4	0	1	0	0	0.0	0.0	0	3%
raw, whole	1 med clove	4	0	1	1	0	0.0	0.0	0	3%
raw, whole	3 med cloves	13	1	3	2	0	0.0	0.0	0	3%
Jarred										
crushed *Gilroy*	1 tsp	8	0	2	4	0	0.0	0.0	0	0%
dehydrated *(Basic American)*	1 oz	86	5	22	8	1	0.1	0.0	0	1%
minced *(Gilroy)*	1 tsp	23	0	2	4	0	1.0	0.0	0	49%
GARLIC BREAD. See under BREAD.										
GARLIC OIL *(Hain)*	1 tbsp	120	0	0	0	0	14.0	3.0	0	100%
GARLIC POWDER										
	1 tbsp	28	1	6	2	1	0.1	0.0	0	2%
	1 tsp	9	0	2	1	0	0.0	0.0	0	2%
(Lawry's)	1/4 tsp	0	0	1	0	na	0.0	0.0	0	0%
(McCormick/Schilling)	1 tsp	10	0	2	2	1	0.0	0.0	0	0%
(Spice Islands)	1 tsp	5	0	1	1	0	0.0	0.0	0	0%
(Tone's)	1 tsp	9	1	2	1	0	0.1	0.0	0	8%
fresh ground *(Durkee)*	1 tsp	10	0	0	0	0	0.0	0.0	0	0%
fresh ground *(Laurel Leaf)*	1 tsp	10	0	0	0	0	0.0	0.0	0	0%
w/parsley *(Lawry's)*	1 tsp	12	1	2	5	0	0.9	0.0	0	42%
GARLIC SALT. See under SEASONING MIX.										
GARLIC TABLETS *(Shaklee)*	2 tablets	5	0	1	0	0	0.0	0.0	0	0%
GATORADE. See under SPORTS AND DIET/NUTRITION DRINKS.										
GEFILTE FISH										
(Mother's)										
in jelled broth, 'Old Fashioned' 24-oz jar	1 ball	70	9	5	0	0	1.0	0.0	0	14%
in jelled broth, 'Old Fashioned' 12-oz jar	1 ball	54	7	4	0	0	0.8	0.0	0	14%
in jelled broth, 'Old World'	1 ball	70	8	7	0	0	1.0	0.0	0	13%
in jelled broth, 'Unsalted'	1 ball	45	5	2	0	0	1.0	0.0	0	24%
in liquid, 'Old Fashioned' 24- or 31-oz jar	1 ball	70	9	7	0	0	1.0	0.0	0	12%
in liquid, 'Old Fashioned' 12-oz'	1 ball	54	7	5	0	0	0.8	0.0	0	13%
sweet, 'Old World'	1 ball	54	6	5	0	0	0.8	0.0	0	14%
(Rokeach)										
hors d'oeuvres	8 balls	60	8	4	0	0	1.0	0.0	0	16%
in jelled broth, 'Old Vienna' 31-oz jar	3 oz	81	9	9	0	0	1.0	0.0	0	11%
in jelled broth, 'Old Vienna' 24-oz jar	2.6 oz	70	8	8	0	0	1.0	0.0	0	12%
in jelled broth, 'Old Vienna' 12-oz jar	2 oz	54	6	6	0	0	1.0	0.0	0	16%
in jelled broth, 'Redi-Jelled'	2 oz	46	6	3	222	0	1.0	0.0	0	20%
in natural broth, 24-oz pkg	4 oz	60	8	4	835	0	1.0	0.0	0	16%
WHITEFISH										
(Mother's)										
in jelled broth, 12-oz jar	1 ball	46	7	3	0	0	0.8	0.0	0	15%
in liquid, 12-oz pkg	1 ball	54	7	5	0	0	0.8	0.0	0	13%
WHITEFISH AND PIKE										
(Mother's)										
in jelled broth	1 ball	60	9	4	0	0	1.0	0.0	0	15%
in jelled broth, 'Old World'	1 ball	54	6	5	0	0	0.8	0.0	0	14%
in liquid	1 ball	70	9	7	0	0	1.0	0.0	0	12%
(Rokeach) in jelled broth	2 oz	46	7	3	0	0	1.0	0.0	0	18%
GELATIN, unflavored *(Knox)*	1 pkt	25	6	0	10	0	0.0	0.0	0	0%
GELATIN DESSERT										
(Estee) all flavors	1/2 cup	8	1	1	0	0	0.0	0.0	0	0%

Food Name	Serving Size	Calories	Prot. gms	Carbs gms	Sod. mgs	Fiber gms	Fat gms	Sat. Fat gms	Chol. mgs	% Fat Cal.
(Jell-O)										
'Berry Blue'	3.5 oz	80	1	18	40	0	0.0	0.0	0	0%
cherry	3.5 oz	80	1	18	40	0	0.0	0.0	0	0%
cherry, sugar-free	1 snack	10	1	0	50	0	0.0	0.0	0	0%
orange, sugar-free	1 snack	10	1	0	50	0	0.0	0.0	0	0%
raspberry, sugar-free	1 snack	10	1	0	50	0	0.0	0.0	0	0%
strawberry	3.5 oz	80	1	18	40	0	0.0	0.0	0	0%
strawberry, sugar-free	1 snack	10	1	0	50	0	0.0	0.0	0	0%
GELATIN DESSERT MIX										
(D-Zerta) all flavors, except strawberry, low-calorie, prepared	1/2 cup	8	2	0	0	0	0.0	0.0	0	0%
(Featherweight) all flavors, except lemon, prepared	1/2 cup	10	2	1	5	0	0.0	0.0	0	0%
APPLE *(Royal)* prepared	1/2 cup	80	2	19	95	0	0.0	0.0	0	0%
BANANA *(Ener-G Foods)* low-fat, gluten free, prepared	1/2 cup	249	0	62	28	1	0.0	0.0	0	0%
BLACK RASPBERRY *(Jell-O)* prepared	1/2 cup	80	2	19	35	0	0.0	0.0	0	0%
BLACKBERRY *(Royal)* prepared	1/2 cup	80	2	19	95	0	0.0	0.0	0	0%
CHERRY										
(Jell-O) sugar-free, prepared	1/2 cup	8	1	0	80	0	0.0	0.0	0	0%
(Royal)										
prepared	1/2 cup	80	2	19	95	0	0.0	0.0	0	0%
sugar-free, mix only	1 serving	8	1	1	90	0	0.0	0.0	0	0%
CHOCOLATE *(Ener-G Foods)* prepared	1/2 cup	231	0	56	47	4	0.6	0.1	0	2%
GRAPE										
(Jell-O) Concord, prepared	1/2 cup	80	2	19	35	0	0.0	0.0	0	0%
(Royal) Concord, prepared	1/2 cup	80	2	19	130	0	0.0	0.0	0	0%
LEMON										
(Ener-G Foods) prepared	1/2 cup	246	0	63	30	1	0.0	0.0	0	0%
(Featherweight) prepared	1/2 cup	10	2	1	4	0	0.0	0.0	0	0%
(Jell-O) sugar-free, prepared	1/2 cup	10	1	0	55	0	0.0	0.0	0	0%
(Royal) prepared	1/2 cup	80	2	19	125	0	0.0	0.0	0	0%
LEMON-LIME *(Royal)* prepared	1/2 cup	80	2	19	95	0	0.0	0.0	0	0%
LIME										
(Jell-O) sugar-free, prepared	1/2 cup	8	1	0	65	0	0.0	0.0	0	0%
(Royal)										
prepared	1/2 cup	80	2	19	125	0	0.0	0.0	0	0%
sugar-free, mix only	1 serving	8	1	1	100	0	0.0	0.0	0	0%
MIXED BERRY *(Royal)* prepared	1/2 cup	80	2	19	90	0	0.0	0.0	0	0%
MIXED FRUIT										
(Jell-O) sugar-free, prepared	1/2 cup	10	1	0	50	0	0.0	0.0	0	0%
(Royal) 'Fruit Punch' prepared	1/2 cup	80	2	19	90	0	0.0	0.0	0	0%
ORANGE										
(Ener-G Foods) prepared	1/2 cup	242	0	60	46	1	0.0	0.0	0	0%
(Jell-O) sugar-free, prepared	1/2 cup	8	1	0	55	0	0.0	0.0	0	0%
(Royal)										
prepared	1/2 cup	80	2	19	95	0	0.0	0.0	0	0%
sugar-free, mix only	1 serving	10	1	1	90	0	0.0	0.0	0	0%
ORANGE-PINEAPPLE *(Jell-O)* prepared	1/2 cup	80	2	19	65	0	0.0	0.0	0	0%
PEACH *(Royal)* prepared	1/2 cup	80	2	19	95	0	0.0	0.0	0	0%
PINEAPPLE *(Royal)* mix only	1 serving	80	2	19	95	0	0.0	0.0	0	0%
RASPBERRY										
(Ener-G Foods) low-fat, prepared	1/2 cup	248	0	62	29	1	0.0	0.0	0	0%
(Jell-O) sugar-free, prepared	1/2 cup	8	1	0	55	0	0.0	0.0	0	0%
(Royal)										
prepared	1/2 cup	80	2	19	125	0	0.0	0.0	0	0%

Food Name	Serving Size	Calories	Prot. gms	Carbs gms	Sod. mgs	Fiber gms	Fat gms	Sat. Fat gms	Chol. mgs	% Fat Cal.
sugar-free, mix only	1 serving	8	1	1	90	0	0.0	0.0	0	0%
STRAWBERRY										
(D-Zerta) low-calorie, prepared	1/2 cup	10	1	0	55	0	0.0	0.0	0	0%
(Jell-O) sugar-free, prepared	1/2 cup	10	1	0	55	0	0.0	0.0	0	0%
(Royal)										
prepared	1/2 cup	80	2	19	105	0	0.0	0.0	0	0%
sugar-free, mix only	1 serving	8	1	1	90	0	0.0	0.0	0	0%
STRAWBERRY-BANANA										
(Jell-O) sugar-free, prepared	1/2 cup	10	1	0	50	0	0.0	0.0	0	0%
(Royal)										
prepared	1/2 cup	80	2	19	105	0	0.0	0.0	0	0%
sugar-free, mix only	1 serving	8	1	1	85	0	0.0	0.0	0	0%
STRAWBERRY-ORANGE *(Royal)* mix only	1 serving	80	2	19	110	0	0.0	0.0	0	0%
TROPICAL FRUIT *(Royal)* mix only	1 serving	80	2	19	110	0	0.0	0.0	0	0%
WATERMELON *(Jell-O)* sugar-free, prepared	1/2 cup	10	1	0	55	0	0.0	0.0	0	0%
GHEE / clarified butter	1 oz	249	0.0	0.0	na	0	28.4	(mq)	(mq)	100%
GIN										
80 proof	1 fl oz	64	0	0	0	0	0.0	0.0	0	0%
86 proof	1 fl oz	70	0	0	0	0	0.0	0.0	0	0%
90 proof	1 fl oz	73	0	0	0	0	0.0	0.0	0	0%
94 proof	1 fl oz	76	0	0	0	0	0.0	0.0	0	0%
100 proof	1 fl oz	82	0	0	0	0	0.0	0.0	0	0%
GINGER										
Dried										
ground	1 tbsp	19	0	4	2	1	0.3	0.1	0	14%
ground	1 tsp	6	0	1	1	0	0.1	0.0	0	14%
ground *(Durkee)*	1 tsp	7	0	0	0	0	0.0	0.0	0	0%
ground *(Laurel Leaf)*	1 tsp	7	0	0	0	0	0.0	0.0	0	0%
ground *(McCormick/Schilling)*	1 tsp	7	0	2	0	0	0.0	0.0	0	0%
ground *(Spice Islands)*	1 tsp	6	0	1	1	0	0.1	0.0	0	15%
ground *(Tone's)*	1 tsp	6	0	1	1	0	0.1	0.1	0	13%
Fresh										
raw, minced	1 tsp	1	0	0	0	0	0.0	0.0	0	9%
raw, sliced, 1-inch diam.	1/4 cup	17	0	4	3	0	0.2	0.0	0	9%
Pickled *(Eden Foods)*	1 tbsp	15	0	3	340	1	0.0	0.0	0	0%
GINGERBREAD MIX. See under CAKE, SNACK, MIX.										
GINKGO NUT										
Canned										
approx 78 kernels	1 cup	172	4	34	476	14	2.5	0.5	0	12%
approx 14 kernels	1 oz	31	1	6	87	3	0.5	0.1	0	12%
Dried	1 oz	99	3	21	4	na	0.6	0.1	0	5%
Fresh, raw	1 oz	52	1	11	2	na	0.5	0.1	0	8%
GLOBE ARTICHOKE. See under ARTICHOKE.										
GLUTEN. See WHEAT GLUTEN.										
GLUTINOUS RICE. See under RICE.										
GNOCCHI, RAW. See under POTATO DISH/ENTRÉE.										
GOA BEAN. See BEAN, WINGED.										
GOAT										
raw	1 oz	31	6	0	23	0	0.7	0.2	16	19%
roasted	3 oz	122	23	0	73	0	2.6	0.8	64	19%
GOATFISH										
raw	1 lb	435	92.5	0.0	(mq)	0	4.5	(mq)	(mq)	10%
raw	1 oz	27	5.8	0.0	(mq)	0	0.3	(mq)	(mq)	10%
GOAT'S MILK. See under MILK.										

Food Name	Serving Size	Calories	Prot. gms	Carbs gms	Sod. mgs	Fiber gms	Fat gms	Sat. Fat gms	Chol. mgs	% Fat Cal.
GOBO. See BURDOCK ROOT.										
GOOSE.										
AVERAGE OF ALL PARTS										
meat and skin, raw	1 oz	105	4.5	0.0	21	0	9.5	2.8	23	83%
meat and skin, roasted	4 oz	346	28.5	0.0	79	0	24.9	7.8	103	66%
meat only, raw	1 oz	46	6.4	0.0	25	0	2.0	0.8	24	41%
meat only, roasted	4 oz	270	32.9	0.0	86	0	14.4	5.2	109	50%
GIBLETS, raw	3.5 oz	156	21.1	0.6	70	0	7.0	2.0	350	42%
GIZZARD, raw	3.5 oz	139	21.4	0.0	65	0	5.3	1.0	145	36%
LIVER. See also PÂTÉ.										
raw	1 med liver	125	15	6	132	0	4.0	1.5	484	29%
GOOSE FAT										
	1 cup	1846	0	0	0	0	204.6	56.8	205	98%
	1 tbsp	115	0	0	0	0	12.8	3.5	13	98%
GOOSEBERRY										
Canned, in light syrup, w/liquid	1 cup	184	2	47	5	6	0.5	0.0	0	2%
Fresh, raw	1 cup	66	1	15	2	6	0.9	0.1	0	11%
GOOSEFISH. See MONKFISH.										
GORDITA, low-fat (La Tortilla)	1 serving	150	4	29	175	2	2.5	0.5	0	15%
GOURD, BOTTLE / calabash gourd / white-flowered gourd										
boiled, drained, cubed	1 cup	22	1	5	3	na	0.0	0.0	0	1%
raw, cubed	1/2 cup	8	0	2	1	na	0.0	0.0	0	1%
raw, whole	1 gourd	108	5	26	15	na	0.2	0.0	0	1%
GOURD, CALABASH. See GOURD, BOTTLE.										
GOURD, DISHCLOTH / loofah gourd / rag gourd / sponge gourd / towelgourd / vegetable sponge										
boiled, drained, chopped, 1-inch pieces	1 cup	100	1	26	37	na	0.6	0.0	0	5%
boiled, drained, sliced, 1-inch slices	1/2 cup	50	1	13	19	na	0.3	0.0	0	5%
raw, chopped, 1-inch pieces	1 cup	19	1	4	3	na	0.2	0.0	0	8%
raw, whole	1 medium	36	2	8	5	na	0.4	0.0	0	8%
GOURD, LOOFAH. See GOURD, DISHCLOTH.										
GOURD, RAG. See GOURD, DISHCLOTH.										
GOURD, SPONGE. See GOURD, DISHCLOTH.										
GOURD, WAX										
boiled, drained, cubed	1 cup	23	1	5	187	2	0.3	0.0	0	13%
raw, cubed	1 cup	17	1	4	147	4	0.3	0.0	0	13%
raw, whole	1 medium	741	23	171	6327	165	11.4	0.9	0	13%
GOURD, WHITE / Chinese watermelon / tunka										
boiled, drained	4 oz	15	0.5	3.4	121	>.6 c	0.2	<.1	0	-10%
boiled, drained, cubed	1/2 cup	11	0.4	2.6	93	>.4 c	0.2	0.0	0	13%
raw, cubed	1 cup	17	0.5	4.0	147	>.7 c	0.3	0.0	0	13%
raw, trimmed	1 oz	4	0.1	0.9	31	.2	0.1	tr	0	18%
raw, untrimmed	1 lb	42	1.3	9.7	358	1.9	0.6	0.1	0	11%
GOURD, WHITE-FLOWERED. See GOURD, BOTTLE.										
GOVERNOR PLUM, trimmed	1 oz	31	0.1	8.4	na	>.1 c	0.0	0.0	0	0%
GRAHAM CRACKER. See under COOKIE.										
GRAHAM CRACKER CRUMBS. See under COOKIE CRUMBS.										
GRAHAM FLOUR, ORGANIC. See under FLOUR.										
GRAIN CAKE										
(Great Cakes)										
w/summer fruits, 'Nature Cake'	4 oz	250	9	45	10	21	3.5	0.0	0	13%
w/tropical fruits, 'Nature Cake'	4 oz	245	9	47	5	21	2.5	0.0	0	9%
carob, 'Nature Cake'	4 oz	255	8	45	10	21	5.0	0.0	0	18%
w/raspberry, 'Nature Cake'	4 oz	235	9	47	5	21	2.5	0.0	0	9%
GRANADILLA. See PASSIONFRUIT.										

Food Name	Serving Size	Calories	Prot. gms	Carbs gms	Sod. mgs	Fiber gms	Fat gms	Sat. Fat gms	Chol. mgs	% Fat Cal.
GRANOLA. See under CEREAL, HOT; CEREAL, READY-TO-EAT.										
GRANOLA/CEREAL BAR										
(Barbara's Bakery)										
apple-filled, nonfat	1 bar	110	2	27	90	2	0.0	0.0	0	0%
blueberry-filled, nonfat	1 bar	110	2	27	90	2	0.0	0.0	0	0%
carob chip, no cholesterol	1 bar	80	2	16	5	2	2.0	0.0	0	20%
cinnamon and oats	1 bar	260	6	31	105	2	15.0	4.0	0	48%
cinnamon-raisin, no cholesterol	1 bar	80	2	16	5	3	2.0	0.0	0	20%
coconut-almond	1 bar	290	6	23	20	3	20.0	8.0	0	61%
oats and honey, no cholesterol	1 bar	80	2	15	5	2	2.0	0.0	0	21%
peanut butter	1 bar	260	9	28	75	3	15.0	4.0	0	48%
peanut butter, no cholesterol	1 bar	80	2	14	5	2	3.0	0.0	0	30%
raspberry-filled, nonfat	1 bar	110	2	27	110	2	0.0	0.0	0	0%
strawberry-filled, nonfat	1 bar	110	2	27	110	2	0.0	0.0	0	0%
(Bear Valley)										
carob-cocoa, food bar, 'Pemmican'	3.75 oz	440	16	68	80	7	12.0	0.0	0	24%
coconut almond, 'Meal Pack'	3.75 oz	400	16	56	80	6	12.0	0.0	0	27%
fruit and nut, 'Pemmican'	3.75 oz	420	17	59	90	9	13.0	0.0	0	28%
sesame lemon, 'Meal Pack'	3.75 oz	410	17	57	85	4	13.0	0.0	0	28%
(Ener-G Foods) gluten-free	1 serving	335	7	29	115	4	21.3	1.5	0	57%
(Glenny's)										
'Bee Pollen Sunrise'	1.5 oz	190	5	22	0	0	8.0	0.0	0	40%
'Ginseng Sunrise'	1.5 oz	160	1	24	0	0	7.0	0.0	0	39%
'Spirulina Sunrise'	1.5 oz	140	3	21	0	0	5.0	0.0	0	32%
almond, toasted, w/oat bran, 'Brown Rice Treats'	1 bar	200	4	34	20	2	5.0	0.0	0	23%
carob mint, w/oat bran, 'Brown Rice Treats'	1 bar	180	3	37	20	2	2.0	0.0	0	10%
cinnamon and raisin, 'Brown Rice Treats'	1.75 oz	170	2	38	30	1	1.0	0.0	0	5%
coconut almandine, 'Moist & Chewy'	1.5 oz	190	3	22	20	0	10.0	0.0	0	47%
oatmeal raisin, 'Moist & Chewy'	1.5 oz	160	3	30	25	0	3.0	0.0	0	17%
peanut and raisin, 'Brown Rice Treats'	2 oz	210	4	39	29	0	5.0	0.0	0	21%
peanut snack, 'Moist & Chewy'	1.5 oz	180	5	24	20	0	7.0	0.0	0	35%
raisin bran, 'Brown Rice Treats'	1.75 oz	170	2	38	17	0	1.0	0.0	0	5%
rice, plain and fancy, 'Brown Rice Treats'	1.25 oz	120	1	28	29	0	1.0	0.0	0	7%
sunflower, 'Moist & Chewy'	1.5 oz	180	5	24	15	0	7.0	0.0	0	35%
(Golden Temple)										
cashew almond, 'Wha Guru Chew Bar'	1 bar	164	3	15	63	1	11.0	1.0	0	58%
peanut cashew, 'Wha Guru Chew Bar'	1 bar	167	4	14	62	1	11.0	1.0	0	58%
sesame almond, 'Wha Guru Chew Bar'	1 bar	160	3	15	61	1	10.0	1.0	0	56%
(Health Valley)										
blueberry apple, nonfat	1 bar	140	3	33	10	4	0.0	0.0	0	0%
blueberry, nonfat	1 bar	140	2	35	5	3	0.0	0.0	0	0%
chocolate chip, nonfat	1 bar	140	2	35	5	3	0.0	0.0	0	0%
date-almond, nonfat	1 bar	140	2	35	5	3	0.0	0.0	0	0%
raisin, nonfat	1 bar	140	2	35	5	3	0.0	0.0	0	0%
strawberry, nonfat	1 bar	140	2	35	5	3	0.0	0.0	0	0%
(Hershey's)										
chocolate chip, chocolate coated	1.2-oz bar	170	2	22	50	0	8.0	0.0	0	43%
cocoa creme, chocolate-coated	1.2-oz bar	180	2	22	50	0	9.0	0.0	5	46%
cookies and creme, chocolate-coated	1.2-oz bar	170	2	22	50	0	8.0	0.0	0	43%
peanut butter, chocolate-coated	1.2-oz bar	180	4	19	65	0	10.0	0.0	5	49%
(Kellogg's)										
almond and brown sugar, low-fat, crunchy	1 bar	80	2	16	60	1	1.5	0.0	0	16%
apple spice, crunchy, low-fat	1 bar	80	2	16	60	1	1.5	0.0	0	16%
raspberry-filled 'Common Sense Smart Start'	1 bar	170	2	28	160	1	6.0	0.0	0	31%

Food Name	Serving Size	Calories	Prot. gms	Carbs gms	Sod. mgs	Fiber gms	Fat gms	Sat. Fat gms	Chol. mgs	% Fat Cal.
(M&M Mars)										
chocolate chip, 'Kudos'	1 bar	180	3	21	60	0	9.0	0.0	0	46%
chocolate chunk, 'Simply Kudos'	1 bar	100	1	13	50	0	4.0	0.0	0	39%
fudge, nutty, 'Kudos'	1 bar	190	4	19	60	0	11.0	0.0	0	52%
honey nut, 'Simply Kudos'	1 bar	100	2	13	55	0	4.0	0.0	0	38%
oatmeal raisin, 'Simply Kudos'	1 bar	90	1	13	55	0	4.0	0.0	0	39%
peanut butter, chocolate coated, 'Kudos'	1.3-oz bar	190	4	18	70	0	12.0	0.0	0	55%
(Nature Valley)										
chocolate chip, crunchy	2 bars	210	4	32	120	2	9.0	1.5	0	36%
cinnamon	2 bars	180	4	29	180	2	6.0	0.5	0	29%
oat bran-honey graham	0.8-oz bar	110	2	16	90	1	4.0	1.0	0	33%
oats and honey	2 bars	180	4	29	180	2	6.0	0.5	0	29%
peanut butter	2 bars	190	5	28	180	2	6.0	1.0	0	29%
(Nature's Choice)										
carob chip	0.75-oz bar	90	2	15	15	0	3.0	0.0	0	28%
cinnamon-raisin	0.75-oz bar	90	2	15	10	0	3.0	0.0	0	28%
oats 'n honey	0.75-oz bar	90	2	15	15	0	3.0	0.0	0	28%
peanut butter	0.75-oz bar	90	2	14	25	0	3.0	0.0	0	30%
(Nutri-Grain)										
blueberry, 'Smart Start'	1.5-oz bar	180	2	26	170	1	8.0	0.0	0	39%
corn, mixed berry-filled, 'Smart Start'	1 bar	170	2	27	160	1	7.0	0.0	0	35%
raisin bran, 'Smart Start'	1.5-oz bar	160	2	28	170	2	5.0	0.0	0	27%
Rice Krispies, w/almonds, 'Smart Start'	1-oz bar	130	2	18	65	1	6.0	0.0	0	40%
strawberry, 'Smart Start'	1.5-oz bar	180	2	26	170	1	8.0	0.0	0	39%
(Quaker)										
apple berry, chewy	1-oz bar	120	2	20	95	0	4.0	0.0	0	29%
Butterfinger, chewy	1 bar	160	2	29	100	1	4.0	2.0	0	23%
caramel apple, chewy low-fat	1 bar	120	2	21	80	1	3.5	1.0	0	26%
caramel nut, 'Granola Dipps'	1-oz bar	148	2	21	81	1	6.4	2.8	2	39%
chocolate chip, 'Chewy'	1 bar	128	2	19	90	1	4.7	1.5	0	33%
chocolate chip, 'Granola Dipps'	1-oz bar	139	2	19	78	1	6.3	2.8	1	41%
chocolate chunk, low-fat, chewy	1 bar	110	1	22	110	1	2.0	0.5	0	16%
chocolate fudge 'Granola Dipps'	1-oz bar	160	2	20	74	0	7.9	0.0	0	45%
crunch, chewy	1 bar	160	2	28	95	1	5.0	2.0	0	27%
honey and oats, 'Chewy'	1-oz bar	125	2	19	95	1	4.4	1.1	1	32%
nut and raisin, chunky, 'Chewy'	1-oz bar	131	3	17	86	2	5.8	1.3	1	40%
peanut butter chocolate chip, 'Chewy'	1-oz bar	131	3	17	112	1	5.7	1.5	0	39%
peanut butter chocolate chip, 'Granola Dipps'	1 bar	174	4	17	102	0	10.0	0.0	0	52%
peanut butter, 'Chewy'	1-oz bar	128	3	18	116	1	4.9	1.3	1	35%
peanut butter, 'Granola Dipps'	1-oz bar	170	4	19	74	1	9.1	3.1	2	48%
raisin cinnamon, 'Chewy'	1-oz bar	128	2	19	92	1	5.0	1.1	0	35%
S'mores, 'Chewy'	1-oz bar	126	2	20	108	1	4.4	1.4	0	31%
trail mix, 'Chewy'	1 oz	130	2	18	105	0	5.0	0.0	0	36%
(Sunbelt)										
apple bar, baked	1.31 oz	130	1	28	130	1	2.0	0.0	0	13%
chocolate chip, chewy	1.25 oz	150	3	23	75	2	7.0	3.0	2	38%
chocolate chip, fudge-dipped, chewy	1.5 oz	210	2	26	55	4	10.0	4.0	2	45%
oats and honey, chewy	1-oz bar	130	2	18	35	0	5.0	0.0	1	36%
oats and honey, fudge-dipped, chewy	1.38-oz bar	190	2	24	55	0	10.0	0.0	1	46%
w/almonds, chewy	1-oz bar	120	3	18	65	0	6.0	0.0	1	39%
w/chocolate chips, chewy	1.75-oz bar	220	4	32	105	0	9.0	0.0	1	36%
w/peanuts, fudge-dipped, chewy	1.38-oz bar	190	2	24	55	0	10.0	0.0	1	46%
w/peanuts, fudge-dipped, chewy	1.5-oz bar	200	4	24	60	4	12.0	4.0	2	49%
w/peanuts, fudge-dipped, chewy	2.25-oz bar	300	6	36	90	0	18.0	0.0	1	49%

Food Name	Serving Size	Calories	Prot. gms	Carbs gms	Sod. mgs	Fiber gms	Fat gms	Sat. Fat gms	Chol. mgs	% Fat Cal.
w/raisins, chewy	1.25-oz bar	150	2	24	65	2	6.0	0.0	0	34%
w/raisins, fudge-dipped, chewy	1.5-oz bar	200	4	24	60	0	12.0	0.0	1	49%

GRANOLA SNACK. See under CEREAL SNACK. Also see GRANOLA/CEREAL BAR.

GRAPE

AMERICAN (Concord, Delaware, Niagara)

Fresh

Food Name	Serving Size	Calories	Prot. gms	Carbs gms	Sod. mgs	Fiber gms	Fat gms	Sat. Fat gms	Chol. mgs	% Fat Cal.
(Dole)	1.5 cup	85	1.0	24.0	3	2.0	0.0	na	na	0%
slipskin, peeled and seeded	1 oz	18	0.2	4.9	<1	>.2 c	0.1	<.1	0	4%
slipskin, trimmed	10 medium	15	0.2	4.1	0	>.2 c	0.1	0.0	0	5%
slipskin, untrimmed	1 lb	165	1.7	45.1	4	>2.0 c	0.9	0.3	0	4%
slipskin, untrimmed	1 cup	58	0.6	15.8	2	>.9 c	0.3	0.1	0	4%

EUROPEAN (Muskat, Tokay, Thompson)

Canned

Food Name	Serving Size	Calories	Prot. gms	Carbs gms	Sod. mgs	Fiber gms	Fat gms	Sat. Fat gms	Chol. mgs	% Fat Cal.
Thompson, seedless, in heavy syrup, w/liquid	1 cup	187	1	50	13	1	0.3	0.1	0	1%
Thompson, seedless, in water, w/liquid	1 cup	98	1	25	15	2	0.3	0.1	0	2%

Fresh

Food Name	Serving Size	Calories	Prot. gms	Carbs gms	Sod. mgs	Fiber gms	Fat gms	Sat. Fat gms	Chol. mgs	% Fat Cal.
adherent skin, w/seeds	1/2 cup	57	0.5	14.2	2	0.6	0.5	0.2	0	7%
adherent skin, w/seeds	1 oz	20	0.2	5.0	1	0.2	0.2	0.1	0	8%
adherent skin, w/o seeds	1/2 cup	57	0.5	14.2	2	0.6	0.5	0.2	0	7%
adherent skin, w/o seeds	1 oz	20	0.2	5.0	1	0.2	0.2	0.1	0	8%
adherent skin, w/o seeds, approx 1.75 oz	10 medium	36	0.3	8.9	1	0.4	0.3	0.1	0	7%

GRAPE DRINK. See under FRUIT DRINK; FRUIT JUICE BLEND; FRUIT JUICE DRINK.

GRAPE JUICE

Canned, bottled, or boxed

Food Name	Serving Size	Calories	Prot. gms	Carbs gms	Sod. mgs	Fiber gms	Fat gms	Sat. Fat gms	Chol. mgs	% Fat Cal.
(Flav-R-Pac)	1 cup	130	0	33	10	0	0.0	0.0	0	0%
(IGA) unsweetened	6 fl oz	120	0	30	5	0	0.0	0.0	0	0%
(J. Hungerford)										
100% juice	9.03 fl oz	155	1	39	11	0	0.0	0.0	0	0%
regular	9.03 fl oz	160	0	40	0	0	0.0	0.0	0	0%
(Juicy Juice)	6 fl oz	90	1	22	5	0	0.0	0.0	0	0%
(Knudsen)										
	8 fl oz	150	1	37	30	na	0.0	0.0	0	0%
Concord	8 fl oz	130	1	32	0	0	0.0	0.0	0	0%
(Kraft) 'Pure 100% Unsweetened'	6 fl oz	104	1	25	0	0	0.0	0.0	0	0%
(Lucky Leaf)	6 fl oz	130	0	32	0	0	0.0	0.0	0	0%
(Minute Maid)	6 fl oz	100	1	24	20	0	1.0	0.0	0	8%
(Pathmark)										
'No Frills'	6 fl oz	113	0	27	10	0	0.0	0.0	0	0%
unsweetened	6 fl oz	120	0	30	10	0	0.0	0.0	0	0%
(S&W) Concord, unsweetened	6 fl oz	100	1	25	9	0	0.0	0.0	0	0%
(Sippin' Pak)	8.45 fl oz	130	1	32	25	0	0.0	0.0	0	0%
(Squeezit 100) 100% natural, 'Caped Grape'	6.75 fl oz	100	0	24	20	0	0.0	0.0	0	0%
(Tree Top) 100%										
	8 fl oz	160	0	38	22	0	0.0	0.0	0	0%
(Tropicana) 'Season's Best'	8 fl oz	160	1	39	25	1	0.0	na	na	0%
(Veryfine) '100%'	8 fl oz	153	1	37	20	0	0.0	0.0	0	0%
(Welch's)										
purple	6 fl oz	120	0	30	10	0	0.0	0.0	0	0%
red	6 fl oz	120	0	30	15	0	0.0	0.0	0	0%
red, sparkling	6 fl oz	128	0	30	30	0	0.0	0.0	0	0%
white	6 fl oz	120	0	30	15	0	0.0	0.0	0	0%
white, sparkling	6 fl oz	120	0	30	30	0	0.0	0.0	0	0%
Refrigerated or frozen										
(Minute Maid)	6 fl oz	90	0	24	0	0	0.0	0.0	0	0%

Food Name	Serving Size	Calories	Prot. gms	Carbs gms	Sod. mgs	Fiber gms	Fat gms	Sat. Fat gms	Chol. mgs	% Fat Cal.
(Sunkist) concentrate, prepared....................	6 fl oz	69	0	17	3	0	0.1	0.0	0	1%
(Welch's)										
purple, concentrate, prepared.....................	6 fl oz	100	0	25	0	0	0.0	0.0	0	0%
white, concentrate, prepared.......................	6 fl oz	100	0	25	0	0	0.0	0.0	0	0%
GRAPE LEAVES										
raw	1 cup	13	1	2	1	2	0.3	0.0	0	19%
raw, whole............................	1 medium	3	0	1	0	0	0.1	0.0	0	19%
whole (Reese)............................	1 leaf	5	0	1	110	0	0.0	0.0	0	0%
GRAPEFRUIT										
PINK										
Fresh										
Arizona, sections, w/juice	1 cup	85	1	22	2	na	0.2	0.0	0	2%
Arizona, whole, approx 3.75-inch diam.............	1/2 fruit	46	1	12	1	na	0.1	0.0	0	2%
California, sections, w/juice........................	1 cup	85	1	22	2	na	0.2	0.0	0	2%
California, whole, approx 3.75-inch diam	1/2 fruit	46	1	12	1	na	0.1	0.0	0	2%
Florida, sections, w/juice..........................	1 cup	69	1	17	0	3	0.2	0.0	0	3%
Florida, whole, approx 3.75-inch diam	1/2 fruit	37	1	9	0	1	0.1	0.0	0	3%
whole, approx 4.5-inch diam	1/2 fruit	53	1	13	0	2	0.2	0.0	0	3%
whole, approx 4-inch diam	1/2 fruit	41	1	10	0	1	0.1	0.0	0	3%
whole, approx 3.5-inch diam......................	1/2 fruit	32	1	8	0	1	0.1	0.0	0	3%
RED										
Fresh										
Arizona, sections, w/juice	1 cup	85	1	22	2	na	0.2	0.0	0	2%
Arizona, whole, approx 3.75-inch diam.............	1/2 fruit	46	1	12	1	na	0.1	0.0	0	2%
California, sections, w/juice........................	1 cup	85	1	22	2	na	0.2	0.0	0	2%
California, whole, approx 3.75-inch diam	1/2 fruit	46	1	12	1	na	0.1	0.0	0	2%
Florida, sections, w/juice..........................	1 cup	69	1	17	0	3	0.2	0.0	0	3%
Florida, whole, approx 3.75-inch diam	1/2 fruit	37	1	9	0	1	0.1	0.0	0	3%
whole, approx 4.5-inch diam	1/2 fruit	53	1	13	0	2	0.2	0.0	0	3%
whole, approx 4-inch diam	1/2 fruit	41	1	10	0	1	0.1	0.0	0	3%
whole, approx 3.5-inch diam......................	1/2 fruit	32	1	8	0	1	0.1	0.0	0	3%
WHITE										
Canned										
sections, in juice, w/liquid	1 cup	92	2	23	17	1	0.2	0.0	0	2%
sections, in light syrup, w/liquid....................	1 cup	152	1	39	5	1	0.3	0.0	0	1%
sections, in water, w/liquid........................	1 cup	88	1	22	5	1	0.2	0.0	0	2%
Fresh										
California, sections, w/juice........................	1 cup	85	2	21	0	na	0.2	0.0	0	2%
California, whole, approx 3.75-inch diam	1/2 fruit	44	1	11	0	na	0.1	0.0	0	2%
Florida, sections, w/juice..........................	1 cup	74	1	19	0	na	0.2	0.0	0	3%
Florida, whole, approx 3.75-inch diam	1/2 fruit	38	1	10	0	na	0.1	0.0	0	3%
whole, approx 4.5-inch diam	1/2 fruit	53	1	13	0	2	0.2	0.0	0	3%
whole, approx 4-inch diam	1/2 fruit	41	1	10	0	1	0.1	0.0	0	3%
whole, approx 3.5-inch diam......................	1/2 fruit	32	1	8	0	1	0.1	0.0	0	3%
GRAPEFRUIT JUICE										
Canned, bottled, or boxed										
(Del Monte)	6 fl oz	70	1	17	10	0	0.0	0.0	0	0%
(Florida's Natural) ruby red, not from concentrate	8 fl oz	100	1	24	0	0	0.0	0.0	0	0%
(J. Hungerford)										
100% juice.	9.03 fl oz	98	1	24	6	0	0.0	0.0	0	0%
regular.......................	9.03 fl oz	120	0	30	0	0	0.0	0.0	0	0%
(Knudsen) pink............................	8 fl oz	100	2	23	35	na	0.0	0.0	0	0%
(Kraft)................................	6 fl oz	70	1	16	0	0	0.0	0.0	0	0%
(Libby's)................................	6 fl oz	70	1	17	0	0	0.0	0.0	0	0%

Food Name	Serving Size	Calories	Prot. gms	Carbs gms	Sod. mgs	Fiber gms	Fat gms	Sat. Fat gms	Chol. mgs	% Fat Cal.
(Minute Maid) 'Juices To Go'	6 fl oz	70	1	17	20	0	0.0	0.0	0	0%
(Mott's)	10 fl oz	124	1	30	5	0	0.0	0.0	0	0%
(Ocean Spray)										
. . . .	6 fl oz	70	1	16	10	0	0.0	0.0	0	0%
'Pink Premium'	6 fl oz	60	1	15	10	0	0.0	0.0	0	0%
'Ruby Red'	6 fl oz	100	0	24	15	0	0.0	0.0	0	0%
(S&W)	6 fl oz	80	1	18	0	0	0.0	0.0	0	0%
(Stokely)	6 fl oz	76	1	18	5	0	1.0	0.0	0	11%
(Sunkist) 'Fresh Squeezed'	8 fl oz	96	1	23	3	0	0.2	0.0	0	2%
(Tree Top) 100%	8 fl oz	104	0	24	32	0	0.0	0.0	0	0%
(TreeSweet)										
pink	6 fl oz	72	0	17	15	0	0.0	0.0	0	0%
regular	6 fl oz	72	0	17	15	0.	0.0	0.0	0	0%
(Tropicana)										
100% pure	6 fl oz	70	1	14	20	0	1.0	0.0	0	13%
golden, 'Pure Premium'	8 fl oz	90	1	23	0	0	0.0	na	na	0%
'Ruby Red' 100% pure	6 fl oz	70	1	14	20	0	1.0	0.0	0	13%
ruby red, 'Pure Premium'	8 fl oz	100	1	23	0	1	0.0	na	na	0%
'Season's Best'	8 fl oz	90	1	22	5	1	0.0	na	na	0%
'100%'	8 fl oz	101	1	23	10	0	0.0	0.0	0	0%
Refrigerated or frozen										
(A&P) concentrate, prepared	6 fl oz	80	1	18	0	0	1.0	0.0	0	11%
(Del Monte)	6 fl oz	70	1	17	10	0	0.0	0.0	0	0%
(Kraft)	6 fl oz	70	1	16	0	0	0.0	0.0	0	0%
(Minute Maid) concentrate, prepared	6 fl oz	80	1	18	0	0	0.0	0.0	0	0%
(Ocean Spray)	6 fl oz	70	1	16	10	0	0.0	0.0	0	0%
(S&W)	6 fl oz	80	1	18	0	0	0.0	0.0	0	0%
(Stokely)	6 fl oz	76	1	18	5	0	1.0	0.0	0	11%
(Sunkist) concentrate, prepared	6 fl oz	56	1	13	1	0	0.2	0.0	0	3%
(TreeSweet)										
. . . .	6 fl oz	72	0	17	15	0	0.0	0.0	0	0%
concentrate, prepared	6 fl oz	78	1	18	15	0	0.0	0.0	0	0%
(Veryfine) '100%'	8 fl oz	101	1	23	10	0	0.0	0.0	0	0%
GRAPESEED OIL										
. . . .	1 cup	1927	0	0	0	0	218.0	20.9	0	100%
. . . .	1 tbsp	120	0	0	0	0	13.6	1.3	0	100%
GRAVY										
AU JUS										
(Franco-American)	1/4 cup	10	1	2	310	0	0.5	0.0	3	27%
(Heinz) 'HomeStyle'	1/4 cup	18	0	2	350	0	1.0	0.0	0	53%
BEEF										
(Franco-American)	1/4 cup	30	1	3	310	0	1.5	0.5	3	46%
(Heinz) nonfat	1/4 cup	15	1	3	330	0	0.0	0.0	0	0%
(Hormel) w/chunky beef. 'Great Beginnings'	5 oz	136	12	7	904	0	7.0	0.0	0	45%
(Pepperidge Farm)										
hearty	1 jar	146	10	21	2145	na	2.4	0.8	17	15%
hearty	1 serving	26	2	4	379	na	0.4	0.1	3	15%
98% fat-free	1/4 cup	25	1	4	360	0	1.0	0.0	5	31%
BROWN										
(Heinz)										
'HomeStyle'	1/4 cup	25	1	3	320	0	1.0	0.0	0	36%
savory, 'HomeStyle'	1/4 cup	24	1	3	352	na	0.8	0.3	2	29%
w/onions, 'HomeStyle'	1/4 cup	25	1	3	330	0	1.0	0.0	0	36%
(La Choy)	1/4 cup	275	3	66	320	0	0.0	0.0	0	0%

Food Name	Serving Size	Calories	Prot. gms	Carbs gms	Sod. mgs	Fiber gms	Fat gms	Sat. Fat gms	Chol. mgs	% Fat Cal.
(McCormick/Schilling)	1/3 cup	30	1	5	417	0	1.0	0.0	0	29%
(Pillsbury)	1/4 cup	10	0	3	270	0	0.0	0.0	0	0%
CHICKEN										
(Franco-American)										
	1/4 cup	40	0	3	240	0	3.0	1.0	3	69%
giblet	1/4 cup	30	1	3	310	0	2.0	0.0	10	53%
(Heinz)										
classic, homestyle	1/4 cup	30	1	3	340	0	1.5	0.0	0	46%
'HomeStyle'	1/4 cup	35	1	3	350	0	2.0	0.0	0	53%
w/mushrooms and onions, 'HomeStyle'	1/4 cup	35	1	3	330	0	2.0	0.4	1	53%
(Hormel) w/chunky chicken, 'Great Beginnings'	5 oz	147	14	5	567	0	8.0	0.0	0	49%
(Pepperidge Farm) golden, 98% fat-free	2 oz	25	1	3	240	0	1.0	0.0	0	36%
(Pillsbury) chicken style	1/4 cup	20	1	4	260	0	0.0	0.0	0	0%
COUNTRY (Heinz) homestyle, 'Blue Ribbon'	1/4 cup	25	0	4	210	1	1.0	0.0	0	36%
CREAM (Franco-American)	2 oz	35	0	4	220	0	2.0	0.0	0	53%
HOMESTYLE (Pillsbury)	1/4 cup	10	0	3	270	0	0.0	0.0	0	0%
MUSHROOM										
(Franco-American) creamy	1/4 cup	20	1	4	310	0	1.0	0.0	3	31%
(Heinz) 'HomeStyle'	1/4 cup	25	1	3	340	0	1.0	0.0	0	36%
PORK										
(Franco-American) golden	1/4 cup	45	1	3	340	1	4.0	1.5	4	69%
(Heinz) 'HomeStyle'	1/4 cup	25	1	3	310	0	1.0	0.0	0	36%
(Hormel) w/chunky pork, 'Great Beginnings'	5 oz	140	14	5	567	0	8.0	0.0	0	49%
SAUSAGE										
(Nestlé)										
country, 'Chef-Mate'	1 pkg	4614	137	187	11313	21	369.1	95.9	625	72%
country, 'Chef-Mate'	1/4 cup	96	3	4	236	0	7.7	2.0	13	72%
TURKEY										
(Franco-American)	1/4 cup	25	1	3	290	0	1.0	0.0	3	39%
(Heinz)										
'HomeStyle'	1/4 cup	25	1	3	370	0	1.0	0.0	0	36%
nonfat	1/4 cup	15	1	3	330	0	0.0	0.0	0	0%
roasted, homestyle	1/4 cup	25	1	3	360	0	1.0	0.0	0	36%
(Hormel) w/chunky turkey, 'Great Beginnings'	5 oz	138	11	7	585	0	8.0	0.0	0	50%
(Pepperidge Farm) seasoned, 98% fat-free	2 oz	25	1	4	320	0	1.0	0.0	0	31%
GRAVY MIX										
AU JUS										
(Custom Foods)										
base, 'Red Label' mix only	16-oz pkg	867	71	104	84548	14	18.2	10.3	27	19%
base, 'Red Label' mix only	1 serving	19	2	2	1862	0	0.4	0.2	1	19%
instant, 'Superb' mix only	4-oz pkg	334	24	45	12501	3	6.8	3.1	7	18%
instant, 'Superb' mix only	1 serving	20	1	3	741	0	0.4	0.2	0	18%
(French's) mix, prepared	1/4 cup	10	0	2	260	0	0.0	0.0	0	0%
(Lawry's) mix, prepared	1 cup	84	6	11	3454	0	1.6	0.0	0	17%
(McCormick/Schilling) mix, prepared	1/4 cup	20	1	4	786	0	0.3	0.0	0	13%
(Nestlé)										
'Trio' mix only	7-oz pkg	554	2	115	26334	2	9.9	3.5	8	16%
'Trio' mix only	1 tsp	8	0	2	399	0	0.1	0.1	0	16%
(Tone's) mix only	1 tsp	10	0	1	680	0	0.5	0.1	1	45%
BEEF										
(Custom Foods)										
instant, 'Superb' mix only	1 serving	25	1	4	349	0	0.6	0.3	1	23%
instant, 'Superb' mix only	16-oz pkg	1675	44	277	23622	20	43.0	22.2	50	23%
(McCormick/Schilling) and herb, mix only	2 tsp	30	1	3	290	0	1.0	0.0	3	36%

Food Name	Serving Size	Calories	Prot. gms	Carbs gms	Sod. mgs	Fiber gms	Fat gms	Sat. Fat gms	Chol. mgs	% Fat Cal.
BISCUIT										
(Custom Foods)										
old-fashioned, 'Superb' mix only	1 pkg	3366	45	369	13416	33	190.6	57.0	20	51%
old-fashioned, 'Superb' mix only	1 serving	48	1	5	191	0	2.7	0.8	0	51%
BROWN										
(Crown Colony) mix only	2 tbsp	15	1	3	310	0	0.0	0.0	0	0%
(Custom Foods)										
instant, 'Superb' mix only	1 pkg	1725	39	271	22941	15	53.8	26.6	54	28%
instant, 'Superb' mix only	1 serving	25	1	4	339	0	0.8	0.4	1	28%
(French's) prepared	1/4 cup	20	1	4	250	0	1.0	0.0	0	31%
(Hain) mix only	1/4 pkg	16	1	3	600	0	0.0	0.0	0	0%
(Lawry's) prepared	1 cup	94	4	17	1500	0	1.4	0.0	0	13%
(Loma Linda) vegetarian, 'Gravy Quik' mix only	1 tbsp	20	1	4	367	0	0.0	0.0	0	7%
(McCormick/Schilling)										
'Lite' prepared	1/4 cup	10	1	2	450	0	1.0	0.0	0	43%
mix only	1 pkg	91	2	14	1251	0	3.0	0.0	0	30%
prepared	1/4 cup	23	1	4	313	0	0.8	0.0	0	31%
(Nestlé)										
'Trio' mix only	16-oz pkg	1839	47	262	19764	16	67.0	19.4	0	33%
'Trio' mix only	1 tbsp	24	1	3	262	0	0.9	0.3	0	33%
'Trio Supreme' mix only	16-oz pkg	1843	45	262	22700	0	68.0	6.8	14	33%
'Trio Supreme' mix only	1 tbsp	24	1	3	300	0	0.9	0.1	0	33%
(Pillsbury)										
mix only	2 tsp	10	0	3	270	0	0.0	0.0	0	0%
prepared w/water	1/4 cup	16	0	3	180	0	0.0	0.0	0	0%
(Tone's) mix only	1 tsp	10	0	2	239	0	0.2	0.1	1	16%
(Weight Watchers)										
prepared	1/4 cup	10	1	2	360	0	0.0	0.0	0	0%
w/mushrooms, prepared	1/4 cup	10	1	2	270	0	0.0	0.0	0	0%
w/onions, prepared	1/4 cup	10	1	2	310	0	0.0	0.0	0	0%
CHICKEN										
(Custom Foods)										
instant, 'Superb' mix only	16-oz pkg	1793	46	257	20907	15	64.6	20.5	159	32%
instant, 'Superb' mix only	1 serving	26	1	4	309	0	1.0	0.3	2	32%
(French's) prepared w/water	1/4 cup	25	1	4	270	0	1.0	0.0	0	31%
(Lawry's) prepared w/water	1 cup	99	3	16	980	0	2.8	0.0	0	26%
(Loma Linda) 'Gravy Quik'	1 tbsp	19	1	3	408	0	0.1	0.0	0	6%
(McCormick/Schilling) prepared w/water	1/4 cup	22	1	4	300	0	0.4	0.0	0	17%
(Nestlé)										
'Trio' mix only	1 pkg	2596	73	405	20833	9	75.6	26.1	179	26%
'Trio' mix only	1 tbsp	32	1	5	260	0	0.9	0.3	2	26%
'Trio Supreme' mix only	1 pkg	2291	63	357	20219	0	67.2	7.0	23	26%
'Trio Supreme' mix only	1 tbsp	32	1	5	285	0	0.9	0.1	0	26%
(Pillsbury)										
mix only	2 tsp	20	1	4	260	0	0.0	0.0	0	0%
prepared w/water	1/4 cup	25	1	4	230	0	1.0	0.0	0	31%
(Tone's) mix only	1 tsp	11	0	2	157	0	0.2	0.2	1	17%
(Weight Watchers) prepared	1/4 cup	10	1	2	410	0	0.0	0.0	0	0%
COUNTRY										
(Custom Foods)										
'Superb' mix only	1 pkg	3271	55	364	15239	33	177.3	70.9	14	49%
'Superb' mix only	1 serving	47	1	5	217	0	2.5	1.0	0	49%
(Loma Linda) 'Gravy Quik'	1 tbsp	22	1	4	249	0	0.6	0.1	0	23%

Food Name	Serving Size	Calories	Prot. gms	Carbs gms	Sod. mgs	Fiber gms	Fat gms	Sat. Fat gms	Chol. mgs	% Fat Cal.
(Nestlé)										
'Trio' mix only	1 pkg	2702	57	405	15968	56	95.3	24.9	37	32%
'Trio' mix only	1 tbsp	35	1	5	205	1	1.2	0.3	0	32%
(Tone's) mix only	1 tsp	12	0	2	114	0	0.5	0.0	1	40%
(Williams) low-fat, low-cholesterol	0.33 oz	40	1	5	320	0	2.0	0.0	0	43%
HOMESTYLE										
(French's) prepared	1/4 cup	20	1	4	250	0	1.0	0.0	0	31%
(McCormick/Schilling) prepared	1/4 cup	24	1	4	295	0	0.8	0.0	0	30%
(Pillsbury)										
mix only	2 tsp	10	0	3	270	0	0.0	0.0	0	0%
prepared w/water, 1/4 cup 2% milk	1/4 cup	25	1	4	170	0	1.0	0.0	0	31%
HERB *(McCormick/Schilling)* prepared	1/4 cup	20	1	3	312	0	0.5	0.0	0	24%
MUSHROOM										
(French's) prepared w/water	1/4 cup	20	1	3	250	0	1.0	0.0	0	36%
(Loma Linda) 'Gravy Quik' mix only	1 tbsp	16	1	3	304	1	0.3	0.1	0	14%
(McCormick/Schilling) mix only	1/4 cup	19	1	3	270	0	0.5	0.0	0	24%
ONION										
(French's) prepared w/water	1/4 cup	25	1	4	270	0	1.0	0.0	0	31%
(Loma Linda) 'Gravy Quik' mix only	1 tbsp	18	1	3	229	1	0.0	0.0	0	0%
(McCormick/Schilling) mix only	2 tsp	20	1	3	340	0	0.5	0.0	0	24%
PORK										
(Custom Foods)										
instant, 'Superb' mix only	16-oz pkg	1648	38	294	20289	11	35.8	17.8	45	20%
instant, 'Superb' mix only	1 serving	24	1	4	299	0	0.5	0.3	1	20%
(French's) prepared w/water	1/4 cup	20	1	4	250	0	1.0	0.0	0	31%
(McCormick/Schilling) prepared w/water	1/4 cup	20	1	4	297	0	0.6	0.0	0	23%
SOUTHERN										
(Nestlé)										
'Trio' mix only	1 pkg	1770	9	223	10672	0	93.7	20.6	7	48%
'Trio' mix only	1 serving	48	0	6	290	0	2.5	0.6	0	48%
TURKEY										
(Custom Foods)										
instant, 'Superb' mix only	16-oz pkg	1857	53	261	18569	17	66.6	22.4	109	32%
instant, 'Superb' mix only	1 serving	27	1	4	274	0	1.0	0.3	2	32%
(Lawry's) prepared w/water	1 cup	102	3	13	1400	0	4.1	0.0	0	37%
(McCormick/Schilling) prepared w/water	1/4 cup	22	1	4	353	0	0.5	0.0	0	20%
(Nestlé)										
'Trio' mix only	1 pkg	2053	49	409	19204	9	24.6	5.6	62	11%
'Trio' mix only	1 serving	29	1	6	271	0	0.3	0.1	1	11%

GREAT NORTHERN BEAN. See BEAN, GREAT NORTHERN.

GREEK SEASONING MIX. See under SEASONING MIX.

GREEN BEAN. See BEAN, FRENCH; BEAN, GREEN; BEAN DISH/ENTRÉE.

GREEN ONION. See SCALLION.

GREEN PEAS. See PEAS, GREEN.

GREEN PEPPER. See PEPPER, BELL.

GREEN PEPPER DISH/ENTRÉE. See PEPPER, BELL, DISH/ENTRÉE.

GREEN TURTLE. See TURTLE, GREEN.

GREENLAND HALIBUT. See under HALIBUT.

GRENADINE SYRUP. See under COCKTAIL MIX.

GRITS

CORN

Instant

(Quaker)										
butter flavor	1 pkt	101	2	21	323	1	1.4	0.3	0	12%
cheddar cheese flavor	1 pkt	102	2	21	522	1	1.6	0.5	1	14%

Food Name	Serving Size	Calories	Prot. gms	Carbs gms	Sod. mgs	Fiber gms	Fat gms	Sat. Fat gms	Chol. mgs	% Fat Cal.
plain.	1 cup	159	4	37	517	2	0.5	0.0	0	3%
plain.	1 pkt	96	2	22	305	1	0.3	0.0	0	3%
w/imitation bacon bits	1 pkt	94	3	21	331	1	0.5	0.1	0	4%
w/imitation ham bits.	1 pkt	92	3	20	510	1	0.5	0.1	0	5%
w/sausage bits	1 serving	100	3	21	480	2	1.0	0.0	0	9%
Quick-cooking										
white, enriched, cooked w/water, w/o salt	1 cup	145	3	31	0	0	0.5	0.1	0	3%
white, enriched, cooked w/water, w/o salt	3/4 cup	109	3	24	0	0	0.4	0.1	0	3%
white, unenriched, cooked w/water, w/o salt	1 cup	145	3	31	0	0	0.5	0.1	0	3%
white, unenriched, cooked w/water, w/o salt	3/4 cup	109	3	24	0	0	0.4	0.1	0	3%
white, unenriched, dry.	1 cup	579	14	124	2	2	1.9	0.3	0	3%
white, unenriched, dry.	1 tbsp	36	1	8	0	0	0.1	0.0	0	3%
yellow, enriched, cooked w/water, w/o salt	1 cup	145	3	31	0	0	0.5	0.1	0	3%
yellow, enriched, cooked w/water, w/o salt	3/4 cup	109	3	24	0	0	0.4	0.1	0	3%
yellow, enriched, dry	1 cup	579	14	124	2	2	1.9	0.3	0	3%
yellow, enriched, dry	1 tbsp	36	1	8	0	0	0.1	0.0	0	3%
yellow, unenriched, cooked w/water, w/o salt	1 cup	145	3	31	0	0	0.5	0.1	0	3%
yellow, unenriched, cooked w/water, w/o salt	3/4 cup	109	3	24	0	0	0.4	0.1	0	3%
yellow, unenriched, dry	1 cup	579	14	124	2	2	1.9	0.3	0	3%
yellow, unenriched, dry	1 tbsp	36	1	8	0	0	0.1	0.0	0	3%
(Arrowhead Mills)										
white, dry.	2 oz	200	5	43	1	2	1.0	0.0	0	4%
yellow, dry.	2 oz	200	5	44	1	2	1.0	0.0	0	4%
(Aunt Jemima) white, enriched, dry.	3 tbsp	101	2	22	1	1	0.2	0.0	0	2%
(Quick) yellow, enriched, dry	3 tbsp	101	2	22	1	1	0.2	0.0	0	2%
(Tone's) yellow, enriched, dry.	1 tsp	12	0	3	0	0	0.1	0.0	0	7%
HOMINY										
Canned										
(Allens)										
golden.	1/2 cup	80	2	16	370	0	1.0	0.0	0	11%
Mexican.	1/2 cup	80	2	16	330	0	1.0	0.0	0	11%
white.	1/2 cup	70	2	16	430	0	1.0	0.0	0	11%
(Bush's Best)										
golden.	1/2 cup	45	1	11	390	0	0.0	0.0	0	0%
white.	1/2 cup	45	1	11	450	0	0.0	0.0	0	0%
(Juanita's) Mexican style	1/2 cup	60	2	10	190	5	0.5	0.0	0	9%
(S&W)										
golden, 'Sun-Vista'	1/2 cup	70	2	19	540	3	0.0	0.0	0	0%
white.	1/2 cup	65	2	18	530	3	0.5	0.0	0	5%
white, 'Sun-Vista'.	1/2 cup	65	2	18	530	3	0.5	0.0	0	5%
(Van Camp's)										
golden.	1 cup	128	3	28	701	1	0.6	0.0	0	4%
golden, w/red and green peppers	1 cup	129	3	29	685	1	0.5	0.0	0	3%
white.	1 cup	138	3	30	708	1	0.7	0.0	0	5%
Instant										
(Albers) 'Hominy Quick Grits'.	1/2 cup	150	4	33	0	0	0.0	0.0	0	0%
(Aunt Jemima) white, enriched, 'Quick'.	3 tbsp	101	2	22	1	1	0.2	0.0	0	2%
(Quaker) w/real cheddar cheese flavor	1 pkt	104	2	22	497	1	1.0	0.0	0	9%
Quick-cooking										
(Aunt Jemima) white, enriched, 'Regular'	3 tbsp	101	2	22	1	1	0.2	0.0	0	2%
(Quaker)										
white.	1/4 cup	130	3	29	0	2	0.5	0.0	0	3%
yellow.	1/3 cup	133	3	30	0	2	0.5	0.0	0	3%

GROUND HUSK TOMATO. See TOMATILLO.

Food Name	Serving Size	Calories	Prot. gms	Carbs gms	Sod. mgs	Fiber gms	Fat gms	Sat. Fat gms	Chol. mgs	% Fat Cal.
GROUPER										
mixed species, baked, broiled, grilled, or microwaved	3 oz	100	21	0	45	0	1.1	0.3	40	10%
mixed species, raw	3 oz	78	16	0	45	0	0.9	0.2	31	10%
GUACAMOLE. See under DIP.										
GUACAMOLE SEASONING. See under SEASONING MIX.										
GUANABANA / soursop										
raw, trimmed	1/2 cup	75	1.1	18.9	16	>1.2 c	0.3	na	0	3%
raw, untrimmed	1 lb	202	3.0	51.2	42	>3.3 c	0.9	na	0	4%
raw, whole, approx 2.1 lb.	1 medium	416	6.3	105.3	87	>6.9 c	1.9	na	0	4%
GUAVA										
raw, chopped.	1 cup	84	1	20	5	9	1.0	0.3	0	10%
raw, whole, trimmed	1 medium	46	1	11	3	5	0.5	0.2	0	10%
GUAVA, STRAWBERRY										
raw, chopped	1 cup	168	1	42	90	13	1.5	0.4	0	7%
raw, whole, trimmed	1 medium	4	0	1	2	0	0.0	0.0	0	7%
GUAVA JUICE										
Frozen *(Welch's)* 'Orchard Tropicals' prepared.	6 fl oz	100	0	25	20	0	0.0	0.0	0	0%
GUINEA HEN										
giblets, raw	3.5 oz	157	20.8	1.2	70	0	7.0	2.0	350	42%
meat and skin, raw	1 lb	567	84.0	0.0	241	0	23.2	6.3	266	38%
meat only, raw.................................	1 oz	31	5.9	0.0	(mq)	0	0.7	(mq)	18	21%
GUM. See under CANDY.										
GUMBO FILE POWDER. See under SEASONING MIX.										

H

Food Name	Serving Size	Calories	Prot. gms	Carbs gms	Sod. mgs	Fiber gms	Fat gms	Sat. Fat gms	Chol. mgs	% Fat Cal.
HADDOCK										
Fresh										
baked, broiled, grilled, or microwaved.................	3 oz	95	21	0	74	0	0.8	0.1	63	7%
raw	3 oz	74	16	0	58	0	0.6	0.1	48	7%
Frozen										
fillet, 'Fishmarket Fresh' *(Gorton's)*	5 oz	110	25	0	120	0	1.0	0.0	0	8%
fillet *(SeaPak)*	4 oz	90	18	0	120	0	1.0	0.0	0	11%
fillet *(Van de Kamp's)*	4 oz	90	21	0	125	0	1.0	0.0	20	10%
Smoked										
fillet	3 oz	99	21	0	649	0	0.8	0.1	65	7%
fillet, boneless	1 oz	33	7	0	216	0	0.3	0.0	22	7%
finnian haddie	4 oz	132	28.6	0.0	865	0	1.1	0.2	87	8%
HADDOCK, NORWAY. See OCEAN PERCH, ATLANTIC.										
HADDOCK DINNER/ENTRÉE										
(Van de Kamp's)										
fillet, battered, frozen.............................	2 pieces	250	12	19	580	0	15.0	3.0	30	52%
fillet, breaded, frozen.............................	2 pieces	270	12	19	290	0	16.0	3.0	25	54%
fillet, light, frozen	1 piece	240	15	21	590	0	11.0	2.0	35	41%
HAKE, SILVER. See WHITING.										
HALIBUT										
ATLANTIC										
Fresh										
baked, broiled, grilled, or microwaved.................	4 oz	159	30.3	0.0	78	0	3.3	0.5	46	20%
baked, broiled, grilled, or microwaved.................	3 oz	119	22.7	0.0	59	0	2.5	0.4	35	20%
raw	1 lb	497	94.4	0.0	245	0	10.4	1.5	146	20%

Food Name	Serving Size	Calories	Prot. gms	Carbs gms	Sod. mgs	Fiber gms	Fat gms	Sat. Fat gms	Chol. mgs	% Fat Cal.
raw	3 oz	94	17.7	0.0	46	0	2.0	0.3	27	20%
raw	1 oz	31	5.9	0.0	15	0	0.6	0.1	9	19%
Frozen, steaks (SeaPak)	6-oz pkg	160	36	0	120	0	1.0	0.0	0	6%
GREENLAND										
baked, broiled, grilled, or microwaved	3 oz	203	15.7	0.0	88	0	15.1	2.6	50	68%
raw	1 lb	845	65.2	0.0	363	0	62.8	11.0	209	68%
raw	3 oz	158	12.2	0.0	68	0	11.8	2.1	39	69%
raw	1 oz	53	4.1	0.0	23	0	3.9	0.7	13	68%
PACIFIC										
Fresh										
baked, broiled, grilled, or microwaved	4 oz	159	30.3	0.0	78	0	3.3	0.5	46	20%
baked, broiled, grilled, or microwaved	3 oz	119	22.7	0.0	59	0	2.5	0.4	35	20%
raw	1 lb	497	94.4	0.0	245	0	10.4	1.5	146	20%
raw	3 oz	94	17.7	0.0	46	0	2.0	0.3	27	20%
raw	1 oz	31	5.9	0.0	15	0	0.6	0.1	9	19%
Frozen										
fillet, boneless, skinless, raw (Peter Pan Seafoods)	3.5 oz	110	21	0	54	0	2.3	0.0	32	20%
loin steaks, raw (Peter Pan Seafoods)	3.5 oz	110	21	0	54	0	2.3	0.0	32	20%
steaks, standard cut, raw (Peter Pan Seafoods)	3.5 oz	110	21	0	54	0	2.3	0.0	32	20%
steaks (SeaPak)	6 oz pkg	160	36	0	120	0	1.0	0.0	0	6%
HALIBUT DINNER/ENTRÉE										
(Van de Kamp's) fillet, battered, frozen	2 pieces	150	8	16	400	0	6.0	1.0	10	36%
HAM. See also HAM SUBSTITUTE; PORK. Also see under LUNCHEON MEAT.										
CANNED										
chopped	1 oz	68	4.6	0.1	387	0	5.3	1.8	14	72%
chopped	0.75-oz slice	50	3.4	0.1	287	0	4.0	1.3	10	72%
cured, extra lean, approx 4% fat, baked	3 oz	116	18.0	0.4	965	0	4.2	1.4	25	34%
cured, extra lean, approx 4% fat, unheated	1 oz	34	5.2	0.0	356	0	1.3	0.4	11	36%
cured, extra lean and regular, baked	3 oz	142	17.8	0.4	908	0	7.2	2.4	35	47%
cured, extra lean and regular, unheated	1 oz	41	5.1	0.0	362	0	2.1	0.7	11	48%
cured, regular, approx 13% fat, baked	3 oz	192	17.5	0.4	800	0	12.9	4.3	53	62%
cured, regular, approx 13% fat, unheated	1 oz	54	4.8	0.0	352	0	3.7	1.2	11	63%
(Armour) chopped	3 oz	190	13	1	1260	0	14.0	0.0	0	69%
(Black Label) 3-lb can	4 oz	140	20	0	1315	0	7.0	0.0	0	44%
(Chi-Chi's) 'Black Label'	1 oz	37	5	2	303	0	1.0	1.0	15	24%
(EXL)										
	4 oz	120	22	0	1382	0	4.0	0.0	0	29%
'Deli Ham' 10-lb can	4 oz	130	20	0	1368	0	6.0	0.0	0	40%
(Holiday Glaze) '3-lb can'	4 oz	130	21	2	0	0	4.0	0.0	0	28%
(Hormel)										
'Bone-In'	4 oz	210	17	1	0	0	15.0	0.0	0	65%
chopped, 12-oz can	2 oz	120	10	0	703	0	9.0	0.0	0	67%
chunk	2.5 oz	110	11	1	780	0	7.0	2.0	35	57%
'Cure/81'	4 oz	160	22	0	1322	0	8.0	0.0	0	45%
'Curemaster'	4 oz	140	22	1	1361	0	5.0	0.0	0	33%
'Light & Lean 97'	2 oz	60	10	1	450	0	2.0	1.0	26	29%
patty	1 patty	180	7	0	456	0	16.0	0.0	0	84%
patty, w/cheese	1 patty	190	7	0	468	0	18.0	0.0	0	85%
roll	4 oz	170	21	0	1338	0	10.0	0.0	0	52%
spiced	3 oz	240	13	1	1093	0	21.0	0.0	0	77%
(JM) '95% Fat-Free'	2 oz	60	10	1	680	0	2.0	0.0	0	29%
(Light & Lean) 'No bone'	2 oz	60	10	0	574	0	2.0	0.0	0	31%
(Oscar Mayer) 'Jubilee'	1 oz	29	5	0	287	0	0.9	0.4	14	28%
(Rath) hickory smoked, 'Black Hawk'	2 oz	60	10	1	720	0	2.0	0.0	0	29%

Food Name	Serving Size	Calories	Prot. gms	Carbs gms	Sod. mgs	Fiber gms	Fat gms	Sat. Fat gms	Chol. mgs	% Fat Cal.
(Swift) patty, 'Premium Brown 'N Serve'	1 patty	130	3	1	260	0	13.0	0.0	0	88%

CURED

(NOTE: TRIMMED = Lean; separable fat removed. UNTRIMMED = Separable fat not removed.)

Bone in, Boston butt, trimmed

Food Name	Serving Size	Calories	Prot. gms	Carbs gms	Sod. mgs	Fiber gms	Fat gms	Sat. Fat gms	Chol. mgs	% Fat Cal.
medium fat, chopped, roasted.	1 cup	340	38.9	0.0	1393	0	19.3	7.0	123	53%
medium fat, roasted	9.8 oz	678	77.6	0.0	2777	0	38.5	13.9	246	53%

Bone in, whole

Food Name	Serving Size	Calories	Prot. gms	Carbs gms	Sod. mgs	Fiber gms	Fat gms	Sat. Fat gms	Chol. mgs	% Fat Cal.
honey glazed, 'Traditional' (Carving Board).	1 slice	50	8	1	560	0	1.5	0.5	25	27%
trimmed, fully cooked, baked	3 oz	133	21.3	0.0	1128	0	4.7	1.6	47	33%
trimmed, fully cooked, unheated.	1 oz	42	6.3	0.0	430	0	1.6	0.5	15	36%
smoked (Carving Board).	1 slice	45	8	0	570	0	1.5	1.5	20	30%
untrimmed, fully cooked, baked	3 oz	207	18.3	0.0	1009	0	14.2	5.1	53	64%
untrimmed, fully cooked, unheated.	1 oz	70	5.2	0.0	364	0	5.3	1.9	16	70%
water added, baked (Carving Board)	1 slice	50	8	1	550	0	1.5	0.5	25	27%

Boneless

Food Name	Serving Size	Calories	Prot. gms	Carbs gms	Sod. mgs	Fiber gms	Fat gms	Sat. Fat gms	Chol. mgs	% Fat Cal.
breakfast, 'Light AM' (Healthy Deli)	1 oz	27	4	1	200	0	0.6	0.0	11	20%
'Breakfast Ham' (Oscar Mayer).	1.5 oz slice	47	7	1	582	0	1.5	0.6	21	29%
center slice, country-style, trimmed, unheated	4 oz	220	31	0	3045	0	9.4	3.1	79	38%
center slice, country style, untrimmed, heated	4 oz	229	23	0	1566	0	14.6	5.2	61	57%
extra lean, approx 5% fat, baked.	3 oz	123	17.8	1.3	1023	0	4.7	1.5	45	36%
extra lean, approx 5% fat, baked, chopped.	1 cup	203	29	2	1684	0	7.7	2.5	74	34%
extra lean, approx 5% fat, unheated	1 oz	37	5.5	0.3	405	0	1.4	0.5	13	35%
extra lean and regular, baked	3 oz	140	18.7	0.4	1177	0	6.5	2.2	48	43%
extra lean and regular, baked, chopped	1 cup	231	31	1	1939	0	10.7	3.7	80	42%
extra lean and regular, unheated	1 oz	46	5.2	0.7	362	0	2.4	0.8	15	48%
extra lean and regular, unheated, chopped	1 cup	227	26	3	1789	0	11.7	3.8	74	47%
extra lean and regular, unheated, 4 x 6 1/4 inch slice. . . .	1 slice	46	5.2	0.7	362	0	2.4	0.8	15	48%
mini (JM)	3 oz	90	17	0	40	0	3.0	0.0	0	28%
regular, approx 11% fat, baked	3 oz	151	19.2	0.0	1275	0	7.7	2.7	50	47%
regular, approx 11% fat, baked, chopped	1 cup	249	32	0	2100	0	12.6	4.4	83	46%
regular, approx 11% fat, unheated	1 oz	52	5.0	0.9	373	0	3.0	1.0	16	53%
steak, dinner sliced (Oscar Mayer)	1 piece	60	10	0	750	0	2.0	0.5	30	31%
steak, unheated.	2 oz	69	11.1	0.0	720	0	2.4	0.8	26	33%
whole (JM).	3 oz	140	17	0	40	0	8.0	0.0	0	51%
w/natural juices, 'EZ Cut' (JM)	2 oz	70	11	1	660	0	3.0	0.0	0	36%
Patty, raw	1 oz	89	4	0	308	0	8.0	2.9	20	81%
Puréed (Bryan Foods)	1/3 cup	160	11	0	75	0	12.0	4.0	40	71%

HAM DINNER/ENTRÉE

Food Name	Serving Size	Calories	Prot. gms	Carbs gms	Sod. mgs	Fiber gms	Fat gms	Sat. Fat gms	Chol. mgs	% Fat Cal.
(Armour) steak, frozen, 'Classics'	10.75 oz	270	15	36	1320	0	7.0	0.0	50	24%
(Banquet) frozen, 'Platters'.	10 oz	400	20	43	1180	0	17.0	0.0	50	38%
(Cook's)										
hickory-smoked, honey, spiral-sliced.	3 oz	150	14	2	850	0	10.0	3.0	30	58%
hickory-smoked, honey, w/glaze, spiral-sliced, ...	3 oz	160	14	4	850	0	10.0	3.0	30	56%
(Hormel) 96% nonfat, water added, cooked, 'Curemaster' . .	3 oz	80	14	0	940	0	3.0	1.0	40	33%
(Le Menu) steak, frozen.	10 oz	300	19	31	1500	0	11.0	0.0	0	33%
(Louis Rich) dinner slices, baked, 98% fat-free	1 slice	80	16	1	1150	0	1.5	0.5	40	17%
(Marie Callender's) steak, honey-smoked, w/macaroni and cheese.	14 oz	490	29	63	2310	5	13.0	7.0	80	24%
(Morton) frozen	10 oz	290	15	49	1400	0	4.0	0.0	45	12%
(Pillsbury) casserole, w/cheese, 'Microwave Classic'	1 pkg	470	18	34	1300	0	29.0	0.0	0	56%
(Stouffer's) w/asparagus	1 entrée	520	16	32	1040	2	36.0	14.0	75	63%
(Swanson) w/scalloped potatoes, 'Homestyle Recipe'. . . .	9 oz	300	19	26	1080	0	13.0	0.0	0	39%
(West Virginia) boneless, no water added, cooked	3 oz	110	15	1	900	0	4.0	1.5	40	36%

HAM SUBSTITUTE

Food Name	Serving Size	Calories	Prot. gms	Carbs gms	Sod. mgs	Fiber gms	Fat gms	Sat. Fat gms	Chol. mgs	% Fat Cal.
(Worthington) meatless, vegetarian, 'Wham'.	1 slice	82	7	1	426	0	5.2	0.8	1	57%

Food Name	Serving Size	Calories	Prot. gms	Carbs gms	Sod. mgs	Fiber gms	Fat gms	Sat. Fat gms	Chol. mgs	% Fat Cal.
HAM SPREAD										
(Libby's) salad, 'Spreadables'	1/3 cup	110	8	8	621	4	4.5	1.0	20	39%
(Hormel)										
deviled.	1 oz	76	4	1	214	0	6.0	2.0	19	73%
deviled.	1 tbsp	35	2	0	108	0	3.0	0.0	0	77%
(Underwood)										
deviled.	2-1/8 oz	220	8	1	430	0	19.0	6.0	50	83%
deviled, 'Light'	2-1/8 oz	120	11	1	250	0	8.0	1.0	35	60%
deviled, smoked	2-1/8 oz	190	9	1	260	0	18.0	6.0	65	80%
HAMBURG PARSLEY. See PARSLEY ROOT.										
HAMBURGER. See under BEEF; BEEF DINNER/ENTRÉE. See also HAMBURGER ENTRÉE MIX.										
HAMBURGER BUN. See BUN, HAMBURGER.										
HAMBURGER ENTRÉE MIX										
(Hamburger Helper)										
beef noodle, mix only	1/5 pkg	140	5	26	1000	0	2.0	0.0	0	13%
beef noodle, prepared	1 cup	320	20	26	1050	0	15.0	0.0	0	42%
beef pasta, prepared.	1 cup	270	20	26	910	1	10.0	4.0	50	33%
beef Romanoff, prepared	1 cup	280	20	27	920	0	10.0	4.0	50	32%
beef taco, prepared.	1 cup	310	20	31	930	1	11.0	4.0	50	33%
beef teriyaki, mix only	1/5 pkg	180	4	38	1110	0	1.0	0.0	0	5%
beef teriyaki, prepared	1 cup	360	20	38	1160	0	14.0	0.0	0	35%
cheddar 'n bacon meal, mix only.	2/3 cup	170	7	25	810	1	5.0	1.5	10	26%
cheddar 'n bacon meal, prepared	1 cup	350	24	28	890	1	16.0	6.0	65	41%
cheeseburger macaroni meal, mix only	1/3 cup	180	5	30	860	1	4.0	1.5	5	20%
cheeseburger macaroni meal, prepared.	1 cup	360	23	33	940	1	15.0	6.0	65	38%
cheesy Italian meal, mix only	1/2 cup	150	5	26	850	1	3.0	1.0	3	18%
cheesy Italian meal, prepared.	1 cup	330	22	29	920	1	14.0	5.0	60	38%
chili macaroni meal, mix only	1/3 cup	140	3	30	820	1	1.0	0.0	0	6%
chili macaroni meal, prepared.	1 cup	290	19	30	870	1	10.0	4.0	55	31%
chili tomato meal, mix only	1/5 pkg	150	5	31	1360	0	1.0	0.0	0	6%
chili tomato meal, prepared.	1 cup	330	20	31	1410	0	14.0	0.0	0	38%
chili w/beans meal, mix only	1/4 pkg	130	5	25	1680	0	1.0	0.0	0	7%
chili w/beans meal, prepared	1-1/4 cup	350	24	25	1740	0	17.0	0.0	0	44%
creamy Stroganoff, prepared w/whole milk.	1 cup	390	22	30	870	0	20.0	0.0	0	46%
creamy Stroganoff, prepared.	1 cup	320	21	30	830	0	13.0	5.0	55	36%
hamburger hash meal, mix only	1/5 pkg	140	3	27	970	0	2.0	0.0	0	13%
hamburger hash meal, prepared.	1 cup	320	18	27	1020	0	15.0	0.0	0	43%
hamburger stew meal, mix only.	1/5 pkg	120	3	25	960	0	1.0	0.0	0	7%
hamburger stew meal, prepared	1 cup	300	18	25	1010	0	14.0	0.0	0	42%
lasagna meal, mix only	2/3 cup	140	4	30	950	0	1.0	0.0	0	6%
lasagna meal, prepared	1 cup	280	19	30	990	0	10.0	4.0	50	31%
meat loaf meal, mix only	1-1/2 tbsp	50	2	10	500	0	0.5	0.0	0	9%
mushroom and wild rice meal, mix only	1/5 pkg	180	4	34	880	0	3.0	0.0	0	15%
mushroom and wild rice meal, prepared.	1 cup	380	21	37	950	0	16.0	0.0	0	38%
nacho cheese meal, mix only	1/2 cup	160	5	28	860	1	2.5	0.5	0	15%
nacho cheese meal, prepared.	1 cup	320	22	30	930	1	13.0	5.0	55	36%
pizza dish meal, mix only	1/5 pkg	180	6	37	960	0	1.0	0.0	0	5%
pizza dish meal, prepared.	1 cup	360	21	37	1010	0	14.0	0.0	0	35%
pizza pasta w/cheese topping, mix only	1/2 cup	150	4	30	700	0	1.5	0.0	0	9%
pizza pasta w/cheese topping, prepared.	1 cup	290	19	31	750	0	10.0	4.0	50	31%
pizzabake, mix only	1 serving	140	3	28	670	1	1.5	0.0	0	10%
pizzabake, prepared	1 serving	270	17	28	720	1	10.0	3.5	45	33%
potato Stroganoff meal, mix only.	2/3 cup	120	2	24	810	2	2.0	0.5	0	15%
potato Stroganoff meal, prepared	1 cup	270	18	25	870	2	12.0	4.5	55	39%

Food Name	Serving Size	Calories	Prot. gms	Carbs gms	Sod. mgs	Fiber gms	Fat gms	Sat. Fat gms	Chol. mgs	% Fat Cal.
potatoes au gratin meal, mix only	2/3 cup	120	3	23	740	2	2.5	0.5	3	18%
potatoes au gratin meal, prepared	1 cup	290	18	24	820	2	14.0	5.0	55	43%
rice Oriental meal, mix only	1/4 cup	160	3	35	1000	0	0.5	0.0	0	3%
rice Oriental meal, prepared	1 cup	310	19	35	1050	0	10.0	4.0	55	29%
sloppy Joe meal, mix only	1/6 pkg	180	5	33	1060	0	3.0	0.0	0	15%
sloppy Joe meal, prepared	5 oz	340	18	33	1100	0	15.0	0.0	0	40%
spaghetti meal, mix only	1/2 cup	150	5	29	890	1	1.0	0.0	0	6%
spaghetti meal, prepared	1 cup	300	21	29	940	1	11.0	4.0	55	33%
Stroganoff meal, mix only	1/5 pkg	190	5	30	800	0	5.0	0.0	0	24%
Stroganoff meal, prepared	2/3 cup	160	5	27	760	0	3.0	1.0	0	17%
taco meal, 'Tacobake' mix only	1/6 pkg	170	4	31	920	0	4.0	0.0	0	20%
taco meal, 'Tacobake' prepared	5.75 oz	320	17	31	940	0	15.0	0.0	0	41%
tamale pie meal, mix only	1/5 pkg	200	4	39	890	0	3.0	0.0	0	14%
tamale pie meal, prepared	1 cup	380	19	39	940	0	16.0	0.0	0	38%
three cheese meal mix, prepared	1/5 pkg	400	24	32	980	0	20.0	0.0	0	45%
three cheese meal, mix only	1/5 pkg	210	7	30	910	0	7.0	0.0	0	30%
zesty Italian meal, mix only	1/3 cup	160	5	34	840	1	1.0	0.0	0	5%
zesty Italian meal, prepared	1 cup	320	21	34	890	1	11.0	4.0	55	31%

HAMBURGER RELISH. See under RELISH.
HAMBURGER SUBSTITUTE. See under BEEF SUBSTITUTE DINNER/ENTRÉE.
HARD ROLL. See under ROLL.
HARICOTS. See under BEAN, FRENCH.
HASH
CORNED BEEF
(Armour)

Food Name	Serving Size	Calories	Prot. gms	Carbs gms	Sod. mgs	Fiber gms	Fat gms	Sat. Fat gms	Chol. mgs	% Fat Cal.
canned	1 pkg	897	43	22	1539	3	71.0	28.2	174	71%
canned	1 serving	498	24	12	854	2	39.4	15.6	97	71%
(Hormel) canned	1 cup	387	21	22	1003	3	24.2	10.2	76	56%
(Libby's)										
	1 cup	470	21	25	1200	8	35.0	16.0	90	63%
	1/4 cup	120	15	0	490	0	7.0	3.0	50	51%
(Nestlé)										
'Chef Mate'	1 pkg	5823	291	348	19108	73	363.7	160.7	1062	56%
'Chef Mate'	1 cup	486	24	29	1594	6	30.3	13.4	89	56%
ROAST BEEF										
(Libby's)	1 cup	460	19	23	1390	3	33.0	13.0	80	64%
(Hormel) canned	1 cup	385	21	23	793	4	23.6	9.9	73	55%

HAWAIIAN YAM. See under YAM.

Food Name	Serving Size	Calories	Prot. gms	Carbs gms	Sod. mgs	Fiber gms	Fat gms	Sat. Fat gms	Chol. mgs	% Fat Cal.
HAWS / hawthorn tree fruit, scarlet, w/skin, raw	3.5 oz	87	2.0	20.8	0	>2.1	0.7	0.0	0	7%

HAZELNUT / cobnut / filbert

Food Name	Serving Size	Calories	Prot. gms	Carbs gms	Sod. mgs	Fiber gms	Fat gms	Sat. Fat gms	Chol. mgs	% Fat Cal.
dried	1 oz	178	4	5	0	3	17.2	1.3	0	81%
dried	10 medium	88	2	2	0	1	8.5	0.6	0	81%
dried, blanched	1 oz	178	4	5	0	3	17.3	1.3	0	81%
dried, chopped	1 cup	722	17	19	0	11	69.9	5.1	0	81%
dried, ground	1 cup	471	11	13	0	7	45.6	3.3	0	81%
dried, whole	1 cup	848	20	23	0	13	82.0	6.0	0	81%
dry-roasted, no salt added	1 oz	183	4	5	0	3	17.7	1.3	0	81%
natural, unsalted *(Flanigan Farms)*	1/4 cup	180	4	4	0	2	18.0	1.5	0	84%
natural, whole *(Oregon Hazelnuts)*	1/2 cup	396	11	12	1	9	36.8	2.5	0	78%

HAZELNUT BUTTER

Food Name	Serving Size	Calories	Prot. gms	Carbs gms	Sod. mgs	Fiber gms	Fat gms	Sat. Fat gms	Chol. mgs	% Fat Cal.
creamy, roasted fresh, no salt added *(Roaster Fresh)*	1 oz	188	4	5	1	0	19.0	2.0	0	83%

HAZELNUT OIL

Food Name	Serving Size	Calories	Prot. gms	Carbs gms	Sod. mgs	Fiber gms	Fat gms	Sat. Fat gms	Chol. mgs	% Fat Cal.
	1 cup	1927	0	0	0	0	218.0	16.1	0	100%
	1 tbsp	120	0	0	0	0	13.6	1.0	0	100%
(International Collection)	1 tbsp	120	0	0	0	0	14.0	1.0	0	100%

Food Name	Serving Size	Calories	Prot. gms	Carbs gms	Sod. mgs	Fiber gms	Fat gms	Sat. Fat gms	Chol. mgs	% Fat Cal.
HAZELNUT SPREAD										
w/milk and cocoa, 'Nutella' (Ferrero)	1 tbsp	80	1	9	10	0	5.0	0.0	0	53%
HEAD CHEESE. See under SAUSAGE.										
HEART NUT. See CASHEW.										
HERB SEASONING MIX. See under SEASONING MIX.										
HEARTS OF PALM. See under PALM.										
HERBAL TEA. See under TEA.										
HERRING										
ATLANTIC										
fillet, baked, broiled, grilled, or microwaved	3 oz	173	20	0	98	0	9.9	2.2	65	52%
fillet, kippered, large, approx 7 x 2.25 x 1/4 inch	1 fillet	141	16	0	597	0	8.0	1.8	53	51%
fillet, kippered, medium, approx 5 x 1.75 x 1/4 inch	1 fillet	87	10	0	367	0	4.9	1.1	33	51%
fillet, kippered, small, approx 2-3/8 x 1-3/8 x 1/4 inch	1 fillet	43	5	0	184	0	2.5	0.6	16	51%
fillet, kippered, boneless	1 oz	62	7	0	260	0	3.5	0.8	23	51%
fillet, kippered, smoked, salt added (Crown Prince)	1/4 cup	110	11	0	230	0	8.0	1.0	35	62%
fillet, kippered, w/naturally smoked wood flavoring										
(Beach Cliff)	3.3 oz	220	17	1	475	0	17.0	0.0	0	68%
pickled	1 cup	367	20	13	1218	0	25.2	3.3	18	62%
pickled, approx 1.75 x 7/8 x 1/2 inch	1 piece	39	2	1	131	0	2.7	0.4	2	62%
pickled, boneless	1 oz	74	4	3	247	0	5.1	0.7	4	62%
raw	3 oz	134	15	0	77	0	7.7	1.7	51	52%
raw, boneless	1 oz	45	5	0	26	0	2.6	0.6	17	52%
snacks, kippered, w/smoke flavoring, drained										
(Beach Cliff)	3.3 oz	220	17	1	350	0	17.0	0.0	0	68%
steaks, in soybean oil, drained (Beach Cliff)	3 oz	240	16	0	350	0	20.0	0.0	0	74%
steaks, in water, drained (Beach Cliff)	3 oz	230	17	1	350	0	18.0	0.0	0	69%
steaks, w/mustard, drained (Beach Cliff)	3 oz	227	13	4	350	0	18.0	0.0	0	70%
steaks, w/tomato, drained (Beach Cliff)	3 oz	210	15	0	350	0	17.0	0.0	0	72%
PACIFIC										
baked, broiled, grilled, or miocrowaved	3 oz	213	18	0	81	0	15.1	3.5	84	64%
raw	3 oz	166	14	0	63	0	11.8	2.8	65	64%
HERRING OIL. See under FISH OIL.										
HICKORY NUT										
dried	1 cup	788	15	22	1	8	77.2	8.4	0	82%
dried	1 oz	186	4	5	0	2	18.2	2.0	0	82%
dried	1 medium	20	0	1	0	0	1.9	0.2	0	82%
HIRITAKE. See MUSHROOM, OYSTER.										
HIZIKI. See under SEA VEGETABLE.										
HOG PLUM. See JOBO.										
HOMINY. See under GRITS.										
HON SHIMEJI. See MUSHROOM, JAPANESE HONEY.										
HONEY										
(Golden Blossom)	1 tbsp	60	0	16	0	0	0.0	0.0	0	0%
(Knott's Berry Farm)	1 tbsp	60	0	17	0	0	0.0	0.0	0	0%
(Sioux)	1 tbsp	60	0	16	0	0	0.0	0.0	0	0%
mesquite, desert, 100%, raw, wild, unblended										
(Trader Joe's)	1 tbsp	60	0	17	0	0	0.0	0.0	0	0%
strained or extracted	1 cup	1031	1	279	14	1	0.0	0.0	0	0%
strained or extracted	1 tbsp	64	0	17	1	0	0.0	0.0	0	0%
HONEY BUTTER (Honey Butter)	1 tbsp	50	1	11	5	0	1.0	0.0	0	16%
HONEY MUSHROOM. See MUSHROOM, JAPANESE HONEY.										
HONEYDEW MELON. See MELON, HONEYDEW.										
HORSE										
raw	1 oz	38	6	0	15	0	1.3	0.4	15	31%

Food Name	Serving Size	Calories	Prot. gms	Carbs gms	Sod. mgs	Fiber gms	Fat gms	Sat. Fat gms	Chol. mgs	% Fat Cal.
roasted	3 oz	149	24	0	47	0	5.1	1.6	58	31%
roasted, boneless, yield from 1 lb raw	11.9 oz	595	96	0	187	0	20.6	6.5	231	31%
HORSE BEAN. See BEAN, FAVA.										
HORSERADISH										
Prepared										
	1 tbsp	7	0	2	47	0	0.1	0.0	0	12%
	1 tsp	2	0	1	16	0	0.0	0.0	0	12%
(Crowley)	1 oz	10	1	2	25	0	1.0	0.0	0	43%
(Gold's) hot	1 tsp	4	1	1	60	0	1.0	0.0	0	53%
(Gold's) red	1 tsp	4	1	1	75	0	0.0	0.0	0	0%
(Gold's) white	1 tsp	4	1	1	55	0	1.0	0.0	0	53%
(Kraft)	1 tbsp	10	0	1	140	0	0.0	0.0	0	0%
(Kraft) cream style	1 tbsp	12	0	1	85	0	0.0	0.0	0	0%
(Silver Spring) cream style	1 tsp	0	0	0	10	0	0.0	0.0	0	0%
Raw	1 lb	288	10.6	65.3	27	>7.9 c	1.0	0.0	0	3%
HORSERADISH, JAPANESE. See WASABI ROOT.										
HORSERADISH SPREAD (Alouette)										
cheese and chive	1 oz	85	2	1	130	0	8.0	0.0	28	86%
HORSERADISH TREE										
leafy tips, boiled, drained, chopped	1 cup	25	2	5	4	1	0.4	0.1	0	13%
leafy tips, raw, chopped	1 cup	13	2	2	2	0	0.3	na	0	18%
pods, boiled, drained, sliced	1 cup	42	2	10	51	5	0.2	0.0	0	4%
pods, raw, sliced	1 cup	37	2	9	42	3	0.2	0.0	0	5%
pods, raw, whole, approx 15 1/3 inch long	1 pod	4	0	1	5	0	0.0	0.0	0	5%
HOT COCOA. See COCOA, HOT, MIX.										
HOT DOG. See FRANKFURTER.										
HOT DOG BUN. See BUN, FRANKFURTER.										
HUBBARD SQUASH. See SQUASH, HUBBARD.										
HUMMUS MIX										
(Fantastic Foods) mix only	2 tbsp	60	3	9	220	2	2.0	0.0	0	27%
(Casbah) prepared	1 oz	160	5	14	180	1	8.0	0.0	0	49%
HUMPBACK SALMON. See under SALMON.										
HUNGARIAN PEPPER. See PEPPER, HUNGARIAN.										
HUSHPUPPY										
(SeaPak) regular, frozen	4 oz	330	6	56	690	0	9.0	0.0	0	25%
(Stilwell) jalapeño, frozen	3 pieces	70	2	4	360	2	5.0	1.0	0	65%
(Stilwell) regular, frozen	3 pieces	140	2	19	310	2	6.0	1.5	0	39%
HUSHPUPPY MIX										
(Golden Dipt)										
deluxe	1.25 oz	120	3	26	520	0	0.0	0.0	0	0%
jalapeño	1.25 oz	120	3	27	570	0	0.0	0.0	0	0%
w/onion	1.25 oz	120	3	27	520	0	0.0	0.0	0	0%
HYACINTH BEAN. See BEAN, HYACINTH.										

I

Food Name	Serving Size	Calories	Prot. gms	Carbs gms	Sod. mgs	Fiber gms	Fat gms	Sat. Fat gms	Chol. mgs	% Fat Cal.
ICE BAR/DESSERT. See also FRUIT BAR, FROZEN; SHERBET; SORBET.										
BAR										
(Cool Creations)										
fruit flavors, nonfat, 'Mickey & Minnie Surprise Pop'	1 pop	60	0	14	5	0	0.0	0.0	0	0%
(Crystal Light) all flavors, nonfat	1 bar	14	0	2	10	0	0.0	0.0	0	0%

Food Name	Serving Size	Calories	Prot. gms	Carbs gms	Sod. mgs	Fiber gms	Fat gms	Sat. Fat gms	Chol. mgs	% Fat Cal.
(Eskimo Pie) vanilla, w/dark chocolate coating	1 bar	166	2	12	34	na	12.1	7.3	14	65%
(Freezer Pleezer) assorted flavors, nonfat.	1 bar	40	0	10	0	0	0.0	0.0	0	0%
(Gold Bond) all flavors, nonfat, 'Twin Pop'	1 bar	60	0	14	0	0	0.0	0.0	0	0%
(Good Humor)										
all flavors, nonfat, 'Ice Stripes'.	1 bar	35	0	9	0	0	0.0	0.0	0	0%
cherry, 'Calippo'.	1 bar	138	0	35	5	0	0.1	0.0	0	1%
cherry, Italian.	6 oz	138	0	34	0	0	0.1	0.0	0	1%
lemon, 'Calippo'.	1 bar	112	0	28	0	0	0.1	0.0	0	1%
orange, 'Calippo'.	1 bar	111	0	27	0	0	0.2	0.0	0	2%
(Jell-O)										
all flavors nonfat, 'Gelatin Pops'	1 bar	35	1	8	25	0	0.0	0.0	0	0%
lemon, nonfat, 'Snowburst Bars'	1 bar	45	0	12	10	0	0.0	0.0	0	0%
orange, nonfat, 'Snowburst Bars'.	1 bar	45	0	12	10	0	0.0	0.0	0	0%
(Klondike Bar) vanilla, w/chocolate coating	1 bar	489	6	36	108	na	35.7	19.4	40	66%
(Kool-Aid)										
all flavors, 'Cream Pops'	1 bar	50	1	9	20	0	2.0	0.0	5	31%
all flavors, 'Kool Pumps'.	1 snack	80	1	16	25	0	1.0	0.0	5	12%
all flavors, nonfat, 'Kool Pops'	1 bar	40	0	10	10	0	0.0	0.0	0	0%
(Mama Tish's)										
Italian ice, cherry, made w/real fruit.	4 oz	120	0	29	0	0	0.0	0.0	0	0%
Italian ice, lemon, made w/real fruit.	4 oz	90	0	24	0	0	0.0	0.0	0	0%
Italian ice, strawberry, made w/real fruit	4 oz	80	1	21	5	0	0.0	0.0	0	0%
Italian ice, tropical, made w/real fruit.	4 oz	110	0	27	0	0	0.0	0.0	0	0%
(Popsicle)										
all flavors, 'All Natural'	1 bar	60	0	14	0	0	0.0	0.0	0	0%
all flavors, except cherry and wildberry, 'Water Ice'.	1 bar	50	0	12	10	0	0.0	0.0	0	0%
cherry, cola/cherry, 'Twister'.	1 piece	45	0	10	0	0	0.0	0.0	0	0%
cherry, 'Water Ice'	1 bar	70	0	17	15	0	0.0	0.0	0	0%
wildberry, 'Water Ice'	1 bar	40	0	10	10	0	0.0	0.0	0	0%
(Push-ups) assorted, orange, cherry, grape, 'Flintstones' . . .	1 tube	100	1	20	25	0	2.0	1.0	5	18%
(Tootsie Pop) assorted, cherry, grape, orange.	1 bar	70	2	13	32	0	1.0	1.0	4	13%
ITALIAN ICE										
(Luigi's)										
cherry	1 cup	120	1	28	10	0	0.0	0.0	0	0%
chocolate fudge.	1 cup	150	1	38	10	0	0.0	0.0	0	0%
grape	1 cup	110	0	26	10	0	0.0	0.0	0	0%
lemon	1 cup	110	1	25	10	0	0.0	0.0	0	0%
strawberry	1 cup	110	1	26	10	0	0.0	0.0	0	0%

ICE CREAM. See also ICE CREAM BAR/DESSERT; ICE CREAM CONE; ICE CREAM MIX; ICE CREAM SUBSTITUTE; ICE CREAM SUBSTITUTE BAR/DESSERT; ICE CREAM SUBSTITUTE MIX; ICE MILK.

Food Name	Serving Size	Calories	Prot. gms	Carbs gms	Sod. mgs	Fiber gms	Fat gms	Sat. Fat gms	Chol. mgs	% Fat Cal.
(Borden)										
butter pecan, 'Lady Borden'	1/2 cup	180	3	16	65	0	12.0	0.0	0	59%
chocolate swirl.	1/2 cup	130	2	18	65	0	6.0	0.0	0	40%
chocolate, Dutch, 'Olde Fashioned Recipe'.	1/2 cup	130	2	16	65	0	6.0	0.0	0	43%
strawberry	1/2 cup	130	2	18	55	0	6.0	0.0	0	40%
strawberry cream, 'Olde Fashioned Recipe'	1/2 cup	130	2	19	55	0	5.0	0.0	0	35%
vanilla, 'Olde Fashioned Recipe'.	1/2 cup	130	2	15	55	0	7.0	0.0	0	48%
(Breyers)										
butter almond	1/2 cup	170	4	15	125	0	10.0	4.0	25	54%
butter pecan	1/2 cup	180	3	15	125	0	12.0	5.0	25	60%
cherry vanilla.	1/2 cup	150	3	17	45	0	7.0	4.0	20	44%
chocolate.	1/2 cup	160	3	20	30	0	8.0	5.0	20	44%
chocolate chip	1/2 cup	170	3	18	45	0	10.0	0.0	35	52%
coffee	1/2 cup	150	3	16	50	0	8.0	5.0	30	49%

Food Name	Serving Size	Calories	Prot. gms	Carbs gms	Sod. mgs	Fiber gms	Fat gms	Sat. Fat gms	Chol. mgs	% Fat Cal.
cookies and cream	1/2 cup	170	3	19	60	0	9.0	5.0	20	48%
mint chocolate chip	1/2 cup	170	3	18	45	0	10.0	6.0	25	52%
mocha almond fudge	1/2 cup	190	4	20	60	0	10.0	0.0	0	48%
peach, natural	1/2 cup	130	2	18	35	0	6.0	3.0	15	40%
strawberry	1/2 cup	130	2	16	40	0	6.0	4.0	20	43%
vanilla	1/2 cup	150	3	15	50	0	8.0	5.0	25	50%
vanilla fudge twirl	1/2 cup	160	3	19	55	0	8.0	4.0	20	45%
vanilla-chocolate	1/2 cup	160	3	17	40	0	8.0	5.0	25	47%
vanilla-chocolate-strawberry	1/2 cup	150	3	17	40	0	8.0	4.0	20	47%
(Darigold)										
chocolate	1/2 cup	140	2	17	70	0	7.0	0.0	0	45%
chocolate, 'Alpine'	1/2 cup	140	2	17	70	0	7.0	0.0	0	45%
chocolate, 'Classic'	1/2 cup	180	3	16	30	0	13.0	0.0	0	61%
vanilla	1/2 cup	130	2	15	50	0	7.0	0.0	0	48%
vanilla, 'Alpine'	1/2 cup	130	2	15	50	0	7.0	0.0	0	48%
vanilla, 'Classic'	1/2 cup	180	2	16	40	0	12.0	0.0	0	60%
(Dreyer's/Edys)										
black cherry vanilla, fat-free	1/2 cup	100	3	22	45	na	0.0	0.0	0	0%
black cherry vanilla, sugar-free	1/2 cup	90	3	12	50	na	3.0	1.5	10	31%
butter pecan, light	1/2 cup	120	3	16	100	na	5.0	2.0	20	37%
caramel cream, dreamy, light	1/2 cup	110	2	18	60	na	3.0	2.0	20	25%
chocolate almond fudge, light	1/2 cup	120	3	16	45	na	5.0	2.0	20	37%
chocolate chip	1/2 cup	150	3	16	40	0	9.0	0.0	30	52%
chocolate fudge, fat-free	1/2 cup	110	3	25	55	na	0.0	0.0	0	0%
chocolate fudge mousse, light	1/2 cup	110	3	17	50	na	3.0	2.0	20	25%
cookie dough, light	1/2 cup	130	3	19	75	na	5.0	2.5	20	34%
cookies and cream	1/2 cup	160	3	18	80	0	9.0	0.0	28	49%
cookies and cream, light	1/2 cup	120	3	17	65	na	4.0	2.0	20	31%
espresso fudge chip, light	1/2 cup	120	3	18	60	na	4.0	2.5	15	30%
'French Silk' light	1/2 cup	120	3	19	55	na	4.0	2.5	15	29%
fudge, marble	1/2 cup	150	3	18	50	0	8.0	0.0	28	46%
marble fudge, fat-free	1/2 cup	110	3	24	55	na	0.0	0.0	0	0%
marble fudge, sugar-free	1/2 cup	90	3	13	60	na	3.0	1.5	10	30%
mint fudge, fat free	1/2 cup	110	3	24	55	na	0.0	0.0	0	0%
mocha fudge, sugar-free	1/2 cup	90	3	13	60	na	3.0	1.5	10	30%
peanut butter cup, light	1/2 cup	130	3	17	55	na	5.0	2.5	20	36%
raspberry vanilla, fat free, sugar-free	1/2 cup	90	3	19	45	na	0.0	0.0	0	0%
rocky road	1/2 cup	170	3	18	30	0	10.0	0.0	30	52%
rocky road, light	1/2 cup	120	3	17	45	na	4.0	2.0	20	31%
strawberry, sugar-free	1/2 cup	80	3	11	50	na	3.0	1.5	10	33%
triple chocolate, sugar-free	1/2 cup	100	3	13	60	Fiber	3.5	1.5	10	33%
vanilla	1/2 cup	160	2	14	30	0	10.0	0.0	40	58%
vanilla, fat-free	1/2 cup	100	3	22	45	na	0.0	0.0	0	0%
vanilla, light	1/2 cup	100	3	15	50	na	3.0	2.0	20	27%
vanilla, sugar-free	1/2 cup	80	3	11	55	na	3.0	1.5	10	33%
vanilla and caramel, sugar-free	1/2 cup	90	3	13	60	na	3.0	1.5	10	30%
vanilla-chocolate, fat free, sugar-free	1/2 cup	100	4	20	50	na	0.0	0.0	0	0%
(Eagle Brand) vanilla, 'Homestyle'	1/2 cup	150	3	16	55	0	9.0	0.0	20	52%
(Eskimo Pie) chocolate chip cone, 'Cookie Dough'	1 cone	280	4	33	103	0	14.0	0.0	14	46%
(Frusen Gladje)										
butter pecan	1/2 cup	280	5	16	160	0	21.0	0.0	85	69%
chocolate chocolate chip	1/2 cup	270	5	21	60	0	18.0	9.0	55	61%
chocolate	1/2 cup	240	5	17	65	0	17.0	9.0	75	63%
chocolate, Swiss candy almond	1/2 cup	270	6	18	60	0	19.0	9.0	55	64%

Food Name	Serving Size	Calories	Prot. gms	Carbs gms	Sod. mgs	Fiber gms	Fat gms	Sat. Fat gms	Chol. mgs	% Fat Cal.
strawberry	1/2 cup	230	4	20	60	0	15.0	10.0	65	58%
vanilla	1/2 cup	230	5	16	70	0	17.0	9.0	65	65%
vanilla Swiss almond	1/2 cup	270	6	18	65	0	19.0	9.0	65	64%
vanilla toffee chunk	1/2 cup	270	5	22	160	0	17.0	0.0	85	59%
(Good Humor)										
vanilla, 'Cup'	3 oz	98	2	12	35	0	5.1	0.0	0	47%
vanilla-chocolate cup, 'Combo'	6 oz	201	4	26	80	0	9.2	0.0	0	41%
(Haagen-Dazs)										
caramel nut sundae	1/2 cup	310	5	26	100	0	21.0	0.0	0	60%
chocolate fudge, deep	1/2 cup	290	5	26	70	0	14.0	0.0	0	50%
chocolate mint	1/2 cup	300	5	26	50	0	20.0	0.0	0	59%
chocolate, deep	1/2 cup	290	5	26	70	0	14.0	0.0	0	50%
chocolate, low-fat	1/2 cup	170	7	29	50	1	2.5	1.5	30	14%
chocolate-peanut butter, deep	1/2 cup	330	7	25	90	0	19.0	0.0	0	57%
coffee fudge, low-fat	1/2 cup	170	5	32	95	0	2.5	1.5	25	13%
'Cookie Dough Dynamo'	4 oz	300	4	31	110	0	18.0	0.0	0	54%
strawberry, low-fat	1/2 cup	150	5	28	40	0	2.0	1.0	15	12%
vanilla, low-fat	1/2 cup	170	7	29	50	0	2.5	1.5	20	14%
vanilla honey	1/2 cup	250	5	22	55	0	16.0	8.0	135	57%
vanilla-peanut butter swirl	1/2 cup	280	5	19	120	0	21.0	8.0	110	66%
(Healthy Choice)										
Black Forest, low-fat	1/2 cup	120	3	23	50	1	2.0	1.0	5	15%
Bordeaux cherry, 'Dairy Dessert'	4 oz	120	3	23	50	0	2.0	1.0	5	15%
Bordeaux cherry chocolate chip 'Dairy Dessert'	4 oz	120	3	23	50	0	2.0	1.0	5	15%
butter pecan crunch, low-fat	1/2 cup	120	3	22	60	1	2.0	1.0	3	15%
cappuccino chocolate chunk, low-fat	1/2 cup	120	3	22	60	1	2.0	1.0	10	15%
cappuccino mocha fudge, low-fat	1/2 cup	120	3	23	50	1	2.0	1.0	3	15%
chocolate, 'Dairy Dessert'	4 oz	130	3	24	70	0	2.0	1.0	5	14%
chocolate chip, 'Dairy Dessert'	4 oz	130	3	24	70	0	2.0	1.0	5	14%
coffee toffee, 'Dairy Dessert'	4 oz	130	3	25	80	0	2.0	1.0	5	14%
cookies and cream, low-fat	1/2 cup	120	3	21	90	1	2.0	1.0	3	16%
double fudge swirl, 'Dairy Dessert'	4 oz	130	3	24	70	0	2.0	1.0	5	14%
fudge brownie, low-fat	1/2 cup	120	3	22	55	1	2.0	1.0	5	15%
fudge brownie à la mode, low-fat	1/2 cup	120	3	22	55	1	2.0	1.0	5	15%
mint chocolate chip, low-fat	1/2 cup	120	3	21	50	1	2.0	1.0	3	16%
Neapolitan, 'Dairy Dessert'	4 oz	120	3	22	60	0	2.0	1.0	5	15%
praline and caramel, low-fat	1/2 cup	130	3	25	70	1	2.0	0.5	3	14%
praline caramel cluster, low-fat	1/2 cup	130	3	25	70	1	2.0	0.5	3	14%
raspberry swirl, 'Dairy Dessert'	4 oz	120	3	23	60	0	2.0	1.0	5	15%
rocky road, 'Dairy Dessert'	4 oz	160	3	32	70	0	2.0	1.0	5	11%
strawberry, 'Dairy Dessert'	4 oz	120	2	23	50	0	2.0	1.0	5	14%
turtle fudge cake, low-fat	1/2 cup	130	3	25	60	2	2.0	1.0	3	15%
vanilla, 'Dairy Dessert'	4 oz	120	4	21	60	0	2.0	1.0	5	15%
vanilla, old fashioned, 'Dairy Dessert'	4 oz	120	4	21	60	0	2.0	1.0	5	15%
(Nutra/Balance) high-calorie and -protein	1 serving	232	7	25	79	0	12.0	7.5	46	46%
(Sealtest)										
butter crunch	1/2 cup	150	2	18	90	0	7.0	4.0	25	44%
butter pecan	1/2 cup	160	3	16	125	0	9.0	4.0	15	52%
chocolate	1/2 cup	140	2	18	50	0	6.0	4.0	20	40%
chocolate chip	1/2 cup	150	2	17	50	0	8.0	0.0	15	49%
chocolate triple stripes	1/2 cup	140	2	17	50	0	7.0	0.0	0	45%
chocolate-marshmallow sundae	1/2 cup	150	2	21	40	0	6.0	4.0	20	37%
coffee	1/2 cup	140	2	16	50	0	7.0	4.0	15	47%
fudge Royale	1/2 cup	140	3	19	55	0	7.0	4.0	15	42%

Food Name	Serving Size	Calories	Prot. gms	Carbs gms	Sod. mgs	Fiber gms	Fat gms	Sat. Fat gms	Chol. mgs	% Fat Cal.
heavenly hash	1/2 cup	150	2	19	50	0	7.0	4.0	15	43%
maple walnut	1/2 cup	160	3	17	40	0	9.0	3.0	20	50%
peanut fudge sundae	1/2 cup	140	3	17	50	0	7.0	4.0	20	44%
strawberry	1/2 cup	130	2	18	40	0	5.0	3.0	15	36%
vanilla	1/2 cup	140	2	16	50	0	7.0	4.0	20	47%
vanilla, French	1/2 cup	140	2	16	50	0	7.0	0.0	35	47%
vanilla-chocolate-strawberry 'Cubic Scoops'	1/2 cup	130	2	17	50	0	6.0	3.0	20	42%
vanilla-chocolate-strawberry	1/2 cup	140	2	18	50	0	6.0	3.0	20	40%
vanilla-orange sherbet, 'Cubic Scoops'	1/2 cup	130	2	22	40	0	4.0	2.0	15	27%
vanilla-red raspberry sherbet, 'Cubic Scoops'	1/2 cup	130	2	22	40	0	4.0	2.0	15	27%
(TCBY Treats)										
all flavors, hand-dipped	1/2 cup	140	2	17	60	0	7.0	4.0	25	45%
all flavors, hand-dipped, low-fat, no added sugar	1/2 cup	100	3	19	60	0	2.5	1.5	10	20%
all flavors, hand-dipped, nonfat	1/2 cup	100	2	23	50	1	0.0	0.0	0	0%
(Weight Watchers)										
chocolate chip, 'ONE-ders'	4 oz	120	3	19	80	0	4.0	0.0	10	29%
'Cookie Dough Craze'	1/2 cup	140	3	24	85	1	3.5	2.0	5	23%
heavenly hash 'ONE-ders'	4 oz	130	4	22	90	0	3.0	2.0	10	21%
'Oh! So Very Vanilla' light	1/2 cup	120	4	20	65	1	2.5	1.5	5	19%
'Positively Praline Crunch' light	1/2 cup	140	3	25	105	0	3.0	1.5	5	19%
pralines and creme, 'ONE-ders'	4 oz	120	3	19	110	0	4.0	0.0	10	29%
'Reckless Rocky Road'	1/2 cup	140	4	23	75	1	3.0	1.5	5	20%
'Triple Chocolate Tornado' light	1/2 cup	150	4	26	80	1	3.5	1.5	5	21%

ICE CREAM BAR/DESSERT
BAR

Food Name	Serving Size	Calories	Prot. gms	Carbs gms	Sod. mgs	Fiber gms	Fat gms	Sat. Fat gms	Chol. mgs	% Fat Cal.
(Baker's)										
chocolate fudge sundae 'Fudgetastic'	1 bar	220	3	23	45	0	15.0	0.0	20	56%
chocolate fudge sundae, crunchy, 'Fudgetastic'	1 bar	230	3	24	40	0	14.0	0.0	20	54%
(Eskimo Pie)										
vanilla, w/dark chocolate coating	1 bar	180	2	16	35	0	12.0	0.0	0	60%
vanilla, w/milk chocolate coating	1 bar	190	5	18	16	0	12.0	0.0	0	54%
vanilla, w/milk chocolate coating, almonds	1 bar	140	3	12	35	0	13.0	0.0	0	66%
vanilla, w/milk chocolate coating, crisp rice	1 bar	150	4	12	40	0	11.0	0.0	0	61%
(Freezer Pleezer) vanilla, w/chocolate flavored coating	1 bar	140	2	13	25	1	9.0	7.0	15	57%
(Good Humor)										
'Fat Frog'	1 bar	154	2	16	36	0	9.2	0.0	0	54%
'Halo Bar'	1 bar	230	4	23	64	0	13.7	0.0	0	54%
'Whammy' assorted flavors	1 bar	95	1	7	17	0	7.2	0.0	0	69%
chip candy crunch	1 bar	255	2	21	40	0	17.9	0.0	0	63%
chocolate éclair	1 bar	188	2	23	54	0	9.9	0.0	0	47%
chocolate fudge cake	1 bar	214	2	18	50	0	15.0	0.0	0	63%
strawberry shortcake	1 bar	176	2	24	88	0	8.2	0.0	0	42%
toasted almond	1 bar	212	2	24	34	0	11.8	0.0	0	50%
vanilla, w/chocolate flavor coating	1 bar	198	2	17	44	0	13.7	0.0	0	62%
(Haagen-Dazs)										
caramel almond, 'Crunch Bar'	1 bar	240	3	17	65	0	18.0	7.0	40	67%
peanut butter, 'Crunch Bar'	1 bar	270	6	16	55	0	21.0	7.0	35	68%
vanilla, 'Crunch Bar'	1 bar	220	3	16	55	0	16.0	6.0	40	65%
vanilla, w/milk chocolate-brittle coating	1 bar	370	5	32	160	0	25.0	0.0	0	60%
(Heath) 1 bar	1 bar	170	3	16	155	0	13.0	0.0	0	61%
(Klondike)										
chocolate	1 bar	270	4	23	60	0	19.0	0.0	0	61%
'Krispy'	1 bar	290	4	26	70	0	19.0	0.0	0	59%
'Lite'	1 bar	140	3	10	45	0	10.0	0.0	10	63%

Food Name	Serving Size	Calories	Prot. gms	Carbs gms	Sod. mgs	Fiber gms	Fat gms	Sat. Fat gms	Chol. mgs	% Fat Cal.
w/chocolate flavored coating, 'Lite'	1 bar	110	3	14	50	0	6.0	5.0	5	44%
(Natural Nectar)										
banana cream, 'Stick Novelties'	1 bar	170	3	22	70	0	8.0	0.0	20	42%
cocoa fudge and cream, 'Stick Novelties'	1 bar	170	3	22	70	0	8.0	0.0	20	42%
strawberries and cream, 'Stick Novelties'	1 bar	120	2	18	40	0	5.0	0.0	15	36%
wildberry cream, 'Stick Novelties'	1 bar	120	2	22	50	0	3.0	0.0	15	22%
(Nestlé)										
chocolate, w/milk chocolate coating, 'Quik'	1 bar	210	3	19	40	0	14.0	0.0	0	59%
milk chocolate, w/almonds, milk chocolate coated	1 bar	350	6	28	45	0	23.0	0.0	5	60%
vanilla, w/chocolate coating, crisp rice, 'Crunch'	1 bar	180	2	15	0	0	13.0	0.0	0	63%
vanilla, w/chocolate coating, crisp rice, 'Crunch Lite'	1 bar	120	2	16	50	0	5.0	0.0	0	38%
vanilla, w/white chocolate coating, 'Alpine Premium'	1 bar	350	6	25	50	0	25.0	0.0	5	64%
(Oh Henry!)										
vanilla, w/caramel peanut, milk chocolate coating	1 bar	320	1	34	75	0	20.0	0.0	0	56%
(Weight Watchers)										
chocolate, 'Treat Bars'	1 bar	100	4	18	75	0	1.0	0.0	0	9%
chocolate fudge, double	1 bar	60	3	12	50	0	1.0	0.0	5	13%
chocolate mousse, sugar-free	1 bar	35	2	9	30	0	1.0	0.0	5	17%
CONE										
(Good Humor)										
'King Cone'	5.5 oz	290	5	41	119	0	12.0	0.0	0	37%
boysenberry, 'King Cone'	5 oz	340	4	52	151	0	13.1	0.0	0	35%
NOVELTY										
(Carnation)										
vanilla nuggets, w/dark chocolate coating, 'Bon Bons'	5 pieces	170	2	15	50	0	11.0	0.0	14	59%
vanilla nuggets, w/milk chocolate coating, 'Bon Bons'	5 pieces	165	2	14	50	0	11.0	0.0	16	61%
(Natural Nectar)										
mocha 'Round Novelties'	4 oz	300	4	40	135	0	14.0	0.0	10	42%
nectar 'Round Novelties'	4 oz	300	4	38	120	0	15.0	0.0	15	45%
SANDWICH										
(Eskimo Pie) vanilla, w/chocolate wafer	1 sandwich	170	4	26	142	0	6.0	0.0	0	31%
(Good Humor)										
vanilla	1 sandwich	191	4	31	155	0	5.7	0.0	0	27%
vanilla, w/chocolate chip cookie	1 sandwich	246	3	35	181	0	10.5	0.0	0	38%
(Klondike)										
vanilla, 'Lite'	1 sandwich	100	2	18	110	0	2.0	1.0	5	18%
vanilla	1 sandwich	230	5	33	220	0	9.0	0.0	0	35%
(Weight Watchers)										
sandwich snack	1 sandwich	90	2	17	120	0	2.0	0.0	0	19%
vanilla	1 sandwich	150	3	28	170	0	3.0	2.0	5	18%
ICE CREAM CONE										
(Bozo)										
cake cup	1 cone	16	1	3	13	0	0.0	0.0	0	0%
sugar	1 cone	53	1	11	29	0	1.0	0.1	0	16%
(Comet)										
sugar	1 cone	50	1	11	40	0	0.0	0.0	0	0%
waffle	1 cone	70	1	14	30	1	0.5	0.0	0	7%
(Ener-G Foods) gluten free	1 cone	154	0	36	1	1	1.1	0.4	0	7%
(Joy)	1 cone	16	1	3	5	0	1.0	1.0	0	36%
(Keebler)										
cup, assorted colors	1 cone	15	1	4	20	0	1.0	1.0	0	31%
cup, large, food service product	1 serving	15	0	4	20	0	0.0	0.0	0	1%
plain	1 cone	15	1	4	20	0	1.0	1.0	0	31%
sugar	1 cone	45	1	11	35	0	1.0	1.0	0	16%

Food Name	Serving Size	Calories	Prot. gms	Carbs gms	Sod. mgs	Fiber gms	Fat gms	Sat. Fat gms	Chol. mgs	% Fat Cal.
sugar, food service product..........................	1 serving	47	1	10	28	0	0.2	0.1	0	4%
waffle bowl, large, food service product	1 serving	60	1	12	20	0	1.5	0.3	1	21%
waffle cone, large, food service product	1 serving	100	2	20	35	0	2.0	0.5	0	17%
(Little Debbie) plain, 'Ice Cream Cup'	1 cone	15	0	3	15	0	0.1	0.0	1	6%
(Nabisco)										
cup	1 cone	18	1	4	5	0	1.0	0.0	0	31%
cup, 'Comet'.	1 cone	18	1	4	5	0	1.0	0.0	0	31%
sugar	1 cone	50	1	11	40	0	1.0	0.0	0	16%
ICE CREAM MIX										
(Salada)										
Dutch chocolate, mix only	1 oz	110	1	26	20	0	0.0	0.0	0	0%
Dutch chocolate, prepared	1 cup	310	4	31	75	0	19.0	0.0	0	55%
peach, vanilla, mix only	1 oz	110	0	27	10	0	0.0	0.0	0	0%
peach, vanilla, prepared	1 cup	310	4	32	60	0	18.0	0.0	0	53%
peach, wild strawberry, mix only	1 oz	110	0	27	10	0	0.0	0.0	0	0%
peach, wild strawberry, prepared	1 cup	310	4	32	60	0	18.0	0.0	0	53%
ICE CREAM SANDWICH. See under ICE CREAM BAR/DESSERT.										
ICE CREAM SUBSTITUTE. See also YOGURT, FROZEN.										
(Freezees Nutcreem)										
butter pecan, nondairy, 100% natural	3 oz	131	4	17	78	0	7.0	0.0	0	43%
cashew vanilla, nondairy, 100% natural	3 oz	131	4	17	78	0	7.0	0.0	0	43%
lemon, nondairy, 100% natural	3 oz	131	4	17	78	0	7.0	0.0	0	43%
orange, nondairy, 100% natural	3 oz	131	4	17	78	0	7.0	0.0	0	43%
peanut, nondairy, 100% natural, 'Delight'	3 oz	131	4	17	78	0	7.0	0.0	0	43%
strawberry, nondairy, 100% natural.	3 oz	131	4	17	78	0	7.0	0.0	0	43%
(Ice Bean)										
almond espresso, nondairy.	4 oz	150	3	13	60	0	10.0	0.0	0	58%
chocolate, nondairy, nonfat, 'Thunder'.	1/2 cup	110	1	27	30	1	0.0	0.0	0	0%
peanut butter carob chip, nondairy	4 oz	200	3	18	100	0	13.0	0.0	0	58%
'Raspberry Patch' nondairy, nonfat	1/2 cup	110	1	27	30	1	0.0	0.0	0	0%
'Vanilla Wavy' nondairy, nonfat	1/2 cup	110	1	27	30	1	0.0	0.0	0	0%
(Living Rightly)										
almond pecan, nondairy	1/2 cup	140	3	21	75	0	5.0	0.0	0	32%
carob peppermint, nondairy	1/2 cup	100	2	21	30	0	1.5	0.0	0	13%
chocolate almond, nondairy	1/2 cup	140	3	21	75	0	5.0	0.0	0	32%
vanilla, nondairy	1/2 cup	110	2	22	15	0	1.0	0.0	0	9%
vanilla Swiss almond, nondairy.	1/2 cup	140	3	21	75	0	5.0	0.0	0	32%
(Low, Lite 'n Luscious)										
chocolate chip.	1/2 cup	100	3	19	80	0	2.0	0.0	4	17%
Jamoca Swiss almond	1/2 cup	90	3	19	100	0	2.0	0.0	4	17%
pineapple coconut.	1/2 cup	90	3	19	70	0	1.0	0.0	3	9%
strawberry	1/2 cup	80	3	17	70	0	1.0	0.0	3	10%
(Mocha Mix)										
strawberry swirl, nondairy, 100% milk-free	1/2 cup	140	1	20	55	0	6.0	1.5	0	39%
vanilla, nondairy, 100% milk-free.	1/2 cup	140	1	18	70	0	7.0	1.5	0	45%
(Rice Dream)										
cappuccino flavor, nondairy.	1/2 cup	130	1	17	80	0	5.0	0.0	0	38%
carob almond, nondairy	1/2 cup	140	1	20	85	2	6.0	0.5	0	39%
carob chip, nondairy	1/2 cup	130	1	20	70	1	6.0	1.0	0	39%
carob, nondairy	1/2 cup	130	1	20	80	0	5.0	0.0	0	35%
cocoa marble fudge, nondairy.	1/2 cup	140	1	19	80	0	6.0	0.0	0	40%
cookies and cream, nondairy	1/2 cup	130	1	21	80	0	5.0	0.0	0	34%
lemon, nondairy	1/2 cup	130	1	17	80	0	5.0	0.0	0	38%
mint carob chip, nondairy	1/2 cup	130	1	20	70	1	6.0	1.0	0	39%

Food Name	Serving Size	Calories	Prot. gms	Carbs gms	Sod. mgs	Fiber gms	Fat gms	Sat. Fat gms	Chol. mgs	% Fat Cal.
Neapolitan, nondairy	1/2 cup	130	1	21	80	0	5.0	0.0	0	34%
peanut butter cup, nondairy	1/2 cup	130	2	21	75	1	6.0	1.0	0	37%
peanut butter fudge, nondairy	1/2 cup	160	3	19	100	0	7.0	0.0	0	42%
vanilla fudge, nondairy	1/2 cup	130	1	20	70	1	5.0	0.5	0	35%
vanilla Swiss almond, nondairy	1/2 cup	130	1	20	70	1	6.0	0.5	0	39%
vanilla, nondairy	1/2 cup	130	1	19	70	1	5.0	0.5	0	36%
wildberry, nondairy	1/2 cup	130	1	17	80	0	5.0	0.0	0	38%
(Sealtest)										
black cherry, nonfat, 'Free'	1/2 cup	100	2	25	45	0	0.0	0.0	0	0%
chocolate, nonfat, 'Free'	1/2 cup	100	3	23	50	0	0.0	0.0	0	0%
peach, nonfat, 'Free'	1/2 cup	100	2	23	45	0	0.0	0.0	0	0%
strawberry, nonfat, 'Free'	1/2 cup	100	2	23	40	0	0.0	0.0	0	0%
vanilla, nonfat, 'Free'	1/2 cup	100	3	24	45	0	0.0	0.0	0	0%
vanilla-chocolate strawberry, nonfat, 'Free'	1/2 cup	100	3	23	40	0	0.0	0.0	0	0%
vanilla-fudge royale, nonfat, 'Free'	1/2 cup	100	3	24	50	0	0.0	0.0	0	0%
vanilla-strawberry royale, nonfat, 'Free'	1/2 cup	100	3	25	35	0	0.0	0.0	0	0%
(Simple Pleasures)										
chocolate	1/2 cup	140	9	25	15	0	1.0	0.3	0	6%
coffee	4 oz	120	8	22	15	0	1.0	0.3	0	7%
peach	4 oz	135	9	24	5	0	1.0	0.3	0	6%
rum raisin	4 oz	130	7	25	10	0	1.0	0.3	0	7%
strawberry	4 oz	120	8	22	55	0	1.0	0.3	11	7%
(Sweet Nothings)										
berry blackberry, nondairy, nonfat	1/2 cup	110	0	26	10	0	0.0	0.0	0	0%
'Black Leopard' nondairy, nonfat	1/2 cup	100	1	23	5	0	0.0	0.0	0	0%
chocolate Mandarin, nondairy, nonfat	1/2 cup	100	1	23	5	0	0.0	0.0	0	0%
chocolate, nondairy, nonfat	1/2 cup	100	1	23	5	0	0.0	0.0	0	0%
espresso fudge, nondairy, nonfat	1/2 cup	110	1	25	5	0	0.0	0.0	0	0%
mango raspberry, nondairy, nonfat	1/2 cup	110	0	26	10	0	0.0	0.0	0	0%
raspberry swirl, nondairy, nonfat	1/2 cup	110	0	26	10	0	0.0	0.0	0	0%
'Tiger Stripes' nondairy, nonfat	1/2 cup	110	1	25	5	0	0.0	0.0	0	0%
vanilla, nondairy, nonfat	1/2 cup	110	1	25	5	0	0.0	0.0	0	0%
(Tofutti)										
all flavors, 'Lite Lite'	1/2 cup	90	2	20	80	0	1.0	0.0	0	9%
all flavors, nondairy, 'Fruitti'	1/2 cup	100	2	20	90	na	0.0	0.0	0	0%
butter pecan, nondairy	1 fl oz	55	0	6	50	0	3.3	0.5	0	56%
chocolate cookie, nondairy, 'Supreme'	1 fl oz	53	1	7	25	0	2.8	0.5	0	46%
chocolate fudge, nondairy, 'Better Than Yogurt'	1/2 cup	120	2	25	98	0	2.0	1.0	0	14%
chocolate supreme, nondairy	1/2 cup	210	3	20	130	0	13.0	3.0	0	56%
coffee marshmallow, nondairy, 'Better Than Yogurt'	1/2 cup	100	1	24	77	0	1.0	0.0	0	8%
passion island fruit, nondairy, 'Better Than Yogurt'	1/2 cup	100	1	21	100	0	1.0	0.0	0	9%
peach mango, nondairy, 'Better Than Yogurt'	1/2 cup	100	1	23	102	0	1.0	0.0	0	9%
strawberry banana, nondairy, 'Better Than Yogurt'	1/2 cup	100	1	23	92	0	1.0	0.0	0	9%
vanilla almond bark, nondairy	1 fl oz	53	1	5	33	0	3.3	0.5	0	55%
vanilla fudge, nondairy, 'Better Than Yogurt'	1/2 cup	120	2	24	90	0	2.0	0.0	0	15%
vanilla, nondairy	1 fl oz	48	1	5	53	0	2.8	0.5	0	53%
'Wildberry Supreme' nondairy	1 fl oz	48	1	6	48	0	2.3	0.5	0	44%
(Weight Watchers)										
'Arctic D'Lights'	1 serving	130	3	14	20	0	7.0	3.5	5	48%
berries 'n creme mousse	1 serving	35	2	4	38	1	0.8	0.0	0	25%
chocolate, nonfat	1/2 cup	80	3	19	75	0	0.0	0.0	5	0%
chocolate swirl, nonfat	1/2 cup	90	3	22	75	0	0.0	0.0	5	0%
chocolate treat	1 serving	100	3	21	150	1	1.0	0.0	10	9%

Food Name	Serving Size	Calories	Prot. gms	Carbs gms	Sod. mgs	Fiber gms	Fat gms	Sat. Fat gms	Chol. mgs	% Fat Cal.
Neapolitan, nonfat	1/2 cup	80	3	19	75	0	0.0	0.0	5	0%
vanilla, nonfat	1/2 cup	80	3	20	75	0	0.0	0.0	5	0%

ICE CREAM SUBSTITUTE BAR/DESSERT. See also YOGURT BAR, FROZEN

BAR

(Crystal Light)

Food Name	Serving Size	Calories	Prot. gms	Carbs gms	Sod. mgs	Fiber gms	Fat gms	Sat. Fat gms	Chol. mgs	% Fat Cal.
Amaretto chocolate swirl, 'Cool N'Creamy'	1 bar	60	2	10	60	0	2.0	0.0	0	27%
chocolate vanilla, 'Cool N'Creamy'	1 bar	50	2	7	55	0	2.0	0.0	0	33%
double chocolate fudge, 'Cool N'Creamy'	1 bar	50	2	7	60	0	2.0	0.0	0	33%
orange vanilla, 'Cool N'Creamy'	1 bar	30	1	5	25	0	1.0	0.0	0	27%
(Freezer Pleezer)										
fudge flavored	1 bar	100	2	20	75	1	1.0	0.5	5	9%
orange cream treats	1 bar	80	1	16	20	1	1.5	1.0	10	17%
(Good Humor)										
chocolate fudge	1 bar	127	4	27	91	0	0.6	0.0	0	4%
'Cool Shark'	1 bar	68	0	17	7	0	0.1	0.0	0	1%
'Jumbo Jet Star'	1 bar	85	0	20	0	0	0.7	0.0	0	7%
'Milky Pop'	1 bar	45	1	8	25	0	0.0	0.0	0	0%
strawberry finger	1 bar	49	0	12	0	0	0.1	0.0	0	2%
(Light n' Lively)										
chocolate mousse, nonfat	1 bar	50	2	12	45	0	0.0	0.0	0	0%
double chocolate fudge, nonfat	1 bar	50	2	11	45	0	0.0	0.0	0	0%
orange vanilla, nonfat	1 bar	40	1	10	15	0	0.0	0.0	0	0%
strawberry, nonfat	1 bar	80	2	12	25	0	0.0	0.0	0	0%
vanilla, chocolate dipped	1 bar	110	2	14	35	0	6.0	0.0	0	46%
(Rice Dream)										
chocolate, nondairy	1 bar	270	1	33	115	0	16.0	0.0	0	51%
chocolate, nutty, nondairy	1 bar	330	5	29	110	0	23.0	0.0	0	60%
strawberry, nondairy	1 bar	260	1	31	110	0	14.8	0.0	0	51%
vanilla, nondairy	1 bar	275	1	33	120	0	15.8	0.0	0	51%
vanilla, nutty, nondairy	1 bar	330	5	29	100	0	23.0	0.0	0	60%
(Sealtest)										
chocolate, w/fudge swirl, nonfat, 'Free'	1 bar	80	3	19	55	0	0.0	0.0	0	0%
vanilla, w/fudge swirl, nonfat, 'Free'	1 bar	80	2	18	55	0	0.0	0.0	0	0%
vanilla, w/strawberry swirl, nonfat, 'Free'	1 bar	70	2	17	60	0	0.0	0.0	0	0%
(Trix)										
assorted flavors, nonfat	1 bar	40	0	10	0	0	0.0	0.0	0	0%
'Fudge N' Fruity'	1 bar	80	2	17	60	0	1.0	0.0	5	11%
(Weight Watchers)										
chocolate dip	1 bar	100	3	21	150	1	1.0	0.0	10	9%
'Crispy Pralines & Creme'	1 bar	120	2	13	45	0	6.0	2.0	5	47%

NOVELTY

(Rice Dream)

Food Name	Serving Size	Calories	Prot. gms	Carbs gms	Sod. mgs	Fiber gms	Fat gms	Sat. Fat gms	Chol. mgs	% Fat Cal.
'Dream Pie' mint, nondairy	1 pie	380	3	47	225	0	19.0	0.0	0	46%
'Dream Pie' vanilla, nondairy	1 pie	380	3	47	225	0	19.0	0.0	0	46%
(Tofutti)										
'Love Drops' cappuccino flavored	1/2 cup	230	3	26	120	0	12.0	3.0	0	48%
'Love Drops' chocolate	1/2 cup	230	3	26	100	0	13.0	5.0	0	50%
'Love Drops' vanilla	1/2 cup	220	3	26	100	0	12.0	3.0	0	48%
'Q's' vanilla, chocolate dipped	1 piece	40	1	4	20	0	2.0	0.0	0	47%
(Weight Watchers)										
'ONE-ders' brownies and creme	4 oz	130	4	20	115	0	4.0	0.0	10	27%
parfait, double fudge brownie	1 serving	190	6	39	170	2	2.5	2.0	5	11%
parfait, praline toffee crunch	1 serving	190	5	40	140	2	3.0	2.0	5	13%
parfait, strawberry royale	1 serving	180	5	35	100	0	2.0	1.0	10	10%

Food Name	Serving Size	Calories	Prot. gms	Carbs gms	Sod. mgs	Fiber gms	Fat gms	Sat. Fat gms	Chol. mgs	% Fat Cal.
SUNDAE										
(Weight Watchers)										
chocolate chip cookie dough	1 serving	180	3	33	115	2	4.0	1.5	5	20%
hot caramel fudge	4.5 oz	160	5	27	140	0	4.0	2.0	15	22%
hot chocolate fudge	4.5 oz	160	6	26	115	0	4.0	2.0	15	22%
hot mocha fudge	4.5 oz	160	5	24	120	0	5.0	2.0	15	28%
ICE CREAM SUBSTITUTE MIX										
(Tofutti)										
soft serve	1 oz	48	1	5	24	0	1.0	0.3	0	29%
soft serve, light	1 oz	23	1	5	20	0	0.3	0.0	0	9%
ICE MILK										
(Borden)										
chocolate	1/2 cup	100	3	18	80	0	2.0	0.0	0	18%
strawberry	1/2 cup	90	2	17	65	0	2.0	0.0	0	19%
vanilla	1/2 cup	90	2	17	60	0	2.0	0.0	0	19%
(Breyers)										
chocolate, 'Light'	1/2 cup	120	3	18	55	0	4.0	2.0	15	30%
chocolate chocolate chip, 'Light'	1/2 cup	140	4	20	55	0	5.0	0.0	25	32%
chocolate fudge twirl, 'Light'	1/2 cup	130	4	21	60	0	4.0	2.0	10	26%
heavenly hash, 'Light'	1/2 cup	150	3	21	55	0	5.0	3.0	10	32%
praline almond, 'Light'	1/2 cup	130	3	19	70	0	5.0	2.0	10	34%
strawberry, 'Light'	1/2 cup	110	3	18	50	0	3.0	2.0	15	24%
Swiss almond fudge twirl	1/2 cup	150	4	21	65	0	6.0	3.0	0	35%
toffee fudge parfait, 'Light'	1/2 cup	140	3	22	90	0	5.0	3.0	10	31%
vanilla, 'Light'	1/2 cup	120	3	18	60	0	4.0	2.0	10	30%
vanilla-chocolate-strawberry, 'Light'	1/2 cup	120	3	18	55	0	4.0	2.0	15	30%
vanilla-raspberry parfait, 'Light'	1/2 cup	130	3	23	50	0	3.0	2.0	15	21%
(Darigold)										
chocolate, 'Lite'	1/2 cup	110	3	19	65	0	3.0	0.0	0	23%
vanilla	1/2 cup	110	2	18	66	0	3.0	0.0	0	25%
(Light n' Lively)										
caramel nut	1/2 cup	120	3	18	85	0	4.0	2.0	10	30%
chocolate chip	1/2 cup	120	3	18	35	0	4.0	3.0	10	30%
coffee	1/2 cup	100	3	16	40	0	3.0	1.0	10	26%
cookies and cream	1/2 cup	110	3	18	65	0	3.0	2.0	10	24%
heavenly hash	1/2 cup	120	3	20	35	0	4.0	2.0	10	28%
vanilla	1/2 cup	100	3	16	40	0	3.0	2.0	10	26%
vanilla, w/chocolate covered almonds	1/2 cup	120	3	17	45	0	4.0	1.0	10	31%
vanilla-chocolate-strawberry	1/2 cup	100	2	17	35	0	3.0	2.0	10	26%
vanilla-fudge twirl	1/2 cup	110	3	18	45	0	3.0	2.0	10	24%
vanilla-raspberry swirl	1/2 cup	110	3	19	35	0	3.0	1.0	10	23%
(Ponderosa)										
chocolate	3.5 oz	152	4	30	70	0	2.9	0.0	22	16%
vanilla	3.5 oz	150	4	30	58	0	2.6	0.0	20	15%
(Weight Watchers)										
chocolate, 'Grand Collection'	1/2 cup	110	4	18	75	0	3.0	2.0	10	23%
chocolate chip, 'Grand Collection'	1/2 cup	120	3	19	75	0	4.0	2.0	10	29%
chocolate swirl, 'Grand Collection'	1/2 cup	120	3	19	75	0	3.0	2.0	5	23%
Neapolitan, 'Grand Collection'	1/2 cup	110	3	18	75	0	3.0	1.0	10	24%
pecan pralines and creme, 'Grand Collection'	1/2 cup	120	3	20	80	0	4.0	3.0	10	28%
vanilla, 'Grand Collection'	1/2 cup	100	3	16	75	0	3.0	1.0	10	26%
ICE MILK BAR/DESSERT										
bar, 'Chocolate Almond Crunch' *(Weight Watchers)*	1 bar	120	2	12	45	0	7.0	2.0	5	53%
cone, w/nuts 'Olde Nut Sundae' *(Gold Bond)*	3 oz	230	5	36	0	0	8.0	0.0	0	31%

Food Name	Serving Size	Calories	Prot. gms	Carbs gms	Sod. mgs	Fiber gms	Fat gms	Sat. Fat gms	Chol. mgs	% Fat Cal.
ICEBERG LETTUCE. See LETTUCE, ICEBERG.										
ICED TEA. See TEA, ICED.										
IMBU. See JOBO.										
INDIAN DATE. See TAMARIND.										
INDIAN FRY BREAD. See under BREAD.										
INFANT FORMULA. See under BABY FOOD, FORMULA.										
IRISH MOSS. See under SEA VEGETABLE.										
ITALIAN BEAN. See BEAN, ITALIAN.										
ITALIAN CHESTNUT. See CHESTNUT, EUROPEAN.										
ITALIAN MUSHROOM. See MUSHROOM, CRIMINI.										
ITALIAN SEASONING. See under SEASONING MIX.										
ITALIAN STONE PINE NUT. See PINE NUT.										

J

Food Name	Serving Size	Calories	Prot. gms	Carbs gms	Sod. mgs	Fiber gms	Fat gms	Sat. Fat gms	Chol. mgs	% Fat Cal.
JACK BEAN. See BEAN, FAVA.										
JACK MACKEREL. See under MACKEREL.										
JACKFRUIT										
Fresh, raw, sliced	1 cup	155	2	40	5	3	0.5	0.1	0	3%
Canned, in syrup, drained	1 cup	164	1	43	20	2	0.2	na	0	1%
JALAPEÑO. See PEPPER, JALAPEÑO.										
JAM AND PRESERVES. See also FRUIT SPREAD.										
(Estee) all flavors	1 tsp	2	0	0	10	0	0.0	0.0	0	0%
(Featherweight) all flavors	1 tsp	4	0	1	0	0	0.0	0.0	0	0%
(Kraft) all flavors	1 tsp	17	0	4	0	0	0.0	0.0	0	0%
(S&W) all flavors, 'Nutradiet'	1 tsp	4	0	1	0	0	0.0	0.0	0	0%
APRICOT										
(Finast)	2 tsp	35	0	9	1	0	0.0	0.0	0	0%
(Knott's Berry Farm) pure preserves	1 tsp	18	0	4	0	0	0.0	0.0	0	0%
(Polaner)	2 tsp	35	0	9	5	0	0.0	0.0	0	0%
(Smucker's) natural ingredients	1 tsp	18	0	4	0	0	0.0	0.0	0	0%
APRICOT-PINEAPPLE										
(Knott's Berry Farm) pure preserves	1 tsp	18	0	4	0	0	0.0	0.0	0	0%
(Knudsen)	2 tsp	35	1	8	0	0	1.0	0.0	0	20%
(Smucker's) natural ingredients	1 tsp	18	0	4	0	0	0.0	0.0	0	0%
BLACK CHERRY (Knudsen)	2 tsp	35	1	8	0	0	1.0	0.0	0	20%
BLACKBERRY										
(Finast)	2 tsp	16	0	4	5	0	0.0	0.0	0	0%
(Knott's Berry Farm) seedless, pure preserves	1 tsp	18	0	4	0	0	0.0	0.0	0	0%
(Knudsen)										
	2 tsp	35	1	8	0	0	1.0	0.0	0	20%
organic	2 tsp	25	1	7	0	0	1.0	0.0	0	22%
(Polaner) seedless	2 tsp	35	0	9	5	0	0.0	0.0	0	0%
(Smucker's) natural ingredients	1 tsp	18	0	4	0	0	0.0	0.0	0	0%
(Stilwell) freezer jam	1 tbsp	36	0	8	0	0	0.0	na	na	0%
BLUEBERRY										
(Finast)	2 tsp	16	0	4	5	0	0.0	0.0	0	0%
(Knott's Berry Farm) pure preserves	1 tsp	18	0	4	0	0	0.0	0.0	0	0%
(Knudsen)										
	2 tsp	35	1	8	0	0	1.0	0.0	0	20%
organic	2 tsp	25	1	7	0	0	1.0	0.0	0	22%

Food Name	Serving Size	Calories	Prot. gms	Carbs gms	Sod. mgs	Fiber gms	Fat gms	Sat. Fat gms	Chol. mgs	% Fat Cal.
(Polaner)	2 tsp	35	0	9	5	0	0.0	0.0	0	0%
(Smucker's) natural ingredients	1 tsp	18	0	4	0	0	0.0	0.0	0	0%
BOYSENBERRY										
(Knott's Berry Farm) pure preserves	1 tsp	18	0	4	0	0	0.0	0.0	0	0%
(Knudsen)	2 tsp	35	1	8	0	0	1.0	0.0	0	20%
(Smucker's) natural ingredients	1 tsp	18	0	4	0	0	0.0	0.0	0	0%
CHERRY										
(Finast)	2 tsp	25	0	9	5	0	0.0	0.0	0	0%
(Knott's Berry Farm)										
Bing, pure preserves	1 tsp	18	0	4	0	0	0.0	0.0	0	0%
red, pure preserves	1 tsp	18	0	4	0	0	0.0	0.0	0	0%
(Smucker's) natural ingredients	1 tsp	18	0	4	0	0	0.0	0.0	0	0%
FIG (Knott's Berry Farm) Kadota, pure preserves	1 tsp	18	0	4	0	0	0.0	0.0	0	0%
GRAPE										
(Finast)										
	2 tsp	35	0	9	5	0	0.0	0.0	0	0%
Concord	2 tsp	35	0	9	5	0	0.0	0.0	0	0%
(Knudsen) Concord	2 tsp	35	1	8	0	0	1.0	0.0	0	20%
(Polaner)	2 tsp	35	0	9	5	0	0.0	0.0	0	0%
(Smucker's) Concord, natural ingredients	1 tsp	18	0	4	0	0	0.0	0.0	0	0%
(Welch's)	2 tsp	35	0	9	5	0	0.0	0.0	0	0%
ORANGE										
(Fifty 50) no sugar added	1 tsp	2	0	1	5	0	0.0	0.0	0	0%
(Finast) marmalade	2 tsp	35	0	9	0	0	0.0	0.0	2	0%
(Knott's Berry Farm) marmalade, w/NutraSweet, 'Light'	1 tsp	8	0	2	0	0	0.0	0.0	0	0%
(Knudsen) marmalade	2 tsp	35	1	8	0	0	1.0	0.0	0	20%
(Smucker's)										
marmalade	1 tsp	18	0	4	0	0	0.0	0.0	0	0%
marmalade, low-sugar	1 tsp	8	0	2	0	0	0.0	0.0	0	0%
marmalade, 'Simply Fruit'	1 tsp	16	0	4	0	0	0.0	0.0	0	0%
marmalade, sweet, natural ingredients	1 tsp	18	0	4	0	0	0.0	0.0	0	0%
(Polaner) marmalade	2 tsp	35	0	9	5	0	0.0	0.0	0	0%
PEACH										
(Bama)	2 tsp	30	0	8	5	0	0.0	0.0	0	0%
(Finast)	2 tsp	35	0	9	1	0	0.0	0.0	0	0%
(Knudsen)	2 tsp	35	1	8	0	0	1.0	0.0	0	20%
(Polaner)	2 tsp	35	0	9	5	0	0.0	0.0	0	0%
(Smucker's) natural ingredients	1 tsp	18	0	4	0	0	0.0	0.0	0	0%
PINEAPPLE										
(Finast)	2 tsp	35	0	9	1	0	0.0	0.0	0	0%
(Polaner)	2 tsp	35	0	9	5	0	0.0	0.0	0	0%
(Smucker's) natural ingredients	1 tsp	18	0	4	0	0	0.0	0.0	0	0%
PLUM										
(Bama) red	2 tsp	30	0	8	5	0	0.0	0.0	0	0%
(Smucker's) natural ingredients	1 tsp	18	0	4	0	0	0.0	0.0	0	0%
RASPBERRY										
(Finast) red	2 tsp	35	0	9	3	0	0.0	0.0	0	0%
(Knott's Berry Farm) seedless, pure preserves	1 tsp	18	0	4	0	0	0.0	0.0	0	0%
(Knudsen)										
red	2 tsp	35	1	8	0	0	1.0	0.0	0	20%
red, organic	2 tsp	25	1	7	0	0	1.0	0.0	0	22%
(Polaner)										
red	2 tsp	35	0	9	5	0	0.0	0.0	0	0%
red, seedless	2 tsp	35	0	9	5	0	0.0	0.0	0	0%

Food Name	Serving Size	Calories	Prot. gms	Carbs gms	Sod. mgs	Fiber gms	Fat gms	Sat. Fat gms	Chol. mgs	% Fat Cal.
(Smucker's)										
black, natural ingredients	1 tsp	18	0	4	0	0	0.0	0.0	0	0%
red, seedless, natural ingredients	1 tsp	18	0	4	0	0	0.0	0.0	0	0%
(Stilwell) freezer jam	1 tbsp	33	0	8	0	0	0.0	na	na	0%
RASPBERRY-APPLE *(Welch's)*	2 tsp	35	0	9	5	0	0.0	0.0	0	0%
STRAWBERRY										
(Bama)	2 tsp	30	0	8	5	0	0.0	0.0	0	0%
(Finast)	2 tsp	35	0	9	3	0	0.0	0.0	0	0%
(Knott's Berry Farm) seedless, pure preserves	1 tsp	18	0	4	0	0	0.0	0.0	0	0%
(Knudsen)										
. . . .	2 tsp	35	1	8	0	0	1.0	0.0	0	20%
organic	2 tsp	25	1	7	0	0	1.0	0.0	0	22%
(Kraft) reduced calorie	1 tsp	6	0	2	5	0	0.0	0.0	0	0%
(Piedmont)	2 tsp	35	0	9	10	0	0.0	0.0	0	0%
(Polaner) strawberry	2 tsp	35	0	9	5	0	0.0	0.0	0	0%
(Smucker's) seedless, natural ingredients	1 tsp	18	0	4	0	0	0.0	0.0	0	0%
(Stilwell) freezer jam	1 tbsp	37	0	9	0	0	0.0	na	na	0%
(Welch's)	2 tsp	35	0	9	5	0	0.0	0.0	0	0%
TOMATO *(Smucker's)* natural ingredients	1 tsp	18	0	4	0	0	0.0	0.0	0	0%
JAMAICAN BREADNUT. See BREADNUT TREE SEEDS.										
JAMBALAYA. See under SHRIMP DISH/ENTRÉE.										
JAMBERRY, fresh *(Frieda's)*	3.5 oz	25	1.4	4.2	na	(mq)	0.5	na	0	17%
JAMBOLAN. See JAVA PLUM.										
JAPANESE HONEY MUSHROOM. See MUSHROOM, JAPANESE HONEY.										
JAPANESE MEDLAR. See LOQUAT.										
JAPANESE WHITE RADISH. See DAIKON.										
JASMINE RICE. See under RICE.										
JAVA PLUM / *jambolan*										
cut up	1 cup	81	1	21	19	na	0.3	na	0	3%
whole	3 med fruits	5	0	1	1	na	0.0	na	0	3%
JELL-O. See under GELATIN DESSERT; GELATIN DESSERT MIX.										
JELLY. See also FRUIT SPREAD; JAM AND PRESERVES.										
(Estee) all flavors	1 tsp	2	0	0	10	0	0.0	0.0	0	0%
(Featherweight) all flavors, except grape	1 tsp	4	0	1	0	0	0.0	0.0	0	0%
(Kraft) all flavors	1 tsp	17	0	4	0	0	0.0	0.0	0	0%
APPLE										
(Bama)	2 tsp	30	0	8	5	0	0.0	0.0	0	0%
(Finast)	2 tsp	35	0	9	2	0	0.0	0.0	0	0%
(Lucky Leaf)	1 oz	80	0	20	5	0	0.0	0.0	0	0%
(Musselman's)	1 oz	80	0	20	5	0	0.0	0.0	0	0%
(Polaner)	2 tsp	35	0	9	5	0	0.0	0.0	0	0%
(Smucker's)										
cinnamon-flavored, natural ingredients	1 tsp	18	0	4	0	0	0.0	0.0	0	0%
mint-flavored, natural ingredients	1 tsp	18	0	4	0	0	0.0	0.0	0	0%
natural ingredients.	1 tsp	18	0	4	0	0	0.0	0.0	0	0%
APPLE BLACKBERRY *(Musselman's)*	1 oz	80	0	19	0	0	0.0	0.0	0	0%
APPLE CHERRY *(Musselman's)*	1 oz	80	0	19	5	0	0.0	0.0	0	0%
APPLE GRAPE										
(Musselman's)	1 oz	80	0	20	5	0	0.0	0.0	0	0%
(Welch's)	2 tsp	35	0	9	5	0	0.0	0.0	0	0%
APPLE RASPBERRY *(Musselman's)*	1 oz	80	0	19	0	0	0.0	0.0	0	0%
APPLE STRAWBERRY *(Musselman's)*	1 oz	80	0	20	5	0	0.0	0.0	0	0%
APRICOT-PINEAPPLE										
(Knott's Berry Farm) w/NutraSweet, 'Light'	1 tsp	8	0	2	0	0	0.0	0.0	0	0%

Food Name	Serving Size	Calories	Prot. gms	Carbs gms	Sod. mgs	Fiber gms	Fat gms	Sat. Fat gms	Chol. mgs	% Fat Cal.
BLACKBERRY										
(Bama)	2 tsp	30	0	8	5	0	0.0	0.0	0	0%
(Knott's Berry Farm) w/NutraSweet, 'Light'	1 tsp	8	0	2	0	0	0.0	0.0	0	0%
(Smucker's) natural ingredients	1 tsp	18	0	4	0	0	0.0	0.0	0	0%
BOYSENBERRY										
(Knott's Berry Farm) w/NutraSweet, 'Light'	1 tsp	8	0	2	0	0	0.0	0.0	0	0%
CHERRY (Smucker's) natural ingredients	1 tsp	18	0	4	0	0	0.0	0.0	0	0%
CRABAPPLE (Smucker's) natural ingredients	1 tsp	18	0	4	0	0	0.0	0.0	0	0%
CURRANT										
(Finast)	2 tsp	35	0	9	2	0	0.0	0.0	0	0%
(Polaner)	2 tsp	35	0	9	5	0	0.0	0.0	0	0%
(Smucker's) natural ingredients	1 tsp	18	0	4	0	0	0.0	0.0	0	0%
ELDERBERRY (Smucker's) natural ingredients	1 tsp	18	0	4	0	0	0.0	0.0	0	0%
GRAPE										
(Bama)	2 tsp	30	0	8	5	0	0.0	0.0	0	0%
(Featherweight)	1 tsp	4	0	1	5	0	0.0	0.0	0	0%
(Finast)	2 tsp	35	0	9	5	0	0.0	0.0	0	0%
(Kraft) reduced calorie	1 tsp	6	0	2	5	0	0.0	0.0	0	0%
(Musselman's)	1 oz	80	0	20	0	0	0.0	0.0	0	0%
(Polaner)	2 tsp	35	0	9	5	0	0.0	0.0	0	0%
(Smucker's) Concord, natural ingredients	1 tsp	18	0	4	0	0	0.0	0.0	0	0%
(Welch's)	2 tsp	35	0	9	5	0	0.0	0.0	0	0%
GREEN PEPPER (Great Impressions)	1 tbsp	50	0	13	1	0	0.0	0.0	0	0%
GUAVA (Smucker's) natural ingredients	1 tsp	18	0	4	0	0	0.0	0.0	0	0%
JALAPEÑO										
(Great Impressions)	1 tbsp	58	0	15	51	0	0.0	0.0	0	0%
(Knott's Berry Farm) pure	1 tsp	18	0	4	0	0	0.0	0.0	0	0%
MINT										
(Finast)	2 tsp	35	0	9	2	0	0.0	0.0	0	0%
(Polaner)	2 tsp	35	0	9	5	0	0.0	0.0	0	0%
MIXED FRUIT (Smucker's) natural ingredients	1 tsp	18	0	4	0	0	0.0	0.0	0	0%
PLUM (Smucker's) natural ingredients	1 tsp	18	0	4	0	0	0.0	0.0	0	0%
QUINCE (Smucker's) natural ingredients	1 tsp	18	0	4	0	0	0.0	0.0	0	0%
RASPBERRY										
(Knott's Berry Farm) red, w/NutraSweet, 'Light'	1 tsp	8	0	2	0	0	0.0	0.0	0	0%
(Polaner) raspberry	2 tsp	35	0	9	5	0	0.0	0.0	0	0%
(Smucker's)										
black, natural ingredients	1 tsp	18	0	4	0	0	0.0	0.0	0	0%
red, natural ingredients	1 tsp	18	0	4	0	0	0.0	0.0	0	0%
RED PEPPER (Great Impressions)	1 tbsp	50	0	13	9	0	0.0	0.0	0	0%
STRAWBERRY										
(Finast)	2 tsp	35	0	9	2	0	0.0	0.0	0	0%
(Knott's Berry Farm) w/NutraSweet, 'Light'	1 tsp	8	0	2	0	0	0.0	0.0	0	0%
(Polaner)	2 tsp	35	0	9	5	0	0.0	0.0	0	0%
(Smucker's) natural ingredients	1 tsp	18	0	4	0	0	0.0	0.0	0	0%
STRAWBERRY APPLE (Polaner)	2 tsp	35	0	9	5	0	0.0	0.0	0	0%

JELLYBEAN. See under CANDY, JELLIED AND GUMMED.

JERKY. See BEEF JERKY; BEEF SUBSTITUTE JERKY; TURKEY JERKY.

JERUSALEM ARTICHOKE. See ARTICHOKE, JERUSALEM.

JEW'S EAR. See CHINESE FUNGUS.

JICAMA / Chinese yam / Mexican potato / sicama / yambean tuber

Food Name	Serving Size	Calories	Prot. gms	Carbs gms	Sod. mgs	Fiber gms	Fat gms	Sat. Fat gms	Chol. mgs	% Fat Cal.
raw, sliced	1 cup	46	1	11	5	6	0.1	0.0	0	2%
raw, trimmed (Frieda of California)	1 oz	13	0	3	0	0	0.1	0.0	0	6%
raw, whole	1 medium	250	5	58	26	32	0.6	0.1	0	2%

Food Name	Serving Size	Calories	Prot. gms	Carbs gms	Sod. mgs	Fiber gms	Fat gms	Sat. Fat gms	Chol. mgs	% Fat Cal.
JOBO / hog plum / imbu / yellow mombin										
seeded	1 oz	20	0.2	3.9	na	0.3	0.6	na	0	25%
JUICE. See FRUIT JUICE BLEND; individual listings.										
JUJUBE, CHINESE										
dried	3.5 oz	287	3.7	73.6	9	3.0	1.1	na	0	3%
dried	1 oz	81	1.0	20.1	3	0.9	0.3	(tr)	0	3%
raw	3.5 oz	79	1.2	20.2	3	1.4	0.1	(tr)	0	2%
raw	1 oz	22	0.3	5.7	1	0.4	0.1	(tr)	0	4%
JUNKET MIX										
CHOCOLATE										
mix only *(Junket)*	3/8 oz	40	1	10	5	0	0.0	0.0	0	0%
prepared w/nonfat milk *(Junket)*	1/2 cup	90	5	15	70	0	0.0	0.0	0	0%
prepared w/whole milk *(Junket)*	1/2 cup	120	5	15	65	0	4.0	0.0	0	31%
RASPBERRY										
mix only *(Junket)*	3/8 oz	40	0	10	0	0	0.0	0.0	0	0%
prepared w/nonfat milk *(Junket)*	1/2 cup	90	4	16	65	0	0.0	0.0	0	0%
prepared w/whole milk *(Junket)*	1/2 cup	120	4	16	60	0	4.0	0.0	0	31%
STRAWBERRY										
mix only *(Junket)*	3/8 oz	40	0	10	0	0	0.0	0.0	0	0%
prepared w/nonfat milk *(Junket)*	1/2 cup	90	4	16	65	0	0.0	0.0	0	0%
prepared w/whole milk *(Junket)*	1/2 cup	120	4	16	60	0	4.0	0.0	0	31%
VANILLA										
mix only *(Junket)*	3/8 oz	40	0	10	5	0	0.0	0.0	0	0%
prepared w/nonfat milk *(Junket)*	1/2 cup	90	4	16	70	0	0.0	0.0	0	0%
prepared w/whole milk *(Junket)*	1/2 cup	120	4	16	65	0	4.0	0.0	0	31%
JUTE POTHERB										
boiled, drained	1 cup	32	3	6	10	2	0.2	0.0	0	5%
raw	1 cup	10	1	2	2	na	0.1	0.0	0	6%

K

Food Name	Serving Size	Calories	Prot. gms	Carbs gms	Sod. mgs	Fiber gms	Fat gms	Sat. Fat gms	Chol. mgs	% Fat Cal.
KAISER ROLL. See under ROLL.										
KALE / borecole / cole / colewort										
Canned, chopped *(Allens)*	1/2 cup	25	2	3	15	0	1.0	0.0	0	31%
Fresh										
boiled, drained	4 oz	36	2.2	6.4	26	>.9 c	0.5	0.1	0	12%
boiled, drained, chopped	1 cup	42	2.5	7.3	30	2.6	0.5	0.1	0	10%
raw, chopped	1 cup	34	2	7	29	1	0.5	0.1	0	12%
raw, chopped *(Dole)*	1/2 cup	17	1	3	15	0	0.5	0.0	0	22%
boiled, drained, chopped	1 cup	36	2	7	30	3	0.5	0.1	0	12%
Frozen										
boiled, drained, chopped	1 cup	39	4	7	20	3	0.6	0.1	0	14%
boiled, drained, chopped or diced	1/2 cup	20	2	3	10	1	0.3	0.0	0	14%
chopped *(Frosty Acres)*	3.3 oz	25	3	5	15	1	0.0	0.0	0	0%
chopped *(Seabrook)*	3.3 oz	25	3	5	14	1	0.0	0.0	0	0%
chopped *(Southern)*	3.5 oz	30	3	5	30	0	0.5	0.0	0	13%
unprepared	10-oz pkg	80	8	14	43	6	1.3	0.2	0	14%
KALE, SCOTCH										
boiled, drained, chopped	1 cup	36	2	7	59	2	0.5	0.1	0	12%
raw, chopped	1 cup	28	2	6	47	1	0.4	0.1	0	12%
KANPYO / dried gourd strips	1/2 cup	70	2	18	4	na	0.2	0.0	0	2%

Food Name	Serving Size	Calories	Prot. gms	Carbs gms	Sod. mgs	Fiber gms	Fat gms	Sat. Fat gms	Chol. mgs	% Fat Cal.
KANTEN										
raw	1 lb	116	2.5	30.6	40	>2.0 c	0.1	<.1	0	1%
raw	1 oz	7	0.2	1.9	3	>.1 c	tr	tr	0	0%
KASHA. See BUCKWHEAT GROATS, ROASTED.										
KATURAY / sesbania flower										
flowers, raw, whole	1 cup	5	0	1	3	na	0.0	na	0	1%
flowers, raw, whole	1 medium	1	0	0	0	na	0.0	na	0	1%
flowers, steamed	1 cup	23	1	5	11	na	0.1	na	0	2%
KEFIR										
black cherry flavored, cultured (Alta Dena)	1 cup	200	9	24	120	0	9.0	0.0	0	38%
boysenberry flavored, cultured (Alta Dena)	1 cup	200	9	24	120	0	9.0	0.0	0	38%
peach flavored, cultured (Alta Dena)	1 cup	200	9	24	120	0	9.0	0.0	0	38%
plain, cultured, including acidophilus (Alta Dena)	1 oz	70	1	1	40	0	6.0	0.0	0	87%
red raspberry flavored, cultured (Alta Dena)	1 cup	200	9	24	120	0	9.0	0.0	0	38%
KELP. See under SEA VEGETABLE.										
KETA SALMON. See under SALMON.										
KETCHUP. See CATSUP.										
KIDNEY BEAN. See BEAN, KIDNEY.										
KIELBASA. See under SAUSAGE.										
KING CRAB. See under CRAB.										
KING MACKEREL. See under MACKEREL.										
KING SALMON. See under SALMON.										
KIWI FRUIT / Chinese gooseberry										
Fresh										
raw, cut up	1 cup	108	2	26	9	6	0.8	0.1	0	6%
raw, peeled	1 large	56	1	14	5	3	0.4	0.0	0	6%
raw, peeled	1 medium	46	1	11	4	3	0.3	0.0	0	6%
KOHLRABI / cabbage turnip										
boiled, drained, sliced	1 cup	48	3	11	35	2	0.2	0.0	0	3%
raw, sliced	1 cup	36	2	8	27	5	0.1	0.0	0	3%
KOMBU. See under SEA VEGETABLE.										
KOLBASSY. See under SAUSAGE.										
KOOL-AID. See under FRUIT DRINK; FRUIT DRINK MIX.										
KOTTERIN MIRIN. See under SEASONING MIX.										
KUMQUAT										
raw, trimmed	1 med fruit	12	0	3	1	1	0.0	0.0	0	1%
raw, w/seeds	1 lb	266	3.8	69.3	25	15.6	0.4	na	0	1%

L

Food Name	Serving Size	Calories	Prot. gms	Carbs gms	Sod. mgs	Fiber gms	Fat gms	Sat. Fat gms	Chol. mgs	% Fat Cal.
LAMB, AUSTRALIAN										
(NOTE: All USDA choice grade. TRIMMED = Lean; separable fat removed. UNTRIMMED = Separable fat not removed.)										
COMPOSITE CUTS										
Trimmed										
cooked	3 oz	171	23	0	68	na	8.2	3.4	74	43%
raw	3 oz	121	17	0	71	na	5.3	2.2	54	39%
raw	1 oz	40	6	0	24	na	1.8	0.7	18	39%
Untrimmed										
cooked	3 oz	218	21	0	65	na	14.3	6.7	74	59%
raw	3 oz	195	15	0	63	na	14.4	7.0	56	67%

Food Name	Serving Size	Calories	Prot. gms	Carbs gms	Sod. mgs	Fiber gms	Fat gms	Sat. Fat gms	Chol. mgs	% Fat Cal.
raw	1 oz	65	5	0	21	na	4.8	2.3	19	67%
LEG / CENTER SLICE										
Trimmed										
center slice, raw	9.8 oz	403	58	0	180	na	17.1	6.8	180	38%
center slice, w/bone, broiled	3 oz	156	23	0	56	na	6.5	2.6	72	38%
center slice, w/bone, raw	1 oz	41	6	0	18	na	1.7	0.7	18	38%
Untrimmed										
center slice, broiled	3 oz	183	22	0	55	na	10.0	4.5	72	49%
center slice, raw	11 oz	616	61	0	193	na	39.7	18.4	205	58%
center slice, w/bone, raw	1 oz	55	5	0	17	na	3.6	1.6	18	58%
LEG / FORESHANK										
Trimmed										
braised	3 oz	140	23	0	85	na	4.4	1.6	78	29%
raw	3 oz	105	18	0	90	na	3.2	1.1	56	28%
raw	1 oz	35	6	0	30	na	1.1	0.4	19	28%
Untrimmed										
braised	3 oz	201	21	0	79	na	12.3	5.8	77	55%
raw	3 oz	166	16	0	82	na	10.8	5.1	57	59%
raw	1 oz	55	5	0	27	na	3.6	1.7	19	59%
LEG / SHANK										
Trimmed										
raw	3 oz	113	17	0	69	na	4.3	1.7	54	35%
raw	1 oz	38	6	0	23	na	1.4	0.6	18	35%
roasted	3 oz	155	23	0	59	na	6.2	2.5	71	36%
Untrimmed										
raw	3 oz	171	16	0	64	na	11.5	5.4	56	60%
raw	1 oz	57	5	0	21	na	3.8	1.8	19	61%
roasted	3 oz	196	21	0	57	na	11.6	5.4	71	53%
LEG / SIRLOIN										
Trimmed										
raw	3 oz	117	17	0	68	na	4.8	2.0	54	37%
raw	1 oz	39	6	0	23	na	1.6	0.7	18	37%
roasted	3 oz	183	24	0	71	na	9.1	3.8	89	45%
Untrimmed										
raw	3 oz	216	15	0	60	na	17.0	8.3	56	71%
raw	1 oz	72	5	0	20	na	5.7	2.8	19	71%
roasted	3 oz	239	21	0	66	na	16.5	7.9	87	62%
LEG /WHOLE										
Trimmed										
raw	3 oz	115	17	0	69	na	4.4	1.8	54	35%
raw	1 oz	38	6	0	23	na	1.5	0.6	18	35%
roasted	3 oz	162	23	0	61	na	6.9	2.8	76	38%
Untrimmed										
raw	3 oz	183	16	0	62	na	12.9	6.2	56	64%
raw	1 oz	61	5	0	21	na	4.3	2.1	19	64%
roasted	3 oz	207	21	0	60	na	12.9	6.0	75	56%
LOIN										
Trimmed										
broiled	3 oz	163	23	0	68	na	7.4	3.1	69	41%
broiled, yield from 1 med chop	3.7 oz	111	15	0	46	na	5.1	2.1	47	41%
raw	3 oz	124	18	0	64	na	5.3	2.3	54	39%
raw	1 oz	41	6	0	21	na	1.8	0.8	18	39%
Untrimmed										
broiled	3 oz	186	22	0	66	na	10.4	4.7	70	50%

Food Name	Serving Size	Calories	Prot. gms	Carbs gms	Sod. mgs	Fiber gms	Fat gms	Sat. Fat gms	Chol. mgs	% Fat Cal.
broiled, yield from 1 med chop	2.2 oz	136	16	0	48	na	7.6	3.5	51	50%
raw	3 oz	173	16	0	60	na	11.4	5.4	56	59%
raw	1 oz	58	5	0	20	na	3.8	1.8	19	59%
RIB										
Trimmed										
raw	3 oz	136	17	0	69	na	7.0	3.0	56	46%
raw	1 oz	45	6	0	23	na	2.3	1.0	19	46%
roasted	3 oz	179	21	0	70	na	9.9	4.3	68	50%
Untrimmed										
raw	3 oz	246	14	0	58	na	20.6	10.1	58	76%
raw	1 oz	82	5	0	19	na	6.9	3.4	19	76%
roasted	3 oz	235	19	0	65	na	17.2	8.3	68	66%
SHOULDER / ARM										
Trimmed										
braised	3 oz	264	25	0	62	na	17.3	8.2	90	59%
braised, yield from 1 med chop	6.5 oz	289	28	0	68	na	19.0	9.0	99	59%
raw	3 oz	116	17	0	71	na	4.9	2.0	53	38%
raw	1 oz	39	6	0	24	na	1.6	0.7	18	38%
Untrimmed										
raw	1 oz	69	5	0	20	na	5.4	2.6	18	70%
raw	3 oz	207	15	0	61	na	16.1	7.8	55	70%
SHOULDER / BLADE										
Trimmed										
broiled	3 oz	196	20	0	80	na	12.2	5.4	72	56%
raw	3 oz	139	16	0	77	na	7.7	3.3	54	50%
raw	1 oz	46	5	0	26	na	2.6	1.1	18	50%
Untrimmed										
broiled	3 oz	247	18	0	75	na	18.7	8.9	71	68%
raw	3 oz	223	14	0	66	na	18.1	8.8	57	73%
raw	1 oz	74	5	0	22	na	6.0	2.9	19	73%
SHOULDER / WHOLE										
Trimmed										
cooked	3 oz	198	22	0	77	na	11.4	5.0	77	52%
raw	3 oz	132	16	0	75	na	6.8	2.9	54	47%
raw	1 oz	44	5	0	25	na	2.3	1.0	18	47%
Untrimmed										
cooked	3 oz	252	20	0	72	na	18.4	8.8	76	66%
raw	3 oz	218	14	0	65	na	17.4	8.4	56	72%
raw	1 oz	73	5	0	22	na	5.8	2.8	19	72%
SIRLOIN CHOP										
Trimmed										
broiled	3 oz	200	22	0	54	na	11.8	5.5	72	53%
broiled, yield from 1 med chop	5.3 oz	247	27	0	67	na	14.5	6.7	89	53%
raw	1 oz	59	5	0	17	na	4.1	2.0	19	62%
Untrimmed										
broiled	3 oz	160	23	0	56	na	6.6	2.7	72	37%
broiled, yield from 1 med chop	5.3 oz	179	26	0	63	na	7.4	3.0	81	37%
raw	1 oz	37	6	0	18	na	1.4	0.6	18	34%
LAMB, NEW ZEALAND										
COMPOSITE CUTS										
Trimmed										
cooked	4 oz	234	33.6	0.0	57	0	10.0	4.4	124	40%
raw	1 oz	36	5.9	0.0	13	0	1.3	0.5	21	33%
Untrimmed										
raw	1 oz	182	2.0	0.0	6	0	19.2	10.0	25	96%

Food Name	Serving Size	Calories	Prot. gms	Carbs gms	Sod. mgs	Fiber gms	Fat gms	Sat. Fat gms	Chol. mgs	% Fat Cal.
LEG/FORESHANK										
Trimmed										
braised	3 oz	158	26.1	0.0	42	0	5.1	2.2	86	31%
braised, diced	1 cup	260	43.1	0.0	69	0	8.5	3.7	141	31%
raw	1 lb	535	94.4	0.0	227	0	14.9	6.3	304	26%
raw	1 oz	33	5.8	0.0	14	0	0.9	0.4	19	26%
stewed	4 oz	211	34.9	0.0	56	0	6.8	3.0	115	31%
stewed, diced	1 cup	260	43.1	0.0	69	0	8.5	3.7	141	31%
Untrimmed										
braised	3 oz	219	22.9	0.0	40	0	13.5	6.7	87	57%
braised, diced	1 cup	361	37.8	0.0	66	0	22.2	10.9	143	57%
raw	1 lb	1012	81.8	0.0	204	0	73.3	37.1	322	67%
raw	1 oz	62	5.1	0.0	13	0	4.5	2.3	20	67%
stewed	4 oz	293	30.6	0.0	53	0	18.0	8.9	116	57%
stewed, diced	1 cup	361	37.8	0.0	66	0	22.2	10.9	143	57%
LEG/WHOLE										
Trimmed										
raw	1 lb	558	94.6	0.0	200	0	17.2	7.3	331	29%
raw	1 oz	34	5.8	0.0	12	0	1.1	0.5	20	30%
roasted	3 oz	154	23.5	0.0	38	0	6.0	2.6	85	37%
roasted, diced	1 cup	253	38.8	0.0	63	0	9.8	4.3	140	36%
Untrimmed										
raw	1 lb	980	83.2	0.0	181	0	69.4	34.8	345	65%
raw	1 oz	60	5.1	0.0	11	0	4.3	2.2	21	66%
roasted	3 oz	209	21.1	0.0	37	0	13.2	6.5	86	59%
roasted, diced	1 cup	344	34.7	0.0	60	0	21.8	10.7	141	59%
LOIN										
Trimmed										
broiled	4 oz	226	33.2	0.0	62	0	9.3	4.1	129	39%
raw	1 oz	36	5.9	0.0	13	0	1.2	0.5	22	31%
roasted	3 oz	169	24.9	0.0	47	0	7.0	3.0	97	39%
Untrimmed										
broiled	3 oz	268	19.9	0.0	42	0	20.3	10.2	95	70%
raw	1 oz	85	4.6	0.0	10	0	7.3	3.7	23	78%
RIB										
Trimmed										
raw	1 lb	644	92.9	0.0	236	0	27.5	11.7	345	40%
raw	1 oz	40	5.7	0.0	15	0	1.7	0.7	21	40%
roasted	3 oz	167	20.8	0.0	41	0	8.6	3.8	80	48%
Untrimmed										
raw	1 lb	1569	67.7	0.0	181	0	142.0	72.5	367	83%
raw	1 oz	97	4.2	0.0	11	0	8.8	4.5	23	83%
roasted	3 oz	289	16.1	0.0	37	0	24.4	12.3	85	77%
SHOULDER / WHOLE										
Trimmed										
braised	3 oz	242	29.0	0.0	48	0	13.2	5.8	108	51%
braised, diced	1 cup	399	47.7	0.0	78	0	21.7	9.5	178	51%
raw	1 lb	612	91.8	0.0	213	0	24.6	10.5	322	38%
raw	1 oz	38	5.8	0.0	13	0	1.5	0.7	20	37%
stewed	6.5 oz	522	62.3	0.0	103	0	28.3	12.5	232	51%
stewed, diced	1 cup	399	47.7	0.0	78	0	21.7	9.5	178	51%
Untrimmed										
braised	3 oz	303	24.0	0.0	43	0	22.3	10.8	106	68%
braised, diced	1 cup	491	40.2	0.0	73	0	35.5	17.1	172	67%
raw	1 lb	1234	75.5	0.0	186	0	100.8	50.9	340	75%

Food Name	Serving Size	Calories	Prot. gms	Carbs gms	Sod. mgs	Fiber gms	Fat gms	Sat. Fat gms	Chol. mgs	% Fat Cal.
stewed	4 oz	398	32.5	0.0	59	0	28.8	13.9	139	67%
stewed, diced	1 cup	491	40.2	0.0	73	0	35.5	17.1	172	67%

LAMB, U.S.
(NOTE: All USDA choice grade. TRIMMED = Lean; separable fat removed. UNTRIMMED = Separable fat not removed.)

BRAIN

Food Name	Serving Size	Calories	Prot. gms	Carbs gms	Sod. mgs	Fiber gms	Fat gms	Sat. Fat gms	Chol. mgs	% Fat Cal.
braised	3 oz	123	10.7	0.0	114	0	8.6	2.2	1737	64%
braised, yield from 1 lb raw	12.25 oz	503	43.5	0.0	465	0	35.3	9.0	7089	65%
pan-fried	3 oz	232	14.4	0.0	133	0	18.9	4.8	2128	75%
raw	4 oz	138	11.8	0.0	127	0	9.7	2.5	1533	65%

COMPOSITE CUTS/LEG AND SHOULDER
Trimmed

Food Name	Serving Size	Calories	Prot. gms	Carbs gms	Sod. mgs	Fiber gms	Fat gms	Sat. Fat gms	Chol. mgs	% Fat Cal.
braised, cubed	3 oz	190	28.6	0.0	59	0	7.5	2.7	92	37%
broiled, cubed	3 oz	158	23.9	0.0	65	0	6.2	2.2	77	37%
broiled, ground	3 oz	241	21.0	0.0	69	na	16.7	6.9	82	64%
raw, cubed	1 lb	608	91.7	0.0	295	0	24.0	8.6	295	37%
raw, cubed	1 oz	38	5.7	0.0	18	0	1.5	0.5	18	37%
raw, ground	1 lb	1279	75.1	0.0	268	na	106.2	46.2	331	76%
raw, ground	1 oz	79	4.6	0.0	17	na	6.6	2.8	20	76%
stewed, cubed	4 oz	253	38.2	0.0	79	0	10.0	3.6	122	37%

GROUND

Food Name	Serving Size	Calories	Prot. gms	Carbs gms	Sod. mgs	Fiber gms	Fat gms	Sat. Fat gms	Chol. mgs	% Fat Cal.
broiled	3 oz	241	21	0	69	0	16.7	6.9	82	63%
raw	4 oz	319	19	0	67	0	26.5	11.5	82	75%
raw	1 oz	80	5	0	17	0	6.6	2.9	21	75%

HEART

Food Name	Serving Size	Calories	Prot. gms	Carbs gms	Sod. mgs	Fiber gms	Fat gms	Sat. Fat gms	Chol. mgs	% Fat Cal.
braised	3 oz	157	21.2	1.6	54	0	6.7	2.7	212	40%
raw	4 oz	138	18.7	0.2	101	0	6.4	2.5	153	43%
simmered	4 oz	210	28.3	2.2	71	0	9.0	3.6	282	40%

KIDNEYS

Food Name	Serving Size	Calories	Prot. gms	Carbs gms	Sod. mgs	Fiber gms	Fat gms	Sat. Fat gms	Chol. mgs	% Fat Cal.
braised	3 oz	116	20.1	0.8	128	0	3.1	1.0	480	25%
raw	4 oz	110	17.8	0.9	177	0	3.3	1.1	382	28%

LEG / FORESHANK
Trimmed

Food Name	Serving Size	Calories	Prot. gms	Carbs gms	Sod. mgs	Fiber gms	Fat gms	Sat. Fat gms	Chol. mgs	% Fat Cal.
braised	3 oz	159	26.4	0.0	63	0	5.1	1.8	88	30%
braised	1 oz	53	8.8	0.0	21	0	1.7	0.6	29	30%
braised, diced	1 cup	262	43.4	0.0	104	0	8.4	3.0	146	30%
broiled, ground	1 cup	328	28.7	0.0	94	0	23.1	9.4	113	64%
broiled, ground	4 oz	321	28.1	0.0	92	0	22.3	9.2	110	64%
raw	1 lb	544	95.6	0.0	358	0	14.9	5.3	313	26%
raw	1 oz	34	5.9	0.0	22	0	0.9	0.3	19	26%
raw, ground	1 cup	637	37.4	0.0	133	0	52.9	23.0	165	76%
stewed	4 oz	212	35.2	0.0	84	0	6.8	2.4	118	30%
stewed	1 oz	53	8.8	0.0	21	0	1.7	0.6	29	30%
stewed, diced	1 cup	262	43.4	0.0	104	0	8.4	3.0	146	30%

Untrimmed

Food Name	Serving Size	Calories	Prot. gms	Carbs gms	Sod. mgs	Fiber gms	Fat gms	Sat. Fat gms	Chol. mgs	% Fat Cal.
braised	3 oz	207	24.1	0.0	61	0	11.4	4.8	90	52%
braised	1 oz	69	8.0	0.0	20	0	3.8	1.6	30	52%
braised, diced	1 cup	340	39.7	0.0	101	0	18.8	7.9	148	52%
raw	1 lb	912	85.8	0.0	327	0	60.7	26.4	327	61%
raw	1 oz	56	5.3	0.0	20	0	3.8	1.6	20	62%
stewed	1 oz	69	8.0	0.0	20	0	3.8	1.6	30	52%
stewed, diced	1 cup	340	39.7	0.0	101	0	18.8	7.9	148	52%

LEG/SHANK
Trimmed

Food Name	Serving Size	Calories	Prot. gms	Carbs gms	Sod. mgs	Fiber gms	Fat gms	Sat. Fat gms	Chol. mgs	% Fat Cal.
raw	1 lb	567	93.1	0.0	277	0	19.0	6.8	290	32%

Food Name	Serving Size	Calories	Prot. gms	Carbs gms	Sod. mgs	Fiber gms	Fat gms	Sat. Fat gms	Chol. mgs	% Fat Cal.
raw	1 oz	35	5.8	0.0	17	0	1.2	0.4	18	32%
roasted	3 oz	153	23.9	0.0	56	0	5.7	2.0	74	35%
roasted	1 oz	51	8.0	0.0	19	0	1.9	0.7	25	35%
roasted, diced	1 cup	252	39.4	0.0	92	0	9.3	3.3	122	35%
Untrimmed										
raw	1 lb	912	84.3	0.0	259	0	61.2	26.3	304	62%
raw	1 oz	56	5.2	0.0	16	0	3.8	1.6	19	62%
roasted	3 oz	191	22.5	0.0	55	0	10.6	4.3	77	52%
roasted	1 oz	64	7.5	0.0	18	0	3.5	1.4	26	51%
roasted, diced	1 cup	315	37.0	0.0	91	0	17.4	7.1	126	51%
LEG / SIRLOIN										
Trimmed										
raw	1 lb	608	93.2	0.0	290	0	23.0	8.3	299	36%
raw	1 oz	38	5.8	0.0	18	0	1.4	0.5	18	35%
roasted	3 oz	173	24.1	0.0	60	0	7.8	2.8	78	42%
roasted	1 oz	58	8.0	0.0	20	0	2.6	0.9	26	42%
roasted, diced	1 cup	286	39.7	0.0	99	0	12.8	4.6	129	42%
Untrimmed										
raw	1 lb	1234	76.8	0.0	254	0	100.3	44.1	327	75%
raw	1 oz	76	4.7	0.0	16	0	6.2	2.7	20	75%
roasted	3 oz	248	20.9	0.0	58	0	17.6	7.4	82	66%
roasted	1 oz	83	7.0	0.0	19	0	5.9	2.5	27	66%
roasted, diced	1 cup	409	34.5	0.0	95	0	28.9	12.2	136	65%
LEG /WHOLE										
Trimmed										
raw	1 lb	581	93.3	0.0	281	0	20.5	7.3	290	33%
raw	1 oz	36	5.8	0.0	17	0	1.3	0.5	18	34%
roasted	3 oz	162	24.1	0.0	58	0	6.6	2.3	76	38%
roasted	1 oz	54	8.0	0.0	19	0	2.2	0.8	25	38%
roasted, diced	1 cup	267	39.6	0.0	95	0	10.8	3.9	125	38%
Untrimmed										
raw	1 lb	1043	81.2	0.0	254	0	77.4	33.7	313	68%
raw	1 oz	64	5.0	0.0	16	0	4.8	2.1	19	68%
roasted	3 oz	219	21.7	0.0	56	0	14.0	5.9	79	59%
roasted	1 oz	73	7.2	0.0	19	0	4.7	2.0	26	60%
roasted, diced	1 cup	361	35.8	0.0	92	0	23.0	9.6	130	59%
LIVER										
braised	3 oz	187	26.0	2.2	48	na	7.5	2.9	426	37%
pan-fried	3 oz	202	21.7	3.2	105	na	10.8	4.2	419	49%
raw	4 oz	158	23.1	2.0	79	na	5.7	2.2	421	34%
LOIN										
Trimmed										
broiled	3 oz	184	25.5	0.0	71	0	8.3	3.0	81	42%
raw	1 oz	40	5.8	0.0	19	0	1.7	0.6	18	40%
roasted	3 oz	172	22.6	0.0	56	0	8.3	3.2	74	45%
Untrimmed										
broiled	3 oz	269	21.4	0.0	65	0	19.6	8.4	85	67%
roasted	3 oz	263	19.2	0.0	54	0	20.0	8.7	81	70%
LUNGS										
braised	3 oz	96	16.9	0.0	71	0	2.6	0.9	241	26%
raw	4 oz	108	18.9	0.0	178	0	3.0	1.0	na	26%
PANCREAS										
braised	3 oz	199	19.4	0.0	44	0	12.8	5.8	340	60%
raw	4 oz	172	16.8	0.0	85	0	11.1	5.0	295	60%

Food Name	Serving Size	Calories	Prot. gms	Carbs gms	Sod. mgs	Fiber gms	Fat gms	Sat. Fat gms	Chol. mgs	% Fat Cal.
RIB										
Trimmed										
broiled	3 oz	200	23.6	0.0	72	0	11.0	4.0	77	51%
raw	1 lb	767	90.6	0.0	327	0	41.9	15.0	299	51%
raw	1 oz	47	5.6	0.0	20	0	2.6	0.9	18	51%
roasted	3 oz	197	22.2	0.0	69	0	11.3	4.1	75	53%
Untrimmed										
broiled	3 oz	307	18.8	0.0	65	0	25.1	10.8	84	75%
raw	1 lb	1687	65.9	0.0	254	0	156.0	68.8	345	84%
raw	1 oz	104	4.1	0.0	16	0	9.6	4.2	21	84%
roasted	3 oz	305	18.0	0.0	62	0	25.3	10.9	82	76%
SHOULDER / ARM										
Trimmed										
braised	3 oz	237	30.2	0.0	65	0	12.0	4.3	103	47%
broiled	3 oz	170	23.5	0.0	70	0	7.7	2.9	78	42%
raw	1 oz	37	5.6	0.0	19	0	1.5	0.5	18	38%
roasted	3 oz	163	21.6	0.0	57	0	7.9	3.0	73	45%
Untrimmed										
braised	3 oz	294	25.8	0.0	61	0	20.4	8.4	102	64%
broiled	3 oz	239	20.8	0.0	65	0	16.6	7.1	82	64%
raw	1 oz	73	4.7	0.0	17	0	5.8	2.6	20	74%
roasted	3 oz	237	19.1	0.0	55	0	17.2	7.4	78	67%
SHOULDER / BLADE										
Trimmed										
braised	1 oz	81	9.1	0.0	22	0	4.7	1.8	33	54%
broiled	3 oz	179	21.7	0.0	75	0	9.6	3.4	77	50%
raw	3 oz	128	16.4	0.0	59	0	6.5	2.3	57	47%
roasted	3 oz	178	20.9	0.0	58	0	9.8	3.7	74	51%
Untrimmed										
braised	3 oz	293	24.2	0.0	64	0	21.0	8.8	99	66%
broiled	3 oz	236	19.6	0.0	70	0	17.0	6.9	81	66%
raw	1 lb	1175	75.4	0.0	281	0	94.6	40.5	327	74%
raw	1 oz	73	4.7	0.0	17	0	5.8	2.5	20	74%
roasted	3 oz	239	18.9	0.0	56	0	17.5	7.3	78	68%
SHOULDER / WHOLE										
Trimmed										
braised	4 oz	321	37.2	0.0	90	0	10.0	7.0	133	38%
braised, diced	1 cup	396	45.9	0.0	111	0	22.2	8.6	164	52%
broiled	4 oz	238	30.8	0.0	94	0	11.9	4.4	105	47%
roasted	4 oz	231	28.3	0.0	77	0	12.2	4.6	99	49%
roasted, diced	1 cup	286	34.9	0.0	95	0	15.1	5.7	122	49%
stewed	4 oz	321	37.2	0.0	90	0	10.0	7.0	133	38%
stewed, diced	1 cup	396	45.9	0.0	111	0	22.2	8.6	164	52%
Untrimmed										
braised, diced	1 cup	482	40.2	0.0	105	0	34.4	14.5	162	66%
broiled	4 oz	315	27.7	0.0	88	0	21.8	9.1	110	64%
broiled, diced	1 cup	389	34.2	0.0	109	0	27.0	11.3	136	64%
roasted	4 oz	313	25.5	0.0	75	0	22.6	9.6	104	67%
roasted, diced	1 cup	386	31.5	0.0	92	0	28.0	11.8	129	67%
stewed	4 oz	390	32.5	0.0	85	0	27.8	11.7	132	66%
stewed, diced	1 cup	482	40.2	0.0	105	0	34.4	14.5	162	66%
SPLEEN										
braised	3 oz	133	22.5	0.0	49	0	4.1	1.3	327	29%
raw	4 oz	115	19.5	0.0	95	0	3.5	1.2	283	29%

Food Name	Serving Size	Calories	Prot. gms	Carbs gms	Sod. mgs	Fiber gms	Fat gms	Sat. Fat gms	Chol. mgs	% Fat Cal.
TONGUE										
braised	3 oz	234	18.3	0.0	57	0	17.2	6.7	161	68%
raw	4 oz	252	17.8	0.0	88	0	19.5	7.5	177	71%
LAMB DINNER/ENTRÉE										
(Stouffer's) shepherd's pie, frozen, food service product	1 oz	36	2	3	122	na	1.8	na	3	46%
LAMB'S QUARTERS										
Fresh										
boiled, drained	4 oz	36	3.6	5.7	(mq)	>2.0 c	0.8	0.1	0	16%
boiled, drained, chopped	1 cup	58	5.8	9.0	52	>3.2 c	1.3	0.1	0	17%
raw	3.5 oz	43	4.2	7.3	43	>4.0	0.8	0.1	0	14%
raw, trimmed	1 lb	195	19.1	33.1	(mq)	>9.5 c	3.6	0.3	0	13%
raw, trimmed	1 oz	12	1.2	2.1	(mq)	>.6 c	0.2	<.1	0	12%
LARD										
	1 cup	1849	0	0	0	0	205.0	80.4	195	100%
	1 tbsp	115	0	0	0	0	12.8	5.0	12	100%
LASAGNA/LASAGNA ENTRÉE										
(Amy's Kitchen)										
tofu and vegetable	1 serving	300	18	41	630	6	10.0	1.0	0	28%
vegetable, w/cheese	1 serving	300	15	39	680	5	10.0	4.0	15	29%
(Banquet)										
frozen, 'Extra Helping'	16.5 oz	645	24	88	1582	0	23.0	0.0	38	32%
w/meat sauce	1 entrée	260	10	38	820	5	8.0	2.0	10	27%
(Bernardi)										
'Solito'	1 cup	380	22	33	760	5	18.0	9.0	60	42%
'Supreme'	1 cup	310	18	32	930	3	13.0	7.0	40	37%
supreme, portioned	1-1/4 cup	369	21	38	1108	4	15.0	8.0	45	36%
vegetable, 'Supreme'	1 cup	360	20	35	870	2	17.0	12.0	65	41%
(Budget Gourmet)										
sausage, Italian	1 entrée	430	20	40	730	4	21.0	9.0	60	44%
three cheese	1 entrée	370	20	38	870	5	16.0	10.0	60	38%
vegetable, 'Light'	1 entrée	290	15	36	780	5	9.0	1.8	15	28%
w/cheese and meat sauce	1 entrée	326	20	35	687	4	12.0	5.6	46	33%
w/Italian sausage	1 entrée	456	21	40	903	3	23.8	8.2	48	47%
w/meat sauce, 'Light'	1 entrée	250	15	31	690	3	7.0	3.0	30	26%
(Buitoni)										
in sauce, frozen, 'Family Style'	7.3 oz	370	13	30	940	0	13.0	7.0	55	40%
meat, frozen, 'Single Serving'	9 oz	580	23	57	820	0	19.0	12.0	110	35%
(Celentano)										
	10-oz tray	400	18	51	650	7	14.0	6.0	80	31%
	1 cup	320	14	41	520	6	11.0	5.0	65	31%
frozen, 14-oz tray	7 oz	280	15	33	660	8	10.0	5.0	75	32%
low-fat, frozen, 'Great Choice'	10-oz tray	260	18	42	650	2	2.5	1.0	20	9%
primavera, 'Great Choice'	10-oz tray	240	17	33	600	0	7.0	0.0	0	24%
primavera, 'Selects'	10-oz tray	220	12	32	510	5	5.0	1.5	5	20%
(Chef Boyardee)										
	1 cup	270	10	41	680	3	8.0	3.0	20	26%
hearty, microwave cup, 'Main Meals'	10.5 oz	290	13	41	0	0	8.0	0.0	0	25%
in garden vegetable sauce, canned, microwave	7.5 oz	170	5	14	940	0	1.0	1.0	3	11%
microwave	7.5 oz	230	7	31	1080	0	9.0	0.0	18	35%
(Contadina)										
chicken, food service product, frozen	1 oz	44	2	3	116	na	2.6	na	6	53%
classic, frozen, food service product	1 oz	39	2	4	119	1	1.6	0.9	8	37%
precut, classic, frozen, food service product	1 oz	39	2	3	88	0	2.2	1.0	5	50%

Food Name	Serving Size	Calories	Prot. gms	Carbs gms	Sod. mgs	Fiber gms	Fat gms	Sat. Fat gms	Chol. mgs	% Fat Cal.
(Dining Lite)										
cheese, frozen	9 oz	260	14	36	800	0	6.0	0.0	30	21%
w/meat sauce, frozen	9 oz	240	13	36	800	0	5.0	0.0	25	19%
(Dinty Moore)										
w/meat sauce, packaged, 'American Classics'	10 oz	320	16	33	870	0	14.0	7.0	35	39%
(Freezer Queen) w/meat sauce, 'Deluxe Family Suppers'	7 oz	200	8	28	730	0	6.0	0.0	0	27%
(Green Giant) frozen, 'Entrées'	12 oz	490	33	44	1660	0	20.0	0.0	0	37%
(Healthy Choice)										
Roma, w/meat sauce	1 entrée	400	26	59	580	9	7.0	2.5	15	16%
w/meat sauce, frozen	10 oz	260	18	37	420	0	5.0	2.0	20	17%
zucchini, frozen	11.5 oz	250	14	41	400	0	3.0	2.0	15	11%
(Hormel) microwave cup	7.5 oz	250	8	25	949	0	13.0	6.0	23	47%
(Le Menu)										
garden vegetable, 'Light Style'	10.5 oz	260	11	35	500	0	8.0	3.0	25	28%
w/meat sauce, frozen, 'LightStyle'	10 oz	290	19	36	510	0	8.0	0.0	30	25%
(Lean Cuisine)										
chicken, scaloppini, frozen, 'Café Classics'	1 pkg	290	20	34	560	4	8.0	2.5	40	25%
classic	1 entrée	290	20	38	560	5	6.0	3.0	30	19%
5-cheese, frozen, food service product	1 oz	27	2	3	68	0	0.7	0.3	3	23%
'Hearty Portions'	1 entrée	440	26	64	830	6	9.0	4.0	30	18%
tuna, w/spinach noodles, frozen	9.75 oz	240	16	29	520	0	7.0	2.0	20	26%
vegetable	1 entrée	260	15	35	590	5	7.0	3.0	20	24%
w/meat sauce	1 entrée	290	20	35	560	6	8.0	4.0	35	25%
w/meat sauce, frozen	10.25 oz	280	20	36	560	6	6.0	3.0	25	19%
(Legume)										
vegetable, w/tofu and sauce	12 oz	240	14	26	520	6	8.0	1.7	0	31%
vegetarian, nondairy, classic, w/organic pasta and tofu	1 serving	340	20	37	560	11	13.0	2.0	0	34%
vegetable, vegetarian, nondairy, w/organic pasta and tofu	1 serving	210	13	24	480	5	7.0	1.5	0	30%
(Libby's) w/meat sauce, microwave cup, 'Diner'	7.75 oz	200	9	29	790	2	5.0	3.0	15	23%
(Lunch Bucket) w/meat sauce, microwave lunch cup	7.5 oz	220	8	38	870	0	4.0	0.0	30	16%
(Lunch Express)										
casserole, cheese	1 entrée	270	14	38	590	5	7.0	2.5	15	23%
w/meat sauce	1 entrée	330	18	42	910	5	10.0	5.0	40	27%
(Marie Callender's)										
extra cheese	1 cup	350	16	36	720	4	16.0	7.0	20	41%
w/meat sauce	15 oz	370	17	34	740	4	18.0	9.0	35	44%
w/meat sauce, frozen, family size	1 cup	350	17	32	770	3	16.0	8.0	50	42%
(Mrs. Paul's) seafood, frozen, 'Light'	9.5 oz	290	14	39	750	0	8.0	3.0	57	25%
(Nalley's) canned	7.5 oz	180	10	24	720	0	5.0	0.0	0	25%
(Smart Ones)										
Alfredo	1 entrée	300	14	46	680	3	7.0	4.0	20	21%
Florentine	1 entrée	200	10	34	590	5	2.0	0.0	10	9%
w/meat sauce	1 entrée	240	13	43	520	4	2.0	0.5	10	7%
(Stouffer's)										
fiesta, w/meat, frozen, food service product	1 oz	43	2	4	105	na	2.0	na	4	42%
frozen, 96-oz pkg.	9-3/5 oz	400	30	37	940	0	14.0	0.0	0	32%
frozen, 10-oz pkg.	10 oz	340	18	40	840	0	12.0	0.0	0	32%
frozen, 21-oz pkg.	10.5 oz	360	28	33	1020	0	13.0	0.0	0	32%
vegetable	1 entrée	450	20	41	980	5	23.0	8.0	40	46%
vegetable, frozen, 96-oz pkg.	9.6 oz	400	23	33	760	0	20.0	0.0	0	45%
w/meat and sauce, frozen	1 pkg	768	52	73	2035	9	29.8	13.0	113	35%
w/meat and sauce	1 serving	277	19	26	735	3	10.8	4.7	41	35%
w/meat and sauce, frozen, food service product	1 entrée	40	3	4	94	0	1.7	0.7	5	39%

Food Name	Serving Size	Calories	Prot. gms	Carbs gms	Sod. mgs	Fiber gms	Fat gms	Sat. Fat gms	Chol. mgs	% Fat Cal.
w/meat sauce	1 entrée	360	27	34	780	5	13.0	5.0	50	32%
w/meat sauce, frozen, food service product	1 oz	39	3	3	95	0	1.6	0.7	5	38%
(Swanson)										
w/meat sauce	1 entrée	340	22	37	940	5	12.0	7.0	30	31%
w/meat sauce, frozen, 'Homestyle Recipe'	10.5 oz	400	26	39	1070	0	15.0	0.0	0	34%
(Top Shelf)										
Italian, packaged	10 oz	350	23	30	840	0	16.0	8.0	60	40%
vegetable, packaged	10.6 oz	275	18	34	1024	0	8.0	0.0	35	26%
(Tyson) frozen 'Gourmet Selection'	11.5 oz	380	20	47	840	0	14.0	0.0	0	32%
(Ultra Slim Fast)										
vegetable	12 oz	240	17	39	730	0	4.0	0.0	15	14%
w/meat sauce	12 oz	330	28	38	980	0	9.0	0.0	55	23%
(Weight Watchers)										
Bolognese	1 entrée	300	16	45	590	4	7.0	3.0	20	21%
cheese, Italian	1 entrée	300	20	38	550	5	8.0	3.5	30	24%
garden	1 entrée	270	14	36	4	5	7.0	3.5	30	24%
w/cheese, meat, and tomato sauce	11-oz entrée	358	22	38	755	4	13.2	6.1	50	33%
w/meat sauce	1 entrée	270	14	38	570	6	7.0	3.0	35	23%

LASAGNA NOODLE. See under PASTA.

LAVER. See under SEA VEGETABLE.

LEEK

Fresh

Food Name	Serving Size	Calories	Prot. gms	Carbs gms	Sod. mgs	Fiber gms	Fat gms	Sat. Fat gms	Chol. mgs	% Fat Cal.
boiled, drained, chopped	1/4 cup	8	0	2	3	0	0.1	0.0	0	5%
boiled, drained, whole	1 medium	38	1	9	12	1	0.2	0.0	0	5%
raw, chopped	1 cup	54	1	13	18	2	0.3	0.0	0	4%
raw, whole	1 medium	54	1	13	18	2	0.3	0.0	0	4%

Freeze-dried

Food Name	Serving Size	Calories	Prot. gms	Carbs gms	Sod. mgs	Fiber gms	Fat gms	Sat. Fat gms	Chol. mgs	% Fat Cal.
bulb/lower leaf portion	1/4 cup	3	0	1	0	0	0.0	0.0	0	6%
bulb/lower leaf portion	1 tbsp	1	0	0	0	0	0.0	0.0	0	5%

LEMON

Fresh

Food Name	Serving Size	Calories	Prot. gms	Carbs gms	Sod. mgs	Fiber gms	Fat gms	Sat. Fat gms	Chol. mgs	% Fat Cal.
raw, sectioned, w/o peel	1 cup	61	2	20	4	6	0.6	0.1	0	9%
raw, sliced, w/o peel, 1/8 of 2-1/8-inch diam lemon	1 wedge	2	0	1	0	0	0.0	0.0	0	9%
raw, whole, w/o peel, 2-1/8-inch diam	1 lemon	17	1	5	1	2	0.2	0.0	0	9%
raw, w/peel, w/o seeds, 2-3/8-inch diam	1 lemon	22	1	12	3	5	0.3	0.0	0	14%

LEMON HERB SEASONING. See under SEASONING MIX.

LEMON JUICE

Canned or bottled

Food Name	Serving Size	Calories	Prot. gms	Carbs gms	Sod. mgs	Fiber gms	Fat gms	Sat. Fat gms	Chol. mgs	% Fat Cal.
	1 cup	51	1	16	51	1	0.7	0.1	0	12%
	1 fl oz	6	0	2	6	0	0.1	0.0	0	12%
	1 tbsp	3	0	1	3	0	0.0	0.0	0	12%
unsweetened, single strength	1 cup	54	1	16	2	1	0.8	0.1	0	12%
unsweetened, single strength	1 fl oz	7	0	2	0	0	0.1	0.0	0	12%
(A&P) reconstituted, natural strength	1 fl oz	6	1	2	0	0	1.0	0.0	0	43%
(Lucky Leaf)	6 fl oz	30	1	6	35	0	0.0	0.0	0	0%
(ReaLemon)										
reconstituted, natural strength	1 fl oz	6	0	2	10	0	0.0	0.0	0	0%
reconstituted, '100%'	1 fl oz	6	0	2	5	0	0.0	0.0	0	0%
Fresh										
	1 cup	61	1	21	2	1	0.0	0.0	0	0%
	1 fl oz	8	0	3	0	0	0.0	0.0	0	0%
juice of 1/8 of 2-1/8-inch-diam lemo	0.2 oz	1	0	1	0	0	0.0	0.0	0	0%
juice of 2-1/8-inch-diam lemon	1.6 oz	12	0	4	0	0	0.0	0.0	0	0%

Food Name	Serving Size	Calories	Prot. gms	Carbs gms	Sod. mgs	Fiber gms	Fat gms	Sat. Fat gms	Chol. mgs	% Fat Cal.
Frozen										
(Minute Maid) concentrate, prepared	6 fl oz	8	0	2	0	0	0.0	0.0	0	0%
(Sunkist)	1 fl oz	7	0	2	1	0	0.1	0.0	0	10%
LEMON PEEL										
raw, grated	1 tbsp	3	0	1	0	1	0.0	0.0	0	6%
raw, grated	1 tsp	1	0	0	0	0	0.0	0.0	0	6%
raw, grated *(Tone's)*	1 tsp	0	0	0	0	0	0.0	0.0	0	0%
LEMON PEPPER. See under SEASONING MIX.										
LEMONADE. See under FRUIT DRINK; FRUIT DRINK MIX.										
LEMONGRASS / citronella										
raw	1 cup	66	1	17	4	na	0.3	0.1	0	4%
raw	1 tbsp	5	0	1	0	na	0.0	0.0	0	4%
LEMON-LIME DRINK. See under FRUIT DRINK.										
LENTIL										
Canned, organic *(Eden Foods)*	1/2 cup	90	8	13	210	4	0.0	0.0	0	0%
Dried										
boiled *(A&P)*	1 cup	210	16	39	0	0	1.0	0.0	0	4%
green, raw *(Arrowhead Mills)*	2 oz	190	13	35	9	9	1.0	0.0	0	4%
mature seeds, boiled	1 cup	230	18	40	4	16	0.8	0.1	0	3%
mature seeds, boiled	1 tbsp	14	1	2	0	1	0.0	0.0	0	3%
mature seeds, raw	1 cup	649	54	110	19	59	1.8	0.3	0	2%
mature seeds, raw	1 tbsp	41	3	7	1	4	0.1	0.0	0	2%
pink, raw	1 cup	664	48	114	13	21	4.2	0.7	0	5%
red, raw *(Arrowhead Mills)*	2 oz	195	14	34	10	9	1.0	0.0	0	4%
Sprouted, raw	1 cup	82	7	17	8	na	0.4	0.0	0	4%
LENTIL DISH/ENTRÉE										
(Casbah) pilaf, prepared	3/4 cup	240	9	38	400	2	0.5	0.0	0	2%
(Health Valley) canned, w/garden vegetables, nonfat,										
canned, 'Fast Menu'	7.5 oz	160	13	18	204	16	4.0	0.0	0	23%
(Natural Touch) lentil rice loaf	1 slice	166	8	16	366	4	8.6	2.6	2	47%
LETTUCE										
BIBB, BOSTON, OR BUTTERHEAD										
leaf, large	1 leaf	2	0	0	1	0	0.0	0.0	0	14%
leaf, medium	1 leaf	1	0	0	0	0	0.0	0.0	0	15%
leaf, small	1 leaf	1	0	0	0	0	0.0	0.0	0	14%
shredded	1 cup	7	1	1	3	1	0.1	0.0	0	14%
whole *(Dole)*	1 med head	21	2	4	8	2	0.1	0.0	0	4%
whole, approx 5-inch diam	1 head	21	2	4	8	2	0.4	0.0	0	14%
COS										
inner leaf, whole	1 med leaf	1	0	0	1	0	0.0	0.0	0	12%
shredded	1/2 cup	4	0	1	2	0	0.1	0.0	0	12%
ICEBERG										
leaf, large	1 leaf	2	0	0	1	0	0.0	0.0	0	13%
leaf, medium	1 leaf	1	0	0	1	0	0.0	0.0	0	13%
leaf, small	1 leaf	1	0	0	0	0	0.0	0.0	0	14%
shredded or chopped	1 cup	7	1	1	5	1	0.1	0.0	0	13%
wedge, 1/6 of med head *(Dole)*	1 wedge	20	1	4	10	1	0.0	0.0	0	0%
whole, approx 6-inch diam	1 head	65	5	11	49	8	1.0	0.1	0	13%
LEAF, shredded *(Dole)*	1.5 cup	12	1	1	40	1	0.0	0.0	0	0%
LOOSELEAF										
leaf, medium	1 leaf	2	0	0	1	0	0.0	0.0	0	14%
shredded	1/2 cup	5	0	1	3	1	0.1	0.0	0	14%
ROMAINE										
inner leaf, whole	1 leaf	1	0	0	1	0	0.0	0.0	0	12%

Food Name	Serving Size	Calories	Prot. gms	Carbs gms	Sod. mgs	Fiber gms	Fat gms	Sat. Fat gms	Chol. mgs	% Fat Cal.
shredded...........	1/2 cup	4	0	1	2	0	0.1	0.0	0	12%
shredded *(Dole)*...........	1.5 cup	18	1	2	40	1	1.0	0.0	0	43%

LICHI. See LITCHI.

LIMA BEAN. See BEAN, LIMA; BEAN DISH/ENTRÉE.

LIME

fresh, raw, peeled and seeded............	1 oz	9	02	3.0	1	>.1 c	0.1	tr	0	7%
fresh, raw, whole, approx 2-inch dia............	1 lime	20	0	7	1	2	0.1	0.0	0	6%

LIME DRINK. See under FRUIT DRINK.

LIME JUICE

Canned or bottled

unsweetened............	1 cup	52	1	16	39	1	0.6	0.1	0	9%
unsweetened............	1 fl oz	6	0	2	5	0	0.1	0.0	0	9%
(ReaLime)										
original, unsweetened............	1 tbsp	0	0	0	0	0	0.0	0.0	0	0%
reconstituted, natural strength............	1 fl oz	6	0	2	10	0	0.0	0.0	0	0%
(Roses)............	1 fl oz	48	0	12	6	0	0.0	0.0	0	0%
(Santa Cruz Natural) organic, 'Cruz'............	8 fl oz	120	1	27	0	0	1.0	0.0	0	7%
Fresh										
....	1 cup	66	1	22	2	1	0.2	0.0	0	3%
....	1 fl oz	8	0	3	0	0	0.0	0.0	0	3%
juice of 2-1/8-inch-diam lime............	1.3 oz	10	0	3	0	0	0.0	0.0	0	3%
juice of 1/8 of 2-1/8-inch-diam lime............	0.2 oz	1	0	0	0	0	0.0	0.0	0	3%

LIMEADE. See under FRUIT DRINK.

LING

baked, broiled, grilled, or microwaved............	3 oz	94	21	0	147	0	0.7	na	43	7%
raw............	3 oz	74	16	0	115	0	0.5	0.1	34	7%

LINGCOD

baked, broiled, grilled, or microwaved............	3 oz	93	19	0	65	0	1.2	0.2	57	11%
raw............	3 oz	72	15	0	50	0	0.9	0.2	44	11%

LINGUINE. See under PASTA.

LINGUINE DISH/ENTRÉE. See under PASTA DISH/ENTRÉE.

LIQUEUR

COFFEE

w/cream, 34 proof............	1 fl oz	102	1	7	29	0	4.9	3.0	5	42%
53 proof............	1 fl oz	117	0	16	3	0	0.1	0.0	0	1%
63 proof............	1 fl oz	107	0	11	3	0	0.1	0.0	0	1%
CRÈME DE MENTHE										
72 proof............	1 fl oz	125	0	14	2	0	0.1	0.0	0	1%

LIQUOR. See individual listings.

LITCHI / lychee

dried............	3.5 oz	277	3.8	70.7	3	>1.4 c	1.2	na	0	4%
dried............	1 oz	79	1.1	20.0	1	4.6	0.3	(tr)	0	3%
dried............	1 medium	7	0	2	0	0	0.0	0.0	0	4%
raw............	1 cup	125	2	31	2	2	0.8	0.2	0	6%
raw, shelled and seeded............	1/2 cup	63	0.8	15.7	1	>.2 c	0.4	tr	0	5%
raw, shelled and seeded............	1 oz	19	0.2	4.7	<1	>.1 c	0.1	(tr)	0	4%
raw, trimmed, approx 0.6 oz............	1 medium	6	0	2	0	0	0.0	0.0	0	6%
raw, untrimmed............	1 lb	179	2.3	45.0	2	>.6 c	1.2	na	0	5%

LIVER. See under individual meat listings. Also see PÂTÉ, CANNED.

LIVERWURST. See under LUNCHEON MEAT.

LOBSTER

NORTHERN

boiled, poached, or steamed............	1 cup	142	29.7	1.9	551	0	0.9	0.2	104	6%
boiled, poached or steamed............	4 oz	111	23.2	1.5	431	0	0.7	0.1	82	6%

Food Name	Serving Size	Calories	Prot. gms	Carbs gms	Sod. mgs	Fiber gms	Fat gms	Sat. Fat gms	Chol. mgs	% Fat Cal.
raw	1 lb	410	85.3	2.3	(mq)	0	4.1	(mq)	432	10%
raw	3 oz	77	16.0	0.4	252	0	0.8	0.2	81	10%
raw	1 oz	26	5.3	0.1	(mq)	0	0.3	(mq)	27	11%
SPINY, MIXED SPECIES										
boiled, poached or steamed	3 oz	122	22.5	2.7	193	0	1.6	0.3	77	13%
raw	1 lb	506	93.4	11.0	803	0	6.9	1.1	318	13%
raw	3 oz	95	17.5	2.1	150	0	1.3	0.2	59	13%
raw	1 oz	32	5.8	0.7	50	0	0.4	0.1	20	12%
LOGANBERRY										
Fresh										
raw, trimmed	1 lb	281	4.5	67.6	5	(mq)	2.7	(mq)	0	8%
raw, trimmed	1 cup	89	1.4	21.5	1	>4.3 c	0.9	(mq)	0	8%
raw, untrimmed	1 lb	267	4.3	64.2	4	(mq)	2.6	(mq)	0	8%
Frozen										
	1 cup	81	2.2	19.1	1	7.2	0.5	na	0	5%
	4 oz	62	1.7	14.8	1	(mq)	0.4	(mq)	0	5%
LONGAN / dragon's eye										
Dried	1 oz	81	1.4	21.0	14	13.4	0.1	(tr)	0	1%
Fresh										
raw, approx 0.2 oz	1 medium	2	<.1	0.5	tr	<.1	tr	(tr)	0	0%
raw, shelled and seeded	1 oz	17	0.4	4.3	tr	>.1 c	<.1	(tr)	0	<5%
raw, untrimmed	1 lb	144	3.2	36.4	1	>1.0 c	0.2	na	0	1%
LONGBEAN										
Fresh										
boiled, drained	4 oz	53	2.9	10.4	5	>1.7 c	0.1	<.1	0	2%
boiled, drained, sliced	1/2 cup	25	1.3	4.8	2	>.8 c	0.1	<.1	0	4%
boiled, drained, 13-1/4 inches long x 1/4 inch diam	1 pod	7	0.4	1.3	1	>.2 c	<.1	tr	0	<12%
raw, sliced	1/2 cup	22	1.3	3.8	2	(mq)	0.2	<.1	0	8%
raw, 13-1/4 inches long x 1/4 inch diam	1 pod	6	0.3	1.0	tr	(mq)	0.1	<.1	0	15%
raw, trimmed	1 oz	13	0.8	2.4	1	(mq)	0.1	<.1	0	7%
raw, untrimmed	1 lb	203	12.1	36.0	17	(mq)	1.7	0.5	0	7%
Dried										
boiled	1/2 cup	102	7.1	18.1	4	>1.4 c	0.4	0.1	0	3%
boiled	4 oz	134	9.4	23.9	6	>1.8 c	0.5	0.1	0	3%
raw	1/2 cup	292	20.4	52.0	14	>4.0 c	1.1	0.3	0	3%
raw	1 oz	98	6.9	17.6	5	>1.4 c	0.4	0.1	0	4%
LOOFAH GOURD. See GOURD, DISHCLOTH.										
LOQUAT / Japanese medlar										
raw, cubed	1 cup	70	1	18	1	3	0.3	0.1	0	4%
raw, whole, large	1 fruit	9	0	2	0	0	0.0	0.0	0	4%
raw, whole, medium	1 fruit	8	0	2	0	0	0.0	0.0	0	4%
raw, whole, small	1 fruit	6	0	2	0	0	0.0	0.0	0	4%
LOTTE. See MONKFISH.										
LOTUS ROOT										
boiled, drained, sliced	1/2 cup	40	1	10	27	2	0.0	0.0	0	1%
raw, whole, 9.5-inch long	1 root	85	3	20	46	6	0.1	0.0	0	1%
LOTUS SEED										
dried	1 cup	106	5	21	2	na	0.6	0.1	0	5%
dried, whole, approx 42 kernels	1 oz	94	4	18	1	na	0.6	0.1	0	5%
raw	1 oz	25	1	5	0	na	0.1	0.0	0	5%
LOX. See under SALMON.										
LUNCH COMBINATION, PACKAGED										
(Eckrich)										
ham and Swiss, crackers, 'Lunch Makers'	1 piece	40	2	2	170	0	2.0	0.0	5	53%

Food Name	Serving Size	Calories	Prot. gms	Carbs gms	Sod. mgs	Fiber gms	Fat gms	Sat. Fat gms	Chol. mgs	% Fat Cal.
turkey and cheddar, crackers, 'Lunch Makers'	1 piece	40	2	2	160	0	2.0	0.0	5	53%
(Hillshire Farm)										
bologna and American, cracker, Snickers, 6-oz drink	1 lunch	590	15	55	1130	0	34.0	0.0	0	52%
bologna and American, cracker, Snickers, w/o drink......	1 lunch	490	15	31	1110	0	34.0	0.0	0	62%
chicken and Monterey Jack, cracker, Snickers	1 lunch	400	19	31	1080	0	23.0	0.0	0	51%
ham and cheddar, cracker, Snickers, w/o drink..........	1 lunch	400	17	32	1010	0	23.0	0.0	0	51%
ham and cheddar, cracker, Snickers, 6 oz drink	1 lunch	500	17	56	1030	0	23.0	0.0	0	41%
ham and Swiss, cracker, Oreo, 'Lunch'n Munch'.........	1 lunch	370	16	30	1160	0	21.0	0.0	0	51%
turkey and cheddar, cracker, brownie	1 lunch	400	17	34	1240	0	22.0	0.0	0	49%
(Louis Rich)										
turkey breast and cheddar cheese, 'Lunch Breaks'.......	1 pkg	410	22	23	1715	0	26.0	0.0	70	57%
turkey ham and Swiss cheese, 'Lunch Breaks'	1 pkg	380	24	25	1875	0	22.0	0.0	75	50%
turkey salami and cheddar cheese, 'Lunch Breaks'	1 pkg	430	22	25	1595	0	29.0	0.0	85	58%
turkey, w/Monterey Jack cheese, 'Lunch Breaks'	1 pkg	400	21	27	1665	0	25.0	0.0	75	54%
(Oscar Mayer)										
bologna and American lunch, 'Lunchables'.............	1 lunch	470	17	22	1670	1	35.0	17.0	90	67%
bologna and wild cherry lunch, 'Lunchables'............	1 lunch	530	12	60	1140	1	28.0	13.0	70	47%
chicken and turkey lunch, 'Deluxe' 'Lunchables'	1 lunch	390	21	25	1830	1	23.0	11.0	70	53%
chicken w/Monterey Jack, cracker, pudding, 'Lunchables'	1 lunch	380	19	32	1200	0	21.0	0.0	45	48%
ham and cheddar lunch, 'Lunchables'.................	1 lunch	360	20	21	1750	1	22.0	11.0	75	55%
ham and Swiss lunch, 'Lunchables'	1 lunch	340	21	20	1780	1	20.0	10.0	70	52%
ham w/American cheese, cracker, pudding, 'Lunchables'	1 lunch	410	19	33	1380	0	23.0	0.0	45	50%
ham w/fruit punch, 'Lunchables'	1 lunch	440	15	54	1270	1	20.0	9.0	50	39%
ham w/Surfer Cooler, low-fat, 'Lunchables'	1 lunch	390	17	58	1350	1	11.0	5.0	35	25%
ham w/Swiss, cracker, cookie, 'Lunchables'	1 lunch	380	18	29	1370	0	23.0	0.0	50	52%
ham w/fruit punch, low-fat, 'Lunchables'	1 lunch	330	17	48	1120	1	9.0	4.5	35	24%
pepperoni pizza, 'Lunchables'.....................	1 lunch	310	15	30	790	2	15.0	7.0	35	43%
pepperoni pizza and orange, 'Lunchables'	1 lunch	460	16	62	830	2	16.0	8.0	35	32%
pizza lunch, extra cheesy, 'Lunchables'..............	1 lunch	300	17	30	690	2	13.0	7.0	30	38%
pizza lunch, extra cheesy, w/fruit punch, 'Lunchables'	1 lunch	450	17	63	720	2	15.0	9.0	30	30%
smokie links sausage, 'Lunchables'	1 lunch	130	5	1	430	0	12.0	4.0	25	82%
turkey, lowfat, w/Pacific Cooler, 'Lunchables'	1 lunch	360	15	56	1190	1	9.0	4.5	30	22%
turkey, w/Pacific Cooler, 'Lunchables'	1 lunch	450	15	54	1340	1	20.0	9.0	50	39%
turkey, w/Surfer Cooler, 'Lunchables'	1 lunch	430	13	61	1250	0	15.0	8.0	45	31%
turkey and cheddar, 'Lunchables'	1 lunch	350	20	22	1760	1	20.0	11.0	70	52%
turkey and ham, deluxe, 'Lunchables'................	1 lunch	370	21	25	1940	1	21.0	10.0	65	51%
turkey w/cheddar, cracker, trail mix.................	1 lunch	460	20	41	1230	0	26.0	0.0	40	49%
turkey w/Monterey Jack, wheat cracker, 'Lunchables'.....	1 lunch	360	21	18	1600	0	22.0	0.0	75	56%
(Star-Kist) 'Charlie's Lunch Kit' w/1 mayo packet..........	4.6 oz	290	24	16	780	0	15.0	0.0	0	46%
LUNCHEON MEAT										
BARBECUE LOAF *(Oscar Mayer)*	1 oz	46	5	2	333	0	2.3	1.0	14	45%
BEEF										
(Boar's Head)										
roast, top round, oven-roasted	1 oz	40	7	1	30	0	1.0	0.0	20	22%
roast, top round, oven-roasted, 'Deluxe'	1 oz	45	7	1	40	0	2.0	0.0	20	36%
(Carl Budding)										
peppered, smoked, sliced, chopped, 'Lean'	1 oz	40	5	1	0	0	2.0	0.0	0	43%
smoked, sliced	1 pkg	99	14	0	1016	0	4.6	1.8	48	42%
smoked, sliced	2 oz	79	11	0	811	0	3.7	1.5	38	42%
smoked, sliced, chopped, 'Lean'	1 oz	40	5	1	0	0	2.0	0.0	0	43%
(Eckrich) 'Slender Sliced'	1 oz	35	6	1	270	0	1.0	0.0	0	24%

Food Name	Serving Size	Calories	Prot. gms	Carbs gms	Sod. mgs	Fiber gms	Fat gms	Sat. Fat gms	Chol. mgs	% Fat Cal.
(Healthy Deli)										
roast	1 oz	30	6	0	130	0	0.4	0.0	13	12%
roast, Italian	1 oz	31	6	0	140	0	0.6	0.0	16	18%
(Hillshire Farm) roast, cured 'Deli Select'	1 oz	31	6	1	270	0	0.5	0.0	0	14%
(Hormel)										
jellied, 'Perma-Fresh'	2 slices	90	14	0	900	0	4.0	0.0	0	39%
smoked, cured	1 oz	50	5	0	315	0	2.0	0.0	0	47%
smoked, cured, dried	1 oz	45	8	0	822	0	1.0	0.0	0	22%
(Oscar Mayer)										
'Deli Thin'	4 slices	60	11	1	530	0	1.5	0.5	25	22%
roast, 'Thin Sliced'	0.4 oz	14	2	0	55	0	0.4	0.2	5	26%
smoked	0.5 oz	14	3	0	173	0	0.3	0.1	7	19%
BOLOGNA										
(Bar-S) chicken, 'Tasty Bolony'	1 slice	70	3	3	330	0	5.0	2.0	30	65%
(Boar's Head)										
beef	1 oz	74	4	1	270	0	7.0	0.0	17	76%
ham	1 oz	40	5	1	0	0	2.0	0.0	15	43%
pork and beef	1 oz	80	4	1	250	0	7.0	0.0	15	76%
(Butterball)										
'Turkey Variety Pak'	3/4 oz	50	3	1	280	0	4.0	0.0	0	69%
turkey 'Deli/Slice 'n Serve'	1 oz	70	4	2	370	0	6.0	0.0	0	69%
turkey, 'Cold Cuts'	1 oz	70	4	2	370	0	6.0	0.0	0	69%
(Eckrich)										
	1 oz	100	3	1	240	0	9.0	0.0	0	84%
beef	1 oz	90	3	1	230	0	8.0	0.0	0	82%
beef, 'Thick Sliced'	1.5 oz	130	4	2	340	0	12.0	0.0	0	82%
garlic	1 oz	90	3	1	230	0	9.0	0.0	0	84%
'German Brand'	1 oz	80	4	1	300	0	7.0	0.0	0	76%
'Lean Supreme'	1 oz	70	4	1	240	0	6.0	0.0	0	73%
'Sandwich'	1 oz	100	3	1	240	0	9.0	0.0	0	84%
'Smorgas Pac'	1 oz	100	3	1	240	0	9.0	0.0	0	84%
thick sliced, 1-lb pkg	1.8 oz	170	5	2	430	0	15.0	0.0	0	83%
w/cheese	1 oz	90	3	1	250	0	9.0	0.0	0	84%
(Empire Kosher)										
chicken, kosher	3 slices	200	7	2	360	0	7.0	2.0	40	64%
turkey, kosher, sliced	3 slices	90	8	3	430	0	5.5	1.5	30	53%
(Grillmaster) chicken	1 slice	70	3	1	350	0	6.0	2.0	30	77%
(Health Valley) chicken	1 slice	85	4	1	329	0	8.0	0.0	13	78%
(Healthy Choice)										
beef, low-fat, 'Cold Cuts'	1 slice	35	4	3	240	0	1.0	0.5	10	24%
low-fat, 'Deli-Thin'	4 slices	60	8	5	480	0	1.5	0.5	30	21%
turkey, pork and beef, low-fat, 'Cold Cuts'	1 slice	30	4	3	240	0	1.0	0.5	15	24%
(Healthy Deli) beef and pork	1 oz	41	4	1	200	0	2.0	0.0	9	45%
(Healthy Favorites) sliced	21 grams	20	3	1	239	0	0.3	0.2	5	14%
(Hebrew National) beef, 'Original Deli Style'	1 oz	90	3	1	330	0	3.0	0.0	15	63%
(Hillshire Farm)										
'Large'	1 oz	90	3	1	0	0	8.0	0.0	0	82%
'Ring'	1 oz	89	3	1	0	0	8.0	0.0	0	82%
(Hormel)										
beef, 'Coarse Ground, 1 lb.'	2 oz	160	8	1	576	0	14.0	0.0	0	78%
beef, 'Perma-Fresh'	2 slices	170	6	1	592	0	16.0	0.0	0	84%
'Fine Ground, 1-lb.'	2 oz	170	7	1	596	0	16.0	0.0	0	82%
'Perma-Fresh'	2 slices	180	7	0	599	0	16.0	0.0	0	84%

Food Name	Serving Size	Calories	Prot. gms	Carbs gms	Sod. mgs	Fiber gms	Fat gms	Sat. Fat gms	Chol. mgs	% Fat Cal.
(JM)										
'German Brand'	1 oz	70	4	1	270	0	6.0	0.0	0	73%
beef	1 oz	90	3	1	350	0	8.0	0.0	0	82%
garlic	1 oz	90	3	1	350	0	8.0	0.0	0	82%
(Kahn's)										
beef	1 slice	90	3	1	300	0	8.0	0.0	0	82%
beef, 'Family Pack'	1 slice	70	2	1	230	0	6.0	0.0	0	82%
beef, 'Giant'	1 slice	90	3	1	300	0	8.0	0.0	0	82%
beef, 'Pounder'	1 slice	90	3	1	300	0	8.0	0.0	0	82%
beef and cheddar	1 slice	90	4	1	320	0	8.0	0.0	0	78%
'Deluxe Club Family Pack'	1 slice	70	2	1	220	0	6.0	0.0	0	82%
'Deluxe Club'	1 slice	90	3	1	290	0	8.0	0.0	0	82%
garlic	1 slice	90	3	1	290	0	8.0	0.0	0	82%
'Giant Deluxe'	1 slice	90	3	1	290	0	8.0	0.0	0	82%
'Giant Thick Deluxe'	1 slice	110	4	1	330	0	10.0	0.0	0	82%
'Thick Deluxe'	1 slice	140	5	1	450	0	13.0	0.0	0	83%
'Thin Sliced Deluxe'	1 slice	60	2	1	190	0	5.0	0.0	0	79%
(Light and Lean)										
	2 slices	140	6	2	0	0	12.0	0.0	0	77%
'Thin Sliced'	2 slices	70	3	1	0	0	6.0	0.0	0	77%
(Longacre) turkey, sliced	1 oz	61	4	0	270	0	5.0	0.0	25	74%
(Louis Rich)										
turkey, mild	1 oz	59	4	1	298	0	4.5	1.5	18	69%
turkey	1 slice	52	3	1	270	0	3.7	1.1	19	65%
(Mr. Turkey) turkey	1 slice	67	3	1	377	0	5.6	1.6	25	74%
(Norbest) turkey, 'Blue Label' 2-2.5 lb.	1 oz	68	4	1	331	0	5.6	0.0	0	76%
(OHSE)										
	1 slice	130	4	1	430	0	11.0	5.0	30	83%
	1 oz	75	3	3	280	0	6.0	0.0	0	69%
beef	1 oz	85	3	1	310	0	8.0	0.0	0	82%
'15% Chicken'	1 oz	90	3	1	320	0	8.0	0.0	0	82%
turkey	1 oz	70	3	2	300	0	6.0	0.0	0	73%
(Oscar Mayer)										
	1 slice	90	3	1	290	0	8.0	3.0	30	82%
beef	1 slice	89	3	1	310	0	8.2	3.6	20	83%
beef, Lebanon	0.8 oz	46	5	0	302	0	2.9	1.4	16	56%
beef, light	1 slice	55	3	2	314	0	4.0	1.6	13	65%
chicken, pork, and beef	1 slice	89	3	1	289	0	8.2	2.9	29	83%
fat-free	1 slice	22	4	2	274	0	0.2	0.1	7	7%
garlic	1 slice	130	5	1	420	0	12.0	4.5	40	82%
light	1 slice	60	3	2	310	0	4.0	1.5	15	64%
pork, chicken, and beef, light	1 slice	56	3	2	312	0	4.1	1.6	15	66%
Wisconsin made ring	1 slice	175	7	1	463	0	15.9	6.2	35	82%
w/cheese	0.8 oz	74	3	1	232	0	6.8	2.6	15	82%
(Pilgrim's Pride)	1 oz	59	4	1	228	0	4.4	0.0	16	69%
(Smok-a-Roma) chicken, pork, and beef	1 slice	80	4	1	340	0	6.0	3.0	20	73%
(Tyson) chicken	1 slice	44	2	4	185	0	0.5	0.0	0	16%
CHICKEN BREAST										
(Carl Budding)										
smoked, sliced, chopped, 'Lean'	1 oz	50	5	1	0	0	3.0	0.0	0	53%
smoked, w/dark meat, sliced	1 pkg	117	13	0	677	0	7.2	1.8	38	55%
smoked, w/dark meat, sliced	2 oz	94	10	0	541	0	5.7	1.5	30	55%
(Healthy Choice)										
roasted, 'Cold Cuts'	1 slice	25	5	2	240	0	0.0	0.0	0	0%

Food Name	Serving Size	Calories	Prot. gms	Carbs gms	Sod. mgs	Fiber gms	Fat gms	Sat. Fat gms	Chol. mgs	% Fat Cal.
roasted, 'Fresh Trak'	1 slice	35	5	2	240	0	1.0	0.5	10	24%
smoked, 'Cold Cuts'	1 slice	30	5	2	240	0	1.0	0.5	15	24%
(Healthy Favorites)										
oven-roasted, fat-free, thin sliced	4 slices	40	9	1	620	0	0.0	0.0	25	0%
oven-roasted, thin sliced	1 slice	12	2	1	110	0	1.0	0.0	5	43%
(Hillshire Farm) smoked, boneless, 'Deli Select'	1 slice	31	6	1	290	0	0.2	0.0	0	6%
(Land O'Frost) smoked, thin sliced	2.5 oz	120	12	0	930	0	7.0	2.0	65	57%
(Longacre) 'Premium'	1 slice	45	4	1	280	0	3.0	0.0	20	57%
(Louis Rich)										
baked, 'Classic Baked Grill'	1 slice	44	9	2	514	0	0.2	0.1	23	5%
baked, thin sliced, 'Classic Baked Grill'	1 slice	22	4	1	251	0	0.1	0.0	11	5%
hickory smoked, boneless	1 slice	30	5	1	356	0	0.8	0.3	14	24%
hickory smoked, boneless, 97% fat-free	1 slice	30	5	1	370	0	1.0	0.0	15	27%
honey glazed, 'Carving Board'	1 slice	23	5	1	265	0	0.3	0.0	13	9%
roasted, 'Cold Cuts'	1 slice	36	5	1	335	0	1.6	0.4	17	39%
roasted, deluxe, 'Cold Cuts'	1 slice	28	5	1	333	0	0.6	0.2	14	18%
roasted, thin sliced, 'Deli Thin'	1 slice	15	2	0	155	0	0.4	0.1	6	25%
(Mr. Turkey)										
boneless	1 slice	32	5	1	242	0	1.1	0.0	9	31%
smoked, 'Deli Cut'	3 slices	28	5	2	357	0	0.1	na	13	2%
(Oscar Mayer)										
honey glazed, roasted	1 slice	57	10	2	721	0	0.7	0.2	28	12%
honey glazed, roasted, thin sliced	1 slice	14	3	1	180	0	0.2	0.1	7	12%
oven-roasted	1 slice	29	5	1	414	0	0.7	0.2	15	21%
roasted, fat-free	1 slice	44	10	1	646	0	0.3	0.1	23	6%
roasted, fat-free, thin sliced	1 slice	11	2	0	161	0	0.1	0.0	6	6%
smoked	1 slice	25	5	0	397	0	0.4	0.1	15	14%
'Thin Sliced'	1 slice	13	2	0	151	0	0.4	0.1	5	27%
(Tyson)										
breast, hickory smoked	1 slice	25	4	1	195	0	1.0	0.0	0	32%
honey flavored	1 slice	25	4	1	0	0	1.0	0.0	0	32%
mesquite, oven-roasted	1 slice	25	4	1	0	0	1.0	0.0	0	32%
oven-roasted	1 slice	25	4	1	185	0	0.5	0.0	0	20%
CHICKEN ROLL										
(Longacre) sliced	1 slice	60	4	1	210	0	5.0	0.0	25	69%
(Pilgrim's Pride)	1 slice	35	5	0	260	0	1.2	0.0	15	33%
(Tyson)	1 slice	26	3	1	153	0	0.5	0.0	0	20%
CORNED BEEF LOAF										
jellied	1 slice	43	6	0	270	0	1.7	0.7	13	36%
(Carl Budding)										
chopped, pressed	1 pkg	101	14	1	953	0	4.8	2.0	46	43%
chopped, pressed	2 oz	81	11	1	761	0	3.9	1.6	37	43%
DUTCH LOAF										
(Eckrich)										
'Lean Supreme'	1 slice	60	4	2	250	0	4.0	0.0	0	60%
'Smorgas Pac'	1 slice	70	3	2	300	0	6.0	0.0	0	73%
(Kahn's)	1 slice	80	3	1	280	0	7.0	0.0	0	80%
HAM										
(Boar's Head)										
boiled, 'Deluxe'	1 oz	28	5	1	275	0	1.0	0.0	15	27%
'Lower Salt'	1 slice	28	5	1	250	0	1.0	0.0	15	27%
(Butterball)										
turkey, 'Cold Cuts'	1 oz	35	5	1	390	0	1.0	0.0	0	27%
turkey, honey cured, chopped 'Cold Cuts'	1 oz	35	5	2	290	0	1.0	0.0	0	24%

Food Name	Serving Size	Calories	Prot. gms	Carbs gms	Sod. mgs	Fiber gms	Fat gms	Sat. Fat gms	Chol. mgs	% Fat Cal.
turkey, honey cured, 'Cold Cuts'	1 oz	35	5	1	380	0	1.0	0.0	0	27%
turkey, honey cured, 'Slice 'n Serve'	1 oz	40	5	1	370	0	2.0	0.0	0	43%
turkey, 'Slice 'n Serve'	1 oz	35	5	1	340	0	2.0	0.0	0	43%
turkey, sliced, 'Deli Thin'	1 oz	35	5	1	390	0	1.0	0.0	0	27%
(Carl Budding)										
honey, smoked, sliced, chopped, 'Lean'	1 slice	50	5	1	0	0	3.0	0.0	0	53%
smoked, sliced	1 pkg	116	13	1	981	0	6.6	2.2	39	51%
smoked, sliced	2 oz	92	10	1	783	0	5.3	1.8	31	51%
smoked, sliced, chopped, 'Lean'	1 slice	50	5	1	0	0	3.0	0.0	0	53%
(Danola)										
Danish, premium, 97% fat-free	1 slice	30	5	1	0	0	1.0	0.0	15	27%
Danish, premium, 97% fat-free, thin sliced	2 slices	45	8	0	650	0	1.0	0.5	25	22%
(Decker) chopped	1 slice	100	6	2	500	0	8.0	3.0	20	69%
(Eckrich)										
chopped	1 slice	45	5	1	350	0	2.0	0.0	0	43%
chopped, 'Lean Supreme'	1 slice	35	10	1	350	0	2.0	0.0	0	29%
smoked, 'Slender Sliced'	1 slice	40	5	1	360	0	2.0	0.0	0	43%
(Healthy Choice)										
baked, water added, 'Cold Cuts'	1 slice	30	5	1	240	0	1.0	0.5	10	27%
cooked, water added, 'Fresh Trak'	1 slice	30	5	1	240	0	1.0	0.5	15	27%
honey, water added, 'Cold Cuts'	1 slice	30	5	1	240	0	1.0	0.5	10	27%
honey, water added, 'Fresh Trak'	1 slice	30	5	1	240	0	1.0	0.5	10	27%
smoked, water added, 'Cold Cuts'	1 slice	30	5	1	240	0	1.0	0.5	10	27%
(Healthy Deli)										
baked, Virginia	1 slice	34	5	2	245	0	0.9	0.0	12	24%
baked, Virginia, less salt	1 slice	32	5	1	19	0	0.9	0.0	13	25%
Black Forest	1 slice	32	6	0	220	0	0.6	0.0	16	18%
cooked, fresh	1 slice	33	6	0	120	0	0.8	0.0	13	23%
'Deluxe'	1 slice	31	5	1	245	0	0.9	0.0	12	26%
honey, 'Honey Valley'	1 slice	31	5	1	26	0	0.8	0.0	10	23%
jalapeño	1 slice	25	4	1	260	0	0.6	0.0	11	23%
'Lessalt'	1 slice	32	5	1	190	0	0.9	0.0	13	25%
'Taverne'	1 slice	31	5	0	210	0	0.8	0.0	15	24%
(Healthy Favorites)										
baked, 98% fat-free	4 slices	50	9	1	600	0	1.0	0.0	25	18%
boiled, thin sliced	1 slice	12	2	1	115	0	1.0	0.0	5	43%
chicken, smoked, w/natural juices, thin sliced	1 slice	13	2	0	116	0	0.4	0.1	7	27%
honey, thin sliced	1 slice	14	2	1	115	0	1.0	0.0	5	43%
honey, water added, 'Breakfast'	1 slice	30	5	1	346	0	0.9	0.4	14	27%
honey baked, 98% fat-free, thin sliced	4 slices	50	9	2	630	0	1.5	0.5	25	23%
smoked, cooked, thin sliced	1 slice	14	2	1	115	0	1.0	0.0	5	43%
(Hormel)										
'Cure 81'	1 slice	89	15	0	872	na	3.0	1.0	43	30%
deli, cooked	1 slice	29	4	1	344	0	1.0	2.0	11	31%
chopped, 'Black Label'	1 slice	70	4	1	326	0	6.0	2.0	16	73%
chopped, 'Perma-Fresh'	2 slices	88	11	0	685	0	5.0	0.0	0	51%
(Jennie-O)										
turkey, cooked, natural smoked flavoring, cured	2 oz	80	8	1	610	0	4.5	1.5	35	53%
turkey, cooked, smoke flavoring, lean, 20% water added	2 oz	70	9	0	670	0	3.5	1.0	40	47%
(JM)										
chopped	1 slice	80	4	1	370	0	7.0	0.0	0	76%
cooked	1 slice	30	4	1	360	0	1.0	0.0	0	31%
'Slice 'n Eat 93% Fat-Free'	2 oz	70	10	1	630	0	3.0	0.0	24	38%

Food Name	Serving Size	Calories	Prot. gms	Carbs gms	Sod. mgs	Fiber gms	Fat gms	Sat. Fat gms	Chol. mgs	% Fat Cal.
'Slice 'n Eat 95% Fat-Free Presliced'	2 slices	60	9	1	620	0	2.0	0.0	30	31%
smoked, golden	2 slices	80	8	1	630	0	5.0	0.0	0	56%
smoked, golden, water added	2 slices	70	8	4	810	0	2.0	0.0	23	27%
(Jones Dairy Farm)										
'Farm'	1 slice	50	9	0	381	0	1.1	0.0	21	22%
'Farm Family Ham'	1 slice	35	6	0	298	0	1.2	0.0	14	32%
hickory smoked, 97% fat-free, 'Lean Choice'	2 slices	50	9	0	420	0	1.5	0.0	30	27%
(Kahn's)										
low-salt	1 slice	30	5	1	290	0	1.0	0.0	0	27%
chopped	1 slice	50	5	1	360	0	3.0	0.0	0	53%
cooked, sliced	1 slice	30	5	1	360	0	1.0	0.0	0	27%
(Light and Lean)										
barbecue	2 slices	50	8	0	0	0	2.0	0.0	0	36%
black peppered	2 slices	50	9	0	0	0	2.0	0.0	0	33%
chopped	2 slices	70	8	0	0	0	4.0	0.0	0	53%
cooked, sliced	2 slices	50	9	0	0	0	2.0	0.0	0	33%
glazed	2 slices	50	9	0	0	0	2.0	0.0	0	33%
red peppered	2 slices	50	9	0	0	0	2.0	0.0	0	33%
smoked, cooked	2 slices	50	9	0	0	0	2.0	0.0	0	33%
(Longacre)										
turkey, chunk	1 oz	37	5	0	360	0	2.0	0.0	25	47%
turkey, lean, lite, 'Deli'	1 oz	37	6	0	150	0	2.0	0.0	25	43%
turkey, sliced	1 oz	33	6	0	310	0	1.0	0.0	20	27%
(Louis Rich)										
baked, dinner slices	1 slice	80	16	1	1150	0	1.5	0.5	40	17%
turkey, chopped	1 oz	46	5	0	289	0	2.8	0.7	19	54%
turkey, cured	1 oz	25	4	1	217	0	0.7	0.2	14	25%
turkey, 'Deli Thin'	1 slice	15	3	0	145	0	0.4	0.1	9	25%
turkey, 15% water added, 'Cold Cuts'	1 slice	45	5	1	300	0	2.5	1.0	20	48%
turkey, honey cured, 'Cold Cuts' 15% water added	1 slice	30	5	1	290	0	1.0	0.0	20	27%
turkey, 96% fat-free, 'Deli-Thin'	1 slice	15	2	1	110	0	1.0	0.0	5	43%
turkey, 96% fat-free, square	1 slice	25	4	1	215	0	1.0	0.0	15	31%
turkey, 'Round'	1 oz	34	5	0	300	0	1.2	0.5	19	32%
turkey, 'Square'	1 slice	24	4	0	213	0	0.7	0.3	14	26%
turkey, 10% water added, 'Cold Cuts'	1 slice	35	5	0	310	0	1.0	0.0	20	31%
turkey, 10% water added, 'Square'	1 serving	32	5	0	316	0	1.1	0.3	19	33%
turkey, thin sliced	1 slice	12	2	0	111	0	0.4	0.1	7	28%
turkey, water added	1 oz	33	5	0	294	0	1.4	0.4	19	37%
turkey, water added, 94% fat-free	1 oz	35	5	1	300	0	2.0	0.0	20	43%
turkey, water added, 95% fat-free, round	1 slice	30	5	0	325	0	1.0	0.0	20	27%
(Mr. Turkey)										
turkey	1 slice	33	5	0	322	0	1.4	0.5	20	39%
turkey, chopped	1 oz	37	5	0	301	0	1.6	0.0	17	39%
turkey, smoked	1 slice	33	5	0	322	0	1.4	0.5	20	39%
turkey, smoked, breakfast	1 oz	33	5	0	306	0	1.3	0.0	16	35%
turkey, smoked, buffet style	1 oz	32	5	0	340	0	1.3	0.0	17	36%
turkey, smoked, 'Chub'	1 oz	32	5	0	340	0	1.3	0.0	17	36%
(Norbest)										
turkey, dark meat, hickory smoked	1 oz	39	5	0	335	0	2.2	0.0	0	51%
turkey, thigh meat, cured, Canadian style	1 oz	35	5	0	331	0	1.4	0.0	0	37%
turkey, thigh meat, cured, 'Gold Label'	1 oz	27	6	0	297	0	0.7	0.0	0	20%
turkey, thigh meat, cured, half, 'Tavern'	1 oz	29	5	1	312	0	0.8	0.0	0	25%
turkey, thigh meat cured, whole, 'Tavern'	1 oz	27	5	0	311	0	0.8	0.0	0	24%

Food Name	Serving Size	Calories	Prot. gms	Carbs gms	Sod. mgs	Fiber gms	Fat gms	Sat. Fat gms	Chol. mgs	% Fat Cal.
(OHSE)										
chopped	1 slice	65	4	1	260	0	5.0	0.0	0	69%
cooked	1 slice	30	5	1	260	0	1.0	0.0	0	27%
pit	1 slice	40	4	1	300	0	2.0	0.0	0	47%
smoked, 95% fat-free	1 slice	30	5	1	310	0	1.0	0.0	0	27%
turkey	1 oz	30	4	2	370	0	1.0	0.0	0	27%
(Oscar Mayer)										
baked	1 slice	21	4	0	238	0	0.5	0.1	11	21%
baked, water added, 96% fat free	1 slice	65	10	1	765	0	2.3	0.5	30	32%
baked, water added, 96% fat free, thin sliced	1 slice	22	3	0	255	0	0.8	0.2	10	32%
black peppered, cracked	1 slice	22	4	0	284	0	0.8	0.3	11	31%
boiled	1 slice	23	4	0	275	0	0.7	0.1	12	27%
boiled, thin sliced	1 slice	13	2	0	157	0	0.4	0.1	7	27%
boiled, water added, thin sliced	4 slices	50	9	0	680	0	2.0	0.5	25	33%
chopped	1 slice	50	4	1	340	0	3.0	1.5	15	57%
chopped, w/natural juice	1 slice	52	5	1	327	0	3.4	1.1	na	58%
honey, thin sliced	1 slice	13	2	0	153	0	0.4	0.2	7	26%
'Jubilee'	1 slice	43	5	0	365	0	2.4	0.8	15	50%
peppered, chopped	1 slice	55	4	1	312	0	3.7	1.3	16	61%
smoked, 40% ham/water product	1 slice	34	7	1	509	0	0.3	0.1	18	9%
smoked, 40% ham/water product, thin sliced	1 slice	12	2	0	173	0	0.1	0.0	6	9%
water added, boiled	1 slice	22	3	0	283	0	0.8	0.3	10	32%
water added, smoked, cooked	1 slice	21	3	0	255	0	0.8	0.3	10	33%
(Pilgrim's Pride) chicken	1 slice	35	4	1	430	0	1.8	0.0	18	46%
(Smok-a-Roma) cooked, 95% fat-free	1 slice	35	5	0	410	0	1.5	0.0	15	40%
(Swift)										
'Premium Hostess'	1 slice	30	5	0	330	0	1.0	0.0	0	31%
'Premium Sugar Plum'	1 slice	30	5	1	280	0	1.0	0.0	0	27%
(Tyson) turkey	1 slice	23	3	1	182	0	0.2	0.0	0	10%
HAM LOAF *(Eckrich)*	1 slice	50	5	1	290	0	4.0	0.0	0	60%
HAM AND CHEESE LOAF										
(Eckrich)	1 oz slice	50	4	1	300	0	4.0	0.0	0	64%
(Hormel)										
canned, 8-lb	3 oz	260	13	1	1135	0	22.0	0.0	0	78%
'Perma-Fresh'	2 slices	110	11	0	668	0	7.0	0.0	0	59%
(Kahn's)	1 slice	70	4	1	310	0	6.0	0.0	0	73%
(Light and Lean)	2 slices	90	8	0	0	0	6.0	0.0	0	63%
(OHSE)	1 oz	65	4	2	190	0	5.0	0.0	0	65%
(Oscar Mayer)	1 slice	66	4	1	358	0	5.0	2.4	19	68%
HEAD CHEESE *(Oscar Mayer)*	1 slice	52	4	0	300	0	3.8	1.2	25	66%
HONEY LOAF										
(Eckrich) 'Smorgas Pac'	1 oz slice	35	4	2	280	0	1.0	0.0	0	27%
(Hormel) 'Perma-Fresh'	2 slices	90	1	0	584	0	5.0	0.0	0	92%
(Kahn's)	1 slice	40	4	1	320	0	2.0	0.0	0	47%
(Oscar Mayer)	1 slice	34	5	1	378	0	1.0	0.4	16	27%
IOWA BRAND LOAF *(Hormel)* 'Perma-Fresh'	2 slices	90	10	0	607	0	6.0	0.0	0	57%
JALAPEÑO LOAF *(Kahn's)*	1 slice	70	3	2	340	0	6.0	0.0	0	73%
LIVER CHEESE										
(JM)	1 oz slice	70	4	1	0	0	6.0	0.0	0	73%
(Oscar Mayer) pork fat wrapped	1 slice	114	6	1	419	0	9.9	3.5	80	78%
LIVER LOAF										
(Hormel) 'Perma-Fresh'	2 slices	160	9	1	704	0	13.0	0.0	0	75%
(Kahn's)	1 slice	170	6	3	370	0	15.0	0.0	0	79%

Food Name	Serving Size	Calories	Prot. gms	Carbs gms	Sod. mgs	Fiber gms	Fat gms	Sat. Fat gms	Chol. mgs	% Fat Cal.
LIVERWURST										
(Hickory Farms)	1 oz	97	4	1	249	0	9.0	0.0	74	80%
(Hormel) canned	0.5 oz	35	2	0	0	0	3.0	0.0	0	77%
(Jones Dairy Farm)										
'Farm Club'	1 oz	80	5	0	254	0	6.3	0.0	43	76%
'Farm Slices'	1 slice	75	4	0	186	0	6.6	0.0	43	81%
(Oscar Mayer)										
Braunschweiger, sliced	1 slice	94	4	1	324	0	8.5	3.1	49	81%
Braunschweiger, tube	1 serving	191	8	1	626	0	17.1	6.1	90	81%
(Underwood) canned	2-1/8 oz	180	8	4	470	0	15.0	0.0	90	74%
LOAF										
(Armour)										
canned, 'Treet'	2 oz	200	6	3	840	0	17.0	0.0	0	81%
low-salt, canned, 'Treet'	2 oz	190	6	3	610	0	16.0	0.0	0	80%
(Hormel)										
pork w/chicken, light, 'Spam'	2 oz	108	9	1	578	na	7.8	2.5	42	65%
pork w/ham, 'Spam'	2 oz	172	7	1	789	na	15.6	5.7	39	82%
pork w/ham, less salt, 'Spam'	2 oz	176	8	1	550	0	15.0	5.0	38	79%
pork w/ham, light, 'Spam'	2 oz	140	8	1	560	0	12.0	4.0	43	75%
pork w/ham, smoke-flavored, 'Spam'	2 oz	170	8	0	774	0	15.0	0.0	0	81%
pork w/ham, w/cheese chunks, 'Spam'	2 oz	170	8	0	811	0	16.0	0.0	0	82%
(JM) 'P&B'	1 slice	70	3	2	330	0	5.0	0.0	0	69%
(Kahn's) 'P&B'	1 slice	40	5	1	270	0	2.0	0.0	0	43%
(OHSE)										
	1 slice	100	5	2	440	0	8.0	3.0	30	72%
	1 oz	75	3	1	320	0	6.0	0.0	0	77%
(Oscar Mayer) spiced	1 slice	70	4	2	340	0	5.0	1.5	20	65%
(Smok-a-Roma)										
	2 slices	90	4	0	200	0	8.0	2.5	10	82%
spiced	1 slice	90	4	2	370	0	7.0	3.0	20	72%
MACARONI AND CHEESE LOAF										
(Eckrich)	1 slice	75	3	3	320	0	6.0	0.0	0	69%
(OHSE)	1 slice	60	4	4	310	0	3.0	0.0	0	46%
OLD FASHIONED LOAF (Oscar Mayer)	1 slice	65	4	2	332	0	4.6	1.6	17	64%
OLIVE LOAF										
(Eckrich)	1 slice	80	3	2	320	0	6.0	0.0	0	73%
(Hormel) 'Perma-Fresh'	2 slices	110	7	5	810	0	7.0	0.0	0	57%
(Oscar Mayer) chicken, pork, turkey	1 slice	74	3	2	369	0	6.1	2.0	20	75%
PASTRAMI										
(Boar's Head) 'Round'	1 slice	40	6	1	270	0	1.5	0.0	16	33%
(Butterball)										
turkey, 'Cold Cuts'	1 oz	30	5	0	290	0	1.0	0.0	0	31%
turkey, 'Slice 'n Serve'	1 oz	35	5	1	320	0	1.0	0.0	0	27%
(Carl Budding)										
beef, smoked, chopped, pressed	1 pkg	100	14	1	750	0	4.6	2.1	46	41%
beef, smoked, chopped, pressed	2 oz	80	11	1	599	0	3.7	1.7	37	41%
smoked, sliced, chopped, 'Lean'	1 slice	40	5	1	0	0	2.0	0.0	0	43%
(Empire Kosher) turkey, kosher, sliced	3 slices	60	9	0	270	1	2.0	0.5	30	33%
(Healthy Deli) 'Deli Round'	1 slice	34	5	1	195	0	1.1	0.0	14	29%
(Longacre) turkey, sliced	1 oz	32	5	0	260	0	1.0	0.0	20	31%
(Louis Rich)										
turkey	1 slice	30	5	0	320	0	1.0	0.0	20	31%
turkey, 96% fat-free, 'Deli-Thin'	1 slice	10	2	1	125	0	1.0	0.0	5	43%
turkey, 96% fat-free, square	1 oz slice	25	4	1	260	0	1.0	0.0	15	31%

Food Name	Serving Size	Calories	Prot. gms	Carbs gms	Sod. mgs	Fiber gms	Fat gms	Sat. Fat gms	Chol. mgs	% Fat Cal.
turkey, 'Round'..................	1 oz	32	5	0	288	0	1.1	0.4	18	31%
turkey, 'Square'.................	1 oz	24	4	0	262	0	0.7	0.1	14	27%
turkey, thin sliced...............	1 oz	11	2	0	125	0	0.4	0.2	7	30%
(Mr. Turkey)										
turkey	1 slice	31	4	1	298	0	1.0	0.3	17	30%
turkey, sliced, 'Deli Cut'........	3 slices	36	5	1	260	0	1.4	0.5	21	35%
(Norbest) turkey, 3 lb	1 oz	29	5	0	302	0	0.8	0.0	0	26%
(Oscar Mayer) thin sliced......	1 slice	16	3	0	217	0	0.3	0.2	7	16%
PEPPERED LOAF										
(Eckrich)...................	1 slice	35	5	2	340	0	1.0	0.0	0	24%
(Kahn's)....................	1 slice	40	5	1	340	0	2.0	0.0	0	43%
(Oscar Mayer)	1 slice	39	5	1	367	0	1.5	0.8	14	35%
PICKLE AND PIMIENTO LOAF										
(Oscar Mayer)										
....	1 slice	80	3	3	360	0	6.0	2.0	20	69%
w/chicken....................	1 serving	75	3	3	357	0	6.0	2.0	22	72%
PICKLE LOAF										
(Eckrich) 'Smorgas Pac'.......	1 slice	80	3	2	270	0	6.0	0.0	0	73%
(Hormel) 'Perma-Fresh'........	2 slices	102	8	3	752	0	7.0	0.0	0	59%
(Kahn's)										
....	1 slice	80	3	2	280	0	7.0	0.0	0	76%
beef 'Family Pack'...........	1 slice	60	2	1	210	0	5.0	0.0	0	79%
'Family Pack'...............	1 slice	70	3	2	220	0	6.0	0.0	0	73%
(Light and Lean).............	2 slices	100	8	3	0	0	6.0	0.0	0	55%
(OHSE)....................	1 oz	60	3	2	330	0	4.0	0.0	0	64%
(Smok-a-Roma) w/turkey and pork ...	1 slice	90	5	4	300	0	6.0	1.5	15	60%
PORK *(Eckrich)* 'Slender Sliced'........	1 oz	45	5	1	320	0	2.0	0.0	0	43%
SALAMI										
(Boar's Head) beef..........	1 oz	60	5	1	288	0	4.0	0.0	20	60%
(Eckrich)										
beer.......................	1 slice	70	4	1	330	0	6.0	0.0	0	73%
cotto	1 slice	70	4	1	380	0	6.0	0.0	0	73%
cotto, beef.................	1.3 oz	100	5	2	460	0	8.0	0.0	0	72%
(Gallo Salame)										
dry, Italian, light, w/turkey, pork, and beef	7 slices	70	8	1	360	0	5.0	1.5	30	56%
(Hebrew National) beef, 'Original Deli Style'	1 oz	80	7	1	230	0	7.0	0.0	15	66%
(Hickory Farms)										
dry or hard.................	1 oz	120	6	0	535	0	10.0	0.0	30	79%
Genoa.....................	1 oz	110	6	0	540	0	10.0	0.0	20	79%
(Hormel)										
beef, 'Perma-Fresh'..........	2 slices	50	3	0	219	0	5.0	0.0	0	79%
cotto, 'Club'	1 oz	100	5	0	385	0	5.0	0.0	0	69%
cotto, 'Perma-Fresh'.........	2 slices	105	9	1	750	0	7.0	0.0	0	61%
dry or hard.................	1 oz	110	7	0	468	0	10.0	0.4	0	76%
dry or hard, 'Homeland'......	1 oz	117	6	2	448	0	10.0	4.0	29	74%
dry or hard, 'National Brand'..	1 oz	120	6	0	463	0	11.0	0.0	0	80%
dry or hard, 'Perma-Fresh'....	2 slices	80	4	0	339	0	7.0	0.0	0	80%
dry or hard, 'Sliced'.........	1 oz	110	6	0	483	0	10.0	0.0	0	79%
Genoa.....................	1 oz	110	6	0	456	0	10.0	0.0	0	79%
Genoa, 'DiLusso'............	1 oz	100	6	0	443	0	8.0	0.0	0	75%
Genoa, 'Gran Valore'........	1 oz	110	6	0	453	0	10.0	0.0	0	79%
Genoa, 'San Remo Brand' ...	1 oz	118	7	0	541	0	10.0	0.0	0	76%
'Party'	1 oz	90	5	0	399	0	8.0	0.0	0	78%
piccolo, 'Stick'.............	1 oz	120	6	0	512	0	11.0	0.0	0	80%

Food Name	Serving Size	Calories	Prot. gms	Carbs gms	Sod. mgs	Fiber gms	Fat gms	Sat. Fat gms	Chol. mgs	% Fat Cal.
(JM)										
cotto	1 oz slice	80	4	2	270	0	6.0	0.0	0	69%
dry or hard	1 oz slice	110	6	1	580	0	9.0	0.0	0	74%
Genoa	1 oz slice	100	6	1	540	0	8.0	0.0	0	72%
(Kahn's)										
beef	1 slice	70	3	1	250	0	6.0	0.0	0	77%
beef, 'Family Pack'	1 slice	60	2	1	190	0	5.0	0.0	0	79%
cooked	1 slice	60	4	1	300	0	4.0	0.0	0	64%
cotto, 'Family Pack'	1 slice	45	3	1	230	0	3.0	0.0	0	63%
(Light and Lean) cotto	2 slices	80	6	0	0	0	6.0	0.0	0	69%
(Mr. Turkey) cotto, turkey	1 slice	49	4	1	239	0	3.3	1.1	21	60%
(OHSE) cooked	1 oz	65	4	1	330	0	5.0	0.0	0	69%
(Oscar Mayer)										
beef, 'Machiaeh Brand'	1 slice	60	3	0	265	0	5.0	0.0	15	79%
beer	1 slice	52	3	0	283	0	4.2	1.5	16	73%
cotto	1 slice	70	3	1	280	0	5.0	2.0	25	74%
cotto, beef	1 slice	47	3	0	301	0	3.6	1.6	19	69%
cotto, beef, pork, and chicken	1 slice	56	3	1	252	0	4.7	1.9	18	75%
Genoa	1 slice	35	2	0	164	0	3.0	1.1	9	77%
hard	1 slice	36	2	0	169	0	2.8	1.0	9	70%
SPICE LOAF										
(Hormel)										
canned	3 oz	280	11	2	1110	0	26.0	0.0	0	82%
'Perma-Fresh'	2 slices	118	9	1	702	0	9.0	0.0	0	67%
(JM)	1 slice	70	4	1	370	0	6.0	0.0	0	73%
(Kahn's)										
beef, 'Family Pack'	1 slice	60	2	1	200	0	5.0	0.0	0	79%
'Family Pack'	1 slice	70	3	1	180	0	6.0	0.0	0	77%
'Luncheon Loaf'	1 slice	80	3	1	240	0	7.0	0.0	0	80%
(Oscar Mayer)	1 serving	66	4	2	343	0	4.7	1.5	19	65%
TURKEY BREAST										
(Boar's Head)										
golden	1 oz	35	6	1	200	0	1.0	0.0	20	24%
golden, skinless	1 oz	30	6	1	0	0	1.0	0.0	10	24%
(Butterball)										
barbecue seasoned, 'Slice 'n Serve'	1 oz	40	5	1	210	0	2.0	0.0	0	43%
'Cold Cuts'	1 oz	30	5	1	230	0	1.0	0.0	0	27%
hickory smoked, 'Slice 'n Serve'	1 oz	35	5	1	250	0	1.0	0.0	0	27%
no salt added, 'Deli'	1 oz	45	7	0	15	0	2.0	0.0	0	39%
'Slice 'n Serve'	1 oz	35	5	1	230	0	1.0	0.0	0	27%
smoked, 'Cold Cuts'	1 oz	35	5	0	190	0	1.0	0.0	0	31%
smoked, 'Turkey Variety Pak'	3/4 oz	25	4	1	160	0	1.0	0.0	0	31%
(Carl Budding)										
and dark meat, smoked, sliced	1 pkg	114	12	1	778	0	6.5	2.2	40	51%
and dark meat, smoked, sliced	2 oz	91	10	1	621	0	5.2	1.8	32	51%
smoked, sliced, chopped, 'Lean'	1 oz	50	5	1	0	0	3.0	0.0	0	53%
(Carving Board)										
hickory-smoked	1 slice	40	9	0	540	0	0.5	0.0	20	11%
traditional	1 slice	40	9	0	540	0	0.5	0.0	20	11%
(Empire Kosher)										
oven prepared, kosher, sliced	3 slices	50	10	1	200	0	0.5	0.0	15	9%
smoked, kosher, sliced	3 slices	40	8	0	350	0	0.0	0.0	15	0%

Food Name	Serving Size	Calories	Prot. gms	Carbs gms	Sod. mgs	Fiber gms	Fat gms	Sat. Fat gms	Chol. mgs	% Fat Cal.
(Healthy Choice)										
and white meat, honey roasted and smoked,										
'Cold Cuts'	1 slice	35	5	2	240	0	1.0	0.5	15	24%
honey roasted and smoked	1 slice	35	6	1	230	0	1.0	1.0	15	24%
honey roasted and smoked, 'Fresh Trak'	1 slice	35	5	2	240	0	1.0	0.5	15	24%
roasted, 'Cold Cuts'	1 slice	30	5	1	240	0	1.0	0.5	15	27%
roasted, 'Fresh Trak'	1 slice	30	5	1	240	0	1.0	0.5	15	27%
roasted, 97% fat-free	1 slice	30	6	1	290	0	1.0	1.0	10	24%
smoked, 'Cold Cuts'	1 slice	30	5	2	240	0	1.0	0.5	15	24%
(Healthy Deli)										
'Gourmet'	1 oz	28	5	1	170	0	0.6	0.0	9	20%
honey	1 oz	28	5	1	170	0	0.5	0.0	9	17%
'Lessalt'	1 oz	25	5	0	140	0	0.5	0.0	9	19%
oven cooked	1 oz	26	5	0	180	0	0.2	0.0	8	8%
smoked 'Gourmet'	1 oz	31	6	0	170	0	0.5	0.0	11	15%
smoked, 3-lb	1 oz	29	5	1	180	0	0.5	0.0	8	18%
(Healthy Favorites)										
oven-roasted	1 slice	12	2	1	100	0	1.0	0.0	5	43%
oven-roasted, fat-free	4 slices	40	8	2	610	0	0.0	0.0	15	0%
smoked	1 slice	12	2	1	80	0	1.0	0.0	5	43%
(Hormel)										
'Perma-Fresh'	2 slices	60	9	0	484	0	2.0	0.0	0	33%
smoked, 'Perma-Fresh'	2 slices	60	10	0	540	0	2.0	0.0	0	31%
(Land O'Frost) smoked, thin sliced	2.5 oz	110	12	0	990	0	7.0	2.0	55	57%
(Light and Lean) breast	2 slices	60	8	0	0	0	2.0	0.0	0	36%
(Longacre)										
and white meat, browned and roasted	1 oz	40	5	1	240	0	2.0	0.0	15	43%
and white meat, 'Deli Chef'	1 oz	35	5	1	240	0	1.0	0.0	15	27%
and white meat, skinless 'Deli Chef'	1 oz	40	4	1	240	0	2.0	0.0	15	47%
browned, glazed, 'Gourmet'	1 oz	35	5	1	240	0	1.0	0.0	15	27%
browned, glazed, 'Premium'	1 oz	30	4	1	300	0	1.0	0.0	10	31%
browned, roasted, 'Gourmet'	1 oz	35	5	1	260	0	1.0	0.0	15	27%
browned, roasted, 'Premium'	1 oz	30	4	1	300	0	1.0	0.0	10	31%
'Catering'	1 oz	35	6	1	280	0	1.0	0.0	15	24%
'Gourmet'	1 oz	35	5	1	300	0	1.0	0.0	15	27%
lean, lite, 'Deli'	1 oz	35	6	0	160	0	1.0	0.0	15	27%
lean, lite, skinless, 'Deli'	1 oz	35	6	0	160	0	1.0	0.0	15	27%
lean, lite, smoked, 'Deli'	1 oz	35	6	0	160	0	1.0	0.0	15	27%
low-salt, 'Gourmet'	1 oz	30	6	1	150	0	1.0	0.0	10	24%
'Premium'	1 oz	30	4	1	250	0	1.0	0.0	10	31%
'Salt Watchers'	1 oz	32	7	0	10	0	1.0	0.0	15	24%
skinless, 'Catering'	1 oz	35	6	1	280	0	1.0	0.0	15	24%
skinless, 'Gourmet'	1 oz	30	5	1	260	0	1.0	0.0	15	27%
skinless, 'Premium'	1 oz	30	4	1	250	0	1.0	0.0	10	31%
sliced	1 oz	30	5	1	280	0	1.0	0.0	10	27%
smoked	1 oz	35	6	0	240	0	1.0	0.0	15	27%
smoked, sliced	1 oz	26	5	1	260	0	1.0	0.0	10	27%
(Louis Rich)										
and white meat, roasted	1 serving	27	5	1	309	0	0.5	0.1	11	17%
and white meat, smoked	1 serving	28	5	1	257	0	0.6	0.2	12	21%
'Carving Board'	22 grams	21	5	0	272	0	0.3	0.1	9	13%
cooked, barbecued, no skin	1 oz	30	6	1	280	0	1.0	0.0	10	24%
hickory smoked	1 slice	60	11	2	640	0	0.0	0.0	0	0%
hickory smoked, nonfat, 'Cold Cuts'	1 slice	25	4	1	300	0	0.0	0.0	0	0%

Food Name	Serving Size	Calories	Prot. gms	Carbs gms	Sod. mgs	Fiber gms	Fat gms	Sat. Fat gms	Chol. mgs	% Fat Cal.
honey roasted, 95% fat-free	1 slice	35	5	1	315	0	1.0	0.0	10	27%
nonfat, 'Deli-Thin'	4 slices	40	8	2	608	0	0.0	0.0	0	0%
oven-roasted	1 oz	31	5	1	323	0	0.8	0.3	11	23%
oven-roasted, 97% fat-free, 'Deli-Thin'	1 slice	10	2	1	125	0	1.0	0.0	5	43%
roasted	1 slice	50	11	1	620	0	0.0	0.0	0	0%
roasted, fat-free	1 slice	24	4	1	334	0	0.2	0.1	9	8%
roasted, nonfat, 'Cold Cuts'	1 slice	25	4	1	330	0	0.0	0.0	0	0%
roasted, thin sliced	1 slice	12	2	0	127	0	0.3	0.1	4	23%
smoked	1 slice	21	5	0	211	0	0.3	0.1	9	13%
smoked, 'Carving Board'	1 slice	21	4	0	264	0	0.2	0.1	9	10%
smoked, 98% fat-free	1 slice	20	4	1	210	0	1.0	0.0	10	31%
smoked, 97% fat-free, 'Deli-Thin'	1 slice	10	2	1	110	0	1.0	0.0	5	43%
smoked, 96% fat-free'	1 oz	35	6	1	270	0	1.0	0.0	10	24%
smoked, thin sliced	0.4 oz slice	11	2	0	111	0	0.1	0.0	5	9%
white, smoked, 'Cold Cuts'	1 slice	30	5	0	280	0	1.0	0.0	15	31%
(Mr. Turkey)										
	1 oz	31	6	0	233	0	0.7	0.0	10	21%
smoked	1 oz	31	6	0	332	0	0.7	0.0	10	20%
honey roasted, 'Deli Cut'	3 slices	30	5	2	309	0	0.5	0.1	15	16%
roasted	1 slice	33	5	2	274	0	0.8	0.3	13	21%
roasted, quartered	3.5 oz	94	15	3	1035	0	2.2	0.7	40	21%
smoked, 'Deli Cut'	3 slices	24	4	2	354	0	0.2	0.1	11	6%
smoked, quartered	3.5 oz	89	17	4	1275	0	0.5	0.2	31	5%
(Norbest)										
and thigh, 'Blue Label'	1 oz	31	6	0	238	0	0.9	0.0	0	25%
skinless, 'Blue Label'	1 oz	24	4	1	253	0	0.3	0.0	0	12%
skinless, 'Orange Label'	1 oz	26	5	1	239	0	0.2	0.0	0	7%
skinless, 'Tan Label'	1 oz	24	4	1	354	0	0.5	0.0	0	19%
skinless, 'Yellow Label'	1 oz	24	4	0	284	0	0.5	0.0	0	19%
skinless, salt-free, 'Blue Label'	1 oz	33	8	0	13	0	0.3	0.0	0	8%
smoked, 'Gold Label'	1 oz	29	6	0	270	0	0.6	0.0	0	17%
w/skin, 'Blue Label'	1 oz	28	5	0	239	0	0.7	0.0	0	23%
w/skin, 'Orange Label'	1 oz	26	5	0	256	0	0.3	0.0	0	11%
w/skin, 'Yellow Label'	1 oz	25	5	0	244	0	0.5	0.0	0	19%
w/skin, prebrowned, 'Orange Label'	1 oz	29	5	0	259	0	0.8	0.0	0	25%
w/skin, salt-free, 'Blue Label'	1 oz	35	8	0	13	0	0.5	0.0	0	13%
w/skin, smoked, 'Orange Label'	1 oz	30	5	1	284	0	0.5	0.0	0	15%
(OHSE)										
oven cooked	1 oz	30	5	1	190	0	1.0	0.0	0	27%
smoked	1 oz	30	5	1	340	0	1.0	0.0	0	27%
(Oscar Mayer)										
cooked, oven-roasted, thin sliced	1 slice	12	2	0	151	0	0.2	0.1	5	15%
smoked	1 slice	20	4	0	300	0	0.2	0.1	9	9%
roasted	4 slices	50	9	2	580	0	1.0	0.0	20	17%
roasted, nonfat	4 slices	40	8	2	670	0	0.0	0.0	0	0%
smoked, fat-free	1 slice	10	2	0	142	0	0.1	0.0	4	7%
smoked, honey roasted	4 slices	60	10	2	520	0	1.0	0.0	20	16%
smoked, nonfat	4 slices	40	8	2	570	0	0.0	0.0	0	0%
white, roasted	1 slice	30	4	1	300	0	1.0	0.0	10	31%
(Tyson) breast	1 slice	20	4	0	136	0	0.4	0.0		17%
TURKEY HAM. See under LUNCHEON MEAT, HAM.										
TURKEY LOAF										
(Louis Rich) 89% fat-free	1 oz	45	5	0	270	0	2.8	0.8	16	56%

Food Name	Serving Size	Calories	Prot. gms	Carbs gms	Sod. mgs	Fiber gms	Fat gms	Sat. Fat gms	Chol. mgs	% Fat Cal.
(Mr. Turkey) spiced	1 oz	51	4	1	292	0	3.6	0.0	11	63%
TURKEY ROLL										
(Norbest)										
	1 oz	31	5	1	346	0	1.1	0.0	0	33%
white and dark meat, 'Orange Label'	1 oz	36	4	0	314	0	2.0	0.0	0	51%
white meat, diced	1 oz	31	4	1	318	0	0.9	0.0	0	27%
white meat, 'Orange Label'	1 oz	29	4	1	299	0	0.9	0.0	0	31%
LUNCHEON MEAT SPREAD										
(Hormel)										
deviled, 'Spam'	1 oz	78	4	2	260	0	7.0	2.0	20	72%
deviled, 'Spam'	1 tbsp	35	2	0	125	0	3.0	0.0	0	77%
LUNCHEON MEAT SUBSTITUTE										
(White Wave)										
chicken style, sandwich sliced *(White Wave)*	1 slice	80	12	8	260	0	0.0	0.0	0	0%
pastrami style, vegetarian, sandwich sliced	1 slice	90	14	8	270	1	0.0	0.0	0	0%
(Worthington)										
bologna style, vegetarian, 'Bolono'	3 slices	79	10	2	717	2	3.3	0.8	2	38%
salami style, vegetarian, 'Meatless Salami'	3 slices	130	12	2	930	2	8.0	1.0	0	55.4%
smoked turkey style slices, vegetarian *(Worthington)*	3 slices	142	10	3	618	3	9.9	1.9	1	63%
vegetarian, 'Numete'	3/8-inch slice	130	6	5	270	3	10.0	2.5	0	69.2%
vegetarian, 'Protose'	3/8-inch slice	131	13	5	283	3	6.7	1.0	0	46%
LUPIN										
mature seeds, boiled	1 cup	198	26	16	7	5	4.8	0.6	0	21%
mature seeds, raw	1 cup	668	65	73	27	na	17.5	2.1	0	22%

M

Food Name	Serving Size	Calories	Prot. gms	Carbs gms	Sod. mgs	Fiber gms	Fat gms	Sat. Fat gms	Chol. mgs	% Fat Cal.
MACADAMIA NUT										
dried, whole, 10–12 kernels	1 oz	204	2	4	1	2	21.5	3.4	0	88%
dried, whole or halves	1 cup	962	11	19	7	12	101.5	16.2	0	88%
dry-roasted, salted, whole, 10-12 kernels	1 oz	203	2	4	75	2	21.6	3.4	0	89%
dry-roasted, salted, whole or halves	1 cup	959	10	17	355	11	101.9	16.0	0	89%
dry-roasted, unsalted, whole, 10-12 kernels	1 oz	204	2	4	1	2	21.6	3.4	0	89%
dry-roasted, unsalted, whole or halves	1 cup	962	10	18	5	11	101.9	16.0	0	89%
salted *(Maunu Loa)*	1 oz	210	2	4	75	0	21.0	0.0	0	89%
shelled, salted *(Maunu Loa)*	1 oz	210	2	4	75	0	21.0	0.0	0	89%
unsalted, natural *(Flanigan Farms)*	1/4 cup	200	2	4	0	1	21.0	3.0	0	89%
MACADAMIA NUT BUTTER										
roasted *(Maranatha Natural)*	2 tbsp	200	2	6	5	0	19.0	0.0	0	84%
roasted, organic *(Maranatha Natural)*	2 tbsp	230	3	5	0	3	24.0	4.0	0	87%
MACARONI. See under PASTA.										
MACARONI DISH/ENTRÉE. See under PASTA DISH ENTRÉE.										
MACE										
ground	1 tbsp	25	0	3	4	1	1.7	0.5	0	57%
ground	1 tsp	8	0	1	1	0	0.6	0.2	0	57%
ground *(Durkee)*	1 tsp	10	0	0	0	0	0.0	0.0	0	0%
ground *(Laurel Leaf)*	1 tsp	10	0	0	0	0	0.0	0.0	0	0%
ground *(McCormick/Schilling)*	1 tsp	8	0	1	2	0	0.4	0.0	0	53%
ground *(Spice Islands)*	1 tsp	10	0	1	1	0	0.7	0.0	0	64%
ground *(Tone's)*	1 tsp	8	0	1	1	0	0.6	0.2	0	57%

Food Name	Serving Size	Calories	Prot. gms	Carbs gms	Sod. mgs	Fiber gms	Fat gms	Sat. Fat gms	Chol. mgs	% Fat Cal.
MACKEREL										
ATLANTIC										
baked, broiled, grilled, or microwaved	4 oz	297	27.0	0.0	94	0	20.2	4.7	85	63%
baked, broiled, grilled, or microwaved	3 oz	223	20.3	0.0	71	0	15.1	3.5	64	63%
raw	1 lb	929	84.4	0.0	408	0	63.0	14.8	318	63%
raw	3 oz	174	15.8	0.0	77	0	11.8	2.8	59	63%
JACK, mixed species										
Canned										
drained	1 cup	296	44.1	0.0	720	0	12.0	3.5	150	38%
drained	4 oz	177	26.3	0.0	430	0	7.1	2.1	90	38%
Fresh										
baked, broiled, grilled, or microwaved	3 oz	171	21.9	0.0	94	0	8.6	2.5	51	47%
raw	1 lb	712	91.0	0.0	391	0	35.8	10.2	213	47%
raw	3 oz	134	17.1	0.0	73	0	6.7	1.9	40	47%
KING										
baked, broiled, grilled, or microwaved	3 oz	114	22.1	0.0	173	0	2.2	0.4	58	18%
raw	1 lb	475	92.0	0.0	717	0	9.1	1.6	242	18%
raw	3 oz	89	17.2	0.0	134	0	1.7	0.3	45	18%
PACIFIC, mixed species										
baked, broiled, grilled, or microwaved	3 oz	171	21.9	0.0	94	0	8.6	2.5	51	47%
raw	1 lb	712	91.0	0.0	391	0	35.8	10.2	213	47%
raw	3 oz	134	17.1	0.0	73	0	6.7	1.9	40	47%
SPANISH										
baked, broiled, grilled, or microwaved	5.1-oz fillet	231	34.4	0.0	96	0	9.2	2.6	107	36%
baked, broiled, grilled, or microwaved	4 oz	179	26.8	0.0	75	0	7.2	2.0	83	36%
baked, broiled, grilled, or microwaved	3 oz	134	20.0	0.0	56	0	5.4	1.5	62	36%
raw	1 lb	631	87.5	0.0	266	0	28.6	8.3	345	41%
raw	3 oz	118	16.4	0.0	50	0	5.3	1.5	65	41%
MAHI MAHI / dolphin fish										
Fresh										
baked, broiled, grilled, or microwaved	3 oz	93	20	0	96	0	0.8	0.2	80	7%
raw	3 oz	72	16	0	75	0	0.6	0.2	62	7%
Frozen *(Peter Pan Seafoods)* fillets, boneless, skinless	3.5 oz	85	19	0	88	0	0.7	0.0	73	8%
MAI TAI. See under COCKTAIL MIX.										
MALABAR SPINACH. See SPINACH, MALABAR.										
MALACCA APPLE, w/o seeds	1 oz	9	0.2	2.3	na	>.2 c	<.1	tr	0	<8%
MALT, dry	1 oz	103	3.7	21.7	22	>1.6 c	0.5	0.0	0	4%
MALT EXTRACT, dried	1 oz	103	1.7	25.0	22	0	0.0	0.0	0	0%
MALT SYRUP. See under SYRUP.										
MALTED MILK FLAVOR DRINK MIX										
CHOCOLATE FLAVOR										
w/added nutrients, powder, mix only	1 cup	279	4	66	463	1	2.7	1.5	4	8%
w/added nutrients, powder, prepared w/milk	8 fl oz	225	9	29	244	0	8.7	5.5	34	35%
w/o added nutrients, powder, mix only	1 envelope	79	1	18	53	0	0.8	0.5	1	9%
w/o added nutrients, powder, prepared w/milk	8 fl oz *(1 cup)*	228	9	30	172	0	9.0	5.5	34	36%
(Kraft) powder, 'Instant' mix only	3 tsp	90	1	18	45	0	1.0	0.0	0	11%
NATURAL FLAVOR										
w/added nutrients, powder, prepared	8 fl oz *(1 cup)*	231	10	28	204	0	8.7	5.4	34	34%
w/oadded nutrients, powder, prepared	8 fl oz *(1 cup)*	236	10	27	223	0	9.8	6.0	37	37%
(Kraft) powder, 'Instant'	3 tsp	90	3	16	100	0	2.0	0.0	0	19%
MAMMY APPLE										
peeled, w/o seeds	1 oz	14	0.1	3.5	4	.9	0.1	na	0	6%
raw	3-1/2 oz	51	0.5	12.5	15	3.0	0.5	na	0	8%

Food Name	Serving Size	Calories	Prot. gms	Carbs gms	Sod. mgs	Fiber gms	Fat gms	Sat. Fat gms	Chol. mgs	% Fat Cal.
raw, trimmed, whole, approx 3.1 lb	1 medium	431	4.2	105.8	127	25.4	4.2	na	0	8%
raw, untrimmed	1 lb	139	1.4	34.0	41	>2.7 c	1.4	na	0	8%

MANDARIN ORANGE. See also TANGERINE.
Canned

Food Name	Serving Size	Calories	Prot. gms	Carbs gms	Sod. mgs	Fiber gms	Fat gms	Sat. Fat gms	Chol. mgs	% Fat Cal.
in juice	1 cup	92	2	24	12	2	0.1	0.0	0	1%
in light syrup	1 cup	154	1	41	15	2	0.3	0.0	0	1%

MANGO
Canned or jarred, sliced, chilled (Sun Fresh)... 3.5 oz — 89, 0.5, 21.0, 11, 1.9, 0.3, 0.1, 1, 3%

Food Name	Serving Size	Calories	Prot. gms	Carbs gms	Sod. mgs	Fiber gms	Fat gms	Sat. Fat gms	Chol. mgs	% Fat Cal.
Canned or jarred, sliced, chilled (Sun Fresh)	3.5 oz	89	0.5	21.0	11	1.9	0.3	0.1	1	3%

Fresh

Food Name	Serving Size	Calories	Prot. gms	Carbs gms	Sod. mgs	Fiber gms	Fat gms	Sat. Fat gms	Chol. mgs	% Fat Cal.
raw, peeled, w/o seed	1 oz	18	0.1	4.8	1	.3	0.1	<.1	0	4%
raw, sliced	1 cup	107	0.8	28.1	3	3.0	0.5	0.1	0	4%
raw, trimmed, whole, medium, approx 10.6 oz	1 mango	135	1.1	35.2	4	3.7	0.6	0.1	0	4%
raw, untrimmed	1 lb	204	1.6	53.2	6	3.4	0.9	0.2	0	4%

MANGOSTEEN
Canned

Food Name	Serving Size	Calories	Prot. gms	Carbs gms	Sod. mgs	Fiber gms	Fat gms	Sat. Fat gms	Chol. mgs	% Fat Cal.
in syrup	1 cup	158	1	39	15	4	1.3	na	0	7%
in syrup, drained	1 cup	143	1	35	14	4	1.1	na	0	7%

MANHATTAN. See under COCKTAIL MIX.

MANICOTTI/MANICOTTI ENTRÉE
(Bernardi)

Food Name	Serving Size	Calories	Prot. gms	Carbs gms	Sod. mgs	Fiber gms	Fat gms	Sat. Fat gms	Chol. mgs	% Fat Cal.
cheese	2 pieces	300	15	27	340	1	14.0	8.0	45	43%
cheese, large	1 piece	170	8	16	230	1	8.0	5.0	45	43%
(Budget Gourmet)										
cheese, w/meat sauce	1 entrée	420	18	38	810	4	22.0	11.0	85	47%
frozen, w/meat sauce, frozen	1 entree	440	20	34	780	5	26.0	12.0	90	52%
(Buitoni) frozen 'Single Serving' one package	9 oz	470	18	45	830	0	14.0	8.0	130	33%
(Celentano)										
	10-oz tray	450	24	41	910	9	21.0	8.0	85	42%
Florentine, 'Great Choice'	10-oz tray	210	15	29	600	5	6.0	2.0	35	23%
Florentine, 'Selects'	10-oz tray	230	14	29	670	4	7.0	1.0	5	27%
mini	4.8 oz	280	17	32	500	13	12.0	6.0	66	36%
w/sauce	8 oz	320	17	28	690	6	15.0	7.0	75	43%
w/o sauce	7 oz	410	20	40	630	7	19.0	11.0	100	42%
(Contadina) cheese, frozen	1 oz	31	2	3	95	0	1.4	0.6	3	42%
(Healthy Choice)										
cheese, frozen	9.25 oz	220	15	34	310	0	3.0	2.0	30	12%
w/three cheeses	1 entrée	300	15	40	550	5	9.0	3.0	35	27%
(Le Menu) three cheese, frozen	11.75 oz	390	19	44	870	0	15.0	0.0	0	35%
(Lean Cuisine) cheese and spinach, 'Hearty Portions'	1 entrée	340	18	52	790	10	7.0	2.5	40	18%
(Legume)										
cheese, w/spinach, tofu, and sauce, frozen	11 oz	260	18	30	650	9	7.0	1.0	0	25%
classic, vegetarian, nondairy, w/organic pasta and tofu	1 serving	360	23	40	510	10	13.0	2.0	0	32%
Florentine, nondairy, w/organic pasta and tofu	1 serving	300	19	39	540	11	8.0	1.0	0	24%
(Stouffer's) cheese	1 entrée	340	18	32	810	7	16.0	7.0	50	42%
(Weight Watchers)										
cheese	1 entree	260	17	31	570	5	7.0	3.5	30	25%
cheese, frozen	9.25 oz	260	17	31	510	0	8.0	3.0	25	27%

MANICOTTI NOODLE. See under PASTA.

MANIOC. See CASSAVA.

MAPLE SYRUP. See under SYRUP.

MARGARINE
coconut, hydrogenated and regular, w/safflower and

Food Name	Serving Size	Calories	Prot. gms	Carbs gms	Sod. mgs	Fiber gms	Fat gms	Sat. Fat gms	Chol. mgs	% Fat Cal.
hydrogenated palm	1 stick	815	1	1	1070	0	91.3	64.5	0	99%

Food Name	Serving Size	Calories	Prot. gms	Carbs gms	Sod. mgs	Fiber gms	Fat gms	Sat. Fat gms	Chol. mgs	% Fat Cal.
coconut, hydrogenated and regular, w/safflower and hydrogenated palm	1 tsp	34	0	0	44	0	3.8	2.7	0	99%
corn, hydrogenated	1 stick	815	1	1	1070	0	91.3	15.0	0	99%
corn, hydrogenated	1 tsp	34	0	0	44	0	3.8	0.6	0	99%
corn, hydrogenated and regular	1 stick	815	1	1	1070	0	91.3	15.9	0	99%
corn, hydrogenated and regular	1 tsp	34	0	0	44	0	3.8	0.7	0	99%
corn, hydrogenated and regular, soft	1 cup	1626	2	1	2449	0	182.5	32.0	0	99%
corn, hydrogenated and regular, soft	1 tsp	34	0	0	51	0	3.8	0.7	0	99%
corn, w/hydrogenated soybean and cottonseed	1 stick	815	1	1	1070	0	91.3	17.0	0	99%
corn, w/hydrogenated soybean and cottonseed	1 tsp	34	0	0	44	0	3.8	0.7	0	99%
corn, w/hydrogenated soybean and cottonseed, unsalted	1 stick	810	1	1	2	0	91.1	17.0	0	99%
corn, w/ hydrogenated soybean and cottonseed, unsalted	1 tsp	34	0	0	0	0	3.8	0.7	0	99%
lard, hydrogenated	1 stick	831	1	1	1070	0	91.3	35.8	58	99%
lard, hydrogenated	1 tsp	34	0	0	44	0	3.8	1.5	2	99%
safflower, hydrogenated and regular	1 cup	1626	2	1	2449	0	182.5	20.9	0	99%
safflower, hydrogenated and regular	1 tsp	34	0	0	51	0	3.8	0.4	0	99%
safflower, w/hydrogenated cottonseed and peanut, soft	1 cup	1626	2	1	2449	0	182.5	30.4	0	99%
safflower, w/hydrogenated cottonseed and peanut, soft	1 tsp	34	0	0	51	0	3.8	0.6	0	99%
safflower, w/hydrogenated soybean	1 stick	815	1	1	1070	0	91.3	15.6	0	99%
safflower, w/hydrogenated soybean	1 tsp	34	0	0	44	0	3.8	0.6	0	99%
safflower, w/hydrogenated soybean and cottonseed	1 stick	815	1	1	1070	0	91.3	15.1	0	99%
safflower, w/hydrogenated soybean and cottonseed	1 tsp	34	0	0	44	0	3.8	0.6	0	99%
soybean, hydrogenated	1 stick	812	1	1	1066	0	91.0	18.9	0	99%
soybean, hydrogenated	1 tsp	34	0	0	44	0	3.8	0.8	0	99%
soybean, hydrogenated and regular	1 stick	815	1	1	1070	0	91.3	14.9	0	99%
soybean, hydrogenated and regular	1 tsp	34	0	0	44	0	3.8	0.6	0	99%
soybean, hydrogenated and regular, soft, salted	1 cup	1626	2	1	2449	0	182.5	30.6	0	99%
soybean, hydrogenated and regular, soft, salted	1 tsp	34	0	0	51	0	3.8	0.6	0	99%
soybean, hydrogenated and regular, soft, unsalted	1 cup	1626	2	2	63	0	182.3	30.6	0	99%
soybean, hydrogenated and regular, soft, unsalted	1 tsp	34	0	0	1	0	3.8	0.6	0	99%
soybean, hydrogenated, w/corn and hydrogenated cottonseed	1 stick	815	1	1	1070	0	91.3	22.5	0	99%
soybean, hydrogenated, w/corn and hydrogenated cottonseed	1 tsp	34	0	0	44	0	3.8	0.9	0	99%
soybean, hydrogenated, w/cottonseed	1 stick	815	1	1	1070	0	91.3	18.5	0	99%
soybean, hydrogenated, w/cottonseed	1 tsp	34	0	0	44	0	3.8	0.8	0	99%
soybean, hydrogenated, w/cottonseed, soft	1 cup	1626	2	1	2449	0	182.5	37.5	0	99%
soybean, hydrogenated, w/cottonseed, soft	1 tsp	34	0	0	51	0	3.8	0.8	0	99%
soybean, hydrogenated, w/hydrogenated and regular palm	1 stick	815	1	1	1070	0	91.3	19.8	0	99%
soybean, hydrogenated, w/hydrogenated and regular palm	1 tsp	34	0	0	44	0	3.8	0.8	0	99%
soybean, hydrogenated, w/hydrogenated and regular palm, soft	1 cup	1626	2	1	2449	0	182.5	38.8	0	99%
soybean, hydrogenated, w/hydrogenated and regular palm, soft	1 tsp	34	0	0	51	0	3.8	0.8	0	99%
soybean, hydrogenated, w/safflower, soft	1 cup	1626	2	1	2449	0	182.5	23.6	0	99%
soybean, hydrogenated, w/safflower, soft	1 tsp	34	0	0	51	0	3.8	0.5	0	99%
soybean and cottonseed, hydrogenated	1 stick	815	1	1	1070	0	91.3	17.1	0	99%
soybean and cottonseed, hydrogenated	1 tsp	34	0	0	44	0	3.8	0.7	0	99%
soybean and cottonseed, hydrogenated, soft	1 cup	1626	2	1	2449	0	182.5	36.5	0	99%
soybean and cottonseed, hydrogenated, soft	1 tsp	34	0	0	51	0	3.8	0.8	0	99%

Food Name	Serving Size	Calories	Prot. gms	Carbs gms	Sod. mgs	Fiber gms	Fat gms	Sat. Fat gms	Chol. mgs	% Fat Cal.
soybean and cottonseed, hydrogenated, soft, salted	1 cup	1626	2	1	2449	0	182.5	32.2	0	99%
soybean and cottonseed, hydrogenated, soft, salted	1 tsp	34	0	0	51	0	3.8	0.7	0	99%
soybean and cottonseed, hydrogenated, soft, unsalted	1 cup	1626	2	2	63	0	182.3	32.0	0	99%
soybean and cottonseed, hydrogenated, soft, unsalted	1 tsp	34	0	0	1	0	3.8	0.7	0	99%
soybean and cottonseed, hydrogenated and regular, liquid	1 cup	1637	4	0	1773	0	183.0	30.0	0	99%
soybean and cottonseed, hydrogenated and regular, liquid	1 tsp	34	0	0	37	0	3.8	0.6	0	99%
soybean and palm, hydrogenated	1 stick	815	1	1	1070	0	91.3	17.1	0	99%
soybean and palm, hydrogenated	1 tsp	34	0	0	44	0	3.8	0.7	0	99%
sunflower, w/hydrogenated cottonseed and peanut, soft	1 cup	1626	2	1	2449	0	182.5	29.1	0	99%
sunflower, w/hydrogenated cottonseed and peanut, soft	1 tsp	34	0	0	51	0	3.8	0.6	0	99%
sunflower, w/hydrogenated soybean and cottonseed	1 stick	815	1	1	1070	0	91.3	13.5	0	99%
sunflower, w/hydrogenated soybean and cottonseed	1 tsp	34	0	0	44	0	3.8	0.6	0	99%
(A&P)										
premium	1 tbsp	100	1	1	110	0	11.0	2.0	0	93%
quarters, corn oil	1 tbsp	100	1	1	105	0	11.0	2.0	0	93%
soft, bowl	1 tbsp	100	1	1	105	0	11.0	2.0	0	93%
(Blue Bonnet)										
soft	1 tbsp	100	0	0	95	0	11.0	2.0	0	100%
stick	1 tbsp	100	0	0	95	0	11.0	2.0	0	100%
whipped, stick	1 tbsp	70	0	0	70	0	7.0	1.0	0	100%
(Cannola) soft	1 tbsp	100	0	0	95	0	11.0	1.0	0	100%
(Canoleo) 100% Canola oil, all natural, dairy-free	1 tbsp	100	0	0	120	0	11.0	1.0	0	100%
(Chiffon)										
soft, cup	1 tbsp	90	0	0	95	0	10.0	1.0	0	100%
soft, stick	1 tbsp	100	0	0	105	0	11.0	2.0	0	100%
soft, unsalted	1 tbsp	90	0	0	0	0	10.0	2.0	0	100%
whipped	1 tbsp	70	0	0	80	0	8.0	1.0	0	100%
(Country Morning)										
light, stick	1 tsp	20	0	0	30	0	2.0	0.0	3	100%
light, tub	1 tsp	20	0	0	25	0	2.0	0.0	3	100%
regular, stick	1 tsp	35	0	0	35	0	4.0	0.0	5	100%
regular, tub	1 tsp	30	0	0	25	0	3.0	0.0	5	100%
unsalted, stick	1 tsp	35	0	0	0	0	4.0	0.0	4	100%
unsalted, tub	1 tsp	30	0	0	0	0	3.0	0.0	5	100%
(Fleischmann's)										
diet, lower calorie	1 tbsp	50	0	0	50	0	6.0	1.0	0	100%
40% corn oil, less fat, stick	1 tbsp	52	0	1	77	0	5.6	1.0	0	95%
'Move Over Butter'	1 tbsp	60	0	0	75	0	6.0	1.0	0	100%
regular, soft	1 tbsp	100	0	0	95	0	11.0	2.0	0	100%
regular, stick	1 tbsp	100	0	0	95	0	11.0	2.0	0	100%
sweet, unsalted, soft	1 tbsp	100	0	0	0	0	11.0	2.0	0	100%
sweet, unsalted, stick	1 tbsp	100	0	0	0	0	11.0	2.0	0	100%
whipped, lightly salted	1 tbsp	70	0	0	60	0	7.0	2.0	0	100%
whipped, unsalted	1 tbsp	70	0	0	0	0	7.0	2.0	0	100%
(Hain)										
safflower	1 tbsp	100	0	0	170	0	11.0	2.0	0	100%
safflower, soft	1 tbsp	100	0	0	170	0	11.0	2.0	0	100%
safflower, unsalted	1 tbsp	100	0	0	5	0	11.0	2.0	0	100%
(Hollywood)										
safflower	1 tbsp	100	0	0	130	0	11.0	5.0	0	100%
safflower, unsalted	1 tbsp	100	0	0	2	0	11.0	2.0	0	100%
(I Can't Believe It's Not Butter)	1 tbsp	90	0	0	0	0	10.0	2.0	0	100%

Food Name	Serving Size	Calories	Prot. gms	Carbs gms	Sod. mgs	Fiber gms	Fat gms	Sat. Fat gms	Chol. mgs	% Fat Cal.
(Imperial)										
lower calorie, 'Diet'	1 tbsp	50	0	0	140	0	6.0	1.0	0	100%
soft	1 tbsp	100	0	0	95	0	11.0	0.0	0	100%
(Land O'Lakes)										
corn oil, premium, stick	1 tbsp	35	0	0	35	0	4.0	1.0	0	100%
regular, stick	1 tsp	35	0	0	35	0	4.0	0.0	0	100%
soy oil, regular, stick	1 tbsp	35	0	0	35	0	4.0	1.0	0	100%
soy oil, soft	1 tbsp	35	0	0	35	0	4.0	1.0	0	100%
tub	1 tsp	35	0	0	35	0	4.0	0.0	0	100%
(Mazola)										
	1 tbsp	100	0	0	100	0	11.0	2.0	0	100%
lower calorie	1 tbsp	50	0	0	135	0	5.5	0.8	0	99%
unsalted	1 tbsp	100	0	0	0	0	11.0	2.0	0	100%
(Miracle Brand)										
whipped, cup	1 tbsp	60	0	0	70	0	7.0	1.0	0	100%
whipped, stick	1 tbsp	70	0	0	65	0	7.0	1.0	0	100%
(Nucoa)										
	1 tbsp	100	0	0	160	0	11.0	2.0	0	100%
'Heart Beat'	1 tbsp	25	0	0	110	0	3.0	1.0	0	100%
soft	1 tbsp	90	0	0	150	0	10.0	2.0	0	100%
unsalted, 'Heart Beat'	1 tbsp	24	0	0	0	0	3.0	1.0	0	100%
(P&Q) quarters, 60% vegetable oil	1 tbsp	80	1	1	105	0	8.0	1.0	0	90%
(Parkay)										
	1 tbsp	100	0	0	105	0	11.0	2.0	0	100%
diet, soft	1 tbsp	50	0	0	110	0	6.0	1.0	0	100%
regular, soft	1 tbsp	100	0	0	105	0	11.0	2.0	0	100%
squeezable	1 tbsp	90	0	0	110	0	10.0	2.0	0	100%
whipped, cup	1 tbsp	70	0	0	70	0	7.0	1.0	0	100%
whipped, stick	1 tbsp	70	0	0	65	0	7.0	1.0	0	100%
(Saffola) soft	1 tbsp	100	0	0	95	0	11.0	1.5	0	100%
(Smart Beat)										
super light	1 tbsp	20	0	0	105	0	2.0	0.0	0	100%
trans fat-free, lactose-free	1 tbsp	20	0	0	105	0	2.0	0.0	0	100%
(Weight Watchers)										
light	1 tbsp	45	0	2	70	0	4.0	1.0	0	82%
stick	1 tbsp	60	0	0	130	0	7.0	1.0	0	100%
tub	1 tbsp	50	0	0	130	0	6.0	1.0	0	100%
unsalted	1 tbsp	50	0	0	0	0	6.0	1.0	0	100%
MARGARINE SPREAD										
margarine-butter blend, 60% corn oil margarine, 40% butter	1 stick	811	1	1	1014	0	91.2	32.1	99	99%
margarine-butter blend, 60% corn oil margarine, 40% butter	1 tsp	36	0	0	45	0	4.0	1.4	4	99%
(Blue Bonnet)										
48% vegetable oil	1 tbsp	60	1	1	115	0	6.0	1.0	5	87%
75% vegetable oil	1 tbsp	90	0	0	95	0	11.0	2.0	0	100%
soft, 'Better Blend'	1 tbsp	90	0	0	95	0	11.0	2.0	0	100%
stick, 'Better Blend'	1 tbsp	90	0	0	95	0	11.0	2.0	0	100%
unsalted, 'Better Blend'	1 tbsp	90	0	0	0	0	11.0	2.0	5	100%
whipped, 60% vegetable oil	1 tbsp	80	0	0	100	0	8.0	1.0	0	100%
(Brummel & Brown)										
58% vegetable oil, 10% yogurt	1 tbsp	70	0	0	95	0	8.0	2.0	0	100%
35% vegetable oil, 25% yogurt	1 tbsp	50	0	0	95	0	5.0	1.0	0	100%

Food Name	Serving Size	Calories	Prot. gms	Carbs gms	Sod. mgs	Fiber gms	Fat gms	Sat. Fat gms	Chol. mgs	% Fat Cal.
(Country Crock)										
48% vegetable oil	1 tbsp	60	0	0	110	0	7.0	1.5	0	100%
48% vegetable oil, churn style	1 tbsp	60	0	0	60	0	7.0	1.5	0	100%
52% vegetable oil	1 tbsp	60	0	0	110	0	7.0	1.0	0	100%
52% vegetable oil, churn style, stick	1 tbsp	80	0	0	55	0	9.0	2.0	0	100%
64% vegetable oil, stick	1 tbsp	80	0	0	110	0	9.0	1.5	0	100%
squeezable	1 tbsp	80	0	0	115	0	9.0	1.5	0	100%
(Fleischmann's)										
'Move Over Butter'	1 tbsp	90	0	0	100	0	10.0	2.0	0	100%
72% vegetable oil w/cream buttermilk, tub, whipped, 'Move Over Butter'	1 tbsp	60	0	0	75	0	7.0	1.5	0	100%
72% vegetable. oil w/sweet cream buttermilk, stick, 'Move Over Butter'	1 tbsp	90	0	0	100	0	10.0	2.0	0	100%
(Hollywood) soft	1 tbsp	90	0	1	135	0	10.0	1.0	0	96%
(I Can't Believe It's Not Butter)										
	1 tbsp	90	0	0	0	0	10.0	2.0	0	100%
40% vegetable oil w/cream buttermilk, tub	1 tbsp	50	0	0	90	0	6.0	1.0	0	100%
52% vegetable oil w/cream buttermilk, quarters	1 tbsp	60	0	0	110	0	7.0	1.0	0	100%
single portion	1 tbsp	90	0	0	95	0	10.0	2.0	0	100%
68% vegetable oil w/buttermilk, squeezable	1 tbsp	90	0	0	90	0	10.0	2.0	0	100%
70% vegetable oil w/cream buttermilk, stick	1 tbsp	90	0	0	90	0	10.0	2.0	0	100%
70% vegetable oil w/cream buttermilk, tub	1 tbsp	90	0	0	95	0	10.0	2.0	0	100%
light	1 tbsp	60	0	0	110	0	7.0	1.0	0	100%
(Imperial) 45% vegetable oil, 'Light'	1 tbsp	60	0	0	110	0	6.0	0.0	0	100%
(Kraft)										
bowl, 'Touch of Butter'	1 tbsp	50	0	0	110	0	6.0	1.0	0	100%
stick, 'Touch of Butter'	1 tbsp	90	0	0	110	0	10.0	2.0	0	100%
(Land O'Lakes)										
w/sweet cream, stick	1 tsp	30	0	0	35	0	4.0	0.0	0	100%
w/sweet cream, tub	1 tsp	25	0	0	25	0	3.0	0.0	0	100%
w/sweet cream, unsalted	1 tsp	30	0	0	0	0	4.0	0.0	0	100%
lightly salted, soft, 'Country Morning Blend'	1 tbsp	30	0	0	25	0	3.0	1.0	5	100%
lightly salted, soft, 'Country Morning Light'	1 tbsp	20	0	0	30	0	3.0	1.0	3	100%
lightly salted, soft, 64% soy oil	1 tbsp	25	0	0	25	0	3.0	1.0	0	100%
lightly salted, soft, w/sweet cream	1 tbsp	25	0	0	25	0	3.0	1.0	0	100%
lightly salted, stick, 'Country Morning Blend'	1 tbsp	35	0	0	35	0	4.0	1.0	5	100%
lightly salted, stick, 'Country Morning Light'	1 tbsp	20	0	0	30	0	3.0	1.0	3	100%
lightly salted, stick, w/sweet cream	1 tbsp	30	0	0	35	0	4.0	1.0	0	100%
unsalted, soft, 'Country Morning Blend'	1 tbsp	30	0	0	0	0	3.0	1.0	5	100%
unsalted, stick, 'Country Morning Blend'	1 tbsp	35	0	0	35	0	4.0	1.0	5	100%
unsalted, stick, w/sweet cream	1 tbsp	30	0	0	0	0	4.0	1.0	0	100%
(Parkay) 50% vegetable oil	1 tbsp	60	0	0	110	0	7.0	1.0	0	100%
(Promise)										
24% vegetable oil, 'Ultra'	1 tbsp	30	0	0	55	0	3.5	0.0	0	100%
40% vegetable oil, soft	1 tbsp	50	0	0	55	0	6.0	1.0	0	100%
40% vegetable oil, stick	1 tbsp	50	0	0	55	0	6.0	1.5	0	100%
68% vegetable oil	1 tbsp	90	0	0	90	0	10.0	2.0	0	100%
extra light	1 tbsp	50	0	0	50	0	6.0	1.0	0	100%
lower calorie	1 tbsp	70	0	0	70	0	7.0	1.5	0	100%
w/Canola oil, 'Ultra'	1 tbsp	35	0	0	50	0	4.0	0.0	0	100%
whipped	1 tbsp	60	0	0	45	0	7.0	1.5	0	100%
(Shedd's Spread) 52% vegetable oil	1 tbsp	60	0	0	110	0	7.0	1.0	0	100%
(Touch of Butter) 47% vegetable oil and dairy spread	1 tbsp	60	0	0	110	0	7.0	1.5	0	100%
(Weight Watchers)										
extra light, sweet, no salt, 'Country Cottage'	1 tbsp	50	0	0	0	0	6.0	1.0	0	100%

Food Name	Serving Size	Calories	Prot. gms	Carbs gms	Sod. mgs	Fiber gms	Fat gms	Sat. Fat gms	Chol. mgs	% Fat Cal.
extra light, tub 'Country Cottage Farms'	1 tbsp	45	0	2	75	0	4.0	1.0	0	82%
light, 'Country Cottage Farms'	1 tbsp	50	0	0	130	0	6.0	1.0	0	100%
light, stick	1 tbsp	60	0	0	130	0	7.0	1.0	0	100%
MARGARINE SUBSTITUTE										
corn, hydrogenated and regular, 40% fat	1 cup	801	1	1	2226	0	90.0	14.8	0	99%
corn, hydrogenated and regular, 40% fat	1 tsp	17	0	0	46	0	1.9	0.3	0	99%
soybean, hydrogenated, 40% fat	1 cup	801	1	1	2226	0	90.0	15.1	0	99%
soybean, hydrogenated, 40% fat	1 tsp	17	0	0	46	0	1.9	0.3	0	99%
soybean, hydrogenated, w/cottonseed, 40% fat	1 cup	801	1	1	2226	0	90.0	19.3	0	99%
soybean, hydrogenated, w/cottonseed, 40% fat	1 tsp	17	0	0	46	0	1.9	0.4	0	99%
soybean, hydrogenated, w/hydrogenated and regular palm, 40% fat	1 cup	801	1	1	2226	0	90.0	23.4	0	99%
soybean, hydrogenated/ w.hydrogenated and regular palm, 40% fat	1 tsp	17	0	0	46	0	1.9	0.5	0	99%
soybean, hydrogenated, w/hydrogenated and regular palm, 60% fat, tub	1 cup	1236	1	0	2276	0	139.2	30.9	0	100%
soybean, hydrogenated, w/hydrogenated and regular palm, 60% fat, tub	1 tsp	26	0	0	48	0	2.9	0.6	0	100%
soybean and cottonseed, hydrogenated, 40% fat	1 cup	801	1	1	2226	0	90.0	16.7	0	99%
soybean and cottonseed, hydrogenated, 40% fat	1 tsp	17	0	0	46	0	1.9	0.3	0	99%
soybean and cottonseed, hydrogenated, 60% fat, tub	1 cup	1236	1	0	2276	0	139.2	27.5	0	100%
soybean and cottonseed, hydrogenated, 60% fat, tub	1 tsp	26	0	0	48	0	2.9	0.6	0	100%
soybean and palm, hydrogenated, 60% fat, stick	1 cup	1236	1	0	2276	0	139.2	32.3	0	100%
soybean and palm, hydrogenated, 60% fat, stick	1 tsp	26	0	0	48	0	2.9	0.7	0	100%
(Promise Ultra) nonfat	1 tbsp	5	0	1	90	0	0.0	0.0	0	0%
MARGARITA. See under COCKTAIL MIX.										
MARINADE										
(DiGiorno) refrigerated	5 oz	110	3	12	680	0	6.0	1.0	5	47%
CALCUTTA MASALA (TAJ Cuisine of India)	4 oz	100	2	13	510	2	5.0	1.0	5	43%
FAJITA										
(Old El Paso)	1/8 jar	14	0	3	450	0	0.0	0.0	0	0%
(Tone's)	1 tsp	9	0	2	963	0	0.1	0.0	0	9%
FOR MEAT (Crown Colony)	1/2 tsp	5	0	1	420	0	0.0	0.0	0	0%
FRENCH (Litehouse) country herb, refrigerated	1 tbsp	54	0	2	196	0	5.0	0.0	0	85%
KASHMIR TANDOOKI (TAJ Cuisine of India)	2 oz	50	2	5	260	1	3.0	0.0	0	49%
Lemon Herb (Golden Dipt)	1 oz	130	0	2	210	0	14.0	2.0	0	94%
LEMON PEPPER (Lawry's)	1 oz	20	0	2	800	0	1.1	0.0	0	51%
MESQUITE (S&W)	1 tbsp	10	0	3	400	0	0.0	0.0	0	0%
OYSTER AND SHRIMP (Caribbean Clipper)	1 tsp	10	0	2	140	na	0.0	na	na	0%
SEAFOOD (Golden Dipt) honey soy, nonfat	1 tbsp	30	0	5	360	0	0.0	0.0	0	0%
STIR-FRY (La Choy) food service product	1 tbsp	25	1	5	672	0	0.1	0.0	0	4%
TERIYAKI										
(Golden Dipt) ginger	1 oz	120	1	12	920	0	7.0	1.0	0	55%
(Kikkoman)										
	1 tbsp	15	1	2	610	0	0.0	0.0	0	0%
light	1 tbsp	15	1	3	320	0	0.0	0.0	0	0%
(LaChoy)	1 oz	30	1	5	1640	0	0.0	0.0	0	0%
(Lawry's)										
	2 tbsp	72	6	11	7100	0	0.4	0.2	0	5%
barbecue	1/4 cup	164	8	27	12330	0	2.3	0.0	0	13%
barbecue	1/8 cup	82	4	14	6115	0	1.1	0.0	0	12%
(S&W)										
	1 tbsp	25	1	5	480	0	0.0	0.0	0	0%
light	1 tbsp	25	1	5	220	0	0.0	0.0	0	0%

Food Name	Serving Size	Calories	Prot. gms	Carbs gms	Sod. mgs	Fiber gms	Fat gms	Sat. Fat gms	Chol. mgs	% Fat Cal.
WHITE WINE DIJON (Golden Dipt)	1 tbsp	10	0	1	100	0	0.0	0.0	0	0%
WINE AND GARLIC (Charcoal Companion) glaze, spray	2 tbsp	40	1	4	230	0	0.0	0.0	0	0%
MARINADE MIX										
BARBECUE (Adolph's) 'Marinade in Minutes'	1/2 tsp	5	0	1	310	0	0.0	0.0	0	0%
BEEF										
(Durkee)	1/2 tsp	0	0	1	220	0	0.0	0.0	0	0%
(Lawry's)	1 pkg	49	1	11	7284	0	0.2	0.0	0	4%
(Marinade Magic)	1/2 tsp	10	1	2	400	1	0.0	0.0	0	0%
CAJUN										
(Adolph's) 'Marinade in Minutes'	1/2 tsp	5	0	1	170	0	0.0	0.0	0	0%
(Luzianne)	1/4 tsp	0	0	0	260	0	0.0	0.0	0	0%
(Tone's)	1 tsp	9	0	2	215	1	0.2	0.1	0	15%
CHICKEN										
(Adolph's)										
	3/4 tsp	5	0	1	291	0	0.0	0.0	0	0%
salt-free	3/4 tsp	5	0	2	0	0	0.0	0.0	0	0%
(McCormick/Schilling) mesquite, 'Sauce Blends'	1 pkg	132	2	24	2068	0	3.0	0.0	0	21%
(Schilling) mesquite	1/6 pkg	20	0	4	460	0	0.0	0.0	0	0%
CITRUS (Lawry's) grill	2 tbsp	34	4	3	3350	0	0.4	0.1	0	11%
FAJITA										
(Marinade Magic)	1/2 tsp	5	1	1	100	0	0.0	0.0	0	0%
(McCormick/Schilling)	2 tsp	15	1	3	280	1	0.0	0.0	0	0%
FOR MEAT										
(Adolph's)										
	1/2 tsp	5	0	1	390	0	0.0	0.0	0	0%
no salt	1/2 tsp	5	0	2	0	0	0.0	0.0	0	0%
(French's)	1/8 pkg	10	0	2	540	0	0.0	0.0	0	0%
(Kikkoman)	1 tsp	10	0	2	590	0	0.0	0.0	0	0%
(McCormick/Schilling)	1 tsp	15	0	2	240	0	0.0	0.0	0	0%
GARLIC										
(Adolph's)										
Dijon, 'Marinade in Minutes'	3/4 tsp	10	0	1	210	0	0.0	0.0	0	0%
'Marinade in Minutes'	1/2 tsp	0	0	1	460	0	0.0	0.0	0	0%
HERB										
(Adolph's)										
Italian, 'Marinade in Minutes'	1/4 tsp	0	0	1	270	0	0.0	0.0	0	0%
lemon, 'Marinade in Minutes'	1/2 tsp	10	0	2	170	0	0.0	0.0	0	0%
Parmesan, 'Marinade in Minutes'	3/4 tsp	10	0	1	230	0	0.0	0.0	0	0%
(Lawry's) herb and garlic, w/lemon	2 tbsp	36	4	4	3688	0	1.0	0.1	0	23%
(Marinade Magic) lemon	1/2 tsp	5	1	1	200	0	0.0	0.0	0	0%
HICKORY (Adolph's) grill, 'Marinade in Minutes'	1 tbsp	20	0	4	200	0	0.5	0.0	0	22%
HOT AND SPICY (Adolph's) 'Marinade in Minutes'	3/4 tsp	5	0	1	130	0	0.0	0.0	0	0%
LEMON GARLIC (Adolph's) 'Marinade in Minutes'	1 tbsp	30	0	2	80	0	2.5	0.0	0	74%
LEMON PEPPER (Adolph's) 'Marinade in Minutes'	1/2 tsp	10	0	2	180	0	0.0	0.0	0	0%
MESQUITE										
(Adolph's)										
'Marinade in Minutes' dry	3/4 tsp	10	0	2	230	0	0.0	0.0	0	0%
'Marinade in Minutes' liquid	1 tbsp	45	0	5	270	0	2.5	0.0	0	53%
(Lawry's)	2 tbsp	24	3	3	4142	0	0.4	0.1	0	13%
SCAMPI (Adolph's) 'Marinade in Minutes'	1/2 tsp	10	0	2	240	0	0.0	0.0	0	0%
STEAK (Adolph's) 'Marinade in Minutes'	1/4 tsp	0	0	1	350	0	0.0	0.0	0	0%
TERIYAKI										
(Adolph's)										
'Marinade in Minutes' dry	1 1/2 tsp	15	0	3	380	0	0.0	0.0	0	0%

Food Name	Serving Size	Calories	Prot. gms	Carbs gms	Sod. mgs	Fiber gms	Fat gms	Sat. Fat gms	Chol. mgs	% Fat Cal.
'Marinade in Minutes' liquid	1 tbsp	20	0	5	740	0	0.0	0.0	0	0%
MARIONBERRY TOPPING (Flav-R-Pac)	2 tbsp	40	0	10	0	2	0.0	0.0	0	0%
MARJORAM										
dried	1 tbsp	5	0	1	1	1	0.1	0.0	0	22%
dried	1 tsp	2	0	0	0	0	0.0	0.0	0	22%
dried (Durkee)	1 tbsp	7	0	0	0	0	0.0	0.0	0	0%
dried (Durkee)	1 tsp	2	0	0	0	0	0.0	0.0	0	0%
dried (Laurel Leaf)	1 tbsp	7	0	0	0	0	0.0	0.0	0	0%
dried (McCormick/Schilling)	1 tsp	4	0	1	1	0	0.0	0.0	0	0%
dried (Laurel Leaf)	1 tsp	2	0	0	0	0	0.0	0.0	0	0%
dried (Spice Islands)	1 tsp	4	0	1	1	0	0.1	0.0	0	20%
dried (Tone's)	1 tsp	2	0	0	1	0	0.1	0.0	0	36%
MARMALADE. See under JAM AND PRESERVES.										
MARMALADE PLUM. See SAPOTE.										
MARROW BEAN. See BEAN, MARROW.										
MARROW SQUASH. See SQUASH, MARROW.										
MARSHMALLOW. See under CANDY.										
MARSHMALLOW TOPPING										
(Finast) creme	1 oz	95	0	23	45	0	0.0	0.0	0	0%
(Kraft) creme	1 oz	90	0	23	20	0	0.0	0.0	0	0%
(Marshmallow Fluff)	1 tsp	59	0	15	12	0	0.0	0.0	0	0%
(Smucker's)	2 tbsp	120	0	29	0	0	0.0	0.0	0	0%
MASA HARINA. See under FLOUR.										
MATAI. See under WATER CHESTNUT.										
MATZO. See under CRACKER.										
MATZO MEAL. See under CRACKER MEAL.										
MAYONNAISE										
(Bama)	1 tbsp	100	0	0	65	0	11.0	0.0	0	100%
(Bennett's) 'Real'	1 tbsp	110	0	1	65	0	12.0	0.0	0	96%
(Best Foods)										
cholesterol-free	1 tbsp	50	0	1	80	0	5.0	1.0	0	92%
light	1 tbsp	50	0	1	115	0	5.0	1.0	5	92%
low-fat	1 tbsp	25	0	4	140	0	1.0	0.0	0	36%
'Real'	1 tbsp	100	0	0	80	0	11.0	1.5	5	100%
(Blue Plate)										
less fat, cholesterol-free	1 tbsp	50	0	1	90	0	5.0	0.5	0	92%
100% natural, no additives	1 tbsp	100	0	0	80	0	11.0	1.5	10	100%
(Cains)	1 tbsp	100	0	0	80	0	11.0	2.0	10	100%
(Estee)										
lower calorie	1 tbsp	50	0	1	80	0	5.0	1.0	0	92%
lower calorie	1 packet	15	0	2	35	0	1.0	na	0	53%
(Featherweight)										
lower calorie	1 tbsp	30	0	3	40	0	2.0	0.0	10	60%
soy, 'Soyamaise'	1 tbsp	100	0	0	3	0	11.0	0.0	5	100%
(Finast)										
	1 tbsp	100	0	0	80	0	11.0	2.0	10	100%
lower calorie, 'Lite'	1 tbsp	40	0	1	100	0	4.0	1.0	5	90%
(Hain)										
Canola	1 tbsp	100	0	1	100	0	11.0	1.0	5	96%
cold processed	1 tbsp	110	0	0	70	0	12.0	2.0	5	100%
less fat, no salt added, 'Real'	1 tbsp	110	0	0	0	0	12.0	2.0	5	100%
lower calorie, low sodium, 'Light'	1 tbsp	60	0	2	95	0	6.0	1.0	10	87%
low-sodium, all natural	1 tbsp	110	0	0	70	0	12.0	2.0	5	100%

Food Name	Serving Size	Calories	Prot. gms	Carbs gms	Sod. mgs	Fiber gms	Fat gms	Sat. Fat gms	Chol. mgs	% Fat Cal.
no salt added, 'Real'	1 tbsp	110	0	0	0	0	12.0	2.0	5	100%
safflower	1 tbsp	110	0	0	70	0	12.0	1.0	5	100%
(Hellmann's)										
cholesterol-free	1 tbsp	50	0	1	80	0	5.0	1.0	0	92%
lower calorie, 'Light'	1 tbsp	50	0	1	115	0	5.0	1.0	5	92%
low-fat	1 tbsp	25	0	4	140	0	1.0	0.0	0	36%
'Real'	1 tbsp	100	0	0	80	0	11.0	1.5	5	100%
(Hollywood)										
	1 tbsp	110	0	0	80	0	12.0	1.0	5	100%
Canola	1 tbsp	100	0	1	100	0	11.0	1.0	5	96%
safflower	1 tbsp	100	0	0	75	0	12.0	1.0	5	100%
(Janet Lee) lower calorie, 'Light'	1 tbsp	50	0	1	115	0	5.0	1.0	5	92%
(JFG)										
'Creamy Velvet'	1 tbsp	100	0	0	70	0	11.0	2.0	10	100%
less fat, cholesterol free	1 tbsp	50	0	0	85	0	5.0	1.0	0	100%
(Kraft)										
light	1 tbsp	50	0	2	90	0	5.0	1.0	5	85%
lower calorie, 'Light'	1 tbsp	50	0	1	110	0	5.0	1.0	0	92%
nonfat	1 tbsp	10	0	2	120	0	0.0	0.0	0	0%
'Real'	1 tbsp	100	0	0	75	0	11.0	1.5	5	100%
w/lime juice, 'Mayonesa'	1 tbsp	64	0	0	60	0	12.0	12.0	10	100%
(Pathmark)										
	1 tbsp	100	0	0	70	0	11.0	2.0	5	100%
lower calorie	1 tbsp	40	0	1	100	0	4.0	1.0	5	90%
low-sodium	1 tbsp	100	0	0	70	0	11.0	2.0	5	100%
'No Frills'	1 tbsp	100	0	0	75	0	11.0	2.0	10	100%
(Rokeach)	1 tbsp	100	0	0	70	0	11.0	2.0	10	100%
(Smart Beat) lower calorie, 'Golden Corn Light'	1 tbsp	40	0	1	110	0	4.0	1.0	0	90%
(Spectrum) Canola, eggless, lite	1 tbsp	35	0	1	60	0	3.0	0.0	0	87%
(Weight Watchers)										
light	1 tbsp	25	0	1	40	0	2.0	0.0	5	82%
lower calorie	1 tbsp	50	0	1	100	0	5.0	1.0	5	92%
lower calorie, low-sodium	1 tbsp	50	0	1	45	0	5.0	1.0	5	92%
(Westbrae)										
	1 tbsp	100	0	0	75	0	11.0	0.0	5	100%
Canola	1 tbsp	100	0	0	75	0	11.0	0.0	5	100%
MAYONNAISE SUBSTITUTE										
(Best Foods) vegetarian	1 tbsp	50	0	2	170	0	5.0	1.0	5	85%
(Hain)										
Canola, lower calorie	1 tbsp	60	0	2	160	0	5.0	0.0	0	85%
eggless, no salt added	1 tbsp	110	0	0	5	0	12.0	2.0	0	100%
(Hellmann's)										
cholesterol-free	1 tbsp	50	0	1	80	0	5.0	1.0	0	92%
vegetarian	1 tbsp	50	0	2	170	0	5.0	1.0	5	85%
(Kraft) vegetarian	1 tbsp	50	0	3	95	0	5.0	1.0	5	79%
(Life) sunflower, all natural	1 tbsp	71	1	1	3	0	8.0	0.0	0	90%
(Nasoya) 'Nayonaise'	1 tbsp	35	1	1	104	0	3.3	0.3	0	82%
(Nayonnaise) vegetable dressing and dip	1 tbsp	35	0	1	100	0	3.0	0.2	0	87%
(Nucoa) 'Heart Beat'	1 tbsp	40	0	1	110	0	4.0	1.0	0	90%
(Weight Watchers) cholesterol-free	1 tbsp	50	0	1	90	0	5.0	1.0	0	92%
MEAT LOAF DINNER/ENTRÉE										
(Banquet) w/tomato sauce, potatoes, carrots in sauce, frozen, 'Extra Helping'	1 pkg	612	29	34	1943	6	40.0	15.5	113	59%

Food Name	Serving Size	Calories	Prot. gms	Carbs gms	Sod. mgs	Fiber gms	Fat gms	Sat. Fat gms	Chol. mgs	% Fat Cal.
(Healthy Choice) traditional, w/potato, vegetable,										
apple praline	1 pkg	316	15	52	459	6	5.0	2.5	37	14%
(Lean Magic) flame broiled	1 piece	148	17	4	400	1	7.2	2.8	41	44%
(Lean Magic 30) flame broiled	1 piece	110	15	4	449	1	3.6	1.2	35	29%
(Stouffer's) w/gravy, frozen, food service product	1 oz	40	3	2	96	0	2.4	0.7	11	54%
MEAT LOAF SEASONING. See under SEASONING MIX.										
MEAT STICKS, SMOKED										
	1 oz	156	6	2	420	na	14.1	5.9	38	81%
	1 stick	109	4	1	293	na	9.8	4.1	26	81%
MEAT SUBSTITUTE. See also individual meat substitute listings.										
(Heartline) vegetarian, unflavored, lite	0.5 oz	22	5	1	135	3	0.0	0.0	0	0%
(Worthington)										
multigrain cutlets, vegetarian	1 slice	99	15	5	384	4	1.8	0.7	0	16%
vegetarian, 'Choplets'	1 slice	94	17	3	500	2	1.6	0.8	0	16%
vegetarian, cutlets	1 slice	66	11	3	340	2	1.1	0.5	0	15%
vegetarian, 'Diced Chik'	1/4 cup	57	5	1	236	1	3.5	0.5	1	56%
vegetarian, 'Numete'	1 slice	132	6	5	272	3	9.6	2.4	0	65%
vegetarian, patties, 'Crispychik'	1 serving	175	8	15	596	4	9.4	1.4	1	48%
MEAT TENDERIZER										
(Adolph's)										
seasoned, '100% Natural'	1/4 tsp	0	0	0	450	0	0.0	0.0	0	0%
sodium-free, '100% Natural'	1/4 tsp	0	0	1	0	0	0.0	0.0	0	0%
spiced, sodium-free, '100% Natural'	1/4 tsp	0	0	1	0	0	0.0	0.0	0	0%
unseasoned, '100% Natural'	1/4 tsp	0	0	0	420	0	0.0	0.0	0	0%
(Tone's)										
seasoned	1 tsp	7	0	1	1650	0	0.2	0.1	0	26%
unseasoned	1 tsp	7	0	1	1760	0	0.2	0.1	0	27%
MEATBALL DINNER/ENTRÉE										
(Armour)										
Swedish, 'Classics'	11.25 oz	330	19	23	1140	0	18.0	0.0	80	49%
Swedish, beef, 'Classics'	11.25 oz	360	20	32	1170	0	17.0	0.0	65	42%
(Banquet) Swedish, beef, frozen	11 oz	440	26	27	770	0	27.0	0.0	85	53%
(Bernardi) meatballs	6 meatballs	270	12	5	630	2	22.0	10.0	65	74%
(Budget Gourmet)										
Swedish, beef, frozen	11.2 oz	450	23	40	1110	0	22.0	0.0	70	44%
Swedish, w/cream sauce and noodles, frozen	1 entrée	550	22	40	1050	3	34.0	16.0	150	55%
(Chef Boyardee) stew, canned	8 oz	350	9	24	1315	0	24.0	0.0	0	62%
(Dinty Moore)										
stew	8 oz	240	11	14	980	0	16.0	7.0	30	59%
stew, microwave cup	7.5 oz	240	11	14	980	0	16.0	7.0	30	59%
(Freezer Queen) Swedish, beef, frozen	10 oz	350	19	26	910	0	19.0	0.0	0	49%
(Healthy Choice)										
Italian style, 'Hearty Handfuls'	1 entrée	320	18	51	590	6	5.0	1.5	15	14%
Swedish, frozen	1 entrée	280	22	35	590	3	6.0	2.5	50	19%
(Lean Cuisine)										
Swedish	1 entrée	280	20	33	590	3	7.0	2.5	50	23%
Swedish, w/pasta, frozen	1 entrée	290	22	32	590	3	8.0	3.0	55	25%
Swedish, w/pasta, frozen	1 pkg	276	22	31	562	3	7.2	2.4	46	24%
(Lunch Express) Swedish, w/pasta, frozen	1 entrée	530	19	41	1010	3	32.0	11.0	65	55%
(Marie Callender's) Swedish, frozen	12.5 oz	520	28	44	1020	3	26.0	10.0	65	45%
(Morton) Swedish, beef, frozen	10 oz	310	11	26	1520	0	17.0	0.0	50	51%
(Smart Ones) Swedish	1 entrée	300	19	33	510	2	10.0	4.0	50	30%
(Stouffer's)										
Swedish, frozen	1 entrée	440	23	36	840	3	23.0	8.0	85	47%

Food Name	Serving Size	Calories	Prot. gms	Carbs gms	Sod. mgs	Fiber gms	Fat gms	Sat. Fat gms	Chol. mgs	% Fat Cal.
Swedish, w/gravy, food service product	1 oz	48	3	2	150	0	3.3	1.3	9	61%
(Swanson) Swedish, beef, frozen	10 oz	350	26	37	700	0	11.0	0.0	0	28%
(Weight Watchers) Swedish, frozen.	1 entrée	280	18	34	510	3	8.0	3.5	30	26%

MEATBALL SEASONING. See under SEASONING MIX.

MEDICAL NUTRITIONALS

CARBOHYDRATE SUPPLEMENT

(Mead Johnson Nutritionals)

Food Name	Serving Size	Calories	Prot. gms	Carbs gms	Sod. mgs	Fiber gms	Fat gms	Sat. Fat gms	Chol. mgs	% Fat Cal.
'Moducal, 100% maltodextrin, powder	1/2 cup	240	0	64	na	na	0.0	na	na	0%

(Ross)

Food Name	Serving Size	Calories	Prot. gms	Carbs gms	Sod. mgs	Fiber gms	Fat gms	Sat. Fat gms	Chol. mgs	% Fat Cal.
'Polycose' for oral or tube feeding (not parenteral use), kosher, gluten- and lactose-free, low-residue, liquid.	100 ml	200	0	50	70	na	0.0	na	na	0%
'Polycose' for oral or tube feeding (not parenteral use), kosher, gluten- and lactose-free, low-residue, powder . . .	100 gm	380	0	94	110	na	0.0	na	na	0%

CRITICAL CARE SUPPORT

(Nestlé Clinical Nutrition)

Food Name	Serving Size	Calories	Prot. gms	Carbs gms	Sod. mgs	Fiber gms	Fat gms	Sat. Fat gms	Chol. mgs	% Fat Cal.
'Crucial' for tube feeding, lactose- and gluten-free, low-residue, ready to use	1000 ml	1500	94	135	1168	na	68.0	na	na	41%
'Crucial' for tube feeding, lactose- and gluten-free, low-residue, ready to use.	250 ml	375	24	34	292	na	16.9	na	na	41%

(Novartis [Sandoz])

Food Name	Serving Size	Calories	Prot. gms	Carbs gms	Sod. mgs	Fiber gms	Fat gms	Sat. Fat gms	Chol. mgs	% Fat Cal.
'Impact' ready to use	1000 ml	1000	56	130	1100	na	28.0	na	na	25%
'Impact' ready to use, 1 can, ...	250 ml	250	14	33	267	na	6.9	na	na	25%
'Impact 1.5' for fluid restriction or high caloric needs, ready to use, ...	1000 ml	1500	80	140	1280	na	69.0	na	na	41%
'Impact 1.5' for fluid restriction or high caloric needs, ready to use, 1 can	250 ml	375	21	35	320	na	17.2	na	na	41%
'Impact with Fiber' ready to use	1000 ml	1000	56	140	1100	na	28.0	na	na	25%
'Impact with Fiber' ready to use, 1 can, ...	250 ml	250	14	34	267	na	6.9	na	na	25%

(Ross)

Food Name	Serving Size	Calories	Prot. gms	Carbs gms	Sod. mgs	Fiber gms	Fat gms	Sat. Fat gms	Chol. mgs	% Fat Cal.
'Perative' for tube feeding (not parenteral use), kosher, gluten- and lactose-free, low-residue, ready to use, ...	1 liter	1300	67	177	1040	na	37.4	na	na	26%
'Perative' for tube feeding (not parenteral use), kosher, gluten- and lactose-free, low-residue, ready to use	8 fl oz	308	16	42	250	na	8.8	na	na	26%

DIABETES/GLUCOSE INTOLERANCE SUPPORT

(Mead Johnson Nutritionals)

Food Name	Serving Size	Calories	Prot. gms	Carbs gms	Sod. mgs	Fiber gms	Fat gms	Sat. Fat gms	Chol. mgs	% Fat Cal.
'Choice DM' for oral or tube feeding, ready to use	1000 ml	1060	45	106	850	14	51.0	na	na	43%
'Choice DM' for oral or tube feeding, ready to use	8 fl oz	250	11	25	200	3	12.0	na	na	43%

(Nestlé Clinical Nutrition)

Food Name	Serving Size	Calories	Prot. gms	Carbs gms	Sod. mgs	Fiber gms	Fat gms	Sat. Fat gms	Chol. mgs	% Fat Cal.
'Glytrol with Fiber' for oral or tube feeding, kosher, sucrose-, lactose-, and gluten-free, ready to use	1000 ml	1000	45	100	740	15	47.5	na	na	43%
'Glytrol with Fiber' for oral or tube feeding, kosher, sucrose-, lactose-, and gluten-free, ready to use	250 ml	250	11	25	185	4	11.9	na	na	43%

(Novartis [Sandoz])

Food Name	Serving Size	Calories	Prot. gms	Carbs gms	Sod. mgs	Fiber gms	Fat gms	Sat. Fat gms	Chol. mgs	% Fat Cal.
'Diabetisource with Fiber' ready to use	1000 ml	1000	50	90	1000	4	49.0	na	na	44%
'Diabetisource with Fiber' ready to use, 1 can.	250 ml	250	13	23	250	1	12.2	na	na	44%
'Resource Diabetic with Fiber' for oral or tube feeding, ready to use	1000 ml	1060	63	99	970	13	47.0	na	na	40%
'Resource Diabetic with Fiber' for oral or tube feeding, ready to use	237 ml	250	15	23	230	3	11.1	na	na	40%

(Ross)

Food Name	Serving Size	Calories	Prot. gms	Carbs gms	Sod. mgs	Fiber gms	Fat gms	Sat. Fat gms	Chol. mgs	% Fat Cal.
'Glucerna with Fiber' for oral or tube feeding (not parenteral use), kosher, gluten- and lactose-free, low-residue, ready to use	1 liter	1000	42	96	930	14	54.4	na	na	49%

Food Name	Serving Size	Calories	Prot. gms	Carbs gms	Sod. mgs	Fiber gms	Fat gms	Sat. Fat gms	Chol. mgs	% Fat Cal.
'Glucerna with Fiber' for oral or tube feeding (not parenteral use), kosher, gluten- and lactose-free, low-residue, ready to use	8 fl oz	237	10	23	220	3	12.9	na	na	49%
ELEMENTAL DIET										
(B. Braun/McGaw)										
'Immun-Aid' for oral or tube feeding, high-nitrogen, powder, prepared, daily dose	2000 ml	2000	160	240	1150	na	44.0	na	na	20%
'Immun-Aid' for oral or tube feeding, high-nitrogen, powder, prepared, 1 serving	500 ml	500	40	60	290	na	11.0	na	na	20%
(Mead Johnson Nutritionals)										
'Criticare HN' high-nitrogen, ready to use	1000 ml	1060	38	220	630	na	5.3	na	na	5%
'Criticare HN' high-nitrogen, ready to use	8 fl oz	250	9	51	150	na	1.3	na	na	5%
(Nestlé Clinical Nutrition)										
'Peptamen' for tube feeding, isotonic, lactose- and gluten-free, low-residue, ready to use	1000 ml	1000	40	127	560	na	39.0	na	na	35%
'Peptamen' for tube feeding, isotonic, lactose- and gluten-free, low-residue, ready to use	250 ml	250	10	32	140	na	9.8	na	na	35%
'Peptamen Oral' oral, lactose- and gluten-free, low-residue, ready to use	1000 ml	1000	40	127	560	na	39.0	na	na	35%
'Peptamen Oral' oral, lactose- and gluten-free, low-residue, ready to use	250 ml	250	10	32	140	na	9.8	na	na	35%
'Peptamen VHP' for tube feeding, very high protein, isotonic, lactose- and gluten-free, low-residue, ready to use	1000 ml	1000	63	105	560	na	39.0	na	na	35%
'Peptamen VHP' for tube feeding, very high protein, isotonic, lactose- and gluten-free, low-residue, ready to use	250 ml	250	16	26	140	na	9.8	na	na	35%
'Peptamen VHP' oral, very high protein, lactose- and gluten-free, low-residue, ready to use	1000 ml	1000	63	105	560	na	39.0	na	na	35%
'Peptamen VHP' oral, very high protein, lactose- and gluten-free, low-residue, ready to use	250 ml	250	16	26	140	na	9.8	na	na	35%
'Reabilan' for tube feeding, lactose and gluten-free, low-residue, ready to use	1000 ml	1000	32	132	700	na	40.5	na	na	36%
'Reabilan' for tube feeding, lactose and gluten-free, low-residue, ready to use	375 ml	375	12	49	262	na	15.2	na	na	36%
'Reabilan HN' for tube feeding, high-nitrogen, lactose- and gluten-free, low-residue, ready to use	1000 ml	1333	58	158	1000	na	54.0	na	na	36%
'Reabilan HN' for tube feeding, high-nitrogen, lactose- and gluten-free, low-residue, ready to use	375 ml	500	22	59	380	na	20.2	na	na	36%
(Novartis [Sandoz])										
'Tolerex' powder, prepared	1000 ml	1000	21	230	470	na	1.5	na	na	1%
'Tolerex' powder, prepared, 1 packet	300 ml	300	6	68	141	na	0.4	na	na	1%
'Vivonex Plus' high-nitrogen, powder, prepared	1000 ml	1000	45	190	610	na	6.7	na	na	6%
'Vivonex Plus' high-nitrogen, powder, prepared	300 ml	300	14	57	183	na	2.0	na	na	6%
'Vivonex T.E.N' for gastrointestinal impairment, powder, prepared	1000 ml	1000	38	210	460	na	2.8	na	na	3%
'Vivonex T.E.N' for gastrointestinal impairment, powder, prepared, 1 packet	300 ml	300	12	62	138	na	0.8	na	na	2%
FAT MALABSORPTION SUPPORT										
(Mead Johnson Nutritionals)										
'Lipisorb' lactose-free, low-residue, powder, prepared	8 fl oz	480	17	56	352	na	23.0	na	na	43%
'Lipisorb' lactose-free, low-residue, ready to use	1000 ml	1350	57	161	1350	na	57.0	na	na	38%
'Lipisorb' lactose-free, low-residue, ready to use	8 fl oz	320	14	38	320	na	13.4	na	na	38%

Food Name	Serving Size	Calories	Prot. gms	Carbs gms	Sod. mgs	Fiber gms	Fat gms	Sat. Fat gms	Chol. mgs	% Fat Cal.
GASTROINTESTINAL SUPPORT										
(Nestlé Clinical Nutrition)										
'Elementra' for oral or tube feeding, elemental protein, powder, 2 scoops.	6.6 gm	25	5	0	10	na	0.3	na	na	12%
(Novartis [Sandoz])										
'Sandosource Peptide' semi-elemental, low-fat, ready to use	1000 ml	1000	50	160	1200	na	17.0	na	na	15%
'Sandosource Peptide' semi-elemental, low-fat, ready to use	250 ml	250	13	41	300	na	4.4	na	na	16%
(Ross)										
'Alitraq' for oral or tube feeding (not parenteral use), kosher, gluten-free, low-residue, powder, prepared	1 liter	1000	53	165	1000	na	15.5	na	na	14%
'Alitraq' for oral or tube feeding (not parenteral use), kosher, gluten-free, low-residue, powder, prepared	300 ml	300	16	50	300	na	4.7	na	na	14%
'Vital High Nitrogen' for oral or tube feeding (not parenteral use), kosher, gluten- and lactose-free, low-residue, powder, prepared	1 liter	1000	42	185	566	na	10.8	na	na	10%
'Vital High Nitrogen' for oral or tube feeding (not parenteral use), kosher, gluten- and lactose-free, low-residue, powder, prepared	300 ml	300	13	55	170	na	3.3	na	na	10%
GENERAL PURPOSE										
(Mead Johnson Nutritionals)										
'Boost' oral, milk-based, cholesterol- and lactose-free	8 fl oz	240	10	41	130	0	4.2	na	na	16%
'Sustacal' oral, milk-based, lactose-free cholesterol-free, powder, prepared	8 fl oz	200	13	36	190	0	0.7	na	na	3%
'Sustacal' oral, milk-based, moderate protein, fiber-free, lactose-free, low-residue, ready to use	8 fl oz	240	15	33	220	0	5.5	na	na	21%
'Sustacal Pudding' lactose-free, fiber-free.	8 fl oz	240	7	32	120	na	9.5	na	na	36%
'Sustacal with Fiber' oral, milk-based, w/fiber, lactose-free, ready to use	8 fl oz	250	11	33	170	3	8.3	na	na	30%
(Novartis [Sandoz])										
'Resource' fruit beverage, low-electrolyte, fat-free	1000 ml	760	37	150	230	na	0.0	na	na	0%
'Resource' fruit beverage, low-electrolyte, fat-free, 1 Brik Pak	237 ml	180	9	36	55	na	0.0	na	na	0%
(Ross)										
'Ensure' for oral or tube feeding (not parenteral use), kosher, gluten- and lactose-free, low-residue, powder, prepared	1 liter	1060	37	145	846	na	37.2	na	na	32%
'Ensure' for oral or tube feeding (not parenteral use), kosher, gluten- and lactose-free, low-residue, powder, prepared	8 fl oz	250	9	34	200	na	8.8	na	na	32%
'Ensure' for oral or tube feeding (not parenteral use), kosher, gluten- and lactose-free, low-residue, ready to use	1 liter	1060	37	169	845	na	25.8	na	na	22%
'Ensure' for oral or tube feeding (not parenteral use), kosher, gluten- and lactose-free, low-residue, ready to use	8 fl oz	250	9	40	200	na	6.1	na	na	22%
'Ensure Pudding' oral, patients w/swallowing impairments, kosher, gluten-free, 9.2 g lactose/serving	5 oz can	250	7	34	240	na	9.7	na	na	35%
'Ensure with Fiber' for oral or tube feeding (not parenteral use), fiber-fortified, kosher, gluten- and lactose-free, low-residue, ready to use.	1 liter	1100	40	162	846	14	37.2	na	na	30%

Food Name	Serving Size	Calories	Prot. gms	Carbs gms	Sod. mgs	Fiber gms	Fat gms	Sat. Fat gms	Chol. mgs	% Fat Cal.
'Ensure with Fiber' for oral or tube feeding (not parenteral use), fiber-fortified, kosher, gluten- and lactose-free, low-residue, ready to use.............	8 fl oz	260	9	38	200	3	8.8	na	na	30%
GERIATRIC										
(Nestlé Clinical Nutrition)										
'Probalance with Fiber' for oral or tube feeding, high-fiber, kosher, lactose- and gluten-free, ready to use	1000 ml	1200	54	156	763	10	40.6	na	na	30%
'Probalance with Fiber' for oral or tube feeding, high-fiber, kosher, lactose- and gluten-free, ready to use	250 ml	300	14	39	191	3	10.2	na	na	31%
HEALING SUPPORT										
(Mead Johnson Nutritionals)										
'Protain XL' for tube feeding, high-protein, w/fiber, ready to use	1000 ml	1000	57	129	920	na	30.0	na	na	27%
'Protain XL' for tube feeding, high-protein, w/fiber, ready to use	8 fl oz	237	14	31	220	na	7.1	na	na	27%
'Traumacal' for oral or tube feeding, high-calorie, high-nitrogen	1000 ml	1500	82	142	1180	na	68.0	na	na	41%
'Traumacal' for oral or tube feeding, high-calorie, high-nitrogen	8 fl oz	355	20	34	280	na	16.2	na	na	41%
(Nestlé Clinical Nutrition)										
'Replete' isotonic, kosher, lactose- and gluten-free, low-residue, ready to use	1000 ml	1000	63	113	876	na	34.0	na	na	31%
'Replete' isotonic, kosher, lactose- and gluten-free, low-residue, ready to use	250 ml	250	16	28	219	na	8.5	na	na	31%
'Replete with Fiber' for oral or tube feeding, isotonic, high-fiber, kosher, lactose- and gluten-free, ready to use	1000 ml	1000	63	113	876	14	34.0	na	na	31%
'Replete with Fiber' for oral or tube feeding, isotonic, high-fiber, kosher, lactose- and gluten-free, ready to use	250 ml	250	16	28	219	4	8.5	na	na	31%
(Ross)										
'Ensure' oral, coffee flavored, canned	8 fl oz	250	9	34	0	0	8.8	0.0	0	31%
'Promote' for oral or tube feeding, high-protein, kosher, gluten- and lactose-free, low-residue, ready to use	1 liter	1000	63	130	1000	na	26.0	na	na	23%
'Promote' for oral or tube feeding, high-protein, kosher, gluten- and lactose-free, low-residue, ready to use	8 fl oz	237	15	31	240	na	6.2	na	na	24%
'Promote with Fiber' for oral or tube feeding, high-protein, kosher, gluten- and lactose-free, low-residue, ready to use	1 liter	1000	63	139	1300	na	28.2	na	na	25%
'Promote with Fiber' for oral or tube feeding, high-protein, kosher, gluten- and lactose-free, low-residue, ready to use	8 fl oz	237	15	33	310	na	6.7	na	na	25%
HEPATIC SUPPORT										
(B. Braun/McGaw)										
'Hepatic-Aid II' for oral or tube feeding, amino acid and calories, powder, prepared	340 ml	400	15	57	na	na	12.3	na	na	28%
(Nestlé Clinical Nutrition)										
'Nutrihep' for oral or tube feeding, kosher, lactose- and gluten-free, ready to use	1000 ml	1500	40	290	320	na	21.2	na	na	13%

Food Name	Serving Size	Calories	Prot. gms	Carbs gms	Sod. mgs	Fiber gms	Fat gms	Sat. Fat gms	Chol. mgs	% Fat Cal.
'Nutrihep' for oral or tube feeding, kosher, lactose- and gluten-free, ready to use	250 ml	375	10	73	80	na	5.3	na	na	13%
HIV/AIDS SUPPORT										
(Ross)										
'Advera with Fiber' for oral or tube feeding (not parenteral use), kosher, gluten- and lactose-free, ready to use	1 liter	1280	60	216	1013	9	22.8	na	na	16%
'Advera with Fiber' for oral or tube feeding (not parenteral use), kosher, gluten- and lactose-free, ready to use	8 fl oz	303	14	51	240	2	5.4	na	na	16%
HYDRATION SUPPORT										
(Ross)										
'Equalyte' enteral rehydration solution	8 fl oz	24	0	7	432	0	0.0	0.0	0	0%
'Equalyte' rehydration solution, for oral or tube feeding (not parenteral use), kosher, gluten- and lactose-free, ready to use	1 liter	100	na	25	1800	na	na	na	na	0%
'Introlite' rehydration solution, for tube feeding (not parenteral use), low calorie, kosher, gluten- and lactose-free, low-residue, ready to use	1 liter	530	22	71	930	na	18.4	na	na	31%
'Pedialyte' for children	8 fl oz	24	0	6	244	0	0.0	0.0	0	0%
HYPEROSMOLAR SENSITIVITY SUPPORT										
(Ross)										
for oral or tube feeding (not parenteral use), kosher, gluten- and lactose-free, low-residue, ready to use	1 liter	1060	37	152	640	na	34.7	na	na	29%
for oral or tube feeding (not parenteral use), kosher, gluten- and lactose-free, low-residue, ready to use	8 fl oz	250	9	36	150	na	8.2	na	na	30%
INTACT PROTEIN DIET										
(Mead Johnson Nutritionals)										
'Comply' for tube feeding, high-calorie, lactose-free, ready to use	1000 ml	1500	60	180	1200	na	61.0	na	na	37%
'Comply' for tube feeding, high-calorie, lactose-free, ready to use	8 fl oz	355	14	43	280	na	14.5	na	na	37%
'Deliver 2.0' for oral or tube feeding, high-calorie, high-nitrogen, lactose-free	1000 ml	2000	75	200	800	na	102.0	na	na	46%
'Deliver 2.0' for oral or tube feeding, high-calorie, high-nitrogen, lactose-free	8 fl oz	470	18	47	190	na	24.0	na	na	46%
'Isocal' for tube feeding, lactose-free, low-residue, ready to use	1000 ml	1060	34	135	530	na	44.0	na	na	37%
'Isocal' for tube feeding, lactose-free, low-residue, ready to use	8 fl oz	250	8	32	125	na	10.5	na	na	38%
'Isocal HN' for tube feeding, high-nitrogen, isotonic, low-residue, ready to use	1000 ml	1060	44	123	930	na	145.0	na	na	123%
'Isocal HN' for tube feeding, high-nitrogen, isotonic, low-residue, ready to use	8 fl oz	250	10	29	220	na	10.7	na	na	39%
'Ultracal with Fiber' for tube feeding, high-nitrogen, w/fiber, ready to use	1000 ml	1060	44	123	930	14	45.0	na	na	38%
'Ultracal with Fiber' for tube feeding, high-nitrogen, w/fiber, ready to use	8 fl oz	250	10	29	220	3	10.7	na	na	39%
(Nestlé Clinical Nutrition)										
'Nubasics' oral, low-sodium, kosher, lactose-, gluten-, and cholesterol-free, low-residue, ready to use	250 ml	250	9	33	219	na	9.2	na	na	33%
'Nubasics Complete Nutrition Bar' oral, low-sodium, kosher, lactose- and gluten-free	1 bar	125	4	17	135	na	4.6	na	na	33%

Food Name	Serving Size	Calories	Prot. gms	Carbs gms	Sod. mgs	Fiber gms	Fat gms	Sat. Fat gms	Chol. mgs	% Fat Cal.
'Nubasics Complete Nutrition Soup' oral, low-cholesterol, lactose- and gluten-free, low-residue, 1 envelope	56 g	250	9	33	390	na	9.2	na	na	33%
Nubasics Decaffeinated Coffee Beverage' oral, kosher, lactose-, gluten-, and cholesterol-free, powder	2 scoops level	125	6	19	120	na	2.8	na	na	20%
'Nubasics Juice Drink' oral, kosher, lactose-, gluten-, and cholesterol-free; low-residue	163 ml	163	6	34	50	na	0.1	na	na	1%
'Nubasics Plus' oral, high-calorie, low-sodium, kosher, lactose-, gluten-, and cholesterol-free, low-residue, ready to use	250 ml	375	13	44	292	na	16.2	na	na	39%
'Nubasics 2.0' oral, very high calorie; kosher, lactose- and gluten-free, low-residue, ready to use	250 ml	500	20	49	325	na	26.5	na	na	48%
'Nubasics VHP' oral, high-protein, low-sodium, kosher, lactose-, gluten-, and cholesterol-free, ready to use	250 ml	250	16	28	219	na	8.3	na	na	30%
'Nubasics with Fiber' oral, high-protein with fiber, low-sodium, kosher, lactose-, gluten-, and cholesterol-free, low-residue, ready to use	250 ml	250	9	33	219	4	9.2	na	na	33%
'Nutren 1.0' for oral or tube feeding, kosher, lactose- and gluten-free, low-residue, ready to use	250 ml	250	10	32	219	na	9.5	na	na	34%
'Nutren 1.0' for oral or tube feeding, kosher, lactose- and gluten-free, low-residue, ready to use	1000 ml	1000	40	127	876	na	38.0	na	na	34%
'Nutren 1.0 with Fiber' for oral or tube feeding, high-fiber, kosher, lactose- and gluten-free, ready to use	1000 ml	1000	40	127	876	14	38.0	na	na	34%
'Nutren 1.0 with Fiber' for oral or tube feeding, high-fiber, kosher, lactose- and gluten-free, ready to use	250 ml	250	10	32	219	4	9.5	na	na	34%
'Nutren 1.5' for oral or tube feeding, high-calorie, kosher, lactose- and gluten-free, low-residue, ready to use	1000 ml	1500	60	169	1170	na	67.6	na	na	41%
'Nutren 1.5' for oral or tube feeding, high-calorie, kosher, lactose- and gluten-free, low-residue, ready to use	250 ml	375	15	42	292	na	16.9	na	na	41%
'Nutren 2.0' for oral or tube feeding, very high calorie, kosher, lactose- and gluten-free, low-residue, ready to use	1000 ml	2000	80	196	1300	na	106.0	na	na	48%
'Nutren 2.0' for oral or tube feeding, very high calorie, kosher, lactose- and gluten-free, low-residue, ready to use	250 ml	500	20	49	325	na	26.5	na	na	48%
(Novartis [Sandoz])										
'Citrotein' fruit-flavored, lactose-free, low-residue, powder, prepared, 1 serving	254 ml	170	11	31	170	na	0.4	na	na	2%
'Citrotein' fruit-flavored, lactose-free, low-residue, powder, prepared	100 ml	670	41	120	670	na	1.6	na	na	2%
'Compleat' for tube feeding, blenderized, ready to use	1000 ml	1070	43	130	1300	4	43.0	na	na	36%
'Compleat' for tube feeding, blenderized, ready to use, 1 can	250 ml	265	11	32	317	1	10.7	na	na	36%
'Compleat Modified with Fiber' for tube feeding, blenderized, lactose-free, isotonic, ready to use	1000 ml	1070	43	140	1000	4	37.0	na	na	31%
'Compleat Modified with Fiber' for tube feeding, blenderized, lactose-free, isotonic, ready to use, 1 can	250 ml	265	11	35	250	1	9.2	na	na	31%

Food Name	Serving Size	Calories	Prot. gms	Carbs gms	Sod. mgs	Fiber gms	Fat gms	Sat. Fat gms	Chol. mgs	% Fat Cal.
'Fibersource HN' for oral or tube feeding, high-fiber, high-nitrogen, lactose- and gluten-free, ready to use....	1000 ml	1200	53	160	1100	7	41.0	na	na	31%
'Fibersource HN' for oral or tube feeding, high-fiber, high-nitrogen, lactose- and gluten-free, ready to use, 1 can........	250 ml	300	13	40	283	2	10.4	na	na	31%
'Fibersource' for oral or tube feeding, high-fiber, lactose- and gluten-free, ready to use	1000 ml	1200	43	170	1100	10	41.0	na	na	31%
'Fibersource' for oral or tube feeding, high-fiber, lactose- and gluten-free, ready to use, 1 can........	250 ml	300	11	42	283	3	10.4	na	na	31%
'Isosource HN' for oral or tube feeding, protein maintenance, lactose-, gluten-, and fiber-free, ready to use	1000 ml	1200	53	160	1100	na	41.0	na	na	31%
'Isosource HN' for oral or tube feeding, protein maintenance, lactose-, gluten-, and fiber-free, ready to use	250 ml	300	13	39	267	na	10.4	na	na	31%
'Isosource 1.5 with Fiber' high-calorie, high-nitrogen, ready to use	1000 ml	1500	170	68	1300	8	65.0	na	na	39%
'Isosource 1.5 with Fiber' high-calorie, high-nitrogen, ready to use, 1 can................	250 ml	375	42	17	322	2	16.2	na	na	39%
'Isosource Standard' for oral or tube feeding, protein maintenance, lactose-, gluten-, and fiber-free, ready to use	1000 ml	1200	43	170	1200	na	41.0	na	na	31%
'Isosource Standard' for oral or tube feeding, protein maintenance, lactose-, gluten-, and fiber-free, ready to use	250	300	11	42	300	na	10.4	na	na	31%
'Isosource VHN with Fiber' for oral or tube feeding, w/fiber, ready to use	1000 ml	1000	62	130	1300	10	29.0	na	na	26%
'Isosource VHN with Fiber' for oral or tube feeding, w/fiber, ready to use	250 ml	250	16	32	320	3	7.2	na	na	26%
'Resource Plus' for oral or tube feeding, high-calorie, lactose- and gluten-free, ready to use	1000 ml	1500	55	200	1300	na	53.0	na	na	32%
'Resource Plus' for oral or tube feeding, high-calorie, lactose- and gluten-free, ready to use, 1 Brik Pak	237 ml	355	13	47	300	na	12.6	na	na	32%
'Resource Standard' maintenance protein and calorie, lactose- and gluten-free, ready to use	1000 ml	1100	37	140	890	na	37.0	na	na	30%
'Resource Standard' maintenance protein and calorie, lactose- and gluten-free, ready to use, 1 Brik Pak	237 ml	250	9	34	210	na	8.8	na	na	32%
(Ross)										
'Ensure High Protein' oral (not parenteral use), kosher, gluten- and lactose-free, low-residue, ready to use	8 fl oz	225	12	31	290	na	6.0	0.6	na	24%
'Ensure Plus' for oral or tube feeding (not parenteral use), high-calorie, kosher, gluten- and lactose-free, low-residue, ready to use	1 liter	1500	55	200	1050	na	53.3	na	na	32%
'Ensure Plus' for oral or tube feeding (not parenteral use), high-calorie, kosher, gluten- and lactose-free, low-residue, ready to use	8 fl oz	355	13	47	250	na	12.6	na	na	32%
'Ensure Plus HN' for oral or tube feeding (not parenteral use), high calorie, kosher, gluten- and lactose-free, low-residue, ready to use.............	1 liter	1500	63	200	1180	na	50.0	na	na	30%
'Ensure Plus HN' for oral or tube feeding (not parenteral use), high calorie, kosher, gluten- and lactose-free, low-residue, ready to use..............	8 fl oz	355	15	47	280	na	11.8	na	na	30%

Food Name	Serving Size	Calories	Prot. gms	Carbs gms	Sod. mgs	Fiber gms	Fat gms	Sat. Fat gms	Chol. mgs	% Fat Cal.
'Jevity with Fiber' for tube feeding (not parenteral use), fiber-fortified, isotonic, kosher, gluten-and lactose-free, low-residue, ready to use..............	1 liter	1060	44	154	930	14	34.7	na	na	29%
'Jevity with Fiber' for tube feeding (not parenteral use), fiber-fortified, isotonic, kosher, gluten-and lactose-free, low-residue, ready to use..............	8 fl oz	250	11	36	220	3	8.2	na	na	30%
'Jevity Plus with Fiber' for tube feeding (not parenteral use), high-nitrogen, kosher, gluten- and lactose-free, ready to use....................................	1 liter	1200	56	175	1350	12	39.3	na	na	29%
'Jevity Plus with Fiber' for tube feeding (not parenteral use), high-nitrogen, kosher, gluten- and lactose-free, ready to use.....................................	8 fl oz	285	13	42	275	3	9.3	na	na	29%
'Osmolite' for oral or tube feeding (not parenteral use), high-nitrogen, isotonic, kosher, gluten- and lactose-free, low-residue, ready to use..............	1 liter	1060	44	144	930	na	34.7	na	na	29%
'Osmolite' for oral or tube feeding (not parenteral use), high-nitrogen, isotonic, kosher, gluten- and lactose-free, low-residue, ready to use..............	8 fl oz	250	11	34	220	na	8.2	na	na	30%
'Osmolite HN Plus' for tube feeding (not parenteral use), high-calorie, high-nitrogen, kosher, gluten- and lactose-free, low-residue, ready to use..........	1 liter	1200	56	158	1420	na	39.3	na	na	29%
'Osmolite HN Plus' for tube feeding (not parenteral use), high-calorie, high-nitrogen, kosher, gluten- and lactose-free, low-residue, ready to use..........	8 fl oz	285	13	38	340	na	9.3	na	na	29%
'Twocal HN' for oral or tube feeding (not parenteral use), high-calorie, high-protein, kosher, gluten- and lactose-free, low-residue, ready to use..............	1 liter	2000	84	217	1456	na	90.9	na	na	41%
'Twocal HN' for oral or tube feeding (not parenteral use), high-calorie, high-protein, kosher, gluten- and lactose-free, low-residue, ready to use..............	8 fl oz	475	20	51	345	na	21.5	na	na	41%
PARENTERAL SUPPORT (NUTRIENT INJECTIONS)										
(B. Braun/McGaw)										
'Freamine HBC' 6.9% amino acids, sterile, nonpyrogenic, hypertonic solution	100 ml	na	na	na	na	na	na	na	na	0%
'Freamine III' 8.5% amino acids, nonpyrogenic, hypertonic solution.............................	100 ml	na	na	na	na	na	na	na	na	0%
'Freamine III' 10% amino acids, sterile, nonpyrogenic, hypertonic solution, w/electrolytes	100 ml	na	na	na	na	na	na	na	na	0%
'Freamine III' with Electrolytes' 8.5% amino acids, sterile, nonpyrogenic, hypertonic solution, w/electrolytes......................................	100 ml	na	na	na	na	na	na	na	na	0%
'Freamine II' 3% amino acids, sterile, nonpyrogenic, slightly hypertonic solution, w/electrolytes	100 ml	na	na	na	0	na	na	na	na	0%
'Hepatamine' 8% amino acids, for patients w/cirrhosis or hepatitis, sterile, nonpyrogenic, hypertonic solution...	500 ml	na	na	na	na	na	na	na	na	0%
'Hepatamine' 8% amino acids, for patients w/hepatic encephalopathy - injection	100 ml	na	na	na	na	na	na	na	na	0%
'Procalamine' 3% amino acids, 3% glycerine, sterile, nonpyrogenic, moderately hypertonic injection, w/electrolytes......................................	100 ml	na	na	na	0	na	na	na	na	0%
'Trophanine' 10% amino acids, sterile, nonpyrogenic, hypertonic solution, w/electrolytes	100 ml	na	na	na	na	na	na	na	na	0%

Food Name	Serving Size	Calories	Prot. gms	Carbs gms	Sod. mgs	Fiber gms	Fat gms	Sat. Fat gms	Chol. mgs	% Fat Cal.
'Trophanine' 6% amino acids, sterile, nonpyrogenic, hypertonic solution, w/electrolytes	100 ml	na	na	na	na	na	na	na	na	0%
PEDIATRIC										
(Mead Johnson Nutritionals)										
'Kindercal with Fiber' for oral or tube feeding, lactose-free, isotonic, ready to use	1000 ml	1060	34	135	370	6	44.0	na	na	37%
'Kindercal with Fiber' for oral or tube feeding, lactose-free, isotonic, ready to use	8 fl oz	250	8	32	88	2	10.5	na	na	38%
'Portagen' for GI disorders, children under 2 years, powder, prepared	5 fl oz	100	4	12	55	na	4.8	na	na	43%
(Nestlé Clinical Nutrition)										
'Nutren Junior' for oral or tube feeding, children 1–10 years, kosher, lactose- and gluten-free, low-residue, ready to use	1000 ml	1000	30	128	460	na	42.0	na	na	38%
'Nutren Junior' for oral or tube feeding, children 1–10 years, kosher, lactose- and gluten-free, low-residue, ready to use	250 ml	250	8	32	115	na	10.5	na	na	38%
'Nutren Junior with Fiber' for oral or tube feeding, children 1–10 years, kosher, lactose- and gluten-free, low-residue, ready to use	1000 ml	1000	30	128	460	6	42.0	na	na	38%
'Nutren Junior with Fiber' for oral or tube feeding, children 1–10 years, kosher, lactose- and gluten-free, low-residue, ready to use	250 ml	250	8	32	115	2	10.5	na	na	38%
'Peptamen Junior' for tube feeding, GI patients, children 1-10 years, lactose- and gluten-free, low-residue, ready to use	1000 ml	1000	30	138	460	na	38.5	na	na	35%
'Peptamen Junior' for tube feeding, GI patients, children 1-10 years, lactose- and gluten-free, low-residue, ready to use	250 ml	250	8	34	115	na	9.6	na	na	35%
'Peptamen Junior Oral' oral, for children 1-10 years, lactose- and gluten-free, low-residue, ready to use	1000 ml	1000	30	138	460	na	38.5	na	na	35%
'Peptamen Junior Oral' oral, for children 1-10 years, lactose- and gluten-free, low-residue, ready to use	250 ml	250	8	34	115	na	9.6	na	na	35%
(Novartis [Sandoz])										
'Vivonex Pediatric' for oral or tube feeding, children 1–10 years, powder, prepared	1000 ml	800	24	130	400	na	24.0	na	na	27%
'Vivonex Pediatric' for oral or tube feeding, children 1–10 years, powder, prepared	250 ml	200	6	32	100	na	5.9	na	na	26%
(Ross)										
'Pediasure with Fiber' for oral or tube feeding (not parenteral use), kosher, gluten- and lactose-free, ready to use, not for children with galactosemia	1 liter	1000	30	114	380	na	49.7	na	na	45%
'Pediasure with Fiber' for oral or tube feeding (not parenteral use), kosher, gluten- and lactose-free, ready to use, not for children with galactosemia	8 fl oz	237	7	27	90	na	11.8	na	na	45%
'Pediasure' for oral or tube feeding (not parenteral use) kosher, gluten- and lactose-free, low-residue, not for children with galactosemia	1 liter	1000	30	110	380	na	49.7	na	na	45%
'Pediasure' for oral or tube feeding (not parenteral use) kosher, gluten- and lactose-free, low-residue, not for children with galactosemia	8 fl oz	237	7	26	90	na	11.8	na	na	45%
PROTEIN SUPPLEMENT										
(Mead Johnson Nutritionals)										
'Casec'	100 gm	380	90	0	100	na	2.0	na	na	5%
(Novartis [Sandoz])										
'Meritene' oral, powder, prepared	1000 ml	1100	69	120	1100	na	34.0	na	na	28%

Food Name	Serving Size	Calories	Prot. gms	Carbs gms	Sod. mgs	Fiber gms	Fat gms	Sat. Fat gms	Chol. mgs	% Fat Cal.
'Meritene' oral, powder, prepared, 1 serving..........	275 ml	275	18	31	280	na	8.8	na	na	29%
(Ross)										
for oral or tube feeding (not parenteral use), powder, gluten-free, low-residue, kosher, 2 scoops............	6.6 gm	28	5	1	15	na	0.6	na	na	19%
PULMONARY SUPPORT										
(Mead Johnson Nutritionals)										
'Respalor' for oral or tube feeding, high-nitrogen, high-calorie, ready to use........................	1000 ml	1520	76	148	1270	na	71.0	na	na	42%
'Respalor' for oral or tube feeding, high-nitrogen, high-calorie, ready to use........................	8 fl oz	360	18	35	300	na	16.8	na	na	42%
(Nestlé Clinical Nutrition)										
'Nutrivent' for tube feeding, kosher, lactose- and gluten-free, low-residue, ready to use	1000 ml	1500	68	100	1170	na	94.0	na	na	56%
'Nutrivent' for tube feeding, kosher, lactose- and gluten-free, low-residue, ready to use	250 ml	375	17	25	292	na	23.7	na	na	57%
(Ross)										
'Pulmocare' for oral or tube feeding (not parenteral use), kosher, gluten- and lactose-free, low-residue, ready to use..................................	1 liter	1500	63	106	1310	na	93.3	na	na	56%
'Pulmocare' for oral or tube feeding (not parenteral use), kosher, gluten- and lactose-free, low-residue, ready to use..................................	8 fl oz	355	15	25	310	na	22.1	na	na	56%
RENAL SUPPORT										
(Mead Johnson Nutritionals)										
'Magnacal' for oral or tube feeding, high-calorie, ready to use...................................	1000 ml	2000	75	200	800	na	101.0	na	na	45%
'Magnacal' for oral or tube feeding, high-calorie, ready to use...................................	8 fl oz	470	18	47	190	na	24.0	na	na	46%
(Nestlé Clinical Nutrition)										
'Renalcal Diet' for oral or tube feeding, patients w/renal failure, high-calorie, kosher, lactose- and gluten-free, low-residue, ready to use	1000 ml	2000	34	290	na	na	82.4	na	na	37%
'Renalcal Diet' for oral or tube feeding, patients w/renal failure, high-calorie, kosher, lactose- and gluten-free, low-residue, ready to use	250 ml	500	9	73	na	na	20.6	na	na	37%
(Ross)										
'Nepro' for oral or tube feeding (not parenteral use), dialzyed patients, kosher, gluten- and lactose-free, low-residue, ready to use	1 liter	2000	70	222	842	na	95.6	na	na	43%
'Nepro' for oral or tube feeding (not parenteral use), dialzyed patients, kosher, gluten- and lactose-free, low-residue, ready to use	8 fl oz	475	17	52	200	na	22.7	na	na	43%
'Suplena' for oral or tube feeding (not parenteral use), predialyzed patients, kosher, gluten- and lactose-free, low-residue, ready to use..............	1 liter	2000	30	255	783	na	95.6	na	na	43%
'Suplena' for oral or tube feeding (not parenteral use), predialyzed patients, kosher, gluten- and lactose-free, low-residue, ready to use..............	8 fl oz	475	7	61	186	na	22.7	na	na	43%
MEDLAR, JAPANESE. See LOQUAT.										
MELBA TOAST. See under CRACKER.										
MELON, CANTALOUPE / muskmelon										
Fresh										
balls..	1 cup	62	2	15	16	1	0.5	0.1	0	7%
balls..	10 balls	48	1	12	12	1	0.4	0.1	0	7%
cubed	1 cup	56	1	13	14	1	0.4	0.1	0	7%

Food Name	Serving Size	Calories	Prot. gms	Carbs gms	Sod. mgs	Fiber gms	Fat gms	Sat. Fat gms	Chol. mgs	% Fat Cal.
diced	1 cup	55	1	13	14	1	0.4	0.1	0	7%
wedges, 1/8 of large melon......................	1 wedge	36	1	9	9	1	0.3	0.1	0	7%
wedges, 1/8 of medium melon	1 wedge	24	1	6	6	1	0.2	0.0	0	7%
wedges, 1/8 of small melon....................	1 wedge	19	0	5	5	0	0.2	0.0	0	7%
whole, large, approx 6-1/2-inch diam	1 melon	285	7	68	73	7	2.3	0.6	0	7%
whole, medium, approx 5-inch diam	1 melon	193	5	46	50	4	1.5	0.4	0	7%
whole, small, approx 4-1/4-inch diam	1 melon	154	4	37	40	4	1.2	0.3	0	7%
Frozen, balls (Flav-R-Pac)......................	3/4 cup	40	1	10	16	0	0.0	0.0	0	0%
MELON, CASABA										
cubed	1 cup	44	2	11	20	1	0.2	0.0	0	3%
sliced, medium	1/10 melon	43	1	10	20	1	0.2	0.0	0	3%
whole, medium	1 melon	426	15	102	197	13	1.6	0.4	0	3%
MELON, HONEYDEW										
Fresh										
balls.......................	1 cup	62	1	16	18	1	0.2	0.0	0	2%
diced	1 cup	60	1	16	17	1	0.2	0.0	0	2%
wedges, 1/8 of 5.25-inch diam melon	1 wedge	44	1	11	13	1	0.1	0.0	0	2%
wedges, 1/8 of 6- to 7-inch diam melon	1 wedge	56	1	15	16	1	0.2	0.0	0	2%
whole, approx 5.25-inch diam	1 melon	350	5	92	100	6	1.0	0.3	0	2%
whole, 6- to 7-inch diam	1 melon	448	6	118	128	8	1.3	0.3	0	2%
Frozen										
balls, (Flav-R-Pac).......................	3/4 cup	45	1	11	16	1	0.0	0.0	0	0%
balls, unthawed	1 cup	57	1	14	54	1	0.4	0.1	0	6%
MENHADEN OIL. See under FISH OIL.										
MENUDO MIX. See under SEASONING MIX.										
MESQUITE SEASONING. See under MARINADE MIX; SEASONING MIX.										
MEXICAN OREGANO. See OREGANO, MEXICAN.										
MEXICAN POTATO. See JICAMA.										
MEXICAN SEASONING. See under SEASONING MIX.										
MEXICAN STYLE DINNER/ENTRÉE. See also individual listings.										
(Amy's Kitchen) tamale pie	1 serving	220	10	41	480	11	3.0	0.0	0	12%
(Banquet)										
combination, frozen...............................	12 oz	520	20	72	1980	0	17.0	0.0	0	29%
frozen	12 oz	490	18	62	2000	0	18.0	0.0	0	34%
(Morton) Mexican style, frozen......................	10 oz	300	9	44	1390	0	10.0	0.0	20	30%
(Patio)										
'Fiesta' frozen	12.25 oz	470	16	55	2040	0	20.0	0.0	30	39%
frozen	13.25 oz	540	15	64	1940	0	25.0	0.0	45	42%
w/tamale, beef enchilada, beans, rice, rice............	1 pkg	508	14	68	1812	8	19.9	6.8	26	35%
(Stouffer's) 'Mexi-Mac' frozen, food service product........	1 oz	26	1	4	142	1	0.9	0.4	3	31%
(Swanson) 'Hungry Man'	1 entree	690	26	87	2170	13	27.0	9.0	35	35%
(Van de Kamp's) frozen	1/2 pkg	220	7	25	640	0	10.0	0.0	0	41%
MILK										
COW										
Canned										
Low-fat										
(Carnation)	1/2 cup	110	9	12	130	0	3.0	0.0	0	24%
Nonfat/skim										
(Carnation)	1/2 cup	100	9	14	147	0	0.3	0.0	0	3%
(Diehl)	1/2 cup	100	9	14	150	0	1.0	0.0	0	9%
(Finast)	1/2 cup	100	9	14	150	0	1.0	0.0	0	9%
(Pathmark)	1/2 cup	100	9	14	15	0	0.0	0.0	0	0%
(Pet)	1/2 cup	100	9	14	150	0	1.0	0.0	10	9%
Whole										
(Carnation)	1/2 cup	110	9	12	130	0	3.0	0.0	0	24%

Food Name	Serving Size	Calories	Prot. gms	Carbs gms	Sod. mgs	Fiber gms	Fat gms	Sat. Fat gms	Chol. mgs	% Fat Cal.
Condensed										
sweetened, canned	1 cup	982	24	166	389	0	26.6	16.8	104	24%
sweetened, canned	1 fl oz	123	3	21	49	0	3.3	2.1	13	24%
sweetened, canned *(Borden)*	1/3 cup	320	7	54	115	0	8.0	0.0	0	23%
sweetened, canned *(Carnation)*	1/3 cup	320	7	56	110	0	8.0	0.0	0	22%
sweetened, canned *(Eagle)*	1/2 cup	320	7	52	120	0	9.0	0.0	0	26%
sweetened, canned, 'Jerzee' *(Diehl)*	1/3 cup	320	7	52	120	0	9.0	0.0	0	26%
sweetened, freeze-dried *(Crystalac)*	1 oz	139	3	22	na	na	3.4	1.9	51	23%
Evaporated										
Low-fat										
(Carnation)	1/2 cup	110	8	12	140	0	3.0	2.0	10	25%
canned *(Pathmark)*	1/2 cup	100	9	14	15	0	0.0	0.0	0	0%
Nonfat/skim										
	1 cup	199	19	29	294	0	0.5	0.3	9	2%
	1/2 cup	100	10	15	147	0	0.3	0.2	5	2%
	1 fl oz	25	2	4	37	0	0.1	0.0	1	2%
(Carnation)	1/2 cup	100	9	14	150	0	1.0	0.2	5	9%
(Pet)	1/2 cup	100	9	14	150	0	1.0	0.0	10	9%
Whole										
	1 cup	339	17	25	267	0	19.1	11.6	74	49%
	1/2 cup	169	9	13	133	0	9.5	5.8	37	49%
	1 fl oz	42	2	3	33	0	2.4	1.4	9	49%
(Finast)	1/2 cup	170	8	12	135	0	10.0	0.0	0	53%
(IGA)	1/2 cup	170	8	12	140	0	10.0	0.0	0	53%
(Pathmark)	1/2 cup	170	8	12	140	0	10.9	0.0	0	55%
(Pet)	1/2 cup	170	8	12	140	0	10.0	0.0	36	53%
canned *(Carnation)*	1/2 cup	170	8	12	135	0	10.0	0.0	0	53%
canned *(Diehl)*	1/2 cup	170	8	12	135	0	10.0	0.0	0	53%
filled *(Pet)*	1/2 cup	150	8	12	140	0	8.0	1.0	5	47%
imitation, filled *(Diehl)*	1/2 cup	150	8	12	135	0	8.0	2.0	5	47%
vitamin A, canned	1/2 cup	169	9	13	133	0	9.5	5.8	37	49%
vitamin A, canned	1 fl oz	42	2	3	33	0	2.4	1.4	9	49%
Dry										
Nonfat/skim										
calcium reduced	1 oz	100	10	15	646	0	0.1	0.0	1	1%
calcium reduced	1/4 lb	400	40	59	2576	0	0.2	0.1	2	1%
extra grade, instant *(Saco Foods)*	5 tbsp	80	8	12	125	0	1.0	0.0	5	10%
instant	1 cup	244	24	35	373	0	0.5	0.3	12	2%
instant	1/3 cup	82	8	12	126	0	0.2	0.1	4	2%
instant *(Carnation)*	5 tbsp	80	8	12	125	0	0.2	0.1	5	2%
instant, 'Dairy Creamer' *(Weight Watchers)*	1 pkt	10	1	1	15	0	0.0	0.0	0	0%
instant, 'Dairy Fresh' *(Sanalac)*	0.8 oz	80	8	12	85	0	0.1	0.1	5	1%
instant, prepared *(Alba)*	8 fl oz	80	8	12	190	0	0.0	0.0	0	0%
low lactose *(Nutra/Balance)*	1/4 cup	20	2	3	31	0	0.1	na	na	5%
regular	1 cup	435	43	62	642	0	0.9	0.6	24	2%
regular	1/4 cup	109	11	16	161	0	0.2	0.1	6	2%
vitamin A	1 cup	435	43	62	642	0	0.9	0.6	24	2%
vitamin A	1/4 cup	109	11	16	161	0	0.2	0.1	6	2%
Whole										
	1 cup	635	34	49	475	0	34.2	21.4	124	47%
	1/4 cup	159	8	12	119	0	8.5	5.4	31	47%
Fresh										
Low-fat, 1% fat										
(Crowley)	1 cup	100	8	11	130	0	2.0	0.0	10	19%
protein fortified *(A&P)*	1 cup	100	8	12	120	0	3.0	0.0	0	25%

Food Name	Serving Size	Calories	Prot. gms	Carbs gms	Sod. mgs	Fiber gms	Fat gms	Sat. Fat gms	Chol. mgs	% Fat Cal.
protein fortified *(Borden)*	1 cup	100	8	11	130	0	2.0	0.0	0	19%
protein fortified *(Crowley)*	1 cup	100	8	11	130	0	2.0	0.0	10	19%
protein fortified *(Darigold)*	1 cup	100	8	13	130	0	2.0	1.6	10	18%
protein fortified 'Nice n' Light' *(Knudsen)*	1 cup	130	10	15	153	0	3.0	0.0	0	21%
protein fortified, calcium added *(Darigold)*	1 cup	100	8	11	130	0	2.0	1.6	10	19%
protein fortified, lactose added, 'Lactaid' *(Crowley)*	1 cup	100	8	11	125	0	2.0	0.0	10	19%
vitamin A	1 quart	409	32	47	493	0	10.3	6.4	39	22%
vitamin A	1 cup	102	8	12	123	0	2.6	1.6	10	22%
vitamin A, protein fortified	1 quart	477	39	54	574	0	11.5	7.2	39	21%
vitamin A, protein fortified	1 cup	119	10	14	143	0	2.9	1.8	10	21%
vitamin A, school milk carton	1/2 pint	102	8	12	123	0	2.6	1.6	10	22%
vitamin A, w/added nonfat milk solids	1 quart	418	34	49	514	0	9.5	5.9	39	20%
vitamin A, w/added nonfat milk solids	1 cup	104	9	12	128	0	2.4	1.5	10	20%
vitamin A and D enriched *(Lucerne)*	1 cup	110	9	13	130	0	2.5	1.5	15	20%
Low-fat, 2% fat										
(Lucerne) vitamin A and D enriched	1 cup	130	8	13	125	0	5.0	3.0	20	35%
protein fortified *(A&P)*	1 cup	120	8	12	120	0	5.0	0.0	0	36%
protein fortified *(Crowley)*	1 cup	120	8	11	125	0	5.0	0.0	15	37%
protein fortified *(Darigold)*	1 cup	120	8	11	130	0	5.0	2.9	18	37%
protein fortified *(Finast)*	1 cup	130	9	12	130	0	5.0	0.0	0	35%
protein fortified *(Knudsen)*	1 cup	140	10	13	150	0	5.0	0.0	0	33%
protein fortified *(Viva)*	1 cup	120	8	11	125	0	5.0	0.0	0	37%
protein fortified, 'Hi-Protein' *(Borden)*	1 cup	140	10	13	150	0	5.0	0.0	0	33%
protein fortified, 'Nutrish Acidophilus' *(Darigold)*	1 cup	120	8	11	130	0	5.0	2.9	18	37%
protein fortified, 'Sweet Acidophilus' *(Knudsen)*	1 cup	140	10	13	150	0	5.0	0.0	0	33%
protein fortified, 'Tone Acidophilus' *(Crowley)*	1 cup	120	8	11	125	0	5.0	0.0	15	37%
vitamin A	1 quart	485	33	47	487	0	18.7	11.7	73	34%
vitamin A	1 cup	121	8	12	122	0	4.7	2.9	18	34%
vitamin A, protein fortified	1 quart	546	39	54	579	0	19.5	12.1	76	31%
vitamin A, protein fortified	1 cup	137	10	14	145	0	4.9	3.0	19	31%
vitamin A, school milk carton	1/2 pint	121	8	12	122	0	4.7	2.9	18	34%
vitamin A, w/added nonfat milk solids	1 quart	500	34	49	514	0	18.8	11.7	74	33%
vitamin A, w/added nonfat milk solids	1 cup	125	9	12	128	0	4.7	2.9	18	33%
w/added nonfat milk solids	1 quart	544	39	54	576	0	19.4	12.1	75	31%
w/added nonfat milk solids	1 cup	136	10	13	144	0	4.9	3.0	19	31%
Nonfat/skim										
	1 quart	343	33	48	510	0	1.8	1.1	20	5%
	1 cup	86	8	12	127	0	0.4	0.3	5	5%
protein fortified *(A&P)*	1 cup	90	8	12	125	0	1.0	0.0	0	10%
protein fortified *(Crowley)*	1 cup	90	9	12	130	0	1.0	0.0	1	10%
protein fortified *(Knudsen)*	1 cup	80	9	12	130	0	0.0	0.0	0	0%
protein fortified *(Weight Watchers)*	1 cup	90	9	13	140	0	1.0	0.0	0	9%
protein fortified, 'Skim-Line' *(Borden)*	1 cup	100	10	13	150	0	1.0	0.0	0	9%
protein fortified, 'Trim' *(Darigold)*	1 cup	80	8	11	130	0	1.0	0.3	4	11%
vitamin A, nonfat	1 quart	342	33	48	505	0	1.8	1.1	18	5%
vitamin A, nonfat	1 cup	86	8	12	126	0	0.4	0.3	4	5%
vitamin A, protein fortified, nonfat	1 quart	400	39	55	578	0	2.5	1.6	20	5%
vitamin A, protein fortified, nonfat	1 cup	100	10	14	144	0	0.6	0.4	5	5%
vitamin A, w/added nonfat milk solids	1 quart	361	35	49	519	0	2.5	1.6	20	6%
vitamin A, w/added nonfat milk solids	1 cup	90	9	12	130	0	0.6	0.4	5	6%
vitamin A and D enriched *(Lucerne)*	1 cup	90	9	13	130	0	0.0	0.0	15	0%
Whole										
(Carnation)	1 cup	150	8	12	120	0	8.0	0.0	33	47%
low-salt	1 quart	594	30	44	24	0	33.8	21.0	133	50%

Food Name	Serving Size	Calories	Prot. gms	Carbs gms	Sod. mgs	Fiber gms	Fat gms	Sat. Fat gms	Chol. mgs	% Fat Cal.
low-salt	1 cup	149	8	11	6	0	8.4	5.3	33	50%
low-sodium (A&P)	1 cup	150	8	11	120	0	8.0	0.0	0	49%
low-sodium (Borden)	1 cup	150	8	11	130	0	8.0	0.0	0	49%
low-sodium (Crowley)	1 cup	150	8	11	125	0	8.0	0.0	30	49%
low-sodium (Darigold)	1 cup	150	8	11	125	0	8.0	4.9	33	49%
low-sodium (Knudsen)	1 cup	160	9	12	180	0	8.0	0.0	0	46%
low-sodium, 'Hi-Calcium' (Borden)	1 cup	150	8	11	130	0	8.0	0.0	0	49%
3.7% fat	1 quart	626	32	45	476	0	35.7	22.2	140	50%
3.7% fat	1 cup	157	8	11	119	0	8.9	5.6	35	50%
3.25% fat	1 quart	600	32	45	478	0	32.6	20.3	133	48%
3.25% fat	1 cup	150	8	11	120	0	8.2	5.1	33	48%
3.25% fat	1 tbsp	9	1	1	7	0	0.5	0.3	2	48%
3.25% fat, school milk carton	1/2 pint	150	8	11	120	0	8.2	5.1	33	48%
vitamin A and D enriched (Lucerne)	1 cup	150	8	12	125	0	8.0	5.0	34	47%
vitamin D, homogenized (Borden)	1 cup	150	8	11	130	0	8.0	0.0	0	49%
vitamin D, homogenized (Trader Joe's)	1 cup	150	8	11	115	0	8.0	5.0	35	49%
GOAT										
Evaporated, canned, undiluted (Meyenberg)	4 fl oz	143	8	10	86	0	7.9	0.0	0	50%
Fresh										
	1 quart	672	35	43	486	0	40.4	26.0	111	53%
	1 cup	168	9	11	122	0	10.1	6.5	28	53%
	1 fl oz	21	1	1	15	0	1.3	0.8	3	53%
INDIAN BUFFALO										
	1 quart	943	37	51	509	0	67.2	44.9	185	63%
	1 cup	236	9	13	127	0	16.8	11.2	46	63%
HUMAN										
	1 cup	171	3	17	42	0	10.8	4.9	34	55%
	1 fl oz	21	0	2	5	0	1.3	0.6	4	55%
SHEEP										
	1 quart	1057	59	53	432	0	68.6	45.1	265	57%
	1 cup	264	15	13	108	0	17.1	11.3	66	57%
MILK SUBSTITUTE. See also RICE BEVERAGE; SOYMILK.										
w/lauric acid oil, fluid	1 quart	600	17	60	764	0	33.3	29.6	2	49%
w/lauric acid oil, fluid	1 cup	150	4	15	191	0	8.3	7.4	0	49%
w/hydrogenated vegetable oils, fluid	1 quart	600	17	60	764	0	33.3	7.5	2	49%
w/hydrogenated vegetable oils, fluid	1 cup	150	4	15	191	0	8.3	1.9	0	49%
w/hydrogenated vegetable oils, fluid	1 fl oz	19	1	2	24	0	1.0	0.2	0	49%
(First Alternative) 1%, lactose-free	1 cup	80	8	6	180	0	2.0	0.5	0	24%
(Ener-G Foods) lactose-free	3 tbsp	85	10	7	4	5	1.6	0.0	0	17%
MILKFISH. See AWA.										
MILKSHAKE										
(Killer Shake)										
banana, 'Bodacious Bananaberry'	1 carton	420	12	62	250	5	14.0	8.0	55	30%
chocolate, 'Totally Chocolate'	1 carton	470	14	65	320	6	17.0	10.0	60	33%
(MicroMagic)										
chocolate, frozen	11.5 fl oz	340	5	55	120	0	8.0	0.0	40	23%
strawberry, frozen	11.5 fl oz	340	5	54	120	0	9.0	0.0	40	26%
vanilla, frozen	11.5 fl oz	380	8	60	150	0	13.0	0.0	45	30%
MILKSHAKE MIX, CHOCOLATE										
chocolate fudge (Weight Watchers)	1 pkt	70	6	11	170	0	1.0	0.0	0	12%
orange sherbet (Weight Watchers)	1 pkt	70	6	11	210	0	0.0	0.0	0	0%
MILLET										
pearl, cooked	1/2 cup	143	4.2	28.4	2	1.6	1.2	0.2	0	8%
pearl, cooked	4 oz	135	4.0	26.8	2	1.5	1.1	0.2	0	7%

Food Name	Serving Size	Calories	Prot. gms	Carbs gms	Sod. mgs	Fiber gms	Fat gms	Sat. Fat gms	Chol. mgs	% Fat Cal.
pearl, raw	1/2 cup	378	11.0	72.9	5	8.5	4.2	0.7	0	10%
pearl, raw	1 oz	107	3.1	20.7	1	2.4	1.2	0.2	0	10%
pearl, raw, hulled (Arrowhead Mills)	1 oz	90	3.0	21.0	1	1.8	1.0	(mq)	0	9%
Proso/hog millet, whole grain	3 1/2 oz	327	9.9	72.9	1	>3.2 c	2.9	1.0	0	7%

MINCEMEAT. See under PIE FILLING.

MISO

	1 cup	567	32	77	10029	15	16.7	2.4	0	25%
barley, mugi, organic (Eden Foods)	1 tbsp	25	2	3	760	1	1.0	0.0	0	31%
barley, pasteurized (Westbrae)	1 tsp	12	1	2	310	0	0.0	0.0	0	0%
brown rice, genmai, organic (Eden Foods)	1 tbsp	25	2	3	810	1	1.0	0.0	0	31%
brown rice, pasteurized (Westbrae)	1 tsp	10	1	2	360	0	0.0	0.0	0	0%
hacho (Westbrae)	1 tsp	14	1	1	240	0	0.0	0.0	0	0%
hacho, organic (Eden Foods)	1 tbsp	35	3	2	600	1	1.5	0.0	0	40%
red, instant (Westbrae)	.35 oz	35	3	3	750	0	1.0	0.0	0	27%
red, pasteurized (Westbrae)	1 tsp	10	1	1	375	0	0.0	0.0	0	0%
rice, kome, organic (Eden Foods)	1 tbsp	25	2	3	850	1	1.0	0.0	0	31%
rice, sweet white shiro, organic (Eden Foods)	1 tbsp	35	2	5	410	1	1.0	0.0	0	24%
soy and rice, red, kome, organic (Eden Foods)	1 tbsp	25	2	3	850	0	1.0	0.0	0	31%
soy, hacho, organic (Eden Foods)	1 tbsp	35	3	2	600	0	2.0	0.0	0	47%
soy, pasteurized (Westbrae)	1 tsp	12	1	1	265	0	0.0	0.0	0	0%
white, instant (Westbrae)	.35 oz	35	2	4	740	0	1.0	0.0	0	27%

MOLASSES

	1 cup	872	0	226	121	0	0.3	0.1	0	0%
	1 tbsp	53	0	14	7	0	0.0	0.0	0	0%
bead (LaChoy)	1/2 tsp	7	1	2	1	0	1.0	0.0	0	43%
blackstrap	1 cup	771	0	199	180	0	0.0	0.0	0	0%
blackstrap	1 tbsp	47	0	12	11	0	0.0	0.0	0	0%
dark (Br'er Rabbit)	1 oz	110	0	28	20	0	0.0	0.0	0	0%
gold (Grandma's)	1 tbsp	70	0	17	28	0	0.0	0.0	0	0%
gold, mild flavor (Grandma's)	1 tbsp	70	0	17	28	0	0.0	0.0	0	0%
green, robust flavor (Grandma's)	1 tbsp	70	0	16	57	0	0.0	0.0	0	0%
light (Br'er Rabbit)	1 oz	110	0	29	15	0	0.0	0.0	0	0%

MOMBIN, YELLOW. See JOBO.

MONKFISH / angler fish / bellyfish / frogfish / goosefish / lotte / sea devil

baked, broiled, grilled, or microwaved	3 oz	82	16	0	20	0	1.7	na	27	18%
raw	3 oz	65	12	0	15	0	1.3	0.3	21	18%

MONOSODIUM GLUTAMATE

flavor enhancer, 'MSG' (Accent)	0.13 tsp	0	0	0	80	0	0.0	0.0	0	0%
flavor enhancer, 'MSG' (Tone's)	1 tsp	0	0	0	638	0	0.0	0.0	0	0%

MOOSE

raw	1 oz	29	6	0	18	0	0.2	0.1	17	7%
roasted	3 oz	114	25	0	59	0	0.8	0.2	66	7%
roasted, boneless, yield from 1 lb raw	11.9 oz	456	100	0	235	0	3.3	1.0	265	7%

MOSTACCIOLI. See under PASTA.

MOSTACCIOLI DISH/ENTRÉE. See under PASTA DISH/ENTRÉE.

MOTH BEAN. See BEAN, MOTH.

MOUNTAIN YAM. See under YAM.

MOUSSE

(Estee) orange chocolate	1/2 cup	70	3	9	50	0	3.0	1.5	0	36%
(Weight Watchers)										
chocolate	1 serving	190	6	31	150	3	5.0	1.5	5	23%
pecan praline	1 serving	170	4	31	140	0	3.5	1.0	0	18%
triple chocolate caramel	1 serving	200	5	34	120	2	4.0	1.0	5	19%
MOUSSE BAR chocolate (Weight Watchers)	1 bar	35	2	9	40	2	0.5	0.3	3	9%

Food Name	Serving Size	Calories	Prot. gms	Carbs gms	Sod. mgs	Fiber gms	Fat gms	Sat. Fat gms	Chol. mgs	% Fat Cal.
MOUSSE MIX										
(Alsa) dark chocolate.	2.5 tbsp	105	2	13	83	na	5.1	3.6	na	44%
(Jell-O)										
chocolate, 'Rich & Luscious' mix only	1 pkg	110	3	18	45	0	3.0	0.0	0	24%
chocolate, 'Rich & Luscious' prepared w/whole milk.	1/2 cup	150	5	21	75	0	6.0	0.0	10	34%
chocolate fudge, 'Rich & Luscious' prepared										
w/whole milk.	1/2 cup	140	5	20	75	0	6.0	0.0	10	35%
chocolate fudge 'Rich & Luscious' mix only.	1 pkg	110	3	18	45	0	4.0	0.0	0	30%
(Sans Sucre de Paris)										
cheesecake, w/NutraSweet, mix only	1/2 cup	60	4	7	80	0	1.5	0.5	5	23%
cheesecake, w/NutraSweet, prepared w/skim milk.	1/2 cup	73	5	10	105	0	1.5	0.5	5	18%
chocolate, w/NutraSweet, mix only	1/2 cup	55	1	6	25	0	3.0	1.0	0	49%
chocolate, w/NutraSweet, prepared w/skim milk.	1/2 cup	75	2	8	45	0	3.0	1.0	0	40%
chocolate cheesecake, w/NutraSweet, prepared										
w/skim milk.	1/2 cup	75	5	10	105	0	1.5	0.5	5	18%
chocolate cheesecake, w/NutraSweet, mix only	1/2 cup	60	4	7	80	0	1.5	0.5	5	23%
key lime, w/NutraSweet, mix only	4 oz	60	1	6	40	0	4.0	2.0	0	56%
key lime w/NutraSweet, prepared w/skim milk	4 oz	75	1	6	40	0	4.0	2.0	0	56%
lemon, w/NutraSweet, mix only.	1/2 cup	50	1	7	25	0	2.0	1.0	0	36%
lemon, w/NutraSweet, prepared w/skim milk	1/2 cup	70	2	9	45	0	2.0	1.0	0	29%
strawberry, w/NutraSweet, mix	1/2 cup	50	1	7	25	0	2.0	1.0	0	36%
strawberry, w/NutraSweet, prepared w/skim milk	1/2 cup	70	2	9	45	0	2.0	1.0	0	29%
(Weight Watchers)										
chocolate, prepared w/nonfat milk.	1/2 cup	60	3	9	45	0	3.0	0.0	0	36%
chocolate cheesecake, prepared w/nonfat milk	1/2 cup	60	4	12	75	0	2.0	0.0	0	22%
chocolate raspberry, prepared w/nonfat milk.	1/2 cup	60	3	12	75	0	3.0	0.0	0	31%
white chocolate, almond, prepared w/nonfat milk	1/2 cup	60	3	6	50	0	3.0	0.0	0	43%
MUFFIN. See also ENGLISH MUFFIN; MUFFIN MIX.										
APPLE										
(Awrey's)										
1.5 oz	1 muffin	130	2	17	210	0	6.0	1.0	20	42%
streusel, 4.2 oz, 'Grande'	1 muffin	340	6	50	540	1	13.0	2.0	35	34%
2.5 oz.	1 muffin	220	3	30	350	1	10.0	2.0	35	41%
(Muffin-A-Day) bran, 'Total Health Muffin'	1 muffin	120	7	31	140	9	0.0	0.0	0	0%
APPLE BANANA NUT										
(Awrey's) 4.2 oz, 'Grande'	1 muffin	260	3	27	160	1	16.0	2.0	40	55%
(Hostess) w/walnuts, mini	5 muffins	160	2	17	90	0	9.0	0.0	0	52%
APPLE SPICE										
(Health Valley) nonfat.	1 muffin	130	4	30	110	5	0.0	0.0	0	0%
(Healthy Choice) frozen, 2.5 oz	1 muffin	190	3	40	90	0	4.0	1.0	0	17%
(Sara Lee) frozen, 2.5 oz.	1 muffin	220	4	36	280	0	8.0	0.0	0	31%
(Weight Watchers) 'Microwave' 2.5 oz	1 muffin	160	3	29	260	0	5.0	1.0	0	26%
BANANA										
(Health Valley) nonfat.	1 muffin	130	4	29	110	5	0.0	0.0	0	0%
(Hostess) bran, low-fat.	1 serving	240	4	47	270	2	3.0	0.5	0	12%
BANANA NUT										
(Break Cake) 5 oz	1 muffin	60	1	7	45	0	3.0	0.5	10	46%
(Healthy Choice) frozen, 2.5 oz	1 muffin	180	3	32	80	0	6.0	1.0	0	28%
(Weight Watchers)	1 muffin	180	3	34	260	5	4.0	1.0	15	20%
BLUEBERRY										
(Awrey's)										
4.2 oz, 'Grande'.	1 muffin	360	5	52	480	2	14.0	2.0	35	36%
1.5 oz.	1 muffin	130	2	18	180	1	5.0	1.0	10	36%
(Break Cake) 5 oz	1 muffin	60	1	8	50	0	3.0	0.5	10	43%

Food Name	Serving Size	Calories	Prot. gms	Carbs gms	Sod. mgs	Fiber gms	Fat gms	Sat. Fat gms	Chol. mgs	% Fat Cal.
(Ener-G Foods) gluten-free	1 muffin	51	1	8	54	0	1.9	0.5	15	33%
(Entenmann's)										
	1 muffin	200	3	29	250	0	8.0	0.0	0	36%
nonfat, no cholesterol	1 muffin	120	2	26	220	1	0.0	0.0	0	0%
(Healthy Choice) frozen, 2.5 oz	1 muffin	190	3	39	110	0	4.0	1.0	0	18%
(Hostess)										
low-fat	1 serving	230	4	47	350	1	2.5	0.5	0	10%
mini, 'Breakfast Bake Shop'	5 muffins	240	3	29	180	1	13.0	2.0	40	48%
(Muffin-A-Day) bran, 'Total Health Muffin'	1 muffin	120	7	31	140	9	0.0	0.0	0	0%
(Natural Ovens) low-fat	1 muffin	160	4	32	190	2	1.0	0.0	0	6%
(Pepperidge Farm) frozen, 'Old Fashioned'	1 muffin	170	2	27	250	1	7.0	1.0	25	35%
(Sara Lee)										
frozen, 'Free & Light'	1 muffin	120	3	28	140	0	0.0	0.0	0	0%
frozen, 2.5 oz	1 muffin	200	3	34	290	0	8.0	0.0	0	33%
(Weight Watchers)	1 muffin	180	3	33	270	2	4.0	1.0	15	20%
BLUEBERRY APPLE (Health Valley) twin pack	1 muffin	140	4	32	100	5	0.0	0.0	0	0%
BRAN										
(Awrey's)										
w/raisins, 1.5 oz	1 muffin	110	2	18	170	1	4.0	1.0	15	31%
w/raisins, 2.5 oz	1 muffin	190	3	30	280	2	7.0	1.0	20	32%
w/raisins, 4.2 oz, 'Grande'	1 muffin	320	5	50	470	3	12.0	2.0	35	33%
(Pepperidge Farm) w/raisins, cholesterol-free, frozen, 'Old Fashioned	1 muffin	170	4	30	280	3	6.0	1.0	0	28%
(Sara Lee) w/raisins, 2.5 oz, frozen	1 muffin	220	4	37	400	0	7.0	0.0	0	28%
(Weight Watchers) 'Harvest Honey'	1 muffin	220	3	42	180	5	4.5	1.0	5	18%
BUTTERMILK (Ener-G Foods) gluten-free	1 muffin	195	4	30	425	4	6.9	1.7	14	32%
CARROT										
(Health Valley) nonfat, twin pack	1 muffin	130	4	30	110	5	0.0	0.0	0	0%
(Muffin-A-Day) 'Total Health Muffin'	1 muffin	120	7	31	140	9	0.0	0.0	0	0%
(Natural Ovens) low-fat	1 muffin	150	4	30	200	2	2.0	0.0	0	12%
CHEESE (Sara Lee) streusel, 2.1 oz	1 muffin	220	4	27	170	0	11.0	0.0	0	44%
CHOCOLATE CHIP										
(Sara Lee) chocolate chunk, frozen, 2.1 oz	1 muffin	220	3	33	210	0	8.0	0.0	0	33%
(Weight Watchers)	1 muffin	200	4	39	250	1	4.0	1.5	5	17%
CINNAMON (Pepperidge Farm) swirl, frozen, 'Old Fashioned'	1 muffin	190	2	30	170	1	6.0	1.0	35	30%
CORN										
(Awrey's) 1.5 oz	1 muffin	130	2	20	270	0	5.0	1.0	15	34%
(Pepperidge Farm) frozen, 'Old Fashioned'	1 muffin	180	3	27	260	2	7.0	1.0	30	34%
(Sara Lee) golden, frozen, 2.5 oz	1 muffin	250	4	31	310	0	13.0	0.0	0	46%
CRANBERRY										
(Awrey's) 1.5 oz	1 muffin	120	2	20	210	0	4.0	0.0	10	29%
(Natural Ovens) low-fat	1 muffin	140	4	26	200	2	2.0	0.0	0	13%
OAT BRAN										
(Awrey's)										
2.75 oz	1 muffin	180	5	27	330	2	7.0	1.0	0	33%
w/pineapple and raisins, 2.75 oz	1 muffin	180	5	26	320	2	6.0	1.0	0	30%
(Health Valley)										
w/almonds and dates	1 muffin	180	4	31	81	8	4.0	0.0	0	20%
w/blueberries	1 muffin	180	4	32	99	8	4.0	0.0	0	20%
w/raisins	1 muffin	180	4	31	90	8	5.0	0.0	0	24%
(Hostess)										
'Breakfast Bake Shop'	1 muffin	160	2	21	150	2	7.0	1.0	0	41%
'Snack Cake'	1 serving	160	2	21	150	1	8.0	1.0	0	44%

Food Name	Serving Size	Calories	Prot. gms	Carbs gms	Sod. mgs	Fiber gms	Fat gms	Sat. Fat gms	Chol. mgs	% Fat Cal.
w/banana and nuts, 'Breakfast Bake Shop'	1 muffin	140	2	20	160	1	5.0	1.0	0	34%
(Pepperidge Farm) w/apple, cholesterol-free, frozen, 'Old Fashioned'	1 muffin	190	3	29	200	2	7.0	1.0	0	33%
(Sara Lee)										
2.5 oz	1 muffin	210	4	35	320	0	8.0	0.0	0	32%
w/apple, 2.5 oz	1 muffin	210	4	35	320	0	8.0	0.0	0	32%
RAISIN										
(Awrey's)										
bran, 1.5 oz	1 muffin	110	2	18	170	1	4.0	1.0	15	31%
bran, 4.2 oz, 'Grande'	1 muffin	320	5	50	470	3	12.0	2.0	35	33%
(Health Valley) spice	1 muffin	140	4	32	100	5	0.0	0.0	0	0%
(Pepperidge Farm) bran, cholesterol-free, frozen, 'Old Fashioned'	1 muffin	170	4	30	280	3	6.0	1.0	0	28%
(Sara Lee) bran, 2.5 oz	1 muffin	220	4	37	400	0	7.0	0.0	0	28%
(Wonder) 'Raisin Rounds'	1 muffin	140	4	27	280	1	2.0	0.0	0	13%
RASPBERRY (Health Valley) nonfat, twin pack	1 muffin	130	4	30	110	5	0.0	0.0	0	0%
RICE BRAN										
(Ener-G Foods) gluten-free	1 serving	257	6	32	605	9	11.8	1.5	22	41%
(Health Valley) w/raisins	1 muffin	215	5	35	124	6	7.0	0.0	0	28%
SOURDOUGH (Wonder)	1 muffin	130	4	27	250	1	1.0	0.0	0	7%
MUFFIN MIX										
(Gluten-Free Pantry) gluten-free	1 serving	100	1	24	120	0	0.0	0.0	0	0%
ALMOND										
(Krusteaz) w/poppyseeds, prepared	1 muffin	167	2	30	242	na	4.0	1.1	0	21%
APPLE										
(Betty Crocker)										
cinnamon, prepared w/egg, 2% milk	1/12 pkg	120	2	18	140	0	4.0	1.0	25	31%
cinnamon, prepared w/egg white, nonfat milk	1/12 pkg	110	2	18	140	0	3.0	1.0	0	25%
streusel, Dutch, prepared w/egg, whole milk	1/12 pkg	200	3	32	240	0	7.0	0.0	0	31%
(General Mills)										
and cinnamon, prepared	1 muffin	100	1	17	130	0	3.0	0.0	0	27%
and cinnamon, prepared w/egg white, nonfat milk	1 muffin	110	2	18	140	0	3.0	0.0	0	25%
and cinnamon, prepared w/2% milk, 1 egg	1 muffin	120	2	18	140	0	4.0	0.0	25	31%
(Krusteaz) and cinnamon, prepared	1 muffin	180	3	36	340	0	3.0	1.0	4	15%
(Martha White) and cinnamon, prepared w/2% milk	1 muffin	140	2	25	250	0	3.0	0.0	2	20%
APPLESAUCE										
(Gold Medal) prepared w/egg, whole milk	1/6 pkg	160	3	26	240	0	5.0	0.0	0	28%
(Robin Hood) prepared w/egg, whole milk	1/6 pkg	160	3	26	240	0	5.0	0.0	0	28%
BANANA										
(Gold Medal) prepared w/egg, whole milk	1/12 pkg	150	3	24	240	0	5.0	0.0	0	29%
(Robin Hood) prepared w/egg, whole milk	1/12 pkg	150	3	24	240	0	5.0	0.0	0	29%
BANANA NUT										
(Betty Crocker)										
prepared w/egg, 2% milk	1/12 pkg	120	2	17	140	0	5.0	1.0	25	37%
prepared w/egg white, nonfat milk	1/12 pkg	110	2	17	140	0	4.0	1.0	0	32%
(General Mills)										
prepared	1 muffin	110	1	17	140	0	4.0	0.0	0	33%
prepared w/egg white, nonfat milk	1 muffin	120	2	18	150	0	4.0	0.0	0	31%
prepared w/2% milk, 1 egg	1 muffin	120	2	18	150	0	4.0	0.0	20	31%
(Martha White) prepared w/2% milk	1 muffin	180	3	23	240	0	8.0	0.0	35	41%
BERRY										
(General Mills)										
wild, prepared	1 muffin	100	1	18	140	0	3.0	0.0	0	26%
wild, 'Light' prepared	1 muffin	90	1	20	140	0	1.0	0.0	0	10%

Food Name	Serving Size	Calories	Prot. gms	Carbs gms	Sod. mgs	Fiber gms	Fat gms	Sat. Fat gms	Chol. mgs	% Fat Cal.
wild, 'Light' prepared w/1 egg	1 muffin	90	2	20	140	0	1.0	0.0	20	9%
wild, prepared w/2% milk, 1 egg	1 muffin	120	2	19	150	0	4.0	0.0	20	30%
wild, prepared w/egg white, skim milk	1 muffin	110	2	19	150	0	3.0	0.0	0	24%
BLACKBERRY *(Martha White)* prepared	1 muffin	140	2	25	250	0	3.0	0.0	2	20%
BLUEBERRY										
(Betty Crocker)										
streusel 'Bake Shop' prepared	1/12 pkg	210	3	31	230	0	8.0	0.0	0	35%
wild, mix only	1 serving	128	2	26	186	na	1.8	0.4	na	13%
wild, prepared w/egg, 2% milk	1/12 pkg	120	2	18	150	0	4.0	1.0	25	31%
wild, prepared w/egg white, skim milk	1/12 pkg	110	2	18	150	0	3.0	1.0	0	25%
(Duncan Hines)										
bakery style, mix only	1 muffin	180	2	32	245	0	5.0	0.0	0	25%
bakery style, prepared	1 muffin	190	2	32	250	0	6.0	0.0	0	28%
regular style, mix only	1 muffin	110	2	21	180	0	2.0	0.0	0	16%
regular style, prepared	1 muffin	120	2	21	185	0	3.0	0.0	0	23%
(General Mills)										
prepared w/egg white, nonfat milk	1 muffin	110	2	18	140	0	3.0	0.0	0	25%
prepared w/2% milk, 1 egg	1 muffin	120	2	18	140	0	4.0	0.0	20	31%
'Twice the Blueberries' prepared	1 muffin	100	1	17	130	0	3.0	0.0	0	27%
'Twice the Blueberries' prepared, cholesterol-free recipe	1 muffin	110	2	18	140	0	3.0	0.0	0	25%
'Twice the Blueberries' prepared w/2% milk, 1 egg	1 muffin	120	2	18	140	0	4.0	0.0	20	31%
(Gold Medal) imitation, mix only	1 serving	127	1	24	205	na	2.7	0.5	na	19%
(Krusteaz) prepared	1 muffin	150	3	27	260	1	4.0	1.0	27	23%
(Lovin' Lites)										
prepared w/water, 1 egg	1/12 pkg	100	2	21	160	0	1.0	0.0	20	9%
prepared w/water, 2 egg whites	1/12 pkg	100	3	21	160	0	1.0	0.0	0	9%
(Martha White)										
artificial flavor	1 serving	162	2	30	343	na	3.5	0.8	na	20%
prepared	1/6 pkg	140	2	25	260	0	3.0	0.0	3	20%
prepared w/2% milk	1 muffin	140	2	25	260	0	3.0	0.0	2	20%
(Robin Hood) 'Pouch Mix' prepared w/egg, whole milk	1/6 pkg	170	3	26	240	0	6.0	0.0	0	32%
BRAN										
(Duncan Hines) and honey, bakery style, prepared	1 muffin	200	2	32	220	0	7.0	0.0	0	32%
(Gold Medal) w/honey, prepared w/egg, whole milk	1/6 pkg	170	5	25	240	0	6.0	0.0	0	31%
(Hodgson Mill) stone ground, whole grain	1/4 cup	130	4	27	150	3	1.0	0.0	0	7%
(Krusteaz) w/honey, prepared	1 muffin	140	3	23	290	3	4.0	0.0	0	26%
(Martha White) prepared w/2% milk	1 muffin	150	3	24	330	0	5.0	0.0	35	29%
(Robin Hood) w/honey, prepared w/egg, whole milk	1/6 pkg	170	5	25	240	0	6.0	0.0	0	31%
CARAMEL										
(Gold Medal) 'Pouch Mix' prepared w/egg, whole milk	1/6 pkg	150	3	23	250	0	5.0	0.0	0	30%
(Robin Hood) 'Pouch Mix', prepared w/egg, whole milk	1/6 pkg	150	3	23	250	0	5.0	0.0	0	30%
CARROT NUT										
(Betty Crocker)										
prepared w/egg, 2% milk	1/12 pkg	150	3	22	160	0	5.0	1.0	25	31%
prepared w/egg white, nonfat milk	1/12 pkg	150	3	22	160	0	5.0	1.0	0	31%
CHOCOLATE CHIP										
(Betty Crocker)										
prepared	1/12 pkg	140	2	22	180	0	5.0	2.0	0	32%
prepared w/egg, 2% milk	1/12 pkg	150	2	22	180	0	6.0	2.0	20	36%
(Krusteaz)										
chocolate, prepared	1 muffin	200	3	36	340	0	5.0	1.0	11	22%
chocolate, prepared	1 muffin	200	3	35	340	0	5.0	1.0	11	23%
CINNAMON										
(Betty Crocker) streusel, prepared w/egg, 2% milk	1/12 pkg	200	3	27	240	0	9.0	2.0	30	40%

Food Name	Serving Size	Calories	Prot. gms	Carbs gms	Sod. mgs	Fiber gms	Fat gms	Sat. Fat gms	Chol. mgs	% Fat Cal.
(Duncan Hines)										
swirl, bakery style, mix only	1 muffin	190	2	32	240	0	6.0	0.0	0	28%
swirl, bakery style, prepared	1 muffin	200	2	32	245	0	7.0	0.0	0	32%
(General Mills)										
'Streusel' prepared	1 muffin	190	2	27	220	0	8.0	0.0	0	38%
'Streusel' prepared w/2% milk, 1 egg	1 muffin	200	3	27	240	0	9.0	0.0	25	40%
CORN										
(Arrowhead Mills) blue, prepared	1 muffin	110	4	15	0	3	4.0	0.0	0	32%
(Dromedary)										
mix only	3 1/2 tbsp	110	1	20	250	0	3.0	0.0	0	24%
prepared	1 muffin	120	3	20	270	0	4.0	0.0	0	28%
(Flako)										
mix only	1/3 cup	160	3	29	380	1	4.0	1.0	0	22%
prepared	1 muffin	116	2	20	351	1	3.3	0.6	0	26%
(Gold Medal) prepared w/egg, whole milk	1/6 pkg	130	3	24	250	0	2.0	0.0	0	14%
(Krusteaz) prepared, 1.48 oz	1 muffin	220	4	36	450	0	7.0	0.0	5	28%
(Martha White) yellow, prepared w/water	1 muffin	160	2	30	230	0	3.0	0.0	1	17%
(Robin Hood) prepared w/egg, whole milk	1/6 pkg	130	3	24	250	0	2.0	0.0	0	14%
CRANBERRY ORANGE NUT										
(Duncan Hines) bakery style, prepared	1 muffin	200	2	30	215	0	8.0	0.0	0	36%
LEMON										
(Martha White) and poppy seed, prepared w/2% milk	1 muffin	200	2	30	260	0	9.0	0.0	35	39%
OAT										
(Gold Medal) prepared w/egg & 2% milk	1/6 pkg	150	4	23	220	0	5.0	1.0	45	29%
(Robin Hood) prepared w/egg & 2% milk	1/6 pkg	150	4	23	220	0	5.0	1.0	45	29%
OAT BRAN										
(Arrowhead Mills)										
w/apple and spice, prepared	1 muffin	120	6	15	0	5	4.0	0.0	0	30%
wheat-free, prepared	1 muffin	100	5	11	0	5	5.0	0.0	0	41%
(Betty Crocker)										
prepared w/egg, 2% milk	1/8 pkg	190	4	25	240	0	8.0	2.0	35	38%
prepared w/egg white, nonfat milk	1/8 pkg	180	4	25	240	0	7.0	2.0	0	35%
w/oatmeal and raisins, prepared w/egg, 2% milk	1/12 pkg	140	3	22	125	0	4.0	1.0	25	26%
(General Mills) prepared	1 muffin	170	3	26	230	0	6.0	0.0	0	32%
prepared w/nonfat milk, egg white	1 muffin	170	4	26	260	0	6.0	0.0	0	31%
prepared w/2% milk, 1 egg	1 muffin	180	4	26	250	0	7.0	0.0	35	34%
(Hain)										
w/apple and cinnamon, prepared	1 muffin	140	4	28	200	5	3.0	0.0	0	17%
w/banana and nuts, prepared	1 muffin	140	4	26	190	4	4.0	0.0	0	23%
w/raspberry and spice, prepared	1 muffin	140	5	27	190	4	3.0	0.0	0	17%
(Krusteaz) prepared	1 muffin	190	3	33	310	4	5.0	1.0	0	24%
OATMEAL										
(Betty Crocker)										
and raisin, prepared w/egg white, nonfat milk	1/12 pkg	130	3	22	125	0	3.0	1.0	0	21%
ORANGE										
(Martha White) and berry, prepared w/2% milk	1 muffin	140	2	25	220	0	3.0	0.0	2	20%
PECAN										
(Duncan Hines) crunch, bakery style, prepared	1 muffin	220	3	27	250	0	11.0	0.0	0	45%
RASPBERRY										
(Martha White) raspberry, prepared w/2% milk	1 muffin	140	2	25	180	0	3.0	0.0	2	20%
STRAWBERRY										
(Arrowhead Mills) wheat bran, prepared	2 muffins	270	10	43	0	11	7.0	0.0	0	23%
(Betty Crocker)										
crown, prepared w/egg, 2% milk	1/10 pkg	150	2	24	170	0	5.0	2.0	25	30%
crown, prepared w/egg white, nonfat milk	1/10 pkg	140	2	24	170	0	4.0	1.0	0	26%

Food Name	Serving Size	Calories	Prot. gms	Carbs gms	Sod. mgs	Fiber gms	Fat gms	Sat. Fat gms	Chol. mgs	% Fat Cal.
(Martha White)										
prepared	1/6 pkg	140	2	25	270	0	3.0	0.0	3	20%
prepared w/2% milk........................	1 muffin	140	2	25	270	0	3.0	0.0	2	20%
WHOLE WHEAT										
(Hodgson Mill) stone ground, whole grain	1/4 cup	130	4	27	560	3	1.0	0.0	0	7%
MULBERRY										
fresh, raw	1 cup	60	2	14	14	2	0.5	0.0	0	8%
fresh, raw	10 medium	6	0	1	2	0	0.1	0.0	0	8%
MULLET, STRIPED										
baked, broiled, grilled, or microwaved................	4 oz	170	28.1	0.0	81	0	5.5	1.6	71	31%
raw	1 lb	530	87.8	0.0	294	0	17.2	5.1	224	31%
raw	3 oz	99	16.5	0.0	55	0	3.2	1.0	42	30%
MUNG BEAN. See BEAN, MUNG.										
MUNGO BEAN. See BEAN, MUNGO.										
MUSHROOM, BUTTON. See MUSHROOM, WHITE.										
MUSHROOM, CRIMINI, brown,										
Italian, fresh, raw	1 piece	3	0	1	1	0	0.0	0.0	0	4%
MUSHROOM, ENOKI										
Fresh										
raw, whole.....................................	1 large	2	0	0	0	0	0.0	0.0	0	10%
raw, whole.....................................	1 medium	1	0	0	0	0	0.0	0.0	0	10%
MUSHROOM, JAPANESE HONEY / hon shimeji										
Fresh										
(Frieda of California) trimmed	1 oz	9	1	1	0	0	0.1	0.0	0	11%
MUSHROOM, OYSTER / abalone / hiritake / shimeji / tree mushroom										
Fresh										
raw *(Frieda of California)*..........................	1 oz	7	1	1	1	0	0.1	0.0	0	11%
raw, whole....................................	1 large	55	6	9	46	4	0.8	na	0	12%
raw, whole....................................	1 small	6	1	1	5	0	0.1	na	0	12%
MUSHROOM, SHIITAKE										
Dried										
whole........................	4 medium	44	1	11	2	2	0.1	0.0	0	3%
whole........................	1 medium	11	0	3	0	0	0.0	0.0	0	3%
Fresh										
cooked, pieces	1 cup	80	2	21	6	3	0.3	0.1	0	3%
cooked, whole.....................	4 medium	40	1	10	3	2	0.2	0.0	0	3%
MUSHROOM, STRAW										
Canned										
in salt water, imported *(Orchids)*.....................	11 med pieces	16	2	2	231	2	0.0	0.0	0	0%
Oriental *(Green Giant)*..........................	2 oz	12	1	2	290	1	0.0	0.0	0	0%
pieces, drained	1 cup	58	7	8	699	5	1.2	0.2	0	18%
pieces, drained	1 med piece	2	0	0	21	0	0.0	0.0	0	18%
whole *(Green Giant)*	1/4 cup	12	1	2	290	1	0.0	0.0	0	0%
MUSHROOM, TREE. See MUSHROOM, OYSTER.										
MUSHROOM, WHITE										
Canned										
(B in B)	1/4 cup	12	1	2	240	1	0.0	0.0	0	0%
caps, drained.......................	8 caps	11	1	2	200	1	0.1	0.0	0	10%
pieces, drained	1 cup	37	3	8	663	4	0.5	0.1	0	10%
pieces, drained	1/2 cup	19	1	4	332	2	0.2	0.0	0	10%
pieces and stems *(Allens)*........................	1/2 cup	20	2	3	450	0	1.0	0.0	0	31%
pieces and stems, broiled in butter, 'BinB'										
(Green Giant)	1/2 cup	30	3	4	460	2	0.0	0.0	0	0%
sliced *(Green Giant)*	1/2 cup	30	3	4	440	2	0.0	0.0	0	0%

Food Name	Serving Size	Calories	Prot. gms	Carbs gms	Sod. mgs	Fiber gms	Fat gms	Sat. Fat gms	Chol. mgs	% Fat Cal.
sliced, broiled in butter, 'BinB' (Green Giant)	1/2 cup	30	3	4	460	2	0.0	0.0	0	0%
slices, drained	10 slices	10	1	2	170	1	0.1	0.0	0	10%
stems and pieces (Brandywine)	1/2 cup	20	2	3	400	1	0.0	0.0	0	0%
w/garlic (B in B)	1/4 cup	12	1	2	200	1	0.0	0.0	0	0%
whole, broiled in butter, 'BinB' (Green Giant)	1 can	30	3	4	460	2	0.0	0.0	0	0%
whole, drained, medium	1 mushroom	3	0	1	51	0	0.0	0.0	0	10%
whole, pieces, and stems (Green Giant)	1/4 cup	12	1	2	220	1	0.0	0.0	0	0%
Fresh										
boiled, drained, chopped	1 tbsp	3	0	1	0	0	0.0	0.0	0	15%
boiled drained, sliced	1 cup	42	3	8	3	3	0.7	0.1	0	15%
boiled, drained, sliced	1/2 cup	21	2	4	2	2	0.4	0.0	0	15%
boiled, drained, whole, medium	1 mushroom	3	0	1	0	0	0.1	0.0	0	14%
raw, pieces or slices	1 cup	18	2	3	3	1	0.2	0.0	0	11%
raw, sliced	1/2 cup	9	1	1	1	0	0.1	0.0	0	11%
raw, whole	1 cup	24	3	4	4	1	0.3	0.0	0	11%
raw, whole, medium	1 mushroom	5	1	1	1	0	0.1	0.0	0	11%
Frozen										
(Freshlike)	3.5 oz	30	3	4	15	0	0.0	0.0	0	0%
(Veg-All)	3.5 oz	30	3	4	15	0	0.0	0.0	0	0%
whole, 'Deluxe' (Birds Eye)	2.6 oz	20	2	4	0	2	0.0	0.0	0	0%
MUSHROOM DISH/ENTRÉE										
(Empire Kosher) breaded, frozen	7 mushrooms	90	4	16	390	1	1.0	0.0	0	10%
(Gardenburger) patty, savory, vegetarian, 'Gourmet'	2.5 oz	120	6	18	270	4	3.0	1.8	9	22%
(Green Giant) creamy, 'Right for Lunch'	9.5 oz	220	6	29	860	4	11.0	6.0	25	41%
(Stilwell)										
battered, 'Quick Krisp'	5 pieces	90	3	13	190	2	2.5	0.5	0	26%
breaded	6 pieces	90	4	17	250	1	0.0	0.0	0	0%
MUSKMELON. See MELON, CANTALOUPE.										
MUSKRAT										
raw	1 oz	46	6	0	23	0	2.3	na	na	45%
roasted	3 oz	199	26	0	81	0	10.0	na	103	45%
roasted, boneless, yield from 1 lb raw	11 oz	732	94	0	297	0	36.7	na	379	45%
MUSSEL, BLUE										
boiled, poached, or steamed	3 oz	146	20	6	314	0	3.8	0.7	48	23%
raw	1 cup	129	18	6	429	0	3.4	0.6	42	23%
raw	3 oz	73	10	3	243	0	1.9	0.4	24	23%
raw, large	1 mussel	17	2	1	57	0	0.4	0.1	6	23%
raw, medium	1 mussel	14	2	1	46	0	0.4	0.1	4	23%
raw, small	1 mussel	9	1	0	29	0	0.2	0.0	3	23%
raw, w/o shell	1 oz	24	3	1	81	0	0.6	0.1	8	23%
MUSTARD, DRY										
(Spice Islands)	1 tsp	9	1	0	1	0	0.6	0.0	0	63%
ground (Durkee)	1 tsp	19	0	0	0	0	0.1	0.0	0	100%
ground (Eden Foods)	1 tsp	0	0	1	65	0	0.0	0.0	0	0%
ground (Laurel Leaf)	1 tsp	19	0	0	0	0	0.1	0.0	0	100%
MUSTARD, PREPARED										
yellow	1 cup	165	10	19	2800	8	7.8	0.4	0	39%
yellow	1 tsp	3	0	0	56	0	0.2	0.0	0	40%
(Dietsource) lower calorie, low sodium	1 serving	15	0	1	na	na	1.0	na	na	69%
(Featherweight)	1 tsp	5	0	0	0	0	0.0	0.0	0	0%
(French's)										
'Bold'n Spicy'	1 tsp	5	0	0	80	0	0.0	0.0	0	0%
Dijon	1 tsp	10	0	0	115	0	0.5	0.0	0	100%
horseradish	1 tsp	0	0	0	85	0	0.0	0.0	0	0%

Food Name	Serving Size	Calories	Prot. gms	Carbs gms	Sod. mgs	Fiber gms	Fat gms	Sat. Fat gms	Chol. mgs	% Fat Cal.
Medford	1 tbsp	16	1	1	240	0	1.0	0.0	0	53%
w/onion	1 tsp	8	0	2	70	0	0.0	0.0	0	0%
yellow	1 tsp	0	0	0	55	0	0.0	0.0	0	0%
(Great Impressions) jalapeño	2 tsp	7	0	1	173	0	0.3	0.0	0	38%
(Grey Poupon)										
Dijon	1 tsp	6	0	1	28	0	0.4	0.0	0	50%
Dijon, country	1 tsp	6	0	0	120	0	0.0	0.0	0	0%
Parisian	1 tsp	6	0	0	55	0	0.0	0.0	0	0%
(Gulden's)										
hot, 'Diablo'	.25 oz	8	0	0	55	0	0.0	0.0	0	0%
mild, yellow, creamy	.25 oz	6	0	0	60	0	0.0	0.0	0	0%
spicy, brown	.25 oz	8	0	0	45	0	0.0	0.0	0	0%
(Hain)										
stone ground	1 tbsp	14	1	1	185	0	1.0	0.0	0	53%
stone ground, no salt added	1 tbsp	14	1	1	10	0	1.0	0.0	0	53%
(Heinz)										
mild, yellow	1 tbsp	8	1	1	175	0	1.0	1.0	0	53%
spicy, brown	1 tbsp	14	1	1	115	0	1.0	0.0	0	53%
yellow	1 tsp	3	0	0	55	0	0.2	0.0	0	53%
(Kraft)										
horseradish	1 tbsp	14	1	1	135	0	1.0	0.0	0	53%
'Pure'	1 tbsp	11	0	1	160	0	1.0	0.0	0	69%
(Westbrae)										
Dijon	1 tbsp	16	1	1	195	0	1.0	0.0	0	53%
'Mt. Fuji'	1 tbsp	16	1	1	195	0	1.0	0.0	0	53%
stone ground, no salt	1 tbsp	16	1	1	195	0	1.0	0.0	0	53%
yellow	1 tbsp	16	1	1	195	0	1.0	0.0	0	53%
MUSTARD BLEND										
(Best Foods/Hellmann's) blend, 'Creamy Dijonniase'	1 tsp	10	0	1	60	0	1.0	0.0	0	69%
(Luzianne) 'Creole' yellow and brown	1 tbsp	10	1	2	320	na	0.0	na	na	0%
MUSTARD FLOUR. See under FLOUR.										
MUSTARD GREENS										
Fresh										
boiled, drained, chopped	1 cup	21	3	3	22	3	0.3	0.0	0	13%
raw, chopped	1 cup	15	2	3	14	2	0.1	0.0	0	6%
Canned, chopped (Allens)	1/2 cup	20	1	2	35	0	1.0	0.0	0	43%
Frozen										
(Frosty Acres)	3.3 oz	20	2	3	20	1	0.0	0.0	0	0%
chopped (Flav-R-Pac)	1/3 cup	25	2	2	15	2	0.0	0.0	0	0%
chopped (Seabrook)	3.3 oz	20	2	3	20	1	0.0	0.0	0	0%
chopped (Southern)	3.5 oz	25	3	4	40	0	0.3	0.0	0	10%
chopped, unprepared	1 cup	29	4	5	42	5	0.4	0.0	0	11%
unprepared	10-oz pkg	57	7	10	82	9	0.8	0.0	0	11%
w/o salt, chopped, drained	1 cup	29	3	5	38	4	0.4	0.0	0	11%
w/o salt, drained	10-oz pkg	40	5	7	53	6	0.5	0.0	0	11%
w/salt, chopped or diced, drained	1/2 cup	14	2	2	196	2	0.2	0.0	0	11%
w/salt, drained	10-oz pkg	40	5	7	553	6	0.5	0.0	0	11%
MUSTARD OIL										
	1 cup	1927	0	0	0	0	218.0	25.2	na	100%
	1 tbsp	124	0	0	0	0	14.0	1.6	na	100%
MUSTARD SEED										
(McCormick/Schilling)	1 tsp	17	1	1	0	0	0.8	0.0	0	53%
yellow	1 tbsp	53	3	4	1	2	3.2	0.2	0	51%
yellow	1 tsp	15	1	1	0	0	0.9	0.0	0	51%

Food Name	Serving Size	Calories	Prot. gms	Carbs gms	Sod. mgs	Fiber gms	Fat gms	Sat. Fat gms	Chol. mgs	% Fat Cal.
MUSTARD SPINACH / tendergreen										
boiled, drained, chopped	1 cup	29	3	5	25	4	0.4	na	0	10%
raw, chopped	1 cup	33	3	6	32	4	0.5	0.0	0	11%
MUTTON TALLOW										
	1 cup	1849	0	0	0	0	205.0	97.0	209	100%
	1 tbsp	115	0	0	0	0	12.8	6.1	13	100%
MUTTONFISH. See OCEAN POUT.										

N

Food Name	Serving Size	Calories	Prot. gms	Carbs gms	Sod. mgs	Fiber gms	Fat gms	Sat. Fat gms	Chol. mgs	% Fat Cal.
NACHO CHIPS. See under CORN CHIPS AND SNACKS.										
NACHO SEASONING. See under SEASONING MIX.										
NAPA. See BOK CHOY.										
NAPOLES										
cooked	1 med pad	4	0	1	6	1	0.0	0.0	0	3%
cooked, sliced	1 cup	22	2	5	30	3	0.1	0.0	0	3%
raw, sliced	1 cup	14	1	3	19	2	0.1	0.0	0	6%
NATAL PLUM. See CARISSA.										
NATTO. See SOYBEAN, FERMENTED.										
NAVY BEAN. See BEAN, NAVY.										
NECTAR. See under FRUIT DRINK.										
NECTARINE										
Fresh										
raw, pitted	1 oz	14	0.3	3.3	tr	.5	0.1	na	0	6%
raw, sliced	1 cup	68	1.3	16.3	0	2.2	0.6	na	0	7%
raw, trimmed, whole, approx 2.5 inch diam	1 nectarine	67	1.3	16.0	0	2.2	0.6	na	0	7%
raw, untrimmed (Dole)	1 medium	70	1.0	16.0	0	3.0	1.0	na	na	12%
raw, whole	1 lb	204	3.9	48.6	1	6.6	1.9	na	0	8%
NEW ZEALAND SPINACH. See SPINACH, NEW ZEALAND.										
NONDAIRY DESSERT, FROZEN. See ICE CREAM SUBSTITUTE; ICE CREAM SUBSTITUTE BAR/DESSERT.										
NONDAIRY DESSERT MIX. See ICE CREAM SUBSTITUTE MIX.										
NOODLE. See also PASTA.										
CELLOPHANE. See under NOODLE, CHINESE.										
CHINESE										
cellophane/long rice, mung bean, dry	1 cup	491	0	121	14	1	0.1	0.0	0	0%
chow mein	1 cup	237	4	26	198	2	13.8	2.0	0	49%
chow mein	1.5 oz	227	4	25	189	2	13.2	1.9	0	49%
rice, cooked	1 cup	192	2	44	33	2	0.4	0.0	0	2%
(China Boy) chow mein	1/2 cup	130	3	16	110	1	5.0	0.1	0	37%
(Chun King)										
chow mein, w/almonds	1/3 cup	140	4	15	380	1	7.0	1.5	0	45%
chow mein, w/sesame bits	1/3 cup	140	3	16	460	1	7.0	1.0	0	45%
(La Choy)										
chow mein, food service product	1/2 cup	140	4	17	209	2	6.1	1.3	0	39%
chow mein, wide, crispy	1 cup	296	5	32	578	2	16.5	3.3	0	50%
rice, canned	1 cup	242	5	43	756	1	6.1	1.2	0	22%
rice, food service product	1/2 cup	122	2	22	362	0	3.1	0.4	0	22%
CHOW MEIN. See under NOODLE, CHINESE.										
EGG										
enriched, cooked	1 cup	213	8	40	11	2	2.4	0.5	53	9%
enriched, dry	1 cup	145	5	27	8	1	1.6	0.3	36	9%

Food Name	Serving Size	Calories	Prot. gms	Carbs gms	Sod. mgs	Fiber gms	Fat gms	Sat. Fat gms	Chol. mgs	% Fat Cal.
enriched, dry	2 oz	217	8	41	12	2	2.4	0.5	54	9%
spinach, enriched, cooked	1 cup	211	8	39	19	4	2.5	0.6	53	10%
spinach, enriched, dry	1 cup	145	6	27	27	3	1.7	0.4	36	10%
spinach, enriched, dry	2 oz	218	8	40	41	4	2.6	0.6	54	10%
unenriched, dry	1 cup	145	5	27	8	1	1.6	0.3	36	9%
(American Beauty)										
extra wide, enriched, dry	2 oz	220	8	42	15	0	3.0	0.0	55	12%
fine, enriched, dry	2 oz	220	8	42	15	0	3.0	0.0	55	12%
medium, enriched, dry	2 oz	220	8	42	15	0	3.0	0.0	55	12%
wide, enriched, dry	2 oz	220	8	42	15	0	3.0	0.0	55	12%
(Borden) kluski, enriched, dry	1 cup	220	8	40	210	1	3.0	1.0	55	12%
(Creamette)										
plain, enriched, dry	2 oz	221	8	40	3	1	2.5	0.8	70	10%
w/pasteurized eggs, wide, 'Fancy' dry	2 oz	220	8	40	20	0	3.0	0.0	70	12%
(De Boles)										
Jerusalem artichoke, dry	2 oz	210	7	41	0	1	1.0	0.0	0	4%
Jerusalem artichoke, garlic and parsley, dry	2 oz	210	7	41	5	2	1.0	0.0	0	4%
(De Cecco) spinach, dry	2 oz	210	7	41	35	0	1.0	0.0	0	4%
(Eden Foods)										
bifun, rice	2 oz	200	5	44	5	0	0.5	0.0	0	2%
fine, dry, 'Herb's'	2 oz	220	10	42	5	2	2.0	0.0	60	8%
kluski, medium, dry, 'Herb's'	2 oz	220	10	42	5	2	2.0	0.0	60	8%
kluski, wide, dry, 'Herb's'	2 oz	220	10	42	5	2	2.0	0.0	60	8%
medium, dry, 'Herb's'	2 oz	220	10	42	5	2	2.0	0.0	60	8%
(Gioia) plain, dry	2 oz	220	8	40	0	0	3.0	0.0	0	12%
(Golden Grain) plain, dry	2 oz	210	8	39	10	2	2.2	0.8	65	9%
(Goodman's) plain, 'Country Style' dry	2 oz	220	8	40	15	0	3.0	0.0	0	12%
(Hodgson Mill)										
spinach, whole wheat, dry	2 oz	190	10	32	45	5	2.0	1.0	30	10%
vegetable, dry	2 oz	200	9	37	25	2	2.0	1.0	35	9%
whole wheat, wide, dry	2 oz	190	10	34	20	4	2.0	1.0	30	9%
(Hospitality) wide, enriched, 'Valu Pack' dry	1 1/4 cup	235	9	43	5	2	2.5	0.5	80	10%
(Mrs. Grass) plain, dry	2 oz	220	8	40	200	0	3.0	0.0	0	12%
(Mueller's)										
kluski, dry	2 oz	220	8	38	10	1	3.0	0.5	65	13%
plain, dry	2 oz	220	8	40	10	0	3.0	0.0	55	12%
(No Yolks) no egg yolks, broad, dry	2 oz	200	8	40	25	0	1.0	0.0	0	4%
(P&R) plain, dry	2 oz	220	8	42	15	0	3.0	0.0	0	12%
(Prince) plain, dry	2 oz	210	8	40	35	0	2.0	0.0	65	9%
(Reames) homestyle, frozen	1/2 cup	170	4	32	10	1	2.0	0.5	85	11%
(Ronzoni)										
very low-sodium, dry, 'Egg Pastina'	2 oz	220	8	42	15	0	3.0	0.0	65	12%
wide, enriched, 'Country Kitchen Style' dry	2 oz	220	8	42	15	0	3.0	0.0	65	12%
(San Giorgio) plain, dry	2 oz	220	8	42	15	0	3.0	0.0	0	12%
JAPANESE										
soba, cooked	1 cup	113	6	24	68	na	0.1	0.0	0	1%
soba, dry	2 oz	192	8	43	451	na	0.4	0.1	0	2%
somen, cooked	1 cup	231	7	48	283	na	0.3	0.0	0	1%
somen, dry	2 oz	203	6	42	1049	2	0.5	0.1	0	2%
(Eden Foods)										
harusame, mung bean, dry	2 oz	190	0	47	5	0	0.0	0.0	0	0%
jinenjo soba, wild yam, dry	2 oz	190	9	37	510	2	0.5	0.0	0	2%
kuzu and sweet potato, dry	2 oz	190	0	47	0	0	0.0	0.0	0	0%
soba, 40% buckwheat	2 oz	190	8	37	490	3	1.0	0.0	0	5%

Food Name	Serving Size	Calories	Prot. gms	Carbs gms	Sod. mgs	Fiber gms	Fat gms	Sat. Fat gms	Chol. mgs	% Fat Cal.
soba, buckwheat, 100% buckwheat, dry	2 oz	200	5	41	30	3	1.5	0.0	0	7%
soba, lotus root	2 oz	190	9	37	470	4	1.0	0.0	0	5%
soba, mugwort	2 oz	190	8	37	550	2	0.5	0.0	0	2%
soba, traditional	2 oz	190	8	37	490	3	1.0	0.0	0	5%
soba, wild yam	2 oz	190	9	37	510	2	0.5	0.0	0	2%
udon, brown rice	2 oz	190	8	38	510	2	1.0	0.0	0	5%
(Westbrae)										
buckwheat, dry	2 oz	190	7	40	5	0	2.0	0.0	0	9%
genmai, dry	2 oz	200	5	41	411	0	1.0	0.0	0	5%
somen, whole wheat, dry	2 oz	200	7	41	375	0	1.0	0.0	0	4%
traditional, dry	2 oz	190	7	41	198	0	2.0	0.0	0	9%
udon, whole wheat, organic, dry	2 oz	200	7	41	375	0	1.0	0.0	0	4%

SOBA. See under NOODLE, JAPANESE.
UDON. See under NOODLE, JAPANESE.

NOODLE DISH/ENTRÉE See also PASTA DISH/ENTRÉE.

Food Name	Serving Size	Calories	Prot. gms	Carbs gms	Sod. mgs	Fiber gms	Fat gms	Sat. Fat gms	Chol. mgs	% Fat Cal.
(Banquet)										
and julienne beef, w/sauce, frozen, 'Family Entrées'	7 oz	170	12	22	0	0	3.0	0.0	0	17%
w/beef gravy, frozen, 'Family Entrées'	8 oz	200	13	22	0	0	7.0	0.0	0	31%
w/chicken, frozen	10 oz	350	10	42	460	0	15.0	0.0	45	39%
w/chicken, frozen, 'Family Favorites'	10 oz	340	11	42	455	0	15.0	0.0	45	39%
(Dinty Moore)										
and chicken, packaged, 'American Classics'	10 oz	230	17	24	1020	0	7.0	3.0	65	28%
tuna noodle casserole, packaged, 'American Classics'	10 oz	240	16	28	1280	0	7.0	4.0	65	26%
(Heinz)										
and chicken, canned	7.5 oz	160	6	19	930	0	7.0	0.0	0	39%
w/beef, in sauce, canned	7.5 oz	170	8	17	825	0	8.0	0.0	0	42%
w/tuna, canned	7.5 oz	170	11	20	950	0	5.0	0.0	0	27%
(Hormel) w/chicken, 'Micro-Cup'	7.5 oz	180	7	18	1000	0	8.0	0.0	20	42%
(Kid's Kitchen) rings and chicken, microwave cup	7.5 oz	150	11	17	840	0	4.0	0.0	25	24%
(La Choy)										
and vegetables	1 cup	131	5	27	1311	3	1.3	0.6	0	9%
chow mein, canned	1 cup	300	6	32	440	2	16.0	2.6	0	49%
w/beef, bi-pack	1 cup	148	12	24	1101	3	1.2	0.6	13	7%
w/beef, vegetables	1 cup	156	7	27	1332	3	3.5	1.5	6	19%
w/chicken, bi-pack	1 cup	161	11	23	1163	4	3.8	1.0	13	20%
w/chicken, vegetables	1 cup	163	10	24	858	1	3.3	1.3	19	18%
(Marie Callender's) w/chicken, escalloped	1 cup	420	13	44	1010	3	21.0	3.5	45	45%
(Nalley's)										
and chicken, canned	7 3/8 oz	150	9	17	1000	0	5.0	0.0	0	30%
and chicken, w/vegetables, canned	7 3/8 oz	160	10	18	1450	0	5.0	0.0	0	29%
(Stouffer's)										
Romanoff	1 entrée	490	18	48	1400	4	25.0	6.0	60	46%
Romanoff, frozen, food service product	1 oz	41	2	4	173	0	2.2	0.4	5	48%
(Swanson) w/chicken, frozen	10.5 oz	280	7	45	740	0	8.0	0.0	0	26%
(Van Camp's) w/franks, canned, 'Noodle Weenee'	1 cup	245	9	33	1245	5	8.5	0.0	0	31%
(Weight Watchers) kung pao	1 entrée	260	8	35	690	5	10.0	1.5	5	34%

NOODLE DISH/ENTRÉE MIX. See also PASTA DISH/ENTRÉE MIX.

Food Name	Serving Size	Calories	Prot. gms	Carbs gms	Sod. mgs	Fiber gms	Fat gms	Sat. Fat gms	Chol. mgs	% Fat Cal.
(Kraft)										
cheese, 'Dinner'	3/4 cup	340	10	37	670	0	17.0	4.0	50	45%
chicken flavor, 'Dinner'	3/4 cup	240	8	32	1050	0	9.0	2.0	45	34%
(Lipton)										
egg noodles Alfredo, mix only	1 cup	389	14	58	1646	na	11.0	4.3	104	25%
egg noodles Alfredo, mix only	1 pkg	518	19	77	2195	na	14.6	5.7	139	25%
egg noodles Alfredo, prepared	1 serving	259	10	39	1097	na	7.3	2.8	69	25%

Food Name	Serving Size	Calories	Prot. gms	Carbs gms	Sod. mgs	Fiber gms	Fat gms	Sat. Fat gms	Chol. mgs	% Fat Cal.
(Mountain House) w/chicken, freeze-dried, prepared	1 cup	270	10	34	201	0	10.0	0.0	0	34%
(Ultra Slim Fast) w/Alfredo sauce, prepared	8 oz	240	9	47	1110	4	4.0	0.0	0	14%

NORI. See under SEA VEGETABLE.

NORTHERN PIKE. See under PIKE.

NORWAY HADDOCK. See OCEAN PERCH, ATLANTIC.

NUT SNACK

(Fisher)

Food Name	Serving Size	Calories	Prot. gms	Carbs gms	Sod. mgs	Fiber gms	Fat gms	Sat. Fat gms	Chol. mgs	% Fat Cal.
crisp, golden, 'Nut 'N Crunchies'	1/4 cup	140	4	15	320	1	7.0	1.5	0	45%
fiesta, 'Nut 'N Crunchies'	1/4 cup	140	4	16	330	1	7.0	1.5	0	44%
honey crunch, 'Nut 'N Crunchies'	1/4 cup	140	4	17	210	1	6.0	1.0	0	39%

NUT TOPPING

(Fisher)

Food Name	Serving Size	Calories	Prot. gms	Carbs gms	Sod. mgs	Fiber gms	Fat gms	Sat. Fat gms	Chol. mgs	% Fat Cal.
fancy	1 oz	170	5	7	60	0	15.0	3.0	0	74%
oil roasted, w/peanuts	1 oz	160	6	7	115	0	14.0	2.0	0	71%
(Planters)	1 oz	180	5	6	0	0	16.0	2.0	0	77%
(Smucker's)										
pecan, in syrup	2 tbsp	130	2	28	0	0	1.0	0.0	0	7%
walnut, in syrup	2 tbsp	130	2	27	0	0	1.0	0.0	0	7%

NUTMEG

Food Name	Serving Size	Calories	Prot. gms	Carbs gms	Sod. mgs	Fiber gms	Fat gms	Sat. Fat gms	Chol. mgs	% Fat Cal.
ground	1 tbsp	37	0	3	1	1	2.5	1.8	0	58%
ground	1 tsp	12	0	1	0	0	0.8	0.6	0	58%
ground *(Durkee)*	1 tsp	12	0	0	0	0	0.0	0.0	0	0%
ground *(Laurel Leaf)*	1 tsp	12	0	0	0	0	0.0	0.0	0	0%
ground *(McCormick/Schilling)*	1 tsp	11	0	1	0	0	0.8	0.0	0	57%
ground *(Spice Islands)*	1 tsp	11	0	1	1	0	0.7	0.0	0	61%

NUTMEG BUTTER OIL

Food Name	Serving Size	Calories	Prot. gms	Carbs gms	Sod. mgs	Fiber gms	Fat gms	Sat. Fat gms	Chol. mgs	% Fat Cal.
....	1 cup	1927	0	0	0	0	218.0	196.2	0	98%
....	1 tbsp	120	0	0	0	0	13.6	12.2	0	98%

NUTS, MIXED

(Eagle)

Food Name	Serving Size	Calories	Prot. gms	Carbs gms	Sod. mgs	Fiber gms	Fat gms	Sat. Fat gms	Chol. mgs	% Fat Cal.
....	1/4 cup	200	6	6	140	2	17.0	3.0	0	76%
lightly salted	1/4 cup	200	6	6	65	2	17.0	3.0	0	76%
w/o peanuts, deluxe	1/4 cup	200	5	8	130	2	14.0	3.0	0	71%
(Fisher)										
cashews, honey-glazed 'Favorites'	1/4 cup	170	6	9	110	2	13.0	2.0	0	66%
cashews, praline-glazed, 'Favorites'	1/4 cup	170	5	11	90	1	12.0	2.0	0	63%
cashews, toffee-glazed, 'Favorites'	1/4 cup	170	5	11	90	2	11.0	2.0	0	61%
cashews, tropical fruit, 'Favorites'	1/4 cup	140	4	14	90	2	8.0	1.0	0	50%
lightly salted	1/4 cup	180	6	5	50	2	16.0	2.5	0	77%
salted	1/4 cup	180	6	5	110	2	16.0	2.5	0	77%
(Flanigan Farms) natural, unsalted	1 oz	180	4	5	2	na	17.0	3.0	0	81%
(Guy's) w/peanuts	1 oz	170	8	3	140	0	14.0	0.0	0	74%
(Planters)										
cashews, almonds, and peanuts, 'Select Mix'	1 oz	170	5	7	100	0	14.0	2.0	0	72%
cashews, almonds, and pecans, 'Select Mix'	1 oz	180	4	6	85	0	16.0	2.0	0	78%
cashews, pecans, and peanuts, 'Select Mix'	1 oz	180	4	6	80	0	16.0	2.0	0	78%

Dry-roasted

Food Name	Serving Size	Calories	Prot. gms	Carbs gms	Sod. mgs	Fiber gms	Fat gms	Sat. Fat gms	Chol. mgs	% Fat Cal.
(Eden Foods) sunflower, peanuts, cashews, almonds......	1 oz	170	8	9	55	3	11.0	1.5	0	59%
(Finast)										
lightly salted	1 oz	170	6	7	0	0	15.0	2.0	0	72%
salted	1 oz	170	6	7	125	0	15.0	2.0	0	72%
salted, w/peanuts, 'No Frills'	1 oz	180	5	7	150	0	14.0	0.0	0	72%
w/peanuts, salted, 'No Frills'	1 oz	180	5	7	150	0	14.0	0.0	0	72%
(Pathmark) w/peanuts, salted, 'No Frills'	1 oz	180	6	7	220	0	14.0	2.0	0	71%

Food Name	Serving Size	Calories	Prot. gms	Carbs gms	Sod. mgs	Fiber gms	Fat gms	Sat. Fat gms	Chol. mgs	% Fat Cal.
(Planters)										
....	1 oz	160	5	7	250	0	14.0	2.0	0	72%
sesame nut mix..........	1 oz	160	5	8	330	0	12.0	3.0	0	68%
unsalted..........	1 oz	170	6	7	0	0	15.0	2.0	0	72%
Honey-roasted										
(Eagle) cashews and peanuts	1/4 cup	180	5	8	130	2	14.0	3.0	0	71%
(Fisher) cashews and peanuts..........	1/4 cup	170	6	8	110	1	13.0	2.0	0	68%
(Planters)										
....	1 oz	170	5	9	140	0	13.0	2.0	0	68%
cashews and peanuts	1 oz	170	5	9	170	0	12.0	2.0	0	66%
Oil-roasted										
(Flavor House)	1 oz	180	5	6	125	0	18.0	0.0	0	79%
(Planters)										
....	1 oz	180	5	6	110	0	16.0	2.0	0	77%
'Deluxe'	1 oz	180	4	6	110	0	17.0	3.0	0	79%
lightly salted	1 oz	180	5	6	80	0	16.0	2.0	0	77%
sesame nut mix..........	1 oz	160	5	8	200	0	13.0	2.0	0	69%
unsalted..........	1 oz	180	5	6	0	0	16.0	2.0	0	77%
(Pathmark)										
w/peanuts, salted, 'No Frills'	1 oz	180	6	5	150	0	15.0	0.0	0	75%
w/o peanuts, salted, fancy, 'No Frills'	1 oz	180	4	7	150	0	15.0	0.0	0	75%

O

Food Name	Serving Size	Calories	Prot. gms	Carbs gms	Sod. mgs	Fiber gms	Fat gms	Sat. Fat gms	Chol. mgs	% Fat Cal.
OAT. See also under CEREAL, HOT.										
....	1 cup	607	26	103	3	17	10.8	1.9	0	15%
steel cut *(Arrowhead Mills)*	2 oz	220	10	37	1	3	4.0	0.0	0	16%
OAT BRAN										
cooked..........	1 cup	88	7	25	2	6	1.9	0.4	0	18%
raw	1 cup	231	16	62	4	14	6.6	1.2	0	24%
OAT FLOUR. See under FLOUR.										
OAT MIX, gluten free *(Ener-G Foods)*	1 cup	376	10	7	276	12	7.7	1.4	0	51%
OAT VEGETABLE OIL										
....	1 cup	1927	0	0	0	0	218.0	42.8	0	100%
....	1 tbsp	120	0	0	0	0	13.6	2.7	0	100%
OCEAN CATFISH. See WOLF FISH.										
OCEAN PERCH, ATLANTIC / Norway haddock / red perch / rose perch										
Fresh										
baked, broiled, or grilled	3 oz	103	20	0	82	0	1.8	0.3	46	16%
raw	3 oz	80	16	0	64	0	1.4	0.2	36	16%
raw, boneless	1 oz	27	5	0	21	0	0.5	0.1	12	16%
Frozen										
(Booth)	4 oz	100	20	0	250	0	1.0	0.0	0	10%
fillet, light *(Van de Kamp's)*	1 piece	280	17	21	450	0	14.0	3.0	35	45%
'Fishmarket Fresh' *(Gorton's)*	5 oz	140	25	2	100	0	3.0	0.0	0	20%
natural *(Van de Kamp's)*	4 oz	130	20	0	65	0	5.0	2.0	40	36%
OCEAN POUT / muttonfish										
baked, broiled, or grilled	3 oz	87	18	0	66	0	1.0	0.3	57	10%
raw	3 oz	67	14	0	52	0	0.8	0.3	44	10%
OCEANIC BONITO. See under TUNA.										

Food Name	Serving Size	Calories	Prot. gms	Carbs gms	Sod. mgs	Fiber gms	Fat gms	Sat. Fat gms	Chol. mgs	% Fat Cal.
OCTOPUS										
common, boiled, poached, or steamed	3 oz	139	25	4	391	0	1.8	0.4	82	11%
common, raw	3 oz	70	13	2	196	0	0.9	0.2	41	11%
OHELOBERRY, RAW										
fresh, raw	1 cup	39	1	10	1	na	0.3	na	0	7%
fresh, raw	10 medium	3	0	1	0	na	0.0	na	0	7%
OKRA										
Fresh										
boiled, drained, sliced	1/2 cup	26	1	6	4	2	0.1	0.0	0	4%
boiled, drained, whole, approx 3-inch long	8 med pods	27	2	6	4	2	0.1	0.0	0	4%
raw, sliced	1 cup	33	2	8	8	3	0.1	0.0	0	3%
raw, whole, approx 3-inch long	8 med pods	31	2	7	8	3	0.1	0.0	0	3%
Frozen										
cut (Flav-R-Pac)	3/4 cup	25	2	4	15	3	0.0	0.0	0	0%
cut (Freshlike)	3.3 oz	25	1	6	5	0	0.0	0.0	0	0%
cut (Pictsweet)	3/4 cup	25	1	5	35	3	0.0	0.0	0	0%
cut (Seabrook)	3.3 oz	25	1	6	3	1	0.0	0.0	0	0%
cut (Southern)	3.5 oz	31	2	7	20	0	0.2	0.0	0	5%
cut (Veg-All)	3.3 oz	25	1	6	5	0	0.0	0.0	0	0%
drained	10-oz pkg	71	5	15	8	7	0.8	0.2	0	9%
sliced, drained	1/2 cup	26	2	5	3	3	0.3	0.1	0	9%
unprepared	10-oz pkg	85	5	19	9	6	0.7	0.2	0	7%
unprepared	3 lb pkg	408	23	90	41	30	3.4	0.9	0	7%
whole (Flav-R-Pac)	9 pieces	35	1	6	15	4	0.5	0.0	0	14%
whole (Freshlike)	3.3 oz	30	2	7	5	0	0.0	0.0	0	0%
whole (Seabrook)	3.3 oz	30	2	7	2	1	0.0	0.0	0	0%
whole (Southern)	3.5 oz	35	2	7	20	0	0.2	0.0	0	5%
whole (Veg-All)	3.3 oz	30	2	7	5	0	0.0	0.0	0	0%
whole, baby (Frosty Acres)	3.3 oz	30	2	7	2	1	0.0	0.0	0	0%
OLD-FASHIONED. See under COCKTAIL MIX.										
OLIVE										
all varieties, all sizes, pickled (S&W)	1 oz	46	0	0	215	0	5.1	0.0	0	100%
mixed sizes, chopped	1 tbsp	10	0	1	73	0	0.9	0.1	0	78%
mixed varieties, pickled, chopped (Lindsay)	1 oz	29	0	2	249	1	2.7	0.5	0	76%
mixed varieties, pickled, pitted (Vlasic)	1 oz	37	0	1	230	0	3.9	0.0	0	90%
mixed varieties, pickled, sliced (Lindsay)	1 oz	29	0	2	249	1	2.7	0.5	0	76%
salad, pickled (Progresso)	1/2 cup	120	1	1	2400	4	15.0	2.0	0	94%
whole, large	1 olive	5	0	0	38	0	0.5	0.1	0	78%
whole, small	1 olive	4	0	0	28	0	0.3	0.0	0	78%
ASCOLANO										
all sizes, pickled, pitted (Lindsay)	1 oz	23	0	2	255	1	1.9	0.3	0	69%
colossal, pickled, pitted (Lindsay)	10 olives	90	1	6	1010	3	7.7	1.3	0	70%
jumbo, pickled, pitted (Lindsay)	10 olives	66	1	5	745	2	5.7	1.0	0	70%
super colossal, pickled, pitted (Lindsay)	10 olives	122	2	9	1365	4	10.4	1.8	0	70%
BLACK										
colossal, w/pits (S&W)	1 piece	15	0	1	80	0	1.5	0.0	0	77%
extra large, pitted (S&W)	3 pieces	25	0	1	110	0	2.5	0.0	0	85%
extra large, pitted, 'Black Pearls' (Musco)	3 olives	25	0	1	95	0	2.0	0.0	0	82%
jumbo, pitted (S&W)	3 pieces	25	0	1	135	0	2.0	0.0	0	82%
medium, pitted, 'Black Pearls' (Musco)	5 olives	25	0	1	95	0	2.0	0.0	0	82%
GREEK										
all sizes, salt-cured, oil-coated, pickled, pitted	1 oz	96	0.6	2.5	932	(mq)	10.2	(mq)	0	88%
extra large, salt-cured, oil-coated, pickled, w/pits	10 olives	89	0.6	2.3	868	(mq)	9.5	(mq)	0	88%

Food Name	Serving Size	Calories	Prot. gms	Carbs gms	Sod. mgs	Fiber gms	Fat gms	Sat. Fat gms	Chol. mgs	% Fat Cal.
extra large, salt-cured, pickled, w/pits	10 olives	89	0.6	2.3	868	(mq)	9.5	(mq)	0	88%
medium, salt-cured, oil-coated, pickled, w/pits	10 olives	65	0.4	1.7	631	(mq)	6.9	(mq)	0	88%
medium, salt-cured, pickled, w/pits	10 olives	65	0.4	1.7	631	(mq)	6.9	(mq)	0	88%
GREEN										
chopped *(Early California)*	14 grams	18	0	1	110	0	2.0	0.0	0	82%
extra large, pitted *(Vlasic)*	14 grams	18	0	1	110	0	2.0	0.0	0	82%
jumbo	1 olive	7	0	0	75	0	0.6	0.1	0	71%
large, pitted *(Vlasic)*	15 grams	25	0	1	115	0	2.5	0.0	0	85%
martini, pimento stuffed *(Santa Barbara Olive Co.)*	0.5 oz	25	0	0	95	0	2.0	0.0	0	100%
medium, pitted *(Vlasic)*	14 grams	18	0	1	110	0	2.0	0.0	0	82%
pimento stuffed *(Golden Gate)*	15 grams	15	0	1	260	0	1.0	0.0	0	69%
pitted, pitted *(Vlasic)*	14 grams	18	0	1	110	0	2.0	0.0	0	82%
queen *(S&W)*	2 olives	20	0	1	220	0	2.0	0.0	0	82%
small, pitted *(Vlasic)*	14 grams	18	0	1	110	0	2.0	0.0	0	82%
Spanish, pimento stuffed *(Star)*	15 grams	15	0	1	260	0	1.0	0.0	0	69%
super colossal	1 olive	12	0	1	136	0	1.0	0.1	0	71%
w/jalapeño *(Santa Barbara Olive Co.)*	0.5 oz	25	0	0	95	0	2.0	0.0	0	100%
MANZANILLA										
all sizes, pickled, pitted *(Lindsay)*	1 oz	32	0	2	247	1	3.0	0.5	0	77%
extra large, pickled, pitted *(Lindsay)*	10 olives	63	1	4	484	2	5.9	1.1	0	77%
large, pickled, pitted *(Lindsay)*	10 olives	50	0	3	388	1	4.8	0.8	0	77%
medium, pickled, pitted *(Lindsay)*	10 olives	44	0	2	336	1	4.1	0.7	0	77%
small, pickled, pitted *(Lindsay)*	10 olives	37	0	2	283	1	3.5	0.6	0	77%
stuffed *(S&W)*	3 olives	25	0	1	240	0	2.0	0.0	0	82%
w/pimento *(S&W)*	3 olives	25	0	1	240	0	2.0	0.0	0	82%
MISSION										
all sizes, pickled, pitted *(Lindsay)*	1 oz	32	0	2	247	1	3.0	0.5	0	77%
extra large, pickled, pitted *(Lindsay)*	10 olives	63	1	4	484	2	5.9	1.1	0	77%
large, pickled, pitted *(Lindsay)*	10 olives	50	0	3	388	1	4.8	0.8	0	77%
medium, pickled, pitted *(Lindsay)*	10 olives	44	0	2	336	1	4.1	0.7	0	77%
small, pickled, pitted *(Lindsay)*	10 olives	37	0	2	283	1	3.5	0.6	0	77%
SEVILLANO										
all sizes, pickled, pitted *(Lindsay)*	1 oz	23	0	2	255	1	1.9	0.3	0	69%
colossal, pickled, pitted *(Lindsay)*	10 olives	90	1	6	1010	3	7.7	1.3	0	70%
jumbo, pickled, pitted *(Lindsay)*	10 olives	66	1	5	745	2	5.7	1.0	0	70%
super colossal, pickled, pitted *(Lindsay)*	10 olives	122	2	9	1365	4	10.4	1.8	0	70%
OLIVE APPETIZER										
(Progresso)										
	1/2 cup	180	1	6	1600	3	21.0	3.0	0	87%
'Condite'	1/2 cup	130	1	5	870	2	14.0	2.0	0	84%
OLIVE SALAD *(Progresso)* drained	2 tbsp	25	0	1	360	1	2.5	0.0	0	85%
OLIVE OIL										
salad or cooking	1 cup	1909	0	0	0	0	216.0	29.2	0	100%
salad or cooking	1 tbsp	119	0	0	0	0	13.5	1.8	0	100%
(Amore)										
'Pure'	1 tbsp	130	0	0	0	0	14.0	2.0	0	100%
extra virgin	1 tbsp	130	0	0	0	0	14.0	2.0	0	100%
(Bertolli)	1 tbsp	120	0	0	0	0	14.0	0.0	0	100%
(Filippo Berio)	1 tbsp	120	0	0	0	0	14.0	2.0	0	100%
(Hain)	1 tbsp	120	0	0	0	0	14.0	2.0	0	100%
(Pope) Italian, cold press, no salt	1 tbsp	120	0	0	0	0	14.0	2.0	0	100%
(Progresso)										
'Riviera Blend'	1 tbsp	120	0	0	0	0	14.0	2.0	0	100%

Food Name	Serving Size	Calories	Prot. gms	Carbs gms	Sod. mgs	Fiber gms	Fat gms	Sat. Fat gms	Chol. mgs	% Fat Cal.
extra mild	1 tbsp	120	0	0	0	0	14.0	2.0	0	100%
extra virgin	1 tbsp	120	0	0	0	0	14.0	2.0	0	100%
oil cured	6 olives	80	0	3	330	1	6.0	0.5	0	82%
(Spectrum) extra virgin, pure pressed, organic	1 tbsp	120	0	0	0	0	14.0	2.0	0	100%
(Wesson)	1 tbsp	122	0	0	0	0	13.6	2.2	0	100%
ONION										
COCKTAIL										
large (S&W)	8 onions	5	0	1	300	0	0.0	0.0	0	0%
lightly spiced (Vlasic)	1 oz	4	0	1	365	0	0.0	0.0	0	0%
small (S&W)	12 onions	5	0	1	300	0	0.0	0.0	0	0%
GREEN. See SCALLION.										
RED, WHITE, OR YELLOW										
Canned										
chopped or diced, w/liquid	1/2 cup	21	1	4	416	1	0.1	0.0	0	4%
sweet (Heinz)	1 oz	40	0	9	165	0	0.0	0.0	0	0%
whole, small (Green Giant)	1/2 cup	35	1	8	410	1	0.0	0.0	0	0%
whole, small (Pathmark)	1/2 cup	35	2	7	280	0	0.0	0.0	0	0%
whole, w/liquid	1 medium	12	1	3	234	1	0.1	0.0	0	4%
Dried										
(Basic American)	1 oz	99	3	22	49	1	0.3	na	0	3%
minced, w/green onion (Lawry's)	1 tsp	7	0	2	1	1	0.2	0.0	0	18%
Fresh										
boiled, drained, chopped	1 cup	92	3	21	6	3	0.4	0.1	0	4%
boiled, drained, chopped	1 tbsp	7	0	2	0	0	0.0	0.0	0	4%
boiled, drained, chopped or diced	1/2 cup	29	1	7	13	2	0.1	0.0	0	3%
boiled, drained, chopped or diced	1 tbsp	4	0	1	2	0	0.0	0.0	0	3%
boiled, drained, whole, medium, approx 2.5-inch diam	1 onion	41	1	10	3	1	0.2	0.0	0	4%
boiled, drained, sliced, medium, 1/8 inch thick	1 slice	5	0	1	0	0	0.0	0.0	0	4%
raw, chopped	1 cup	61	2	14	5	3	0.3	0.0	0	4%
raw, chopped	1 tbsp	4	0	1	0	0	0.0	0.0	0	4%
raw, sliced	1 cup	44	1	10	3	2	0.2	0.0	0	4%
raw, sliced, medium, 1/8-inch thick	1 slice	5	0	1	0	0	0.0	0.0	0	3%
raw, whole, medium, approx 2.5-inch diam	1 onion	42	1	9	3	2	0.2	0.0	0	4%
Frozen										
chopped (Ore-Ida)	2 oz	20	0	4	10	0	1.0	0.0	0	36%
chopped (Seabrook)	1 oz	8	0	2	2	0	0.0	0.0	0	0%
diced (Flav-R-Pac)	2/3 cup	30	1	6	30	1	0.0	0.0	0	0%
diced (Freshlike)	3.3 oz	8	0	2	0	0	0.0	0.0	0	0%
diced (Veg-All)	3.3 oz	8	0	2	0	0	0.0	0.0	0	0%
unprepared	10-oz pkg	82	2	19	34	5	0.3	0.0	0	3%
whole (Freshlike)	3.3 oz	35	1	8	10	0	0.0	0.0	0	0%
whole (Veg-All)	3.3 oz	35	1	8	10	0	0.0	0.0	0	0%
whole, small (Birds Eye)	4 oz	40	1	10	10	2	0.0	0.0	0	0%
whole, small (Flav-R-Pac)	1/2 cup	25	1	7	15	2	0.0	0.0	0	0%
whole, small (Seabrook)	3.3 oz	35	1	8	9	1	0.0	0.0	0	0%
WELSH										
trimmed	1 lb	160	8.0	28.8	na	4.8	1.6	1.6	0	10%
trimmed	1 oz	10	0.5	1.8	na	0.3	0.1	0.1	0	10%
ONION DISH MIX (Vidalia Sweet) rings,										
all purpose	1/4 cup	100	3	21	690	1	na	na	na	0%
ONION FLAKES										
dehydrated	1 tbsp	17	0	4	1	0	0.0	0.0	0	1%
dehydrated	1/4 cup	49	1	12	3	1	0.1	0.0	0	1%

Food Name	Serving Size	Calories	Prot. gms	Carbs gms	Sod. mgs	Fiber gms	Fat gms	Sat. Fat gms	Chol. mgs	% Fat Cal.
minced *(Lawry's)*	1 tsp	7	0	2	1	1	0.2	0.0	0	18%
ONION POWDER										
	1 tbsp	23	1	5	3	0	0.1	0.0	0	3%
	1 tsp	7	0	2	1	0	0.0	0.0	0	3%
ground *(Durkee)*	1 tsp	8	0	0	0	0	0.0	0.0	0	0%
ground *(Laurel Leaf)*	1 tsp	8	0	0	0	0	0.0	0.0	0	0%
ground *(McCormick/Schilling)*	1 tsp	10	0	2	2	0	0.0	0.0	0	0%
ground *(Spice Islands)*	1 tsp	8	0	2	1	0	0.1	0.0	0	11%
ground *(Tone's)*	1 tsp	5	0	2	1000	0	0.1	0.0	0	10%
ONION SALT										
(Schilling) 'California blend'	1/4 tsp	0	0	0	170	0	0.0	0.0	0	0%
(Tone's)	1 tsp	1	0	0	1599	0	0.0	0.0	0	0%
ONION SNACK *(Wise)* rings	1 oz	130	1	21	360	0	5.0	0.0	0	34%
OPOSSUM										
roasted	3 oz	188	26	0	49	0	8.7	1.0	110	42%
roasted, boneless, yield from 1 lb raw	14 oz	882	120	0	231	0	40.7	4.8	515	42%
roasted, diced	1 cup	309	42.3	0.0	(mq)	0	14.3	(mq)	(mq)	43%
ORANGE										
ALL VARIETIES										
raw, peeled, sections	1 cup	85	2	21	0	4	0.2	0.0	0	2%
raw, peeled, whole, large, approx 3-1/16 inch diam	1 orange	86	2	22	0	4	0.2	0.0	0	2%
raw, peeled, whole, medium, approx 2-5/8 inch diam	1 orange	62	1	15	0	3	0.2	0.0	0	2%
raw, peeled, whole, small, approx 2-3/8 inch diam	1 orange	45	1	11	0	2	0.1	0.0	0	2%
raw, w/peel	1 cup	68	2	26	3	8	0.5	0.1	0	7%
raw, medium, w/peel, w/o seeds	1 orange	64	2	25	3	7	0.5	0.1	0	7%
CALIFORNIA										
Navel										
peeled, raw, sections, w/o membranes	1 cup	76	2	19	2	4	0.1	0.0	0	2%
peeled, raw, whole, medium, approx 2-7/8 inch diam	1 orange	64	1	16	1	3	0.1	0.0	0	2%
Valencia										
peeled, raw, sections, w/o membranes	1 cup	88	2	21	0	5	0.5	0.1	0	5%
peeled, raw, whole, medium, approx 2-5/8 inch diam	1 orange	59	1	14	0	3	0.4	0.0	0	5%
FLORIDA										
raw, whole, peeled, medium, approx 2-11/16 inch diam	1 orange	69	1	17	0	4	0.3	0.0	0	4%
raw, whole, peeled, medium, approx 2-5/8 inch diam	1 orange	65	1	16	0	3	0.3	0.0	0	4%
raw, sections, peeled, w/o membranes	1 cup	85	1	21	0	4	0.4	0.0	0	4%
ORANGE DRINK. See under FRUIT DRINK; FRUIT JUICE DRINK.										
ORANGE JUICE										
canned or boxed	1 cup	105	1	25	5	0	0.3	0.0	0	3%
fresh squeezed	1 cup	112	2	26	2	0	0.5	0.1	0	4%
fresh squeezed	1 fl oz	14	0	3	0	0	0.1	0.0	0	4%
fresh squeezed, juice from 1 med fruit	3 oz	39	1	9	1	0	0.2	0.0	0	4%
(A&P) frozen concentrate, prepared	6 fl oz	80	1	19	0	0	1.0	0.0	0	10%
(Citrus Hill)										
'Plus Calcium'	6 fl oz	90	1	20	10	0	1.0	0.0	0	10%
'Select'	6 fl oz	90	1	20	10	0	1.0	0.0	0	10%
(Crowley)	8 fl oz	110	2	26	5	0	0.0	0.0	0	0%
(Del Monte) canned or boxed, 'Unsweetened'	6 fl oz	80	1	19	10	0	0.0	0.0	0	0%
(Donald Duck)										
100% orange juice, from concentrate	8 fl oz	120	1	29	0	0	0.0	0.0	0	0%
100% pure, from concentrate	6 fl oz	90	1	22	0	0	0.0	0.0	0	0%
(Flav-R-Pac)	1 cup	120	1	29	0	0	0.0	0.0	0	0%

Food Name	Serving Size	Calories	Prot. gms	Carbs gms	Sod. mgs	Fiber gms	Fat gms	Sat. Fat gms	Chol. mgs	% Fat Cal.
(Florida's Natural)										
homestyle, Florida fruit, not from concentrate	8 fl oz	120	1	29	0	0	0.0	0.0	0	0%
(Knudsen)										
	8 fl oz	100	2	23	35	na	0.0	0.0	0	0%
float	8 fl oz	120	2	27	0	0	0.0	0.0	0	0%
(Kraft) chilled, 'Pure 100% Unsweetened'	6 fl oz	80	1	19	0	0	0.0	0.0	0	0%
(Minute Maid)										
calcium-fortified	6 fl oz	80	1	20	20	0	0.0	0.0	0	0%
calcium-fortified, frozen concentrate, prepared	6 fl oz	80	1	20	0	0	0.0	0.0	0	0%
country style	6 fl oz	80	1	20	20	0	0.0	0.0	0	0%
country style, frozen concentrate, prepared	6 fl oz	80	1	20	0	0	0.0	0.0	0	0%
premium choice	6 fl oz	90	1	21	0	0	0.0	0.0	0	0%
pulp-free	6 fl oz	80	1	20	20	0	0.0	0.0	0	0%
pulp-free, frozen concentrate, prepared	6 fl oz	80	1	20	0	0	0.0	0.0	0	0%
reduced acid, frozen concentrate, prepared	6 fl oz	80	1	20	0	0	0.0	0.0	0	0%
regular	6 fl oz	80	1	20	20	0	0.0	0.0	0	0%
regular, frozen concentrate, prepared	6 fl oz	80	1	20	0	0	0.0	0.0	0	0%
(Ocean Spray)	6 fl oz	80	0	19	15	0	0.0	0.0	0	0%
(S&W)	6 fl oz	90	1	22	0	0	0.0	0.0	0	0%
(Sippin' Pak)	8.45 fl oz	110	1	26	25	0	0.0	0.0	0	0%
(Stokely) canned or boxed, 'Unsweetened'	6 fl oz	89	1	21	5	0	1.0	0.0	0	9%
(Sunkist)										
	6 fl oz	84	1	20	2	0	0.1	0.0	0	1%
8–16 servings per pkg, frozen concentrate, prepared	6 fl oz	112	2	27	3	0	0.1	0.0	0	1%
'Fresh Squeezed'	6 fl oz	77	1	18	2	0	0.3	0.0	0	3%
(Tree Top) 100%	8 fl oz	120	0	28	24	0	0.0	0.0	0	0%
(TreeSweet)										
	6 fl oz	78	1	18	15	0	0.0	0.0	0	0%
frozen concentrate, prepared	6 fl oz	84	1	20	15	0	0.0	0.0	0	0%
(Tropicana)										
from concentrate	60 ml	110	1	27	5	1	0.0	na	na	0%
homestyle, 'Season's Best'	8 fl oz	110	1	27	5	0	0.0	na	na	0%
plus calcium, 'Pure Premium'	8 fl oz	110	2	26	0	na	0.0	0.0	0	0%
plus calcium, 'Season's Best'	8 fl oz	110	1	27	5	0	0.0	na	na	0%
plus fiber, 'Pure Premium'	8 fl oz	120	1	30	0	3	0.0	na	na	0%
plus vitamins, 'Pure Premium'	8 fl oz	110	2	26	0	na	0.0	0.0	0	0%
plus vitamins, 'Season's Best'	8 fl oz	110	1	27	5	0	0.0	na	na	0%
'Pure Premium'	8 fl oz	110	1	26	0	0	0.0	0.0	0	0%
reconstituted, 100% pure	6 fl oz	80	1	16	20	0	1.0	0.0	0	12%
(Veryfine)										
blend, '100%'	8 fl oz	120	1	30	35	0	0.0	0.0	0	0%
'100%'	8 fl oz	121	2	24	10	0	0.0	0.0	0	0%
ORANGE JUICE BLEND. See under FRUIT JUICE BLEND.										
ORANGE PEEL										
grated, raw	1 tbsp	6	0	2	0	1	0.0	0.0	0	2%
grated, raw	1 tsp	2	0	1	0	0	0.0	0.0	0	2%
ORANGE ROUGHY / slimehead										
baked, broiled, or grilled	3 oz	76	16	0	69	0	0.8	0.0	22	9%
raw	3 oz	59	12	0	54	0	0.6	0.0	17	9%
ORANGEADE. See under FRUIT DRINK.										
OREGANO										
(McCormick/Schilling)	1 tsp	6	0	1	1	1	0.0	0.0	0	0%
dried *(Golden Dipt)*	2 grams	6	0	1	88	0	0.0	0.0	0	0%
dried *(Spice Islands)*	1 tsp	6	0	1	1	0	0.1	0.0	0	16%

Food Name	Serving Size	Calories	Prot. gms	Carbs gms	Sod. mgs	Fiber gms	Fat gms	Sat. Fat gms	Chol. mgs	% Fat Cal.
dried *(Tone's)*	1 tsp	5	0	1	1	0	0.2	0.1	0	27%
ground	1 tbsp	14	0	3	1	2	0.5	0.1	0	28%
ground	1 tsp	5	0	1	0	1	0.2	0.0	0	28%
ground *(Durkee)*	1 tsp	5	0	0	0	0	0.0	0.0	0	0%
ground *(Laurel Leaf)*	1 tsp	5	0	0	0	0	0.0	0.0	0	0%
OREGANO, MEXICAN *(McCormick/Schilling)*	1 tsp	4	0	1	0	0	0.0	0.0	0	0%
ORIENTAL STYLE DINNER/ENTRÉE. See also individual listings.										
(Le Menu) Empress, w/seasoned rice, frozen,	8.25 oz	210	16	26	690	0	5.0	1.0	30	21%
(Pasta Roni) stir-fry	1 serving	131	3	17	452	1	5.4	0.5	0	38%
(Rice A Roni) stir-fry, 'Fast Cook'	2.5 oz	164	3	24	525	1	5.6	1.1	0	31%
ORIENTAL RADISH. See DAIKON.										
ORIENTAL SEASONING MIX. See under SEASONING MIX.										
OYSTER										
ALL SPECIES										
Canned										
(Bumble Bee)	1 cup	218	25	15	185	0	5.3	0.0	0	23%
(S&W)	2 oz	70	8	2	160	2	3.0	0.0	20	40%
'Fancy' *(S&W)*	2 oz	95	12	4	0	0	3.0	0.0	0	30%
cherrywood smoked, petite, in cottonseed oil, w/salt *(Reese)*	2 oz	110	8	6	220	0	6.0	3.5	50	49%
salt and water added, whole *(Crown Prince)*	3 pieces	70	7	4	150	0	3.0	2.0	35	38%
smoked *(S&W)*	2 oz	100	10	6	210	4	6.0	2.0	40	46%
smoked, whole, in cottonseed oil *(Crown Prince)*	1 can	170	14	8	280	1	9.0	4.0	20	48%
EASTERN										
Canned										
	3 oz	59	6	3	95	0	2.1	0.5	47	32%
	1 medium	6	1	0	9	0	0.2	0.1	4	32%
drained	1 oz	16	2	1	26	0	0.6	0.1	13	32%
drained	1 cup	112	11	6	181	0	4.0	1.0	89	32%
w/liquid	12 oz	188	19	11	305	0	6.7	1.7	150	32%
w/liquid	1 cup	171	18	10	278	0	6.1	1.6	136	32%
Fresh										
breaded and fried	3 oz	167	7	10	354	na	10.7	2.7	69	58%
breaded and fried	6 medium	173	8	10	367	na	11.1	2.8	71	58%
farmed, cooked	3 oz	67	6	6	139	0	1.8	0.6	32	24%
farmed, cooked	6 medium	47	4	4	96	0	1.3	0.4	22	24%
farmed, raw	3 oz	50	4	5	151	0	1.3	0.4	21	24%
farmed, raw	6 medium	50	4	5	150	0	1.3	0.4	21	24%
wild, cooked, dry heat	3 oz	61	7	4	207	0	1.6	0.5	42	24%
wild, cooked, dry heat	6 medium	42	5	3	144	0	1.1	0.3	29	24%
wild, cooked, moist heat	3 oz	116	12	7	359	0	4.2	1.3	89	32%
wild, cooked, moist heat	6 medium	58	6	3	177	0	2.1	0.6	44	32%
wild, raw	1 cup	169	17	10	523	0	6.1	1.9	131	33%
wild, raw	6 medium	57	6	3	177	0	2.1	0.6	45	33%
PACIFIC										
cooked	3 oz	139	16	8	180	0	3.9	0.9	85	25%
cooked	1 medium	41	5	2	53	0	1.1	0.3	25	25%
raw	3 oz	69	8	4	90	0	2.0	0.4	43	26%
raw	1 medium	41	5	2	53	0	1.1	0.3	25	26%
OYSTER DISH/ENTRÉE										
(Campbell's) stew, canned, condensed, prepared	8 oz	70	2	5	840	0	5.0	0.0	25	62%
OYSTER MUSHROOM. See MUSHROOM, OYSTER.										
OYSTER PLANT. See SALSIFY.										

P

Food Name	Serving Size	Calories	Prot. gms	Carbs gms	Sod. mgs	Fiber gms	Fat gms	Sat. Fat gms	Chol. mgs	% Fat Cal.
PACIFIC COD. See COD, PACIFIC.										
PACIFIC MACKEREL. See MACKEREL, PACIFIC.										
PACIFIC ROCKFISH. See ROCKFISH, PACIFIC.										
PAD THAI SEASONING. See under SEASONING MIX.										
PAK-CHOI. See BOK CHOY.										
PALM, HEARTS OF										
Canned										
....	1 cup	41	4	7	622	4	0.9	0.2	0	19%
....	1 med piece	9	1	2	141	1	0.2	0.0	0	19%
Brazilian (Reese).........	1/3 cup	15	2	1	420	2	1.0	0.0	0	43%
PALM KERNEL OIL / babassu oil										
....	1 cup	1879	0	0	0	0	218.0	177.7	0	100%
....	1 tbsp	117	0	0	0	0	13.6	11.1	0	100%
....	2 tbsp	234	0	0	0	0	27.2	22.2	0	100%
PALM OIL										
....	1 cup	1909	0	0	0	0	216.0	106.5	0	100%
....	1 tbsp	120	0	0	0	0	13.6	6.7	0	100%
PANCAKE										
(Aunt Jemima)										
homestyle, frozen......	3 pancakes	210	6	40	560	2	3.5	0.5	20	15%
low-fat, frozen......	3 pancakes	150	5	30	530	8	1.5	0.0	3	9%
original, frozen, microwave......	3 pancakes	211	6	40	801	2	3.6	0.0	0	15%
(Downyflake) frozen......	3 pancakes	280	5	45	920	0	9.0	0.0	0	29%
(Krusteaz) mini, frozen, microwave......	6 pancakes	120	3	21	280	0	2.0	0.0	4	16%
(Pillsbury) original, frozen, microwave......	3 pancakes	240	6	47	550	0	4.0	0.0	0	15%
BLUEBERRY										
(Aunt Jemima) frozen......	3 pancakes	210	6	40	590	2	3.5	0.5	20	15%
(Downyflake) frozen......	3 pancakes	290	5	48	920	0	9.0	0.0	0	28%
(Krusteaz) frozen, 4.5-oz serving......	3 pancakes	280	8	49	710	0	5.0	1.3	14	16%
(Pillsbury) frozen, microwave......	3 pancakes	250	5	49	540	0	4.0	0.0	0	14%
BUTTERMILK										
(Aunt Jemima)										
frozen, microwave......	3 pancakes	210	6	40	600	2	3.5	1.0	20	15%
frozen, microwave, 'Lite'......	3 pancakes	140	7	28	660	0	3.0	0.0	0	16%
(Downyflake) frozen......	3 pancakes	280	5	45	920	0	9.0	0.0	0	29%
(Krusteaz)										
frozen, 4.75-oz serving......	3 pancakes	290	8	53	900	0	5.0	1.3	14	16%
mini, frozen, microwave......	1 serving	116	4	22	290	na	1.6	0.2	na	13%
(Pillsbury)										
frozen, microwave......	3 pancakes	260	6	51	590	0	4.0	0.0	0	14%
mini, frozen, microwave......	11 pancakes	230	5	44	550	1	4.0	1.0	10	16%
(Weight Watchers) frozen, microwave, 2.5-oz serving......	1/2 pkg	140	5	22	270	0	3.0	1.0	10	20%
WHOLE WHEAT										
(Krusteaz) whole, and honey, frozen, 4.75-oz serving......	3 pancakes	250	8	45	990	1	4.0	0.0	12	15%
(Pillsbury) harvest, frozen, microwave......	3 pancakes	240	6	48	420	0	4.0	0.0	0	14%
PANCAKE BATTER										
(Aunt Jemima)										
blueberry, frozen......	3.6 oz	204	5	39	688	2	4.0	0.7	27	17%
buttermilk, frozen......	3.6 oz	180	6	36	778	2	2.3	0.7	27	11%
plain, frozen......	3.6 oz	183	6	37	763	2	2.4	0.6	19	11%

Food Name	Serving Size	Calories	Prot. gms	Carbs gms	Sod. mgs	Fiber gms	Fat gms	Sat. Fat gms	Chol. mgs	% Fat Cal.
PANCAKE DISH/MEAL										
(Aunt Jemima)										
and sausages, frozen, 'Homestyle'	6 oz	420	12	57	1140	0	16.0	0.0	0	34%
breakfast, lite, w/lite syrup, frozen, 'Homestyle'	6 oz	260	10	53	860	0	3.0	0.0	0	10%
w/lite links, lite, frozen, 'Homestyle'	6 oz	310	14	43	970	0	10.0	0.0	0	28%
(Downyflake) and sausages, frozen	5.5 oz	430	11	47	1170	0	23.0	0.0	0	47%
(Great Starts)										
silver dollar sized, w/sausage	1 meal	340	9	36	670	1	18.0	9.0	70	47%
w/bacon	1 meal	400	12	42	1030	1	20.0	7.0	100	45%
w/sausage	1 meal	490	14	52	950	3	25.0	11.0	90	46%
(Swanson) whole wheat, w/lite links, 'Great Starts'	5.5 oz	350	15	39	600	0	16.0	0.0	0	40%
PANCAKE MIX. See also PANCAKE/WAFFLE MIX.										
(Betty Crocker) complete, mix only	1/3 cup	200	6	39	540	1	3.0	1.0	10	13%
(Gluten Free Pantry) gluten-free, mix only	1 serving	130	3	28	270	1	1.0	0.0	5	7%
(Sweet 'n Low) low-salt and -cholesterol, w/Sweet 'n Low prepared, 3-inch diam	5 pancakes	160	4	32	20	1	2.0	0.6	0	11%
BUCKWHEAT										
(Hodgson Mill) whole grain, stone ground, mix only	1/3 cup	190	5	40	560	3	1.0	0.0	0	5%
BUTTERMILK										
(Aunt Jemima) lower calorie, complete, mix only	1/3 cup	131	7	28	477	5	1.4	0.5	14	8%
(Betty Crocker) complete, mix only	1/3 cup	200	5	39	540	1	2.5	0.5	10	11%
(Hungry Jack)										
complete, mix only	1/3 cup	160	4	32	561	1	1.5	0.0	3	9%
mix only	1/3 cup	160	4	33	651	1	1.5	0.0	0	8%
(MET-RX Caffe) mix only	1/2 cup	200	12	33	590	2	3.0	3.0	0	13%
(Robin Hood) mix only	1/3 cup	180	5	31	510	1	3.0	1.0	0	16%
WHOLE WHEAT *(Hodgson Mill)* w/buttermilk, mix only	1/3 cup	120	4	28	550	4	1.0	0.0	0	7%
PANCAKE SYRUP. See under SYRUP.										
PANCAKE/WAFFLE MIX										
(Arrowhead Mills)										
'Griddle Lite' mix only	1/2 cup	260	8	50	0	0	3.0	0.0	0	10%
original style, mix only	1/4 cup	130	4	24	180	0	2.0	0.0	0	14%
(Aunt Jemima)										
'Original' prepared, 4-inch diam	3 pancakes	116	3	25	609	1	0.8	0.1	0	6%
complete, mix only	1/3 cup	165	5	34	408	1	1.7	0.4	13	9%
(Bisquick) 'Shake 'n Pour' prepared, 4-inch diam	3 pancakes	260	6	48	850	0	5.0	0.0	0	17%
(Downyflake) plain, prepared, 'Crisp & Healthy'	1 waffle	80	2	16	180	1	1.0	0.0	0	11%
(Estee) prepared, 3-inch diam	3 pancakes	100	3	21	130	0	0.0	0.0	0	0%
(Featherweight) prepared, 4-inch diam	3 pancakes	140	6	24	90	0	2.0	0.0	5	13%
(Gold Medal) 'Pouch Mix' prepared w/egg	1/8 pouch	100	3	17	280	0	2.0	0.0	0	18%
(Hungry Jack)										
'Panshakes' prepared, 4-inch diam	3 pancakes	250	7	43	880	0	6.0	0.0	0	21%
light, complete, 'Extra Lights' mix only	1/17 pkg	180	4	38	730	1	3.0	0.0	0	14%
light, complete, 'Extra Lights' prepared w/water, 4-inch diam	3 pancakes	180	4	38	730	1	3.0	0.0	0	14%
light, complete, 'Extra Lights' prepared, 4-inch diam	3 pancakes	190	4	37	700	0	2.0	0.0	0	10%
light, prepared w/3/4 cup skim milk, 2 tbsp oil, 2 egg whites, 4-inch diam	3 pancakes	170	6	28	500	1	4.0	1.0	0	21%
light, regular, 'Extra Lights' mix only	1/17 pkg	180	4	38	730	1	3.0	0.0	0	14%
light, regular, 'Extra Lights' prepared w/3/4 cup 2% milk, 2 tbsp oil, 1 egg, 4-inch diam	3 pancakes	190	5	28	490	1	6.0	1.0	55	29%
light, regular, 'Extra Lights' prepared w/nonfat milk, 2 egg whites, 4-inch diam	3 pancakes	170	6	28	500	1	4.0	1.0	0	21%

Food Name	Serving Size	Calories	Prot. gms	Carbs gms	Sod. mgs	Fiber gms	Fat gms	Sat. Fat gms	Chol. mgs	% Fat Cal.
light, regular, 'Extra Lights' prepared w/water,										
4-inch diam	3 pancakes	180	4	38	730	1	3.0	0.0	0	14%
light, regular, 'Extra Lights' prepared, 4-inch diam	3 pancakes	210	6	30	490	0	7.0	0.0	0	30%
pre-measured, mix only	1/2 pkt	200	5	38	780	1	3.5	1.0	0	15%
pre-measured, prepared w/water, 4-inch diam	3 pancakes	180	4	33	650	0	3.0	1.0	0	15%
regular, mix only	1/3 cup	150	3	32	640	1	1.5	0.0	0	9%
(Martha White)										
'FlapStax' prepared w/water	1 pancake	80	3	17	320	0	1.0	0.0	0	10%
'Light Crust' mix only	2 oz	120	4	20	290	0	3.0	0.0	25	22%
(Robin Hood) 'Pouch Mix' prepared w/egg	1/8 pouch	100	3	17	280	0	2.0	0.0	0	18%
APPLE CINNAMON										
(Bisquick) 'Shake 'n Pour 4', prepared	3 pancakes	270	6	49	870	0	5.0	0.0	0	17%
(Downyflake) 'Crisp & Healthy'	1 waffle	80	2	16	180	1	1.0	0.0	0	11%
CORN Arrowhead Mills) blue corn, mix only	1/3 cup	150	4	28	130	0	2.0	0.0	0	12%
BLUEBERRY										
(Hungry Jack)										
microwave, mix only	3/4 pkg	230	5	47	550	1	4.0	1.0	10	15%
prepared, 4-inch diam	3 pancakes	320	6	41	820	0	15.0	0.0	0	42%
wild, mix only	1/5 pkg	170	3	38	780	0	1.0	0.0	0	5%
wild, prepared w/1-1/4 cup milk, 1/4 cup oil, 1 egg,										
4-inch diam	3 pancakes	320	6	41	820	0	14.0	3.0	45	40%
(Krusteaz) imitation, prepared, 4 inch diam	3 pancakes	205	5	39	660	0	4.0	0.0	14	17%
BUCKWHEAT										
(Arrowhead Mills) mix only	1/2 cup	270	11	53	0	0	2.0	0.0	0	7%
(Aunt Jemima) mix only	1/4 cup	105	4	24	488	3	0.9	0.0	0	6%
(Don's Chuck Wagon) buckwheat, compete, mix only	1/3 cup	160	5	33	550	1	1.0	0.0	0	6%
(Krusteaz) buckwheat, prepared, 4-inch diam	3 pancakes	215	8	40	770	6	3.0	0.0	9	12%
BUTTERMILK										
(Aunt Jemima)										
complete, 'Lite' prepared, 4-inch diam	3 pancakes	130	7	25	570	0	2.0	0.0	0	12%
complete, mix only	1/3 cup	162	5	32	408	2	1.7	0.4	93	9%
original, prepared, 4-inch diam	3 pancakes	122	4	26	698	1	0.7	0.1	1	5%
(Betty Crocker)										
complete, prepared, 4-inch diam	3 pancakes	210	5	41	500	0	3.0	0.0	0	13%
original, mix only	1/2 cup	170	4	36	760	0	1.0	0.0	0	5%
original, prepared, 4-inch diam	3 pancakes	210	5	41	500	0	3.0	0.0	0	13%
original, prepared w/2/3 cup milk, 1 tbsp oil, egg,										
4-inch diam	3 pancakes	280	8	39	810	0	10.0	0.0	0	32%
(Bob's Red Mill) mix only	1/2 cup	190	4	11	26	1	1.0	0.0	2	13%
(Downyflake) 'Jumbo'	2 waffles	170	4	30	630	0	4.0	1.0	0	21%
(Health Valley) 'Biscuit & Pancake' mix only	1 oz	100	4	20	170	3	1.0	0.0	0	9%
(Hungry Jack) complete, mix only	1/17 pkg	180	5	38	720	1	1.0	0.0	5	5%
complete, packets, prepared, 4-inch diam	3 pancakes	180	4	35	680	0	3.0	0.0	0	15%
complete, prepared, 4-inch diam	3 pancakes	180	4	39	710	0	1.0	0.0	0	5%
complete, prepared w/water, 4-inch diam	3 pancakes	180	5	38	720	1	1.0	1.0	5	5%
microwave, mix ony	3/4 pkg	260	5	51	590	1	4.0	1.0	10	14%
original, mix only	1/25 pkg	120	3	26	530	1	0.0	0.0	0	0%
original, prepared, 4-inch diam	3 pancakes	240	7	29	570	0	11.0	0.0	0	41%
original, prepared w/2/3 cup 2% milk, 2 tbsp oil,										
1 egg, 4-inch diam	3 pancakes	210	6	28	560	1	9.0	2.0	55	37%
original, prepared w/2/3 cup nonfat milk, 2 tbsp oil,										
2 egg whites, 4-inch diam	3 pancakes	200	6	28	570	1	7.0	1.0	0	32%
(Krusteaz) prepared, 4-inch diam	3 pancakes	200	5	39	770	0	3.0	1.0	10	13%

Food Name	Serving Size	Calories	Prot. gms	Carbs gms	Sod. mgs	Fiber gms	Fat gms	Sat. Fat gms	Chol. mgs	% Fat Cal.
MULTIGRAIN (Arrowhead Mills) mix only............	1/2 cup	350	12	70	0	1	2.0	0.0	0	5%
OAT BRAN										
(Arrowhead Mills) oat bran, mix only..............	1/2 cup	200	9	64	0	2	2.0	0.0	0	6%
(Bisquick) 'Shake 'n Pour' prepared, 4-inch diam.........	3 pancakes	240	7	45	580	1	4.0	0.0	0	15%
(Hungry Jack) microwave, mix onlry	3/4 pkg	230	6	45	580	3	4.0	1.0	10	15%
(Krusteaz) 'Lite' prepared, 4-inch diam	3 pancakes	130	5	36	370	10	1.0	0.0	0	5%
WHOLE WHEAT										
(Aunt Jemima)										
mix only.................................	1/4 cup	120	6	26	519	3	0.5	0.0	0	3%
prepared, 4-inch diam....................	3 pancakes	161	7	35	892	4	1.0	0.2	0	5%
(Hungry Jack) harvest, microwave, mix only	3/4 pkg	230	6	46	560	3	4.0	1.0	10	15%
(Krusteaz) w/honey, prepared, 4-inch diam...........	3 pancakes	215	8	42	630	5	1.0	0.0	9	4%
(Stone-Buhr) mix only	1/4 cup	120	5	28	330	3	1.0	0.0	0	6%
PAPAYA										
raw, cubed......................................	1 cup	55	1	14	4	3	0.2	0.1	0	3%
raw, mashed	1 cup	90	1	23	7	4	0.3	0.1	0	3%
raw, whole, large, 5.75 inch long, 3.25 inch diam........	1 papaya	148	2	37	11	7	0.5	0.2	0	3%
raw, whole, medium, 5 1/8 inch long, 3 inch diam........	1 papaya	119	2	30	9	5	0.4	0.1	0	3%
raw, whole, small, 4.5 inch long, 2.75 inch diam........	1 papaya	59	1	15	5	3	0.2	0.1	0	3%
PAPAYA DRINK. See under FRUIT DRINK; FRUIT JUICE DRINK.										
PAPAYA JUICE (Knudsen) creamed	8 fl oz	160	0	40	40	na	0.0	0.0	0	0%
PAPRIKA										
ground..	1 tbsp	20	1	4	2	1	0.9	0.1	0	38%
ground...	1 tsp	6	0	1	1	0	0.3	0.0	0	38%
ground (Durkee)	1 tsp	8	0	0	0	0	0.0	0.0	0	0%
ground (Laurel Leaf)	1 tsp	8	0	0	0	0	0.0	0.0	0	0%
ground (McCormick/Schilling)	1 tsp	9	0	1	2	1	0.4	0.0	0	36%
ground (Spice Islands)	1 tsp	7	0	1	1	0	0.2	0.0	0	24%
PARANUT. See BRAZIL NUT.										
PARROTFISH / pollyfish										
raw	1 lb	390	87.5	0.0	(mq)	0	1.8	(mq)	(mq)	4%
raw	1 oz	24	5.5	0.0	(mq)	0	0.1	(mq)	(mq)	4%
PARSLEY										
dried	1 tbsp	4	0	1	6	0	0.1	0.0	0	14%
dried	1 tsp	1	0	0	1	0	0.0	0.0	0	13%
dried (McCormick/Schilling)	1 tsp	2	0	0	2	0	0.0	0.0	0	0%
freeze-dried...................................	1/4 cup	4	0	1	5	0	0.1	na	0	16%
freeze-dried...................................	1 tbsp	1	0	0	2	0	0.0	na	0	16%
fresh, raw	1 cup	22	2	4	34	2	0.5	0.1	0	18%
fresh, raw	10 sprigs	4	0	1	6	0	0.1	0.0	0	18%
fresh, raw	1 tbsp	1	0	0	2	0	0.0	0.0	0	18%
PARSLEY FLAKES										
(Spice Islands)	1 tsp	4	0	1	6	0	0.1	0.0	0	22%
ground (Durkee)	1 tsp	1	0	0	0	0	0.0	0.0	0	0%
ground (Laurel Leaf)	1 tsp	1	0	0	0	0	0.0	0.0	0	0%
PARSLEY ROOT / Hamburg parsley / turnip-rooted parsley										
fresh	1 lb	50	12.7	10.4	454	5.9	2.7	na	0	21%
fresh	1 oz	3	0.8	0.7	28	0.4	0.2	(tr)	0	23%
PARSLEY SEASONING. See under SEASONING MIX.										
PARSNIP										
boiled, drained, sliced..........................	1/2 cup	63	1	15	8	3	0.2	0.0	0	3%
boiled, drained, whole, approx 9 inch long	1 parsnip	130	2	31	16	6	0.5	0.1	0	3%
raw, sliced....................................	1 cup	100	2	24	13	7	0.4	0.1	0	3%

Food Name	Serving Size	Calories	Prot. gms	Carbs gms	Sod. mgs	Fiber gms	Fat gms	Sat. Fat gms	Chol. mgs	% Fat Cal.
PARTY MIX										
(Michael Season's)										
spicy, low-fat, original	1 oz	110	2	23	280	1	1.5	0.0	0	12%
traditional, low-fat	1 oz	120	3	23	320	1	1.5	0.0	0	11%
PASSIONFRUIT / granadilla										
purple, raw, sliced	1 cup	229	5	55	66	25	1.7	0.1	0	6%
purple, raw, whole, trimmed	1 fruit	17	0	4	5	2	0.1	0.0	0	6%
PASSIONFRUIT JUICE										
purple	1 cup	126	1	34	15	0	0.1	0.0	0	1%
purple	1 fl oz	16	0	4	2	0	0.0	0.0	0	1%
yellow	1 cup	148	2	36	15	0	0.4	0.0	0	3%
yellow	1 fl oz	19	0	4	2	0	0.1	0.0	0	3%
PASTA. See also NOODLE.										
(NOTE: 2 ounces uncooked pasta = approximately 1 cup cooked.)										
(Al Dente) wild mushroom, dry	2 oz	220	8	40	20	0	2.0	0.0	0	9%
(Creamette)										
dry	2 oz	210	7	42	0	0	1.0	0.0	0	4%
rainbow, dry	2 oz	210	8	42	5	1	1.0	0.0	0	4%
vegetable, dry	2 oz	210	8	42	5	1	1.0	0.0	0	4%
w/egg, dry	2 oz	221	8	40	3	1	2.5	0.8	7	10%
(De Boles)										
rainbow, dry, 'Primavera'	2 oz	200	8	41	8	0	1.0	0.0	0	4%
vegetable, dry, 'Primavera' dry	2 oz	200	8	41	8	0	1.0	0.0	0	4%
(Golden Grain) dry	2 oz	203	8	41	26	0	0.7	0.1	0	3%
(Misura) whole wheat, w/bran, dry	2 oz	197	6	40	16	0	1.0	0.0	0	5%
(Mueller's) 'Super Shapes' dry	2 oz	210	7	42	0	1	1.0	0.0	0	4%
(Pastamania!)										
beet, spinach, and tomato	2 oz	200	8	40	10	1	1.0	0.0	0	4%
oat bran, natural, gourmet, dry	2 oz	209	8	41	7	2	1.0	0.0	0	4%
(Ronzoni) dry	2 oz	210	7	41	5	0	1.0	0.0	0	4%
ACINI PEPE *(Ronzoni)* enriched, dry	2 oz	210	7	42	0	0	1.0	0.0	0	4%
AGNOLOTTI *(Contadina)* refrigerated, 'Fresh'	3 oz	270	13	38	230	0	7.0	2.0	40	24%
ANGEL HAIR										
(American Beauty) 100% durum wheat semolina, dry	2 oz	210	7	42	0	0	1.0	0.0	0	4%
(Contadina)	1 1/4 cup	240	10	43	30	2	3.0	1.0	90	11%
(Creamette) enriched, dry	2 oz	210	7	42	0	2	1.0	0.0	0	4%
(De Boles)										
Jerusalem artichoke, dry	2 oz	210	7	41	0	1	1.0	0.0	0	4%
Jerusalem artichoke, garlic and parsley, dry	2 oz	210	7	41	5	2	1.0	0.0	0	4%
Jerusalem artichoke, tomato and basil, dry	2 oz	210	7	41	0	2	1.0	0.0	0	4%
Jerusalem artichoke, tomato and lemon pepper, dry	2 oz	200	8	40	10	1	1.0	0.0	0	4%
Jerusalem artichoke, whole wheat, dry	2 oz	210	7	40	0	5	2.0	0.0	0	9%
(DiGiorno) refrigerated, uncooked	3 oz	250	11	47	140	0	3.0	0.0	0	10%
(Hodgson Mill) 100% durum whole wheat flour, dry	2 oz	190	9	34	10	6	1.0	0.0	0	5%
(Westbrae) corn, dry	2 oz	210	4	46	10	0	2.0	0.0	0	8%
BOW TIE										
(De Cecco) farfelle, enriched, dry	2 oz	210	7	41	0	0	1.0	0.0	0	4%
(Garden Time) four-color, dry	2 oz	203	8	41	1	1	1.0	0.0	0	4%
(Hodgson Mill) whole wheat, dry	2 oz	190	9	34	10	6	1.0	0.0	0	5%
(Mueller's) dry	2 oz	220	8	38	10	1	3.0	0.5	65	13%
(Pasta Perfect) dry	1 cup	140	5	26	20	3	2.0	0.4	25	13%
(Ronzoni) enriched, dry	2 oz	210	7	42	0	0	1.0	0.0	0	4%
(Westbrae) vegetable, dry	2 oz	190	9	39	10	5	2.0	0.0	0	9%

Food Name	Serving Size	Calories	Prot. gms	Carbs gms	Sod. mgs	Fiber gms	Fat gms	Sat. Fat gms	Chol. mgs	% Fat Cal.
CAPELLINI										
(American Beauty) 100% durum wheat semolina, dry	2 oz	210	7	42	0	0	1.0	0.0	0	4%
CORN (Westbrae) corn, dry	2 oz	210	4	46	10	0	2.0	0.0	0	8%
CURLS (Ancient Harvest) quinoa, wheat-free, dry	2 oz	180	5	35	5	3	2.0	0.0	0	10%
FARFALLE. See PASTA, BOW TIE.										
FETTUCCINE										
(Al Dente)										
basil, dry	2 oz	220	8	40	20	0	2.0	0.0	0	9%
curry, dry	2 oz	220	8	40	20	0	2.0	0.0	0	9%
dill, dry	2 oz	220	8	40	20	0	2.0	0.0	0	9%
spinach, dry	2 oz	220	8	40	20	0	2.0	0.0	0	9%
tarragon, dry	2 oz	220	8	40	20	0	2.0	0.0	0	9%
whole wheat, dry	2 oz	210	8	42	10	0	1.0	0.0	0	4%
(American Beauty)										
spinach and egg, enriched, dry, 'Florentine'	2 oz	220	8	42	35	0	3.0	0.0	65	12%
(Antoine's) egg, enriched, dry	2 oz	210	7	41	0	0	1.0	0.0	0	4%
(Contadina)										
	1-1/4 cup	250	10	45	30	2	3.5	1.0	85	13%
cholesterol-free	1 cup	240	9	46	16	2	3.0	0.0	0	11%
(De Boles)										
cholesterol-free, low-sodium, low-fat	2 oz	210	7	41	0	2	1.0	0.0	0	4%
Jerusalem artichoke, dry	2 oz	210	7	41	0	1	1.0	0.0	0	4%
Jerusalem artichoke, spinach, dry	2 oz	210	9	41	5	0	1.0	0.0	0	4%
Jerusalem artichoke, tomato and lemon pepper, dry	2 oz	200	6	40	10	1	1.0	0.0	0	5%
Jerusalem artichoke, tomato and pesto, dry	2 oz	210	7	41	5	2	1.0	0.0	0	4%
(De Cecco) egg, dry, 'Home-Style'	2 oz	210	8	40	35	0	3.0	0.0	0	12%
(DiGiorno)										
dry, approx 1 1/3 cups cooked	3 oz	250	11	47	140	0	3.0	0.0	0	10%
spinach, dry, approx 1 1/3 cups cooked	3 oz	250	12	46	140	0	3.0	0.0	0	10%
(Eden Foods)										
bell pepper basil, dry, 'Herb's'	2 oz	220	10	42	5	2	2.0	0.0	60	8%
parsley garlic, dry, 'Herb's'	2 oz	220	10	42	5	2	2.0	0.0	60	8%
spinach, dry, 'Herb's'	2 oz	220	10	42	5	2	2.0	0.0	60	8%
(Hodgson Mill) whole wheat, dry	2 oz	190	9	34	10	6	1.0	0.0	0	5%
(Pastamania!)										
durum wheat, dry	2 oz	200	8	38	20	1	2.0	1.0	30	9%
garlic and parsley, dry	2 oz	200	8	38	20	1	2.0	1.0	30	9%
garlic, parsley, and basil, dry	2 oz	200	8	38	20	1	2.0	1.0	30	9%
spinach and durum wheat, dry	2 oz	200	8	38	30	1	2.0	1.0	35	9%
w/lemon and pepper, dry	2 oz	220	8	40	15	2	3.0	1.0	35	12%
w/mushrooms, dry	2 oz	210	8	41	15	2	2.0	1.0	35	8%
w/Jerusalem artichoke	2 oz	210	8	41	10	2	2.0	na	na	8%
(Ronzoni) egg, extra long, enriched, dry	2 oz	220	8	42	15	0	3.0	0.0	65	12%
(Rummo) nested, dry	2 oz	210	7	41	4	0	1.0	0.0	0	4%
FUSILLI										
(Antoine's)										
rainbow, dry	2 oz	210	7	41	20	0	1.0	0.0	0	4%
tricolor, dry	2 oz	210	7	41	20	0	1.0	0.0	0	4%
tricolor, vegetable, enriched, dry	2 oz	210	7	41	25	2	1.0	0.0	0	4%
vegetable, dry	2 oz	210	7	41	20	0	1.0	0.0	0	4%
(De Cecco)										
enriched, dry	2 oz	210	7	41	0	0	1.0	0.0	0	4%
spinach, enriched, dry	2 oz	210	7	41	5	0	1.0	0.0	0	4%
(Pastamania!) tomato and spinach, tre colore, dry	2 oz	200	7	40	20	2	1.0	0.0	0	5%

Food Name	Serving Size	Calories	Prot. gms	Carbs gms	Sod. mgs	Fiber gms	Fat gms	Sat. Fat gms	Chol. mgs	% Fat Cal.
GEMELLI										
(Antoine's) macaroni, enriched, dry	2 oz	210	7	41	0	0	1.0	0.0	0	4%
LASAGNA										
(American Beauty) 100% durum wheat semolina, dry	2 oz	210	7	42	0	0	1.0	0.0	0	4%
(Bernardi)										
sheets	1 piece	250	9	47	15	2	3.0	1.0	5	11%
sheets, wavy	1 piece	310	12	60	20	2	2.5	1.0	5	7%
(Creamette) 100% semolina, enriched, dry	2 oz	210	7	42	0	0	1.0	0.0	0	4%
(De Boles)										
Jerusalem artichoke, dry	2 oz	210	7	41	0	1	1.0	0.0	0	4%
whole wheat, dry	2 oz	210	9	40	0	0	2.0	0.0	0	8%
(De Cecco) 100% semolina, dry	2 oz	210	7	41	0	0	1.0	0.0	0	4%
(Ener-G Foods) gluten-free, dry	2 oz	214	4	42	1	2	0.1	0.0	1	0%
(Health Valley)										
whole wheat, dry	2 oz	170	9	40	10	7	1.0	0.0	0	4%
whole wheat, spinach, dry	2 oz	170	9	40	15	7	1.0	0.0	0	4%
(Hodgson Mill) whole wheat, dry	2 oz	190	9	34	10	6	1.0	1.0	0	5%
(Mueller's) dry	2 oz	210	7	42	0	1	1.0	0.0	0	4%
(Ronzoni) curly edge, enriched, dry	2 oz	210	7	42	0	0	1.0	0.0	0	4%
(Westbrae)										
spinach, whole wheat, no egg, dry	2 oz	210	8	40	0	6	2.0	0.0	0	9%
whole wheat, no egg, dry	2 oz	210	8	40	0	7	2.0	0.0	0	9%
LINGUINE										
(Ancient Harvest) quinoa, wheat-free, dry	2 oz	180	5	35	5	3	2.0	0.0	0	10%
(Creamette) enriched, dry	2 oz	210	7	42	0	0	1.0	0.0	0	4%
(De Boles) Jerusalem artichoke, dry	2 oz	210	7	41	0	1	1.0	0.0	0	4%
(De Cecco) enriched, dry	2 oz	210	7	41	0	0	1.0	0.0	0	4%
(DiGiorno)										
dry, approx 1-1/3 cups cooked	3 oz	250	11	46	135	0	3.0	0.0	0	11%
refrigerated, uncooked	3 oz	250	11	47	140	0	3.0	0.0	0	10%
(Pastamania!) durum wheat, dry	2 oz	200	8	38	20	1	2.0	1.0	30	9%
(Quinoa) quinoa, wheat-free, dry	2 oz	180	5	35	5	3	2.0	0.0	0	10%
(Ronzoni) enriched, dry	2 oz	210	7	42	0	0	1.0	0.0	0	4%
MACARONI										
	2 oz	211	7	43	4	1	0.9	0.1	0	4%
elbows, enriched, cooked	1 cup	197	7	40	1	2	0.9	0.1	0	4%
elbows, enriched, dry	1 cup	390	13	78	7	3	1.7	0.2	0	4%
elbows, unenriched, cooked	1 cup	197	7	40	1	2	0.9	0.1	0	4%
elbows, unenriched, dry	1 cup	390	13	78	7	3	1.7	0.2	0	4%
elbows, whole wheat, cooked	1 cup elbows	174	7	37	4	4	0.8	0.1	0	4%
elbows, whole wheat, dry	1 cup elbows	198	8	43	5	5	0.8	0.1	0	3%
small shells, dry	1 cup	345	12	69	7	2	1.5	0.2	0	4%
spirals, enriched, cooked	1 cup	189	6	38	1	2	0.9	0.1	0	4%
spirals, enriched, dry	1 cup	312	11	63	6	2	1.3	0.2	0	4%
spirals, vegetable, enriched, dry	1 cup spirals	209	7	43	25	2	0.6	0.1	0	2%
spirals, whole wheat, dry	1 cup spirals	365	15	79	8	9	1.5	0.3	0	3%
vegetable, enriched, cooked	1 cup	172	6	36	8	6	0.1	0.0	0	1%
vegetable, enriched, dry	1 cup	308	11	63	36	4	0.9	0.1	0	2%
(American Beauty)										
elbows, 100% durum wheat semolina, dry	2 oz	210	7	42	0	0	1.0	0.0	0	4%
100% durum wheat semolina, dry, 'Curly-Roni'	2 oz	210	7	42	0	0	1.0	0.0	0	4%
(Ancient Harvest)										
elbows, quinoa, wheat-free, dry	2 oz	180	5	36	5	3	2.0	0.0	0	10%
elbows, wheat-free, gluten-free	2 oz	180	5	35	5	3	2.0	0.0	0	10%

Food Name	Serving Size	Calories	Prot. gms	Carbs gms	Sod. mgs	Fiber gms	Fat gms	Sat. Fat gms	Chol. mgs	% Fat Cal.
(Creamette) elbows, enriched, dry	2 oz	210	7	42	0	0	1.0	0.0	0	4%
(De Boles)										
elbows, corn, wheat-free, dry	2 oz	210	5	45	0	1	1.0	0.0	0	4%
elbows, dry, 'Primavera'	2 oz	210	9	41	0	0	1.0	0.0	0	4%
elbows, Jerusalem artichoke, dry	2 oz	210	7	41	0	1	1.0	0.0	0	4%
elbows, whole wheat and Jerusalem artichoke, dry	2 oz	210	7	40	0	5	2.0	0.0	0	9%
(Delmonico) dry	2 oz	210	7	42	0	0	1.0	0.0	0	4%
(Eden Foods)										
elbows, whole wheat, vegetable	2 oz	210	7	42	10	2	1.0	0.0	0	4%
elbows, whole-grain, organic, dry	2 oz	210	10	39	0	6	1.5	0.0	0	6%
(Eden Foods) elbows, whole-grain, organic, dry	2 oz	210	10	39	0	6	1.5	0.0	0	6%
(Ener-G Foods)										
brown rice, gluten-free, dry	2 oz	212	4	44	1	2	0.1	0.0	0	1%
rice, gluten-free, dry	2 oz	214	4	42	1	2	0.1	0.0	1	0%
shells, rice, gluten free, dry	2 oz	214	4	42	1	2	0.1	0.0	0	0%
(Gioia) dry	2 oz	210	7	41	0	0	1.0	0.0	0	4%
(Hodgson Mill) elbows, whole wheat, dry	2 oz	190	9	34	10	6	1.0	0.0	na	5%
(Hospitality) elbows, enriched, dry, 'Valu Pack'	1/2 cup	240	8	48	0	2	0.5	0.0	0	2%
(P&R) dry	2 oz	210	7	42	0	0	1.0	0.0	0	4%
(Prince) dry	2 oz	210	7	43	5	0	1.0	0.0	0	4%
(Quinoa) elbows, quinoa, wheat-free, dry	2 oz	180	5	36	5	3	2.0	0.0	0	10%
(Ronzoni) dry	2 oz	210	7	41	5	0	1.0	0.0	0	4%
(San Giorgio) dry, 'Italian/American Style'	2 oz	210	7	42	0	0	1.0	0.0	0	4%
(Westbrae) elbows, corn, dry	2 oz	210	4	46	10	0	2.0	0.0	0	8%
MANICOTTI (Ronzoni) extra fancy, enriched, dry	2 oz	210	7	42	0	0	1.0	0.0	0	4%
MOSTACCIOLI										
(American Beauty)										
100% durum wheat semolina, dry	2 oz	210	7	42	0	0	1.0	0.0	0	4%
tricolor, 'Italiano' dry	2 oz	210	7	42	0	0	1.0	0.0	0	4%
(Creamette) enriched, dry	2 oz	210	7	42	0	2	1.0	0.0	0	4%
(Ronzoni) enriched, dry	2 oz	210	9	40	0	2	1.0	0.0	0	4%
ORZO (Ronzoni) enriched, dry	2 oz	210	7	42	0	0	3.0	0.0	0	12%
PAGODAS										
(Ancient Harvest)										
garden	2 oz	180	5	35	5	3	2.0	0.0	0	10%
garden, gluten-free	2 oz	180	5	35	5	3	2.0	0.0	0	10%
PENNE (Hodgson Mill) whole wheat, dry	2 oz	190	9	34	10	6	1.0	0.0	0	5%
PENNE RIGATI										
(Antoine's) uncooked	2 oz	210	7	41	0	0	1.0	0.0	0	4%
(De Cecco) macaroni, enriched, dry	2 oz	210	7	41	0	0	1.0	0.0	0	4%
PENNONI (De Cecco) macaroni, enriched, dry	2 oz	210	7	41	0	0	1.0	0.0	0	4%
RADIATORE										
(Antoine's) macaroni, enriched, dry	2 oz	210	7	41	0	0	1.0	0.0	0	4%
(Hodgson Mill)										
four colors	2 oz	200	8	41	15	1	1.0	0.0	0	4%
whole wheat, dry	2 oz	190	9	34	10	6	1.0	1.0	0	5%
(Ronzoni) tomato and spinach, tri-color, macaroni, dry	2 oz	210	7	42	30	0	1.0	0.0	0	4%
RIBBON										
(Creamette)										
spinach, enriched, dry	2 oz	210	7	42	70	0	1.0	0.0	0	4%
yolk-free, dry, 'Dutch'	2 oz	210	7	42	0	0	1.0	0.0	0	4%
(De Boles) whole wheat and Jerusalem artichoke, dry	2 oz	210	7	40	0	5	2.0	0.0	0	9%
(Eden Foods)										
extra fine, organic, dry	2 oz	220	8	44	0	3	1.0	1.0	0	4%

Food Name	Serving Size	Calories	Prot. gms	Carbs gms	Sod. mgs	Fiber gms	Fat gms	Sat. Fat gms	Chol. mgs	% Fat Cal.
mixed vegetable, dry, 'Herb's'	2 oz	220	10	42	5	2	2.0	0.0	60	8%
paella, organic, dry	2 oz	220	8	44	0	3	1.0	0.0	0	4%
paella, wheat, w/saffron, organic, dry	2 oz	228	8	44	0	0	1.0	0.0	0	4%
parsley garlic, organic, dry	2 oz	220	8	44	0	3	1.0	0.0	0	4%
pesto, organic, dry	2 oz	220	8	44	0	3	1.0	0.0	0	4%
wheat, parsley garlic, organic, dry	2 oz	228	8	44	0	0	1.0	0.0	0	4%
whole grain, dry, 'Herb's' dry	2 oz	200	8	40	10	7	1.5	0.0	0	7%
whole grain, spinach, organic, dry	2 oz	200	8	40	10	7	1.5	0.0	0	7%
(Hodgson Mill) whole wheat, dry	2 oz	190	10	34	15	5	1.0	1.0	0	5%
RIGATONI										
(Creamette) enriched, dry	2 oz	210	7	42	0	0	1.0	0.0	0	4%
(De Boles)										
Jerusalem artichoke, dry	2 oz	210	7	41	0	1	1.0	0.0	0	4%
Jerusalem artichoke, dry, 'Primavera'	2 oz	210	7	41	0	1	1.0	0.0	0	4%
(De Cecco) enriched, dry	2 oz	210	7	41	0	0	1.0	0.0	0	4%
(Ronzoni) enriched, dry	2 oz	210	7	42	0	0	1.0	0.0	0	4%
ROTELLE										
(American Beauty) 100% durum wheat semolina, dry	2 oz	210	7	42	30	0	1.0	0.0	0	4%
(Ancient Harvest) quinoa, wheat-free, dry	2 oz	180	5	35	5	3	2.0	0.0	0	10%
(Creamette) enriched, dry	2 oz	210	7	42	0	0	1.0	0.0	0	4%
(De Cecco) enriched, dry	2 oz	210	7	41	0	0	1.0	0.0	0	4%
(Pastamania!) beet, spinach, and tomato, dry	2 oz	200	8	40	10	1	1.0	0.0	0	4%
(Quinoa)										
quinoa, dry	2 oz	210	10	40	11	8	1.0	0.0	0	4%
quinoa, wheat-free, dry	2 oz	180	5	35	5	3	2.0	0.0	0	10%
(Ronzoni) enriched, dry	2 oz	210	9	40	0	2	1.0	0.0	0	4%
ROTINI										
(American Beauty)										
100% durum wheat semolina, dry	2 oz	210	7	42	0	0	1.0	0.0	0	4%
quinoa, dry	2 oz	210	10	40	11	8	1.0	0.0	0	4%
tricolor, 'Italiano' dry	2 oz	210	7	42	0	0	1.0	0.0	0	4%
wheat and quinoa, organic, low-salt, no cholesterol	2 oz	210	10	42	8	7	1.0	0.0	0	4%
(Bernardi) vegetable	1 1/4 cup	220	9	44	15	2	1.0	0.5	0	4%
(Creamette) enriched, dry	2 oz	210	7	42	0	0	1.0	0.0	0	4%
(De Boles)										
Jerusalem artichoke, dry	2 oz	210	7	41	0	1	1.0	0.0	0	4%
Jerusalem artichoke, garlic and parsley, dry	2 oz	210	7	41	5	2	1.0	0.0	0	4%
Jerusalem artichoke, tomato and basil, dry	2 oz	210	7	41	0	2	1.0	0.0	0	4%
vegetable, dry, 'Primavera'	2 oz	210	9	41	0	0	1.0	0.0	0	4%
(Eden Foods) mixed vegetable	2 oz	210	7	42	10	2	1.0	0.0	0	4%
(Hodgson Mill) vegetable, four flavors, dry	2 oz	200	8	na	15	1	1.0	0.0	0	22%
(Pasta Perfect)										
	1 cup	140	5	28	0	1	0.0	0.0	0	0%
spinach	1 cup	140	5	27	0	1	0.0	0.0	0	0%
RUFFLE										
(Mueller's) trio, dry	2 oz	210	7	42	10	1	1.0	0.0	0	4%
SHELLS										
(American Beauty)										
100% durum wheat semolina, dry	2 oz	210	9	40	0	2	1.0	0.0	0	4%
100% durum wheat semolina, macaroni, dry	2 oz	210	7	42	0	0	1.0	0.0	0	4%
large, durum wheat semolina, dry	2 oz	210	7	42	0	0	1.0	0.0	0	4%
medium, durum wheat semolina, dry	2 oz	210	7	42	0	0	1.0	0.0	0	4%
tricolor, 'Italiano' dry	2 oz	210	7	42	0	0	1.0	0.0	0	4%
(Ancient Harvest) quinoa, wheat-free, dry	2 oz	180	5	35	5	3	2.0	0.0	0	10%

Food Name	Serving Size	Calories	Prot. gms	Carbs gms	Sod. mgs	Fiber gms	Fat gms	Sat. Fat gms	Chol. mgs	% Fat Cal.
(Creamette) medium, enriched, dry	2 oz	210	7	42	0	0	1.0	0.0	0	4%
(De Boles)										
	2 oz	210	7	41	0	1	1.0	0.0	0	4%
corn, wheat-free, dry	2 oz	210	5	45	0	0	1.0	0.0	0	4%
dry, 'Primavera'	2 oz	210	9	41	0	0	1.0	0.0	0	4%
whole wheat and Jerusalem artichoke, dry	2 oz	210	7	40	0	5	2.0	0.0	0	9%
(Eden Foods)										
vegetable, organic, dry	2 oz	210	8	42	10	2	1.0	0.0	0	4%
w/mixed vegetable, dry, 'Herb's'	2 oz	210	7	42	10	2	1.0	0.0	0	4%
wheat, vegetable, no eggs, organic, dry	2 oz	228	8	44	0	0	1.0	0.0	0	4%
(Hodgson Mill) whole wheat, medium	2 oz	190	9	34	10	6	1.0	0.0	0	5%
(Mueller's)										
dry	2 oz	210	7	42	0	1	1.0	0.0	0	4%
jumbo, dry	2 oz	210	7	42	0	1	1.0	0.0	0	4%
(Pasta Perfect)	1 cup	140	5	28	0	1	0.0	0.0	0	0%
(Pastamania!) tomato and spinach, dry	2 oz	200	8	40	10	1	1.0	0.0	0	4%
(Quinoa) quinoa 'Supergrain Wheat-free' dry	2 oz	180	5	35	5	3	2.0	0.0	0	10%
(Ronzoni)										
enriched, dry	2 oz	210	7	42	0	0	1.0	0.0	0	4%
extra fancy, enriched, dry	2 oz	210	7	42	0	0	1.0	0.0	0	4%
jumbo, enriched, dry	2 oz	210	7	42	0	0	1.0	0.0	0	4%
(Westbrae) corn, dry	2 oz	210	4	46	10	0	2.0	0.0	0	8%
SPAGHETTI										
enriched, cooked	1 cup	197	7	40	1	2	0.9	0.1	0	4%
protein-fortified, cooked	1 cup	230	11	44	7	2	0.3	0.0	0	1%
unenriched, cooked	1 cup	197	7	40	1	2	0.9	0.1	0	4%
(Al Dente) pepper, 'Three Pepper Pasta' dry	2 oz	220	8	40	20	0	2.0	0.0	0	9%
(American Beauty) 100% durum wheat semolina, dry	2 oz	210	7	42	0	0	1.0	0.0	0	4%
(Ancient Harvest) quinoa, wheat-free, dry	2 oz	180	5	35	5	3	2.0	0.0	0	10%
(Creamette)										
dry	2 oz	210	7	42	5	0	1.0	0.0	0	4%
enriched, thin, dry	2 oz	210	7	42	0	0	1.0	0.0	0	4%
spinach, w/egg, uncooked	2 oz	220	8	40	65	1	3.0	0.0	70	12%
(De Boles)										
corn, wheat-free, dry	2 oz	210	5	45	0	0	1.0	0.0	0	4%
Jerusalem artichoke, dry	2 oz	210	7	41	0	1	1.0	0.0	0	4%
Jerusalem artichoke, spinach	2 oz	200	7	41	30	2	1.0	0.0	0	4%
whole wheat and Jerusalem artichoke, dry	2 oz	210	7	40	0	5	2.0	0.0	0	9%
(DiGiorno) uncooked, approx 1-1/3 cups cooked	3 oz	250	11	47	140	0	3.0	0.0	0	10%
(Eden Foods)										
durum wheat, organic, dry	2 oz	210	8	42	10	2	1.0	0.0	0	4%
kamut, whole grain, organic, dry	2 oz	210	10	38	0	6	1.5	0.0	0	7%
parsley garlic, organic, dry	2 oz	210	7	42	10	2	1.0	0.0	0	4%
whole grain, organic, dry	2 oz	210	10	39	0	6	1.5	0.0	0	6%
(Ener-G Foods)										
brown rice, gluten-free, dry	2 oz	212	4	44	1	2	0.1	0.0	0	1%
rice, gluten-free, dry	2 oz	214	4	42	1	2	0.1	0.0	1	0%
(Health Valley)										
amaranth, dry	2 oz	170	7	40	10	9	1.0	0.0	0	5%
oat bran, dry	2 oz	120	4	23	2	4	1.0	0.0	0	8%
whole wheat, dry	2 oz	170	9	40	10	7	1.0	0.0	0	4%
whole wheat, spinach, dry	2 oz	170	9	40	10	7	1.0	0.0	0	4%
(Hodgson Mill)										
durum whole wheat, thin, dry	2 oz	190	9	34	25	6	1.0	0.0	0	5%

Food Name	Serving Size	Calories	Prot. gms	Carbs gms	Sod. mgs	Fiber gms	Fat gms	Sat. Fat gms	Chol. mgs	% Fat Cal.
whole wheat, spinach, dry.........................	2 oz	190	9	35	25	5	2.0	0.0	0	9%
(Hospitality) enriched, 100% semolina, dry..............	2 oz	210	7	42	0	2	0.5	0.0	0	2%
(Quinoa) quinoa, 'Supergrain'.........................	2 oz	210	10	40	11	8	1.0	0.0	0	4%
(Ronzoni)										
enriched, dry..................................	2 oz	210	7	42	0	0	1.0	0.0	0	4%
enriched, thin, dry..............................	2 oz	210	7	42	0	0	1.0	0.0	0	4%
(Rummo) dry...................................	2 oz	210	7	41	10	0	1.0	0.0	0	4%
(Westbrae)										
corn, dry.....................................	2 oz	210	4	46	10	0	2.0	0.0	0	8%
whole wheat, no egg, dry........................	2 oz	210	8	40	0	7	2.0	0.0	0	9%
whole wheat, spinach, no egg, dry..................	2 oz	210	8	40	0	6	2.0	0.0	0	9%
SPAGHETTINI (De Cecco) enriched, dry.............	2 oz	210	7	41	0	0	1.0	0.0	0	4%
SPIRAL										
(American Beauty)										
rainbow, 100% durum wheat semolina, dry............	2 oz	210	7	42	30	0	1.0	0.0	0	4%
(Antoine's) spicy, uncooked.........................	2 oz	210	7	41	40	0	1.0	0.0	0	4%
(Eden Foods)										
kamut, whole grain, organic, dry...................	2 oz	210	10	38	0	6	1.5	0.0	0	7%
sesame rice, whole grain, organic, dry..............	2 oz	200	10	37	0	6	2.0	0.0	0	9%
vegetable, whole grain, organic, dry...............	2 oz	210	10	39	0	6	1.5	0.0	0	6%
wheat, sesame rice, organic, dry..................	2 oz	212	10	40	0	0	1.0	0.0	0	4%
wheat, vegetable, no eggs, organic, dry............	2 oz	228	8	44	0	0	1.0	0.0	0	4%
(Hodgson Mill) whole wheat, whole grain, dry..........	2 oz	190	9	34	10	6	1.0	1.0	0	5%
(Mueller's) 'Twist Trio' dry.........................	2 oz	210	7	42	10	1	1.0	0.0	0	4%
TAGLIATELLE										
(Contadina) spinach..............................	1 1/4 cup	270	12	46	110	4	4.0	1.0	105	13%
(Ener-G Foods)										
brown rice, gluten-free, dry.......................	2 oz	212	4	44	1	2	0.1	0.0	0	1%
rice, gluten-free, dry............................	2 oz	214	4	42	1	2	0.1	0.0	1	0%
TAGLIERINI (Pastamania!) tomato and spinach, dry........	2 oz	210	8	40	20	2	2.0	1.0	35	9%
TRICOLOR										
(Creamette) dry.................................	2 oz	210	8	42	5	1	1.0	0.0	0	4%
TRICOLOR PASTA, PRIMAVERA										
(De Boles) tricolor, 'Primavera' dry....................	2 oz	200	8	41	8	0	1.0	0.0	0	4%
WAGON WHEEL (Hodgson Mill) four flavors, dry..........	2 oz	200	8	41	15	1	1.0	0.0	0	4%
VERMICELLI										
(American Beauty) 100% durum wheat semolina, dry.....	2 oz	210	7	42	0	0	1.0	0.0	0	4%
(Creamette) enriched, extra thin, dry...................	2 oz	210	7	42	0	0	1.0	0.0	0	4%
(Ener-G Foods) rice, gluten-free, dry..................	2 oz	214	4	42	1	2	0.1	0.0	0	0%
(Ronzoni) enriched, dry............................	2 oz	210	7	42	0	0	1.0	0.0	0	4%
WHEAT										
(De Boles) whole wheat 'Natural Gourmet' dry..........	2 oz	200	7	40	0	6	1.0	0.0	0	5%
ZITI										
(De Boles)										
	2 oz	210	7	41	0	1	1.0	0.0	0	4%
Jerusalem artichoke, dry..........................	2 oz	210	7	41	0	1	1.0	0.0	0	4%
(Ronzoni) enriched, dry............................	2 oz	210	7	42	0	0	1.0	0.0	0	4%
PASTA CHIPS										
(Bachman) pasta snack chip 'Pastapazazz'..............	1 oz	150	2	15	340	0	9.0	0.0	0	54%
PASTA DISH/ENTRÉE. See also LASAGNA/LASAGNA ENTRÉE; MANICOTTI/MANICOTTI ENTRÉE; RAVIOLI DISH/ENTRÉE; TORTELLINI DISH/ENTRÉE.										
(Budget Gourmet)										
w/chicken, in wine and mushroom sauce w/chicken......	1 entrée	280	15	40	890	3	7.0	2.0	25	22%
(Celentano) and cheese, baked, frozen................	6 oz	290	12	29	350	0	13.0	0.0	0	42%

Food Name	Serving Size	Calories	Prot. gms	Carbs gms	Sod. mgs	Fiber gms	Fat gms	Sat. Fat gms	Chol. mgs	% Fat Cal.
(Chef Boyardee)										
rings and franks, microwave	7.5 oz	190	7	31	980	3	5.0	2.0	20	23%
rings and meatballs, microwave	7.5 oz	220	8	33	990	4	8.0	3.0	25	31%
(Contadina) chicken, herb, w/tomato sauce, frozen	1 oz	27	2	4	54	na	0.6	na	3	20%
(Green Giant)										
Dijon, frozen, 'Microwave Garden Gourmet'	1 pkg	300	7	24	560	3	20.0	0.0	0	59%
Parmesan, w/sweet peas, frozen, 'One Serving'	5.5 oz	160	9	21	420	3	5.0	3.0	10	27%
(Healthy Choice)										
primavera, microwave	11 oz	280	11	51	360	0	3.0	2.0	15	10%
vegetable, Italiano	1 entrée	250	9	48	480	6	3.0	1.5	10	11%
w/chicken, teriyaki, frozen, 'Classics'	12.6 oz	350	24	58	370	0	3.0	1.0	45	8%
w/shrimp, frozen, 'Classics'	12.5 oz	270	16	44	490	0	4.0	2.0	50	13%
(Lean Cuisine)										
cheddar bake	1 entrée	220	12	29	560	3	6.0	2.0	20	25%
w/chicken and herb tomato sauce, frozen	9.5 oz	270	17	38	460	0	6.0	2.0	35	20%
w/turkey, Dijon sauce, frozen, 'Lunch Express'	9 7/8 oz	290	18	39	540	0	7.0	2.0	35	22%
(Lunch Bucket)										
chicken, Italian, lunch cup, 'Light'n Healthy'	7.5 oz	130	7	23	630	0	1.0	0.0	10	7%
(Lunch Express)										
and tuna, casserole	1 entrée	280	18	39	590	4	6.0	2.0	20	19%
and turkey, Dijon	1 entrée	270	16	37	570	6	6.0	1.5	30	20%
(Marie Callender's)										
frozen, 'Callender's Deluxe'	1 cup	350	31	4	610	5	23.0	9.0	30	60%
primavera, w/chicken, frozen	1 cup	310	12	22	450	3	19.0	8.0	25	56%
w/beef and broccoli	15 oz	570	35	73	1160	6	15.0	4.0	70	24%
(MET-RX) café pasta meal	1 cup	190	19	27	45	0	1.0	0.0	0	5%
(Smart Ones)										
and spinach, Romano	1 entrée	260	12	35	510	4	8.0	3.0	15	28%
Portafino, in wine sauce, frozen	9.5 oz	160	8	30	220	0	1.0	1.0	0	6%
(Tyson) trio, frozen, 'Gourmet Selection'	11 oz	450	21	53	890	0	17.0	0.0	0	34%
(Weight Watchers)										
and spinach, Romano	1 entrée	240	11	32	510	4	8.0	3.5	5	30%
Italiano, frozen, 'Ultimate 200'	8 oz	190	17	19	450	0	4.0	2.0	5	20%
w/tomato basil sauce	1 entrée	260	12	33	360	5	9.0	3.5	10	31%
ANGEL HAIR										
(Budget Gourmet)	1 entrée	230	8	38	430	3	5.0	1.5	10	20%
(Lean Cuisine) frozen	1 entrée	220	8	41	420	6	3.0	0.5	0	12%
(Marie Callender's) w/sausage and breadstick, frozen	1 entrée	370	14	43	630	4	15.0	4.0	10	37%
(Smart Ones)	1 entrée	170	8	29	520	7	2.0	0.0	0	11%
BOW TIES										
(Marie Callender's)										
Alfredo	13 oz	620	20	40	1080	8	42.0	19.0	80	61%
and meat sauce	13 oz	480	25	44	970	3	22.0	10.0	45	42%
marinara	13 oz	430	18	46	930	6	19.0	7.0	30	40%
(Lean Cuisine) and chicken, 'Cafe Classic'	1 entrée	270	19	34	550	5	6.0	1.5	60	20%
(Pasta Perfect) w/vegetables	1/2 cup	110	5	19	55	na	1.0	na	15	9%
(Weight Watchers) Marsala	1 entrée	280	13	36	560	5	9.0	3.5	10	29%
CANNELLONI										
(Bernardi) w/beef	1 piece	200	9	19	290	1	10.0	5.0	25	45%
(Celentano) Florentine, frozen	12 oz	350	21	48	620	0	8.0	0.0	0	21%
(Dining Lite) cheese, frozen	9 oz	310	19	38	650	0	9.0	0.0	70	26%
(Lean Cuisine)										
beef, w/tomato sauce, frozen	9 5/8 oz	200	14	28	490	0	3.0	1.0	25	14%
cheese	1 entrée	240	19	29	590	4	5.0	3.0	22	19%

Food Name	Serving Size	Calories	Prot. gms	Carbs gms	Sod. mgs	Fiber gms	Fat gms	Sat. Pat gms	Chol. mgs	% Fat Cal.
cheese, w/tomato sauce, frozen	9 1/8 oz	270	23	27	590	0	8.0	4.0	25	26%
CAVATELLI (Celentano)	2/3 cup	400	16	79	15	9	1.5	0.5	15	3%
FETTUCCINE										
(Armour) chicken, frozen, 'Classics'	11 oz	260	17	28	660	0	9.0	0.0	50	31%
(Banquet)										
Alfredo	1 entrée	350	11	40	850	4	16.0	7.0	25	41%
Alfredo, four cheeses, frozen	1 entrée	480	20	48	1120	3	24.0	13.0	55	44%
chicken, frozen, 'Healthy Balance'	11.25 oz	320	17	47	650	0	7.0	3.0	35	20%
w/meat sauce, frozen	10 oz	290	16	34	980	0	10.0	0.0	25	31%
(Budget Gourmet) primavera, w/chicken	1 entrée	280	14	38	650	3	8.0	3.5	30	26%
(Contadina) grilled chicken, frozen, food service product	1 oz	42	2	3	113	0	2.7	1.4	10	57%
(Dining Lite) w/broccoli, frozen	9 oz	290	12	33	1020	0	12.0	0.0	35	38%
(Green Giant)										
primavera, frozen	1 pkg	230	13	26	610	6	8.0	3.0	25	32%
primavera, 'Microwave Garden Gourmet'	1 pkg	260	17	25	640	6	13.0	0.0	0	41%
(Hain) Alfredo, 'Pasta & Sauce'	1/4 pkg	180	5	27	420	0	4.0	0.0	0	22%
(Healthy Choice)										
Alfredo	1 entrée	250	11	39	480	3	5.0	2.0	15	18%
chicken, Alfredo	1 entrée	280	22	35	410	3	7.0	2.5	40	22%
chicken, frozen	8.5 oz	240	22	29	370	0	4.0	2.0	45	15%
(Kraft) Alfredo, 'Pasta & Cheese' prepared	1/2 cup	180	7	19	590	0	9.0	3.0	30	44%
(Lean Cuisine)										
Alfredo, frozen	9 oz	280	14	41	570	0	7.0	3.0	15	22%
chicken	1 entrée	270	22	33	580	2	6.0	2.5	45	20%
chicken, Alfredo sauce, frozen 'Lunch Express'	10.25 oz	240	16	31	540	0	6.0	2.0	35	22%
chicken, frozen	9 oz	280	23	33	500	0	6.0	3.0	35	19%
primavera, frozen	10 oz	260	14	32	510	0	8.0	3.0	45	28%
(Lunch Express) primavera	1 entrée	420	15	33	690	6	25.0	12.0	95	54%
(Marie Callender's)										
Alfredo, frozen	1 cup	190	10	29	400	2	21.0	9.0	45	55%
Alfredo, supreme	1 cup	450	15	35	680	4	27.0	12.0	80	55%
Alfredo, w/bread	14 oz	800	23	71	1270	5	47.0	19.0	95	53%
primavera, w/torellini	1 cup	430	11	35	670	4	27.0	12.0	35	57%
w/broccoli and chicken	13 oz	410	16	32	550	4	24.0	10.0	45	53%
(Michelinas) w/creamy pesto sauce 'Lean 'n' Tasty'	1 entrée	250	10	38	590	3	6.0	3.5	20	22%
(Right Course) chicken, Italiano, w/vegetables, frozen	9 5/8 oz	280	24	29	560	0	8.0	2.0	45	25%
(Stouffer's)										
Alfredo	1 entrée	580	14	42	810	4	39.0	21.0	120	61%
chicken, 'Homestyle'	1 entrée	390	31	32	1250	3	15.0	4.0	65	35%
chicken, homestyle, w/vegetable medley, frozen	9.5 oz	350	23	27	780	0	17.0	0.0	0	43%
(Ultra Slim Fast)	12 oz	390	31	38	980	0	12.0	0.0	65	28%
(Weight Watchers)										
Alfredo, w/broccoli	1 entrée	230	10	34	450	3	6.0	3.0	20	23%
chicken	1 entrée	290	19	39	590	4	7.0	2.0	50	21%
LINGUINE										
(Banquet) w/meat sauce, frozen, 'Healthy Balance'	11.5 oz	290	11	49	560	0	6.0	3.0	25	18%
(Budget Gourmet)										
w/shrimp, frozen	10 oz	330	15	33	1250	0	15.0	0.0	75	41%
w/shrimp and clams, 'Light'	1 entrée	280	14	38	800	3	8.0	5.0	70	26%
w/tomato sauce, sausage, 'Special Selections'	1 entrée	360	15	43	610	5	14.0	4.0	25	35%
(Healthy Choice) w/shrimp, frozen	9.5 oz	230	13	40	420	0	2.0	1.0	60	8%
(Lean Cuisine)										
w/clam sauce, frozen	9 5/8 oz	280	17	36	560	0	8.0	2.0	30	25%
w/meatballs, frozen, food service product	1 oz	25	2	3	78	1	0.8	0.3	3	29%

Food Name	Serving Size	Calories	Prot. gms	Carbs gms	Sod. mgs	Fiber gms	Fat gms	Sat. Fat gms	Chol. mgs	% Fat Cal.
(Marie Callender's) and Italian sausage	15 oz	710	26	70	1330	8	36.0	16.0	30	46%
(Top Shelf) w/clam sauce, packaged	1 serving	330	12	30	1420	0	18.0	0.0	85	49%
MACARONI										
(Amy's Kitchen)										
and cheese	1 serving	390	17	50	550	4	14.0	8.0	40	32%
and soy cheese	1 serving	360	16	42	500	4	14.0	1.0	0	35%
(Banquet)										
and beef, shells, frozen	10 oz	340	20	34	985	0	14.0	0.0	35	37%
and cheese	1 entree	320	11	44	970	4	11.0	3.5	20	31%
and cheese, frozen	10 oz	420	14	46	450	0	20.0	0.0	30	43%
and cheese, frozen, 'Family Entrees'	8 oz	290	12	32	0	0	13.0	0.0	0	40%
(Budget Gourmet)										
and cheese	1 entrée	270	10	45	520	2	6.0	2.5	10	20%
and cheese, frozen, 'Side Dish'	5.3 oz	210	9	23	370	0	8.0	0.0	25	36%
and cheese, frozen, 'Special Selections'	1 entree	400	17	38	1320	4	20.0	12.0	45	45%
(Chef Boyardee)										
and cheese, canned	7.5 oz	170	7	33	970	2	2.0	1.0	25	10%
and cheese, w/shells, canned	7.5 oz	150	6	31	930	0	1.0	1.0	0	6%
and chicken, canned	7.5 oz	180	10	30	850	1	2.0	1.0	15	10%
canned, 'Roller Coasters'	7.5 oz	230	7	28	1070	3	10.0	3.0	19	39%
dinosaurs, in tomato and cheese sauce	1 cup	210	6	45	830	4	0.0	0.0	0	0%
dinosaurs, w/mini meatballs, in tomato sauce	1 cup	270	9	38	930	4	9.0	4.0	25	30%
elbows w/beef, in sauce, microwave	7.5 oz	210	8	29	1000	0	7.0	0.0	15	30%
in cheese sauce, canned, 'ABC's & 123's'	8.6 oz	200	6	42	1020	0	1.0	1.0	2	4%
in cheese sauce, canned, 'Sharks'	7.5 oz	170	5	34	780	0	1.0	1.0	2	5%
in cheese sauce, canned, 'Smurfs'	7.5 oz	150	6	29	830	3	1.0	0.0	2	6%
in cheese sauce, canned, 'Tic Tac Toes'	8.6 oz	190	5	41	1080	0	1.0	0.0	0	5%
in cheese sauce, canned, 'Tic Tac Toes'	7.5 oz	160	5	31	870	3	1.0	1.0	1	6%
in cheese sauce, microwave, 'ABC's & 123's'	7.5 oz	180	5	37	940	3	1.0	1.0	3	5%
in cheese sauce, microwave, 'Dinosaurs'	7.5 oz	180	6	36	880	3	1.0	1.0	3	5%
in cheese sauce, microwave, 'Tic Tac Toes'	7.5 oz	170	5	36	930	2	1.0	1.0	2	5%
in chicken sauce, canned, 'Pac Man'	7.5 oz	170	6	22	905	0	7.0	0.0	0	36%
in sauce, canned 'ABC's & 123's'	7.5 oz	160	5	31	830	3	1.0	1.0	2	6%
in sauce, canned 'Turtles'	7.5 oz	150	4	31	830	0	1.0	0.0	0	6%
in sauce, microwave, 'Turtles'	7.5 oz	160	5	33	870	2	1.0	0.0	3	6%
in tomato and cheese sauce, 'Street Sharks'	1 cup	210	6	47	750	4	0.0	0.0	0	0%
in tomato sauce, canned, 'Pac Man'	7.5 oz	150	6	30	830	0	1.0	1.0	2	6%
mini bites, canned	7.5 oz	260	8	30	1020	1	12.0	2.0	17	42%
shells, in meat sauce, canned	7.5 oz	190	7	31	810	4	6.0	1.0	5	26%
shells, in meat sauce, microwave	7.5 oz	210	8	32	1090	0	6.0	0.0	15	25%
shells, in mushroom sauce, microwave	7.5 oz	170	6	35	1080	0	1.0	1.0	2	5%
'Teenage Mutant Ninja Turtles'	1 pkg	227	8	34	840	3	6.8	3.0	21	27%
w/beef, canned, 'Beefaroni'	1 cup	260	10	37	870	5	7.0	3.0	25	25%
w/beef, microwave, 'Beefaroni'	7.5 oz	220	7	31	1145	2	7.0	1.0	18	29%
w/meatballs, canned, 'ABC's & 123's'	8.6 oz	280	9	35	1090	0	11.0	0.0	23	36%
w/meatballs, canned, 'Dinosaurs'	8.6 oz	280	9	36	1131	0	11.0	0.0	21	35%
w/meatballs, canned, 'Pac Man'	7.5 oz	230	7	32	880	5	9.0	3.0	17	34%
w/meatballs, canned, 'Smurfs'	7.5 oz	240	8	31	900	2	9.0	2.0	19	34%
w/meatballs, canned, 'Tic Tac Toes'	7.5 oz	240	8	31	1000	0	9.0	0.0	18	34%
w/meatballs, canned, 'Tic Tac Toes'	8.6 oz	290	8	39	1045	0	11.0	1.0	0	34%
w/meatballs, canned, 'Turtles'	7.5 oz	220	7	30	940	0	8.0	0.0	20	33%
w/meatballs, in sauce, canned, 'Zooroni'	7.5 oz	240	8	33	970	0	8.0	0.0	17	31%
w/meatballs, 'Street Sharks' *(Chef Boyardee)*	1 cup	250	8	37	940	4	8.0	3.5	25	29%
(Franco-American) and cheese	1 cup	210	8	29	1060	4	7.0	3.0	10	30%

Food Name	Serving Size	Calories	Prot. gms	Carbs gms	Sod. mgs	Fiber gms	Fat gms	Sat. Fat gms	Chol. mgs	% Fat Cal.
(Green Giant)										
and cheese, frozen, 'One Serving'	5.7 oz	230	9	28	590	0	9.0	4.0	25	35%
(Healthy Choice)										
and cheese	1 entrée	290	15	50	580	4	7.0	2.5	25	20%
and cheese, meatless	1 entrée	320	15	50	580	4	7.0	2.5	25	20%
(Heinz)										
and cheese, canned	7.5 oz	190	5	26	1105	0	8.0	0.0	0	37%
w/beef, in tomato sauce, canned.	7.5 oz	200	8	23	850	0	8.0	0.0	0	37%
(Hormel) and cheese, micro cup	7.5 oz	189	7	26	874	0	6.0	0.0	17	29%
(Kid Cuisine)										
and cheese, frozen, 'Mega Meal'	12.45 oz	470	14	75	1270	0	13.0	0.0	0	25%
and cheese, w/apples, corn, fudge brownie, frozen	1 meal	310	7	54	710	6	7.0	2.5	15	21%
and cheese, w/mini franks, frozen.	9 oz	380	9	55	1000	0	14.0	0.0	40	33%
(Kid's Kitchen)										
beefy, microwave cup	7.5 oz	200	11	25	780	0	6.0	2.0	25	27%
and cheese, microwave cup	7.5 oz	260	12	28	650	0	11.0	6.0	45	38%
(Lean Cuisine)										
and beef	1 entrée	280	13	40	550	3	8.0	2.0	25	25%
and beef, frozen, food service product	1 oz	27	2	3	71	0	0.9	0.2	4	30%
and beef, in tomato sauce, frozen.	1 pkg	249	14	37	563	3	5.4	1.6	23	19%
and cheese	1 entrée	290	13	43	590	4	7.0	4.0	20	22%
and cheese, frozen, food service product	1 oz	33	2	4	85	0	1.1	0.5	3	30%
(Libby's) and cheese, microwave cup, 'Diner'	7.5 oz	360	14	27	1020	2	22.0	9.0	35	55%
(Lipton) and cheese, w/shells, 'Hearty Ones'.	11 oz	367	15	60	1406	0	7.4	0.0	14	18%
(Lunch Bucket) and cheese, microwave lunch cup	7.5 oz	210	9	24	990	0	9.0	0.0	0	38%
(Lunch Express) and cheese, w/broccoli.	1 entrée	240	12	35	460	5	6.0	3.0	15	22%
(Marie Callender's)										
and beef, w/tomatoes and soft breadstick, frozen.	1 entrée	310	12	40	680	5	11.0	4.0	15	32%
and cheese	13.5 oz	510	22	65	2020	5	18.0	9.0	35	32%
and cheese, frozen, 'Marie's Special'	1 cup	420	20	47	1410	3	17.0	9.0	40	36%
(Michelinas)										
and beef, 'Lean n Tasty'.	1 entrée	230	12	34	830	2	6.0	2.0	20	23%
and cheese, 'Lean n Tasty'	1 entrée	270	12	41	620	2	6.0	3.5	20	20%
(Morton) and cheese casserole, frozen.	6.5 oz	290	8	30	760	0	14.0	0.0	0	45%
(Myers) and cheese, frozen.	3.5 oz	168	7	16	516	0	9.0	0.0	0	47%
(Nalley's) w/beef.	7.5 oz	180	9	29	900	0	3.0	0.0	0	15%
(Nestlé)										
and cheese, canned, 'Chef Mate'	1 pkg	3397	130	425	16105	39	131.9	74.3	334	35%
and cheese, canned, 'Chef Mate'	1 cup	283	11	35	1343	3	11.0	6.2	28	35%
(Pathmark) w/beef, in tomato sauce, canned, 'No Frills'	7.5 oz	200	9	22	880	0	8.0	0.0	0	37%
(Smart Ones) and cheese	1 entrée	220	9	42	640	4	2.0	0.5	5	8%
(Stouffer's)										
and beef	1 entrée	420	19	40	1530	5	20.0	8.0	50	43%
and beef, w/tomato	10 oz	270	15	43	590	4	4.0	1.5	25	13%
and cheese	6 oz	330	14	31	940	2	17.0	6.0	30	46%
and cheese, frozen, food service product	1 oz	39	2	4	105	0	1.6	0.7	3	37%
(Swanson)										
and beef, frozen	12 oz	370	12	48	930	0	15.0	0.0	0	36%
and cheese, frozen	12.25 oz	370	13	43	1070	0	15.0	0.0	0	38%
and cheese, frozen	7 oz	200	7	24	740	0	8.0	0.0	0	37%
and cheese, frozen, 'Homestyle Recipe'.	10 oz	390	17	37	1150	0	19.0	0.0	0	44%
(Tyson)										
and cheese, frozen, 'Tweety'.	8 oz	340	12	49	650	0	10.0	0.0	28	27%
frozen, 'Bugs Bunny/Tazmanian Devil'	8 oz	290	13	41	420	0	8.0	0.0	0	25%

Food Name	Serving Size	Calories	Prot. gms	Carbs gms	Sod. mgs	Fiber gms	Fat gms	Sat. Fat gms	Chol. mgs	% Fat Cal.
frozen, 'Daffy Duck & Elmer Fudd'	8 oz	270	11	40	430	0	7.0	0.0	0	24%
frozen, 'Foghorn Leghorn/Henry Hawk'	8 oz	230	9	39	320	0	4.0	0.0	0	16%
frozen, 'Looney Tunes Sylvester & Tweety'	8 oz	250	13	41	380	0	4.0	0.0	0	14%
(Weight Watchers)										
and beef	1 entree	220	13	32	560	4	4.5	1.5	10	18%
in tomato sauce, frozen	1 pkg	282	16	45	492	7	4.6	1.6	13	15%
and cheese	1 entree	280	13	42	590	4	7.0	3.5	25	22%
MOSTACCIOLI										
(Banquet) w/meat sauce, frozen, 'Family Entrees'	7 oz	170	7	28	0	0	3.0	0.0	0	16%
(Contadina) w/meat sauce, frozen, food service product	1 oz	35	1	5	119	1	1.2	0.4	3	31%
PENNE										
(Budget Gourmet)										
w/tomato sauce, Italian sausage, frozen	10 oz	320	12	53	520	0	9.0	2.0	5	24%
w/tomato and sausage, 'Special Selections'	1 entrée	330	17	49	530	6	8.0	2.5	10	21%
(Healthy Choice) w/roasted tomato sauce	1 entrée	230	9	36	490	5	5.0	1.0	10	20%
(Marie Callender's) and pepperoni	15 oz	800	29	74	1780	11	43.0	17.0	30	48%
(Michelinas) w/mushrooms, 'Lean n Tasty'	1 entrée	250	10	38	650	3	6.0	3.5	20	22%
(Weight Watchers)										
and ricotta, spicy	1 entrée	280	12	45	370	5	6.0	2.0	5	19%
pollo	1 entrée	290	22	40	620	3	5.0	2.0	35	15%
w/sun dried tomatoes	1 entrée	290	13	40	560	5	9.0	3.0	10	28%
RIGATONI										
(Chef Boyardee)										
canned, 'Special Recipe' 'Ragatoni'	7.5 oz	210	9	33	1040	4	6.0	2.0	20	24%
microwave 'Ragatoni'	7.5 oz	210	8	31	1080	0	6.0	0.0	17	26%
(Budget Gourmet)										
tomato sauce, frozen, 'Special Selections'	1 entree	420	16	41	620	2	22.0	8.0	65	46%
w/broccoli and chicken, in cream sauce, frozen	10.8 oz	290	19	44	710	0	7.0	3.0	30	20%
w/broccoli, white chicken, in cream sauce	1 entrée	250	10	37	530	1	7.0	3.5	20	25%
(Healthy Choice)										
in meat sauce, frozen	9.5 oz	260	16	34	540	0	6.0	2.0	30	21%
w/chicken, frozen, 'Classics'	12.5 oz	360	31	50	430	0	4.0	2.0	60	10%
(Lean Cuisine)										
	1 entrée	180	10	25	560	4	4.0	1.5	20	20%
jumbo, w/meatballs, 'Hearty Portions'	1 entrée	440	27	62	780	8	9.0	4.5	40	19%
(Marie Callender's)										
Parmigiana, family size, frozen	1 cup	320	15	32	670	4	14.0	7.0	25	40%
Parmigiana, w/breadstick, frozen	1 cup + bread	300	12	32	650	3	14.0	6.0	25	42%
(Stouffer's) w/meat sauce, homestyle, frozen	12 oz	400	21	49	860	0	13.0	0.0	0	29%
ROTINI										
(Green Giant)										
cheddar cheese, 'Microwave Garden Gourmet'	1 pkg	230	9	32	570	5	10.0	6.0	20	35%
(Mrs. Paul's) seafood, frozen, 'Light'	9 oz	240	12	34	570	0	6.0	2.0	25	23%
(Norpac)										
w/spinach rotini and vegetables, 'Pasta Perfect'	1/2 cup	100	4	19	15	na	0.0	0.0	0	0%
w/vegetables, vegetarian, 'Pasta Perfect'	1/2 cup	110	5	20	60	3	1.0	0.0	0	8%
(Weight Watchers) three cheese, w/vegetables, frozen	9 oz	270	14	34	500	0	8.0	3.0	5	27%
SHELLS										
(Bernardi)										
cheese stuffed	2 pieces	240	12	25	330	1	11.0	7.0	60	40%
cheese stuffed, large	1 piece	160	8	13	250	1	9.0	5.0	50	49%
Florentine	1 piece	190	11	17	340	1	8.0	5.0	30	39%
(Buitoni) shells, stuffed, frozen, 'Single Serving'	9 oz	460	18	46	840	0	13.0	7.0	80	31%

Food Name	Serving Size	Calories	Prot. gms	Carbs gms	Sod. mgs	Fiber gms	Fat gms	Sat. Fat gms	Chol. mgs	% Fat Cal.
(Celentano)										
broccoli stuffed, frozen, 'Great Choice'	10 oz	190	12	31	520	0	4.0	0.0	0	17%
stuffed, frozen	8 oz	330	18	41	680	0	11.0	0.0	0	30%
stuffed, lowfat, frozen 'Great Choice'.	10 oz	250	16	41	675	0	2.0	0.0	0	7%
stuffed, w/sauce, frozen	10 oz	410	23	51	850	0	14.0	0.0	0	30%
stuffed, w/sauce, frozen	6.25 oz	340	17	31	420	0	16.0	0.0	0	43%
(Healthy Choice)										
stuffed, in tomato sauce, frozen, 'Classics'	12 oz	330	24	53	470	0	3.0	2.0	35	8%
(Le Menu) stuffed, 3-cheese, frozen 'LightStyle'	10 oz	280	17	34	690	0	8.0	0.0	25	26%
(Lean Cuisine) cheese stuffed, frozen	1 oz	25	1	3	65	0	0.8	0.4	3	29%
(Norpac)										
seashells w/vegetables, vegetarian, 'Pasta Perfect'	1/2 cup	130	6	25	65	na	1.0	na	0	7%
(Stouffer's) cheese, w/tomato sauce, frozen	9.25 oz	300	17	28	820	0	13.0	0.0	0	39%
SPAGHETTI										
(Banquet)										
w/meat sauce, frozen, 'Casserole'	8 oz	270	14	35	1250	0	8.0	0.0	0	27%
w/meatballs, frozen	10 oz	290	11	44	580	0	10.0	0.0	30	29%
(Budget Gourmet)										
marinara	1 entrée	290	10	50	790	4	6.0	1.5	5	18%
w/tomato and meat sauce, 'Special Selections'	1 entrée	320	15	49	470	4	7.0	2.5	5	20%
(Buitoni) and meatballs, in sauce, canned.	7.5 oz	190	9	21	940	0	8.0	6.0	20	38%
(Chef Boyardee)										
and beef, in tomato sauce, canned.	7.5 oz	240	7	30	1120	0	9.0	0.0	0	35%
and meatballs	1 cup	250	9	32	950	3	10.0	4.0	25	35%
and meatballs, in tomato sauce, canned.	1 pkg	442	16	60	1666	4	15.3	6.8	38	31%
and meatballs, in tomato sauce, canned.	1 serving	250	9	34	941	2	8.6	3.9	22	31%
and meatballs, canned, 'Microwave'	7.5 oz	230	7	29	1060	0	10.0	0.0	20	38%
w/beef, 'Beefagetti'	1 cup	250	8	37	990	4	7.0	3.0	25	26%
(Dining Lite) w/beef, frozen	9 oz	220	12	25	440	0	8.0	0.0	20	33%
(Estee) meatballs, canned.	7.5 oz	240	9	19	130	0	14.0	6.0	30	53%
(Featherweight) and meatballs, canned.	7.5 oz	160	12	23	400	0	3.0	0.0	20	16%
(Finast) rings, in tomato sauce, canned.	7.5 oz	150	4	31	480	0	1.0	0.0	0	6%
(Franco-American)										
in tomato and cheese sauce	1 cup	210	7	41	1020	3	2.0	1.0	5	9%
in tomato and cheese sauce, 'Spaghettio's'	1 cup	190	5	36	990	2	2.0	0.5	5	10%
in tomato sauce.	1 cup	270	11	35	1060	4	10.0	5.0	30	33%
w/meatballs, 'Spaghettio's'	1 cup	260	11	31	1150	5	11.0	5.0	20	37%
w/sliced frankfurters, 'Spaghettio's'	1 cup	250	10	32	1210	4	11.0	5.0	25	37%
(Freezer Queen) w/meat sauce, frozen 'Single Serve'	10 oz	350	14	47	610	0	12.0	0.0	0	31%
(Healthy Choice) Bolognese, frozen	1 serving	255	14	43	473	5	2.9	1.0	17	10%
(Kid Cuisine) w/meat sauce, frozen.	9.25 oz	310	9	43	690	0	12.0	0.0	35	34%
(Le Menu)										
w/beef, sauce, and mushrooms, frozen, 'LightStyle'	9 oz	280	12	45	450	0	6.0	1.0	15	19%
(Lean Cuisine)										
. . . .	1 entrée	290	11	50	570	7	5.0	1.5	20	16%
w/meat sauce	1 entrée	290	14	45	550	4	6.0	1.5	20	19%
w/meat sauce, frozen	1 entrée	313	14	51	610	6	5.9	1.4	13	17%
w/meatballs.	1 entrée	290	17	40	520	4	7.0	2.0	30	22%
w/meatballs and sauce, frozen	1 entrée	299	18	40	465	5	7.5	2.1	5	23%
(Legume)										
and neatballs, vegetarian	1 serving	330	28	46	650	7	4.0	0.5	0	11%
w/organic pasta and tofu, vegetarian	1 serving	240	13	23	660	6	11.0	2.0	0	41%
w/veggie protein cutlet, vegetarian	1 serving	380	25	47	650	9	10.0	1.5	0	24%
(Lunch Express) w/meat sauce	1 entrée	320	15	43	580	5	10.0	3.5	30	28%

Food Name	Serving Size	Calories	Prot. gms	Carbs gms	Sod. mgs	Fiber gms	Fat gms	Sat. Fat gms	Chol. mgs	% Fat Cal.
(Marie Callender's)										
and meat sauce, w/garlic bread	1 cup	380	16	51	700	5	13.0	4.0	10	30%
marinara, w/cheese garlic bread	1 cup	410	13	61	680	6	13.0	4.0	20	28%
(Michelinas)										
and meatballs, w/Pomodoro sauce, low-fat, frozen	1 pkg	312	14	49	1011	6	7.1	2.2	14	20%
and meatballs, w/Pomodoro sauce, low-fat, frozen	1 serving	312	14	49	1011	6	7.1	2.2	14	20%
(Morton) w/meatballs, frozen	10 oz	200	6	39	1090	0	3.0	0.0	10	13%
(Nalley's) and meatballs, canned	7.5 oz	190	10	29	950	0	4.0	0.0	0	19%
(Pathmark)										
w/meatballs, in tomato sauce, canned 'No Frills'	7.5 oz	200	9	22	860	0	8.0	0.0	0	37%
(Stouffer's)										
and meatballs	1 entrée	420	19	51	680	5	15.0	4.0	45	33%
Parmesan, w/Italian-style green beans, frozen	10.25 oz	240	10	30	810	0	9.0	0.0	0	34%
w/meat sauce, frozen	12 7/8 oz	320	16	38	560	0	12.0	0.0	0	33%
(Swanson)										
w/Italian meatballs, frozen, 'Homestyle Recipe'	13 oz	490	23	60	940	0	18.0	0.0	0	33%
w/meatballs, frozen	12.5 oz	390	14	46	1100	0	17.0	0.0	0	39%
(Top Shelf)										
spaghettini, packaged	1 serving	240	13	35	1020	0	5.0	0.0	5	19%
w/meat sauce	10 oz	260	14	37	980	0	6.0	2.0	20	21%
(Tyson) w/meatballs, frozen, 'Daffy Duck'	8.65 oz	340	11	49	570	0	10.0	0.0	20	27%
(Ultra Slim Fast) w/beef and mushroom sauce	12 oz	370	20	49	990	0	10.0	0.0	25	25%
(Van Camp's) w/franks, canned, 'Spaghettee Weenee'	1 cup	243	9	35	1128	1	7.4	0.0	0	27%
(Weight Watchers)										
marinara	1 entrée	280	9	46	690	5	7.0	1.5	5	22%
w/meat sauce	1 entrée	290	14	45	560	5	6.0	1.5	15	19%
SPIRALS *(Chef Boyardee)* canned, spirals, in pizza sauce . . .	7.5 oz	180	5	35	1080	3	3.0	1.0	5	14%
ZITI										
(Budget Gourmet) Parmesano	1 entrée	260	11	39	550	4	7.0	2.0	10	24%
(Healthy Choice)										
w/zesty tomato sauce, frozen, 'Classics'	12 oz	350	16	59	530	0	5.0	2.0	30	13%
(Weight Watchers) w/mozzarella	1 entrée	280	11	45	430	4	6.0	1.5	5	19%
PASTA DISH/ENTRÉE MIX. See also NOODLE DISH/ENTRÉE MIX.										
(Fantastic Foods)										
salad, Italian herb, prepared	1 cup	170	7	34	380	2	1.5	0.5	0	8%
salad, Oriental, spicy, prepared	1 cup	200	7	37	420	3	3.0	0.0	0	13%
(Kraft) salad, Italian, 97% fat free, prepared	3/4 cup	190	8	35	740	2	2.0	1.0	3	9%
(Lunch Bucket)										
'Pasta 'n Chicken' microwave lunch cup	7.5 oz	180	9	22	860	0	6.0	0.0	45	30%
w/beef, in wine sauce, micro cup, 'Light'n Healthy'	7.5 oz	130	5	21	600	0	3.0	0.0	10	21%
(Pasta Roni) Parmesano pasta, 'Tenderthin' prepared	1 serving	226	7	28	536	1	9.6	2.5	6	38%
(Suddenly Salad)										
salad, classic, mix only	3/4 cup	190	7	38	910	2	1.5	0.0	0	7%
salad, classic, prepared	3/4 cup	250	7	38	910	2	8.0	1.0	0	29%
(Ultra Slim Fast)										
w/beef flavored sauce, prepared	8 oz	230	8	45	1070	4	3.0	0.0	0	11%
w/chicken flavored sauce, prep	8 oz	220	8	45	980	4	3.0	0.0	0	11%
w/tomato herb sauce, prep	8 oz	220	8	46	1090	5	3.0	0.0	0	11%
w/zesty cheese sauce, prepared	8 oz	230	9	44	770	4	4.0	0.0	0	15%
ANGEL HAIR										
(Golden Saute)										
w/chicken and broccoli, mix only	1/3 pkg	220	8	44	840	2	1.0	0.0	0	4%
w/chicken and broccoli, prepared	1 cup	270	8	44	910	2	7.0	1.0	0	23%
w/Parmesan, mix only	1/4 pkg	130	5	21	470	0	3.0	0.0	0	21%
w/Parmesan, prepared	1/2 cup	160	5	21	500	0	6.0	0.0	0	34%

Food Name	Serving Size	Calories	Prot. gms	Carbs gms	Sod. mgs	Fiber gms	Fat gms	Sat. Fat gms	Chol. mgs	% Fat Cal.
(Pasta Roni)										
w/Parmesan cheese, prepared	1 serving	145	4	18	404	1	6.5	1.4	2	40%
w/herb sauce, prepared	1 serving	145	4	19	379	1	6.3	1.1	2	38%
CORKSCREW										
(Pasta Roni)										
w/creamy garlic sauce, prepared	1 serving	190	4	18	456	1	11.1	2.3	2	53%
w/four cheese sauce, prepared	1 serving	231	7	28	587	1	10.2	2.8	6	40%
FETTUCINE										
(Pasta Roni)										
broccoli au gratin, prepared	1 serving	164	6	22	480	1	5.6	2.0	23	31%
cheddar, prepared	1 serving	169	6	23	500	1	5.9	2.0	6	32%
chicken, prepared	1 serving	181	6	23	576	1	7.6	1.4	3	37%
Romanoff, prepared	1 serving	231	7	27	604	1	10.7	3.1	6	42%
Stroganoff, prepared	1 serving	209	8	27	6	1	7.9	2.0	6	34%
w/Alfredo sauce, prepared	1 serving	265	6	27	627	1	14.1	3.4	6	50%
LINGUINE										
(Pasta Roni)										
linguine w/chicken and broccoli sauce, prepared	1 serving	209	6	28	565	2	9.0	2.3	3	37%
w/creamy chicken, Parmesan sauce, prepared	1 serving	231	7	26	621	1	10.4	2.5	3	41%
MACARONI										
(De Boles)										
and cheddar, w/artichoke pasta shells, mix only	2 oz	210	9	40	160	0	2.0	0.0	0	8%
and cheddar, w/artichoke pasta shells, prepared	3/4 cup	220	8	31	140	0	7.0	0.0	0	29%
and cheese, w/artichoke pasta elbows, 'Mac & Cheese' mix only	2 oz	210	9	40	160	0	2.0	0.0	0	8%
and cheese, w/artichoke pasta elbows, 'Mac & Cheese' prepared	3/4 cup	200	7	27	120	0	8.0	0.0	0	35%
and cheese, w/artichoke pasta elbows, mix only	1/2 cup	200	8	33	390	1	3.5	2.0	10	16%
and cheese, w/artichoke pasta elbows, prepared	3/4 cup	250	8	33	390	1	8.5	3.0	10	32%
and cheese, w/artichoke pasta shells, mix only	1/2 cup	200	8	33	390	1	3.5	2.0	10	16%
and cheese, w/artichoke pasta shells, prepared	3/4 cup	250	8	33	390	1	8.5	3.0	10	32%
and cheese, w/wheat pasta elbows, mix only	1/2 cup	200	8	32	390	3	4.0	2.0	10	18%
and cheese, w/wheat pasta elbows, prepared	3/4 cup	250	8	32	390	3	9.0	3.0	10	34%
elbows, w/cheese sauce, mix only	2 oz	210	9	40	160	0	2.0	0.0	0	8%
(Fantastic Foods)										
shells, w/curry, 'Tofu Classics' mix only	1/2 cup	200	8	40	500	5	1.5	0.0	0	7%
(Hodgson Mill)										
and cheese, w/whole wheat pasta, mix only	1 pkg	774	29	143	1259	16	9.7	2.8	16	11%
and cheese, w/whole wheat pasta, mix only	2.5 oz	263	10	48	428	5	3.3	1.0	6	11%
(Hormel) and cheese, micro cup	7.5 oz	189	7	26	874	0	6.0	0.0	17	29%
(Kraft)										
and cheese, 'Deluxe Dinner' prepared	3/4 cup	260	11	36	590	0	8.0	4.0	20	28%
and cheese, 'Dinner' prepared	3/4 cup	290	9	34	530	0	13.0	3.0	5	40%
and cheese, 'Dinomac Dinner' prepared	3/4 cup	310	9	36	560	0	14.0	3.0	10	41%
and cheese, 'Family Size Dinner' prepared	3/4 cup	290	9	34	490	0	13.0	3.0	5	40%
and cheese, original flavor, mix only	1 serving	259	11	48	561	1	2.6	1.3	10	9%
and cheese, 'Original' prepared	1 cup	410	12	49	750	1	18.0	4.5	10	40%
and cheese, 'Teddy Bears Dinner' prepared	3/4 cup	310	9	36	560	0	14.0	3.0	10	41%
and cheese, 'Wild Wheels Dinner' prepared	3/4 cup	310	9	36	560	0	14.0	3.0	10	41%
and cheese, w/spirals, 'Dinner' prepared	3/4 cup	340	9	36	600	0	18.0	4.0	10	47%
shells w/Velveeta, 'Original'	1 cup	360	16	44	1030	1	13.0	8.0	40	33%
(Libby's) and cheese, microwave cup, 'Diner'	7.5 oz	360	14	27	1020	2	22.0	9.0	35	55%
(Lipton) and cheese, w/shells, 'Hearty Ones'	11 oz	367	15	60	1406	0	7.4	0.0	14	18%
(Lunch Bucket)										
and cheese, microwave lunch cup	7.5 oz	210	9	24	990	0	9.0	0.0	0	38%

Food Name	Serving Size	Calories	Prot. gms	Carbs gms	Sod. mgs	Fiber gms	Fat gms	Sat. Fat gms	Chol. mgs	% Fat Cal.
and vegetables, micro cup, 'Light'n Healthy'	7.5 oz	150	4	30	630	0	1.0	0.0	0	6%
elbows, in tomato sauce, microwave lunch cup	7.5 oz	190	4	38	860	0	2.0	0.0	0	10%
(Nestlé) shells, w/sausage, canned, 'Chef-Mate'	1 cup	382	15	19	987	1	27.6	8.8	53	65%
(Pasta Roni) shells w/white cheddar, prepared	1 serving	220	7	27	649	1	9.0	2.5	8	38%
(Ultra Slim Fast) and cheese, prepared	1 cup	230	9	46	700	4	3.0	0.0	0	11%
PENNE										
(Golden Saute)										
stir-fry, w/chicken, mix only	1/2 cup	220	7	45	850	2	2.0	0.0	0	8%
stir fry, w/chicken, prepared	1 cup	270	7	45	920	2	8.0	1.0	0	26%
(Pasta Roni) w/herb and butter sauce	1 serving	194	4	19	339	1	11.1	2.5	0	52%
RIGATONI										
(Pasta Roni)										
w/tomato basil sauce, prepared	1 serving	81	2	12	237	1	3.0	0.3	0	34%
w/white cheddar and broccoli sauce, prepared	1 serving	181	5	22	415	1	8.6	2.3	5	42%
ROTINI										
(Golden Saute)										
w/chicken, herbs, and Parmesan, mix only	1 cup	280	8	45	900	3	9.0	2.5	5	28%
SPAGHETTI										
(Chef Boyardee)										
w/condensed meat sauce, 'Dinner' prepared	3.25 oz	250	12	37	595	0	6.0	0.0	0	22%
w/meat sauce, 'Dinner' prepared	7.9 oz	240	12	42	1155	0	3.0	0.0	0	11%
w/mushroom sauce, 'Dinner' prepared	7.9 oz	210	11	41	1085	0	1.0	0.0	0	4%
(Fantastic Foods) w/whole wheat noodles, low-fat,										
'All-O-Round' prepared	10 oz	211	10	45	275	2	2.0		4	8%
(Hormel) w/meatballs, micro cup	7.5 oz	210	10	27	930	0	7.0	3.0	20	30%
(Kid's Kitchen)										
rings, microwave cup, mix only	7.5 oz	180	8	35	930	0	1.0	1.0	10	5%
rings and franks, w/tomato sauce, micro cup, mix only	7.5 oz	290	12	33	960	0	12.0	0.0	30	38%
w/meatballs, microwave cup	7.5 oz	220	11	26	880	0	8.0	4.0	20	33%
(Kraft)										
mild, 'American Style Dinner' prepared	1 cup	300	10	50	630	0	7.0	2.0	0	21%
tangy, 'Italian Style Dinner' prepared	1 cup	310	11	49	670	0	8.0	2.0	5	23%
w/meat sauce, 'Dinner' prepared	1 cup	360	12	47	880	0	14.0	4.0	15	35%
(Libby's) w/meatballs, in sauce, 'Diner' micro cup	7.75 oz	190	10	31	870	2	3.0	1.0	15	14%
(Lunch Bucket) and meat sauce' microwave lunch cup	7.5 oz	240	9	39	870	0	5.0	0.0	30	19%
(Mountain House)										
w/meat and sauce, freeze-dried, prepared	1 cup	260	12	41	0	0	5.0	0.0	0	18%
VERMICELLI										
(Pasta Roni) w/garlic and olive oil sauce, prepared	1 serving	203	5	27	570	1	8.8	1.4	0	38%
PASTA SAUCE. See under SAUCE.										
PASTA SEASONING. See under SEASONING MIX.										
PASTRY. See also CAKE, SNACK; PASTRY, TOASTER.										
(Tio Pepe's) churro, original	1 serving	140	2	14	180	0	9.0	2.0	10	56%
(Entenmann's) Danish ring	1.5 oz	180	3	18	160	0	10.0	0.0	0	52%
APPLE										
(Aunt Fanny's)										
cinnamon roll, old-fashioned, individual	2 oz	180	4	34	125	2	1.0	1.5	5	6%
strudel, individual	3 oz	330	4	38	210	0	18.0	7.0	0	49%
(Awrey's)										
filled Danish, 2.75 oz, 'Round'	1 piece	270	3	34	310	1	14.0	3.0	5	46%
filled Danish, 4.5 oz, 'Round'	1 piece	390	4	50	390	1	20.0	4.0	10	45%
filled Danish, 3 oz, 'Square'	1 piece	220	3	34	230	1	8.0	2.0	10	33%
filled Danish, 1.7 oz, miniature	1 piece	160	2	21	170	1	8.0	2.0	5	44%
(Break Cake)										
roll, sweet, 1.4 oz, multi-pak	1 roll	120	2	24	150	0	2.0	0.5	0	15%

Food Name	Serving Size	Calories	Prot. gms	Carbs gms	Sod. mgs	Fiber gms	Fat gms	Sat. Fat gms	Chol. mgs	% Fat Cal.
roll, sweet, 4.5 oz	2 rolls	380	8	75	460	0	5.0	1.6	0	12%
(Entenmann's)										
'Apple Puffs'	1 puff	280	4	39	320	0	13.0	0.0	0	40%
strudel, old-fashioned	1.5 oz	120	1	17	110	0	5.0	0.0	0	38%
(Hormel) 'Apple Dulcita'	4 oz	290	5	44	350	0	10.0	0.0	0	31%
(Hostess) filled Danish, fried, 'Breakfast Bake Shop'	1 piece	400	4	46	340	2	22.0	10.0	20	50%
(Pepperidge Farm)										
crisp, 'Berkshire'	1 ramekin	250	2	43	130	1	8.0	4.0	4	29%
Danish, 2-1/4 oz	1 piece	220	2	35	130	0	8.0	0.0	0	33%
fruit square	1 piece	220	2	27	170	0	12.0	0.0	0	48%
turnover, frozen	1 piece	300	3	34	210	0	17.0	0.0	0	51%
turnover, ready to bake	1 serving	284	4	31	176	2	16.0	4.0	na	51%
(Pillsbury)										
cinnamon roll, w/icing, ready to bake	1 roll	140	2	21	310	1	5.0	1.5	0	33%
pocket	1 piece	240	4	25	520	0	13.0	3.0	0	50%
turnover, refrigerated	1 piece	170	2	23	320	0	8.0	2.0	0	42%
(Sara Lee)										
Danish twist	1/8 pkg	190	3	22	200	0	10.0	0.0	10	47%
Danish, 'Free & Light'	1/8 pkg	130	2	30	120	0	0.0	0.0	0	0%
Danish, 'Individual' 1.3 oz	1 piece	120	2	15	120	0	6.0	0.0	0	44%
(Tastykake) pocket	3 oz	323	4	38	222	2	17.6	4.0	11	48%
(Tio Pepe's) churro, apple filled, regular size	1 serving	160	2	22	115	1	7.0	1.5	15	40%
(Weight Watchers)										
crisp, 'Sweet Celebrations'	1/2 pkg	190	1	40	190	0	5.0	1.0	0	22%
roll, sweet 'Microwave'	1/2 pkg	160	3	27	100	0	4.0	1.0	5	23%
APRICOT										
(Entenmann's) Danish twist, fat-free, cholesterol-free	1 slice	150	3	34	110	1	0.0	0.0	0	0%
(Tio Pepe's) filled churro, regular size	1 serving	170	2	25	130	1	7.0	1.5	15	37%
BAVARIAN CREAM										
(Entenmann's)	1.3 oz	80	2	20	90	0	0.0	0.0	0	0%
(Rich's) cream puff	1 piece	150	2	17	70	0	8.0	0.0	25	49%
(Tio Pepe's) filled churro, regular size	1 serving	160	2	22	120	0	7.0	1.5	15	40%
BLACK FOREST (Entenmann's) fat-free, cholesterol-free	1 slice	130	3	32	115	2	0.0	0.0	0	0%
BLUEBERRY, turnover (Pepperidge Farm)	1 piece	310	3	32	230	0	19.0	0.0	0	55%
CARAMEL (Pillsbury) w/nuts	1 piece	160	2	19	240	0	8.0	2.0	0	46%
CHEESE										
(Awrey's)										
filled Danish, 4.5 oz, 'Round'	1 piece	420	5	52	530	1	22.0	5.0	15	46%
filled Danish, 2.75 oz, 'Round'	1 piece	280	3	34	350	1	15.0	3.0	10	48%
filled Danish, 2.5 oz, 'Square'	1 piece	210	4	25	300	1	11.0	3.0	15	46%
filled Danish, miniature 1.7 oz	1 piece	170	2	21	200	4	9.0	2.0	5	47%
(Pepperidge Farm) Danish, 2-1/4 oz	1 piece	240	3	25	230	0	14.0	0.0	0	53%
(Sara Lee)										
Danish, 'Individual' 1.3 oz	1 piece	130	2	13	130	0	8.0	0.0	0	55%
Danish twist	1/8 pkg	200	3	21	270	0	12.0	0.0	15	53%
(Tastykake) pocket	3 oz	325	4	41	231	1	16.7	3.9	11	45%
CHERRY										
(Aunt Fanny's) strudel, individual	3 oz	320	4	39	190	0	16.0	6.5	5	46%
(Hormel) 'Cherry Dulcita'	4 oz	300	5	48	345	0	9.0	0.0	0	28%
(Pepperidge Farm) turnover	1 piece	310	3	32	280	0	19.0	0.0	0	55%
(Pillsbury) turnover	1 piece	170	2	23	320	0	8.0	2.0	0	42%
CHOCOLATE										
Fresh										
churro, creme filled, regular size (Tio Pepe's)	1 serving	180	2	28	140	0	7.0	2.0	15	34%

Food Name	Serving Size	Calories	Prot. gms	Carbs gms	Sod. mgs	Fiber gms	Fat gms	Sat. Fat gms	Chol. mgs	% Fat Cal.
fudge tart, frosted *(Toastettes)*	1 serving	190	2	34	280	1	5.0	1.5	0	24%
Frozen or refrigerated										
éclair *(Weight Watchers)*	1 serving	150	2	25	160	2	4.0	1.0	30	25%
éclair, 'Sweet Celebrations' *(Weight Watchers)*	2.1 oz	150	3	26	110	0	4.0	2.0	15	24%
éclair, triple chocolate *(Weight Watchers)*	1 serving	160	3	25	190	1	5.0	1.0	30	29%
éclair, 2 oz *(Rich's)*	1 piece	210	2	27	110	0	10.0	0.0	35	44%
CINNAMON										
(Awrey's) cinnamon-walnut Danish, 'Round' 2.75 oz	1 piece	300	4	31	290	1	18.0	3.0	5	54%
(Entenmann's) filbert ring	1.5 oz	190	3	19	160	0	12.0	0.0	0	55%
(Tio Pepe's) churro	1 churro	110	1	14	100	2	5.0	1.5	15	43%
CINNAMON-RAISIN										
(Awrey's)										
filled Danish, 3 oz, 'Square'	1 piece	290	3	41	280	1	12.0	3.0	15	38%
filled Danish, miniature 1.5 oz	1 piece	160	2	21	150	1	8.0	2.0	5	44%
(Entenmann's) bun, nonfat, no cholesterol	1 serving	160	3	36	125	1	0.0	0.0	0	0%
(Pepperidge Farm) Danish, 2-1/4 oz	1 piece	250	3	35	170	0	11.0	0.0	0	39%
(Pillsbury) Danish, w/icing	1 piece	150	2	20	230	0	7.0	2.0	0	42%
(Sara Lee) Danish, individual, 1.3 oz	1 piece	150	2	17	140	0	8.0	0.0	0	49%
DATE NUT *(Awrey's)* 1 piece	1.6 oz	230	2	35	150	1	10.0	2.0	15	38%
ÉCLAIR *(Tasty-Klair)* custard-filled, prepared	1 pie	296	7	27	381	1	17.7	4.7	144	54%
LEMON										
(Entenmann's)										
lemon Danish twist	1.2 oz	140	2	17	140	0	7.0	0.0	0	45%
twist, fat-free, cholesterol-free	1 slice	130	3	31	140	1	0.0	0.0	0	0%
NUT										
(Flanigan Farms)										
and fruit, almond, raisin, date, sunflower seed, no salt	1/4 cup	130	4	12	0	1	8.0	0.5	0	53%
peanut, raisin, and sunflower seed, no salt	1/4 cup	130	5	11	4	1	10.0	1.0	0	58%
ORANGE *(Pillsbury)* Danish, w/icing	1 piece	150	2	19	250	0	7.0	2.0	0	43%
PEACH *(Pepperidge Farm)* turnover	1 piece	310	3	34	260	0	18.0	0.0	0	52%
PECAN *(Entenmann's)* Danish ring	1.5 oz	190	3	19	130	0	12.0	0.0	0	55%
PINEAPPLE *(Awrey's)* filled Danish, miniature, 1.7 oz	1 piece	157	2	21	180	1	8.0	2.0	5	44%
RASPBERRY										
(Awrey's) filled Danish, 3 oz, 'Square'	1 piece	260	3	45	210	1	8.0	2.0	10	27%
(Entenmann's)										
cheese, fat-free, cholesterol-free	1 slice	140	3	32	110	1	0.0	0.0	0	0%
Danish twist	1.2 oz	140	2	18	120	0	7.0	0.0	0	44%
(Hostess) raspberry-filled Danish, fried	1 piece	390	4	49	290	2	20.0	10.0	20	46%
(Pepperidge Farm)										
raspberry Danish, 2 1/4 oz	1 piece	220	3	31	140	0	9.0	0.0	0	37%
turnover	1 piece	310	4	36	260	0	17.0	0.0	0	49%
(Sara Lee) raspberry Danish twist, 1/8 pkg	1/8 pkg	200	3	25	220	0	9.0	0.0	15	42%
(Tio Pepe's) churro, regular size	1 serving	160	2	23	125	1	7.0	1.5	15	39%
STRAWBERRY										
(Awrey's)										
filled Danish, 4.5 oz, 'Round'	1 piece	400	4	53	410	1	20.0	4.0	10	44%
filled Danish, 2.75 oz, 'Round'	1 piece	270	3	34	320	1	14.0	3.0	5	46%
filled Danish, miniature, 1.7 oz	1 piece	160	2	21	180	0	8.0	2.0	5	44%
WALNUT *(Entenmann's)* Danish ring	1.5 oz	190	3	19	130	0	12.0	0.0	0	55%
PASTRY, TOASTER										
APPLE										
(Auburn Farms)										
cinnamon, nonfat	1 pastry	157	2	36	162	1	0.5	0.0	0	3%
cinnamon, 'Toast 'n Jammers'	1 pastry	180	3	42	200	4	0.0	0.0	0	0%

Food Name	Serving Size	Calories	Prot. gms	Carbs gms	Sod. mgs	Fiber gms	Fat gms	Sat. Fat gms	Chol. mgs	% Fat Cal.
(Kellogg's)										
cinnamon, frosted, low-fat, 'Pop Tarts'	1 pastry	191	2	40	206	1	2.9	0.6	0	13%
cinnamon, 'Pop Tarts'	1 pastry	205	2	37	174	1	5.3	0.9	0	23%
cinnamon Danish, 'Pastry Swirls' 'Pop Tarts'	1 pastry	256	3	37	190	1	11.0	3.0	0	39%
(Pepperidge Farm)										
cinnamon, 'Croissant Toaster Tarts'	1 pastry	170	3	25	120	0	7.0	2.0	0	36%
(Pastry Poppers) fruit juice sweetened, low-sodium	2 oz	212	3	38	115	0	5.4	0.0	0	23%
(Pillsbury)										
'Danish' 'Toaster Strudel'	1 pastry	197	3	25	188	1	9.8	1.5	21	44%
spice, 'Muffins' 'Toaster Strudel'	1 pastry	130	2	21	100	0	5.0	0.0	0	33%
'Toaster Strudel'	1 pastry	180	3	9	190	1	7.0	1.5	5	57%
(Toastettes)										
'Frosted Tarts'	1 pastry	190	2	35	170	1	5.0	1.0	0	23%
'Tarts'	1 pastry	190	2	36	170	1	5.0	1.0	0	23%
BANANA NUT										
(Pillsbury)										
'Muffins' 'Toaster Strudel'	1 pastry	130	2	19	85	0	6.0	0.0	0	39%
'Strudel Breakfast Pastries' 'Toaster Strudel'	1 pastry	190	2	28	190	0	8.0	0.0	0	38%
BERRY *(Kellogg's)* wild, frosted, 'Pop Tarts'	1 pastry	210	2	39	168	1	5.0	1.4	0	21%
BLUEBERRY										
(Auburn Farms) nonfat	1 pastry	165	3	38	189	2	0.5	0.0	0	3%
(Howard Johnson's) frozen, ready to eat, 'Toasties'	1 serving	235	5	32	408	na	9.7	1.5	21	37%
(Kellogg's)										
frosted, 'Pop Tarts'	1 pastry	203	2	37	207	1	5.2	1.0	0	23%
low-fat, 'Pop Tarts'	1 pastry	192	2	40	222	1	2.9	0.6	0	13%
plain, 'Pop Tarts'	1 pastry	212	2	36	207	1	6.9	1.1	0	29%
(Pastry Poppers) fruit juice sweetened, low-sodium	2 oz	212	3	38	115	0	4.5	0.0	0	20%
(Pillsbury)										
	1 pastry	180	3	9	200	1	7.0	1.5	5	57%
'Strudel Breakfast Pastries' 'Toaster Strudel'	1 pastry	190	2	28	200	0	8.0	0.0	0	38%
'Toaster Strudel'	1 pastry	190	3	26	210	0	9.0	2.0	5	41%
wild, Maine, 'Toaster Strudel'	1 pastry	120	2	23	135	0	3.0	0.0	0	21%
(Toastettes)										
'Frosted Tarts'	1 pastry	190	2	35	190	1	5.0	1.5	0	23%
'Tarts'	1 pastry	190	2	35	200	1	5.0	1.0	0	23%
BRAN *(Thomas')* 'Toast-r-Cakes'	1 pastry	103	2	18	163	0	2.9	0.0	0	25%
BROWN SUGAR CINNAMON										
(Kellogg's)										
frosted, 'Pop Tarts'	1 pastry	211	3	34	185	1	7.4	1.1	0	32%
frosted w/cinnamon, low-fat, 'Pop Tarts'	1 pastry	188	2	39	210	1	2.8	0.6	0	13%
plain, 'Pop Tarts'	1 pastry	219	3	32	214	1	9.2	1.0	0	38%
CHEESE										
(Kellogg's) Danish, 'Pastry Swirls' 'Pop Tarts'	1 pastry	252	3	37	180	0	11.0	3.0	1	39%
(Pepperidge Farm) 'Croissant Toaster Tarts'	1 pastry	190	5	22	180	0	10.0	3.0	10	45%
(Pillsbury)										
cream cheese	1 pastry	190	3	9	230	0	10.0	3.5	15	65%
cream cheese, w/blueberry	1 pastry	190	3	9	220	1	9.0	3.0	10	63%
cream cheese, w/strawberry	1 pastry	190	3	9	220	1	9.0	3.0	10	63%
CHERRY										
(Kellogg's)										
low-fat, 'Pop Tarts'	1 pastry	192	2	40	222	1	2.9	0.6	0	13%
plain, 'Pop Tarts'	1 pastry	204	2	37	220	1	5.4	0.9	0	24%
(Pastry Poppers) fruit juice sweetened, low-sodium	2 oz	212	3	38	115	0	4.5	0.0	0	20%

Food Name	Serving Size	Calories	Prot. gms	Carbs gms	Sod. mgs	Fiber gms	Fat gms	Sat. Fat gms	Chol. mgs	% Fat Cal.
(Pillsbury)										
....	1 pastry	180	3	9	200	1	7.0	1.5	5	57%
'Strudel Breakfast Pastries' 'Toaster Strudel'	1 pastry	190	2	26	200	0	9.0	0.0	0	42%
'Toaster Strudel'	1 pastry	190	3	26	200	1	8.0	1.5	5	38%
(Toastettes)										
'Frosted Tarts'	1 pastry	190	2	35	180	1	5.0	1.5	0	23%
'Tarts'	1 pastry	190	2	35	200	1	5.0	1.0	0	23%
CHOCOLATE FUDGE										
(Kellogg's)										
fudge, frosted, 'Pop Tarts'	1 pastry	201	3	37	203	1	4.8	1.0	0	22%
fudge, frosted, low-fat, 'Pop Tarts'	1 pastry	190	3	40	249	1	3.0	0.5	0	14%
milk chocolate, 'Pop Tarts' *(Kellogg's)*	1 pastry	205	3	36	227	1	5.8	1.5	0	26%
vanilla creme, frosted, 'Pop Tarts'	1 pastry	203	3	37	229	1	5.3	1.0	0	23%
CINNAMON										
(Pillsbury)										
....	1 pastry	190	3	9	200	1	8.0	1.5	5	60%
'Danish' 'Toaster Strudel'	1 pastry	214	4	24	197	1	11.9	3.0	11	49%
'Strudel Breakfast Pastries' 'Toaster Strudel'	1 pastry	190	2	26	200	0	8.0	0.0	0	39%
'Toaster Strudel'	1/6 pkg	200	5	23	200	0	10.0	2.0	5	45%
(Toastettes) frosted, brown sugar cinnamon	1 pastry	190	2	35	180	1	5.0	1.5	0	23%
CORN										
(Pillsbury) old-fashioned, 'Muffins' 'Toaster Strudel'	1 pastry	120	2	17	200	0	5.0	0.0	0	37%
(Oroweat) toaster biscuit	1 biscuit	200	5	39	230	1	3.0	1.0	5	13%
FRENCH TOAST *(Pillsbury)*	1 pastry	190	3	9	200	1	7.0	1.5	5	57%
FRUIT PUNCH *(Toastettes)* 'Frosted Tarts'	1 pastry	190	2	35	200	1	5.0	1.0	0	23%
GRAPE *(Kellogg's)* frosted, 'Pop Tarts'	1 pastry	203	2	38	198	1	5.1	0.9	0	23%
LEMON *(Pillsbury)* 'Danish' 'Toaster Strudel'	1 pastry	197	3	25	188	1	9.8	1.5	21	44%
OAT BRAN *(Awrey's)* w/raisins, 'Toastums'	1 pastry	130	3	17	310	1	5.0	1.0	0	36%
PEACH-APRICOT										
(Pastry Poppers) fruit juice sweetened, low-salt	2 oz	212	3	38	115	0	4.5	0.0	0	20%
RAISIN										
RAISIN BRAN										
(Pillsbury)										
bran, 'Muffins' 'Toaster Strudel'	1 pastry	120	3	16	220	0	5.0	0.0	0	37%
'Danish' 'Toaster Strudel'	1 pastry	197	3	25	188	1	9.8	1.5	21	44%
RASPBERRY										
(Auburn Farms)										
nonfat	1 pastry	180	3	42	200	4	0.0	0.0	0	0%
'Toast 'n Jammers' *(Auburn Farms)*	1 pastry	180	3	42	200	3	0.0	0.0	0	0%
(Kellogg's) frosted, 'Pop Tarts'	1 pastry	205	2	37	211	1	5.5	1.0	0	24%
(Pastry Poppers) fruit juice sweetened, low-sodium	2 oz	212	3	38	115	0	4.5	0.0	0	20%
(Pillsbury)										
....	1 pastry	180	3	9	200	1	7.0	1.5	5	57%
'Danish' 'Toaster Strudel'	1 pastry	197	3	25	188	1	9.8	1.5	21	44%
'Strudel Breakfast Pastries' 'Toaster Strudel'	1 pastry	190	2	27	200	0	8.0	0.0	0	38%
'Toaster Strudel'	1 pastry	180	3	26	200	1	7.0	1.5	5	35%
S'MORES *(Kellogg's)* 'Pop Tarts'	1 pastry	204	3	36	199	1	5.5	1.5	0	24%
STRAWBERRY										
(Auburn Farms) nonfat	1 pastry	180	3	42	200	4	0.0	0.0	0	0%
(Kellogg's)										
frosted, 'Pop Tarts'	1 pastry	203	2	38	169	1	5.0	1.4	0	22%
frosted, low-fat, 'Pop Tarts'	1 pastry	191	2	40	201	1	3.0	0.6	0	14%
low-fat, 'Pop Tarts'	1 pastry	192	2	40	220	1	2.9	0.6	0	13%
'Pastry Swirls' 'Pop Tarts'	1 pastry	254	3	37	170	1	11.0	3.0	0	39%

Food Name	Serving Size	Calories	Prot. gms	Carbs gms	Sod. mgs	Fiber gms	Fat gms	Sat. Fat gms	Chol. mgs	% Fat Cal.
'Pop Tarts'	1 pastry	210	2	37	200	0	6.0	0.0	0	26%
(Pastry Poppers) fruit juice sweetened, low-sodium	2 oz	212	3	38	115	0	4.5	0.0	0	20%
(Pepperidge Farm) 'Croissant Toaster Tarts'	1 pastry	190	3	28	120	0	7.0	2.0	0	34%
(Pillsbury)	1 pastry	180	3	9	200	1	7.0	1.5	5	57%
'Danish' 'Toaster Strudel'	1 pastry	197	3	25	188	1	9.8	1.5	21	44%
'Strudel Breakfast Pastries' 'Toaster Strudel'	1 pastry	190	2	27	200	0	8.0	0.0	0	38%
'Toaster Strudel'	1 pastry	180	3	26	200	1	7.0	1.5	5	35%
(Toast N' Jammers) 100% juice sweetened, whole wheat	1 pastry	165	3	38	189	2	0.5	0.0	0	3%
(Toastettes) frosted	1 pastry	190	2	35	190	1	5.0	1.5	0	23%
PASTRY FLOUR. See under FLOUR.										
PÂTÉ, CANNED										
chicken liver	1 oz	57	4	2	109	0	3.7	1.1	111	59%
chicken liver	1 tbsp	26	2	1	50	0	1.7	0.5	51	59%
goose liver, de foie gras, smoked	1 oz	131	3	1	198	0	12.4	4.1	43	86%
goose liver, de foie gras, smoked	1 tbsp	60	1	1	91	0	5.7	1.9	20	86%
liver (Sells)	2.25 oz	190	8	3	460	0	16.0	0.0	0	77%
PATTYPAN SQUASH. See SQUASH, SCALLOP.										
PEACH										
Canned										
extra light, halves or slices, w/liquid	1 cup	104	1	27	12	2	0.2	0.0	0	2%
halves (Hunt's)	1/2 cup	100	1	24	10	1	0.0	0.0	0	0%
in extra heavy syrup, halves or slices, w/liquid	1 cup	252	1	68	21	3	0.1	0.0	0	0%
in heavy syrup, halves, w/liquid	1/2 med fruit	73	0	20	6	1	0.1	0.0	0	1%
in heavy syrup, slices, w/liquid	1 cup	194	1	52	16	3	0.3	0.0	0	1%
in juice, halves, w/liquid	1/2 fruit	43	1	11	4	1	0.0	0.0	0	1%
in juice, halves or slices, w/liquid	1 cup	109	2	29	10	3	0.1	0.0	0	1%
in light syrup, halves, w/liquid	1/2 fruit	53	0	14	5	1	0.0	0.0	0	0%
in light syrup, halves or slices, w/liquid	1 cup	136	1	37	13	3	0.1	0.0	0	0%
in water, halves, w/liquid	1/2 fruit	24	0	6	3	1	0.1	0.0	0	2%
in water, halves or slices, w/liquid	1 cup	59	1	15	7	3	0.1	0.0	0	2%
sliced (Hunt's)	1/2 cup	100	1	24	10	1	0.0	0.0	0	0%
spiced, in heavy syrup, whole, w/liquid	1 cup	182	1	49	10	3	0.2	0.0	0	1%
Dried										
sulfured, stewed	1 cup	322	5	83	10	na	1.0	0.1	0	3%
sulfured, uncooked	1 cup	377	6	96	12	na	1.2	0.1	0	3%
sulfured, uncooked, halves	1 cup	382	6	98	11	13	1.2	0.1	0	3%
sulfured, uncooked, halves	1/2 medium	31	0	8	1	1	0.1	0.0	0	3%
sulfured, w/added sugar	1 cup	278	3	72	5	6	0.6	0.1	0	2%
sulfured, w/o added sugar	1 cup	199	3	51	5	7	0.6	0.1	0	3%
Fresh										
raw, sliced	1 cup	73	1	19	0	3	0.2	0.0	0	2%
raw, whole, large, 2.75 inch diam, 2.5 per lb	1 peach	68	1	17	0	3	0.1	0.0	0	2%
raw, whole, medium, 2.5 inch diam, 4 per lb	1 peach	42	1	11	0	2	0.1	0.0	0	2%
raw, whole, small, 2 inch diam, 5 per lb	1 peach	34	1	9	0	2	0.1	0.0	0	2%
Frozen										
in syrup, sliced (Flav-R-Pac)	2/3 cup	100	1	25	0	1	0.0	0.0	0	0%
sliced (Flav-R-Pac)	2/3 cup	50	1	13	0	2	0.0	0.0	0	0%
sliced, thawed	1 cup	235	2	60	15	5	0.3	0.0	0	1%
sweetened, sliced	10-oz pkg	267	2	68	17	5	0.4	0.0	0	1%
sweetened, sliced	10 med slices	146	1	37	9	3	0.2	0.0	0	1%
PEACH BUTTER, nonfat (Smucker's)	1 tsp	15	0	4	0	0	0.0	0.0	0	0%
PEACH DRINK. See under FRUIT DRINK; FRUIT JUICE BLEND; FRUIT JUICE DRINK; PEACH JUICE.										
PEACH JUICE										
(Dole) orchard blend, 'Pure & Light'	6 fl oz	90	0	24	10	0	0.0	0.0	0	0%

Food Name	Serving Size	Calories	Prot. gms	Carbs gms	Sod. mgs	Fiber gms	Fat gms	Sat. Fat gms	Chol. mgs	% Fat Cal.
(Mountain Sun) 'Mountain Peach' organic	8 fl oz	112	0	27	0	0	0.0	0.0	0	0%
(Smucker's) 'Naturally 100%'	8 fl oz	120	1	30	10	0	0.0	0.0	0	0%
PEANUT										
ALL TYPES										
lightly salted, shelled (Eagle)	1 oz	180	7	5	65	2	15.0	3.0	0	74%
salted (Frito-Lay's)...........................	1 oz	170	6	6	170	0	15.0	0.0	0	74%
salted in shell, shelled (Fisher)	1/4 cup	170	7	6	170	2	14.0	2.0	0	71%
salted, shelled (Little Debbie)	1.25 oz	230	10	5	90	0	18.0	0.0	1	73%
shelled (Beer Nuts)	1 oz	180	7	7	60	0	14.0	0.0	0	69%
shelled (Weight Watchers)	1 pouch	100	8	4	50	0	7.0	0.0	0	57%
shelled, 'Ballpark' (Eagle)	1 oz	180	8	5	110	1	15.0	3.0	0	72%
shelled, 'Sweet & Crunchy' (Pathmark).......	1 oz	140	4	15	30	0	8.0	0.0	0	49%
shelled, 'Sweet-N-Crunchy' (Planters).......	1 oz	140	4	15	20	0	8.0	1.0	0	49%
spicy, hot, shelled, 'Heat' (Planters)........	1 oz	170	7	5	190	0	14.0	2.0	0	72%
spicy, mild, shelled, 'Heat' (Planters).......	1 oz	170	7	5	130	0	14.0	2.0	0	72%
unsalted, shelled (Little Debbie)	1.25 oz	230	10	5	1	0	18.0	0.0	0	73%
Dry roasted										
lightly salted (Finast)........................	1 oz	160	8	6	120	0	14.0	0.0	0	69%
lightly salted (Fisher)........................	1 oz	160	7	6	100	0	14.0	2.0	0	71%
lightly salted (Planters)	1 oz	170	7	5	110	0	15.0	2.0	0	74%
salted (Fisher)...............................	1 oz	160	7	6	210	0	14.0	2.0	0	71%
salted (Flavor House)	1 oz	180	8	5	200	0	14.0	0.0	0	71%
salted (Frito-Lay's)..........................	1 1/8 oz	190	7	7	300	0	16.0	0.0	0	72%
salted (Guy's)	1 oz	170	8	3	310	0	14.0	0.0	0	74%
salted (Pathmark)	1 oz	170	7	5	150	0	14.0	0.0	0	72%
salted (Planters)	1 oz	160	7	6	250	0	14.0	2.0	0	71%
unsalted (Finast)	1 oz	160	7	5	15	0	14.0	0.0	0	72%
unsalted (Flavor House)	1 oz	180	8	5	0	0	14.0	0.0	0	71%
unsalted (Pathmark)	1 oz	170	7	5	0	0	14.0	0.0	0	72%
unsalted (Planters)	1 oz	170	7	5	0	0	15.0	2.0	0	74%
unsalted, natural (Flanigan Farms)	1 oz	170	7	6	1	na	14.0	na	0	71%
unsalted, 'No Frills' (Pathmark)	1 oz	180	8	5	0	0	14.0	2.0	0	71%
Golden roasted										
(Fisher)	1/4 cup	160	7	10	220	2	12.0	2.0	0	61%
barbecue, crunchy (Fisher)	1/4 cup	160	7	10	210	2	11.0	2.0	0	59%
Honey roasted										
(Fisher)	1/4 cup	170	6	7	110	1	13.0	2.5	0	69%
(Flavor House)...............................	1 oz	160	6	9	120	0	11.0	0.0	0	62%
(Little Debbie)	1.13 oz	190	8	9	15	0	13.0	0.0	1	63%
(Pathmark)	1 oz	170	6	8	75	0	13.0	0.0	0	68%
(Planters)....................................	1 oz	170	6	8	180	0	13.0	2.0	0	68%
(Weight Watchers)	1 pouch	100	8	4	50	0	7.0	0.0	0	57%
'Honey Roast' (Eagle)	1 oz	170	7	7	140	0	13.0	0.0	0	68%
unsalted (Fisher).............................	1 oz	150	7	4	0	0	13.0	2.0	0	73%
Oil roasted										
(Fisher)	1/4 cup	170	7	5	130	2	15.0	2.5	0	74%
(Planters)....................................	1 oz	170	7	5	110	0	14.0	2.0	0	72%
lightly salted (Planters)	1 oz	170	7	5	80	0	14.0	2.0	0	72%
lightly salted	1 oz	160	7	6	65	0	14.0	0.0	0	71%
redskin (Planters)	1 oz	170	7	5	150	0	15.0	5.0	0	74%
salted (Flavor House)	1 oz	170	7	5	125	0	15.0	0.0	0	74%
salted (Pathmark)	1 oz	180	8	5	150	0	14.0	0.0	0	71%
salted (Planters)	1 oz	170	7	5	160	0	15.0	3.0	0	74%

Food Name	Serving Size	Calories	Prot. gms	Carbs gms	Sod. mgs	Fiber gms	Fat gms	Sat. Fat gms	Chol. mgs	% Fat Cal.
salted, cocktail (Planters)	1 oz	170	7	5	160	0	15.0	3.0	0	74%
unsalted (Planters)	1 oz	170	7	5	0	0	14.0	2.0	0	72%
unsalted, cocktail (Planters)	1 oz	170	7	5	0	0	15.0	3.0	0	74%
Raw										
	1 cup	828	38	24	26	12	71.9	10.0	0	73%
	1 oz	161	7	5	5	2	14.0	1.9	0	73%
Roasted										
salted, in shell (Planters)	1.5 oz	170	7	5	240	0	14.0	2.0	0	72%
unsalted, in shell (Planters)	1.5 oz	170	7	5	0	0	14.0	2.0	0	72%
Yogurt coated (Harmony)	17 pieces	210	4	21	30	1	13.0	6.0	0	54%
SPANISH										
shelled, salted (Guy's)	1 oz	170	8	3	170	0	14.0	0.0	0	74%
Dry roasted (Planters)	1 oz	160	7	6	200	0	14.0	3.0	0	71%
Oil roasted										
(Flavor House)	1 oz	170	7	5	125	0	15.0	0.0	0	74%
(Planters)	1 oz	170	7	5	100	0	15.0	5.0	0	74%
Raw										
	1 cup	832	38	23	32	14	72.4	11.2	0	73%
	1 oz	162	7	4	6	3	14.1	2.2	0	73%
(Planters)	1 oz	160	7	5	5	0	14.0	2.0	0	72%
salted (Fisher)	1 oz	160	7	5	0	0	14.0	2.0	0	72%
Roasted										
salted (Eagle)	1 oz	180	7	5	135	2	15.0	2.0	0	74%
salted (Fisher)	1/4 cup	180	5	6	130	2	16.0	2.5	0	77%
VALENCIA										
Oil roasted										
unsalted	1 cup	848	39	23	1112	13	73.8	11.4	0	73%
unsalted	1 oz	167	8	5	219	3	14.5	2.2	0	73%
Raw										
unsalted	1 cup	832	37	31	1	13	69.5	10.7	0	70%
unsalted	1 oz	162	7	6	0	2	13.5	2.1	0	70%
VIRGINIA										
Oil roasted										
unsalted	1 cup	827	37	28	619	13	69.5	9.1	0	70%
unsalted	1 oz	164	7	6	123	3	13.8	1.8	0	70%
Raw										
unsalted	1 cup	822	37	24	15	12	71.2	9.3	0	72%
unsalted	1 oz	160	7	5	3	2	13.8	1.8	0	72%
PEANUT BUTTER										
chunky	1 cup	1520	62	56	1254	17	128.8	24.7	0	71%
chunky	2 tbsp	188	8	7	156	2	16.0	3.1	0	71%
chunky, no salt added	1 cup	1520	62	56	44	17	128.8	24.7	0	71%
chunky, no salt added	2 tbsp	188	8	7	5	2	16.0	3.1	0	71%
smooth	1 cup	1530	65	50	1205	15	131.7	26.7	0	72%
smooth	2 tbsp	190	8	6	149	2	16.3	3.3	0	72%
smooth, no salt added	1 cup	1530	65	50	44	15	131.7	26.7	0	72%
smooth, no salt added	2 tbsp	190	8	6	5	2	16.3	3.3	0	72%
(Arrowhead Mills)										
chunky	2 tbsp	190	9	6	1	5	16.0	0.0	0	71%
creamy	2 tbsp	190	9	6	1	5	16.0	0.0	0	71%
(Bama)										
chunky	2 tbsp	200	7	6	115	0	17.0	0.0	0	75%
creamy	2 tbsp	200	7	6	140	0	17.0	0.0	0	75%
crunchy	2 tbsp	200	7	6	115	0	17.0	0.0	0	75%
smooth	2 tbsp	200	7	6	140	0	17.0	0.0	0	75%

Food Name	Serving Size	Calories	Prot. gms	Carbs gms	Sod. mgs	Fiber gms	Fat gms	Sat. Fat gms	Chol. mgs	% Fat Cal.
(Estee)										
chunky	2 tbsp	200	8	6	0	0	18.0	2.0	0	74%
creamy	2 tbsp	200	8	6	0	0	18.0	2.0	0	74%
(Featherweight)										
chunky	1 tbsp	90	4	2	5	0	7.0	0.0	0	72%
smooth	1 tbsp	90	4	2	3	0	7.0	0.0	0	72%
(Finast)										
chunky, 'Crunchy'	2 tbsp	195	9	6	175	0	17.0	0.0	0	72%
smooth	2 tbsp	195	9	6	175	0	17.0	0.0	0	72%
(Health Valley)										
chunky, no salt added	2 tbsp	180	8	6	2	3	14.0	0.0	0	69%
creamy, no salt added	2 tbsp	180	8	6	2	3	14.0	0.0	0	69%
(Hollywood)										
chunky	1 tbsp	35	2	1	25	1	3.0	0.0	0	69%
creamy	1 tbsp	35	2	1	25	1	3.0	0.0	0	69%
no salt added	1 tbsp	35	2	1	0	1	3.0	0.0	0	69%
(JFG)										
creamy	2 tbsp	200	7	8	150	2	16.0	3.0	0	71%
creamy, 50% less salt	2 tbsp	200	7	8	75	2	16.0	3.0	0	71%
crunchy	2 tbsp	200	7	8	140	2	16.0	3.0	0	71%
(Jif)										
creamy	2 tbsp	190	8	7	150	2	16.0	3.0	0	71%
creamy, 'Simply Jif'	2 tbsp	190	8	6	65	2	16.0	3.0	0	72%
crunchy, 'Simply Jif'	2 tbsp	190	8	7	50	2	16.0	3.0	0	71%
extra crunchy	2 tbsp	190	8	7	130	2	16.0	3.0	0	71%
smooth	2 tbsp	190	9	6	155	0	16.0	3.0	0	71%
(Maranatha Natural) crunchy	2 tbsp	190	8	7	5	0	15.0	0.0	0	69%
(Pathmark)										
chunky, 'Super Chunky'	2 tbsp	200	7	6	140	0	17.0	0.0	0	75%
'Natural'	2 tbsp	200	9	5	130	0	17.0	0.0	0	73%
smooth, 'Creamy'	2 tbsp	200	7	6	170	0	17.0	0.0	0	75%
smooth, 'No Frills'	2 tbsp	200	7	6	170	0	17.0	0.0	0	75%
(Peter Pan)										
creamy	2 tbsp	189	8	7	152	2	16.0	3.3	0	71%
creamy, low salt	2 tbsp	197	8	6	10	2	17.5	2.5	0	74%
creamy, whipped	2 tbsp	148	6	5	120	2	12.6	2.6	0	71%
crunchy	2 tbsp	188	8	6	119	2	15.9	3.2	0	71%
crunchy, low salt	2 tbsp	197	8	6	9	2	17.3	2.3	0	73%
crunchy, salt-free	2 tbsp	190	9	5	0	2	17.0	2.0	0	73%
crunchy, whipped	2 tbsp	148	7	5	94	2	12.5	2.5	0	71%
smooth, no salt added	2 tbsp	195	9	5	1	0	17.1	2.4	0	73%
(Real Brand)										
creamy	2 tbsp	189	10	5	94	3	16.4	3.0	0	72%
crunchy	2 tbsp	189	9	5	92	4	16.3	3.0	0	72%
(Reese) creamy	2 tbsp	204	8	6	105	2	16.1	3.2	0	71%
(Roaster Fresh) gourmet	1 oz	166	8	5	2	0	14.0	2.4	0	71%
(S&W) 'Nutradiet'	1 tbsp	93	3	2	10	0	8.0	0.0	0	78%
(Skippy)										
chunky, roasted honey nut	2 tbsp	190	7	6	120	2	17.0	3.5	0	75%
chunky, 'Super Chunk'	2 tbsp	190	8	5	140	2	17.0	3.5	0	75%
creamy	2 tbsp	190	8	5	150	2	17.0	3.5	0	75%
creamy, roasted honey nut	2 tbsp	190	7	6	120	2	17.0	3.5	0	75%
(Smucker's)										
chunky, 'Chunky Natural'	2 tbsp	200	8	6	120	0	16.0	3.0	0	72%
honey sweetened	2 tbsp	200	7	7	150	0	16.0	3.0	0	72%

Food Name	Serving Size	Calories	Prot. gms	Carbs gms	Sod. mgs	Fiber gms	Fat gms	Sat. Fat gms	Chol. mgs	% Fat Cal.
no salt added, 'Natural'	2 tbsp	200	8	6	10	0	16.0	3.0	0	72%
smooth, 'Natural'	2 tbsp	200	8	6	120	0	16.0	3.0	0	72%
smooth, no salt added, 'Natural'	2 tbsp	200	8	6	10	0	17.0	1.0	0	73%
(Westbrae)										
crunchy, no salt added, 'Natural'	2 tbsp	190	8	7	0	0	16.0	0.0	0	71%
crunchy, w/salt, 'Natural'	2 tbsp	190	8	7	5	0	16.0	0.0	0	71%
smooth, no salt added, 'Natural'	2 tbsp	190	8	7	0	0	16.0	0.0	0	71%
(Woodstock) smooth, unsalted, 'Old Fashioned'	2 tbsp	200	9	6	3	0	16.0	0.0	0	71%
PEANUT BUTTER CHIPS										
for baking, 'Reese's' (Hershey's)	1.5 oz	230	9	19	90	0	13.0	0.0	5	51%
PEANUT BUTTER SPREAD										
(Bama) w/jelly	2 tbsp	150	3	20	75	0	7.0	0.0	0	41%
(Bama) w/jelly	2 tbsp	150	3	20	75	0	7.0	0.0	0	41%
(Jif) creamy, less fat	2 tbsp	190	8	15	250	2	12.0	2.5	0	54%
(Peter Pan) creamy, less fat	2 tbsp	180	8	15	188	2	11.0	2.2	0	52%
(Peter Pan) crunchy, less fat	2 tbsp	195	8	15	153	2	11.7	1.6	0	54%
(Skippy) chunky, less fat	2 tbsp	180	8	13	170	2	12.4	2.4	0	57%
(Skippy) creamy, less fat	2 tbsp	190	9	13	200	1	12.5	2.5	0	56%
(Smucker's) w/grape jelly, 'Goober Grape'	2 tbsp	180	5	18	120	0	10.0	2.0	0	49%
(Smucker's) w/strawberry jelly, 'Goober Strawberry'	2 tbsp	180	5	18	120	0	10.0	2.0	0	49%
PEANUT BUTTER TOPPING, w/caramel (Smucker's)	2 tbsp	150	3	29	120	0	2.0	0.0	0	12%
PEANUT OIL										
	1 cup	1909	0	0	0	0	216.0	36.5	0	100%
	1 tbsp	119	0	0	0	0	13.5	2.3	0	100%
(Hain)	1 tbsp	120	0	0	0	0	14.0	2.0	0	100%
(Wesson)	1 tbsp	122	0	0	0	0	13.6	2.5	0	100%
100% pure (Hollywood)	1 tbsp	120	0	0	0	0	14.0	2.0	0	100%
100% pure (Planters)	1 tbsp	120	0	0	0	0	14.0	2.0	0	100%
pure pressed, organic (Spectrum)	1 tbsp	120	0	0	0	0	14.0	2.0	0	100%
PEAR										
Canned										
in extra heavy syrup, halves, w/liquid	1 cup	258	1	67	13	4	0.3	0.0	0	1%
in extra heavy syrup, halves, w/1.75 tbsp liquid	1 med half	77	0	20	4	1	0.1	0.0	0	1%
in extra light syrup, halves, w/liquid	1 cup	116	1	30	5	4	0.2	0.0	0	2%
in extra light syrup, halves, w/liquid	1 med half	36	0	9	2	1	0.1	0.0	0	2%
in heavy syrup, w/liquid	1 cup	197	1	51	13	4	0.3	0.0	0	1%
in heavy syrup, w/liquid	1 med half	56	0	15	4	1	0.1	0.0	0	1%
in juice, halves, w/liquid	1 cup	124	1	32	10	4	0.2	0.0	0	1%
in juice, halves, w/liquid	1 med half	38	0	10	3	1	0.1	0.0	0	1%
in light syrup, halves, w/liquid	1 cup	143	0	38	13	4	0.1	0.0	0	0%
in light syrup, halves, w/liquid	1/2 fruit	43	0	12	4	1	0.0	0.0	0	0%
in water, halves, w/liquid	1 cup	71	0	19	5	4	0.1	0.0	0	1%
in water, halves, w/liquid	1 med half	22	0	6	2	1	0.0	0.0	0	1%
Dried										
sulfured, stewed, halves	1 cup	324	2	86	8	16	0.8	0.0	0	2%
sulfured, uncooked, halves	1 cup	472	3	125	11	14	1.1	0.1	0	2%
sulfured, uncooked, halves	1 med half	47	0	13	1	1	0.1	0.0	0	2%
Fresh										
sliced	1 cup	97	1	25	0	4	0.7	0.0	0	6%
whole, large, 2 per lb	1 pear	123	1	32	0	5	0.8	0.0	0	6%
whole, medium, 2.5 per lb	1 pear	98	1	25	0	4	0.7	0.0	0	6%
whole, small, 3 per lb	1 pear	82	1	21	0	3	0.6	0.0	0	6%
PEAR JUICE										
(Knudsen)	8 fl oz	110	1	28	0	0	0.0	0.0	0	0%

Food Name	Serving Size	Calories	Prot. gms	Carbs gms	Sod. mgs	Fiber gms	Fat gms	Sat. Fat gms	Chol. mgs	% Fat Cal.
(Mountain Sun) organic, 'Mountain pear'	8 fl oz	102	0	25	0	0	0.0	0.0	0	0%
(Santa Cruz Natural) organic, 'Cruz'	8 fl oz	135	1	32	0	0	1.0	0.0	0	6%

PEAR NECTAR. See under FRUIT JUICE DRINK.
PEAS, BLACK-EYED. See BLACK-EYED PEAS.
PEAS, CROWDER. See under BLACK-EYED PEAS.
PEAS, FIELD
Canned

Food Name	Serving Size	Calories	Prot. gms	Carbs gms	Sod. mgs	Fiber gms	Fat gms	Sat. Fat gms	Chol. mgs	% Fat Cal.
'Fresh' *(Allens)*	1/2 cup	100	7	18	370	0	1.0	0.0	0	8%
tiny, w/snaps 'Fresh' *(Allens)*	1/2 cup	70	6	13	340	0	1.0	0.0	0	11%
w/snaps *(Bush's Best)*	1/2 cup	80	6	16	550	3	0.0	0.0	0	0%
w/snaps, 'Fresh' *(Allens)*	1/2 cup	100	5	20	370	0	1.0	0.0	0	8%
w/snaps, seasoned w/pork *(Luck's)*	1/2 cup	130	7	19	320	4	3.0	1.0	3	21%

PEAS, GREEN
Canned

Food Name	Serving Size	Calories	Prot. gms	Carbs gms	Sod. mgs	Fiber gms	Fat gms	Sat. Fat gms	Chol. mgs	% Fat Cal.
dry, early June *(Allens)*	1/2 cup	80	5	15	320	0	1.0	0.0	0	10%
early *(A&P)*	1/2 cup	70	4	15	350	0	1.0	0.0	0	11%
early *(Stokely)*	1/2 cup	60	4	12	320	0	0.0	0.0	0	0%
early, 'LeSueur' *(Green Giant)*	1/2 cup	60	4	12	380	3	0.0	0.0	0	0%
early, 50% less sodium, 'LeSueur' *(Green Giant)*	1/2 cup	60	4	11	190	4	0.0	0.0	0	0%
early June *(Green Giant)*	1/2 cup	50	3	12	330	3	0.0	0.0	0	0%
early June, 'Petit Pois' *(S&W)*	1/2 cup	70	4	12	330	0	0.0	0.0	0	0%
early June *(Veg-All)*	1/2 cup	50	4	10	370	0	0.0	0.0	0	0%
early June, medium *(TenderSweet)*	1/2 cup	70	4	11	370	3	0.5	0.0	0	7%
early June, medium, no salt added *(TenderSweet)*	1/2 cup	50	4	10	10	0	0.0	0.0	0	0%
early June, 'Sun-Vista' *(S&W)*	1/2 cup	80	6	18	510	5	0.0	0.0	0	0%
early June, tiny, party *(Stokely)*	1/2 cup	60	4	10	360	3	0.0	0.0	0	0%
early, very young, small *(Green Giant)*	1/2 cup	50	3	12	390	3	0.0	0.0	0	0%
mixed, no salt or sugar added *(IGA)*	1/2 cup	50	4	10	10	0	0.0	0.0	0	0%
mixed sizes *(A&P)*	1/2 cup	60	4	12	350	0	1.0	0.0	0	12%
no salt added, w/liquid *(Del Monte)*	1/2 cup	60	3	11	10	0	0.0	0.0	0	0%
no salt or sugar added *(Stokely)*	1/2 cup	50	4	9	5	0	0.0	0.0	0	0%
seasoned, w/liquid *(Del Monte)*	1/2 cup	60	3	11	355	0	0.0	0.0	0	0%
small, w/liquid *(Del Monte)*	1/2 cup	50	3	9	355	0	0.0	0.0	0	0%
sweet *(Featherweight)*	1/2 cup	70	5	12	10	0	0.0	0.0	0	0%
sweet *(Finast)*	1/2 cup	70	4	13	300	0	1.0	0.0	0	12%
sweet *(Green Giant)*	1/2 cup	60	4	11	390	4	0.0	0.0	0	0%
sweet *(Stokely)*	1/2 cup	70	4	11	370	3	0.5	0.0	0	7%
sweet *(Veg-All)*	1/2 cup	50	4	10	370	0	0.0	0.0	0	0%
sweet, 50% less sodium *(Green Giant)*	1/2 cup	60	4	11	195	3	0.0	0.0	0	0%
sweet, 50% less sodium, 'LeSueur' *(Green Giant)*	1/2 cup	60	4	11	190	4	0.0	0.0	0	0%
sweet, garden *(Freshlike)*	1/2 cup	50	4	10	350	0	0.0	0.0	0	0%
sweet, garden, no salt added *(Freshlike)*	1/2 cup	50	4	10	10	0	0.0	0.0	0	0%
sweet, garden, fancy *(Pathmark)*	1/2 cup	70	4	12	350	0	1.0	0.0	0	12%
sweet, large, tender *(Pathmark)*	8 fl oz	70	4	12	350	0	1.0	0.0	0	12%
sweet, 'LeSueur' *(Green Giant)*	8 fl oz	60	4	12	380	3	0.0	0.0	0	0%
sweet, 'Little Gem' *(Pathmark)*	1/2 cup	70	4	12	350	0	1.0	0.0	0	12%
sweet, mini, in brine *(Green Giant)*	1/2 cup	60	4	12	240	4	1.0	0.0	0	12%
sweet, mixed sizes *(Veg-All)*	1/2 cup	50	4	10	370	0	0.0	0.0	0	0%
sweet, mixed sizes, no salt added *(Pathmark)*	1/2 cup	50	4	10	10	0	0.0	0.0	0	0%
sweet, no salt added *(Finast)*	1/2 cup	60	4	12	10	0	0.0	0.0	0	0%
sweet, 'No Frills' *(Pathmark)*	1 cup	120	8	25	640	0	1.0	0.0	0	6%
sweet, 'Nutradiet' *(S&W)*	1/2 cup	40	3	8	5	0	0.0	0.0	0	0%
sweet, 'Perfection' *(S&W)*	1/2 cup	70	4	12	330	0	0.0	0.0	0	0%
sweet, small *(Freshlike)*	1/2 cup	50	4	10	350	0	0.0	0.0	0	0%

Food Name	Serving Size	Calories	Prot. gms	Carbs gms	Sod. mgs	Fiber gms	Fat gms	Sat. Fat gms	Chol. mgs	% Fat Cal.
sweet, small *(Pathmark)*	1/2 cup	70	4	12	350	0	1.0	0.0	0	12%
sweet, small *(Veg-All)*	1/2 cup	50	4	10	370	0	0.0	0.0	0	0%
sweet, tiny, early June *(IGA)*	1/2 cup	70	4	12	340	0	0.0	0.0	0	0%
sweet, very young, small *(Green Giant)*	1/2 cup	50	4	12	390	4	0.0	0.0	0	0%
sweet, very young, tender *(Green Giant)*	1/2 cup	50	4	11	390	4	0.0	0.0	0	0%
sweet, water packed, no sugar or salt added *(Freshlike)*	1/2 cup	50	4	10	10	0	0.0	0.0	0	0%
very young, sweet, 'LeSueur' *(Green Giant)*	1/2 cup	50	4	12	390	0	0.0	0.0	0	0%
w/liquid *(Del Monte)*	1/2 cup	60	3	10	355	0	0.0	0.0	0	0%
Freeze-dried, prepared *(Mountain House)*	1/2 cup	70	4	12	21	0	1.0	0.0	0	12%
Fresh										
boiled, drained	1 cup	134	9	25	5	9	0.4	0.1	0	2%
boiled, drained	1/2 cup	62	4	11	70	4	0.2	0.0	0	3%
raw	1 cup	117	8	21	7	7	0.6	0.1	0	4%
Frozen										
(Birds Eye)	3.3 oz	80	5	13	130	4	0.0	0.0	0	0%
(Flav-R-Pac)	2/3 cup	70	5	12	105	4	0.5	0.0	0	6%
(Freshlike)	3.3 oz	80	5	13	75	0	0.0	0.0	0	0%
(Frosty Acres)	3.3 oz	80	5	13	91	2	0.0	0.0	0	0%
(Health Valley)	1/2 cup	65	4	11	70	3	0.0	0.0	0	0%
(Seabrook)	3.3 oz	80	5	13	91	2	0.0	0.0	0	0%
(Southern)	3.5 oz	79	6	14	130	0	0.5	0.0	0	5%
(Veg-All)	3.3 oz	80	5	13	75	0	0.0	0.0	0	0%
boiled, drained	10-oz pkg	197	13	36	220	14	0.7	0.1	0	3%
early, baby, 'LeSueur Select' *(Green Giant)*	1/2 cup	60	4	13	115	4	0.0	0.0	0	0%
early, very young, small, 50% less sodium , 'LeSueur' *(Green Giant)*	1/2 cup	60	4	11	190	4	0.0	0.0	0	0%
early June, 'Harvest Fresh' *(Green Giant)*	1/2 cup	60	4	12	140	3	1.0	0.0	0	12%
LeSueur style, 'Valley Combinations' *(Green Giant)*	1/2 cup	70	4	12	400	2	2.0	0.0	0	22%
no salt added *(Flav-R-Pac)*	2/3 cup	70	5	12	15	4	0.5	0.0	0	6%
petite *(C&W)*	2/3 cup	70	5	12	105	4	0.5	0.0	0	6%
petite *(Flav-R-Pac)*	2/3 cup	70	5	12	105	4	0.5	0.0	0	6%
petite *(Southern)*	3.5 oz	64	5	11	50	0	0.4	0.0	0	5%
petite, no salt added *(C&W)*	2/3 cup	70	5	12	10	4	0.5	0.0	0	6%
'Portion Pack' *(Birds Eye)*	3 oz	70	5	12	120	4	0.0	0.0	0	0%
'Singles' *(Stokely)*	3 oz	65	4	12	95	0	1.0	0.0	0	12%
sweet *(Finast)*	3.3 oz	80	5	13	125	0	0.0	0.0	0	0%
sweet *(Green Giant)*	1/2 cup	50	4	11	95	4	0.0	0.0	0	0%
sweet, baby, 'LeSueur Select' *(Green Giant)*	2/3 cup	60	5	11	150	5	0.0	0.0	0	0%
sweet, 'Harvest Fresh' *(Green Giant)*	1/2 cup	50	4	12	135	3	0.0	0.0	0	0%
sweet, no salt added *(Del Monte)*	1/2 cup	60	3	11	10	4	0.0	0.0	0	0%
sweet 'Plain Polybag' *(Green Giant)*	2/3 cup	70	4	13	135	4	0.0	0.0	0	0%
tender, tiny, 'Deluxe' *(Birds Eye)*	3.3 oz	60	4	11	120	4	0.0	0.0	0	0%
tiny *(Freshlike)*	3.3 oz	60	4	11	75	0	0.0	0.0	0	0%
tiny *(Frosty Acres)*	3.3 oz	60	4	11	127	2	0.0	0.0	0	0%
tiny *(Seabrook)*	3.3 oz	60	4	11	127	2	0.0	0.0	0	0%
tiny *(Veg-All)*	3.3 oz	60	4	11	75	0	0.0	0.0	0	0%
Sprouted, mature seeds, raw	1 cup	154	11	34	24	na	0.8	0.1	0	4%
PEAS, GREEN, DISH/ENTRÉE										
(A&P)										
and carrots, frozen	3.3 oz	60	3	11	75	0	1.0	0.0	0	14%
early June, and carrots, canned, no salt added	1/2 cup	60	4	12	10	0	1.0	0.0	0	12%
mixed sizes, and carrots, canned	1/2 cup	60	4	12	10	0	1.0	0.0	0	12%
sweet, and carrots, frozen	1/2 cup	80	5	13	90	0	1.0	0.0	0	11%
(Allens) creamed, 'Fresh'	1/2 cup	90	7	14	440	0	1.0	0.0	0	10%

Food Name	Serving Size	Calories	Prot. gms	Carbs gms	Sod. mgs	Fiber gms	Fat gms	Sat. Fat gms	Chol. mgs	% Fat Cal.
(Birds Eye)										
and pearl onions, frozen, 'Combination Vegetables'	3.3 oz	70	5	13	440	3	0.0	0.0	0	0%
(Budget Gourmet)										
w/water chestnuts, Oriental, 'Side Dish'	5 oz	120	5	15	240	0	3.0	0.0	5	25%
(Del Monte) and carrots, canned, w/liquid	1/2 cup	50	2	10	355	0	0.0	0.0	0	0%
(Finast) and carrots, canned	1/2 cup	55	3	9	315	0	0.0	0.0	0	0%
(Flav-R-Pac)										
and carrots, frozen	2/3 cup	50	3	9	75	3	0.0	0.0	0	0%
and pearl onions, frozen	2/3 cup	70	4	12	95	4	0.5	0.0	0	7%
(Freshlike)										
and carrots, frozen	3.3 oz	60	3	11	60	0	0.0	0.0	0	0%
and onions, frozen	3.3 oz	70	4	13	100	0	0.0	0.0	0	0%
sweet, and diced carrots, canned, in water, no salt added	1/2 cup	50	3	12	30	0	0.0	0.0	0	0%
sweet, and diced carrots, canned, in water, no sugar added	1/2 cup	50	3	12	30	0	0.0	0.0	0	0%
sweet, and sliced carrots, canned	1/2 cup	50	3	12	340	0	0.0	0.0	0	0%
sweet, and tiny onions, canned	1/2 cup	60	4	12	440	0	0.0	0.0	0	0%
(Frosty Acres)										
and carrots, frozen	3.3 oz	60	3	11	75	1	0.0	0.0	0	0%
and pearl onions, frozen	3.3 oz	70	4	13	80	0	0.0	0.0	0	0%
(Green Giant) and pearl onions, canned, w/liquid	1/2 cup	50	4	11	510	4	0.0	0.0	0	0%
(Kohl's) and carrots, canned	1/2 cup	50	3	20	330	0	1.0	0.0	0	9%
(Pathmark) and carrots, canned	1/2 cup	60	3	18	330	0	1.0	0.0	0	10%
(S&W) and carrots, canned, 'Nutradiet'	1/2 cup	35	2	7	5	0	0.0	0.0	0	0%
(Seabrook)										
and carrots, frozen	3.3 oz	60	3	11	75	1	0.0	0.0	0	0%
and onions, frozen	3.3 oz	70	4	13	0	0	0.0	0.0	0	0%
(Southern) and carrots, frozen	3.5 oz	64	3	12	80	0	0.0	0.0	0	0%
(Stokely)										
and carrots, canned	1/2 cup	50	3	9	320	0	0.0	0.0	0	0%
and diced carrots, no salt or sugar added	1/2 cup	45	3	8	20	0	0.0	0.0	0	0%
and sliced carrots, no salt or sugar added	1/2 cup	45	3	8	25	0	0.0	0.0	0	0%
(Veg-All)										
and carrots, frozen	3.3 oz	60	3	11	60	0	0.0	0.0	0	0%
and onions, frozen	3.3 oz	70	4	13	100	0	0.0	0.0	0	0%
sweet, and diced carrots, canned	1/2 cup	50	3	12	340	0	0.0	0.0	0	0%
sweet, and sliced carrots, canned	1/2 cup	50	3	12	340	0	0.0	0.0	0	0%
PEAS, PIGEON										
immature seeds, boiled, drained	1 cup	170	9	30	8	9	2.1	0.6	0	10%
immature seeds, raw	1 cup	209	11	37	8	8	2.5	0.5	0	10%
immature seeds, raw	10 seeds	5	0	1	0	0	0.1	0.0	0	10%
red gram, mature seeds, boiled	1 cup	203	11	39	8	11	0.6	0.1	0	3%
red gram, mature seeds, raw	1 cup	703	44	129	35	31	3.1	0.7	0	4%
PEAS, PURPLE HULLED										
canned, 'Fresh' *(Allens)*	1/2 cup	100	6	16	370	0	1.0	0.0	0	9%
frozen *(Frosty Acres)*	3.3 oz	130	9	23	6	0	0.0	0.0	0	0%
PEAS, SNAP										
sugar snap *(Green Giant)*	1/2 cup	30	2	8	0	2	0.0	0.0	0	0%
sugar snap, 'Deluxe' *(Birds Eye)*	2.6 oz	45	2	9	5	4	0.0	0.0	0	0%
sugar snap, frozen *(Flav-R-Pac)*	3/4 cup	30	2	7	10	2	0.0	0.0	0	0%
sugar snap, 'Harvest Fresh' *(Green Giant)*	1/2 cup	30	2	8	100	2	0.0	0.0	0	0%
sugar snap, 'Select' *(Green Giant)*	1/2 cup	30	2	8	0	2	0.0	0.0	0	0%

Food Name	Serving Size	Calories	Prot. gms	Carbs gms	Sod. mgs	Fiber gms	Fat gms	Sat. Fat gms	Chol. mgs	% Fat Cal.
PEAS, SNOW / Chinese pea pods										
Fresh										
edible-podded, boiled, drained	1 cup	67	5	11	6	4	0.4	0.1	0	5%
edible-podded, raw, whole	10 pods	14	1	3	1	1	0.1	0.0	0	4%
edible-podded, raw, chopped	1 cup	41	3	7	4	3	0.2	0.0	0	4%
edible-podded, raw, whole	1 cup	26	2	5	3	2	0.1	0.0	0	4%
Frozen										
(Chun King)	1.5 oz	20	1	3	10	0	0.0	0.0	0	0%
(Flav-R-Pac)	1 cup	50	2	6	10	2	0.0	0.0	0	0%
(Seabrook)	2 oz	20	2	4	0	0	0.0	0.0	0	0%
baby, pods (C&W)	2/3 cup	40	3	7	45	3	0.0	0.0	0	0%
'Deluxe' (Birds Eye)	3 oz	35	2	6	0	3	0.0	0.0	0	0%
edible-podded, drained	1 cup	83	6	14	8	5	0.6	0.1	0	6%
edible-podded, drained	1/2 cup	42	3	7	4	2	0.3	0.1	0	6%
edible-podded, drained	10 oz pkg	132	9	23	13	8	1.0	0.2	0	6%
edible-podded, unprepared	10-oz pkg	119	8	20	11	9	0.9	0.2	0	6%
edible-podded, unprepared	1/2 cup	30	2	5	3	2	0.2	0.0	0	6%
pods, food service product (La Choy)	1 cup	41	2	9	9	3	0.0	0.0	0	0%
PEAS, SPLIT										
boiled (A&P)	1 cup	220	16	40	15	0	1.0	0.0	0	4%
green, raw (Arrowhead Mills)	2 oz	200	14	35	14	8	1.0	0.0	0	4%
mature seeds, boiled	1 cup	231	16	41	4	16	0.8	0.1	0	3%
mature seeds, boiled	1 tbsp	14	1	3	0	1	0.0	0.0	0	3%
mature seeds, raw	1 cup	672	48	119	30	50	2.3	0.3	0	3%
PEAS AND CARROTS. See under PEAS, GREEN, DISH/ENTRÉE.										
PECAN										
Dried										
chopped	1 cup	822	11	16	0	11	85.6	7.3	0	87%
halves	1 cup	746	10	15	0	10	77.7	6.7	0	87%
halves, approx 20 pieces	1 oz	196	3	4	0	3	20.4	1.8	0	87%
Dry roasted										
unsalted	1 oz	201	3	4	0	3	21.1	1.8	0	88%
salted	1 oz	201	3	4	109	3	21.1	1.8	0	88%
Honey roasted (Planters)	1 oz	200	2	8	80	0	18.0	2.0	0	80%
Oil roasted										
salted	1 cup	787	10	14	432	10	82.8	8.0	0	88%
salted, halves, approx 15 pieces	1 oz	203	3	4	111	3	21.3	2.1	0	88%
unsalted	1 cup	787	10	14	1	10	82.8	8.0	0	88%
unsalted, halves, approx 15 pieces	1 oz	203	3	4	0	3	21.3	2.1	0	88%
Raw										
(Fisher)	1 oz	190	2	5	0	0	19.0	2.0	0	86%
chips (Planters)	1 oz	190	2	5	0	0	20.0	2.0	0	87%
halves (Planters)	1 oz	190	2	5	0	0	20.0	2.0	0	87%
pieces (Planters)	1 oz	190	2	5	0	0	20.0	2.0	0	87%
Roasted										
chipped pieces, shelled (Azar)	2 oz	370	4	10	4	0	38.0	3.0	0	86%
chopped, shelled (Fisher)	1 oz	190	2	5	0	0	19.0	2.0	0	86%
ground, shelled (Fisher)	1 oz	190	2	5	0	0	19.0	2.0	0	86%
halves, pieces, or chips, shelled (Planters)	1 oz	190	2	5	0	0	20.0	2.0	0	87%
halves and pieces, shelled, (Azar)	2 oz	370	4	10	4	0	38.0	3.0	0	86%
pieces, shelled (Azar)	2 oz	370	4	10	4	0	38.0	3.0	0	86%
pieces, shelled, natural, unsalted (Flanigan Farms)	1 oz	190	3	4	4	na	20.0	2.0	0	87%
shelled, natural, unsalted (Flanigan Farms)	1/4 cup	190	2	5	0	2	19.0	1.5	0	86%

Food Name	Serving Size	Calories	Prot. gms	Carbs gms	Sod. mgs	Fiber gms	Fat gms	Sat. Fat gms	Chol. mgs	% Fat Cal.
PECAN BUTTER roasted, organic										
(Maranatha Natural)	2 tbsp	220	3	7	0	3	21.0	1.5	0	83%
PECTIN MIX, unsweetened	1.75 oz	163	0	45	100	4	0.1	0.0	0	0%
PENNE. See under PASTA.										
PENNE DISH/ENTRÉE. See under PASTA DISH/ENTRÉE.										
PEPITAS										
dried, in shell	1 lb	1817	82.4	59.8	59	>7.5 c	153.9	29.1	0	71%
dried, shelled	1 cup	747	33.9	24.6	24	>3.1 c	63.3	12.0	0	71%
dried, shelled, approx 142 kernels	1 oz	154	7.0	5.1	5	>.6 c	13.0	2.5	0	71%
natural, unsalted (Flanigan Farms)	1/4 cup	150	7	5	5	4	13.0	2.5	0	71%
roasted, shelled	1 cup	1184	74.8	30.5	40	>4.1 c	95.6	18.1	0	67%
roasted, shelled	1 oz	148	9.4	3.8	5	>.5 c	12.0	2.2	0	67%
roasted, whole, in shell	1 cup	285	11.9	34.4	12	>23.0 c	12.4	2.3	0	38%
roasted, whole, in shell, approx 85 seeds	1 oz	127	5.3	15.3	5	>10.2 c	5.5	1.0	0	38%
shelled, salted	1 cup	285	11.9	34.4	368	>23.0 c	12.4	2.3	0	38%
shelled, salted	1 lb	2021	84.1	243.8	2608	>162.8 c	88.0	16.6	0	38%
shelled, salted	1 oz	127	5.3	15.3	163	>10.2 c	5.5	1.0	0	38%
PEPEAO. See CHINESE FUNGUS.										
PEPPER, ANCHO, dried, whole	1 medium	48	2	9	7	4	1.4	0.1	0	24%
PEPPER, BANANA										
Canned or jarred, hot (Vlasic)	1 oz	5	0	1	480	0	0.0	0.0	0	0%
Fresh										
raw, chopped	1 cup	33	2	7	16	4	0.6	0.1	0	14%
raw, whole, small, approx 4-inch long	1 pepper	9	1	2	4	1	0.1	0.0	0	14%
raw, whole, medium, approx 4.5-inch long	1 pepper	12	1	2	6	2	0.2	0.0	0	14%
raw, whole, large, approx 5-inch long	1 pepper	20	1	4	10	3	0.3	0.0	0	14%
PEPPER, BELL / green pepper / red pepper / sweet pepper / yellow pepper										
Canned or jarred										
California roasted (Mezzetta)	1 oz	8	0	0	129	1	0.0	0.0	0	0%
fried (Progresso)	1/2 jar	37	1	4	17	1	3.0	1.0	0	57%
green, halves, w/liquid	1 cup	25	1	5	1917	2	0.4	0.1	0	14%
red, halves, w/liquid	1 cup	25	1	5	1917	2	0.4	0.1	0	14%
red, halves, w/liquid	1/2 cup	13	1	3	958	1	0.2	0.0	0	14%
roasted (Progresso)	1/2 cup	20	1	5	2	2	1.0	1.0	0	27%
'Sweet Pepper Mementos' (Heinz)	1 oz	6	0	1	320	0	0.0	0.0	0	0%
Freeze-Dried										
	1/4 cup	5	0	1	3	0	0.0	0.0	0	8%
	1 tbsp	1	0	0	1	0	0.0	0.0	0	8%
red	1/4 cup	5	0	1	3	0	0.0	0.0	0	8%
red	1 tbsp	1	0	0	1	0	0.0	0.0	0	8%
Fresh										
(Dole)	1 medium	25	1	5	0	2	1.0	0.0	0	27%
green, boiled, drained, chopped	1/2 cup	19	1	5	1	1	0.1	0.0	0	6%
green, boiled, drained, minced	1 tbsp	3	0	1	0	0	0.0	0.0	0	6%
green, boiled, drained, strips	1 cup	38	1	9	3	2	0.3	0.0	0	6%
green, raw, chopped	1 cup	40	1	10	3	3	0.3	0.0	0	6%
green, raw, minced	1 tbsp	3	0	1	0	0	0.0	0.0	0	6%
green, raw, rings, 3-inch diam, 1/4-inch thick	1 ring	3	0	1	0	0	0.0	0.0	0	6%
green, raw, sliced	1 cup	25	1	6	2	2	0.2	0.0	0	6%
green, raw, strips	10 strips	7	0	2	1	0	0.1	0.0	0	6%
green, raw, whole, approx 2.75-inch long, 2.5-inch diam	1 pepper	32	1	8	2	2	0.2	0.0	0	6%
green, raw, whole, approx 3.75-inch long, 3-inch diam	1 pepper	44	1	11	3	3	0.3	0.0	0	6%
red, boiled, drained, chopped	1/2 cup	19	1	5	1	1	0.1	0.0	0	6%

Food Name	Serving Size	Calories	Prot. gms	Carbs gms	Sod. mgs	Fiber gms	Fat gms	Sat. Fat gms	Chol. mgs	% Fat Cal.
red, boiled, drained, minced	1 tbsp	3	0	1	0	0	0.0	0.0	0	6%
red, boiled, drained, strips.	1 cup	38	1	9	3	2	0.3	0.0	0	6%
red, raw	1 small	20	1	5	1	1	0.1	0.0	0	6%
red, raw, chopped	1 cup	40	1	10	3	3	0.3	0.0	0	6%
red, raw, minced	1 tbsp	3	0	1	0	0	0.0	0.0	0	6%
red, raw, rings, 3-inch diam, 1/4-inch thick	1 ring	3	0	1	0	0	0.0	0.0	0	6%
red, raw, sliced	1 cup	25	1	6	2	2	0.2	0.0	0	6%
red, raw, whole, approx 2.75-inch long, 2.5-inch diam.	1 medium	32	1	8	2	2	0.2	0.0	0	6%
red, raw, whole, approx 3.75-inch long, 3-inch diam	1 large	44	1	11	3	3	0.3	0.0	0	6%
yellow, raw, strips	10 strips	14	1	3	1	0	0.1	0.0	0	7%
yellow, whole, approx 3.75-inch long, 30-inch diam	1 pepper	50	2	12	4	2	0.4	0.1	0	7%
Frozen										
green (Seabrook)	1 oz	6	0	1	1	0	0.0	0.0	0	0%
green, chopped, unprepared.	10-oz pkg	57	3	13	14	5	0.6	0.1	0	9%
green, diced (Flav-R-Pac).	3/4 cup	20	1	4	10	2	0.0	0.0	0	0%
red (Seabrook)	1 oz	8	0	1	0	0	0.0	0.0	0	0%
red, chopped, unprepared.	10-oz pkg	57	3	13	14	5	0.6	0.1	0	9%
red, chopped, unprepared.	1 oz	6	0	1	1	0	0.1	0.0	0	9%
red, diced (Flav-R-Pac)	3/4 cup	20	1	4	10	2	0.0	0.0	0	0%
red, strips (Flav-R-Pac)	3/4 cup	20	1	4	10	2	0.0	0.0	0	0%
strips (Flav-R-Pac)	3/4 cup	20	1	4	10	2	0.0	0.0	0	0%
PEPPER, BELL, DISH/ENTRÉE										
(Celentano) red, sweet, stuffed, frozen	13 oz	350	28	28	810	0	20.0	0.0	0	45%
(Lean Cuisine) red, stuffed, frozen, 'Salsa'lito'	1 oz	26	1	4	80	na	0.6	na	1	21%
(Stouffer's)										
stuffed, frozen.	1 entrée	200	9	24	900	1	8.0	1.5	25	35%
stuffed, w/beef, in tomato sauce	1 pkg	378	16	42	1155	11	16.2	5.4	44	39%
stuffed, w/beef, in tomato sauce	1 serving	189	8	21	579	5	8.1	2.7	22	39%
stuffed, w/sauce, frozen, food service product	1 oz	25	1	3	122	0	1.1	0.3	3	39%
stuffed, w/o sauce, food service product.	1 oz	31	2	3	125	1	1.4	0.5	5	41%
PEPPER, CHERRY										
Canned or jarred										
diced, drained (Progresso)	2 tbsp	30	0	2	30	1	2.0	0.0	0	69%
diced, fried (Progresso).	2 tbsp	60	0	3	60	1	5.0	0.5	0	79%
hot (Progresso).	1/2 cup	190	0	3	130	1	20.0	3.0	0	94%
hot (Vlasic).	1 oz	10	0	2	480	0	0.0	0.0	0	0%
hot, pickled (Progresso)	1/2 cup	130	0	3	110	1	12.0	2.0	0	90%
hot, whole (Progresso)	1 med pepper	15	0	3	250	0	0.0	0.0	0	0%
hot or mild, rings (Vlasic).	1 oz	5	0	1	480	0	0.0	0.0	0	0%
mild (Vlasic).	1 oz	10	0	2	480	0	0.0	0.0	0	0%
PEPPER, CHILI / chile										
Canned or jarred										
green (Santiago)	2 oz	13	0	3	122	1	0.1	0.0	0	6%
green, chopped (Old El Paso).	2 tbsp	8	1	2	70	0	1.0	0.0	0	43%
green, chopped, no seeds, w/liquid.	1/2 cup	14	1	3	798	1	0.1	0.0	0	4%
green, diced (Pancho Villa)	2 tbsp	5	0	1	110	1	0.0	0.0	0	0%
green, diced (Rosarita)	2 tbsp	6	0	1	85	1	0.1	0.0	0	10%
green, diced, food service product (Rosarita)	2 tbsp	6	0	1	85	1	0.1	0.0	0	10%
green, diced, w/liquid (Del Monte).	1/2 cup	20	0	5	690	0	0.0	0.0	0	0%
green, strips, food service product (Rosarita)	1/4 cup	4	0	1	74	1	0.1	0.0	0	11%
green, whole (Old El Paso)	1 med pepper	8	1	1	105	0	1.0	0.0	0	53%
green, whole (Rosarita).	2 tbsp	4	0	1	74	1	0.1	0.0	0	11%
green, whole, diced, sliced, or strips (Ortega)	1 oz	10	0	3	20	0	0.0	0.0	0	0%
green, whole, food service product (Rosarita)	2 tbsp	4	0	1	74	1	0.1	0.0	0	11%

Food Name	Serving Size	Calories	Prot. gms	Carbs gms	Sod. mgs	Fiber gms	Fat gms	Sat. Fat gms	Chol. mgs	% Fat Cal.
green, whole, no seeds, w/liquid	1 med pepper	15	1	4	856	1	0.1	0.0	0	4%
green, whole, w/liquid (Del Monte)	1/2 cup	20	0	5	690	0	0.0	0.0	0	0%
hot, diced (Ortega)	1 oz	8	0	2	0	0	0.0	0.0	0	0%
hot, whole (Ortega)	1 oz	8	0	2	0	0	0.0	0.0	0	0%
hot, tiny, Mexican (Vlasic)	1 oz	6	0	2	430	0	0.0	0.0	0	0%
red, chopped, no seeds, w/liquid	1/2 cup	14	1	3	798	1	0.1	0.0	0	4%
red, whole, no seeds, w/liquid	1 med pepper	15	1	4	856	1	0.1	0.0	0	4%
Fresh										
green, chopped or diced	1/2 cup	30	2	7	5	1	0.1	0.0	0	4%
green, raw, whole	1 med pepper	18	1	4	3	1	0.1	0.0	0	4%
red, chopped or diced	1/2 cup	30	2	7	5	1	0.1	0.0	0	4%
red, raw, whole	1 med pepper	18	1	4	3	1	0.1	0.0	0	4%
Frozen										
green (Santiago)	2 oz	15	1	3	13	0	0.2	0.0	0	11%
green, chopped (Old El Paso)	2 tbsp	5	0	1	110	1	0.0	0.0	0	0%
hot, roasted, peeled, chopped (Baca's)	2 tbsp	5	0	1	5	0	0.0	0.0	0	0%
Sun-dried										
hot, chopped	1 cup	120	4	26	34	11	2.1	0.3	0	15%
hot, whole	1 med pepper	2	0	0	0	0	0.0	0.0	0	15%
PEPPER, GREEN. See PEPPER, BELL.										
PEPPER, GROUND										
BLACK										
	1 tbsp	16	1	4	3	2	0.2	0.1	0	11%
	1 dash	0	0	0	0	0	0.0	0.0	0	10%
(Durkee)	1 tsp	8	0	0	0	0	0.0	0.0	0	0%
(Laurel Leaf)	1 tsp	8	0	0	0	0	0.0	0.0	0	0%
(McCormick/Schilling)	1 tsp	7	0	1	0	0	0.0	0.0	0	0%
(Spice Islands)	1 tsp	9	0	2	1	0	0.2	0.0	0	21%
coarse grind, 'Mr. Pepper' (Tone's)	1 tsp	8	0	2	1	1	0.1	0.1	0	9%
fine grind, 'Mr. Pepper' (Tone's)	1 tsp	8	0	2	1	0	0.1	0.1	0	9%
CAYENNE (Spice Islands)	1 tsp	9	0	1	1	1	0.3	0.0	0	33%
CHILI										
(Spice Islands)	1 tsp	9	0	1	1	0	0.3	0.0	0	31%
fresh ground (Durkee)	1 tsp	11	0	0	0	0	0.0	0.0	0	0%
fresh ground (Laurel Leaf)	1 tsp	11	0	0	0	0	0.0	0.0	0	0%
red (McCormick/Schilling)	1 tsp	10	0	1	1	1	0.4	0.0	0	36%
RED										
(Spice Islands)	1 tsp	9	0	1	1	1	0.3	0.0	0	33%
fresh-ground (Durkee)	1 tsp	8	0	0	0	0	0.0	0.0	0	0%
fresh-ground (Laurel Leaf)	1 tsp	8	0	0	0	0	0.0	0.0	0	0%
WHITE										
	1 tbsp	21	1	5	0	2	0.2	0.0	0	6%
	1 tsp	7	0	2	0	1	0.1	0.0	0	6%
(Durkee)	1 tsp	9	0	0	0	0	0.0	0.0	0	0%
(Laurel Leaf)	1 tsp	9	0	0	0	0	0.0	0.0	0	0%
(McCormick/Schilling)	1 tsp	8	0	2	0	0	0.0	0.0	0	0%
(Spice Islands)	1 tsp	9	0	2	1	0	0.2	0.0	0	20%
PEPPER, HUNGARIAN, raw	1 med pepper	8	0	2	0	na	0.1	0.0	0	12%
PEPPER, JALAPEÑO										
Canned or jarred										
(Old El Paso)	2 tbsp	16	1	4	100	1	0.0	0.0	0	0%
chopped, w/liquid	1 cup	37	1	6	2273	4	1.3	0.1	0	29%
diced (Ortega)	1 oz	10	0	3	20	0	0.0	0.0	0	0%

Food Name	Serving Size	Calories	Prot. gms	Carbs gms	Sod. mgs	Fiber gms	Fat gms	Sat. Fat gms	Chol. mgs	% Fat Cal.
diced (Rosarita)	2 tbsp	5	0	1	121	1	0.2	0.0	0	26%
for nachos (La Victoria)	14 pieces	5	0	1	330	0	0.0	0.0	0	0%
for nachos (La Victoria)	1 tbsp	2	1	1	335	0	1.0	0.0	0	53%
hot (Vlasic)	1/4 cup	10	0	2	490	0	0.0	0.0	0	0%
marinated (La Victoria)	1 tbsp	4	1	1	251	0	1.0	0.0	0	53%
marinated (La Victoria)	1.5 pieces	10	0	2	300	0	0.0	0.0	0	0%
nacho sliced (Rosarita)	2 tbsp	4	0	1	448	1	0.1	0.0	0	18%
nacho sliced, food service product (Rosarita)	2 tbsp	4	0	1	448	1	0.1	0.0	0	18%
pickled (Old El Paso)	2 peppers	5	0	1	380	0	0.0	0.0	0	0%
sliced, w/liquid (Del Monte)	1/2 cup	30	1	6	1690	0	1.0	0.0	0	24%
sliced, w/liquid	1 cup	28	1	5	1738	3	1.0	0.1	0	29%
slices, pickled (Old El Paso)	2 tbsp	15	0	3	400	1	0.0	0.0	0	0%
whole (Old El Paso)	2 peppers	14	0	1	480	0	1.0	0.0	0	69%
whole (Ortega)	1 oz	10	0	3	20	0	0.0	0.0	0	0%
whole (Rosarita)	2 tbsp	8	1	1	430	1	0.1	0.0	0	14%
whole, food service product (Rosarita)	2 peppers	6	0	1	568	1	0.1	0.0	0	18%
whole, w/escabeche (Rosarita)	1.16 oz	8	1	1	430	1	0.2	0.0	0	18%
whole, w/liquid	1 med pepper	6	0	1	368	1	0.2	0.0	0	29%
whole, w/liquid (Del Monte)	1/2 cup	30	1	6	1690	0	1.0	0.0	0	24%
Fresh										
raw, whole	1 pepper	4	0	1	0	0	0.1	0.0	0	17%
raw, sliced	1 cup	27	1	5	1	3	0.6	0.1	0	17%
PEPPER, PEPPERONCINI										
(Progresso) Tuscan	1/2 cup	20	0	7	5	1	0.0	0.0	0	0%
(Vlasic)	1 oz	5	0	1	440	0	0.0	0.0	0	0%
PEPPER, PERSIL, dried	1 medium	24	1	4	6	2	1.1	na	0	38%
PEPPER, RED. See PEPPER, BELL.										
PEPPER, SERRANO										
Fresh										
raw, chopped	1 cup	34	2	7	11	4	0.5	0.1	0	12%
raw, whole	1 medium	2	0	0	1	0	0.0	0.0	0	12%
PEPPER, SWEET. See PEPPER, BELL.										
PEPPER, TUSCAN, canned or jarred,										
drained (Progresso)	3 medium	10	0	1	330	1	0.0	0.0	0	0%
PEPPER, YELLOW. See PEPPER, BANANA, PEPPER, BELL.										
PEPPER DISH/ENTRÉE. See PEPPER, BELL, DISH/ENTRÉE.										
PEPPER DILL SEASONING. See under SEASONING MIX.										
PEPPERMINT										
fresh, raw, whole	2 leaves	0	0	0	0	0	0.0	0.0	0	12%
fresh, raw, chopped	2 tbsp	2	0	0	1	0	0.0	0.0	0	11%
PEPPERONCINI. See PEPPER, PEPPERONCINI.										
PEPPERONI. See under SAUSAGE.										
PERCH										
Fresh										
mixed species, baked, broiled, grilled, or microwaved	3 oz	99	21	0	67	0	1.0	0.2	98	9%
mixed species, raw	3 oz	77	16	0	53	0	0.8	0.2	77	9%
Frozen										
(Booth)	4 oz	100	20	0	90	0	1.0	0.0	0	10%
(SeaPak)	4 oz	100	19	0	80	0	2.0	0.0	0	19%
fillet, battered (Van de Kamp's)	2 pieces	310	12	18	500	0	21.0	4.0	30	61%
PERSIL PEPPER. See PEPPER, PERSIL.										
PERSIMMON										
dried, organic (Flanigan Farms)	1 pkg	90	1	20	10	1	0.0	0.0	0	0%
dried, whole, trimmed, medium, approx 2.5 inch diam	1 fruit	93	0	25	1	5	0.2	na	0	2%

Food Name	Serving Size	Calories	Prot. gms	Carbs gms	Sod. mgs	Fiber gms	Fat gms	Sat. Fat gms	Chol. mgs	% Fat Cal.
raw, Japanese, whole, medium, approx 2.5 inch diam	1 fruit	118	1	31	2	6	0.3	0.0	0	2%
raw, native, trimmed, medium, approx 2.5 inch diam	1 fruit	32	0	8	0	na	0.1	na	0	3%

PESTO. See under SAUCE.

PE-TSAI. See BOK CHOY.

PHEASANT

Food Name	Serving Size	Calories	Prot. gms	Carbs gms	Sod. mgs	Fiber gms	Fat gms	Sat. Fat gms	Chol. mgs	% Fat Cal.
breast, meat only, raw	6.4 oz	242	44	0	60	0	5.9	2.0	106	22%
leg, meat only, raw, 1 medium	3.5 oz	133	22	0	45	0	4.3	1.4	79	29%
leg, meat only, raw, 1 medium, boneless/skinless	3.3 oz	143	24	0	48	0	4.6	1.6	86	29%

PHYLLO DOUGH

Food Name	Serving Size	Calories	Prot. gms	Carbs gms	Sod. mgs	Fiber gms	Fat gms	Sat. Fat gms	Chol. mgs	% Fat Cal.
	1 oz	85	2	15	137	1	1.7	0.4	0	18%
frozen, ready-to-use (Apollo)	1 oz	80	3	18	200	0	0.4	0.0	0	4%

PICCALILLI. See under RELISH.

PICKLE

BREAD AND BUTTER

(Claussen)

Food Name	Serving Size	Calories	Prot. gms	Carbs gms	Sod. mgs	Fiber gms	Fat gms	Sat. Fat gms	Chol. mgs	% Fat Cal.
chips	4 slices	20	0	4	170	0	0.0	0.0	0	0%
sandwich slices	2 slices	25	0	5	210	0	0.0	0.0	0	0%
(Heinz) slices 'Cucumber Slices'	1 oz	25	0	6	170	0	0.0	0.0	0	0%
(Mrs. Fanning's) slices	2 slices	16	0	3	140	0	0.0	0.0	0	0%
(Vlasic)										
chunks, 'Old-Fashion'	1 oz	25	0	6	120	0	0.0	0.0	0	0%
'Deli'	1 oz	25	0	6	120	0	0.0	0.0	0	0%
'Sandwich Stackers'	1 oz	25	0	6	170	na	0.0	0.0	0	0%
sweet, 'Sweet Butter Chips'	1 oz	30	0	7	160	0	0.0	0.0	0	0%
sweet, 'Sweet Butter Stix'	1 oz	18	0	5	110	0	0.0	0.0	0	0%

DILL

(Claussen)

Food Name	Serving Size	Calories	Prot. gms	Carbs gms	Sod. mgs	Fiber gms	Fat gms	Sat. Fat gms	Chol. mgs	% Fat Cal.
halves, kosher	1 oz	5	0	1	330	0	0.0	0.0	0	0%
miniature, kosher	1 piece	5	0	1	300	0	0.0	0.0	0	0%
no garlic	1 piece	17	1	3	895	0	0.3	0.0	0	17%
sandwich slices, kosher	2 slices	5	0	1	440	0	0.0	0.0	0	0%
whole, kosher	1 oz	5	0	1	330	0	0.0	0.0	0	0%
(Featherweight) whole	1 piece	4	0	1	5	0	0.0	0.0	0	0%
(Heinz)										
baby	1 oz	4	0	1	285	0	0.0	0.0	0	0%
chips	1 oz	4	0	1	275	0	0.0	0.0	0	0%
halves, 'Deli Style'	1 oz	4	0	1	280	0	0.0	0.0	0	0%
hamburger slices	1 oz	2	0	0	405	0	0.0	0.0	0	0%
spears, kosher	1 oz	4	0	1	295	0	0.0	0.0	0	0%
spears, Polish style	1 oz	4	0	1	285	0	0.0	0.0	0	0%
whole, 'Genuine'	1 oz	2	0	0	420	0	0.0	0.0	0	0%
whole, kosher	1 oz	4	0	1	295	0	0.0	0.0	0	0%
whole, kosher, 'Old Fashioned'	1 oz	4	0	1	280	0	0.0	0.0	0	0%
whole, Polish style	1 oz	4	0	1	285	0	0.0	0.0	0	0%
whole, processed	1 oz	2	0	0	435	na	0.0	0.0	0	0%
(Steinfeld)										
baby, kosher	1 oz	5	0	1	300	0	0.0	0.0	0	0%
hamburger chips	1 oz	5	0	1	300	0	0.0	0.0	0	0%
(Vlasic)										
baby, whole, kosher	1 oz	5	0	1	220	0	0.0	0.0	0	0%
chunks, Polish, snack	1 oz	4	0	1	300	0	0.0	0.0	0	0%
chunks, zesty, snacks	1 oz	4	0	1	290	0	0.0	0.0	0	0%
crunchy	1 oz	4	0	1	210	0	0.0	0.0	0	0%
crunchy, half salt	1 oz	4	0	1	125	0	0.0	0.0	0	0%

Food Name	Serving Size	Calories	Prot. gms	Carbs gms	Sod. mgs	Fiber gms	Fat gms	Sat. Fat gms	Chol. mgs	% Fat Cal.
crunchy, zesty	1 oz	4	0	1	250	0	0.0	0.0	0	0%
gherkins	1 oz	4	0	1	210	0	0.0	0.0	0	0%
hamburger chips, half salt	1 oz	2	0	1	175	0	0.0	0.0	0	0%
original	1 oz	5	0	1	390	0	0.0	0.0	0	0%
'Sandwich Stackers' kosher	1 oz	5	0	1	210	0	0.0	0.0	0	0%
'Sandwich Stackers' Polish	1 oz	5	0	1	280	0	0.0	0.0	0	0%
'Sandwich Stackers' zesty	1 oz	5	0	1	280	0	0.0	0.0	0	0%
spears, deli style	1 oz	5	0	1	310	0	0.0	0.0	0	0%
spears, half salt	1 oz	4	0	1	120	0	0.0	0.0	0	0%
spears, kosher	1 oz	4	0	1	175	0	0.0	0.0	0	0%
spears, no garlic	1 oz	4	0	1	210	0	0.0	0.0	0	0%
spears, Polish	1 oz	5	0	1	280	na	0.0	0.0	0	0%
spears, zesty	1 oz	4	0	1	230	0	0.0	0.0	0	0%
HOT AND SPICY *(Vlasic)* garden, mixed	1 oz	4	0	1	380	0	0.0	0.0	0	0%
KOSHER. See also PICKLE, DILL.										
(Heinz)										
chips, 'Old Fashioned'	1 oz	4	0	1	270	0	0.0	0.0	0	0%
halves, 'Old Fashioned Deli Halves'	1 oz	4	0	1	275	0	0.0	0.0	0	0%
(Vlasic) chunks, snack	2 pieces	5	0	1	220	0	0.0	0.0	0	0%
SOUR *(Claussen)* halves, deli style	1 oz	5	0	1	260	0	0.0	0.0	0	0%
SWEET										
(Featherweight) sliced	3.5 pieces	24	0	6	5	0	0.0	0.0	0	0%
(Heinz)										
cubes, salad	1 oz	30	0	7	270	0	0.0	0.0	0	0%
'Cucumber Stix'	1 oz	25	0	6	145	0	0.0	0.0	0	0%
gherkins	1 oz	35	0	8	210	0	0.0	0.0	0	0%
mixed, low-sodium	1 oz	40	0	9	200	0	0.0	0.0	0	0%
sliced	1 oz	35	0	8	205	0	0.0	0.0	0	0%
sliced, 'Cucumber Slices'	1 oz	20	0	5	195	0	0.0	0.0	0	0%
(Steinfeld) chips	1 oz	30	0	8	110	0	0.0	0.0	0	0%
(Vlasic)	1 oz	35	0	9	170	na	0.0	0.0	0	0%
PICKLING SPICE. See under SEASONING MIX.										
PIE										
APPLE										
(Amy's Kitchen) single serving	1 pie	220	2	35	130	2	8.0	4.5	25	33%
(Banquet)										
'Family Size'	1/6 pie	250	2	37	290	0	11.0	0.0	0	39%
frozen, ready to bake	1 serving	292	3	41	361	1	13.2	5.7	9	41%
(Entenmann's)										
beehive, nonfat, cholesterol free	1 piece	270	2	65	330	2	0.0	0.0	0	0%
homestyle	2.1 oz	140	1	21	150	0	7.0	0.0	0	42%
(McMillin's)	4 oz	430	4	51	340	0	23.0	0.0	0	48%
(Mrs. Smith's)										
'Pie In Minutes'	1/8 pie	210	2	29	250	0	9.0	2.0	0	40%
less fat, frozen	1 slice	250	2	43	290	1	8.0	1.5	0	29%
(Pet-Ritz)	1/16 pie	330	2	53	385	0	12.0	0.0	0	33%
(Sara Lee)										
'Homestyle'	1/10 pie	280	2	42	220	0	12.0	0.0	0	38%
'Homestyle High'	1/10 pie	400	3	46	450	0	23.0	0.0	0	51%
streusel, frozen, 'Free & Light'	1/8 pie	170	1	36	140	0	2.0	0.0	0	11%
BANANA CREAM										
(Banquet)	1/6 pie	180	2	21	150	0	10.0	0.0	0	49%
(Mrs. Smith's)	1 slice	280	2	37	170	1	14.0	4.0	0	45%
(Pet-Ritz)	1/6 pie	170	2	22	155	0	9.0	0.0	0	46%

Food Name	Serving Size	Calories	Prot. gms	Carbs gms	Sod. mgs	Fiber gms	Fat gms	Sat. Fat gms	Chol. mgs	% Fat Cal.
BERRY *(McMillin's)*.	4 oz	430	3	52	410	0	23.0	0.0	0	48%
BLACKBERRY *(Banquet)* frozen, 'Family Size'	1/6 pie	270	3	40	350	0	11.0	0.0	0	37%
BLUEBERRY										
(Banquet) 'Family Size'	1/6 pie	270	3	40	350	0	11.0	0.0	0	37%
(Mrs. Smith's) 'Pie In Minutes'	1/8 pie	220	2	32	240	0	9.0	2.0	0	37%
(Pet-Ritz)	1/6 pie	370	3	50	330	0	12.0	0.0	0	34%
(Sara Lee) 'Homestyle'.	1/10 pie	300	2	45	210	0	12.0	0.0	0	36%
CHERRY										
(Banquet) frozen, 'Family Size'	1/6 pie	250	3	36	260	0	11.0	0.0	0	39%
(Entenmann's) beehive, nonfat, cholesterol free	1 piece	270	3	64	310	1	0.0	0.0	0	0%
(Mrs. Smith's)										
frozen, 'Pie In Minutes'	1/8 pie	220	2	32	200	0	9.0	2.0	0	37%
less fat, frozen	1 slice	250	2	44	310	1	8.0	1.5	0	28%
(Pet-Ritz) frozen	1/6 pie	300	3	48	330	0	12.0	0.0	0	35%
(Sara Lee)										
frozen, 'Homestyle'	1/10 pie	270	2	37	270	0	13.0	0.0	0	43%
streusel, frozen, 'Free & Light'	1/10 pie	160	2	34	140	0	2.0	0.0	0	11%
CHOCOLATE										
(Banquet) cream, frozen	1/6 pie	190	2	24	110	0	10.0	0.0	0	46%
(McMillin's) pudding	4 oz	420	3	54	350	0	21.0	0.0	0	45%
(Pet-Ritz) cream, frozen.	1/6 pie	190	1	27	145	0	8.0	0.0	0	39%
(Weight Watchers)										
Mississippi mud.	1 serving	160	4	24	120	0	5.0	1.5	5	29%
mocha.	1 serving	170	6	31	125	2	4.0	1.0	5	20%
COCONUT										
(Banquet) cream, frozen	1/6 pie	190	2	22	120	0	11.0	0.0	0	51%
(Entenmann's) custard	1.8 oz	140	3	16	160	0	8.0	0.0	0	49%
(McMillin's) pudding	4 oz	450	4	50	420	0	26.0	0.0	0	52%
(Pet-Ritz) cream, frozen.	1/6 pie	190	2	27	145	0	8.0	0.0	0	38%
EGG CUSTARD *(Pet-Ritz)* frozen.	1/6 pie	200	5	28	0	0	8.0	0.0	0	35%
KEY LIME *(Mrs. Smith's)*	1 slice	380	5	58	240	0	14.0	5.0	15	33%
LEMON										
(Banquet) cream, frozen	1/6 pie	170	2	23	120	0	9.0	0.0	0	45%
(McMillin's).	4 oz	450	4	52	330	0	25.0	0.0	0	50%
(Mrs. Smith's) meringue, frozen	1/8 pie	210	2	38	130	0	5.0	0.0	0	22%
(Pet-Ritz) cream, frozen.	1/6 pie	190	2	26	150	0	9.0	0.0	0	42%
MINCEMEAT										
(Banquet) frozen, 'Family Size'	1/6 pie	260	3	38	370	0	11.0	0.0	0	38%
(Mrs. Smith's) frozen	1 slice	300	2	48	400	2	11.0	2.0	0	33%
(Pet-Ritz) frozen.	1/6 pie	280	2	48	0	0	9.0	0.0	0	29%
(Sara Lee) frozen, 'Homestyle'.	1/10 pie	300	3	43	340	0	13.0	0.0	0	39%
NEAPOLITAN *(Pet-Ritz)* cream, frozen	1/6 pie	180	1	17	185	0	10.0	0.0	0	56%
PEACH										
(Banquet) frozen, 'Family Size'	1/6 pie	245	3	35	280	0	11.0	0.0	0	39%
(McMillin's).	4 oz	430	4	52	370	0	24.0	0.0	0	49%
(Pet-Ritz) frozen.	1/6 pie	320	2	51	320	0	12.0	0.0	0	34%
(Sara Lee) frozen, 9-inch, 'Homestyle'.	1/10 pie	280	2	41	170	0	12.0	0.0	0	39%
PECAN										
(Mrs. Smith's) frozen	1 slice	520	5	73	450	1	23.0	4.0	70	40%
(Sara Lee) frozen, 'Homestyle'.	1/10 pie	400	4	56	290	0	18.0	0.0	55	40%
PUMPKIN										
(Banquet) frozen, 'Family Size'	1/6 pie	200	3	29	350	0	8.0	0.0	0	36%
(Mrs. Smith's) frozen	1 slice	270	5	44	350	1	8.0	2.0	45	27%
(Pet-Ritz) custard, frozen.	1/6 pie	250	4	39	0	0	9.0	0.0	0	32%

Food Name	Serving Size	Calories	Prot. gms	Carbs gms	Sod. mgs	Fiber gms	Fat gms	Sat. Fat gms	Chol. mgs	% Fat Cal.
(Sara Lee) frozen, 'Homestyle'.	1/10 pie	240	4	34	250	0	10.0	0.0	40	37%
RASPBERRY *(Sara Lee)* frozen, 'Homestyle'	1/10 pie	280	2	39	150	0	13.0	0.0	0	42%
STRAWBERRY										
(Banquet) cream, frozen	1/6 pie	170	2	22	120	0	9.0	0.0	0	46%
(McMillin's).	4 oz	400	3	50	370	0	20.0	0.0	0	46%
(Mrs. Smith's) frozen	1 slice	280	2	45	190	1	11.0	2.5	0	34%
(Pet-Ritz) cream, frozen	1/6 pie	170	2	20	145	0	9.0	0.0	0	48%
STRAWBERRY RHUBARB *(Mrs. Smith's)* frozen	1 slice	280	2	44	380	0	11.0	2.0	0	35%
SWEET POTATO PIE										
(Mrs. Smith's) frozen	1 slice	280	4	43	220	1	11.0	2.5	40	34%
(Pet-Ritz) frozen.	1/6 pie	150	2	21	110	0	7.0	0.0	0	41%
PIE, SNACK										
(Tastykake) 'Klair'.	1 piece	402	6	51	315	2	20.1	3.8	56	44%
APPLE										
(Break Cake) 'Fried Pie' 4.5 oz.	2 pies	430	5	63	370	0	18.0	4.5	0	37%
(Drake's).	1 piece	210	2	29	135	0	10.0	2.0	0	42%
(Hostess)										
French.	1 piece	430	3	60	390	2	20.0	9.0	15	42%
'Snack Cake'	1 serving	480	3	67	390	2	22.0	9.0	158	41%
(Little Debbie)										
Dutch apple, 2.5 oz.	1 piece	270	2	48	170	0	8.0	0.0	1	26%
Dutch apple, 2.17 oz.	1 piece	230	2	42	150	0	8.0	0.0	1	29%
(Tastykake)										
.	1 piece	296	3	46	339	3	12.3	2.6	0	36%
French, 4.2 oz.	1 piece	353	3	63	225	2	10.7	2.5	0	27%
(Weight Watchers).	1/2 pkg	200	2	39	280	0	5.0	1.0	5	22%
BANANA CREAM *(Tastykake)* 4.2 oz.	1 piece	382	5	54	428	2	16.1	5.7	26	38%
BLACKBERRY *(Hostess)*.	1 piece	420	4	59	360	2	18.0	9.0	15	39%
BLUEBERRY										
(Drake's) w/apple.	1 piece	210	2	30	135	0	10.0	2.0	0	41%
(Hostess) 'Snack Cake'.	1 serving	480	3	70	460	2	21.0	10.0	20	39%
(Tastykake).	1 piece	308	3	55	410	2	9.4	2.1	0	27%
CHERRY										
(Break Cake) 'Fried Pie'.	2 pies	410	5	64	370	0	16.0	4.3	0	34%
(Drake's) w/apple.	1 piece	220	2	30	135	0	10.0	2.0	0	41%
(Hostess) 'Snack Cake'.	1 serving	470	3	65	470	1	22.0	11.0	20	42%
(McMillin's).	4 oz	430	3	51	350	0	24.0	0.0	0	50%
(Tastykake).	1 piece	298	3	49	306	2	9.7	2.2	0	30%
CHOCOLATE										
(Hostess) pudding.	1 piece	490	5	76	439	0	19.0	0.0	21	35%
(Pepperidge Farm)										
Mississippi mud, 'American Collection'.	1 ramekin	310	3	23	60	0	23.0	12.0	45	67%
(Tastykake) pudding.	1 piece	443	6	68	0	0	16.2	0.0	0	33%
COCONUT *(Tastykake)* creme.	1 piece	377	5	46	416	2	20.2	5.2	65	47%
LEMON										
(Break Cake) 'Fried Pie'.	2 pies	490	5	66	370	0	23.0	3.4	0	42%
(Drake's).	1 piece	210	2	27	115	0	11.0	2.0	0	46%
(Hostess) 'Snack Cake'.	1 serving	500	3	66	430	0	24.0	11.0	20	44%
(Tastykake).	1 piece	319	4	48	375	2	13.2	2.9	39	36%
LEMON-LIME *(Tastykake)*.	1 piece	310	3	54	329	0	8.8	0.0	55	26%
OATMEAL										
(Little Debbie)										
cream, 2.75 oz.	1 piece	350	4	51	260	0	14.0	0.0	1	36%
cream, 1.33 oz.	1 piece	160	2	25	125	0	6.0	0.0	1	33%

Food Name	Serving Size	Calories	Prot. gms	Carbs gms	Sod. mgs	Fiber gms	Fat gms	Sat. Fat gms	Chol. mgs	% Fat Cal.
PEACH										
(Hostess) 'Snack Cake'	1 serving	480	3	68	460	1	21.0	10.0	25	40%
(Tastykake)	1 piece	310	3	54	329	0	8.8	0.0	55	26%
PECAN										
(Little Debbie)										
3 oz	1 piece	280	3	60	340	0	3.0	0.0	1	10%
1.83 oz	1 piece	170	2	37	200	0	2.0	0.0	1	10%
PINEAPPLE CHEESE (Tastykake)	1 piece	343	5	54	405	2	13.2	3.3	19	34%
PUMPKIN (Tastykake)	1 piece	324	5	47	520	2	14.2	4.1	28	39%
STRAWBERRY										
(Hostess)	1 piece	410	4	56	360	2	19.0	9.0	15	42%
(Tastykake)	1 piece	342	3	57	303	1	11.4	2.7	0	30%
PIE CRUST										
(Keebler)										
shell, chocolate, food service product, 'Ready Crust'	1 slice	100	1	13	95	1	4.5	1.0	0	42%
tart shell, graham, food service product, 'Ready Crust'	1 serving	120	1	15	150	1	6.0	1.0	0	46%
(Mrs. Smith's)										
shell, 8-inch	1/8 shell	80	1	8	105	0	5.0	1.0	0	56%
shell, 9-inch	1/8 shell	90	1	10	125	0	5.0	1.0	0	51%
shell, 9-5/8 inch	1/8 shell	120	2	12	160	0	7.0	2.0	0	53%
shell, less fat, frozen, 9-inch	1 slice	100	1	13	95	0	5.0	1.0	0	45%
(Nabisco)										
chocolate cookie crumb, 'Oreo'	1 slice	140	1	18	180	1	7.0	1.5	0	45%
vanilla wafer crumb, 'Nilla'	1 slice	144	1	18	63	0	7.6	1.4	3	48%
(Oronoque)										
deep dish, 9-inch	1/8 crust	100	2	8	95	0	7.0	1.5	0	61%
deep dish, 9-inch, frozen	1/6 shell	130	2	11	130	0	9.0	2.0	0	61%
deep dish, 10-inch	1/8 crust	130	2	10	120	0	8.0	2.0	0	60%
regular, 9-inch	1/8 crust	90	1	7	80	0	6.0	1.5	0	63%
regular, 9-inch, frozen	1/6 shell	120	2	9	115	0	8.0	2.0	0	62%
regular, 6-inch	1/4 crust	110	2	9	105	0	7.0	1.5	0	59%
tart shell, 3-inch	1 tart	140	2	11	130	0	9.0	2.0	0	61%
(Pet-Ritz)										
	1/6 shell	110	1	11	110	0	7.0	0.0	7	57%
all vegetable shortening	1/6 shell	110	2	10	60	0	8.0	2.0	0	60%
deep dish	1/6 shell	130	1	12	120	0	8.0	0.0	7	58%
deep dish, whole grain	1/6 shell	130	1	14	125	0	8.0	0.0	0	55%
deep dish, w/vegetable shortening	1/6 shell	140	2	12	75	0	9.0	2.0	0	59%
graham cracker	1/6 shell	110	1	8	80	0	6.0	0.0	7	60%
9-5/8-inch	1/6 shell	170	2	15	180	0	11.0	0.0	7	59%
tart shell, 3-inch	1 shell	150	3	12	150	0	10.0	0.0	7	60%
(Pillsbury)	1 slice	110	1	12	140	0	7.0	3.0	5	56%
PIE CRUST MIX										
(Betty Crocker)										
	1 serving	110	1	9	150	0	8.0	2.0	0	64%
stick	1/8 stick	120	1	10	140	0	8.0	2.0	0	62%
(Flako)										
mix only	1/4 cup	130	2	13	170	1	8.0	3.0	5	55%
prepared	1 serving	247	4	24	393	1	15.0	4.5	9	55%
(General Mills) mix only	1/16 pkg	120	1	10	150	0	8.0	0.0	0	62%
(Krusteaz) prepared	1/8 shell	90	1	10	120	0	5.0	0.0	0	51%
(Nabisco)										
chocolate cookie crumbs, 'Oreo' mix only	2 tbsp	80	1	13	140	0	3.0	1.0	0	33%
graham cracker crumbs 'Honey Maid' mix only	2-1/2 tbsp	70	1	13	90	0	2.0	1.0	0	24%

Food Name	Serving Size	Calories	Prot. gms	Carbs gms	Sod. mgs	Fiber gms	Fat gms	Sat. Fat gms	Chol. mgs	% Fat Cal.
vanilla wafer crumbs, 'Nilla' mix only	2 tbsp	70	1	12	55	0	2.0	1.0	5	26%
(Pillsbury)										
mix only	2 tbsp	100	1	10	150	0	6.0	1.5	0	55%
prepared w/water	1/8 pkg	200	3	20	300	0	13.0	3.0	0	56%
PIE FILLING. See also PUDDING/PIE FILLING MIX.										
APPLE PIE FILLING										
(Comstock)										
canned	3.5 oz	120	0	30	15	0	0.0	0.0	0	0%
canned, 'Lite'	3.5 oz	80	0	20	10	0	0.0	0.0	0	0%
(Lucky Leaf)										
canned	4 oz	120	0	30	60	0	0.0	0.0	0	0%
canned, 'Deluxe'	4 oz	120	0	35	40	0	0.0	0.0	0	0%
canned, 'Plus'	4 oz	121	0	30	24	0	0.0	0.0	0	0%
turnover, diced, canned	4 oz	120	0	30	60	0	0.0	0.0	0	0%
(Musselman's)										
canned	4 oz	120	0	30	60	0	0.0	0.0	0	0%
canned, 'Deluxe'	4 oz	120	0	35	40	0	0.0	0.0	0	0%
canned, 'Plus'	4 oz	121	0	30	24	0	0.0	0.0	0	0%
turnover, diced, canned	4 oz	120	0	30	60	0	0.0	0.0	0	0%
(Pathmark) canned 'No Frills'	4 oz	130	0	33	60	0	0.0	0.0	0	0%
(White House) canned	3.5 oz	121	0	29	44	0	1.0	0.0	0	7%
APRICOT										
(Comstock) canned	3.5 oz	110	0	29	100	0	0.0	0.0	0	0%
(Lucky Leaf) canned	4 oz	150	0	39	90	0	0.0	0.0	0	0%
(Musselman's) canned	4 oz	150	0	39	90	0	0.0	0.0	0	0%
BANANA *(Comstock)* canned	3.5 oz	110	1	22	300	1	2.0	0.0	0	16%
BLACKBERRY										
(Lucky Leaf)										
canned	4 oz	120	1	31	140	0	0.0	0.0	0	0%
canned, 'Plus'	4 oz	121	1	30	20	0	0.0	0.0	0	0%
(Musselman's)										
canned	4 oz	120	1	31	140	0	0.0	0.0	0	0%
canned 'Plus'	4 oz	121	1	30	20	0	0.0	0.0	0	0%
BLUEBERRY										
(Comstock)										
canned	3.5 oz	110	0	28	15	1	0.0	0.0	0	0%
canned, 'Lite'	3.5 oz	75	0	17	15	1	0.0	0.0	0	0%
(Lucky Leaf)										
canned, cultivated	4 oz	120	1	31	150	0	0.0	0.0	0	0%
canned, 'Plus'	4 oz	145	0	35	17	0	0.0	0.0	0	0%
(Musselman's)										
canned, cultivated	4 oz	120	1	31	150	0	0.0	0.0	0	0%
canned 'Plus'	4 oz	145	0	35	17	0	0.0	0.0	0	0%
(White House) canned	3.5 oz	118	0	28	48	0	1.0	0.0	0	7%
BOYSENBERRY										
(Lucky Leaf) canned	4 oz	120	1	31	140	0	0.0	0.0	0	0%
(Musselman's) canned	4 oz	120	1	31	140	0	0.0	0.0	0	0%
CHERRY										
(Comstock)										
canned	3.5 oz	110	0	28	15	0	0.0	0.0	0	0%
canned, 'Lite'	3.5 oz	75	0	19	15	0	0.0	0.0	0	0%
(Lucky Leaf) canned	4 oz	120	1	29	50	0	0.0	0.0	0	0%
(Musselman's)										
canned	4 oz	120	1	29	50	0	0.0	0.0	0	0%

Food Name	Serving Size	Calories	Prot. gms	Carbs gms	Sod. mgs	Fiber gms	Fat gms	Sat. Fat gms	Chol. mgs	% Fat Cal.
canned, 'Plus'	4 oz	108	1	26	10	0	0.2	0.0	0	2%
(Pathmark) canned 'No Frills'	4 oz	130	0	33	60	0	0.0	0.0	0	0%
(White House) canned	3.5 oz	141	0	33	54	0	1.0	0.0	0	6%
CHOCOLATE										
(Comstock) canned	3.5 oz	130	1	26	240	0	3.0	0.0	0	20%
(Royal) mousse, 'No-Bake'	1/8 pie	130	3	21	190	0	4.0	0.0	0	27%
COCONUT (Comstock) canned	3.5 oz	120	1	22	290	0	3.0	0.0	0	23%
GOOSEBERRY										
(Lucky Leaf) canned	4 oz	180	0	45	30	0	0.0	0.0	0	0%
(Musselman's) canned	4 oz	180	0	45	30	0	0.0	0.0	0	0%
LEMON										
(Comstock) canned	3.5 oz	140	0	34	110	0	1.0	0.0	0	6%
(Lucky Leaf) canned	4 oz	200	0	48	235	0	2.0	0.0	0	9%
(Lucky Leaf) canned, 'French'	4 oz	180	0	42	140	0	1.0	0.0	0	5%
(Musselman's) canned	4 oz	200	0	48	235	0	2.0	0.0	0	9%
(Musselman's) canned, 'French'	4 oz	180	0	42	140	0	1.0	0.0	0	5%
MINCEMEAT										
(Comstock) canned	3.5 oz	150	0	39	180	1	1.0	0.0	0	5%
(Lucky Leaf) canned	4 oz	190	0	48	145	0	1.0	0.0	0	4%
(Musselman's) canned	4 oz	190	0	48	145	0	1.0	0.0	0	4%
(None Such)										
canned	1/3 cup	200	1	48	280	0	1.0	0.0	0	4%
canned, condensed	1/4 pkg	220	1	50	310	0	2.0	0.0	0	8%
w/brandy and rum, canned	1/3 cup	220	1	48	260	0	2.0	0.0	0	8%
(S&W)	1/4 cup	180	1	43	210	4	2.5	1.5	0	11%
PEACH										
(Comstock) canned	3.5 oz	110	0	26	20	0	0.0	0.0	0	0%
(Lucky Leaf)										
canned	4 oz	150	0	37	65	0	0.0	0.0	0	0%
canned, 'Plus'	4 oz	113	1	27	16	0	0.0	0.0	0	0%
(Musselman's)										
canned	4 oz	150	0	37	65	0	0.0	0.0	0	0%
canned 'Plus'	4 oz	113	1	27	16	0	0.0	0.0	0	0%
(White House) canned	3.5 oz	117	0	28	30	0	1.0	0.0	0	7%
PINEAPPLE										
(Comstock) canned	3.5 oz	100	0	28	65	0	0.0	0.0	0	0%
(Lucky Leaf) canned	4 oz	110	0	30	65	0	0.0	0.0	0	0%
(Musselman's) canned	4 oz	110	0	30	65	0	0.0	0.0	0	0%
PUMPKIN										
(Comstock) canned	3.5 oz	100	0	24	180	0	0.0	0.0	0	0%
(Libby's)										
canned	1 cup	260	2	64	440	0	0.3	0.0	0	1%
canned	1/2 cup	100	1	25	150	2	0.0	0.0	0	0%
(Lucky Leaf) canned	4 oz	170	1	33	200	0	4.0	0.0	0	21%
(Musselman's) canned	4 oz	170	1	33	200	0	4.0	0.0	0	21%
(Stokely) canned	1/2 cup	170	1	44	420	0	0.0	0.0	0	0%
RAISIN										
(Comstock) canned	3.5 oz	120	0	32	80	0	0.0	0.0	0	0%
(Lucky Leaf) canned	4 oz	130	1	34	120	0	1.0	0.0	0	6%
(Musselman's) canned	4 oz	130	1	34	120	0	1.0	0.0	0	6%
RASPBERRY										
(Lucky Leaf) black, canned	4 oz	190	0	43	50	0	0.0	0.0	0	0%
(Lucky Leaf) red, canned	4 oz	190	0	46	80	0	0.0	0.0	0	0%
(Musselman's) black, canned	4 oz	190	0	43	50	0	0.0	0.0	0	0%

Food Name	Serving Size	Calories	Prot. gms	Carbs gms	Sod. mgs	Fiber gms	Fat gms	Sat. Fat gms	Chol. mgs	% Fat Cal.
(Musselman's) red, canned	4 oz	190	0	46	80	0	0.0	0.0	0	0%
STRAWBERRY										
(Comstock) canned	3.5 oz	100	0	25	20	1	0.0	0.0	0	0%
(Lucky Leaf)										
canned	4 oz	120	0	30	75	0	0.0	0.0	0	0%
canned, 'Plus'	4 oz	138	1	34	17	0	0.0	0.0	0	0%
(Musselman's)										
canned	4 oz	120	0	30	75	0	0.0	0.0	0	0%
canned, 'Plus'	4 oz	138	1	34	17	0	0.0	0.0	0	0%
STRAWBERRY-RHUBARB										
(Lucky Leaf) canned	4 oz	120	0	31	95	0	0.0	0.0	0	0%
(Musselman's) canned	4 oz	120	0	31	95	0	0.0	0.0	0	0%
VANILLA CREME										
(Lucky Leaf)	4 oz	150	0	32	145	0	3.0	0.0	0	17%
(Musselman's)	4 oz	150	0	32	145	0	3.0	0.0	0	17%
PIE MIX										
BANANA CREAM										
(Jell-O)										
'No Bake' prepared	1/8 pie	240	3	27	300	0	14.0	0.0	30	51%
'No Bake' mix only	1 pkg	140	1	25	190	0	5.0	0.0	0	30%
'No Bake' prepared w/whole milk	1/8 pie	240	3	27	300	0	14.0	0.0	30	51%
CHOCOLATE PIE MIX, MOUSSE										
(Jell-O)										
mousse, 'No Bake' mix only	1 pkg	160	2	22	320	0	7.0	0.0	0	40%
mousse, 'No Bake' prepared	1/8 pie	260	4	25	430	0	17.0	0.0	30	57%
mousse, 'No Bake' prepared w/whole milk	1/8 pie	260	4	25	430	0	17.0	0.0	30	57%
(Royal)										
mint, 'No-Bake' prepared	1/8 pie	260	5	25	280	0	15.0	0.0	0	53%
mousse, 'No Bake' prepared	1/8 pie	230	4	27	260	0	12.0	0.0	0	47%
COCONUT CREAM										
(Jell-O)										
'No Bake' mix only	1 pkg	160	1	25	200	0	7.0	0.0	0	38%
'No Bake' prepared	1/8 pie	260	3	27	300	0	16.0	0.0	30	55%
'No Bake' prepared w/whole milk	1/8 pie	260	3	27	300	0	16.0	0.0	30	55%
LEMON MERINGUE										
(Royal) 'No Bake' prepared	1/8 pie	310	3	50	250	0	11.0	0.0	0	32%
PUMPKIN										
(Jell-O)										
'No Bake' mix only	1 pkg	140	1	28	330	0	3.0	0.0	0	19%
'No Bake' prepared	1/8 pie	250	4	31	450	0	13.0	0.0	30	46%
'No Bake' prepared w/whole milk	1/8 pie	250	4	31	450	0	13.0	0.0	30	46%
(Libby's) prepared	1/6 pie	390	7	53	380	0	17.0	5.0	70	39%
PIEROGI										
(Mrs. T's)										
potato and American cheese filled	3 pierogies	220	9	32	540	1	6.0	3.5	20	25%
potato and onion filled	3 pierogies	180	6	34	340	2	2.0	0.0	15	10%
sauerkraut filled	3 pierogies	160	6	32	850	3	1.5	0.0	10	8%

PIGEON. See SQUAB.

PIGEON PEA. See PEAS, PIGEON.

PIGNOLI NUT. See PINE NUT.

PIG'S EAR. See under PORK.

PIG'S FEET. See under PORK.

PIG'S HEART. See under PORK.

PIG'S JOWL. See under PORK.

Food Name	Serving Size	Calories	Prot. gms	Carbs gms	Sod. mgs	Fiber gms	Fat gms	Sat. Fat gms	Chol. mgs	% Fat Cal.
PIG'S KNUCKLES. See under PORK.										
PIG'S TAIL. See under PORK.										
PIG'S TONGUE. See under PORK.										
PIKE										
NORTHERN										
baked, broiled, grilled, or microwaved	3 oz	96	21	0	42	0	0.7	0.1	43	7%
raw	3 oz	75	16	0	33	0	0.6	0.1	33	7%
WALLEYE										
baked, broiled, grilled, or microwaved	3 oz	101	21	0	55	0	1.3	0.3	94	12%
raw	3 oz	79	16	0	43	0	1.0	0.2	73	12%
PILAF ENTRÉE										
(Health Valley)										
oat bran, w/garden vegetables 'Fast Menu'	7.5 oz	210	8	31	445	6	7.0	0.0	0	29%
(Weight Watchers) Florentine	1 entrée	290	9	47	550	6	7.0	2.0	5	22%
PILI NUT, CANARY TREE										
dried	1 cup	863	13	5	4	na	95.5	37.4	0	93%
dried, approx 15 kernels	1 oz	204	3	1	1	na	22.6	8.8	0	93%
PIMIENTO										
Canned or jarred										
	1 cup	44	2	10	27	4	0.6	0.1	0	11%
all varieties, drained *(Dromedary)*	1 oz	10	0	2	5	0	0.0	0.0	0	0%
chopped	1 tbsp	3	0	1	2	0	0.0	0.0	0	11%
sliced	1 slice	<1	0	0	0	0	0.0	0.0	0	11%
whole	1 whole pimiento	15	1	3	9	1	0.2	0.0	0	11%
PIMIENTO SPREAD *(Price's)*	1 oz	80	3	2	0	0	6.0	0.0	0	73%
PIÑA COLADA. See under COCKTAIL; COCKTAIL MIX.										
PINE NUT / Colorado pinyon / Italian stone pine nut / pignoli / pinnochio /piñon										
(Progresso)	1 oz jar	170	0	2	0	0	13.0	1.0	0	94%
dried	1 cup	770	33	19	5	6	69.0	10.6	0	75%
dried	1 oz	160	7	4	1	1	14.4	2.2	0	75%
dried	1 tbsp	49	2	1	0	0	4.4	0.7	0	75%
dried	10 med nuts	10	0	0	0	0	0.9	0.1	0	75%
natural, unsalted *(Flanigan Farms)*	1/4 cup	150	7	4	0	1	14.0	2.0	0	74%
PINEAPPLE										
Canned										
chunks, in extra heavy syrup, w/liquids	1 cup	216	1	56	3	2	0.3	0.0	0	1%
chunks, in heavy syrup, w/liquid	1 cup	198	1	51	3	2	0.3	0.0	0	1%
chunks, in juice, w/liquid	1 cup	149	1	39	2	2	0.2	0.0	0	1%
chunks, in light syrup, w/liquid	1 cup	131	1	34	3	2	0.2	0.0	0	2%
chunks, in water, w/liquid	1 cup	79	1	20	2	2	0.2	0.0	0	2%
crushed, in extra heavy syrup, w/liquids	1 cup	216	1	56	3	2	0.3	0.0	0	1%
crushed, in heavy syrup, w/liquid	1 cup	198	1	51	3	2	0.3	0.0	0	1%
crushed, in juice, w/liquid	1 cup	149	1	39	2	2	0.2	0.0	0	1%
crushed, in light syrup, w/liquid	1 cup	131	1	34	3	2	0.3	0.0	0	2%
crushed, in water, w/liquid	1 cup	79	1	20	2	2	0.2	0.0	0	2%
rings, in heavy syrup, 3-inch diam, w/liquid	1 ring	38	0	10	0	0	0.1	0.0	0	1%
rings, in juice, 3-inch diam, w/liquid	1 ring w/liqid	28	0	7	0	0	0.0	0.0	0	1%
rings, in light syrup, 3-inch diam, w/liquid	1 ring w/liqid	25	0	6	0	0	0.1	0.0	0	2%
rings, in water, 3-inch diam, w/liquid	1 ring w/liqid	15	0	4	0	0	0.0	0.0	0	2%
sliced *(S&W)*	1 slice	90	0	23	10	1	0.0	0.0	0	0%
sliced, in extra heavy syrup, w/liquids	1 cup	216	1	56	3	2	0.3	0.0	0	1%
sliced, in heavy syrup, w/liquid	1 cup	198	1	51	3	2	0.3	0.0	0	1%
sliced, in juice, w/liquid	1 cup	149	1	39	2	2	0.2	0.0	0	1%
sliced, in light syrup, w/liquid	1 cup	131	1	34	3	2	0.3	0.0	0	2%

Food Name	Serving Size	Calories	Prot. gms	Carbs gms	Sod. mgs	Fiber gms	Fat gms	Sat. Fat gms	Chol. mgs	% Fat Cal.
sliced, in water, w/liquid............................	1 cup	79	1	20	2	2	0.2	0.0	0	2%
Fresh										
raw, diced	1 cup	76	1	19	2	2	0.7	0.1	0	7%
raw, sliced, 3.5 inch diam, 1/2 inch thick..............	1 slice	27	0	7	1	1	0.2	0.0	0	7%
raw, sliced, 3.5 inch diam, 3/4 inch thick..............	1 slice	41	0	10	1	1	0.4	0.0	0	7%
raw, whole, trimmed	1 med fruit	231	2	58	5	6	2.0	0.2	0	7%
Frozen										
chunks (Flav-R-Pac).............................	2/3 cup	75	0	19	0	0	0.0	0.0	0	0%
chunks, sweetened	1 cup	208	1	54	5	3	0.2	0.0	0	1%

PINEAPPLE DRINK. See under FRUIT DRINK; FRUIT JUICE DRINK.

PINEAPPLE JUICE. See also under FRUIT JUICE BLEND; FRUIT JUICE DRINK.

Can, bottle, box, or carton

Food Name	Serving Size	Calories	Prot. gms	Carbs gms	Sod. mgs	Fiber gms	Fat gms	Sat. Fat gms	Chol. mgs	% Fat Cal.
unsweetened, w/added ascorbic acid	1 cup	140	1	34	3	1	0.2	0.0	0	1%
unsweetened, w/o added ascorbic acid	1 cup	140	1	34	3	1	0.2	0.0	0	1%
(Del Monte)										
. . . .	8 fl oz	110	1	29	15	2	0.0	0.0	0	0%
unsweetened...............................	6 fl oz	100	0	25	10	0	0.0	0.0	0	0%
(Dole)	6 fl oz	103	1	25	2	0	0.2	0.0	0	2%
(IGA) unsweetened	6 fl oz	100	0	25	10	0	0.0	0.0	0	0%
(J. Hungerford)										
100% juice.	9.03 fl oz	124	1	31	9	0	0.0	0.0	0	0%
regular.	9.03 fl oz	114	0	29	0	0	0.0	0.0	0	0%
(Knudsen)	8 fl oz	110	1	25	0	0	0.0	0.0	0	0%
(Minute Maid).	6 fl oz	90	1	23	20	0	0.0	0.0	0	0%
(Mott's)	9.5 fl oz	169	0	42	0	0	0.0	0.0	0	0%
(Pathmark)										
'Hawaiian'	6 fl oz	100	0	25	10	0	0.0	0.0	0	0%
unsweetened, 'No Frills'	6 fl oz	100	0	25	0	0	0.0	0.0	0	0%
(S&W)										
. . . .	8 fl oz	110	0	29	15	2	0.0	0.0	0	0%
unsweetened...............................	6 fl oz	90	0	23	10	2	0.0	0.0	0	0%
(Veryfine) '100%'	8 fl oz	125	1	31	10	0	0.0	0.0	0	0%
Frozen or chilled										
concentrate, prepared......................	1 cup	130	1	32	3	1	0.1	0.0	0	0%
concentrate, unprepared....................	6 fl oz	387	3	96	6	2	0.2	0.0	0	0%
(Minute Maid).	6 fl oz	90	1	23	0	0	0.0	0.0	0	0%

PINEAPPLE TOPPING

Food Name	Serving Size	Calories	Prot. gms	Carbs gms	Sod. mgs	Fiber gms	Fat gms	Sat. Fat gms	Chol. mgs	% Fat Cal.
(Kraft)	1 tbsp	50	0	13	0	0	0.0	0.0	0	0%
(Smucker's)	2 tbsp	130	0	32	0	0	0.0	0.0	0	0%

PINK BEAN. See BEAN, PINK.

PINK GRAPEFRUIT JUICE. See under GRAPEFRUIT JUICE.

PINK SALMON. See under SALMON.

PINNOCHIO. See PINE NUT.

PIÑON. See PINE NUT.

PINTO BEAN. See BEAN, PINTO.

PISTACHIO

Food Name	Serving Size	Calories	Prot. gms	Carbs gms	Sod. mgs	Fiber gms	Fat gms	Sat. Fat gms	Chol. mgs	% Fat Cal.
in shell (Dole)	1 oz	90	3	3	250	0	7.0	0.0	0	72%
natural (Blue Diamond).	1 oz	140	6	4	210	3	12.0	2.0	0	73%
natural, in shell (Fisher).	1 oz	170	5	7	85	0	14.0	2.0	0	72%
natural, unsalted (Flanigan Farms)	1/4 cup	180	6	8	0	3	14.0	2.0	0	69%
red (Blue Diamond).	1 oz	140	6	3	230	3	12.0	2.0	0	75%
red (Fisher)	1/4 cup	111	3	4	33	1	9.8	1.6	0	75%
Dried										
raw	1 cup	705	26	37	1	13	55.3	6.8	0	66%

Food Name	Serving Size	Calories	Prot. gms	Carbs gms	Sod. mgs	Fiber gms	Fat gms	Sat. Fat gms	Chol. mgs	% Fat Cal.
raw	30 nuts	99	4	5	0	2	7.8	1.0	0	66%
raw, approx 47 kernels	1 oz	156	6	8	0	3	12.2	1.5	0	66%
Dry roasted										
(Dole)	1 oz	163	6	7	2	0	14.0	0.0	0	71%
natural or red (Planters)	1 oz	170	6	6	250	0	14.0	2.0	0	72%
salted	1 cup	726	27	35	545	13	58.5	7.1	0	68%
salted, approx 47 kernels	1 oz	161	6	8	121	3	13.0	1.6	0	68%
unsalted	1 cup	730	27	36	13	13	58.5	7.1	0	67%
unsalted, approx 47 kernels	1 oz	162	6	8	3	3	13.0	1.6	0	67%
Roasted, (David's) salted	1 pkg	270	9	11	250	4	21.0	2.5	0	70%
PISTACHIO BUTTER, roasted										
(Maranatha Natural)	2 tbsp	170	6	7	5	0	13.0	0.0	0	69%
PITA. See under BREAD.										
PITANGA / Surinam cherry										
raw	1 cup	57	1.4	13.0	5	>1.0 c	0.7	na	0	10%
raw, trimmed	1/2 cup	29	0.7	6.5	3	>.5 c	0.3	(tr)	0	9%
raw, trimmed	1 oz	9	0.2	2.1	1	>.2 c	0.1	(tr)	0	9%
raw, trimmed, approx .3 oz	1 medium	2	0.1	0.5	0	tr	0.0	na	0	0%
raw, untrimmed	1 lb	132	3.2	29.9	11	>2.4 c	1.6	na	0	10%
PIZZA										
(Banquet)										
cheese, on French bread, frozen, 'Zap'	4.5 oz	310	14	41	800	0	10.0	0.0	35	29%
deluxe, on French bread, frozen, 'Zap'	4.8 oz	330	13	39	890	0	13.0	0.0	25	36%
pepperoni, 'Pizza Pie'	1 pizza	470	11	45	970	0	27.0	0.0	35	52%
pepperoni, on French bread, 'Zap'	4.5 oz	350	15	36	1060	0	16.0	0.0	40	41%
sausage, 'Pizza Pie'	6 oz	500	11	48	860	0	29.0	0.0	35	53%
sausage and pepperoni, 'Pizza Pie'	6 oz	470	12	43	930	0	27.0	0.0	40	52%
(Celentano)										
cheese, 5.5 oz	2 1/4 slices	340	14	46	440	4	11.0	5.0	25	29%
thick crust, 6.5 oz	1/2 pizza	390	18	62	840	8	12.0	8.0	25	25%
(Celeste)										
cheese, individual	1 pizza	420	18	42	830	3	20.0	10.0	35	43%
cheese, large	1 slice	320	14	32	590	3	16.0	8.0	25	44%
four cheese, individual, 'Original'	1 pizza	480	22	41	920	4	26.0	11.0	45	48%
four cheese, zesty, individual	1 pizza	470	21	44	970	4	24.0	12.0	40	45%
individual, 'Deluxe'	1 pizza	470	18	46	1140	5	25.0	9.0	25	47%
large, 'Deluxe'	1 slice	350	14	35	880	4	18.0	6.0	20	45%
pepperoni, individual	1 pizza	470	16	41	1100	4	27.0	9.0	20	52%
pepperoni, large	1 slice	350	13	33	990	3	20.0	7.0	20	49%
sausage	1/4 pizza	375	16	30	900	3	22.0	7.0	15	52%
sausage, individual sized	1 pizza	530	23	52	1400	5	27.0	9.0	25	45%
sausage, w/green and red peppers, mushrooms, frozen, 'Deluxe'	1 pkg	1538	67	133	3050	na	82.6	32.4	147	48%
sausage, w/green and red peppers, mushrooms, frozen, 'Deluxe'	1 serving	386	17	33	765	na	20.7	8.1	37	48%
suprema, individual	1 pizza	500	22	49	1290	6	27.0	9.0	25	46%
suprema, large	1 slice	290	13	27	770	3	16.0	5.0	15	47%
vegetable, individual sized	1 pizza	420	17	46	1120	5	21.0	7.0	5	43%
(Crisp 'N Tasty)										
combination	1/2 serving	280	10	27	680	1	15.0	4.0	15	48%
pepperoni	1/2 serving	280	10	28	710	1	15.0	4.0	15	47%
sausage	1/2 serving	280	10	27	640	1	15.0	3.0	10	48%
(Empire Kosher)										
kosher	1 piece	150	7	15	390	0	5.0	2.5	15	34%

Food Name	Serving Size	Calories	Prot. gms	Carbs gms	Sod. mgs	Fiber gms	Fat gms	Sat. Fat gms	Chol. mgs	% Fat Cal.
kosher, on English muffin	1 muffin	130	7	15	390	1	5.0	2.5	15	34%
kosher, 3 pack.	1 pizza	210	10	23	630	7	9.0	4.0	20	38%
kosher, 10 oz.	1/2 pizza	340	18	38	970	2	13.0	7.0	30	34%
(Graindance Pizza)										
cheese, whole wheat crust, all natural	1 slice	200	9	23	400	0	8.0	0.0	0	36%
(Healthy Choice)										
cheese, on French bread	1 entrée	340	22	51	480	5	5.0	1.5	15	13%
deluxe, on French bread, frozen	6.25 oz	330	23	41	490	0	8.0	3.0	35	22%
pepperoni, on French bread	1 entrée	340	24	49	580	6	5.0	1.5	20	13%
sausage, on French bread	1 entrée	320	21	48	580	5	5.0	1.5	25	14%
supreme, on French bread	1 entrée	330	21	51	580	6	5.0	1.5	20	14%
vegetable, on French bread	1 entrée	280	17	45	480	5	4.0	1.5	10	13%
(Jack's)										
pepperoni, frozen, 'Jack's Original'	1 pkg	1288	60	118	2440	na	64.2	24.8	160	45%
pepperoni, frozen, 'Jack's Original'	1 serving	323	15	30	612	na	16.1	6.2	40	45%
sausage and pepperoni, 'Great Combinations'	1 pkg	1389	69	120	2828	na	70.0	26.4	175	45%
sausage and pepperoni, 'Great Combinations'	1 serving	348	17	30	708	na	17.5	6.6	44	45%
(Jeno's)										
cheese, microwave, individual	1 serving	240	10	25	530	1	11.0	3.5	15	41%
combination, microwave, individual	1 serving	310	11	25	720	1	18.0	4.5	15	53%
pepperoni, 'Pizza Pocket'	1 serving	370	12	35	790	0	20.0	6.0	25	49%
pepperoni, frozen, 'Crisp 'n Tasty'	1 pkg	516	19	46	1221	3	28.8	6.5	23	50%
pepperoni, individual, microwave	1 serving	280	10	25	710	1	16.0	3.5	15	51%
sausage, individual	1 serving	280	10	25	650	1	16.0	4.0	10	51%
sausage, 'Pizza Pocket'	1 serving	360	11	35	660	0	19.0	7.0	15	48%
sausage and pepperoni, 'Crisp 'n Tasty'	1 pkg	491	17	52	1239	3	24.2	5.7	26	44%
sausage and pepperoni, 'Pizza Pocket'	1 serving	360	12	35	710	0	20.0	7.0	20	49%
supreme, 'Pizza Pocket'	1 serving	370	12	36	720	0	19.0	7.0	20	47%
(Kashi) spicy Southwest, vegetarian, frozen	1 slice	210	9	28	380	11	7.0	0.0	9	30%
(Kid Cuisine)										
cheese	6.85 oz	380	11	57	390	0	12.0	0.0	25	28%
hamburger	6.85 oz	330	11	50	700	0	10.0	0.0	15	27%
(Lean Cuisine)										
cheese, on French bread	1 entrée	350	22	48	400	4	8.0	4.0	20	20%
deluxe, on French bread	1 entrée	330	23	45	560	5	6.0	2.5	30	17%
pepperoni, on French bread	1 entrée	330	20	46	590	4	7.0	3.0	25	19%
sausage, on French bread, frozen	6 oz	350	22	42	600	0	10.0	4.0	35	26%
(Mrs. Paterson's)										
supreme, hand held, frozen, 'Aussie Pie'	5.5 oz	470	12	44	880	0	27.0	10.0	75	52%
(Nature's Hilights)										
Italian cheese	1/2 pizza	360	18	46	640	2	12.0	7.0	30	30%
soy cheese	1/2 pizza	290	16	52	430	2	1.5	0.0	0	5%
(Oven Lovin')										
cheese, microwave	1/2 pizza	250	11	24	430	0	12.0	4.0	10	44%
cheese, on French bread, frozen, microwave	1 serving	350	17	40	700	0	14.0	5.0	15	36%
combination, microwave	1/2 pizza	310	13	26	580	0	18.0	7.0	20	51%
combination, on French bread, frozen, microwave	1 serving	420	18	41	910	0	21.0	10.0	30	44%
pepperoni, microwave	1/2 pizza	300	13	25	620	0	17.0	6.0	25	50%
pepperoni, on French bread, frozen, microwave	1 serving	410	18	40	980	0	21.0	8.0	35	45%
sausage, microwave	1/2 pizza	290	12	26	510	0	16.0	7.0	15	49%
sausage, on French bread, frozen, microwave	1 serving	400	18	41	830	0	20.0	10.0	25	43%
supreme, microwave	1/2 pizza	310	13	27	570	0	18.0	7.0	20	50%
(Pappalo's)										
cheese, on French bread, frozen	1 piece	360	16	40	830	0	15.0	0.0	0	38%

Food Name	Serving Size	Calories	Prot. gms	Carbs gms	Sod. mgs	Fiber gms	Fat gms	Sat. Fat gms	Chol. mgs	% Fat Cal.
combination, on French bread, frozen	1 piece	430	19	41	1120	0	21.0	0.0	0	44%
pepperoni, deep dish	1 slice	340	17	37	720	2	14.0	6.0	30	37%
pepperoni, deep dish, individual, frozen, 'For One'	1 pizza	525	23	65	983	3	19.5	7.3	38	33%
pepperoni, on French bread, frozen	1 piece	410	16	41	1130	0	20.0	0.0	0	44%
pepperoni, pan pizza	1/5 pizza	350	22	40	720	3	11.0	6.0	50	29%
pepperoni, pizzeria style, 12 inch	1 slice	380	18	38	840	2	17.0	8.0	40	41%
pepperoni, traditional crust, 9 inch	1/2 pizza	390	23	47	870	4	14.0	6.0	45	31%
sausage, deep dish	1 slice	330	16	36	600	2	13.0	8.0	25	36%
sausage, on French bread, frozen	1 piece	410	18	41	1000	0	18.0	0.0	0	41%
sausage, pan pizza	1/5 pizza	350	22	39	530	3	11.0	5.0	40	29%
sausage, pizzeria style crust, 12 inch	1 slice	370	18	38	710	2	16.0	10.0	30	39%
sausage, traditional crust, 9 inch	1/2 pizza	380	22	47	680	4	13.0	6.0	40	30%
sausage and pepperoni, deep dish	1 slice	330	16	36	650	2	14.0	8.0	25	38%
sausage and pepperoni, pan pizza	1/5 pizza	360	22	40	630	3	12.0	6.0	45	30%
sausage and pepperoni, pizzeria style, 12 inch	1 slice	380	18	39	780	2	17.0	9.0	35	40%
sausage and pepperoni, traditional crust, 9 inch	1/2 pizza	390	23	45	650	4	15.0	7.0	45	33%
supreme, pan pizza	1/5 pizza	340	22	37	610	3	12.0	6.0	45	31%
supreme, traditional crust, 12 inch	1/4 pizza	350	22	38	640	4	12.0	6.0	45	31%
supreme, traditional crust, 9 inch	1/2 pizza	400	25	46	700	4	16.0	7.0	45	34%
three cheese, pan	1/5 pizza	310	20	39	490	3	8.0	5.0	30	23%
three cheese, traditional crust, 12 inch	1/4 pizza	310	20	41	440	4	7.0	4.0	30	21%
three cheese, traditional crust, 9 inch	1/2 pizza	350	21	47	640	4	11.0	6.0	30	27%
(Pepperidge Farm)										
cheese, on croissant pastry	1 pizza	430	15	41	640	0	23.0	0.0	0	48%
deluxe, on croissant pastry	1 pizza	440	16	43	790	0	23.0	0.0	0	47%
pepperoni, on croissant pastry	1 pizza	420	14	43	690	0	22.0	0.0	0	46%
(Pillsbury)										
cheese, on French bread, frozen, 'Microwave'	1 piece	370	18	41	680	0	15.0	0.0	0	36%
pepperoni, on French bread, frozen, 'Microwave'	1 piece	430	19	45	940	0	19.0	0.0	0	40%
sausage, on French bread, frozen, 'Microwave'	1 piece	410	18	48	860	0	16.0	0.0	0	35%
sausage combo, w/pepperoni, on French bread, frozen, 'Microwave'	1 piece	450	19	47	950	0	21.0	0.0	0	42%
(Pizsoy)										
cheese, w/tofu mozzarella, whole wheat crust, original	1 slice	165	12	28	206	0	5.0	0.0	0	22%
(Red Baron)										
cheese	1/5 pizza	350	16	33	680	2	17.0	8.0	30	44%
cheese, 'Deep Dish Singles'	1 pizza	460	15	41	760	2	23.0	9.0	20	48%
cheese, sausage, mushrooms, pepperoni, and vegetable	1/5 pizza	340	14	31	690	2	18.0	7.0	25	47%
pepperoni, 'Deep Dish Singles'	1 pizza	530	18	47	90	2	31.0	11.0	35	52%
pepperoni, frozen, 'Premium Deep Dish Singles'	1 pkg	961	32	96	1777	na	50.1	16.4	57	47%
pepperoni, frozen, 'Premium Deep Dish Singles'	1 serving	480	16	48	889	na	25.0	8.2	29	47%
pepperoni, frozen	1 pkg	1788	73	146	4137	na	101.5	36.6	150	51%
pepperoni, frozen	1 serving	442	18	36	1023	na	25.1	9.0	37	51%
sausage	1/5 pizza	340	15	32	700	2	18.0	7.0	25	46%
sausage, ham, and pepperoni, 'Deep Dish Singles'	1 pizza	490	16	41	970	2	26.0	9.0	25	51%
sausage, pepperoni, mushroom, pepper, and onion	1/5 pizza	360	15	33	730	2	19.0	7.0	25	47%
supreme, w/sausage, mushrooms, pepperoni, frozen	1 pkg	1736	69	161	3725	na	91.2	30.7	117	47%
supreme, w/sausage, mushrooms, pepperoni, frozen	1 serving	344	14	32	738	na	18.1	6.1	23	47%
two cheese, w/sausage, pepperoni, onions, 'Deluxe'	1 pkg	1746	62	166	3653	na	92.3	32.5	127	48%
two cheese, w/sausage, pepperoni, onions, 'Deluxe'	1 serving	337	12	32	704	na	17.8	6.3	25	48%
(Smart Ones) combo, deluxe, pizza	1 entrée	380	23	47	550	6	11.0	6.0	40	26%
(Soypreme)										
cheese, w/tofu mozzarella, whole wheat crust	1 slice	209	10	22	300	0	7.0	0.0	0	33%

Food Name	Serving Size	Calories	Prot. gms	Carbs gms	Sod. mgs	Fiber gms	Fat gms	Sat. Fat gms	Chol. mgs	% Fat Cal.
cheese, w/tofu mozzarella, whole wheat crust, 'Garden Patch'	1 slice	211	10	24	362	0	7.0	0.0	0	32%
(Stouffer's)										
bacon cheddar, on French bread	1 entrée	440	16	44	940	4	22.0	7.0	30	45%
Canadian bacon, on French bread	5.5 oz	370	18	40	1070	0	15.0	0.0	0	37%
cheese, on French bread	1/2 pizza	350	15	42	660	3	14.0	5.0	15	36%
cheeseburger, on French bread	1/2 pizza	440	21	31	1110	5	26.0	9.0	55	53%
deluxe, w/sausage, pepperoni, mushroom, on French bread, frozen	1 pkg	858	32	89	1680	7	41.3	12.7	67	43%
deluxe, w/sausage, pepperoni, mushroom, on French bread, frozen	1 serving	429	16	44	840	4	20.6	6.4	33	43%
double cheese, on French bread	1/2 pizza	420	19	44	790	5	19.0	7.0	30	40%
hamburger, on French bread, frozen	1 pkg	410	23	39	650	0	18.0	0.0	0	40%
on French bread, 'Deluxe'	1/2 pizza	440	19	42	980	5	22.0	7.0	35	45%
pepperoni, on French bread	1/2 pizza	420	18	42	930	3	20.0	6.0	35	43%
pepperoni, w/mushrooms, on French bread	1/2 pizza	430	17	43	1000	3	21.0	6.0	30	44%
sausage, on French bread	1/2 pizza	420	19	41	900	4	20.0	5.0	35	43%
sausage and pepperoni, on French bread	1/2 pizza	490	22	45	1130	4	25.0	7.0	4	46%
vegetable, deluxe, on French bread	1/2 pizza	400	18	43	830	5	17.0	6.0	25	39%
w/sausage and pepperoni, on French bread, frozen	1 pkg	896	35	87	1720	5	45.0	14.3	74	45%
w/sausage and pepperoni, on French bread, frozen	1 serving	448	18	44	860	2	22.5	7.1	37	45%
(Tombstone)										
bacon, Canadian style, 12 inch, 'Original'	3.6 oz	230	12	23	580	0	10.0	4.0	25	39%
bacon cheeseburger, 12 inch, 'Special Order'	4.7 oz	330	17	29	730	0	16.0	7.0	40	44%
cheese, microwave, 7 inch	7.7 oz	500	25	45	940	0	24.0	8.0	40	44%
cheese, original, 12 inch	3.4 oz	230	11	23	460	0	10.0	4.0	25	40%
cheese, original, 9 inch	5.6 oz	380	18	40	730	0	17.0	7.0	35	40%
cheese, sausage, and mushroom, original, 12 inch	3.8 oz	240	13	23	570	0	11.0	4.0	30	41%
cheese, w/hamburger, original, 12 inch	3.7 oz	250	13	23	570	0	12.0	5.0	30	43%
cheese, w/pepperoni, 'Italian Thincrust'	3 oz	230	11	15	540	0	14.0	5.0	25	55%
cheese, w/sausage, 12' 'Original'	3.7 oz	240	13	23	590	0	11.0	4.0	30	41%
cheese and hamburger, original, 9 inch	6.3 oz	440	22	41	960	0	21.0	8.0	50	43%
cheese and pepperoni, microwave, 7 inch	7.5 oz	550	27	38	1240	0	32.0	11.0	55	53%
cheese and pepperoni, original, 9 inch	6.3 oz	480	21	40	1100	0	26.0	10.0	50	49%
cheese and sausage 'Italian Thincrust'	3.2 oz	220	11	15	490	0	13.0	5.0	30	53%
cheese and sausage, original, 9 inch	6.3 oz	420	22	41	1000	0	19.0	7.0	50	40%
chicken, deluxe, light,	1/2 pizza	180	13	23	440	2	4.0	1.0	15	20%
chicken, light, 8 inch	4.5 oz	240	17	28	450	0	8.0	3.0	25	29%
deluxe, original, 12 inch	1 slice	310	15	29	690	3	14.0	6.0	30	42%
double cheese, w/pepperoni, double top, 12 inch	4.8 oz	360	20	24	920	0	20.0	8.0	50	51%
four cheese, 'Special Order'	4.3 oz	300	15	28	630	0	14.0	6.0	35	42%
four meat, 'Special Order'	4.6 oz	320	17	28	810	0	15.0	6.0	40	43%
four meat, 9 inch, 'Special Order'	3.9 oz	280	14	24	670	0	14.0	6.0	35	45%
Italian sausage, 'Special Order'	4.5 oz	300	17	28	740	0	13.0	6.0	40	39%
Italian sausage, microwave, 7 inch	8.0 oz	550	28	38	1210	0	32.0	10.0	65	52%
pepperoni and sausage, original, 9 inch	6.6 oz	490	24	40	1230	0	26.0	10.0	60	48%
pepperoni and sausage, original, frozen	1 pkg	952	40	82	2184	5	51.7	18.9	96	49%
pepperoni and sausage, original, frozen	1 serving	317	13	27	728	2	17.2	6.3	32	49%
pepperoni, 'Special Order'	4.4 oz	320	16	28	780	0	16.0	7.0	40	45%
pepperoni, 8 inch, 'Light'	4.0 oz	250	16	27	630	0	10.0	4.0	20	34%
pepperoni, 9 inch, 'Special Order'	3.7 oz	280	13	24	650	0	14.0	6.0	30	46%
pepperoni, original, 12 inch	1 slice	400	19	35	930	3	21.0	9.0	40	47%
pepperoni, original, frozen, 12 inch	1 pkg	938	44	85	1659	na	47.3	18.1	95	45%
pepperoni, original, frozen, 12 inch	1 serving	312	14	28	551	na	15.7	6.0	32	45%

Food Name	Serving Size	Calories	Prot. gms	Carbs gms	Sod. mgs	Fiber gms	Fat gms	Sat. Fat gms	Chol. mgs	% Fat Cal.
pepperoni, original, frozen, 9 inch	1 pkg	1659	71	155	3489	na	83.6	31.5	165	45%
pepperoni, original, frozen, 9 inch	1 serving	413	18	39	869	na	20.8	7.8	41	45%
pepperoni, thin crust	1 slice	400	18	25	920	2	25.0	11.0	50	57%
ranchero, deluxe, 'Mexican Style Thincrust'	3.4 oz	230	11	16	530	0	13.0	5.0	40	52%
sausage, double top, w/double cheese, 12 inch	4.8 oz	330	21	24	860	0	16.0	6.0	50	44%
sausage and mushroom, original	1 pkg	1496	70	152	3509	na	67.1	24.8	129	40%
sausage and mushroom, original	1 serving	306	14	31	718	na	13.7	5.1	26	40%
sausage and pepperoni, double top, 12 inch	4.8 oz	340	21	24	910	0	18.0	7.0	50	47%
sausage and pepperoni, microwave, 7 inch	8 oz	570	32	39	1430	0	32.0	11.0	70	50%
sausage and pepperoni, original	1 pkg	1635	72	153	3944	11	81.7	30.4	156	45%
sausage and pepperoni, original	1 serving	328	14	31	790	2	16.4	6.1	31	45%
sausage and pepperoni, original, 12 inch	3.7 oz	260	13	23	640	0	13.0	5.0	30	45%
supreme, 'Italian Style Thincrust'	3.38 oz	230	11	16	520	0	14.0	5.0	30	54%
supreme, 'Special Order'	4.4 oz	320	17	29	800	0	15.0	6.0	40	42%
supreme, 9 inch, 'Special Order'	4.0 oz	280	13	24	640	0	14.0	6.0	35	46%
supreme, light	1 slice	270	17	30	720	3	9.0	3.5	20	30%
supreme, microwave, 7 inch	8.5 oz	550	27	40	1260	0	31.0	10.0	55	51%
supreme, original, 12 inch	3.8 oz	270	12	24	630	0	14.0	5.0	30	47%
supreme, thin crust	1 slice	380	18	26	840	2	22.0	10.0	45	53%
taco, microwave, 7 inch	8.4 oz	590	28	41	1460	0	34.0	13.0	100	53%
three sausage, 9 inch, 'Special Order'	3.8 oz	260	14	24	600	0	12.0	5.0	35	42%
vegetable, light	1 slice	240	14	31	500	3	7.0	2.5	10	26%
(Tony's)										
pepperoni, w/Italian style pastry crust, frozen	1 pkg	1232	45	110	2531	na	67.9	23.2	96	50%
pepperoni, w/Italian style pastry crust, frozen	1 serving	406	15	36	834	na	22.4	7.6	32	50%
sausage, deep dish, frozen, 'D'Primo'	1 pkg	1576	50	164	3351	na	80.2	23.2	63	46%
sausage, deep dish, frozen, 'D'Primo'	1 serving	391	12	41	830	na	19.9	5.7	16	46%
sausage and pepperoni, w/Italian style pastry crust	1 pkg	1319	46	126	2186	na	70.2	20.9	72	48%
sausage and pepperoni, w/Italian style pastry crust	1 serving	434	15	41	719	na	23.1	6.9	24	48%
supreme, w/sausage, pepperoni, mushroom, peppers, onion, Italian crust	1 pkg	1213	48	118	2341	na	60.6	20.9	85	45%
supreme, w/sausage, pepperoni, mushroom, peppers, onion, Italian crust	1 serving	400	16	39	772	na	20.0	6.9	28	45%
taco style, w/sausage, sauce, corn style crust	1 pkg	1326	43	130	2293	na	70.5	23.5	84	48%
taco style, w/sausage, sauce, corn style crust	1 serving	437	14	43	756	na	23.3	7.7	28	48%
(Totino's)										
baconburger, on French bread, 'Party'	1/2 pizza	370	15	33	880	2	20.0	4.5	15	48%
Canadian bacon, 'Party'	1/2 pizza	320	14	33	900	2	15.0	2.5	10	42%
cheese, 'Pan Pizza'	1/6 pizza	290	15	35	440	0	10.0	4.0	20	31%
cheese, family size, 'Party Pizza'	1/3 pizza	320	14	43	580	2	11.0	3.0	15	30%
cheese, microwaveable, individual	1 pizza	240	10	25	530	1	11.0	3.5	15	41%
cheese, on French bread, 'Party'	1/2 pizza	320	15	33	630	2	14.0	5.0	20	40%
combination, 'Party'	1/2 pizza	390	15	34	910	2	21.0	4.5	20	49%
combination, family size, 'Party Pizza'	1/3 pizza	400	17	47	990	3	18.0	4.0	20	39%
combination, microwaveable, individual	1 pizza	310	11	25	720	1	18.0	4.5	15	53%
hamburger, 'Party'	1/2 pizza	350	15	33	860	2	18.0	4.0	20	46%
Mexican, zesty, 'Party'	1/2 pizza	370	15	34	750	2	19.0	4.5	15	47%
pepperoni, 'Pan Pizza'	1/6 pizza	330	16	35	620	0	15.0	6.0	30	40%
pepperoni, 'Party Pizza Family Size'	1/3 pizza	410	16	44	1060	3	20.0	4.0	20	43%
pepperoni, crisp crust, frozen	1 pkg	728	26	69	1946	na	38.9	7.6	23	48%
pepperoni, crisp crust, frozen	1 serving	364	13	35	973	na	19.4	3.8	12	48%
pepperoni, microwaveable, individual	1 pizza	280	10	25	710	1	16.0	3.5	15	51%
pepperoni, zesty	1/2 pizza	380	14	33	920	2	21.0	5.0	20	50%
sausage, 'Pan Pizza'	1/6 pizza	320	16	35	500	0	13.0	7.0	20	36%

Food Name	Serving Size	Calories	Prot. gms	Carbs gms	Sod. mgs	Fiber gms	Fat gms	Sat. Fat gms	Chol. mgs	% Fat Cal.
sausage, 'Party'	1/2 pizza	380	15	34	870	2	20.0	4.5	15	48%
sausage, family size, 'Party Pizza'	1/3 pizza	410	16	48	870	4	18.0	4.0	15	39%
sausage, individual, microwaveable	1 pizza	280	10	25	650	1	16.0	4.0	10	51%
sausage and pepperoni, 'Pan Pizza'	1/6 pizza	330	16	35	560	0	15.0	7.0	25	40%
sausage and pepperoni, crisp crust	1 pkg	769	28	72	2082	na	40.7	8.8	24	48%
sausage and pepperoni, crisp crust	1 serving	385	14	36	1041	na	20.4	4.4	12	48%
(Tyson)										
hamburger, 'Looney Tunes Wile E. Coyote'	6 oz	310	12	40	630	0	11.0	0.0	13	32%
pepperoni, 'Looney Tunes Foghorn Leghorn'	6.35 oz	400	13	57	610	0	13.0	0.0	18	29%
(Weight Watchers)										
cheese	6.03 oz	300	24	36	310	0	7.0	2.0	10	21%
combination, 'Deluxe'	1 serving	380	23	47	550	6	11.0	3.5	40	26%
extra cheese	1 serving	390	23	49	590	6	12.0	4.0	35	27%
pepperoni	1 serving	390	23	46	650	4	12.0	4.0	45	28%
(Wolfgang-Puck's)										
chicken, spicy, 'Pizza California'	1/2 pizza	360	19	36	620	5	16.0	7.0	45	40%
mushroom and spinach, 'Pizza California'	1/2 pizza	270	14	36	380	5	8.0	3.0	10	26%
PIZZA CRUST										
(Boboli) cheese, 6 inch	1/2 crust	150	6	25	305	na	3.5	na	1	20%
(Ener-G Foods) gluten-free, 10 inch	1 slice	134	1	20	132	1	5.7	0.6	0	38%
(Pillsbury) 'All Ready'	1/8 crust	90	3	16	170	0	1.0	0.0	0	11%
PIZZA CRUST DOUGH *(Rhodes)* frozen	1 slice	130	5	23	280	1	2.0	0.0	0	14%
PIZZA CRUST MIX										
(Chef Boyardee) 'Quick & Easy' mix only	1/6 pkg	150	6	26	300	0	2.0	0.0	0	12%
(French Meadow) spelt, organic, yeast-free, prepared	1/6 crust	90	3	10	110	2	2.0	0.0	0	26%
(Gold Medal)										
just add water, prepared	1/4 crust	160	5	32	340	1	2.0	0.5	0	11%
'Pouch Mix' mix only	1/6 pkg	110	3	22	220	0	1.0	0.0	0	8%
(Martha White)										
deep dish, prepared w/water	1 slice	110	3	23	110	0	1.0	0.0	0	8%
regular, prepared w/water	1 slice	100	2	19	125	0	2.0	0.0	0	18%
(Robin Hood) 'Pouch Mix' mix only	1/6 pkg	110	3	22	220	0	1.0	0.0	0	8%
PIZZA DINNER/ENTRÉE										
(Kid Cuisine)										
cheese, 'Mega Meal'	9.7 oz	430	17	75	700	0	7.0	0.0	0	15%
w/hamburger, apples, corn, chocolate pudding	1 meal	330	12	50	440	5	9.0	2.5	20	25%
PIZZA KIT										
(Chef Boyardee)										
cheese, 'Complete'	1/4 pkg	230	9	36	740	0	6.0	0.0	0	23%
cheese, '2 Complete'	1/8 pkg	210	10	31	650	0	5.0	0.0	0	22%
pepperoni, 'Complete'	1/4 pkg	250	13	31	870	0	9.0	0.0	0	32%
pepperoni, '2 Complete'	1/8 pkg	210	10	31	595	0	7.0	0.0	0	28%
plain	1/4 pkg	180	6	32	640	0	3.0	0.0	0	15%
sausage	1/4 pkg	270	14	34	930	0	10.0	0.0	0	32%
(Contadina)										
cheese	4.94 oz	320	16	41	850	0	10.0	4.0	20	28%
pepperoni	4.94 oz	370	18	38	980	0	16.0	6.0	30	39%
PIZZA SNACK										
(Jenny's Cuisine) puffs, cheese, w/vegetables, thick crust	1 puff	252	9	34	504	2	8.5	3.1	9	30%
(Totino's)										
roll, hamburger, frozen	1 pkg	577	23	66	1041	na	24.4	na	na	38%
roll, hamburger, frozen	1 serving	231	9	26	417	na	9.8	na	na	38%
roll, pepperoni, frozen	1 pkg	579	22	59	1302	3	28.4	7.5	47	44%
roll, pepperoni, frozen	1 serving	385	14	39	866	2	18.9	5.0	31	44%
roll, sausage, frozen	1 pkg	528	21	60	950	4	22.5	5.2	36	38%

Food Name	Serving Size	Calories	Prot. gms	Carbs gms	Sod. mgs	Fiber gms	Fat gms	Sat. Fat gms	Chol. mgs	% Fat Cal.
roll, sausage, frozen	1 serving	351	14	40	632	3	14.9	3.5	24	38%
PLANTAIN										
cooked, mashed	1 cup	232	2	62	10	5	0.4	0.1	0	1%
cooked, sliced	1 cup	179	1	48	8	4	0.3	0.1	0	1%
raw, sliced	1 cup	181	2	47	6	3	0.5	0.2	0	3%
raw, whole	1 medium	218	2	57	7	4	0.7	0.3	0	3%
PLUM										
Canned										
purple, in heavy syrup, w/liquid	1 medium	41	0	11	9	0	0.0	0.0	0	1%
purple, in juice, w/liquid	1 medium	27	0	7	0	0	0.0	0.0	0	0%
purple, in light syrup, w/liquid	1 medium	29	0	7	9	0	0.0	0.0	0	1%
purple, in water, w/liquid	1 medium	19	0	5	0	0	0.0	0.0	0	0%
purple, pitted, in extra heavy syrup, w/liquid	1 cup	264	1	69	50	3	0.3	0.0	0	1%
purple, pitted, in heavy syrup, w/liquid	1 cup	230	1	60	49	3	0.3	0.0	0	1%
purple, pitted, in juice, w/liquid	1 cup	146	1	38	3	3	0.1	0.0	0	0%
purple, pitted, in light syrup, w/liquid	1 cup	159	1	41	50	3	0.3	0.0	0	1%
purple, pitted, in water, w/liquid	1 cup	102	1	27	2	2	0.0	0.0	0	0%
Fresh										
raw, sliced	1 cup	91	1	21	0	2	1.0	0.1	0	9%
raw, whole, approx 2-1/8 inch diam	1 plum	36	1	9	0	1	0.4	0.0	0	9%
PLUM, JAPANESE. See UMEBOSHI.										
POI										
	1 cup	269	1	65	29	1	0.3	0.1	0	1%
crumbles (Ener-G Foods)	1 cup	376	1	75	21	3	8.0	0.5	0	19%
POKEBERRY SHOOT										
boiled, drained	1 cup	33	4	5	30	2	0.7	0.2	0	17%
boiled, drained	1 tbsp	2	0	0	2	0	0.0	0.0	0	17%
raw	1 cup	37	4	6	37	3	0.6	na	0	15%
POLENTA MIX (Fantastic Foods)										
'Polenta' prepared	1/2 cup	106	3	18	246	0	2.0	0.0	0	18%
POLISH SAUSAGE. See under SAUSAGE.										
POLLACK										
ALASKAN										
baked, broiled, grilled, or microwaved	4 oz	128	26.7	0.0	132	0	1.3	0.3	109	10%
raw	1 lb	365	77.9	0.0	449	0	3.6	0.7	323	9%
raw	1 oz	23	4.9	0.0	28	0	0.2	<.1	20	8%
ATLANTIC										
baked, broiled, grilled, or microwaved	3 oz	100	21	0	94	0	1.1	0.1	77	10%
raw	3 oz	78	17	0	73	0	0.8	0.1	60	10%
WALLEYE										
baked, broiled, grilled, or microwaved	3 oz	96	20	0	99	0	1.0	0.2	82	9%
raw	3 oz	69	15	0	84	0	0.7	0.1	60	9%
POLLYFISH. See PARROTFISH.										
POMEGRANATE / Chinese apple										
raw, trimmed	1 oz	19	0.3	4.9	1	>.1 c	0.1	na	0	4%
raw, untrimmed	1 lb	172	2.4	43.6	8	>.5 c	0.8	na	0	4%
raw, whole, medium, approx 3-3/8 inch diam	1 pomegranate	105	1.5	26.4	5	.9	0.5	na	0	4%
POMEGRANATE JUICE										
(Knudsen)	8 fl oz	85	1	21	0	0	0.0	0.0	0	0%
(Knudsen) fruit juice sweetened	8 fl oz	150	1	37	10	0	0.0	0.0	0	0%
POMELO / pummelo										
raw, sections	1/2 cup	36	0.7	9.1	1	1.0	<.1	(tr)	0	<1%
raw, trimmed	1 oz	11	0.2	2.7	1	>.1 c	<.1	(tr)	0	<1%
raw, untrimmed	1 lb	95	1.9	24.4	3	>.5 c	0.1	(tr)	0	1%

Food Name	Serving Size	Calories	Prot. gms	Carbs gms	Sod. mgs	Fiber gms	Fat gms	Sat. Fat gms	Chol. mgs	% Fat Cal.
raw, whole, medium, approx 5-1/2 inches diam, 2.4 lbs . . .	1 pomelo	228	4.6	58.6	7	6.1	0.2	(tr)	0	1%
POMFRET										
raw	1 lb	663	78.4	0.0	401	0	36.4	(mq)	295	51%
raw	1 oz	41	4.9	0.0	25	0	2.3	(mq)	18	51%
POMPANO, FLORIDA										
baked, broiled, grilled, or microwaved	3 oz	179	20	0	65	0	10.3	3.8	54	52%
raw	3 oz	139	16	0	55	0	8.1	3.0	43	52%
raw, boneless	1 oz	46	5	0	18	0	2.7	1.0	14	52%
POP. See SOFT DRINKS AND MIXERS.										
POPCORN										
(NOTE: All popcorn is popped unless otherwise noted.)										
(Act II)										
artificial butter flavor, 'Butter Lovers' unpopped	3 tbsp	170	3	19	340	4	11.0	2.5	0	53%
butter flavor, microwave, unpopped	3 tbsp	170	3	19	400	4	11.0	2.5	0	53%
natural, microwave, unpopped	3 tbsp	180	3	19	260	4	12.0	2.5	0	55%
(Auburn Farms) caramel, nonfat	2/3 cup	120	0	28	140	1	0.0	0.0	0	0%
(Bachman)										
. . . .	0.5 oz	80	1	7	160	0	6.0	0.0	0	63%
cheese flavor	0.5 oz	90	1	7	165	0	6.0	0.0	0	63%
'Lite'	0.5 oz	50	1	10	35	2	1.0	0.0	0	17%
white cheddar cheese flavor	0.5 oz	70	1	7	150	0	4.0	0.0	0	53%
(Bearitos)										
buttery	1 cup	60	1	4	47	1	4.0	0.7	0	66%
cheese flavor, 'Organic'	1 oz	137	3	13	122	2	8.0	0.0	0	52%
herb, lite, organic	3.5 cups	140	3	20	230	1	6.0	0.5	0	37%
no salt, no oil	1 cup	30	1	6	3	1	0.5	0.1	0	15%
no salt, organic	1 oz	108	4	22	1	1	0.8	0.0	0	7%
'Organic Lite'	1 oz	132	3	15	39	3	6.9	0.0	0	47%
'Organic Traditional'	1 oz	140	2	12	85	3	9.2	0.0	0	59%
(Betty Crocker)										
butter flavor, microwave, 'Pop Secret'	3 cups	100	2	11	170	2	6.0	1.0	0	51%
butter flavor, microwave, 'Pop Secret By Request'	3 cups	60	2	12	160	0	1.0	0.0	0	14%
butter flavor, microwave, 'Pop Secret Light'	3 cups	70	2	12	115	2	3.0	1.0	0	33%
butter flavor, no salt, 'Pop Secret'	3 cups	100	2	11	5	2	6.0	0.0	0	51%
butter flavor, original, microwave, 'Pop Secret'	1 cup	35	1	4	50	1	2.5	0.5	0	53%
butter flavor, 'Pop Secret'	1/4 bag	120	2	13	250	2	8.0	0.0	0	55%
butter flavor, 'Pop Secret Light'	1/4 bag	90	2	13	160	2	4.0	0.0	0	38%
butter flavor, 'Pop Secret Pop Qwiz'	1 bag	110	2	11	210	2	7.0	0.0	0	55%
butter flavor, 'Pop Secret Pop Qwiz'	2 3/4 cups	80	1	9	130	2	5.0	0.0	0	53%
butter flavor, salt-free, 'Pop Secret'	1/4 bag	120	2	13	5	2	7.0	0.0	0	51%
butter flavor, singles 'Pop Secret Light'	1 bag	180	4	28	310	4	8.0	0.0	0	36%
butter flavor, singles, 'Pop Secret Light'	6 cups	140	3	23	190	4	6.0	0.0	0	34%
butter flavor, singles, 'Pop Secret'	1 bag	250	4	27	460	4	16.0	0.0	0	54%
butter flavor, singles, 'Pop Secret'	6 cups	200	3	23	310	4	12.0	0.0	0	51%
buttery burst, microwave, 'Pop Secret'	1 cup	35	1	4	50	1	2.5	0.5	0	53%
buttery burst, light, microwave, 'Pop Secret'	1 cup	25	1	4	45	1	1.0	0.0	0	31%
cheese flavor, microwave, 'Pop Secret' 1/3 pkg.	3 cups	170	3	15	260	2	11.0	0.0	0	58%
natural, 'Pop Secret'	1/4 bag	120	2	13	250	2	8.0	0.0	0	55%
natural, 'Pop Secret Light'	1/4 bag	90	2	13	200	2	4.0	0.0	0	38%
natural, 'Pop Secret Pop Qwiz'	2 3/4 cups	80	1	9	140	2	5.0	0.0	0	53%
natural, 'Pop Secret Pop Qwiz'	1 bag	110	2	11	220	2	7.0	0.0	0	55%
natural, microwave, 'Pop Secret'	3 cups	100	2	11	170	2	6.0	2.0	0	51%
natural, microwave, 'Pop Secret By Request'	3 cups	60	2	12	170	0	1.0	0.0	0	14%
natural, microwave, 'Pop Secret Light'	3 cups	70	2	12	160	2	3.0	1.0	0	33%

Food Name	Serving Size	Calories	Prot. gms	Carbs gms	Sod. mgs	Fiber gms	Fat gms	Sat. Fat gms	Chol. mgs	% Fat Cal.
natural, singles, 'Pop Secret Light'	1 bag	170	4	26	440	4	7.0	0.0	0	34%
natural, singles 'Pop Secret Light'	6 cups	150	4	23	320	4	6.0	0.0	0	33%
(Bonnie Lee)										
air popped, salted	1 qt	109	3	20	1	0	1.0	0.0	0	9%
oil popped, salted	1 qt	172	3	20	230	0	8.0	0.0	0	44%
(Cape Cod)										
all natural.	3.5 cups	160	3	18	200	3	9.0	2.0	0	49%
butter, old fashioned	3 cups	170	3	16	220	2	10.0	3.0	5	54%
white cheddar cheese flavor	0.5 oz	80	2	6	150	0	5.0	0.0	0	58%
(Clover Club) white cheddar cheese flavor	0.5 oz	70	1	6	140	0	5.0	0.0	0	62%
(Country Grown) no added fat or salt, microwave	3 cups	85	3	17	0	4	1.0	0.0	0	11%
(Cracker Jack)										
butter toffee, w/almonds, pecans, 'Nutty Delux'.	1 oz	130	1	19	135	1	6.0	2.0	5	40%
caramel, w/peanuts.	1/2 cup	120	2	23	70	1	2.0	0.0	0	15%
(Estee) caramel coated, bag	1 oz	140	3	25	55	0	3.0	1.5	5	19%
(Featherweight)										
butter flavor, low-salt, microwave.	3 cups	100	3	14	70	0	3.0	0.0	0	28%
natural, low-salt, microwave	3 cups	80	3	14	0	0	1.0	0.0	0	12%
(Frito-Lay's)										
. . . .	0.5 oz	70	1	9	200	0	3.0	0.0	0	40%
cheese flavor.	0.5 oz	80	1	7	180	0	5.0	0.0	0	58%
(Good Health) butterscotch, 100% natural.	30-g pkg	110	1	24	220	1	0.0	0.0	0	0%
(Healthy Choice) natural flavor.	1 cup	15	1	4	25	1	0.0	0.0	0	0%
(Jiffy Pop)										
butter flavor 'Pan Popcorn'	4 cups	130	3	16	270	2	6.0	0.0	0	42%
butter flavor, microwave.	4 cups	140	3	17	270	3	7.0	0.0	0	44%
microwave.	4 cups	140	3	17	270	3	7.0	0.0	0	44%
'Pan Popcorn'	4 cups	130	3	16	270	2	6.0	0.0	0	42%
(Jolly Time)										
butter flavored, light, microwave	3 cups	60	2	12	105	3	2.0	0.5	0	24%
butter flavored, microwave	3 cups	90	2	13	95	3	5.0	1.0	0	43%
cheddar flavor, microwave.	3 cups	155	3	17	220	4	10.0	1.0	0	53%
natural flavor, light, microwave	3 cups	70	2	13	110	3	2.0	0.6	0	23%
natural flavor, microwave.	3 cups	120	2	15	125	3	7.0	1.5	0	48%
white, air-popped.	3 cups	60	2	15	2	4	1.0	0.0	0	12%
white, unsalted	4 cups	75	3	20	2	5	1.0	0.0	0	9%
yellow, air-popped	3 cups	60	2	14	2	4	1.0	0.0	0	12%
yellow, unsalted.	4 cups	75	3	19	2	5	1.0	0.0	0	9%
(Keebler)										
honey caramel, 'Pop Deluxe'	1 oz	120	1	22	180	0	3.0	1.0	0	23%
white cheddar cheese flavor	1 oz	140	1	13	270	0	10.0	2.0	5	62%
(Kettle Poppins)										
brewer's yeast	0.5 oz	70	2	8	40	1	2.5	0.5	0	36%
lightly salted	0.5 oz	70	2	9	40	1	2.5	0.5	0	34%
white cheddar	0.5 oz	70	2	9	120	1	2.5	0.5	1	34%
(Lapidus Popcorn Company)										
herb, organic	2 cups	170	3	15	650	4	11.0	1.0	0	58%
white cheddar, organic	2 cups	180	3	13	15	2	13.0	1.5	5	65%
(Laura Scudder's)										
'Tender Baby White Corn'	0.5 oz	80	1	6	140	0	6.0	0.0	0	66%
white cheddar cheese flavor	0.5 oz	70	1	6	140	0	5.0	0.0	0	62%
(Louise's)										
nonfat	1 oz	100	1	24	80	1	0.0	0.0	0	0%
toffee caramel, buttery, nonfat.	1 oz	100	1	24	80	1	0.0	0.0	0	0%

Food Name	Serving Size	Calories	Prot. gms	Carbs gms	Sod. mgs	Fiber gms	Fat gms	Sat. Fat gms	Chol. mgs	% Fat Cal.
(Nature's Choice)										
caramel, original	1 oz	108	1	25	0	0	1.0	0.0	0	8%
caramel, w/peanuts	1 oz	114	1	23	0	0	1.0	0.0	0	9%
(Orville Redenbacher)										
butter flavored, light, microwave, 'Gourmet'	3 cups	80	2	14	250	3	4.0	0.9	0	36%
butter flavored, light, microwave, snack size	3 cups	70	2	11	90	0	3.0	0.0	0	34%
butter flavored, microwave, 'Gourmet'	3 cups	110	2	12	300	3	8.0	1.9	0	56%
butter flavored, microwave, 'Smart Pop'	3 cups	50	2	11	100	0	1.0	0.0	0	15%
butter flavored, microwave, snack size	3 cups	100	2	11	140	0	6.0	0.0	0	51%
butter flavored, salt-free, microwave, 'Gourmet'	3 cups	110	2	12	0	3	8.0	1.9	0	56%
butter toffee, microwave, 'Gourmet'	2 1/2 cups	210	2	26	85	2	12.0	3.0	1	49%
caramel, 'Ready-to-Eat'	1 oz	112	1	22	65	3	3.5	0.7	1	25%
caramel, microwave, 'Gourmet'	2 1/2 cups	240	2	29	90	2	14.0	3.4	1	50%
cheddar cheese, microwave, 'Gourmet'	3 cups	130	2	14	280	3	8.0	1.8	2	53%
cheddar cheese, microwave, 'Gourmet'	3 cups	150	3	13	370	3	10.0	2.2	2	58%
hot air, 'Gourmet'	3 cups	40	1	10	0	3	1.0	0.0	0	17%
hot air, unpopped	2 tbsp	92	4	24	3	6	0.8	0.1	0	6%
natural, light, microwave, 'Gourmet'	3 cups	80	2	14	290	3	4.0	0.9	0	36%
natural, microwave, 'Gourmet'	3 cups	110	2	12	550	3	8.0	1.9	0	56%
natural, salt-free, microwave 'Gourmet'	3 cups	110	2	12	0	3	8.0	1.9	0	56%
original, 'Gourmet'	3 cups	80	1	10	0	3	4.0	0.0	0	45%
regular	1 oz	138	3	17	3	5	8.7	1.3	0	49%
sour cream and onion, microwave, 'Gourmet'	3 cups	180	3	16	320	3	13.0	2.9	1	61%
white cheddar cheese, 'Ready-to-Eat'	1.06 oz	139	3	17	285	4	8.6	1.2	1	49%
white, 'Gourmet'	3 cups	80	1	10	0	3	4.0	0.0	0	45%
(Painted Desert) microwave	1 cup	27	1	6	0	0	1.0	0.0	0	26%
(Pillsbury)										
butter flavor, frozen, microwave	3 cups	210	3	20	480	0	13.0	0.0	0	56%
original, frozen, microwave	3 cups	210	3	20	420	0	13.0	0.0	0	56%
salt-free, frozen, microwave	3 cups	170	3	23	0	0	7.0	0.0	0	38%
(Planters)										
butter flavor, microwave	3 cups	140	2	13	560	0	10.0	1.0	0	60%
natural, microwave	3 cups	140	2	14	560	0	9.0	1.0	0	56%
(Pop Weaver's)										
butter flavor, microwave	4 cups	140	3	20	230	4	8.0	0.0	0	44%
natural, microwave	3 cups	140	3	20	230	4	8.0	0.0	0	44%
(Pops-Rite)										
butter flavor, microwave	3 cups	90	2	13	140	0	5.0	0.0	0	43%
microwave, 'Natural'	3 cups	90	2	13	190	0	5.0	0.0	0	43%
white, air popped, no salt	1 oz	100	3	20	0	1	2.0	0.0	0	16%
white, oil popped, unsalted	1 oz	220	3	20	0	1	15.0	0.0	0	59%
yellow, air popped, no salt	1 oz	100	2	21	0	1	2.0	0.0	0	16%
yellow, oil popped, unsalted	1 oz	220	2	21	0	1	15.0	0.0	0	59%
(Smartfood) white cheddar cheese flavor	0.5 oz	80	2	7	150	0	5.0	0.0	0	56%
(Tone's)	1 cup	30	1	6	1	2	0.4	0.1	0	11%
(Ultra Slim Fast) butter flavor, 'Lite 'N Tasty'	0.5 oz	60	2	10	150	2	2.0	0.0	0	27%
(Vic's)										
caramel, lite, 'Gourmet'	1/2 cup	60	1	10	50	0	2.0	0.0	0	29%
white cheddar cheese, lite, 'Gourmet'	2/3 cup	40	1	4	50	0	2.0	0.0	1	47%
white, lite, 'Gourmet'	1 cup	35	1	6	15	0	2.0	0.0	0	39%
yellow cheddar cheese, lite, 'Gourmet'	2/3 cup	40	1	4	60	0	2.0	0.0	1	47%
(Weight Watchers)										
butter	0.66 oz	90	2	13	100	0	3.0	0.0	0	31%
caramel	1 serving	100	1	22	45	1	1.0	0.0	0	9%

Food Name	Serving Size	Calories	Prot. gms	Carbs gms	Sod. mgs	Fiber gms	Fat gms	Sat. Fat gms	Chol. mgs	% Fat Cal.
'Lightly Salted'	0.66 oz	80	2	12	65	0	4.0	0.0	0	39%
microwave	1 oz pkg	100	4	22	5	0	1.0	0.0	0	8%
white cheddar cheese flavor	0.66 oz pkg	100	2	10	85	0	6.0	0.0	0	53%
(Wise)										
butter flavor	1 cup	80	1	7	140	0	5.0	0.0	0	58%
'Tender Baby White Corn'	0.5 oz	80	1	6	140	0	6.0	0.0	0	66%
'Tender Eating Baby Popcorn'	0.5 oz	70	1	4	120	0	6.0	0.0	0	73%
white cheddar cheese flavor	0.5 oz	70	1	6	140	0	5.0	0.0	0	62%
POPCORN OIL										
(Orville Redenbacher) and topping oil	1 tbsp	120	0	0	0	0	13.5	1.9	0	100%
(Planters)	1 tbsp	120	0	0	0	0	14.0	2.0	0	100%
(Wesson)										
buttery flavor	1 tbsp	120	0	0	0	0	13.5	2.0	0	100%
popping and topping oil, food service product	1 tbsp	122	0	0	0	0	13.5	2.0	0	100%
POPCORN SEASONING. See under SEASONING MIX.										
POPPY SEED										
	1 tbsp	47	2	2	2	1	3.9	0.4	0	70%
	1 tsp	15	1	1	1	0	1.3	0.1	0	70%
(McCormick/Schilling)	1 tsp	17	1	1	0	1	1.2	0.0	0	63%
(Spice Islands)	1 tsp	13	1	1	1	0	0.9	0.0	0	59%
whole (Durkee)	1 tsp	15	0	0	0	0	0.0	0.0	0	0%
whole (Laurel Leaf)	1 tsp	15	0	0	0	0	0.0	0.0	0	0%
POPPY SEED FILLING (Solo) 'Sokal'	2 tbsp	119	2	21	27	na	3.2	0.4	na	24%
POPPY SEED OIL										
	1 cup	1927	0	0	0	0	218.0	29.4	0	100%
	1 tbsp	120	0	0	0	0	13.6	1.8	0	100%
PORK. See also HAM.										
(NOTE: TRIMMED = Lean; separable fat removed. UNTRIMMED = Separable fat not removed.)										
BACKFAT										
Fresh										
wholesale cuts, raw	1 lb	3683	13.3	0.0	50	0	402.3	146.1	259	99%
wholesale cuts, raw	1 oz	230	0.8	0.0	3	0	25.1	9.1	16	99%
BACKRIB										
Fresh										
Untrimmed										
raw	1 lb	1279	73.1	0.0	340	0	107.0	39.6	367	77%
raw	1 oz	80	4.6	0.0	21	0	6.7	2.5	23	77%
raw 'Gourmet' (JM)	5.5 oz	220	15.0	0.0	50	0	18.0	(mq)	(mq)	73%
roasted	3 oz	315	20.6	0.0	86	0	25.1	9.3	100	73%
BELLY										
Fresh										
wholesale cuts, raw	1 lb	2350	42.4	0.0	145	0	240.5	87.7	327	93%
wholesale cuts, raw	1 oz	147	2.7	0.0	9	0	15.0	5.5	20	93%
BRAIN										
Fresh										
braised	3 oz	117	10.3	0.0	77	0	8.1	1.8	2169	64%
in milk gravy (Armour)	2.75 oz	110	7.0	1.0	400	na	8.0	na	na	69%
raw	1 oz	36	2.9	0.0	34	0	2.6	0.6	622	67%
CENTER LOIN										
Fresh										
Trimmed										
chop, bone in, braised	3 oz	172	25	0.0	53	0	7.1	2.6	72	37%
chop, bone in, broiled	3 oz	172	26	0.0	51	0	6.9	2.5	70	36%
chop, bone in, pan fried	3 oz	197	27	0.0	73	0	8.9	3.1	78	41%

Food Name	Serving Size	Calories	Prot. gms	Carbs gms	Sod. mgs	Fiber gms	Fat gms	Sat. Fat gms	Chol. mgs	% Fat Cal.
roast, bone in, roasted	3 oz	169	23	0.0	56	0	7.7	2.8	67	41%
Untrimmed
chop, bone in, braised	3 oz	210	24	0.0	50	0	12.0	4.5	73	52%
chop, bone in, broiled	3 oz	204	24	0.0	49	0	11.1	4.1	70	49%
chop, bone in, pan fried	3 oz	235	25	0.0	68	0	14.1	5.1	78	54%
roast, bone in, roasted	3 oz	199	22	0.0	54	0	11.4	4.3	68	52%
CENTER RIB
Fresh
Trimmed
chop, bone in, braised	3 oz	179	24	0.0	35	0	8.6	3.4	60	43%
chop, bone in, broiled	3 oz	186	26	0.0	55	0	8.3	2.9	69	40%
chop, bone in, pan-fried	3 oz	185	24	0.0	44	0	9.2	3.4	60	45%
roast, bone in, roasted	3 oz	182	24	0.0	43	0	8.6	3.0	71	43%
Untrimmed
chop, bone in, braised	3 oz	217	22	0.0	34	0	13.4	5.2	62	56%
chop, bone in, broiled	3 oz	224	24	0.0	53	0	13.2	4.8	70	53%
chop, bone in, pan-fried	3 oz	225	22	0.0	43	0	14.4	5.4	62	58%
roast, bone in, roasted	3 oz	217	23	0.0	39	0	13.0	5.0	62	54%
CHITTERLINGS
Fresh
raw	1 oz	71	2.8	0.1	10	0	6.5	2.3	45	84%
simmered	3 oz	258	8.7	0.0	33	0	24.4	8.6	122	86%
CHOP
Refrigerated or frozen
boneless, 'America's Cut' (JM)	6 oz	330	38.0	0.0	90	0	20.0	(mq)	(mq)	54%
center cut, 'Always Tender' (Hormel)	4 oz	187	21	1.0	424	na	10.8	4.0	59	52%
center cut, 'Always Tender' (Hormel)	1 oz	47	5	0.0	107	na	2.7	1.0	15	52%
COMPOSITE CUTS
Canned
(Hormel)	3 oz	240	11.0	2.0	1056	0	21.0	(mq)	(mq)	78%
chopped (Hormel)	3 oz	200	12.0	2.0	1073	0	16.0	(mq)	(mq)	72%
Fresh
Trimmed
leg, loin, and shoulder, cooked	3 oz	180	25	0.0	50	0	8.2	2.9	73	41%
leg, loin, and shoulder, raw	1 oz	41	6	0.0	16	0	1.7	0.6	17	37%
loin and shoulder, cooked	3 oz	179	25.0	0.0	48	0	8.0	2.8	72	42%
loin and shoulder, raw	1 oz	41	6.0	0.0	15	0	1.7	0.6	17	39%
retail cuts, cooked	3 oz	232	23.4	0.0	53	0	14.6	5.3	77	58%
retail cuts, raw	1 lb	980	86.0	0.0	249	0	67.8	24.0	304	64%
retail cuts, raw	1 oz	61	5.4	0.0	16	0	4.2	1.5	19	64%
roasted	3 oz	180	24.9	0.0	50	0	8.2	2.9	73	43%
Untrimmed
leg, loin, shoulder, spareribs, cooked	3 oz	232	23	0.0	53	0	14.6	5.3	77	57%
leg, loin, shoulder, spareribs, raw	1 oz	64	5	0.0	15	0	4.7	1.6	20	65%
loin and shoulder, cooked	3 oz	214	23.6	0.0	48	0	12.6	4.5	73	55%
loin and shoulder, raw	1 lb	907	88.6	0.0	231	0	58.5	20.3	290	60%
loin and shoulder, raw	1 oz	57	5.5	0.0	14	0	3.7	1.3	18	60%
raw	1 lb	1030	82.8	0.0	245	0	74.8	26.2	313	67%
raw	1 oz	64	5.2	0.0	15	0	4.7	1.6	20	67%
EAR
Fresh
raw	1 oz	66	6	0	54	0	4.3	1.5	23	58%
simmered	1 medium	184	18	0	185	0	12.0	4.3	100	59%

Food Name	Serving Size	Calories	Prot. gms	Carbs gms	Sod. mgs	Fiber gms	Fat gms	Sat. Fat gms	Chol. mgs	% Fat Cal.
FEET										
Fresh										
raw	1 oz	75	6	0	18	0	5.3	1.8	30	64%
simmered	3 oz	165	16	0	26	0	10.5	3.6	85	58%
Pickled										
approx 6 oz *(Penrose)*	1 piece	220	19	2	2890	0	15.0	0.0	0	62%
cured	1 oz	58	4	0	262	0	4.6	1.6	26	72%
GROUND										
Fresh										
cooked	3 oz	252	21.8	0.0	62	0	17.6	6.6	80	65%
raw	4 oz	297	19	0	63	0	23.9	8.9	81	73%
Refrigerated or frozen *(JM)*	3 oz	190	15.0	0.0	40	0	14.0	(mq)	(mq)	68%
HEART										
Fresh										
braised	1 cup	215	34	1	51	0	7.3	1.9	320	31%
braised	1 medium	191	30	1	45	0	6.5	1.7	285	31%
raw	1 medium	267	39	3	127	0	9.9	2.6	296	33%
raw	1 oz	33	5	0	16	0	1.2	0.3	37	33%
HOCKS, refrigerated, hickory smoked *(Cook's)*	3 oz	270	17	5	1150	0	20.0	6.0	55	67%
JOWL										
Fresh										
raw	4 oz	740	7	0	28	0	78.7	28.5	102	96%
raw	1 oz	186	2	0	7	0	19.7	7.2	26	96%
KIDNEYS										
Fresh										
braised	1 cup	211	35.6	0.0	112	0	6.6	2.1	672	29%
braised	3 oz	128	21.6	0.0	68	0	4.0	1.3	408	29%
raw	1 oz	28	4.7	0.0	34	0	0.9	0.3	90	30%
KNUCKLES, jarred, pickled, approx 6 oz *(Penrose)*	1 piece	290	23	1	2380	0	21.0	0.0	0	66%
LEG, RUMP HALF										
Fresh										
Trimmed										
raw	1 lb	621	96.3	0.0	313	0	23.5	8.1	277	35%
raw	1 oz	39	6.0	0.0	20	0	1.5	0.5	17	36%
roasted	3 oz	175	26.3	0.0	55	0	6.9	2.4	82	37%
roasted, diced	1 cup	278	41.8	0.0	88	0	11.0	3.9	130	37%
Untrimmed										
raw	1 lb	1007	85.0	0.0	277	0	71.2	24.7	299	65%
raw	1 oz	63	5.3	0.0	17	0	4.4	1.5	19	65%
roasted	3 oz	214	24.5	0.0	53	0	12.1	4.5	82	53%
roasted	1.5 oz	117	11.3	0.0	26	0	7.6	2.7	40	60%
roasted, diced	1 cup	340	39.0	0.0	84	0	19.3	7.1	130	53%
LEG, SHANK HALF										
Fresh										
Trimmed										
raw	1 lb	631	93.5	0.0	304	0	25.5	8.8	272	38%
raw	1 oz	39	5.8	0.0	19	0	1.6	0.6	17	38%
roasted	3 oz	183	24.0	0.0	54	0	8.9	3.1	78	46%
roasted, diced	1 cup	290	38.1	0.0	86	0	14.2	4.9	124	46%
Untrimmed										
raw	1 lb	1193	77.5	0.0	249	0	95.4	33.1	308	74%
raw	1 oz	75	4.8	0.0	16	0	6.0	2.1	19	74%
roasted	3 oz	246	21.5	0.0	50	0	17.0	6.3	78	64%
roasted	1.5 oz	129	10.3	0.0	25	0	9.4	3.4	39	67%

Food Name	Serving Size	Calories	Prot. gms	Carbs gms	Sod. mgs	Fiber gms	Fat gms	Sat. Fat gms	Chol. mgs	% Fat Cal.
roasted, diced	1 cup	390	34.2	0.0	80	0	27.1	9.9	124	64%
LEG, WHOLE										
Fresh										
Trimmed										
raw	1 lb	617	92.9	0.0	249	0	24.5	8.5	308	37%
raw	1 oz	39	5.8	0.0	16	0	1.5	0.5	19	37%
roasted	3 oz	179	25.0	0.0	54	0	8.0	2.8	80	42%
roasted	1.5 oz	94	12.0	0.0	27	0	4.7	1.6	40	47%
roasted	1 cup	285	39.7	0.0	86	0	12.7	4.5	127	42%
Untrimmed										
raw	1 lb	1111	79.1	0.0	213	0	85.6	29.7	331	71%
raw	1 oz	69	4.9	0.0	13	0	5.3	1.9	21	71%
roasted	3 oz	232	22.8	0.0	51	0	15.0	5.5	80	60%
roasted	1.5 oz	125	10.6	0.0	25	0	8.8	3.2	40	65%
roasted, diced	1 cup	369	36.2	0.0	81	0	23.8	8.7	127	60%
LIVER										
Fresh										
braised	3 oz	140	22.1	3.2	42	0	3.7	1.2	302	25%
fried	3 oz	205	25.4	2.1	94	0	9.8	2.9	372	45%
raw	1 oz	38	6.1	0.7	25	0	1.0	0.3	85	25%
LOIN										
Fresh										
Trimmed										
blade, braised	3 oz	191	21.3	0.0	53	0	11.1	4.0	71	54%
blade, broiled	3 oz	199	21.6	0.0	68	0	11.8	4.3	71	55%
blade, pan-fried	3 oz	205	21.0	0.0	66	0	12.8	4.4	70	58%
blade, pan-fried in vegetable oil	4 oz	321	27.6	0.0	84	0	22.5	7.7	110	65%
blade, roasted	3 oz	210	22.6	0.0	25	0	12.6	4.5	79	56%
ribs, country-style, braised	3 oz	199	22.1	0.0	54	0	11.6	4.2	73	54%
ribs, country-style, raw	1 oz	45	5.5	0.0	19	0	2.3	0.8	18	49%
ribs, country-style, roasted	3 oz	210	22.6	0.0	25	0	12.6	4.5	79	56%
whole, braised	3 oz	173	24.3	0.0	43	0	7.8	2.9	67	42%
whole, broiled	3 oz	178	24.3	0.0	54	0	8.3	3.1	67	44%
whole, chopped, braised	1 cup	382	46.2	0.0	105	0	20.4	7.1	147	50%
whole, chopped, broiled	1 cup	360	39.0	0.0	105	0	21.4	7.4	133	55%
whole, chopped, roasted	1 cup	336	37.7	0.0	97	0	19.5	6.7	126	54%
whole, raw	1 oz	44	5.9	0.0	18	0	2.1	0.7	17	45%
whole, roasted	3 oz	178	24.3	0.0	49	0	8.2	3.0	69	43%
Untrimmed										
blade, braised	3 oz	275	18.6	0.0	47	0	21.6	8.1	72	72%
blade, broiled	3 oz	272	19.1	0.0	59	0	21.1	7.9	73	71%
blade, pan-fried	3 oz	291	18.3	0.0	57	0	23.6	8.6	72	74%
blade, pan-fried in vegetable oil	4 oz	469	21.3	0.0	69	0	41.9	15.1	108	82%
blade, roasted	3 oz	275	20.2	0.0	25	0	20.9	7.8	79	70%
ribs, country-style, braised	3 oz	252	20.3	0.0	50	0	18.3	6.8	74	67%
ribs, country-style, raw	1 oz	68	4.8	0.0	16	0	5.3	1.8	20	71%
ribs, country-style, roasted	3 oz	279	19.9	0.0	44	0	21.5	7.8	78	71%
whole, braised	3 oz	203	23	0.0	41	0	11.6	4.3	68	51%
whole, broiled	3 oz	206	23.2	0.0	53	0	11.8	4.4	68	53%
whole, roasted	3 oz	211	23.0	0.0	50	0	12.4	4.6	70	55%
Refrigerated or frozen										
boneless, 'Always Tender' (Hormel)	1 oz	41	5	0.0	100	na	2.0	0.8	14	44%
boneless, 'Always Tender' (Hormel)	4 oz	163	21	1.0	400	na	8.0	3.2	55	44%
whole or half, center cut, boneless (JM)	3 oz	190	16	0.0	50	0	13.0	0.0	0	65%

Food Name	Serving Size	Calories	Prot. gms	Carbs gms	Sod. mgs	Fiber gms	Fat gms	Sat. Fat gms	Chol. mgs	% Fat Cal.
LUNGS										
Fresh										
braised	3 oz	84	14.1	0.0	69	0	2.6	0.9	329	29%
raw	1 oz	24	4.0	0.0	43	0	0.8	0.3	91	31%
PANCREAS										
Fresh										
braised	3 oz	186	24.2	0.0	36	0	9.2	3.2	268	46%
raw	4 oz	225	21	0.0	50	0	15.0	5.2	218	60%
SHOULDER										
Fresh										
Trimmed										
arm picnic, braised	3 oz	211	27.4	0.0	87	0	10.4	3.5	97	46%
arm picnic, raw	1 oz	40	5.6	0.0	23	0	1.8	0.6	18	42%
arm picnic, roasted	3 oz	194	22.7	0.0	68	0	10.7	3.7	81	52%
Boston blade, braised	3 oz	232	26.4	0.0	64	0	13.2	4.7	99	53%
Boston blade, broiled	3 oz	193	22.7	0.0	63	0	10.7	3.8	80	52%
Boston blade, raw	1 oz	47	5.4	0.0	20	0	2.6	0.9	19	52%
Boston blade, roasted	3 oz	197	20.6	0.0	75	0	12.2	4.4	72	57%
whole, chopped, roasted	1 cup	341	35.5	0.0	107	0	21.0	7.2	135	57%
whole, raw	1 lb	671	88.7	0.0	345	0	32.4	11.2	304	45%
whole, raw	1 oz	42	5.5	0.0	22	0	2.0	0.7	19	45%
whole, roasted	3 oz	195	21.5	0.0	64	0	11.5	4.1	77	55%
whole, roasted, diced	1 cup	310	34.2	0.0	101	0	18.3	6.5	122	55%
Untrimmed										
arm picnic, braised	3 oz	280	24	0.0	75	0	19.7	7.2	93	64%
arm picnic, braised, diced	1 cup	444	38	0.0	119	0	31.3	11.5	147	64%
arm picnic, raw	1 oz	72	5	0.0	19	0	5.7	2.0	20	72%
arm picnic, roasted	3 oz	269	20.0	0.0	59	0	20.4	7.5	80	70%
arm picnic, roasted, diced	1 cup	428	32	0.0	95	0	32.4	11.9	127	68%
Boston blade, braised	3 oz	271	24.4	0.0	59	0	18.5	6.8	96	63%
Boston blade, broiled	3 oz	220	21.7	0.0	59	0	14.1	5.1	81	59%
Boston blade, raw	1 lb	989	80.1	0.0	286	0	71.8	24.9	322	67%
Boston blade, roasted	3 oz	229	19.6	0.0	57	0	16.0	5.9	73	65%
whole, raw	1 oz	67	4.9	0.0	18	0	5.1	1.8	20	70%
whole, roasted	3 oz	248	19.8	0.0	58	0	18.2	6.7	77	67%
whole, roasted, diced	1 cup	394	31.4	0.0	92	0	28.9	10.6	122	67%
SIRLOIN										
Fresh										
Trimmed										
chop, bone in, braised	3 oz	167	23.0	0.0	45	0	7.7	2.7	69	43%
chop, bone in, broiled	3 oz	181	24.2	0.0	61	0	8.6	3.1	72	44%
chop, boneless, braised	3 oz	149	23.0	0.0	39	0	5.6	2.0	69	35%
chop, boneless, broiled	3 oz	164	26.5	0.0	48	0	5.7	1.9	78	33%
chop, boneless, raw	1 lb	581	95.5	0.0	231	0	19.1	6.6	286	31%
chop or roast, raw	1 oz	43	6.0	0.0	14	0	1.9	0.7	18	42%
roast, bone in, roasted	3 oz	184	24.5	0.0	54	0	8.8	3.1	73	45%
roast, boneless, roasted	3 oz	168	24.5	0.0	48	0	7.0	2.5	73	39%
Untrimmed										
chop, bone in, braised	3 oz	208	21.6	0.0	43	0	12.8	4.7	70	57%
chop, bone in, broiled	3 oz	220	22.6	0.0	58	0	13.7	5.0	73	58%
chop, boneless, braised	3 oz	161	22.6	0.0	39	0	7.1	2.6	69	41%
chop, boneless, broiled	3 oz	177	25.9	0.0	48	0	7.3	2.5	77	39%
chop or roast, raw	1 oz	78	4.9	0.0	12	0	6.3	2.3	20	74%
roast, bone in, roasted	3 oz	222	23.1	0.0	51	0	13.6	4.8	74	57%

Food Name	Serving Size	Calories	Prot. gms	Carbs gms	Sod. mgs	Fiber gms	Fat gms	Sat. Fat gms	Chol. mgs	% Fat Cal.
roast, boneless, roasted	3 oz	176	24.2	0.0	48	0	8.0	2.9	73	43%
SPARERIBS										
Fresh										
Untrimmed										
braised	3 oz	337	24.7	0.0	79	0	25.8	9.4	103	70%
raw	1 oz	81	4.8	0.0	22	0	6.7	2.5	22	76%
Refrigerated or frozen, raw, 'Gourmet' (JM)	4.5 oz	250	14.0	0.0	70	0	22.0	(mq)	(mq)	78%
SPLEEN										
Fresh										
braised	3 oz	127	24.0	0.0	91	0	2.7	0.9	428	20%
raw	1 oz	28	5.1	0.0	28	0	0.7	0.2	103	24%
STOMACH										
Fresh										
raw	4 oz	177	19	0.0	59	0	10.8	3.8	218	55%
raw	1 oz	45	4.7	0.0	15	0	2.7	na	55	56%
TAIL										
Fresh										
raw	4 oz	427	20	0	71	0	37.9	13.2	110	80%
raw	1 oz	107	5	0	18	0	9.5	3.3	28	80%
simmered	3 oz	337	14	0	21	0	30.4	10.6	110	82%
TENDERLOIN										
Fresh										
Trimmed										
broiled	3 oz	159	25.9	0.0	55	0	5.4	1.9	80	32%
raw	1 lb	544	95.2	0.0	227	0	15.5	5.3	295	27%
raw	1 oz	34	5.9	0.0	14	0	1.0	0.3	18	28%
roasted	3 oz	139	23.9	0.0	48	0	4.1	1.4	67	28%
roasted, chopped or diced	1 cup	232	40.3	0.0	94	0	6.7	2.3	130	27%
Untrimmed										
broiled	3 oz	171	25.4	0.0	54	0	6.9	2.5	80	38%
raw	1 oz	39	5.8	0.0	14	0	1.5	0.5	19	37%
roasted	3 oz	147	23.6	0.0	47	0	5.1	1.8	67	33%
Refrigerated, boneless (JM)	3 oz	120	17.0	0.0	40	0	5.0	(mq)	(mq)	40%
TONGUE										
Canned, cured, '8-lb. can' (Hormel)	3 oz	190	17	0	966	0	13.0	0.0	0	63%
Fresh										
braised	3 oz	230	20	0	93	0	15.8	5.5	124	62%
raw	4 oz	254	18	0	124	0	19.4	6.7	114	69%
raw	1 oz	64	5	0	31	0	4.9	1.7	29	69%
TOP LOIN										
Fresh										
Trimmed										
chop or roast, raw	1 oz	46	6.2	0.0	13	0	2.1	0.7	16	43%
chop, boneless, braised	3 oz	172	24.7	0.0	36	0	7.3	2.7	62	40%
chop, boneless, broiled	3 oz	173	26.5	0.0	55	0	6.6	2.3	68	36%
chop, boneless, pan-fried in vegetable oil	4 oz	291	31.7	0.0	57	0	17.4	6.0	92	55%
chop, boneless, pan-fried	3 oz	191	25.9	0.0	48	0	8.9	3.1	65	44%
roast, boneless, raw	1 oz	40	6.2	0.0	13	0	1.5	0.5	16	35%
roast, boneless, roasted	3 oz	165	25.7	0.0	38	0	6.1	2.2	66	35%
roast, boneless, roasted, chopped	1 cup	343	39.5	0.0	64	0	19.3	6.7	111	52%
Untrimmed										
chop, boneless, braised	3 oz	198	23.6	0.0	36	0	10.8	4.0	64	51%
chop, boneless, broiled	3 oz	195	25.5	0.0	54	0	9.6	3.4	69	46%
chop, boneless, pan-fried in vegetable oil	3 oz	337	18.5	0.0	39	0	28.6	10.3	72	78%

Food Name	Serving Size	Calories	Prot. gms	Carbs gms	Sod. mgs	Fiber gms	Fat gms	Sat. Fat gms	Chol. mgs	% Fat Cal.
chop, boneless, pan-fried	3 oz	218	24.7	0.0	47	0	12.6	4.5	66	53%
chop or roast, boneless, raw	1 oz	54	5.7	0.0	12	0	3.3	1.1	17	57%
roast, boneless, roasted	3 oz	192	24.5	0.0	37	0	9.7	3.5	66	47%
roast, boneless, roasted, chopped	1 cup	462	33.9	0.0	62	0	35.2	12.7	115	70%
PORK, SALT										
cured (Hormel)	2 oz	320	4	0.0	1800	0	33.0	10.0	40	95%
cured, raw	8 oz	1698	11	0.0	3232	0	182.7	66.7	195	97%
cured, raw	1 oz	212	1	0.0	404	0	22.8	8.3	24	97%
PORK AND BEANS. See under BAKED BEANS, CANNED.										
PORK DINNER/ENTRÉE										
(Armour) brain, in milk gravy	2.75 oz	110	7.0	1.0	400	na	8.0	na	na	69%
(Banquet) cutlet	1 entrée	420	11	38	1060	4	25.0	7.0	35	53%
(Bryan Foods) puréed	1/3 cup	140	11	0	30	0	11.0	4.0	40	69%
(Chun King) sweet and sour, frozen	13 oz	400	11	78	1460	0	5.0	0.0	0	11%
(Cook's) picnic, smoked, whole, super trim, water added	3 oz	160	11	1	1570	0	13.0	3.0	40	71%
(Healthy Choice) patty, grilled, glazed	1 entrée	300	16	44	380	6	6.0	2.0	20	18%
(Hormel)										
loin fillet, lemon garlic, 'Always Tender'	1 oz	33	5	1	165	na	1.2	0.4	12	32%
loin fillet, lemon garlic, 'Always Tender'	4 oz	132	20	2	661	na	4.7	1.6	47	32%
steak, breaded, frozen	3 oz	220	12	11	0	0	15.0	0.0	0	59%
tenderlion, peppercorn, 'Always Tender'	4 oz	123	19	2	666	na	4.3	1.3	53	31%
tenderloin, teriyaki, 'Always Tender'	4 oz	134	20	5	462	na	3.4	1.2	52	23%
(John Morrell)										
back rib, barbecued, frozen 'Classics'	4.75 oz	240	12	8	480	0	17.0	0.0	62	66%
chop, center cut, barbecued, frozen	4.5 oz	230	29	7	410	0	9.0	0.0	90	36%
loin, thin sliced, barbecued, frozen	5 slices	150	17	5	440	0	6.0	0.0	52	38%
tenderloin, barbecued, frozen, 'Pork Classics'	3 oz	130	18	3	220	0	5.0	0.0	53	35%
(La Choy)										
chow mein, bi-pack	1 cup	78	7	9	1183	2	2.2	0.9	10	24%
sweet and sour, frozen, food service product	1 cup	241	5	43	1733	4	6.2	2.6	7	22%
(Lloyds)										
baby back rib, w/barbecue sauce, fully cooked	3 ribs	350	20	17	770	2	23.0	9.0	50	58%
sparerib, w/barbecue sauce, fully cooked	3 ribs	380	22	13	920	1	27.0	11.0	60	63%
(Marie Callender's) chop, country fried	15 oz	550	26	50	2240	9	27.0	9.0	65	44%
(Pierre)										
nuggets, breaded, frozen, product 1921	1 piece	42	2	2	62	0	2.8	0.7	7	60%
patty, country fried, frozen, product 1920	1 piece	279	14	14	432	1	18.7	5.0	30	60%
patty, country fried, frozen, product 3701	1 piece	241	14	13	424	1	15.0	3.9	30	56%
patty, country fried, frozen, product 3801	1 piece	242	14	13	414	1	15.0	4.1	28	56%
steak, country fried, frozen, product 3700	1 piece	293	16	15	483	0	18.7	5.0	46	57%
steak, country fried, frozen, product 3800	1 piece	370	19	17	532	0	25.0	6.8	57	61%
(Swanson) loin, frozen	10.75 oz	280	20	27	790	0	12.0	0.0	0	36%
(Tyson)										
patty, deluxe, frozen, 'Looney Tunes Porky Pig'	6.5 oz	370	14	48	490	0	14.0	0.0	35	34%
(Wonderbites)										
and turkey, barbecue, flame broiled, product 9119, 'Lean Magic 30'	1 piece	132	16	8	560	1	4.1	1.4	37	28%
barbecue, flame broiled, product 1830	1 piece	207	11	3	383	1	16.2	6.2	36	71%
barbecue, flame broiled, product 3734	1 piece	153	15	3	399	1	8.6	3.2	44	51%
barbecue, flame broiled, product 3735	1 piece	36	4	1	94	0	2.0	0.8	10	51%
barbecue, flame broiled, product 3834	1 piece	152	14	3	394	1	9.0	3.4	37	53%
barbecue, flame broiled, product 3835, 'Dippers'	1 piece	41	3	1	95	0	2.9	1.1	9	63%
barbecue, flame broiled, product 9800	1 piece	184	16	3	442	1	11.8	4.4	43	57%
barbecue, flame broiled, product 9966, 'Dippers'	1 piece	44	4	1	107	0	2.9	1.1	10	59%

Food Name	Serving Size	Calories	Prot. gms	Carbs gms	Sod. mgs	Fiber gms	Fat gms	Sat. Fat gms	Chol. mgs	% Fat Cal.
barbecue, flame broiled, w/100 serving trays, product 9968	1 piece	50	3	1	110	0	3.6	1.4	10	66%
barbecue, less fat, flame broiled, product 3730	1 piece	35	4	1	99	0	1.8	0.7	9	47%
barbecue, less fat, flame broiled, product 3731	1 piece	140	15	3	401	1	7.4	2.7	37	47%
barbecue, ready to cook, product 1190	1 piece	224	10	4	438	1	18.7	6.4	39	75%
barbecue, ready to cook, product 1330	1 piece	267	12	5	502	1	22.7	7.8	45	76%
Oriental crunch, flame-broiled, frozen, 'Dippers'	1 piece	90	4	5	154	1	6.2	1.6	10	61%
Oriental crunch, product 3702	1 piece	87	4	5	143	0	5.9	1.4	12	61%
rib, barbecue, flame broiled, frozen, product 3736	1 piece	40	4	2	132	0	1.8	0.7	9	42%
rib, barbecue, flame broiled, product 1805, 'Lean Magic'	1 piece	160	17	8	568	1	6.7	2.5	38	37%
rib, barbecue, flame broiled, product 1809, 'Lean Magic'	1 piece	47	4	2	142	0	2.6	1.0	10	50%
rib, flame broiled, frozen, product 3831, 'Lean Magic'	1 piece	132	15	3	402	1	6.3	2.3	37	43%
(Rib-B-Q) rib, barbecue, flame broiled, product 3830, 'Lean Magic'	1 piece	39	3	1	102	0	2.5	0.9	10	57%
teriyaki, flame broiled, product 3759	1 piece	45	4	2	135	0	2.3	0.9	12	47%

PORK FAT

Food Name	Serving Size	Calories	Prot. gms	Carbs gms	Sod. mgs	Fiber gms	Fat gms	Sat. Fat gms	Chol. mgs	% Fat Cal.
leaf, raw	1 oz	243	0	0.0	1	0	26.7	12.8	31	99%
leaf, fresh	4 oz	968	2	0.0	6	0	106.4	51.1	124	99%
separable fat from fully cooked ham, roasted	1 oz	167	2.2	0.0	177	0	17.5	6.4	24	95%
separable fat from fully cooked ham, unheated	1 oz	164	1.6	<.1	143	0	17.4	6.4	19	96%
separable fat from ham and arm picnic, roasted	3 oz	502	6.5	0.0	530	0	52.6	19.3	73	95%
separable fat from ham and arm picnic, roasted	1 oz	168	2.2	0.0	177	0	17.5	6.4	24	95%
separable fat from ham and arm picnic, unheated	1 oz	164	1.6	0.0	143	0	17.4	6.4	19	96%

PORK SEASONING. See under SEASONING MIX.

PORK SEASONING AND COATING MIX. See under SEASONING AND COATING MIX.

PORK SKINS

Food Name	Serving Size	Calories	Prot. gms	Carbs gms	Sod. mgs	Fiber gms	Fat gms	Sat. Fat gms	Chol. mgs	% Fat Cal.
barbecue	1 oz	153	16	0	756	na	9.0	3.3	33	53%
barbecue	1/2 oz	76	8	0	378	na	4.5	1.6	16	53%
plain	1 oz	155	17	0	521	0	8.9	3.2	27	52%
plain	1/2 oz	77	9	0	261	0	4.4	1.6	13	52%

PORK SUBSTITUTE

Food Name	Serving Size	Calories	Prot. gms	Carbs gms	Sod. mgs	Fiber gms	Fat gms	Sat. Fat gms	Chol. mgs	% Fat Cal.
(Worthington) vegetarian, 'Choplets'	2 slices	90	17	3	500	2	1.5	1.0	0	15.0%

POT ROAST SEASONING. See under SEASONING MIX.

POTATO

Canned

Food Name	Serving Size	Calories	Prot. gms	Carbs gms	Sod. mgs	Fiber gms	Fat gms	Sat. Fat gms	Chol. mgs	% Fat Cal.
(Stokely)	1/2 cup	50	2	11	360	0	0.0	0.0	0	0%
(Veg-All)	1/2 cup	60	1	13	260	0	0.0	0.0	0	0%
diced (Bush's Best)	1/2 cup	40	1	8	340	0	0.0	0.0	0	0%
diced (Taylor's Brand)	1 cup	90	3	25	292	0	0.0	0.0	0	0%
new, extra small, whole (IGA)	1/2 cup	45	2	9	310	0	0.0	0.0	0	0%
new, small, whole (IGA)	1/2 cup	45	2	9	300	0	0.0	0.0	0	0%
new, whole, drained (Hunt's)	4 oz	70	2	15	230	1	1.0	0.0	0	12%
sliced (Bush's Best)	1/2 cup	40	1	8	340	0	0.0	0.0	0	0%
sliced (Taylor's Brand)	1 cup	90	3	25	292	0	0.0	0.0	0	0%
sliced, w/liquid (Del Monte)	1/2 cup	45	1	10	355	0	0.0	0.0	0	0%
white, diced (Allens)	1/2 cup	45	2	10	360	0	1.0	0.0	0	16%
white, double diced (Allens)	1/2 cup	45	2	10	540	0	1.0	0.0	0	16%
white, sliced (A&P)	1/2 cup	45	2	11	320	0	1.0	0.0	0	15%
white, sliced (Allens)	1/2 cup	45	2	10	360	0	1.0	0.0	0	16%
white, sliced, no salt added (Pathmark)	1 cup	100	3	20	15	0	0.0	0.0	0	0%
white, small, sliced (Finast)	1/2 cup	55	1	13	375	0	0.0	0.0	0	0%

Food Name	Serving Size	Calories	Prot. gms	Carbs gms	Sod. mgs	Fiber gms	Fat gms	Sat. Fat gms	Chol. mgs	% Fat Cal.
white, small, whole (Finast)	1/2 cup	55	1	13	375	0	0.0	0.0	0	0%
white, whole (A&P)	1/2 cup	45	2	11	320	0	1.0	0.0	0	15%
white, whole, no salt added (Pathmark)	1 cup	100	3	20	15	0	0.0	0.0	0	0%
whole (Bush's Best)	1/2 cup	40	1	8	340	0	0.0	0.0	0	0%
whole (Stokely)	2/3 cup	70	2	14	450	1	0.0	0.0	0	0%
whole, w/liquid (Del Monte)	1/2 cup	45	1	10	355	0	0.0	0.0	0	0%
Dried, slices and dices, rehydrated (Basic American)	1/2 cup	72	2	16	240	2	0.1	0.0	0	1%
Fresh										
baked, flesh and skin, 2 1/3 x 4 3/4 inch	1 potato	220	5	51	16	5	0.2	0.1	0	1%
baked, flesh only	1/2 cup	57	1	13	3	1	0.1	0.0	0	1%
baked, flesh only, 2 1/3 x 4 3/4 inch	1 potato	145	3	34	8	2	0.2	0.0	0	1%
boiled, cooked in skin, flesh only	1/2 cup	68	1	16	3	1	0.1	0.0	0	1%
boiled, cooked in skin, flesh only, 2.5 inch diam	1 potato	118	3	27	5	2	0.1	0.0	0	1%
boiled, cooked w/o skin, flesh only	1/2 cup	67	1	16	4	1	0.1	0.0	0	1%
boiled, cooked w/o skin, flesh only, 2.5 inch diam	1 potato	116	2	27	7	2	0.1	0.0	0	1%
Finnish yellow, raw (Frieda's)	3.5 oz	100	3.3	22.0	na	(mq)	na	na	0	0%
microwaved, cooked in skin, flesh and skin, 2.5 inch diam	1 potato	212	5	49	16	5	0.2	0.1	0	1%
microwaved, cooked in skin, flesh and skin	1/2 cup	78	2	18	5	1	0.1	0.0	0	1%
microwaved, cooked in skin, flesh/skin, 2 1/3 x 4.75 inch	1 potato	156	3	36	11	2	0.2	0.0	0	1%
raw, diced, flesh and skin	1/2 cup	59	2	13	5	1	0.1	0.0	0	1%
raw, sliced	1 cup	142	4	32	46	2	0.3	0.1	0	2%
raw, whole, large, 3–4.25 inch diam, flesh and skin	1 potato	145	4	33	11	3	0.2	0.0	0	1%
raw, whole, long, 2 1/3 x 4 3/4 inch, flesh and skin	1 potato	160	4	36	12	3	0.2	0.1	0	1%
raw, whole, medium, 2.25–3 inch diam, flesh and skin	1 potato	96	3	22	7	2	0.1	0.0	0	1%
raw, whole, small, 1.75–2.25 inch diam, flesh and skin	1 potato	73	2	17	6	1	0.1	0.0	0	1%
skin, baked	1 skin	115	2	27	12	5	0.1	0.0	0	0%
skin, boiled	1 skin	27	1	6	5	1	0.0	0.0	0	1%
skin, microwaved	1 skin	77	3	17	9	3	0.1	0.0	0	1%
skin, raw	1 skin	22	1	5	4	1	0.0	0.0	0	1%
Frozen										
red, whole, 2 to 3 potatoes (C&W)	85 grams	60	1	15	30	1	0.0	0.0	0	0%
redskin, diced, frozen (Flav-R-Pac)	3/4 cup	60	1	16	35	1	0.0	0.0	0	0%
redskin, tri-cut, frozen (Flav-R-Pac)	2/3 cup	60	1	15	30	1	0.0	0.0	0	0%
redskin, wedges, frozen (Flav-R-Pac)	3/4 cup	60	1	15	30	1	0.0	0.0	0	0%
skin, baked (Tato Skins)	1 oz	150	1	17	160	0	8.0	1.0	0	50%
white, whole (Southern)	3.5 oz	69	2	15	20	0	0.1	0.0	0	1%
white, whole, boiled (Seabrook)	3.2 oz	60	2	13	5	0	0.0	0.0	0	0%
whole, small (Ore-Ida)	3 oz	70	2	16	45	0	1.0	0.0	0	11%
POTATO CHIPS AND SNACKS										
CHIPS										
(Auburn Farms)										
barbecue, nonfat	1 oz	100	3	23	140	1	0.0	0.0	0	0%
Cajun, nonfat	1 oz	99	3	23	227	1	0.0	0.0	0	0%
cheddar cheese, 96% fat free, Spudbakes'	1 oz	100	2	22	105	1	1.0	0.5	0	9%
cheddar, nonfat	1 oz	99	3	22	168	1	0.0	0.0	0	0%
mesquite barbecue, 98% fat free, Spudbakes'	1 oz	110	2	25	75	1	0.5	0.0	0	4%
original, nonfat	1 oz	99	3	23	138	1	0.0	0.0	0	0%
sour cream and onion, 98% fat free, Spudbakes'	1 oz	100	2	21	110	2	0.5	0.0	0	5%
sour cream and onion, nonfat	1 oz	99	3	22	138	1	0.0	0.0	0	0%
(Bachman)										
barbecue flavor	1 oz	150	2	14	280	0	9.0	0.0	0	56%
barbecue flavor, hot	1 oz	150	2	14	200	0	9.0	0.0	0	56%

Food Name	Serving Size	Calories	Prot. gms	Carbs gms	Sod. mgs	Fiber gms	Fat gms	Sat. Fat gms	Chol. mgs	% Fat Cal.
'Kettle Cooked'	1 oz	140	2	16	115	0	8.0	0.0	0	50%
plain	1 oz	160	2	14	270	0	10.0	0.0	0	58%
'Ridge'	1 oz	160	2	14	260	0	10.0	0.0	0	58%
'Ruffled'	1 oz	160	2	14	260	0	10.0	0.0	0	58%
Saratoga style, 'Kettle Cooked'	1 oz	140	2	16	115	0	8.0	0.0	0	50%
sour cream and onion flavor	1 oz	150	2	14	200	0	9.0	0.0	0	56%
unsalted	1 oz	160	2	14	5	0	10.0	0.0	0	58%
vinegar flavor	1 oz	150	2	15	610	0	9.0	0.0	0	54%
(Barbara's Bakery)										
herb and garlic, 'True Blues'	1 oz	140	2	15	120	0	9.0	0.0	0	54%
no salt added	1 1/4 cup	150	2	15	20	1	10.0	1.0	0	57%
plain	1 1/4 cup	150	2	15	180	1	10.0	1.0	0	57%
rippled	1-1/4 cup	150	2	15	180	1	10.0	1.0	0	57%
yogurt and green onion	1-1/4 cup	150	2	15	240	1	9.0	1.0	0	54%
yogurt and green onion, no salt added	1-1/4 cup	150	2	15	20	1	9.0	1.0	0	54%
(Barrel O'Fun) plain	1 oz	150	2	14	160	0	10.0	0.0	0	58%
(Cape Cod)										
dill and sour cream flavor	1 oz	150	2	16	160	0	8.0	0.0	0	50%
dill and sour cream flavor, no salt added	1 oz	150	2	16	15	0	8.0	0.0	0	50%
no salt added	1 oz	150	2	16	0	0	8.0	0.0	0	50%
plain	1 oz	150	2	16	120	0	8.0	0.0	0	50%
plain, 'Selects'	1 oz (19 chips)	130	2	18	110	1	6.0	0.5	0	40%
sea salt and vinegar, approx 18 chips	1 oz	150	2	17	130	1	8.0	2.0	0	49%
sour cream and chives, approx 18 chips	1 oz	150	2	15	160	1	9.0	2.0	0	54%
'Waves'	1 oz	150	2	16	120	0	8.0	0.0	0	50%
(Cottage Fries) no salt added	1 oz	160	2	14	5	0	11.0	0.0	0	61%
(Eagle)										
barbecue flavor, 'Extra Crunchy'	1 oz	150	2	16	220	0	8.0	0.0	0	50%
barbecue flavor, 'Extra Crunchy Louisiana'	1 oz	150	2	16	140	0	8.0	0.0	0	50%
barbecue flavor, 'Thins'	1 oz	150	2	15	220	0	10.0	0.0	0	57%
cheddar and sour cream, rippled, crispy	1 oz	160	2	14	200	2	11.0	1.0	0	61%
'Eagle Thins'	1 oz	150	2	15	220	0	10.0	0.0	0	57%
'Extra Crunchy'	1 oz	150	2	16	180	0	8.0	0.0	0	50%
extra crunchy, 'Hawaiian Kettle'	1 oz	150	2	17	150	1	8.0	2.0	0	49%
Idaho russet	1 oz	150	2	16	180	0	8.0	0.0	0	50%
Idaho russet, dark and crunchy	1 oz	140	2	17	150	1	7.0	1.5	0	45%
mesquite BBQ, rippled	1 oz	160	2	15	170	1	10.0	2.0	0	57%
'Ridged Thins'	1 oz	150	2	15	220	0	10.0	0.0	0	57%
ripple chips	1 oz	150	2	14	170	1	10.0	2.5	0	58%
sour cream and onion flavor, 'Ridged'	1 oz	150	2	15	280	0	10.0	0.0	0	57%
sour cream and onion flavor, thins	1 oz	160	2	14	180	1	10.0	2.0	5	58%
spicy, fiesta thins	1 oz	160	2	15	220	1	9.0	2.5	0	54%
thins, no salt added	1 oz	150	2	14	0	1	10.0	2.5	0	58%
(Featherweight) low salt	1 oz	160	2	14	4	0	11.0	0.0	0	61%
(Great Snackers)										
barbecue flavor	1 serving	60	1	8	170	0	3.0	0.0	0	43%
cheddar cheese flavor	1 serving	60	1	8	170	0	3.0	0.0	0	43%
sour cream and onion	0.5 oz	70	1	10	140	0	3.0	1.0	0	38%
toasted onion flavor	1 serving	60	1	8	120	0	3.0	0.0	0	43%
(Guiltless Gourmet)										
baked, less salt	1 oz	110	2	22	180	1	1.5	0.0	0	12%
baked, seasoned salt	1 oz	110	2	22	230	1	1.5	0.0	0	12%
barbecue, baked	1 oz	110	2	22	200	1	1.5	0.0	0	12%
sour cream and onion	1 oz	110	2	22	200	1	1.5	0.0	0	12%

Food Name	Serving Size	Calories	Prot. gms	Carbs gms	Sod. mgs	Fiber gms	Fat gms	Sat. Fat gms	Chol. mgs	% Fat Cal.
(Health Valley)										
'Country Dip'	1 oz	160	2	15	60	1	10.0	0.0	0	57%
'Country Ripple'	1 oz	160	2	15	60	1	10.0	0.0	0	57%
'Country'	1 oz	160	2	15	60	1	10.0	0.0	0	57%
'Natural'	1 oz	160	2	15	60	1	10.0	0.0	0	57%
no salt added, 'Country Dip'	1 oz	160	2	15	1	1	10.0	0.0	0	57%
no salt added, 'Country Natural'	1 oz	160	2	15	1	1	10.0	0.0	0	57%
no salt added, 'Country Ripple'	1 oz	160	2	15	1	1	10.0	0.0	0	57%
no salt added, 'Country'	1 oz	160	2	15	1	1	10.0	0.0	0	57%
(Keebler)										
lightly seasoned	1 oz	140	1	18	190	0	7.0	1.0	0	45%
sour cream and onion	1 oz	140	2	17	260	0	7.0	1.0	0	45%
(Kettle Chips)										
jalapeño Jack	1 oz	150	2	15	110	0	9.0	1.0	0	54%
lightly salted	1 oz	150	2	15	80	0	9.0	1.0	0	54%
New York cheddar	1 oz	150	2	15	100	0	9.0	1.0	0	54%
no salt added	1 oz	150	2	15	10	0	9.0	1.0	0	54%
organically grown, w/sea salt	1 oz	150	2	15	80	0	9.0	1.0	0	54%
salsa w/mesquite	1 oz	150	2	15	120	0	9.0	1.0	0	54%
sea salt and vinegar	1 oz	150	2	15	120	0	9.0	1.0	0	54%
yogurt and green onion	1 oz	150	2	15	120	0	9.0	1.0	0	54%
(King Kold)										
'Rip-L'	1 oz	150	2	16	150	0	9.0	0.0	0	53%
au gratin flavor	1 oz	150	2	15	220	0	8.0	0.0	0	51%
barbecue flavor 'BBQ'	1 oz	140	2	16	360	0	8.0	0.0	0	50%
dill flavor	1 oz	150	2	16	340	0	8.0	0.0	0	50%
onion-garlic flavor	1 oz	150	2	15	420	0	9.0	0.0	0	54%
plain	1 oz	150	2	16	160	0	9.0	0.0	0	53%
sour cream and onion flavor	1 oz	150	2	15	220	0	10.0	0.0	0	57%
(Lay's)										
au gratin, wavy	1 oz	150	2	14	200	1	10.0	3.0	3	58%
baked, low-fat	1 oz	110	2	23	150	2	1.5	0.0	0	12%
barbecue flavor, approx. 15-20 chips	1 oz	150	1	15	270	1	9.0	0.0	0	56%
barbecue flavor, baked, low-fat, 'KC Masterpiece'	1 oz	120	2	22	210	2	3.0	0.0	0	22%
barbecue flavor, 'KC Masterpiece'	1 oz	160	2	15	200	1	10.0	3.0	0	57%
Cajun flavor, 'Crunch Tators Amazin Cajun'	1 oz	150	2	17	150	1	8.0	0.0	0	49%
cheddar cheese flavor, 15–20 chips	1 oz	150	2	14	1	1	10.0	0.0	0	58%
cheddar, deli style	1 oz	150	2	16	190	1	10.0	3.0	0	56%
chili, deli style	1 oz	150	2	16	210	1	10.0	3.0	0	56%
deli style	1 oz	150	1	16	180	1	10.0	3.0	0	57%
'Flamin' Hot' 15–20 chips	1 oz	150	2	15	190	1	9.0	0.0	0	54%
jalapeño flavor, 'Crunch Tators Hoppin' Jalapeño'	1 oz	140	1	18	200	1	7.0	0.0	0	45%
mesquite barbecue flavor 'Crunch Tators Mighty Mesquite'	1 oz	150	2	17	135	1	8.0	0.0	0	49%
original	1 oz	150	2	15	180	1	10.0	3.0	0	57%
original, 'Crunch Tators' approx 16 chips	1 oz	150	2	17	120	1	8.0	0.0	0	49%
ranch flavor, wavy	1 oz	160	2	14	150	1	11.0	3.0	0	61%
salt and vinegar flavor	1 oz	150	2	15	340	1	10.0	2.5	0	57%
sour cream and onion	1 oz	150	2	15	180	1	9.0	2.5	0	54%
sour cream and onion, baked, lowfat	1 oz	120	2	21	210	2	3.0	0.0	0	23%
tangy ranch flavor, approx 15–20 chips	1 oz	160	2	15	210	1	10.0	0.0	0	57%
unsalted	1 oz	150	2	15	10	0	10.0	0.0	0	57%
wavy	1 oz	160	2	15	210	1	10.0	2.5	0	57%

Food Name	Serving Size	Calories	Prot. gms	Carbs .gms	Sod. mgs	Fiber gms	Fat gms	Sat. Fat gms	Chol. mgs	% Fat Cal.
(Louise's)										
barbecue, nonfat	1 oz	110	3	23	180	2	0.0	0.0	0	0%
Maui onion, nonfat	1 oz	110	3	24	180	2	0.0	0.0	0	0%
mesquite barbecue flavor	1 oz	100	2	23	200	0	1.0	0.0	0	8%
nonfat, no salt added	1 oz	110	3	24	10	2	0.0	0.0	0	0%
original	1 oz	100	2	23	200	0	1.0	0.0	0	8%
original, nonfat	1 oz	110	3	23	180	2	0.0	0.0	0	0%
vinegar and salt flavor	1 oz	100	2	23	200	0	1.0	0.0	0	8%
vinegar and salt, nonfat	1 oz	110	3	23	300	2	0.0	0.0	0	0%
(Michael Season's)										
baked, less salt	1 oz	110	3	21	130	1	1.5	0.0	0	12%
French onion flavor, baked	1 serving	110	3	21	150	1	1.5	0.0	0	12%
hickory barbecue, baked	1 oz	110	3	21	180	1	1.5	0.0	0	12%
honey barbecue	1 oz	140	2	20	250	1	6.0	1.0	0	38%
honey barbecue, 40% less fat	1 oz	140	2	20	250	1	6.0	1.0	0	38%
less fat, rippled	1 oz	140	2	17	120	1	6.7	1.0	0	44%
lightly salted, 40% less fat	1 oz	130	2	17	80	1	6.0	1.0	0	42%
no salt added, 40% less fat	1 oz	130	2	17	5	1	6.0	1.0	0	42%
yogurt and green onion, 40% lower fat	1 oz	130	2	17	105	1	6.0	1.0	0	42%
(Mr. Phipps)										
barbecue, tater crisps	0.5 oz	60	1	10	160	0	2.0	1.0	0	29%
sour cream 'n onion, tater crisps	0.5 oz	60	1	10	150	0	2.0	1.0	0	29%
(Munchos) plain, approx 16 chips	1 oz	160	1	15	230	0	10.0	0.0	0	58%
(Nabisco)										
baked, baked, snack chips, 'Zings'	0.5 oz	70	1	10	115	0	3.0	1.0	0	38%
cheese, cheddar, baked, cracker chips, 'Zings'	0.5 oz	70	1	9	140	0	3.0	1.0	2	40%
cheese, cheddar, cracker chips, 'Zings'	15 pieces	70	1	9	130	0	3.0	0.0	0	40%
ranch, baked, cracker chips, 'Zings'	0.5 oz	70	1	9	140	0	3.0	1.0	2	40%
(O'Boisies)										
plain	1 oz	150	1	16	180	0	9.0	2.0	0	54%
sour cream and onion flavor	1 oz	150	2	15	190	0	9.0	2.0	0	54%
(Pacific Grain)										
'Rancho-O's'	1 oz	130	2	22	55	0	1.0	0.0	0	9%
baked, 100% natural	1 oz	120	2	23	230	0	1.0	0.0	0	8%
BBQ, baked, 100% natural	1 oz	120	2	23	150	0	2.0	0.0	0	15%
(Poore Brothers)										
barbecue	1 oz	150	2	15	60	2	10.0	2.0	0	57%
Cajun	1 oz	140	2	16	55	2	8.0	1.0	0	50%
dill pickle	1 oz	140	2	16	95	2	8.0	1.0	0	50%
grilled steak and onion	1 oz	140	2	15	110	2	8.0	1.0	0	51%
jalapeño	1 oz	140	2	16	100	2	9.0	2.0	0	53%
Parmesan and garlic	1 oz	140	2	16	80	2	9.0	2.0	0	53%
regular	1 oz	140	2	17	40	2	8.0	1.0	0	49%
salt and vinegar	1 oz	140	2	15	125	1	9.0	2.0	0	54%
unsalted	1 oz	140	2	17	5	2	8.0	1.0	0	49%
(Pringle's)										
barbecue flavor, 'Light'	1 oz	150	2	17	125	0	8.0	0.0	0	49%
barbecue flavor, 'Right Crisp'	1 oz	140	2	18	160	1	7.0	2.0	0	44%
cheddar and sour cream, 'Ridges'	1 oz	150	1	15	201	1	10.0	2.5	0	58%
'Cheez Ums'	1 oz	150	2	14	190	1	10.0	2.5	0	58%
French onion flavor, 'Idaho Rippled'	1 oz	170	2	13	175	0	12.0	0.0	0	64%
'Idaho Rippled'	1 oz	170	2	13	150	0	12.0	0.0	0	64%
'Light'	1 oz	150	2	17	120	0	8.0	0.0	0	49%
mesquite barbecue, 'Ridges'	1 oz	150	1	15	150	1	10.0	2.5	0	58%

Food Name	Serving Size	Calories	Prot. gms	Carbs gms	Sod. mgs	Fiber gms	Fat gms	Sat. Fat gms	Chol. mgs	% Fat Cal.
mesquite barbecue, ridged	1 oz	150	1	15	220	1	10.0	2.5	0	58%
original flavor, 1/3 less fat	16 chips	140	1	19	135	1	7.0	2.0	0	44%
ranch flavor, 'Light'	1 oz	150	2	17	135	0	8.0	0.0	0	49%
ranch	1 oz	150	2	15	130	1	10.0	2.5	0	57%
ranch, 'Right Crisp'	1 oz	140	2	18	160	1	7.0	2.0	0	44%
'Right Crisp'	1 oz	140	2	19	135	1	7.0	2.0	0	43%
sour cream and onion	1 oz	160	2	15	135	1	10.0	2.5	0	57%
sour cream and onion, 'Right Crisp'	1 oz	140	2	18	120	1	7.0	2.0	0	44%
taco and cheddar flavor, 'Idaho Rippled'	1 oz	170	2	13	160	0	12.0	0.0	0	64%
(Ruffles)										
barbecue flavor	1 oz	150	1	16	320	0	9.0	0.0	0	54%
barbecue, mesequite, 'KC Masterpiece'	1 oz	150	2	15	190	1	9.0	2.5	0	54%
Cajun flavor, 'Cajun Spice'	1 oz	150	1	15	240	0	10.0	0.0	0	58%
cheddar and sour cream	1 oz	160	2	14	190	1	10.0	3.0	0	58%
40% less fat 'Choice' approx 16 chips	1 oz	130	2	18	130	1	6.0	1.0	0	40%
French onion flavor	1 oz	150	2	15	180	1	10.0	3.0	0	57%
low-fat	1 oz	130	2	18	160	1	6.7	1.0	0	43%
mesquite barbecue flavor, 'Mesquite Grille'	1 oz	160	2	14	260	0	10.0	0.0	0	58%
1/3 less fat, 'Light Choice'	1 oz	130	2	19	140	0	6.0	0.0	0	39%
original	1 serving	150	2	14	180	1	10.0	2.5	0	58%
ranch flavor	1 oz	150	2	15	280	1	9.0	2.5	0	54%
sour cream and onion flavor	1 oz	150	2	15	240	0	9.0	0.0	0	54%
(Snacktime)										
jalapeño flavor, 'Krunchers!'	1 oz	150	2	16	270	0	9.0	0.0	0	53%
'Krunchers!'	1 oz	150	2	16	170	0	9.0	0.0	0	53%
mesquite barbecue flavor, 'Krunchers!'	1 oz	150	2	16	200	0	9.0	0.0	0	53%
(Spicer's)										
barbecue wheat, for weight control	1 oz	100	5	12	75	9	5.0	0.0	0	40%
dietetic, natural, for weight control	1 oz	100	4	11	65	9	4.0	0.0	0	38%
sour cream and onion, for weight control	1 oz	100	4	12	150	6	4.0	0.0	0	36%
(Tato Skins)										
cheese and bacon flavor, potato skins	1 oz	150	1	17	180	0	8.0	1.0	0	50%
sour cream n' chives flavor, potato skins	1 oz	150	1	17	180	0	8.0	1.0	0	50%
(Westbrae)										
potato chips, no salt added	1 oz	150	2	16	10	0	8.0	0.0	0	50%
'Ripple'	1 oz	150	2	16	100	0	8.0	0.0	0	50%
salted	1 oz	160	2	15	100	0	10.0	0.0	0	57%
(Wise)										
barbecue flavor	1 oz	150	2	14	240	0	10.0	0.0	0	58%
barbecue flavor, 'Ridgies'	1 oz	150	2	14	240	0	10.0	0.0	0	58%
hot	1 oz	160	2	14	290	0	11.0	0.0	0	61%
'New York Deli'	1 oz	160	2	14	120	0	11.0	0.0	0	61%
onion-garlic flavor	1 oz	150	2	14	250	0	10.0	0.0	0	58%
'Plain'	1 oz	150	2	14	190	0	10.0	0.0	0	58%
'Ridgies Super Crispy'	1 oz	150	2	14	220	0	10.0	0.0	0	58%
'Ridgies'	1 oz	150	2	14	190	0	10.0	0.0	0	58%
'Rippled'	1 oz	150	2	14	190	0	10.0	0.0	0	58%
sour cream and onion flavor 'Ridgies'	1 oz	160	2	14	240	0	11.0	0.0	0	61%
(Zapp's)										
Cajun flavor, 'Lite Kettle'	1 oz	150	2	16	94	0	8.0	0.0	0	50%
Cajun flavor, 'Original Kettle'	1 oz	150	2	16	94	0	8.0	0.0	0	50%
jalapeño flavor, 'Original Kettle'	1 oz	150	2	16	85	0	8.0	0.0	0	50%
'Lite Kettle'	1 oz	150	2	16	45	0	8.0	0.0	0	50%
mesquite barbecue flavor, 'Lite Kettle'	1 oz	150	2	16	87	0	8.0	0.0	0	50%

Food Name	Serving Size	Calories	Prot. gms	Carbs gms	Sod. mgs	Fiber gms	Fat gms	Sat. Fat gms	Chol. mgs	% Fat Cal.
mesquite barbecue flavor, 'Original Kettle'	1 oz	150	2	16	87	0	8.0	0.0	0	50%
no salt added, 'Lite Kettle'	1 oz	150	2	16	1	0	8.0	0.0	0	50%
no salt added, 'Original Kettle'	1 oz	150	2	16	1	0	8.0	0.0	0	50%
'Original Kettle'	1 oz	150	2	16	45	0	8.0	0.0	0	50%
sour cream and onion flavor 'Lite'	1 oz	150	2	16	79	0	8.0	0.0	0	50%
STICKS										
(Allens)										
shoestring, canned	1 oz	140	2	16	190	0	8.0	0.0	0	50%
shoestring, no salt added, canned	1 oz	140	1	16	10	0	8.0	0.0	0	51%
(Flavor Tree) sour cream and onion	1/4 cup	127	3	13	360	0	8.3	0.0	0	55%
(Planters)										
	1 oz	160	1	15	170	0	10.0	2.0	0	58%
barbecue flavor	1 oz	160	1	15	220	0	10.0	2.0	0	58%
(S&W)										
fabulous fries, 'Pik-Nik'	2/3 cup	150	2	16	120	1	9.0	2.0	0	53%
ketchup and fries, 'Pik-Nik'	2/3 cup	160	2	17	160	1	10.0	2.0	0	54%
shoestring, 'Pik-Nik'	2/3 cup	280	2	26	180	2	18.0	4.0	0	59%
shoestring, 50% less salt, 'Pik-Nik'	3/4 cup	165	2	16	60	1	12.0	3.0	0	60%
shoestring, Sante Fe BBQ, 'Pik-Nik'	2/3 cup	180	2	18	240	2	12.0	3.0	0	57%
shoestring, sour cream and cheddar, 'Pik-Nik'	2/3 cup	180	2	17	130	2	13.0	3.0	0	61%
POTATO DISH/ENTRÉE										
(A&P)										
fried, crinkle cut	3.5 oz	140	2.0	25.0	25	(mq)	4.0	(mq)	0	25%
fried, regular	3.5 oz	140	2.0	25.0	25	(mq)	4.0	(mq)	0	25%
fried, shoestring	3.5 oz	170	2.0	24.0	50	(mq)	6.0	(mq)	0	34%
fried, steak fries	3.5 oz	140	2.0	24.0	30	(mq)	4.0	(mq)	0	26%
hash brown	3.5 oz	80	2.0	17.0	20	(mq)	0.0	0.0	0	0%
morsels	3.5 oz	140	2.0	23.0	30	(mq)	4.0	(mq)	0	27%
(Basic American)										
au gratin, 'Classic Casseroles'	3 oz	81	2	13	354	1	2.6	0.7	1	28%
hash brown, 'Golden Grill'	1/2 cup	118	1	13	144	1	6.8	0.6	0	52%
hash brown, 'ReddiShred'	1/2 cup	134	2	16	161	2	6.8	0.6	0	46%
scalloped, 'Classic Casseroles'	3 oz	81	2	13	283	1	2.3	0.6	1	26%
(Bernardi) gnocchi, uncooked	2/3 cup	281	9	56	601	3	2.0	1.0	10	6%
(Budget Gourmet)										
w/broccoli, cheese sauce, frozen, 'Light and Healthy'	10.5 oz	300	13	40	740	0	10.0	4.0	30	30%
(Crispy Crowns) puffs, frozen, prepared	10 puffs	133	2	18	448	2	6.4	3.1	0	40%
(Empire Kosher)										
potato pancake, triangle, latkes w/onions, frozen	2 oz	77	1.0	13.0	108	na	2.4	na	na	28%
(Healthy Choice)										
casserole, frozen, 'Garden Style'	1 meal	200	11	30	520	6	4.0	1.5	10	18%
cheddar broccoli, w/cheese Sauce, frozen	1 pkg	328	13	53	551	6	7.0	3.0	27	19%
garden casserole	1 serving	220	11	30	520	6	6.0	2.0	10	25%
w/broccoli and cheddar cheese	1 entrée	330	13	53	550	6	7.0	3.0	25	19%
(Heinz)										
fried, crinkle cut 'Deep Fries'	3 oz	150	2.0	22.0	30	(mq)	6.0	3.0	0	36%
fried 'Deep Fries'	3 oz	160	2.0	23.0	20	(mq)	6.0	3.0	0	35%
fried, shoestring 'Deep Fries'	3 oz	200	2.0	25.0	20	(mq)	10.0	5.0	0	46%
hash brown, w/butter and onions 'Deep Fries'	3 oz	110	1.0	14.0	80	(mq)	7.0	4.0	5	51%
(Hormel) scalloped, w/ham, microwaveable	1 cup	240	7	20	920	2	14.0	6.0	35	54%
(Joan of Arc)										
salad, German style, canned	1/2 cup	120	2.0	23.0	550	1.6	3.0	(mq)	na	21%
salad, homestyle, canned	1/2 cup	340	4.0	32.0	1070	3.0	22.0	(mq)	na	58%
(Lean Cuisine)										
baked, w/broccoli and cheddar, frozen	10 3/8 oz	290	14	37	590	0	9.0	4.0	20	28%

Food Name	Serving Size	Calories	Prot. gms	Carbs gms	Sod. mgs	Fiber gms	Fat gms	Sat. Fat gms	Chol. mgs	% Fat Cal.
baked, w/sour cream, frozen..............	10 3/8 oz	230	9	38	570	0	5.0	2.0	15	19%
cheddar, 'Deluxe'....................	1 entrée	230	13	32	570	6	6.0	2.5	20	23%
roasted, w/broccoli, cheddar cheese sauce	1 entrée	260	12	39	590	7	6.0	3.5	15	21%
scalloped.....................	1 entrée	250	10	38	590	6	6.0	2.5	25	22%
(Lunch Bucket) scalloped, microwave cup..............	7.5 oz	160	4	20	770	0	7.0	0.0	35	40%
(MicroMagic)										
fried......................	3 oz	290	3.0	40.0	30	(mq)	13.0	(mq)	na	41%
fried, skinny.................	3 oz	350	4.0	49.0	40	(mq)	15.0	(mq)	na	39%
sticks, 'Tater Sticks'................	4 oz	390	2.0	43.0	620	(mq)	22.0	(mq)	na	52%
(Mountain House) hash brown, freeze-dried, prepared.....	1 cup	150	2.0	36.0	(mq)	(mq)	0.0	0.0	na	0%
(Ore-Ida)										
fried, cottage cut.............	3 oz	120	2.0	19.0	25	(mq)	5.0	2.0	0	35%
fried, 'Country Style Dinner Fries'..........	3 oz	110	2.0	19.0	30	(mq)	3.0	2.0	0	24%
fried, crinkle cut, 'Golden Crinkles'..........	3 oz	120	2.0	19.0	35	(mq)	4.0	2.0	0	30%
fried, crinkle cut, 'Lites'.............	3 oz	90	1.0	16.0	35	(mq)	2.0	(mq)	0	21%
fried, crinkle cut, microwave............	3.5 oz	180	2.0	26.0	35	(mq)	8.0	4.0	0	39%
fried, crinkle cut, 'Pixie Crinkles'............	3 oz	140	2.0	21.0	40	(mq)	6.0	3.0	0	37%
fried, 'Crisp Crowns'............	3 oz	160	2.0	20.0	525	(mq)	9.0	4.0	0	48%
fried, 'Crispers!'............	3 oz	230	2.0	25.0	545	(mq)	15.0	8.0	0	56%
fried, French, extra crispy 'Nacho Crispers'........	3 oz	180	2.0	21.0	280	na	10.0	na	0	50%
fried, French, 'Fast Fries'...........	3 oz	150	2.0	23.0	230	na	7.0	na	0	39%
fried, 'Golden Fries'............	3 oz	120	2.0	19.0	35	(mq)	4.0	2.0	0	30%
fried, 'Lites'..................	3 oz	90	2.0	16.0	30	(mq)	2.0	<1.0	0	20%
fried, shoestring.............	3 oz	140	2.0	21.0	30	(mq)	6.0	3.0	0	37%
fried, shoestring, 'Lites'............	3 oz	90	1.0	15.0	25	(mq)	4.0	2.0	0	36%
fried, wedges, 'Home Style Potato Wedges'......	3 oz	100	2.0	17.0	45	(mq)	3.0	1.0	0	26%
fried, w/onions, 'Crispy Crowns'............	3 oz	170	1.0	20.0	570	(mq)	9.0	5.0	0	49%
hash brown, 'Golden Patties'........	2.5 oz	140	1.0	15.0	295	(mq)	8.0	4.0	0	53%
hash brown, microwave............	2 oz	130	1.0	12.0	170	(mq)	8.0	4.0	0	58%
hash brown, shredded............	3 oz	70	1.0	15.0	40	(mq)	<1.0	na	0	<12%
hash brown, 'Southern Style'........	3 oz	70	1.0	16.0	35	(mq)	<1.0	na	0	<12%
hashbrown, w/cheddar, 'Cheddar Browns'........	3 oz	90	2.0	13.0	415	(mq)	2.0	1.0	10	23%
puffs, bacon flavored 'Tater Tots'.......	3 oz	140	2.0	19.0	625	(mq)	6.0	3.0	0	39%
puffs 'Tater Tots'............	3 oz	140	1.0	19.0	550	(mq)	7.0	3.0	0	44%
puffs, microwave, 'Tater Tots'........	4 oz	200	2.0	29.0	670	(mq)	9.0	4.0	0	40%
puffs, w/onion, 'Tater Tots'............	3 oz	140	2.0	19.0	715	(mq)	6.0	3.0	0	39%
(Pik-Nik) shoestring................	1 oz	160	1	15	103	1	10.3	2.3	0	59%
(Quick 'n Crispy)										
fried, crinkle cut................	4 oz	370	3.0	44.0	50	(mq)	19.0	(mq)	na	48%
fried, shoestring.............	4 oz	390	3.0	48.0	50	(mq)	20.0	(mq)	na	47%
fried, thin cuts.............	4 oz	370	3.0	44.0	50	(mq)	19.0	(mq)	na	48%
wedges..................	4 oz	280	3.0	36.0	40	(mq)	13.0	(mq)	na	43%
(Read)										
salad, German style, canned............	1/2 cup	120	2.0	23.0	550	1.6	3.0	(mq)	na	21%
salad, homestyle, canned............	1/2 cup	340	4.0	32.0	1070	3.0	22.0	(mq)	na	58%
(Seabrook)										
fried....................	3 oz	120	2.0	20.0	25	(mq)	4.0	(mq)	na	29%
fried, cottage cut..............	2.8 oz	110	1.0	17.0	14	(mq)	4.0	(mq)	na	33%
fried, crinkle cut..............	3 oz	120	2.0	20.0	24	(mq)	4.0	(mq)	na	29%
fried, shoestring............	3 oz	140	2.0	20.0	45	(mq)	6.0	(mq)	na	38%
(Stouffer's)										
au gratin...............	1/2 cup	130	4	15	590	1	6.0	2.5	15	42%
au gratin, frozen, food service product............	1 oz	32	1	4	130	0	1.3	0.4	3	36%
scalloped...............	1/2 cup	140	4	17	450	2	6.0	1.0	3	39%
scalloped, frozen, food service product............	1 oz	31	1	4	109	0	1.3	0.1	1	38%

Food Name	Serving Size	Calories	Prot. gms	Carbs gms	Sod. mgs	Fiber gms	Fat gms	Sat. Fat gms	Chol. mgs	% Fat Cal.
(Weight Watchers)										
baked, vegetable primavera, frozen	11.15 oz	320	11	49	500	0	9.0	2.0	5	25%
baked, w/broccoli and ham, frozen	11.5 oz	240	19	30	520	0	5.0	3.0	15	19%
baked, w/turkey, homestyle, frozen	11.25 oz	230	17	27	510	0	7.0	3.0	45	26%
w/broccoli and cheese	1 serving	250	12	35	590	6	7.0	2.0	10	25%
POTATO DISH/ENTRÉE MIX										
(Arrowhead Mills) Western, flakes	2 oz	140	5.0	44.0	24	na	0.0	0.0	0	0%
(Barbara's Bakery)										
mashed, mix only	1/3 cup	70	2	17	10	1	0.0	0.0	0	0%
Western, mix only	4 oz	389	7.0	89.0	63	na	1.0	na	1	2%
(Betty Crocker)										
au gratin, prepared w/margarine and skim milk	1/2 cup	150	4.0	21.0	600	(mq)	5.0	(mq)	(mq)	31%
hash brown, mix only	1/2 cup	120	3	30	35	3	0.0	0.0	0	0%
hash brown, w/onions, prepared w/margarine	1/2 cup	160	2.0	24.0	100	(mq)	6.0	(mq)	na	34%
hash brown, w/onions, prepared	1/6 pkg	110	2.0	24.0	40	(mq)	1.0	na	na	8%
mashed, cheddar cheese, 'Potato Buds' mix only	1/12 pkg	110	2.0	20.0	440	na	2.0	na	na	17%
mashed, cheddar cheese, 'Potato Buds' prepared	1/2 cup	180	3.0	21.0	510	na	9.0	na	na	46%
mashed, cheddar cheese, 'Potato Buds' reduced fat recipe, mix only	1/12 pkg	140	3.0	21.0	480	na	5.0	na	na	32%
mashed, 'Potato Buds' mix only	1/3 cup	80	2	18	20	1	0.0	0.0	0	0%
mashed, 'Potato Buds' prepared w/o added salt	1/2 cup	130	3.0	17.0	90	(mq)	6.0	(mq)	(mq)	40%
mashed, 'Potato Buds' prepared	1/2 cup	130	3.0	17.0	360	(mq)	6.0	(mq)	(mq)	40%
scalloped, cheesy, mix only	1/6 pkg	90	2.0	19.0	500	(mq)	1.0	na	na	10%
scalloped, cheesy, prepared	1/2 cup	140	3.0	20.0	560	(mq)	5.0	(mq)	(mq)	33%
scalloped, mix only	1/6 pkg	90	2.0	19.0	520	(mq)	1.0	na	na	10%
scalloped, prepared	1/2 cup	140	3.0	20.0	580	(mq)	5.0	(mq)	(mq)	33%
scalloped, sour cream and chives, mix only	1/6 pkg	100	2.0	19.0	460	(mq)	2.0	(mq)	na	18%
scalloped, sour cream and chives, prepared	1/2 cup	140	3.0	21.0	520	(mq)	5.0	(mq)	(mq)	32%
scalloped, w/ham, mix only	1/5 pkg	100	2.0	20.0	470	(mq)	1.0	(mq)	(mq)	9%
scalloped, w/ham, prepared	1/2 cup	160	4.0	22.0	540	(mq)	6.0	(mq)	(mq)	34%
stuffed, butter, herbed, 'Twice Baked' prepared	1/2 cup	220	5.0	20.0	540	(mq)	13.0	(mq)	(mq)	54%
stuffed, butter, herbed, 'Twice Baked' mix only	1/6 pkg	100	2.0	18.0	440	(mq)	2.0	(mq)	na	18%
stuffed, cheddar, mild, w/onion, 'Twice Baked' mix only	1/6 pkg	100	2.0	18.0	540	(mq)	2.0	(mq)	na	18%
stuffed, cheddar, mild, w/onion, 'Twice Baked' prepared	1/2 cup	190	5.0	19.0	640	(mq)	11.0	(mq)	(mq)	51%
stuffed, sour cream and chives, 'Twice Baked,' mix only	1/6 pkg	90	2.0	17.0	480	(mq)	2.0	(mq)	na	19%
stuffed, sour cream and chives, 'Twice Baked' prepared	1/2 cup	200	5.0	19.0	570	(mq)	11.0	(mq)	(mq)	51%
stuffed, w/bacon and cheddar, 'Twice Baked' mix only	1/6 pkg	110	3.0	19.0	500	(mq)	2.0	(mq)	na	17%
stuffed, w/bacon and cheddar, 'Twice Baked' prepared	1/2 cup	210	6.0	21.0	600	(mq)	11.0	(mq)	(mq)	48%
(Country Store) mashed, prepared	1/3 cup	70	1.0	16.0	10	(mq)	0.0	0.0	0	0%
(Ener-G Foods) mix, gluten-free	1 cup	878	0	226	420	0	0.0	0.0	0	0%
(Fantastic Foods)										
au gratin, prepared w/whole milk	1/2 cup	156	6.0	25.0	440	(mq)	4.0	(mq)	(mq)	23%
au gratin, prepared w/whole milk and salted butter	1/2 cup	196	6.0	25.0	495	(mq)	8.0	(mq)	(mq)	37%
country style, prepared	1/2 cup	85	3.0	19.0	316	(mq)	0.3	na	na	3%
country style, prepared w/salted butter	1/2 cup	118	3.0	19.0	362	(mq)	4.0	(mq)	(mq)	29%
(French's)										
au gratin, tangy, prepared	1/2 cup	130	4.0	20.0	480	(mq)	5.0	(mq)	na	32%
casserole, cheddar and bacon, prepared	1/2 cup	130	4.0	18.0	390	(mq)	5.0	(mq)	na	34%
scalloped, creamy Italian, prepared	1/2 cup	120	4.0	19.0	430	(mq)	3.0	(mq)	na	23%
scalloped, crispy top, w/savory onion, prepared	1/2 cup	140	3.0	20.0	430	na	5.0	(mq)	na	33%

Food Name	Serving Size	Calories	Prot. gms	Carbs gms	Sod. mgs	Fiber gms	Fat gms	Sat. Fat gms	Chol. mgs	% Fat Cal.
scalloped, real cheese, prepared	1/2 cup	140	4.0	19.0	380	(mq)	5.0	(mq)	na	33%
scalloped, sour cream and chives, prepared	1/2 cup	150	3.0	19.0	550	(mq)	7.0	(mq)	na	42%
Western, creamy, prepared	1/2 cup	130	3.0	20.0	520	(mq)	4.0	(mq)	na	28%
(General Mills)										
au gratin, mix only	1/6 pkg	100	2.0	20.0	520	na	1.0	na	na	9%
au gratin, prepared w/margarine and 2% milk	1/2 cup	150	3.0	21.0	580	na	6.0	na	na	36%
au gratin, w/broccoli, homestyle, mix only	1/6 pkg	90	2.0	18.0	490	na	1.0	na	na	10%
au gratin, w/broccoli, homestyle, prepared w/margarine and 2% milk	1/2 cup	140	3.0	19.0	550	na	6.0	na	na	38%
hash brown	1/6 pkg	110	2.0	24.0	25	na	<1.0	na	na	<8%
hash brown, prepared w/margarine	1/2 cup	160	2.0	24.0	100	na	6.0	na	na	34%
julienne, mix only	1/6 pkg	90	2.0	17.0	520	na	1.0	na	na	11%
julienne, prepared w/margarine and 2% milk	1/2 cup	130	3.0	19.0	580	na	5.0	na	na	34%
mashed, American cheese, homestyle, mix only	1/6 pkg	100	2.0	20.0	560	na	1.0	na	na	9%
mashed, American cheese, homestyle, prepared w/margarine and 2% milk	1/2 cup	150	3.0	21.0	620	na	6.0	na	na	36%
mashed, cheddar and bacon, mix only	1/6 pkg	100	2.0	20.0	480	na	1.0	na	na	9%
mashed, cheddar and bacon, prepared w/margarine and 2% milk	1/2 cup	150	3.0	21.0	540	na	6.0	na	na	36%
mashed, cheddar cheese, homestyle, mix only	1/6 pkg	90	2.0	19.0	470	na	1.0	na	na	10%
mashed, cheddar cheese, homestyle, prepared w/margarine and 2% milk	1/2 cup	150	3.0	21.0	530	na	6.0	na	na	36%
scalloped, mix only	1/6 pkg	90	2.0	19.0	510	na	1.0	na	na	10%
scalloped, prepared w/margarine and 2% milk	1/2 cup	140	3.0	20.0	570	na	5.0	na	na	33%
scalloped, smoky cheddar, mix only	1/6 pkg	100	2.0	20.0	520	na	1.0	na	na	9%
scalloped, smoky cheddar, prepared w/margarine and 2% milk	1/2 cup	140	3.0	21.0	580	na	5.0	na	na	32%
scalloped, sour cream and chive	1/6 pkg	100	2.0	19.0	460	na	2.0	na	na	18%
scalloped, sour cream and chive, prepared w/margarine and 2% milk	1/2 cup	150	3.0	20.0	520	na	6.0	na	na	37%
scalloped, w/ham, mix only	1/5 pkg	100	2.0	20.0	550	na	1.0	na	na	9%
scalloped, w/ham, prepared w/margarine and 2% milk	1/2 cup	170	4.0	22.0	620	na	7.0	na	na	38%
Western, cheesy, homestyle, mix only	1/6 pkg	100	2.0	19.0	500	na	2.0	na	na	18%
Western, cheesy, homestyle, prepared w/margarine and 2% milk	1/2 cup	150	3.0	20.0	560	na	6.0	na	na	37%
Western, potato buds, mix only	1/8 pkg	70	2.0	16.0	20	na	0.0	na	na	0%
Western, potato buds, prepared w/o salt	1/2 cup	130	3.0	17.0	90	na	6.0	na	na	40%
Western, potato buds, prepared	1/2 cup	130	3.0	17.0	360	na	6.0	na	na	40%
(Hungry Jack)										
mashed, 'Flakes' prepared	1/2 cup	140	3.0	17.0	380	(mq)	7.0	(mq)	na	44%
Western, flakes	13.3 oz	70	1.0	16.0	25	1.0	0.0	0.0	0	0%
Western, flakes, prepared w/margarine, 2% milk, salt, water	1/2 cup	130	2.0	17.0	260	1.0	6.0	1.0	0	42%
Western, flakes, prepared w/margarine, 2% milk, water	1/2 cup	130	2.0	17.0	85	1.0	6.0	1.0	0	42%
(Idaho) potato pancake, prepared, 3 inch diam	3 pancakes	90	3	16	420	0	2.0	0.0	0	19%
(Idaho Spuds)										
potato pancake, prepared, 3 inch diam	3 cakes	90	3.0	16.0	420	(mq)	2.0	(mq)	na	19%
Western, flakes	13.3 oz	70	1.0	15.0	40	1.0	0.0	0.0	0	0%
Western, granules	13.3 oz	60	1.0	14.0	30	1.0	0.0	0.0	0	0%
Western, granules, prepared	1/2 cup	130	2.0	16.0	320	(mq)	6.0	(mq)	na	43%
Western, granules, prepared w/margarine, 2% milk, water	1/2 cup	120	2.0	16.0	85	1.0	5.0	0.0	0	39%
Western, granules, prepared w/margarine, 2% milk, salt, water	1/2 cup	120	2.0	16.0	190	1.0	5.0	0.0	0	39%

Food Name	Serving Size	Calories	Prot. gms	Carbs gms	Sod. mgs	Fiber gms	Fat gms	Sat. Fat gms	Chol. mgs	% Fat Cal.
(Idaho Spuds)										
Western, flakes, prepared	1/2 cup	140	3.0	17.0	380	(mq)	7.0	(mq)	na	44%
Western, flakes, prepared w/margarine, 2% milk, water	1/2 cup	130	3.0	16.0	105	1.0	6.0	1.0	0	42%
Western, flakes, prepared w/margarine, 2% milk, salt, water	1/2 cup	130	3.0	16.0	370	1.0	6.0	1.0	0	42%
(Idahoan)										
au gratin, prepared	1/2 cup	130	3.0	18.0	475	(mq)	5.0	(mq)	(mq)	35%
hash brown, herb and butter, mix only	1/6 pkg	90	2.0	16.0	425	(mq)	2.0	(mq)	na	20%
hash brown, prepared w/unsalted butter	1/2 cup	140	2.0	18.0	50	(mq)	7.0	(mq)	na	44%
hash brown, 'Quick One-Pan' prepared	1/2 cup	140	2.0	18.0	400	(mq)	7.0	(mq)	na	44%
mashed, cheddar, spicy, mix only	1/6 pkg	90	2.0	17.0	450	(mq)	1.0	na	na	11%
mashed, cheddar, spicy, prepared	1/2 cup	140	3.0	21.0	500	(mq)	5.0	(mq)	(mq)	32%
scalloped, prepared	1/2 cup	140	3.0	20.0	425	(mq)	5.0	(mq)	(mq)	33%
scalloped, prepared w/o added salt, w/unsalted butter	1/2 cup	140	3.0	16.0	55	(mq)	7.0	(mq)	(mq)	45%
scalloped, sour cream and chives, mix only	1/6 pkg	90	2.0	15.0	340	(mq)	2.0	(mq)	na	21%
scalloped, sour cream and chives, prepared	1/2 cup	130	2.0	18.0	400	(mq)	5.0	(mq)	(mq)	36%
Western, 'Complete' mix only	1/3 cup	100	2.0	19.0	310	2.0	2.0	0.5	0	18%
Western, mix only	1/3 cup	80	2.0	18.0	15	2.0	0.0	0.0	0	0%
(Ore-Ida)										
mashed, natural butter flavor, prepared w/2% milk	1/2 cup	170	4.0	23.0	230	na	5.0	na	5	29%
mashed, natural butter flavor, unprepared	2.25 oz	100	1.0	14.0	140	na	3.0	na	5	31%
(Pillsbury)										
au gratin, tangy, 'Specially' mix only	1/6 pkg	90	2.0	19.0	470	1.0	1.0	0.0	0	10%
au gratin, tangy, prepared w/butter and whole milk	1/2 cup	140	3.0	20.0	520	1.0	6.0	3.0	15	37%
mashed, cheddar and bacon, 'Specialty' mix only	1/6 pkg	90	2.0	18.0	430	1.0	1.0	0.0	0	10%
mashed, cheddar and bacon, 'Specialty' prepared w/butter and whole milk	1/2 cup	140	3.0	19.0	480	1.0	6.0	3.0	15	38%
potato pancake, 'Specialty'	1/8 pkg	70	2.0	16.0	400	1.0	0.0	0.0	0	0%
potato pancake, 'Specialty' prepared w/water and egg, 3 inch diam each	3 cakes	90	3.0	16.0	420	1.0	2.0	0.0	55	19%
scalloped, sour cream and chives, 'Specialty,' mix only	1/6 pkg	100	2.0	18.0	450	1.0	2.0	1.0	0	18%
scalloped, sour cream and chives, 'Specialty,' prepared w/butter and whole milk	1/2 cup	150	3.0	20.0	500	1.0	6.0	4.0	15	37%
Western, cheesy, 'Specialty' mix only	1/6 pkg	100	2.0	19.0	490	1.0	2.0	0.0	0	18%
Western, cheesy, 'Specialty,' prepared w/butter, whole milk	1/2 cup	150	3.0	20.0	540	1.0	6.0	3.0	15	37%
Western, creamy white sauce, 'Specialty,' mix only	1/6 pkg	100	2.0	19.0	410	1.0	2.0	0.0	0	18%
POTATO JUICE, bottled *(Biotta)*	6 fl oz	144	2	31	222	0	0.1	0.0	0	1%
POTATO SALAD. See under POTATO DISH/ENTRÉE.										
POTATO SALAD DRESSING. See under SALAD DRESSING.										
POTATO SALAD SEASONING. See under SEASONING MIX.										
POTATO SEASONING. See under SEASONING MIX.										
POTATO STARCH *(Featherweight)*	1 cup	620	0	154	51	0	1.0	0.0	0	1%
POTTED MEAT SPREAD										
(Armour)	1.83 oz	100	7	1	550	0	7.0	0.0	0	66%
(Hormel)	1 oz	53	4	2	280	0	4.0	2.0	23	60%
(Libby's)	1/4 cup	110	10	0	440	0	7.0	2.0	30	61%
POULTRY SEASONING. See under SEASONING MIX.										
POWER BAR. See under SPORTS AND DIET/NUTRITION BARS.										
PRESERVES. See JAM AND PRESERVES.										
PRETZEL										
(A & Eagle)	1 oz	110	3	22	570	0	2.0	0.0	0	15%

Food Name	Serving Size	Calories	Prot. gms	Carbs gms	Sod. mgs	Fiber gms	Fat gms	Sat. Fat gms	Chol. mgs	% Fat Cal.
(Bachman)										
hard	1 oz	110	3	23	290	0	1.0	0.0	0	8%
hard, unsalted	1 oz	110	3	23	50	0	1.0	0.0	0	8%
logs	1 oz	110	3	21	470	0	2.0	0.0	0	16%
'Nutzels'	1 oz	110	3	21	470	0	2.0	0.0	0	16%
'Petite'	1 oz	110	3	21	410	0	2.0	0.0	0	16%
rings	1 oz	110	3	21	240	0	2.0	0.0	0	16%
rod	1 oz	110	3	21	2	0	2.0	0.0	0	16%
sodium-free, 'Petite'	1 oz	110	3	21	410	0	2.0	0.0	0	16%
thin	1 oz	110	3	21	410	0	2.0	0.0	0	16%
thin, 'Thin'n Light'	1 oz	110	3	21	410	0	2.0	0.0	0	16%
treats	1 oz	110	3	21	410	0	2.0	0.0	0	16%
twist	1 oz	110	3	21	410	0	2.0	0.0	0	16%
(Barbara's Bakery)										
Bavarian	2 pretzels	100	5	20	170	3	1.5	0.0	0	12%
Bavarian, no salt added	2 pretzels	100	5	20	20	3	1.5	0.0	0	12%
mini, no salt added	18 pretzels	100	5	21	30	4	1.5	0.0	0	11%
mini, no salt added, 17 pretzels	1 oz	110	4	21	10	0	1.0	0.0	0	8%
none-grain	2 pretzels	100	4	20	180	3	1.5	0.0	0	12%
(Bearitos) stick, thin, organic	30 grams	110	3	24	350	1	0.5	0.0	0	4%
(Benzel's Bretzles) tiny, thin	1 oz	104	3	23	470	1	0.0	0.0	0	0%
(Cape Cod) multigrain, no fat	30 pretzels	110	3	25	310	3	0.0	0.0	0	0%
(Delicious)										
party	1 oz	110	3	23	500	0	1.0	0.0	0	8%
stick	1 oz	110	3	23	500	0	1.0	0.0	1	8%
twist	1 oz	110	3	23	500	0	1.0	0.0	0	8%
(Eagle)										
Bavarian, sourdough, no fat	1 oz	110	3	24	430	1	0.0	0.0	0	0%
Bavarian, sourdough, no fat, no salt added	1 oz	110	3	24	60	1	0.0	0.0	0	0%
mini bites, low-fat	1 oz	110	3	22	470	1	10.0	1.0	0	47%
stick, low-fat	1 oz	110	3	24	470	1	1.0	0.0	0	8%
twist, thin, low-fat	1 oz	110	3	22	470	1	10.0	1.0	0	47%
twist, thin, no fat	1 oz	100	3	22	470	1	0.0	0.0	0	0%
(Estee)										
Dutch style, unsalted	2 pretzels	110	3	23	30	0	1.0	1.0	0	8%
unsalted	15 pretzels	75	2	16	5	0	1.0	1.0	0	11%
unsalted	5 pretzels	25	1	5	5	1	1.0	1.0	0	27%
(Featherweight) low-salt	20 pieces	110	3	23	30	0	1.0	0.0	0	8%
(Harmony) yogurt coated	1/3 cup	140	2	21	210	0	5.0	4.0	0	33%
(J&J Snack Foods)										
Bavarian, soft	1 pretzel	180	6	34	360	1	2.5	0.5	0	12%
Bavarian, twist, soft	1 pretzel	210	8	41	430	2	3.0	0.5	0	12%
cheese-filled, soft, 'Superpretzel'	1 pretzel	380	14	61	937	4	7.0	3.0	3	17%
cinnamon-raisin, soft, king size, 'Superpretzel'	1 pretzel	390	12	76	570	3	4.0	0.5	0	9%
cinnamon-raisin, soft, regular size, 'Superpretzel'	1 pretzel	190	6	38	290	2	2.0	0.0	0	9%
cinnamon-raisin, w/icing, soft, king size, 'Superpretzel'	1 pretzel	420	12	85	580	3	4.0	0.5	0	8%
cinnamon-raisin, w/icing, soft, regular size, 'Superpretzel'	1 pretzel	210	6	43	290	2	2.0	0.0	0	8%
jalapeño, soft, 'Superpretzel'	1 pretzel	360	13	78	460	4	0.0	0.0	0	0%
rod, sweet dough, soft	1 pretzel	300	8	60	230	2	3.0	0.5	0	9%
soft, all natural, regular size	1 pretzel	190	8	41	160	2	0.0	0.0	0	0%
soft, king size, 'Superpretzel'	1 pretzel	390	14	83	320	4	0.0	0.0	0	0%
soft, no salt, frozen, 'Superpretzel'	1 pretzel	170	6	37	140	2	0.0	0.0	0	0%

Food Name	Serving Size	Calories	Prot. gms	Carbs gms	Sod. mgs	Fiber gms	Fat gms	Sat. Fat gms	Chol. mgs	% Fat Cal.
stick, cheese-filled, nacho, 'Superpretzel'	2 softstix	140	5	24	270	1	2.5	1.5	10	16%
stick, cheese-filled, pizza, 'Superpretzel'	2 softstix	140	5	24	250	1	2.5	1.5	10	16%
stick, sweet dough, soft	1 pretzel	170	5	34	130	1	1.5	0.0	0	8%
(Keebler)										
braids, 'Butter Pretzels'	1 oz	110	3	21	620	0	1.0	1.0	0	9%
knots, 'Butter Pretzels'	1 oz	110	3	21	530	0	1.0	1.0	0	9%
(Louise's) sourdough, nonfat	1 oz	90	1	19	470	1	0.0	0.0	0	0%
(M&M Mars) w/cheddar, 'Combos'	10 combos	139	3	20	335	na	5.1	na	2	33%
(Michael Season's) mini	18 pretzels	120	3	21	30	1	1.0	0.0	na	9%
(Mister Salty)										
Dutch style	2 pretzels	120	3	25	580	1	1.0	0.0	0	7%
'Juniors'	1 oz	110	2	22	500	0	2.0	0.0	0	16%
rings	1 oz	110	3	21	510	0	2.0	0.0	0	16%
rings, butter flavor	1 oz	110	3	21	570	0	2.0	0.0	0	16%
stick	1 oz	110	3	23	380	1	1.0	1.0	5	8%
stick, butter flavor	1 oz	110	3	22	620	0	1.0	0.0	0	8%
stick, nonfat	47 stick	110	3	23	370	1	0.0	0.0	0	0%
stick, very thin, approx 92 pieces	1 oz	110	3	22	600	1	3.0	0.0	0	21%
twist, nonfat	9 pieces	110	3	23	380	1	0.0	0.0	0	0%
(Mr. Phipps)										
less salt	16 pretzels	120	2	21	410	1	2.5	0.0	0	20%
original, nonfat	16 pretzels	100	2	22	630	1	0.0	0.0	0	0%
(Mr. Salty)										
30% less sodium	88 stick	110	3	25	400	1	0.0	0.0	0	0%
nonfat	16 pretzels	100	2	22	621	1	0.0	0.0	0	0%
(Nabisco) chips, sesame	8 pieces	60	1	10	250	0	2.0	0.0	0	29%
(Pepperidge Farm) 'Snack Stick'	8 pieces	120	3	23	430	1	3.0	0.0	0	21%
(Quinlan)										
beer	1 oz	110	3	22	446	0	1.4	0.0	0	12%
logs	1 oz	103	3	22	388	0	0.8	0.0	0	7%
oat bran	1 oz	115	4	22	156	0	1.5	0.0	0	12%
rice bran, no salt	1 oz	101	3	20	52	2	2.3	0.0	0	19%
stick	1 oz	105	3	22	538	0	0.6	0.0	0	5%
thin	1 oz	104	3	22	765	0	0.6	0.0	0	5%
thin, 'Ultra Thin'	1 oz	106	3	23	618	0	0.6	0.0	0	5%
tiny, thin	1 oz	109	3	21	601	0	1.5	0.0	0	12%
tiny, thin, no salt	1 oz	115	3	22	10	0	1.6	0.0	0	13%
(Rokeach)										
Dutch style	1 oz	110	3	24	0	0	0.0	0.0	0	0%
Dutch style, unsalted	1 oz	110	2	20	30	0	0.0	0.0	0	0%
'Party'	1 oz	110	2	23	0	0	1.0	0.0	0	8%
unsalted, 'Baldies'	1 oz	110	2	20	30	0	0.0	0.0	0	0%
(Rold Gold)										
baked, 33% less sodium	10 pretzels	110	3	23	340	1	0.0	0.0	0	0%
Bavarian, 3 pretzels	1 oz	120	3	22	430	0	2.0	0.0	0	15%
rod	1 oz	110	3	22	370	1	1.0	0.0	0	8%
stick	1 oz	110	2	23	760	0	1.0	0.0	0	8%
stick, nonfat	1 oz	110	3	23	530	1	0.0	0.0	0	0%
thin twist	1 oz	110	3	23	420	1	1.0	0.0	0	8%
thin, baked, 33% less sodium, fat-free'	1 oz	110	3	23	340	1	0.0	0.0	0	0%
tiny, twist, nonfat	1 oz	100	3	23	420	1	0.0	0.0	0	0%
'Tiny Tim'	1 oz	110	2	23	610	0	1.0	0.0	0	8%
twist, thin, 10 twists	1 oz	110	2	23	470	0	1.0	0.0	0	8%

Food Name	Serving Size	Calories	Prot. gms	Carbs gms	Sod. mgs	Fiber gms	Fat gms	Sat. Fat gms	Chol. mgs	% Fat Cal.
(Seyfert's) rod, butter flavor	1 oz	110	3	21	530	0	1.0	0.0	0	9%
(Snyder's) pieces, buttermilk ranch, sourdough	1 oz	130	2	19	250	0	5.0	1.0	0	35%
(Ultra Slim Fast) twist	1 oz	100	2	21	460	3	1.0	0.0	0	9%
PRICKLY PEAR										
raw, sliced	1 cup	61	1	14	7	5	0.8	0.1	0	10%
raw, whole, trimmed	1 medium	42	1	10	5	4	0.5	0.1	0	10%
PROTEIN BAR. See under SPORTS AND DIET/NUTRITION BARS.										
PRUNE										
Canned										
in heavy syrup, w/liquid	1 cup	246	2	65	7	9	0.5	0.0	0	2%
in heavy syrup, w/liquid	5 medium	90	1	24	3	3	0.2	0.0	0	2%
Dried										
low-moisture, stewed	1 cup	316	3	83	6	na	0.7	0.1	0	2%
low-moisture, uncooked	1 cup	447	5	118	7	na	1.0	0.1	0	2%
pitted, stewed	1 cup	265	3	70	5	16	0.6	0.0	0	2%
pitted, uncooked	1 cup	406	4	107	7	12	0.9	0.1	0	2%
uncooked	1 medium	20	0	5	0	1	0.0	0.0	0	2%
PRUNE JUICE										
Canned or bottled										
	1 cup	182	2	45	10	3	0.1	0.0	0	0%
	1 fl oz	23	0	6	1	0	0.0	0.0	0	0%
(Del Monte) unsweetened	6 fl oz	120	1	33	10	0	0.0	0.0	0	0%
(J. Hungerford) 100% juice	9.03 fl oz	178	2	44	10	3	0.0	0.0	0	0%
(Knudsen) organic	8 fl oz	170	1	42	0	0	0.0	0.0	0	0%
(Lucky Leaf)	6 fl oz	150	0	36	0	0	0.0	0.0	0	0%
(Mott's)										
	6 fl oz	130	1	32	8	0	0.0	0.0	0	0%
country style	6 fl oz	130	1	32	7	0	0.0	0.0	0	0%
(Pathmark)										
'All Natural'	6 fl oz	120	1	30	10	0	0.0	0.0	0	0%
w/prune pulp, 'Homestyle'	6 fl oz	130	1	32	10	0	0.0	0.0	0	0%
(S&W) unsweetened	6 fl oz	120	1	31	20	0	0.0	0.0	0	0%
(SunSweet)	6 fl oz	130	1	33	20	0	0.0	0.0	0	0%
PSYLLIUM FIBER, smooth texture (Metamucil)	1 heaping tsp	20	0	5	na	3	0.0	na	na	0%
PUDDING. See also PUDDING MIX; PUDDING/PIE FILLING MIX.										
ALMOND										
(Imagine Foods) nondairy, low-fat, 'Dream Pudding'	4 oz	150	1	31	30	0	2.0	0.0	0	12%
BANANA										
(Del Monte) 'Pudding Cup'	5 oz	180	3	30	285	0	5.0	0.0	0	25%
(Hunt's) 'Snack Pack'	1/2 cup	158	2	25	163	0	5.8	1.7	0	33%
(Imagine Foods) nondairy, 'Dream Pudding'	4 oz	120	1	30	5	0	0.0	0.0	0	0%
(Lucky Leaf)	4 oz	150	2	24	110	0	5.0	0.0	0	30%
(Musselman's)	4 oz	150	2	24	110	0	5.0	0.0	0	30%
BUTTERSCOTCH										
(Crowley)	4.5 oz	150	3	27	210	0	3.0	0.0	10	18%
(Del Monte) 'Pudding Cup'	5 oz	180	3	31	285	0	5.0	0.0	0	25%
(Featherweight)	1/2 cup	100	0	21	160	0	1.0	0.0	0	10%
(Hunt's) 'Snack Pack'	4 oz	153	2	24	211	0	5.7	1.7	1	34%
(Imagine Foods) nondairy	1 cup	150	1	31	45	0	3.0	0.0	0	17%
(Lucky Leaf)	4 oz	170	2	26	135	0	7.0	0.0	0	36%
(Musselman's)	4 oz	170	2	26	135	0	7.0	0.0	0	36%
(Rich's) frozen	3 oz	130	2	18	130	0	6.0	0.0	0	40%

Food Name	Serving Size	Calories	Prot. gms	Carbs gms	Sod. mgs	Fiber gms	Fat gms	Sat. Fat gms	Chol. mgs	% Fat Cal.
(Ultra Slim Fast) 'Lite 'N Tasty'	4 oz	100	2	21	230	2	1.0	0.0	0	9%
(White House)	3.5 oz	113	1	20	195	0	3.0	0.0	0	24%
BUTTERSCOTCH-CHOCOLATE-VANILLA										
(Jell-O) swirl	4 oz	180	3	28	140	0	5.0	0.0	0	27%
CARAMEL *(Hershey's)* caramello	4 oz	180	3	28	170	0	6.0	0.0	0	30%
CAROB										
(Imagine Foods) nondairy, nonfat, 'Dream Pudding'	4 oz	130	1	31	30	0	0.0	0.0	0	0%
CHOCOLATE										
(Crowley)	4.5 oz	190	4	29	100	0	3.0		10	17%
(Del Monte)										
'Pudding Cup'	5 oz	190	4	31	280	0	6.0	0.0	0	28%
'Pudding Snack Light'	4.25 oz	100	2	19	85	0	1.0	0.0	0	10%
fudge, 'Pudding Cup'	5 oz	190	4	31	260	0	6.0	0.0	0	28%
(Estee)	1/2 cup	70	5	12	85	0	1.0	1.0	2	12%
(Featherweight)	1/2 cup	100	1	21	110	0	1.0	0.0	0	9%
(Hershey's)										
	4 oz	180	3	29	260	0	5.0	0.0	0	26%
fudge, 'Snack Pack'	4 oz	158	2	24	178	0	5.9	1.7	0	34%
'Hershey's Special Dark'	4 oz	180	4	30	135	0	5.0	0.0	0	25%
'Light' 'Snack Pack'	4 oz	100	3	20	120	0	2.0	0.0	0	16%
milk chocolate variety, 'Snack Pack'	4 oz	166	2	26	166	0	5.9	1.5	1	32%
nonfat, 'Snack Pack'	4 oz	96	2	21	212	0	0.4	0.0	0	4%
'Snack Pack'	4 oz	161	2	25	178	0	5.9	1.5	0	33%
(Imagine Foods) nondairy	1 cup	170	1	36	65	1	3.0	0.0	0	15%
(Jell-O)										
	4 oz	170	3	28	130	0	6.0	0.0	0	30%
fat free	1 serving	102	3	23	192	1	0.5	0.3	2	4%
fudge	4 oz	170	3	28	130	0	6.0	0.0	0	30%
fudge, 'Light Pudding Snacks'	4 oz	100	3	22	125	0	1.0	0.0	5	8%
fudge, 'Pudding Snacks'	4 oz	170	3	28	130	0	6.0	0.0	0	30%
fudge-milk chocolate swirl	4 oz	170	3	28	135	0	6.0	0.0	0	30%
'Light Pudding Snacks'	4 oz	100	3	21	125	0	2.0	0.0	5	16%
milk chocolate 'Pudding Snacks'	4 oz	170	4	29	135	0	6.0	0.0	0	29%
nonfat	1 serving	100	3	23	190	1	0.0	0.0	0	0%
nonfat, 'Free'	4 oz	100	3	24	200	0	0.0	0.0	0	0%
(Lucky Leaf)										
	4 oz	180	2	27	100	0	7.0	0.0	0	35%
fudge	4 oz	180	2	25	105	0	8.0	0.0	0	40%
(Musselman's)										
	4 oz	180	2	27	100	0	7.0	0.0	0	35%
fudge	4 oz	180	2	25	105	0	8.0	0.0	0	40%
(Pathmark) 'No Frills'	5 oz	200	2	30	140	0	8.0	0.0	0	36%
(Rich's) frozen	3 oz	140	2	18	135	0	7.0	0.0	0	44%
(Swiss Miss)										
fudge	4 oz	175	3	28	207	0	5.6	1.6	1	29%
fudge, 'Light'	4 oz	100	3	20	120	0	1.0	0.3	0	9%
fudge, nonfat	1/2 cup	103	2	23	151	0	0.3	0.0	1	3%
milk chocolate variety	4 oz	166	2	26	166	0	2.9	1.5	1	19%
nonfat	1/2 cup	100	2	22	154	0	0.4	0.0	1	3%
sundae	4 oz	220	2	36	140	0	7.0	1.7	5	29%
(Ultra Slim Fast) chocolate	4 oz	100	2	21	240	2	1.0	0.0	0	9%
(White House) chocolate	3.5 oz	120	2	22	130	0	4.0	0.0	0	27%
CHOCOLATE ALMOND *(Hershey's)*	4 oz	180	3	29	210	0	6.0	0.0	0	30%

Food Name	Serving Size	Calories	Prot. gms	Carbs gms	Sod. mgs	Fiber gms	Fat gms	Sat. Fat gms	Chol. mgs	% Fat Cal.
CHOCOLATE AND VANILLA										
(Hershey's)										
'Kisses'	4 oz	180	3	29	210	0	6.0	0.0	0	30%
'Kisses-Free'	4 oz	100	2	22	180	0	0.0	0.0	0	0%
(Jell-O)										
'Light Pudding Snacks'	4 oz	100	3	21	125	0	2.0	0.0	5	16%
nonfat	1 serving	100	3	23	210	1	0.0	0.0	0	0%
swirl	4 oz	170	3	28	135	0	6.0	0.0	0	30%
swirl, 'Free'	4 oz	100	3	24	220	0	0.0	0.0	0	0%
swirl, 'Pudding Snacks'	4 oz	180	3	28	140	0	6.0	0.0	0	30%
swirl, variety pack	1 snack	100	3	23	190	0	0.0	0.0	0	0%
(Swiss Miss)										
parfait, 'Light'	4 oz	100	2	20	110	0	1.0	0.3	0	9%
nonfat	1/2 cup	104	2	23	171	0	0.3	0.0	1	3%
chocolate-vanilla-chocolate swirl	4 oz	172	3	27	163	0	6.0	1.6	1	31%
variety	4 oz	171	2	27	162	0	6.0	1.5	1	32%
CHOCOLATE-CARAMEL										
(Hunt's) swirl, 'Snack Pack'	4 oz	165	3	25	178	0	5.9	1.5	1	32%
(Jell-O) swirl, 'Pudding Snacks'	4 oz	170	3	28	130	0	6.0	0.0	0	30%
CHOCOLATE MARSHMALLOW										
(Hunt's)										
'Snack Pack'	4 oz	155	2	23	124	0	5.9	1.9	0	34%
s'mores, 'Snack Pack'	4 oz	154	1	25	129	0	5.6	1.5	1	33%
CHOCOLATE MINT										
(Hershey's) 'York Peppermint Pattie'	4 oz	180	3	29	210	0	6.0	0.0	0	30%
(Jell-O) swirl, 'Free'	4 oz	100	3	24	220	0	0.0	0.0	0	0%
CHOCOLATE PEANUT BUTTER										
(Hunt's) chocolate peanut butter swirl, 'Snack Pack'	4 oz	169	2	26	173	0	6.3	1.6	1	34%
CHOCOLATE RASPBERRY *(Healthy Choice)*	1 cup	110	2	22	125	0	2.0	0.5	0	16%
COCONUT										
(Imagine Foods) nondairy, low-fat, 'Dream Pudding'	4 oz	150	1	32	10	0	2.0	0.0	0	12%
LEMON										
(Imagine Foods) nondairy	1 cup	150	1	33	50	1	3.0	0.0	0	17%
(Hunt's) 'Snack Pack'	4 oz	138	0	28	85	0	2.8	0.8	0	18%
(White House)	3.5 oz	152	0	37	65	0	1.0	0.0	0	6%
RICE										
(Crowley)	4.5 oz	125	4	22	80	0	2.0	0.0	10	15%
(Lucky Leaf)	4 oz	120	3	20	95	0	3.0	0.0	0	23%
(Musselman's)	4 oz	120	3	20	95	0	3.0	0.0	0	23%
(White House)	3.5 oz	111	1	20	135	0	3.0	0.0	0	24%
TAPIOCA										
(Crowley)	4.5 oz	135	4	27	70	0	1.0	0.0	5	7%
(Del Monte) 'Pudding Cup'	5 oz	180	3	30	250	0	4.0	0.0	0	21%
(Healthy Choice) French creme	1 cup	110	1	21	125	0	2.0	0.5	0	17%
(Hunt's)										
nonfat, 'Snack Pack'	1/2 cup	95	2	21	185	0	0.3	0.0	0	3%
'Snack Pack'	4 oz	151	2	23	134	0	5.7	1.1	1	34%
'Snack Pack Light'	4 oz	100	2	18	105	0	2.0	0.0	0	18%
(Jell-O)	4 oz	170	3	27	140	0	4.0	0.0	0	23%
(Lucky Leaf)	4 oz	140	1	20	95	0	6.0	0.0	0	39%
(Musselman's)	4 oz	140	1	20	95	0	6.0	0.0	0	39%
(Swiss Miss)										
'Light'	4 oz	100	2	18	105	0	2.0	0.0	0	18%
nonfat	1/2 cup	99	2	22	151	0	0.3	0.0	1	3%

Food Name	Serving Size	Calories	Prot. gms	Carbs gms	Sod. mgs	Fiber gms	Fat gms	Sat. Fat gms	Chol. mgs	% Fat Cal.
(White House)	3.5 oz	131	1	19	105	0	6.0	0.0	0	40%
VANILLA										
(Crowley)	4.5 oz	140	3	26	130	0	3.0	0.0	10	19%
(Del Monte)										
'Pudding Cup'	5 oz	180	3	32	285	0	5.0	0.0	0	24%
'Pudding Snack Light'	4.25 oz	100	1	19	200	0	1.0	0.0	0	10%
(Estee)	1/2 cup	70	4	12	65	0	1.0	1.0	2	12%
(Featherweight)	1/2 cup	100	0	20	150	0	2.0	0.0	0	18%
(Healthy Choice) French	1 cup	110	2	20	125	0	2.0	0.5	0	17%
(Hunt's)										
'Snack Pack'	4 oz	158	2	25	141	0	5.7	1.5	0	33%
'Snack Pack Light'	4 oz	93	2	21	167	0	0.4	0.0	1	4%
(Jell-O)										
	4 oz	180	3	28	140	0	7.0	0.0	0	34%
fat free	1 serving	104	2	23	241	0	0.2	0.2	2	2%
'Free'	4 oz	100	3	23	250	0	0.0	0.0	0	0%
'Light Pudding Snacks'	4 oz	100	3	20	130	0	2.0	0.0	5	16%
pudding snack	1 serving	100	2	23	240	0	0.0	0.0	0	0%
(Lucky Leaf)	4 oz	170	2	25	135	0	7.0	0.0	0	37%
(Musselman's)	4 oz	170	2	25	135	0	7.0	0.0	0	37%
(Pathmark) 'No Frills'	5 oz	200	2	28	150	0	8.0	0.0	0	38%
(Rich's) frozen	3 oz	130	2	18	160	0	6.0	0.0	0	40%
(Swiss Miss)										
'Light'	4 oz	100	2	18	110	0	2.0	0.0	0	18%
nonfat	1/2 cup	99	2	22	162	0	0.4	0.0	1	4%
sundae	4 oz	175	2	27	174	0	6.8	1.7	1	35%
(Ultra Slim Fast) 'Lite 'N Tasty'	4 oz	100	2	21	230	2	1.0	0.0	0	9%
(White House)	3.5 oz	111	1	20	135	0	3.0	0.0	0	24%
PUDDING BAR, FROZEN										
(Jell-O)										
chocolate fudge, 'Pudding Pops'	1 bar	80	2	13	90	0	2.0	0.0	0	23%
chocolate-peanut butter swirl 'Pudding Pops'	1 bar	80	2	12	75	0	3.0	0.0	0	33%
chocolate-vanilla swirl, 'Pudding Pops'	1 bar	80	2	13	70	0	2.0	0.0	0	23%
double chocolate swirl, 'Pudding Pops'	1 bar	80	2	13	90	0	2.0	0.0	0	23%
milk chocolate, 'Pudding Pops'	1 bar	80	2	13	90	0	2.0	0.0	0	23%
PUDDING MIX. See also PUDDING/PIE FILLING MIX.										
BANANA										
(Jell-O)										
cream, instant, prepared w/whole milk	1/2 cup	160	4	28	410	0	4.0	0.0	15	22%
cream, microwave, prepared w/whole milk	1/2 cup	150	4	25	220	0	4.0	0.0	15	24%
instant, sugar-free, prepared w/2% milk	1/2 cup	80	4	11	390	0	2.0	0.0	10	23%
(Royal)										
cream, instant, prepared w/whole milk	1/2 cup	180	4	29	390	0	5.0	0.0	0	25%
cream, prepared w/whole milk	1/2 cup	160	4	27	210	0	4.0	0.0	0	23%
BUTTER ALMOND										
(Royal) toasted, instant, prepared w/whole milk	1/2 cup	170	4	30	350	0	4.0	0.0	0	21%
BUTTER PECAN (Jell-O) instant, prepared w/whole milk	1/2 cup	170	4	28	410	0	5.0	0.0	15	26%
BUTTERSCOTCH										
(D-Zerta) low-calorie, prepared w/nonfat milk	1/2 cup	70	4	12	65	0	0.0	0.0	0	0%
(Featherweight)										
instant, prepared w/whole milk	1/2 cup	100	4	19	190	0	0.0	0.0	5	0%
prepared as directed	1/2 cup	12	0	3	6	0	0.0	0.0	0	0%
(Jell-O)										
cook and serve	1 serving	80	0	20	5	0	0.0	0.0	0	0%

Food Name	Serving Size	Calories	Prot. gms	Carbs gms	Sod. mgs	Fiber gms	Fat gms	Sat. Fat gms	Chol. mgs	% Fat Cal.
instant, prepared w/whole milk	1/2 cup	160	4	28	450	0	4.0	0.0	15	22%
instant, sugar-free, prepared w/2% milk	1/2 cup	90	4	12	390	0	2.0	0.0	10	22%
microwave, prepared w/whole milk	1/2 cup	170	4	28	180	0	4.0	0.0	15	22%
prepared, w/whole milk	1/2 cup	170	4	30	190	0	4.0	0.0	15	21%
(Royal)										
instant, prepared w/whole milk	1/2 cup	180	4	29	390	0	5.0	0.0	0	25%
instant, sugar-free, prepared w/2% milk	1/2 cup	100	4	16	470	0	2.0	0.0	0	18%
prepared, w/whole milk	1/2 cup	160	4	27	210	0	4.0	0.0	0	23%
CHOCOLATE										
(D-Zerta) lower calorie	1 serving	20	0	5	0	1	0.0	0.0	0	0%
(Featherweight)										
instant, prepared	1/2 cup	110	5	22	190	0	0.0	0.0	5	0%
prepared	1/2 cup	12	0	3	0	0	0.0	0.0	15	0%
(Jell-O)										
cook and serve, sugar-free, mix only	1/2 cup	30	1	7	100	0	0.0	0.0	0	0%
cook and serve, sugar-free, prepared w/nonfat milk	1/2 cup	70	5	13	160	0	3.0	0.0	0	27%
cook and serve, sugar-free, prepared w/2% milk	1/2 cup	90	5	13	160	0	3.0	0.0	10	27%
fudge, instant, sugar-free, prepared w/2% milk	1/2 cup	100	5	14	330	0	3.0	0.0	10	26%
fudge, instant, sugar-free, prepared w/whole milk	1/2 cup	180	5	31	440	0	5.0	0.0	15	24%
fudge, prepared w/whole milk	1/2 cup	160	5	28	170	0	4.0	0.0	15	21%
instant, prepared w/whole milk	1/2 cup	180	4	31	480	0	4.0	0.0	15	20%
instant, sugar-free, prepared w/2% milk	1/2 cup	90	4	13	380	0	3.0	0.0	10	28%
microwave, prepared w/whole milk	1/2 cup	170	5	28	190	0	5.0	0.0	15	25%
milk chocolate, instant, prepared w/whole milk	1/2 cup	180	5	31	470	0	5.0	0.0	15	24%
milk chocolate, microwave, prepared w/whole milk	1/2 cup	160	4	27	190	0	5.0	0.0	15	27%
milk chocolate, prepared w/whole milk	1/2 cup	160	4	28	170	0	4.0	0.0	15	22%
prepared w/whole milk	1/2 cup	160	5	28	170	0	4.0	0.0	15	21%
(Royal)										
chocolate chip, prepared w/whole milk	1/2 cup	190	4	35	390	0	4.0	0.0	0	19%
dark and sweet, prepared w/whole milk	1/2 cup	190	4	35	390	0	4.0	0.0	0	19%
instant, prepared w/whole milk	1/2 cup	190	4	35	390	0	4.0	0.0	0	19%
instant, sugar-free, prepared w/2% milk	1/2 cup	110	5	17	480	0	3.0	0.0	0	23%
prepared w/whole milk	1/2 cup	180	5	33	150	0	4.0	0.0	0	19%
(Weight Watchers) instant, prepared w/nonfat milk	1/2 cup	90	6	18	420	0	1.0	0.0	0	9%
CHOCOLATE MINT										
(Royal) instant, prepared w/whole milk	1/2 cup	190	4	35	390	0	4.0	0.0	0	19%
COCONUT										
(Jell-O) cream, instant, prepared w/whole milk	1/2 cup	180	4	27	320	0	6.0	0.0	15	30%
(Royal) toasted, instant, prepared w/whole milk	1/2 cup	170	4	30	350	0	4.0	0.0	0	21%
CUSTARD										
(Jell-O)										
egg, golden, 'Americana' prepared w/whole milk	1/2 cup	160	5	23	200	0	5.0	0.0	80	29%
(Royal) prepared w/whole milk	1/2 cup	150	4	22	115	0	5.0	0.0	0	30%
FLAN										
(Jell-O) prepared w/whole milk	1/2 cup	150	4	26	65	0	4.0	0.0	15	23%
(Royal) w/caramel sauce, prepared w/whole milk	1/2 cup	150	4	22	115	0	5.0	0.0	0	30%
KEY LIME *(Royal)* prepared w/whole milk	1/2 cup	160	1	30	120	0	3.0	0.0	0	18%
LEMON										
(Featherweight) custard, prepared w/whole milk	1/2 cup	40	1	8	40	0	0.0	0.0	0	0%
(French's) prepared	1/2 cup	110	1	22	110	0	1.0	0.0	0	9%
(Jell-O) instant, prepared w/whole milk	1/2 cup	170	4	29	360	0	4.0	0.0	15	21%
(Royal)										
instant, prepared w/whole milk	1/2 cup	180	1	29	350	0	5.0	0.0	0	27%
lemon, prepared w/whole milk	1/2 cup	160	1	30	120	0	3.0	0.0	0	18%

Food Name	Serving Size	Calories	Prot. gms	Carbs gms	Sod. mgs	Fiber gms	Fat gms	Sat. Fat gms	Chol. mgs	% Fat Cal.
PISTACHIO										
(Jell-O)										
instant, prepared w/whole milk	1/2 cup	170	4	28	410	0	5.0	0.0	15	26%
instant, sugar-free, prepared w/2% milk	1/2 cup	90	4	12	390	0	3.0	0.0	10	30%
(Royal) instant, prepared w/whole milk	1/2 cup	170	4	30	350	0	4.0	0.0	0	21%
RASPBERRY										
(Salada) and pie glaze, prepared w/whole milk	1/2 cup	130	0	32	5	0	0.0	0.0	0	0%
RICE *(Jell-O)* rice 'Americana' prepared w/whole milk	1/2 cup	170	5	30	160	0	4.0	0.0	15	20%
STRAWBERRY										
(Salada) and pie glaze, prepared w/whole milk	1/2 cup	130	0	32	5	0	0.0	0.0	0	0%
TAPIOCA										
(Jell-O) vanilla, 'Americana' prepared w/whole milk	1/2 cup	160	4	27	170	0	4.0	0.0	15	23%
(Minute) mix only	1 1/2 tsp	20	0	5	0	0	0.0	0.0	0	0%
(Royal) vanilla, prepared w/whole milk	1/2 cup	160	4	27	150	0	4.0	0.0	0	23%
VANILLA										
(D-Zerta) low-calorie, prepared w/nonfat milk	1/2 cup	70	4	12	65	0	0.0	0.0	0	0%
(Featherweight)										
instant, prepared	1/2 cup	100	4	19	190	0	0.0	0.0	5	0%
custard, prepared w/whole milk	1/2 cup	40	1	8	40	0	0.0	0.0	0	0%
(Jell-O)										
cook and serve, sugar-free, prepared w/skim milk	1/2 cup	60	4	11	200	0	2.0	0.0	0	23%
cook and serve, sugar-free, prepared w/2% milk	1/2 cup	80	4	11	200	0	2.0	0.0	10	23%
cook and serve, sugar-free, mix only	1/2 cup	20	0	5	140	0	0.0	0.0	0	0%
French, instant, prepared w/whole milk	1/2 cup	160	4	28	400	0	4.0	0.0	15	22%
instant, prepared w/whole milk	1/2 cup	170	4	29	410	0	4.0	0.0	15	21%
instant, sugar-free, prepared w/2% milk	1/2 cup	90	4	12	390	0	2.0	0.0	10	22%
microwave, prepared w/whole milk	1/2 cup	160	4	26	180	0	4.0	0.0	15	23%
prepared w/whole milk	1/2 cup	160	4	26	200	0	4.0	0.0	15	23%
(Royal)										
instant, prepared w/whole milk	1/2 cup	180	4	29	390	0	5.0	0.0	0	25%
instant, sugar-free, prepared w/2% milk	1/2 cup	100	4	16	470	0	2.0	0.0	0	18%
prepared w/whole milk	1/2 cup	160	4	27	210	0	4.0	0.0	0	23%
PUDDING/PIE FILLING MIX. See also PUDDING MIX.										
BANANA										
(Jell-O)										
cream, instant, prepared w/whole milk	1/2 cup	160	4	28	410	0	4.0	0.0	15	22%
cream, mix only	1 pkg	50	0	14	120	0	0.0	0.0	0	0%
cream, prepared w/whole milk	1/6 pkg	100	3	17	160	0	3.0	0.0	10	25%
instant, sugar-free, mix only	1 pkg	25	0	6	330	0	0.0	0.0	0	0%
instant, sugar-free, prepared w/2% milk	1/2 cup	80	4	11	390	0	2.0	0.0	10	23%
microwave, cream, mix only	1 pkg	80	0	19	160	0	0.0	0.0	0	0%
microwave, cream, prepared w/whole milk	1/2 cup	150	4	25	220	0	4.0	0.0	15	24%
(Royal)										
cream, instant, mix only	1 serving	90	0	22	390	0	0.0	0.0	0	0%
cream, mix only	1 serving	80	0	20	110	0	0.0	0.0	0	0%
BUTTER PECAN *(Jell-O)* instant, prepared w/whole milk	1/2 cup	170	4	28	410	0	5.0	0.0	15	26%
BUTTERSCOTCH										
(D-Zerta)										
lower calorie, mix only	1 pkg	25	0	6	0	0	0.0	0.0	0	0%
lower calorie, prepared	1/2 cup	70	4	12	65	0	0.0	0.0	0	0%
(Jell-O)										
instant, sugar-free, mix only	1 pkg	25	0	6	330	0	0.0	0.0	0	0%
instant, sugar-free, prepared w/2% milk	1/2 cup	90	4	12	390	0	2.0	0.0	10	22%

Food Name	Serving Size	Calories	Prot. gms	Carbs gms	Sod. mgs	Fiber gms	Fat gms	Sat. Fat gms	Chol. mgs	% Fat Cal.
instant, prepared w/whole milk	1/2 cup	160	4	28	450	0	4.0	0.0	15	22%
microwave, mix only	1 pkg	90	0	23	120	0	0.0	0.0	0	0%
microwave, prepared w/whole milk	1/2 cup	170	4	28	180	0	4.0	0.0	15	22%
regular, mix only	1 pkg	90	0	24	130	0	0.0	0.0	0	0%
regular, prepared w/whole milk	1/2 cup	170	4	30	190	0	4.0	0.0	15	21%
(My-T-Fine) prepared	1/2 cup	90	0	22	190	0	0.0	0.0	0	0%
(Royal)										
instant, mix only	1 serving	90	0	22	400	0	0.0	0.0	0	0%
prepared	1/2 cup	90	0	23	180	0	0.0	0.0	0	0%
CHERRY VANILLA (Royal) instant, mix only	1 serving	90	0	23	300	0	0.0	0.0	0	0%
CHOCOLATE										
(D-Zerta)										
lower calorie, mix only	1 pkg	20	0	5	0	0	0.0	0.0	0	0%
lower calorie, prepared	1/2 cup	60	5	11	70	0	0.0	0.0	0	0%
(Jell-O)										
cook and serve, nonfat, lower calorie	1 serving	90	0	23	107	0	0.3	0.1	0	3%
cook and serve, sugar-free, prepared	1 serving	31	1	7	109	1	0.3	0.2	0	9%
fat-free, sugar-free, prepared	1 serving	34	1	8	318	1	0.3	0.1	0	7%
fudge, instant, mix only	1 pkg	100	1	25	380	0	1.0	0.0	0	8%
fudge, instant, prepared w/whole milk	1/2 cup	180	5	31	440	0	5.0	0.0	15	24%
fudge, instant, sugar-free, mix only	1 pkg	35	1	8	270	0	1.0	0.0	0	20%
fudge, mix only	1 pkg	90	1	22	110	0	0.0	0.0	0	0%
instant, mix only	1 pkg	100	0	25	420	0	0.0	0.0	0	0%
instant, mix only	1 serving	99	0	25	414	1	0.3	0.1	0	3%
instant, prepared w/whole milk	1/2 cup	180	4	31	480	0	4.0	0.0	15	20%
instant, sugar-free, mix only	1 pkg	30	0	7	320	0	0.0	0.0	0	0%
instant, sugar-free, prepared w/2% milk	1/2 cup	100	5	14	330	0	3.0	0.0	10	26%
instant, sugar-free, prepared w/2% milk	1/2 cup	90	4	13	380	0	3.0	0.0	10	28%
microwave, mix only	1 pkg	90	1	22	130	0	1.0	0.0	0	9%
microwave, prepared w/whole milk	1/2 cup	170	5	28	190	0	5.0	0.0	15	25%
milk chocolate, instant, mix only	1 pkg	100	1	25	410	0	1.0	0.0	0	8%
milk chocolate, instant, prepared w/whole milk	1/2 cup	180	5	31	470	0	5.0	0.0	15	24%
milk chocolate, microwave, mix only	1 pkg	90	0	21	130	0	1.0	0.0	0	10%
milk chocolate, microwave, prepared w/whole milk	1/2 cup	160	4	27	190	0	5.0	0.0	15	27%
milk chocolate, mix only	1 pkg	90	0	22	110	0	0.0	0.0	0	0%
milk chocolate, prepared w/whole milk	1/2 cup	160	4	28	170	0	4.0	0.0	15	22%
sugar-free, mix only,	1 pkg	30	1	7	100	0	0.0	0.0	0	0%
prepared w/whole milk	1/2 cup	160	5	28	170	0	4.0	0.0	15	21%
sugar-free, prepared w/2% milk	1/2 cup	90	5	13	160	0	3.0	0.0	10	27%
(My-T-Fine)										
fudge, prepared	1/2 cup	100	1	24	140	1	0.0	0.0	0	0%
prepared	1/2 cup	100	1	23	135	0	0.0	0.0	0	0%
(Royal)										
chocolate chip, instant, mix only	1 serving	110	1	26	390	0	1.0	0.0	0	8%
dark and sweet, prepared	1/2 cup	90	1	22	95	1	0.0	0.0	0	0%
instant, mix only	1 serving	110	1	27	450	0	0.0	0.0	0	0%
instant, sugar-free, prepared	1/2 cup	50	0	11	420	0	0.0	0.0	0	0%
prepared	1/2 cup	90	1	22	90	0	0.0	0.0	0	0%
CHOCOLATE ALMOND										
(My-T-Fine) prepared	1/2 cup	100	1	23	135	0	1.0	0.0	0	9%
(Royal) instant, prepared	1/2 cup	120	0	26	440	0	1.0	0.0	0	8%
CHOCOLATE PEANUT BUTTER CHIP										
(Royal) instant, mix only	1 serving	110	1	26	480	0	1.0	0.0	0	8%

Food Name	Serving Size	Calories	Prot. gms	Carbs gms	Sod. mgs	Fiber gms	Fat gms	Sat. Fat gms	Chol. mgs	% Fat Cal.
COCONUT										
(Jell-O)										
cream, mix only	1 pkg	60	0	12	100	0	2.0	0.0	0	27%
cream, prepared w/whole milk	1/6 pkg	110	3	16	140	0	4.0	0.0	10	32%
cream, instant, prepared w/whole milk	1/2 cup	180	4	27	320	0	6.0	0.0	15	30%
(Royal) toasted, instant	1/2 cup	100	0	20	450	0	2.0	0.0	0	18%
CUSTARD *(Royal)*	1/2 cup	60	0	16	75	0	0.0	0.0	0	0%
FLAN										
(Jell-O)										
flan, mix only	1 pkg	80	0	20	5	0	0.0	0.0	0	0%
flan, prepared w/whole milk	1/2 cup	150	4	26	65	0	4.0	0.0	15	23%
(Royal) caramel, prepared	1/2 cup	60	0	15	55	0	0.0	0.0	0	0%
KEY LIME *(Royal)* mix only	1 serving	50	0	13	120	0	0.0	0.0	0	0%
LEMON										
(Jell-O)										
instant, mix only	1 pkg	90	0	23	300	0	0.0	0.0	0	0%
instant, prepared w/whole milk	1/2 cup	170	4	29	360	0	4.0	0.0	15	21%
mix only	1 pkg	50	0	13	70	0	0.0	0.0	0	0%
prepared	1/6 pkg	170	2	38	95	0	2.0	0.0	90	10%
(My-T-Fine) mix only	1 serving	90	0	22	170	0	0.0	0.0	0	0%
(Royal)										
instant, mix only	1 serving	90	0	23	320	0	0.0	0.0	0	0%
meringue, 'No-Bake'	1/8 pie	210	3	38	170	0	5.0	0.0	0	22%
mix only	1 serving	50	0	13	120	0	0.0	0.0	0	0%
PISTACHIO										
(Jell-O)										
instant, mix only	1 pkg	100	0	22	350	0	1.0	0.0	0	9%
instant, prepared w/whole milk	1/2 cup	170	4	28	410	0	5.0	0.0	15	26%
instant, sugar-free, mix only	1 pkg	30	0	6	330	0	1.0	0.0	0	27%
instant, sugar-free, prepared w/2% milk	1/2 cup	90	4	12	390	0	3.0	0.0	10	30%
(Royal) instant, mix only	1 serving	90	0	22	360	0	1.0	0.0	0	9%
STRAWBERRY *(Royal)* instant, mix only	1 serving	100	0	24	330	0	0.0	0.0	0	0%
TAPIOCA *(My-T-Fine)* mix only	1 serving	80	0	19	160	0	0.0	0.0	0	0%
VANILLA										
(D-Zerta)										
lower calorie, mix only	1 pkg	25	0	6	0	0	0.0	0.0	0	0%
lower calorie, prepared	1/2 cup	70	4	12	65	0	0.0	0.0	0	0%
(Jell-O)										
cook and serve, nonfat, lower calorie	1 serving	86	0	22	138	0	0.0	0.0	0	0%
cook and serve, sugar-free, prepared	1 serving	21	0	5	113	0	0.0	0.0	0	1%
fat-free, sugar-free, prepared	1 serving	26	0	6	332	0	0.1	0.0	0	2%
French, instant, mix only	1 pkg	90	0	23	350	0	0.0	0.0	0	0%
French, instant, prepared w/whole milk	1/2 cup	160	4	28	400	0	4.0	0.0	15	22%
French, mix only	1 pkg	90	0	24	125	0	0.0	0.0	0	0%
French, prepared w/whole milk	1/2 cup	170	4	30	190	0	4.0	0.0	15	21%
instant, mix only	1 pkg	94	0	23	353	0	0.2	0.1	0	2%
instant, prepared w/whole milk	1/2 cup	170	4	29	410	0	4.0	0.0	15	21%
instant, sugar-free, mix only	1 pkg	25	0	6	330	0	0.0	0.0	0	0%
instant, sugar-free, prepared w/2% milk	1/2 cup	90	4	12	390	0	2.0	0.0	10	22%
microwave, mix only	1 pkg	80	0	21	120	0	0.0	0.0	0	0%
microwave, prepared w/whole milk	1/2 cup	160	4	26	180	0	4.0	0.0	15	23%
mix only	1 pkg	80	0	21	140	0	0.0	0.0	0	0%
prepared w/whole milk	1/2 cup	160	4	26	200	0	4.0	0.0	15	23%

Food Name	Serving Size	Calories	Prot. gms	Carbs gms	Sod. mgs	Fiber gms	Fat gms	Sat. Fat gms	Chol. mgs	% Fat Cal.
sugar-free, mix only	1 pkg	20	0	5	140	0	0.0	0.0	0	0%
sugar-free, prepared w/2% milk	1/2 cup	80	4	11	200	0	2.0	0.0	10	23%
(My-T-Fine)										
mix only	1 serving	80	0	20	160	0	0.0	0.0	0	0%
prepared	1/2 cup	90	0	22	120	0	0.0	0.0	0	0%
(Nutra/Balance) low-lactose	1 serving	242	8	36	94	0	7.5	0.7	3	27%
(Royal)										
chocolate chip, instant, mix only	1 serving	90	0	22	350	0	1.0	0.0	0	9%
(Royal) instant, mix only	1 serving	90	0	23	325	0	0.0	0.0	0	0%
PUERTO RICAN CHERRY. See ACEROLA.										
PUFF PASTRY										
ready-to-bake, frozen, baked	1 oz	158	2	13	72	0	10.9	1.6	0	62%
ready-to-bake, frozen, unprepared	1 oz	156	2	13	71	0	10.8	2.7	0	62%
(Pepperidge Farm)										
sheet, frozen	1/4 sheet	260	4	22	290	0	17.0	0.0	0	60%
shell, mini, frozen	1 shell	50	1	4	40	0	4.0	0.0	0	64%
shell, patty, frozen	1 shell	210	3	16	180	0	15.0	0.0	0	64%
PUMMELO, RAW. See POMELO.										
PUMPKIN										
Fresh										
boiled, drained, mashed	1 cup	49	2	12	2	3	0.2	0.1	0	3%
raw, cubed, 1-inch cubes	1 cup	30	1	8	1	1	0.1	0.1	0	3%
Canned										
	1 cup	83	3	20	590	7	0.7	0.4	0	7%
(Del Monte)	1/2 cup	35	1	9	10	0	0.0	0.0	0	0%
solid pack (Libby's)	1/2 cup	40	2	9	5	5	0.5	0.0	0	9%
(Stokely)	1/2 cup	40	2	10	15	0	0.0	0.0	0	0%
PUMPKIN FLOWER										
boiled, drained	1 cup	20	1	4	8	1	0.1	0.1	0	4%
raw	1 cup	5	0	1	2	na	0.0	0.0	0	4%
raw, whole	1 medium	<1	0	0	0	na	0.0	0.0	0	3%
PUMPKIN LEAF										
boiled, drained	1 cup	15	2	2	6	2	0.2	0.1	0	9%
raw	1 cup	7	1	1	4	na	0.2	0.1	0	18%
PUMPKIN PIE SPICE. See under SEASONING MIX.										
PUMPKIN SEED										
dried, kernels	1 cup	747	34	25	25	5	63.3	12.0	0	71%
dried, kernels, hulled, approx 142 seeds	1 oz	153	7	5	5	1	13.0	2.5	0	71%
dry roasted, w/tamari, garlic, and cayenne										
(Eden Foods)	1 oz	170	11	5	80	3	11.0	2.5	0	61%
roasted, kernels	1 cup	1185	75	30	41	9	95.6	18.1	0	68%
roasted, kernels	1 oz	148	9	4	5	1	11.9	2.3	0	68%
roasted, salted (David's)	1 pkg	320	15	6	17	2	25.0	5.0	0	73%
roasted, whole	1 cup	285	12	34	12	na	12.4	2.3	0	36%
roasted, whole, approx 85 seeds	1 oz	126	5	15	5	na	5.5	1.0	0	36%
PUMPKINFISH. See SUNFISH.										
PUNCH. See under FRUIT DRINK; FRUIT DRINK MIX; FRUIT JUICE DRINK.										
PURPLE HULLED PEAS. See PEAS, PURPLE HULLED.										
PURSLANE / pussley										
boiled, drained	1 cup	21	2	4	51	na	0.2	na	0	9%
boiled, drained	1/2 cup	10	0.9	2.1	26	>.5 c	0.1	na	0	7%
raw	1 cup	7	0.6	1.5	19	>.3 c	0.0	na	0	0%
raw	1/2 cup	4	0.3	0.7	10	>.2 c	<.1	(tr)	0	<18%
PUSSLEY. See PURSLANE.										

Q

Food Name	Serving Size	Calories	Prot. gms	Carbs gms	Sod. mgs	Fiber gms	Fat gms	Sat. Fat gms	Chol. mgs	% Fat Cal.
QUAIL. / bobwhite										
breast, meat only, raw	1 oz	35	6.4	0.0	16	0	0.8	0.2	(mq)	22%
giblets, raw	3.5 oz	176	21.8	6.7	70	0	6.2	2.0	350	33%
meat and skin, raw	1 oz	54	5.6	0.0	15	0	3.4	1.0	(mq)	58%
meat only, raw	1 oz	34	6.0	0.0	29	0	0.9	0.1	24	25%
QUEEN CRAB. See under CRAB.										
QUICHE										
(Nancy's)										
broccoli-cheddar, frozen, microwave, 'French Baked'	1 quiche	490	17	33	750	2	33.0	16.0	165	60%
Monterey Jack, w/Swiss and bacon, 'Classic French'	1 quiche	520	21	30	670	1	37.0	18.0	210	62%
(Stilwell)										
bacon and onion	1/6 carton	210	12	4	480	1	16.0	12.0	185	69%
broccoli and cheese	1/6 carton	180	10	4	270	1	14.0	8.0	180	69%
ham	1/6 carton	190	12	4	330	0	15.0	11.0	200	68%
spinach and onion	1/6 carton	190	10	7	280	1	13.0	10.0	200	63%
three cheese	1/6 carton	200	13	4	310	1	16.0	12.0	190	68%
QUINCE										
raw, trimmed	1 medium	52	0.4	14.1	4	1.8	0.1	0.0	0	2%
raw, trimmed	1 oz	16	0.1	4.3	1	>.5 c	<.1	tr	0	<5%
raw, untrimmed	1 lb	158	1.1	42.3	11	>4.7 c	0.3	<.1	0	2%
QUINOA										
flakes, steam-rolled, uncooked *(Ancient Harvest)*	1/3 cup	105	3	23	5	3	1.0	0.0	0	8%
flakes, steam-rolled, uncooked *(Quinoa)*	1/3 cup	105	3	23	5	3	1.0	0.0	0	8%
organic, uncooked *(Arrowhead Mills)*	1/4 cup	140	5	25	0	4	2.0	0.0	0	13%
uncooked *(Eden Foods)*	2 oz	200	8	38	30	4	4.0	0.0	0	16%
uncooked	1 cup	636	22	117	36	10	9.9	1.0	0	13%
whole grain, uncooked *(Ancient Harvest)*	1/4 cup	159	5	28	8	6	2.0	0.0	0	12%
whole grain, uncooked *(Quinoa)*	1/4 cup	159	5	28	8	6	2.0	0.0	0	12%
QUINOA FLOUR. See under FLOUR.										
QUINOA SEED										
(Arrowhead Mills)	2 oz	200	9	35	3	5	3.0	0.0	0	13%
wild, uncooked *(Eden Foods)*	1/4 cup	170	7	31	0	3	2.5	0.0	0	13%

R

Food Name	Serving Size	Calories	Prot. gms	Carbs gms	Sod. mgs	Fiber gms	Fat gms	Sat. Fat gms	Chol. mgs	% Fat Cal.
RABBIT										
domesticated, composite cuts, raw	1 oz	39	6	0	12	0	1.6	0.5	16	37%
domesticated, composite cuts, roasted	3 oz	167	25	0	40	0	6.8	2.0	70	37%
domesticated, composite cuts, stewed	3 oz	175	26	0	31	0	7.1	2.1	73	37%
wild, raw	1 oz	32	6	0	14	0	0.7	0.2	23	18%
wild, stewed	3 oz	147	28	0	38	0	3.0	0.9	105	18%
RACCOON, roasted	3 oz	217	25	0	67	0	12.3	3.5	82	51%
RADICCHIO										
fresh, raw, leaf	1 med leaf	2	0	0	2	0	0.0	0.0	0	9%
fresh, raw, shredded	1 cup	9	1	2	9	0	0.1	0.0	0	9%
RADISH										
fresh, raw, sliced	1 cup	23	1	4	28	2	0.6	0.0	0	23%

Food Name	Serving Size	Calories	Prot. gms	Carbs gms	Sod. mgs	Fiber gms	Fat gms	Sat. Fat gms	Chol. mgs	% Fat Cal.
fresh, raw, sliced	1/2 cup	12	0	2	14	1	0.3	0.0	0	23%
fresh, raw, whole *(Dole)*	7 med radishes	20	0	3	35	0	0.0	0.0	0	0%
fresh, raw, whole, large, 1–1.25-inch diam	1 radish	2	0	0	2	0	0.0	0.0	0	23%
fresh, raw, whole, medium, 3/4–1-inch diam	1 radish	1	0	0	1	0	0.0	0.0	0	22%
fresh, raw, whole, small, under 3/4-inch diam	1 radish	<1	0	0	0	0	0.0	0.0	0	23%
BLACK / winter radish										
raw, trimmed	1 lb	77	4.5	16.3	82	(mq)	0.5	(mq)	0	5%
raw, trimmed	1 oz	5	0.3	1.0	5	(mq)	<.1	tr	0	<15%
ORIENTAL. See DAIKON.										
RED										
fresh, raw, sliced	1 cup	23	1	4	28	2	0.6	0.0	0	23%
fresh, raw, sliced	1/2 cup	12	0	2	14	1	0.3	0.0	0	23%
fresh, raw, whole *(Dole)*	7 med radishes	20	0	3	35	0	0.0	0.0	0	0%
fresh, raw, whole, large, 1–1.25-inch diam	1 radish	2	0	0	2	0	0.0	0.0	0	23%
fresh, raw, whole, medium, 3/4–1-inch diam	1 radish	1	0	0	1	0	0.0	0.0	0	22%
fresh, raw, whole, small, under 3/4-inch diam	1 radish	<1	0	0	0	0	0.0	0.0	0	23%
WHITE ICICLE										
raw, sliced	1/2 cup	7	0.6	1.3	8	>.4 c	0.1	0.0	0	11%
raw, trimmed	1 oz	4	0.3	0.7	5	>.2 c	<.1	tr	0	<18%
raw, untrimmed	1 lb	41	3.2	7.7	47	>2.1 c	0.3	0.1	0	6%
raw, whole, approx 7-inch long	1 medium	2	0.2	0.5	3	>.1 c	0.0	0.0	0	0%
RADISH JUICE, bottled *(Biotta)*	6 fl oz	39	2	8	101	0	0.1	0.0	0	2%
RADISH LEAVES, trimmed	1 oz	15	0.8	2.8	(mq)	>.4 c	0.1	tr	0	6%
RADISH SEED										
sprouted	1 lb	186	17.3	13.9	28	(mq)	11.5	3.5	0	45%
sprouted	1 oz	12	1.1	0.9	2	(mq)	0.7	0.2	0	44%
sprouted, raw	1 cup	16	1	1	2	na	1.0	0.3	0	49%
sprouted, raw	1/2 cup	8	0.7	0.7	1	>.4 c	0.5	0.2	0	45%
RAG GOURD. See GOURD, DISHCLOTH.										
RAINBOW SMELT. See SMELT, RAINBOW.										
RAISIN										
Golden										
seedless	1 cup packed	498	6	131	20	7	0.8	0.2	0	1%
seedless	1 cup	438	5	115	17	6	0.7	0.2*	0	1%
seedless *(S&W)*	1/4 cup	130	1	31	10	2	0.0	0.0	0	0%
seedless *(Sun-Maid)*	1/4 cup	130	1	31	10	3	0.0	0.0	0	0%
Dark										
seeded	1 cup packed	488	4	129	46	11	0.9	0.3	0	2%
seeded	1 cup	429	4	114	41	10	0.8	0.3	0	2%
seedless	1 cup packed	495	5	131	20	7	0.8	0.2	0	1%
seedless	1 cup	435	5	115	17	6	0.7	0.2	0	1%
seedless	50 medium	78	1	21	3	1	0.1	0.0	0	1%
seedless *(S&W)*	1/4 cup	130	1	31	10	2	0.0	0.0	0	0%
seedless, for baking *(Sun-Maid)*	1/4 cup	124	1	30	7	2	0.0	na	0	0%
seedless, mini-box	0.5 oz	42	0	11	2	1	0.1	0.0	0	1%
seedless, natural *(Sun-Maid)*	1/4 cup	130	1	31	10	3	0.0	0.0	0	0%
RAMBUTAN										
canned, in syrup	1 cup	175	1	45	24	2	0.4	na	0	2%
canned, in syrup	1 medium	7	0	2	1	0	0.0	na	0	2%
canned, in syrup, drained	1 cup	123	1	31	17	1	0.3	na	0	2%
RASPBERRY / bramble										
Canned, in heavy syrup, w/liquid	1 cup	233	2	60	8	8	0.3	0.0	0	1%
Fresh										
raw	1 pint	153	3	36	0	21	1.7	0.1	0	9%

Food Name	Serving Size	Calories	Prot. gms	Carbs gms	Sod. mgs	Fiber gms	Fat gms	Sat. Fat gms	Chol. mgs	% Fat Cal.
raw	1 cup	60	1	14	0	8	0.7	0.0	0	9%
raw	10 medium	9	0	2	0	1	0.1	0.0	0	9%
Frozen										
(Flav-R-Pac)	1 cup	50	1	11	0	2	0.0	0.0	0	0%
in syrup (Flav-R-Pac)	2/3 cup	230	1	57	40	4	0.0	0.0	0	0%
red, sweetened	10-oz pkg	293	2	74	3	12	0.5	0.0	0	1%
red, sweetened, unthawed	1 cup	258	2	65	3	11	0.4	0.0	0	1%
RASPBERRY JUICE (Smucker's) red, 'Naturally 100%'	8 fl oz	120	0	30	10	0	0.0	0.0	0	0%
RASPBERRY SYRUP. See under SYRUP.										
RASPBERRY TOPPING										
(Flav-R-Pac)	2 tbsp	45	0	11	0	2	0.0	0.0	0	0%
(Knudsen) pourable	1 oz	75	0	18	0	0	1.0	0.0	0	11%
(Smucker's) nonfat, 'Light'	2 tbsp	55	0	14	0	0	0.0	0.0	0	0%
RAVIOLI DISH/ENTRÉE										
(Amy's Kitchen)										
cheese, in sauce, organic, frozen	8-oz entrée	340	15	44	580	6	12.0	3.0	20	31%
cheese, organic, frozen	1 cup	215	12	26	346	3	5.0	0.0	7	23%
(Bernardi)										
beef, breaded	1 cup	270	11	43	660	2	6.0	2.0	25	20%
beef, jumbo, round	1 cup	450	22	48	930	3	19.0	9.0	135	38%
beef, square	1 cup	280	14	37	530	2	9.0	4.5	65	28%
beef ravioletti, square	1 cup	330	13	47	540	2	10.0	4.5	30	27%
cheese, jumbo	1 cup	380	26	47	400	2	9.0	4.5	210	22%
cheese, round, jumbo	1 cup	410	21	48	570	2	15.0	9.0	50	33%
cheese, square	1 cup	260	14	36	320	2	7.0	4.0	40	24%
cheese ravioletti	1 cup	280	13	40	360	2	8.0	4.0	15	25%
chicken, jumbo, round	1 cup	450	21	52	420	2	17.0	10.0	115	34%
Espanol, breaded	1 cup	290	13	43	840	2	6.0	3.0	25	19%
Florentine, round, jumbo	1 cup	370	21	53	440	3	10.0	6.0	60	23%
pesto, round, jumbo	1 cup	480	21	57	510	4	19.0	11.0	110	35%
seafood, round, jumbo	1 cup	440	18	57	790	3	15.0	9.0	120	31%
vegetable, jumbo, round	1 cup	430	15	59	440	2	15.0	8.0	90	31%
(Buitoni)										
cheese, frozen	4 oz	360	12	31	220	0	8.0	5.0	65	30%
cheese, in sauce, canned	7.5 oz	190	7	27	790	0	6.0	2.0	5	28%
meat, in sauce, canned	7.5 oz	180	7	28	890	0	4.0	1.0	5	20%
(Celentano)										
cheese, mini	12 ravioli	270	13	42	150	2	6.0	3.0	30	20%
cheese, round	6 raviolis	400	21	61	390	11	9.0	5.0	100	20%
frozen	6.5 oz	380	21	50	510	0	11.0	0.0	0	26%
frozen, 'Great Choice'	6 ravioli	360	12	69	700	1	4.0	2.0	35	10%
mini, frozen	4 oz	250	13	39	210	0	5.0	0.0	0	18%
(Chef Boyardee)										
beef, canned, microwave	7.5 oz	190	7	31	1160	2	4.0	2.0	11	19%
beef, canned 'Sir Chomps'	7.5 oz	170	7	32	690	4	3.0	1.0	15	15%
beef, in tomato and meat sauce, canned	1 pkg	400	15	64	2044	6	9.4	4.3	26	21%
beef, in tomato and meat sauce, canned	1 cup	230	9	37	1150	4	5.0	2.5	20	20%
beef, microwave cup, 'Main Meals'	10.5 oz	290	12	52	0	0	4.0	0.0	0	12%
beef, mini, in tomato and meat sauce	1 pkg	404	15	69	2019	6	8.0	3.0	30	18%
beef, mini, in tomato and beef sauce	1 cup	240	8	37	1180	3	6.0	2.5	20	23%
beef, w/meat sauce, canned, 'Smurfs'	7.5 oz	230	9	38	1160	0	5.0	0.0	11	19%
beef and cheese, in tomato sauce	1 cup	220	9	38	1110	4	3.0	1.5	15	13%
cheese, canned 'Sir Chomps'	7.5 oz	170	6	38	740	6	1.0	1.0	5	5%

Food Name	Serving Size	Calories	Prot. gms	Carbs gms	Sod. mgs	Fiber gms	Fat gms	Sat. Fat gms	Chol. mgs	% Fat Cal.
cheese, in meat sauce, canned, microwave	7.5 oz	200	6	37	1010	0	3.0	0.0	10	14%
cheese, in tomato sauce	1 cup	210	7	44	860	4	0.0	0.0	0	0%
chicken, canned	7.5 oz	180	7	29	1100	0	4.0	0.0	13	20%
chicken, mini, canned	7.5 oz	220	7	29	1090	0	8.0	0.0	0	33%
(Contadina)										
beef, refrigerated, 'Fresh'	3 oz	270	13	30	250	0	11.0	3.0	75	37%
beef and garlic.	1-1/4 cup	350	17	39	350	3	14.0	5.0	110	36%
cheese.	1 cup	280	13	31	350	2	12.0	6.0	31	38%
cheese, light	1 cup	240	13	35	340	2	5.0	2.0	60	19%
chicken, refrigerated, 'Fresh'	3 oz	260	11	32	310	0	10.0	2.0	80	34%
chicken and rosemary.	1-1/4 cup	330	13	43	420	3	12.0	4.0	85	33%
garden vegetable, light	1-1/4 cup	290	15	43	370	3	6.0	3.5	65	19%
(DiGiorno)										
cheese, w/herb, Italian, refrigerated, cooked	1 cup	280	12	35	490	0	10.0	4.0	35	32%
sausage, Italian, refrigerated, cooked.	1 cup	270	13	34	520	0	9.0	4.0	40	30%
(Estee) beef, canned	7.5 oz	230	8	25	100	0	11.0	4.0	10	43%
(Finast) beef, in sauce, canned	7.5 oz	250	7	33	1165	0	10.0	0.0	0	36%
(Franco-American) beef, in meat sauce.	1 cup	280	11	38	1160	2	9.0	4.0	20	29%
(Healthy Choice) cheese, Parmigiana	1 entrée	260	11	44	290	6	5.0	2.5	20	17%
(Hormel) beef, in tomato sauce, micro cup	7.5 oz	247	8	28	951	0	11.0	0.0	21	41%
(Kid Cuisine)										
cheese, mini, frozen	8.75 oz	250	6	52	730	0	2.0	0.0	20	7%
cheese, mini, w/applesauce, corn, and brownie, frozen . . .	1 meal	310	7	61	750	5	4.0	1.0	10	12%
(Kid's Kitchen)										
mini, microwave cup	7.5 oz	230	10	34	870	0	6.0	3.0	15	23%
(Lean Cuisine) cheese.	1 entrée	270	11	40	580	5	7.0	3.0	45	24%
(Libby's) beef, in sauce, microwave cup, 'Diner'.	7.75 oz	240	13	35	890	2	5.0	4.0	15	19%
(Lucca)										
beef.	1 cup	190	9	28	370	4	5.0	1.5	45	23%
chicken, w/savory herbs	1 cup	180	11	26	450	4	4.0	0.0	55	20%
Italian sausage, w/herbs and seasonings.	1 cup	200	9	29	520	4	6.0	1.5	55	26%
(Lunch Express) cheese	1 entrée	360	15	43	700	7	14.0	5.0	60	35%
(Marie Callender's)										
w/marinara sauce and 1 oz garlic bread, frozen.	1 serving	370	14	47	520	4	14.0	5.0	35	34%
(Nalley's) beef, canned	7.5 oz	180	8	30	1040	0	3.0	0.0	0	15%
(Pathmark)										
beef, bite size, in tomato sauce, 'No Frills'	7.5 oz	180	7	28	890	0	4.0	0.0	0	20%
cheese in tomato sauce, canned, 'No Frills'	7.5 oz	185	7	27	790	0	6.0	0.0	0	28%
(Progresso)										
beef, frozen.	1 cup	260	9	45	940	4	5.0	2.0	5	17%
cheese, frozen.	1 cup	220	9	43	930	4	2.0	1.0	5	8%
(Smart Ones) Florentine	1 entrée	220	9	43	490	4	2.0	0.5	5	8%
(Weight Watchers) cheese, baked, frozen.	9 oz	240	18	27	370	0	6.0	2.0	30	23%

RED BEAN. See BEAN, RED.

RED CABBAGE. See CABBAGE, RED.

RED CURRANT. See under CURRANT.

RED CURRY BASE. See under SEASONING MIX.

RED PEPPER. See PEPPER, BELL. See also under PEPPER, CHILI; PEPPER, GROUND.

RED PERCH. See OCEAN PERCH, ATLANTIC.

RED SALMON. See under SALMON.

REFRIED BEANS. See under BEAN DISH/ENTRÉE.

RELISH

| CORN, canned *(Green Giant)* . . . . | 1 tbsp | 20 | 0 | 5 | 40 | 0 | 0.0 | 0.0 | 0 | 0% |

Food Name	Serving Size	Calories	Prot. gms	Carbs gms	Sod. mgs	Fiber gms	Fat gms	Sat. Fat gms	Chol. mgs	% Fat Cal.
CRANBERRY-ORANGE, for chicken, canned										
(Ocean Spray)	1/4 cup	120	0	29	35	1	0.0	0.0	0	0%
DILL, nonfat (Vlasic)	1 oz	2	0	1	415	0	0.0	0.0	0	0%
HAMBURGER (Heinz)	1 oz	40	0	9	255	0	0.0	0.0	0	0%
HOT DOG (Vlasic)	1 oz	40	0	8	255	0	1.0	0.0	0	22%
INDIA (Heinz)	1 oz	35	0	9	215	0	0.0	0.0	0	0%
PICCALILLI										
(Heinz)	1 oz	30	0	7	145	0	0.0	0.0	0	0%
(Progresso)	1/2 cup	190	1	4	220	1	20.0	3.0	0	90%
not (Vlasic)	1 oz	35	0	8	165	0	0.0	0.0	0	0%
PICKLE										
dill (Vlasic)	1 tbsp	5	0	1	240	1	0.0	0.0	0	0%
hot dog (Heinz)	1 tbsp	15	0	4	105	0	0.0	0.0	0	0%
India (Vlasic)	1 tbsp	15	0	4	140	0	0.0	0.0	0	0%
sweet (Claussen)	1 tbsp	15	0	3	85	0	0.0	0.0	0	0%
sweet (Heinz)	1 tbsp	15	0	4	110	0	0.0	0.0	0	0%
sweet (Vlasic)	1 tbsp	15	0	4	140	0	0.0	0.0	0	0%
RENNIN, enzyme tablet, unsweetened	0.35 oz	8	0	2	2579	0	0.0	0.0	0	1%
RHUBARB										
Fresh										
raw, whole	1 med stalk	11	0	2	2	1	0.1	0.0	0	8%
raw, diced	1 cup	26	1	6	5	2	0.2	0.1	0	8%
Frozen										
(Flav-R-Pac)	1 cup	30	1	5	0	2	0.5	0.0	0	16%
w/sugar, cooked	1 cup	278	1	75	2	5	0.1	0.0	0	0%
uncooked, diced	1 cup	29	1	7	3	2	0.2	0.0	0	4%
RICE										
ARBORIO										
(Colavita) dry	1 oz	100	2	22	5	0	0.0	0.0	0	0%
(Fantastic Foods) dry, 'Elegant Grains'	1/4 cup	210	4	45	0	1	0.0	0.0	0	0%
BASMATI										
(Arrowhead Mills)										
brown, long-grain, dry	2 oz	200	4	44	3	3	1.0	0.0	0	4%
white, long grain, dry	1/4 cup	150	3	33	0	2	1.0	0.0	0	6%
(Fantastic Foods)										
brown, cooked, w/1 tbsp salted butter	1/2 cup	115	3	22	20	0	2.0	0.0	0	15%
brown, dry, 'Elegant Grains'	1/4 cup	170	3	36	0	1	1.5	0.0	0	8%
white, cooked, prep w/1 tbsp salted butter	1/2 cup	116	2	23	18	0	1.0	0.0	0	8%
white, dry, 'Elegant Grains'	1/4 cup	180	3	38	0	1	0.0	0.0	0	0%
(Texmati) white, long-grain, cooked w/o salt or butter	1/2 cup	82	3	31	0	0	0.0	0.0	0	0%
BROWN										
long grain, cooked	1 cup	216	5	45	10	4	1.8	0.4	0	7%
long grain, raw	1 cup	685	15	143	13	6	5.4	1.1	0	7%
medium grain, cooked	1 cup	218	5	46	2	4	1.6	0.3	0	6%
medium grain, raw	1 cup	688	14	145	8	6	5.1	1.0	0	6%
(Arrowhead Mills)										
long grain, raw	2 oz	200	4	44	3	3	1.0	0.0	0	4%
medium grain, raw	2 oz	200	4	44	3	3	1.0	0.0	0	4%
short grain, raw	2 oz	200	4	44	3	3	1.0	0.0	0	4%
Spanish, quick, dry	1/3 cup	150	4	30	250	2	1.0	0.0	0	6%
vegetable, quick, dry	1/3 cup	150	4	30	160	3	1.0	0.0	0	6%
wild, dry	1/3 cup	140	4	28	220	3	1.0	0.0	0	7%
(Carolina) long grain, cooked, no salt or butter	1/2 cup	110	2	23	0	0	0.0	0.0	0	0%

Food Name	Serving Size	Calories	Prot. gms	Carbs gms	Sod. mgs	Fiber gms	Fat gms	Sat. Fat gms	Chol. mgs	% Fat Cal.
(Eden Foods)										
traditional	1/2 cup	200	8	38	80	3	2.0	0.0	0	9%
udon, organic, traditional, dry	1/2 cup	200	8	38	80	3	2.0	0.0	0	9%
(Fantastic Foods)										
cooked	1 cup	240	7	55	650	2	2.0	0.0	0	7%
w/miso, dry	1/2 cup	250	7	55	570	1	3.0	0.0	0	10%
(Lundberg Family)										
golden rose, organic	1/4 cup	160	3	34	0	1	2.0	0.0	0	11%
long grain, cooked	1 cup	232	5	50	0	3	1.2	0.0	0	5%
(Mahatma) long grain, cooked, no salt or butter	1/2 cup	110	2	23	10	0	0.0	0.0	0	0%
(Minute) instant	1/2 cup	120	3	25	5	0	1.0	0.0	0	7%
(River) long grain, cooked, no salt or butter	1/2 cup	110	2	23	0	0	0.0	0.0	0	0%
(S&W)										
long grain, cooked, no salt or butter	3.5 oz	110	2	25	0	0	0.0	0.0	0	0%
long grain, dry	1/4 cup	150	3	32	0	1	1.0	0.0	0	6%
(Uncle Ben's)										
instant, original, dry	1/4 cup	170	4	37	0	1	1.5	0.2	0	8%
long grain, cooked, no salt or butter	2/3 cup	130	3	27	0	0	1.0	0.0	0	7%
precooked, prepared, no salt or butter	1/2 cup	90	2	21	11	1	1.0	0.0	0	9%
GLUTINOUS										
white, cooked	1 cup	169	4	37	9	2	0.3	0.1	0	2%
white, raw	1 cup	685	13	151	13	5	1.0	0.2	0	1%
JASMINE *(Fantastic Foods)* uncooked, 'Elegant Grains'	1/4 cup	170	3	38	0	1	0.0	0.0	0	0%
WHITE										
long grain, cooked	1 cup	205	4	45	2	1	0.4	0.1	0	2%
long grain, dry	1 cup	675	13	148	9	2	1.2	0.3	0	2%
long grain, parboiled, cooked	1 cup	200	4	43	5	1	0.5	0.1	0	2%
long grain, parboiled, dry	1 cup	686	13	151	9	3	1.0	0.3	0	1%
long grain, precooked or instant, enriched, dry	1 cup	360	7	79	6	2	0.3	0.1	0	1%
long grain, precooked or instant, enriched, prepared	1 cup	162	3	35	5	1	0.3	0.1	0	1%
medium grain, cooked	1 cup	242	4	53	0	1	0.4	0.1	0	1%
medium grain, dry	1 cup	702	13	155	2	3	1.1	0.3	0	1%
short grain, cooked	1 cup	242	4	53	0	na	0.4	0.1	0	1%
short grain, dry	1 cup	716	13	158	2	6	1.0	0.3	0	1%
(Botan) long grain, Calrose	1/4 cup	150	3	33	0	0	0.0	0.0	0	0%
(Carolina)										
long grain, cooked, w/o salt, butter	1/2 cup	100	2	22	10	0	0.0	0.0	0	0%
long grain, instant, cooked, w/o salt, butter	1/2 cup	110	2	23	0	0	0.0	0.0	0	0%
(Dynasty) long grain, enriched	1 oz	118	2	26	0	0	0.0	0.0	0	0%
(Finast) long grain, cooked, w/o salt, butter	1/2 cup	115	2	26	0	0	0.0	0.0	0	0%
(Mahatma) long grain, cooked, w/o salt, butter	1/2 cup	110	2	23	0	0	0.0	0.0	0	0%
(Minute)										
long grain, cooked, w/o salt, butter	2/3 cup	120	3	27	0	0	0.0	0.0	0	0%
long grain, cooked, w/o salt, butter	1/2 cup	90	2	20	0	0	0.0	0.0	0	0%
long grain, 'Premium' cooked, w/o salt, butter	2/3 cup	120	3	27	0	0	0.0	0.0	0	0%
'Original'	2/3 cup	120	3	27	5	0	0.0	0.0	0	0%
(River) long grain, cooked, w/o salt, butter	1/2 cup	100	2	22	10	0	0.0	0.0	0	0%
(S&W) long grain, cooked, w/o salt, butter	3.5 oz	106	2	23	0	0	0.0	0.0	0	0%
(Success) long grain, enriched, cooked, w/o salt, butter	1/2 cup	100	2	21	0	0	0.0	0.0	0	0%
(Uncle Ben's)										
long grain, cooked, w/o salt and butter	2/3 cup	130	3	28	0	0	1.0	0.0	0	7%
long grain, cooked, w/o salt, butter	1/2 cup	90	2	20	10	0	1.0	0.0	0	9%
long grain, instant, cooked, w/salt and butter	2/3 cup	130	3	27	310	0	2.0	0.0	0	13%
long grain, instant, cooked, w/o salt, butter	2/3 cup	120	3	27	10	0	1.0	0.0	0	7%

Food Name	Serving Size	Calories	Prot. gms	Carbs gms	Sod. mgs	Fiber gms	Fat gms	Sat. Fat gms	Chol. mgs	% Fat Cal.
long grain, 'Natural' cooked, w/salt, butter	2/3 cup	150	3	28	420	0	3.0	0.0	0	18%
long grain, parboiled, cooked, w/salt, butter	2/3 cup	140	2	28	410	0	2.0	0.0	0	13%
long grain, parboiled, cooked, w/o salt, butter	2/3 cup	120	2	28	0	0	1.0	0.0	0	7%
(Water Maid) long grain, cooked, w/o salt, butter	1/2 cup	100	2	22	10	0	0.0	0.0	0	0%
RICE, WILD										
cooked (Fantastic Foods)	1/2 cup	83	3	18	0	0	0.0	0.0	0	0%
cooked.	1 cup	166	7	35	5	3	0.6	0.1	0	3%
extra fancy, prepared (Gourmet House)	1 oz	107	4	22	8	1	0.3	0.1	0	3%
giant, prepared (Gourmet House).	1 oz	106	4	22	3	1	0.3	0.1	0	2%
raw	1 cup	571	24	120	11	10	1.7	0.3	0	3%
select, prepared (Gourmet House)	1 oz	106	4	22	14	1	0.3	0.1	0	3%
RICE AND BEANS. See under RICE DISH/ENTRÉE.										
RICE BEVERAGE										
(Amazake Light) nondairy, original flavor.	1 cup	90	2	20	75	2	0.0	0.0	0	0%
(Don Jose)										
original flavor, 'Horchata'	8 fl oz	70	1	6	95	0	4.0	0.0	0	56%
strawberry flavor, 'Horchata'	8 fl oz	70	1	7	95	0	3.5	0.0	0	50%
(Eden Foods) original flavor, organic, w/soy	8 fl oz	120	7	16	85	0	3.0	0.5	0	23%
(Grainaissance)										
almond flavor, sweet brown rice, 'Amazake'	8 fl oz	198	4	37	20	0	4.0	0.0	0	18%
apricot flavor, sweet brown rice, 'Amazake'.	8 fl oz	158	3	36	20	0	0.0	0.0	0	0%
cocoa-almond flavor, brown rice, 'Amazake'	8 fl oz	198	4	36	20	0	4.0	0.0	0	18%
mocha java flavor, sweet brown rice, 'Amazake'	8 fl oz	178	3	37	20	0	2.0	0.0	0	10%
original flavor, brown rice, 'Amazake'	8 fl oz	148	2	34	20	0	0.0	0.0	0	0%
sesame flavor, sweet brown rice, 'Amazake'.	8 fl oz	198	4	37	20	0	1.0	0.0	0	5%
vanilla pecan flavor, brown rice, 'Amazake'.	8 fl oz	198	4	37	20	0	4.0	0.0	0	18%
(Imagine Foods)										
carob flavor, brown rice, nondairy, 'Rice Dream Lite'	8 fl oz	150	1	32	80	0	3.0	0.0	0	17%
carob flavor, nondairy, 'Rice Dream'	8 fl oz	150	1	32	100	0	2.5	0.0	0	15%
chocolate flavor, brown rice, nondairy, 'Rice Dream'.	8 fl oz	190	1	44	80	0	3.0	0.0	0	13%
chocolate flavor, enriched, nondairy, 'Rice Dream'	8 fl oz	170	1	36	115	0	3.0	0.0	0	15%
chocolate flavor, nondairy, 'Rice Dream'	8 fl oz	160	1	35	100	0	2.5	0.0	0	14%
nondairy, 'Rice Dream'	8 fl oz	130	1	28	90	0	2.0	0.0	0	13%
original flavor, enriched, nondairy, 'Rice Dream'	8 fl oz	120	1	25	90	0	2.0	0.0	0	15%
vanilla flavor, brown rice, nondairy, 'Rice Dream Lite'	8 fl oz	120	1	28	80	0	2.0	0.0	0	13%
vanilla flavor, enriched, nondairy, 'Rice Dream'.	8 fl oz	130	1	28	90	0	2.0	0.0	0	13%
(Sovex) original vanilla flavor, 'Better Than Milk'	2 tbsp	72	1	17	90	0	0.0	0.0	0	0%
(Westbrae Naturals)										
plain.	8 fl oz	100	1	18	70	0	3.0	0.5	0	26%
vanilla flavor	8 fl oz	120	1	22	70	0	3.0	0.5	0	23%
RICE BEVERAGE MIX										
(Devan Sweet) made from organic brown rice.	1 1/2 tsp	25	0	2	0	0	0.0	0.0	0	0%
RICE BRAN, crude.	1 cup	373	16	59	6	25	24.6	4.9	0	55%
RICE BRAN OIL										
. . . .	1 cup	1927	0	0	0	0	218.0	42.9	0	100%
. . . .	1 tbsp	120	0	0	0	0	13.6	2.7	0	100%
(Hain)	1 tbsp	120	0	0	0	0	14.0	3.0	0	100%
RICE CAKE										
(Lundberg Family)										
all flavors, sodium-free	1 cake	60	1	14	3	0	0.5	0.0	0	7%
all flavors, very low sodium	1 cake	60	1	14	30	0	0.5	0.0	0	7%
APPLE CINNAMON										
(Hain)	1 serving	50	1	11	10	0	0.0	0.0	0	0%
(Quaker) nonfat.	1 cake	40	1	9	0	0	0.0	0.0	0	0%

Food Name	Serving Size	Calories	Prot. gms	Carbs gms	Sod. mgs	Fiber gms	Fat gms	Sat. Fat gms	Chol. mgs	% Fat Cal.
BROWN RICE										
. . . .	1 cake	35	1	7	29	0	0.3	0.1	0	6%
buckwheat.	1 cake	34	1	7	10	0	0.3	0.1	0	8%
buckwheat, unsalted.	1 cake	34	1	7	0	na	0.3	0.1	0	8%
corn.	1 cake	35	1	7	26	0	0.3	0.1	0	7%
multigrain.	1 cake	35	1	7	23	0	0.3	0.1	0	8%
multigrain, unsalted.	1 cake	35	1	7	0	na	0.3	0.1	0	8%
unsalted.	1 cake	35	1	7	2	0	0.3	0.1	0	6%
rye.	1 cake	35	1	7	10	0	0.3	0.1	0	8%
w/sesame seed.	1 cake	35	1	7	20	0	0.3	0.0	0	8%
w/sesame seed, unsalted. . .	1 cake	35	1	7	0	na	0.3	0.0	0	8%
(Lundberg) unsalted.	1 cake	70	1	16	0	2	0.0	0.0	0	0%
HONEY NUT *(Hain)*. . . .	1 serving	50	1	11	25	0	0.0	0.0	0	0%
BARBECUE *(Hain)* mini. . . .	0.5 oz	70	1	10	50	0	3.0	0.0	0	38%
CARAWAY RYE *(Lundberg)*. . . .	1 cake	60	1	14	120	2	0.0	0.0	0	0%
CAROB COATED										
(Carafection)										
'Mint Rice Crisps'.	1 oz	139	2	17	26	0	7.0	0.0	0	45%
'Rice Crisps'.	1 oz	139	2	17	26	0	7.0	0.0	0	45%
CHEESE										
(Hain)										
mini.	0.5 oz	60	1	10	80	0	2.0	0.0	0	29%
nacho, mini.	0.5 oz	70	1	10	90	0	2.0	0.0	5	29%
(Lundberg Family)										
mini.	5 cakes	57	1	13	116	0	1.0	0.0	1	14%
mini.	5 cakes	57	1	13	116	0	1.0	0.0	1	14%
CINNAMON										
(Quaker) crunch.	1 serving	50	1	11	25	0	0.0	0.0	0	0%
(Chico-San) sugar, mini. . . .	5 cakes	50	1	12	0	0	0.0	0.0	0	0%
CORN *(Quaker)*.	1 cake	35	1	7	53	0	0.2	0.0	0	5%
DILL *(Lundberg Family)* creamy, mini. . .	5 cakes	60	1	13	57	0	1.0	0.0	2	14%
HONEY NUT *(Chico-San)* unglazed, mini . . .	4 cakes	60	1	2	35	0	1.0	0.0	0	43%
MUGWORT *(Grainaissance)* bake and serve, 'Mochi' . . .	2 oz	140	3	29	2	0	1.3	0.0	0	8%
MULTIGRAIN										
(Chico-San) very low sodium. . . .	1 cake	35	1	8	30	0	0.0	0.0	0	0%
(Hain) five grain.	1 cake	40	1	8	10	0	1.0	0.0	0	20%
(Pritikin)										
sodium-free *(Pritikin)*. . . .	1 cake	35	1	7	0	0	0.0	0.0	0	0%
very low sodium	1 cake	35	1	7	30	0	0.0	0.0	0	0%
(Quaker).	0.32 oz	34	1	7	29	0	0.4	0.1	0	10%
PLAIN										
(Chico-San) nonfat, original. . . .	1 cake	35	1	8	30	0	0.0	0.0	0	0%
(Grainaissance) organic, bake and serve, 'Mochi' . . .	2 oz	140	3	29	2	0	1.3	0.0	0	8%
(Hain)										
. . . .	1 cake	40	1	8	10	0	1.0	0.0	0	20%
mini.	0.5 oz	60	1	12	20	0	1.0	0.0	0	15%
mini, unsalted.	0.5 oz	60	1	12	5	0	1.0	0.0	0	15%
unsalted.	1 cake	40	1	8	5	0	1.0	0.0	0	20%
unsalted, mini.	0.5 oz	60	1	12	5	0	1.0	0.0	0	15%
(Konriko) unsalted, original. . . .	1 cake	30	0	7	1	0	0.0	0.0	0	0%
(Koyo)										
organic, lightly salted. . . .	1 cake	40	1	8	80	0	0.0	0.0	0	0%
organic, no added salt. . . .	1 cake	40	1	8	0	0	0.0	0.0	0	0%
(Lundberg Family) organic, lightly salted. . . .	1 cake	60	1	14	140	0	0.5	0.0	0	7%

Food Name	Serving Size	Calories	Prot. gms	Carbs gms	Sod. mgs	Fiber gms	Fat gms	Sat. Fat gms	Chol. mgs	% Fat Cal.
(Pritikin)										
sodium-free	1 cake	35	1	7	0	0	0.0	0.0	0	0%
very low sodium	1 cake	35	1	7	35	0	0.0	0.0	0	0%
(Quaker)										
. . . .	0.32 oz	35	1	7	36	0	0.3	0.1	0	8%
lightly salted	1 cake	35	1	7	35	0	0.0	0.0	0	0%
unsalted.	1 cake	35	1	7	0	0	0.3	0.1	0	8%
RAISIN										
(Grainaissance) cinnamon, bake and serve, 'Mochi'	2 oz	143	3	30	77	0	1.2	0.0	0	8%
RYE *(Quaker)*	1 cake	34	1	7	12	0	0.4	0.1	0	10%
SESAME										
(Chico-San) original	1 cake	35	1	8	0	0	0.0	0.0	0	0%
(Grainaissance) garlic, bake and serve, 'Mochi'	2 oz	143	3	28	25	0	1.9	0.0	0	12%
(Hain)										
unsalted.	1 cake	40	1	8	5	0	1.0	0.0	0	20%
. . . .	1 cake	40	1	8	10	0	1.0	0.0	0	20%
(Pritikin)										
nonfat, sodium-free	1 cake	35	1	7	0	0	0.0	0.0	0	0%
nonfat, very low sodium.	1 cake	35	1	7	35	0	0.0	0.0	0	0%
(Quaker)	0.32 oz	35	1	7	36	0	0.3	0.1	0	8%
(Westbrae)										
double sesame	0.28 oz	30	1	6	65	0	1.0	0.0	0	24%
garlic	0.28 oz	30	1	6	55	0	1.0	0.0	0	24%
TERIYAKI										
(Hain) mini	0.5 oz	50	1	12	75	0	1.0	0.0	0	15%
(Westbrae)	0.28 oz	30	1	6	45	0	1.0	0.0	0	24%
WHEAT *(Quaker)*	1 cake	34	1	7	52	1	0.3	0.1	0	8%
WHOLE GRAIN, herb and garlic *(American Grains)*	0.5 oz	60	1	11	92	0	1.7	0.0	0	24%
RICE CHIPS, brown rice *(Eden Foods)*	1-oz bag	130	2	19	197	0	5.0	0.0	0	35%
RICE DISH/ENTRÉE										
(Bearitos)										
rice and beans, Cajun style.	1 cup	140	7	26	490	5	1.0	0.0	0	6%
rice and beans, Cuban style	1 cup	150	7	27	490	5	1.0	0.0	0	6%
rice and beans, Mexican style.	1 cup	160	7	30	490	4	1.0	0.0	0	6%
(Lean Cuisine)										
Mexican style, w/chicken, frozen, 'Lunch Express'	9 1/8 oz	270	12	43	580	0	5.0	1.0	20	17%
(Lunch Express) stir-fry, w/chicken	1 entrée	280	11	39	590	3	9.0	1.0	15	29%
(Marie Callender's) w/chicken and broccoli, cheesy	12 oz	390	24	44	1220	6	13.0	9.0	55	30%
(Smart Ones) Santa Fe style rice and beans.	1 entrée	290	12	43	590	6	8.0	4.0	20	25%
(Suzi Wan) sweet and sour	1 cup	268	5	46	754	1	6.9	1.4	0	23%
(Weight Watchers)										
and vegetables, Hunan style.	1 entrée	250	7	39	630	8	7.0	2.0	5	26%
and vegetables, Peking style.	1 entrée	270	7	48	640	3	6.0	1.0	5	20%
paella.	1 entrée	280	7	48	680	5	7.0	1.0	5	22%
rice and beans, Santa Fe style, 'Smart Ones'	1 entrée	290	12	41	670	10	9.0	4.0	5	28%
risotto, w/cheese and mushrooms	1 entrée	290	11	44	540	4	8.0	4.0	20	25%
RICE DISH/ENTRÉE MIX										
(Casbah)										
pilaf, nutted, prepared	3/4 cup	190	5	35	500	1	2.0	0.0	0	10%
pilaf, prepared	3/4 cup	210	9	38	390	1	0.5	0.0	0	2%
Spanish pilaf *(Casbah)* prepared	3/4 cup	200	4	40	430	1	0.5	0.0	0	2%
tabbouleh rice, mix only	1 oz	90	3	20	350	1	1.0	0.0	0	9%
(Ener-G Foods)										
brown rice pilaf, 'Old World' prepared	1 cup	364	9	76	418	6	3.0	0.6	0	7%

Food Name	Serving Size	Calories	Prot. gms	Carbs gms	Sod. mgs	Fiber gms	Fat gms	Sat. Fat gms	Chol. mgs	% Fat Cal.
gluten-free, low-sodium, mix only	1 cup	507	9	111	6	3	2.0	0.5	0	4%
gluten-free, mix only	1 cup	528	9	97	283	3	1.8	0.3	0	4%
(Fantastic Foods)										
rice and beans, Caribbean, mix only	1 serving	230	10	44	480	6	1.5	0.0	0	6%
rice and beans, northern Italian, mix only	1 serving	240	8	49	460	4	1.5	0.0	0	6%
rice and beans, Szechuan, mix only	1 serving	210	7	41	480	3	2.0	0.0	0	9%
rice and pinto beans, Tex-Mex, mix only	2.3 oz	240	8	48	590	6	2.5	0.5	0	9%
rice and red beans, Cajun, mix only	2.3 oz	230	10	46	480	8	3.0	0.0	0	11%
(La Choy) fried, prepared	1 cup	236	5	53	1024	2	1.1	0.2	0	4%
(Lundberg Family)										
blend, brown and white, mix only	1/4 cup	150	4	35	0	3	1.5	0.0	0	8%
brown rice picante, prepared, 'Spanish Fiesta' 'Quick'	1 cup	260	6	53	670	5	2.5	0.5	na	9%
brown rice, exotic wild rice, and mushrooms, prepared, 'Quick'	1 cup	260	6	53	800	4	3.0	1.0	na	10%
(Minute)										
long grain and wild, mix only	1/2 cup	120	3	25	530	0	0.0	0.0	0	0%
long grain and wild, prepared w/salted butter	1/2 cup	150	3	25	570	0	4.0	0.0	10	24%
(Rice A Roni)										
beef flavored, 1/3 less sodium, prepared	2.5 oz	158	4	30	423	1	2.8	0.6	0	16%
beef flavored, prepared	2.5 oz	169	5	27	598	na	4.5	na	na	24%
chicken flavored, 'Fast Cook' prepared	2.5 oz	141	3	23	519	1	3.7	0.8	3	24%
chicken flavored, 1/3 less sodium, prepared	2.5 oz	158	4	30	390	1	2.8	0.6	0	16%
chicken flavored, prepared	2.5 oz	181	4	29	618	1	5.4	0.6	0	27%
fried, 1/3 less sodium, prepared	2.5 oz	147	3	29	525	1	2.0	0.3	0	12%
fried, prepared	2.5 oz	181	3	29	900	1	6.2	1.1	0	30%
herb and butter, prepared	2.5 oz	175	3	30	655	1	5.1	0.8	3	26%
long grain and wild, original, prepared	2.5 oz	164	4	28	700	2	4.8	0.8	0	25%
long grain and wild, w/chicken, almond, prepared	2.5 oz	164	4	28	700	2	4.8	0.8	0	25%
pilaf, long grain and wild, prepared	2.5 oz	135	3	24	514	1	3.1	0.6	0	20%
pilaf, prepared	2.5 oz	175	3	30	621	1	5.1	0.6	0	26%
Spanish, 'Fast Cook' prepared	2.5 oz	141	3	25	567	1	3.1	0.6	0	20%
Spanish, prepared	2 oz	122	3	21	546	1	3.6	0.5	0	26%
Stroganoff, prepared	2.5 oz	203	5	28	587	1	8.2	2.0	3	36%
w/chicken, broccoli, prepared	2.5 oz	164	4	29	793	1	4.2	0.6	0	23%
white cheddar and herb, prepared	2.5 oz	192	4	28	553	1	7.9	2.3	3	36%

RICE FLOUR. See under FLOUR.

RICE SEASONING. See under SEASONING MIX.

Food Name	Serving Size	Calories	Prot. gms	Carbs gms	Sod. mgs	Fiber gms	Fat gms	Sat. Fat gms	Chol. mgs	% Fat Cal.
RICE STICK, wild rice *(Golden Flavor)* wild	1 oz	150	5	17	170	2	7.0	1.0	0	42%

RICE SYRUP. See under SYRUP.

RISOTTO. See under RICE DISH/ENTRÉE.

ROAST BEEF HASH. See under HASH.

ROCKFISH, PACIFIC

Food Name	Serving Size	Calories	Prot. gms	Carbs gms	Sod. mgs	Fiber gms	Fat gms	Sat. Fat gms	Chol. mgs	% Fat Cal.
baked, broiled, grilled, or microwaved	3 oz	103	20	0	65	0	1.7	0.4	37	15%
raw	3 oz	80	16	0	51	0	1.3	0.3	30	15%

ROE

Food Name	Serving Size	Calories	Prot. gms	Carbs gms	Sod. mgs	Fiber gms	Fat gms	Sat. Fat gms	Chol. mgs	% Fat Cal.
mixed species, cooked	3 oz	173	24	2	99	0	7.0	1.6	407	36%
mixed species, cooked	1 oz	58	8	1	33	0	2.3	0.5	136	36%
mixed species, raw	3 oz	119	19	1	77	0	5.5	1.2	318	41%
mixed species, raw	1 oz	40	6	0	26	0	1.8	0.4	106	41%

ROLL. See also BREAD; BUN; CROISSANT; ENGLISH MUFFIN; ROLL, SWEET.

Food Name	Serving Size	Calories	Prot. gms	Carbs gms	Sod. mgs	Fiber gms	Fat gms	Sat. Fat gms	Chol. mgs	% Fat Cal.
(Brownberry) assorted, 'Hearth'	1 roll	124	4	24	247	2	2.3	0.0	7	16%
(Country Oven) enriched, brown and serve	1 roll	80	2	13	140	0	2.0	0.0	0	23%
(King's Hawaiian Bread) ready-to-eat	1 roll	90	3	15	80	1	2.0	5.0	10	20%
(Pepperidge Farm) brown and serve, 'Hearth'	1 roll	50	2	10	100	0	1.0	0.0	0	16%

Food Name	Serving Size	Calories	Prot. gms	Carbs gms	Sod. mgs	Fiber gms	Fat gms	Sat. Fat gms	Chol. mgs	% Fat Cal.
(Wonder)										
gem style, brown and serve	1 roll	80	2	13	140	1	2.0	0.0	0	23%
plain pan	1 roll	80	2	14	140	1	1.0	0.0	0	12%
CLUB *(Pepperidge Farm)* brown and serve, 'Deli Classic'	1 roll	100	3	19	190	1	1.0	0.0	0	9%
CRESCENT *(Pepperidge Farm)* butter, 'Deli Classic'	1 roll	110	2	13	150	0	6.0	3.0	15	47%
DINNER										
(Arnold) '24 Dinner Party'	1 roll	51	2	9	81	1	1.2	0.0	1	19%
(Awrey's)										
'Black Forest'	1 roll	50	2	10	110	0	1.0	0.0	0	16%
cracked wheat	1 roll	50	2	10	120	0	1.0	0.0	0	16%
crusty	1 roll	70	2	12	150	0	1.0	0.0	0	14%
plain	1 roll	60	2	11	115	0	1.0	0.0	0	15%
w/poppy seed	1 roll	59	2	11	115	0	1.0	0.0	0	15%
w/sesame seed	1 roll	60	2	11	115	0	1.0	0.0	0	15%
(Ener-G Foods) tapioca, gluten-free	1 serving	151	2	24	6	1	5.7	0.3	0	33%
(Home Pride)										
wheat	1 roll	70	3	12	140	1	1.0	0.0	0	13%
white	1 roll	80	2	14	170	1	2.0	0.0	0	22%
(Pepperidge Farm)										
country style, 'Classic'	1 roll	50	2	9	90	0	1.0	0.0	0	17%
'Old Fashioned'	1 roll	50	2	7	85	0	2.0	1.0	5	33%
'Party'	1 roll	30	1	5	50	0	1.0	0.0	0	27%
(Pillsbury)										
butterflake	1 serving	130	3	19	530	1	5.0	1.0	0	34%
hot	1 serving	130	4	21	220	1	3.0	0.5	15	21%
(Roman Meal)	1 roll	69	3	13	140	1	1.2	0.0	0	15%
(Wonder)										
	1 roll	80	2	14	140	1	1.0	0.0	0	12%
brown and serve	1 serving	80	2	13	150	0	2.0	0.5	0	23%
EGG *(Levy's)* 'Old Country Deli'	1 roll	146	5	28	431	2	2.8	0.0	11	16%
FINGER w/poppy seeds	1 roll	50	2	8	80	0	2.0	0.0	5	31%
FRENCH										
(Du Jour) petite, brown and serve	1 roll	230	9	45	490	2	2.0	0.0	0	8%
(Francisco) 'International'	1 roll	108	4	21	285	1	1.5	0.0	0	12%
(Pepperidge Farm)										
brown and serve, 'Deli Classic'	1/2 roll	120	4	24	250	1	1.0	0.0	0	7%
'Deli Classic' 4 per pkg	1/2 piece	120	4	22	250	1	2.0	0.0	0	15%
'Deli Classic' 9 per pkg	1 roll	100	4	20	230	1	1.0	0.0	0	9%
sourdough	1 piece	100	4	19	240	1	1.0	0.0	0	9%
HARD, including Kaiser	1 oz	83	3	15	154	1	1.2	0.2	0	13%
HOAGIE										
(Wonder)	1 roll	400	13	73	800	3	7.0	0.0	0	15%
(Pepperidge Farm) soft, 'Deli Classic'	1 roll	210	8	34	320	1	5.0	1.0	0	21%
ITALIAN *(Du Jour)* crusty, brown and serve	1 roll	80	3	16	200	1	1.0	0.0	0	11%
KAISER										
(Arnold) 'Francisco'	1 roll	184	7	35	338	2	2.9	0.0	5	13%
(Brownberry) 'Hearth'	1 roll	152	5	29	318	2	2.8	0.0	9	15%
(Holsum) 'Big'	1 bun	200	5	38	320	0	3.0	0.0	0	14%
LUIGI 'Twin Pack' *(Colombo Brand)*	2 oz piece	146	8	25	334	0	1.6	0.0	0	10%
ONION										
(Holsum) 'Big'	1 bun	190	6	32	190	0	4.0	0.0	0	19%
(Levy's) 'Old Country Deli'	1 roll	153	6	31	380	2	1.9	0.0	11	10%
(Pepperidge Farm) w/poppy seeds, sandwich	1 roll	150	5	26	260	1	3.0	1.0	0	18%

Food Name	Serving Size	Calories	Prot. gms	Carbs gms	Sod. mgs	Fiber gms	Fat gms	Sat. Fat gms	Chol. mgs	% Fat Cal.
PARKER HOUSE										
(Bridgford)	1 roll	85	3	16	172	0	1.3	0.0	0	14%
(Pepperidge Farm)	1 roll	60	2	9	80	0	1.0	0.0	5	17%
POTATO										
(Mrs. Wright's) Dutch style, long	1 roll	150	4	27	250	1	2.5	0.0	0	15%
(Pepperidge Farm)										
	1 roll	160	4	28	260	1	4.0	1.0	0	22%
'Hearty Classic'	1 roll	90	2	14	125	0	3.0	0.0	0	30%
SANDWICH										
(Arnold) w/egg, 'Dutch'	1 roll	123	5	22	203	2	3.3	0.0	1	22%
(Awrey's) oat bran	1 roll	120	4	22	250	1	2.0	0.0	0	15%
(Pepperidge Farm)										
'Deli Classic'	1 roll	110	4	16	150	0	4.0	0.0	10	31%
w/sesame seeds	1 roll	140	5	23	230	1	3.0	1.0	0	19%
SOFT (Pepperidge Farm) 'Family'	1 roll	100	4	18	190	1	2.0	1.0	0	17%
SOUR (Colombo Brand) 'Sour '49er'	1.2-oz roll	90	5	16	189	0	0.6	0.0	0	6%
SWEET (Colombo Brand) 'Sweet '49er'	1.2-oz roll	96	5	15	196	0	1.8	0.0	0	17%
STEAK										
(Colombo Brand)										
sour	2.6-oz roll	200	10	35	413	0	2.2	0.0	0	10%
sweet	2.6-oz roll	206	10	34	439	0	3.3	0.0	0	14%
TWIST (Pepperidge Farm) golden, 'Heat 'n Serve'	1 piece	110	2	14	150	0	5.0	2.0	5	41%
WHEAT										
(Country Oven) w/honey, brown and serve	1 roll	70	2	13	240	0	2.0	0.0	0	23%
(King's Hawaiian Bread) w/honey, ready-to-eat	1 roll	90	3	15	80	1	2.0	0.5	8	20%
ROLL, SWEET. See also BUN, SWEET; PASTRY.										
CARAMEL NUT (Aunt Fanny's) individual	2 oz	190	4	33	125	1	6.0	2.0	5	27%
CHEESE (Weight Watchers) frozen, microwave	1/2 pkg	180	5	32	210	0	4.0	1.0	5	20%
CHERRY										
(Break Cake)										
4.5 oz	2 rolls	400	8	79	390	0	3.0	1.8	0	7%
multi-pak, 1.4 oz	1 roll	130	2	25	125	0	2.0	0.6	0	14%
CINNAMON										
(Aunt Fanny's)										
11-oz size, rectangular	2 oz	181	4	34	83	0	3.0	1.0	8	15%
individual	1.9 oz	180	4	32	150	1	5.0	1.5	5	24%
(Awrey's)										
homestyle	1 piece	240	4	40	200	1	7.0	1.0	5	26%
swirl, 'Grande'	1 piece	340	4	46	370	1	16.0	3.0	10	42%
(Break Cake)										
4.5 oz	2 rolls	420	9	73	430	0	10.0	2.5	0	22%
multi pak, 1.3 oz	1 roll	120	3	22	125	0	3.0	0.8	0	21%
nut, 3 oz	2 rolls	330	5	52	220	0	11.0	2.0	0	30%
(Hostess Snack Cake)	1 serving	210	3	34	190	0	7.0	2.5	10	30%
(Hungry Jack) iced, refrigerated	2 pieces	290	3	37	570	0	14.0	0.0	0	44%
(Pillsbury)										
iced, refrigerated	1 piece	110	1	17	260	0	5.0	1.0	0	38%
raisin, w/icing	1 serving	180	2	26	310	1	7.0	1.5	0	36%
w/icing	1 serving	140	2	21	330	0	5.0	1.5	0	33%
(Sara Lee) all butter	2 oz piece	230	3	31	220	0	11.0	0.0	0	42%
(Weight Watchers) glazed	1 serving	200	4	33	200	2	5.0	1.5	5	23%
FRUIT (Aunt Fanny's) Dixie, individual	2 oz	180	3	34	120	1	4.0	1.5	5	20%
ORANGE (Hostess) swirl, 'Breakfast Bake Shop'	1 piece	230	3	26	150	1	12.0	6.0	10	48%

Food Name	Serving Size	Calories	Prot. gms	Carbs gms	Sod. mgs	Fiber gms	Fat gms	Sat. Fat gms	Chol. mgs	% Fat Cal.
PECAN										
(Aunt Fanny's) 11-oz size, rectangular	2 oz	184	4	32	79	0	4.0	1.0	8	20%
(Break Cake) multi pak, 1.3 oz	1 roll	120	2	22	120	0	3.0	0.6	0	22%
(Hostess) caramel swirl, 'Breakfast Bake Shop'	1 piece	240	3	23	160	2	15.0	7.0	10	56%
(Hostess) spinner, 'Breakfast Bake Shop'	1 piece	220	3	30	135	1	10.0	2.0	5	41%
RAISIN (Break Cake) cinnamon, multi pak, 1.25 oz.	1 roll	120	2	21	110	0	3.0	0.7	0	23%
STRAWBERRY										
(Aunt Fanny's) 11-oz size, rectangular	2 oz	190	4	35	140	0	4.0	0.0	5	19%
(Weight Watchers) frozen, microwave	1/2 pkg	170	3	29	90	0	5.0	1.0	20	26%
ROLL, SWEET, DOUGH										
(Pillsbury)										
apple cinnamon, w/icing, refrigerated, prepared	1 roll	140	2	21	310	1.0	5.0	1.5	0	33%
cinnamon raisin, w/icing, refrigerated, prepared	1 roll	180	2	26	310	1.0	7.0	1.5	0	36%
cinnamon, w/icing, refrigerated, prepared	1 roll	150	2	24	334	na	5.0	1.3	na	30%
ROLL DOUGH										
(Mrs. Wright's) crescent, refrigerated	1 roll	80	2	13	250	1	3.0	1.0	0	31%
(Pillsbury)										
butterflake, refrigerated	1 roll	140	3	20	530	0	5.0	1.0	0	33%
crescent, cheese, refrigerated	2 rolls	210	4	21	600	1	12.0	3.0	5	52%
(Rhodes)										
cinnamon, frozen	1 roll	236	4	35	238	1	9.6	na	12	36%
nonfat, no preservatives, 'Lite'	1 roll	89	3	18	135	1	0.4	0.0	0	4%
Parker House style, frozen	1 oz	90	2	14	156	0	2.0	0.0	0	22%
wheat, flaked, frozen	1 roll	140	6	24	210	3	3.0	0.0	0	18%
white, frozen	1 roll	98	3	17	141	1	2.1	0.0	0	18%
white, Texas style, frozen	1 roll	156	5	28	224	1	3.3	0.0	0	18%
whole wheat, Texas style, frozen	1 roll	140	7	24	210	4	3.0	0.0	0	18%
ROLL MIX										
(Dromedary)										
hot, mix only	1/8 pkg	209	6	41	363	0	2.0	0.0	0	9%
hot, prepared	2 pieces	239	6	41	410	0	5.0	0.0	0	19%
(Krusteaz) hot, prepared	1 roll	150	3	28	190	0	3.0	0.0	0	18%
(Pillsbury)										
hot	1/4 cup	110	3	21	200	1	1.0	0.0	0	9%
'Hot Roll Mix' prepared	1/16 pkg	120	4	21	210	0	2.0	0.0	15	15%
ROMAN BEAN. See BEAN, CRANBERRY.										
ROOT BEER. See under SOFT DRINKS AND MIXERS.										
ROSE COCO BEAN. See BEAN, CRANBERRY.										
ROSE PERCH. See OCEAN PERCH, ATLANTIC.										
ROSELLE										
raw, trimmed	1 cup	28	0.6	6.4	3	>.7 c	0.4	na	0	11%
trimmed	1 oz	14	0.3	3.2	2	>.3 c	0.2	(tr)	0	11%
untrimmed	1 lb	136	2.7	31.3	16	>3.2 c	1.8	na	0	11%
ROSEMARY										
Dried										
	1 tbsp	11	0	2	2	1	0.5	0.2	0	38%
	1 tsp	4	0	1	1	1	0.2	0.1	0	39%
(McCormick/Schilling)	1 tsp	6	0	1	0	1	0.0	0.0	0	0%
(Spice Islands)	1 tsp	5	0	1	1	0	0.2	0.0	0	33%
Fresh										
	1 tbsp	2	0	0	0	0	0.1	0.0	0	38%
	1 tsp	1	0	0	0	0	0.0	0.0	0	37%
Ground										
(Durkee)	1 tsp	5	0	0	0	0	0.0	0.0	0	0%

Food Name	Serving Size	Calories	Prot. gms	Carbs gms	Sod. mgs	Fiber gms	Fat gms	Sat. Fat gms	Chol. mgs	% Fat Cal.
(Laurel Leaf)	1 tsp	5	0	0	0	0	0.0	0.0	0	0%

ROTINI. See under PASTA.
ROTINI DISH/ENTRÉE. See under PASTA DISH/ENTRÉE.
ROTINI DISH/ENTRÉE MIX. See under PASTA DISH/ENTRÉE MIX.
RUCOLA. See ARUGULA.
RUGULA. See ARUGULA.
RUM

Food Name	Serving Size	Calories	Prot. gms	Carbs gms	Sod. mgs	Fiber gms	Fat gms	Sat. Fat gms	Chol. mgs	% Fat Cal.
80 proof	1 fl oz	64	0	0	0	0	0.0	0.0	0	0%
86 proof	1 fl oz	70	0	0	0	0	0.0	0.0	0	0%
90 proof	1 fl oz	73	0	0	0	0	0.0	0.0	0	0%
94 proof	1 fl oz	76	0	0	0	0	0.0	0.0	0	0%
100 proof	1 fl oz	82	0	0	0	0	0.0	0.0	0	0%

RUM RUNNER. See under COCKTAIL MIX.
RUTABAGA
Fresh

Food Name	Serving Size	Calories	Prot. gms	Carbs gms	Sod. mgs	Fiber gms	Fat gms	Sat. Fat gms	Chol. mgs	% Fat Cal.
boiled, drained, cubed	1 cup	66	2	15	34	3	0.4	0.0	0	5%
boiled, drained, mashed	1 cup	94	3	21	48	4	0.5	0.1	0	5%
raw, cubed	1 cup	50	2	11	28	4	0.3	0.0	0	5%
raw, whole	1 medium	139	5	31	77	10	0.8	0.1	0	5%
Canned, diced (Allens)	1/2 cup	20	1	4	260	0	1.0	0.0	0	31%

RYE

Food Name	Serving Size	Calories	Prot. gms	Carbs gms	Sod. mgs	Fiber gms	Fat gms	Sat. Fat gms	Chol. mgs	% Fat Cal.
	1 cup	566	25	118	10	25	4.2	0.5	0	6%
flakes, rolled (Arrowhead Mills)	1/3 cup	110	4	24	0	4	0.5	0.0	0	4%
whole-grain (Arrowhead Mills)	2 oz	190	7	42	1	8	1.0	0.0	0	4%
RYE CAKE (Quaker) 'Grain Cakes'	.32 oz piece	35	1	7	52	1	0.3	0.0	0	8%

RYE FLOUR. See under FLOUR.
RYE WHISKEY. See WHISKEY.

S

Food Name	Serving Size	Calories	Prot. gms	Carbs gms	Sod. mgs	Fiber gms	Fat gms	Sat. Fat gms	Chol. mgs	% Fat Cal.
SABLEFISH. See COD, ALASKAN.										
SACCHARIN. See under SUGAR SUBSTITUTE.										
SAFFLOWER OIL										
expeller pressed (Hollywood)	1 tbsp	120	0	0	0	0	14.0	1.0	0	100%
'Hi-Oleic' (Hain)	1 tbsp	120	0	0	0	0	14.0	1.0	0	100%
100% pure pressed (Loriva')	1 tbsp	120	0	0	0	0	12.0	1.0	0	100%
over 70% oleic	1 cup	1927	0	0	0	0	218.0	21.3	0	100%
over 70% oleic	1 tbsp	124	0	0	0	0	14.0	1.4	0	100%
pure pressed, organic (Spectrum)	1 tbsp	120	0	0	0	0	14.0	1.0	0	100%
salad or cooking, over 70% linoleic	1 cup	1927	0	0	0	0	218.0	13.5	0	100%
salad or cooking, over 70% linoleic	1 tbsp	120	0	0	0	0	13.6	0.8	0	100%
salad or cooking, over 70% oleic	1 cup	1927	0	0	0	0	218.0	13.5	0	100%
salad or cooking, over 70% oleic	1 tbsp	120	0	0	0	0	13.6	0.8	0	100%
SAFFLOWER SEED, kernels, dried	1 oz	147	5	10	1	na	10.9	1.0	0	62%
SAFFLOWER SEED MEAL, partially defatted	1 oz	97	10	14	1	na	0.7	0.1	0	6%
SAFFRON										
dried	1 tbsp	7	0	1	3	0	0.1	0.0	0	16%
dried	1 tsp	2	0	0	1	0	0.0	0.0	0	16%
SAGE										
ground	1 tbsp	6	0	1	0	1	0.3	0.1	0	34%
ground	1 tsp	2	0	0	0	0	0.1	0.0	0	34%

Food Name	Serving Size	Calories	Prot. gms	Carbs gms	Sod. mgs	Fiber gms	Fat gms	Sat. Fat gms	Chol. mgs	% Fat Cal.
ground *(Durkee)*	1 tbsp	9	0	0	0	0	0.0	0.0	0	0%
ground *(Durkee)*	1 tsp	3	0	0	0	0	0.0	0.0	0	0%
ground *(Laurel Leaf)*	1 tbsp	9	0	0	0	0	0.0	0.0	0	0%
ground *(Laurel Leaf)*	1 tsp	3	0	0	0	0	0.0	0.0	0	0%
ground *(McCormick/Schilling)*	1 tsp	4	0	0	0	0	0.0	0.0	0	0%
ground *(Spice Islands)*	1 tsp	4	0	1	1	0	0.1	0.1	0	24%
SALAD DRESSING										
(Estee) regular	1 tbsp	4	0	1	13	0	0.0	0.0	0	0%
(Johnny's) lite	2 tbsp	70	0	14	380	0	2.0	0.0	0	24%
(Ott's) lower calorie, 'Famous'	1 tbsp	26	0	4	60	0	1.3	0.0	0	43%
BACON										
(Estee) and tomato	1 tbsp	8	1	1	35	0	1.0	1.0	5	53%
(Kraft)										
and tomato	2 tbsp	140	1	2	280	0	14.0	2.5	3	93%
and tomato, reduced calorie	1 tbsp	30	0	2	150	0	2.0	0.0	0	69%
creamy, lower calorie	1 tbsp	30	0	2	150	0	2.0	0.0	0	69%
(T. Marzetti) buttermilk, refrigerated	1 tbsp	93	0	0	127	0	10.0	0.0	2	100%
BLUE CHEESE										
(Estee)	1 tbsp	8	1	1	50	0	1.0	1.0	0	53%
(Featherweight) 'Neu Bleu'	1 tbsp	4	0	1	110	0	0.0	0.0	0	0%
(Hidden Valley Ranch)										
	2 tbsp	20	0	4	270	0	0.0	0.0	0	0%
low-fat'	1 tbsp	10	0	3	140	0	0.0	0.0	0	0%
(Kraft)										
	2 tbsp	45	0	11	360	1	0.0	0.0	0	0%
chunky	1 tbsp	60	1	2	230	0	6.0	1.0	5	82%
chunky, lower calorie	1 tbsp	30	0	2	240	0	2.0	1.0	5	69%
(La Martinique) vinaigrette	2 tbsp	160	2	0	450	0	17.0	6.0	5	95%
(Lawry's) 'Classic' 1 oz	1 tbsp	186	0	2	385	0	2.0	0.0	0	69%
(Litehouse)										
and dip, refrigerated, 'Lite'	1 tbsp	33	1	1	86	0	3.0	0.0	0	77%
and dip, refrigerated, 'Original'	1 tbsp	77	1	0	82	0	8.0	0.0	0	95%
country, and dip, refrigerated	1 tbsp	76	1	0	84	0	8.0	0.0	0	95%
(Roka)										
	1 tbsp	60	1	1	170	0	6.0	1.0	10	87%
lower calorie	1 tbsp	16	1	1	280	0	1.0	1.0	5	53%
(S&W) 'Nutradiet'	1 tbsp	25	0	2	200	0	2.0	0.0	0	69%
(T. Marzetti)										
	1 tbsp	90	1	1	180	0	9.0	0.0	2	91%
buttermilk, refrigerated	1 tbsp	90	1	1	161	0	10.0	0.0	5	92%
chunky, refrigerated	1 tbsp	78	1	1	159	0	8.0	0.0	14	90%
'Light'	1 tbsp	90	1	1	180	0	9.0	0.0	2	91%
refrigerated, 'Lite'	1 tbsp	45	0	0	150	0	5.0	0.0	5	100%
(Walden Farms) calorie-free	2 tbsp	0	0	0	260	0	0.0	0.0	0	0%
(Wish-Bone)										
chunky	1 tbsp	75	0	1	149	0	7.9	1.2	1	94%
chunky, light	2 tbsp	80	1	2	410	0	8.0	0.0	0	86%
BUTTERMILK										
(Hain) buttermilk, 'Old Fashioned'	1 tbsp	70	0	0	100	0	7.0	0.0	0	100%
(Hollywood) 'Old Fashioned'	1 tbsp	75	0	1	40	0	8.0	1.0	0	95%
(Kraft)										
creamy	1 tbsp	80	0	1	120	0	8.0	1.0	5	95%
creamy, lower calorie	1 tbsp	30	0	1	125	0	3.0	0.0	5	87%

Food Name	Serving Size	Calories	Prot. gms	Carbs gms	Sod. mgs	Fiber gms	Fat gms	Sat. Fat gms	Chol. mgs	% Fat Cal.
(Seven Seas) 'Buttermilk Recipe'	1 tbsp	80	0	1	130	0	8.0	1.0	5	95%
(T. Marzetti) and herbs	1 tbsp	95	0	0	150	0	10.0	0.0	3	100%
CAESAR										
(Cardini's)	2 tbsp	80	0	1	100	1	8.0	1.0	9	95%
(Cook's Classics)	1 tbsp	50	1	1	30	0	5.0	0.9	0	85%
(Estee)	2 tbsp	8	1	1	130	0	1.0	0.0	2	53%
(Hain)										
creamy	1 tbsp	60	0	1	220	0	6.0	0.0	5	93%
creamy, low-salt	1 tbsp	60	0	1	15	0	6.0	0.0	5	93%
(Hollywood)	1 tbsp	70	1	2	65	0	7.0	1.0	0	84%
(Johnny's) 'Great Caesar'	2 tbsp	170	1	1	260	0	18.0	1.5	1	95%
(Kraft) golden	1 tbsp	70	0	1	180	0	7.0	1.0	0	94%
(Lawry's) 'Classic'	1 tbsp	130	1	1	337	0	13.5	1.8	0	94%
(Litehouse) and dip, refrigerated	1 tbsp	57	0	0	84	0	6.0	0.0	0	100%
(T. Marzetti)										
	1 tbsp	80	0	1	170	0	8.0	0.0	2	95%
light, 50% less fat	2 tbsp	80	1	1	370	0	7.0	1.0	10	91%
refrigerated	1 tbsp	75	0	0	178	0	8.0	0.0	0	100%
house	1 tbsp	75	1	1	180	0	8.0	0.0	1	90%
(Walden Farms) calorie-free	2 tbsp	0	0	0	360	0	0.0	0.0	0	0%
(Weight Watchers)										
nonfat	1 tbsp	5	0	1	195	0	0.0	0.0	0	0%
(Weight Watchers) nonfat, 'Single Serve'	1 tbsp	6	0	1	270	0	0.0	0.0	0	0%
(Wish-Bone)										
	1 tbsp	77	0	1	248	0	8.0	1.2	1	93%
w/olive oil	2 tbsp	100	0	2	400	0	10.0	1.5	0	92%
w/olive oil, 'Lite'	2 tbsp	60	1	3	410	0	5.0	1.0	0	74%
CATALINA *(Kraft)* Catalina, nonfat	2 tbsp	35	0	8	320	1	0.0	0.0	0	0%
CELERY SEED										
(T. Marzetti)										
and onion	1 tbsp	75	0	9	90	0	6.0	0.0	0	60%
refrigerated	1 tbsp	72	0	5	101	0	5.0	0.0	0	69%
CHEESE										
(Bernstein's) 'Cheese Fantastico Parmesan'	2 tbsp	30	1	5	360	0	1.0	0.0	0	27%
(Featherweight)	1 tbsp	20	0	1	70	0	2.0	0.0	0	82%
(Hollywood)	1 tbsp	80	0	2	60	0	8.0	1.0	0	90%
(Lawry's) creamy, w/Parmesan, 'Classic'	1 oz	156	0	5	178	0	15.1	2.1	0	88%
(Wish-Bone)	1 tbsp	89	0	1	170	0	9.2	1.3	1	95%
CILANTRO *(Paula's)* and tomato, 'Herb Garden'	0.5 oz	54	0	1	26	0	6.0	0.0	0	93%
CITRUS *(Hain)* tangy, 'Canola'	1 tbsp	50	0	1	75	0	5.0	0.0	0	92%
COLESLAW										
(Best Foods) 'One Step'	2 tbsp	160	0	4	180	0	16.0	2.5	5	90%
(Hellmann's) 'One Step'	2 tbsp	160	0	4	180	0	16.0	2.5	5	90%
(Blue Plate)	2 tbsp	140	0	5	240	0	13.0	2.0	15	85%
(JFG)	2 tbsp	140	0	5	240	0	13.0	2.0	15	85%
(Kraft)	1 tbsp	70	0	4	200	0	6.0	1.0	10	77%
(Litehouse) refrigerated	1 tbsp	80	0	2	41	0	8.0	0.0	0	90%
(T. Marzetti)										
light	1 tbsp	50	0	6	240	0	3.0	0.0	0	53%
original	1 tbsp	79	1	3	180	0	7.0	0.0	14	80%
'South Recipe'	1 tbsp	66	0	6	93	0	5.0	0.0	9	65%
(Hidden Valley Ranch) coleslaw, nonfat	2 tbsp	35	0	9	200	1	0.0	0.0	0	0%
CREAMY										
(Estee) nonfat	1 tbsp	4	0	1	13	0	0.0	0.0	0	0%

Food Name	Serving Size	Calories	Prot. gms	Carbs gms	Sod. mgs	Fiber gms	Fat gms	Sat. Fat gms	Chol. mgs	% Fat Cal.
(Hain)										
....	1 tbsp	80	0	0	100	0	8.0	0.0	0	100%
no salt added........................	1 tbsp	80	0	1	25	0	8.0	0.0	0	95%
(Hollywood) creamy....................	1 tbsp	90	0	2	140	0	9.0	1.0	0	91%
(Kraft)										
house,...............................	1 tbsp	60	0	1	115	0	6.0	1.0	0	93%
house, lower calorie	1 tbsp	30	0	1	115	0	2.0	0.0	0	82%
lower calorie	1 tbsp	25	0	1	120	0	2.0	0.0	0	82%
nonfat, no oil, lower calorie	1 tbsp	4	0	1	220	0	0.0	0.0	0	0%
w/real sour cream	1 tbsp	50	0	1	120	0	5.0	1.0	0	92%
zesty	1 tbsp	50	0	1	260	0	5.0	1.0	0	92%
zesty, lower calorie	1 tbsp	20	0	1	230	0	2.0	0.0	0	82%
(Life) creamy, egg-free, 'All Natural' ..	1 tbsp	39	1	2	4	0	4.0	0.0	0	75%
(Pathmark)										
....	1 tbsp	70	0	1	260	0	7.0	1.0	0	94%
zesty	1 tbsp	70	0	1	370	0	8.0	1.0	0	95%
zesty, nonfat, lower calorie	1 tbsp	6	0	1	190	0	0.0	0.0	0	0%
(Rancher's Choice)										
....	1 tbsp	90	0	1	140	0	10.0	1.0	5	96%
lower calorie	1 tbsp	30	0	1	150	0	3.0	0.0	5	87%
(S&W)										
nonfat, no oil	1 tbsp	2	0	0	290	0	0.0	0.0	0	0%
'Nutradiet'	1 tbsp	10	0	1	180	0	1.0	0.0	0	69%
(Seven Seas) creamy..................	1 tbsp	70	0	1	240	0	7.0	1.0	0	94%
(Weight Watchers) creamy, nonfat, 'Single Serve'..........	1 tbsp	9	0	2	430	0	0.0	0.0	0	0%
(Wish-Bone)										
....	1 tbsp	56	0	2	149	0	5.5	0.9	1	89%
herbal, 'Classics'	1 tbsp	70	0	1	228	0	7.3	0.0	0	93%
'Lite'	1 tbsp	26	0	2	148	0	2.0	0.4	1	68%
CUCUMBER										
(Featherweight) creamy, nonfat	1 tbsp	4	0	1	80	0	0.0	0.0	0	0%
(Hain) dill, creamy	1 tbsp	80	0	0	210	0	8.0	0.0	5	100%
(Herb Magic) creamy, no oil..........	2 tbsp	15	0	4	270	na	0.0	na	0	0%
(Kraft)										
creamy	1 tbsp	70	0	1	190	0	8.0	1.0	0	95%
creamy, less fat, lower calorie	1 tbsp	25	0	1	220	0	2.0	0.0	0	82%
DIJON										
(Estee) creamy......................	1 tbsp	8	1	1	100	0	1.0	1.0	5	53%
(Featherweight) creamy..............	1 tbsp	20	0	1	80	0	2.0	0.0	0	82%
(Great Impressions) mustard.........	1 tbsp	57	0	0	103	0	6.1	0.0	18	95%
(Cook's Classics) oil-free...........	1 tbsp	8	0	2	100	0	0.0	0.0	0	0%
(Pritikin) w/balsamic vinegar, nonfat ..	2 tbsp	30	0	6	125	0	0.0	0.0	0	0%
DILL										
(Nasoya) creamy	2 tbsp	63	1	3	145	0	5.4	0.4	0	76%
(Hain) cucumber, creamy.............	1 tbsp	80	0	0	210	0	8.0	0.0	5	100%
(Paula's) and garlic, 'Herb Garden' ..	0.5 oz	54	0	1	28	0	6.0	0.0	0	93%
FRENCH										
(Catalina)										
....	1 tbsp	60	0	4	180	0	5.0	1.0	0	74%
reduced calorie	1 tbsp	18	0	3	120	0	1.0	0.0	0	43%
(Cook's Classics) 'Country French' ..	1 tbsp	10	0	3	80	0	0.0	0.0	0	0%
(Estee)										
....	1 tbsp	4	0	1	10	0	0.0	0.0	0	0%
creamy	2 tbsp	10	0	2	130	0	0.0	0.0	0	0%

Food Name	Serving Size	Calories	Prot. gms	Carbs gms	Sod. mgs	Fiber gms	Fat gms	Sat. Fat gms	Chol. mgs	% Fat Cal.
(Featherweight)	1 tbsp	14	0	3	15	0	0.0	0.0	0	0%
(Great Impressions) w/green pepper, low-calorie	1 tbsp	64	0	4	188	0	5.2	0.0	0	73%
(Hain)										
creamy	1 tbsp	60	0	1	80	0	6.0	0.0	0	93%
spicy mustard, 'Canola'	1 tbsp	50	1	1	190	0	5.0	0.0	5	85%
(Hollywood) creamy	1 tbsp	70	0	2	45	0	7.0	1.0	0	89%
(Kraft)										
	1 tbsp	60	0	2	125	0	6.0	1.0	0	87%
'Miracle'	1 tbsp	70	0	3	240	0	6.0	1.0	0	82%
reduced calorie	1 tbsp	20	0	3	120	0	1.0	0.0	0	43%
(Litehouse) country herb, and marinade, refrigerated	1 tbsp	54	0	2	196	0	5.0	0.0	0	85%
(Pathmark)										
creamy	1 tbsp	60	0	2	90	0	5.0	1.0	0	85%
reduced calorie	1 tbsp	20	0	3	160	0	1.0	0.0	0	43%
(Pritikin)										
sodium-free	1 tbsp	10	0	3	0	0	0.0	0.0	0	0%
(S&W) 'Nutradiet'	1 tbsp	18	0	3	120	0	0.0	0.0	0	0%
(Seven Seas)										
creamy	1 tbsp	60	0	2	240	0	6.0	1.0	0	87%
'French! Light'	1 tbsp	35	0	2	210	0	3.0	0.0	0	77%
(T. Marzetti)										
California French	1 tbsp	90	1	5	100	0	6.0	0.0	4	69%
California, 'Light'	1 tbsp	40	0	3	180	0	3.0	0.0	2	69%
country	1 tbsp	72	0	4	110	0	6.0	0.0	6	77%
fat-free, 'California French'	1 tbsp	16	1	4	140	0	0.0	0.0	0	0%
'Frenchette'	1 tbsp	10	0	3	140	0	0.0	0.0	0	0%
honey, blue, refrigerated	1 tbsp	70	0	5	122	0	6.0	0.0	1	73%
honey, refrigerated	1 tbsp	74	0	5	115	0	6.0	0.0	0	73%
honey, refrigerated, 'Lite'	1 tbsp	48	0	5	118	0	3.0	0.0	0	57%
'Light'	1 tbsp	16	0	3	160	0	1.0	0.0	0	43%
(Ultra Slim Fast) cholesterol-free	1 tbsp	20	0	4	105	0	1.0	0.0	0	36%
(Weight Watchers) low-calorie	1 tbsp	10	0	2	170	0	0.0	0.0	0	0%
(Wish-Bone)										
'Deluxe Food Service'	1 tbsp	61	0	2	86	0	5.6	0.0	0	83%
'Deluxe'	1 tbsp	60	0	2	83	0	5.4	0.8	0	84%
garlic, creamy	1 tbsp	55	0	2	158	0	5.3	0.0	0	86%
'Lite'	1 tbsp	31	0	2	70	0	2.5	0.0	0	73%
'Lite Sweet 'n Spicy'	1 tbsp	18	0	3	110	0	0.5	0.0	0	26%
low-calorie, 'Lite'	1 tbsp	30	0	2	67	0	2.5	0.1	0	74%
red, low-calorie, 'Lite'	1 tbsp	17	0	3	155	0	0.4	0.0	0	21%
'Sweet'n Spicy'	1 tbsp	63	0	3	156	0	5.7	0.8	0	81%
FRUIT SALAD										
(Knott's Berry Farm)	1 tbsp	50	2	3	75	0	5.0	0.0	0	69%
(Great Impressions) orange marmalade	1 tbsp	87	0	5	48	0	7.1	0.0	11	74%
GARLIC										
(Cook's Classics) 'Garlic Lover's'	1 tbsp	50	0	1	95	0	5.0	0.8	0	92%
(Estee) creamy, nonfat	1 tbsp	2	0	0	10	0	0.0	0.0	0	0%
(Hain) and sour cream	1 tbsp	70	0	0	100	0	7.0	0.0	0	100%
(Kraft)										
creamy	2 tbsp	110	0	2	360	0	11.0	2.0	0	93%
creamy	1 tbsp	50	0	1	170	0	5.0	1.0	0	92%
(Life) w/tofu, and dip, 'All Natural'	1 tbsp	70	1	1	0	0	7.1	0.0	75	87%
(Pritikin) herb, nonfat, sodium-free	1 tbsp	6	0	2	0	0	0.0	0.0	0	0%

Food Name	Serving Size	Calories	Prot. gms	Carbs gms	Sod. mgs	Fiber gms	Fat gms	Sat. Fat gms	Chol. mgs	% Fat Cal.
(Wish-Bone) creamy	1 tbsp	74	0	1	158	1	8.0	0.0	0	97%
HERB										
(Featherweight)										
	1 tbsp	25	0	2	65	0	2.0	0.0	0	69%
nonfat	1 tbsp	6	0	1	5	0	0.0	0.0	0	0%
(Hain) savory, 'No Salt Added'	1 tbsp	90	0	0	25	0	10.0	0.0	0	100%
(Nasoya)										
garden	2 tbsp	62	1	3	149	0	5.4	0.0	0	77%
garlic, 'Vegi-Dressing'	1 tbsp	40	1	1	50	0	3.0	0.0	0	77%
(Pritikin) garlic and, nonfat, sodium-free	1 tbsp	6	0	2	0	0	0.0	0.0	0	0%
(Seven Seas)										
and spice, 'Viva'	1 tbsp	60	0	1	170	0	6.0	1.0	0	93%
'Viva Herbs and Spices! Light'	1 tbsp	30	0	1	200	0	3.0	0.0	0	87%
HOMESTYLE										
(Dorothy Lynch)										
	1 tbsp	55	0	5	85	0	3.8	0.5	0	63%
lower calorie	1 tbsp	30	0	7	80	0	1.0	0.0	0	24%
HONEY (Hain) and sesame	1 tbsp	60	0	2	210	0	5.0	0.0	0	85%
HONEY MUSTARD										
(Cook's Classics) apple	1 tbsp	50	0	2	80	0	6.0	1.0	0	87%
(Knott's Berry Farm) 'Peggy Jane's'	1 tbsp	60	0	2	40	0	6.0	0.0	0	87%
(Kraft) Dijon, nonfat	2 tbsp	45	0	10	330	1	0.0	0.0	0	0%
(Litehouse) and dip, refrigerated	1 tbsp	67	0	2	55	0	7.0	0.0	0	89%
(Marzetti) Dijon, peppercorn	2 tbsp	150	0	7	250	0	13.0	2.0	20	81%
(Pritikin) Dijon	2 tbsp	45	0	11	130	1	0.0	0.0	0	0%
(T. Marzetti)										
Dijon	1 tbsp	67	0	3	51	0	6.0	0.0	7	82%
Dijon, light	1 tbsp	24	0	6	69	0	0.0	0.0	0	0%
Dijon, refrigerated	1 tbsp	68	0	3	103	0	6.0	0.0	9	82%
Dijon ranch	1 tbsp	89	1	1	100	0	9.0	0.0	14	91%
(Weight Watchers) Dijon, nonfat	1 tbsp	23	0	6	75	0	0.0	0.0	0	0%
(Wish-Bone) Dijon, 'Healthy Sensation!'	1 tbsp	25	0	5	140	0	0.0	0.0	0	0%
ITALIAN										
(Bernstein's) herb and garlic, creamy	1 tbsp	60	0	1	135	0	6.0	0.0	5	93%
(Best Foods) creamy, homestyle	2 tsp	60	0	0	80	0	7.0	1.0	5	100%
(Cardini's)	2 tbsp	130	0	1	195	0	14.0	2.0	0	97%
(Cook's Classics) garlic gusto, oil free	1 tbsp	6	0	1	90	0	0.0	0.0	0	0%
(Estee)										
creamy	2 tbsp	14	1	2	130	0	1.0	0.0	0	43%
nonfat	2 tbsp	4	0	1	130	0	0.0	0.0	0	0%
(Featherweight) nonfat	1 tbsp	4	0	1	120	0	0.0	0.0	0	0%
(Hain)										
'Canola'	1 tbsp	50	0	1	150	0	5.0	0.0	0	92%
no oil	1 tbsp	2	0	1	170	0	0.0	0.0	0	0%
no salt added, 'Traditional'	1 tbsp	60	0	1	20	0	6.0	0.0	0	93%
Thousand Island, no oil	1 tbsp	12	0	3	150	0	0.0	0.0	1	0%
'Traditional'	1 tbsp	80	0	0	330	0	8.0	0.0	0	100%
(Herb Magic) no oil	2 tbsp	10	0	2	260	na	0.0	na	na	0%
(Hidden Valley Ranch) parmesan, lowfat	1 tbsp	16	0	3	140	0	1.0	0.0	0	43%
(Hollywood)	1 tbsp	90	0	1	300	0	9.0	1.0	0	95%
(Kraft)										
creamy, 'Deliciously Light'	1 tbsp	25	0	1	120	0	2.0	0.0	0	82%
creamy, 'Reduce-Calorie'	1 tbsp	25	0	1	120	0	2.0	0.0	0	82%
creamy, w/real sour cream	1 tbsp	50	0	1	120	0	5.0	1.0	0	92%

Food Name	Serving Size	Calories	Prot. gms	Carbs gms	Sod. mgs	Fiber gms	Fat gms	Sat. Fat gms	Chol. mgs	% Fat Cal.
'Deliciously Light'	1 tbsp	35	0	1	115	0	3.0	0.0	0	87%
house	1 tbsp	60	0	1	115	0	6.0	1.0	0	93%
house, reduced calorie	1 tbsp	30	0	1	115	0	2.0	0.0	0	82%
nonfat	2 tbsp	20	0	4	430	0	0.0	0.0	0	0%
nonfat, 'Free'	2 tbsp	20	0	4	430	0	0.3	0.2	1	13%
nonfat, 'Healthy Sensation'	2 tbsp	15	0	2	280	0	0.0	0.0	0	0%
nonfat, oil-free 'Reduce-Calorie'	1 tbsp	4	0	1	220	0	0.0	0.0	0	0%
'Presto'	1 tbsp	70	0	1	150	0	7.0	1.0	0	94%
zesty	2 tbsp	109	0	2	505	0	11.1	1.2	0	92%
zesty	1 tbsp	50	0	1	260	0	5.0	1.0	0	92%
zesty, reduced calorie	1 tbsp	20	0	1	230	0	2.0	0.0	0	82%
(Litehouse) creamy, and dip, refrigerated	1 tbsp	60	0	0	76	0	6.0	0.0	0	100%
(Nasoya)										
creamy	2 tbsp	61	1	3	188	0	5.2	0.4	0	76%
'Vegi-Dressing'	1 tbsp	40	1	1	50	0	3.0	0.0	0	77%
(Ott's)	1 tbsp	80	0	0	87	0	9.1	0.0	1	99%
(Pritikin)										
sodium-free, nonfat	1 tbsp	8	0	2	0	0	0.0	0.0	0	0%
zesty, nonfat	2 tbsp	20	0	5	115	0	0.0	0.0	0	0%
(Seven Seas)										
creamy	2 tbsp	120	0	1	510	0	12.0	2.0	0	96%
nonfat	2 tbsp	50	0	12	330	1	0.0	0.0	0	0%
nonfat, 'Free Viva'	1 tbsp	4	0	1	220	0	0.0	0.0	0	0%
'Viva Creamy Italian! Light'	1 tbsp	45	0	1	230	0	4.0	1.0	0	90%
'Viva Italian! Light'	1 tbsp	30	0	1	230	0	3.0	0.0	0	87%
'Viva'	1 tbsp	50	0	1	240	0	5.0	1.0	0	92%
(T. Marzetti)										
creamy	1 tbsp	80	0	1	100	0	8.0	0.0	4	95%
garlic, refrigerated	1 tbsp	81	0	1	73	0	9.0	0.0	9	95%
gusto	1 tbsp	58	0	0	204	0	8.0	0.0	0	100%
'Light'	1 tbsp	35	0	1	300	0	3.0	0.0	0	87%
nonfat, 'Fat-Free'	1 tbsp	5	0	1	270	0	0.0	0.0	0	0%
nonfat, 'Frenchette'	1 tbsp	6	0	2	280	0	0.0	0.0	0	0%
'Olde Venice'	2 tbsp	130	0	2	490	0	13.0	2.0	0	94%
Romano cheese, refrigerated	1 tbsp	77	1	1	183	0	8.0	0.0	3	90%
Romano	1 tbsp	80	0	0	135	0	8.0	0.0	2	100%
w/olive oil	1 tbsp	60	0	1	220	0	7.0	0.0	0	94%
(Ultra Slim Fast) cholesterol-free	1 tbsp	6	0	1	105	0	1.0	0.0	0	69%
(Walden Farms)										
calorie-free	2 tbsp	0	0	0	350	0	0.0	0.0	0	0%
country, calorie-free	2 tbsp	0	0	0	260	1	0.0	0.0	0	0%
w/sun-dried tomatoes, calorie-free	2 tbsp	0	0	0	390	0	0.0	0.0	0	0%
(Weight Watchers)										
	1 tbsp	2	0	0	140	0	0.0	0.0	0	0%
creamy	1 tbsp	3	0	1	180	0	0.0	0.0	0	0%
creamy, nonfat	1 tbsp	12	0	3	85	0	0.0	0.0	0	0%
creamy, whipped	1 tbsp	50	0	2	80	0	5.0	5.0	5	85%
nonfat	1 tbsp	6	0	1	200	0	0.0	0.0	0	0%
nonfat, 'Single Serve'	0.75 oz	8	0	2	270	0	0.0	0.0	0	0%
(Wish-Bone)										
	1 tbsp	46	0	2	280	0	4.5	0.6	0	87%
'Lite'	1 tbsp	7	0	1	212	0	0.3	0.0	0	38%
nonfat, 'Healthy Sensation!'	1 tbsp	6	0	1	140	0	0.0	0.0	0	0%
olive oil, 'Classic'	1 tbsp	34	0	2	190	0	3.0	0.4	0	80%

Food Name	Serving Size	Calories	Prot. gms	Carbs gms	Sod. mgs	Fiber gms	Fat gms	Sat. Fat gms	Chol. mgs	% Fat Cal.
'Robusto'	1 tbsp	47	0	2	288	0	4.5	0.6	0	84%
MAYONNAISE TYPE										
(A&P)	1 tbsp	70	1	2	100	0	7.0	1.0	0	84%
(Bama)	1 tbsp	50	0	3	105	0	4.0	0.0	0	75%
(Blue Plate)	1 tbsp	70	0	2	105	0	7.0	1.0	5	89%
(Finast)	1 tbsp	70	0	2	90	0	7.0	0.0	0	89%
(Hain) eggless, no salt added	1 tbsp	110	0	0	0	0	12.0	1.5	0	100%
(JFG)	1 tbsp	50	0	2	125	0	5.0	1.0	5	85%
(Kraft)										
light	1 tbsp	50	0	1	120	0	4.9	0.8	5	89%
'Miracle Whip'	1 tbsp	70	0	2	85	0	7.0	1.0	5	89%
'Miracle Whip Light'	1 tbsp	45	0	2	125	0	4.0	1.0	0	82%
nonfat	1 tbsp	11	0	2	120	0	0.4	0.1	2	35%
nonfat, 'Miracle Whip-Free'	1 tbsp	20	0	5	210	0	0.0	0.0	0	0%
(Ott's) 'Famous'	1 tbsp	40	0	4	195	0	2.7	0.0	1	59%
(P&Q)	1 tbsp	50	1	3	110	0	5.0	1.0	8	74%
(Pathmark) 'No Frills'	1 tbsp	50	0	3	120	0	5.0	1.0	5	79%
(Spin Blend)										
	1 tbsp	60	0	3	110	0	5.0	1.0	10	79%
cholesterol-free	1 tbsp	40	0	2	110	0	4.0	1.0	0	82%
(Weight Watchers)										
whipped	1 tbsp	45	0	3	100	0	4.0	1.0	0	75%
whipped, low-sodium	1 tbsp	50	0	1	45	0	5.0	1.0	5	92%
whipped, nonfat	1 tbsp	12	0	4	125	0	0.0	0.0	0	0%
ONION										
(Kraft) and chives, creamy	1 tbsp	70	0	1	150	0	7.0	1.0	0	94%
(Paula's) toasted, nonfat	2 tbsp	10	0	3	80	0	0.0	0.0	0	0%
(Wish-Bone) and chives, 'Lite'	1 tbsp	37	0	2	164	0	3.3	0.0	0	80%
ORIENTAL STYLE (Featherweight)	1 tbsp	20	0	1	75	0	2.0	0.0	0	82%
PARMESAN (T. Marzetti) peppercorn, refrigerated	1 tbsp	81	1	1	129	0	9.0	0.0	6	91%
PEANUT (A Taste of Thai) spicy	1 tbsp	40	1	6	360	1	1.5	0.5	0	33%
PEPPERCORN										
(Litehouse) and dip, refrigerated	1 tbsp	67	0	0	66	0	7.0	0.0	0	100%
(T. Marzetti) cracked, refrigerated	1 tbsp	62	0	0	135	0	7.0	0.0	13	100%
(Weight Watchers) creamy, nonfat	1 tbsp	8	0	2	85	0	0.0	0.0	0	0%
PESTO (Cardini's) pasta, w/basil	2 tbsp	140	0	0	195	0	14.0	6.0	0	100%
POPPYSEED										
(Great Impressions)	2 tbsp	131	0	8	130	0	11.0	0.0	0	75%
(Hain) Natural Classics	2 tbsp	140	1	3	250	0	14.0	2.0	5	90%
(Knott's Berry Farm)										
	2 tbsp	120	0	10	190	0	9.0	1.5	0	67%
Peggy Jane's'	1 tbsp	60	0	4	90	0	5.0	0.0	0	74%
(La Martinique)	2 tbsp	170	0	8	330	0	15.0	4.0	na	81%
(Litehouse) and dip, refrigerated	1 tbsp	65	0	3	83	0	6.0	0.0	0	82%
(T. Marzetti) refrigerated	1 tbsp	72	1	5	146	0	6.0	0.0	8	69%
POTATO SALAD										
(Best Foods) One Step	2 tbsp	160	0	2	370	0	17.0	2.5	5	95%
(Blue Plate)	2 tbsp	130	0	1	380	0	14.0	2.5	15	97%
(Hellmann's) One Step	2 tbsp	160	0	2	370	0	17.0	2.5	5	95%
(JFG)	2 tbsp	130	0	1	380	0	14.0	2.5	15	97%
(T. Marzetti)	1 tbsp	80	0	3	170	0	7.0	0.0	9	84%
RANCH										
(Bernstein's) Parmesan garlic	2 tbsp	45	2	7	280	0	1.0	0.5	5	20%

Food Name	Serving Size	Calories	Prot. gms	Carbs gms	Sod. mgs	Fiber gms	Fat gms	Sat. Fat gms	Chol. mgs	% Fat Cal.
(Best Foods)										
homestyle	2 tsp	70	0	1	120	0	7.0	0.0	0	94%
homestyle, light,	1 1/3 tbsp	70	0	2	200	0	7.0	1.0	0	89%
(Hellmann's)										
homestyle	2 tsp	70	0	1	120	0	7.0	0.0	0	94%
light, homestyle	1 1/3 tbsp	70	0	2	200	0	7.0	1.0	0	89%
(Herb Magic) no oil	2 tbsp	15	1	4	270	na	0.0	na	0	0%
(Hidden Valley Ranch)										
94% fat-free	2 tbsp	40	0	5	320	0	2.0	0.0	0	47%
honey Dijon	2 tbsp	35	1	7	270	0	0.0	0.0	0	0%
honey Dijon, low-fat	1 tbsp	20	0	3	140	0	1.0	0.0	0	43%
original, 'Light'	1 tbsp	40	0	2	140	0	4.0	0.0	5	82%
(Kraft)										
	2 tbsp	148	0	1	287	0	15.6	2.4	8	95%
buttermilk	2 tbsp	150	0	1	240	0	16.0	2.5	3	97%
cucumber	2 tbsp	140	0	2	220	0	15.0	2.0	0	94%
light, 'Light Done Right!'	2 tbsp	77	0	3	303	0	6.8	0.6	8	80%
nonfat	2 tbsp	48	0	11	354	0	0.3	0.1	0	7%
nonfat, 'Healthy Sensation'	2 tbsp	40	0	9	280	0	0.0	0.0	0	0%
peppercorn, nonfat	2 tbsp	45	0	11	330	1	0.0	0.0	0	0%
w/salsa	2 tbsp	130	0	1	320	0	13.0	2.0	10	97%
(Litehouse)										
and dip, refrigerated	1 tbsp	59	0	1	67	0	6.0	0.0	0	93%
and dip, refrigerated, 'Lite'	1 tbsp	35	1	1	80	0	3.0	0.0	0	77%
country, and dip, refrigerated	1 tbsp	61	0	1	75	0	7.0	0.0	0	94%
jalapeño, and dip, refrigerated	1 tbsp	60	0	1	80	0	6.0	0.0	0	93%
(Pritikin) sodium-free, nonfat	1 tbsp	16	0	4	0	0	0.0	0.0	0	0%
(Seven Seas)										
'Buttermilk Recipe Ranch! Light'	1 tbsp	50	0	1	135	0	5.0	1.0	0	92%
nonfat	2 tbsp	45	0	11	330	1	0.0	0.0	0	0%
'Viva Ranch! Light'	1 tbsp	50	0	2	125	0	5.0	1.0	5	85%
'Viva'	1 tbsp	80	0	1	135	0	8.0	1.0	5	95%
(T. Marzetti)										
(T. Marzetti)	1 tbsp	90	0	0	92	0	2.0	0.0	3	100%
buttermilk, refrigerated	1 tbsp	93	0	0	127	0	10.0	0.0	2	100%
buttermilk, refrigerated, 'Lite'	1 tbsp	45	0	1	135	0	5.0	0.0	3	92%
Caesar	1 tbsp	95	1	1	150	0	10.0	0.0	3	92%
fat-free	1 tbsp	12	1	3	220	0	0.0	0.0	0	0%
garden	1 tbsp	100	0	1	165	0	10.0	0.0	2	96%
honey Dijon	1 tbsp	89	1	1	100	0	9.0	0.0	14	91%
'Light'	1 tbsp	40	0	2	166	0	4.0	0.0	2	82%
Parmesan, refrigerated	1 tbsp	86	0	1	120	0	9.0	0.0	6	95%
peppercorn	1 tbsp	85	0	1	13	0	9.0	0.0	4	95%
peppercorn, fat-free	1 tbsp	14	0	3	173	0	0.0	0.0	0	0%
(Walden Farms) calorie-free	2 tbsp	0	0	0	360	1	0.0	0.0	0	0%
(Weight Watchers)										
creamy, nonfat	1 tbsp	25	0	6	100	0	0.0	0.0	0	0%
creamy, nonfat, 'Single Serve'	1 pkt	35	0	8	140	0	0.0	0.0	0	0%
(Wish-Bone)										
	1 tbsp	78	0	1	156	0	8.3	1.2	4	94%
and salsa, 'Santa Fe'	2 tbsp	150	0	3	220	0	15.0	2.5	5	92%
lite	2 tbsp	100	0	5	300	0	9.0	2.0	5	80%
nonfat, 'Healthy Sensation!'	1 tbsp	16	0	3	140	0	0.0	0.0	0	0%

Food Name	Serving Size	Calories	Prot. gms	Carbs gms	Sod. mgs	Fiber gms	Fat gms	Sat. Fat gms	Chol. mgs	% Fat Cal.
RASPBERRY										
(Walden Farms) diet	2 tbsp	<1	0	0	380	0	0.0	0.0	0	0%
(Pritikin) vinaigrette, w/olive oil	2 tbsp	45	0	11	70	0	0.0	0.0	0	0%
RUSSIAN										
(Kraft)										
	1 tbsp	60	0	4	130	0	5.0	1.0	0	74%
creamy	1 tbsp	60	0	2	150	0	5.0	1.0	5	85%
reduced calorie	1 tbsp	30	0	4	130	0	1.0	0.0	0	36%
w/pure honey, low-calorie	1 tbsp	60	0	4	130	0	5.0	1.0	0	74%
(Featherweight) nonfat	1 tbsp	6	0	1	125	0	0.0	0.0	0	0%
(S&W) Russian, 'Nutradiet'	1 tbsp	25	0	4	120	0	1.0	0.0	0	36%
(Weight Watchers) whipped	1 tbsp	50	0	2	80	0	5.0	1.0	5	85%
(Wish-Bone)										
	1 tbsp	46	0	6	147	0	2.5	0.4	0	48%
'Food Service'	1 tbsp	47	0	6	147	0	2.5	0.0	0	48%
'Lite'	1 tbsp	22	0	4	126	0	0.6	0.1	0	25%
SAN FRANCISCO (Lawry's) w/Romano cheese, 'Classic'	1 oz	136	1	2	547	0	14.0	1.9	0	92%
SESAME										
(Hain) honey and	1 tbsp	60	0	2	210	0	5.0	0.0	0	85%
(Nasoya) garlic	2 tbsp	63	1	3	137	0	5.4	0.5	0	76%
SOUR CREAM										
(Crowley) nondairy	1 oz	40	1	1	5	0	4.0	0.0	0	82%
(Friendship) 'Sour Treat'	1 oz	36	1	2	15	0	3.0	0.0	0	69%
SPINACH SALAD (T. Marzetti) refrigerated	1 tbsp	35	0	2	100	0	10.0	0.0	0	92%
SWEET AND SOUR										
(Herb Magic) no oil	2 tbsp	35	0	9	240	na	0.0	na	0	0%
(Old Dutch) oil-, fat-, and cholesterol-free	2 tbsp	50	0	13	480	na	0.0	na	0	0%
(T. Marzetti)										
'Fat-Free'	1 tbsp	20	0	5	130	0	0.0	0.0	0	0%
'Light'	1 tbsp	45	0	5	105	0	3.0	0.0	0	57%
refrigerated	1 tbsp	72	0	5	99	0	6.0	0.0	0	73%
THOUSAND ISLAND										
(Best Foods) homestyle	1 1/3 tbsp	80	0	3	200	0	8.0	1.0	0	86%
(Estee)	1 tbsp	8	0	2	30	0	0.0	0.0	0	0%
(Featherweight)	1 tbsp	18	0	3	70	0	0.0	0.0	0	0%
(Hain)	1 tbsp	50	0	0	85	0	5.0	0.0	0	100%
(Hollywood)	1 tbsp	60	0	3	15	0	6.0	1.0	5	82%
(Kraft)										
	1 tbsp	60	0	2	150	0	5.0	1.0	5	85%
'Free'	1 tbsp	20	0	5	135	0	0.0	0.0	0	0%
reduced calorie	1 tbsp	20	0	3	135	0	1.0	0.0	0	43%
w/bacon	1 tbsp	60	0	2	100	0	6.0	1.0	0	87%
(Litehouse) and dip, refrigerated	1 tbsp	65	0	1	99	0	7.0	0.0	0	94%
(S&W) 'Nutradiet'	1 tbsp	25	0	2	105	0	2.0	0.0	0	69%
(Seven Seas)										
creamy	1 tbsp	50	0	2	150	0	5.0	1.0	5	85%
'Thousand Island! Light'	1 tbsp	30	0	3	160	0	2.0	0.0	5	60%
(T. Marzetti)										
	1 tbsp	74	0	2	120	0	7.0	0.0	5	89%
fat-free	1 tbsp	17	0	4	172	0	0.0	0.0	0	0%
'Frenchette'	1 tbsp	20	0	3	155	0	0.0	0.0	4	0%
light	1 tbsp	35	0	3	155	0	3.0	0.0	4	69%
refrigerated	1 tbsp	82	0	6	93	0	5.0	0.0	0	65%
(Ultra Slim Fast) cholesterol-free	1 tbsp	18	0	4	95	0	1.0	0.0	0	36%

Food Name	Serving Size	Calories	Prot. gms	Carbs gms	Sod. mgs	Fiber gms	Fat gms	Sat. Fat gms	Chol. mgs	% Fat Cal.
(Walden Farms)	2 tbsp	0	0	0	290	1	0.0	0.0	0	0%
(Weight Watchers) whipped	1 tbsp	50	0	2	80	0	5.0	1.0	5	85%
(Wish-Bone)										
	1 tbsp	63	0	3	158	0	5.6	0.8	7	80%
'Lite'	1 tbsp	36	0	2	99	0	3.0	0.4	9	76%
TOMATO										
(Cook's Classics) basil	1 tbsp	12	1	1	115	0	1.0	0.2	0	53%
(Featherweight) zesty, nonfat	1 tbsp	2	0	0	5	0	0.0	0.0	0	0%
TUNA SALAD										
(Best Foods) 'One Step'	2 tbsp	140	0	4	270	0	14.0	2.0	5	89%
(Blue Plate)	2 tbsp	130	0	1	290	0	13.0	2.0	10	97%
(Hellmann's) 'One Step'	2 tbsp	140	0	4	270	0	14.0	2.0	5	89%
(JFG)	2 tbsp	130	0	1	290	0	13.0	2.0	10	97%
VINAIGRETTE										
(Great Impressions) balsamic vinegar and oil	1 tbsp	67	1	2	367	0	6.5	0.0	0	82%
(Hain)										
cheese	1 tbsp	55	0	0	130	0	6.0	0.0	5	100%
Dijon	1 tbsp	50	0	0	180	0	5.0	0.0	5	100%
Dijon, creamy, 'Natural Classics'	2 tbsp	130	0	3	280	0	13.0	2.0	3	91%
Swiss cheese	1 tbsp	60	0	0	160	0	7.0	0.0	5	100%
tomato, garden, 'Canola'	1 tbsp	60	0	1	150	0	6.0	0.0	0	93%
(Herb Magic) no oil	2 tbsp	10	0	3	270	na	0.0	na	0	0%
(Hollywood) Dijon	1 tbsp	60	0	2	40	0	6.0	1.0	0	87%
(Knott's Berry Farm) w/sun dried tomato	1 tbsp	45	0	1	100	0	4.0	0.0	0	90%
(Kraft) oil and vinegar	1 tbsp	70	0	1	210	0	8.0	1.0	0	95%
(La Martinique) French	2 tbsp	170	0	0	430	na	19.0	5.0	na	100%
(Lawry's)										
Chinese vinegar, w/sesame and ginger, 'Classic'	1 tbsp	145	0	2	325	0	15.0	2.1	0	93%
(Litehouse) sour cream and chives, refrigerated	1 tbsp	63	0	1	72	0	7.0	0.0	0	94%
(Marie's)										
herb, 'Lite and Zesty'	1 tbsp	16	0	4	130	0	0.0	0.0	0	0%
Italian, 'Lite and Zesty'	1 tbsp	16	0	4	135	0	0.0	0.0	0	0%
(Newman's Own) olive oil and vinegar	2 tbsp	150	0	1	150	0	16.0	2.5	0	97%
(Pritikin)										
herb, sodium-free	1 tbsp	8	0	2	0	0	0.0	0.0	0	0%
olive oil, raspberry	2 tbsp	45	0	11	70	0	0.0	0.0	0	0%
(S&W)										
balsamic wine, 'Vintage Lites'	2 tbsp	35	0	8	460	0	0.0	0.0	0	0%
mango key lime, 'Vintage Lites'	2 tbsp	30	0	7	390	0	0.0	0.0	0	0%
Oriental rice wine, 'Vintage Lites'	2 tbsp	30	0	8	280	0	0.0	0.0	0	0%
raspberry blush, 'Vintage Lites'	2 tbsp	40	0	10	410	0	0.0	0.0	0	0%
red wine w/herb, 'Vintage Lites'	2 tbsp	40	0	11	440	0	0.0	0.0	0	0%
white wine w/herb, 'Vintage Lites'	2 tbsp	40	0	10	450	0	0.0	0.0	0	0%
(Seven Seas) red wine vinegar	2 tbsp	15	0	3	410	0	0.0	0.0	0	0%
(Simply Delicious)										
ginger plum, 'Un-Dressing'	1 tbsp	36	0	1	199	0	4.0	0.0	0	90%
herb garlic, 'Un-Dressing'	1 tbsp	43	0	1	132	0	4.0	0.0	0	90%
honey mustard, 'Un-Dressing'	1 tbsp	41	0	2	122	0	4.0	0.0	0	82%
lemon tahini, 'Un-Dressing'	1 tbsp	43	0	1	170	0	4.0	0.0	9	90%
lime cilantro, 'Un-Dressing'	1 tbsp	41	0	1	116	0	4.0	0.0	0	90%
pink peppercorn, 'Un-Dressing'	1 tbsp	40	0	1	148	0	4.0	0.0	0	90%
(Walden Farms)										
balsamic, diet	2 tbsp	0	0	0	380	0	0.0	0.0	0	0%
honey Dijon	2 tbsp	0	0	0	270	1	0.0	0.0	0	0%

Food Name	Serving Size	Calories	Prot. gms	Carbs gms	Sod. mgs	Fiber gms	Fat gms	Sat. Fat gms	Chol. mgs	% Fat Cal.
(Weight Watchers) tomato	1 tbsp	8	0	2	150	0	0.0	0.0	0	0%
(Wish-Bone)										
Dijon, 'Classic'	1 tbsp	60	0	1	171	0	6.1	0.9	1	92%
Dijon, lite	2 tbsp	60	0	3	410	0	5.0	1.0	0	79%
olive oil	1 tbsp	28	0	2	111	0	2.3	0.0	0	74%
olive oil, 'Lite'	1 tbsp	16	0	2	111	0	0.9	0.1	0	50%
red wine	1 tbsp	51	0	4	216	0	3.8	0.5	0	67%
VEGETABLE *(T. Marzetti)* and dip, refrigerated	1 tbsp	88	0	1	120	0	10.0	0.0	2	96%
WINE VINEGAR										
(Estee) red wine, nonfat	1 tbsp	2	0	0	10	0	0.0	0.0	0	0%
(Featherweight) red wine, nonfat	1 tbsp	6	0	1	100	0	0.0	0.0	0	0%
(Great Impressions)										
red wine, and oil	1 tbsp	64	1	3	277	0	6.1	0.0	0	80%
white wine, and oil	1 tbsp	63	1	1	242	0	6.6	0.0	0	89%
(Kraft)										
red wine, and oil	1 tbsp	60	0	4	200	0	4.0	1.0	0	69%
red wine, nonfat	2 tbsp	15	0	3	400	0	0.0	0.0	0	0%
(Lawry's)										
red wine, w/Cabernet, 'Classics'	1 tbsp	138	0	5	178	0	13.7	1.0	0	86%
vintage, w/sherry wine, 'Classics'	1 tbsp	110	4	3	415	0	10.5	2.1	0	78%
white wine, w/Chardonnay, 'Classic'	1 tbsp	153	0	3	178	0	15.7	2.0	0	93%
(Marie's) white wine, nonfat, 'Lite and Zesty'	1 tbsp	20	0	5	135	0	0.0	0.0	0	0%
(Pathmark) red wine, and oil	1 tbsp	70	0	2	235	0	7.0	1.0	0	89%
(Seven Seas)										
red wine, and oil, 'Viva Red Wine!'	1 tbsp	45	0	1	190	0	4.0	1.0	0	90%
red wine, and oil, 'Viva'	1 tbsp	70	0	1	290	0	7.0	1.0	0	94%
SALAD DRESSING MIX										
BACON *(Lawry's)* mix only	1 pkg	65	5	9	1820	1	0.8	0.0	0	11%
BLUE CHEESE										
(Best Foods) blue cheese, homestyle, mix only	2 tsp	45	0	1	130	0	4.5	1.0	10	91%
(Good Seasons)										
and herbs, mix only	1 pkg	4	0	1	150	0	0.0	0.0	0	0%
and herbs, prepared	1 tbsp	70	0	1	150	0	8.0	0.0	0	95%
(Hain) 'No Oil' prepared	1 tbsp	14	1	1	180	0	1.0	0.0	5	53%
(Hidden Valley Ranch)										
mix only	1.1 oz	112	4	19	1931	0	2.0	0.0	0	16%
prepared	1 tbsp	58	0	1	95	0	6.0	0.0	2	93%
(Tone's) blue cheese, mix only	1 tsp	13	0	2	146	0	0.2	0.0	0	14%
(Weight Watchers) mix only	1 tbsp	8	0	1	110	0	0.0	0.0	0	0%
BUTTERMILK										
(Good Seasons)										
'Farm Style' prepared	1 tbsp	60	1	1	135	0	6.0	0.0	5	87%
nonfat, 'Farm Style' mix only	1 pkg	4	0	1	95	0	0.0	0.0	0	0%
(Hain) 'No Oil' prepared	1 tbsp	11	1	1	150	0	1.0	0.0	0	53%
(Hidden Valley Ranch) original recipe, prepared	1 tbsp	58	0	1	110	0	3.0	0.0	4	87%
(Tone's) mix only	1 tsp	10	0	2	389	1	0.2	0.1	0	16%
CAESAR										
(Good Seasons) gourmet, prepared	2 tbsp	150	0	3	300	0	16.0	2.5	0	92%
(Hain) 'No Oil' prepared	1 tbsp	6	0	1	200	0	1.0	0.0	0	69%
(Lawry's) mix only	1 pkg	75	3	9	1962	0	3.1	0.0	0	37%
CHEESE										
(Good Seasons)										
garlic, mix only	1 serving	40	0	8	2640	0	0.0	0.0	0	0%
garlic, prepared	2 tbsp	140	0	1	330	0	16.0	2.5	0	97%

Food Name	Serving Size	Calories	Prot. gms	Carbs gms	Sod. mgs	Fiber gms	Fat gms	Sat. Fat gms	Chol. mgs	% Fat Cal.
Italian, mix only	1 pkg	4	0	1	130	0	0.0	0.0	0	0%
CHICKEN SALAD (Kikkoman) Chinese, mix only	1 tbsp	30	1	6	500	0	0.0	0.0	0	0%
DILL										
(Good Seasons)										
'Classic' mix only.	1 tbsp	2	0	0	150	0	0.0	0.0	0	0%
'Classic' prepared	1 tbsp	70	0	1	150	0	8.0	0.0	0	95%
(Knorr) and dip, mix only	1 tbsp	2	1	1	65	0	1.0	0.0	0	53%
FRENCH										
(Hain) 'No Oil' prepared	1 tbsp	12	0	3	340	0	0.0	0.0	0	0%
(Weight Watchers) mix only	1 tbsp	3	0	1	150	0	0.0	0.0	0	0%
GARLIC										
(Good Seasons)										
and herb, mix only.	1 serving	40	0	8	2720	0	0.0	0.0	0	0%
and herb, prepared	1 tbsp	70	0	1	190	0	8.0	0.0	0	95%
(Hain) and cheese, 'No Oil' prepared	1 tbsp	6	1	1	180	0	1.0	0.0	0	53%
HERB										
(Good Seasons)										
'Classic' mix only.	1 pkg	2	0	0	150	0	0.0	0.0	0	0%
'Classic' prepared	1 tbsp	70	0	1	150	0	8.0	0.0	0	95%
zesty, lowfat recipe, prepared	1 tbsp	12	0	1	150	0	1.0	0.0	0	69%
zesty, mix only.	1 tbsp	6	0	1	130	0	0.0	0.0	0	0%
zesty, nonfat recipe, prepared	1 tbsp	6	0	1	150	0	0.0	0.0	0	0%
(Hain) 'No Oil' prepared	1 tbsp	2	0	1	140	0	0.0	0.0	0	0%
(Hidden Valley Ranch)										
creamy, mix only.	0.9 oz	76	3	16	1931	0	0.0	0.0	0	0%
creamy, prepared	1 tbsp	58	0	1	100	0	6.0	0.0	5	93%
HONEY MUSTARD										
(Good Seasons)										
low-fat recipe, prepared.	1 tbsp	18	0	2	130	0	1.0	0.0	0	53%
nonfat recipe, mix only	1 serving	160	0	40	2240	0	0.0	0.0	0	0%
nonfat recipe, prepared.	1 tbsp	10	0	2	130	0	0.0	0.0	0	0%
prepared	1 tbsp	80	0	2	125	0	8.0	0.0	0	90%
ITALIAN										
(Good Seasons)										
cheese, 'Lite' mix only	1 tbsp	25	0	1	135	0	3.0	0.0	0	87%
cheese, mix only	1 pkg	4	0	1	130	0	0.0	0.0	0	0%
cheese, prepared	1 tbsp	70	0	1	130	0	8.0	0.0	0	95%
creamy, fat-free recipe, prepared	1 tbsp	8	0	2	140	0	0.0	0.0	0	0%
creamy, low-fat recipe, prepared.	1 tbsp	16	0	2	150	0	1.0	0.0	0	53%
creamy, nonfat, mix only	1 serving	80	0	24	2160	0	0.0	0.0	0	0%
lemon and herbs, mix only	1 tbsp	70	0	1	140	0	8.0	0.0	0	95%
lemon and herbs, prepared.	1 tbsp	70	0	1	140	0	8.0	0.0	0	95%
'Lite' mix only.	1 tbsp	25	0	1	180	0	3.0	0.0	0	87%
mild, mix only	1 serving	80	0	16	2960	0	0.0	0.0	0	0%
mild, prepared	1 tbsp	70	0	1	190	0	8.0	0.0	0	95%
mix only.	1 serving	40	0	8	2560	0	0.0	0.0	0	0%
mix only	1 tbsp	6	0	1	170	0	0.0	0.0	0	0%
'No Oil' mix only	1 tbsp	6	0	2	30	0	0.0	0.0	0	0%
nonfat, mix only.	1 serving	80	0	24	2320	0	0.0	0.0	0	0%
nonfat, prepared	2 tbsp	10	0	3	290	0	0.0	0.0	0	0%
prepared w/o oil.	1 tbsp	6	0	2	30	0	0.0	0.0	0	0%
prepared	1 tbsp	70	0	1	170	0	8.0	0.0	0	95%
prepared	2 tbsp	140	0	1	320	0	15.0	2.0	0	97%
zesty, 'Lite' mix only.	1 tbsp	25	0	1	135	0	3.0	0.0	0	87%

Food Name	Serving Size	Calories	Prot. gms	Carbs gms	Sod. mgs	Fiber gms	Fat gms	Sat. Fat gms	Chol. mgs	% Fat Cal.
zesty, 'Lite' prepared	1 tbsp	25	0	1	135	0	3.0	0.0	0	87%
zesty, mix only	1 pkg	2	0	1	120	0	0.0	0.0	0	0%
zesty, mix only	1 serving	40	0	8	1760	0	0.0	0.0	0	0%
zesty, prepared	1 tbsp	70	0	1	120	0	8.0	0.0	0	95%
(Lawry's)										
mix only	1 pkg	45	2	9	2255	0	0.2	0.0	0	4%
w/cheese, mix only	1 pkg	74	2	12	1624	0	2.1	0.0	0	26%
(Tone's)										
creamy, mix only	1 tsp	13	0	3	251	0	0.1	0.0	0	7%
mix only	1 tsp	12	0	3	323	0	0.1	0.0	0	7%
LEMON										
(Good Seasons)										
and herbs, Italian, prepared	1 tbsp	70	0	1	140	0	8.0	0.0	0	95%
and herbs, Italian, mix only	1 pkg	2	0	1	140	0	0.0	0.0	0	0%
RANCH										
(Good Seasons)										
'Lite' prepared	1 tbsp	30	1	2	115	0	2.0	0.0	5	60%
Italian, 'Lite' prepared	1 tbsp	30	1	2	115	0	2.0	0.0	5	60%
Italian, prepared	1 tbsp	60	0	1	110	0	6.0	0.0	5	93%
lower calorie, mix only	1 serving	160	0	32	3202	0	0.0	0.0	0	0%
mix only	1 serving	80	0	16	2243	0	0.0	0.0	0	0%
prepared	1 tbsp	60	0	1	110	0	6.0	0.0	5	93%
(Hidden Valley Ranch)										
lower calorie, mix only	1.1 oz	98	3	17	2301	0	2.0	0.0	0	18%
lower calorie, prepared	1 tbsp	35	0	2	120	0	3.0	0.0	4	77%
original, mix only	1 oz	93	3	18	2211	0	1.0	0.0	0	10%
original, prepared	1 tbsp	58	0	1	105	0	6.0	0.0	5	93%
w/bacon, mix only	1.2 oz	118	7	1	1953	0	2.0	0.0	0	36%
w/bacon, prepared	1 tbsp	58	0	1	135	0	6.0	0.0	5	93%
RUSSIAN *(Weight Watchers)* mix only	1 tbsp	4	0	1	120	0	0.0	0.0	0	0%
SESAME, Oriental *(Good Seasons)* mix only	1/8 envelope	15	0	3	360	0	0.0	0.0	0	0%
SOY SESAME *(Kikkoman)* mix only	2 tsp	15	1	3	270	0	1.0	0.0	0	39%
THOUSAND ISLAND										
(Best Foods) homestyle, mix only	2 tsp	40	0	1	110	0	4.0	1.0	0	90%
(Weight Watchers) nonfat, mix only	1 tbsp	4	0	1	140	0	0.0	0.0	0	0%
VINAIGRETTE Oriental *(Kikkoman)* mix only	2 tsp	20	0	3	230	0	0.0	0.0	0	0%
SALAD MIX										
(Suddenly Salad)										
Caesar, mix only	2/3 cup	150	5	30	580	1	1.0	0.0	0	6%
Caesar, prepared	3/4 cup	220	5	30	580	1	9.0	1.5	0	37%
ranch, and bacon, prepared	3/4 cup	330	7	30	480	1	20.0	3.0	15	55%
ranch, and bacon, low-fat, prepared	3/4 cup	180	7	30	530	1	2.0	0.0	3	11%
SALAD SEASONING. See under SEASONING MIX.										
SALAD TOPPING										
(Produce Partners) seasoned	1 tbsp	30	2	3	40	0	1.0	0.0	0	31%
(Salad Crispins)										
bacon and onion, 'American Style'	1 tbsp	35	1	4	125	0	1.0	0.0	0	31%
cheddar and onion	1 tbsp	35	1	4	115	0	1.0	0.0	0	31%
Italian style, w/Parmesan cheese	1 tbsp	35	1	4	95	0	1.0	0.0	0	31%
ranch	1 tbsp	35	1	4	125	0	1.0	0.0	0	31%
(Salad Nibbler)										
buttermilk ranch, crouton topping	1 oz	128	7	13	241	0	5.0	0.0	2	36%
cheddar, seasoned, crouton topping	1 oz	129	6	13	224	0	6.0	0.0	2	42%
(Schilling) seasoned	1 tbsp	35	1	2	95	0	1.5	0.0	0	53%

Food Name	Serving Size	Calories	Prot. gms	Carbs gms	Sod. mgs	Fiber gms	Fat gms	Sat. Fat gms	Chol. mgs	% Fat Cal.
(Special Edition)										
garlic and cheese, sesame, nuggets.................	1 tbsp	40	1	3	130	0	2.5	0.0	0	58%
sesame, nuggets..................................	1 tbsp	35	1	3	115	0	2.5	0.0	0	58%
(Tone's) 'American'...............................	1 tsp	7	1	1	34	0	0.3	0.1	1	38%
SALISBURY STEAK. See under BEEF DINNER/ENTRÉE.										
SALMON										
ATLANTIC										
Fresh										
farmed, baked, broiled, grilled, or microwaved	3 oz	175	19	0	52	0	10.5	2.1	54	54%
farmed, raw.....................................	3 oz	156	17	0	50	0	9.2	1.9	50	53%
wild, baked, broiled, grilled, or microwaved.............	3 oz	155	22	0	48	0	6.9	1.1	60	40%
wild, raw	3 oz	121	17	0	37	0	5.4	0.8	47	40%
BLUEBACK. See under SOCKEYE.										
CHINOOK / king										
Fresh										
baked, broiled, grilled, or microwaved.................	3 oz	196	22	0	51	0	11.4	2.7	72	52%
raw...	3 oz	153	17	0	40	0	8.9	2.1	56	52%
Smoked										
....	3 oz	99	16	0	666	0	3.7	0.8	20	33%
boneless......................................	1 oz	33	5	0	222	0	1.2	0.3	7	33%
flaked..	1 cup	159	25	0	1066	0	5.9	1.3	31	33%
lox...	3 oz	99	16	0	1700	0	3.7	0.8	20	33%
lox...	1 oz	33	5	0	567	0	1.2	0.3	7	33%
CHUM / keta										
Canned										
(Bumble Bee)	1 cup	306	47	0	0	0	11.4	0.0	0	35%
(Libby's).....................................	3.7 oz	130	20	0	450	0	6.0	2.0	40	40%
drained, w/bone...............................	3 oz	120	18	0	414	0	4.7	1.3	33	35%
drained, w/bone, no salt added....................	3 oz	120	18	0	64	0	4.7	1.3	33	35%
w/liquid *(Bumble Bee)*.........................	3.5 oz	160	20	0	490	0	8.0	2.0	60	47%
Fresh										
baked, broiled, grilled, or microwaved.................	3 oz	131	22	0	54	0	4.1	0.9	81	28%
raw	3 oz	102	17	0	43	0	3.2	0.7	63	28%
Frozen										
(Peter Pan Seafoods) fillet portion, raw...............	3.5 oz	120	20	0	50	0	3.8	0.0	74	30%
(Peter Pan Seafoods) side, pinbone in, raw	3.5 oz	120	20	0	50	0	3.8	0.0	74	30%
(Peter Pan Seafoods) steak, raw..................	3.5 oz	120	20	0	50	0	3.8	0.0	74	30%
COHO / silver										
Canned										
meat only *(Deming's)*	1/2 cup	140	22	0	450	0	5.0	0.0	0	34%
Fresh										
farmed, baked, broiled, grilled, or microwaved	3 oz	151	21	0	44	0	7.0	1.7	54	42%
farmed, raw....................................	3 oz	136	18	0	40	0	6.5	1.5	43	43%
wild, baked, broiled, grilled, or microwaved.............	3 oz	118	20	0	49	0	3.7	0.9	47	28%
wild, boiled or poached..........................	3 oz	156	23	0	45	0	6.4	1.4	48	37%
wild, raw......................................	3 oz	124	18	0	39	0	5.0	1.1	38	37%
HUMPBACK. See PINK.										
KETA. See COHO.										
KING. See CHINOOK.										
MIXED SPECIES										
Canned, boneless, skinless *(Libby's)*..................	3.25 oz	110	16	1	420	0	4.0	1.0	50	35%
Frozen, steak, w/o seasoning mix *(SeaPak)*	8-oz pkg	270	46	0	115	0	9.0	0.0	170	31%
Smoked, Nova, sliced *(Lascco)*......................	3 oz	120	18	0	1070	0	6.0	2.0	35	43%

Food Name	Serving Size	Calories	Prot. gms	Carbs gms	Sod. mgs	Fiber gms	Fat gms	Sat. Fat gms	Chol. mgs	% Fat Cal.
PINK / humpback										
Canned										
(Captains Choice)	3 oz	110	16	0	420	0	5.0	1.0	55	41%
Alaska, w/liquid (Deming's)	1/2 cup	140	20	0	450	0	6.0	1.0	65	40%
Alaskan, fancy (Crown Prince)	3.5 oz	140	20	0	450	0	6.0	2.0	40	40%
Alaskan, fresh packed (Libby's)	3.7 oz	130	20	0	450	0	6.0	2.0	40	40%
boneless, skinless (Chicken of the Sea)	2 oz	60	10	0	280	0	2.0	0.5	20	31%
boneless, skinless, w/liquid (Bumble Bee)	3.5 oz	120	17	0	420	0	5.0	1.0	25	40%
chunk, boneless, skinless, w/liquid (Deming's)	3.25 oz	120	17	0	420	0	5.0	0.0	0	40%
drained, w/bones	3 oz	118	17	0	64	0	5.1	1.3	47	39%
w/bones and liquid	3 oz	118	17	0	471	0	5.1	1.3	47	39%
w/liquid (Bumble Bee)	1 cup	310	45	0	851	0	13.0	0.0	0	39%
w/liquid (Bumble Bee)	3.5 oz	160	20	0	490	0	8.0	2.0	50	47%
w/liquid (Del Monte)	1/2 cup	160	22	0	660	0	7.0	0.0	0	42%
w/liquid (Featherweight)	2 oz	70	11	0	45	0	3.0	0.0	20	38%
w/liquid (Libby's)	7.75 oz	310	45	0	790	0	13.0	0.0	0	39%
Fresh										
baked, broiled, grilled, or microwaved	3 oz	127	22	0	73	0	3.8	0.6	57	27%
raw	3 oz	99	17	0	57	0	2.9	0.5	44	27%
RED. See SOCKEYE.										
SILVER. See COHO.										
SOCKEYE / red										
Canned										
(Bumble Bee)	1 cup	376	45	0	1148	0	20.5	0.0	0	51%
(Libby's)	7.75 oz	380	45	0	760	0	21.0	0.0	0	51%
(S&W)	3 oz	152	18	0	369	0	8.8	2.0	56	53%
Alaska (Deming's)	1/2 cup	170	20	0	450	0	9.0	2.0	65	50%
Alaska, medium (Deming's)	1/2 cup	150	21	0	450	0	7.0	2.0	65	43%
blueback (Rubinstein's)	1/2 cup	170	20	0	450	0	9.0	2.0	0	50%
blueback, 'Fancy' (S&W)	1/2 cup	190	25	0	590	0	10.0	0.0	0	47%
boneless, skinless, w/liquid (Bumble Bee)	3.5 oz	130	17	0	420	0	6.0	1.0	30	44%
drained, w/bone	3 oz	130	17	0	457	0	6.2	1.4	37	43%
drained, w/bone, no salt added	3 oz	130	17	0	64	0	6.2	1.4	37	43%
'Nutradiet' (S&W)	1/2 cup	188	22	0	47	0	11.0	0.0	0	53%
w/liquid (Bumble Bee)	3.5 oz	180	20	0	490	0	10.0	2.0	60	53%
w/liquid (Del Monte)	1/2 cup	180	23	0	660	0	9.0	0.0	0	47%
Fresh										
baked, broiled, grilled, or microwaved	3 oz	184	23	0	56	0	9.3	1.6	74	46%
raw	3 oz	143	18	0	40	0	7.3	1.3	53	46%
SALMON OIL. See under FISH OIL.										
SALMON SUBSTITUTE (Mox Lox) smoked	1.5 oz	25	2	3	380	0	1.0	0.0	5	31%
SALSA. See also under SAUCE.										
(Arizona Cactus Ranch)										
cactus fruit or prickly pear, organic	2 tbsp	15	1	4	120	0	0.0	0.0	0	0%
(Chi-Chi's)										
hot	1 oz	8	2	2	153	0	2.0	2.0	2	53%
medium	1 oz	7	2	2	135	0	2.0	2.0	2	53%
mild	1 oz	7	2	2	116	0	2.0	2.0	2	53%
(Del Monte)										
burrito, can or jar	1/4 cup	20	0	4	355	0	0.0	0.0	0	0%
green chili, mild	1/4 cup	20	0	3	590	0	0.0	0.0	0	0%
roja, mild	1/4 cup	20	0	4	510	0	0.0	0.0	0	0%
(Eagle)										
medium	2 tbsp	10	3	2	250	1	0.0	0.0	0	0%

Food Name	Serving Size	Calories	Prot. gms	Carbs gms	Sod. mgs	Fiber gms	Fat gms	Sat. Fat gms	Chol. mgs	% Fat Cal.
mild	2 tbsp	10	3	2	250	1	0.0	0.0	0	0%
w/cheese, medium	2 tbsp	40	1	3	300	0	3.0	1.0	5	63%
(Enrico's)										
hot, chunky style	2 tbsp	8	1	2	34	0	0.0	0.0	0	0%
hot, chunky style, no salt added	2 tbsp	8	1	2	10	0	0.0	0.0	0	0%
mild, chunky style	2 tbsp	8	1	2	34	0	0.0	0.0	0	0%
mild, chunky style, no salt added	2 tbsp	8	1	2	10	0	0.0	0.0	0	0%
(Garden of Eden)										
nonfat, organic, 'Great Garlic/Hot Habenero'	2 tbsp	10	0	2	95	0	0.0	0.0	0	0%
(Guiltless Gourmet)										
medium	2 tbsp	10	0	2	140	0	0.0	0.0	0	0%
red pepper, roasted	2 tbsp	10	0	2	120	0	0.0	0.0	0	0%
Southwestern grill	2 tbsp	10	0	2	150	0	0.0	0.0	0	0%
tomatillo	2 tbsp	10	0	2	160	1	0.0	0.0	0	0%
(Hain)										
green chili, hot	1/4 cup	22	1	4	480	0	0.0	0.0	0	0%
mild	1/2 cup	20	1	4	410	0	0.0	0.0	0	0%
(Heluva Good)										
hot	2 tbsp	10	0	2	180	0	0.0	0.0	0	0%
mild	2 tbsp	10	0	2	180	0	0.0	0.0	0	0%
(Hot Cha Cha) 'Texas'	1 oz	6	0	3	2	0	0.0	0.0	0	0%
(Kaukauna)										
Mexican, medium	2 tbsp	15	0	3	170	0	0.0	0.0	0	0%
Mexican, mild	2 tbsp	15	0	3	170	0	0.0	0.0	0	0%
(La Victoria)										
'Brava'	1 tbsp	6	1	1	100	0	1.0	0.0	0	53%
'Casera'	1 tbsp	4	1	1	80	0	1.0	0.0	0	53%
chili dip, chunky	2 tbsp	9	0	2	148	0	0.0	na	na	5%
green chili	2 tbsp	10	0	2	150	0	0.0	0.0	0	0%
green chili, mild	2 tbsp	8	0	1	175	0	0.1	na	na	9%
green jalapeño	1 tbsp	4	1	1	105	0	1.0	0.0	0	53%
green jalapeño	2 tbsp	10	0	1	181	0	0.3	na	0	31%
hot	1 tbsp	2	0	0	33	0	0.1	na	0	25%
hot	2 tbsp	9	0	2	171	0	0.1	na	0	9%
hot, 'Victoria'	2 tbsp	7	0	1	163	0	0.1	na	0	10%
hot, thick and chunky	2 tbsp	9	0	1	133	0	0.1	na	0	11%
jalapeña	2 tbsp	12	0	2	148	0	0.2	na	0	13%
medium	2 tbsp	8	0	1	150	0	0.1	na	0	11%
medium, 'Suprema'	2 tbsp	8	0	1	166	0	0.1	na	0	9%
medium, thick and chunky	2 tbsp	8	0	1	160	0	0.1	na	0	12%
mild	2 tbsp	8	0	1	182	0	0.1	na	0	10%
mild, 'Suprema'	2 tbsp	8	0	2	179	0	0.1	na	0	10%
mild, thick and chunky	2 tbsp	8	0	1	157	0	0.1	na	0	10%
omelet	1 tbsp	6	1	1	95	0	1.0	0.0	0	53%
'Ranchera'	1 tbsp	6	1	1	85	0	1.0	0.0	0	53%
red jalapeño	1 tbsp	6	1	1	95	0	1.0	0.0	0	53%
'Suprema'	2 tbsp	10	0	2	220	0	0.0	0.0	0	0%
'Victoria'	1 tbsp	4	1	1	80	0	1.0	0.0	0	53%
(Litehouse) medium, 'Zesty'	1 tbsp	4	0	1	110	0	0.0	0.0	0	0%
(Mi Ranchito)										
hot, restaurant style	2 tbsp	10	0	2	120	0	0.0	0.0	0	0%
mild, fat-free, restaurant style	2 tbsp	10	0	2	120	0	0.0	0.0	0	0%
(Millina's Finest) hot, mild or garlic, fat-free, organic	2 tbsp	10	0	2	60	0	0.0	0.0	0	0%

Food Name	Serving Size	Calories	Prot. gms	Carbs gms	Sod. mgs	Fiber gms	Fat gms	Sat. Fat gms	Chol. mgs	% Fat Cal.
(Mission)										
hot....................	2 tbsp	5	0	2	70	0	0.0	0.0	0	0%
mild..................	2 tbsp	5	0	2	70	0	0.0	0.0	0	0%
'Poco Picante'.............	2 tbsp	5	0	2	70	0	0.0	0.0	0	0%
(Nabisco)										
green chili, hot...........	1 tbsp	6	0	2	190	0	0.0	0.0	0	0%
green chili, medium...........	1 tbsp	6	0	1	190	0	0.0	0.0	0	0%
green chili, mild..........	1 tbsp	8	0	2	190	0	0.0	0.0	0	0%
taco, hot, can or jar, 'Thick & Smooth'.............	1 tbsp	8	0	2	105	0	0.0	0.0	0	0%
taco, medium, can or jar, 'Thick & Smooth'.............	1 tbsp	8	0	2	105	0	0.0	0.0	0	0%
taco, mild, can or jar, 'Thick & Smooth'.............	1 tbsp	8	0	2	115	0	0.0	0.0	0	0%
(Old El Paso)										
green chili, medium...........	2 tbsp	10	0	2	110	1	0.0	0.0	0	0%
green chili, 'Thick 'n Chunky'...........	2 tbsp	3	0	1	270	0	0.0	0.0	0	0%
homestyle, medium...........	2 tbsp	5	0	1	110	0	0.0	0.0	0	0%
homestyle, mild...........	2 tbsp	5	0	1	110	0	0.0	0.0	0	0%
hot, 'Pico de Gallo'...........	2 tbsp	5	0	2	260	1	0.0	0.0	0	0%
hot, 'Thick n' Chunky'...........	2 tbsp	10	0	2	130	0	0.0	0.0	0	0%
medium, 'Pico de Gallo'...........	2 tbsp	5	0	2	260	1	0.0	0.0	0	0%
medium, 'Salsa Verde'...........	2 tbsp	10	0	2	95	0	0.0	0.0	0	0%
medium, 'Thick n'Chunky'...........	2 tbsp	10	0	2	140	0	0.0	0.0	0	0%
mild or medium, chunky...........	2 tbsp	15	1	3	230	1	0.0	0.0	0	0%
mild, 'Thick n' Chunky'...........	2 tbsp	10	0	2	140	0	0.0	0.0	0	0%
taco, hot...........	1 tbsp	5	0	1	90	0	0.0	0.0	0	0%
taco, medium...........	1 tbsp	5	0	1	70	0	0.0	0.0	0	0%
taco, mild...........	1 tbsp	5	0	1	85	0	0.0	0.0	0	0%
taco, mild, extra chunky...........	1 tbsp	5	0	1	80	0	0.0	0.0	0	0%
verde, 'Thick 'n Chunky'...........	2 tbsp	10	1	2	135	0	1.0	0.0	0	43%
(Ortega)										
green chili, hot...........	1 oz	10	0	2	180	0	0.0	0.0	0	0%
green chili, medium...........	1 oz	8	0	2	180	0	0.0	0.0	0	0%
green chili, mild...........	1 oz	8	0	2	180	0	0.0	0.0	0	0%
medium, thick and chunky...........	1 tbsp	4	0	1	150	0	0.0	0.0	0	0%
ranchera...........	1 oz	12	0	3	250	0	0.0	0.0	0	0%
taco, hot, can or jar...........	1 oz	10	0	2	300	0	0.0	0.0	0	0%
taco, mild, can or jar...........	1 oz	10	0	2	290	0	0.0	0.0	0	0%
(Pablo's)										
hot, 'Deli Style'...........	1 oz	10	1	2	250	0	0.0	0.0	0	0%
mild, 'Deli Style'...........	1 oz	10	1	2	250	0	0.0	0.0	0	0%
(Pace)										
medium, thick and chunky...........	2 tbsp	4	1	1	101	0	1.0	0.0	0	53%
mild, thick and chunky...........	2 tbsp	4	1	1	101	0	1.0	0.0	0	53%
salsa dip, medium, 'Chunky'...........	2 tbsp	4	1	1	102	0	1.0	0.0	0	53%
salsa dip, mild, 'Chunky'...........	2 tbsp	4	1	1	101	0	1.0	0.0	0	53%
(Parrot Brand)										
black bean, medium, organic, nonfat...........	2 tbsp	10	0	2	115	1	0.0	0.0	0	0%
hot, fat-free, organic...........	2 tbsp	10	1	2	72	1	0.0	0.0	0	0%
pinto bean, medium, fat-free, organic...........	2 tbsp	9	0	2	64	10	0.0	0.0	0	0%
tomatillo, spicy, all natural, 'Green Verde'...........	2 tbsp	17	0	2	91	1	0.0	0.0	0	0%
(Pritikin) very low-sodium...........	1/4 cup	25	1	5	15	0	0.0	0.0	0	0%
(Progresso)										
Italian, hot...........	2 tbsp	10	1	2	170	1	0.0	0.0	0	0%
Italian, medium...........	2 tbsp	10	1	2	170	1	0.0	0.0	0	0%
Italian, mild...........	2 tbsp	10	1	2	170	1	0.0	0.0	0	0%

Food Name	Serving Size	Calories	Prot. gms	Carbs gms	Sod. mgs	Fiber gms	Fat gms	Sat. Fat gms	Chol. mgs	% Fat Cal.
(Rosarita)										
green chile, mild, food service product	2 tbsp	7	0	2	167	0	0.1	0.0	0	14%
green chili, extra chunky, 'de Mexico Style'	2 tbsp	30	1	7	280	0	1.0	0.0	0	22%
green chili, mild	1.09 oz	7	0	2	167	0	0.1	0.0	0	11%
green tomatillo, 'de Mexico Style'	2 tbsp	20	1	4	190	0	1.0	0.0	0	31%
green tomatillo, medium	2 tbsp	8	0	2	188	1	0.2	0.0	0	22%
hot, chunky	3 tbsp	25	1	6	300	1	1.0	0.0	0	24%
jalapeño picante, hot	2 tbsp	8	0	2	240	0	0.1	0.0	0	8%
jalapeño picante, medium	2 tbsp	8	0	2	240	0	0.1	0.0	0	8%
jalapeño picante, mild	2 tbsp	8	0	2	239	0	0.1	0.0	0	8%
medium, chunky	3 tbsp	25	1	6	350	1	1.0	0.0	0	24%
medium, extra chunky	2 tbsp	7	0	1	228	0	0.2	0.0	0	22%
mild, 'Casa Mamita'	1.13 oz	7	0	1	170	0	0.1	0.0	0	12%
mild, chunky	3 tbsp	25	1	6	340	1	1.0	0.0	0	24%
picante, food service product	2 tbsp	26	0	6	342	0	0.1	0.0	0	3%
roasted, mild	2 tbsp	10	0	2	232	1	0.3	0.0	0	26%
taco, medium, chunky	3 tbsp	25	1	6	310	1	1.0	0.0	0	24%
taco, mild	2 oz	27	1	6	304	0	0.1	0.0	1	3%
taco, mild, chunky	3 tbsp	25	1	6	300	1	1.0	0.0	0	24%
traditional, 'de Mexico Style'	2 tbsp	12	1	3	350	0	0.0	0.0	0	0%
traditional, medium	2 tbsp	7	0	2	234	1	0.1	0.0	0	12%
traditional, mild	2 tbsp	7	1	1	248	1	0.1	0.0	0	11%
(S&W)										
hot, 'Sun-Vista'	2 tbsp	5	0	2	170	1	0.0	0.0	0	0%
medium, 'Ready Cut'	1/4 cup	20	1	4	190	1	0.0	0.0	0	0%
mild, 'Ready Cut'	1/4 cup	20	1	4	190	1	0.0	0.0	0	0%
w/chipotle, 'Ready Cut'	1/4 cup	20	1	4	190	1	0.0	0.0	0	0%
w/cilantro, 'Ready Cut'	1/4 cup	20	1	4	190	1	0.0	0.0	0	0%
(Santiago) chunky	1 fl oz	10	0	2	232	0	0.1	0.0	0	9%
(Sun Vista) hot	2 tbsp	5	0	2	170	1	0.0	0.0	0	0%
(Territorial House) green chili	0.5 oz	4	1	1	80	0	1.0	0.0	0	53%
(Timpone's) tomato, fresh roasted, 'Salsa Muy Rica'	2 tbsp	10	0	2	110	0	0.0	0.0	0	0%
(Tostitos)										
con queso	4 tbsp	80	2	10	560	1	5.0	2.0	5	48%
con queso, low-fat	4 tbsp	80	2	8	560	1	3.0	2.0	5	40%
medium or hot	4 tbsp	30	2	6	520	2	0.0	0.0	0	0%
mild	4 tbsp	30	2	6	520	2	0.0	0.0	0	0%
'Ultimate Garden'	4 tbsp	30	2	6	460	2	0.0	0.0	0	0%
SALSIFY / oyster plant / vegetable oyster										
boiled, drained, sliced	1 cup	92	4	21	22	4	0.2	0.1	0	2%
boiled, drained, sliced	1/2 cup	46	1.9	10.5	11	2.1	0.1	na	0	2%
raw, sliced	1 cup	109	4	25	27	4	0.3	na	0	2%
raw, sliced	1/2 cup	55	2.2	12.5	13	2.2	0.1	na	0	2%
SALSIFY, BLACK / scorzonera										
raw	1 lb	372	15.0	84.4	91	(mq)	0.1	(tr)	0	0%
raw	1 oz	23	0.9	5.3	6	(mq)	tr	(tr)	0	0%
SALT										
iodized *(Morton)*	1 tsp	0	0	0	2300	0	0.0	0.0	0	0%
kosher *(Morton)*	1 tsp	0	0	0	1880	0	0.0	0.0	0	0%
'Nature's Seasons' *(Morton)*	1 tsp	3	0	1	1400	0	0.1	0.0	0	17%
non-iodized *(Morton)*	1 tsp	0	0	0	2300	0	0.0	0.0	0	0%
sea *(Hain)*	1 tsp	0	0	0	2255	0	0.0	0.0	0	0%
sea *(Tone's)*	1 tsp	0	0	0	2132	0	0.0	0.0	0	0%
table	1 cup	0	0	0	113173	0	0.0	0.0	0	0%

Food Name	Serving Size	Calories	Prot. gms	Carbs gms	Sod. mgs	Fiber gms	Fat gms	Sat. Fat gms	Chol. mgs	% Fat Cal.
table	1 dash	0	0	0	155	0	0.0	0.0	0	0%
table	1 tbsp	0	0	0	6976	0	0.0	0.0	0	0%
table	1 tsp	0	0	0	2325	0	0.0	0.0	0	0%
SALT PORK. See PORK, SALT.										
SALT SEASONING. See under SEASONING MIX.										
SALT SUBSTITUTE										
(Featherweight)	1/4 tsp	0	0	0	0	0	0.0	0.0	0	0%
(Morton)	1 tsp	1	0	0	1	0	0.0	0.0	0	0%
'Chef Shaker' (Diamond Crystal)..............	1/2 tsp	0	0	0	0	na	0.0	0.0	0	0%
extra spicy (Mrs. Dash)	0.13 tsp	2	0	0	1	na	0.0	na	0	14%
'Lite' (Lawry's)	1 tsp	8	0	2	357	0	0.1	0.0	0	10%
lite, 1/2 the salt of regular salt (Morton)	1/4 tsp	0	0	0	290	0	0.0	0.0	0	0%
'Lite Salt' (Morton)........................	1 tsp	1	0	0	1100	0	0.0	0.0	0	0%
'Salt-Free' (Lawry's).......................	1 tsp	10	0	2	2	0	0.2	0.0	0	18%
'Salt-It' (Estee)...........................	1/8 tsp	0	0	0	0	0	0.0	0.0	0	0%
seasoned (Adolph's)	1/4 tsp	0	0	0	0	0	0.0	0.0	0	0%
seasoned (Featherweight)...................	1/4 tsp	0	0	0	0	0	0.0	0.0	0	0%
seasoned (Morton)	1 tsp	2	0	1	1	0	0.1	0.0	0	27%
seasoned (Mrs. Dash).....................	0.13 tsp	2	0	0	1	na	0.0	na	0	4%
seasoned, 'Instead of Salt' (Health Valley)	1 tsp	11	1	2	3	0	0.5	0.0	0	36%
seasoned, 'Salt-Free' (Lawry's)	1 tsp	3	0	1	7	0	0.1	0.0	0	24%
SAND PEAR. See ASIAN PEAR.										
SANDWICH										
BEEF										
(Healthy Choice) Philly beef steak, 'Hearty Handfuls'	1 entrée	290	16	47	550	5	5.0	1.5	15	15%
(Hot Pockets)										
beef and cheddar stuffed sandwich, frozen.............	1 pkg	403	16	39	906	na	20.2	8.8	53	45%
pocket, w/cheddar, frozen	5 oz	370	17	36	1390	0	17.0	0.0	60	42%
pocket, w/cheese, no gravy, 'Beef & Cheddar'	1 pocket	524	17	36	620	1	34.8	10.9	42	60%
(Igor's Piroshki) pocket, w/cheddar	1 sandwich	370	15	31	630	2	20.0	6.0	45	49%
(Kid Cuisine)										
double patty w/cheese, frozen, 'Mega Meal'............	9.1 oz	480	20	55	1040	0	20.0	0.0	0	38%
patty w/cheese, frozen	6.25 oz	400	12	47	550	0	19.0	0.0	40	42%
(Lean Pockets) pocket, w/broccoli, frozen	1 pkg	250	11	30	760	0	8.0	0.0	0	31%
(Manwich)										
'Chili Fixin's'...................................	1 cup	290	20	20	980	5	14.0	5.4	65	44%
extra thick and chunky, prepared....................	1 sandwich	330	17	36	870	3	13.0	4.7	50	36%
Mexican, prepared	1 sandwich	310	17	30	690	2	13.0	4.7	50	38%
'sloppy Joe', prepared.........................	1 sandwich	310	17	31	620	1	13.0	4.7	50	38%
(MicroMagic)										
burger, w/cheese, frozen........................	4.75 oz	450	17	29	790	0	25.0	0.0	80	55%
hamburger, frozen................................	4 oz	350	13	26	500	0	18.0	0.0	55	51%
(Mrs. Paterson's)										
steak, w/mushroom, pocket, hand held, 'Aussie Pie'	5.5 oz	410	14	43	820	0	20.0	8.0	80	44%
(Pierre)										
submarine, flame-broiled.........................	1 piece	152	16	2	294	1	8.9	3.5	41	53%
submarine, flame-broiled, 'Hot Diggity Sub'	1 piece	158	16	2	291	1	9.5	3.8	41	54%
(Tyson) barbecue, no bone, frozen, microwave	1 sandwich	200	15	29	600	0	2.7	0.0	30	12%
CALZONE										
(Amy's Kitchen) cheese, pocket, organic, frozen..........	1 sandwich	290	14	38	390	3	9.0	4.0	20	28%
CANADIAN BACON										
(Quick Meal)										
Canadian bacon, w/egg and cheese, on muffin	4.5 oz	250	16	29	680	0	8.0	4.0	115	29%

Food Name	Serving Size	Calories	Prot. gms	Carbs gms	Sod. mgs	Fiber gms	Fat gms	Sat. Fat gms	Chol. mgs	% Fat Cal.
CHICKEN										
(*Banquet*) breast patty, bun, microwave.	4 oz	310	16	31	664	0	14.0	0.0	0	40%
(*BestFresh*)										
breast, teriyaki, charbroiled.	1 sandwich	490	34	45	1030	6	20.0	4.0	60	36%
w/cucumber yogurt dressing.	1 sandwich	390	24	38	960	1	15.0	4.0	70	35%
(*Hot Pockets*)										
w/broccoli, cheese, stuffed, 'Croissant Pockets'	1 pkg	602	23	78	1303	3	22.0	6.7	74	33%
chicken, w/cheddar, pocket, frozen	5 oz	310	16	38	720	0	11.0	0.0	0	31%
(*Kid Cuisine*) chicken, dinner.	8.2 oz	470	16	61	830	0	17.0	0.0	40	33%
(*Lean Pockets*)										
fajita, pocket, frozen	1 pocket	250	13	36	810	0	6.0	2.0	30	22%
Oriental, pocket, frozen.	1 pkg	250	14	35	840	0	6.0	0.0	0	22%
supreme, glazed, frozen	1 pkg	464	20	68	1119	na	12.5	3.8	46	24%
supreme, glazed, frozen	1 serving	233	10	34	562	na	6.3	1.9	23	24%
w/Parmesan, pocket, frozen	1 pkg	270	19	35	750	0	6.0	0.0	0	20%
(*MicroMagic*) frozen.	4.5 oz	390	13	42	650	0	16.0	0.0	35	40%
(*Quick Meal*)										
. . . .	4.3 oz	320	16	40	640	0	11.0	2.0	65	31%
biscuit	4.2 oz	310	13	36	900	0	13.0	0.0	50	37%
grilled.	4.7 oz	300	21	35	620	0	9.0	0.0	60	27%
(*Tyson*)										
barbecue, frozen, microwave	4 oz	230	16	27	510	0	6.0	0.0	0	24%
breast, frozen, microwave	3.5 oz	275	14	27	0	0	12.0	0.0	0	40%
breast, grilled, boneless	3.5 oz	150	17	2	400	0	8.0	0.0	44	49%
breast, grilled, microwave	1 entrée	210	13	25	460	2	6.0	1.5	25	26%
grilled, boneless	3.5 oz	200	15	25	470	0	5.0	0.0	32	22%
mini, frozen, microwave.	3.5 oz	230	12	39	0	0	5.0	0.0	0	18%
(*Weight Watchers*)										
grilled, 'Ultimate 200'.	4 oz	200	18	22	420	0	5.0	2.0	20	22%
w/broccoli, cheese, pocket sandwich, 'On-The-Go'.	1 pkg	266	13	40	388	na	6.1	1.8	14	20%
EGG (*Great Starts*) w/bacon and cheese, muffin.	1 sandwich	290	14	25	750	2	15.0	6.0	95	46%
ENGLISH MUFFIN (*Weight Watchers*).	1 sandwich	210	13	28	420	2	5.0	3.0	20	22%
FISH										
(*Fisher Boy*) burger, crunchy.	1 burger	180	15	18	870	0	6.0	0.0	0	29%
(*Quick Meal*)	5.2 oz	430	16	56	910	0	16.0	4.0	68	33%
HAM										
(*Hot Pockets*)										
and cheese, pocket, frozen	5 oz	360	19	36	1320	0	16.0	0.0	90	40%
and cheese, stuffed	1 pkg	681	30	77	1331	na	28.4	11.6	100	38%
and cheese, stuffed.	1 serving	340	15	38	666	na	14.2	5.8	50	38%
w/cheese, no gravy, pocket, 'Ham 'n Cheese'.	1 pocket	524	17	36	620	1	34.8	10.9	42	60%
(*Igor's Piroshki*) and cheese, pocket	1 sandwich	370	14	46	880	3	15.0	6.0	35	36%
(*Owens*) and cheese, refrigerated, 'Border Breakfasts'	2 oz	150	7	14	600	0	6.0	0.0	0	39%
(*Red Baron*)										
and cheese, 'Premium Pockets'	1 pkg	721	30	73	2128	na	34.2	12.5	83	43%
and cheese, 'Premium Pockets'.	1 serving	356	15	36	1052	na	16.9	6.2	41	43%
(*Swanson*)										
and cheese, on bagel, refrigerated, 'Great Starts'	3 oz	240	12	28	600	0	8.0	0.0	0	31%
(*Weight Watchers*)										
and cheese, on bagel	3 oz	210	13	28	460	0	6.0	2.0	15	25%
and cheese, pocket, frozen, 'Ultimate 200'	4 oz	200	14	24	490	0	6.0	2.0	5	26%
HOT DOG										
(*Kid Cuisine*) w/bun	6.7 oz	450	13	27	880	0	19.0	0.0	40	52%
(*Kid Cuisine*) w/bun, 'Mega Meal'.	8.25 oz	500	16	52	1260	0	25.0	0.0	0	45%

Food Name	Serving Size	Calories	Prot. gms	Carbs gms	Sod. mgs.	Fiber gms	Fat gms	Sat. Fat gms	Chol. mgs	% Fat Cal.
PIZZA										
(Hot Pockets)										
pepperoni, pocket, frozen	5 oz	380	17	40	1240	0	17.0	0.0	45	40%
pepperoni, stuffed, frozen	1 pkg	735	27	77	1352	na	35.3	13.3	82	43%
pepperoni, stuffed, frozen	1 serving	367	14	39	676	na	17.7	6.6	41	43%
sausage, pocket, frozen	5 oz	360	15	40	590	0	16.0	0.0	65	40%
(Igor's Piroshki) pepperoni and sausage, pocket	1 sandwich	400	18	39	590	3	19.0	7.0	40	43%
(Lean Pockets)										
pocket, frozen, 'Deluxe'	1 pkg	280	14	34	500	0	9.0	0.0	0	30%
sausage and pepperoni, pocket, frozen, 'Deluxe'	1 pocket	300	13	37	670	0	11.0	5.0	35	33%
(Weight Watchers) pocket, 'Deluxe' 'Ultimate 200'	4 oz	200	15	25	400	0	5.0	3.0	5	22%
PORK										
(Quick Meal) barbecue	4.3 oz	350	16	40	550	0	14.0	5.0	65	36%
(Swanson) rib, hot, smothered	10.25 oz	340	13	50	690	0	10.0	0.0	25	26%
SUBMARINE *(BestFresh)* 'Deluxe'	1 sandwich	790	39	59	2070	8	44.0	17.0	105	50%
TURKEY										
(BestFresh) smoked	1 sandwich	580	39	49	1770	7	26.0	10.0	80	40%
(Healthy Deli)										
w/corned beef, 'Doubledecker'	1 oz	30	5	1	195	0	0.7	0.0	12	22%
w/ham, 'Doubledecker'	1 oz	30	5	1	185	0	0.9	0.0	11	27%
(Hot Pockets) w/ham and cheese, frozen	5 oz	320	17	37	780	0	11.0	0.0	0	31%
(Igor's Piroshki) and Swiss, w/broccoli, frozen	1 sandwich	320	15	41	580	3	11.0	3.5	20	31%
(Lean Pockets) w/broccoli and cheese, frozen	1 pocket	260	13	32	680	0	9.0	3.0	30	31%
VEGGIE										
(Ken & Robert's)										
barbecue style, 'Truly Amazing'	5 oz	320	11	50	560	2	10.0	0.6	0	27%
broccoli cheddar, 'Truly Amazing'	5 oz	275	11	37	540	0	9.0	0.7	0	30%
Greek style, 'Truly Amazing'	5 oz	270	11	35	500	0	10.0	1.0	0	33%
Indian style, 'Truly Amazing'	5 oz	300	10	41	500	1	12.0	1.0	0	35%
Oriental style, 'Truly Amazing'	5 oz	295	10	41	572	1	12.0	0.9	0	35%
pizza style, 'Truly Amazing'	5 oz	315	12	42	620	1	12.0	1.0	0	33%
Tex Mex style, 'Truly Amazing'	5 oz	310	11	43	595	0	11.0	1.0	0	31%
(Morningstar Farms)										
burger and cheese style, 'Stuffed Sandwiches'	1 sandwich	290	14	10	400	2	8.0	3.5	10	24.8%
ham and cheese style, 'Stuffed Sandwiches'	1 sandwich	300	15	45	520	1	7.0	2.5	10	21.0%
pepperoni pizza style, 'Stuffed Sandwiches'	1 sandwich	280	12	42	420	5	7.0	3.0	5	22.5%
SANDWICH FILLING MIX										
(French's) sloppy Joe, mix only	1/8 pkg	16	0	4	390	0	0.0	0.0	0	0%
(Hunt's)										
sloppy Joe, barbecue, 'Manwich' mix only	1/4 cup	57	1	14	887	1	0.2	0.1	0	3%
sloppy Joe, bold, 'Manwich' mix only	1/4 cup	63	1	13	802	na	1.1	0.0	0	15%
sloppy Joe, Mexican, 'Manwich' mix only	1/4 cup	27	1	5	552	1	0.2	0.0	0	6%
sloppy Joe, original, 'Manwich' mix only	1/4 cup	32	1	6	365	1	0.4	0.0	0	12%
sloppy Joe, thick and chunky, 'Manwich'	1/4 cup	44	1	9	737	1	0.5	0.0	0	9%
(McCormick/Schilling) sloppy Joe, mix only	1 tsp	15	0	3	360	0	0.0	0.0	0	0%
(Schilling) sloppy Joe, mix only	1/4 pkg	26	1	6	750	0	0.5	0.0	0	15%
(Tone's) sloppy Joe, mix only	1 tsp	14	0	3	347	0	0.1	0.0	0	6%
SANDWICH SPREAD. See also LUNCHEON MEAT SPREAD; POTTED MEAT SPREAD.										
(Best Foods)	1 tbsp	50	0	3	170	0	5.0	1.0	3	79%
(Blue Plate)	1 tbsp	75	0	3	105	0	7.0	1.0	5	84%
(Hellmann's)	1 tbsp	50	0	3	170	0	5.0	1.0	3	79%
(JFG)	1 tbsp	60	0	3	150	0	5.0	1.0	7	79%
(Oscar Mayer)										
	2 oz	130	4	8	460	0	10.0	4.0	25	65%

Food Name	Serving Size	Calories	Prot. gms	Carbs gms	Sod. mgs	Fiber gms	Fat gms	Sat. Fat gms	Chol. mgs	% Fat Cal.
pork, chicken, and beef.................	1 serving	71	2	5	246	0	5.0	1.7	14	63%
SAPODILLA										
fresh, raw, pulp..................	1 cup	200	1	48	29	13	2.7	0.5	0	11%
fresh, raw, whole.................	1 medium	141	1	34	20	9	1.9	0.3	0	11%
SAPOTE / marmalade plum										
fresh, raw, trimmed..............	1 oz	38	0.6	9.6	3	>.5 c	0.2	na	0	4%
fresh, raw, trimmed, whole, approx 11.2 oz..........	1 medium	302	5	76	23	6	1.4	na	0	4%
fresh, raw, untrimmed.............	1 lb	431	6.8	108.7	31	>6.1 c	1.9	na	0	4%
SARDINE										
ATLANTIC										
Canned										
in oil, drained, w/bone..............	1 oz	59	7	0	143	0	3.2	0.4	40	50%
in oil, drained, w/bone..............	2 medium	50	6	0	121	0	2.7	0.4	34	50%
in oil, drained, w/bone..............	1 cup	310	37	0	752	0	17.1	2.3	212	50%
BRISLING / Norwegian										
Canned										
(S&W).............	3 oz	257	16	0	306	0	20.9	5.6	96	75%
in mild sardine oil, drained (Empress)..	3.75 oz	260	19	1	0	0	20.0	0.0	0	69%
in mustard sauce (Crown Prince)......	3.75 oz	240	18	2	450	0	18.0	0.0	0	67%
smoked, in oil (Crown Prince)........	3.75 oz	260	19	1	120	0	42.0	0.0	0	83%
w/liquid (Underwood).............	3.75 oz	260	19	1	450	0	20.0	0.0	0	69%
MAINE										
Canned										
in mustard, drained (Beach Cliff)......	3 oz	227	13	4	350	0	18.0	0.0	0	70%
in soybean oil, drained (Beach Cliff)...	3 oz	240	16	0	20	0	20.0	0.0	0	74%
in tomato sauce, drained (Beach Cliff)...	3 oz	210	15	0	350	0	17.0	0.0	0	72%
in water, drained (Beach Cliff)........	3 oz	230	17	1	350	0	18.0	0.0	0	69%
MIXED SPECIES										
Canned										
boneless, skinless (S&W)...........	3 oz	177	21	0	443	0	10.6	1.8	35	53%
in mustard sauce (Underwood)........	3.75 oz	220	16	2	650	0	16.0	0.0	0	67%
in oil (Featherweight).............	1 1/8 oz	130	19	1	65	0	10.0	0.0	45	53%
in olive oil, boneless, skinless (Crown Prince)	1 pkg	230	24	0	300	1	15.0	6.0	40	58%
in soya oil, drained (Underwood)..	3.75 oz	230	16	1	400	0	18.0	0.0	0	70%
in Tabasco sauce, drained (Underwood)..	3 oz	220	16	1	400	0	16.0	0.0	0	68%
in tomato sauce (Del Monte).........	1/2 cup	360	19	45	540	0	12.0	0.0	0	30%
in tomato sauce (Underwood)........	3.75 oz	220	16	2	500	0	16.0	0.0	0	67%
in tomato sauce, drained, w/bone......	1 cup	158	15	0	368	0	10.7	2.7	54	61%
in tomato sauce, drained, w/bone......	1 medium	68	6	0	157	0	4.6	1.2	23	61%
in water (Featherweight)...........	1 1/8 oz	95	9	1	65	0	7.0	0.0	20	61%
kippered, 'Kippered Snacks' (Brunswick)...	3.5 oz	185	16	1	610	0	14.0	0.0	0	65%
NORWEGIAN. See BRISLING.										
SARDINE OIL. See under FISH OIL.										
SAUCE										
ALFREDO SAUCE										
(Bernardi)...................	1/2 cup	180	6	10	500	1	13.0	9.0	35	65%
(Contadina)										
	1/2 cup	400	7	8	510	0	38.0	21.0	80	85%
frozen, food service product......	1 oz	67	1	3	142	0	5.7	1.5	11	77%
light........................	1/2 cup	190	3	10	550	0	13.0	7.0	40	69%
pouch, food service product.......	1 oz	70	1	2	181	0	6.1	2.0	10	78%
refrigerated 'Fresh'..............	6 oz	540	9	10	620	0	53.0	0.0	85	86%
(DiGiorno)										
light........................	1/4 cup	140	5	9	600	0	9.0	6.0	30	59%

Food Name	Serving Size	Calories	Prot. gms	Carbs gms	Sod. mgs	Fiber gms	Fat gms	Sat. Fat gms	Chol. mgs	% Fat Cal.
reduced-fat, 'Lighter Varieties'.	1/4 cup	180	5	15	580	0	11.0	6.0	35	55%
refrigerated .	2 oz	200	4	2	490	0	20.0	12.0	55	88%
(Five Brothers)										
.	1/4 cup	120	2	2	430	0	11.0	7.0	40	86%
w/mushrooms .	1/4 cup	80	2	3	490	0	7.0	4.0	30	76%
(Progresso) canned, 'Authentic Pasta Sauces' .	1/2 cup	340	13	6	1080	0	30.0	19.0	95	78%
APPLE-APRICOT										
(Lucky Leaf) 'Fruit n' Sauce'.	4 oz	90	0	22	20	0	0.0	0.0	0	0%
(Musselman's) 'Fruit n' Sauce'.	4 oz	90	0	22	20	0	0.0	0.0	0	0%
APPLE-CHERRY										
(Lucky Leaf) 'Fruit n' Sauce'.	4 oz	100	0	24	20	0	0.0	0.0	0	0%
(Musselman's) 'Fruit n' Sauce'.	4 oz	100	0	24	20	0	0.0	0.0	0	0%
APPLE-CRANBERRY *(Lucky Leaf)* .	4 oz	80	0	19	15	0	0.0	0.0	0	0%
APPLE-PEACH										
(Lucky Leaf) 'Fruit n' Sauce'	4 oz	90	0	22	20	0	0.0	0.0	0	0%
(Musselman's) 'Fruit n' Sauce'.	4 oz	90	0	22	20	0	0.0	0.0	0	0%
APPLE-PINEAPPLE										
(Lucky Leaf) 'Fruit n' Sauce' .	4 oz	110	0	26	20	0	0.0	0.0	0	0%
(Musselman's) 'Fruit n' Sauce'.	4 oz	110	0	26	20	0	0.0	0.0	0	0%
APPLE-STRAWBERRY										
(Lucky Leaf) 'Fruit n' Sauce' .	4 oz	100	0	24	20	0	0.0	0.0	0	0%
(Musselman's) 'Fruit n' Sauce'.	4 oz	100	0	24	20	0	0.0	0.0	0	0%
BARBECUE										
(Bull's Eye)										
regular.	0.5 oz	22	0	5	47	0	0.0	0.0	0	0%
Ridge's .	2 tbsp	63	0	15	302	na	0.1	na	na	1%
(Cattleman's)										
classic .	2 tbsp	70	0	15	410	0	0.0	0.0	0	0%
mild .	1 tbsp	25	0	5	260	0	0.0	0.0	0	0%
smoky .	1 tbsp	25	0	5	300	0	0.0	0.0	0	0%
(Enrico's)										
'Original' .	1 tbsp	18	1	3	4	0	1.0	0.0	0	36%
mesquite .	1 tbsp	18	1	3	4	0	1.0	0.0	0	36%
(Estee) regular.	1 tbsp	18	1	3	5	0	1.0	1.0	0	36%
(Golden Dipt) Cajun style.	1 oz	90	0	5	360	0	8.0	0.0	0	78%
(Hain) honey .	1 tbsp	14	0	1	120	0	1.0	0.0	0	69%
(Healthy Choice)										
hickory.	1.13 oz	26	0	6	229	1	0.2	0.0	0	7%
hot and spicy.	1.13 oz	25	0	6	229	1	0.2	0.0	0	7%
original.	1.13 oz	25	0	6	229	1	0.2	0.0	0	7%
(Heinz)										
Cajun style .	1 tbsp	15	0	3	108	0	0.1	0.0	0	6%
chunky, 'Thick & Rich' .	1 tbsp	24	0	5	230	0	0.0	0.0	0	0%
Hawaiian style.	1 tbsp	19	0	4	108	0	0.1	0.0	0	5%
Hawaiian style, 'Thick & Rich' .	1 oz	40	0	10	210	0	0.0	0.0	0	0%
hickory smoke .	1 tbsp	19	0	4	56	0	0.1	0.0	0	5%
hickory smoke, 'Thick & Rich' .	1 tbsp	20	0	5	220	0	0.0	0.0	0	0%
hickory, 'Select' .	1 oz	35	0	8	260	0	0.0	0.0	0	0%
hot, 'Thick & Rich' .	1 tbsp	20	0	5	220	0	0.0	0.0	0	0%
mesquite smoke, 'Thick & Rich'.	1 oz	30	0	7	380	0	0.0	0.0	0	0%
mushroom .	1 tbsp	14	0	3	219	0	0.1	0.0	0	6%
mushroom, 'Thick & Rich' .	1 tbsp	20	0	5	220	0	0.0	0.0	0	0%
'Old Fashioned' .	1 tbsp	18	0	4	180	0	0.1	0.0	0	5%
old fashioned, 'Thick & Rich' .	1 oz	35	0	8	350	0	0.0	0.0	0	0%

Food Name	Serving Size	Calories	Prot. gms	Carbs gms	Sod. mgs	Fiber gms	Fat gms	Sat. Fat gms	Chol. mgs	% Fat Cal.
onion	1 tbsp	15	0	3	255	0	0.1	0.0	0	6%
onion, 'Thick & Rich'	1 tbsp	20	0	5	200	0	0.0	0.0	0	0%
original, 'Thick & Rich'	1 tbsp	20	0	5	230	0	0.0	0.0	0	0%
'Select'	1 tbsp	18	0	4	60	0	0.1	0.0	0	5%
Texas style, hot, 'Thick & Rich'	1 tbsp	15	0	3	210	0	0.2	0.0	0	11%
(Hunt's)										
'Chicken Sensations'	1 tbsp	35	0	3	308	0	2.7	0.3	0	67%
country style	1.2 oz	39	0	9	399	0	0.3	0.0	0	7%
hickory	1 tbsp	20	1	5	160	1	1.0	0.0	0	27%
hickory, 'Light'	1.13 oz	27	1	6	245	1	0.2	0.0	0	6%
homestyle	1.23 oz	41	1	10	381	1	0.1	0.0	0	2%
Kansas City style	1.23 oz	43	0	10	220	1	0.2	0.0	0	4%
New Orleans style	1.23 oz	41	1	9	383	1	0.2	0.0	0	4%
original recipe	2 tbsp	40	0	9	410	1	0.0	0.0	0	0%
Southern style	1.2 oz	40	1	9	361	1	0.4	0.0	0	9%
Texas style	1.23 oz	42	0	10	305	1	0.1	0.0	0	2%
western style	1.23 oz	41	0	10	394	1	0.2	0.0	0	4%
(Kraft)										
chunky, 'Thick 'N Spicy'	2 tbsp	60	0	13	420	0	1.0	0.0	0	15%
hickory smoke	2 tbsp	39	0	9	418	0	0.1	0.0	0	2%
hickory smoke, 'Thick 'N Spicy'	2 tbsp	50	0	12	450	0	0.0	0.0	0	0%
hickory smoke, w/onion bits	2 tbsp	50	0	11	340	0	1.0	0.0	0	17%
honey, 'Thick 'N Spicy'	2 tbsp	60	0	13	360	0	0.0	0.0	0	0%
hot	2 tbsp	40	0	9	520	0	0.0	0.0	0	0%
Kansas City style	2 tbsp	50	0	11	310	0	0.0	0.0	0	0%
Kansas City style, 'Thick 'N Spicy'	2 tbsp	60	0	14	310	0	0.0	0.0	0	0%
mesquite smoke	2 tbsp	40	0	9	420	0	0.0	0.0	0	0%
mesquite smoke, 'Thick 'N Spicy'	2 tbsp	50	0	12	440	0	0.0	0.0	0	0%
original	2 tbsp	39	0	9	424	0	0.1	0.0	0	2%
original, 'Thick 'N Spicy'	2 tbsp	50	0	12	440	0	0.0	0.0	0	0%
roasted garlic	2 tbsp	50	0	12	360	0	0.0	0.0	0	0%
salsa style	2 tbsp	45	0	9	420	0	0.0	0.0	0	0%
w/Italian seasonings	2 tbsp	50	0	10	280	0	1.0	0.0	0	18%
w/onion bits	2 tbsp	45	0	11	360	0	0.0	0.0	0	0%
(LaChoy) Oriental	1 tbsp	16	1	4	304	1	0.1	0.0	0	5%
(Lawry's)										
Dijon and honey	1/2 cup	203	5	27	1768	0	1.2	0.0	0	8%
orange juice, 'California Grill'	1/4 cup	34	4	3	3846	0	0.7	0.0	0	18%
(Libby's) w/beef, 'Sloppy Joe'	1/3 cup	110	5	7	190	0	7.0	0.0	0	57%
(Luzianne) mustard base, 'Cajun'	2 tbsp	110	0	19	350	0	4.0	1.0	0	32%
(Marzetti) original, 'Texas Best'	2 tbsp	42	1	4	315	na	2.7	0.6	0	57%
(Maull's) smoky	1 tbsp	20	1	4	139	1	1.0	0.0	1	31%
(Open Pit)										
hickory	2 tbsp	50	0	11	430	0	0.5	0.0	0	9%
original	2 tbsp	50	0	11	415	0	0.5	0.0	0	9%
(Open Range)										
hickory	1.2 oz	37	1	9	423	1	0.2	0.0	0	5%
hickory, food service product	2 tbsp	37	0	9	424	1	0.2	0.0	0	5%
original	1.2 oz	38	1	9	333	1	0.2	0.0	0	4%
original, food service product	2 tbsp	38	1	9	332	1	0.2	0.0	0	5%
(Ott's)										
regular	1 tbsp	14	0	3	147	0	0.1	0.0	1	6%
smoky	1 tbsp	14	0	3	149	0	0.1	0.0	1	6%
(Woodys) sweet and sour	2 tbsp	70	0	17	610	1	0.0	0.0	0	0%

Food Name	Serving Size	Calories	Prot. gms	Carbs gms	Sod. mgs	Fiber gms	Fat gms	Sat. Fat gms	Chol. mgs	% Fat Cal.
BASIL-HERB										
(Golden Dipt) 'Nature Bay'	2 grams	8	0	1	36	0	0.0	0.0	0	0%
(Nature Bay)	2 grams	8	0	1	36	0	0.0	0.0	0	0%
BEARNAISE (Great Impressions)	2 tbsp	192	1	0	148	0	21.0	0.0	48	99%
BEEF										
(Ragu)										
barbecue, 'Beef Tonight'	4 oz	70	2	15	580	0	1.0	0.0	0	12%
skillet lasagna, 'Beef Tonight'	4 oz	60	3	9	630	0	1.0	0.0	5	16%
stroganoff, 'Beef Tonight'	4 oz	130	1	6	770	0	12.0	10.0	10	79%
(Simmer Chef) Stroganoff, family style	1/2 cup	110	2	8	760	1	7.0	5.0	5	61%
BOLOGNESE										
(Contadina)										
	5 oz	130	8	0	500	0	7.0	1.0	25	66%
refrigerated, 'Fresh'	7.5 oz	230	22	12	600	0	11.0	0.0	50	42%
(Progresso) canned, 'Authentic Pasta Sauces'	1/2 cup	150	10	12	520	3	8.0	2.0	20	45%
BROCCOLI (Simmer Chef) creamy	1/2 cup	110	1	9	670	2	8.0	3.0	5	64%
BROWNING (Gravymaster)	1 tsp	12	1	2	1	0	0.0	0.0	0	0%
CACCIATORE										
(Recipe Sauces)	3.9 oz	40	1	9	570	0	1.0	0.0	0	18%
(Simmer Chef) old country	1/2 cup	110	2	15	540	2	4.0	1.0	0	35%
CARBONARA (DiGiorno) refrigerated	2 oz	200	4	3	380	0	19.0	9.0	40	86%
CHARDONNAY (Golden Dipt)	1 oz	60	0	1	160	0	6.0	0.0	0	93%
CHEESE										
(Contadina)										
four cheese, refrigerated 'Fresh'	6 oz	470	12	8	500	0	45.0	0.0	147	84%
four cheese, w/white wine & shallots	1/2 cup	320	8	8	240	0	28.0	14.0	70	80%
(DiGiorno) four cheese	1/4 cup	160	5	3	410	0	15.0	7.0	30	81%
(J. Hungerford)										
cheddar, 'Stadium'	2 oz	80	1	6	500	0	5.0	1.5	4	62%
nacho	2.01 oz	120	2	7	440	0	9.0	2.0	5	69%
nacho, 'Stadium'	2.01 oz	80	1	6	410	0	5.0	1.5	4	62%
(Kaukauna)										
nacho	1 oz	80	3	4	330	0	6.0	0.0	8	66%
nacho, medium, microwaveable	2 tbsp	90	3	4	330	0	7.0	2.0	10	69%
nacho, mild, microwaveable	2 tbsp	90	3	4	330	0	7.0	2.0	10	69%
(Kraft)										
jalapeño pepper, pasteurized process, 'Cheez Whiz'	2 tbsp	90	4	3	510	0	7.0	5.0	25	69%
pasteurized process, 'Cheez Whiz'	2 tbsp	90	4	3	540	0	7.0	5.0	20	69%
salsa, mild, pasteurized process, 'Cheez Whiz'	2 tbsp	100	4	3	530	0	7.0	5.0	25	69%
(La Victoria)										
cheddar	1/4 cup	105	1	6	633	0	8.5	2.3	2	73%
nacho, w/jalapeno peppers	1/4 cup	122	1	7	547	0	9.7	2.7	4	71%
(Lucky Leaf)										
cheddar	4 oz	220	3	12	1000	0	18.0	0.0	0	73%
cheddar, aged	4 oz	240	5	11	920	0	20.0	0.0	0	74%
cheddar, mild, aged	4 oz	200	5	9	790	0	18.0	0.0	0	74%
cheddar, sharp, aged	4 oz	230	9	6	850	0	17.0	0.0	0	72%
nacho	4 oz	220	4	11	1010	0	18.0	0.0	0	73%
(Musselman's)										
cheddar	4 oz	220	3	12	1000	0	18.0	0.0	0	73%
cheddar, aged	4 oz	240	5	11	920	0	20.0	0.0	0	74%
cheddar, mild, aged	4 oz	200	5	9	790	0	18.0	0.0	0	74%
cheddar, sharp, aged	4 oz	230	9	6	850	0	17.0	0.0	0	72%
nacho	4 oz	220	4	11	1010	0	18.0	0.0	0	73%

Food Name	Serving Size	Calories	Prot. gms	Carbs gms	Sod. mgs	Fiber gms	Fat gms	Sat. Fat gms	Chol. mgs	% Fat Cal.
(Nestlé)										
cheddar, 'Chef Mate'	1 cup	327	7	32	1885	0	18.8	6.3	25	52%
cheddar, 'Chef Mate'	1/4 cup	82	2	8	471	0	4.7	1.6	6	52%
cheddar, sharp, 'Chef Mate'	1 cup	532	22	7	1893	3	46.0	18.3	91	78%
cheddar, sharp, 'Chef Mate'	1/4 cup	133	5	2	473	1	11.5	4.6	23	78%
con queso, 'Que Bueno'	1 cup	335	15	14	2220	0	24.1	11.7	63	65%
con queso, 'Que Bueno'	1/4 cup	84	4	4	555	0	6.0	2.9	16	65%
golden, 'Chef-Mate'	1 cup	554	27	9	2006	3	45.5	22.3	116	74%
golden, 'Chef-Mate'	1/4 cup	139	7	2	501	1	11.4	5.6	29	74%
jalapeño, 'Que Bueno'	1 pkg	3876	96	370	27255	0	224.2	86.2	301	52%
jalapeño, 'Que Bueno'	1/4 cup	81	2	8	571	0	4.7	1.8	6	52%
nacho, mild, 'Que Bueno'	1 cup	476	18	10	1968	2	40.5	16.9	81	77%
nacho, mild, 'Que Bueno'	1/4 cup	119	5	3	492	1	10.1	4.2	20	77%
nacho, 'Que Bueno'	1 cup	512	21	16	2318	2	40.4	23.2	116	71%
nacho, 'Que Bueno'	1/4 cup	128	5	4	580	0	10.1	5.8	29	71%
(Pablo's)										
jalapeño, 'Deli Style'	1 oz	59	2	4	470	0	4.0	1.0	5	60%
nacho, 'Deli Style'	1 oz	59	2	4	470	0	4.0	1.0	5	60%
(Snow's) Welsh rarebit	1/2 cup	170	9	10	460	0	11.0	0.0	0	57%
(Weight Watchers) cheddar, sharp	2 tbsp	70	4	7	190	0	3.0	2.0	10	38%
(White House)										
cheddar, aged	3.5 oz	213	4	10	810	0	18.0	0.0	0	74%
jalapeño	3.5 oz	193	3	10	890	0	16.0	0.0	0	73%
nacho	3.5 oz	193	3	10	890	0	16.0	0.0	0	73%
CHICKEN										
(Hunt's) Southwestern, 'Chicken Sensations'	1 tbsp	27	0	1	281	0	2.6	0.3	0	81%
(Ragu)										
cacciatore, 'Chicken Tonight'	4 oz	70	1	12	490	0	2.0	0.0	0	26%
French, country, 'Chicken Tonight'	4 oz	140	1	6	730	0	12.0	0.0	5	79%
herbed, w/wine, 'Chicken Tonight'	4 oz	100	2	13	610	0	4.0	0.0	5	38%
honey mustard, light, 'Chicken Tonight'	4 oz	50	1	12	420	0	1.0	0.0	0	15%
Italian, primavera, 'Light'	4 oz	50	2	9	540	0	1.0	0.0	0	17%
primavera, creamy, 'Chicken Tonight'	4 oz	90	1	9	650	0	6.0	0.0	5	57%
sweet and sour, 'Chicken Tonight'	4 oz	80	0	19	280	0	0.0	0.0	0	0%
sweet and spicy, light, 'Chicken Tonight'	4 oz	50	2	10	390	0	1.0	0.0	0	16%
w/mushrooms, creamy, 'Chicken Tonight'	4 oz	110	1	5	650	0	10.0	0.0	5	79%
CHILI										
(Chef Boyardee) hot dog, w/beef	1 oz	30	1	4	140	0	1.0	0.0	0	31%
(Del Monte)	1 tbsp	20	0	5	480	0	0.0	0.0	0	0%
(El Molino) green, mild	2 tbsp	10	0	2	210	0	0.0	0.0	0	0%
(Featherweight)	1 tbsp	8	0	2	10	0	0.0	0.0	0	0%
(Gebhardt) hot dog	2 tbsp	20	1	2	150	0	1.0	0.0	0	43%
(Heinz)	1 oz	30	0	7	430	0	0.0	0.0	0	0%
(Just Rite) hot dog sauce	2.19 oz	50	2	5	265	2	2.9	1.3	2	47%
(Las Palmas) red	1/2 cup	25	1	3	670	0	1.0	0.0	0	36%
(Manwich) 'Chili Fixin's'	5.3 oz	110	6	20	900	5	1.0	0.0	0	8%
(Open Range) hot dog	2.22 oz	61	3	6	255	2	3.5	1.5	4	46%
(S&W)										
'Chili Makin's'	1/2 cup	100	5	20	782	0	1.0	0.0	0	8%
steakhouse	1 tbsp	15	0	4	180	0	0.0	0.0	0	0%
(Wolf Brand) hot dog	1.25 oz	44	2	4	199	0	2.3	0.0	0	47%
CHOCOLATE *(Chocolate Mountain)*	2 tbsp	120	1	20	80	0	4.0	0.0	4	30%
CLAM										
(Buitoni) red, canned	5 oz	190	8	28	560	0	6.0	1.0	20	27%

Food Name	Serving Size	Calories	Prot. gms	Carbs gms	Sod. mgs	Fiber gms	Fat gms	Sat. Fat gms	Chol. mgs	% Fat Cal.
(Contadina)										
red, refrigerated, 'Fresh'	7.5 oz	120	7	15	800	0	4.0	0.0	35	29%
white, refrigerated, 'Fresh'	6 oz	290	8	13	800	0	23.0	0.0	94	71%
(Ferrara)										
red, canned	4 oz	70	5	8	320	0	2.0	0.0	10	26%
white, canned	4 oz	80	5	4	570	0	5.0	1.0	10	56%
(Progresso)										
red, canned	1/2 cup	70	5	7	560	0	3.0	0.0	0	36%
white, canned	1/2 cup	110	9	1	280	0	8.0	0.0	0	64%
COCKTAIL										
(Del Monte)	1/4 cup	100	1	24	910	0	0.0	0.0	0	0%
(Estee)	1 tbsp	10	1	2	35	0	1.0	1.0	0	43%
(Golden Dipt)										
extra hot	1 tbsp	20	0	5	210	0	0.0	0.0	0	0%
regular	1 tbsp	20	0	5	210	0	0.0	0.0	0	0%
(Great Impressions)										
	1 tbsp	21	0	5	182	0	0.1	0.0	0	4%
'Brandy Glow'	1 tbsp	68	0	2	106	0	6.7	0.0	10	89%
low-salt	1 tbsp	21	0	5	6	0	0.1	0.0	0	4%
(Heinz)	1/4 cup	60	1	14	680	1	0.0	0.0	0	0%
(S&W)	1 tsp	20	0	5	220	0	0.0	0.0	0	0%
(Sauceworks)	1 tbsp	14	0	3	170	0	0.0	0.0	0	0%
(Stokely)	1 tbsp	18	0	5	90	0	0.0	0.0	0	0%
CRANBERRY-ORANGE										
(Ocean Spray) crushed, for chicken, 'CranFruit'	2 oz	90	0	23	10	0	0.0	0.0	0	0%
CRANBERRY-RASPBERRY										
(Ocean Spray) crushed, for chicken, 'CranFruit'	2 oz	90	0	23	10	0	0.0	0.0	0	0%
CRANBERRY-STRAWBERRY										
(Ocean Spray) crushed, for chicken, 'CranFruit'	2 oz	90	0	22	10	0	0.0	0.0	0	0%
CREOLE										
(Enrico's) Cajun, 'Light'	4 oz	76	2	9	284	0	2.8	0.0	0	36%
(Golden Dipt) cooking sauce	1 oz	20	0	2	190	0	1.0	0.0	0	53%
(Nestlé)										
'Chef Mate'	1 cup	99	4	15	1357	3	2.8	0.3	0	25%
'Chef Mate'	1/4 cup	25	1	4	339	1	0.7	0.1	0	25%
CURRY										
(Flavor of the Rain Forest) ginger, stir-fry	1 tbsp	15	1	2	173	0	1.0	0.0	0	43%
(TAJ Cuisine of India) Bombay	4 oz	90	2	10	470	2	5.0	0.0	0	48%
DIABLE *(Escoffier)* nonfat	1 tbsp	20	0	4	160	0	0.0	0.0	0	0%
DIJONAISSE *(Golden Dipt)*	1 oz	52	0	2	130	0	4.0	0.0	0	82%
ENCHILADA										
(Del Monte)										
hot	1/2 cup	45	1	11	1090	0	0.0	0.0	0	0%
mild	1/2 cup	45	1	11	1150	0	0.0	0.0	0	0%
(El Molino) hot	2 tbsp	16	0	2	100	0	1.0	0.0	0	53%
(Gebhardt)	1/4 cup	35	1	4	218	1	2.0	0.9	0	52%
(La Victoria)										
	1 cup	80	1	10	1520	0	5.0	0.0	0	51%
	1/4 cup	20	0	3	397	0	0.9	na	0	40%
(Las Palmas) hot	1/2 cup	25	1	3	670	0	1.0	0.0	0	36%
(Nestlé)										
'Que Bueno'	1 pkg	1928	56	259	9946	39	76.3	11.2	0	36%
'Que Bueno'	2 tbsp	15	0	2	77	0	0.6	0.1	0	36%

Food Name	Serving Size	Calories	Prot. gms	Carbs gms	Sod. mgs	Fiber gms	Fat gms	Sat. Fat gms	Chol. mgs	% Fat Cal.
(Old El Paso)										
green	2 tbsp	11	1	3	200	0	0.0	0.0	0	0%
green chili	1/4 cup	30	1	3	330	0	1.5	na	0	49%
hot	1/4 cup	30	1	4	250	0	1.0	0.0	0	31%
mild	1/4 cup	25	0	4	160	0	1.0	na	0	36%
(Ortega)										
hot	1 oz	12	0	3	280	0	0.0	0.0	0	0%
mild	1 oz	12	0	3	280	0	0.0	0.0	0	0%
(Rosarita)										
	1/4 cup	23	1	3	409	0	1.1	0.1	0	43%
food service product	1/4 cup	23	1	3	5	0	1.1	0.1	0	43%
mild	2.5 oz	25	1	3	230	1	1.0	1.0	0	36%
(Santiago)	1 fl oz	11	0	2	138	0	0.1	0.0	0	9%
FAJITA										
(S&W) Southwestern	1 tbsp	10	0	2	230	1	0.0	0.0	0	0%
(Tio Sancho) 'Skillet Sauce'	1 oz	14	1	2	590	0	0.5	0.0	0	33%
FORESTIERA *(Contadina)* refrigerated, 'Fresh'	7.5 oz	270	6	15	830	0	9.0	0.0	15	49%
GARLIC										
(A Taste of Thai) chili pepper	1 tbsp	10	0	2	220	0	0.0	0.0	0	0%
(Golden Dipt) herb, nonfat, 'Nature Bay'	2 grams	8	0	1	87	0	0.0	0.0	0	0%
(Hunt's) Italian, 'Chicken Sensations'	1 tbsp	30	0	1	326	1	2.7	0.2	0	80%
GINGER										
(Flavor of the Rain Forest) curry, stir-fry	1 tbsp	15	1	2	173	0	1.0	0.0	0	43%
(Mr. Spice) stir fry, fat-free, salt-free	1 tbsp	11	1	3	0	0	0.0	0.0	0	0%
HERB *(Lawry's)* and garlic, w/lemon juice	1/4 cup	36	4	4	3688	0	0.4	0.0	0	11%
HOISIN *(Dynasty)*	2 tbsp	80	1	15	540	1	1.5	0.0	0	17%
HOLLANDAISE *(Great Impressions)*	2 tbsp	192	1	0	107	0	21.0	0.0	48	98%
HONEY MUSTARD										
(Ragu) light, Chicken Tonight'	4 oz	50	1	12	420	0	0.5	0.0	0	8%
(Simmer Chef)	1/2 cup	150	1	30	400	1	2.0	0.0	0	13%
HORSERADISH										
(Great Impressions)	1 tbsp	74	0	1	199	0	7.6	0.0	1	92%
(Heinz)	1 tbsp	74	0	2	113	0	7.4	0.0	0	88%
(Life) strong, 'All Natural'	1/2 tbsp	7	1	1	2	0	1.0	0.0	0	53%
(Sauceworks)	1 tbsp	50	0	2	105	0	5.0	1.0	5	85%
HOT DOG										
(Chili Bowl) chili, w/beef	1/4 cup	100	3	6	260	3	7.0	5.0	10	64%
(Gebhardt)										
chili, food service product	1/4 cup	61	3	6	255	2	3.5	1.5	4	46%
chili, w/beef	1/4 cup	57	3	6	262	2	3.2	1.4	12	45%
(Hunt's) chili, w/beef	1/4 cup	61	3	6	255	2	3.5	1.5	4	46%
(Just Rite)	1/4 cup	50	2	5	265	2	2.9	1.3	2	47%
(Nestlé)										
chili, w/beef, 'Chef-Mate'	1 pkg	3368	131	449	19382	83	115.7	47.2	214	31%
chili, w/beef, 'Chef-Mate'	1/4 cup	69	3	9	399	2	2.4	1.0	4	31%
Coney Island, 'Chef-Mate'	1 cup	303	9	23	1533	6	19.7	3.6	7	59%
Coney Island, 'Chef-Mate'	1/4 cup	76	2	6	383	1	4.9	0.9	2	59%
HOT SAUCE										
(Gebhardt) pepper, 'Louisiana Style'	1/2 tsp	0	0	0	45	0	0.0	0.0	0	0%
(Tabasco) pepper	1 tsp	1	0	0	30	0	0.0	0.0	0	53%
(Tabasco) pepper	1/4 tsp	1	0	1	9	0	0.0	0.0	0	0%
(Gebhardt)	1 tsp	1	0	0	89	0	0.0	0.0	0	31%
HUNTER *(McCormick/Schilling)*	1 tbsp	25	1	4	270	0	0.0	0.0	0	0%

Food Name	Serving Size	Calories	Prot. gms	Carbs gms	Sod. mgs	Fiber gms	Fat gms	Sat. Fat gms	Chol. mgs	% Fat Cal.
ITALIAN										
(Nestlé) 'Chef-Mate'	1 cup	125	2	24	627	2	2.4	0.3	0	17%
(Nestlé) 'Chef-Mate'	1/4 cup	61	1	11	304	1	1.2	0.2	0	17%
JALAPEÑO (Tabasco)	1 tsp	0	0	0	70	0	0.0	0.0	0	0%
KUNG PAO (Dynasty) spicy hot	2 tbsp	50	1	6	600	1	2.5	0.0	0	45%
LEMON										
(Nestlé) 'Chef-Mate'	1 pkg	2849	5	679	170	0	12.5	1.5	0	4%
(Nestlé) 'Chef-Mate'	2 tbsp	43	0	10	3	0	0.2	0.0	0	4%
LEMON BUTTER DILL (Golden Dipt)	1 oz	100	0	4	190	0	9.0	0.0	0	84%
LEMON DILL (Golden Dipt) 'Nature Bay'	1 oz	110	0	3	150	0	11.0	0.0	0	89%
LEMON HERB (Hunt's) 'Chicken Sensations'	1 tbsp	31	0	2	378	0	2.7	0.2	0	76%
LOBSTER SAUCE (Progresso) rock	1/2 cup	120	4	11	430	2	8.0	1.0	10	55%
MARINARA. See also SAUCE, PASTA.										
(Angela Mia) food service product	1/2 cup	47	2	9	503	4	0.3	0.0	0	6%
(Bernardi)	1/2 cup	120	2	20	480	2	4.0	1.0	0	29%
(Buitoni)	1/2 cup	70	1	11	570	0	3.0	1.0	0	36%
(Contadina)										
	1 cup	145	3	17	938	3	7.0	1.1	0	44%
	1/2 cup	73	2	9	469	2	3.5	0.6	0	44%
frozen, food service product	1 oz	18	0	2	88	1	0.9	0.1	0	47%
(Five Brothers) w/burgundy wine	1/2 cup	80	2	9	480	2	4.0	0.5	0	45%
(Hunt's) chunky	1/2 cup	60	1	12	526	2	1.6	1.6	5	21%
(Millina's Finest)										
organic	4 oz	48	2	9	210	0	0.5	0.0	0	9%
Zinfandel, organic	4 oz	44	2	9	215	0	0.5	0.0	0	9%
(Pathmark)										
'All Natural'	1/2 cup	80	2	12	710	0	2.0	0.0	0	24%
'No Frills'	1/2 cup	80	1	12	620	0	3.0	0.0	0	34%
(Prego)	1/2 cup	110	2	12	670	3	6.0	1.5	0	49%
(Progresso)										
	1/2 cup	90	4	9	520	0	5.0	1.0	1	46%
'Authentic Pasta Sauces'	1/2 cup	110	4	10	250	2	6.0	1.5	4	49%
(Ragu) 'Old World Style'	1/2 cup	90	2	9	820	3	5.0	1.0	0	51%
(Rokeach)	3 oz	60	1	9	257	0	2.0	0.0	0	31%
(Westbrae)										
	4 oz	40	2	7	370	0	1.0	0.0	0	20%
w/mushrooms	4 oz	50	2	7	380	0	29.0	0.0	0	88%
MESQUITE										
(Lawry's) w/lime juice	1/4 cup	24	3	3	4142	0	0.4	0.0	0	13%
(S&W) and marinade	1 tbsp	10	0	3	400	0	0.0	0.0	0	0%
MEXICAN (S&W) mild, 'Tomato Garden'	1/4 cup	20	1	4	190	1	0.0	0.0	0	0%
MOLE POBLANO (La Victoria)	2 oz	240	8	28	1847	9	10.3	na	0	39%
MUSHROOM (Simmer Chef) and herb, creamy	1/2 cup	110	0	7	580	0	9.0	2.0	5	74%
NEWBURG (Snow's) canned, w/sherry	1/3 cup	120	3	10	520	0	8.0	1.0	0	58%
ONION (Simmer Chef) and mushroom, hearty	1/2 cup	50	1	9	670	1	1.0	0.0	0	18%
ORANGE DIJON (Golden Dipt) 'Nature Bay'	1 oz	110	0	6	200	0	9.0	0.0	0	77%
ORANGE (LaChoy) Mandarin	1 tbsp	24	0	6	38	0	0.0	0.0	0	0%
OREGANO HERB (Golden Dipt) 'Nature Bay'	2 grams	6	0	1	88	0	0.0	0.0	0	0%
PARMIGIANA (Betty Crocker) 'Recipe Sauces'	3.9 oz	50	2	9	430	0	1.0	1.0	0	17%
PASTA / spaghetti. See also SAUCE, MARINARA; SAUCE, TOMATO.										
(Angela Mia)	1/2 cup	49	2	11	607	3	0.5	0.0	0	8%
(Campbell's)										
extra garlic and onion	4 oz	50	2	12	320	2	1.0	0.0	0	14%
'Homestyle'	4 oz	40	2	10	360	2	0.0	0.0	0	0%

Food Name	Serving Size	Calories	Prot. gms	Carbs gms	Sod. mgs	Fiber gms	Fat gms	Sat. Fat gms	Chol. mgs	% Fat Cal.
Italian style	4 oz	50	2	12	360	2	0.0	0.0	0	0%
mushroom	4 oz	50	2	11	330	2	1.0	0.0	0	15%
traditional, 'Healthy Request'	4 oz	50	2	12	360	2	0.0	0.0	0	0%
w/fresh mushrooms, 'Healthy Request'	4 oz	50	2	11	330	2	1.0	0.0	0	15%
(Chef Boyardee)										
meat flavor	3.75 oz	80	2	11	650	0	3.0	0.0	0	34%
meat flavor, 'Original'	3.75 oz	120	3	13	650	0	6.0	0.0	0	46%
meatless, 'Jars'	4 oz	60	1	11	790	0	1.0	0.0	0	16%
mushroom flavor	3.75 oz	60	1	11	790	0	1.0	0.0	0	16%
mushroom flavor, 'Jars'	4 oz	70	1	11	655	0	2.0	0.0	0	27%
mushroom flavor, 'Original'	3.75 oz	80	1	13	680	0	3.0	0.0	0	33%
w/ground beef, 'Jars'	4 oz	90	2	14	605	0	3.0	0.0	0	30%
(Classico) sun-dried tomato, 'Di Capri'	1/2 cup	80	2	8	430	2	4.5	1.0	0	50%
(Contadina)										
meat flavored, 'Original Recipe'	1/2 cup	100	3	17	430	0	3.2	1.1	2	27%
mushroom, 'Original Recipe'	1/2 cup	90	2	18	430	0	2.3	0.4	0	21%
traditional, 'Original Recipe'	1/2 cup	90	2	17	440	0	2.3	0.0	0	21%
(Del Monte) flavored w/meat	1/2 cup	70	2	9	440	0	2.0	0.0	0	29%
traditional	1/2 cup	70	1	11	430	0	2.0	0.0	0	27%
w/garlic and onion	1/2 cup	70	1	10	430	0	2.0	0.0	0	29%
w/mushrooms	1/2 cup	70	1	11	440	0	2.0	0.0	0	27%
(DiGiorno) plum tomato and mushroom, refrigerated	5 oz	100	3	20	240	0	1.0	0.0	0	9%
(Eden Foods)										
and pizza sauce, organic	4 oz	80	3	10	320	0	3.0	0.0	0	34%
organic, no salt added	4 oz	80	3	14	0	0	2.0	0.0	0	21%
(Enrico's)										
all natural, no salt added	4 oz	60	2	9	30	0	1.0	0.0	0	17%
garlic and sun-dried tomatoes, all natural	3.5 oz	62	2	9	474	2	2.0	0.0	2	29%
Italian style, all natural	3.5 oz	53	2	11	333	1	1.0	0.0	9	15%
mushroom and green pepper, all natural	4 oz	60	2	9	345	0	1.0	0.0	0	17%
mushroom and green pepper, no salt added	4 oz	60	2	9	30	0	1.0	0.0	0	17%
mushroom flavor	4 oz	60	2	9	0	0	1.0	0.0	0	17%
organic tomatoes, 'Hot & Spicy Arabiati'	3.5 oz	60	2	9	464	3	1.8	0.0	0	27%
original, all natural	4 oz	60	2	9	345	0	1.0	0.0	0	17%
peppers and mushrooms, all natural	4 oz	60	2	9	345	0	1.0	0.0	0	17%
w/fresh mushrooms	4 oz	60	2	9	336	0	1.0	0.0	0	17%
(Featherweight) mushroom flavor	4 oz	60	2	11	310	0	1.0	0.0	0	15%
(Five Brothers)										
garden vegetable primavera	1/2 cup	70	2	9	500	2	3.0	0.0	0	38%
tomato basil	1/2 cup	60	2	8	470	2	2.0	0.0	0	31%
w/sautéed mushrooms	1/2 cup	90	2	10	460	3	4.0	0.5	0	43%
(Healthy Choice)										
garlic and herb	4 oz	40	2	9	390	0	1.0	0.0	0	17%
garlic and herb, original	1/2 cup	50	2	10	390	2	0.0	0.0	0	0%
garlic and onion	1/2 cup	40	2	9	390	2	0.0	0.0	0	0%
garlic and onion, chunky	4 oz	40	2	10	350	0	0.0	0.0	0	0%
Italian vegetable, chunky	4.41 oz	50	2	11	331	3	0.6	0.0	0	10%
mushroom and green pepper, super chunky	1/2 cup	45	2	9	390	2	0.0	0.0	0	0%
mushroom, chunky	4 oz	45	2	10	350	0	0.0	0.0	0	0%
mushroom, super chunky	1/2 cup	40	2	9	390	2	0.0	0.0	0	0%
traditional	4 oz	40	2	9	380	0	1.0	0.0	0	17%
vegetable primavera, super chunky	1/2 cup	45	2	9	390	2	0.0	0.0	0	0%
w/chunky mushrooms, nonfat	4 oz	45	2	10	350	0	0.0	0.0	0	0%
w/mushrooms	4 oz	40	2	9	390	0	1.0	0.0	0	17%

Food Name	Serving Size	Calories	Prot. gms	Carbs gms	Sod. mgs	Fiber gms	Fat gms	Sat. Fat gms	Chol. mgs	% Fat Cal.
w/vegetables, Italian style, chunky	4 oz	40	1	9	350	0	0.0	0.0	0	0%
(Hunt's)										
'Homestyle'	4 oz	60	2	10	530	2	2.0	0.3	0	27%
'Traditional'	4 oz	70	2	12	530	0	2.0	0.0	0	24%
100% natural, 'Old Country'	4 oz	60	2	8	560	0	2.0	0.0	0	31%
garlic and herb, 'Classic'	4.41 oz	58	2	10	598	2	2.1	0.3	0	29%
garlic and herb, 'Light'	4.41 oz	39	2	7	379	3	0.8	0.1	0	16%
garlic and herb, 'Old Country'	1/2 cup	63	2	9	522	3	2.7	0.4	0	35%
garlic and onion, 'Classic Italian'	1/2 cup	58	2	10	598	2	2.1	0.3	0	29%
Italian sausage	1/2 cup	77	2	12	596	2	2.7	0.5	2	30%
Italian style vegetable, chunky	1/2 cup	63	2	13	528	2	1.0	0.1	0	13%
Italian vegetable, 'Old Country'	1/2 cup	64	2	9	616	3	2.6	0.4	0	34%
light meat	4.41 oz	45	2	8	437	3	1.2	0.6	2	21%
meat flavor	4 oz	70	2	12	570	0	2.0	0.0	0	24%
meat flavored, 'Home Style'	1/2 cup	57	2	7	596	2	2.6	1.2	2	39%
meat flavored, 'Old Country'	1/2 cup	56	2	7	474	3	2.6	0.6	0	38%
meat flavored, 'Original'	1/2 cup	65	2	11	604	2	2.3	0.6	3	29%
meat	4.44 oz	65	2	11	604	2	2.3	0.6	3	29%
meat, 'Homestyle'	4.41 oz	56	2	7	596	2	2.6	1.2	2	39%
mushroom flavor	4 oz	70	2	12	560	0	2.0	0.0	0	24%
mushroom	4.44 oz	65	2	11	604	2	2.3	0.3	0	29%
mushroom, 'Home Style'	1/2 cup	57	2	7	586	2	2.6	0.4	0	39%
mushroom, light	4.41 oz	39	2	7	379	3	0.8	0.1	0	16%
mushroom, 'Old Country'	1/2 cup	53	2	7	542	3	2.7	0.4	0	40%
mushroom, 'Original'	1/2 cup	65	2	11	604	2	2.3	0.3	0	29%
Parmesan, 'Classic Italian'	1/2 cup	50	2	8	634	2	2.1	0.3	0	33%
spaghetti, cheese and garlic, Italian style	1/2 cup	65	3	9	690	2	2.4	0.6	1	31%
spaghetti, chunky	4 oz	50	1	12	470	2	1.0	0.0	0	15%
spaghetti, tomato basil, 'Classic'	4.41 oz	48	2	8	613	4	2.1	0.3	0	34%
spaghetti, tomato, garlic, and onion, chunky	1/2 cup	61	1	13	526	2	1.0	0.1	0	14%
spaghetti, w/tomato chunks, 'Chunky Style'	4 oz	50	1	12	470	0	1.0	0.0	0	15%
tomato and basil, 'Classic Italian'	1/2 cup	48	2	8	613	4	2.1	0.3	0	34%
traditional ,'Light'	4 oz	40	2	9	360	0	0.0	0.0	0	0%
traditional, 'Home Style'	1/2 cup	57	2	7	596	2	2.6	0.4	0	39%
traditional, 'Old Country'	1/2 cup	53	2	7	542	3	2.7	0.4	0	40%
traditional, 'Original'	1/2 cup	65	2	11	621	4	2.3	0.3	0	29%
w/meat	4 oz	70	2	12	570	2	2.0	0.3	2	24%
w/mushrooms	4 oz	70	2	12	560	2	2.0	0.3	0	24%
w/mushrooms, 'Light'	4 oz	40	2	9	330	0	0.0	0.0	0	0%
(McCormick/Schilling) herb and garlic	1 tbsp	20	1	2	500	0	0.0	0.0	0	0%
(Millina's Finest)										
sweet pepper and onion, nonfat organic	4 oz	41	2	7	305	0	0.5	0.0	0	11%
tomato and mushroom, nonfat, organic	4 oz	45	2	9	200	0	0.0	0.0	0	0%
tomato basil, nonfat, organic	4 oz	46	2	9	232	0	0.5	0.0	0	9%
(Nestlé)	1/2 cup	70	2	12	563	2	1.6	0.2	0	21%
(P&Q)										
meat flavor	1/2 cup	70	1	11	510	0	2.0	0.0	0	27%
meatless	1/2 cup	70	1	14	540	0	1.0	0.0	0	13%
mushroom flavor	1/2 cup	70	1	14	580	0	1.0	0.0	0	13%
(Pastorelli) 'Italian Chef'	4 oz	81	3	11	430	1	3.0	0.0	0	33%
(Pathmark)										
meat flavor, 'All Natural'	1/2 cup	80	2	11	790	0	3.0	0.0	0	34%
meat flavor, 'No Frills'	1/2 cup	90	2	11	620	0	5.0	0.0	0	46%
meatless, 'All Natural'	1/2 cup	70	2	11	710	0	2.0	0.0	0	26%

Food Name	Serving Size	Calories	Prot. gms	Carbs gms	Sod. mgs	Fiber gms	Fat gms	Sat. Fat gms	Chol. mgs	% Fat Cal.
meatless, 'No Frills'	1/2 cup	80	1	11	583	0	3.0	0.0	0	36%
mushroom flavor, 'All Natural'	1/2 cup	70	2	11	730	0	2.0	0.0	0	26%
(Prego)										
. . . .	1/2 cup	110	2	19	420	3	3.0	0.5	0	24%
garden combination.	4 oz	80	2	14	420	0	2.0	0.0	0	22%
garden combination, chunky.	1/2 cup	100	2	19	480	3	2.0	1.0	0	18%
garlic and cheese, extra chunky	1/2 cup	130	3	22	610	3	3.5	1.0	0	24%
low-salt	1/2 cup	110	2	11	25	3	6.0	1.5	0	51%
meat flavored.	1/2 cup	140	3	21	500	3	6.0	1.5	5	36%
mushroom	1/2 cup	150	2	23	670	3	5.0	1.5	0	31%
mushroom, extra chunky, extra spicy	1/2 cup	120	2	19	510	3	4.0	0.0	0	30%
mushroom, w/onion, extra chunky.	1/2 cup	110	2	18	500	3	3.0	1.0	5	25%
mushroom, w/tomato, chunky	1/2 cup	110	2	19	510	3	3.0	1.0	0	24%
mushroom and green pepper, chunky.	1/2 cup	120	2	18	430	6	4.5	1.0	5	34%
mushroom flavor	4 oz	130	2	20	630	0	5.0	0.0	0	34%
onion, tomato-based, 'Extra Chunky'	4 oz	110	2	14	490	0	5.0	0.0	0	41%
onion, w/garlic	1/2 cup	110	2	19	420	3	3.0	0.5	0	24%
sausage, w/peppers, extra chunky	1/2 cup	180	4	22	570	3	9.0	2.5	10	44%
spaghetti, traditional, '100% Natural'.	2 tbsp	136	2	21	557	4	5.0	1.1	0	34%
three cheese	1/2 cup	100	3	18	460	3	2.0	1.0	5	18%
tomato and onion, w/garlic, extra chunky	1/2 cup	110	2	19	480	3	3.5	1.0	0	27%
traditional.	1/2 cup	140	2	23	610	2	4.5	1.5	0	29%
(Pritikin)										
garden style, chunky.	1/2 cup	50	2	11	30	0	0.0	0.0	0	0%
original.	1/2 cup	60	2	14	35	0	1.0	0.0	0	12%
(Progresso)										
meat flavor.	1/2 cup	110	4	13	660	0	5.0	1.0	5	40%
mushroom flavor	1/2 cup	110	3	13	630	0	5.0	1.0	5	41%
primavera, creamy, 'Authentic Pasta Sauces'	1/2 cup	190	5	8	410	1	17.0	10.0	54	75%
Sicilian, 'Authentic Pasta Sauces'	1/2 cup	30	1	2	660	1	2.5	1.0	0	65%
spaghetti	1/2 cup	110	3	13	660	0	5.0	1.0	2	41%
(Ragu)										
beef flavored, 'Hearty'	1/2 cup	130	4	19	580	3	4.5	1.0	3	31%
'Fresh Italian'	4 oz	90	2	13	490	0	3.0	0.0	0	31%
garden, 'Light'	1/2 cup	50	2	11	390	3	0.0	0.0	0	0%
garden harvest, 'Today's Recipe'.	4 oz	50	2	8	370	0	1.0	0.0	0	18%
'Gardenstyle Chunky'	1/2 cup	120	2	18	540	3	4.0	0.5	0	31%
green and red pepper, 'Gardenstyle Chunky'	1/2 cup	120	2	19	570	2	4.0	0.5	0	30%
'Homestyle'	4 oz	50	2	6	390	0	2.0	0.0	0	36%
Italian garden combination, 'Chunky Gardenstyle'	4 oz	110	2	15	500	0	5.0	0.0	0	40%
Italian tomato, 'Hearty'.	1/2 cup	120	3	19	580	3	3.0	0.5	0	23%
meat flavored, 'Old World Style'	1/2 cup	90	3	9	820	3	5.0	1.0	3	48%
mushroom, 'Old World Style'	1/2 cup	80	2	10	820	3	3.5	0.5	0	40%
mushroom, chunky, 'Light'	1/2 cup	50	3	11	390	2	0.0	0.0	0	0%
mushroom, chunky, 'Today's Recipe'.	4 oz	50	2	8	370	0	1.0	0.0	0	18%
no sugar added, 'Light'	1/2 cup	60	3	9	390	3	1.5	0.0	0	22%
Parmesan, 'Hearty'	1/2 cup	120	4	18	630	2	4.0	1.0	3	29%
smooth, traditional 'Old World'.	1/2 cup	80	2	12	756	3	2.6	0.4	na	30%
spaghetti, 'Chunky Gardenstyle'	4 oz	70	2	10	440	0	3.0	0.0	0	36%
spaghetti, 'Slow Cooked Homestyle'	4 oz	110	2	15	510	0	5.0	0.0	0	40%
'Thick & Hearty'	4 oz	100	2	15	460	0	3.0	0.0	0	28%
tomato, garlic, and onion, 'Gardenstyle Chunky'	1/2 cup	120	2	19	550	3	4.0	0.5	0	30%
tomato, Italian, 100% natural, ...	1/2 cup	120	3	19	580	3	3.0	0.5	0	23%
tomato and herbs, 'Today's Recipe'.	4 oz	50	2	8	370	0	1.0	0.0	0	18%

Food Name	Serving Size	Calories	Prot. gms	Carbs gms	Sod. mgs	Fiber gms	Fat gms	Sat. Fat gms	Chol. mgs	% Fat Cal.
traditional, 'Old World Style'	1/2 cup	80	2	10	820	3	3.5	0.5	0	40%
vegetable primavera, 'Gardenstyle Super'	1/2 cup	110	2	17	480	4	4.0	0.5	0	32%
w/meat, 'Homestyle'	4 oz	110	2	15	510	0	5.0	0.0	2	40%
w/mushrooms, 'Gardenstyle Super'	1/2 cup	120	3	19	540	3	4.0	0.5	0	29%
w/mushrooms, 'Homestyle'	4 oz	110	2	15	530	0	2.0	0.0	0	21%
w/mushrooms, 'Thick & Hearty'	4 oz	100	2	15	460	0	3.0	0.0	0	28%
w/mushrooms and green peppers, 'Gardenstyle Chunky'	1/2 cup	120	2	18	570	3	4.0	0.5	0	31%
w/mushrooms and onions, 'Gardenstyle Chunky'	1/2 cup	120	2	19	560	3	4.0	0.5	0	30%
w/sautéed onion and garlic, 100% natural, 'Hearty'	1/2 cup	130	3	19	530	3	5.0	0.5	0	34%
w/sautéed onion and mushroom, 'Hearty'	1/2 cup	110	3	17	550	3	4.0	0.5	0	31%
w/tomato and herbs, 'Homestyle'	4 oz	110	2	15	510	0	5.0	0.0	0	40%
w/tomato and herbs, 'Ragu Fine Italian'	4 oz	90	2	13	490	0	3.0	0.0	0	31%
(S&W) 'Ready Cut'	1/4 cup	20	1	4	210	1	0.0	0.0	0	0%
(Sutter Home) Zinfandel wine	1/2 cup	100	2	11	520	0	5.0	0.0	0	46%
(Timpone's) fresh garlic and basil, 'Mom's Sauce'	4.5 oz	70	2	7	490	1	4.0	0.5	0	50%
(Weight Watchers)										
meat flavor	1/3 cup	50	2	9	440	0	1.0	0.0	0	17%
mushroom flavor, nonfat	1/3 cup	40	1	9	430	0	0.0	0.0	0	0%
(Westbrae)										
primavera	4 oz	60	2	7	490	0	3.0	0.0	0	43%
primavera, nonfat, no salt added	4 oz	40	2	7	105	0	0.0	0.0	0	0%
PEANUT										
(Mr. Spice) Thai, nonfat, salt-free	1 tbsp	19	1	3	0	0	1.0	0.0	0	36%
(San-J) Thai	1 tbsp	30	1	3	311	1	1.3	0.2	0	38%
PEPPER DILL (Golden Dipt) 'Nature Bay'	2 grams	8	0	1	96	0	0.0	0.0	0	0%
PEPPER										
(Hunt's) homestyle, hot	1 tsp	1	0	0	205	0	0.0	0.0	0	33%
(Hunt's) orignal homestyle, original	1 tsp	1	0	0	205	0	0.0	0.0	0	33%
PEPPER STEAK (Betty Crocker) 'Recipe Sauces'	3.8 oz	50	1	8	270	0	2.0	0.0	0	33%
PEPPERCORN (McCormick/Schilling) green, blend	2 tsp	20	1	3	360	0	0.0	0.0	0	0%
PESTO										
(Christopher Ranch) basil and garlic	1/4 cup	230	4	4	325	3	23.0	4.0	0	87%
(Contadina)										
frozen, food service product	1 oz	66	3	2	109	1	5.4	1.3	7	73%
refrigerated, 'Fresh'	2.33 oz	350	6	6	420	0	34.0	0.0	10	86%
w/basil	1/4 cup	310	6	5	440	0	30.0	5.0	10	86%
w/sun-dried tomatoes	1/4 cup	250	3	6	520	3	24.0	4.0	0	86%
(DiGiorno) refrigerated	2.3 oz	340	8	5	430	0	32.0	6.0	20	85%
PICANTE										
(Azteca) mild	1 tbsp	4	0	1	85	0	0.0	0.0	0	0%
(Chi-Chi's)										
hot	1 oz	10	2	2	268	0	2.0	2.0	2	53%
medium	1 oz	8	2	2	192	0	2.0	2.0	2	53%
mild	1 oz	9	2	2	198	0	2.0	2.0	2	53%
(Del Monte)										
hot	1/2 cup	20	0	4	385	0	0.0	0.0	0	0%
hot, chunky	1/4 cup	15	0	3	405	0	0.0	0.0	0	0%
(Estee)	2 tbsp	8	1	2	60	0	0.0	0.0	0	0%
(Gebhardt)	1 tbsp	4	0	1	120	0	0.0	0.0	0	0%
(Guiltless Gourmet)										
hot	2 tbsp	8	0	1	133	1	0.0	0.0	0	0%
medium	2 tbsp	8	0	1	133	1	0.0	0.0	0	0%
mild	2 tbsp	8	0	1	133	1	0.0	0.0	0	0%

Food Name	Serving Size	Calories	Prot. gms	Carbs gms	Sod. mgs	Fiber gms	Fat gms	Sat. Fat gms	Chol. mgs	% Fat Cal.
(Hunt's) mild, 'Homestyle'	1.09 oz	11	1	2	256	1	0.2	0.0	0	15%
(La Victoria)										
medium	2 tbsp	5	0	1	180	0	0.0	0.0	0	0%
mild	2 tbsp	10	1	2	230	0	0.0	0.0	0	0%
(LaCasita) mild, chunky	2 oz	16	1	4	226	0	0.0	0.0	0	0%
(Nestlé)										
'Que Bueno'	1 pkg	1311	47	257	32382	0	8.9	0.8	0	6%
'Que Bueno'	2 tbsp	10	0	2	252	0	0.1	0.0	0	6%
(Old El Paso)										
'Thick 'n Chunky'	2 tbsp	6	1	1	310	1	0.0	0.0	0	0%
all varieties, 'Chunky'	2 tbsp	7	0	2	270	0	0.0	0.0	0	0%
all varieties	2 tbsp	8	1	2	310	0	1.0	0.0	0	43%
hot	2 tbsp	10	0	2	230	0	0.0	0.0	0	0%
hot, 'Thick n' Chunky'	2 tbsp	10	0	2	160	0	0.0	0.0	0	0%
medium	2 tbsp	10	0	2	230	0	0.0	0.0	0	0%
medium, 'Thick n' Chunky'	2 tbsp	10	0	2	140	0	0.0	0.0	0	0%
mild	2 tbsp	10	0	2	230	0	0.0	0.0	0	0%
mild, 'Thick n' Chunky'	2 tbsp	10	0	2	130	0	0.0	0.0	0	0%
(Ortega) picante, can or jar	1 oz	10	0	2	300	0	0.0	0.0	0	0%
(Pace)										
extra mild, 'Thick & Chunky'	2 tsp	3	0	1	111	0	0.1	0.0	0	22%
hot, 'Thick & Chunky'	2 tsp	3	0	1	111	0	0.1	0.0	0	22%
medium, 'Thick & Chunky'	2 tsp	3	0	1	111	0	0.1	0.0	0	22%
mild, 'Thick & Chunky'	2 tsp	3	0	1	111	0	0.1	0.0	0	22%
(Rosarita)										
	1.09 oz	7	0	1	247	0	0.1	0.0	0	12%
hot, chunky	3 tbsp	18	1	4	515	1	1.0	0.0	0	31%
jalapeño, hot, zesty	1.09 oz	8	0	2	246	1	0.2	0.0	0	18%
jalapeño, medium, zesty	1.09 oz	9	0	2	254	1	0.2	0.0	0	18%
jalapeño, mild, zesty	1.09 oz	8	1	2	239	1	0.1	0.0	0	9%
jalapeño, zesty, 'de Mexico Style'	2 tbsp	12	1	3	370	0	0.0	0.0	0	0%
mild	3.5 oz	45	2	9	1015	0	1.0	0.0	0	17%
mild, chunky	3 tbsp	25	1	5	630	1	1.0	0.0	0	27%
(S&W) hot, 'Sun-Vista'	2 tbsp	10	0	2	260	0	0.0	0.0	0	0%
(Santiago)	1 fl oz	10	0	2	216	0	0.1	0.0	0	5%
(Sun Vista) hot	2 tbsp	10	0	2	260	0	0.0	0.0	0	0%
(Sun Vista) mild	2 tbsp	5	0	2	200	0	0.0	0.0	0	0%
(Wise)	2 tbsp	12	0	3	130	0	0.0	0.0	0	0%
PIZZA										
(Angela Mia)										
food service product	1/4 cup	63	1	4	251	2	0.5	0.0	0	19%
super heavy, food service product	1/4 cup	29	2	6	36	3	0.5	0.0	0	13%
super heavy, 'Premium Choice'	2.26 oz	28	3	6	36	3	0.5	0.0	0	12%
(Chef Boyardee)										
w/cheese	2.63 oz	70	1	7	385	0	4.0	0.0	0	53%
w/cheese, 'Jars'	3.88 oz	90	1	10	565	0	6.0	0.0	0	55%
(Contadina)										
	1/4 cup	25	1	4	30	1	0.5	0.0	0	18%
deluxe	1/4 cup	34	1	5	117	1	0.7	0.3	2	19%
original, 'Quick & Easy'	1/4 cup	30	1	5	330	0	1.0	0.0	0	27%
pepperoni flavor	1/4 cup	30	1	4	360	1	1.0	0.0	0	31%
'Pizza Squeeze'	1/4 cup	30	1	5	330	0	1.0	0.0	0	27%
w/Italian cheese	1/4 cup	30	1	4	350	1	1.0	0.0	0	31%
(Eden Foods) and pasta sauce, organic	4 oz	80	3	10	320	0	3.0	0.0	0	34%

Food Name	Serving Size	Calories	Prot. gms	Carbs gms	Sod. mgs	Fiber gms	Fat gms	Sat. Fat gms	Chol. mgs	% Fat Cal.
(Enrico's) all natural, no salt added, 'Homemade Style'	4 oz	60	2	9	30	0	1.0	0.0	0	17%
(Hunt's)										
....	2.36 oz	32	2	5	416	2	1.1	0.0	0	27%
fully prepared	2.22 oz	21	1	4	251	2	0.5	0.0	0	18%
(Nestlé) deluxe	1 pkg	1623	66	261	5559	60	34.6	13.8	90	19%
(Pastorelli) 'Italian Chef'	4 oz	90	3	12	430	0	3.0	0.0	0	31%
(Pizza Quick) traditional	3 tbsp	35	1	3	330	0	2.0	0.0	0	53%
PLUM										
(Dynasty) nonfat	2 tbsp	80	1	18	210	0	0.0	0.0	0	0%
(La Choy)										
....	1 tbsp	25	0	6	4	0	0.1	0.0	0	3%
food service product	1 tbsp	25	0	6	5	0	0.0	0.0	0	1%
PRIMAVERA										
(McCormick/Schilling) blend	1 tbsp	30	0	4	490	0	1.0	0.0	3	36%
(Ragu) Italian, light, 'Chicken Tonight'	4 oz	50	2	9	540	0	1.0	0.0	0	17%
RIB (Dip n'Joy) 'Saucy Rib'	1 oz	60	0	14	250	0	0.0	0.0	0	0%
RIGOLETTO (DiGiorno) refrigerated	5 oz	110	2	9	660	0	8.0	1.0	0	62%
ROBERT (Escoffier) 'Sauce Robert'	1 tbsp	20	0	5	70	0	0.0	0.0	0	0%
SANDWICH										
(Hunt's)										
barbecue flavored, 'Manwich'	1/4 cup	60	1	14	890	1	0.0	0.0	0	0%
bold flavor, 'Manwich'	2.22 oz	62	1	13	802	1	1.1	0.0	0	15%
extra thick and chunky, 'Manwich'	2.5 oz	60	1	15	640	0	1.0	0.0	0	12%
'Manwich'	2.26 oz	32	1	6	365	1	0.4	0.0	0	11%
Mexican, 'Manwich'	2.26 oz	26	1	5	552	1	0.2	0.0	0	7%
nonfat, 'Manwich'	2.5 oz	40	1	10	390	0	0.0	0.0	0	0%
thick and chunky, 'Manwich'	2.29 oz	44	1	9	737	1	0.5	0.0	0	10%
SAUSAGE AND BELL PEPPER (Contadina) spicy Italian	1/2 cup	100	4	9	540	3	5.0	1.0	40	46%
SEAFOOD										
(Great Impressions)										
Creole	1 tbsp	21	0	5	182	0	0.1	0.0	0	4%
dipping	1 tbsp	17	1	2	129	0	0.7	0.0	0	36%
Polynesian, dipping	1 tbsp	38	1	10	127	0	1.0	0.0	0	18%
(Progresso) mixed	1/2 cup	110	5	12	445	2	6.0	1.0	11	44%
SEASONING										
(A Taste of Thai)	1 tbsp	15	2	1	1760	0	0.0	0.0	0	0%
(Cajun Sunshine) hot pepper	1 tsp	0	0	0	160	na	0.0	na	na	0%
(Dragon Sauce) rice, vegetables, and stir fry	1 tsp	5	1	1	260	na	0.0	na	na	0%
(Eden Foods)										
carob, 'EdenBlend'	8 oz	150	6	23	105	0	4.0	0.5	0	24%
original, 'EdenBlend'	8 oz	120	7	16	85	0	3.0	0.5	0	23%
original, 'Edensoy'	8 oz	130	10	13	105	0	4.0	0.5	0	28%
original extra, 'EdenBlend'	8 oz	130	10	13	105	0	4.0	0.5	0	28%
(Maggi) Asian	1 tsp	0	1	0	410	0	0.0	0.0	0	0%
(Tennessee Sunshine)	1 tsp	0	0	0	160	na	0.0	na	na	0%
(Tiger Sauce) meat, seafood, and poultry	1 tsp	10	0	2	140	na	0.0	na	na	0%
(Yucatan Sunshine) habanero pepper	1 tsp	0	0	0	125	na	0.0	na	na	0%
SHRIMP (Tone's) 'Craboil'	1 tsp	10	0	1	1	0	0.6	0.1	1	47%
SHOYU. See under Soy Sauce, below.										
SLOPPY JOE										
(Del Monte)										
hickory flavor	1/4 cup	70	1	18	700	0	0.0	0.0	0	0%
Italian recipe	2.5 oz	60	1	14	650	0	0.0	0.0	0	0%
original recipe	1/4 cup	70	1	16	680	0	0.0	0.0	0	0%

Food Name	Serving Size	Calories	Prot. gms	Carbs gms	Sod. mgs	Fiber gms	Fat gms	Sat. Fat gms	Chol. mgs	% Fat Cal.
(Hormel) 'Not-so-Sloppy-Sloppy Joe'	2.24 oz	70	1	16	730	0	1.0	0.0	5	12%
(Libby's)	1/3 cup	45	1	10	430	1	0.0	0.0	0	0%
SOY										
from hydrolyzed vegetable protein	1/4 cup	24	1	4	3300	0	0.0	0.0	0	2%
from hydrolyzed vegetable protein	1 tbsp	7	0	1	1024	0	0.0	0.0	0	2%
from hydrolyzed vegetable protein	1 tsp	2	0	0	341	0	0.0	0.0	0	2%
shoyu, from soy and wheat	1 cup	150	20	20	13885	2	0.1	0.0	0	1%
shoyu, from soy and wheat	1 tbsp	9	1	1	871	0	0.0	0.0	0	1%
shoyu, from soy and wheat	1 tsp	3	0	0	289	0	0.0	0.0	0	1%
shoyu, from soy and wheat, low-sodium	1 cup	135	13	22	8499	2	0.2	0.0	0	1%
shoyu, from soy and wheat, low-sodium	1 tbsp	10	1	2	600	0	0.0	0.0	0	1%
shoyu, from soy and wheat, low-sodium	1 tsp	3	0	0	177	0	0.0	0.0	0	1%
tamari, from soy	1 tbsp	11	2	1	1005	0	0.0	0.0	0	1%
tamari, from soy	1 tsp	4	1	0	335	0	0.0	0.0	0	1%
(Angostura)	1 tbsp	10	1	1	390	na	0.0	0.0	0	0%
(Eden Foods)										
shoyu, from soy and wheat, organic	1/2 tsp	2	0	0	140	0	0.0	0.0	0	0%
shoyu, naturally brewed	1/2 tsp	2	0	0	140	0	0.0	0.0	0	0%
shoyu, reduced-sodium, organic	1/2 tsp	2	0	0	80	0	0.0	0.0	0	0%
tamari, wheat-free, organic	1/2 tsp	2	0	0	160	0	0.0	0.0	0	0%
(Golden Dipt) honey, 'Nature Bay'	1 oz	90	0	5	250	0	8.0	0.0	0	78%
(Kikkoman)										
'Lite'	1 tbsp	10	1	1	605	0	0.0	0.0	0	0%
naturally brewed	1 tbsp	10	2	0	920	0	0.0	0.0	0	0%
(La Choy)										
	1 tbsp	11	2	1	1227	0	0.0	0.0	0	3%
food service product	1 tbsp	11	1	1	1315	0	0.0	0.0	0	2%
light	1 tbsp	15	2	2	542	0	0.0	0.0	0	2%
light, food service product	1 tbsp	15	1	2	505	0	0.0	0.0	0	1%
shoyu	1 tsp	1	0	0	429	0	0.0	0.0	0	0%
shoyu, 'Lite'	1 tsp	1	0	0	220	0	0.0	0.0	0	0%
(San-J) tamari, less salt	1 tbsp	16	2	1	607	0	0.0	0.0	0	0%
(Westbrae)										
low-salt	1/2 tsp	2	1	1	170	0	0.0	0.0	0	0%
mild	1/2 tsp	2	1	1	85	0	0.0	0.0	0	0%
organic	1/2 tsp	2	1	1	105	0	0.0	0.0	0	0%
wheat-free	1/2 tsp	3	1	1	140	0	0.0	0.0	0	0%
STEAK										
(A.1.)										
bold	1 tbsp	18	0	4	160	0	0.0	0.0	0	0%
regular	1 tbsp	18	0	4	160	0	0.0	0.0	0	0%
(Adolph's) '100% Natural'	1/4 tsp	0	0	0	310	0	0.0	0.0	0	0%
(Angostura)										
regular	1 tbsp	12	0	3	90	na	0.0	0.0	0	0%
salsa flavor	1 tbsp	8	0	2	85	na	0.0	0.0	0	0%
(Bullfighter) and burger	1 tbsp	15	0	4	220	na	0.0	na	na	0%
(Heinz 57)										
hickory smoke, '57'	1 tbsp	16	0	4	180	0	0.0	0.0	0	0%
traditional	1 tbsp	12	0	3	200	0	0.0	0.0	0	0%
(Hunt's)	1 tbsp	10	0	2	256	0	0.1	0.0	0	10%
(Kikkoman)	1 tbsp	20	0	5	290	0	0.0	0.0	0	0%
(Lea & Perrins)	1 oz	40	1	10	220	0	1.0	0.0	0	17%
STIR-FRY										
(Dynasty) Chinese	2 tbsp	60	1	5	1000	0	3.0	0.5	0	53%

Food Name	Serving Size	Calories	Prot. gms	Carbs gms	Sod. mgs	Fiber gms	Fat gms	Sat. Fat gms	Chol. mgs	% Fat Cal.
(Flavor of the Rain Forest)										
ginger, curry	1 tbsp	15	1	2	173	0	1.0	0.0	0	43%
honey hibiscus	1 tbsp	45	0	2	106	0	4.0	0.0	0	82%
lime coconut, for seafood	1 tbsp	49	0	1	121	0	5.0	0.0	3	92%
'Mango Grille'	1 tbsp	13	0	2	136	0	1.0	0.0	0	53%
papaya pepper	1 tsp	3	0	1	50	0	0.0	0.0	0	0%
savory	1 tsp	4	0	1	90	0	0.0	0.0	0	0%
(Kikkoman)	1 tbsp	15	1	3	530	0	0.0	0.0	0	0%
(La Choy)										
and marinade, food service product	1 tbsp	25	1	5	672	0	0.1	0.0	0	4%
Mandarin soy	1/4 cup	35	1	8	426	1	0.1	0.0	0	3%
Szechwan	1/4 cup	42	1	9	312	0	0.1	0.0	0	2%
(Lawry's)	1/4 cup	120	2	20	1128	0	3.8	0.0	0	28%
(Mr. Spice) ginger, fat-free, salt-free	1 tbsp	11	1	3	0	0	0.0	0.0	0	0%
(Nestlé) all-purpose, 'Chef-Mate'	1 tbsp	16	0	2	233	0	0.6	0.1	0	36%
(S&W) Oriental	1 tbsp	20	1	5	390	0	0.0	0.0	0	0%
STROGANOFF *(Betty Crocker)* 'Recipe Sauces'	4 oz	60	1	6	540	0	4.0	0.0	10	56%
SUKIYAKI *(Kikkoman)*	1 tbsp	20	1	4	460	0	0.0	0.0	0	0%
SWEET AND SOUR										
(A Taste of Thai) tangy, hot	2 tbsp	30	0	8	95	0	0.0	0.0	0	0%
(Betty Crocker) 'Recipe Sauces'	4.1 oz	130	1	32	360	0	0.0	0.0	0	0%
(Contadina)	2 tbsp	40	0	8	110	0	1.0	0.0	0	22%
(Dynasty)	2 tbsp	70	0	14	125	0	1.0	0.0	0	14%
(Great Impressions)										
Hawaiian	2 tbsp	102	0	26	1	0	0.0	0.0	0	0%
hot	2 tbsp	102	0	26	1	0	0.0	0.0	0	0%
regular	2 tbsp	102	0	26	1	0	0.0	0.0	0	0%
(Hickory Farms)										
Hawaiian	2 tbsp	102	0	26	2	0	0.0	0.0	0	0%
regular	2 tbsp	102	0	26	1	0	0.0	0.0	0	0%
(Kikkoman)	2 tbsp	35	0	9	190	0	0.0	0.0	0	0%
(La Choy)										
	1/4 cup	69	1	18	377	1	0.0	0.0	0	0%
	1 tbsp	29	0	7	52	0	0.1	0.0	0	3%
duck sauce	1 tbsp	31	0	7	64	0	0.1	0.0	0	2%
food service product	2 tbsp	58	0	14	121	0	0.1	0.0	0	1%
(Lawry's)	1/4 cup	549	3	12	4056	0	7.5	0.0	0	53%
(Nestlé) glaze, 'Chef-Mate'	2 tbsp	51	0	12	229	0	0.0	0.0	0	0%
(Ragu) 'Chicken Tonight'	4 oz	80	0	19	280	0	0.0	0.0	0	0%
(Sauceworks)	1 tbsp	25	0	5	50	0	0.0	0.0	0	0%
(Simmer Chef) Oriental	1/2 cup	110	0	23	280	0	1.0	0.0	0	9%
SZECHUAN										
(LaChoy) hot and spicy	1 oz	48	0	12	141	0	0.2	0.0	0	4%
(Nestle) 'Chef-Mate'	2 tbsp	42	0	6	436	0	1.8	0.2	0	39%
(San-J)	1 tbsp	15	1	2	473	0	0.1	na	0	9%
TACO										
(Chi-Chi's)										
hot	1 oz	18	2	4	254	0	2.0	2.0	1	43%
thick, chunky	1 oz	12	2	3	140	0	2.0	2.0	2	47%
(Del Monte)										
hot	1/4 cup	15	0	4	440	0	0.0	0.0	0	0%
mild	1/2 cup	15	0	4	480	0	0.0	0.0	0	0%
(El Molino) red, mild	2 tbsp	10	0	2	170	0	0.0	0.0	0	0%
(Enrico's) mild, no salt added	2 tbsp	14	1	3	25	0	0.0	0.0	0	0%

Food Name	Serving Size	Calories	Prot. gms	Carbs gms	Sod. mgs	Fiber gms	Fat gms	Sat. Fat gms	Chol. mgs	% Fat Cal.
(Estee)	2 tbsp	14	1	3	25	0	0.0	0.0	0	0%
(Hain) and dip	4 tbsp	25	1	5	350	0	1.0	0.0	5	27%
(Heinz)										
medium	1 tbsp	6	0	1	0	0	0.0	0.0	0	0%
mild	1 tbsp	6	0	1	0	0	0.0	0.0	0	0%
(La Victoria)										
green	1 tbsp	0	0	1	90	0	0.0	0.0	0	0%
green, medium	1 tbsp	5	0	1	96	0	0.1	na	0	11%
green, mild	1 tbsp	5	0	1	96	0	0.1	na	0	11%
mild	1 tbsp	7	0	1	103	0	0.1	na	0	9%
red	1 tbsp	5	0	1	80	0	0.0	0.0	0	0%
red, medium	1 tbsp	7	0	1	103	0	0.1	na	0	9%
(Lawry's)										
chunky	1/4 cup	22	1	4	549	0	0.4	0.0	0	16%
'Sauce'n Seasoner'	1/4 cup	40	1	8	636	0	0.6	0.0	0	14%
(Manwich) seasoning	1/4 cup	30	1	6	620	1	0.0	0.0	0	0%
(Old El Paso)										
canned	2 tbsp	15	1	3	300	1	0.0	0.0	0	0%
hot	2 tbsp	10	1	2	130	0	1.0	0.0	0	43%
medium	2 tbsp	10	1	2	130	0	1.0	0.0	0	43%
mild or medium, extra chunky	1 tbsp	5	0	1	80	0	0.0	0.0	0	0%
mild	2 tbsp	10	1	2	130	0	1.0	0.0	0	43%
(Ortega)										
hot	1 oz	12	0	3	210	0	0.0	0.0	0	0%
mild	1 oz	12	0	3	220	0	0.0	0.0	0	0%
Western style	1 oz	8	0	2	180	0	0.0	0.0	0	0%
(Pancho Villa) mild	2 tbsp	15	0	3	170	0	0.0	0.0	0	0%
(Rosarita)										
	0.18 oz	2	0	0	40	0	0.0	0.0	0	0%
food service product	1 tbsp	2	0	0	40	0	0.0	0.0	0	9%
(Santiago)	1 fl oz	13	0	3	164	0	0.2	0.0	0	14%
TAMARI. See under Soy Sauce, above.										
TANGY, nonfat, salt-free *(Mr. Spice)*	1 tsp	4	1	1	0	0	0.0	0.0	0	0%
TARTAR										
(Best Foods)										
	2 tbsp	140	0	1	260	na	16.0	2.5	10	99%
low-fat	2 tbsp	40	0	7	360	na	1.5	0.0	0	33%
(Golden Dipt)										
	1 tbsp	70	0	2	100	0	7.0	1.0	10	89%
'Lite'	1 tbsp	50	0	4	40	0	4.0	1.0	5	69%
(Great Impressions)	1 tbsp	86	0	1	76	0	9.0	0.0	10	94%
(Heinz)	1 tbsp	71	0	2	124	0	7.2	0.0	0	89%
(Hellmann's)										
	1 tbsp	70	0	0	220	0	8.0	1.0	5	100%
low-fat	2 tbsp	40	0	7	360	na	1.5	0.0	0	33%
(Kraft) nonfat, 'Free'	1 tbsp	10	0	3	120	0	0.0	0.0	0	0%
(Life) egg-free, all-natural	1 tbsp	38	1	1	2	0	4.0	0.0	0	82%
(Sauceworks)										
	1 tbsp	50	0	2	85	0	5.0	1.0	5	85%
lemon and herb flavor, natural	1 tbsp	70	0	0	85	0	8.0	1.0	5	100%
(Weight Watchers)	1 tbsp	35	0	3	80	0	3.0	1.0	5	69%
TEMPURA, dipping sauce *(Kikkoman)*	1 tsp	5	0	1	340	0	0.0	0.0	0	0%
TERIYAKI										
(Angostura)	1 tbsp	10	0	2	260	na	0.0	0.0	0	0%

Food Name	Serving Size	Calories	Prot. gms	Carbs gms	Sod. mgs	Fiber gms	Fat gms	Sat. Fat gms	Chol. mgs	% Fat Cal.
(Betty Crocker) 'Recipe Sauces'	3.9 oz	60	2	13	860	0	1.0	0.0	0	13%
(Golden Dipt) ginger	1 oz	120	1	12	920	0	7.0	1.0	0	55%
(Kikkoman)										
baste and glaze	2 tbsp	50	1	11	810	0	0.0	0.0	0	0%
baste and glaze, w/honey and pineapple	2 tbsp	80	1	18	770	0	0.0	0.0	0	0%
(La Choy)										
	1/4 cup	47	1	11	577	1	0.1	0.0	0	1%
	1 tbsp	17	1	3	917	1	0.1	0.0	0	5%
basting	1.23 oz	37	1	8	1524	0	0.0	0.0	0	0%
hot	1 tbsp	17	2	3	994	0	0.4	0.0	0	18%
light	1 tbsp	18	1	4	439	0	0.0	0.0	0	1%
'Sauce & Marinade'	1 oz	30	1	5	1640	0	0.0	0.0	0	0%
thick and rich	1 oz	41	1	9	509	0	0.1	0.1	1	2%
(Lawry's)										
barbecue	1/8 cup	82	4	14	6115	0	1.1	0.0	0	12%
w/pineapple juice	1/4 cup	72	6	11	7100	0	0.4	0.0	0	5%
(Nestlé) 'Chef-Mate'	1 tbsp	21	0	4	159	0	0.6	0.1	0	25%
(S&W)										
and marinade	1 tbsp	25	1	5	480	0	0.0	0.0	0	0%
and marinade, light	1 tbsp	25	1	5	220	0	0.0	0.0	0	0%
TOMATO										
(S&W)										
herb and garlic, Italian	1 tbsp	15	0	2	150	0	1.0	0.0	0	53%
original, 'Tomato Garden'	1/4 cup	20	0	4	200	1	0.0	0.0	0	0%
(Simmer Chef) Mexicali, zesty	1/2 cup	90	2	16	400	1	3.0	1.0	5	27%
TONKATSU *(Kikkoman)*	1 tbsp	20	0	5	290	0	0.0	0.0	0	0%
VEGETABLE *(Contadina)* garden, 'Light'	0.5 oz	50	2	10	620	0	0.0	0.0	0	0%
WHITE *(Golden Dipt)* French	1 oz	55	0	3	210	0	4.0	0.0	0	75%
WORCESTERSHIRE										
(Angostura)	1 tsp	5	0	1	20	0	0.0	0.0	0	0%
(French's)										
regular	1 tsp	0	0	1	55	0	0.0	0.0	0	0%
smoky	1 tsp	0	0	1	55	0	0.0	0.0	0	0%
(Heinz)	1 tbsp	6	0	1	170	0	0.0	0.0	0	0%
(Lea & Perrins)										
	1 tsp	5	1	1	55	0	1.0	0.0	0	53%
white wine	1 tsp	3	1	1	42	0	1.0	0.0	0	53%
(Life) 'All Natural'	1/2 tbsp	5	1	1	2	0	1.0	0.0	0	53%
(Wine & Pepper) w/sherry, hot pepper	1 tsp	0	0	1	90	na	0.0	na	na	0%
SAUCE MIX										
ALFREDO										
(French's) 'Pasta Toss' mix only	2 tsp	25	1	2	310	0	2.0	0.0	0	60%
(Lawry's) 'Pasta Alfredo' mix only	1 pkg	226	8	19	3222	1	13.3	0.0	0	52%
(Schilling) 'Pasta Prima' mix only	1/4 envelope	40	2	3	410	0	2.5	1.5	10	53%
(Knorr) CPC, mix only	2 tbsp	62	2	7	730	na	2.7	1.7	5	40%
BARBECUE										
(Blue Plate) concentrate	2 tbsp	110	0	19	350	0	4.0	1.0	0	32%
(Woody's) concentrate, 'Cook-in' Sauce'	2 tbsp	50	1	4	490	1	4.0	0.5	0	64%
BEEF SAUCE										
(Lipton) sauté, golden, mix only	1/6 pkg	120	3	24	520	0	2.0	0.0	0	14%
(Lipton) sauté, golden, prepared w/2 tsp butter	1/2 cup	180	3	24	570	0	8.0	0.0	0	40%
CHEESE										
(Custom Foods)										
cheddar, 'Superb' mix only	1 serving	60	1	8	685	1	2.6	1.5	4	39%

Food Name	Serving Size	Calories	Prot. gms	Carbs gms	Sod. mgs	Fiber gms	Fat gms	Sat. Fat gms	Chol. mgs	% Fat Cal.
nacho, 'Superb' mix only	1 serving	60	1	8	733	0	2.6	1.5	3	39%
(Durkee) mix only	1/4 cup	25	1	4	260	0	1.5	1.0	2	40%
(French's) prepared w/whole milk	1/4 cup	80	3	7	430	0	4.0	0.0	0	47%
(McCormick/Schilling)										
mix only	1/4 pkg	35	2	4	477	0	1.5	0.0	0	38%
nacho, mix only	1/4 pkg	42	3	5	409	0	1.5	0.0	0	31%
(Nestlé)										
nacho, 'Trio' mix only	2 tbsp	51	1	8	338	0	1.9	0.8	2	33%
supreme, 'Trio' mix only	2 tbsp	54	1	7	361	0	2.4	1.3	4	41%
'Trio' mix only	2 tbsp	54	1	7	310	0	2.3	0.8	2	39%
CHICKEN										
(McCormick/Schilling)										
cacciatore 'Sauce Blends' mix only	1 pkg	132	4	28	1092	0	4.8	0.0	0	25%
Creole 'Sauce Blends' mix only	1 pkg	140	2	24	1084	0	4.8	0.0	0	29%
curry 'Sauce Blends' mix only	1 pkg	152	2	24	1288	0	5.6	0.0	0	32%
Dijon 'Sauce Blends' mix only	1 pkg	156	3	20	1414	0	6.8	0.0	0	40%
mesquite marinade, 'Sauce Blends' mix only	1 pkg	132	2	24	2068	0	3.0	0.0	0	21%
teriyaki, 'Sauce Blends' mix only	1 pkg	172	7	28	1380	0	3.6	0.0	0	19%
CURRY										
(S&B)										
golden, hot, mix only	1/5 pkt	120	1	11	810	1	7.0	3.0	5	57%
golden, medium hot, mix only	1/5 pkt	120	1	10	790	1	7.0	3.0	5	59%
ENCHILADA										
(Old El Paso) mix only	2 tsp	10	0	2	540	1	0.0	0.0	0	0%
(Tio Sancho) 'Dinner Kit' mix only	3 oz	278	5	62	4058	2	1.5	0.0	0	5%
HOLLANDAISE										
(McCormick/Schilling) mix only	1/4 pkg	51	1	4	170	0	3.8	0.0	0	66%
(Tone's) mix only	1 tsp	15	0	1	60	0	1.0	0.0	0	58%
ITALIAN										
(Custom Foods) all purpose, 'Red Label' mix only	1 serving	19	0	4	359	0	0.2	0.0	0	9%
LEMON BUTTER Weight Watchers) mix only	1 tbsp	6	1	1	90	0	0.0	0.0	0	0%
PASTA / spaghetti										
(Estee) prepared w/margarine and nonfat milk	4 oz	60	2	9	30	0	1.0	1.0	0	17%
(Featherweight) prepared w/margarine and nonfat milk	4 oz	60	2	11	310	0	1.0	0.0	0	15%
(French's)										
cheese and garlic, 'Pasta Toss' mix only	2 tsp	25	1	2	320	0	2.0	0.0	0	60%
Italian, 'Pasta Toss' mix only	2 tsp	25	1	2	340	0	2.0	0.0	0	60%
Romanoff 'Pasta Toss' mix only	2 tsp	30	1	1	310	0	2.0	0.0	0	69%
w/mushrooms, prepared	5/8 cup	100	2	13	1050	0	4.0	0.0	0	38%
(Lawry's)										
'Rich & Thick' mix only	1 pkg	147	4	28	2172	1	2.2	0.0	0	14%
w/imported mushrooms, mix only	1 pkg	143	5	26	2015	2	1.5	0.0	0	10%
(McCormick/Schilling) mix only	1/4 pkg	32	1	6	615	0	0.3	0.0	0	9%
(Prego) prepared w/margarine and nonfat milk	4 oz	130	2	20	630	0	5.0	0.0	0	34%
(Ragu) prepared w/margarine and nonfat milk	4 oz	80	2	9	740	0	4.0	0.0	0	45%
PEANUT (A Taste of Thai) mix only	2 tbsp	25	1	4	115	0	0.5	0.0	0	18%
PESTO (French's) 'Pasta Toss' mix only	2 tsp	20	1	1	280	0	1.0	0.0	0	53%
SANDWICH (Manwich) mix only	0.25 oz	22	0	5	351	0	0.1	0.0	0	4%
SEAFOOD (Old Bay) 'Old Bay Seas'n' mix only	1/5 pkg	30	0	4	160	0	0.0	0.0	0	0%
SOUR CREAM (McCormick/Schilling) mix only	1/4 pkg	44	1	4	272	0	2.8	0.0	0	54%
SPAGHETTI. See SAUCE, PASTA.										
STROGANOFF										
(Lawry's) mix only	1 pkg	123	5	26	2814	1	0.3	0.0	0	2%
(McCormick/Schilling) mix only	2 tsp	15	1	3	350	0	0.0	0.0	0	0%

Food Name	Serving Size	Calories	Prot. gms	Carbs gms	Sod. mgs	Fiber gms	Fat gms	Sat. Fat gms	Chol. mgs	% Fat Cal.
(Natural Touch) prepared as directed	4 oz	90	4	10	0	0	3.0	0.0	0	33%
SWEET AND SOUR										
(Kikkoman) mix only	1-1/2 tbsp	60	0	14	220	0	0.0	0.0	0	0%
(Sun Bird) Oriental, mix only	1/2 tbsp	15	0	4	110	0	0.0	0.0	0	0%
TACO *(Tio Sancho)* 'Dinner Kit' prepared	2 oz	62	2	13	750	1	0.2	0.0	0	3%
TAHINI *(Casbah)* prepared	1/4 cup	160	5	10	160	1	13.0	0.0	0	66%
TERIYAKI *(Kikkoman)* mix only	2 tsp	20	0	5	640	0	0.0	0.0	0	0%
SAUERKRAUT										
Canned										
(A&P) w/liquid	1/2 cup	20	1	5	800	0	1.0	0.0	0	27%
(Allens) shredded, w/liquid	1/2 cup	21	1	5	880	0	1.0	0.0	0	27%
(Bush's Best)										
'Bavarian Kraut'	1/2 cup	60	1	15	400	3	0.0	0.0	0	0%
chopped, 'Kraut'	1/2 cup	20	1	5	680	0	0.0	0.0	0	0%
kosher, deli-style, 'Kraut'	1/2 cup	20	1	5	680	0	0.0	0.0	0	0%
shredded, 'Kraut'	1/2 cup	20	1	5	680	0	0.0	0.0	0	0%
(Del Monte)										
	2 tbsp	0	0	1	180	1	0.0	0.0	0	0%
w/liquid	1/2 cup	25	1	6	775	0	0.0	0.0	0	0%
(Eden Foods) organic	1/2 cup	25	2	4	580	3	1.0	0.0	0	27%
(Finast) w/liquid	1/2 cup	30	1	6	800	0	0.0	0.0	0	0%
(Libby's)										
Bavarian style, w/caraway seeds	2 tbsp	15	0	3	180	1	0.0	0.0	0	0%
crispy	2 tbsp	5	0	1	190	1	0.0	0.0	0	0%
(Pathmark) w/liquid	1/2 cup	20	0	4	880	0	0.0	0.0	0	0%
(S&W)	2 tbsp	5	0	2	180	0	0.0	0.0	0	0%
(Silver Floss) Bavarian style	1/2 cup	35	1	7	500	0	0.0	0.0	0	0%
(Snow Floss) w/liquid	1/2 cup	28	1	4	780	1	0.0	0.0	0	0%
(Stokely)										
Bavarian style, w/caraway seeds, mild	1/2 cup	35	0	7	860	3	0.0	0.0	0	0%
Bavarian style, w/liquid	1/2 cup	30	1	7	780	0	0.0	0.0	0	0%
shredded and chopped, w/liquid	1/2 cup	20	1	4	810	0	0.0	0.0	0	0%
shredded, traditional	2 tbsp	5	0	1	190	1	0.0	0.0	0	0%
extra mild	1/2 cup	80	0	18	850	3	0.0	0.0	0	0%
(Vlasic) w/liquid, 'Old Fashioned'	1/2 cup	4	0	1	280	0	0.0	0.0	0	0%
Frozen or refrigerated										
(Claussen)	1/4 cup	5	0	1	210	1	0.0	0.0	0	0%
(S&W)	2 tbsp	5	0	1	220	0	0.0	0.0	0	0%
SAUERKRAUT JUICE, canned or bottled *(Biotta)*	6 fl oz	21	1	4	1482	0	0.1	0.0	0	4%
SAUSAGE										
(Armour) links, 'Premium Smokee'	2 links	150	6	2	480	0	13.0	5.0	40	79%
(Eckrich) minced, roll	1 oz slice	80	4	1	300	0	7.0	0.0	0	76%
(Hickory Farms) 'Safari'	1 oz	98	5	1	343	0	9.0	0.0	14	77%
(JM)										
patty, cooked	1 patty	70	2	1	170	0	6.0	0.0	0	82%
patty, raw	1 oz	130	3	1	180	0	14.0	0.0	0	89%
raw, 'Tasty Link'	2 links	220	6	1	340	0	21.0	0.0	0	87%
(Jones Dairy Farm)										
patty	1 patty	155	6	0	281	0	14.4	0.0	36	85%
patty, 'Golden Brown'	1 patty	155	5	0	250	0	14.7	0.0	29	88%
patty, spicy, 'Golden Brown'	1 link	100	3	0	159	0	9.5	0.0	18	88%
roll, 'Cello Roll'	1 slice	105	4	0	200	0	9.6	0.0	24	85%
(Oscar Mayer) link, 'Smokie Links'	1 serving	130	5	1	433	0	11.7	4.0	27	81%

Food Name	Serving Size	Calories	Prot. gms	Carbs gms	Sod. mgs	Fiber gms	Fat gms	Sat. Fat gms	Chol. mgs	% Fat Cal.
BEEF										
(Eckrich)										
	1 oz	100	3	1	270	0	9.0	0.0	0	84%
'Lean Supreme'	1 oz	80	4	1	230	0	7.0	0.0	0	76%
'Smok-Y-Links'	2 links	160	6	2	350	0	14.0	0.0	0	80%
(Hillshire Farm)										
'Flavorseal'	2 oz	180	7	2	490	0	16.0	0.0	0	80%
hot links	1 serving	260	10	2	650	0	24.0	11.0	60	82%
(Jones Dairy Farm) 'Golden Brown'	1 link	75	4	0	159	0	6.1	0.0	18	78%
(Oscar Mayer) 'Smokies'	1 serving	128	5	1	425	0	11.5	4.8	28	81%
(Pemmican) Tabasco	1.1 oz	120	5	2	410	0	10.0	0.0	0	76%
BEERWURST										
beef, 4-inch diam, 1/8 inch slice	1 slice	76	3	0	236	0	6.9	3.0	14	82%
beef, 2.5-inch diam, 1/4 inch slice	1 slice	20	1	0	62	0	1.8	0.8	4	82%
pork, 4-inch diam, 1/8 inch slice	1 slice	55	3	0	285	0	4.3	1.4	14	71%
pork, 2.5-inch diam, 1/4 inch slice	1 slice	14	1	0	74	0	1.1	0.4	4	71%
BERLINER										
pork and beef	1 oz	65	4	1	368	0	4.9	1.7	13	67%
pork and beef, 2.5-inch diam, 1/4 inch slice	1 slice	53	4	1	298	0	4.0	1.4	11	67%
BLOOD SAUSAGE										
	1 oz	107	4	0	193	0	9.8	3.8	34	82%
5 x 4-5/8 x 1/16 inch slice	1 slice	95	4	0	170	0	8.6	3.3	30	82%
BOCKWURST										
pork, veal, milk, and eggs	1 oz	87	4	0	313	0	7.8	2.9	17	81%
pork, veal, milk, and eggs, 7 links per lb.	1 link	200	9	0	718	0	17.9	6.6	38	81%
BRATWURST										
pork, cooked	1 oz	85	4	1	158	0	7.3	2.6	17	78%
pork, cooked, 4 per 12-oz pkg.	1 link	256	12	2	473	0	22.0	7.9	51	78%
(Eckrich)	1 link	310	11	1	820	0	30.0	0.0	0	85%
(Hickory Farms)										
'Brotwurst'	1 oz	90	4	1	277	0	8.0	0.0	8	78%
cheddar, 'Cheddy Brots'	1 oz	98	4	1	259	0	9.0	0.0	7	80%
hot, 'Hot Brots'	1 oz	96	4	1	269	0	9.0	0.0	8	80%
(Johnsonville) w/real Wisconsin beef	1 link	300	14	1	800	0	27.0	10.0	70	80%
(Kahn's)	1 link	190	7	2	490	0	17.0	0.0	0	81%
BRAUNSCHWEIGER										
	1 oz	102	4	1	324	0	9.1	3.1	44	81%
2.5-inch diam, 1/4-inch slice	1 slice	65	2	1	206	0	5.8	2.0	28	81%
(Hormel)	1 oz	80	4	0	322	0	7.0	0.0	0	80%
(JM)	1 oz	80	3	2	260	0	6.0	0.0	0	73%
(Oscar Mayer)										
	1 oz	100	4	1	230	0	9.0	0.0	50	80%
	1 slice	100	4	1	320	0	9.0	3.0	50	80%
'German Brand'	1 oz	96	4	1	329	0	8.7	3.0	45	81%
'Tube'	1 oz	97	4	1	301	0	8.7	3.0	47	81%
BREAKFAST										
(Green Giant)										
links, frozen	3 links	110	12	5	340	4	5.0	0.5	0	40%
patties, frozen	2 patties	100	10	5	280	3	4.0	0.5	0	38%
(Healthy Choice)										
links	2 links	50	7	3	300	0	1.5	0.5	15	25%
patties	2 patties	50	7	3	300	0	1.5	0.5	15	25%
(Hudson) turkey, ground	1 oz	65	4	0	180	0	5.3	0.0	0	74%

Food Name	Serving Size	Calories	Prot. gms	Carbs gms	Sod. mgs	Fiber gms	Fat gms	Sat. Fat gms	Chol. mgs	% Fat Cal.
(Louis Rich)										
turkey, 85% fat-free	1 oz	55	6	1	230	0	3.0	0.0	25	49%
turkey, ground, cooked	1 oz	56	6	0	215	0	3.5	1.5	22	56%
(Mr. Turkey) turkey	2.5 oz	190	17	0	665	0	13.4	3.9	92	64%
(The Turkey Store) links, mild	2 oz	140	8	1	360	0	11.0	3.0	45	73%
BROWN AND SERVE										
(Eckrich) 'Lean Supreme'	2 links	120	7	1	440	0	10.0	0.0	0	74%
(Hormel)										
link, uncooked	2 links	180	7	0	411	0	17.0	0.0	0	85%
link, cooked	2 links	140	6	0	430	0	13.0	0.0	0	83%
(Jones Dairy Farm) link, 'Light'	1 link	60	4	1	150	0	4.1	0.0	16	67%
(Swift)										
link, 'Country Recipe'	1 link	130	4	1	240	0	12.0	0.0	0	84%
link, 'Premium Original'	1 link	130	3	1	260	0	12.0	0.0	0	87%
link, beef, 'Premium Brown 'N Serve'	1 link	120	4	1	250	0	12.0	0.0	0	84%
link, maple flavored	1 link	120	3	1	260	0	12.0	0.0	0	87%
link, microwave	1 link	120	4	1	270	0	12.0	0.0	0	84%
link, smoked flavor	1 link	120	4	1	280	0	11.0	0.0	0	83%
link, w/bacon	1 link	120	4	1	270	0	11.0	0.0	0	83%
link, w/ham	1 link	130	3	1	260	0	13.0	0.0	0	88%
patty, 'Country Recipe'	1 patty	130	4	1	240	0	12.0	0.0	0	84%
patty, 'Premium Original'	1 patty	120	4	1	270	0	12.0	0.0	0	84%
CAPOCOLLO *(Hormel)*	1 oz	80	5	0	273	0	6.0	0.0	0	73%
CERVELAT										
(Hillshire Farm) Thuringer	2 oz	180	9	1	650	0	15.0	0.0	0	77%
(Hormel)										
Thuringer, 'Old Smokehouse Chub'	1 oz	100	5	0	332	0	9.0	0.0	0	80%
Thuringer, 'Old Smokehouse Sliced'	1 oz	100	5	0	321	0	9.0	0.0	0	80%
Thuringer, 'Old Smokehouse'	1 oz	90	4	1	328	0	8.0	0.0	0	78%
Thuringer, 'Viking Club Cervelat'	1 oz	90	5	0	325	0	8.0	0.0	0	78%
(JM)										
Thuringer, beef	1 oz slice	80	5	1	340	0	7.0	0.0	0	72%
Thuringer, 'Cervalot'	1 oz slice	70	4	1	260	0	6.0	0.0	0	73%
(Oscar Mayer)										
Thuringer, beef	1 serving	142	7	1	655	0	12.4	5.4	37	79%
Thuringer, beef, sliced	1 slice	71	3	0	328	0	6.2	2.7	18	79%
Thuringer, beef and pork	1 oz	95	4	0	352	0	8.4	3.4	21	80%
Thuringer, beef and pork, 4-inch diam, 1/8-inch slice	1 slice	77	4	0	286	0	6.8	2.8	17	80%
CHEESE										
(Eckrich)										
'Smok-Y-Links'	2 links	160	6	2	360	0	14.0	0.0	0	80%
hot, 'Smok-Y-Links'	2 links	150	6	1	360	0	14.0	0.0	0	82%
maple flavored, 'Smok-Y-Links'	2 links	160	6	2	390	0	14.0	0.0	0	80%
original, 'Smok-Y-Links'	2 links	160	6	2	340	0	14.0	0.0	0	80%
w/ham, 'Smok-Y-Links'	2 links	160	6	2	500	0	15.0	0.0	0	81%
(Hillshire Farm)										
bun size, 'Cheddarwurst'	2 oz	200	8	1	480	0	18.0	0.0	0	82%
hot, 'Flavorseal'	2 oz	180	7	2	510	0	16.0	0.0	0	80%
links, 'Cheddarwurst'	2 oz	190	8	1	480	0	17.0	0.0	0	81%
smoked, 'Cheddarwurst'	1 serving	260	11	3	900	0	23.0	12.0	50	79%
(Hormel) 'Smokie Cheezers'	2 links	168	9	1	623	0	15.0	0.0	0	77%
(Louis Rich)										
turkey, and cheddar, smoked, 90% fat-free	1 oz	45	5	1	270	0	3.0	0.0	20	53%
turkey, w/cheese, smoked	1 oz	47	5	1	269	0	2.8	0.8	18	54%

Food Name	Serving Size	Calories	Prot. gms	Carbs gms	Sod. mgs	Fiber gms	Fat gms	Sat. Fat gms	Chol. mgs	% Fat Cal.
(Oscar Mayer)										
pork and turkey, little, 'Smokies'	1 link	28	1	0	93	0	2.5	1.0	6	81%
'Smokies'	1 serving	130	6	1	450	0	11.7	4.4	30	81%
CHORIZO										
pork and beef	1 oz	129	7	1	350	0	10.8	4.1	25	76%
pork and beef, 4-inch link	1 link	273	14	1	741	0	23.0	8.6	53	76%
(Carmelita)										
beef	2.5 oz	250	8	5	510	0	23.0	11.0	80	80%
pork	2.5 oz	250	8	3	500	0	23.0	9.0	110	82%
GERMAN STYLE *(Hickory Farms)*	1 oz	100	5	1	385	0	8.0	0.0	20	75%
HEAD CHEESE *(Oscar Mayer)*	1 slice	50	5	0	360	0	4.0	1.5	25	64%
HONEY ROLL										
beef	1 oz	52	5	1	375	0	3.0	1.2	14	52%
beef, 4-inch diam, 1/8-inch slice	1 slice	42	4	1	304	0	2.4	0.9	12	52%
HOT										
(JM)										
patty, cooked	1 patty	70	2	1	170	0	6.0	0.0	0	82%
patty, raw	1 oz	130	3	1	180	0	14.0	0.0	0	89%
(OHSE) 'Hot Links'	1 oz	80	4	4	310	0	3.0	0.0	0	46%
JALAPENO *(Bar-S)* smoked	2 oz	180	7	2	630	0	16.0	5.0	40	80%
ITALIAN STYLE										
pork, cooked, 5 links per lb.	1 link	216	13	1	618	0	17.2	6.1	52	72%
pork, cooked, 4 links per lb.	1 link	268	17	1	765	0	21.3	7.5	65	72%
pork, raw, 7 links per lb	1 link	315	13	1	665	0	28.5	10.3	69	82%
pork, raw, 4 links per lb	1 link	391	16	1	826	0	35.4	12.7	86	82%
(Hillshire Farm) smoked, 'Flavorseal'	2 oz	200	7	1	500	0	18.0	0.0	0	84%
(Johnsonville)										
hot	1 link	300	14	1	800	0	27.0	10.0	70	80%
mild	1 link	300	14	1	800	0	27.0	10.0	70	80%
(Shelton's) turkey	1 serving	160	7	0	310	0	16.0	5.0	30	84%
(The Turkey Store) turkey, hot	3 oz	140	15	2	681	0	9.0	2.5	45	54%
KIELBASA										
pork and beef	1 oz	88	4	1	305	0	7.7	2.8	19	79%
(Eckrich)										
light, 'Lean Supreme Polska'	1 oz	72	4	1	224	0	6.0	0.0	0	73%
w/o skin, 'Polska'	1 link	180	7	2	420	0	16.0	0.0	0	80%
(Healthy Choice) low-fat	2 oz	70	7	6	480	0	1.5	0.5	20	21%
(Hillshire Farm) bun size	1 serving	180	7	2	660	0	16.0	7.0	40	80%
(Hormel)										
'Kolbase'	3 oz	220	12	1	904	0	19.0	0.0	0	77%
w/o skin	1/2 link	180	12	1	826	0	14.0	0.0	0	71%
(Louis Rich) turkey, smoked, 90% fat-free	1 oz	40	5	1	250	0	2.0	0.0	20	43%
(Mr. Turkey) 'Polska Kielbasa'	1 oz	59	4	1	264	0	4.4	0.0	15	67%
KNOCKWURST										
pork and beef	1 oz	87	3	0	286	0	7.9	2.9	16	81%
pork and beef, 4-inch x 1-1/8-inch diam	1 link	209	8	1	687	0	18.9	6.9	39	81%
(Hebrew National) beef, 1 link	3 oz	263	10	1	877	0	25.0	0.0	26	83%
LIVER. See SAUSAGE, BRAUNSCHWEIGER.										
LUNCHEON										
pork and beef	1 oz	74	4	0	335	0	5.9	2.2	18	73%
pork and beef, 4-inch diam, 1/8-inch slice	1 slice	60	4	0	272	0	4.8	1.8	15	73%
MILD *(Jones Dairy Farm)* 'Golden Brown'	1 link	100	3	0	150	0	9.8	0.0	18	89%
MORTADELLA										
beef and pork	1 oz	88	5	1	353	0	7.2	2.7	16	74%

Food Name	Serving Size	Calories	Prot. gms	Carbs gms	Sod. mgs	Fiber gms	Fat gms	Sat. Fat gms	Chol. mgs	% Fat Cal.
beef and pork, 15 per 8-oz pkg	1 slice	47	2	0	187	0	3.8	1.4	8	74%
NEW ENGLAND STYLE										
pork and beef	1 oz	46	5	1	346	0	2.1	0.7	14	42%
pork and beef, 4-inch diam, 1/8-inch slice	1 slice	37	4	1	281	0	1.7	0.6	11	42%
(Eckrich) New England brand	1 oz slice	35	5	1	370	0	1.0	0.0	0	27%
(Light & Lean) New England brand	2 slices	90	10	0	0	0	6.0	0.0	0	57%
(Oscar Mayer)	1 slice	60	8	1	570	0	2.5	1.0	25	38%
PEPPERONI										
pork and beef, 10 1/4 inch long x 1 3/8 inch diam	1 sausage	1247	53	7	5120	0	110.4	40.5	198	80%
pork and beef, 1 3/8 inch diam, 1/8-inch slice	1 slice	27	1	0	112	0	2.4	0.9	4	80%
(Gallo Salame)										
deli style	11 slices	160	7	0	610	0	14.0	5.0	30	82%
pizza style	9 slices	140	6	0	550	0	13.0	4.0	30	83%
(Hickory Farms)	1 oz	140	6	1	578	0	13.0	0.0	23	81%
(Hormel)										
	1 oz	140	6	0	462	0	13.0	0.0	0	83%
bits	1 tbsp	35	2	0	0	0	3.0	0.0	0	77%
'Chunk'	1 oz	140	6	0	423	0	12.0	0.0	0	82%
'Leoni Brand'	1 oz	130	6	0	508	0	12.0	0.0	0	82%
'Perma-Fresh'	2 slices	80	3	0	281	0	7.0	0.0	0	84%
'Rosa'	1 oz	140	6	0	626	0	13.0	0.0	0	83%
'Rosa Grande'	1 oz	140	6	0	512	0	13.0	0.0	0	83%
turkey, 'Pillow Pak'	1 serving	74	9	1	557	na	3.5	0.9	37	42%
(JM) sliced	8 slices	70	3	1	290	0	6.0	0.0	0	77%
(Oscar Mayer)	15 slices	140	6	0	550	0	13.0	5.0	25	83%
PICKLED										
(Penrose)										
beer	1 link	40	2	1	220	0	3.0	0.0	0	69%
firecracker	1 link	40	2	1	220	0	3.0	0.0	0	69%
firecracker, giant	1 link	170	9	1	870	0	14.0	0.0	0	76%
hot	1 link	40	2	1	220	0	3.0	0.0	0	69%
red hot	1 link	40	2	1	220	0	3.0	0.0	0	69%
POLISH STYLE. See also KIELBASA.										
pork	1 oz	92	4	0	248	0	8.1	2.9	20	79%
pork, 10-inch long x 1.25-inch diam	1 sausage	740	32	4	1989	0	65.2	23.4	159	79%
(Hormel)	2 links	170	9	0	574	0	14.0	0.0	0	78%
(OHSE)										
hot	1 oz	70	4	3	270	0	5.0	0.0	0	62%
	1 oz	80	4	1	290	0	7.0	0.0	0	76%
(Penrose) pickled	1 link	40	2	1	220	0	3.0	0.0	0	69%
(Pilgrim's Pride)	3 oz	131	13	2	780	0	7.7	0.0	72	53%
PORK										
link, 4-inch long x 1 1/8 inch diam	1 link	265	15	1	1020	0	21.6	7.7	46	74%
link, fresh, cooked, 4-inch long x 7/8-inch diam										
before cooking	1 link	48	3	0	168	0	4.1	1.4	11	76%
link, fresh, raw, 7/8-inch diam x 4-inch long	1 link	117	3	0	187	0	11.3	4.1	19	87%
link, 2-inch long x 3/4-inch diam	1 link	62	4	0	240	0	5.1	1.8	11	74%
patty, fresh, cooked, 3 7/8 inch diam x 1/4 inch thick										
before cooking		100	5	0	349	0	8.4	2.9	22	76%
patty, fresh, raw 3 7/8 inch diam x 1/4 inch thick	1 patty	238	7	1	380	0	23.0	8.2	39	87%
(Hormel)										
links, 'Midget Links'	2 links	143	7	0	327	0	13.0	0.0	0	81%
links, 'Little Sizzlers'	2 links	103	6	0	172	0	9.0	0.0	0	77%

Food Name	Serving Size	Calories	Prot. gms	Carbs gms	Sod. mgs	Fiber gms	Fat gms	Sat. Fat gms	Chol. mgs	% Fat Cal.
(Jimmy Dean)										
hot	2 oz	250	10	0	540	0	24.0	8.0	50	84%
'Light'	1.2 oz	80	6	1	230	0	7.0	0.0	25	69%
links	2 links	180	7	1	380	0	17.0	0.0	0	83%
patties	1 patty	140	5	1	300	0	13.0	0.0	0	83%
regular, cooked	1 oz	120	4	1	240	0	11.0	0.0	0	83%
sage	2 oz	250	10	0	540	0	24.0	8.0	50	84%
(JM)										
and bacon, cooked, 'Tasty Link'	2 links	100	6	1	240	0	9.0	0.0	0	74%
cooked, 'Tasty Link'	2 links	190	6	1	290	0	18.0	0.0	0	85%
raw, 'Tasty Link'	2 links	260	6	1	380	0	26.0	0.0	0	89%
(Jones Dairy Farm)										
	1 link	140	3	0	176	0	13.7	0.0	24	91%
'Golden Brown Light'	1 link	55	3	1	132	0	4.2	0.0	16	71%
'Light'	1 link	70	4	1	232	0	5.0	0.0	21	68%
(Oscar Mayer)										
(Oscar Mayer) link	2 links	170	9	1	410	0	15.0	5.0	40	77%
(Oscar Mayer) link, cooked	1 link	82	4	0	201	0	7.3	2.6	18	80%
link, 'Little Friers' cooked	1 link	82	3	0	219	0	7.5	2.7	17	82%
(Owens)										
country style	2 oz	290	10	0	420	0	27.0	10.0	20	86%
country style, hot	2 oz	290	10	0	460	0	27.0	9.0	15	86%
country style, sage	2 oz	250	11	1	310	0	23.0	8.0	20	81%
(Pierre)										
link, all meat, product 3755	1 piece	85	8	0	232	0	5.3	2.0	27	56%
patty, all meat, product 3750	1 piece	85	8	0	232	0	5.3	2.0	27	56%
patty, all meat, product 3751	1 piece	174	17	1	473	0	10.8	4.0	55	56%
patty, all meat, product 3850	1 piece	95	8	1	231	0	6.6	2.5	27	62%
patty, all meat, product 3851	1 piece	193	16	1	469	0	13.4	5.0	55	62%
(Tyson) country, whole hog	3.5 oz	320	13	1	905	0	29.0	0.0	49	82%
PORK AND BEEF										
link, 4-inch long x 1-1/8-inch diam	1 link	228	9	1	643	0	20.6	7.2	48	81%
link, fresh, cooked, 4-inch long x 7/8-inch diam										
before cooking	1 link	51	2	0	105	0	4.7	1.7	9	83%
link, 2-inch long x 3/4-inch diam	1 link	54	2	0	151	0	4.9	1.7	11	81%
patty, fresh, cooked, 3-7/8-inch diam x 1/4-inch thick										
before cooking	1 patty	107	4	1	217	0	9.8	3.5	19	83%
PORK AND TURKEY *(Oscar Mayer)* little, 'Smokies'	1 link	27	1	0	92	0	2.4	0.8	6	81%
SAGE *(Jimmy Dean)* cooked	1 oz	120	4	1	240	0	11.0	0.0	0	83%
SALAMI. See also under LUNCHEON MEAT.										
beef and pork, cooked	1 oz	71	4	1	302	0	5.7	2.3	18	73%
beef and pork, cooked, 4-inch diam, 1/8 inch slice	1 slice	58	3	1	245	0	4.6	1.9	15	73%
beef, cooked	1 oz	74	4	1	333	0	5.9	2.6	18	71%
beef, cooked, 4-inch diam, 1/8 inch slice	1 slice	60	3	1	270	0	4.8	2.1	15	71%
pork, dry or hard, 3-1/8-inch diam, 1/16-inch slice	1 slice	41	2	0	226	0	3.4	1.2	8	75%
pork and beef, dry or hard, 3-1/8-inch diam, 1/16-inch slice	1 slice	42	2	0	186	0	3.4	1.2	8	74%
SCRAPPLE *(Jones Dairy Farm)*	1 slice	65	3	4	165	0	3.7	0.0	24	55%
SMOKED										
(Eckrich)										
'Lean Supreme'	1 oz	70	4	1	230	0	6.0	0.0	0	73%
'No skin'	1 link	180	7	2	420	0	16.0	0.0	0	80%
(Healthy Choice) low-fat	2 oz	70	7	6	480	0	1.5	0.5	20	21%
(Hillshire Farm)										
'Flavorseal'	2 oz	190	7	1	500	0	17.0	0.0	0	83%

Food Name	Serving Size	Calories	Prot. gms	Carbs gms	Sod. mgs	Fiber gms	Fat gms	Sat. Fat gms	Chol. mgs	% Fat Cal.
original, bun size	1 serving	180	7	2	660	0	16.0	7.0	40	80%
(Hormel) 'Smokies'	2 links	160	9	2	597	0	14.0	0.0	0	74%
(OHSE)	1 oz	80	4	1	320	0	7.0	0.0	0	76%
(Oscar Mayer) link 'Big & Juicy'	2.7 oz	227	9	1	757	0	20.5	7.0	48	81%
(Pilgrim's Pride)	3 oz	144	13	3	890	0	9.1	0.0	64	57%
SUMMER										
(Eckrich)	1 oz slice	80	4	1	320	0	7.0	0.0	0	76%
(Hormel)										
beef, 'Beefy'	1 oz	100	5	0	313	0	9.0	0.0	0	80%
'Perma-Fresh'	2 slices	140	10	0	706	0	11.0	0.0	0	71%
'Tangy, Chub'	1 oz	90	5	0	317	0	7.0	0.0	0	76%
'Thuringer'	1 oz	90	4	0	332	0	9.0	0.0	0	84%
(Lean & Lite)	1 oz	43	6	1	0	0	2.3	0.0	18	42%
(Light & Lean)	2 slices	100	6	0	0	0	8.0	0.0	0	75%
(Louis Rich)										
turkey	1 oz slice	55	5	0	326	0	3.9	1.2	21	63%
turkey, 85% fat-free	1 oz slice	55	5	1	325	0	4.0	0.0	25	60%
(OHSE)										
	1 oz	75	5	2	340	0	5.0	0.0	0	62%
beef	1 oz	80	5	1	330	0	6.0	0.0	0	69%
(Oscar Mayer) sliced	1 slice	69	4	0	331	0	6.1	2.7	19	79%
SWEDISH STYLE (Hickory Farms)	1 oz	100	5	0	380	0	9.0	0.0	20	80%
TURKEY										
(Butterball)	1 oz	50	4	1	250	0	4.0	0.0	0	64%
(Jimmy Dean) 'Light'	1.2 oz	80	6	1	230	0	7.0	0.0	25	69%
(Louis Rich)										
link, cooked	1 link	46	5	0	234	0	2.7	1.5	18	52%
link, cooked, 85% fat-free	0.84 oz	45	6	1	235	0	3.0	0.0	20	49%
original or hot	2.5 oz	120	12	1	430	0	8.0	2.5	55	58%
smoked	1 serving	90	8	2	515	0	5.4	1.5	36	54%
(Norbest) 'Tasti-Lean, Chub or Links'	1 oz	53	5	0	179	0	2.8	0.0	0	56%
(Shelton's)										
links	1 serving	140	6	0	260	0	14.0	5.0	30	84%
patty	1 serving	140	10	0	370	0	11.0	3.0	45	71%
VEGETARIAN										
(Boca) breakfast patty, vegetarian	1 patty	70	9	4	300	2	3.0	0.0	0	34%
(Garden Sausage) garden sausage, meatless, soy-free	1 oz	95	4	18	65	4	1.0	0.5	0	9%
(Heartline)										
Italian style, cooked	2 oz	176	19	9	680	0	7.0	0.0	0	36%
pepperoni style, lite	0.5 oz	22	5	1	135	3	0.0	0.0	0	0%
(Loma Linda)										
breakfast links, vegetarian	2 links	93	8	3	226	1	5.6	0.8	1	54%
'Linketts'	1 link	70	7	1	160	1	4.5	0.5	0	57.9%
'Little Links'	2 links	90	8	1	230	2	6.0	1.0	0	60.0%
(Morningstar Farms)										
'Breakfast Links'	2 links	60	8	2	340	2	2.0	0.5	0	30.0%
'Breakfast Patties'	1 patty	80	10	3	270	2	3.0	0.5	0	33.7%
'Sausage Style Recipe Crumbles'	2/3 cup	90	11	5	370	2	3.0	0.0	0	30.0%
(Worthington)										
breakfast links, vegetarian	2 links	63	8	2	338	2	2.4	0.5	1	35%
breakfast patty, vegetarian	1 pkg	8531	1065	399	27839	212	297.6	54.7	82	31%
breakfast patty, vegetarian	1 patty	79	10	4	259	2	2.8	0.5	1	31%
'Leanies'	1 link	100	7	2	430	1	7.0	1.0	0	63.0%
'Low Fat Veja-Links'	1 link	40	5	1	190	0	1.5	0.0	0	33.8%

Food Name	Serving Size	Calories	Prot. gms	Carbs gms	Sod. mgs	Fiber gms	Fat gms	Sat. Fat gms	Chol. mgs	% Fat Cal.
'Prosage Links'	2 links	63	8	2	338	2	2.4	0.5	1	35%
'Prosage Patties'	1 patty	96	10	3	296	2	3.2	0.5	1	36%
'Prosage' roll, frozen	5/8-inch slice	142	10	2	392	2	10.4	2.0	1	66%
'Saucettes'	2 slices	86	6	1	205	1	6.5	1.1	1	68%
'Super Links'	1 link	110	7	2	350	1	8.0	1.0	0	65.5%
'Veja-Links'	1 link	49	5	1	192	0	3.0	0.6	1	55%
VIENNA										
beef and pork, canned, 7/8-inch diam x 2-inch long	1 sausage	45	2	0	152	0	4.0	1.5	8	81%
(Armour)										
chicken, in beef stock, lite, canned, 'Premium'	2 oz	150	6	1	400	0	13.0	0.0	0	81%
hot and spicy, canned	2.5 oz	190	6	3	860	0	17.0	0.0	0	81%
in barbecue sauce, canned	2.5 oz	190	6	4	760	0	17.0	0.0	0	79%
in beef stock, canned	2 oz	180	5	1	530	0	17.0	0.0	0	86%
in beef stock, lite, canned	2 oz	150	6	1	400	0	13.0	0.0	0	81%
smoked, canned	2 oz	180	5	1	530	0	17.0	0.0	0	86%
(Hormel)										
canned	1 oz	69	3	2	225	0	7.0	2.0	15	76%
chicken, canned	1 oz	56	3	1	220	0	5.0	1.0	27	74%
no broth, canned	4 links	200	7	1	479	0	18.0	0.0	0	84%
(Libby's)										
chicken, in beef broth, canned	2 oz	130	7	3	560	0	10.0	0.0	0	69%
in barbecue sauce, canned	2.5 oz	180	8	2	420	0	15.0	0.0	0	77%
in beef broth, canned, approx. 3 1/2 links	2 oz	160	6	1	330	0	15.0	0.0	0	83%
SAUSAGE STICK										
(Hickory Farms) stick, 'Sportsman Stick'	1 oz	138	9	4	1075	0	10.0	0.0	40	63%
(Slim Jim) smoked, 'Giant Slim'	1.1 oz	180	7	2	470	0	16.0	0.0	0	80%
(Slim Jim) Tabasco, 'Handi-Paks'	0.31 oz	50	2	1	130	0	4.0	0.0	0	75%
(Slim Jim) smoked, 'Jumbo Jim'	1 oz	150	8	2	430	0	12.0	0.0	0	73%
(Slim Jim) smoked, pepperoni 'Handi-Paks'	0.31 oz	50	2	1	130	0	4.0	0.0	0	75%
(Slim Jim) smoked, spicy 'Handi-Paks'	0.31 oz	50	2	1	130	0	4.0	0.0	0	75%
SAVORY										
ground	1 tbsp	12	0	3	1	2	0.3	0.1	0	18%
ground	1 tsp	4	0	1	0	1	0.1	0.0	0	18%
ground (Durkee)	1 tsp	5	0	0	0	0	0.0	0.0	0	0%
ground (Laurel Leaf)	1 tsp	5	0	0	0	0	0.0	0.0	0	0%
ground (McCormick/Schilling)	1 tsp	7	0	2	0	1	0.0	0.0	0	0%
ground (Spice Islands)	1 tsp	5	0	1	1	0	0.1	0.0	0	17%
summer, ground (Tone's)	1 tsp	4	0	1	1	0	0.1	0.0	0	17%
SAVOY CABBAGE. See CABBAGE, SAVOY.										
SCALLION										
Fresh										
raw, chopped (Dole)	1 tbsp	2	0	0	0	0	0.1	0.0	0	36%
raw, tops and bulb, chopped	1 cup	32	2	7	16	3	0.2	0.0	0	5%
raw, tops and bulb, chopped	1 tbsp	2	0	0	1	0	0.0	0.0	0	5%
raw, tops and bulb, whole, large, 5-1/4 inch long	1 scallion	8	0	2	4	1	0.0	0.0	0	5%
raw, tops and bulb, whole, medium, 4-1/8-inch long	1 scallion	5	0	1	2	0	0.0	0.0	0	5%
raw, tops and bulb, whole, small, 3-inch long	1 scallion	2	0	0	1	0	0.0	0.0	0	5%
Freeze dried										
(McCormick/Schilling)	1 tsp	4	0	1	3	0	0.0	0.0	0	0%
SCALLOP										
mixed species, breaded and fried	2 large	67	6	3	144	na	3.4	0.8	19	45%
mixed species, raw	2 large	26	5	1	48	0	0.2	0.0	10	8%
mixed species, raw	3 oz	75	14	2	137	0	0.6	0.1	28	8%
SCALLOP SQUASH. See SQUASH, SCALLOP.										

Food Name	Serving Size	Calories	Prot. gms	Carbs gms	Sod. mgs	Fiber gms	Fat gms	Sat. Fat gms	Chol. mgs	% Fat Cal.
SCALLOP SUBSTITUTE										
made from Surimi	3 oz	84	11	9	676	0	0.3	0.1	19	4%
vegetarian, 'Skallops' *(Worthington)*	1/2 cup	86	15	3	412	3	1.4	0.5	0	15%
SCORZONERA. See SALSIFY, BLACK.										
SCOTCH KALE. See KALE, SCOTCH.										
SCRAPPLE. See under SAUSAGE.										
SCROD ENTRÉE										
(Gorton's) frozen, baked 'Microwave Entrees'	1 pkg	320	22	17	420	0	18.0	4.0	80	51%
SCUP / sea bream										
baked, broiled, grilled, or microwaved	3 oz	115	21	0	46	0	3.0	na	57	23%
raw	1 cup	174	31	0	70	0	4.5	1.1	86	23%
raw	3 oz	89	16	0	36	0	2.3	0.5	44	23%
raw, boneless	1 oz	30	5	0	12	0	0.8	0.2	15	23%
SEA BASS. See BASS, SEA.										
SEA BREAM. See SCUP.										
SEA DEVIL. See MONKFISH.										
SEA PERCH. See OCEAN PERCH, ATLANTIC.										
SEA TROUT. See under TROUT.										
SEA VEGETABLE										
AGAR, raw	2 tbsp	3	0	1	1	0	0.0	0.0	0	1%
ALARIA, dry *(Maine Coast)*	1/3 cup	18	1	3	301	3	0.0	0.0	0	0%
DULSE										
dry *(Maine Coast)*	1/3 cup	18	2	3	122	2	0.0	0.0	0	0%
raw	3.5 oz	<1	0.0	0.0	2085	>1.2 c	3.2	0.0	0	0%
HIZIKI, dry *(Eden Foods)*	1/2 cup	30	0	6	160	6	0.0	0.0	0	0%
IRISH MOSS, raw	2 tbsp	5	0	1	7	0	0.0	0.0	0	3%
KELP										
dry *(Maine Coast)*	1/3 cup	17	1	3	312	3	0.0	0.0	0	0%
raw	2 tbsp	4	0	1	23	0	0.1	0.0	0	11%
KOMBU, wild, 7-inch pieces *(Eden Foods)*	1/2 piece	10	0	2	90	1	0.0	0.0	0	0%
LAVER										
raw	10 sheets	9	2	1	12	0	0.1	0.0	0	7%
raw	2 tbsp	4	1	1	5	0	0.0	0.0	0	7%
NORI										
dry *(Maine Coast)*	1/3 cup	22	2	3	113	3	0.0	0.0	0	0%
dry *(Eden Foods)*	1 piece	10	1	1	5	1	0.0	0.0	0	0%
dry, for sushi *(Eden Foods)*	1 sheet	10	1	1	5	1	0.0	0.0	0	0%
WAKAME										
dry *(Eden Foods)*	1/2 cup	25	2	4	660	4	0.0	0.0	0	0%
flakes, instant *(Eden Foods)*	1 tsp	3	0	0	72	0	0.0	0.0	0	0%
raw	2 tbsp	5	0	1	87	0	0.1	0.0	0	12%
SEA VEGETABLE CHIPS *(Eden Foods)*	1 oz	130	1	22	200	0	5.0	0.0	0	33%
SEAFOOD DINNER/ENTRÉE. See also individual listings.										
(Armour) w/natural herbs, frozen, 'Classics Lite'	10 oz	190	13	29	1020	0	2.0	0.0	35	10%
(Budget Gourmet)										
Newburg, frozen	10 oz	350	17	43	660	0	12.0	0.0	70	31%
shrimp w/scallops, frozen, 'Mariner'	11.5 oz	320	16	43	690	0	9.0	0.0	70	26%
(Cajun Cookin') gumbo, frozen	17 oz	330	16	51	1330	0	7.0	0.0	0	19%
(Mrs. Paul's)										
shrimp and clams, w/linguini, frozen, 'Light'	10 oz	240	12	36	750	0	5.0	2.0	40	19%
(Pillsbury) casserole, frozen, 'Microwave Classic'	1 pkg	420	15	37	950	0	24.0	0.0	0	51%
(Swanson) Creole, w/rice, frozen, 'Homestyle Recipe'	9 oz	240	7	40	810	0	6.0	0.0	0	22%
SEAFOOD SEASONING. See under SEASONING MIX.										
SEASONING AND COATING MIX. See also MARINADE; MARINADE MIX.										

Food Name	Serving Size	Calories	Prot. gms	Carbs gms	Sod. mgs	Fiber gms	Fat gms	Sat. Fat gms	Chol. mgs	% Fat Cal.
ALL-PURPOSE										
(Golden Dipt) breading	1 oz	90	3	20	630	0	0.0	0.0	0	0%
(Shake 'N Bake) country mild recipe	1/4 pkt	80	1	10	500	0	4.0	0.0	0	45%
CHICKEN										
(Don's Chuck Wagon) frying mix, super crispy	1/4 cup	95	3	21	850	1	0.0	0.0	0	0%
(Golden Dipt)										
	1 oz	90	2	20	1430	0	0.0	0.0	0	0%
frying mix	1 oz	90	2.0	20.0	1430	(mq)	0.0	0.0	0	0%
(Luzianne) Cajun coating, bake, fry, or microwave	2 tbsp	100	3	20	1260	1	0.5	0.0	0	5%
(Oven Fry)										
extra crispy recipe	1 serving	60	2	10	420	0	1.0	0.0	0	16%
home style flour recipe	1 serving	40	1	7	470	0	1.0	0.0	0	23%
(Shake 'N Bake)										
barbecue	1 serving	45	0	9	410	0	1.0	0.0	0	20%
hot and spicy	1/4 pkt	80	2	15	380	0	2.0	0.0	0	21%
original	1 serving	40	1	7	220	0	1.0	0.0	0	22%
'Original Barbecue Recipe'	1/4 pkt	90	1	18	840	0	2.0	0.0	0	19%
(Tone's) Cajun, batter seasoning	1 tsp	12	0	3	75	0	0.1	0.1	0	7%
FISH										
(Tone's) Cajun	1 tsp	12	0	3	49	0	0.1	0.1	0	7%
(Don's Chuck Wagon) no MSG	1/4 cup	95	4	21	940	1	0.0	0.0	0	0%
(Shake 'N Bake) original	1 serving	70	1	14	420	1	1.5	0.0	0	18%
FLOUR, seasoned, all-purpose, dry (Kentucky Kernel)	1/4 cup	90	3	20	1360	0	0.0	0.0	0	0%
PORK										
(Oven Fry) extra crispy recipe	1 serving	60	2	11	340	0	1.5	0.0	0	21%
(Shake 'N Bake)										
	1 serving	45	0	9	410	0	1.0	0.0	0	20%
hot and spicy	1/8 pkt	45	1	8	220	0	1.0	0.0	0	20%
'Original Recipe'	1/8 pkt	40	1	8	310	0	1.0	0.0	0	20%
SEAFOOD										
(Don's Chuck Wagon) seasoned, no MSG	1/4 cup	95	2	21	990	1	0.0	0.0	0	0%
(Golden Dipt)										
fish fry, Cajun style, mix only	2/3 oz	60	2	14	470	0	0.0	0.0	0	0%
fish fry, mix only	2/3 oz	60	2	14	430	0	0.0	0.0	0	0%
mix only	2/3 oz	60	1	14	600	0	0.0	0.0	0	0%
(Luzianne) bake, fry, or microwave, Cajun, mix only	2 tbsp	100	2	22	1200	1	0.5	0.0	0	4%
SEASONING MIX										
ALL-PURPOSE										
(Knorr)	1 gram	5	0	0	240	0	0.0	0.0	0	0%
(Mrs. Dash) table blend	0.13 tsp	2	0	0	1	na	0.0	na	0	9%
(Praise Allah) for steak, meats, stews, and gravies	1/4 tsp	0	0	0	105	na	0.0	na	na	0%
(Spike All Purpose) all natural	1/4 tsp	1	0	0	161	0	0.0	0.0	0	0%
(Trader Joe's) salt-free, '21 Seasoning Salute'	1/4 tsp	0	0	0	0	0	0.0	0.0	0	0%
APPLE PIE SPICE (Tone's)	1 tsp	9	0	2	1	1	0.2	0.1	0	15%
BARBECUE SPICE (Tone's)	1 tsp	9	0	1	713	0	0.4	0.1	0	35%
BEEF										
(Adolph's) stew, 'Meal Makers'	1 tbsp	20	1	4	750	0	0.0	0.0	0	0%
(Bag 'n Season)										
pot roast	1 tsp	10	1	1	390	na	0.0	0.0	0	0%
Swiss steak	1 tsp	15	0	2	430	na	0.0	0.0	0	0%
(French's) w/onions, ground	1/4 pkg	25	1	6	440	0	0.0	0.0	0	0%
(Kikkoman) broccoli beef stir-fry	2 tsp	15	1	3	480	0	0.0	0.0	0	0%
(Lawry's)										
pot roast, 'Seasoning Blends'	1 pkg	122	4	25	4008	1	0.7	0.0	0	5%

Food Name	Serving Size	Calories	Prot. gms	Carbs gms	Sod. mgs	Fiber gms	Fat gms	Sat. Fat gms	Chol. mgs	% Fat Cal.
stew, 'Seasoning Blends'	1 pkg	131	5	26	3181	1	0.7	0.0	0	5%
(McCormick/Schilling) stew	2 tsp	15	1	3	410	0	0.0	0.0	0	0%
(Schilling)										
pot roast, 'Bag'n Season'	1 pkg	55	4	9	3030	0	0.6	0.0	0	10%
steak, 'Montreal LaGrille'	1/4 tsp	0	0	0	150	0	0.0	0.0	0	0%
steak, broiled, 'Spice Blends'	1/4 tsp	1	0	0	273	0	0.0	0.0	0	0%
stew	1/2 pkg	33	1	6	806	0	0.3	0.0	0	8%
stew, 'Bag'n Season'	1 pkg	87	8	11	4320	0	1.0	0.0	1	11%
stew, 'Bag'n Season'	1 tsp	15	1	1	670	na	0.0	0.0	0	0%
Stroganoff	1/4 pkg	32	1	6	1078	0	0.3	0.0	0	9%
Swiss steak, 'Bag'n Season'	1 pkg	81	2	17	2651	0	0.4	0.0	1	5%
(Sun Bird) beef and broccoli, Oriental	3/4 tbsp	20	0	5	140	0	0.0	0.0	0	0%
(Tone's) steak, blackened	1 tsp	9	0	2	486	0	0.3	0.0	0	25%
BURRITO										
(Lawry's) 'Seasoning Blends'	1 pkg	132	6	23	2516	1	1.7	0.0	0	12%
(Old El Paso)	2 tsp	20	1	3	290	1	0.0	0.0	0	0%
(Tio Sancho) 'Dinner Kit'	3.25 oz	265	12	49	5031	6	2.1	0.0	0	7%
CAJUN										
(Luzianne)	1/4 tsp	0	0	0	260	0	0.0	0.0	0	0%
(Tone's)	1 tsp	9	0	2	215	1	0.2	0.1	0	15%
CHICKEN										
(Featherweight)	1/4 pkg	18	1	8	30	0	0.0	0.0	0	0%
(Kikkoman) roast	1 tbsp	25	1	4	1980	0	0.0	0.0	0	0%
(Lawry's) Southwest, 'Seasoning Blends'	1 pkg	71	1	16	3947	0	0.3	0.0	0	4%
(Schilling)										
'Bag'n Season'	1 pkg	134	3	19	4771	0	5.0	0.0	1	34%
barbecue, tangy	2 tsp	20	0	3	400	0	0.0	0.0	0	0%
fried chicken	1/4 tsp	1	0	0	132	0	0.1	0.0	0	43%
rotisserie style	3/4 tsp	0	0	1	340	0	0.0	0.0	0	0%
CHILI										
(Carroll Shelby's) Texas brand, original	3 tbsp	80	2	14	1600	0	1.5	0.0	0	17%
(Gebhardt)										
'Chili Quik'	1 tbsp	14	0	3	204	0	0.3	0.1	0	16%
'Chili Quik' food service product	1 tbsp	18	1	4	407	1	0.4	0.1	0	16%
(Hain)										
hot	1/4 pkg	30	1	5	370	0	1.0	0.0	0	27%
medium	1/4 pkg	30	1	5	300	0	1.0	0.0	0	27%
mild	1/2 pkg	30	1	5	330	0	1.0	0.0	0	27%
(Lawry's) 'Seasoning Blends'	1 pkg	143	5	27	2291	2	1.8	0.0	0	11%
(McCormick/Schilling) original	1 tbsp	25	1	4	240	2	0.5	0.0	0	20%
(Old El Paso)	1 tbsp	25	1	4	770	1	0.5	0.0	0	18%
(Schilling)	1/4 pkg	27	1	5	290	0	0.5	0.0	0	17%
(Tio Sancho)	1.23 oz	109	4	6	832	4	2.2	0.0	0	33%
(Tone's)	1 tsp	12	0	2	231	0	0.3	0.1	0	20%
(Wick Fowler's)										
mild, 'False Alarm'	2 tbsp	50	2	9	980	0	1.5	0.0	0	23%
'2 Alarm'	3 tbsp	60	2	10	980	0	1.5	0.0	0	22%
CHILI POWDER										
	1 tbsp	24	1	4	76	3	1.3	0.2	0	45%
	1 tsp	8	0	1	26	1	0.4	0.1	0	45%
(Gebhardt)	1 tbsp	3	0	1	1	0	0.2	0.0	0	36%
(Tone's)										
hot	1 tsp	8	0	1	25	1	0.4	0.1	0	35%
mild	1 tsp	8	0	1	25	1	0.4	0.1	0	35%

Food Name	Serving Size	Calories	Prot. gms	Carbs gms	Sod. mgs	Fiber gms	Fat gms	Sat. Fat gms	Chol. mgs	% Fat Cal.
CHOP SUEY (Sun Bird) Oriental	1 tbsp	20	0	5	550	0	0.0	0.0	0	0%
CHOW MEIN (Kikkoman)	1 tbsp	20	1	3	570	0	0.0	0.0	0	0%
CREOLE, no MSG (Tony Chachere's)	1/4 tsp	0	0	0	310	0	0.0	0.0	0	0%
CURRY										
(A Taste of Thai)										
panang curry base	1 tbsp	25	0	2	180	0	2.0	1.0	0	69%
red curry base	1 tbsp	20	0	1	430	0	1.5	0.5	0	77%
CURRY POWDER										
	1 tbsp	20	1	4	3	2	0.9	0.1	0	36%
	1 tsp	7	0	1	1	1	0.3	0.0	0	36%
(Tone's)	1 tsp	6	0	1	1000	0	0.3	0.1	0	31%
DILL (Schilling) 'Parsley Patch It's a Dilly'	1 tsp	11	0	2	5	0	0.4	0.0	0	27%
ENCHILADA										
(Lawry's) 'Seasoning Blends'	1 pkg	152	5	30	1723	1	1.2	0.0	0	7%
(Old El Paso)	1/8 pkg	6	0	1	80	0	0.0	0.0	0	0%
FAJITA										
(Crown Colony)	1/2 tsp	5	0	1	95	0	0.0	0.0	0	0%
(Lawry's) 'Seasoning Blends'	1 pkg	63	2	14	2118	1	0.4	0.0	0	5%
FISH (Featherweight)	1/4 pkg	18	1	8	10	0	0.0	0.0	0	0%
FIVE-SPICE (Tone's) Oriental	1 tsp	9	0	2	2	1	0.3	0.1	0	23%
FRENCH FRY (Tone's)	1 tsp	5	0	1	1551	0	0.1	0.1	0	16%
GARLIC										
(Golden Dipt)	2 grams	8	0	1	87	0	0.0	0.0	0	0%
(Lawry's) concentrate	1 tbsp	15	0	0	21	0	1.6	0.0	0	95%
(Schilling)										
'Parsley Patch'	1 tsp	13	1	2	1	0	0.5	0.0	0	31%
'Season All'	1/4 tsp	2	0	0	163	0	0.0	0.0	0	0%
spread	1/2 tbsp	45	0	1	140	0	4.0	1.0	0	90%
GARLIC AND HERB										
(Cook's Classics) spread	1 tbsp	100	1	0	90	0	11.0	na	na	96%
(Mrs. Dash) seasoning	0.13 tsp	2	0	0	0	na	0.0	na	0	5%
(Schilling) spread	1/2 tbsp	45	0	1	125	0	4.5	1.0	0	91%
GARLIC BREAD										
(Gran' Mere's) spread, all-purpose	1 oz	90	0	2	135	0	9.0	1.0	0	91%
(Lawry's) spread	1/2 tbsp	47	0	1	15	0	4.6	0.0	0	90%
(Molly McButter) garlic butter flavored	1/2 tsp	3	0	1	37	0	0.0	na	0	8%
(Schilling) 'Garlic Bread Sprinkle'	1/4 tsp	5	0	0	25	0	0.4	0.0	0	82%
(Tone's) 'Garlic Bread Sprinkle'	1 tsp	17	0	1	167	0	1.6	0.4	1	80%
GARLIC PEPPER (Lawry's)	1/4 tsp	0	0	0	70	0	0.0	0.0	0	0%
GARLIC SALT										
(Good Day)	1/4 tsp	0	0	0	520	0	0.0	0.0	0	0%
(Lawry's)	1/4 tsp	0	0	0	240	0	0.0	0.0	0	0%
(Morton)	1 tsp	3	1	1	1300	0	0.1	0.0	0	10%
(Schilling)	1/4 tsp	0	0	0	490	0	0.0	0.0	0	0%
(Tone's)	1 tsp	2	0	0	1706	0	0.0	0.0	0	0%
GREEK (Cavender's) all purpose	1/4 tsp	0	0	0	241	0	0.0	0.0	0	0%
GUACAMOLE										
(Lawry's) 'Seasoning Blend'	1 pkg	60	2	13	1495	1	0.4	0.0	0	6%
(Old El Paso)	1/7 pkg	7	0	2	240	0	0.0	0.0	0	0%
GUMBO (Tone's) file powder	1 tsp	8	0	2	1	1	0.2	0.1	0	19%
HERB										
(Lawry's) mixed, 'Pinch of Herbs'	1 tsp	9	0	1	259	0	0.5	0.0	0	48%
(Schilling) Italian, 'Bag'n Season'	1 pkg	94	2	21	1367	0	0.2	0.0	0	2%

Food Name	Serving Size	Calories	Prot. gms	Carbs gms	Sod. mgs	Fiber gms	Fat gms	Sat. Fat gms	Chol. mgs	% Fat Cal.
ITALIAN										
(Tone's)	1 tsp	3	0	1	1	0	0.1	0.1	0	22%
(Trader Joe's) salt-free	1/4 tsp	0	0	0	0	0	0.0	0.0	0	0%
LEMON DILL (Schilling) 'Bag'n Season'	1 pkg	161	3	15	2035	0	11.0	0.0	0	58%
LEMON HERB										
(Mrs. Dash)	0.13 tsp	2	0	0	1	na	0.0	na	0	4%
(Schilling) 'Spice Blends'	1/4 tsp	1	0	0	154	0	0.1	0.0	0	43%
LEMON PEPPER										
(Lawry's)										
. . . .	1/4 tsp	<1	0	0	80	0	0.0	0.0	0	0%
'Spice Blends'	1 tsp	6	0	1	340	0	0.1	0.0	0	14%
(Schilling)										
'Parsley Patch'	1 tsp	13	0	1	2	0	0.6	0.0	0	49%
salt-free	1/4 tsp	0	0	0	0	0	0.0	0.0	0	0%
'Spice Blends'	1 tsp	7	0	1	618	0	0.0	0.0	0	0%
(Tone's)										
. . . .	1 tsp	6	0	1	1086	1	0.2	0.1	0	31%
coarse ground, 'Mr. Pepper'	1 tsp	12	0	3	1	0	0.1	0.1	0	7%
fine ground, 'Mr. Pepper'	1 tsp	12	0	3	1	0	0.1	0.1	0	7%
(Trader Joe's) salt-free	1/4 tsp	0	0	0	0	0	0.0	0.0	0	0%
KOTTERIN MIRIN (Kikkoman) sweet	1 tbsp	40	0	10	15	0	0.0	0.0	0	0%
MEAT LOAF										
(Adolph's) 'Meal Makers'	1 tbsp	30	1	7	360	1	0.0	0.0	0	0%
(Bag 'n Season)	2 tsp	15	1	2	390	1	0.0	0.0	0	0%
(French's)	1/8 pkg	20	1	5	620	0	0.0	0.0	0	0%
(Lawry's) 'Seasoning Blends'	1 pkg	355	16	65	6547	2	1.2	0.0	0	3%
(Schilling) 'Bag'n Season'	1 pkg	111	1	26	3090	0	0.7	0.0	1	6%
MEATBALL										
(French's)	1/4 pkg	35	1	7	830	0	0.0	0.0	0	0%
(Schilling) Swedish	1/6 pkg	45	1	4	790	0	1.0	0.0	0	31%
MENUDO (Gebhardt)	1 tsp	4	0	1	182	0	0.2	0.0	0	36%
MESQUITE (Tone's)	1 tsp	13	0	3	467	0	0.1	0.0	0	6%
MEXICAN (Tone's)	1 tsp	6	0	1	4185	0	0.1	0.1	0	12%
NACHO (Lawry's) 'Seasoning Blends'	1 pkg	141	7	15	2168	2	6.8	0.0	0	41%
ORIENTAL (Schilling) 'Bag'n Season'	1 pkg	152	5	31	1912	0	8.0	0.0	0	33%
PAD THAI (Kikkoman)	2 tsp	20	0	4	430	0	0.0	0.0	0	0%
PARSLEY (Schilling) all purpose 'Parsley Patch'	1 tsp	6	0	1	3	0	0.0	0.0	0	0%
PASTA										
(Tone's) spaghetti	1 tsp	11	0	3	469	0	0.1	0.0	0	8%
(Trader Joe's) salt-free	1/4 tsp	0	0	0	0	0	0.0	0.0	0	0%
PEPPER										
(Lawry's)	1/4 tsp	0	0	1	0	na	0.0	0.0	0	0%
(Schilling) seasoned, 'All Pepper'	1/4 tsp	1	0	0	106	0	0.0	0.0	0	0%
PEPPER DILL (Golden Dipt)	2 grams	8	0	1	96	0	0.0	0.0	0	0%
PICKLING SPICE (Tone's)	1 tsp	10	0	1	1	0	0.6	0.1	0	47%
POPCORN										
(Tone's)	1 tsp	0	0	0	2455	0	0.0	0.0	0	0%
(McCormick/Schilling) 'Parsley Patch'	1 tsp	10	1	3	4	0	0.1	0.0	0	6%
PORK										
(Bag 'n Season)										
chop	2 tsp	15	0	4	590	na	0.0	0.0	0	0%
spare rib	1 tbsp	30	1	6	590	1	0.0	0.0	0	0%
(Schilling)										
chop, 'Bag'n Season'	1 pkg	103	1	24	3126	0	0.4	0.0	0	4%

Food Name	Serving Size	Calories	Prot. gms	Carbs gms	Sod. mgs	Fiber gms	Fat gms	Sat. Fat gms	Chol. mgs	% Fat Cal.
spare rib, 'Bag'n Season'	1 pkg	185	0	42	3690	0	1.5	0.0	2	7%
POTATO										
(Perfect Potatoes) herb and garlic	1/6 pkt	20	0	5	370	0	0.0	0.0	0	0%
(Potato Shakers)										
cheddar, zesty	8 grams	30	1	5	500	0	1.0	0.0	0	27%
Parmesan and herb	8 grams	25	1	5	740	0	0.5	0.0	0	16%
(Shake 'N Bake) herb and garlic	1/8 pkt	20	0	5	370	0	0.0	0.0	0	0%
POTATO SALAD (Tone's)	1 tsp	5	0	0	1498	0	0.2	0.1	0	47%
PROTEIN (Bragg) liquid aminos	1/2 tsp	2	0.265	0	121	0	0.0	0.0	0	0%
PUMPKIN PIE										
	1 tbsp	19	0	4	3	1	0.7	0.4	0	31%
	1 tsp	6	0	1	1	0	0.2	0.1	0	31%
RICE										
(Kikkoman) fried	1 1/3 tbsp	30	1	6	490	0	0.0	0.0	0	0%
(Lawry's) Mexican, 'Seasoning Blends'	1 pkg	94	4	17	3246	2	2.0	0.0	0	18%
(McCormick/Schilling) fried, w/chicken	1 tbsp	35	1	6	780	1	0.0	0.0	0	0%
(Sun Bird) fried	1/2 tbsp	12	0	3	380	0	0.0	0.0	0	0%
SALAD										
(Lawry's) taco, 'Seasoning Blends'	1 pkg	124	4	25	1451	2	0.9	0.0	0	7%
(Schilling) 'Salad Supreme'	1 tsp	11	1	1	2807	0	0.1	0.0	0	16%
SALT										
(Estee) 'Seasoned Salt-It'	1/8 tsp	0	0	0	0	0	0.0	0.0	0	0%
(Good Day)	1/4 tsp	0	0	0	400	0	0.0	0.0	0	0%
(Lawry's)										
	1/4 tsp	0	0	0	380	0	0.0	0.0	0	0%
'Hot n' Spicy'	1 tsp	3	0	2	79	0	0.1	0.0	0	12%
no MSG	1/4 tsp	0	0	0	380	0	0.0	0.0	0	0%
(Morton) seasoned	1 tsp	4	1	1	1300	0	0.1	0.0	0	10%
(Schilling)										
'California style'	1/4 tsp	0	0	0	250	0	0.0	0.0	0	0%
no MSG, 'Home Style'	1/4 tsp	0	0	0	370	0	0.0	0.0	0	0%
no MSG, 'Season All'	1/4 tsp	0	0	0	340	0	0.0	0.0	0	0%
SAUSAGE (Tone's) pork	1 tsp	12	0	3	1	1	0.3	0.2	0	18%
SEAFOOD										
(Golden Dipt)										
all purpose	1/4 tsp	2	0	0	85	0	0.0	0.0	0	0%
blackened redfish	1/4 tsp	2	0	0	140	0	0.0	0.0	0	0%
broiled fish	1/4 tsp	2	0	0	125	0	0.0	0.0	0	0%
lemon pepper	1/4 tsp	8	1	1	115	0	0.0	0.0	0	0%
shrimp and crab, Cajun style	1/4 tsp	2	0	0	200	0	0.0	0.0	0	0%
(Old Bay) seafood, poultry, meat seasoning	1/2 tsp	0	0	0	330	0	0.0	0.0	0	0%
(Schilling) Chesapeake Bay	1/2 tsp	2	0	0	202	0	0.1	0.0	0	43%
(Tone's)										
	1 tsp	10	1	1	1	0	0.7	0.1	0	53%
Chesapeake	1 tsp	8	0	1	1032	0	0.3	0.1	0	34%
SESAME										
(Eden Foods)										
garlic, shake, organic	1/2 tsp	10	0	0	35	1	1.5	0.0	0	100%
shake, organic	1/2 tsp	10	0	0	40	1	0.5	0.0	0	100%
seaweed, shake, organic	1/2 tsp	10	0	0	35	1	0.5	0.0	0	100%
(Maranatha Natural) sesame salt	7 grams	200	7	7	460	0	16.0	0.0	0	72%
(Schilling) all-purpose, 'Parsley Patch'	1 tsp	15	1	1	2	0	1.0	0.0	0	58%
SLOPPY JOE (Lawry's) 'Seasoning Blends'	1 pkg	126	3	28	3442	1	0.4	0.0	0	3%
SOUR CREAM FLAVORED (Molly McButter)	1/2 tsp	4	0	1	65	0	0.1	na	0	13%

Food Name	Serving Size	Calories	Prot. gms	Carbs gms	Sod. mgs	Fiber gms	Fat gms	Sat. Fat gms	Chol. mgs	% Fat Cal.
STIR-FRY										
(Adolph's) teriyaki flavor, 'Meal Makers'	1 tbsp	30	1	7	1170	0	0.0	0.0	0	0%
(Gilroy)	1 tsp	6	0	1	5	0	0.0	0.0	0	0%
(Kikkoman)										
. . . .	1 tbsp	30	1	6	680	0	0.0	0.0	0	0%
shrimp, Szechwan	1-1/3 tbsp	30	1	5	640	0	0.5	0.0	0	17%
tomato-beef	2 tsp	20	0	4	400	0	0.0	0.0	0	0%
(McCormick/Schilling)	2 tsp	20	1	3	490	0	0.0	0.0	0	0%
(Sun Bird) Oriental	1/2 tbsp	15	0	3	310	0	0.0	0.0	0	0%
TACO										
(Hain)	1/10 pkg	10	1	2	200	0	0.0	0.0	0	0%
(Lawry's) 'Seasoning Blends'	1 pkg	118	3	24	1441	1	1.1	0.0	0	8%
(McCormick/Schilling) mild	2 tsp	20	1	4	460	1	0.0	0.0	0	0%
(Nabisco) mild, mix for one taco	1 serving	90	2	18	999	0	1.0	0.0	0	10%
(Old El Paso)										
. . . .	2 tsp	20	0	5	550	0	0.0	0.0	0	0%
40% less sodium	2 tsp	20	0	4	330	0	0.0	0.0	0	0%
(Ortega) meat	1 oz	90	2	18	1970	0	1.0	0.0	0	10%
(Pancho Villa)	2 tsp	20	0	5	550	0	0.0	0.0	0	0%
(Schilling)	1/4 pkg	31	1	6	675	0	0.5	0.0	0	14%
(Tio Sancho)										
. . . .	1.25 oz	104	2	21	2500	2	1.4	0.0	0	12%
'Dinner Kit'	1.51 oz	132	3	26	2623	2	1.7	0.0	0	12%
TURKEY *(Schilling)* roast, 'Bag'n Season'	1 pkg	146	6	20	1935	0	5.0	0.0	0	30%
TERIYAKI *(Golden Dipt)* ginger	1 oz	120	1	12	920	0	7.0	0.0	0	55%
SEAWEED. See SEA VEGETABLE.										
SEITAN										
Philly steak slices, vegetarian *(White Wave)*	3 slices	60	14	2	105	0	0.0	0.0	0	0%
traditional, vegetarian *(White Wave)*	1 piece	140	31	4	240	1	0.0	0.0	0	0%
turkey style, vegetarian, sandwich sliced *(White Wave)* . . .	1 slice	80	13	7	400	1	0.0	0.0	0	0%
SEITAN MIX										
quick, flavored *(Arrowhead Mills)* mix only	1/3 cup	150	21	14	20	2	1.0	0.0	0	6%
SELTZER. See under SOFT DRINKS AND MIXERS.										
SEMOLINA										
enriched	1 cup	601	21	122	2	7	1.8	0.3	0	2%
unenriched	1 cup	601	21	122	2	7	1.8	0.3	0	2%
whole grain	1 cup	602	21.2	121.6	2	6.5	1.8	0.3	0	3%
whole grain	1 oz	102	3.6	20.6	<1	1.1	0.3	<.1	0	3%
SERRANO PEPPER. See PEPPER, SERRANO.										
SESAME BUTTER / tahini. See also TAHINI MIX.										
. . . .	1 tbsp	95	3	4	2	1	8.1	1.1	0	72%
made from raw and stone ground kernels	1 oz	162	5	7	21	3	13.6	1.9	0	70%
made from raw and stone ground kernels	1 tbsp	86	3	4	11	1	7.2	1.0	0	70%
made from roasted and toasted kernels	1 oz	169	5	6	33	3	15.2	2.1	0	76%
made from roasted and toasted kernels	1 tbsp	89	3	3	17	1	8.1	1.1	0	76%
made from unroasted kernels, hulls removed	1 oz	172	5	5	0	3	16.0	2.2	0	78%
made from unroasted kernels, hulls removed	1 tbsp	85	3	3	0	1	7.9	1.1	0	78%
(Arrowhead Mills) organic	1 oz	170	6	4	5	0	17.0	0.0	0	79%
(Erewhon) 'Sesame Tahini'	2 tbsp	200	6	3	65	0	18.0	0.0	0	82%
(Maranatha Natural)										
raw, 'Sesame Tahini'	2 tbsp	210	8	3	5	0	19.0	0.0	0	80%
roasted, 'Sesame Tahini'	2 tbsp	210	8	3	20	0	19.0	0.0	0	80%
(Roaster Fresh)										
gourmet	1 oz	168	5	6	3	0	15.0	2.2	0	75%

Food Name	Serving Size	Calories	Prot. gms	Carbs gms	Sod. mgs	Fiber gms	Fat gms	Sat. Fat gms	Chol. mgs	% Fat Cal.
roasted, w/o salt, creamy	1 oz	168	5	6	3	0	15.0	2.0	0	75%
(Westbrae)										
Mid-Eastern, organic, no salt added	2 tbsp	220	9	3	0	0	20.0	0.0	0	79%
organic, 'Natural'	2 tbsp	220	6	6	35	0	19.0	0.0	0	78%
original, no salt added	2 tbsp	210	8	1	0	na	19.0	na	0	83%
raw, organic	2 tbsp	210	8	1	0	0	19.0	0.0	0	83%
toasted, organic, no salt added	2 tbsp	220	8	3	0	0	19.0	0.0	0	80%
SESAME MEAL, partially defatted	1 oz	161	5	7	11	na	13.6	1.9	0	71%
SESAME OIL										
	1 cup	1927	0	0	0	0	218.0	31.0	0	100%
	1 tbsp	120	0	0	0	0	13.6	1.9	0	100%
(Hain)	1 tbsp	120	0	0	0	0	14.0	2.0	0	100%
100% pure *(Dynasty)*	1 tbsp	130	0	0	0	0	14.0	2.0	0	100%
100% pure, extra virgin *(Loriva')*	1 tbsp	120	0	0	0	0	14.0	0.0	0	100%
hot pepper *(Eden Foods)*	1 tbsp	120	0	0	0	0	14.0	2.0	0	100%
pure pressed, organic *(Spectrum)*	1 tbsp	120	0	0	0	0	14.0	2.0	0	100%
toasted *(Eden Foods)*	1 tbsp	130	0	0	0	0	14.0	2.0	0	100%
toasted *(International Collection)*	1 tbsp	120	0	0	0	0	14.0	2.0	0	100%
toasted, pure pressed, organic *(Spectrum)*	1 tbsp	120	0	0	0	0	14.0	2.0	0	100%
unrefined *(Eden Foods)*	1 tbsp	120	0	0	0	0	14.0	2.0	0	100%
SESAME SEED / sim sim										
Dried										
hulled	1 cup	882	40	14	60	17	82.2	11.5	0	78%
hulled	1 tbsp	47	2	1	3	1	4.4	0.6	0	78%
hulled	1 tsp	16	1	0	1	0	1.5	0.2	0	78%
hulled *(Arrowhead Mills)*	1 oz	160	6	4	3	4	14.0	0.0	0	76%
whole	1 cup	825	26	34	16	17	71.5	10.0	0	73%
whole	1 tbsp	52	2	2	1	1	4.5	0.6	0	73%
whole *(Arrowhead Mills)*	1 oz	160	5	6	4	3	14.0	0.0	0	74%
Raw										
(McCormick/Schilling)	1 tsp	21	1	0	7	0	1.6	0.0	0	75%
hulled, natural, unsalted *(Flanigan Farms)*	1/4 cup	160	5	7	0	3	14.0	2.0	0	72%
whole *(Durkee)*	1 tsp	13	0	0	0	0	0.0	0.0	0	0%
whole *(Laurel Leaf)*	1 tsp	13	0	0	0	0	0.0	0.0	0	0%
whole *(Spice Islands)*	1 tsp	9	1	1	1	1	0.4	0.0	0	39%
Roasted and toasted, whole	1 oz	160	5	7	3	4	13.6	1.9	0	71%
Toasted										
hulled, salted	1 cup	726	22	33	753	22	61.4	8.6	0	71%
hulled, salted	1 oz	161	5	7	167	5	13.6	1.9	0	71%
hulled, unsalted	1 cup	726	22	33	50	22	61.4	8.6	0	71%
hulled, unsalted	1 oz	161	5	7	11	5	13.6	1.9	0	71%
SESAME STICKS										
wheat-based, unsalted	1 oz	153	3	13	8	na	10.4	1.8	0	59%
wheat-based, unsalted	2 oz	307	6	26	16	na	20.8	3.7	0	59%
wheat-based, unsalted	1 oz	153	3	13	422	1	10.4	1.8	0	59%
wheat-based, unsalted	2 oz	307	6	26	844	2	20.8	3.7	0	59%
SESBANIA FLOWER. See KATURAY.										
SHAD, AMERICAN										
baked, broiled, grilled, or microwaved	3 oz	214	18	0	55	0	15.0	na	82	63%
raw	3 oz	167	14	0	43	0	11.7	2.7	64	63%
SHALLOT										
Freeze-dried										
chopped	1/4 cup	13	0	3	2	na	0.0	0.0	0	1%
chopped	1 tbsp	3	0	1	1	na	0.0	0.0	0	1%

Food Name	Serving Size	Calories	Prot. gms	Carbs gms	Sod. mgs	Fiber gms	Fat gms	Sat. Fat gms	Chol. mgs	% Fat Cal.
chopped *(McCormick/Schilling)*	1 tsp	2	0	0	0	0	0.0	0.0	0	0%
Fresh										
raw	3.5 oz	72	2.5	16.8	12	>.7 c	0.1	0.0	0	1%
raw, chopped	1 tbsp	7	0	2	1	na	0.0	0.0	0	1%
raw, trimmed	1 oz	20	0.7	4.8	3	>.2 c	<.1	tr	0	<4%
raw, untrimmed	1 lb	287	10.0	67.1	48	>2.8 c	0.4	0.1	0	1%
SHARK										
MAKO, frozen, steak, boneless, raw *(Peter Pan Seafoods)*	3.5 oz	87	19	0	79	0	1.2	0.0	51	12%
MIXED SPECIES, fresh										
batter dipped, fried	3 oz	194	16	5	104	0	11.7	2.7	50	55%
raw	3 oz	110	17.8	0.0	67	0	3.8	0.8	43	32%
SHEA NUT OIL										
	1 cup	1927	0	0	0	0	218.0	101.6	0	98%
	1 tbsp	120	0	0	0	0	13.6	6.3	0	98%
SHEEPSHEAD / fathead										
baked, broiled, grilled, or microwaved	3 oz	107	22	0	62	0	1.4	0.3	54	12%
raw	3 oz	92	17	0	60	0	2.0	0.5	43	20%
SHELLIE BEAN. See BEAN, SHELLY.										
SHELLY BEAN. See BEAN, SHELLY.										
SHERBET. See also FRUIT BAR, FROZEN; ICE BAR/DESSERT; SHERBET BAR, FROZEN; SORBET.										
(Borden) orange	1/2 cup	110	1	25	40	0	1.0	0.0	0	8%
(Darigold) orange	1/2 cup	120	1	26	25	0	1.0	0.0	0	8%
(Dreyers)										
strawberry kiwi	1/2 cup	120	1	27	30	na	1.0	0.5	5	7%
Swiss orange	1/2 cup	150	1	30	45	na	2.5	2.0	5	15%
(Edys)										
strawberry kiwi	1/2 cup	120	1	27	30	na	1.0	0.5	5	7%
Swiss orange	1/2 cup	150	1	30	45	na	2.5	2.0	5	15%
(Sealtest) all flavors	1/2 cup	130	1	28	30	0	1.0	0.0	5	7%
SHERBET BAR, FROZEN										
(Creamsicle) all flavors, w/cream, sugar-free	1 bar	25	1	5	20	0	1.0	0.0	0	27%
(Fudgsicle)										
all flavors, fat-free	1 bar	70	2	14	45	0	0.0	0.0	0	0%
all flavors, sugar-free	1 bar	35	2	6	50	0	1.0	0.0	5	22%
chocolate	1 bar	70	2	12	70	0	1.0	0.0	0	14%
chocolate, w/nuts, no sugar, 'Fudge Nut Dip'	1 bar	130	2	12	40	0	8.0	0.0	5	56%
SHERRY										
(Gallo)										
	2 fl oz	64	0	2	0	0	0.0	0.0	0	0%
cream, 'Livingston Cellars'	2 fl oz	78	0	6	0	0	0.0	0.0	0	0%
very dry, 'Livingston Cellars'	2 fl oz	60	0	1	0	0	0.0	0.0	0	0%
(Italian Swiss Colony)										
cream	2 fl oz	85	0	7	4	0	0.0	0.0	0	0%
dry	2 fl oz	63	0	1	4	0	0.0	0.0	0	0%
straight	2 fl oz	67	0	2	4	0	0.0	0.0	0	0%
SHIITAKE. See MUSHROOM, SHIITAKE.										
SHIMEJI. See MUSHROOM, OYSTER.										
SHORTENING										
For baking										
hydrogenated soybean oil w/ palm and cottonseed oils	1 cup	1812	0	0	0	0	205.0	59.1	0	100%
hydrogenated soybean oil w/ palm and cottonseed oils	1 tbsp	113	0	0	0	0	12.8	3.7	0	100%
For bread										
hydrogenated soybean oil w/cottonseed oil	1 cup	1812	0	0	0	0	205.0	45.1	0	100%
hydrogenated soybean oil w/cottonseed oil	1 tbsp	113	0	0	0	0	12.8	2.8	0	100%

Food Name	Serving Size	Calories	Prot. gms	Carbs gms	Sod. mgs	Fiber gms	Fat gms	Sat. Fat gms	Chol. mgs	% Fat Cal.
For cake and frosting										
hydrogenated soybean oil	1 cup	1812	0	0	0	0	205.0	41.0	0	100%
hydrogenated soybean oil	1 tbsp	113	0	0	0	0	12.8	2.6	0	100%
For cake mix										
hydrogenated soybean and cottonseed oils	1 cup	1812	0	0	0	0	205.0	55.8	0	100%
hydrogenated soybean and cottonseed oils	1 tbsp	113	0	0	0	0	12.8	3.5	0	100%
For confectionery										
fractionated palm oil	1 cup	1927	0	0	0	0	218.0	142.8	0	98%
fractionated palm oil	1 tbsp	120	0	0	0	0	13.6	8.9	0	98%
hydrogenated coconut and/or palm kernel oil	1 cup	1812	0	0	0	0	205.0	187.2	0	100%
hydrogenated coconut and/or palm kernel oil	1 tbsp	113	0	0	0	0	12.8	11.7	0	100%
For frying										
heavy-duty, beef tallow and cottonseed oil	1 cup	1845	0	0	0	0	205.0	92.0	205	100%
heavy-duty, beef tallow and cottonseed oil	1 tbsp	115	0	0	0	0	12.8	5.7	13	100%
heavy-duty, hydrogenated palm oil	1 cup	1812	0	0	0	0	205.0	97.4	0	100%
heavy-duty, hydrogenated palm oil	1 tbsp	113	0	0	0	0	12.8	6.1	0	100%
heavy-duty, hydrogenated soybean (under 1% linoleic)	1 cup	1812	0	0	0	0	205.0	43.3	0	100%
heavy-duty, hydrogenated soybean (under 1% linoleic)	1 tbsp	113	0	0	0	0	12.8	2.7	0	100%
heavy-duty, hydrogenated soybean (30% linoleic), w/stabilizers	1 cup	1812	0	0	0	0	205.0	37.7	0	100%
heavy-duty, hydrogenated soybean (30% linoleic), w/stabilizers	1 tbsp	113	0	0	0	0	12.8	2.4	0	100%
hydrogenated soybean and cottonseed oils	1 cup	1812	0	0	0	0	205.0	31.6	0	100%
hydrogenated soybean and cottonseed oils	1 tbsp	113	0	0	0	0	12.8	2.0	0	100%
Household										
hydrogenated soybean and cottonseed oils	1 cup	1812	0	0	0	0	205.0	51.3	0	100%
hydrogenated soybean and cottonseed oils	1 tbsp	113	0	0	0	0	12.8	3.2	0	100%
hydrogenated soybean oil w/ palm oil	1 cup	1812	0	0	0	0	205.0	51.3	0	100%
hydrogenated soybean oil w/ palm oil	1 tbsp	113	0	0	0	0	12.8	3.2	0	100%
lard and vegetable oil	1 cup	1845	0	0	0	0	205.0	82.6	115	100%
lard and vegetable oil	1 tbsp	115	0	0	0	0	12.8	5.2	7	100%
(Crisco)										
vegetable oil	1 tbsp	110	0	0	0	0	12.0	3.0	0	100%
(Finast)										
vegetable oil	1 tbsp	110	0	0	0	0	13.0	0.0	0	100%
vegetable oil, butter flavor	1 tbsp	110	0	0	0	0	12.0	3.0	0	100%
(Wesson) vegetable oil	1 tbsp	109	0	0	0	0	12.1	2.7	0	100%
Industrial										
hydrogenated soybean oil w/cottonseed oil	1 cup	1812	0	0	0	0	205.0	52.5	0	100%
hydrogenated soybean oil w/cottonseed oil	1 tbsp	113	0	0	0	0	12.8	3.3	0	100%
lard and vegetable oil	1 cup	1845	0	0	0	0	205.0	73.2	115	100%
lard and vegetable oil	1 tbsp	115	0	0	0	0	12.8	4.6	7	100%
(Wesson)										
'Crystal'	1 tbsp	122	0	0	0	0	13.5	2.0	0	100%
low-melt	1 tbsp	122	0	0	0	0	13.5	3.8	0	100%
'Super'	1 tbsp	122	0	0	0	0	13.5	3.6	0	100%
'Wesgold'	1 tbsp	122	0	0	0	0	13.5	2.6	0	100%
'Wespour'	1 tbsp	122	0	0	0	0	13.5	2.5	0	100%
Multipurpose										
hydrogenated soybean and palm oils	1 cup	1812	0	0	0	0	205.0	62.4	0	100%
hydrogenated soybean and palm oils	1 tbsp	113	0	0	0	0	12.8	3.9	0	100%
(Quest)										
'Cirol'	1 oz	256	0	2	0	na	28.4	5.4	0	97%

Food Name	Serving Size	Calories	Prot. gms	Carbs gms	Sod. mgs	Fiber gms	Fat gms	Sat. Fat gms	Chol. mgs	% Fat Cal.
'Durola Select'	1 oz	256	0	0	0	0	28.4	2.6	0	100%
'Duromel'	1 oz	256	0	0	0	0	28.4	8.2	0	100%

SHOYU. See under SAUCE.

SHRIMP. See also SHRIMP DISH/ENTRÉE.

Canned

Food Name	Serving Size	Calories	Prot. gms	Carbs gms	Sod. mgs	Fiber gms	Fat gms	Sat. Fat gms	Chol. mgs	% Fat Cal.
medium, deveined, in water and salt (S&W)	1/4 cup	45	10	0	650	0	0.0	0.0	115	0%
mixed species	1 cup	154	30	1	216	0	2.5	0.5	221	15%
mixed species	10 medium	38	7	0	54	0	0.6	0.1	55	15%
mixed species	3 oz	102	20	1	144	0	1.7	0.3	147	15%
mixed species, cooked	1 oz	34	7	0	48	0	0.6	0.1	49	15%
mixed species, drained (Louisiana Brand)	2 oz	58	12	0	0	0	1.0	0.0	0	16%
mixed species, large, drained (ShopRite)	2 oz	50	10	0	720	0	1.0	0.0	0	18%
peeled, broken (Crown Prince)	1/2 can	60	13	1	360	0	0.5	0.0	145	7%
small, deveined, in water and salt (S&W)	1/4 cup	45	10	0	650	0	0.0	0.0	115	0%
tiny, peeled (Crown Prince)	1/2 can	60	13	1	360	0	0.5	0.0	145	7%

Fresh

Food Name	Serving Size	Calories	Prot. gms	Carbs gms	Sod. mgs	Fiber gms	Fat gms	Sat. Fat gms	Chol. mgs	% Fat Cal.
mixed species, boiled, poached, or steamed	3 oz	84	18	0	190	0	0.9	0.2	166	10%
mixed species, large, boiled, poached, or steamed	4 shrimp	22	5	0	49	0	0.2	0.1	43	10%
mixed species, raw	3 oz	90	17	1	126	0	1.5	0.3	129	15%
mixed species, raw, large	4 shrimp	30	6	0	41	0	0.5	0.1	43	15%
mixed species, raw, medium	1 shrimp	6	1	0	9	0	0.1	0.0	9	15%
mixed species, raw, small	1 shrimp	5	1	0	7	0	0.1	0.0	8	15%

Frozen

Food Name	Serving Size	Calories	Prot. gms	Carbs gms	Sod. mgs	Fiber gms	Fat gms	Sat. Fat gms	Chol. mgs	% Fat Cal.
butterfly, 'Specialty' (Gorton's)	4 oz	160	19	16	540	0	1.0	0.0	0	6%
cooked, peeled, deveined, tail off, 250/300 count (Contessa)	3 oz	40	10	0	420	0	0.0	0.0	95	0%
w/tails (Harvest Of The Sea)	3 oz	70	17	0	280	0	0.0	0.0	0	0%

SHRIMP COCKTAIL. See under SHRIMP DISH/ENTRÉE.

SHRIMP DISH/ENTRÉE

(Armour)

Food Name	Serving Size	Calories	Prot. gms	Carbs gms	Sod. mgs	Fiber gms	Fat gms	Sat. Fat gms	Chol. mgs	% Fat Cal.
baby bay, frozen, 'Classics Lite'	9.75 oz	220	12	31	890	0	6.0	0.0	105	24%
Creole, frozen, 'Classics Lite'	11.25 oz	260	6	53	900	0	2.0	0.0	45	7%

(Booth)

Food Name	Serving Size	Calories	Prot. gms	Carbs gms	Sod. mgs	Fiber gms	Fat gms	Sat. Fat gms	Chol. mgs	% Fat Cal.
Alfredo, w/fettucini, frozen	10 oz	260	19	28	620	0	8.0	0.0	0	28%
cocktail, w/garlic butter sauce and vegetable rice	10 oz	400	13	40	750	(mq)	25.0	(mq)	(mq)	52%
New Orleans, w/wild rice, frozen	10 oz	230	13	35	950	0	5.0	0.0	0	19%
Oriental, w/pineapple rice, frozen	10 oz	190	11	30	950	0	3.0	0.0	0	14%
primavera, w/fettuccini, frozen	10 oz	200	16	28	760	0	3.0	0.0	0	13%
w/garlic butter sauce and vegetable rice, frozen	10 oz	400	13	40	750	0	25.0	0.0	0	51%

(Budget Gourmet)

Food Name	Serving Size	Calories	Prot. gms	Carbs gms	Sod. mgs	Fiber gms	Fat gms	Sat. Fat gms	Chol. mgs	% Fat Cal.
cocktail, w/fettuccine, frozen	9.5 oz	375	10	38	660	(mq)	20.0	(mq)	145	48%
mariner, frozen, 'Light & Healthy'	1 dinner	230	11	40	550	0	6.0	2.0	55	21%

(Cajun Cookin')

Food Name	Serving Size	Calories	Prot. gms	Carbs gms	Sod. mgs	Fiber gms	Fat gms	Sat. Fat gms	Chol. mgs	% Fat Cal.
Creole, frozen	12 oz	390	17	55	1130	0	11.0	0.0	0	26%
etouffée, frozen	17 oz	360	19	52	1170	0	9.0	0.0	0	22%
jambalaya, frozen	12 oz	450	20	43	800	0	20.0	0.0	0	42%

(Gorton's)

Food Name	Serving Size	Calories	Prot. gms	Carbs gms	Sod. mgs	Fiber gms	Fat gms	Sat. Fat gms	Chol. mgs	% Fat Cal.
breaded, w/original seasoning	6 shrimp	229	10	18	549	1	13.0	2.5	80	51%
crisps, frozen, 'Specialty'	4 oz	280	9	26	740	0	15.0	0.0	0	49%
crunchy, frozen, microwave, 'Crunchy Shrimp'	1/2 pkg	160	7	12	380	0	9.0	0.0	40	52%
crunchy, whole, frozen, 'Microwave Specialty'	5 oz	380	14	35	870	0	20.0	3.0	65	48%
popcorn	1 cup	260	9	21	600	1	16.0	3.0	60	55%
scampi, baked	6 shrimp	250	9	18	409	1	16.0	3.0	70	57%

Food Name	Serving Size	Calories	Prot. gms	Carbs gms	Sod. mgs	Fiber gms	Fat gms	Sat. Fat gms	Chol. mgs	% Fat Cal.
scampi, frozen, 'Microwave Entrees'	1 pkg	390	10	21	470	0	30.0	0.0	0	69%
(Healthy Choice)										
Creole, frozen	11.25 oz	210	8	42	560	0	1.0	1.0	65	4%
marinara	1 entree	250	10	44	360	5	4.0	2.0	55	14%
w/vegetables	1 entree	270	15	39	580	6	6.0	3.0	50	20%
(Hudson) stir-fry, complete meal kit, frozen	1 3/4 cup	210	15	35	990	3	2.0	0.0	83	8%
(LaChoy)										
chow mein	1 cup	53	3	10	948	2	0.9	0.3	9	13%
chow mein, canned	3/4 cup	35	4	4	940	2	1.0	0.3	50	22%
cocktail, w/lobster sauce, 'Fresh & Lite'	10 oz	240	12	36.4	946	2.8	6.2	(mq)	118	22%
(Longacre)										
salad, 'Saladfest'	1 oz	45	2.0	2.0	150	na	3.0	(mq)	25	63%
salad, w/seafood, 'Saladfest'	1 oz	42	2.0	2.0	160	na	3.0	(mq)	15	63%
(Marie Callender's) over angel hair pasta, frozen	1 cup	300	11	37	470	3	12.0	2.0	30	36%
(Mrs. Paul's)										
breaded, fried, frozen	3 oz	200	9	16	430	0	11.0	0.0	0	50%
Cajun style, frozen, 'Light'	9 oz	230	9	37	740	0	5.0	1.0	60	20%
cocktail, w/clams and linguini, 'Light'	10 oz	240	12	36	750	(mq)	5.0	2.0	40	19%
primavera, frozen 'Light'	9.5 oz	180	11	28	840	0	3.0	1.0	125	15%
(Right Course) primavera, frozen	9 5/8 oz	240	12	32	590	0	7.0	1.0	50	26%
(Sau-Sea) cocktail	4 oz	113	7	19	1020	na	1.0	(mq)	102	8%
(SeaPak)										
battered, frozen, 'Shrimp 'n Batter'	4 oz	260	11	20	470	0	15.0	0.0	20	52%
breaded, butterfly, frozen, 'Mikado'	4 oz	160	12	26	170	0	1.0	0.0	110	6%
breaded, butterfly/round, frozen	4 oz	150	14	20	0	0	1.0	0.0	0	6%
cocktail, 'Super Valu' heat and serve	4 oz	210	12	30	730	(mq)	4.0	(mq)	80	18%
w/crab meat stuffing, battered, frozen	4 oz	260	8	27	780	0	13.0	0.0	0	46%
(Shanghai) stir-fry, frozen	10.3 oz	170	18	19	1200	0	2.0	0.0	55	11%
(Smart Ones)										
marinara	1 entrée	200	8	37	590	4	2.0	0.0	40	9%
marinara, w/linguini, frozen	8 oz	150	8	26	390	0	1.0	1.0	60	6%
(Ultra Slim Fast)										
Creole, frozen	12 oz	240	12	45	730	0	4.0	0.0	80	14%
marinara, frozen	12 oz	290	17	53	880	0	3.0	0.0	70	9%
SHRIMP PASTE, canned	1 tsp	13	1.5	0.1	10	0	0.7	0.4	12	50%
SHRIMP SALAD. See under SHRIMP DISH/ENTRÉE.										
SHRIMP SUBSTITUTE, made from surimi	3 oz	86	11	8	599	0	1.3	0.2	31	13%
SICAMA. See JICAMA										
SILVER HAKE. See WHITING.										
SILVER SALMON. See under SALMON.										
SIM SIM. See SESAME SEED.										
SISYMBRIUM SEED										
dried, whole	1 cup	235	9	43	68	na	3.4	0.7	0	12%
dried, whole	1 oz	90	3	17	26	na	1.3	0.3	0	12%
SKIL. See COD, ALASKAN.										
SKIPJACK. See under TUNA.										
SKUNK CABBAGE. See CABBAGE, SKUNK.										
SLIMEHEAD. See ORANGE ROUGHY.										
SLOPPY JOE MIX. See under SANDWICH FILLING MIX.										
SLOPPY JOE SEASONING. See under SEASONING MIX.										
SMELT, RAINBOW										
baked, broiled, grilled, or microwaved	3 oz	105	19	0	65	0	2.6	0.5	77	23%
raw	3 oz	82	15	0	51	0	2.1	0.4	60	23%

Food Name	Serving Size	Calories	Prot. gms	Carbs gms	Sod. mgs	Fiber gms	Fat gms	Sat. Fat gms	Chol. mgs	% Fat Cal.
SNACK BAR. See also BREAKFAST BAR; CAKE, SNACK; FRUIT BAR; GRANOLA/CEREAL BAR; SPORTS AND DIET/NUTRITION BARS.										
(Barbara's Bakery)										
apple-filled, whole grain, organic.....................	1.3 oz bar	120	1	29	55	2	0.0	0.0	0	0%
blueberry-filled, whole grain, organic	1.3 oz bar	120	1	29	55	2	0.0	0.0	0	0%
raspberry-filled, whole grain, organic, nonfat	1 bar	110	1	28	26	2	0.0	0.0	0	0%
strawberry-filled, whole grain, organic, nonfat..........	1.3 oz bar	120	1	29	55	2	0.0	0.0	0	0%
(Bear Valley)										
carob cocoa, food bar, 'Pemmican'	3.75 oz	440	16	68	80	7	12.0	0.0	0	24%
coconut almond, food bar, 'Meal Pack'	3.75 oz	400	13	56	80	6	12.0	0.0	0	28%
fruit and nut, food bar, 'Pemmican'	3.75 oz	420	17	59	90	9	13.0	0.0	0	28%
sesame lemon, food bar, 'Meal Pack'	3.75 oz	410	17	57	85	4	13.0	0.0	0	28%
(Clif)										
chocolate chip, '100% Natural Endurance'	2.4 oz	250	4	51	45	3	3.0	0.5	0	11%
dark chocolate, '100% Natural Endurance'	2.4 oz	250	5	52	20	2	2.0	0.5	0	7%
(Earth Grains)										
banana apple walnut, 'Bagel Power Bar'.............	1 bar	270	12	45	280	0	6.0	0.0	0	19%
citrus almond, w/mixed fruit 'Bagel Power Bar'	1 bar	260	12	45	280	0	4.0	0.0	0	14%
fruit and nut, 'Bagel Power Bar'	1 bar	240	9	48	280	0	3.0	0.0	0	11%
(Edgebar) chocolate crunch.................	1 bar	234	11	46	95	0	2.0	1.0	5	7%
(Fruit Boosters)										
apple, low-fat.............................	1 bar	130	1	27	0	1	2.0	0.0	0	14%
blueberry, low-fat...........................	1 bar	130	1	27	0	1	2.0	0.0	0	14%
(General Mills) date	1/32 pkg	60	1	9	35	0	2.0	0.0	0	31%
(Glenny's)										
apple-cinnamon............................	1.25 oz	120	1	28	15	0	1.0	0.0	0	7%
caramel	1.25 oz	120	1	29	65	0	1.0	0.0	0	7%
chocolate................................	1.25 oz	120	1	28	20	0	1.0	0.0	0	7%
raspberry................................	1.25 oz	120	1	29	15	0	1.0	0.0	0	7%
(Golden Temple)										
original, 100% natural, 'Wha Guru Chew'	1.13 oz	166	5	14	0	0	9.0	0.0	0	52%
sesame almond, 100% natural, 'Wha Guru Chew'	1.13 oz	162	4	11	0	0	11.0	0.0	0	62%
(Great Cakes)										
all natural 'Summer Fruits'.........................	3 oz	190	7	35	7	16	2.5	0.0	0	12%
all natural 'Tropical Fruits'	3 oz	185	7	35	4	16	2.0	0.0	0	10%
(Health Valley)										
apple, 'Bakes'	1 serving	100	2	16	27	3	3.0	0.0	0	27%
'Date Bakes'	1 serving	100	3	16	25	3	3.0	0.0	0	26%
fruit, 'Fruit & Fitness	2 bars	200	4	39	234	5	3.0	0.0	0	14%
fruit-nut, 'Oat Bran Jumbo Fruit Bars'	1 serving	150	4	29	11	8	4.0	0.0	0	21%
oat bran, 'Fig & Nut Bakes'	1 serving	110	2	19	18	3	3.0	0.0	0	24%
oat bran, 'Oat Bran Jumbo Fruit Bars'.................	1 serving	170	4	28	9	7	5.0	0.0	0	26%
oat bran, raisin and cinnamon.....................	1 serving	140	3	32	12	6	2.0	0.0	0	11%
'Oat Bran Apricot Bakes'.........................	1 serving	100	2	19	18	3	2.0	0.0	0	18%
'Raisin Bakes'	1 serving	100	2	16	19	3	3.0	0.0	0	27%
rice bran, almond, and date	1 serving	190	4	29	6	6	6.0	0.0	0	29%
(Kellogg's)										
apple-cinnamon, wheat, whole-grain oats, fruit..........	1 bar	140	2	26	65	1	4.0	1.0	0	24%
wheat, whole-grain oats, fruit	1 bar	140	2	26	65	1	4.0	1.0	0	24%
(Kudos)										
peaches and cream, 'Pan Squares'..................	1 sq.	150	2	22	105	2	6.0	0.0	0	36%
peanut butter and chocolate chip, 'Pan Squares'	1 sq.	170	3	20	105	2	9.0	0.0	0	47%
strawberry and cream cheese, 'Pan Squares'...........	1 sq.	150	2	22	105	2	6.0	0.0	0	36%
(Marin)										
fig, honey sweetened, organic......................	1 bar	120	2	21	100	3	3.0	1.0	0	23%

Food Name	Serving Size	Calories	Prot. gms	Carbs gms	Sod. mgs	Fiber gms	Fat gms	Sat. Fat gms	Chol. mgs	% Fat Cal.
fig, organic	1 bar	70	1	16	100	2	0.0	0.0	0	0%
(Natural Nectar)										
almond, 'Treat Yourself Right'	1 bar	150	3	22	40	5	5.0	0.0	0	31%
apple, 'Original Fruit Bar'	1 bar	100	2	15	15	4	3.0	1.0	0	28%
apple-cinnamon, low-fat, 'Fi-Bar'	1 bar	90	1	22	65	2	1.0	0.0	0	9%
apple-oatmeal spice 'Fi-Bar A.M.'	1 bar	150	3	27	25	5	3.0	0.0	0	18%
banana nut, 'Fi-Bar A.M.'	1 bar	150	2	26	20	5	4.0	0.0	0	24%
chocolate, 'Fi-Bar Lite'	2.5 oz	190	4	29	140	0	6.0	0.0	5	29%
cocoa-almond crunch, 'Fi-Bar'	1 bar	130	3	21	20	4	4.0	0.0	0	27%
cocoa-almond, whole grain, 'Fi-Bar Chewy & Nutty'	1 bar	140	3	23	25	2	4.5	2.0	0	28%
cocoa peanut butter crunch, 'Chewy & Nutty'	1 bar	130	3	20	20	2	4.0	1.0	0	28%
cocoa peanut, 'Fi-Bar Chewy & Nutty'	1 bar	130	3	20	20	4	1.0	0.0	0	9%
coconut	1 bar	120	2	20	30	6	4.0	1.0	0	29%
cranberry, w/wild berries, 'Original Fruit Bar'	1 bar	120	2	23	15	4	2.0	0.0	0	15%
lemon, 'Original Fruit Bar'	1 bar	100	2	15	15	4	3.0	1.0	0	28%
Mandarin orange 'Original Fruit Bar'	1 bar	100	2	15	15	4	3.0	1.0	0	28%
peanut butter	1 bar	130	3	20	30	6	4.0	1.0	0	28%
peanut butter, 'Treat Yourself Right'	1 bar	150	4	18	55	5	5.0	0.0	0	34%
raisin nut bran, 'Fi-Bar A.M.'	1 bar	150	3	26	30	5	4.0	0.0	0	24%
raspberry, 'Canadian'	1 bar	120	2	21	15	3	3.0	1.0	0	23%
raspberry, 'Original Fruit Bar'	1 bar	120	2	23	15	4	2.0	0.0	0	15%
strawberry, 'Canadian'	1 bar	120	2	21	15	3	3.0	1.0	0	23%
strawberry, 'Original Fruit Bar'	1 bar	120	2	23	15	4	2.0	0.0	0	15%
strawberry-oatmeal, w/almonds, 'Fi-Bar A.M.'	1 bar	150	3	24	30	5	4.0	0.0	0	25%
vanilla almond, 'Fi-Bar Chewy & Nutty'	1 bar	130	3	21	20	4	4.0	0.0	0	27%
vanilla almond crunch, 'Canadian Chewy & Nutty'	1 bar	130	3	21	20	2	4.0	1.0	0	27%
vanilla peanut, 'Fi-Bar Chewy & Nutty'	1 bar	130	3	20	20	4	4.0	0.0	0	28%
(Pemmican) carob cocoa, meatless	1 pkg	440	16	68	80	7	12.0	2.0	0	24%
SNACK BAR MIX. See also CAKE, SNACK, MIX.										
(Betty Crocker)										
caramel oatmeal, 'Supreme Dessert' mix only	1/32 pkg	90	1	15	50	0	3.0	0.0	0	30%
caramel oatmeal, 'Supreme Dessert' prepared w/margarine	1 bar	110	1	15	65	0	5.0	0.0	0	41%
chocolate and toffee, 'Supreme Dessert' mix only	1/32 pkg	90	1	17	55	0	2.0	0.0	0	20%
chocolate and toffee, 'Supreme Dessert' prepared	1 bar	110	1	17	55	0	4.0	0.0	10	33%
chocolate peanut butter 'Supreme Dessert' prepared	1 bar	110	1	14	100	0	5.0	0.0	10	43%
chocolate peanut butter, 'Supreme Dessert' mix only	1/32 pkg	100	1	14	85	0	4.0	0.0	0	38%
date, 'Classic' prepared	1 bar	60	1	9	35	0	2.0	1.0	0	31%
M&M's cookie bars, 'Supreme Dessert' mix only	1/32 pkg	100	1	16	60	0	3.0	1.0	0	28%
M&M's cookie bars, 'Supreme Dessert' prepared	1 bar	110	1	16	80	0	5.0	1.0	10	40%
raspberry, 'Supreme Dessert' mix only	1/32 pkg	100	1	16	80	0	3.0	1.0	0	28%
raspberry, 'Supreme Dessert' prepared	1/32 pkg	100	1	16	95	0	4.0	1.0	0	35%
Sunkist lemon, 'Supreme Dessert' mix only	1/32 pkg	100	1	17	55	0	3.0	0.0	0	27%
Sunkist lemon, 'Supreme Dessert' prepared w/4 eggs	1 bar	110	1	17	65	0	4.0	0.0	30	33%
SNACK CHIPS. See also BAGEL CHIPS, BANANA CHIPS; CARROT CHIPS; CORN CHIPS AND SNACKS; PASTA CHIPS; POTATO CHIPS AND SNACKS; RICE CHIPS; SEA VEGETABLE CHIPS; SNACK MIX; TARO CHIPS; TORTILLA CHIPS; VEGETABLE CHIPS; WASABI CHIPS.										
(Bake-Itos) pico de gallo	1 oz	110	3	23	59	0	0.9	0.0	0	7%
(Bugles)										
nacho flavor	1 1/3 cup	160	2	18	300	0	9.0	7.0	0	50%
original flavor	1 1/3 cup	160	1	18	310	1	9.0	8.0	0	52%
ranch flavor	1 1/3 cup	160	2	18	310	1	9.0	8.0	0	50%
(Frito-Lay's)										
'Funyuns'	1 oz	140	2	18	270	1	7.0	1.5	0	44%
'Munchos'	1 oz	160	1	16	260	1	10.0	2.0	0	57%

Food Name	Serving Size	Calories	Prot. gms	Carbs gms	Sod. mgs	Fiber gms	Fat gms	Sat. Fat gms	Chol. mgs	% Fat Cal.
(Sun Chips)										
French onion	1 oz	140	2	19	115	2	6.0	1.0	0	39%
harvest cheddar	1 oz	140	2	19	115	2	6.0	1.0	0	39%
original	1 oz	140	2	19	115	2	6.0	1.0	0	39%
SNACK MIX										
(Burns & Ricker) nonfat, 'Party Mix'	3/4 cup	120	4	23	210	1	0.0	0.0	0	0%
(Eagle) 'Snack Mix'	1/2 cup	150	4	17	270	1	7.0	1.0	0	43%
(Flavor Tree)										
no salt, 'Party Mix'	1-1/2 cups	163	4	13	8	0	10.8	0.0	0	59%
original, 'Party Mix'	1/4 cup	163	3	12	407	0	11.0	0.0	0	61%
(General Mills)										
barbecue flavor, 'Chex'	1 oz	130	3	18	380	0	5.0	0.0	0	35%
cheese, 'Chex'	2/3 cup	120	3	18	288	2	4.9	1.6	0	35%
cool sour cream and onion flavor, 'Chex'	2/3 cup	130	3	19	300	0	5.0	0.0	0	34%
golden cheddar, 'Chex'	2/3 cup	130	3	19	300	0	5.0	0.0	0	34%
nacho cheese, 'Chex'	2/3 cup	130	3	19	430	0	5.0	0.0	0	34%
(Harmony)										
Oriental, party mix	1/4 cup	150	5	11	270	2	10.0	1.5	0	58%
'Swiss Mix'	1/4 cup	190	4	27	15	2	8.0	4.0	0	37%
(Nabisco)										
original flavor, 'Doo Dads'	1/2 cup	129	3	18	360	2	5.2	1.0	0	35%
traditional, baked, 'Ritz'	1 oz	130	2	18	310	0	6.0	1.0	0	40%
(Pepperidge Farm)										
'Classic'	1 oz	140	4	14	360	1	8.0	1.0	0	50%
lightly smoked	1 oz	150	4	13	350	1	9.0	1.0	0	54%
spicy	1 oz	140	4	14	340	1	8.0	2.0	5	50%
super cheddar, 'Goldfish Party Mix'	1 oz	140	4	15	330	0	7.0	1.0	15	45%
w/cashews and almonds, 'Nutty Deluxe' 'Goldfish'	1/2 cup	180	5	20	330	2	9.0	1.5	25	45%
w/honey roasted peanuts, original, 'Goldfish'	1/2 cup	170	5	21	360	2	8.0	1.5	5	41%
(Super Snax)	1 oz	137	3	17	207	0	6.5	0.0	0	42%
SNACK STICKS, sesame and cheese, 'Twigs' *(Nabisco)*	15 sticks	150	4	17	300	1	7.0	1.5	0	43%
SNAP BEAN. See BEAN, GREEN.										
SNAP PEAS. See PEAS, SNAP.										
SNAPPER										
mixed species, baked, broiled, grilled, or microwaved	3 oz	109	22	0	48	0	1.5	0.3	40	12%
mixed species, raw	3 oz	85	17	0	54	0	1.1	0.2	31	12%
SOBA NOODLE. See under NOODLE, JAPANESE.										
SOCKEYE SALMON. See under SALMON.										
SODA. See under SOFT DRINKS AND MIXERS.										
SOFT DRINKS AND MIXERS. See also WATER, FLAVORED.										
(A&W)										
cream	1 fl oz	14	0	4	2	0	0.0	0.0	0	0%
cream, diet	1 fl oz	1	0	0	4	0	0.1	0.0	0	69%
root beer	1 fl oz	15	0	4	5	0	0.1	0.0	0	6%
root beer, diet	1 fl oz	1	0	0	4	0	0.0	0.0	0	0%
(Canada Dry)										
Collins mixer	8 fl oz	80	0	20	17	0	0.0	0.0	0	0%
ginger ale	8 fl oz	90	0	21	7	0	0.0	0.0	0	0%
ginger ale, 'Golden'	8 fl oz	100	0	24	24	0	0.0	0.0	0	0%
grape, 'Concord'	8 fl oz	130	0	32	21	0	0.0	0.0	0	0%
tonic water	8 fl oz	90	0	22	7	0	0.0	0.0	0	0%
whiskey sour mixer	8 fl oz	90	0	22	17	0	0.0	0.0	0	0%
(Coca-Cola)										
'Caffeine-Free Coke'	12 fl oz	145	0	41	13	0	0.0	0.0	0	0%

Food Name	Serving Size	Calories	Prot. gms	Carbs gms	Sod. mgs	Fiber gms	Fat gms	Sat. Fat gms	Chol. mgs	% Fat Cal.
'Caffeine-Free Diet Coke'	12 fl oz	2	0	0	6	0	0.0	0.0	0	0%
'Classic Coke'	12 fl oz	145	0	41	13	0	0.0	0.0	0	0%
'Coke'	6 fl oz	77	0	20	4	0	0.0	0.0	0	0%
'Diet Cherry Coke'	6 fl oz	1	0	0	4	0	0.0	0.0	0	0%
'Diet Coke'	12 fl oz	2	0	0	6	0	0.0	0.0	0	0%
'Tab'	6 fl oz	1	0	0	4	0	0.0	0.0	0	0%
(Dr. Diablo) cola	12 fl oz	140	0	38	14	0	0.0	0.0	0	0%
(Dr. Pepper)										
'Caffeine-Free Diet Dr. Pepper'	12 fl oz	3	0	0	18	0	0.0	0.0	0	0%
cola	12 fl oz	150	0	38	18	0	0.0	0.0	0	0%
cola, caffeine-free	12 fl oz	150	0	38	18	0	0.0	0.0	0	0%
'Diet 'Dr. Pepper'	12 fl oz	3	0	0	18	0	0.0	0.0	0	0%
(Fresca) citrus	6 fl oz	2	0	0	0	0	0.0	0.0	0	0%
(Health Valley)										
ginger ale	12 fl oz	153	1	35	30	0	1.0	0.0	0	6%
root beer, 'Old Fashioned'	12 fl oz	120	1	26	12	0	1.0	0.0	0	8%
root beer, sarsaparilla	12 fl oz	153	1	35	27	0	1.0	0.0	0	6%
wild berry	12 fl oz	142	1	33	27	0	1.0	0.0	0	6%
(Hires)										
cream, caffeine-free	6 fl oz	90	1	24	40	0	1.0	0.0	0	8%
cream, diet, caffeine-free	6 fl oz	2	1	1	45	0	1.0	0.0	0	53%
root beer, caffeine-free	6 fl oz	90	1	23	55	0	1.0	0.0	0	9%
root beer, caffeine-free, diet, w/NutraSweet	6 fl oz	2	1	1	70	0	1.0	0.0	0	53%
(Jolt) cola	6 fl oz	85	0	21	10	0	0.0	0.0	0	0%
(Mello Yello)										
citrus	6 fl oz	87	0	22	14	0	0.0	0.0	0	0%
citrus, diet	6 fl oz	3	0	0	1	0	0.0	0.0	0	0%
(Mug) root beer, diet	12 fl oz	4	0	1	39	0	0.0	0.0	0	0%
(Natural 90 Diet) all flavors	6 fl oz	2	0	1	10	0	0.0	0.0	0	0%
(Pathmark) cola, sugar-free, 'No Frills'	8 fl oz	0	0	0	0	0	0.0	0.0	0	0%
(Pepsi-Cola)										
'Light'	12 fl oz	1	0	0	2	0	0.0	0.0	0	0%
'Wild Cherry'	12 fl oz	163	0	43	2	0	0.0	0.0	0	0%
'Diet Crystal'	6 fl oz	0	0	0	35	0	0.0	0.0	0	0%
'Caffeine-Free Diet Pepsi'	12 fl oz	1	0	0	2	0	0.0	0.0	0	0%
(Santa Cruz Natural) ginger ale, organic, 'Sparkling'	8 fl oz	155	1	36	0	0	1.0	0.0	0	6%
(Schweppes)										
bitter lemon	6 fl oz	82	0	20	13	0	0.0	0.0	0	0%
blackberry, 'Royal'	6 fl oz	35	0	8	5	0	0.0	0.0	0	0%
citrus, tropical, 'Royal'	6 fl oz	35	0	8	5	0	0.0	0.0	0	0%
club soda	6 fl oz	0	0	0	25	0	0.0	0.0	0	0%
Collins mixer	6 fl oz	75	0	18	51	0	0.0	0.0	0	0%
ginger ale	6 fl oz	65	0	16	10	0	0.0	0.0	0	0%
ginger ale, sugar-free	6 fl oz	2	0	1	39	0	0.0	0.0	0	0%
grape	6 fl oz	95	0	23	15	0	0.0	0.0	0	0%
grapefruit	6 fl oz	80	0	20	28	0	0.0	0.0	0	0%
kiwi-passionfruit, 'Royal'	6 fl oz	35	0	8	5	0	0.0	0.0	0	0%
lemon-lime	6 fl oz	72	0	18	30	0	0.0	0.0	0	0%
orange, sparkling	6 fl oz	88	0	22	17	0	0.0	0.0	0	0%
peaches and cream, 'Royal'	6 fl oz	35	0	8	5	0	0.0	0.0	0	0%
raspberry ginger ale, diet	6 fl oz	2	0	1	55	0	0.0	0.0	0	0%
root beer	6 fl oz	76	0	19	17	0	0.0	0.0	0	0%
seltzer, all flavors	6 fl oz	0	0	0	5	0	0.0	0.0	0	0%
seltzer, low-sodium	6 fl oz	0	0	0	7	0	0.0	0.0	0	0%

Food Name	Serving Size	Calories	Prot. gms	Carbs gms	Sod. mgs	Fiber gms	Fat gms	Sat. Fat gms	Chol. mgs	% Fat Cal.
sour lemon	6 fl oz	79	0	19	12	0	0.0	0.0	0	0%
strawberry-banana, 'Royal'	6 fl oz	35	0	8	5	0	0.0	0.0	0	0%
tonic water	6 fl oz	64	0	16	8	0	0.0	0.0	0	0%
tonic water, diet	6 fl oz	2	0	1	45	0	0.0	0.0	0	0%
vanilla bean, 'Royal'	6 fl oz	35	0	8	5	0	0.0	0.0	0	0%
Vichy water	6 fl oz	0	0	0	76	0	0.0	0.0	0	0%
wild cherry, 'Royal'	6 fl oz	35	0	8	5	0	0.0	0.0	0	0%
wild raspberry, 'Royal'	6 fl oz	35	0	8	5	0	0.0	0.0	0	0%
(7-Up)										
cherry citrus	12 fl oz	148	0	39	32	0	0.0	0.0	0	0%
cherry citrus, diet	12 fl oz	4	0	0	32	0	0.0	0.0	0	0%
lemon-lime	12 fl oz	144	0	36	32	0	0.0	0.0	0	0%
lemon-lime, diet	12 fl oz	4	0	0	32	0	0.0	0.0	0	0%
(Shasta)										
black cherry	12 fl oz	162	0	44	29	0	0.0	0.0	0	0%
cherry cola	12 fl oz	140	0	38	22	0	0.0	0.0	0	0%
citrus mist	12 fl oz	170	0	46	19	0	0.0	0.0	0	0%
club soda	12 fl oz	0	0	0	46	0	0.0	0.0	0	0%
cola	12 fl oz	147	0	40	3	0	0.0	0.0	0	0%
Collins mixer	12 fl oz	118	0	32	23	0	0.0	0.0	0	0%
'Creme'	12 fl oz	154	0	42	23	0	0.0	0.0	0	0%
fruit punch	12 fl oz	173	0	47	32	0	0.0	0.0	0	0%
ginger ale	12 fl oz	120	0	33	23	0	0.0	0.0	0	0%
grape	12 fl oz	177	0	48	34	0	0.0	0.0	0	0%
lemon-lime	12 fl oz	146	0	39	19	0	0.0	0.0	0	0%
'Luigi Berry'	8 fl oz	130	0	32	30	0	0.0	0.0	0	0%
'Mario Punch'	8 fl oz	130	0	31	40	0	0.0	0.0	0	0%
orange	12 fl oz	177	0	48	28	0	0.0	0.0	0	0%
'Princess Toadstool Cherry'	8 fl oz	130	0	31	30	0	0.0	0.0	0	0%
red berry	12 fl oz	158	0	43	20	0	0.0	0.0	0	0%
root beer	12 fl oz	154	0	42	31	0	0.0	0.0	0	0%
strawberry	12 fl oz	147	0	40	36	0	0.0	0.0	0	0%
tonic water	12 fl oz	121	0	33	17	0	0.0	0.0	0	0%
'Yoshi Apple'	8 fl oz	130	0	31	30	0	0.0	0.0	0	0%
(Slice) orange, 'Diet'	12 fl oz	12	0	2	2	0	0.0	0.0	0	0%
(Soda-Licious)										
cherry cola	1 pouch	100	1	22	20	0	1.0	0.0	0	9%
fruit punch, red	1 pouch	100	1	22	20	0	1.0	0.0	0	9%
grape	1 pouch	100	1	22	20	0	1.0	0.0	0	9%
lemon-lime	1 pouch	100	1	22	20	0	1.0	0.0	0	9%
orange	1 pouch	100	1	22	20	0	1.0	0.0	0	9%
root beer	1 pouch	100	1	22	20	0	1.0	0.0	0	9%
(Spree)										
cherry-lime	12 fl oz	158	0	43	2	0	0.0	0.0	0	0%
cola	12 fl oz	147	0	40	1	0	0.0	0.0	0	0%
ginger ale	12 fl oz	120	0	33	1	0	0.0	0.0	0	0%
grapefruit	12 fl oz	154	0	42	1	0	0.0	0.0	0	0%
lemon-lime	12 fl oz	154	0	42	1	0	0.0	0.0	0	0%
lemon-tangerine	12 fl oz	165	0	45	1	0	0.0	0.0	0	0%
lime, Mandarin	12 fl oz	154	0	42	1	0	0.0	0.0	0	0%
root beer	12 fl oz	154	0	42	2	0	0.0	0.0	0	0%
tropical blend	12 fl oz	146	0	41	2	0	0.0	0.0	0	0%
(Squirt)										
citrus	1 fl oz	13	0	3	2	0	0.0	0.0	0	0%

Food Name	Serving Size	Calories	Prot. gms	Carbs gms	Sod. mgs	Fiber gms	Fat gms	Sat. Fat gms	Chol. mgs	% Fat Cal.
citrus, 'Diet'	1 fl oz	1	0	0	1	0	0.0	0.0	0	0%
citrus berry, 'Ruby Red'	8 fl oz	120	0	30	25	0	0.0	0.0	0	0%
(Vernors)										
ginger ale	3.5 fl oz	40	0	10	4	0	0.1	0.0	0	2%
ginger ale, 'Diet'	3.5 fl oz	1	0	0	7	0	0.1	0.0	0	53%
(Wink) grapefruit	8 fl oz	120	0	30	19	0	0.0	0.0	0	0%
SOLE										
Fresh										
baked, broiled, grilled, or microwaved	3 oz	99	20.5	0.0	89	0	1.3	0.3	58	13%
raw	3 oz	77	16.0	0.0	69	0	1.0	0.2	41	12%
Frozen										
Atlantic *(Booth)*	4 oz	90	19	0	180	0	1.0	0.0	0	11%
fillet *(SeaPak)*	4 oz	90	20	0	135	0	1.0	0.0	0	10%
fillet, lightly breaded *(Van de Kamp's)*	1 serving	220	14	17	410	0	11.0	2.0	40	44%
fillet, 'Natural' *(Van de Kamp's)*	4 oz	100	22	0	105	0	2.0	1.0	35	17%
'Fishmarket Fresh' *(Gorton's)*	5 oz	110	24	1	140	0	1.0	0.0	0	8%
SOLE DISH/ENTRÉE										
(Gorton's)										
fillet, stuffed, frozen, 'Select' approx 5 oz	1 fillet	160	16	18	730	0	3.0	1.0	50	17%
in lemon butter, frozen, 'Microwave Entrees'	1 pkg	380	25	17	560	0	24.0	11.0	120	56%
(Healthy Choice)										
au gratin, frozen	11 oz	270	16	40	470	0	5.0	3.0	55	17%
w/lemon butter sauce, frozen	8.25 oz	230	16	33	430	0	4.0	2.0	45	16%
SOMEN NOODLE. See under NOODLE, JAPANESE.										
SORBET. See also SHERBET.										
(Cascadian Farm)										
blackberry sorbet, all-fruit, organic, nonfat	1/2 cup	90	0	22	76	1	0.0	0.0	0	0%
blackberry, nonfat	1 oz	25	1	21	0	0	0.1	0.0	0	1%
blackberry, w/vanilla ice cream, organic	1/2 cup	110	2	21	30	1	2.0	1.5	10	16%
orange, w/vanilla ice cream, organic	1/2 cup	110	2	21	30	0	2.0	1.5	10	16%
raspberry, all-fruit, organic, nonfat	1/2 cup	90	0	21	55	1	0.0	0.0	0	0%
raspberry, nonfat	1 oz	28	1	21	0	0	0.2	0.0	0	2%
raspberry, w/vanilla ice cream, organic	1/2 cup	110	2	21	30	1	2.0	1.5	10	16%
strawberry, all-fruit, organic, nonfat	1/2 cup	70	1	17	41	1	0.0	0.0	0	0%
strawberry, nonfat	1 oz	26	1	22	0	0	0.1	0.0	0	1%
(Diamond Crystal) lower calorie, all flavors	1 serving	30	0	7	30	na	0.0	0.0	0	0%
(Dole)										
Mandarin orange, nonfat	4 oz	110	1	28	9	0	0.1	0.0	0	1%
peach, nonfat	4 oz	120	1	28	11	0	0.6	0.0	0	5%
pineapple, nonfat	4 oz	120	1	28	11	0	0.1	0.0	0	1%
raspberry, nonfat	4 oz	110	1	28	12	0	0.1	0.0	0	1%
strawberry, nonfat	4 oz	110	1	28	1	0	0.1	0.0	0	1%
(Frusen Gladje) raspberry, nonfat	1/2 cup	140	0	36	10	0	0.0	0.0	0	0%
(Haagen-Dazs)										
blueberry, w/vanilla ice cream	1/2 cup	190	3	25	35	0	8.0	0.0	0	39%
key lime, w/vanilla ice cream	1/2 cup	200	2	29	30	0	7.0	0.0	0	34%
lemon, 'Ice Cream Shop'	4 oz	140	1	34	5	0	0.0	0.0	0	0%
orange, 'Ice Cream Shop'	4 oz	113	1	30	7	0	0.0	0.0	0	0%
raspberry	1/2 cup	120	0	29	5	1	0.0	0.0	0	0%
raspberry, nonfat, 'Ice Cream Shop'	4 oz	93	0	22	7	0	0.0	0.0	0	0%
strawberry	1/2 cup	130	0	33	0	1	0.0	0.0	0	0%
(Real Fruit)										
red raspberry, chunky, nonfat	1/2 cup	100	0	25	5	0	0.0	0.0	0	0%
tropical blend, chunky, nonfat	1/2 cup	100	0	26	5	1	0.0	0.0	0	0%

Food Name	Serving Size	Calories	Prot. gms	Carbs gms	Sod. mgs	Fiber gms	Fat gms	Sat. Fat gms	Chol. mgs	% Fat Cal.
wildberry, chunky, nonfat	1/2 cup	100	0	25	10	1	0.0	0.0	0	0%
(TCBY Treats) all flavors, soft serve, nonfat	1/2 cup	100	0	24	30	0	0.0	0.0	0	0%
SORGHUM										
broomcorn, whole grain	3.5 oz	327	9.9	72.9	1	>3.2 c	2.9	1.0	0	7%\
whole grain . . . .'.	1 cup	651	21.7	143.3	na	>4.6 c	6.3	0.9	0	8%
whole grain	1 oz	96	3.2	21.2	na	>.7 c	0.9	0.1	0	8%
SORGHUM SYRUP. See under SYRUP.										
SORREL										
boiled, drained	4 oz	23	2.1	3.3	3	>.8 c	0.7	(tr)	0	23%
raw, trimmed	1 oz	6	0.6	0.9	1	>.2 c	0.2	(tr)	0	23%
raw, trimmed, chopped	1/2 cup	15	1.3	2.1	3	1.9	0.5	(tr)	0	25%
raw, untrimmed	1 lb	70	6.4	10.2	13	>2.5 c	2.2	na	0	23%
SOUP. See also SOUP MIX.										
ASPARAGUS, CREAM OF										
Canned, condensed										
prepared w/milk	1 cup	161	6	16	1042	1	8.2	3.3	22	45%
prepared w/water	1 cup	85	2	11	981	0	4.1	1.0	5	42%
unprepared	10.75-oz can	210	6	26	2385	1	9.9	2.5	12	42%
unprepared	1 cup	173	5	21	1963	1	8.2	2.1	10	42%
Frozen										
(Kettle Ready)	3/4 cup	62	1	5	406	0	4.3	1.5	0	62%
(Myers)	9.75 oz	152	11	10	992	0	8.0	0.0	0	46%
(Soup Supreme)	1 cup	160	4	17	920	1	9.0	3.0	0	49%
BARLEY W/MUSHROOM										
Canned, condensed (Rokeach) prepared	1 cup	85	3	17	904	0	0.2	0.0	0	2%
BARLEY BEAN, frozen (Tabatchnick)	7.5 oz	130	6	22	217	0	2.0	0.0	0	14%
BEAN AND HAM, heat and serve (Healthy Choice)	1 cup	160	12	29	480	5	1.5	0.5	2	8%
BEAN										
Canned, condensed										
w/frankfurter, prepared	1 cup	188	10	22	1093	na	7.0	2.1	13	33%
w/frankfurter, unprepared	11.25-oz can	453	24	53	2651	15	16.9	5.1	29	33%
w/frankfurter, unprepared	1 cup	373	20	44	2186	12	14.0	4.2	24	33%
w/pork, prepared	1 cup	172	8	23	951	9	5.9	1.5	3	31%
w/pork, unprepared	11.5-oz can	421	19	55	2311	19	14.4	3.7	7	30%
w/pork, unprepared	1 cup	347	16	46	1907	16	11.9	3.1	5	31%
(Campbell's)										
'Homestyle' prepared	1 cup	130	6	25	700	0	1.0	0.0	0	7%
w/bacon, 'Healthy Request' unprepared	1/2 cup	150	7	26	480	7	2.0	1.0	5	12%
(Stouffer's) navy bean, classic, food service product,										
prepared	1 cup	128	6	18	951	4	3.2	0.8	7	23%
Canned, ready to use										
w/ham, chunky, commercial product	19.25-oz can	519	28	61	2184	25	19.1	7.5	49	33%
w/ham, chunky, commercial product	1 cup	231	13	27	972	11	8.5	3.3	22	33%
(Grandma Brown's)	1 cup	190	9	31	700	10	3.4	0.0	1	16%
(Health Valley) five bean vegetable, nonfat	7.5 oz	100	8	14	260	3	0.0	0.0	0	0%
(Hormel) w/ham, 'Hearty Soups'	7.5 oz	190	9	29	640	0	4.0	1.0	23	19%
Frozen										
(Kettle Ready)										
w/beef, vegetable	3/4 cup	85	4	11	448	0	3.0	0.6	0	31%
w/ham	3/4 cup	113	7	20	459	0	3.6	1.0	0	23%
(Soup Supreme)										
royal navy, food service product	1 cup	140	7	24	1110	5	2.0	0.0	0	13%
w/ham, food service product	1 cup	140	8	23	910	5	2.0	1.0	10	13%
(Tabatchnick) Northern bean	7.5 oz	164	8	29	240	0	2.0	0.0	0	11%

Food Name	Serving Size	Calories	Prot. gms	Carbs gms	Sod. mgs	Fiber gms	Fat gms	Sat. Fat gms	Chol. mgs	% Fat Cal.
BEEF										
Canned, condensed										
(Campbell's)										
prepared	1 cup	80	5	10	830	0	2.0	0.0	10	23%
w/bouillon, prepared	1 cup	16	3	1	820	0	0.0	0.0	0	0%
w/broth, prepared	1 cup	16	3	1	820	0	0.0	0.0	0	0%
Canned, ready to use										
chunky	19-oz can	383	26	44	1946	3	11.5	5.7	32	27%
chunky	1 cup	170	12	20	866	1	5.1	2.5	14	27%
(Campbell's)										
'Chunky'	10.75-oz can	200	15	24	1100	0	5.0	0.0	0	22%
Stroganoff style, 'Chunky'	10.75-oz can	320	15	28	1230	0	16.0	0.0	0	46%
w/vegetables and pasta, 'Home Cookin'	10.75-oz can	140	12	18	1060	0	2.0	0.0	0	13%
(College Inn) w/broth, ready to serve	1 cup	18	2	1	1280	0	0.0	0.0	0	0%
(Health Valley) w/broth, no salt added	7.5 oz	17	1	2	0	0	1.0	0.0	1	43%
(Healthy Choice) 'Hearty Beef'	7.5 oz	120	9	17	580	0	2.0	1.0	20	15%
(Progresso)										
	10.5-oz can	180	15	17	840	0	6.0	0.0	35	30%
hearty	9.5 oz	160	15	15	820	0	4.0	2.0	35	23%
w/broth, seasoned	1/2 cup	10	2	1	380	0	1.0	0.0	0	43%
w/minestrone	10.5-oz can	180	15	18	1000	0	6.0	0.0	35	29%
(Swanson) w/broth, ready to serve	7.25 oz	18	2	0	750	0	1.0	0.0	0	53%
BEEF AND POTATO										
Canned, ready to use *(Healthy Choice)*	1 cup	110	10	17	450	5	1.0	0.0	5	8%
BEEF BARLEY										
Canned, ready to use										
(Progresso)										
	10.5-oz can	150	13	16	870	3	5.0	0.0	30	28%
low-fat, 'Healthy Classics'	1 cup	142	11	20	470	3	1.9	0.7	19	12%
BEEF BROTH/BOUILLON										
Canned, condensed										
prepared	1 cup	23	3	0	969	na	1.3	na	1	50%
unprepared	10.5-oz can	72	13	4	1550	0	0.0	0.0	0	0%
unprepared	1 cup	59	11	4	1279	0	0.0	0.0	0	0%
Canned, ready to use										
	14-oz can	28	5	0	1294	0	0.9	0.4	0	28%
	10.5-oz can	41	7	0	1910	0	1.3	0.6	0	28%
	1 cup	17	3	0	782	0	0.5	0.3	0	28%
and tomato juice	5.5-oz can	62	1	14	220	0	0.2	0.1	0	2%
and tomato juice	1 oz	11	0	3	40	0	0.0	0.0	0	2%
(College Inn)	7 oz	16	3	1	960	0	0.0	0.0	0	0%
(Health Valley)										
no salt added	6.9 oz	10	1	2	5	0	0.0	0.0	0	0%
nonfat	1 cup	20	5	0	160	0	0.0	0.0	0	0%
regular	6.9 oz	10	1	2	290	0	0.0	0.0	0	0%
(Swanson) clear	1 cup	20	2	1	820	0	1.0	0.5	0	43%
BEEF MUSHROOM										
Canned, condensed										
prepared	1 cup	73	6	6	942	0	3.0	1.5	7	37%
unprepared	10.75-oz can	186	14	16	2358	1	7.3	3.7	15	35%
unprepared	1 cup	153	12	13	1940	1	6.0	3.0	13	35%
BEEF NOODLE										
Canned, condensed										
prepared	1 cup	83	5	9	952	1	3.1	1.1	5	33%

Food Name	Serving Size	Calories	Prot. gms	Carbs gms	Sod. mgs	Fiber gms	Fat gms	Sat. Fat gms	Chol. mgs	% Fat Cal.
unprepared	10.75-oz can	204	12	22	2315	2	7.5	2.8	12	33%
unprepared	1 cup	168	10	18	1905	2	6.2	2.3	10	33%
(Campbell's) 'Homestyle' prepared	1 cup	80	5	7	810	0	4.0	0.0	20	43%
Canned, ready to use (Progresso)	9.5 oz	170	15	18	1030	0	4.0	0.0	40	21%
BEEF VEGETABLE										
Canned, condensed										
(Campbell's) 'Healthy Request' unprepared	1/2 cup	70	5	9	490	0	2.0	0.0	5	24%
(Progresso) and rotini, prepared	1 cup	120	11	10	830	3	3.5	1.5	20	27%
Canned, ready to use										
country, chunky	1 cup	153	12	16	868	na	4.4	1.3	24	26%
w/barley, prepared	1 cup	77	5	10	898	na	1.8	0.6	8	21%
(Healthy Choice) 'Vegetable Beef'	7.5 oz	130	8	21	530	0	1.0	1.0	15	7%
(Hormel)										
'Hearty Soups'	7.5 oz	90	6	15	730	0	1.0	2.0	5	10%
micro cup, 'Hearty Soups'	1 container	71	5	12	811	0	1.0	0.0	9	12%
(Lipton) 'Hearty Ones'	11-oz container	229	10	40	921	0	3.0	0.0	29	12%
(Progresso)	10.5-oz can	170	17	18	880	0	3.0	0.0	40	16%
BERRY										
Canned, ready to use (Great Impressions) 'Three Berry'	3/4 cup	107	1	26	90	0	0.2	0.0	0	2%
BLACK BEAN										
Canned, condensed										
prepared	1 cup	116	6	20	1198	4	1.5	0.4	0	12%
unprepared	11-oz can	284	15	48	3026	21	4.1	1.1	0	13%
unprepared	1 cup	234	12	40	2493	17	3.4	0.9	0	13%
(Stouffer's) prepared	1 cup	192	9	30	847	14	3.2	1.6	7	16%
Canned, ready to use										
(Health Valley)										
	7.5 oz	160	7	24	285	17	3.0	0.0	0	18%
and vegetable, nonfat	1 cup	110	11	24	280	12	0.0	0.0	0	0%
no salt added	7.5 oz	160	7	24	20	17	3.0	0.0	0	18%
Frozen										
(Kettle Ready) w/ham	3/4 cup	154	8	23	613	0	6.2	1.3	0	31%
(Soup Supreme) Southern style, food service product	1 cup	150	9	23	1450	7	3.0	0.0	5	17%
BLUEBERRY, canned, ready to use (Great Impressions)	3/4 cup	95	0	23	92	0	0.3	0.0	0	3%
BORSCHT										
Canned, ready to use										
(Gold's)										
	1 cup	100	4	21	1280	0	0.0	0.0	0	0%
low-calorie	1 cup	20	1	5	1160	0	1.0	0.0	0	27%
(Manischewitz)										
low-calorie	1 cup	20	1	4	725	0	0.0	0.0	0	0%
w/beets	1 cup	80	1	20	660	0	0.0	0.0	0	0%
(Rokeach)										
	1 cup	96	1	23	985	0	0.3	0.0	0	3%
'Diet'	1 cup	29	1	6	897	1	0.2	0.0	0	6%
'Unsalted'	1 cup	103	1	23	50	1	0.3	0.0	0	3%
BROCCOLI										
Canned, ready to use (Health Valley) carotene, nonfat	1 cup	70	6	16	240	7	0.0	0.0	0	0%
BROCCOLI CREAM OF										
Canned, condensed										
(Campbell's)										
'Healthy Request' unprepared	1/2 cup	70	2	9	480	1	2.0	1.0	5	29%
prepared w/whole milk	1 cup	140	5	14	850	0	7.0	0.0	0	45%
unprepared	1/2 cup	80	2	12	730	1	3.0	1.0	3	33%

Food Name	Serving Size	Calories	Prot. gms	Carbs gms	Sod. mgs	Fiber gms	Fat gms	Sat. Fat gms	Chol. mgs	% Fat Cal.
(Stouffer's) prepared w/whole milk	1 cup	272	9	17	783	2	19.2	10.4	48	63%
Canned, ready to use										
(Andersen's)	.5 oz	170	5	20	670	0	8.0	0.0	0	42%
(Stouffer's) food service product	1 cup	288	10	13	903	2	21.6	8.0	43	68%
(Progresso) 'Healthy Classics'	1 cup	88	2	13	578	2	2.8	0.7	5	29%
Frozen										
(Kettle Ready)	6 oz	94	1	6	417	0	7.2	2.6	0	69%
(Myers)	9.75 oz	174	8	11	905	0	11.0	0.0	0	57%
(Soup Supreme)										
food service product	1 cup	180	6	16	760	2	11.0	4.0	5	53%
w/cheese, food service product	1 cup	190	6	16	890	1	12.0	4.0	15	55%
(Tabatchnick)	7.5 oz	90	4	10	285	0	4.0	0.0	4	39%
CABBAGE SOUP, frozen *(Tabatchnick)*	7.5 oz	110	2	21	185	0	2.0	0.0	0	16%
CAULIFLOWER, CREAM OF, frozen *(Kettle Ready)*	3/4 cup	93	2	6	445	0	7.0	3.1	0	67%
CELERY, CREAM OF										
Canned, condensed										
prepared w/milk	1 cup	164	6	15	1009	1	9.7	3.9	32	52%
prepared w/water	1 cup	90	2	9	949	1	5.6	1.4	15	54%
unprepared	10.75-oz can	220	4	21	2309	2	13.6	3.4	34	55%
unprepared	1 cup	181	3	18	1900	2	11.2	2.8	28	55%
(Campbell's)										
'Healthy Request' unprepared	1/2 cup	70	2	11	480	1	2.0	0.5	5	26%
prepared w/water	1 cup	100	2	8	820	0	7.0	0.0	5	61%
CHEDDAR CAULIFLOWER										
Frozen *(Soup Supreme)* food service product	1 cup	130	4	13	1100	2	8.0	2.5	5	51%
CHEDDAR VEGETABLE										
Frozen, *(Soup Supreme)* food service product	1 cup	140	4	14	1110	2	8.0	2.5	5	50%
CHEESE										
Canned, condensed										
prepared w/milk	1 cup	231	9	16	1019	1	14.6	9.1	48	55%
prepared w/water	1 cup	156	5	11	958	1	10.5	6.7	30	59%
unprepared	11-oz can	378	13	26	2331	2	25.4	16.2	72	59%
unprepared	1 cup	311	11	21	1920	2	20.9	13.3	59	59%
(Campbell's)										
nacho, prepared w/water	1 cup	110	4	8	740	0	8.0	0.0	0	60%
nacho, prepared w/whole milk	1 cup	180	8	13	800	0	12.0	0.0	0	56%
Frozen										
(Kettle Ready)										
cheddar, cream of	3/4 cup	158	4	7	616	0	12.5	6.1	0	71%
cheddar, cream of, w/broccoli	3/4 cup	137	4	5	533	0	11.3	5.2	0	75%
(Myers) and broccoli	9.75 oz	325	12	19	1257	0	23.0	0.0	0	63%
(Soup Supreme) cheddar, club, food service product	1 cup	240	8	17	1280	1	16.0	6.0	20	59%
CHERRY, canned, ready to use *(Great Impressions)*	3/4 cup	123	1	30	88	0	0.2	0.0	0	1%
CHICKEN										
Canned, condensed										
w/dumplings, prepared	10.5-oz can	234	14	15	2092	1	13.4	3.2	82	51%
w/dumplings, prepared	1 cup	96	6	6	860	0	5.5	1.3	34	51%
w/dumplings, unprepared	10.5-oz can	235	14	15	2095	1	13.4	3.2	80	51%
w/dumplings, unprepared	1 cup	194	11	12	1729	1	11.1	2.6	66	51%
(Stouffer's) prepared	1 cup	104	2	12	1111	1	4.8	0.8	16	43%
Canned, ready to use										
chunky	19-oz can	383	27	37	1908	3	14.2	4.3	65	33%
chunky	10.75-oz can	217	15	21	1080	2	8.1	2.4	37	33%
chunky	1 cup	178	13	17	889	2	6.6	2.0	30	33%

Food Name	Serving Size	Calories	Prot. gms	Carbs gms	Sod. mgs	Fiber gms	Fat gms	Sat. Fat gms	Chol. mgs	% Fat Cal.
(Campbell's) 'Chunky Old Fashioned'	10-3/4 oz	180	12	21	1220	0	5.0	0.0	0	25%
(Healthy Choice) hearty	1 cup	130	9	18	460	3	2.5	1.0	10	17%
(Progresso)										
'Homestyle'	9.5 oz	110	11	12	740	0	3.0	0.0	20	23%
spicy, w/penne	1 cup	120	8	13	680	0	4.0	1.0	20	30%
w/meatballs, 'Chickarina'	9.5 oz	130	8	13	820	0	5.0	0.0	20	35%
Frozen *(Tabatchnick)*	7.5 oz	65	2	10	255	0	2.0	0.0	0	27%
CHICKEN, CREAM OF										
Canned, condensed										
prepared w/milk	10.75-oz can	464	18	36	2540	1	27.8	11.3	66	53%
prepared w/milk	1 cup	191	7	15	1047	0	11.5	4.6	27	53%
prepared w/water	10.75-oz can	285	8	23	2396	1	17.9	5.0	24	56%
prepared w/water	1 cup	117	3	9	986	0	7.4	2.1	10	56%
unprepared	10.75-oz can	284	8	23	2397	1	17.9	5.1	24	56%
unprepared	1 cup	233	7	19	1973	1	14.7	4.2	20	56%
(Campbell's)										
'Healthy Request' prepared w/water	1 cup	70	2	11	490	0	2.0	0.0	10	26%
'Healthy Request' unprepared	1/2 cup	80	2	12	480	0	2.0	1.0	10	24%
98% nonfat, unprepared	1/2 cup	80	3	9	910	0	3.0	1.0	10	36%
Canned, ready to use *(Progresso)*	9.5 oz	190	10	12	970	0	11.0	0.0	35	53%
Frozen										
(Kettle Ready)	3/4 cup	98	6	5	668	0	6.2	2.3	0	57%
(Soup Supreme)	1 cup	160	8	14	910	2	8.0	2.0	15	45%
CHICKEN AND BROCCOLI, CREAM OF										
Canned, condensed										
(Campbell's)										
'Healthy Request' unprepared	1/2 cup	80	3	10	480	1	2.5	1.0	5	30%
prepared	1 cup	110	3	9	710	0	7.0	0.0	10	57%
CHICKEN BARLEY										
Canned, condensed *(Campbell's)* prepared	1 cup	70	3	10	850	0	2.0	0.0	0	26%
Canned, ready to use *(Progresso)*	9.25 oz	100	10	12	740	4	2.0	0.0	20	17%
CHICKEN BROTH/BOUILLON										
Canned, condensed										
prepared	1 cup	38	5	1	763	0	1.4	0.4	0	32%
unprepared	10.75-oz can	95	13	2	1909	0	3.2	0.9	3	30%
unprepared	1 cup	78	11	2	1571	0	2.6	0.8	3	30%
(Campbell's) prepared	1 cup	30	1	2	710	0	2.0	0.0	0	60%
Canned, ready to use										
(Campbell's)										
'Healthy Request'	1 cup	16	3	1	470	0	0.0	0.0	0	0%
low-salt	1 cup	40	4	2	140	0	2.0	1.0	5	43%
nonfat, 'Healthy Request'	1 cup	16	3	1	470	0	0.0	0.0	0	0%
(College Inn)										
. . . .	1 cup	35	1	0	1320	0	3.0	0.0	0	87%
lower salt	7 oz	20	1	0	550	0	2.0	1.0	5	82%
(Hain)										
. . . .	8.75 oz	70	2	0	870	0	6.0	0.0	5	87%
'No Salt Added'	8.75 oz	60	3	0	75	0	5.0	0.0	5	79%
(Health Valley)										
. . . .	7.5 oz	35	4	1	410	0	2.0	0.0	2	47%
no salt added	7.5 oz	35	4	1	0	0	2.0	0.0	2	47%
nonfat	1 cup	30	6	0	170	0	0.0	0.0	0	0%
(Pritikin) defatted	1 cup	18	3	1	160	0	1.0	0.0	0	36%
(Progresso) nonfat	1/2 cup	8	2	0	360	0	0.0	0.0	5	0%

Food Name	Serving Size	Calories	Prot. gms	Carbs gms	Sod. mgs	Fiber gms	Fat gms	Sat. Fat gms	Chol. mgs	% Fat Cal.
(Shelton's)										
nonfat	1 cup	10	2	0	60	0	0.0	0.0	0	0%
w/salt and pepper	1 cup	35	2	0	580	0	2.5	0.5	2	74%
(Swanson) clear	1 cup	30	2	1	1000	0	2.0	0.5	0	60%
CHICKEN CORN CHOWDER										
Canned, ready to use *(Healthy Choice)*	1 cup	160	8	26	470	4	2.5	1.0	5	14%
CHICKEN GUMBO										
Canned, condensed										
prepared	1 cup	56	3	8	954	2	1.4	0.3	5	23%
unprepared	10.75-oz can	137	6	20	2321	5	3.5	0.8	9	23%
unprepared	1 cup	113	5	17	1910	4	2.9	0.7	8	23%
Frozen										
(Kettle Ready)	3/4 cup	94	4	12	473	0	3.5	0.7	0	34%
(Soup Supreme)										
food service product	1 cup	90	5	11	1300	1	2.5	0.5	10	26%
spicy, Southern style, food service product	1 cup	110	6	14	960	1	3.0	1.0	15	25%
Canned, ready to use										
(Campbell's) w/sausage, 'Home Cookin'	10.75-oz can	140	11	15	1090	0	4.0	0.0	0	26%
CHICKEN MINESTRONE										
Canned, ready to use										
(Campbell's) 'Home Cookin'	10-3/4 oz	180	15	17	950	0	6.0	0.0	0	30%
(Progresso)	10.5 oz	140	12	14	1060	0	4.0	0.0	20	26%
CHICKEN MUSHROOM										
Canned, condensed										
prepared	1 cup	132	4	9	942	0	9.2	2.4	10	63%
unprepared	10.75-oz can	332	11	23	2358	1	22.3	5.9	24	60%
unprepared	1 cup	274	9	19	1940	1	18.3	4.8	20	60%
Canned, ready to use										
chowder, chunky	1 cup	192	7	17	814	3	10.6	2.8	14	50%
(Campbell's) creamy, 'Chunky'	10.5 oz	270	12	13	1280	0	19.0	0.0	0	63%
CHICKEN NOODLE										
Canned, condensed										
prepared	1 cup	75	4	9	1106	1	2.5	0.7	7	29%
unprepared	10.5-oz can	182	10	23	2256	2	5.5	1.5	15	27%
unprepared	1 cup	150	8	19	1862	1	4.6	1.2	12	27%
(Campbell's)										
creamy, prepared w/2% milk	1 cup	180	8	16	850	0	9.0	0.0	0	46%
creamy, prepared w/water	1/2 cup	120	4	10	800	0	7.0	0.0	0	53%
'Healthy Request' unprepared	1/2 cup	70	3	9	480	0	2.0	0.5	15	27%
Teddy bear pasta in chicken broth, prepared	1 cup	60	2	11	770	0	1.0	0.0	5	15%
unprepared	10.75-oz can	156	8	21	2291	2	4.6	1.5	27	26%
(Progresso) prepared	1 cup	80	9	8	730	1	2.0	0.5	20	21%
Canned, ready to use										
chunky	19-oz can	393	29	38	1908	9	13.5	3.1	43	30%
chunky	1 cup	175	13	17	850	4	6.0	1.4	19	30%
w/celery and carrots, homestyle	1 cup	95	6	9	985	na	3.4	0.9	21	32%
w/meatballs, chunky	20-oz can	227	19	19	2376	na	8.2	2.4	23	32%
w/meatballs, chunky	1 cup	99	8	8	1039	na	3.6	1.1	10	32%
(Campbell's)										
'Chunky'	10-3/4 oz	200	14	20	1140	0	7.0	0.0	0	32%
hearty, 'Healthy Request'	1 cup	100	5	14	480	1	3.0	1.0	15	26%
'Home Cookin'	10-3/4 oz	140	13	12	1150	0	4.0	0.0	0	26%
low-salt	1 cup	170	11	18	120	2	5.0	1.5	50	28%

Food Name	Serving Size	Calories	Prot. gms	Carbs gms	Sod. mgs	Fiber gms	Fat gms	Sat. Fat gms	Chol. mgs	% Fat Cal.
(Hain)										
. . . .	9.5 oz	120	9	11	980	0	4.0	0.0	20	31%
low-salt, low-fat, 'Homestyle Naturals'.	1 cup	80	7	8	100	1	2.0	1.0	15	23%
(Healthy Choice)										
old-fashioned.	1 cup	150	8	23	480	1	2.5	1.0	15	15%
w/pasta	1 cup	120	8	17	470	1	2.5	1.0	5	18%
(Hormel)										
'Hearty Soups'.	7.5 oz	110	7	14	690	0	3.0	1.0	18	24%
micro cup, 'Hearty Soups'	1 container	108	7	14	686	0	3.0	0.0	22	24%
(Lipton) 'Hearty Ones Homestyle'	11 oz	227	10	37	989	0	4.0	0.0	37	16%
(Lunch Bucket) microwave cup	7.25 oz	90	4	13	810	0	2.0	0.0	25	21%
(Pritikin) w/ribbon pasta	1 cup	80	6	13	180	1	1.0	0.0	5	11%
(Progresso)										
'Healthy Classics'	1 cup	76	6	9	460	1	1.6	0.4	19	19%
w/rotini, hearty.	1 cup	90	10	8	860	0	2.0	0.5	20	20%
(Weight Watchers)										
. . . .	10.5 oz	80	6	9	1230	0	2.0	0.0	0	23%
microwave cup	7.5 oz	90	8	13	450	0	1.0	0.0	15	10%
Frozen										
(Kettle Ready)	3/4 cup	94	5	12	569	0	3.0	0.6	0	28%
(Myers).	9.75 oz	87	8	5	1046	0	5.0	0.0	0	46%
(Soup Supreme)										
food service product	1 cup	120	7	15	1050	1	3.0	1.0	20	23%
seasoned, food service product	1 cup	100	3	16	1120	1	2.5	0.5	10	23%
CHICKEN RICE										
Canned, condensed										
prepared	10.5-oz can	147	9	17	1981	2	4.6	1.1	18	28%
prepared	1 cup	60	4	7	815	1	1.9	0.5	7	28%
unprepared	10.5-oz can	146	9	17	1982	1	4.6	1.1	15	29%
unprepared	1 cup	121	7	14	1636	1	3.8	0.9	12	29%
(Campbell's)										
'Healthy Request' unprepared.	1/2 cup	60	2	10	480	1	2.5	1.0	15	32%
'Healthy Request' prepared.	1 cup	60	2	7	480	0	3.0	0.0	10	43%
(Progresso) and vegetable, prepared	1 cup	110	7	12	790	1	3.0	1.0	15	26%
Canned, ready to use										
chunky.	19-oz can	286	28	29	1994	2	7.2	2.2	27	23%
chunky.	1 cup	127	12	13	888	1	3.2	1.0	12	23%
(Campbell's)										
hearty, 'Healthy Request'.	1 cup	110	5	15	480	0	3.0	0.0	10	25%
microwave.	10.5 oz	120	5	20	1130	2	2.5	1.0	10	18%
(Healthy Choice)	7.5 oz	140	5	18	510	1	4.0	1.0	15	28%
(Hormel) 'Hearty Soup'	7.5 oz	110	5	17	890	0	2.0	1.0	6	17%
(Progresso)										
. . . .	10.5 oz	120	9	12	990	0	4.0	0.0	25	30%
. . . .	9.5 oz	130	9	16	750	0	3.0	0.0	25	21%
wild rice.	9.5 oz	120	6	17	850	0	3.0	1.0	20	23%
wild rice, w/vegetables	1 cup	93	6	12	784	na	2.2	0.6	14	21%
w/vegetables, 'Healthy Classics'	1 cup	88	6	13	459	1	1.5	0.4	17	15%
Frozen										
(Soup Supreme)										
w/white and wild rice, food service product.	1 cup	210	8	17	1230	0	12.0	2.5	20	52%
CHICKEN VEGETABLE										
Canned, condensed										
prepared	10.5-oz can	182	9	21	2297	2	6.9	2.1	23	34%

Food Name	Serving Size	Calories	Prot. gms	Carbs gms	Sod. mgs	Fiber gms	Fat gms	Sat. Fat gms	Chol. mgs	% Fat Cal.
prepared	1 cup	75	4	9	945	1	2.8	0.8	10	34%
unprepared	10.5-oz can	182	9	21	2298	2	6.9	2.1	21	33%
unprepared	1 cup	150	7	17	1897	2	5.7	1.7	17	33%
(Campbell's) 'Healthy Request' unprepared	1/2 cup	80	3	12	480	1	2.0	0.5	5	23%
Canned, ready to use										
chunky.	19-oz can	372	28	42	2399	na	10.8	3.2	38	26%
chunky.	1 cup	166	12	19	1068	na	4.8	1.4	17	26%
(Campbell's)										
'Chunky'	9.5 oz	170	10	19	1080	0	6.0	0.0	25	32%
hearty, 'Healthy Request'.	1 cup	120	7	16	420	0	3.0	0.0	10	23%
'Home Cookin'.	10-3/4 oz	180	11	25	970	0	4.0	0.0	0	20%
low-sodium, 'Chunky'	10-3/4 oz	240	15	21	95	0	11.0	0.0	10	41%
(Hain)										
	9.5 oz	120	8	14	930	0	4.0	0.0	15	29%
no salt added.	9.5 oz	130	8	14	100	0	4.0	0.0	20	29%
(Health Valley)										
chunky.	7.5 oz	125	7	20	425	4	2.0	0.0	11	14%
chunky, no salt added	7.5 oz	125	7	20	60	4	2.0	0.0	11	14%
(Hormel) and rice, micro cup, 'Hearty Soups'	1 container	114	5	16	1025	0	3.0	0.0	7	24%
(Pritikin)	1 cup	70	5	12	150	2	1.0	1.0	5	12%
(Progresso)	9.5 oz	140	9	17	800	0	4.0	0.0	25	26%
CHILI BEEF										
Canned, condensed										
prepared	1 cup	170	7	21	1035	10	6.6	3.4	13	35%
unprepared	11.25-oz can	412	16	52	2514	23	16.0	8.0	32	35%
unprepared	1 cup	339	13	43	2072	19	13.2	6.6	26	35%
(Campbell's) prepared.	1 cup	140	5	20	840	0	5.0	0.0	10	31%
(Stouffer's) w/beans, food service product, prepared	1 cup	144	8	19	583	6	3.2	0.8	10	21%
Canned, ready to use										
(Campbell's)										
'Chunky'	11 oz	290	21	37	1120	0	7.0	0.0	0	21%
'Microwave'	7.5 oz	190	7	32	870	0	4.0	0.0	0	19%
(Healthy Choice)	1 cup	170	15	29	440	6	1.5	0.5	3	7%
Frozen										
(Kettle Ready)										
jalapeño.	3/4 cup	173	11	15	531	0	8.0	2.1	0	41%
traditional.	3/4 cup	161	12	14	454	0	6.5	2.0	0	36%
(Soup Supreme)										
panhandle, food service product.	1 cup	200	14	16	1100	4	10.0	4.0	35	43%
w/beans, classic, food service product	1 cup	250	19	23	1020	7	10.0	4.0	45	35%
w/beans, grande, food service product	1 cup	250	18	23	1080	6	10.0	4.0	45	35%
CLAM CHOWDER										
Canned, condensed										
Manhattan, prepared.	10.75-oz can	190	5	30	1405	4	5.4	0.9	6	26%
Manhattan, prepared.	1 cup	78	2	12	578	1	2.2	0.4	2	26%
Manhattan, unprepared.	10.75-oz can	186	5	30	1394	4	5.4	0.9	6	26%
Manhattan, unprepared.	1 cup	153	4	24	1147	3	4.4	0.8	5	26%
New England, prepared w/milk.	10.75-oz can	397	23	40	2408	4	16.0	7.2	54	36%
New England, prepared w/milk.	1 cup	164	9	17	992	1	6.6	3.0	22	36%
New England, prepared w/water.	10.75-oz can	231	12	30	2224	4	7.0	1.0	12	27%
New England, prepared w/water.	1 cup	95	5	12	915	1	2.9	0.4	5	27%
New England, unprepared	10.75-oz can	214	13	27	2266	2	6.1	0.9	12	25%
New England, unprepared	1 cup	176	11	22	1865	2	5.0	0.8	10	25%

Food Name	Serving Size	Calories	Prot. gms	Carbs gms	Sod. mgs	Fiber gms	Fat gms	Sat. Fat gms	Chol. mgs	% Fat Cal.
(Campbell's)										
Manhattan style, 'Seashore Soups' unprepared	1/2 cup	70	2	10	820	0	2.0	0.0	5	27%
New England, prepared w/whole milk	1 cup	150	7	17	930	0	7.0	0.0	0	40%
New England, 'Seashore Soups' unprepared	1/2 cup	80	3	12	870	0	3.0	0.0	5	31%
(Doxsee) Manhattan, prepared	7.5 oz	70	3	11	780	0	2.0	0.0	0	24%
(Gorton's)										
New England, prepared w/whole milk	1/4 can	140	7	17	740	0	5.0	0.0	15	32%
New England, unprepared	3.75 oz	70	3	12	670	0	1.0	0.0	5	13%
(Snow's)										
Manhattan, prepared	7.5 oz	70	3	11	780	0	2.0	0.0	0	24%
Manhattan, unprepared	3.75 oz	70	3	9	630	0	2.0	0.0	0	27%
New England, prepared w/whole milk	7.5 oz	140	8	13	670	0	6.0	0.0	0	39%
New England, unprepared	3.75 oz	70	5	8	620	0	2.0	0.0	0	26%
(Stouffer's)										
Boston, food service product, prepared w/milk	1 cup	208	9	20	919	2	10.4	4.0	32	45%
Manhattan, food service product, prepared	1 cup	80	4	10	823	2	2.4	0.4	8	27%
New England, food service product, prepared w/whole milk	1 cup	248	11	21	999	2	13.6	6.4	40	49%
Canned, ready to use										
Manhattan, chunky	19-oz can	302	16	42	2248	6	7.6	4.7	32	23%
Manhattan, chunky	1 cup	134	7	19	1001	3	3.4	2.1	14	23%
(Campbell's)										
New England, 'Healthy Request'	1 cup	100	4	14	490	0	3.0	0.0	10	27%
New England, 'Home Cookin''	10-3/4 oz	260	8	15	1240	0	18.0	0.0	0	64%
(Gorton's)	7.5 oz	140	7	17	720	0	5.0	0.0	20	32%
(Hain) New England, ready to serve	9.25 oz	180	8	26	780	0	4.0	0.0	25	21%
(Health Valley)										
Manhattan	7.5 oz	110	6	15	510	13	2.0	0.0	15	18%
Manhattan, no salt added	7.5 oz	110	6	15	60	13	2.0	0.0	15	18%
(Healthy Choice) New England	1 cup	120	7	22	480	3	1.0	0.5	5	7%
(Hormel)										
New England, 'Hearty Soup'	7.5 oz	130	5	16	790	0	5.0	2.0	30	35%
New England, micro cup, 'Hearty Soups'	1 container	118	5	15	882	0	5.0	0.0	30	36%
(Progresso)										
Manhattan	1 cup	110	12	11	710	3	2.0	0.0	10	16%
New England	1 cup	180	6	17	850	2	10.0	3.0	15	49%
New England, 'Healthy Classics'	1 cup	117	5	20	529	1	2.0	0.5	5	15%
(Stouffer's)										
Boston, food service product, 'Heat 'N Serve'	1 cup	192	10	20	975	2	8.0	3.2	34	37%
New England, food service product, 'Heat 'N Serve'	1 cup	184	10	23	871	2	5.6	2.4	25	27%
(Weight Watchers) New England	7.5 oz	90	5	16	450	0	0.0	0.0	5	0%
Frozen										
(Kettle Ready)										
Boston	3/4 cup	131	4	13	417	0	7.3	1.5	0	50%
Manhattan	3/4 cup	69	4	8	549	0	2.6	0.5	0	34%
New England	3/4 cup	116	3	11	373	0	6.5	2.4	0	50%
(Myers) New England	9.75 oz	152	7	21	910	0	5.0	0.0	0	29%
(Soup Supreme)										
Boston, food service product	1 cup	200	11	17	940	1	10.0	3.0	30	45%
New England, food service product	1 cup	180	9	22	730	1	6.0	2.5	15	30%
(Stouffer's) New England	1 cup	180	8	16	790	0	9.0	0.0	0	46%
(Tabatchnick) New England	3/4 cup	98	6	14	255	0	2.0	0.0	0	18%
CONSOMMÉ										
Canned, condensed *(Campbell's)* beef, w/gelatin, prepared	1 cup	25	4	2	750	0	0.0	0.0	0	0%

Food Name	Serving Size	Calories	Prot. gms	Carbs gms	Sod. mgs	Fiber gms	Fat gms	Sat. Fat gms	Chol. mgs	% Fat Cal.
CORN AND BROCCOLI CHOWDER										
Frozen *(Kettle Ready)*	3/4 cup	102	1	13	323	0	5.0	1.8	0	44%
CORN										
Canned, condensed										
(Campbell's)										
golden, cream, prepared w/2% milk	1 cup	160	6	23	760	0	5.0	0.0	10	28%
golden, cream, prepared w/water	1 cup	110	2	18	700	0	3.0	0.0	5	25%
golden, cream, unprepared	1/2 cup	110	2	18	700	0	3.0	0.0	5	25%
Canned, ready to use										
(Health Valley)										
country, and vegetable	7.5 oz	70	4	13	290	3	0.0	0.0	0	0%
country, and vegetable, nonfat	1 cup	70	5	17	135	7	0.0	0.0	0	0%
CORN CHOWDER										
Canned, condensed										
(Snow's)										
New England, prepared w/milk	7.5 oz	150	5	18	640	0	6.0	0.0	0	37%
New England, unprepared	3.75 oz	80	2	13	590	0	2.0	0.0	0	23%
(Stouffer's) food service product, prepared w/whole milk	1 cup	264	7	28	1055	2	13.6	4.0	16	47%
Canned, ready to use										
(Progresso)	9.25 oz	200	5	22	840	0	10.0	0.0	10	45%
(Stouffer's) 'Heat 'N Serve'	1 cup	280	6	21	791	2	20.0	2.4	5	63%
Frozen *(Soup Supreme)* Captain's	1 cup	200	6	29	770	2	7.0	2.0	5	31%
CRAB										
Canned, condensed										
(Stouffer's) Maryland, food service product, prepared	1 cup	80	3	10	735	3	2.4	0.8	18	28%
Canned, ready to use										
	13-oz can	114	8	16	1867	1	2.3	0.6	15	18%
	1 cup	76	5	10	1235	1	1.5	0.4	10	18%
CREOLE										
Canned, ready to use *(Campbell's)* 'Chunky'	10-3/4 oz	240	11	31	910	0	8.0	0.0	0	30%
Frozen *(Soup Supreme)* Southern style	1 cup	110	4	20	1660	2	3.0	0.5	5	22%
ESCAROLE										
Canned, ready to use										
	19.5-oz can	61	3	4	8616	na	4.0	1.2	6	60%
	1 cup	27	2	2	3864	na	1.8	0.5	2	60%
(Progresso) in chicken broth	9.25 oz	30	2	2	1100	0	1.0	0.0	5	36%
FISH CHOWDER										
Canned, condensed										
(Snow's)										
New England, prepared w/whole milk	7.5 oz	130	9	11	620	0	6.0	0.0	0	40%
New England, unprepared	3.75 oz	60	5	6	560	0	2.0	0.0	0	29%
GARLIC AND PASTA										
Canned, ready to use *(Progresso)* 'Healthy Classics'	1 cup	100	4	18	450	3	1.3	0.3	5	12%
GAZPACHO										
Canned, ready to use										
	13-oz can	70	11	7	1118	1	0.4	0.0	0	5%
	1 cup	46	7	4	739	0	0.2	0.0	0	5%
GREEN PEA										
Canned, condensed										
prepared w/milk	11.25-oz can	579	31	78	2353	7	17.1	9.7	43	26%
prepared w/milk	1 cup	239	13	32	970	3	7.0	4.0	18	26%
prepared w/water	1 cup	165	9	27	918	3	2.9	1.4	0	16%
unprepared	11.25-oz can	399	21	64	2227	7	7.1	3.4	0	16%
unprepared	1 cup	329	17	53	1836	6	5.9	2.8	0	16%

Food Name	Serving Size	Calories	Prot. gms	Carbs gms	Sod. mgs	Fiber gms	Fat gms	Sat. Fat gms	Chol. mgs	% Fat Cal.
HAM AND BEAN										
Canned, ready to use										
(Campbell's) w/butter beans, 'Chunky'.	10-3/4 oz	280	12	34	1180	0	10.0	0.0	0	33%
(Progresso)	9.5 oz	140	11	28	950	8	2.0	0.0	10	10%
ITALIAN STYLE WEDDING										
Canned, condensed										
(Stouffer's) food service product, prepared	1 cup	216	10	25	1790	na	8.0	na	29	34%
LEMON, canned, ready to use (Great Impressions)	3/4 cup	90	0	22	109	0	1.0	0.0	0	9%
LENTIL										
Canned, ready to use										
w/ham	20-oz can	318	21	46	3016	na	6.3	2.6	17	18%
w/ham	1 cup	139	9	20	1319	na	2.8	1.1	7	18%
(Hain)										
.	9.5 oz	160	9	25	690	0	3.0	0.0	5	17%
no salt added.	9.5 oz	160	9	24	65	0	3.0	0.0	5	17%
(Health Valley)										
.	7.5 oz	170	9	28	435	17	2.0	0.0	0	11%
and carrot, nonfat	1 cup	90	10	25	220	14	0.0	0.0	0	0%
no salt added.	7.5 oz	170	9	28	25	17	2.0	0.0	0	11%
(Healthy Choice)	1 cup	140	9	28	470	4	1.0	0.0	0	6%
(Progresso)										
.	1 cup	140	9	22	750	7	2.0	0.0	0	13%
'Healthy Classics'	1 cup	126	8	20	443	6	1.5	0.3	0	11%
w/sausage.	9.5 oz	170	8	21	840	5	8.0	0.0	20	38%
Frozen (Tabatchnick)	7.5 oz	170	11	27	240	0	2.0	0.0	0	11%
MACARONI AND BEAN										
Canned, ready to use (Progresso)	10-1/2 oz	150	9	27	1020	8	4.0	0.0	0	20%
MENUDO, canned, ready to use (Old El Paso)	1/2 can	476	15	14	770	2	52.0	21.0	176	80%
MINESTRONE										
Canned, condensed										
prepared	10.5-oz can	199	10	27	2215	2	6.1	1.3	6	27%
prepared	1 cup	82	4	11	911	1	2.5	0.6	2	27%
unprepared	10.5-oz can	203	10	27	2217	2	6.1	1.3	3	27%
unprepared	1 cup	167	9	23	1830	2	5.0	1.1	2	27%
(Campbell's) 'Healthy Request' unprepared.	1/2 cup	90	4	17	480	2	1.0	0.5	0	10%
(Stouffer's) food service product, prepared	1 cup	104	4	16	959	2	2.4	0.8	4	22%
Canned, ready to use										
chunky.	19-oz can	286	11	47	1940	13	6.3	3.3	11	20%
chunky.	1 cup	127	5	21	864	6	2.8	1.5	5	20%
(Campbell's) hearty, 'Healthy Request'	1 cup	120	4	24	480	3	2.0	0.5	3	14%
(Hain)										
.	9.5 oz	170	8	27	1060	0	2.0	0.0	0	11%
no salt added.	9.5 oz	160	7	28	35	0	4.0	0.0	0	20%
(Health Valley)										
.	7.5 oz	130	6	19	637	13	3.0	0.0	0	21%
no salt added.	7.5 oz	130	6	19	80	13	3.0	0.0	0	21%
nonfat	1 cup	80	8	21	210	11	0.0	0.0	0	0%
(Healthy Choice)	1 cup	110	4	24	480	5	1.0	0.0	0	7%
(Hormel)										
'Hearty Soups'.	7.5 oz	100	5	17	460	0	1.0	2.0	5	9%
micro cup, 'Hearty Soups'	1 container	104	7	15	903	0	2.0	0.0	10	17%
(Lipton) 'Hearty Ones'	11 oz	189	8	36	821	0	3.2	0.0	6	14%
(Progresso)										
.	1 cup	130	6	22	960	5	2.5	0.5	0	17%
chunky, hearty.	9.25 oz	110	7	16	740	0	2.0	0.0	5	16%

Food Name	Serving Size	Calories	Prot. gms	Carbs gms	Sod. mgs	Fiber gms	Fat gms	Sat. Fat gms	Chol. mgs	% Fat Cal.
chunky, zesty	9.5 oz	150	7	19	1130	4	8.0	0.0	10	41%
'Healthy Classics'	1 cup	123	5	20	470	1	2.5	0.4	0	19%
(Stouffer's) food service product, 'Heat 'N Serve'	1 cup	80	3	10	871	2	2.4	0.8	5	28%
Frozen										
(Kettle Ready) hearty	3/4 cup	104	3	15	577	0	4.4	1.1	0	35%
(Soup Supreme) food service product	1 cup	70	3	11	1030	2	2.5	0.0	0	29%
(Tabatchnick)	7.5 oz	137	8	24	265	0	2.0	0.0	0	12%
MUSHROOM										
Canned, condensed										
w/beef stock, prepared	10.75-oz can	208	8	23	2354	2	9.8	3.8	18	42%
w/beef stock, prepared	1 cup	85	3	9	969	1	4.0	1.6	7	42%
w/beef stock, unprepared	10.75-oz can	207	8	23	2358	0	9.8	3.8	18	42%
w/beef stock, unprepared	1 cup	171	6	19	1940	0	8.1	3.1	15	42%
(Campbell's)										
beefy, prepared	1 cup	60	4	5	960	0	3.0	0.0	10	43%
w/ground beef, prepared	1 cup	90	4	10	820	0	4.0	0.0	25	39%
MUSHROOM, CREAM OF										
Canned, condensed										
prepared w/milk	10.75-oz can	494	15	36	2227	1	33.0	12.5	48	59%
prepared w/milk	1 cup	203	6	15	918	0	13.6	5.1	20	59%
prepared w/water	10.75-oz can	314	6	23	2141	1	21.8	5.9	6	61%
prepared w/water	1 cup	129	2	9	881	0	9.0	2.4	2	61%
unprepared	10.75-oz can	314	5	23	2111	1	23.1	6.3	3	65%
unprepared	1 cup	259	4	19	1737	1	19.0	5.1	3	65%
(Campbell's)										
'Healthy Request' unprepared	1/2 cup	70	1	10	480	0	2.5	1.0	10	34%
98% nonfat, unprepared	1/2 cup	70	1	9	830	0	3.0	1.0	3	40%
Canned, ready to use										
(Campbell's) low-sodium	10 1/2 oz	210	3	18	55	0	14.0	0.0	0	60%
(Hain) creamy	9.25 oz	110	4	16	740	0	4.0	0.0	15	31%
(Progresso)	9.25 oz	160	4	14	1120	0	10.0	0.0	15	56%
(Weight Watchers)	10 1/2 oz	90	3	14	1250	0	2.0	0.0	0	21%
Frozen										
(Kettle Ready)	3/4 cup	85	1	6	371	0	6.4	2.4	0	68%
(Soup Supreme) food service product	1 cup	200	4	13	940	1	15.0	4.0	10	67%
(Tabatchnick)	3/4 cup	75	3	11	325	0	2.0	0.0	3	24%
MUSHROOM BARLEY										
Canned, condensed										
prepared	10.75-oz can	178	5	28	2164	2	5.5	1.1	0	28%
prepared	1 cup	73	2	12	891	1	2.3	0.4	0	28%
unprepared	10.75-oz can	186	5	29	2227	na	5.5	1.1	0	27%
unprepared	1 cup	153	4	24	1832	na	4.5	0.9	0	27%
Canned, ready to use										
(Hain)	9.5 oz	100	4	17	600	0	2.0	0.0	10	18%
(Health Valley)										
	7.5 oz	100	5	16	394	9	2.0	0.0	0	18%
no salt added	7.5 oz	100	5	16	20	9	2.0	0.0	0	18%
Frozen										
(Tabatchnick)										
	7.5 oz	92	2	16	234	0	2.0	0.0	0	20%
'No Salt'	7.5 oz	97	4	18	77	0	1.0	0.0	0	9%
ONION										
Canned, condensed										
prepared	10.5-oz can	141	9	20	2561	2	4.2	0.6	0	26%
prepared	1 cup	58	4	8	1053	1	1.7	0.3	0	26%

Food Name	Serving Size	Calories	Prot. gms	Carbs gms	Sod. mgs	Fiber gms	Fat gms	Sat. Fat gms	Chol. mgs	% Fat Cal.
unprepared	10.5-oz can	137	9	20	2563	2	4.2	0.6	0	26%
unprepared	1 cup	113	8	16	2116	2	3.5	0.5	0	26%
(Stouffer's) French, food service product, prepared	1 cup	72	1	9	1551	2	2.4	0.8	4	35%
Frozen										
(Kettle Ready) French	3/4 cup	42	1	5	562	0	2.2	0.4	0	46%
(Soup Supreme) French, food service product	1 cup	80	2	11	1110	1	4.0	0.5	0	41%
ONION, CREAM OF										
Canned, condensed										
prepared w/milk	10.75-oz can	452	16	45	2438	2	22.8	9.8	78	44%
prepared w/milk	1 cup	186	7	18	1004	1	9,4	4.0	32	44%
prepared w/water	10.75-oz can	261	7	31	2253	2	12.8	3.6	36	43%
prepared w/water	1 cup	107	3	13	927	1	5,3	1.5	15	43%
unprepared	10.75-oz can	268	7	32	2318	1	12.8	3.6	37	42%
unprepared	1 cup	221	6	26	1908	1	10.5	2.9	30	42%
(Campbell's)										
prepared w/4 oz soup, 2 oz whole milk, 2 oz water	1 cup	140	4	15	860	0	7.0	0.0	0	45%
PEA										
Frozen										
(Kettle Ready) tortellini, in tomato	3/4 cup	122	4	15	447	0	5.4	1.3	0	40%
(Tabatchnick)										
	7.5 oz	175	10	31	290	0	1.0	0.0	0	5%
'No Salt'	7.5 oz	175	10	31	79	0	1.0	0.0	0	5%
PEPPER POT										
Canned, condensed										
prepared	1 cup	104	6	9	971	0	4.6	2.0	10	40%
prepared	10.5-oz can	252	15	23	2362	1	11.3	5.0	23	40%
unprepared	10.5-oz can	250	15	23	2360	1	11.3	5.0	24	41%
unprepared	1 cup	207	13	19	1948	1	9.3	4.1	20	41%
POT ROAST										
Frozen (Soup Supreme) Yankee, food service product	1 cup	90	6	13	730	2	1.5	0.0	15	15%
POTATO, CREAM OF										
Canned, condensed										
prepared w/milk	10.75-oz can	361	14	42	2577	1	15.7	9.2	54	38%
prepared w/milk	1 cup	149	6	17	1061	0	6.4	3.8	22	38%
prepared w/water	10.75-oz can	178	4	28	2431	1	5.8	3.0	12	28%
prepared w/water	1 cup	73	2	11	1000	0	2.4	1.2	5	28%
unprepared	10.75-oz can	180	4	28	2431	1	5.7	3.0	15	28%
unprepared	1 cup	148	3	23	2000	1	4.7	2.4	13	28%
(Campbell's) prepared w/tofu, 1 tbsp oil	1 cup	120	3	15	900	0	4.0	0.0	0	33%
(Stouffer's) food service product, prepared										
w/whole milk	1 cup	264	9	28	1127	2	12.8	5.6	32	44%
Frozen (Soup Supreme) food service product	1 cup	190	5	22	750	1	9.0	3.0	5	43%
Canned, ready to use										
(Andersen's)	7.5 oz	200	4	25	630	0	10.0	0.0	0	44%
(Stouffer's) food service product, 'Heat 'N Serve'	1 cup	240	10	28	1031	2	9.6	3.2	22	36%
POTATO-LEEK										
Canned, ready to use										
(Health Valley)										
	7.5 oz	130	4	23	360	7	2.0	0.0	0	14%
no salt added	7.5 oz	130	4	23	20	7	2.0	0.0	0	14%
RED BEAN AND RICE, (Norpac) lowfat, 'Soup Supreme'	1 cup	130	5	26	770	5	1.5	0.0	0	10%
SCHAV, canned, ready to serve (Gold's)	1 cup	25	2	4	1380	0	0.0	0.0	15	0%
SCOTCH BROTH										
Canned, condensed										
prepared	10.5-oz can	193	12	23	2461	3	6.4	2.7	12	30%

Food Name	Serving Size	Calories	Prot. gms	Carbs gms	Sod. mgs	Fiber gms	Fat gms	Sat. Fat gms	Chol. mgs	% Fat Cal.
prepared	1 cup	80	5	9	1012	1	2.6	1.1	5	30%
unprepared	10.5-oz can	197	12	23	2461	3	6.4	2.7	12	29%
unprepared	1 cup	162	10	19	2032	2	5.3	2.2	10	29%
(Campbell's) prepared	1 cup	80	4	9	870	0	3.0	0.0	10	34%
SEAFOOD BISQUE, frozen *(Myers)*	9.75 oz	163	9	13	1393	0	8.0	0.0	0	45%
SEAFOOD CHOWDER										
Canned, condensed										
(Snow's)										
New England, prepared w/whole milk	7.5 oz	140	8	14	670	0	6.0	0.0	0	38%
New England, unprepared	3.75 oz	60	4	6	640	0	2.0	0.0	0	31%
SEAFOOD GUMBO										
Frozen *(Soup Supreme)* food service product	1 cup	90	5	14	900	1	1.5	0.0	20	15%
SHRIMP AND OKRA GUMBO										
Frozen										
(Soup Supreme) Southern style, food service product	1 cup	110	5	16	1660	1	3.0	0.5	20	24%
SHRIMP, CREAM OF										
Canned, condensed										
prepared w/milk	10.75-oz can	397	17	34	2516	1	22.6	14.0	84	51%
prepared w/milk	1 cup	164	7	14	1037	0	9.3	5.8	35	51%
unprepared	10.75-oz can	220	7	20	2373	1	12.6	7.9	40	51%
unprepared	1 cup	181	6	16	1953	1	10.4	6.5	33	51%
(Campbell's)										
'Seashore Soups' prepared w/2% milk	1/2 cup	140	5	13	810	0	10.0	3.0	20	56%
'Seashore Soups' prepared w/whole milk	1 cup	160	5	13	860	0	10.0	0.0	0	56%
'Seashore Soups' unprepared	1/2 cup	90	2	8	810	0	6.0	2.0	20	57%
SIRLOIN BURGER										
Canned, ready to use *(Campbell's)* 'Chunky'	10-3/4 oz	220	12	23	1240	0	9.0	0.0	0	37%
SPINACH, CREAM OF										
Frozen										
(Myers)	9.75 oz	174	9	10	905	0	11.0	0.0	0	57%
(Stouffer's)	3/4 cup	210	7	12	1020	0	15.0	0.0	0	64%
(Tabatchnick)	3/4 cup	85	5	12	200	0	2.0	0.0	4	21%
SPLIT PEA										
Canned, condensed										
w/ham, prepared w/milk	11.5-oz can	461	25	68	2444	6	10.7	4.3	18	21%
w/ham, prepared w/water	1 cup	190	10	28	1007	2	4.4	1.8	8	21%
w/ham, unprepared	11.5-oz can	460	25	68	2445	6	10.7	4.3	20	21%
w/ham, unprepared	1 cup	379	21	56	2018	5	8.8	3.5	16	21%
(Campbell's) w/ham and bacon, prepared w/water	1 cup	160	9	24	780	0	4.0	0.0	5	21%
(Rokeach) w/egg barley, prepared w/water	1 cup	132	8	24	757	0	0.5	0.0	0	3%
(Stouffer's) w/ham, food service product, prepared w/water	1 cup	176	11	29	1103	6	1.6	0.4	7	8%
Canned, ready to use										
w/ham, chunky	19-oz can	415	25	60	2167	9	8.9	3.6	16	19%
w/ham, chunky	1 cup	185	11	27	965	4	4.0	1.6	7	19%
(Andersen's) nonfat	7.5 oz	130	9	24	770	0	0.0	0.0	0	0%
(Campbell's) low-salt	1 cup	240	12	38	50	5	4.0	3.0	5	15%
(Grandma Brown's)	1 cup	208	12	31	522	6	4.1	0.0	1	18%
(Hain)										
	9.5 oz	170	11	28	970	0	1.0	0.0	0	5%
no salt added	9.5 oz	170	11	29	40	0	1.0	0.0	0	5%
(Health Valley)										
and carrot, nonfat	1 cup	110	8	17	230	4	0.0	0.0	0	0%
green	7.5 oz	190	11	34	276	15	0.3	0.0	0	1%
no salt added	7.5 oz	190	11	34	25	15	0.3	0.0	0	1%

Food Name	Serving Size	Calories	Prot. gms	Carbs gms	Sod. mgs	Fiber gms	Fat gms	Sat. Fat gms	Chol. mgs	% Fat Cal.
(Healthy Choice) and ham............................	1 cup	160	13	25	480	3	1.5	1.0	3	8%
(Progresso)										
green..	10 1/2 oz	201	12	31	920	0	3.0	0.0	0	14%
'Healthy Classics'.................................	1 cup	180	10	30	420	5	2.3	0.8	5	12%
w/ham...	1 cup	160	9	20	830	5	4.0	1.5	15	24%
Frozen										
(Kettle Ready) w/ham............................	3/4 cup	155	11	25	483	0	4.4	1.3	0	21%
(Soup Supreme) w/ham, food service product	1 cup	120	9	18	1030	6	1.5	0.0	5	11%
STOCKPOT										
Canned, condensed										
prepared	11-oz can	240	12	28	2544	na	9.5	2.1	12	36%
prepared	1 cup	99	5	11	1047	na	3.9	0.9	5	36%
unprepared	11-oz can	243	12	28	2546	na	9.5	2.1	9	35%
unprepared	1 cup	200	10	23	2097	na	7.8	1.7	8	35%
TOMATO										
Canned, condensed										
prepared w/milk....................................	10.75-oz can	391	15	54	1806	7	14.6	7.0	42	32%
prepared w/milk....................................	1 cup	161	6	22	744	3	6.0	2.9	17	32%
prepared w/water	10.75-oz can	208	5	40	1690	1	4.7	0.9	0	20%
prepared w/water	1 cup	85	2	17	695	0	1.9	0.4	0	20%
unprepared	10.75-oz can	207	5	40	1690	1	4.7	0.9	0	20%
unprepared	1 cup	171	4	33	1391	1	3.8	0.7	0	20%
(Campbell's)										
'Healthy Request' unprepared......................	1/2 cup	90	1	18	460	1	1.5	0.5	0	15%
'Healthy Request' prepared w/1/2 cup 2% milk..........	1 cup	140	5	22	490	0	3.0	0.0	5	20%
'Healthy Request' prepared w/water	1 cup	90	1	17	430	0	2.0	0.0	0	20%
'Healthy Request' prepared w/whole milk..............	1 cup	150	5	22	490	0	4.0	0.0	10	25%
(Stouffer's)										
hearty, food service product, prepared w/water	1 cup	96	3	13	1031	2	3.2	1.2	4	31%
Canned, ready to use										
(Campbell's) w/tomato pieces, low-salt.................	1 cup	170	4	28	60	2	6.0	2.5	10	30%
(Health Valley)										
....	7.5 oz	100	2	17	450	1	3.0	0.0	0	26%
no salt added..	7.5 oz	100	2	17	40	1	3.0	0.0	0	26%
(Healthy Choice) garden	1 cup	100	5	19	420	5	1.5	0.5	0	12%
(Progresso)										
....	9.5 oz	120	4	20	1100	0	3.0	0.0	0	22%
garden, 'Healthy Classics'...........................	1 cup	99	3	19	480	4	1.0	0.2	0	9%
(Stouffer's)										
garden, food service product, 'Heat 'N Serve'...........	1 cup	112	2	10	863	3	7.2	0.8	14	56%
Frozen										
(Soup Supreme)										
basil, vegetarian, low-fat, food service product..........	1 cup	100	3	15	690	1	3.0	1.5	5	27%
Florentine, food service product	1 cup	90	3	16	1000	2	1.5	0.0	0	15%
TOMATO, CREAM OF										
Canned, condensed										
(Campbell's)										
'Healthy Request' prepared w/nonfat milk.............	1/2 cup	130	5	22	490	0	2.0	0.0	5	14%
'Homestyle' prepared w/water.......................	1 cup	110	1	20	810	0	3.0	0.0	5	24%
'Homestyle' prepared w/whole milk...................	1 cup	180	5	25	860	0	7.0	0.0	0	34%
prepared w/whole milk..............................	1 cup	150	5	22	740	0	4.0	0.0	0	25%
zesty, prepared w/water	1 cup	100	1	20	760	0	2.0	0.0	0	18%
TOMATO BEEF										
Canned, condensed										
w/noodles, prepared	10.75-oz can	338	11	51	2230	4	10.4	3.9	12	28%

Food Name	Serving Size	Calories	Prot. gms	Carbs gms	Sod. mgs	Fiber gms	Fat gms	Sat. Fat gms	Chol. mgs	% Fat Cal.
w/noodles, prepared	1 cup	139	4	21	917	1	4.3	1.6	5	28%
w/noodles, unprepared	10.75-oz can	342	11	51	2230	4	10.4	3.9	9	27%
w/noodles, unprepared	1 cup	281	9	42	1835	3	8.6	3.2	8	27%
Canned, ready to use (Progresso) w/rotini	9.5 oz	170	12	18	930	0	6.0	0.0	30	31%
TOMATO BISQUE										
Canned, condensed										
prepared w/milk	11-oz can	481	15	71	2692	1	16.0	7.6	55	29%
prepared w/milk	1 cup	198	6	29	1109	1	6.6	3.1	23	29%
unprepared	11-oz can	300	5	58	2546	2	6.1	1.3	12	18%
unprepared	1 cup	247	5	47	2097	2	5.0	1.1	10	18%
TOMATO RICE										
Canned, condensed										
prepared	11-oz can	288	5	53	1980	4	6.6	1.3	6	20%
prepared	1 cup	119	2	22	815	1	2.7	0.5	2	20%
unprepared	1 cup	239	4	44	1632	3	5.4	1.0	3	20%
unprepared	11-oz can	290	5	53	1981	4	6.6	1.2	3	20%
Frozen (Tabatchnick)	3/4 cup	73	2	14	300	0	1.0	0.0	0	12%
TOMATO TORTELLINI, canned, ready to use (Progresso)	1 cup	120	5	13	910	2	5.0	1.5	10	38%
TOMATO VEGETABLE										
Canned, ready to use (Health Valley) nonfat	1 cup	80	6	17	240	5	0.0	0.0	0	0%
TORTELLINI										
Canned, ready to use										
(Progresso)										
	9.5 oz	90	5	11	930	0	3.0	0.0	10	30%
creamy	9.25 oz	240	5	17	910	0	16.0	8.5	35	62%
TURKEY										
Canned, condensed										
prepared	10.75-oz can	166	9	21	1981	2	4.9	1.4	12	26%
prepared	1 cup	68	4	9	815	1	2.0	0.6	5	26%
unprepared	10.75-oz can	168	9	21	1983	2	4.8	1.3	12	26%
unprepared	1 cup	138	8	17	1632	2	4.0	1.1	10	26%
Canned, ready to use										
chunky	18.75-oz can	303	23	32	2080	na	9.9	2.8	21	29%
chunky	1 cup	135	10	14	923	na	4.4	1.2	9	29%
TURKEY RICE										
Canned, ready to use										
(Hain)										
	9.5 oz	100	8	10	970	0	3.0	0.0	20	27%
no salt added	9.5 oz	120	7	13	85	0	4.0	0.0	15	31%
(Healthy Choice) white and wild rice	1 cup	90	7	14	415	2	2.0	0.5	3	18%
TURKEY VEGETABLE										
Canned, condensed										
prepared	10.5-oz can	176	8	21	2203	1	7.4	2.2	6	38%
prepared	1 cup	72	3	9	906	0	3.0	0.9	2	38%
unprepared	10.5-oz can	179	8	21	2202	1	7.4	2.2	3	37%
unprepared	1 cup	148	6	17	1818	1	6.1	1.8	2	37%
Canned, ready to use										
(Campbell's) 'Chunky'	9 3/1 cup	150	9	16	1060	0	6.0	0.0	0	35%
(Weight Watchers)	10 1/2 oz	70	4	10	1020	0	2.0	0.0	0	24%
VEGETABLE										
Canned, condensed										
(Campbell's)										
'Healthy Request' unprepared	1/2 cup	90	3	16	480	2	1.0	0.0	5	11%
'Homestyle' prepared	1 cup	60	2	9	880	0	2.0	0.0	0	29%
vegetarian	1/2 cup	60	2	14	720	2	0.0	0.0	0	0%

Food Name	Serving Size	Calories	Prot. gms	Carbs gms	Sod. mgs	Fiber gms	Fat gms	Sat. Fat gms	Chol. mgs	% Fat Cal.
w/pasta, 'Healthy Request' unprepared	1/2 cup	90	2	18	830	2	1.0	0.0	0	10%
w/pasta, hearty, prepared	1 cup	70	3	15	800	0	1.0	0.0	0	11%
(Stouffer's) vegetarian, food service product, prepared	1 cup	96	2	14	783	3	2.4	0.4	0	24%
Canned, ready to use										
chunky	19-oz can	275	8	43	2269	3	8.3	1.2	0	27%
chunky	1 cup	122	4	19	1010	1	3.7	0.6	0	27%
(Campbell's)										
hearty, 'Healthy Request'	1 cup	100	3	20	470	2	1.0	0.0	0	9%
Mediterranean, 'Chunky' ready to serve	9.5 oz	170	4	24	1010	0	6.0	0.0	0	33%
(Hain)										
Italian, w/pasta	9.5 oz	160	4	25	910	0	5.0	0.0	20	28%
Italian, w/pasta, low-sodium	9.5 oz	140	4	22	90	0	6.0	0.0	20	34%
vegetarian	9.5 oz	140	4	22	920	0	4.0	0.0	0	26%
vegetarian, no salt added	9.5 oz	150	5	23	45	0	5.0	0.0	0	29%
(Health Valley)										
	7.5 oz	110	4	20	296	4	1.0	0.0	0	9%
5-bean, chunky, no salt added	7.5 oz	110	4	21	56	11	2.0	0.0	0	15%
5-bean, nonfat	1 cup	140	10	32	250	13	0.0	0.0	0	0%
no salt added	7.5 oz	110	4	20	40	4	1.0	0.0	0	9%
power carotene	1 cup	70	5	17	240	6	0.0	0.0	0	0%
(Healthy Choice)										
country	1 cup	100	5	22	430	5	0.5	0.0	0	4%
garden	1 cup	120	6	24	480	3	1.0	0.0	0	7%
(Hormel)										
country, 'Hearty Soups'	7.5 oz	90	4	14	730	0	2.0	2.0	2	20%
country, micro cup, ' Hearty Soups'	1 container	89	5	13	865	0	2.0	0.0	1	20%
(Lunch Bucket) country, microwave cup	7.25 oz	70	1	15	740	0	1.0	0.0	0	12%
(Norpac) vegetarian, low-fat, 'Soup Supreme'	1 cup	70	3	13	560	3	1.5	0.0	0	17%
(Progresso)										
	9.5 oz	80	4	15	1190	4	2.0	0.0	5	19%
'Healthy Classics'	1 cup	81	4	13	466	1	1.3	0.3	5	14%
(Stouffer's)										
vegetarian, food service product, 'Heat 'N Serve'	1 cup	96	3	16	823	4	2.4	0.8	0	22%
(Westbrae)										
Sante Fe, nonfat	1 cup	115	6	23	570	4	0.0	0.0	0	0%
Southwest, spicy, nonfat	1 cup	70	4	15	500	2	0.0	0.0	0	0%
(Weight Watchers)										
vegetarian, chunky	10 1/2 oz	100	3	18	1250	0	2.0	0.0	0	18%
w/beef stock	10 1/2 oz	90	4	13	1370	0	2.0	0.0	0	21%
Frozen										
(Kettle Ready) garden	3/4 cup	85	3	12	296	0	3.0	0.5	0	31%
(Soup Supreme)										
harvest, food service product	1 cup	90	3	17	960	3	1.5	0.5	0	14%
Italian, zesty, food service product	1 cup	70	3	14	720	2	1.0	0.0	0	12%
(Tabatchnick)										
	7.5 oz	97	4	18	190	0	1.0	0.0	0	9%
no salt	7.5 oz	92	2	16	77	0	2.0	0.0	0	20%
VEGETABLE BARLEY										
Canned, ready to use *(Health Valley)* nonfat	1 cup	90	6	19	210	4	0.0	0.0	0	0%
VEGETABLE BEEF										
Canned, condensed										
prepared	10.5-oz can	199	7	32	1969	1	4.6	1.1	6	21%
prepared	1 cup	82	3	13	810	0	1.9	0.4	2	21%
unprepared	10.5-oz can	197	7	32	1970	4	4.6	1.1	3	21%

Food Name	Serving Size	Calories	Prot. gms	Carbs gms	Sod. mgs	Fiber gms	Fat gms	Sat. Fat gms	Chol. mgs	% Fat Cal.
unprepared	1 cup	162	6	26	1626	3	3.8	0.9	2	21%
(Campbell's)										
'Healthy Request' prepared	1 cup	70	4	10	470	0	2.0	0.0	10	24%
'Healthy Request' unprepared	1/2 cup	80	5	11	480	2	2.0	1.0	5	22%
(Stouffer's) w/barley, food service product, prepared	1 cup	144	4	12	1103	2	8.8	2.4	11	55%
Canned, ready to use										
(Campbell's)										
hearty, 'Healthy Request'	1 cup	140	9	20	480	3	2.5	1.0	20	16%
low-salt, 'Chunky'	1 cup	160	13	11	95	4	4.5	1.5	80	30%
old-fashioned, 'Chunky'	10-3/4 oz	190	13	20	1100	0	6.0	0.0	25	29%
(Stouffer's) w/barley, 'Heat 'N Serve'	1 cup	144	6	11	943	2	8.8	0.8	9	54%
(Weight Watchers) microwave cup	7.5 oz	90	8	13	450	0	1.0	0.0	10	10%
Frozen										
(Myers)	9.75 oz	120	9	8	1030	0	6.0	0.0	0	44%
(Soup Supreme)										
food service product	1 cup	80	5	14	1020	2	1.5	0.0	10	15%
w/barley, food service product	1 cup	90	5	14	830	2	2.0	1.0	10	19%
VEGETABLE BROTH										
Canned, ready to use										
(Hain)										
	9.5 oz	45	1	10	1180	0	0.0	0.0	0	0%
low-sodium	9.5 oz	40	1	8	85	0	1.0	0.0	0	20%
(Swanson) canned	1 cup	20	2	3	1000	0	1.0	0.0	0	31%
WILD RICE										
Canned, ready to use										
(Hain) 99% fat free, 'Healthy Naturals'	1 cup	80	2	15	480	1	2.0	0.5	0	21%
ZUCCHINI, frozen *(Tabatchnick)*	3/4 cup	80	3	12	285	0	2.0	0.0	3	23%
SOUP MIX										
ASPARAGUS, CREAM OF, prepared	1 cup	58	2	9	800	na	1.7	0.1	0	26%
BEAN										
w/bacon, prepared	1 cup	106	5	16	927	9	2.1	1.0	3	18%
(Bean Cuisine)										
'Island Black Bean' bag, prepared	1 cup	160	9	29	15	9	1.0	0.0	0	6%
'Island Black Bean' box, prepared	1 cup	126	7	24	7	8	1.0	1.0	0	7%
'Mesa Maise & Bean' prepared	1 cup	180	10	32	20	10	1.5	0.0	0	7%
'Rocky Mountain Red Bean' prepared	1 cup	190	11	35	15	12	1.5	0.0	0	7%
13-bean bouillabaisse, bag, prepared	1 cup	110	7	19	15	7	0.5	0.0	0	4%
13-bean bouillabaisse, box, prepared	1 cup	99	6	18	5	5	1.0	0.0	0	9%
'White Bean Provencal' bag, prepared	1 cup	180	10	32	15	11	1.0	0.0	0	5%
'White Bean Provencal' box, prepared	1 cup	103	6	19	7	6	1.0	0.0	0	8%
(Fantastic Foods) 5-bean, 'Hearty Soups' mix only	2.3 oz	230	12	43	480	10	1.0	0.0	0	4%
(Hodgson Mill) choice, no barley, mix only	1/4 cup	150	9	27	5	11	0.0	0.0	0	0%
(Hormel) w/ham, chowder 'Micro-Cup Hearty Soups' prepared	1 container	191	10	31	664	0	3.0	0.0	30	14%
BEEF										
broth, cubed, mix only	1 cube	9	1	1	611	0	0.3	0.2	0	34%
broth, dried, prepared	1 cup	19	1	2	1359	0	0.7	0.3	1	34%
(American Institutional) stock, concentrated, mix only	2 tsp	20	2	2	570	0	0.0	0.0	0	0%
(Soup Starter) hearty, 'Homestyle' mix only	27 grams	90	2	20	740	0	1.0	0.0	0	9%
(Tone's) base, mix only	1 tsp	11	0	1	1	0	0.6	0.0	0	49%
(Ultra Slim Fast) w/noodles, prepared	6 oz	45	5	7	700	2	1.0	0.0	5	16%
BEEF NOODLE										
prepared	1 cup	40	2	6	1042	1	0.8	0.3	3	18%

Food Name	Serving Size	Calories	Prot. gms	Carbs gms	Sod. mgs	Fiber gms	Fat gms	Sat. Fat gms	Chol. mgs	% Fat Cal.
(Campbell's)										
w/vegetables, prepared	6 oz	220	7	44	1600	0	2.0	0.0	0	8%
microwave cup, prepared	1.35 oz	130	6	23	1270	0	2.0	0.0	0	13%
'Ramen Noodle' prepared	6 oz	160	5	32	890	0	1.0	0.0	0	6%
(Estee) prepared	6 oz	20	1	3	140	0	1.0	1.0	1	36%
(Lipton)										
'Cup-A-Soup' prepared	6 oz	44	2	8	746	0	0.7	0.0	0	14%
hearty, prepared	6 oz	107	4	20	698	0	1.4	0.0	0	12%
BEEF VEGETABLE *(Soup Starter)* 'Homestyle' mix only	26 grams	90	3	18	790	0	1.0	0.0	0	10%
BOUILLON										
Beef flavor										
(Diamond Crystal) dried, instant, low-salt, mix only	1 serving	10	0	2	10	0	0.0	0.0	0	0%
(Featherweight) dried, instant, mix only	1 tsp	18	0	2	10	0	1.0	0.0	5	53%
(Herb-Ox)										
cubed, mix only	1 cube	5	0	1	900	0	0.0	0.0	0	0%
cubed, low-salt, mix only	1 cube	10	0	2	5	0	0.0	0.0	0	0%
granulated, mix only	1 tsp	5	0	1	1020	0	0.0	0.0	0	0%
(Lite-Line) dried, instant, low-sodium, mix only	1 tsp	12	1	2	5	0	1.0	0.0	0	43%
(Steero)										
cubed, mix only	1 cube	6	1	1	930	0	1.0	0.0	0	53%
dried, instant, mix only	1 tsp	6	1	1	930	0	1.0	0.0	0	53%
(Weight Watchers) dried, instant, 'Broth Mix' mix only	1 pkt	8	1	1	930	0	0.0	0.0	0	0%
(Wyler's)										
cubed, mix only	1 cube	6	1	1	930	0	1.0	0.0	0	53%
dried, mix only	1 tsp	5	0	1	900	0	0.0	0.0	0	0%
dried, instant, mix only	1 tsp	6	1	1	930	0	1.0	0.0	0	53%
dried, low-salt, mix only	1 tsp	10	0	2	10	0	0.0	0.0	0	0%
Brown										
(G. Washington's) dried, 'Seasoning & Broth' mix only	0.14 oz	6	0	1	1015	0	0.0	0.0	0	0%
Chicken flavor										
(Diamond Crystal) dried, instant, low-salt, mix only	1 serving	10	0	2	20	0	0.0	0.0	0	0%
(Featherweight) dried, instant, mix only	1 tsp	18	0	2	5	0	1.0	0.0	5	53%
(Herb-Ox)										
cubed, mix only	1 cube	5	0	1	1100	0	0.0	0.0	0	0%
cubed, low-salt	1 cube	10	0	2	5	0	0.0	0.0	0	0%
granulated, mix only	1 tsp	5	0	1	1100	0	0.0	0.0	0	0%
(Lite-Line) dried, instant, low-sodium, mix only	1 tsp	12	1	2	5	0	1.0	0.0	0	43%
(Steero)										
cubed, mix only	1 cube	8	1	1	990	0	1.0	0.0	0	53%
dried, instant, mix only	1 tsp	8	1	1	990	0	1.0	0.0	0	53%
(Weight Watchers) dried, instant 'Broth Mix' mix only	1 pkt	8	1	1	990	0	0.0	0.0	0	0%
(Wyler's)										
cubed, mix only	1 cube	8	1	1	900	0	1.0	0.0	0	53%
dried, instant, mix only	1 tsp	8	1	1	900	0	1.0	0.0	0	53%
dried, low-salt, mix only	1 tsp	10	0	2	0	0	0.0	0.0	0	0%
Golden										
(G. Washington's)										
dried, kosher, 'Seasoning & Broth' mix only	0.13 oz	6	0	1	1015	0	0.0	0.0	0	0%
dried, 'Seasoning & Broth' mix only	0.13 oz	6	0	1	935	0	0.0	0.0	0	0%
Onion flavor										
(G. Washington's) dried, 'Seasoning & Broth' mix only	0.11 cup	12	1	2	695	0	0.0	0.0	0	0%
(Wyler's) dried, instant, mix only	1 tsp	10	1	1	670	0	1.0	0.0	0	53%
Vegetable										
(G. Washington's) dried, 'Seasoning & Broth' mix only	0.11 cup	12	1	2	715	0	0.0	0.0	0	0%

Food Name	Serving Size	Calories	Prot. gms	Carbs gms	Sod. mgs	Fiber gms	Fat gms	Sat. Fat gms	Chol. mgs	% Fat Cal.
(Herb-Ox) cubed, mix only	1 cube	5	0	1	980	0	0.0	0.0	0	0%
(Wyler's) dried, instant, mix only	1 tsp	6	1	1	910	0	1.0	0.0	0	53%
BROCCOLI										
(Fantastic Foods) and cheddary, creamy, mix only	1.4 oz	160	7	26	590	2	3.0	2.0	10	17%
(Lipton)										
and cheese, 'Cup-A-Soup' mix only	1 serving	67	2	9	545	1	2.9	0.8	3	39%
creamy, 'Cup-A-Soup Food Service' prepared	6 oz	62	2	9	658	0	2.3	0.0	0	33%
creamy, 'Cup-A-Soup' prepared	6 oz	62	1	9	610	0	2.4	0.0	0	35%
golden, 'Cup-A-Soup Lite' prepared	6 oz	42	1	16	427	0	1.2	0.0	1	13%
(Ultra Slim Fast) creamy, prepared	6 oz	75	5	14	800	2	1.0	0.0	0	11%
CAULIFLOWER, prepared	1 cup	69	3	11	843	na	1.7	0.3	0	22%
CELERY, prepared	1 cup	64	3	10	838	na	1.6	0.3	0	23%
CHEESE										
(Fantastic Noodles) cheddar, creamy, w/noodles, prepared	6 oz	178	7	21	578	0	8.0	0.0	0	39%
(Hain)										
'Savory Soup & Sauce Mix' prepared	6 oz	250	6	20	890	0	16.0	0.0	0	58%
and broccoli, prepared	6 oz	310	7	19	980	0	22.0	0.0	0	66%
CHICKEN										
broth, cubed, mix only	1 cube	11	1	1	743	0	0.6	0.1	1	47%
broth, dried, mix only	1 tsp	5	0	0	372	0	0.3	0.1	0	47%
broth, dried, prepared	6 fl oz	16	1	1	1115	0	0.8	0.2	1	47%
(American Institutional) stock, concentrated, mix only	2 tsp	15	1	1	620	0	0.0	0.0	0	0%
(Campbell's) w/white meat, creamy, prepared	6 oz	90	3	12	1020	0	4.0	0.0	0	38%
(Lipton)										
broth, 'Cup-A-Soup' prepared	1 serving	18	1	3	442	0	0.1	0.0	0	7%
Florentine, 'Lite' prepared	6 oz	42	10	8	481	0	0.5	0.0	6	6%
lemon, 'Cup-A-Soup Lite' prepared	6 oz	48	2	9	419	0	0.4	0.0	4	8%
w/pasta, fat-free, 'Cup-A-Soup' prepared	1 serving	44	2	8	449	0	0.3	0.0	0	7%
w/pasta, beans, 'Kettle Creations' prepared	1 serving	106	5	19	699	3	1.3	0.3	6	11%
w/corn, 'Country' prepared	6 oz	133	3	18	704	0	5.5	0.0	0	37%
hearty, supreme, 'Cup-A-Soup' prepared	1 serving	90	1	14	635	1	3.8	1.4	1	37%
CHICKEN, CREAM OF										
(Lipton)										
'Cup-A-Soup' mix only	1 envelope	68	1	12	636	1	2.2	0.3	1	29%
'Food Service' prepared	6 oz	84	2	9	840	0	4.4	0.0	0	47%
w/vegetables, prepared	6 oz	93	2	14	708	0	3.1	0.0	0	30%
hearty, 'Country Style' prepared	6 oz	69	4	11	688	0	1.1	0.0	0	14%
CHICKEN LEEK *(Ultra Slim Fast)* creamy, prepared	6 oz	50	5	7	1070	2	1.0	0.0	2	16%
CHICKEN NOODLE										
prepared	1 cup	58	2	9	578	0	1.4	0.3	10	21%
(Campbell's)										
'Lowfat Block' prepared	1 cup	160	5	32	940	0	1.0	0.0	0	6%
microwave cup, mix only	1.35 oz	140	7	22	1340	0	3.0	0.0	0	19%
'Ramen Noodle' prepared	1 cup	190	5	26	970	0	8.0	0.0	0	37%
w/vegetables, prepared	1 cup	270	6	38	1470	0	10.0	0.0	0	34%
w/vegetables, low-fat, prepared	1 cup	220	7	44	1500	0	2.0	0.0	0	8%
w/white meat, prepared	6 oz	90	6	12	770	0	2.0	0.0	0	20%
(Estee) 'Instant' prepared	6 oz	25	1	4	135	0	1.0	1.0	1	31%
(Lipton)										
and rice, prepared	6 oz	47	2	8	667	0	0.8	0.0	0	15%
'Cup-A-Soup' prepared	6 oz	48	3	7	635	0	1.1	0.0	0	21%
hearty, 'Cup-A-Soup' mix only	1 envelope	61	3	10	591	0	1.2	0.4	14	17%
prepared w/water	1 cup	81	4	12	792	0	1.8	0.0	0	20%

Food Name	Serving Size	Calories	Prot. gms	Carbs gms	Sod. mgs	Fiber gms	Fat gms	Sat. Fat gms	Chol. mgs	% Fat Cal.
real chicken broth, 'Soup Secrets' prepared	1 serving	62	2	9	724	0	1.9	0.6	14	28%
'Soup Secrets' prepared	1 serving	77	3	11	690	0	2.0	0.6	15	23%
supreme, prepared	6 oz	107	2	12	757	0	5.9	0.0	0	50%
w/diced white meat, prepared	1 cup	81	4	12	795	0	1.8	0.0	0	20%
w/meat, 'Cup-A-Soup' prepared	1 serving	381	16	62	4177	2	8.0	2.9	88	19%
w/vegetables, 'Cup' prepared	6 oz	47	3	8	566	0	0.6	0.0	8	12%
w/vegetable, hearty, prepared	1 cup	75	3	12	687	0	1.6	0.0	0	19%
(Mrs. Grass) 'Chickeny Rich' mix only	1/4 pkg	70	2	10	900	0	2.0	0.0	0	27%
(Soup Starter) 'Homestyle' mix only	21 grams	70	2	15	770	0	1.0	0.0	10	12%
(Ultra Slim Fast) prepared	6 oz	45	5	6	970	2	1.0	0.0	5	17%
CHICKEN RICE, prepared w/water	1 cup	58	2	9	931	1	1.4	0.3	2	21%
CHICKEN VEGETABLE, prepared w/water	1 cup	49	3	8	803	0	0.8	0.2	3	15%
CHILI (Fantastic Foods) 'Cha Cha Chili' 'Hearty Soups'										
mix only	2.4 oz	220	18	37	470	13	1.0	0.0	0	4%
CHILI PEPPER (A Taste of Thai) hot and sour, prepared	1 cup	40	0	5	1330	0	2.0	1.0	0	47%
CLAM CHOWDER										
(Golden Dipt)										
Manhattan, mix only	1/4 pkg	80	2	13	700	0	2.0	1.0	3	23%
Manhattan, prepared	1 cup	95	3	13	745	1	3.7	0.6	1	34%
New England, mix only	1/4 pkg	70	2	12	680	0	2.0	1.0	2	24%
CONSOMMÉ w/gelatin, prepared	1 cup	17	2	2	3301	0	0.0	0.0	0	1%
CORN CHOWDER										
(Bean Cuisine) 'Sante Fe' prepared	1 cup	112	6	21	9	6	1.0	0.0	0	8%
(Fantastic Foods) and potato, creamy, mix only	1.6 oz	170	6	34	440	3	2.0	0.0	5	10%
COUSCOUS-LENTIL										
(Fantastic Foods) 'Hearty Soups' mix only	2.3 oz	230	12	44	480	7	1.0	0.0	0	4%
CRAB (Kikkoman) Chinese style, mix only	1 tbsp	25	1	5	920	0	0.0	0.0	0	0%
EGG FLOWER										
(Kikkoman)										
corn, Chinese style, mix only	1 tbsp	50	2	11	850	0	0.0	0.0	0	0%
hot and sour, Chinese style, mix only	2 tsp	30	1	6	880	0	0.0	0.0	0	0%
vegetable, Chinese style, mix only	1-1/2 tbsp	45	1	7	920	0	2.0	0.0	0	36%
GINGER (A Taste of Thai) tangy coconut, prepared	1 cup	250	3	3	1050	0	1.5	0.5	0	36%
GREEN PEA										
prepared w/water	1 cup	133	8	23	1220	3	1.6	0.4	3	11%
(Hain) 'Savory Soup Mix' prepared	6 oz	310	4	16	940	0	10.0	0.0	0	53%
(Lipton)										
'Cup-A-Soup' prepared	6 oz	113	4	14	553	0	4.2	0.0	0	34%
'Cup-A-Soup Food Service' prepared	6 oz	115	4	15	635	1	4.5	0.0	0	35%
Virginia, 'Country Style' prepared	6 oz	148	5	17	828	1	6.4	0.0	0	39%
Virginia, prepared	6 oz	113	5	15	664	0	4.1	0.0	1	32%
HERB										
(Lipton)										
Fiesta, 'Recipe Secrets' prepared	1 serving	29	1	6	559	0	0.3	0.1	1	11%
savory, w/garlic 'Recipe Secrets' prepared	1 serving	31	1	6	477	0	0.4	0.1	1	12%
LEEK										
prepared	1 cup	71	2	11	965	3	2.1	1.0	3	25%
(Ultra Slim Fast) creamy, prepared	6 oz	80	5	15	780	2	1.0	0.0	0	10%
LENTIL										
(Bean Cuisine) 'Lots of Lentil' prepared	1 cup	230	9	20	0	10	0.0	0.0	0	0%
(Fantastic Foods) country, 'Hearty Soups' mix only	2.3 oz	230	15	41	480	12	1.0	0.0	0	4%
(Hain) 'Savory Soup Mix' prepared w/water	6 oz	130	4	20	810	0	2.0	0.0	0	16%
(Legumes Plus)										
Cajun, w/brown rice, mix only	1/5 cup	190	10	34	170	3	1.0	0.0	0	5%

Food Name	Serving Size	Calories	Prot. gms	Carbs gms	Sod. mgs	Fiber gms	Fat gms	Sat. Fat gms	Chol. mgs	% Fat Cal.
meatless, mix only	1/4 cup	190	15	31	460	15	1.0	0.0	0	5%
minestrone style, mix only	1/3 cup	150	9	28	530	2	0.5	0.0	0	3%
pasta-pasta, mix only	1/3 cup	180	11	33	420	4	1.0	0.0	0	5%
red curry, mix only	1/5 cup	200	13	34	410	2	1.0	0.5	0	5%
robust bacon flavor, mix only	1/4 cup	170	12	26	450	11	2.0	1.0	0	11%
subtly seasoned, mix only	1/3 cup	190	14	31	470	15	1.0	0.0	0	5%
w/barley, hearty, mix only	1/4 cup	140	8	26	390	8	1.0	0.0	0	6%
w/country vegetable, mix only	1/3 cup	180	12	34	470	6	0.0	0.0	0	0%
w/herbs and rice, mix only	1/6 cup	150	7	29	470	2	1.0	0.0	0	6%
w/wagon wheel pasta, mix only	1/3 cup	190	13	34	450	5	0.5	0.0	0	2%
w/wild rice and herbs, mix only	1/4 cup	160	6	31	440	10	1.0	0.0	0	6%
zesty tomato, mix only	1/4 cup	180	13	29	250	12	1.0	0.0	0	5%
(Lipton) homestyle, 'Kettle Creations' prepared	1 serving	127	7	22	753	5	1.2	0.1	0	8%
LOBSTER BISQUE (Golden Dipt) mix only	1/4 pkg	30	1	5	560	0	1.0	0.0	2	27%
MINESTRONE										
(Cous-cous) tomato, prepared	10 oz	200	9	41	590	0	0.0	0.0	0	0%
(Fantastic Foods) hearty, mix only	1.5 oz	150	6	29	480	4	1.0	0.0	0	6%
(Hain) 'Savory Soup Mix' prepared	6 oz	110	4	20	870	0	1.0	0.0	0	9%
(Manischewitz) prepared	6 oz	50	3	9	160	0	1.0	0.0	0	16%
MISO										
(Kikkoman)										
red, prepared	1 serving	35	2	4	790	0	1.0	0.0	0	27%
shiro, white, prepared	1 serving	35	3	4	820	0	1.0	0.0	0	24%
tofu, prepared	1 serving	35	3	4	740	0	1.0	0.0	0	24%
tofu-spinach	1 serving	35	3	4	790	0	1.0	0.0	0	24%
MUSHROOM										
(Estee) 'Instant' prepared	6 oz	40	1	3	115	0	2.0	1.0	10	53%
(Fantastic Foods) garlic, creamy, mix only	1.5 oz	160	7	28	480	2	3.0	1.0	10	16%
(Hain)										
no salt added, 'Savory Soup & Recipe Mix' prepared	6 oz	250	5	15	180	0	20.0	0.0	0	69%
'Savory Soup & Recipe Mix' prepared	6 oz	210	4	11	710	0	15.0	0.0	0	69%
(Lipton)										
beef flavor, prepared	1 cup	38	2	7	763	0	0.5	0.0	0	12%
beefy, 'Recipe Secrets' prepared	1 serving	33	1	7	645	0	0.4	0.1	0	10%
MUSHROOM, CREAM OF										
(Lipton) 'Cup-A-Soup' prepared	6 oz	71	1	9	756	0	3.2	0.0	0	41%
NOODLE										
(Campbell's)										
double noodle, in chicken broth, mix only	1.71 oz	200	8	36	770	0	2.0	0.0	0	9%
hearty, 'Quality Soup & Recipe' prepared	1 cup	90	4	15	840	0	1.0	0.0	0	11%
Oriental, 'Ramen Noodle Lowfat Block' prepared	1 cup	150	5	31	940	0	1.0	0.0	0	6%
Oriental, 'Ramen Noodle' prepared	1 cup	190	5	26	930	0	8.0	0.0	0	37%
'Quality Soup & Recipe' prepared	1 cup	110	5	19	700	0	2.0	0.0	0	16%
w/chicken broth, microwave cup, mix only	1.35 oz	130	6	23	1360	0	2.0	0.0	0	13%
w/vegetables, Oriental, 'Cup-A-Ramen Lowfat' prepared	1 cup	220	7	44	1400	0	2.0	0.0	0	8%
w/vegetables, Oriental, 'Cup-A-Ramen' prepared	1 cup	270	6	38	1210	0	10.0	0.0	0	34%
(Fantastic Foods)										
curry ramen, mix only	1.5 oz	140	6	28	490	3	1.0	0.0	0	6%
vegetable miso ramen, mix only	1.3 oz	130	5	25	540	2	1.0	0.0	0	7%
(Kikkoman) memmi, noodle soup base, mix only	2 tbsp	40	2	7	2020	0	0.0	0.0	0	0%
(Lipton)										
giggle noodle, 'Soup Secrets' prepared	1 serving	74	3	11	736	0	2.1	0.7	18	26%
ring noodle, 'Cup-A-Soup' prepared	1 serving	53	2	9	557	0	1.1	0.4	12	19%

Food Name	Serving Size	Calories	Prot. gms	Carbs gms	Sod. mgs	Fiber gms	Fat gms	Sat. Fat gms	Chol. mgs	% Fat Cal.
ring noodle, 'Soup Secrets' prepared	1 serving	66	2	10	724	0	2.0	0.6	16	27%
w/extra noodle, 'Soup Secrets' prepared.	1 serving	86	3	15	681	1	1.6	0.6	23	16%
(Oodles of Noodles) Oriental, prepared.	1 cup	390	10	49	1660	0	18.0	0.0	0	41%
(Top Ramen) Oriental, mix only	1 serving	190	4	28	487	na	7.2	3.2	na	34%
Beef flavor										
(Cup O'Noodles) prepared.	1 cup	290	8	33	1490	0	14.0	0.0	0	43%
(Oodles of Noodles) prepared	1 cup	390	9	49	1810	0	18.0	0.0	0	41%
(Top Ramen) prepared.	1 cup	390	9	49	1810	0	18.0	0.0	0	41%
Chicken flavor										
(Campbell's)										
'Cup 2 Minute Soup' prepared.	6 oz	90	4	15	910	0	2.0	0.0	0	19%
double noodle, prepared.	1 cup	200	8	36	770	0	2.0	0.0	0	9%
(Cup O'Noodles)										
country, 'Hearty' prepared.	1 cup	300	8	35	1210	0	14.0	0.0	0	42%
prepared	1 cup	300	9	32	1790	0	16.0	0.0	0	47%
(Oodles of Noodles) prepared	1 cup	400	10	48	1910	0	18.0	0.0	0	41%
(Top Ramen) individual package, mix only	1 container	296	6	37	1434	na	14.1	6.3	na	43%
Pork flavor										
(Campbell's)										
'Ramen Noodle' prepared	1 cup	200	5	26	860	0	8.0	0.0	0	37%
'Ramen Noodle Lowfat Block' prepared	1 cup	150	4	31	1140	0	1.0	0.0	0	6%
w/vegetables, microwave, mix only.	1.7 oz	180	7	32	1320	0	2.0	0.0	0	10%
(Cup O'Noodles)										
vegetable beef, 'Hearty' prepared	1 cup	290	8	36	1150	0	15.0	0.0	0	43%
w/old fashioned vegetables, 'Hearty' prepared	6 oz	290	6	34	1250	0	15.0	0.0	0	46%
w/seafood, savory, 'Hearty' prepared	1 cup	300	7	34	1170	0	15.0	0.0	0	45%
w/shrimp, prepared	1 cup	300	10	32	1480	0	14.0	0.0	0	43%
(Oodles of Noodles) prepared	1 cup	390	10	51	2060	0	20.0	0.0	0	42%
(Top Ramen) prepared.	1 cup	390	10	51	2060	0	20.0	0.0	0	42%
ONION										
prepared	1 cup	27	1	5	849	1	0.6	0.1	0	18%
(Estee) prepared	6 oz	25	1	4	140	0	1.0	1.0	0	31%
(Hain)										
'Savory Soup, Dip & Recipe Mix' no salt, prepared.	6 oz	50	1	9	470	0	1.0	0.0	0	18%
'Savory Soup, Dip & Recipe Mix' prepared	6 oz	50	2	6	900	0	2.0	0.0	0	36%
(Lipton)										
'Recipe Secrets' prepared.	1 serving	18	0	4	610	0	0.1	0.0	0	7%
beefy, 'Recipe Secrets' prepared.	1 serving	25	1	5	607	0	0.6	0.1	0	23%
(Mrs. Grass) 'Soup & Dip Mix' mix only	1/4 pkg	35	1	6	1070	0	1.0	0.0	0	24%
(Ultra Slim Fast) creamy, prepared	6 oz	45	5	7	1180	2	1.0	0.0	0	16%
ONION MUSHROOM (Lipton) 'Recipe Secrets' prepared	1 serving	32	1	6	626	0	0.8	0.1	0	22%
ORIENTAL (Lipton) 'Cup-A-Soup Lite' prepared.	6 oz	45	2	6	457	0	1.7	0.0	3	34%
OSUIMONO (Kikkoman) Japanese clear broth, prepared	1 serving	0	0	1	660	0	0.0	0.0	0	0%
OXTAIL, prepared.	1 cup	71	3	9	1210	1	2.6	1.3	3	32%
PASTA (Lipton) spirals, 'Soup Secrets' prepared	1 serving	64	2	11	657	0	0.9	0.3	2	12%
PASTA AND BEAN										
(Bean Cuisine)										
'Ultima Pasta E Fagioli' bag, prepared	1 cup	190	11	34	15	10	1.0	0.0	5	5%
'Ultima Pasta E Fagioli' box, prepared.	1 cup	117	7	22	8	4	1.0	0.0	0	7%
(Lipton) homestyle, 'Kettle Creations' prepared	1 serving	125	6	23	693	4	1.4	0.3	0	10%
POTATO LEEK (Hain) 'Savory Soup Mix' prepared	6 oz	260	4	20	690	0	18.0	0.0	0	63%
SCALLOP (Kikkoman) Chinese style, mix only	1 tbsp	35	1	7	1020	0	0.0	0.0	0	0%
SEAFOOD CHOWDER (Golden Dipt) mix only	1/4 pkg	70	2	12	730	0	2.0	1.0	2	24%

Food Name	Serving Size	Calories	Prot. gms	Carbs gms	Sod. mgs	Fiber gms	Fat gms	Sat. Fat gms	Chol. mgs	% Fat Cal.
SHRIMP										
(Campbell's)										
w/vegetables 'Cup-A-Ramen' prepared	1 cup	280	6	40	1190	0	10.0	0.0	0	33%
w/vegetables, low-fat, prepared	1 cup	230	7	45	1290	0	2.0	0.0	0	8%
(Kikkoman) Chinese style, mix only	1 tbsp	30	1	5	830	0	0.5	0.0	3	16%
SHRIMP BISQUE *(Golden Dipt)* mix only	1/4 pkg	30	1	5	570	0	1.0	0.0	2	27%
SPLIT PEA										
(Bean Cuisine)										
'Thick As Fog Split Pea' bag, prepared	1 cup	140	9	24	10	10	0.5	0.0	0	3%
'Thick As Fog Split Pea' box, prepared	1 cup	116	8	21	13	1	1.0	0.0	0	7%
(Legumes Plus)										
green, traditional, mix only	1/4 cup	180	11	32	490	12	1.0	0.0	0	5%
yellow, mix only	1/4 cup	170	16	30	740	10	2.5	1.0	0	11%
(Manischewitz) green, prepared w/water	6 oz	45	3	9	320	0	1.0	0.0	0	16%
TOMATO										
prepared	1 cup	103	2	19	943	1	2.4	1.1	0	20%
(Estee) 'Instant' prepared	6 oz	40	1	5	95	0	1.0	1.0	0	27%
(Hain) 'Savory Soup & Recipe Mix' prepared	6 oz	220	3	19	770	0	14.0	0.0	0	59%
(Lipton) 'Cup-A-Soup' mix only	1 envelope	95	2	20	506	1	0.9	0.4	2	8%
(Ultra Slim Fast) creamy, prepared	6 oz	60	5	10	990	2	1.0	0.0	0	13%
TOMATO RICE PARMESANO										
(Fantastic Foods) creamy, mix only	1 serving	200	6	41	550	2	2.0	0.0	0	9%
TOMATO VEGETABLE										
prepared	1 cup	56	2	10	1146	1	0.9	0.4	0	14%
(Fantastic Foods)										
ramen noodle, mix only	1.5 oz	150	5	31	490	3	1.0	0.0	0	6%
w/noodles, prepared	7 oz	158	5	20	434	0	8.0	0.0	0	42%
VEGETABLE										
(American Institutional) stock, concentrated, mix only	2 tsp	15	0	3	510	0	0.0	0.0	0	0%
(Campbell's) nonfat, 'Quality Soup & Recipe' prepared	1 cup	40	1	8	710	0	0.0	0.0	0	0%
(Cous-cous) parmesan, prepared	10 oz	200	9	35	550	0	3.0	0.0	0	13%
(Hain)										
no salt added, 'Savory Soup Mix' prepared	6 oz	80	2	13	330	0	1.0	0.0	0	13%
'Savory Soup Mix' prepared	6 oz	80	2	13	730	0	1.0	0.0	0	13%
(Lipton)										
'Cup-A-Soup' mix only	1 serving	52	1	10	518	0	1.0	0.4	10	18%
'Recipe Secrets' mix only	1 serving	28	1	6	603	1	0.2	0.0	0	8%
spring, 'Cup-A-Soup' mix only	1 envelope	47	2	8	497	1	1.0	0.2	8	19%
(Manischewitz) prepared	6 oz	50	3	9	65	0	1.0	0.0	0	16%
(Ultra Slim Fast) hearty, prepared	6 oz	45	5	5	850	2	1.0	0.0	0	18%
VEGETABLE, CREAM OF, prepared	1 cup	107	2	12	1170	1	5.7	1.4	0	47%
VEGETABLE BARLEY										
(Fantastic Foods) hearty, mix only	1.5 oz	150	6	29	470	6	0.5	0.0	0	3%
VEGETABLE BEEF, prepared	1 cup	57	3	9	1066	0	1.2	0.6	1	19%
WAKAME *(Kikkoman)* prepared	1 serving	15	1	3	700	0	0.0	0.0	0	0%
SOUR CREAM										
cultured	1 cup	493	7	10	123	0	48.2	30.0	102	86%
cultured	1 tbsp	26	0	1	6	0	2.5	1.6	5	86%
half and half, less fat, cultured	1 cup	326	7	10	98	0	29.0	18.1	93	78%
half and half, less fat, cultured	1 tbsp	20	0	1	6	0	1.8	1.1	6	78%
(Alta Dena) pasteurized, 100% natural	1 oz	60	1	1	15	0	6.0	0.0	0	87%
(Bison)	2 tbsp	50	1	1	15	0	5.0	0.0	20	85%
(Breakstone's)										
half and half, 'Light Choice'	1 tbsp	25	1	1	10	0	2.0	1.0	5	69%

Food Name	Serving Size	Calories	Prot. gms	Carbs gms	Sod. mgs	Fiber gms	Fat gms	Sat. Fat gms	Chol. mgs	% Fat Cal.
less fat	2 tbsp	47	1	2	18	0	3.7	2.4	16	71%
nonfat	2 tbsp	29	2	5	23	0	0.4	0.3	3	13%
regular	1 tbsp	30	0	1	5	0	3.0	2.0	10	87%
(Crowley)										
French onion	2 tbsp	50	1	1	130	0	5.0	0.0	20	85%
light	2 tbsp	30	1	2	25	0	2.0	0.0	5	60%
regular	2 tbsp	50	1	1	15	0	5.0	0.0	20	85%
(Darigold)	1 tbsp	23	1	1	5	0	2.8	1.8	5	76%
(Friendship)										
low-fat, 'Lite Delite'	2 tbsp	35	1	2	25	0	2.0	0.0	8	60%
regular	2 tbsp	55	1	1	15	0	5.0	0.0	42	85%
(Knudsen)										
light	2 tbsp	40	1	2	20	0	3.0	2.0	10	69%
nonfat	2 tbsp	35	2	6	25	0	0.0	0.0	0	0%
regular, 'Hampshire'	2 tbsp	60	1	1	10	0	6.0	3.0	20	87%
(Land O'Lakes)										
'Light'	2 tbsp	40	2	4	35	0	2.0	1.0	5	43%
nonfat	2 tbsp	30	1	5	35	0	0.0	0.0	0	0%
w/chives, 'Light'	2 tbsp	40	2	4	150	0	2.0	1.0	5	43%
(Naturally Yours) no fat, 'Real Dairy'	2 tbsp	15	3	1	15	0	0.0	0.0	0	0%
(Sealtest)										
half and half, 'Light'	1 tbsp	25	1	1	10	0	2.0	1.0	5	69%
regular	1 tbsp	30	0	1	5	0	3.0	2.0	10	87%
(Tone's) w/chives, topping	1 tsp	16	0	1	1	0	1.2	0.4	57	66%
(Weight Watchers) light	2 tbsp	35	2	2	40	0	2.0	0.0	0	53%
SOUR CREAM SUBSTITUTE										
cultured	1 cup	479	6	15	235	0	44.9	40.9	0	82%
cultured	1 oz	59	1	2	29	0	5.5	5.0	0	82%
(Crowley) nondairy	1 oz	40	1	1	5	0	4.0	0.0	0	82%
(IMO)	1 tbsp	30	0	0	15	0	3.0	2.6	0	100%
(Light n' Lively) nonfat, cultured	1 tbsp	10	1	1	30	0	0.0	0.0	10	0%
(Pet)	1 tbsp	25	1	1	25	0	2.0	0.0	1	69%
(Tofutti) no cholesterol, 'Sour Supreme'	1 tbsp	25	1	1	60	na	2.5	1.0	0	85%
SOURSOP. See GUANABANA.										
SOY BEVERAGE										
(Ah Soy)										
carob	6 fl oz	160	4	30	120	0	3.0	0.0	0	17%
chocolate	6 fl oz	160	4	29	120	0	3.0	0.0	0	17%
vanilla	6 fl oz	160	5	23	140	0	5.0	0.0	0	29%
(Eden Foods)										
'Edensoy'	8 fl oz	150	6	23	90	0	3.0	0.0	0	19%
'Edensoy' carob, natural	8.45 fl oz	160	6	30	125	0	5.0	0.0	0	24%
'Edensoy' original, natural, organic, dairy-free	8.45 fl oz	140	10	14	120	0	4.0	0.6	0	27%
'Edensoy' vanilla, natural	8.45 fl oz	150	8	25	140	0	3.0	0.4	0	17%
'Edensoy Extra'	8 fl oz	150	6	24	95	0	3.0	0.0	0	18%
'Edensoy Extra' vanilla, dairy-free	8.45 fl oz	150	8	25	95	3	3.0	0.4	0	17%
(Health Valley) nonfat, 'Soy Moo'	8 fl oz	110	6	22	60	1	0.0	0.0	0	0%
(Pacific Foods)										
'Pacific Lite' plain	8 fl oz	100	4	14	115	0	2.5	0.0	0	24%
'Pacific Lite' vanilla	8 fl oz	110	4	18	115	0	2.0	0.0	0	17%
'Pacific Select' plain	8 fl oz	100	4	14	115	0	3.0	0.0	0	27%
'Pacific Select' vanilla	8 fl oz	120	4	17	115	0	3.0	0.0	0	24%
(Sovex) 'Better Than Milk' original, premixed	8 fl oz	90	2	15	85	0	2.0	0.0	0	21%

Food Name	Serving Size	Calories	Prot. gms	Carbs gms	Sod. mgs	Fiber gms	Fat gms	Sat. Fat gms	Chol. mgs	% Fat Cal.
(Vitasoy)										
carob supreme	8 fl oz	210	8	32	160	1	6.0	1.0	0	25%
cocoa, light	8 fl oz	130	4	25	130	1	2.0	0.5	0	13%
cocoa, rich	8 fl oz	210	8	32	180	1	6.0	1.0	0	25%
original, creamy	8 fl oz	160	9	14	180	1	7.0	1.0	0	41%
original, light	8 fl oz	90	4	15	95	1	2.0	0.5	0	19%
vanilla delite	8 fl oz	190	7	27	130	1	6.0	1.0	0	28%
vanilla, light	8 fl oz	110	4	20	95	1	2.0	0.5	0	16%
(Westbrae Natural Foods)										
'WestSoy' almond malted, lite	6 fl oz	160	5	26	140	0	4.0	0.0	0	23%
'WestSoy' almond malted, natural	6 fl oz	250	7	31	140	0	11.0	0.0	0	39%
'WestSoy' banana, creamy, lite	6 fl oz	160	5	26	140	0	3.0	0.0	0	18%
'WestSoy' carob malted, natural	6 fl oz	270	7	37	120	0	11.0	0.0	0	36%
'WestSoy' carob, malted, lite	6 fl oz	160	5	27	140	0	3.0	0.0	0	17%
'WestSoy' cocoa, lite	8 fl oz	140	3	27	95	0	2.0	0.0	10	13%
'WestSoy' cocoa-mint malted, nondairy, frozen	6 fl oz	270	6	37	140	0	11.0	0.0	0	37%
'WestSoy' cocoa-mint, lite	6 fl oz	160	5	26	140	0	3.0	0.0	0	18%
'WestSoy' java malted, natural	6 fl oz	270	7	37	140	0	11.0	0.0	0	36%
'WestSoy' original, natural	8 fl oz	150	7	18	115	0	5.0	0.0	0	31%
'WestSoy' plain, lite	8 fl oz	100	4	16	100	0	2.0	1.0	0	18%
'WestSoy' unsweetened, natural	8 fl oz	100	7	5	40	0	5.0	0.0	0	48%
'WestSoy' vanilla malted, natural	6 fl oz	250	7	31	140	0	11.0	0.0	0	39%
'WestSoy' vanilla royale, lite	6 fl oz	160	5	26	140	0	3.0	0.0	0	18%
'WestSoy' vanilla, lite	8 fl oz	110	3	20	80	0	2.0	0.0	0	16%
'WestSoy' vanilla, natural	8 fl oz	120	4	22	140	0	2.5	0.5	0	18%
'WestSoy Plus' carob	8 fl oz	160	6	21	80	0	5.0	0.0	0	29%
'WestSoy Plus' plain	8 fl oz	150	6	18	140	0	5.0	0.0	0	32%
'WestSoy Plus' vanilla	8 fl oz	150	6	20	120	0	5.0	0.0	0	30%
SOY BEVERAGE MIX										
(Better Than Milk)										
(Darifree) fat free	3 tbsp	90	0	21	115	0	0.0	0.0	0	0%
(Snoe Tofu) lactose & cholesterol free	3 tbsp	90	2	10	160	0	5.0	1.0	0	48%
(Solait)										
chocolate	2 tbsp	114	5	18	120	2	3.0	0.0	0	23%
original	3 tbsp	90	4	13	80	2	2.0	0.0	0	21%
vanilla bean	3 tbsp	98	3	16	60	1	2.0	0.0	0	19%
(Sovex)										
'Better Than Milk'	2 tbsp	98	1	19	173	0	2.0	0.0	0	18%
'Better Than Milk' carob, nondairy	1 fl oz	130	2	20	175	0	5.0	0.0	0	34%
'Better Than Milk' light	2 tbsp	70	2	14	105	0	0.5	0.0	0	7%
'Better Than Milk' natural, light, nondairy	2 tbsp	80	2	15	120	0	1.0	0.0	0	12%
'Better Than Milk' original	2 tbsp	100	2	16	100	0	2.5	0.0	0	24%
(Soy Moo)	8 fl oz	125	9	11	55	0	5.0	0.0	0	36%
SOY CHEESE. See under CHEESE SUBSTITUTE.										
SOY MEAL										
defatted, raw	1 cup	414	55	49	4	na	2.9	0.3	0	6%
defatted, raw, crude protein basis Nx6.25	1 cup	411	60	44	4	na	2.9	0.3	0	6%
SOY PROTEIN CONCENTRATE										
produced by acid wash	1 oz	94	16	9	255	2	0.1	0.0	0	1%
produced by alcohol extraction	1 oz	94	16	9	1	2	0.1	0.0	0	1%
SOY PROTEIN ISOLATE										
	1 oz	96	23	2	285	2	1.0	0.1	0	8%
K type	1 oz	92	23	3	14	2	0.1	0.1	0	1%
K type, crude protein basis Nx6.25	1 oz	91	25	1	14	1	0.1	0.0	0	1%

Food Name	Serving Size	Calories	Prot. gms	Carbs gms	Sod. mgs	Fiber gms	Fat gms	Sat. Fat gms	Chol. mgs	% Fat Cal.
(Protein Technologies)										
'ProPlus'	1 oz	108	24	0	11	na	1.1	0.1	0	9%
'Supro'	1 oz	110	25	0	337	na	1.1	0.2	0	9%
SOY SAUCE. See under SAUCE.										
SOYBEAN										
Dried										
mature, boiled.....................	1 cup	298	29	17	2	10	15.4	2.2	0	43%
mature, boiled.....................	1 tbsp	19	2	1	0	1	1.0	0.1	0	43%
mature, dry-roasted....................	1 cup	774	68	56	3	14	37.2	5.4	0	40%
mature, raw.....................	1 cup	774	68	56	4	17	37.1	5.4	0	40%
mature, roasted.....................	1 cup	810	61	58	7	30	43.7	6.3	0	45%
mature, sprouted, raw.....................	1/2 cup	43	5	3	5	0	2.3	0.3	0	46%
mature, sprouted, raw.....................	10 sprouts	12	1	1	1	0	0.7	0.1	0	46%
mature, sprouted, steamed.....................	1 cup	76	8	6	9	1	4.2	0.6	0	46%
raw *(Arrowhead Mills)*	2 oz	230	19	19	2	13	10.0	0.0	0	37%
roasted halves *(Solnuts)*	1 oz	146	13	8	10	3	6.8	1.3	0	42%
Green										
boiled, drained.....................	1 cup	254	22	20	25	8	11.5	1.3	0	38%
raw.....................	1 cup	376	33	28	38	11	17.4	2.0	0	39%
SOYBEAN, FERMENTED / natto	1 cup	371	31	25	12	9	19.3	2.8	0	43%
SOYBEAN CURD. See TOFU.										
SOYBEAN FLAKES *(Arrowhead Mills)*	2 oz	250	20	18	2	8	11.0	0.0	0	39%
SOYBEAN OIL										
salad or cooking	1 cup	1927	0	0	0	0	218.0	31.4	0	100%
salad or cooking	1 tbsp	120	0	0	0	0	13.6	2.0	0	100%
salad or cooking, hydrogenated	1 cup	1927	0	0	0	0	218.0	32.5	0	100%
salad or cooking, hydrogenated	1 tbsp	120	0	0	0	0	13.6	2.0	0	100%
(Crisco)	1 tbsp	120	0	0	0	0	14.0	2.0	0	100%
(Hain) salad or cooking	1 tbsp	120	0	0	0	0	14.0	2.0	0	100%
(IGA) salad or cooking.....................	1 tbsp	120	0	0	0	0	14.0	2.0	0	100%
SOYBEAN-COTTONSEED OIL										
salad or cooking, hydrogenated	1 cup	1927	0	0	0	0	218.0	39.2	0	100%
salad or cooking, hydrogenated	1 tbsp	120	0	0	0	0	13.6	2.4	0	100%
SOYBEAN-LECITHIN OIL										
....	1 cup	1663	0	0	0	0	218.0	32.7	0	100%
....	1 tbsp	104	0	0	0	0	13.6	2.0	0	100%
SOYMILK										
....	1 cup	81	7	4	29	3	4.7	0.5	0	48%
....	1 fl oz	10	1	1	4	0	0.6	0.1	0	48%
SOYMILK MIX, powder *(Soyamel)*	8 oz	130	7	10	210	0	7.0	1.0	0	48%
SOYNUT										
dry-roasted *(Karen's Kitchen)*	1 oz	90	12	7	200	8	4.0	na	0	32%
dry-roasted, honey-coated *(Nature's Select)*.....................	1 oz	130	12	13	180	8	4.0	na	0	26%
SPAGHETTI. See under PASTA										
SPAGHETTI DISH/ENTRÉE. See under PASTA DISH/ENTRÉE.										
SPAGHETTI SQUASH. See SQUASH, SPAGHETTI.										
SPANISH MACKEREL. See under MACKEREL.										
SPANISH PEANUT. See under PEANUT.										
SPEARMINT										
dried	1 tbsp	5	0	1	6	0	0.1	0.0	0	18%
dried	1 tsp	1	0	0	2	0	0.0	0.0	0	18%
dried *(McCormick/Schilling)*	1 tsp	2	0	0	2	0	0.0	0.0	0	0%
fresh	2 tbsp	5	0	1	3	1	0.1	0.0	0	14%

Food Name	Serving Size	Calories	Prot. gms	Carbs gms	Sod. mgs	Fiber gms	Fat gms	Sat. Fat gms	Chol. mgs	% Fat Cal.
SPINACH. See also SPINACH DISH/ENTRÉE.										
Canned										
(Allens)	1/2 cup	28	2	3	35	0	1.0	0.0	0	31%
(Finast)	1/2 cup	25	3	4	360	0	0.0	0.0	0	0%
(Stokely)	1/2 cup	30	2	3	420	0	0.0	0.0	0	0%
chopped (Allens)	1/2 cup	28	2	3	330	0	1.0	0.0	0	31%
chopped (Bush's Best)	1/2 cup	25	2	4	330	0	0.0	0.0	0	0%
chopped, w/liquid (Del Monte)	1/2 cup	25	2	4	355	0	0.0	0.0	0	0%
cut (Freshlike)	1/2 cup	20	2	4	340	0	0.0	0.0	0	0%
cut (Veg-All)	1/2 cup	20	2	4	340	0	0.0	0.0	0	0%
cut, w/butter sauce (Green Giant)	1/2 cup	40	2	5	280	2	1.5	1.0	3	33%
cut, water packed, no salt added (Freshlike)	1/2 cup	20	2	4	20	0	0.0	0.0	0	0%
cut, water packed, no sugar or salt added (Freshlike)	1/2 cup	20	2	4	20	0	0.0	0.0	0	0%
drained	1 cup	49	6	7	58	5	1.1	0.2	0	18%
no salt, w/liquid	1 cup	44	5	7	176	5	0.9	0.1	0	16%
no salt added (Finast)	1/2 cup	25	3	4	110	0	0.0	0.0	0	0%
no salt added (Pathmark)	1/2 cup	30	2	4	35	0	1.0	0.0	0	27%
'Premium Northwest' (S&W)	1/2 cup	25	2	3	395	0	0.0	0.0	0	0%
regular pack, w/liquid	1 cup	44	5	7	746	4	0.9	0.1	0	16%
sliced (Allens)	1/2 cup	28	2	3	330	0	1.0	0.0	0	31%
whole leaf (Allens)	1/2 cup	28	2	3	330	0	1.0	0.0	0	31%
whole leaf (Featherweight)	1/2 cup	35	2	4	30	0	1.0	0.0	0	27%
whole leaf (Pathmark)	1/2 cup	30	2	4	370	0	1.0	0.0	0	27%
whole leaf, 'No Frills' (Pathmark)	1 cup	45	5	8	700	0	1.0	0.0	0	15%
whole leaf, w/liquid (Del Monte)	1/2 cup	25	2	4	355	0	0.0	0.0	0	0%
whole leaf, w/liquid, no salt added (Del Monte)	1/2 cup	25	2	4	35	0	0.0	0.0	0	0%
Fresh										
raw	1 cup	7	1	1	24	1	0.1	0.0	0	13%
raw	1 med leaf	2	0	0	8	0	0.0	0.0	0	13%
raw (Dole)	3 oz	9	3	0	107	8	0.3	0.0	0	18%
Frozen										
chopped (A&P)	3.3 oz	20	3	4	90	0	1.0	0.0	0	24%
chopped (Birds Eye)	3.3 oz	20	3	3	90	3	0.0	0.0	0	0%
chopped (C&W)	1/3 cup	20	2	2	115	2	0.0	0.0	0	0%
chopped (Finast)	3.3 oz	20	3	3	70	0	0.0	0.0	0	0%
chopped (Flav-R-Pac)	1/3 cup	20	2	2	115	2	0.0	0.0	0	0%
chopped (Frosty Acres)	3.3 oz	20	3	3	70	1	0.0	0.0	0	0%
chopped (Seabrook)	3.3 oz	20	3	3	70	1	0.0	0.0	0	0%
chopped (Southern)	3.5 oz	25	3	4	100	0	0.3	0.0	0	9%
chopped or leaf, boiled, drained	10-oz pkg	62	7	12	708	7	0.5	0.1	0	6%
chopped or leaf, boiled, drained	1/2 cup	27	3	5	306	3	0.2	0.0	0	6%
chopped or leaf, no salt added, drained	10-oz pkg	62	7	12	189	7	0.5	0.1	0	6%
chopped or leaf, no salt added, drained	1/2 cup	27	3	5	82	3	0.2	0.0	0	6%
chopped or leaf, unprepared	10-oz pkg	68	8	11	210	9	0.9	0.1	0	11%
chopped or leaf, unprepared	1 cup	37	5	6	115	5	0.5	0.1	0	11%
cut (Freshlike)	3.3 oz	20	3	4	75	0	0.0	0.0	0	0%
cut (Green Giant)	3/4 cup	25	3	3	65	3	0.0	0.0	0	0%
cut (Seabrook)	3.3 oz	20	3	4	77	1	0.0	0.0	0	0%
cut (Veg-All)	3.3 oz	20	3	4	75	0	0.0	0.0	0	0%
'Harvest Fresh' (Green Giant)	1/2 cup	25	3	3	240	2	0.0	0.0	0	0%
'Plain Polybag' (Green Giant)	1/2 cup	25	3	6	100	5	0.0	0.0	0	0%
whole leaf (A&P)	3.3 oz	25	3	4	100	0	1.0	0.0	0	24%
whole leaf (Birds Eye)	3.3 oz	20	3	4	90	3	0.0	0.0	0	0%
whole leaf (Finast)	3.3 oz	20	3	4	75	0	0.0	0.0	0	0%

Food Name	Serving Size	Calories	Prot. gms	Carbs gms	Sod. mgs	Fiber gms	Fat gms	Sat. Fat gms	Chol. mgs	% Fat Cal.
whole leaf (Flav-R-Pac)	1/3 cup	20	2	2	115	2	0.0	0.0	0	0%
whole leaf (Frosty Acres)	3.3 oz	20	3	4	75	1	0.0	0.0	0	0%
whole leaf (Southern)	3.5 oz	25	3	4	100	0	0.3	0.0	0	9%
whole leaf, 'Portion Pack' (Birds Eye)	3.2 oz	20	3	3	70	2	0.0	0.0	0	0%
SPINACH, MALABAR										
cooked	1 med bunch	4	1	0	9	0	0.1	na	0	28%
cooked	1 cup	10	1	1	24	1	0.3	na	0	28%
SPINACH, NEW ZEALAND										
boiled, drained, chopped	1 cup	22	2	4	193	na	0.3	0.0	0	12%
raw, chopped	1 cup	8	1	1	73	na	0.1	0.0	0	12%
SPINACH, VINE / basella										
raw	1 lb	86	8.2	15.4	(mq)	>3.2	1.4	(mq)	0	12%
raw	3.5 oz	19	1.8	3.4	24	>0.7	0.3	na	0	12%
SPINACH DISH/ENTRÉE										
(Birds Eye) creamed, 'Combination Vegetables'	3 oz	60	2	5	310	1	4.0	0.0	0	56%
(Budget Gourmet) au gratin, frozen	1 pkg	222	7	11	654	2	16.6	7.6	42	67%
(Green Giant) creamed	1/2 cup	80	4	10	520	2	3.0	1.5	0	33%
(Stouffer's)										
cream of, side dish	1/2 cup	160	4	8	380	2	12.0	4.0	15	69%
creamed	1 pkg	336	7	18	670	5	26.3	7.4	32	70%
creamed, food service product	1 oz	46	1	2	102	1	3.8	0.7	7	75%
soufflé, side dish	1/2 cup	150	6	9	480	0	10.0	2.0	120	60%
SPINY LOBSTER. See under LOBSTER.										
SPIRULINA. See under ALGAE.										
SPLIT PEAS. See PEAS, SPLIT.										
SPONGE GOURD. See GOURD, DISHCLOTH.										
SPORTS AND DIET/NUTRITION BARS										
(Advantage Bar)										
almond brownie, 'Atkins Diet Food Bar'	1 bar	230	20	3	223	2	10.0	3.0	3	49%
chocolate coconut, 'Atkins Diet Food Bar'	1 bar	250	18	2	197	1	13.0	8.0	5	59%
chocolate peanut butter, 'Atkins Diet Food Bar'	1 bar	218	19	3	124	1	13.0	6.0	1	57%
praline crunch, 'Atkins Diet Food Bar'	1 bar	221	21	3	180	na	13.0	5.0	1	55%
(Bally BFIT)										
chocolate covered chocolate energy bar	1 bar	240	12	37	144	2	5.0	2.0	10	19%
chocolate covered peanut energy bar	1 bar	240	12	37	220	2	5.0	2.0	10	19%
wafer snack, 'Trim Fat'	2 wafers	25	na	5	0	1	0.0	na	na	0%
(Bear Valley)										
coconut almond food bar, 'Meal Pack'	1 pkg	400	16	56	80	6	12.0	2.0	0	27%
sesame lemon food bar, 'Meal Pack'	1 pkg	410	17	57	85	4	13.0	2.0	0	28%
(Biochem Ultimate)										
chocolate brownie nut food bar, low-carbohydrate	1 bar	240	23	2	260	na	7.0	1.0	na	39%
chocolate chip protein bar	1 bar	290	30	19	35	na	5.0	4.0	na	19%
honey almond food bar, low-carbohydrate	1 bar	240	25	2	230	na	7.0	1.0	na	37%
(BIOX)										
chocolate and peanut butter protein bar	1 bar	300	21	37	160	1	7.0	4.0	15	21%
chocolate chip protein bar	1 bar	330	27	48	120	3	3.0	2.0	21	8%
chocolate protein bar	1 bar	290	21	40	140	2	5.0	4.0	15	16%
triple chocolate chip protein bar	1 bar	330	27	48	120	3	4.0	2.0	20	11%
(Biozone) 'Food Bar'	1 bar	180	15	20	na	na	4.0	na	na	20%
(Boulder Bar)										
apple cinnamon energy bar	1 bar	190	8	37	70	4	2.0	0.0	0	9%
berry energy bar	1 bar	190	8	37	70	4	2.0	0.0	0	9%
chocolate energy bar	1 bar	200	8	40	60	4	3.0	1.0	0	12%
peanut butter energy bar	1 bar	210	8	37	45	3	4.0	1.0	0	17%

Food Name	Serving Size	Calories	Prot. gms	Carbs gms	Sod. mgs	Fiber gms	Fat gms	Sat. Fat gms	Chol. mgs	% Fat Cal.
(Clif)										
apple cherry, '100% Natural Endurance'	2.4 oz	250	4	52	100	2	2.0	0.5	0	7%
apricot, '100% Natural Endurance'	2.4 oz	250	6	50	55	2	2.0	0.5	0	7%
(Clif Bar)										
apple cherry energy bar	1 bar	250	4	52	100	5	2.0	1.0	0	7%
apricot energy bar	1 bar	250	6	50	55	5	2.0	1.0	0	7%
carrot cake energy bar	1 bar	240	9	42	50	5	4.0	1.0	0	15%
chocolate almond fudge energy bar	1 bar	250	10	39	40	6	5.0	1.0	0	19%
chocolate chip energy bar	1 bar	250	4	51	45	3	3.0	1.0	0	11%
chocolate chip peanut energy bar	1 bar	250	12	40	110	5	6.0	1.0	0	21%
chocolate espresso energy bar	1 bar	250	4	51	100	5	3.0	1.0	0	11%
chocolate pecan nutrition bar, for women, 'Luna'	1 bar	180	10	24	125	1	5.0	3.0	0	25%
cookies 'n cream energy bar	1 bar	250	9	42	80	5	5.0	1.0	0	18%
lemon zest nutrition bar, for women, 'Luna'	1 bar	180	10	26	50	1	4.0	3.0	0	20%
peanut butter energy bar, crunchy	1 bar	250	10	45	150	4	4.0	1.0	0	14%
real berry energy bar	1 bar	250	4	52	100	5	2.0	1.0	0	7%
(Complete Bar)										
chocolate, '40/30/30 Bar'	1 bar	190	14	21	160	0	6.0	3.0	0	28%
graham, '40/30/30 Bar'	1 bar	190	14	21	160	0	6.0	3.0	0	28%
peanut butter, '40/30/30 Bar'	1 bar	190	14	21	160	0	6.0	3.0	0	28%
(Complete Protein Diet) 'Complete Protein Diet Bar'	1 bar	190	22	2	120	1	5.0	3.0	0	32%
(Energx)										
chocolate protein cookie, all natural	2 cookies	200	15	28	150	5	3.0	1.0	0	14%
oatmeal raisin protein cookie, all natural	2 cookies	200	15	31	180	4	2.0	0.0	0	9%
peanut butter protein cookie, all natural	2 cookies	200	15	31	190	4	3.0	1.0	0	13%
(Fi-Bar) strawberry, oatmeal, almond 'A.M. snack bar'	1 bar	150	3	24	30	5	4.0	0.0	0	25%
(Figurines)										
chocolate caramel, '100'	1 bar	100	2	10	55	0	6.0	0.0	0	53%
chocolate caramel, w/8 oz nonfat milk	2 bars	280	13	33	250	2	12.0	3.0	5	37%
chocolate peanut butter, w/8 oz nonfat milk	2 bars	290	14	31	230	2	12.0	3.0	5	38%
chocolate, w/8 oz nonfat milk	2 bars	280	12	34	230	2	11.0	3.0	5	35%
S'mores, w/8 oz nonfat milk	2 bars	290	12	34	230	2	11.0	3.0	5	35%
vanilla, w/8 oz nonfat milk	2 bars	290	13	33	230	2	12.0	3.0	5	37%
(Gatorade Bar) peanut butter energy bar	1 bar	260	7	47	180	1	5.0	1.0	0	17%
(Genisoy)										
apple spice protein bar, yogurt-coated, soy	1 bar	220	14	32	130	1	4.0	3.0	0	16%
café mocha protein bar, soy	1 bar	220	14	34	150	1	3.5	2.5	0	14%
café mocha protein bar, soy	1 bar	220	14	34	150	1	4.0	3.0	0	16%
chocolate coated protein bar, soy	1 bar	220	14	33	190	1	3.5	2.5	0	14%
chocolate mint protein bar, soy	1 bar	220	14	33	150	2	4.0	3.0	0	16%
chocolate protein bar, uncoated, soy	1 bar	210	14	36	160	2	0.0	0.0	0	0%
peanut butter fudge protein bar, soy	1 bar	230	14	31	160	2	5.0	3.0	0	20%
(Jenny Craig)										
chocolate peanut nutrition meal	1 bar	220	10	33	240	1	5.0	4.0	na	21%
lemon meringue nutrition meal	1 bar	210	10	31	130	na	5.0	3.0	na	22%
oatmeal raisin nutrition meal	1 bar	210	10	35	75	3	3.0	0.0	0	13%
(Jog Mate) muscle recovery protein supplement	1 tube	100	10	8	230	na	3.0	2.0	10	27%
(Kashi) chocolate and peanut butter high-protein bar, 'Golean'	1 bar	280	13	50	150	7	6.0	3.0	0	18%
(Lean Body)										
coconut cream meal replacement	1 bar	300	30	19	35	0	7.0	6.0	5	24%
mint chocolate chip meal replacement	1 bar	300	30	19	35	1	7.0	4.0	5	24%
(Maxxbar) chocolate chip energy bar	1 bar	170	10	25	75	1	4.0	0.0	0	20%

Food Name	Serving Size	Calories	Prot. gms	Carbs gms	Sod. mgs	Fiber gms	Fat gms	Sat. Fat gms	Chol. mgs	% Fat Cal.
(MET-RX)										
apple caramel energy bar, 'Sourceone'	1 bar	190	15	30	80	1	3.0	3.0	0	13%
apple cinnamon oatmeal cereal bar, 'Caffe'	1 pkt	290	25	43	35	4	3.0	1.0	0	9%
chocolate cheesecake energy bar, 'Sourceone'	1 bar	190	15	30	40	1	3.0	3.0	0	13%
chocolate chip cookie dough energy bar	1 bar	340	27	50	110	0	4.0	2.0	0	10%
chocolate chip graham cracker energy bar	1 bar	320	27	48	95	1	3.0	2.0	0	8%
chocolate peanut energy bar, 'Sourceone'	1 bar	190	15	30	95	1	3.0	2.0	0	13%
chocolate raspberry energy bar, 'Sourceone'	1 bar	180	15	31	65	1	3.0	3.0	0	13%
devil's food energy bar, 'Sourceone'	1 bar	190	15	30	90	1	3.0	3.0	0	13%
extreme chocolate nutrition bar	1 bar	240	38	18	384	3	8.0	1.0	24	24%
extreme vanilla nutrition bar	1 bar	320	27	48	110	0	3.0	1.0	0	8%
fudge brownie nutrition bar	1 bar	320	26	52	110	2	3.0	1.0	0	8%
high-protein bar, 'Protein Plus'	1 bar	290	32	15	85	1	8.0	3.0	5	28%
oatmeal raisin energy bar, iced, 'Sourceone'	1 bar	180	15	33	60	0	3.0	3.0	0	12%
peanut butter cookie dough energy bar	1 bar	340	27	50	110	0	4.0	2.0	0	10%
traditional flavor oatmeal cereal bar, 'Caffe'	1 pkt	280	27	35	15	5	4.0	1.0	0	13%
(MLO Hardbody)										
chocolate truffle energy bar, 'Vita-Ox Formula'	1 bar	280	11	41	140	3	7.0	4.0	0	23%
honey almond energy bar, 'Vita-Ox Formula'	1 bar	280	7	46	100	3	7.0	3.0	0	23%
peanut butter energy bar, 'Vita-Ox Formula'	1 bar	290	7	46	120	3	7.0	3.0	0	23%
pineapple coconut energy bar, 'Vita-Ox Formula'	1 bar	280	9	46	120	2	7.0	3.0	0	22%
(Myoplex)										
chocolate fudge food bar	1 bar	340	24	44	140	2	7.0	2.0	5	19%
chocolate nutrition bar, deluxe, 'Plus'	1 bar	340	24	42	144	2	7.0	2.0	6	19%
chocolate peanut butter nutrition bar, deluxe, 'Plus'	1 bar	340	12	45	240	0	7.0	2.0	6	22%
chocolate peanut butter precision nutrition bar, deluxe, 'Plus'	1 bar	340	24	44	230	0	7.0	2.0	4	19%
chocolate precision nutrition bar, deluxe	1 bar	340	24	43	150	2	7.0	2.0	5	19%
(Nature's Plus) high-protein wafers, all flavors 'Spirutein'	6 wafers	99	14	9	0	2	1.0	0.0	0	9%
(Nextra) apple protein crunch energy bar	1 pkg	140	17	14	180	2	2.0	1.0	10	13%
(Nutrablast) 'Nutrablast Her for Women'	1 bar	190	11	27	240	1	6.0	4.0	na	26%
(Odwalla Bar)										
'C Monster Food Bar'	1 bar	230	4	52	35	4	2.0	0.0	0	7%
carrot raisin food bar, organic	1 bar	230	6	51	55	5	2.0	1.0	0	7%
chocolate raspberry food bar	1 bar	240	7	45	40	5	5.0	2.0	0	18%
cranberry citrus food bar	1 bar	240	5	52	55	4	2.0	1.0	0	7%
peanut crunch food bar	1 bar	260	9	44	220	4	7.0	2.0	0	23%
'Super Protein Food Bar'	1 bar	260	9	44	220	4	7.0	2.0	0	23%
(Peak Bar)										
chocolate chip energy bar	1 bar	314	5	58	202	3	6.0	1.0	23	18%
chocolate malt energy bar	1 bar	290	6	62	200	2	4.0	1.0	20	12%
fruit mania energy bar	1 bar	284	5	58	202	3	5.0	1.0	23	15%
peanut chocolate chunk energy bar	1 bar	295	7	56	200	3	7.0	1.0	10	20%
(PowerBar)										
apple crisp, 'Harvest'	1 bar	240	7	45	80	4	4.0	1.0	0	15%
apple-cinnamon	1 bar	230	10	45	96	3	3.0	1.0	0	11%
banana	1 bar	230	9	45	96	3	2.0	1.0	0	8%
blueberry, 'Harvest'	1 bar	240	7	45	80	4	4.0	1.0	0	15%
cherry crunch, 'Harvest'	1 bar	240	7	45	80	4	4.0	1.0	0	15%
chocolate energy gel	1 pack	120	0	28	50	0	2.0	1.0	0	14%
chocolate	1 bar	230	10	45	90	3	2.0	1.0	0	8%
chocolate, 'Essentials'	1 bar	180	10	28	105	3	4.0	2.0	0	19%
chocolate, 'Harvest'	1 bar	240	7	45	80	4	4.0	1.0	0	15%
chocolate, 'Protein Plus'	1 bar	290	24	38	290	3	5.0	4.0	5	15%

Food Name	Serving Size	Calories	Prot. gms	Carbs gms	Sod. mgs	Fiber gms	Fat gms	Sat. Fat gms	Chol. mgs	% Fat Cal.
lemon lime energy gel	1 pack	110	0	28	50	0	0.0	0.0	0	0%
malt nut	1 bar	230	10	45	90	3	3.0	1.0	0	11%
mocha	1 bar	230	10	45	90	3	3.0	1.0	0	11%
oatmeal raisin	1 bar	230	10	45	120	3	3.0	1.0	0	11%
peanut butter	1 bar	230	10	45	110	3	3.0	1.0	0	11%
peanut butter w/chocolate chips, 'Harvest'	1 bar	240	7	45	72	4	5.0	1.0	0	18%
strawberry, 'Harvest'	1 bar	240	7	45	80	4	4.0	1.0	0	15%
tropical fruit energy gel	1 pack	110	0	28	50	0	0.0	0.0	0	0%
vanilla energy gel	1 pack	110	0	28	50	0	0.0	0.0	0	0%
vanilla yogurt, 'Protein Plus'	1 bar	290	24	38	190	2	5.0	4.0	5	15%
wild berry	1 bar	230	10	45	90	3	3.0	1.0	0	11%
(PR Bar)										
Bavarian mint nutrition bar, '40-30-30'	1 bar	190	13	21	144	2	7.0	3.0	0	32%
carrot cake food bar	1 bar	200	13	23	105	na	6.0	2.0	na	27%
chocolate peanut nutrition bar	1 bar	190	14	19	130	na	6.0	3.0	0	29%
granola food bar	1 bar	180	14	21	125	2	6.0	1.0	0	28%
iced brownie food bar	1 bar	200	13	22	170	1	6.0	3.0	0	28%
strawberry yogurt food bar	1 bar	200	13	23	100	na	6.0	3.0	na	27%
(Pure Protein Bar)										
chocolate chip protein bar	1 bar	190	20	11	25	1	4.0	3.0	3	23%
white chocolate protein bar	1 bar	180	21	11	25	0	3.0	2.0	3	17%
(Sci Fit)										
chocolate protein bar	1 bar	334	35	22	70	1	5.0	4.0	5	16%
cinnamon protein bar	1 bar	334	35	22	40	1	6.0	4.0	5	19%
oatmeal protein bar	1 bar	330	35	24	35	1	6.0	4.0	5	19%
(Shaklee)										
'Carbo Crunch'	1 bar	180	9	27	85	0	4.0	1.0	0	20%
'Fiber Blend Tablets'	5 tablets	6	1	1	10	3	0.5	0.0	0	43%
(Slim Fast)										
chocolate chip crunch	1 bar	120	2	16	25	2	4.0	2.0	0	33%
Dutch chocolate	1 bar	140	5	20	80	2	5.0	2.0	3	31%
peanut butter	1 bar	150	6	19	80	2	5.0	3.0	3	31%
(Sportpharma Promax)										
double fudge brownie protein bar	1 bar	270	20	34	190	2	5.0	4.0	14	17%
Dutch chocolate protein bar	2 scoops	270	50	2	220	na	2.0	2.0	85	8%
lemon chiffon protein bar	1 bar	270	20	41	125	1	4.0	3.0	5	13%
(Sweet Success) oatmeal raisin, chewy	1 bar	120	2	23	30	3	4.0	2.0	3	26%
(Tiger's Milk)										
peanut butter and honey snack, carob coated	1 bar	160	6	23	90	0	5.0	0.0	0	28%
(Trek Barr)										
apple raisin cinnamon energy bar	1 bar	130	3	29	25	2	1.0	0.0	0	7%
chocolate extreme energy bar	1 bar	130	3	29	20	3	2.0	1.0	0	12%
java express energy bar	1 bar	130	3	29	20	3	2.0	0.0	0	12%
mountain berry energy bar	1 bar	130	3	29	20	3	2.0	0.0	0	12%
peach apricot energy bar	1 bar	130	3	29	20	2	1.0	0.0	0	7%
peanut butter chocolate chip energy bar	1 bar	130	3	26	50	2	2.0	1.0	0	13%
(Twinlab)										
apple sports bar, 'Protein Fuel'	1 bar	340	35	12	250	0	5.0	4.0	0	19%
chocolate food bar, 'Soy Sensations'	1 bar	180	15	22	200	5	6.0	3.0	0	27%
chocolate sports bar, 'Protein Fuel'	1 bar	320	35	12	250	2	5.0	4.0	0	19%
lemon food bar, 'Soy Sensations'	1 bar	180	15	23	200	5	5.0	2.0	0	23%
peanut butter sports bar, 'Protein Fuel'	1 bar	340	35	12	280	0	5.0	1.0	0	19%
peanut food bar, 'Soy Sensations'	1 bar	170	15	23	230	7	5.0	1.0	0	23%
peanut nutrition bar, creamy, 'Ironman'	1 bar	230	16	23	280	0	8.0	2.0	0	32%

Food Name	Serving Size	Calories	Prot. gms	Carbs gms	Sod. mgs	Fiber gms	Fat gms	Sat. Fat gms	Chol. mgs	% Fat Cal.
(Ultra Slim Fast)										
apple breakfast	1 bar	160	2	38	250	1	0.0	0.0	0	0%
blueberry breakfast	1 bar	170	1	39	170	2	0.0	0.0	0	0%
brownie	1 bar	120	2	20	45	1	4.0	1.0	0	29%
caramel crunch, chewy	1 bar	120	1	22	45	2	3.5	2.0	3	26%
choco almond crunch	1 bar	120	2	20	35	1	4.0	2.0	0	29%
chocolate chip crunch snack	1 bar	120	2	19	30	3	4.0	0.0	0	30%
fig breakfast	1 bar	160	2	37	270	2	0.0	0.0	0	0%
peanut butter crunch	1 bar	120	2	19	45	2	4.0	2.0	0	30%
peanut caramel crunch	1 bar	120	1	22	35	2	4.0	2.0	3	28%
strawberry breakfast	1 bar	170	2	39	190	2	0.0	0.0	0	0%
vanilla crunch	1 bar	120	2	20	30	1	4.0	2.0	0	29%
(Viactiv) apple crunch, 'Energy Bar for Women'	1 bar	180	6	29	90	na	5.0	4.0	na	24%
(Weider)										
'Sportsfood Enerquench Bar'	1 bar	200	6	44	80	0	1.0	0.0	0	4%
chewable, 'Victory Explosive Workout'	6 wafers	30	1	6	60	0	0.0	0.0	0	0%
protein bar, 'Sportsfood'	1 bar	160	10	21	140	0	4.0	0.0	0	23%
(Weight Watchers)										
chocolate brownie, chewy, 'Sweet Success'	1 bar	120	2	23	45	3	4.0	2.0	3	26%
chocolate chip, chewy 'Sweet Success'	1 bar	120	2	23	40	3	4.0	2.0	3	26%
chocolate peanut butter, chewy 'Sweet Success'	1 bar	120	2	23	35	3	4.0	2.0	3	26%
(Zone Perfect)										
apple cinnamon crunch nutrition bar, '40-30-30'	1 bar	210	14	23	340	1	7.0	4.0	0	30%
strawberry yogurt nutrition bar, '40-30-30'	1 bar	210	14	24	320	1	7.0	4.0	na	29%

SPORTS AND DIET/NUTRITION DRINKS. See SPORTS AND DIET/NUTRITION DRINK MIX.

Food Name	Serving Size	Calories	Prot. gms	Carbs gms	Sod. mgs	Fiber gms	Fat gms	Sat. Fat gms	Chol. mgs	% Fat Cal.
(All Sport)										
fruit punch	8 fl oz	70	0	20	55	na	0.0	0.0	0	0%
grape, caffeine-free, 'Thirst Quencher'	8 fl oz	70	0	20	55	0	0.0	0.0	0	0%
lemon-lime, 'Thirst quencher, caffeine-free	8 fl oz	70	0	19	55	0	0.0	0.0	0	0%
orange, caffeine-free, 'Thirst Quencher'	8 fl oz	70	0	19	55	0	0.0	0.0	0	0%
(Clinical Resource) yogurt, flavored	8 fl oz	250	9	44	65	na	4.2	na	na	15%
(Dannon) yogurt drink, all flavors, 'Dan'up'	8 fl oz	190	6	32	110	0	4.0	0.0	10	19%
(Endurox) 'Endurox R4'	12 fl oz	280	14	53	230	na	2.0	1.0	10	6%
(Ensure)										
black walnut flavor liquid nutrition	8 fl oz	250	9	34	0	0	8.8	0.0	0	31%
chocolate liquid nutrition	8 fl oz	250	9	34	200	0	8.8	0.0	5	31%
chocolate liquid nutrition, 'Plus'	8 fl oz	355	14	47	250	0	12.6	0.0	5	32%
chocolate liquid nutrition, w/fiber	8 fl oz	260	10	38	200	0	8.8	0.0	5	29%
eggnog flavor liquid nutrition	8 fl oz	250	9	34	0	0	8.8	0.0	0	31%
strawberry flavor liquid nutrition	8 fl oz	250	9	34	200	0	8.8	0.0	5	31%
strawberry flavor liquid nutrition, 'Plus'	8 fl oz	355	13	47	250	0	12.6	0.0	5	32%
vanilla liquid nutrition	8 fl oz	250	9	34	200	0	8.8	0.0	5	31%
vanilla liquid nutrition, 'Plus'	8 fl oz	355	13	47	250	0	12.6	0.0	5	32%
vanilla liquid nutrition, w/fiber	8 fl oz	260	9	38	200	0	8.8	0.0	5	29%
(Gatorade)										
fruit punch, low-sodium, no caffeine	8 fl oz	50	0	14	110	0	0.0	0.0	0	0%
grape, low-sodium, no caffeine	8 fl oz	50	0	14	110	0	0.0	0.0	0	0%
lemon and tea	8 fl oz	50	0	14	110	0	0.0	0.0	0	0%
lemon-lime, 'Thirst Quencher'	8 fl oz	50	0	14	110	0	0.0	0.0	0	0%
lemon-lime, 'Thirst Quencher Light'	8 fl oz	25	0	7	80	0	0.0	0.0	0	0%
orange, 'Thirst Quencher'	8 fl oz	50	0	14	110	0	0.0	0.0	0	0%
original, 'Thirst Quencher'	8 fl oz	50	0	14	110	0	0.0	0.0	0	0%
pineapple-citrus, 'Thirst Quencher Light'	8 fl oz	25	0	7	80	0	0.0	0.0	0	0%
tropical fruit, 'Thirst Quencher'	8 fl oz	50	0	14	110	0	0.0	0.0	0	0%

Food Name	Serving Size	Calories	Prot. gms	Carbs gms	Sod. mgs	Fiber gms	Fat gms	Sat. Fat gms	Chol. mgs	% Fat Cal.
(Genesis Nutrition)										
'Super Carbo Charge'	1 serving	348	0	87	0	na	0.0	0.0	0	0%
'Super Metabolic Optimizer'	1 serving	260	15	48	65	na	1.0	na	0	3%
'Super Weight Gain 1800'	1 serving	1800	40	284	na	na	24.0	na	na	14%
'Super Workout Pak'	1 serving	0	0	0	na	0	0.0	0.0	0	0%
(Go Healthy)										
chocolate nutrition drink	8 fl oz	235	14	40	210	na	3.0	na	na	11%
mocha nutrition drink	8 fl oz	235	14	40	210	na	3.0	na	na	11%
orange cream nutrition drink	8 fl oz	220	14	36	200	na	3.0	na	na	12%
strawberry-banana nutrition drink	8 fl oz	220	14	36	200	na	3.0	na	na	12%
vanilla nutrition drink	8 fl oz	220	14	36	200	na	3.0	na	na	12%
(Knudsen)										
fruit juice sweetened, all flavors	8 fl oz	70	1	18	25	0	0.0	0.0	0	0%
'Lemon Recharge'	1 cup	70	0	18	25	na	0.0	0.0	0	0%
'Orange Recharge'	1 cup	70	0	18	25	na	0.0	0.0	0	0%
'Tropical Recharge'	1 cup	70	0	18	25	na	0.0	0.0	0	0%
'Vita Juice Fortified Blend'	8 fl oz	120	2	29	35	na	0.0	0.0	0	0%
(Nutra/Balance)										
'Nutra/Shake Free'	4 fl oz	200	7	25	75	na	8.0	na	18	36%
'Nutra/Shake with Fiber'	4 fl oz	200	7	40	73	3	1.3	na	0	6%
'Nutra/Shake'	4 fl oz	229	7	35	63	na	6.9	na	21	27%
(Nutrament)										
chocolate shake, meal replacement	12 fl oz	360	16	52	250	0	10.0	0.0	0	25%
vanilla shake, meal replacement	12 fl oz	360	16	52	250	0	10.0	0.0	0	25%
(Opti-Carb 140)										
grape	16 fl oz	140	0	35	9	0	0.0	0.0	0	0%
orange	16 fl oz	140	0	35	9	0	0.0	0.0	0	0%
(Power Burst)										
lemonade, advanced performance beverage	8 fl oz	50	0	14	25	0	0.0	0.0	0	0%
(Powerade)										
fruit punch	16 fl oz	144	0	38	56	0	0.0	0.0	0	0%
grape	16 fl oz	146	0	38	56	0	0.0	0.0	0	0%
lemon-lime	16 fl oz	144	0	38	56	0	0.0	0.0	0	0%
'Mountain Blast'	16 fl oz	146	0	38	56	0	0.0	0.0	0	0%
orange	16 fl oz	144	0	38	56	0	0.0	0.0	0	0%
(Pro-formance)										
fruit punch	8 fl oz	99	0	26	0	0	0.0	0.0	0	0%
grape	8 fl oz	99	0	26	0	0	0.0	0.0	0	0%
lemon-lime	8 fl oz	99	0	26	0	0	0.0	0.0	0	0%
orange	8 fl oz	99	0	26	0	0	0.0	0.0	0	0%
(Resource)										
chocolate health shake	4 fl oz	190	6	32	110	0	4.0	0.7	5	19%
vanilla health shake	4 fl oz	190	6	32	100	0	4.0	0.7	5	19%
(Sego)										
chocolate, 'Lite'	10 fl oz	150	11	20	480	0	3.0	0.0	5	18%
chocolate, 'Very Chocolate'	10 fl oz	225	11	43	450	0	1.0	0.0	5	4%
chocolate malt, 'Very Chocolate'	10 fl oz	225	11	43	450	0	1.0	0.0	5	4%
Dutch chocolate, 'Lite'	10 fl oz	150	11	20	480	0	3.0	0.0	5	18%
French vanilla, 'Lite'	10 fl oz	150	11	17	390	0	4.0	0.0	5	24%
strawberry, 'Lite'	10 fl oz	150	11	17	390	0	4.0	0.0	5	24%
strawberry, 'Very Strawberry'	10 fl oz	225	11	34	360	0	5.0	0.0	5	20%
vanilla, plain, 'Lite'	10 fl oz	150	11	17	390	0	4.0	0.0	5	24%
vanilla, 'Very Vanilla'	10 fl oz	225	11	34	360	0	5.0	0.0	5	20%

Food Name	Serving Size	Calories	Prot. gms	Carbs gms	Sod. mgs	Fiber gms	Fat gms	Sat. Fat gms	Chol. mgs	% Fat Cal.
(Shasta)										
lemon-lime, caffeine-free, 'Body Works'	8 fl oz	60	0	15	95	0	0.0	0.0	0	0%
orange, caffeine-free, 'Body Works'	8 fl oz	60	0	15	95	0	0.0	0.0	0	0%
(Slim Fast)										
chocolate shake	8 fl oz	190	13	33	240	2	1.3	0.8	9	6%
chocolate shake, 'Nutra Start'	1 shake	210	10	40	370	5	2.5	0.5	0	10%
strawberry shake	8 fl oz	190	13	33	264	2	0.7	0.6	9	3%
vanilla shake, 'Nutra Start'	1 shake	210	10	38	350	5	2.5	0.5	3	10%
(Sustacal)										
chocolate, liquid food, nutritionally complete	8 fl oz	240	15	33	220	0	5.5	0.0	0	21%
vanilla, liquid food, nutritionally complete	8 fl oz	240	15	33	220	0	5.5	0.0	0	21%
(Weight Watchers)										
chocolate mocha, w/phenylalanine, 'Sweet Success'	10 fl oz	200	11	32	230	6	3.0	0.0	0	14%
chocolate, w/phenylalanine, 'Sweet Success'	10 fl oz	200	12	38	240	6	3.0	1.0	5	12%
dark chocolate fudge, 'Sweet Success'	10 fl oz	200	11	32	210	6	3.0	0.0	0	14%
milk chocolate, creamy, 'Sweet Success'	10 fl oz	200	11	32	230	6	3.0	0.0	0	14%
vanilla, w/phenylalanine, 'Sweet Success'	10 fl oz	200	11	32	230	6	3.0	0.0	0	14%
(Ultra Slim Fast)										
'Chocolate Fantasy'	8 fl oz	270	11	51	288	8	1.9	1.0	9	7%
chocolate fudge shake	1 shake	220	10	42	180	5	3.0	1.0	10	11%
chocolate royale shake	1 shake	220	10	38	330	5	3.0	1.0	5	12%
coffee shake	1 shake	220	10	38	300	5	3.0	0.5	5	12%
French vanilla	12 fl oz	220	13	38	240	5	1.0	0.0	0	4%
milk chocolate shake	1 shake	220	10	42	330	5	3.0	1.0	5	11%
strawberry shake	1 shake	220	10	42	460	5	3.0	1.0	10	11%
vanilla shake	1 shake	220	10	38	460	5	3.0	1.0	10	12%
(Yogloo)										
yogurt, fruit basket, nonfat	10 fl oz	170	3	40	80	0	0.0	0.0	0	0%
yogurt, original, nonfat	10 fl oz	170	3	40	80	0	0.0	0.0	0	0%
yogurt, peach, nonfat	10 fl oz	170	3	40	80	0	0.0	0.0	0	0%
yogurt, strawberry, nonfat	10 fl oz	170	3	40	80	0	0.0	0.0	0	0%
SPORTS AND DIET/NUTRITION DRINK MIX										
(Alba)										
milkshake mix, double fudge, sugar-free, mix only	0.75 oz	60	6	10	135	0	0.0	0.0	0	0%
milkshake mix, strawberry, sugar-free, mix only	0.75 oz	60	5	11	130	0	0.0	0.0	0	0%
milkshake mix, vanilla flavor, no sugar, mix only	0.75 oz	70	6	11	160	0	0.0	0.0	0	0%
(Alba '77)										
'Fit'N' chocolate marshmallow, prepared	6 fl oz	346	28	52	690	1	3.6	0.0	0	9%
'Fit'N' chocolate, prepared	6 fl oz	346	26	56	709	1	2.5	0.0	0	6%
'Fit'N' frosty double fudge, prepared	6 fl oz	346	28	52	728	1	3.3	0.0	0	8%
'Fit'N' strawberry, prepared	6 fl oz	333	25	55	805	0	1.7	0.0	0	5%
'Fit'N' vanilla, prepared	6 fl oz	333	26	55	810	0	1.4	0.0	0	4%
(Amerifit) 'Heavy Weight Bulk Up' prepared	12 fl oz	71	4	14	71	0	0.3	0.2	8	4%
(Balance Drink) meal replacement, '40-30-30' mix only	2 scoops	180	14	19	300	na	6.0	1.0	5	29%
(Bally)										
muscle growth supplement, whey, mix only	1 scoop	100	19	3	55	na	2.0	1.0	15	17%
protein supplement, soy	2 scoops	80	16	1	150	na	1.0	na	na	12%
'Mass Builder' vanilla	4 scoops	750	25	163	420	2	1.0	1.0	10	1%
(BFIT-RX)										
meal replacement, chocolate, light, mix only	1 pkt	190	20	26	290	1	1.0	0.0	5	5%
meal replacement, vanilla, mix only	1 pkt	290	40	27	430	1	2.0	1.0	10	6%
meal replacement for women, mix only	1 pkt	220	20	33	288	0	1.0	0.0	6	4%
(Bio-Design X) vanilla, whey, mix only	20 grams	77	16	1	45	na	1.0	na	15	12%
(BIOX) protein drink, chocolate, mix only	1 pkg	130	19	12	180	2	1.0	1.0	15	7%

Food Name	Serving Size	Calories	Prot. gms	Carbs gms	Sod. mgs	Fiber gms	Fat gms	Sat. Fat gms	Chol. mgs	% Fat Cal.
(Champion Nutrition)										
'Heavyweight Gainer 900' prepared	1 serving	650	30	105	120	na	12.0	na	na	17%
(Complete Protein Diet)										
complete protein diet, chocolate, mix only	1 pkt	200	35	3	70	0	5.0	2.0	20	23%
(EAS Precision)										
whey protein, 'Muscle Builder' mix only	3 tbsp	100	20	3	50	1	1.0	1.0	15	9%
(Gatorade)										
'Thirst Quencher' fruit punch, prepared.	8 fl oz	60	0	15	110	0	0.0	0.0	0	0%
'Thirst Quencher' lemonade, prepared	8 fl oz	60	0	15	110	0	0.0	0.0	0	0%
'Thirst Quencher' lemon-lime, mix only	3/4 scoop	58	0	15	96	na	0.0	na	na	0%
(Genesis Nutrition)										
milk and egg protein drink, mix only	1 tbsp	39	8	2	na	na	0.0	0.0	0	0%
'Super Trim Fast' mix only	1 serving	90	7	15	na	3	0.5	na	na	5%
'Super Trim Fast' prepared	1 serving	198	17	27	na	3	2.0	na	na	9%
(Genisoy)										
protein shake, chocolate, ultra soy protein, mix only	1 scoop	120	14	16	150	2	0.0	0.0	0	0%
(Knox)										
gelatin drink, orange flavor, mix only	1 envelope	39	6	4	17	0	0.1	0.0	0	2%
gelatin drink, orange flavor, w/aspartame, mix only	1 envelope	41	7	3	18	na	0.1	0.1	0	2%
(Labrada)										
'Kwik Size XXXL' mix only	5 scoops	740	30	150	130	3	2.0	1.0	30	2%
'Proplex+' mix only	1 scoop	90	17	3	35	0	1.0	1.0	30	10%
(Lean Body)										
chocolate peanut butter, mix only	1 pkt	300	45	28	250	1	2.0	1.0	25	6%
vanilla, mix only.	1 pkt	300	45	28	200	1	2.0	1.0	25	6%
(MET-RX)										
apple pie a la mode, mix only	1 pkt	250	37	22	370	1	2.0	2.0	15	7%
extreme chocolate, mix only	1 pkt	240	38	18	384	3	1.0	2.0	0	4%
milk chocolate, w/protein, mix only	3 scoops	220	46	7	120	1	2.0	1.0	15	8%
original flavor, mix only	1 pkt	250	37	22	370	1	2.0	2.0	15	7%
peach, mix only.	1 pkt	250	37	22	370	1	2.0	2.0	15	7%
strawberry cream, w/protein, mix only.	3 scoops	210	46	3	115	0	1.0	1.0	15	4%
vanilla butter cream, w/protein, mix only	3 scoops	210	46	3	115	0	1.0	1.0	15	4%
white chocolate mocha, mix only	1 pkt	250	37	22	370	1	2.0	2.0	15	7%
(MLO)										
'MUS-L Blast 2000' chocolate, mix only	4 scoops	580	20	118	350	3	3.0	2.0	51	5%
'MUS-L Blast 2000' strawberry and banana, mix only.	4 scoops	570	20	118	370	na	3.0	2.0	50	5%
'MUS-L Blast 2000' vanilla, mix only	4 scoops	570	20	118	370	na	3.0	2.0	50	5%
(Myoplex)										
'Mass Drink' chocolate cream, mix only	1 pkt	500	33	75	570	2	7.0	2.0	10	13%
'Mass Drink' strawberry cream, light, mix only	1 pkt	280	42	24	330	1	2.0	1.0	15	6%
'Mass Drink' strawberry cream, mix only.	1 pkt	500	33	76	570	1	7.0	1.0	10	13%
'Mass Drink' vanilla cream, light, mix only.	1 pkt	280	42	24	330	1	2.0	1.0	15	6%
'Mass Drink' vanilla cream, mix only	1 pkt	500	33	75	570	1	7.0	1.0	10	13%
nutrition drink, chocolate cream, light, mix only	1 pkt	190	25	20	450	0	2.0	1.0	5	9%
nutrition drink, chocolate cream, mix only.	1 pkt	280	42	24	330	1	2.0	1.0	15	6%
nutrition drink, chocolate, deluxe, mix only	1 pkt	280	42	24	336	1	2.0	1.0	15	6%
(Nature's Plus)										
'Carrot-tein' mix only	1 scoop	97	14	11	120	0	0.0	0.0	0	0%
'Fruitein' mix only	1 scoop	96	10	14	120	0	0.0	0.0	0	0%
high-protein drink, banana, mix only.	1 scoop	94	14	10	120	2	0.0	0.0	0	0%
high-protein drink, cappuccino, mix only	1 scoop	100	14	11	120	2	0.0	0.0	0	0%
high-protein drink, chocolate, vanilla, mix only	1 scoop	87	14	8	120	2	0.0	0.0	0	0%
'Oxy-Nectar' mix only	1 scoop	107	10	17	0	0	0.0	0.0	0	0%

Food Name	Serving Size	Calories	Prot. gms	Carbs gms	Sod. mgs	Fiber gms	Fat gms	Sat. Fat gms	Chol. mgs	% Fat Cal.
(Olympian Labs)										
carbohydrate loading recovery drink, mix only	3 scoops	336	1	80	0	3	1.0	0.0	0	3%
100% egg white w/complex carbs, vanilla, mix only	2 scoops	120	15	15	240	0	1.0	0.0	0	7%
(Opti-Lean)										
chocolate, mix only	1 pkt	170	20	20	60	0	1.0	na	10	5%
vanilla, mix only	1 pkt	170	20	20	60	0	1.0	na	10	5%
(Scandishake)										
chocolate shake, instant, mix only	3 oz	440	4	58	120	2	21.0	9.0	0	43%
chocolate shake, instant, lactose-free, mix only	3 oz	190	7	55	70	3	21.0	9.0	0	43%
weight-gain shake, instant, lactose-free, mix only	3 oz	440	7	55	116	0	21.0	8.0	0	43%
weight-gain shake, instant, sweetened w/aspartame, mix only	3 oz	440	7	55	100	0	21.0	4.0	0	43%
weight-gain shake, instant, vanilla or strawberry, mix only	3 oz	440	4	58	90	0	21.0	9.0	0	43%
(Shaklee)										
'After Exercise Energizer'	1/3 cup	180	12	33	90	0	0.5	0.0	3	2%
'Daily Blend' mix only	1 1/2 tbsp	40	1	13	0	5	0.0	0.0	0	0%
'Fiber Blend' 25% soluble/75% insoluble, mix only	1 tbsp	20	1	5	0	3	1.0	0.0	0	27%
'Fiber Plan' fruit-flavored, mix only	2 tbsp	90	0	22	5	5	0.0	0.0	0	0%
'Fiber Plan' unflavored, mix only	2 tsp	20	0	5	0	4	0.0	0.0	0	0%
'Meal Shake' Bavarian cocoa, mix only	1/4 cup	120	7	23	70	3	0.5	0.0	3	4%
'Meal Shake' Bavarian cocoa, prepared w/low-fat milk	8 fl oz prep	230	15	32	200	3	5.0	0.0	20	19%
'Meal Shake' French vanilla, mix only	1/4 cup	120	7	23	80	3	0.5	0.0	3	4%
'Meal Shake' French vanilla, prepared w/low-fat milk	8 fl oz	230	15	32	200	3	5.0	0.0	20	19%
'Physique' mix only	1/2 cup	210	14	38	80	0	0.5	0.0	3	2%
'Physique' prepared w/2 oz mix, 8 oz nonfat milk	1 serving	300	22	50	205	0	1.0	1.0	6	3%
'Physique' prepared w/3 oz mix, 8 oz water	1 serving	320	21	57	120	0	1.0	1.0	3	3%
protein drink, cocoa flavor, mix only	1/2 cup	110	16	8	140	0	1.0	0.0	0	9%
protein drink, instant, mix only.	1/4 cup	100	16	8	140	0	0.5	0.0	0	4%
'Slim Plan' high fiber, low-fat, low-sodium, mix only	1/2 cup	210	15	33	370	4	3.0	0.0	3	12%
(Slim Fast)										
chocolate malt shake, prepared w/skim milk.	8 fl oz	190	13	33	240	2	1.0	0.8	9	5%
vanilla shake, prepared w/skim milk	1 cup	190	14	33	264	2	0.7	0.6	9	3%
(Sportpharma)										
'Actisyn' strawberry flavor, mix only.	1 pkt	150	27	8	220	1	1.0	1.0	10	6%
'Just Whey' vanilla cream, mix only.	1 oz	110	23	2	105	2	1.0	0.0	10	8%
'Musclemax' chocolate, mix only.	3 scoops	450	25	85	100	1	1.0	1.0	10	2%
'Nutriforce' chocolate royale, mix only.	1 pkt	250	40	21	210	2	2.0	2.0	0	7%
'Nutriforce' French vanilla, mix only.	1 pkt	260	40	21	230	0	2.0	2.0	0	7%
(Strength Systems) 'USA Diet Octane" prepared.	8 fl oz	127	21	9	50	2	1.0	0.5	0	7%
(Weight Watchers)										
'Sweet Success' chocolate almond, mix only	1 scoop	90	7	12	150	6	2.0	0.0	0	19%
'Sweet Success' chocolate almond, prepared.	8 fl oz	180	15	24	280	6	2.0	0.0	0	10%
'Sweet Success' chocolate, mix only.	1 scoop	90	7	19	210	6	1.5	1.0	5	11%
'Sweet Success' dark chocolate fudge, mix only.	1 scoop	90	7	11	150	6	2.0	0.0	0	20%
'Sweet Success' dark chocolate fudge, prepared	8 fl oz	180	15	23	280	6	2.0	0.0	0	11%
(Tiger's Milk)										
'Breakfast Booster' mix only	2 tbsp	70	2	14	20	0	1.0	0.0	0	12%
'Energy Booster' mix only	3 round tbsp	120	0	28	10	0	1.0	0.0	0	7%
'Energy Booster' prepared w/8 oz nonfat milk.	8 fl oz	200	8	40	135	0	1.0	0.0	0	4%
'Protein Booster' Dutch chocolate, mix only	3 round tbsp	90	8	12	140	0	1.0	0.0	0	10%
'Protein Booster' Dutch chocolate, prepared w/skim milk.	8 fl oz	200	20	28	270	0	1.0	0.0	0	4%
'Protein Booster' vanilla-orange creme, mix only	3 round tbsp	90	8	12	140	0	1.0	0.0	0	10%

Food Name	Serving Size	Calories	Prot. gms	Carbs gms	Sod. mgs	Fiber gms	Fat gms	Sat. Fat gms	Chol. mgs	% Fat Cal.
'Protein Booster' vanilla-orange creme, prepared w/nonfat milk	8 fl oz	200	20	28	270	0	1.0	0.0	0	4%
(Turbo Nutrition)										
protein powder, chocolate, prepared w/low-fat milk	8 fl oz	330	36	34	450	0	6.0	0.0	0	16%
protein powder, strawberry flavored, mix only	2 oz	210	28	22	300	0	1.0	0.0	0	4%
protein powder, strawberry flavored, prepared w/whole milk	8 fl oz	360	36	33	420	0	9.0	0.0	0	23%
weight gain protein powder, chocolate, mix only	2 oz	210	28	22	320	0	1.0	0.0	0	4%
(Twinlab)										
'Fuel Plex' whey protein, chocolate, mix only	1 pkt	300	45	25	310	0	2.0	1.0	40	6%
'Fuel Plex' whey protein, strawberry, mix only	1 pkt	300	45	25	310	0	2.0	1.0	40	6%
'Fuel Plex' whey protein, vanilla, mix only	1 pkt	300	45	25	310	0	2.0	1.0	40	6%
(Ultra Slim Fast)										
'Cafe Mocha' mix only	1 scoop	100	5	24	130	6	1.0	0.0	0	7%
'Cafe Mocha' prepared w/nonfat milk	8 fl oz	200	15	38	280	6	1.0	0.0	0	4%
'Chocolate Fantasy' 'Plus' mix only	1.41 oz	120	3	33	140	8	1.0	0.0	0	6%
chocolate fudge shake, prepared w/skim milk	8 fl oz	200	13	36	216	5	2.6	1.2	9	11%
chocolate malt shake, prepared w/skim milk	8 fl oz	200	13	36	216	5	1.3	0.8	9	6%
'Chocolate Royale' shake, prepared w/skim milk	8 fl oz	200	13	36	264	6	1.3	1.0	9	6%
French vanilla, mix only	1 scoop	100	5	24	120	4	1.0	0.0	0	7%
French vanilla, prepared w/8 oz nonfat milk	1 serving	190	14	36	250	4	1.0	0.0	0	4%
milk chocolate shake, prepared w/skim milk	8 fl oz	210	13	36	240	6	1.3	0.2	9	6%
'Mixes w/Fruit Juice' mix only	1 scoop	90	10	17	75	6	0.0	0.0	0	0%
'Mixes w/Fruit Juice' prepared w/orange juice	8 fl oz	200	11	43	80	6	1.0	0.0	0	4%
'Plus' chocolate, mix only	1 scoop	120	3	33	140	8	1.0	0.0	0	6%
'Plus' chocolate, prepared w/nonfat milk	12 fl oz	250	15	50	330	8	2.0	0.0	0	6%
'Plus' pina colada flavor, mix only	1.16 oz	90	5	24	120	6	1.0	0.0	0	7%
'Plus' pina colada flavor, prepared w/nonfat milk	8 fl oz	190	15	38	260	6	1.0	0.0	0	4%
'Plus' strawberry jubilee, mix only	1 scoop	110	3	32	140	8	1.0	0.0	0	6%
'Plus' strawberry jubilee, prepared w/nonfat milk	12 fl oz	240	15	50	330	8	2.0	0.0	0	6%
strawberry shake, prepared w/skim milk	8 fl oz	200	13	36	264	4	1.3	0.6	9	6%
vanilla shake, prepared w/skim milk	8 fl oz	200	13	33	264	6	0.7	0.4	9	3%
(Weider)										
beef protein drink, mix only	1 cup	420	66	39	781	0	0.0	0.0	0	0%
beef protein drink, prepared w/nonfat milk	8 fl oz	165	23	19	293	0	0.0	0.0	0	0%
'Big' chocolate malt, sugar-free, mix only	4 scoops	320	18	58	370	0	2.0	0.0	0	6%
'Big' chocolate malt, sugar-free, prepared w/milk	16 fl oz	620	34	81	610	0	18.0	0.0	0	26%
'Carbo Energizer' orange flavor, mix only	4 scoops	230	0	58	40	0	0.0	0.0	0	0%
'Crash Weight Gain No. 7' vanilla, mix only	4 round tbsp	300	6	61	84	0	3.0	0.0	0	9%
'Crash Weight Gain No. 7' vanilla, prepared w/milk	16 fl oz	610	22	83	0	0	21.0	0.0	0	31%
'Dynamic Body Shaper' Dutch chocolate, mix only	2 scoops	110	13	12	170	0	1.0	0.0	0	8%
'Dynamic Body Shaper' Dutch chocolate, mix only	2 scoops	190	21	24	320	0	1.0	0.0	0	5%
'Dynamic Body Shaper' mix only	1 cup	420	39	66	631	3	1.5	0.0	0	3%
'Dynamic Body Shaper' prepared w/nonfat milk	8 fl oz	173	16	26	251	1	0.7	0.0	3	4%
'Dynamic Muscle Builder' chocolate, mix only	2 scoops	200	26	21	300	0	1.0	0.0	0	5%
'Dynamic Muscle Builder' chocolate, natural, mix only	2 scoops	120	18	9	170	0	1.0	0.0	0	8%
'Dynamic Muscle Builder' chocolate, prepared	11 fl oz	220	18	36	260	0	1.0	0.0	0	4%
'Dynamic Muscle Builder' mix only	1/3 cup	190	18	27	160	1	0.0	0.0	0	0%
'Dynamic Muscle Builder' mix only	3 heaping tbsp	100	18	6	116	0	0.0	0.0	0	0%
'Dynamic Muscle Builder' prepared w/ whole milk	8 fl oz	250	26	17	116	0	9.0	0.0	0	32%
'Dynamic Muscle Builder' prepared w/skim milk	8 fl oz	206	20	29	214	1	0.3	0.6	3	1%
'Dynamic Muscle Builder' vanilla, natural, mix only	2 scoops	120	18	9	180	0	1.0	0.0	0	8%
'Dynamic Protein' vanilla, mix only	2 scoops	100	16	10	150	0	0.0	0.0	0	0%

Food Name	Serving Size	Calories	Prot. gms	Carbs gms	Sod. mgs	Fiber gms	Fat gms	Sat. Fat gms	Chol. mgs	% Fat Cal.
'Dynamic Protein' vanilla, prepared w/skim milk	8 fl oz	190	24	22	280	0	1.0	0.0	0	5%
'Dynamic Weight Gainer 1250' milkshake, prepared w/water	16 fl oz	330	18	61	400	0	1.0	0.0	0	3%
'Dynamic Weight Gainer 1250' milkshake, prepared w/whole milk	16 fl oz	630	34	84	640	0	17.0	0.0	0	24%
'Dynamic Weight Gainer 1250' milkshake, prepared w/whole milk	32 fl oz	1250	68	168	1280	0	34.0	0.0	0	24%
'Dynamic Weight Gainer' chocolate, prepared	11 fl oz	280	18	48	320	0	2.0	0.0	0	6%
'Dynamic Weight Gainer' Dutch chocolate, mix only	4 scoops	320	18	61	400	0	1.0	0.0	0	3%
'Dynamic Weight Gainer' mix only	1 cup	660	36	124	820	0	1.0	0.0	0	1%
'Dynamic Weight Gainer' peanut butter, mix only	4 scoops	330	18	61	390	0	2.0	0.0	0	5%
'Dynamic Weight Gainer' prepared w/whole milk	1 cup	252	14	34	260	0	6.6	22.9	26	24%
'Dynamic Weight Gainer' vanilla, mix only	4 tbsp	310	20	54	183	0	2.0	0.0	0	6%
'Dynamic Weight Gainer' vanilla, prepared w/milk	16 fl oz	630	36	76	0	0	20.0	0.0	0	29%
'Dynamic' vanilla, natural, prepared w/skim milk	16 fl oz	200	26	21	310	0	1.0	0.0	0	5%
egg protein drink, mix only	1 cup	360	60	27	931	0	0.0	0.0	0	0%
egg protein drink, prepared w/nonfat milk	8 fl oz	150	21	16	330	0	0.0	0.0	0	0%
'Fat Burner System' mix only	1/3 cup	110	13	11	170	3	1.0	0.0	0	9%
'Fat Burner System' prepared w/skim milk	8 fl oz	146	16	17	221	2	1.1	na	3	7%
'Giant Mega Mass 4000' mix only	1 cup	547	27	106	400	0	1.3	0.7	16	2%
'Giant Mega Mass 4000' prepared w/low-fat milk	8 fl oz	336	18	59	260	0	3.0	1.8	17	8%
'Mass 1000' mix only	1 cup	513	23	104	340	2	0.7	na	27	1%
'Mass 1000' prepared w/low-fat milk	8 fl oz	290	15	51	215	1	2.9	na	22	9%
'90% Plus Protein' chocolate malt, mix only	3 heaping tbsp	180	33	12	0	0	1.0	0.0	0	5%
'90% Plus Protein' chocolate malt, sugar-free, mix only	3 heaping tbsp	100	24	0	293	0	0.0	0.0	0	0%
'90-Plus Protein' vanilla, sugar-free, mix only	2 scoops	100	25	1	150	0	0.0	0.0	0	0%
'90-Plus Protein' vanilla, sugar-free, prepared w/skim milk	8 fl oz	190	33	13	280	0	1.0	0.0	0	5%
'Nitro-Fire' protein blend, mix only	2 tbsp	110	8	17	100	0	1.0	0.0	0	8%
'Nitro-Fire' protein blend, prepared w/skim milk	8 fl oz	190	16	29	230	0	1.0	0.0	0	5%
'Performance Builder' mix only	1 cup	601	54	93	751	3	3.0	0.0	0	4%
'Performance Builder' prepared w/skim milk	8 fl oz	218	20	32	281	na	1.1	0.0	3	4%
'Performance Shaper' mix only	1 cup	450	45	66	721	3	1.5	0.0	0	3%
'Performance Shaper' prepared w/skim milk	1 cup	180	17	26	274	1	0.7	na	3	3%
'Performance Weight Gainer' mix only	1 cup	585	27	117	375	0	1.5	0.8	0	2%
'Performance Weight Gainer' prepared w/low-fat milk	8 fl oz	306	16	54	223	0	0.9	na	11	3%
'Protein Blast' chocolate, prepared	11.5 fl oz	270	22	44	240	0	1.0	0.0	0	3%
'Signature Line Dynamic Muscle Builder' mix only	2 scoops	120	18	9	180	0	1.0	0.0	0	8%
'Sports Food Enerquench' lemon-lime, prepared	8 fl oz	60	0	15	0	0	0.0	0.0	0	0%
'Sports Food Enerquench' orange flavor, prepared	8 fl oz	60	0	15	0	0	0.0	0.0	0	0%
'Sports Foods Gainer' chocolate supreme, prepared w/water	1 serving	300	14	53	110	0	3.0	0.0	0	9%
'Sports Foods Gainer' chocolate, prepared w/skim milk	1 serving	460	30	77	390	0	3.0	0.0	0	6%
'Sports Foods Gainer' vanilla frost, prepared w/water	1 serving	300	14	53	150	0	3.0	0.0	0	9%
'Sports Foods Gainer' vanilla, prepared w/skim milk	1 serving	460	30	77	430	0	3.0	0.0	0	6%
'Sports Foods Gainer' wild strawberry, prepared w/skim milk	1 serving	460	30	77	430	0	3.0	0.0	0	6%
'Sports Foods Gainer' wild strawberry, prepared w/water	1 serving	300	14	53	150	0	3.0	0.0	0	9%
'Sports Gainer' French vanilla, prepared w/skim milk	12 fl oz	460	30	77	390	0	3.0	0.0	0	6%
'Sports Gainer' French vanilla, prepared w/water	12 fl oz	300	14	53	110	0	3.0	0.0	0	9%
'Sports Gainer' strawberry, prepared w/skim milk	16 fl oz	460	30	77	430	0	3.0	0.0	0	6%

Food Name	Serving Size	Calories	Prot. gms	Carbs gms	Sod. mgs	Fiber gms	Fat gms	Sat. Fat gms	Chol. mgs	% Fat Cal.
'Sports Gainer' strawberry, prepared w/water	12 fl oz	300	14	53	150	0	3.0	0.0	0	9%
'Sports Line Power Shake' Dutch chocolate, prepared	11 fl oz	220	15	37	150	0	1.0	0.0	0	4%
'Super Mega Mass 2000' banana, mix only	1 cup	547	27	106	400	0	1.5	0.9	15	3%
'Super Mega Mass 2000' banana, prepared w/low-fat milk	8 fl oz	334	18	59	261	0	3.1	na	17	8%
'Super Mega Mass 2000' chocolate, mix only	1 cup	547	27	106	400	0	1.5	0.9	15	3%
'Super Mega Mass 2000' chocolate, prepared w/low-fat milk	8 fl oz	334	18	59	261	0	3.1	na	17	8%
'Super Mega Mass 2000' strawberry, mix only	1 cup	547	27	106	400	0	1.5	0.9	15	3%
'Super Mega Mass 2000' strawberry, prepared w/low-fat milk	8 fl oz	334	18	59	261	0	3.1	na	17	8%
'Super Mega Mass 2000' vanilla, mix only	1 cup	547	27	106	400	0	1.5	0.9	15	3%
'Super Mega Mass 2000' vanilla, prepared w/low-fat milk	8 fl oz	334	18	59	261	0	3.1	na	17	8%
vegetable protein drink, mix only	1 cup	390	45	42	721	0	0.0	0.0	0	0%
vegetable protein drink, prepared w/nonfat milk	8 fl oz	158	17	20	278	0	0.0	0.0	0	0%
'Victory CarboFire' prepared w/water	8 fl oz	250	0	62	50	0	0.0	0.0	0	0%
'Victory Explosive Workout' citrus, mix only	4 tbsp	190	0	48	50	0	0.0	0.0	0	0%
'Victory Mass 1000' vanilla, prepared w/low-fat milk	16 fl oz	1020	51	180	760	0	11.0	0.0	0	10%
'Victory Mass 1000' vanilla, prepared w/water	16 fl oz	770	35	156	520	0	1.0	0.0	0	1%
'Victory Mega Mass 2000' prepared w/low-fat milk	24 fl oz	2000	106	351	1510	0	19.0	0.0	0	9%
'Victory Mega Mass 2000' prepared w/water	16 fl oz	1090	55	211	800	0	3.0	0.0	0	2%
'Victory Mega Mass 2000' prepared w/water	24 fl oz	1640	82	317	1200	0	5.0	0.0	0	3%
'Victory Mega Mass 2000' prepared w/water	8 fl oz	550	27	106	400	0	2.0	0.0	0	3%
(Weight Watchers)										
'Sweet Success' chocolate raspberry, mix only	1 scoop	90	7	11	150	6	2.0	1.0	5	20%
'Sweet Success' vanilla flavor, mix only	1 scoop	90	7	20	180	6	0.5	0.0	5	4%
SPOT										
baked, broiled, grilled, or microwaved	3 oz	134	20	0	31	0	5.3	1.6	65	36%
raw	3 oz	105	16	0	25	0	4.2	1.2	51	36%
SPRING ONION. See SCALLION.										
SQUAB										
average of all parts, meat and skin, raw	3 oz	252	16	0	46	0	20.4	7.2	81	73%
average of all parts, meat only, raw	3 oz	122	15	0	44	0	6.4	1.7	77	48%
light meat, meat only, raw	3 oz	115	19	0	47	0	3.9	1.0	77	30%
SQUASH. See also ZUCCHINI.										
ACORN										
baked, cubed	1 cup	115	2	30	8	9	0.3	0.1	0	2%
boiled, mashed	1 cup	83	2	22	7	6	0.2	0.0	0	2%
raw, approx 4-inch diam	1 squash	172	3	45	13	6	0.4	0.1	0	2%
raw, cubed	1 cup	56	1	15	4	2	0.1	0.0	0	2%
raw, cubed *(Frieda of California)*	1 oz	16	1	4	3	0	0.1	0.0	0	5%
BANANA, baked *(Frieda of California)*	1 oz	18	1	4	3	0	0.1	0.0	0	4%
BUTTERNUT										
Fresh										
baked, cubed	1 cup	82	2	22	8	na	0.2	0.0	0	2%
raw, cubed	1 cup	63	1	16	6	na	0.1	0.0	0	2%
Frozen										
boiled, mashed	1 cup	94	3	24	5	na	0.2	0.0	0	2%
unprepared	12-oz pkg	194	6	49	7	4	0.3	0.1	0	1%
unprepared	4-lb pkg	1034	32	261	36	24	1.8	0.4	0	1%
unprepared *(Flav-R-Pac)*	1/3 cup	30	1	8	5	2	0.0	0.0	0	0%
CROOKNECK										
Canned, yellow *(Allens)*	1/2 cup	16	1	3	230	0	1.0	0.0	0	36%

Food Name	Serving Size	Calories	Prot. gms	Carbs gms	Sod. mgs	Fiber gms	Fat gms	Sat. Fat gms	Chol. mgs	% Fat Cal.
Frozen										
cooked (Kohl's)	4 oz	45	1	11	0	0	1.0	0.0	0	16%
yellow (Seabrook)	3.3 oz	18	1	4	1	1	0.0	0.0	0	0%
yellow (Southern)	3.5 oz	21	2	4	20	0	0.1	0.0	0	4%
HUBBARD										
Fresh										
baked, cubed	1 cup	103	5	22	16	na	1.3	0.3	0	10%
boiled, mashed	1 cup	71	3	15	12	7	0.9	0.2	0	10%
raw, cubed	1 cup	46	2	10	8	na	0.6	0.1	0	10%
MARROW / vegetable marrow										
raw, trimmed	1 oz	4	0.2	1.0	na	>.1 c	<.1	tr	0	<16%
SCALLOP										
boiled, mashed	1 cup	38	2	8	2	5	0.4	0.1	0	9%
boiled, sliced	1 cup	29	2	6	2	3	0.3	0.1	0	9%
raw, sliced	1 cup	23	2	5	1	na	0.3	0.1	0	9%
SPAGHETTI										
boiled or baked, drained	1 cup	42	1	10	28	2	0.4	0.1	0	8%
raw, cubed	1 cup	31	1	7	17	na	0.6	0.1	0	15%
SUMMER. See also ZUCCHINI.										
Canned										
crookneck or straightneck, no salt added, mashed, drained	1 cup	31	1	7	12	3	0.2	0.0	0	5%
crookneck or straightneck, no salt added, diced, drained	1 cup	27	1	6	11	3	0.1	0.0	0	5%
crookneck or straightneck, no salt added, drained	1 cup	28	1	6	11	3	0.2	0.0	0	5%
Fresh										
all varieties, boiled, drained, sliced	1 cup	36	2	8	2	3	0.6	0.1	0	13%
all varieties, raw, sliced	1 cup	23	1	5	2	2	0.2	0.1	0	9%
all varieties, raw, whole	1 large	65	4	14	6	6	0.7	0.1	0	9%
all varieties, raw, whole	1 medium	39	2	9	4	4	0.4	0.1	0	9%
all varieties, raw, whole	1 small	24	1	5	2	2	0.2	0.1	0	9%
crookneck or straightneck, boiled, drained, sliced	1 cup	36	2	8	2	3	0.6	0.1	0	13%
crookneck or straightneck, drained, solid, sliced	1/2 cup	18	1	4	1	1	0.3	0.1	0	13%
crookneck or straightneck, raw, sliced	1 cup	25	1	5	3	2	0.3	0.1	0	11%
Frozen										
crookneck or straightneck, drained, sliced	1 cup	48	2	11	12	3	0.4	0.1	0	7%
crookneck or straightneck, sliced, unprepared	1 cup	26	1	6	7	2	0.2	0.0	0	6%
WINTER										
Fresh										
all varieties, baked, cubed	1 cup	80	2	18	2	6	1.3	0.3	0	14%
all varieties, raw, cubed	1 cup	43	2	10	5	2	0.3	0.1	0	5%
Frozen										
cooked (Birds Eye)	4 oz	45	1	11	0	2	0.0	0.0	0	0%
cooked (Seabrook)	4 oz	45	1	11	2	1	0.0	0.0	0	0%
YELLOW, frozen, sliced (Flav-R-Pac) sliced	2/3 cup	15	1	2	15	1	0.0	0.0	0	0%
SQUASH DISH/ENTRÉE										
(Stouffer's) casserole, frozen, food service product	1 oz	35	2	2	91	0	2.1	0.5	7	55%
SQUASH SEED										
dried, kernels	1 cup	747	34	25	25	5	63.3	12.0	0	71%
dried, kernels, hulled, approx 142 seeds	1 oz	153	7	5	5	1	13.0	2.5	0	71%
roasted, kernels	1 cup	1185	75	30	41	9	95.6	18.1	0	68%
roasted, kernels	1 oz	148	9	4	5	1	11.9	2.3	0	68%
roasted, whole	1 cup	285	12	34	12	na	12.4	2.3	0	36%

Food Name	Serving Size	Calories	Prot. gms	Carbs gms	Sod. mgs	Fiber gms	Fat gms	Sat. Fat gms	Chol. mgs	% Fat Cal.
roasted, whole, approx 85 seeds	1 oz	126	5	15	5	na	5.5	1.0	0	36%
SQUID / calamari										
mixed species, fried	3 oz	149	15	7	260	0	6.4	1.6	221	38%
mixed species, raw	3 oz	78	13	3	37	0	1.2	0.3	198	14%
mixed species, raw, boneless	1 oz	26	4	1	12	0	0.4	0.1	66	14%
SQUIRREL										
raw	1 oz	34	6	0	29	0	0.9	0.1	24	24%
roasted	3 oz	147	26	0	101	0	4.0	0.7	103	24%
STAR FRUIT / carambola										
raw, cubed.	1 cup	45	1	11	3	4	0.5	0.0	0	9%
raw, sliced	1 cup	36	1	8	2	3	0.4	0.0	0	9%
raw, whole, large, approx 4.5-inch long	1 fruit	42	1	10	3	3	0.4	0.0	0	9%
raw, whole, medium, approx 3-5/8-inch long.	1 fruit	30	0	7	2	2	0.3	0.0	0	9%
raw, whole, small, approx 3-inch long	1 fruit	23	0	5	1	2	0.2	0.0	0	9%
STEAK SAUCE. See under SAUCE.										
STEW. See also under individual types of dinner/entrée listings.										
(Stouffer's) Cajun seasoned, frozen, food service product . .	1 oz	24	1	2	99	1	1.4	0.3	6	52%
STIR-FRY ENTRÉE KIT										
(Tyson)										
. . . .	9 oz	230	22	15	480	0	9.0	0.0	80	35%
'Yoshida Oriental Sauce'	1.6 oz	100	2	22	1260	0	1.0	0.0	0	9%
STIR-FRY SEASONING. See under SEASONING MIX.										
STRAW MUSHROOM. See MUSHROOM, STRAW.										
STRAWBERRY										
Canned, in heavy syrup, w/liquid	1 cup	234	1	60	10	4	0.7	0.0	0	2%
Fresh										
raw, halved	1 cup	46	1	11	2	3	0.6	0.0	0	10%
raw, puréed	1 cup	70	1	16	2	5	0.9	0.0	0	10%
raw, sliced	1 cup	50	1	12	2	4	0.6	0.0	0	10%
raw, trimmed	1 pint	107	2	25	4	8	1.3	0.1	0	10%
raw, whole	1 cup	43	1	10	1	3	0.5	0.0	0	10%
raw, whole, extra large, approx 1-5/8 inch diam.	1 berry	8	0	2	0	1	0.1	0.0	0	10%
raw, whole, large, approx 1-3/8 inch diam.	1 berry	5	0	1	0	0	0.1	0.0	0	10%
raw, whole, medium, approx 1-1/4 inch diam	1 berry	4	0	1	0	0	0.0	0.0	0	10%
raw, whole, small, approx 1 inch diam.	1 berry	2	0	0	0	0	0.0	0.0	0	10%
Frozen										
sliced (Flav-R-Pac)	1/2 cup	150	1	33	0	2	1.5	1.0	0	9%
sliced, sweetened	10-oz pkg	273	2	74	9	5	0.4	0.0	0	1%
sliced, sweetened, thawed	1 cup	245	1	66	8	5	0.3	0.0	0	1%
whole (Flav-R-Pac)	1 cup	50	1	13	5	2	1.0	0.0	0	14%
whole, sweetened	10-oz pkg	222	1	60	3	5	0.4	0.0	0	2%
whole, sweetened, thawed	1 cup	199	1	54	3	5	0.4	0.0	0	2%
whole, unsweetened	1 med berry	4	0	1	0	0	0.0	0.0	0	3%
whole, unsweetened	20 oz pkg	198	2	52	11	12	0.6	0.0	0	3%
whole, unsweetened, thawed	1 cup	77	1	20	4	5	0.2	0.0	0	3%
whole, unsweetened, unthawed	1 cup	52	1	14	3	3	0.2	0.0	0	3%
STRAWBERRY COLADA. See under COCKTAIL MIX.										
STRAWBERRY DRINK. See under FRUIT DRINK; FRUIT JUICE BLEND; FRUIT JUICE DRINK.										
STRAWBERRY GUAVA. See GUAVA, STRAWBERRY.										
STRAWBERRY TOPPING										
. . . .	1 cup	864	1	225	71	3	0.3	0.0	0	0%
. . . .	2 tbsp	107	0	28	9	0	0.0	0.0	0	0%
(Flav-R-Pac).	2 tbsp	40	0	10	0	0	0.0	0.0	0	0%
(Knudsen) pourable	1 oz	75	0	18	0	0	1.0	0.0	0	11%

Food Name	Serving Size	Calories	Prot. gms	Carbs gms	Sod. mgs	Fiber gms	Fat gms	Sat. Fat gms	Chol. mgs	% Fat Cal.
(Kraft) nonfat	1 tbsp	50	0	14	5	0	0.0	0.0	0	0%
(Smucker's)										
nonfat	2 tbsp	120	0	30	0	0	0.0	0.0	0	0%
nonfat, 'Light'	2 tbsp	55	0	14	0	0	0.0	0.0	0	0%
STRING BEAN. See BEAN, GREEN.										
STRIPED BASS. See BASS, STRIPED.										
STRIPED MULLET. See MULLET, STRIPED.										
STROGANOFF ENTRÉE. See under BEEF DINNER/ENTRÉE; BEEF SUBSTITUTE DINNER/ENTRÉE MIX.										
STUFFING										
(Stouffer's) frozen , food service product, 'Old Fashion Stuff'n'	1 oz	70	1	7	142	1	4.0	0.7	1	51%
STUFFING MIX										
(Brownberry) sage and onion, mix only	1 serving	255	9	47	1126	4	3.4	0.6	na	12%
(Pepperidge Farm)										
apple and raisin, mix only	1/2 cup	140	4	27	520	2	1.5	0.0	0	10%
country garden and herb, mix only	1/2 cup	150	4	22	360	2	5.0	1.0	0	30%
harvest vegetable and herb, mix only	1/2 cup	140	5	23	300	2	3.0	0.4	0	19%
(Stove Top)										
chicken-flavored, 'Flexible Serving' prepared	1/2 cup	120	3	19	460	1	3.0	0.0	0	23%
chicken flavored, 'Flexible Serving' prepared w/margarine	1/2 cup	170	4	20	510	1	9.0	1.5	0	46%
cornbread, 'Flexible Serving' prepared	1/2 cup	110	3	19	500	1	2.5	0.0	0	20%
cornbread, 'Flexible Serving' prepared w/margarine	1/2 cup	170	3	21	580	1	8.0	1.5	0	43%
for beef, prepared w/margarine	1/2 cup	180	4	22	540	1	9.0	1.5	0	44%
for turkey, prepared w/margarine	1/2 cup	170	4	20	530	1	9.0	1.5	0	46%
STURGEON										
mixed species, baked, broiled, grilled, or microwaved	3 oz	115	18	0	59	0	4.4	1.0	65	35%
mixed species, baked, broiled, grilled, or microwaved, flaked	1 cup	184	28	0	94	0	7.0	1.6	105	35%
mixed species, raw	3 oz	89	14	0	46	0	3.4	0.8	51	35%
mixed species, smoked	3 oz	147	27	0	628	0	3.7	0.9	68	23%
mixed species, smoked	1 oz	49	9	0	210	0	1.2	0.3	23	23%
SUCCOTASH. See under VEGETABLE DISH/ENTRÉE.										
SUCKER, WHITE										
baked, broiled, grilled, or microwaved	3 oz	101	18	0	43	0	2.5	0.5	45	23%
raw	3 oz	78	14	0	34	0	2.0	0.4	35	23%
SUET										
beef, raw	4 oz	965	2	0	8	0	106.2	59.1	77	99%
beef, raw	1 oz	242	0	0	2	0	26.6	14.8	19	99%
SUGAR										
BEET										
granulated (Crystal)	1 tsp	16	0	4	0	0	0.0	0.0	0	0%
granulated juice, organic (Sucanat)	1 tsp	12	0	3	0	0	0.0	0.0	0	0%
CANE										
Brown										
dark brown 'Old Fashioned' (Domino)	1 tsp	16	0	4	0	0	0.0	0.0	0	0%
golden brown, Hawaiian (C&H)	1 tsp	16	0	4	0	0	0.0	0.0	0	0%
granulated	1 tsp	12	0	3	1	0	0.0	0.0	0	0%
light brown, golden, packed (Domino)	1 tsp	16	0	4	0	0	0.0	0.0	0	0%
light brown, granulated, 'Brownulated' (Domino)	1 tsp	12	0	3	0	0	0.0	0.0	0	0%
packed	1 cup	827	0	214	86	0	0.0	0.0	0	0%
packed	1 tsp	17	0	4	2	0	0.0	0.0	0	0%
unpacked	1 cup	545	0	141	57	0	0.0	0.0	0	0%
unpacked	1 tsp	11	0	3	1	0	0.0	0.0	0	0%

Food Name	Serving Size	Calories	Prot. gms	Carbs gms	Sod. mgs	Fiber gms	Fat gms	Sat. Fat gms	Chol. mgs	% Fat Cal.
White										
confectioner's, sifted, 10-X powdered *(Domino)*	1/2 cup	240	0	60	0	0	0.0	0.0	0	0%
confectioner's/powdered	1 tsp	10	0	2	0	0	0.0	0.0	0	0%
confectioner's/powdered, unsifted	1 cup	467	0	119	1	0	0.1	0.0	0	0%
confectioner's/powdered, unsifted	1 tbsp	31	0	8	0	0	0.0	0.0	0	0%
cubes	1 cube	19	0	5	0	0	0.0	0.0	0	0%
cubes, 'Dots' *(Domino)*	1 cube	8	0	2	0	0	0.0	0.0	0	0%
granulated	1 cup	774	0	200	2	0	0.0	0.0	0	0%
granulated	1 tsp	16	0	4	0	0	0.0	0.0	0	0%
granulated *(Crystal)*	1 tsp	16	0	4	0	0	0.0	0.0	0	0%
granulated *(Domino)*	1 tsp	16	0	4	0	0	0.0	0.0	0	0%
granulated, 'Packets' *(Domino)*	1 pkt	16	0	4	0	0	0.0	0.0	0	0%
granulated juice, organic *(Succanat)*	1 tsp	12	0	3	0	0	0.0	0.0	0	0%
superfine, instant-dissolving *(Domino)*	1 tsp	16	0	4	0	0	0.0	0.0	0	0%
MAPLE										
	1 oz	100	0	26	3	0	0.1	0.0	0	0%
	1 tsp	11	0	3	0	0	0.0	0.0	0	0%
approx 1.75 x 1.25 x 1/2 inch pieces	1 piece	99	0	25	3	0	0.1	0.0	0	0%
TURBINADO *(Hain)*	1 tbsp	50	0	12	0	0	0.0	0.0	0	0%
SUGAR APPLE / sweetsop										
raw, pulp	1 cup	235	5	59	23	11	0.7	0.1	0	3%
raw, whole, approx 2 7/8 inch diam	1 fruit	146	3	37	14	7	0.4	0.1	0	3%
SUGAR CANE BATON										
(Frieda of California)	1 oz	21	0	50	0	0	0.1	0.0	0	0%
(Sprinkle Sweet)	1 tsp	2	0	1	19	0	0.0	0.0	0	0%
SUGAR SNAP PEAS. See PEAS, SNAP.										
SUGAR SUBSTITUTE										
(Featherweight)										
liquid	3 drops	0	0	0	0	0	0.0	0.0	0	0%
saccharin grain tablet	1/4 tablet	0	0	0	2	0	0.0	0.0	0	0%
(Nutra Taste) w/o saccharin	1 pkt	4	0	1	0	0	0.0	0.0	0	0%
(NutraSweet)										
w/aspartame, 'Equal'	1 pkt	4	0	1	0	0	0.0	0.0	0	1%
w/aspartame, 'Equal'	1 tsp	12	0	3	0	0	0.0	0.0	0	0%
(S&W) liquid, 'Nutradiet'	1/8 tsp	0	0	0	0	0	0.0	0.0	0	0%
(Splenda)	1 tsp	2	0	1	0	0	0.0	0.0	0	0%
(Sprinkle Sweet)	1 tsp	2	0	1	0	0	0.0	0.0	0	0%
(Sucanat) juice, organic	1 tsp	12	0	3	0	0	0.0	0.0	0	0%
(Sugar Twin)										
w/saccharin	1 pkt	4	0	1	0	0	0.0	0.0	0	0%
w/saccharin, 'Plus'	1 pkt	3	0	1	0	0	0.0	0.0	0	0%
(Superose)										
liquid	1 tsp	0	0	0	0	0	0.0	0.0	0	0%
	1 tsp	4	0	1	4	0	0.0	0.0	0	0%
(Sweet 'N Low) saccharin-based	1 pkt	4	0	1	0	0	0.0	0.0	0	0%
(Sweet 10)										
	1/8 tsp	0	0	0	2	0	0.0	0.0	0	0%
liquid	1 tsp	0	0	0	0	0	0.0	0.0	0	0%
(Sweet One)	1 pkt	4	0	1	0	0	0.0	0.0	0	0%
(Sweet Plus) w/saccharin, equivalent to 2 tsp sugar	1 pkt	4	0	1	0	0	0.0	0.0	0	0%
(TKI Foods) w/aspartame, 'Superose Plus'	1 serving	0	0	1	0	0	0.0	0.0	0	0%
(Weight Watchers) 'Sweet'ner'	1 pkt	4	0	1	30	0	0.0	0.0	0	0%

SUMMER SQUASH. See under SQUASH. See also ZUCCHINI.

SUNCHOKE. See JERUSALEM ARTICHOKE.

Food Name	Serving Size	Calories	Prot. gms	Carbs gms	Sod. mgs	Fiber gms	Fat gms	Sat. Fat gms	Chol. mgs	% Fat Cal.
SUNDAE. See under ICE CREAM BAR/DESSERT; ICE CREAM SUBSTITUTE BAR/DESSERT.										
SUNFISH / calico bass / crappie / pumpkinfish										
baked, broiled, grilled, or microwaved	3 oz	97	21	0	88	0	0.8	0.2	73	7%
raw	3 oz	76	16	0	68	0	0.6	0.1	57	7%
SUN-DRIED TOMATO. See under TOMATO.										
SUNFLOWER BUTTER										
	1 oz	164	6	8	147	na	13.5	1.4	0	69%
	1 tbsp	93	3	4	83	na	7.6	0.8	0	69%
unsalted	1 oz	164	6	8	1	na	13.5	1.4	0	69%
unsalted	1 tbsp	93	3	4	0	na	7.6	0.8	0	69%
(Maranatha Natural) roasted	2 tbsp	170	4	8	5	0	14.0	0.0	0	72%
(Roaster Fresh)										
gourmet	1 oz	160	6	5	1	0	13.6	1.6	0	74%
roasted, w/o salt, creamy	1 oz	160	6	5	1	0	14.0	2.0	0	74%
SUNFLOWER SEED										
Dried										
(Frito-Lay's)	1 oz	160	7	6	265	0	14.0	0.0	0	71%
kernels (Arrowhead Mills)	1 oz	160	7	6	3	4	13.0	0.0	0	69%
kernels	1 cup	821	33	27	4	15	71.4	7.5	0	73%
kernels, in shell	1 cup	262	10	9	1	5	22.8	2.4	0	73%
kernels, shelled (National Sunflower)	1/4 cup	205	8	6	1	4	18.0	2.2	0	74%
natural, unsalted (Flanigan Farms)	1/4 cup	160	6	5	0	4	14.0	1.5	0	74%
salted, in shell (Fisher)	1 oz	170	6	6	110	0	14.0	1.0	0	72%
salted, in shell, 15–16 shelled seeds (Fisher)	1 oz	160	6	6	100	0	14.0	1.0	0	72%
unsalted (Fisher)	1 oz	170	6	6	0	0	14.0	1.0	0	72%
Dry-roasted										
(Fisher)	1 oz	170	6	6	200	0	15.0	2.0	0	74%
(Planters)	1 oz	160	6	6	170	0	14.0	2.0	0	72%
in shell (Fisher)	1 oz	170	6	6	110	0	15.0	1.0	0	74%
kernels (Flavor House)	1 oz	180	8	4	200	0	15.0	0.0	0	74%
kernels (Pathmark)	1 oz	180	5	7	150	0	14.0	0.0	0	72%
kernels, hulled, unsalted	1 cup	745	25	31	4	14	63.7	6.7	0	72%
kernels, salted	1 cup	745	25	31	998	12	63.7	6.7	0	72%
kernels, salted	1 oz	165	5	7	221	3	14.1	1.5	0	72%
kernels, shelled (Pathmark)	1 oz	180	5	7	150	0	14.0	0.0	0	72%
kernels, unsalted	1 oz	165	5	7	1	3	14.1	1.5	0	72%
w/tamari (Eden Foods)	1 oz	170	8	9	50	3	11.0	1.5	0	59%
Oil-roasted										
(Fisher)	1 oz	170	6	4	170	0	16.0	2.0	0	78%
(Planters)	1 oz	170	6	5	135	0	15.0	4.0	0	75%
kernels, salted	1 cup	830	29	20	814	9	77.6	8.1	0	78%
kernels, salted	1 oz	174	6	4	171	2	16.3	1.7	0	78%
kernels, shelled, salted	1 cup	830	29	20	814	9	77.6	8.1	0	78%
kernels, unsalted	1 cup	830	29	20	4	9	77.6	8.1	0	78%
kernels, unsalted	1 oz	174	6	4	1	2	16.3	1.7	0	78%
Roasted										
barbecue, salted, w/shell (David's)	3/4 cup	190	7	5	1350	2	15.0	1.5	0	74%
barbecue, salted, shelled (David's)	3/4 cup	190	7	5	130	2	15.0	1.5	0	74%
salted, shelled (David's)	3/4 cup	190	7	5	130	2	15.0	1.5	0	74%
salted, w/shell (David's)	3/4 cup	190	7	5	1350	2	15.0	1.5	0	74%
salted (Harmony)	1/4 cup	170	9	11	290	3	13.0	3.0	0	59%
Toasted										
kernels, salted	1 cup	829	23	28	821	15	76.1	8.0	0	77%
kernels, salted	1 oz	175	5	6	174	3	16.1	1.7	0	77%

Food Name	Serving Size	Calories	Prot. gms	Carbs gms	Sod. mgs	Fiber gms	Fat gms	Sat. Fat gms	Chol. mgs	% Fat Cal.
kernels, unsalted	1 cup	829	23	28	4	15	76.1	8.0	0	77%
kernels, unsalted	1 oz	175	5	6	1	3	16.1	1.7	0	77%
SUNFLOWER SEED OIL										
(Hain)	1 tbsp	120	0	0	0	0	14.0	2.0	0	100%
(IGA)	1 tbsp	120	0	0	0	0	14.0	2.0	0	100%
(Kroger)	1 tbsp	122	0	0	0	0	13.6	1.7	0	100%
(Pathmark)	1 tbsp	130	0	0	0	0	14.0	2.0	0	100%
at least 60% linoleic	1 cup	1927	0	0	0	0	218.0	22.5	0	100%
at least 60% linoleic	1 tbsp	120	0	0	0	0	13.6	1.4	0	100%
less than 60% linoleic	1 cup	1927	0	0	0	0	218.0	22.0	0	100%
less than 60% linoleic	1 tbsp	120	0	0	0	0	13.6	1.4	0	100%
linoleic, hydrogenated	1 cup	1927	0	0	0	0	218.0	28.3	0	100%
linoleic, hydrogenated	1 tbsp	120	0	0	0	0	13.6	1.8	0	100%
pure pressed, organic (Spectrum)	1 tbsp	120	0	0	0	0	14.0	1.5	0	100%

SURIMI. See under CRAB SUBSTITUTE; SCALLOP SUBSTITUTE.

SURINAM CHERRY. See PITANGA.

SWAMP CABBAGE. See CABBAGE, SKUNK.

SWEET CHESTNUT. See CHESTNUT, EUROPEAN.

SWEET PEPPER. See PEPPER, BELL.

SWEET POTATO

Food Name	Serving Size	Calories	Prot. gms	Carbs gms	Sod. mgs	Fiber gms	Fat gms	Sat. Fat gms	Chol. mgs	% Fat Cal.
Fresh										
baked in skin	1 cup	206	3	49	20	6	0.2	0.0	0	1%
baked in skin	1 large	185	3	44	18	5	0.2	0.0	0	1%
baked in skin	1 medium	117	2	28	11	3	0.1	0.0	0	1%
baked in skin	1 small	62	1	15	6	2	0.1	0.0	0	1%
boiled, w/o skin	1 medium	159	2	37	20	3	0.5	0.1	0	2%
boiled, w/o skin, mashed	1 cup	344	5	80	43	6	1.0	0.2	0	2%
raw, approx 5-inch long	1 potato	137	2	32	17	4	0.4	0.1	0	2%
raw, cubed	1 cup	140	2	32	17	4	0.4	0.1	0	2%
Canned										
cut, in water (Allens)	1/2 cup	70	1	16	20	0	1.0	0.0	0	12%
mashed	1 cup	258	5	59	191	4	0.5	0.1	0	2%
mashed (Joan of Arc)	1/2 cup	90	1	24	45	0	0.0	0.0	0	0%
mashed (Princella)	1/2 cup	90	1	24	45	0	0.0	0.0	0	0%
mashed (Royal Prince)	1/2 cup	90	1	24	45	0	0.0	0.0	0	0%
mashed, vacuum pack	1 cup	232	4	54	135	5	0.5	0.1	0	2%
pieces, vacuum pack	1 cup	182	3	42	106	4	0.4	0.1	0	2%
syrup pack, drained	1 cup	212	3	50	76	6	0.6	0.1	0	2%
syrup pack, w/liquid	1 cup	203	2	48	100	6	0.5	0.1	0	2%
whole, vacuum pack (Taylor's Brand)	1 cup	210	4	55	56	0	0.0	0.0	0	0%
Frozen										
cubes	1 cup	169	3	39	11	3	0.3	0.1	0	2%
whipped, food service product (Stouffer's)	1 oz	40	0	7	92	1	1.4	0.3	0	31%

SWEET POTATO LEAF

Food Name	Serving Size	Calories	Prot. gms	Carbs gms	Sod. mgs	Fiber gms	Fat gms	Sat. Fat gms	Chol. mgs	% Fat Cal.
Fresh										
raw, whole, 12.25-inch leaf	1 leaf	6	1	1	1	0	0.0	0.0	0	7%
raw, chopped	1 cup	12	1	2	3	1	0.1	0.0	0	7%
steamed, chopped	1 cup	22	1	5	8	1	0.2	0.0	0	7%

SWEETBREAD. See BEEF, PANCREAS; BEEF, THYMUS; LAMB, PANCREAS; VEAL, PANCREAS; VEAL, THYMUS.

SWEETENER. See BARLEY MALT; CORN SYRUP; HONEY; SUGAR, BEET; SUGAR, CANE; SUGAR, MAPLE; SUGAR SUBSTITUTE; SYRUP.

SWEETSOP. See SUGAR APPLE.

SWISS CHARD / chard

Food Name	Serving Size	Calories	Prot. gms	Carbs gms	Sod. mgs	Fiber gms	Fat gms	Sat. Fat gms	Chol. mgs	% Fat Cal.
Fresh										
boiled, drained, chopped	1 cup	35	3	7	313	4	0.1	0.0	0	3%

Food Name	Serving Size	Calories	Prot. gms	Carbs gms	Sod. mgs	Fiber gms	Fat gms	Sat. Fat gms	Chol. mgs	% Fat Cal.
raw, chopped...............................	1 cup	7	1	1	77	1	0.1	0.0	0	9%
raw, whole................................	1 med leaf	9	1	2	102	1	0.1	0.0	0	9%
SWORDFISH										
Fresh										
baked, broiled, grilled, or microwaved.............	3 oz	132	22	0	98	0	4.4	1.2	43	30%
raw...................................	3 oz	103	17	0	77	0	3.4	0.9	33	30%
Frozen										
steaks, boneless, raw (Peter Pan Seafoods)...........	3.5 oz	118	19	0	102	0	4.0	0.0	39	32%
steaks, w/o seasoning mix (SeaPak)...............	6-oz pkg	210	34	0	155	0	7.0	0.0	70	32%
SYRUP										
BLACKBERRY (Knott's Berry Farm)...................	1 oz	120	0	30	0	0	0.0	0.0	0	0%
BLUEBERRY										
(Estee) 'Breakfast'........................	1 tbsp	12	0	3	10	0	0.0	0.0	0	0%
(Featherweight)...........................	1 tbsp	16	0	4	35	0	0.0	0.0	0	0%
(Knott's Berry Farm)										
....	1 oz	120	0	30	0	0	0.0	0.0	0	0%
'Light'.................................	1 oz	50	0	12	0	0	0.0	0.0	0	0%
(Knudsen)..............................	1 oz	75	1	19	0	0	1.0	0.0	0	10%
(S&W) lower calorie.......................	1/4 cup	60	0	15	105	0	0.0	0.0	0	0%
BOYSENBERRY										
(Knott's Berry Farm)										
....	1 oz	120	0	30	0	0	0.0	0.0	0	0%
'Light'.................................	1 oz	50	0	12	0	0	0.0	0.0	0	0%
BUTTER FLAVOR (S&W) lower calorie...............	1/4 cup	60	0	15	105	0	0.0	0.0	0	0%
CHOCOLATE										
(Estee) 'Choco-Syp'.......................	1 tbsp	20	0	5	5	0	0.0	0.0	0	0%
(Hershey's) light, genuine chocolate	2 tbsp	50	1	12	48	1	0.1	0.1	0	3%
(Nestlé) 'Quik'..........................	2 tbsp	100	1	23	30	1	0.5	0.0	0	4%
(Smucker's)............................	2 tbsp	130	1	27	35	0	2.0	0.0	0	14%
FRUIT (Smucker's) all flavors......................	2 tbsp	100	0	26	0	0	0.0	0.0	0	0%
MALT										
....	1 cup	1221	23.8	273.8	134	0	0.0	na	0	0%
....	1 tbsp	76	1.5	17.1	8	0	0.0	na	0	0%
(Eden Foods) barley, organic, w/sprouted barley..........	1 tbsp	60	1	14	0	0	0.0	0.0	0	0%
MAPLE										
....	1 cup	825	0	212	28	0	0.6	0.1	0	1%
....	1 tbsp	52	0	13	2	0	0.0	0.0	0	1%
(Estee) 'Breakfast'	1 tbsp	12	0	3	35	0	0.0	0.0	0	0%
(Knudsen) 'Fruit 'N Maple'...................	1 oz	105	1	26	0	0	1.0	0.0	0	8%
(Maple House)										
100% pure............................	1 oz	100	0	61	4	0	0.0	0.0	0	0%
no sugar.............................	2 tbsp	110	0	27	50	0	0.0	0.0	0	0%
(Maple Valley) no sugar, 'Lite'.................	2 tbsp	60	0	16	60	0	0.0	0.0	0	0%
(Pillsbury)										
butter...............................	1/4 cup	210	0	52	90	0	0.0	0.0	0	0%
butter, lite............................	1/4 cup	100	0	24	180	1	0.0	0.0	0	0%
lite.................................	1/4 cup	100	0	24	180	1	0.0	0.0	0	0%
regular..............................	1/4 cup	210	0	52	90	0	0.0	0.0	0	0%
(S&W) no sugar, Saccharin sweetened.................	1 tsp	4	0	1	25	0	0.0	0.0	0	0%
MAPLE FLAVOR (S&W) lower calorie.................	1/4 cup	60	0	15	105	0	0.0	0.0	0	0%
PANCAKE										
cane and maple, 15% maple.............	1 cup	879	0	237	328	0	0.3	0.1	0	0%
cane and maple, 15% maple.............	1 tbsp	56	0	15	21	0	0.0	0.0	0	0%
cane and maple, 2% maple..............	1 cup	835	0	219	192	0	0.3	0.1	0	0%

Food Name	Serving Size	Calories	Prot. gms	Carbs gms	Sod. mgs	Fiber gms	Fat gms	Sat. Fat gms	Chol. mgs	% Fat Cal.
cane and maple, 2% maple.................	1 tbsp	53	0	14	12	0	0.0	0.0	0	0%
(Aunt Jemima)										
'Butter Rich'............................	1/4 cup	210	0	52	170	0	0.0	0.0	0	0%
'Butterlite'.............................	1/4 cup	100	0	26	150	0	0.0	0.0	0	0%
'Lite'.................................	1 oz	54	0	13	92	0	0.1	0.0	0	2%
lite, lower calorie, 3% real maple syrup........	1/4 cup	100	0	27	160	0	0.0	0.0	0	0%
'Original' rich maple taste.................	1 oz	100	0	26	60	0	0.0	0.0	0	0%
pancake/waffle........................	1/4 cup	210	0	53	120	0	0.0	0.0	0	0%
(Br'er Rabbit)										
dark................................	1 oz	120	0	31	0	0	0.0	0.0	0	0%
light................................	1 oz	120	0	31	0	0	0.0	0.0	0	0%
(Cary's) sugar-free, lower calorie, artificial maple.........	1/4 cup	35	0	9	105	0	0.0	0.0	0	0%
(Estee).............................	1 tbsp	4	0	1	25	0	0.0	0.0	0	0%
(Featherweight)......................	1 tbsp	16	0	4	25	0	0.0	0.0	0	0%
(Hungry Jack)										
....	2 tbsp	100	0	26	25	0	0.0	0.0	0	0%
light, microwaveable....................	1/4 cup	100	0	24	180	1	0.0	0.0	0	0%
lite.................................	2 tbsp	50	0	14	105	0	0.0	0.0	0	0%
microwaveable........................	1/4 cup	210	0	52	90	0	0.0	0.0	0	0%
(Karo).............................	4 tbsp	234	0	59	83	0	0.0	0.0	0	0%
(Knott's Berry Farm)										
....	1 oz	110	0	28	0	0	0.0	0.0	0	0%
'Country'.............................	1 oz	110	0	27	0	0	0.0	0.0	0	0%
'Light' microwaveable...................	1 oz	45	0	11	70	0	0.0	0.0	0	0%
lower calorie, microwave, 'Heat & Pour'........	1 oz	45	0	11	70	0	0.0	0.0	0	0%
microwave, 'Heat & Pour'.................	1 oz	110	0	28	90	0	0.0	0.0	0	0%
w/30% real maple, microwaveable...........	1 oz	110	0	28	90	0	0.0	0.0	0	0%
(Log Cabin)										
butter flavor, 'Country Kitchen'.............	1 oz	100	0	27	100	0	0.0	0.0	0	0%
'Country Kitchen'.......................	1 oz	100	0	26	20	0	0.0	0.0	0	0%
lite, lower calorie......................	1 oz	50	0	13	90	0	0.0	0.0	0	0%
'Pancake & Waffle'.....................	1 oz	100	0	26	35	0	0.0	0.0	0	0%
syrup product 'Country Kitchen Lite'.........	1 oz	50	0	13	85	0	0.0	0.0	0	0%
(Mrs. Butterworth's)										
lower calorie.........................	1/4 cup	100	0	25	100	0	0.0	0.0	0	0%
thick and rich, 'Lite'...................	2 tbsp	60	0	15	65	0	0.0	0.0	0	0%
(S&W)										
butter flavor, reduced calorie.............	1/4 cup	60	0	15	105	na	0.0	0.0	0	0%
maple flavor, reduced calorie.............	1/4 cup	60	0	15	105	na	0.0	0.0	0	0%
(Vermont Maid)......................	1 tbsp	50	0	13	5	0	0.0	0.0	0	0%
(Weight Watchers) lower calorie..........	1 tbsp	25	0	7	40	0	0.0	0.0	0	0%
RASPBERRY *(Knudsen)*.................	1 oz	75	1	18	0	0	1.0	0.0	0	11%
RICE *(Lundberg Family)* organic 'Sweet Dreams'.......	1 tbsp	42	1	10	2	0	1.0	0.0	0	17%
SORGHUM										
....	1 cup	957	0	247	26	0	0.0	0.0	0	0%
....	1 tbsp	61	0	16	2	0	0.0	0.0	0	0%
STRAWBERRY										
(Knott's Berry Farm)..................	1 oz	120	0	30	0	0	0.0	0.0	0	0%
(Knudsen & Sons)....................	1 oz	75	1	18	0	0	1.0	0.0	0	11%
(Nestlé) 'Quik'......................	2 tbsp	110	0	27	0	0	0.0	0.0	0	0%
(S&W)										
lower calorie.........................	1/4 cup	60	0	15	105	0	0.0	0.0	0	0%
w/Saccharin.........................	1 tsp	4	0	1	25	0	0.0	0.0	0	0%

T

Food Name	Serving Size	Calories	Prot. gms	Carbs gms	Sod. mgs	Fiber gms	Fat gms	Sat. Fat gms	Chol. mgs	% Fat Cal.
TABBOULEH MIX. See under RICE DISH/ENTRÉE MIX.										
TACO										
(Owens)										
ham, refrigerated, 'Border Breakfasts'	2.17 oz	90	7	13	430	0	6.0	0.0	50	40%
sausage, refrigerated, 'Border Breakfasts'	2.17 oz	190	7	11	345	0	12.0	0.0	65	60%
TACO DINNER/ENTRÉE KIT										
(Pancho Villa)										
w/2 shells, seasoning, and sauce, mix only	1 serving	150	2	20	790	2	8.0	1.5	0	45%
prepared	2 tacos	270	2	20	840	4	13.0	5.0	60	57%
(Tio Sancho)										
taco sauce, 'Dinner Kit'	2 oz	62	2	13	750	1	0.2	0.0	0	3%
taco seasoning, 'Dinner Kit'	1.25 oz	104	2	21	2500	2	1.4	0.0	0	12%
taco shell, 'Dinner Kit'	1 shell	64	1	8	1	1	3.1	0.0	0	43%
TACO FILLING										
(Hunt's) 'Manwich'	1/4 cup	31	1	7	587	1	0.1	0.0	0	3%
(Chili Bowl) beef	1/4 cup	150	8	4	240	2	11.0	5.0	15	67%
(McCarty) chicken	1.29 oz	80	7	1	181	0	5.1	1.4	75	58%
TACO MIX										
(Del Monte) starter	8 oz	140	3	28	2180	0	1.0	0.0	0	7%
(Natural Touch)										
	3 tbsp	60	8	5	585	3	0.9	0.2	0	14%
vegetarian	2 tbsp	90	10	6	0	0	2.0	0.0	0	22%
(Old El Paso) prepared	1 taco	67	2	8	423	0	3.0	0.0	0	40%
(Ortega) meat, prepared	1 oz	60	4	1	105	0	4.0	2.0	20	64%
(Tio Sancho) 'Dinner Kit'	1 shell	64	1	8	1	1	3.1	0.0	0	43%
TACO SALAD SEASONING. See under SEASONING MIX.										
TACO SEASONING MIX. See under SEASONING MIX.										
TACO SHELL										
baked	1 oz	133	2	18	104	2	6.4	0.9	0	43%
baked, large, 6.5-inch dia.	1 shell	98	2	13	77	2	4.7	0.7	0	43%
baked, medium, 5-inch diam	1 shell	62	1	8	49	1	3.0	0.4	0	43%
baked, mini, 3-inch diam	1 shell	23	0	3	18	0	1.1	0.2	0	43%
baked, no salt added	1 oz	133	2	18	4	2	6.4	0.9	0	43%
baked, no salt added, medium, 5-inch diam	1 shell	61	1	8	2	1	2.9	0.4	0	43%
baked, no salt added, mini, 3-inch diam	1 shell	23	0	3	1	0	1.1	0.2	0	43%
(Azteca)										
corn	1 shell	60	1	7	65	0	3.0	0.0	0	46%
flour, for salad	1 shell	200	3	18	130	0	12.0	0.0	0	56%
(Bearitos) blue corn	1 serving	130	3	17	0	na	7.0	na	0	44%
(Chi-Chi's)	0.96 oz	140	2	17	5	0	7.0	0.0	0	45%
(Gebhardt)	1 shell	52	1	6	2	1	2.8	0.8	0	47%
(Lawry's)										
	1 shell	50	1	8	123	0	2.1	0.0	0	35%
'Super'	1 shell	86	1	13	210	0	3.6	0.0	0	36%
(Old El Paso)										
mini	3 shells	70	1	7	60	1	4.0	0.0	0	53%
'Super'	2 shells	190	3	21	150	2	12.0	2.0	0	53%
'Super Size'	1 shell	100	1	11	95	2	6.0	0.0	0	53%
(Ortega)	1 shell	50	0	8	5	0	2.0	0.0	0	36%
(Pancho Villa)	3 shells	190	2	19	0	3	11.0	2.5	0	54%
(Rosarita)	1 serving	52	1	6	2	1	2.8	0.8	0	47%

Food Name	Serving Size	Calories	Prot. gms	Carbs gms	Sod. mgs	Fiber gms	Fat gms	Sat. Fat gms	Chol. mgs	% Fat Cal.
(Tio Sancho)										
....	1 shell	64	1	8	1	1	3.1	0.0	0	43%
'Super'	1 shell	94	2	11	2	1	4.7	0.0	0	45%
TAFFY. See under CANDY.										
TAHINI. See SESAME BUTTER.										
TAHINI MIX										
(Arrowhead Mills) organic	1 oz	170	6	4	1	3	17.0	0.0	0	79%
(Westbrae)										
Mid-Eastern, organic................................	2 tbsp	220	9	3	0	0	20.0	0.0	0	79%
raw, organic........................	2 tbsp	210	8	1	0	0	19.0	0.0	0	83%
toasted, organic........................	2 tbsp	220	8	3	0	0	19.0	0.0	0	80%
TAMALE DINNER/ENTRÉE										
(Amy's Kitchen) pie, organic, frozen, 'Mexican'	8-oz pie	220	10	41	480	11	3.0	0.0	0	12%
(Dennison's) in chili gravy, canned, 'Tamalito'	7.5 oz	310	6	37	1395	0	16.0	0.0	0	46%
(Derby)										
beef, canned............................	6.561 oz	253	7	21	1034	4	17.4	8.2	23	58%
beef, canned............................	2 tamales	160	8	15	570	1	7.0	3.0	24	41%
(Gebhardt)										
....	2 tamales	290	5	19	730	2	22.0	8.0	54	67%
canned	5.75 oz	269	5	19	770	3	20.7	9.5	28	67%
jumbo, canned..............	6.949 oz	332	6	24	930	3	25.2	11.6	34	66%
jumbo, canned..............	1 serving	166	3	12	465	2	12.6	5.8	17	66%
(Hormel)										
beef, canned.............	2 pieces	140	4	8	550	0	10.0	0.0	0	65%
beef, canned, 'Hot'N Spicy'.................	2 pieces	140	4	9	612	0	10.0	0.0	0	63%
beef, frozen................	1 piece	140	6	13	555	0	7.0	0.0	0	45%
canned	7.5 oz	280	6	19	990	0	20.0	0.0	35	64%
hot-spicy, canned............	7.5 oz	280	6	19	990	0	20.0	0.0	35	64%
(Libby's) beef, w/sauce, canned...........	7.5 oz	408	9	26	1200	0	30.2	13.2	43	66%
(Old El Paso) canned.......................	2 pieces	190	5	16	380	0	12.0	0.0	20	56%
(Patio) frozen.......................	13 oz	470	12	58	1850	0	21.0	0.0	35	40%
(Van Camp's) w/sauce, canned..............	1 cup	293	8	29	1132	2	16.2	0.0	0	50%
(Wolf Brand) canned	7.75 oz	328	8	25	1181	2	24.5	0.0	0	62%
TAMARI. See under SAUCE.										
TAMARIND / Indian date										
Fresh										
raw, pulp	1 cup	287	3	75	34	6	0.7	0.3	0	2%
raw, whole, approx 1 x 3 inches	1 fruit	5	0	1	1	0	0.0	0.0	0	2%
'Tamarindos' *(Frieda of California)*.	3.5 oz	239	3	63	51	0	0.6	0.0	0	2%
TANGERINE. See also MANDARIN ORANGE										
Fresh										
raw, sections	1 cup	86	1	22	2	4	0.4	0.0	0	4%
raw, whole, large, approx 2.5-inch diam	1 fruit	43	1	11	1	2	0.2	0.0	0	4%
raw, whole, medium, approx 2-3/8 inch diam	1 fruit	37	1	9	1	2	0.2	0.0	0	4%
raw, whole, small, approx 2.25 inch diam	1 fruit	31	0	8	1	2	0.1	0.0	0	4%
TANGERINE JUICE										
canned, sweetened...........................	1 cup	125	1	30	2	0	0.5	0.0	0	3%
canned, sweetened...........................	1 fl oz	16	0	4	0	0	0.1	0.0	0	3%
chilled, 'Pure & Light Mandarin Tangerine' *(Dole)*	6 fl oz	97	1	25	20	0	0.1	0.0	0	1%
fresh, raw	1 cup	106	1	25	2	0	0.5	0.1	0	4%
fresh, raw	1 fl oz	13	0	3	0	0	0.1	0.0	0	4%
frozen concentrate, diluted	1 cup	111	1	27	2	na	0.3	0.0	0	2%
frozen concentrate, diluted	1 fl oz	14	0	3	0	na	0.0	0.0	0	2%
frozen concentrate, undiluted	6 fl oz	345	3	83	6	1	0.8	0.1	0	2%

Food Name	Serving Size	Calories	Prot. gms	Carbs gms	Sod. mgs	Fiber gms	Fat gms	Sat. Fat gms	Chol. mgs	% Fat Cal.
frozen or chilled (Minute Maid)	6 fl oz	90	1	23	0	0	0.0	0.0	0	0%
TANNIA. See YAUTIA.										
TAPIOCA. See also under PUDDING.										
pearl, dry	1 cup	544	0	135	2	1	0.0	0.0	0	0%
pearl, dry	1 oz	97	<0.1	25.1	tr	0.3	tr	(tr)	0	0%
TAQUITO beef, crispy, shredded										
(Prima Rosa by Ruiz)	5 taquitos	330	14	35	480	9	15.0	3.0	35	41%
TARO										
cooked, sliced	1 cup	187	1	46	20	7	0.1	0.0	0	1%
raw, sliced	1 cup	116	2	28	11	4	0.2	0.0	0	1%
Tahitian, cooked, sliced	1 cup	60	6	9	74	na	0.9	0.2	0	13%
Tahitian, raw, sliced	1 cup	55	3	9	63	na	1.2	0.2	0	18%
TARO CHIPS										
	1 oz	141	1	19	97	2	7.1	1.8	0	44%
	10 chips	115	1	16	79	2	5.7	1.5	0	44%
salted (Ray's)	1 oz	139	2	20	167	0	6.0	0.0	0	38%
unsalted (Ray's)	1 oz	139	2	20	15	0	6.0	0.0	0	38%
TARO LEAF										
raw, chopped	1 cup	12	1	2	1	1	0.2	0.0	0	15%
raw, whole, 11x6.5-inch leaf	1 leaf	4	0	1	0	0	0.1	0.0	0	15%
steamed, chopped	1 cup	35	4	6	3	3	0.6	0.1	0	14%
TARO SHOOT										
cooked, sliced	1 cup	20	1	4	3	na	0.1	0.0	0	5%
raw, whole	1 med shoot	9	1	2	1	na	0.1	0.0	0	7%
raw, sliced	1/2 cup	5	0	1	0	na	0.0	0.0	0	7%
TARRAGON										
dried (McCormick/Schilling)	1 tsp	2	0	0	0	0	0.0	0.0	0	0%
ground	1 tbsp	14	1	2	3	0	0.3	0.1	0	21%
ground	1 tsp	5	0	1	1	0	0.1	0.0	0	21%
ground (Spice Islands)	1 tsp	5	0	1	1	0	0.1	0.0	0	18%
ground, fresh (Durkee)	1 tsp	10	0	0	0	0	0.0	0.0	0	0%
ground, fresh (Laurel Leaf)	1 tsp	10	0	0	0	0	0.0	0.0	0	0%
TEA										
BLACK										
Brewed										
decaffeinated, prepared w/tap water	6 fl oz	2	0	1	5	0	0.0	0.0	0	0%
decaffeinated, prepared w/tap water	8 fl oz	2	0	1	7	0	0.0	0.0	0	0%
regular, prepared w/distilled water	6 fl oz	2	0	1	0	0	0.0	0.0	0	0%
regular, prepared w/tap water	6 fl oz	2	0	1	5	0	0.0	0.0	0	0%
regular, prepared w/tap water	8 fl oz	2	0	1	7	0	0.0	0.0	0	0%
(Bigelow)										
Darjeeling	5.25 fl oz	1	0	0	1	0	0.0	0.0	0	0%
'Earl Grey'	5.25 fl oz	1	0	0	1	0	0.0	0.0	0	0%
'English Teatime'	5.25 fl oz	1	0	0	0	0	0.0	0.0	0	0%
(Celestial Seasonings)										
'Classic English Breakfast'	8 fl oz	3	0	0	1	0	0.0	0.0	0	0%
decaffeinated	8 fl oz	4	0	1	5	0	0.0	0.0	0	0%
'Extraordinary Earl Grey'	8 fl oz	3	0	1	1	0	0.0	0.0	0	0%
(Exotica)										
'Assam Breakfast'	8 fl oz	0	0	0	0	0	0.0	0.0	0	0%
'Ceylon Earl Grey'	8 fl oz	0	0	0	0	0	0.0	0.0	0	0%
'Champagne Oolong'	8 fl oz	0	0	0	0	0	0.0	0.0	0	0%
'China White'	8 fl oz	0	0	0	0	0	0.0	0.0	0	0%
'Darjeeling'	8 fl oz	0	0	0	0	0	0.0	0.0	0	0%

Food Name	Serving Size	Calories	Prot. gms	Carbs gms	Sod. mgs	Fiber gms	Fat gms	Sat. Fat gms	Chol. mgs	% Fat Cal.
'Dragonwell'	8 fl oz	0	0	0	0	0	0.0	0.0	0	0%
'Osmanthus'	8 fl oz	0	0	0	0	0	0.0	0.0	0	0%
'Reserve Blend'	8 fl oz	0	0	0	0	0	0.0	0.0	0	0%
'Silver Jasmine'	8 fl oz	0	0	0	0	0	0.0	0.0	0	0%
(Lipton)										
black, regular	6 fl oz	0	0	0	0	0	0.0	0.0	0	0%
black, w/lemon flavor	6 fl oz	3	0	1	1	0	0.0	0.0	0	0%
(Stash's)										
'American'	8 fl oz	0	0	0	0	0	0.0	0.0	0	0%
'China Black'	8 fl oz	0	0	0	0	0	0.0	0.0	0	0%
'Earl Grey' decaffeinated	8 fl oz	0	0	0	0	0	0.0	0.0	0	0%
'English Breakfast' decaffeinated	8 fl oz	0	0	0	0	0	0.0	0.0	0	0%
'English Breakfast'	8 fl oz	0	0	0	0	0	0.0	0.0	0	0%
'Oolong'	8 fl oz	0	0	0	0	0	0.0	0.0	0	0%
'Orange Pekoe'	8 fl oz	0	0	0	0	0	0.0	0.0	0	0%
Instant										
powder, unsweetened	1 tsp	2	0	0	1	0	0.0	0.0	0	1%
powder, unsweetened, prepared	8 fl oz	2	0	0	7	0	0.0	0.0	0	0%
(Lipton) decaffeinated, prepared	6 fl oz	0	0	0	0	0	0.0	0.0	0	0%
GREEN, brewed *(Bigelow)* 'Chinese Fortune'	5.25 fl oz	1	0	0	1	0	0.0	0.0	0	0%
HERBAL/FLAVORED										
Bagged										
(Good Earth)										
'Good Night' caffeine-free	1 bag	1	0	1	0	0	0.0	0.0	0	0%
apple and spice, caffeine-free	1 bag	1	0	1	5	0	0.0	0.0	0	0%
chamomile, caffeine-free	1 bag	1	0	0	0	0	0.0	0.0	0	0%
fruit and spice, caffeine-free	1 bag	1	0	1	0	0	0.0	0.0	0	0%
ginseng, caffeine-free	1 bag	1	0	0	0	0	0.0	0.0	0	0%
lemon twist, caffeine-free	1 bag	2	0	1	0	0	0.0	0.0	0	0%
orange spice, caffeine-free	1 bag	1	0	1	0	0	0.0	0.0	0	0%
original flavor, caffeine-free	1 bag	4	0	0	0	0	0.0	0.0	0	0%
original spice, caffeine-free	1 bag	4	0	1	0	0	0.0	0.0	0	0%
(Super Dieters Tea)										
apricot, caffeine-free	1 bag	3	1	1	5	0	1.0	0.0	0	53%
cinnamon spice, caffeine-free	1 bag	3	1	1	5	0	1.0	0.0	0	53%
lemon mint, caffeine-free	1 bag	0	0	0	0	0	0.0	0.0	0	0%
original flavor, caffeine-free	1 bag	3	1	1	5	0	1.0	0.0	0	53%
peppermint, caffeine-free	1 bag	3	1	1	5	0	1.0	0.0	0	53%
Brewed										
chamomile, brewed	6 fl oz	2	0	0	2	0	0.0	0.0	0	0%
chamomile, brewed	8 fl oz	2	0	0	2	0	0.0	0.0	0	0%
herbal, all types, except chamomile, brewed	6 fl oz	2	0	0	2	0	0.0	0.0	0	0%
herbal, all types, except chamomile, brewed	8 fl oz	2	0	0	2	0	0.0	0.0	0	0%
(Bigelow)										
almond orange	5 fl oz	1	0	0	1	0	0.0	0.0	0	0%
'Apple Orchard'	5.25 fl oz	5	0	1	1	0	0.0	0.0	0	0%
apple spice	5 fl oz	1	0	0	1	0	0.0	0.0	0	0%
chamomile	5 fl oz	1	0	0	2	0	0.0	0.0	0	0%
chamomile mint	5 fl oz	1	0	0	1	0	0.0	0.0	0	0%
cinnamon orange	5 fl oz	1	0	0	1	0	0.0	0.0	0	0%
'Cinnamon Stick'	5.25 fl oz	1	0	0	1	0	0.0	0.0	0	0%
'Constant Comment'	5.25 fl oz	1	0	0	1	0	0.0	0.0	0	0%
cranberry apple	5 fl oz	1	0	0	1	0	0.0	0.0	0	0%
'Fruit & Almond'	5.25 fl oz	1	0	0	1	0	0.0	0.0	0	0%

Food Name	Serving Size	Calories	Prot. gms	Carbs gms	Sod. mgs	Fiber gms	Fat gms	Sat. Fat gms	Chol. mgs	% Fat Cal.
grains, roasted, w/carob	5 fl oz	3	0	1	1	0	0.0	0.0	0	0%
hibiscus, w/rose hips	5 fl oz	1	0	0	1	0	0.0	0.0	0	0%
'I Love Lemon'	5.25 fl oz	1	0	0	1	0	0.0	0.0	0	0%
'Lemon & C'	5 fl oz	1	0	0	1	0	0.0	0.0	0	0%
'Lemon Lift'	5.25 fl oz	1	0	0	1	0	0.0	0.0	0	0%
'Mint Blend'	5 fl oz	1	0	0	3	0	0.0	0.0	0	0%
'Mint Medley'	5.25 fl oz	1	0	0	1	0	0.0	0.0	0	0%
'Orange & C'	5 fl oz	1	0	0	1	0	0.0	0.0	0	0%
'Orange & Spice'	5.25 fl oz	1	0	0	1	0	0.0	0.0	0	0%
peppermint	5 fl oz	1	0	0	2	0	0.1	0.0	0	53%
'Plantation Mint'	5.25 fl oz	1	0	0	1	0	0.0	0.0	0	0%
'Raspberry Royale'	5.25 fl oz	1	0	0	1	0	0.0	0.0	0	0%
red raspberry	5 fl oz	1	0	0	1	0	0.0	0.0	0	0%
spearmint	5 fl oz	1	0	0	1	0	0.0	0.0	0	0%
'Specially Strawberry'	5 fl oz	1	0	0	1	0	0.0	0.0	0	0%
'Sweet Dreams'	5.25 fl oz	1	0	0	1	0	0.0	0.0	0	0%
'Take-A-Break'	5.25 fl oz	1	0	1	1	0	0.0	0.0	0	0%
(Celestial Seasonings)										
'Almond Sunset'	8 fl oz	3	0	1	2	0	0.0	0.0	0	0%
'Amaretto Nights'	8 fl oz	3	0	1	1	0	0.0	0.0	0	0%
apple spice, 'Fruit & Tea'	8 fl oz	3	0	0	1	0	0.0	0.0	0	0%
'Bavarian Chocolate Orange'	8 fl oz	7	0	2	5	0	0.0	0.0	0	0%
chamomile	8 fl oz	2	0	1	5	0	0.0	0.0	0	0%
'Cinnamon Apple Spice'	8 fl oz	3	0	0	1	0	0.0	0.0	0	0%
'Cinnamon Rose'	8 fl oz	2	0	1	1	0	0.0	0.0	0	0%
'Cinnamon Vienna'	8 fl oz	2	0	0	2	0	0.0	0.0	0	0%
'Country Peach Spice'	8 fl oz	3	0	1	3	0	0.0	0.0	0	0%
'Cranberry Cove'	8 fl oz	3	0	1	1	0	0.0	0.0	0	0%
'Darjeeling Gardens'	8 fl oz	3	0	1	1	0	0.0	0.0	0	0%
'Emperor's Choice'	8 fl oz	4	0	1	2	0	0.1	0.0	0	18%
'Ginseng Plus'	8 fl oz	3	0	1	4	0	0.0	0.0	0	0%
'Grandma's Tummy Mint'	8 fl oz	2	0	0	7	0	0.0	0.0	0	0%
'Irish Cream Mist'	8 fl oz	3	0	1	1	0	0.0	0.0	0	0%
lemon, 'Fruit & Tea'	8 fl oz	3	0	1	1	0	0.0	0.0	0	0%
'Lemon Mist'	8 fl oz	2	0	1	3	0	0.0	0.0	0	0%
'Lemon Zinger'	8 fl oz	4	0	1	1	0	0.0	0.0	0	0%
'Mandarin Orange Spice'	8 fl oz	5	0	1	2	0	0.0	0.0	0	0%
'Mellow Mint'	8 fl oz	2	0	0	4	0	0.0	0.0	0	0%
'Mint Magic'	8 fl oz	1	0	0	3	0	0.0	0.0	0	0%
'Mo's 24'	8 fl oz	2	0	0	4	0	0.0	0.0	0	0%
'Morning Thunder'	8 fl oz	3	0	0	1	0	0.0	0.0	0	0%
orange spice, 'Fruit & Tea'	8 fl oz	3	0	0	1	0	0.0	0.0	0	0%
'Orange Zinger'	8 fl oz	5	0	1	1	0	0.0	0.0	0	0%
peppermint	8 fl oz	2	0	1	8	0	0.0	0.0	0	0%
raspberry, 'Fruit & Tea'	8 fl oz	2	0	1	1	0	0.0	0.0	0	0%
'Raspberry Patch'	8 fl oz	4	0	1	1	0	0.0	0.0	0	0%
'Red Zinger'	8 fl oz	4	0	1	2	0	0.0	0.0	0	0%
'Roastaroma'	8 fl oz	11	0	2	4	0	0.1	0.0	0	10%
'Sleepytime'	8 fl oz	5	0	1	2	0	0.0	0.0	0	0%
spearmint	8 fl oz	5	0	0	6	0	0.1	0.0	0	43%
'Strawberry Fields'	8 fl oz	4	0	1	1	0	0.0	0.0	0	0%
'Sunburst C'	8 fl oz	3	0	1	6	0	0.0	0.0	0	0%
'Swiss Mint'	8 fl oz	3	0	0	1	0	0.0	0.0	0	0%
'Wild Forest Blackberry'	8 fl oz	2	0	2	1	0	0.0	0.0	0	0%

Food Name	Serving Size	Calories	Prot. gms	Carbs gms	Sod. mgs	Fiber gms	Fat gms	Sat. Fat gms	Chol. mgs	% Fat Cal.
(Glenny's) ginseng, 100% natural	42 grams	180	2	58	20	4	7.0	2.0	0	21%
(Lipton)										
'Almond Pleasure'	8 fl oz	4	0	1	0	0	0.0	0.0	0	0%
chamomile	8 fl oz	4	0	1	0	0	0.0	0.0	0	0%
cinnamon apple	8 fl oz	2	0	1	0	0	0.0	0.0	0	0%
'Citrus Sunset'	8 fl oz	4	0	1	0	0	0.0	0.0	0	0%
'Gentle/Tangy Orange'	8 fl oz	4	0	1	0	0	0.0	0.0	0	0%
'Lemon Soother'	8 fl oz	4	0	1	0	0	0.0	0.0	0	0%
'Toasty Spice'	8 fl oz	6	0	1	0	0	0.0	0.0	0	0%
(Stash's)										
'Apple Cinnamon'	8 fl oz	0	0	0	0	0	0.0	0.0	0	0%
'Black Currant Ice'	8 fl oz	0	0	0	0	0	0.0	0.0	0	0%
'Caravan'	8 fl oz	0	0	0	0	0	0.0	0.0	0	0%
'Chamomile'	8 fl oz	0	0	0	0	0	0.0	0.0	0	0%
'Citrus Spice'	8 fl oz	0	0	0	0	0	0.0	0.0	0	0%
'Crepe Faire'	8 fl oz	0	0	0	0	0	0.0	0.0	0	0%
'Estate'	8 fl oz	0	0	0	0	0	0.0	0.0	0	0%
'Herbal Peach'	8 fl oz	0	0	0	0	0	0.0	0.0	0	0%
'Irish Breakfast'	8 fl oz	0	0	0	0	0	0.0	0.0	0	0%
'Jasmine Spice'	8 fl oz	0	0	0	0	0	0.0	0.0	0	0%
'Lemon Blossom'	8 fl oz	0	0	0	0	0	0.0	0.0	0	0%
'Lemon Spice'	8 fl oz	0	0	0	0	0	0.0	0.0	0	0%
'Licorice Spice'	8 fl oz	0	0	0	0	0	0.0	0.0	0	0%
'Moroccan Mint'	8 fl oz	0	0	0	0	0	0.0	0.0	0	0%
'Orange Spice' decaffeinated	8 fl oz	0	0	0	0	0	0.0	0.0	0	0%
'Orange Spice'	8 fl oz	0	0	0	0	0	0.0	0.0	0	0%
'Oregon Mint'	8 fl oz	0	0	0	0	0	0.0	0.0	0	0%
'Oriental Rose'	8 fl oz	0	0	0	0	0	0.0	0.0	0	0%
'Peach'	8 fl oz	0	0	0	0	0	0.0	0.0	0	0%
'Peppermint'	8 fl oz	0	0	0	0	0	0.0	0.0	0	0%
'Premium Green'	8 fl oz	0	0	0	0	0	0.0	0.0	0	0%
'Ruby Mist'	8 fl oz	0	0	0	0	0	0.0	0.0	0	0%
'Sandman'	8 fl oz	0	0	0	0	0	0.0	0.0	0	0%
'Tangerine'	8 fl oz	0	0	0	0	0	0.0	0.0	0	0%
'Tropical Fruit'	8 fl oz	0	0	0	0	0	0.0	0.0	0	0%
'Tropical Mist'	8 fl oz	0	0	0	0	0	0.0	0.0	0	0%
'Wild Black Currant'	8 fl oz	0	0	0	0	0	0.0	0.0	0	0%
'Wild Raspberry'	8 fl oz	0	0	0	0	0	0.0	0.0	0	0%
'Wintermint'	8 fl oz	0	0	0	0	0	0.0	0.0	0	0%
(Tetley)										
'Apple Freeze'	8 fl oz	79	0	20	1	0	0.0	0.0	0	0%
'Classic'	8 fl oz	69	0	17	1	0	0.0	0.0	0	0%
'Classic Lemon'	8 fl oz	108	0	27	1	0	0.0	0.0	0	0%
'Diet Lemon Frost'	8 fl oz	10	0	2	1	0	0.0	0.0	0	0%
'Diet Raspberry Blizzard'	8 fl oz	10	0	2	1	0	0.0	0.0	0	0%
'Lemon Frost'	8 fl oz	89	0	22	1	0	0.0	0.0	0	0%
'Orange Glazier'	8 fl oz	79	0	20	1	0	0.0	0.0	0	0%
'Peach Chiller'	8 fl oz	79	0	20	1	0	0.0	0.0	0	0%
'Raspberry Blizzard'	8 fl oz	95	0	24	1	0	0.0	0.0	0	0%
Instant										
(Nature's Plus)										
Chinese herbal, citrus-flavored	1 tsp	24	0	6	0	0	0.0	0.0	0	0%
Chinese herbal, decaffeinated, citrus-flavored, 'Chi'	1 tsp	24	0	6	0	0	0.0	0.0	0	0%

Food Name	Serving Size	Calories	Prot. gms	Carbs gms	Sod. mgs	Fiber gms	Fat gms	Sat. Fat gms	Chol. mgs	% Fat Cal.
TEA, ICED										
BLACK										
(Clinical Resource) 'Lemon Iced Tea'	8 fl oz	180	9	36	70	na	0.0	0.0	0	0%
(Lipton)										
regular, w/natural lemon flavor	8.45 fl oz	96	2	24	20	0	0.3	0.0	0	3%
w/lemon, sugar-free	8 fl oz	1	0	0	10	0	0.0	0.0	0	0%
(Nestea)										
diet	8 fl oz	4	0	1	35	0	0.0	0.0	0	0%
regular	8 fl oz	90	0	22	35	0	0.0	0.0	0	0%
sweetened	16 fl oz	97	0	27	0	0	0.0	0.0	0	0%
w/lemon, sugar-free	8 fl oz	2	0	1	0	0	0.0	0.0	0	0%
w/lemon, sugar-sweetened	8 fl oz	70	0	17	0	0	0.0	0.0	0	0%
natural	16 fl oz	180	2	44	50	0	0.0	0.0	0	0%
natural	6 fl oz	66	1	17	18	0	0.0	0.0	0	0%
(Shasta)	12 fl oz	124	0	34	28	0	0.0	0.0	0	0%
(10-K)	8 fl oz	60	0	15	55	0	0.0	0.0	0	0%
(Tetley)										
regular	8 fl oz	74	0	19	20	0	0.0	0.0	0	0%
sweetened	8 fl oz	74	0	19	20	0	0.0	0.0	0	0%
w/lemon	8 fl oz	74	0	19	20	0	0.0	0.0	0	0%
(Thick & Easy)										
honey consistency	1/2 cup	70	0	17	20	0	0.0	0.0	0	0%
nectar consistency	1/2 cup	60	0	16	15	0	0.0	0.0	0	0%
(Veryfine) w/lemon	8 fl oz	80	1	16	10	0	0.0	0.0	0	0%
HERBAL/FLAVORED										
(Fruitopia)										
'Born Raspberry'	16 fl oz	162	0	44	0	0	0.0	0.0	0	0%
'Lemon Berry Intuition'	16 fl oz	166	0	44	0	0	0.0	0.0	0	0%
'Peaceable Peach'	16 fl oz	162	0	44	0	0	0.0	0.0	0	0%
(Knudsen)										
hibiscus, 'Iced Tea Cooler'	1 cup	90	0	23	40	0	0.0	0.0	0	0%
blacklemon, 'Iced Tea Cooler'	1 cup	90	0	23	40	0	0.0	0.0	0	0%
blackmango, 'Iced Tea Cooler'	1 cup	90	0	23	40	0	0.0	0.0	0	0%
blackorange, 'Iced Tea Cooler'	1 cup	90	0	23	40	0	0.0	0.0	0	0%
blackraspberry, 'Iced Tea Cooler'	1 cup	90	0	23	40	0	0.0	0.0	0	0%
(Nestea)										
apple spice	16 fl oz	180	2	44	50	0	0.0	0.0	0	0%
apple spice	6 fl oz	66	1	17	18	0	0.0	0.0	0	0%
peach	16 fl oz	180	2	44	50	0	0.0	0.0	0	0%
peach	6 fl oz	66	1	17	18	0	0.0	0.0	0	0%
raspberry	16 fl oz	180	2	44	50	0	0.0	0.0	0	0%
raspberry	6 fl oz	66	1	17	18	0	0.0	0.0	0	0%
tropical	16 fl oz	180	2	44	50	0	0.0	0.0	0	0%
tropical	6 fl oz	66	1	17	18	0	0.0	0.0	0	0%
(Wyler's) 'Fruit Tea Punch'	12 fl oz	118	0	30	1	0	0.0	0.0	0	0%
TEA, ICED, MIX										
BLACK										
(Crystal Light)										
decaffeinated, sugar-free, prepared	8 fl oz	4	0	0	0	0	0.0	0.0	0	0%
sugar-free, prepared	8 fl oz	4	0	0	0	0	0.0	0.0	0	0%
(Lipton)										
decaffeinated, sugar-free, prepared	8 fl oz	1	0	0	5	0	0.0	0.0	0	0%
lemon flavor, decaffeinated, prepared	6 fl oz	55	0	14	1	0	0.0	0.0	0	0%
lemon flavor, prepared	6 fl oz	55	0	14	1	0	0.0	0.0	0	0%

Food Name	Serving Size	Calories	Prot. gms	Carbs gms	Sod. mgs	Fiber gms	Fat gms	Sat. Fat gms	Chol. mgs	% Fat Cal.
lemon flavor, w/NutraSweet, prepared	8 fl oz	5	0	1	2	0	0.0	0.0	0	0%
sugar-free, prepared	8 fl oz	1	0	0	6	0	0.0	0.0	0	0%
sweet, no lemon, mix only	1 2/3 tbsp	70	0	17	0	0	0.0	0.0	0	0%
sweet, sugar-free, no lemon, mix only	1 tbsp	0	0	1	0	0	0.0	0.0	0	0%
(Nestea)										
decaffeinated, '100%' prepared	8 fl oz	0	0	0	0	0	0.0	0.0	0	0%
lemon flavor, decaffeinated, sugar-free, mix only	2 tsp	6	0	1	0	0	0.0	0.0	0	0%
lemon flavor, sugar-free, prepared	8 fl oz	4	0	1	0	0	0.0	0.0	0	0%
'100%' mix only	1 tsp	2	0	0	0	0	0.0	0.0	0	0%
'100%' prepared	8 fl oz	2	0	0	0	0	0.0	0.0	0	0%
sugar-free, prepared	8 fl oz	6	0	1	5	0	0.0	0.0	0	0%
w/sugar and lemon, prepared	8 fl oz	70	0	19	0	0	0.0	0.0	0	0%
(Pathmark)										
lemon flavor, mix only	1 tsp	6	0	1	0	0	0.0	0.0	0	0%
lemon flavor, artificially sweetened, mix only	1 tsp	4	0	1	20	0	0.0	0.0	0	0%
lemon flavor, decaffeinated, low-calorie, prepared	8 fl oz	4	0	1	0	0	0.0	0.0	0	0%
lemon flavor, decaffeinated, sugar-sweetened, mix only	2 tbsp	80	0	20	0	0	0.0	0.0	0	0%
lemon flavor, low-calorie, prepared	8 fl oz	4	0	1	0	0	0.0	0.0	0	0%
'No Frills' mix only	0.75 oz	70	0	21	75	0	0.0	0.0	0	0%
HERBAL/FLAVORED										
(Lipton)										
tropical flavor, sugar-free, mix only	1 tbsp	5	0	1	0	0	0.0	0.0	0	0%
tropical flavor, w/sugar, mix only	1 2/3 tbsp	90	0	22	0	0	0.0	0.0	0	0%
(Nestea) all flavors, 'Ice Teasers' prepared	8 fl oz	6	0	1	0	0	0.0	0.0	0	0%
(Soothing Moments)										
cinnamon apple, caffeine-free, mix only	1/2 tsp	5	0	1	0	0	0.0	0.0	0	0%
gentle orange, caffeine-free, mix only	1/2 tsp	5	0	1	0	0	0.0	0.0	0	0%
lemon soother, caffeine-free, mix only	1/2 tsp	5	0	1	0	0	0.0	0.0	0	0%
TEASEED OIL										
	1 cup	1927	0	0	0	0	218.0	46.0	0	100%
	1 tbsp	120	0	0	0	0	13.6	2.9	0	100%
TEFF FLOUR. See under FLOUR.										
TEFF SEED (Arrowhead Mills)	2 oz	200	7	41	6	8	1.0	0.0	0	4%
TEMPEH										
	1 cup	320	31	16	15	na	17.9	3.7	0	47%
(White Wave)										
5-grain, vegetarian	1 piece	140	12	15	0	4	4.0	0.5	0	25%
original, soy, vegetarian	1 piece	150	16	10	0	6	6.0	1.0	0	34%
sea veggie, vegetarian	1 piece	120	12	11	25	8	3.0	0.5	0	23%
soy rice, vegetarian	1 piece	140	12	13	0	5	5.0	0.5	0	31%
wild rice, vegetarian	1 piece	140	13	12	10	6	4.0	0.5	0	26%
TENDERGREEN. See MUSTARD SPINACH.										
TEQUILA										
80 proof	1 fl oz	65	0	0	0	0	0.0	0.0	0	0%
86 proof	1 fl oz	70	0	0	0	0	0.0	0.0	0	0%
90 proof	1 fl oz	74	0	0	0	0	0.0	0.0	0	0%
94 proof	1 fl oz	77	0	0	0	0	0.0	0.0	0	0%
100 proof	1 fl oz	83	0	0	0	0	0.0	0.0	0	0%
TERIYAKI STIR-FRY ENTRÉE (Lunch Express)	1 entrée	260	15	39	550	4	5.0	1.0	30	17%
TERRAPIN, diamondback, raw	100 gm	111	18.6	0.0	50	0	3.5	0.0	50	30%
THYME, DRIED										
dried (McCormick/Schilling)	1 tsp	17	0	1	0	0	0.0	0.0	0	0%
fresh	1 tsp	1	0	0	0	0	0.0	0.0	0	13%

Food Name	Serving Size	Calories	Prot. gms	Carbs gms	Sod. mgs	Fiber gms	Fat gms	Sat. Fat gms	Chol. mgs	% Fat Cal.
fresh	1/2 tsp	0	0	0	0	0	0.0	0.0	0	15%
ground *(Spice Islands)*	1 tsp	5	0	1	1	0	0.1	0.0	0	17%
ground	1 tbsp	12	0	3	2	2	0.3	0.1	0	22%
ground	1 tsp	4	0	1	1	1	0.1	0.0	0	23%
ground, fresh *(Durkee)*	1 tsp	5	0	0	0	0	0.0	0.0	0	0%
ground, fresh *(Laurel Leaf)*	1 tsp	5	0	0	0	0	0.0	0.0	0	0%
TILEFISH										
baked, broiled, grilled, or microwaved.	3 oz	125	21	0	50	0	4.0	0.7	54	29%
raw	3 oz	82	15	0	45	0	2.0	0.4	43	22%
TOASTER BISCUIT. See BISCUIT, TOASTER.										
TOASTER PASTRY. See PASTRY, TOASTER.										
TOFU										
fried	1 oz	77	5	3	5	1	5.7	0.8	0	62%
fuyu, salted and fermented	1 block	13	1	1	316	na	0.9	0.1	0	58%
fuyu, salted and fermented, prepared w/calcium sulfate. . .	1 block	13	1	1	316	na	0.9	0.1	0	58%
okara	1 cup	94	4	15	11	na	2.1	0.2	0	19%
(Nasoya)										
five-spice	1 piece	70	8	0	70	0	4.0	0.5	0	53%
French country	1 piece	70	8	0	130	0	4.0	0.5	0	53%
(White Wave) less fat	1 piece	90	10	4	5	2	4.0	0.0	0	39%
EXTRA FIRM										
w/nigari	1/5 block	87	9	2	9	0	5.7	0.8	0	54%
(Azumaya) Chinese style.	3.5 oz	0	11	2	5	0	4.0	0.5	0	0%
(Mori-Nu)										
silken	1 slice	46	6	2	53	0	1.6	0.3	0	31%
silken	3 oz	55	7	2	60	1	2.0	0.0	0	33%
silken, light	1 slice	32	6	1	82	0	0.6	0.1	0	17%
silken, light	3 oz	35	6	1	80	na	1.0	0.0	0	24%
(Nasoya)	1 piece	93	9	1	9	0	5.0	0.7	0	52%
FIRM										
nigan	1/2 cup	97	10	4	10	1	5.6	0.8	0	48%
prepared w/calcium sulfate	1/2 cup	183	20	5	18	3	11.0	1.6	0	50%
(Azumaya) Japanese style.	3.5 oz	70	7	4	5	0	2.5	0.4	0	34%
(Kikkoman).	3 oz	50	6	2	30	0	2.5	0.0	0	41%
(Mori-Nu)										
silken.	1/2 pkg	90	10	4	50	0	4.0	0.0	0	39%
silken	1 slice	52	6	2	30	0	2.3	0.3	0	39%
silken	3 oz	50	6	2	30	1	2.5	0.0	0	41%
silken, light	3 oz	35	5	1	70	1	1.0	0.0	0	27%
silken, light	1 slice	31	5	1	71	0	0.7	0.1	0	19%
(Nasoya)	1 piece	76	9	2	8	0	3.8	0.6	0	45%
FREEZE-DRIED / koyadofu	1 oz	136	13.6	4.1	2	>0.1	8.6	1.2	0	52%
REGULAR, prepared w/calcium sulfate	1/2 cup	94	10	2	9	0	5.9	0.9	0	53%
SOFT										
(Azumaya) Kinugoshi.	3.5 oz	50	4	5	5	0	4.0	0.3	0	50%
(Kikkoman).	3 oz	45	4	2	5	0	2.5	0.0	0	48%
(Mori-Nu)										
silken	1/2 pkg	80	7	4	10	0	4.0	0.0	0	45%
silken	1 slice	46	4	2	4	0	2.3	0.3	0	44%
silken.	3 oz	45	4	2	5	1	2.5	0.0	0	48%
(Nasoya)										
. . . .	1 piece	64	7	2	7	0	3.0	0.4	0	43%
silken.	1 piece	48	5	2	12	0	2.2	0.3	0	42%
nigan	1 cubic inch	11	1	0	1	0	0.6	0.1	0	51%

Food Name	Serving Size	Calories	Prot. gms	Carbs gms	Sod. mgs	Fiber gms	Fat gms	Sat. Fat gms	Chol. mgs	% Fat Cal.
TOFU SPREAD										
(Natural Touch)										
green chili, canned, 'Tofu Topper'	2 tbsp	50	2	2	0	0	4.0	0.0	0	69%
herb and spice, canned, 'Tofu Topper'	2 tbsp	50	2	2	0	0	4.0	0.0	0	69%
Mexican, canned, 'Tofu Topper'	2 tbsp	60	2	2	0	0	5.0	0.0	0	74%
TOM COLLINS. See under COCKTAIL; COCKTAIL MIX.										
TOMATILLO / ground husk tomato										
raw, chopped or diced	1/2 cup	21	1	4	1	1	0.7	0.1	0	27%
raw, whole	1 medium	11	0	2	0	1	0.3	0.0	0	27%
TOMATO. See also TOMATO DISH.										
Canned										
(A&P)	1/2 cup	25	1	6	220	0	1.0	0.0	0	24%
(Featherweight)	1/2 cup	20	1	4	1	0	0.0	0.0	0	0%
'Choice Cut' *(Hunt's)*	1/2 cup	22	1	5	325	1	0.2	0.0	0	7%
chopped, food service product *(Angela Mia)*	1/2 cup	24	2	4	254	1	0.4	0.0	0	14%
crushed *(Angela Mia)*	1/2 cup	27	2	6	380	2	0.2	0.0	0	4%
crushed *(Contadina)*	1/4 cup	20	1	4	150	1	0.0	0.0	0	0%
crushed *(Hunt's)*	1/2 cup	29	1	7	286	2	0.3	0.0	0	6%
crushed *(Pathmark)*	1/2 cup	40	1	9	210	0	0.0	0.0	0	0%
crushed *(Progresso)*	1/4 cup	20	1	4	95	1	0.0	0.0	0	0%
crushed *(S&W)*	1/4 cup	20	1	4	95	1	0.0	0.0	0	0%
crushed, 'No Frills' *(Pathmark)*	1 cup	90	3	20	510	0	0.0	0.0	0	0%
crushed, chunky, food service product *(Angela Mia)*	1/2 cup	26	2	5	317	2	0.3	0.0	0	8%
crushed, concentrated, food service product *(Angela Mia)*	1/4 cup	30	2	6	25	1	0.4	0.0	0	11%
crushed, food service product *(Angela Mia)*	1/2 cup	32	1	7	317	1	0.4	0.0	0	9%
crushed, Italian flavored *(Hunt's)*	1/2 cup	40	2	9	460	1	1.0	0.0	0	17%
crushed, organic, no salt added *(Eden Foods)*	1/2 cup	35	2	6	0	0	0.0	0.0	0	0%
cut, peeled, 'Ready-Cut' *(S&W)*	1/2 cup	25	1	6	220	0	0.0	0.0	0	0%
diced, in juice *(Hunt's)*	1/2 cup	20	1	4	477	1	0.1	0.0	0	5%
diced, in juice, no salt added *(Hunt's)*	1/2 cup	20	1	4	8	1	0.1	0.0	0	4%
diced, in purée, food service product *(Hunt's)*	1/2 cup	23	1	5	304	1	0.1	0.0	0	4%
diced, in rich purée *(S&W)*	1/2 cup	35	1	8	290	0	0.0	0.0	0	0%
diced, Italian style *(Muir Glen)*	1/2 cup	25	1	4	190	1	0.0	0.0	0	0%
diced, organic *(Eden Foods)*	1/2 cup	30	1	6	5	2	0.0	0.0	0	0%
diced, peeled *(Libby's)*	1/2 cup	25	1	4	300	1	0.0	0.0	0	0%
diced, w/green chilies *(Eden Foods)*	1/2 cup	30	2	5	35	2	0.0	0.0	0	0%
diced, w/green chilies *(Ro-Tel)*	1/2 cup	20	0	4	370	1	0.0	0.0	0	0%
diced, w/Italian herbs, 'Choice Cut' *(Hunt's)*	1/2 cup	24	1	5	600	1	0.0	0.0	0	0%
diced, w/roasted garlic, 'Choice Cut' *(Hunt's)*	1/2 cup	24	1	5	505	1	0.0	0.0	0	0%
dried, chopped, marinated *(Parmalat)*	3 pieces	35	1	3	5	1	2.5	0.0	0	58%
in aspic, supreme *(S&W)*	1/2 cup	60	1	16	860	0	0.0	0.0	0	0%
in juice, no salt added *(S&W)*	1/2 cup	25	1	4	30	1	0.0	0.0	0	0%
Italian style *(Contadina)*	1/2 cup	35	1	8	250	0	1.0	0.0	0	20%
Mexican style *(S&W)*	1/2 cup	40	1	8	360	0	0.0	0.0	0	0%
'No Frills' *(Pathmark)*	1 cup	50	2	11	440	0	0.0	0.0	0	0%
organic, diced *(Muir Glen)*	1/2 cup	25	1	4	170	1	0.0	0.0	0	0%
'Pasta Ready' *(Contadina)*	1/2 cup	40	1	5	620	1	2.0	0.0	0	43%
pear-shaped *(Hunt's)*	1/2 cup	20	1	4	360	1	0.1	0.0	0	4%
pear-shaped, Italian flavored *(Hunt's)*	1/2 cup	20	1	5	320	1	1.0	0.0	0	27%
peeled *(Contadina)*	1/2 cup	25	1	4	220	1	0.0	0.0	0	0%
peeled, 'Choice Cut' *(Hunt's)*	1/2 cup	20	1	5	460	1	1.0	0.0	0	27%
peeled, whole, in juice *(DiNapoli)*	1/2 cup	25	1	6	220	0	0.0	0.0	0	0%
plum, w/basil sauce *(Contadina)*	1/2 cup	70	2	8	450	3	3.0	1.0	0	40%

Food Name	Serving Size	Calories	Prot. gms	Carbs gms	Sod. mgs	Fiber gms	Fat gms	Sat. Fat gms	Chol. mgs	% Fat Cal.
primavera 'Pasta Ready' (Contadina)	1/2 cup	50	1	8	600	1	1.5	0.0	0	27%
'Recipe Ready' (Contadina)	1/2 cup	25	1	5	200	1	0.0	0.0	0	0%
sliced (A&P)	1/2 cup	35	1	8	350	0	1.0	0.0	0	20%
sliced (Finast)	1/2 cup	35	1	9	355	0	0.0	0.0	0	0%
sliced (Pathmark)	1/2 cup	35	1	9	360	0	0.0	0.0	0	0%
sliced (S&W)	1/2 cup	35	1	9	355	0	0.0	0.0	0	0%
sliced, Italian (S&W)	1/2 cup	35	1	9	355	0	0.0	0.0	0	0%
w/basil, peeled (Progresso)	1/2 cup	25	1	4	220	1	0.0	0.0	0	0%
w/crushed red pepper 'Pasta Ready' (Contadina)	1/2 cup	60	1	8	690	1	3.0	0.5	0	43%
w/green chilies (Old El Paso)	1/4 cup	14	0	3	480	0	0.0	0.0	0	0%
w/jalapeños (Contadina)	1/2 cup	35	1	8	250	0	1.0	0.0	0	20%
w/jalapeños (Ortega)	1 oz	8	0	1	120	0	0.0	0.0	0	0%
w/mushrooms 'Pasta Ready' (Contadina)	1/2 cup	50	1	9	640	1	1.5	0.0	0	25%
w/olives 'Pasta Ready' (Contadina)	1/2 cup	60	1	8	638	1	3.0	0.5	0	43%
w/three cheeses 'Pasta Ready' (Contadina)	1/2 cup	70	1	8	650	1	4.0	0.0	1	50%
wedges, w/liquid (Del Monte)	1/2 cup	30	1	8	355	0	0.0	0.0	0	0%
whole (Hunt's)	2 tomatoes	22	2	4	404	1	0.1	0.0	0	4%
whole (Stokely)	1/2 cup	25	1	5	190	0	0.0	0.0	0	0%
whole, 'Nutradiet' (S&W)	1/2 cup	25	1	5	20	0	0.0	0.0	0	0%
whole, Italian flavored (Hunt's)	1/2 cup	25	1	6	420	1	1.0	0.0	0	24%
whole, no salt added (Hunt's)	2 tomatoes	22	1	5	3	1	0.5	0.0	0	17%
whole, peeled (Finast)	1/2 cup	25	1	6	195	0	0.0	0.0	0	0%
whole, peeled (Hunt's)	4.83 oz	21	2	4	373	1	0.1	0.0	0	4%
whole, peeled (Libby's)	1/2 cup	25	1	4	220	1	0.0	0.0	0	0%
whole, peeled (Progresso)	1/2 cup	25	1	4	220	1	0.0	0.0	0	0%
whole, peeled (S&W)	1/2 cup	20	2	4	90	1	0.0	0.0	0	0%
whole, peeled, food service product (Hunt's)	1 serving	11	1	2	202	0	0.1	0.0	0	4%
whole, peeled, no salt added (Hunt's)	4.83 oz	21	2	4	9	1	0.1	0.0	0	4%
whole, peeled, no salt added (Pathmark)	1/2 cup	25	1	6	20	0	0.0	0.0	0	0%
whole, peeled, organic (Muir Glen)	1/2 cup	30	1	5	260	1	0.0	0.0	0	0%
whole, peeled, w/liquid (Del Monte)	1/2 cup	25	1	5	220	0	0.0	0.0	0	0%
whole, peeled, w/tomato juice (Pathmark)	1/2 cup	25	1	6	220	0	0.0	0.0	0	0%
Dried (Melissa's)	5 pieces	55	3	10	15	2	0.5	0.0	0	8%
Fresh, raw, ripe										
cherry, red, ripe, June–October	1 cup	31	1	7	13	2	0.5	0.1	0	13%
cherry, red, ripe, June–October, medium	1 tomato	4	0	1	2	0	0.1	0.0	0	13%
cherry, red, ripe, November–May	1 cup	31	1	7	13	2	0.5	0.1	0	13%
cherry, red, ripe, November–May, medium	1 tomato	4	0	1	2	0	0.1	0.0	0	13%
cherry, red, ripe, year-round average	1 cup	31	1	7	13	2	0.5	0.1	0	13%
cherry, red, ripe, year-round average, medium	1 tomato	4	0	1	2	0	0.1	0.0	0	13%
green, raw, chopped	1 cup	43	2	9	23	2	0.4	0.1	0	7%
green, raw, whole, large	1 tomato	44	2	9	24	2	0.4	0.1	0	7%
green, raw, whole, medium	1 tomato	30	1	6	16	1	0.2	0.0	0	7%
green, raw, whole, small	1 tomato	22	1	5	12	1	0.2	0.0	0	7%
orange, raw, chopped	1 cup	25	2	5	66	1	0.3	0.0	0	10%
orange, raw, whole, medium	1 tomato	18	1	4	47	1	0.2	0.0	0	10%
plum, red, ripe, raw, June–October, medium	1 tomato	13	1	3	6	1	0.2	0.0	0	13%
plum, red, ripe, raw, November–May, medium	1 tomato	13	1	3	6	1	0.2	0.0	0	13%
plum, red, ripe, raw, year-round average, whole, medium	1 tomato	13	1	3	6	1	0.2	0.0	0	13%
plum/Italian, raw, June–October, medium	1 tomato	13	1	3	6	1	0.2	0.0	0	13%
red, ripe, boiled	1 cup	65	3	14	26	2	1.0	0.1	0	13%
red, ripe, boiled, medium	2 tomatoes	66	3	14	27	2	1.0	0.1	0	13%
red, ripe, raw, June–October, chopped	1 cup	38	2	8	16	2	0.6	0.1	0	13%

Food Name	Serving Size	Calories	Prot. gms	Carbs gms	Sod. mgs	Fiber gms	Fat gms	Sat. Fat gms	Chol. mgs	% Fat Cal.
red, ripe, raw, June–October, medium	1 tomato	26	1	6	11	1	0.4	0.1	0	13%
red, ripe, raw, June–October, 1/2-inch slices, medium	1 slice	6	0	1	2	0	0.1	0.0	0	13%
red, ripe, raw, June–October, 1/4-inch slices, medium	1 slice	4	0	1	2	0	0.1	0.0	0	13%
red, ripe, raw, June–October, quartered, medium	1/4 tomato	7	0	1	3	0	0.1	0.0	0	13%
red, ripe, raw, June–October, whole, 3 inch diam	1 tomato	38	2	8	16	2	0.6	0.1	0	13%
red, ripe, raw, June–October, whole, 2-3/5 inch diam	1 tomato	26	1	6	11	1	0.4	0.1	0	13%
red, ripe, raw, June–October, whole, 2-2/5 inch diam	1 tomato	19	1	4	8	1	0.3	0.1	0	13%
red, ripe, raw, November–May, chopped or sliced	1 cup	38	2	8	16	2	0.6	0.1	0	13%
red, ripe, raw, November–May, medium	1 tomato	26	1	6	11	1	0.4	0.1	0	13%
red, ripe, raw, November–May, quartered, medium	1/4 tomato	7	0	1	3	0	0.1	0.0	0	13%
red, ripe, raw, November–May, 1/2 inch slices, medium	1 slice	6	0	1	2	0	0.1	0.0	0	13%
red, ripe, raw, November–May, 1/4 inch slices, medium	1 slice	4	0	1	2	0	0.1	0.0	0	13%
red, ripe, raw, November–May, whole, 3 inch diam	1 large	38	2	8	16	2	0.6	0.1	0	13%
red, ripe, raw, November–May, whole, 2-3/5 inch diam	1 tomato	26	1	6	11	1	0.4	0.1	0	13%
red, ripe, raw, year-round average, chopped or sliced	1 cup	38	2	8	16	2	0.6	0.1	0	13%
red, ripe, raw, year-round average, quartered, medium	1/4 tomato	7	0	1	3	0	0.1	0.0	0	13%
red, ripe, raw, year-round average, 1/2 inch slices, medium	1 slice	6	0	1	2	0	0.1	0.0	0	13%
red, ripe, raw, year-round average, 1/4 inch slices, medium	1 slice	4	0	1	2	0	0.1	0.0	0	13%
red, ripe, raw, year-round average, whole, 3-inch diam	1 large	38	2	8	16	2	0.6	0.1	0	13%
red, ripe, raw, year-round average, whole, 2-3/5-inch diam	1 tomato	26	1	6	11	1	0.4	0.1	0	13%
red, ripe, raw, year-round average, whole, 2-2/5-inch diam	1 tomato	19	1	4	8	1	0.3	0.0	0	13%
red, ripe, stewed	1 cup	80	2	13	460	2	2.7	0.5	0	31%
yellow, raw, chopped	1 cup	21	1	4	32	1	0.4	0.1	0	14%
yellow, raw, whole, medium	1 tomato	32	2	6	49	1	0.6	0.1	0	15%
Pickled (Claussen) kosher, in jars, approx. 1.7 oz	1 piece	9	0	2	571	0	0.0	0.0	0	0%
Sun-dried										
	1 cup	139	8	30	1131	7	1.6	0.2	0	10%
	1 piece	5	0	1	42	0	0.1	0.0	0	10%
in oil and herbs (Bella Sun Luci)	2/3 oz	60	2	6	20	2	3.0	0.0	0	46%
packed in oil, drained	1 cup	234	6	26	293	6	15.5	2.1	0	55%
packed in oil, drained	1 piece	6	0	1	8	0	0.4	0.1	0	55%
sun-ripened, 2-3 pieces (Mezzetta)	1/5 oz	15	1	3	5	1	0.0	0.0	0	0%
yellow, in olive oil, 3 pieces (Trader Joe's)	1/5 oz	15	1	3	5	1	0.0	0.0	0	0%
TOMATO DISH										
(Contadina)										
stewed, canned	1/2 cup	40	1	9	250	1	0.0	0.0	0	0%
stewed, Italian style, canned	1/2 cup	40	1	8	260	1	0.0	0.0	0	0%
stewed, Mexican style, canned	1/2 cup	40	1	9	220	1	0.0	0.0	0	0%
(Del Monte)										
stewed, canned	1/2 cup	35	1	8	355	0	0.0	0.0	0	0%
stewed, no salt added, canned	1/2 cup	35	1	8	45	0	0.0	0.0	0	0%
stewed, original recipe, no salt added, canned	1/2 cup	35	1	9	50	2	0.0	0.0	0	0%
(Green Giant)										
stewed, classic recipe, canned	1/2 cup	35	1	7	360	2	0.0	0.0	0	0%
stewed, Italian recipe, canned	1/2 cup	30	1	7	360	2	0.0	0.0	0	0%
stewed, Mexican recipe, canned	1/2 cup	35	1	7	400	2	0.0	0.0	0	0%
(Hunt's)										
stewed, canned	1/2 cup	33	1	7	357	2	0.3	0.0	0	7%

Food Name	Serving Size	Calories	Prot. gms	Carbs gms	Sod. mgs	Fiber gms	Fat gms	Sat. Fat gms	Chol. mgs	% Fat Cal.
stewed, canned, food service product.	1/2 cup	29	1	7	262	1	0.1	0.0	0	2%
stewed, Italian flavored, canned	1/2 cup	35	1	8	400	1	1.0	0.0	0	20%
stewed, no salt added, canned	1/2 cup	29	1	7	21	1	0.1	0.0	0	3%
stewed, no salt added, canned	1/2 cup	33	1	7	31	2	0.3	0.0	0	7%
(Muir Glen) whole, stewed, organic, canned	1/2 cup	25	1	4	190	1	0.0	0.0	0	0%
(S&W)										
stewed, 50% reduced salt, canned	1/2 cup	35	1	9	180	0	0.0	0.0	0	0%
stewed, no salt	1/2 cup	35	1	7	15	2	0.0	0.0	0	0%
(Stokely) stewed, canned.	1/2 cup	35	1	8	220	0	0.0	0.0	0	0%
TOMATO JUICE. See also FRUIT JUICE BLEND.										
canned	1 cup	41	2	10	877	1	0.1	0.0	0	3%
canned	6 fl oz	31	1	8	657	1	0.1	0.0	0	3%
canned, no salt added.	1 cup	41	2	10	24	2	0.1	0.0	0	3%
canned, no salt added.	6 fl oz	31	1	8	18	1	0.1	0.0	0	3%
canned, no salt added.	1 fl oz	5	0	1	3	0	0.0	0.0	0	3%
(A&P)	6 fl oz	30	1	7	550	0	0.0	0.0	0	0%
(Biotta)	6 fl oz	28	1	6	277	0	0.1	0.0	0	3%
(Campbell's).	8 fl oz	50	2	9	860	1	0.0	0.0	0	0%
(Del Monte)										
	8 fl oz	40	3	7	550	0	0.0	0.0	0	0%
from concentrate	8 fl oz	50	2	10	760	1	0.0	0.0	0	0%
(Featherweight)	6 fl oz	35	1	8	10	0	0.0	0.0	0	0%
(Hunt's)										
	8 fl oz	34	2	8	689	2	0.3	0.0	0	8%
food service product	8 fl oz	35	2	7	610	1	0.1	0.0	0	2%
no salt added.	8 fl oz	34	2	8	12	2	0.3	0.0	0	8%
(Knudsen) organic	8 fl oz	50	1	10	0	0	0.0	0.0	0	0%
(Libby's)										
bottled or canned	6 fl oz	35	2	7	500	0	0.0	0.0	0	0%
canned	5.5 fl oz	35	2	6	460	0	0.0	0.0	0	0%
(Pathmark)										
	6 fl oz	30	1	6	510	0	0.0	0.0	0	0%
frozen, diluted	6 fl oz	35	1	8	450	0	0.0	0.0	0	0%
(S&W)										
	5.5 fl oz	30	2	5	380	0	0.0	0.0	0	0%
'California'	6 fl oz	35	1	8	600	0	0.0	0.0	0	0%
'Nutradiet'	6 fl oz	35	1	8	20	0	0.0	0.0	0	0%
(Stokely).	4 fl oz	20	1	4	330	0	0.0	0.0	0	0%
(Welch's)	6 fl oz	35	1	7	550	0	0.0	0.0	0	0%
TOMATO PASTE										
. . . .	6-oz can	139	6	33	1343	7	0.9	0.1	0	6%
. . . .	1/2 cup	107	5	25	1035	5	0.7	0.1	0	6%
no salt added.	1 cup	215	10	51	231	11	1.4	0.2	0	6%
no salt added.	6-oz can	139	6	33	150	7	0.9	0.1	0	6%
no salt added.	1 tbsp	13	1	3	14	1	0.1	0.0	0	6%
(Contadina)										
. . . .	2 tbsp	30	2	6	20	1	0.0	0.0	0	0%
Italian style	2 tbsp	40	1	7	320	1	1.0	0.0	0	22%
(Hunt's) no salt added	2 tbsp	30	1	6	7	2	0.5	0.0	0	14%
(Progresso)	2 tbsp	30	2	6	20	1	0.0	0.0	0	0%
(S&W)	2 tbsp	30	2	6	20	1	0.0	0.0	0	0%
TOMATO PURÉE										
. . . .	1 cup	100	4	24	998	5	0.4	0.1	0	3%
no salt added.	1 cup	100	4	24	85	5	0.4	0.1	0	3%

Food Name	Serving Size	Calories	Prot. gms	Carbs gms	Sod. mgs	Fiber gms	Fat gms	Sat. Fat gms	Chol. mgs	% Fat Cal.
(Angela Mia)	2.19 oz	16	1	3	21	0	0.3	0.0	0	15%
(Contadina)										
	1/4 cup	20	1	4	15	1	0.0	0.0	0	0%
w/crushed tomatoes	1/2 cup	30	1	6	350	0	1.0	0.0	0	24%
(Hunt's)										
	1/4 cup	24	1	5	98	2	0.3	0.0	0	11%
food service product	1/4 cup	26	3	5	22	1	0.4	0.0	0	9%
(Progresso) thick style	1/4 cup	25	1	5	15	1	0.0	0.0	0	0%
TOMATO SAUCE										
(A&P) canned	1/2 cup	45	2	9	600	0	1.0	0.0	0	17%
(Buitoni) marinara	1/2 cup	70	1	11	570	0	3.0	1.0	0	36%
(Contadina)										
	1/4 cup	20	1	4	280	1	0.0	0.0	0	0%
chunky, light	1/2 cup	45	2	8	470	2	0.5	0.0	0	10%
four-cheese	4 oz	300	8	7	400	0	27.0	14.0	80	80%
garden vegetable	5 oz	80	2	9	580	0	3.0	1.0	0	38%
Italian sausage	5 oz	110	5	8	570	0	6.0	2.0	15	51%
Italian style	1/4 cup	15	1	4	320	1	0.0	0.0	0	0%
marinara, refrigerated, 'Fresh'	7.5 oz	100	4	12	700	0	4.0	0.0	0	36%
pesto	2.33 oz	350	7	5	440	0	34.0	5.0	10	86%
plum	5 oz	80	2	8	420	0	4.0	1.0	5	47%
plum, w/basil, refrigerated, 'Fresh'	7.5 oz	100	3	14	700	0	4.0	0.0	5	35%
refrigerated, 'Light'	0.5 oz	50	2	9	570	0	0.0	0.0	0	0%
thick and zesty	1/4 cup	20	1	3	340	1	0.0	0.0	0	0%
(Del Monte)										
canned	1 cup	70	3	16	1330	0	1.0	0.0	0	11%
no salt added	1 cup	70	3	16	50	0	1.0	0.0	0	11%
no salt added	1/4 cup	20	0	4	20	1	0.0	0.0	0	0%
w/onions	1 cup	100	3	23	1150	0	1.0	0.0	0	8%
(Eden Foods) lightly seasoned, organic	1/4 cup	25	1	5	45	1	0.0	0.0	0	0%
(Finast)										
	1/2 cup	45	2	9	650	0	0.0	0.0	0	0%
no salt added	8 oz	90	4	18	10	0	0.0	0.0	0	0%
(Health Valley)										
	1 cup	70	2	13	460	0	0.5	0.0	0	7%
no salt added	1 cup	70	2	13	43	0	0.5	0.0	0	7%
(Hunt's)										
	1/4 cup	16	1	3	366	1	0.2	0.0	0	10%
canned 'Special'	4 oz	35	1	8	320	1	0.0	0.0	0	0%
canned	4 oz	30	1	7	730	0	0.0	0.0	0	0%
'Casera'	2.19 oz	22	1	5	293	1	0.1	0.0	0	4%
chunky tomato	2.19 oz	13	1	3	405	1	0.1	0.0	0	6%
food service product	1/4 cup	15	1	3	360	1	0.2	0.0	0	10%
hot, 'Maya'	1.06 oz	6	0	1	174	0	0.2	0.0	0	24%
Italian style	1/4 cup	33	1	5	210	1	1.2	0.0	0	30%
Italian style	4 oz	60	2	11	520	0	2.0	0.0	0	26%
'Meatloaf Fixin's'	2 oz	20	1	5	580	1	1.0	0.0	0	27%
no salt added	1/4 cup	16	1	3	12	1	0.2	0.0	0	10%
w/garlic	4 oz	70	2	10	480	1	2.0	0.3	0	27%
w/herbs	1/4 cup	32	1	5	271	1	1.0	0.0	0	27%
w/mushrooms	4 oz	25	1	6	710	2	1.0	0.0	0	24%
w/onions	4 oz	40	1	9	650	2	1.0	0.0	0	18%
w/tomato bits	4 oz	30	1	7	620	2	1.0	0.0	0	22%

Food Name	Serving Size	Calories	Prot. gms	Carbs gms	Sod. mgs	Fiber gms	Fat gms	Sat. Fat gms	Chol. mgs	% Fat Cal.
(Old El Paso)										
w/green chilies	1/4 cup	14	1	3	480	0	1.0	0.0	0	36%
w/jalapeños	1/4 cup	11	1	2	150	0	1.0	0.0	0	43%
(Pathmark)										
	1/2 cup	40	2	9	620	0	0.0	0.0	0	0%
marinara, 'No Frills'	1/2 cup	80	1	12	620	0	3.0	0.0	0	34%
no salt added	1/2 cup	45	2	9	25	0	0.0	0.0	0	0%
(Progresso)	1/4 cup	20	1	4	260	1	0.0	0.0	0	0%
(Rokeach)										
Italian style	3 oz	60	1	8	243	0	2.0	0.0	0	33%
low-sodium	3 oz	50	1	8	124	0	2.0	0.0	0	33%
marinara	3 oz	60	1	9	257	0	2.0	0.0	0	31%
(S&W)	1/4 cup	20	1	4	300	1	0.0	0.0	0	0%
(Stokely)	1/2 cup	30	2	7	810	0	0.0	0.0	0	0%
TOMATO SEED OIL										
	1 cup	1927	0	0	0	0	218.0	42.9	0	100%
	1 tbsp	120	0	0	0	0	13.6	2.7	0	100%

TONIC WATER. See under SOFT DRINKS AND MIXERS.

TOPPING. See individual listings.

TORSK. See CUSK.

TORTELLINI DISH/ENTRÉE

Food Name	Serving Size	Calories	Prot. gms	Carbs gms	Sod. mgs	Fiber gms	Fat gms	Sat. Fat gms	Chol. mgs	% Fat Cal.
(Bernardi)										
cheese	1 cup	260	13	40	400	4	6.0	2.5	20	20%
cheese, w/spinach pasta	1 cup	280	13	40	320	2	8.0	5.0	30	25%
cheese, tortelloni	1 cup	260	13	40	400	4	6.0	2.5	20	20%
meat filled, precooked	1 cup	250	11	38	490	2	6.0	3.5	40	22%
meat filled, w/raw pasta	1 cup	280	12	41	460	1	8.0	3.5	20	25%
(Contadina)										
cheese	3/4 cup	261	13	39	331	3	6.0	2.5	45	21%
cheese and basil	1 cup	360	16	49	380	3	11.0	4.0	65	28%
chicken and prosciutto, tortelloni	1 cup	360	15	46	440	3	13.0	4.0	75	32%
chicken and vegetable	3/4 cup	259	10	39	219	2	7.0	2.0	45	24%
garlic and cheese, light	1 cup	280	15	50	390	3	5.0	2.5	55	15%
sausage and bell pepper, tortelloni, spicy	1 cup	330	13	47	290	3	10.0	4.0	90	27%
(Mona's) cheese, frozen	1 cup	370	17	50	490	1	11.0	5.0	30	27%
(Weight Watchers) cheese, frozen	9 oz	310	14	50	570	0	6.0	1.0	15	17%
(Stouffer's) cheese, w/Alfredo sauce, frozen	8 7/8 oz	580	26	35	830	0	37.0	0.0	0	58%
(Tofutti) meatless, frozen	2 oz	220	12	38	110	0	2.0	0.0	0	8%

TORTELLONI ENTRÉE. See under TORTELLINI DISH/ENTRÉE.

TORTILLA

Food Name	Serving Size	Calories	Prot. gms	Carbs gms	Sod. mgs	Fiber gms	Fat gms	Sat. Fat gms	Chol. mgs	% Fat Cal.
corn, no salt added, ready to bake or fry	1 oz	63	2	13	3	1	0.7	0.1	0	9%
corn, no salt added, ready-to-bake or fry, 6-inch diam	1 tortilla	58	1	12	3	1	0.7	0.1	0	9%
corn, ready-to-bake or fry	1 oz	63	2	13	46	1	0.7	0.1	0	9%
corn, ready-to-bake or fry, 6-inch diam	1 tortilla	58	1	12	42	1	0.7	0.1	0	9%
flour, ready to bake or fry, 12-inch diam	1 tortilla	380	10	65	559	4	8.3	2.0	0	19%
flour, ready to bake or fry, 10-inch diam	1 tortilla	234	6	40	344	2	5.1	1.3	0	19%
flour, ready to bake or fry, 7–8-inch diam	1 tortilla	159	4	27	234	2	3.5	0.9	0	19%
flour, ready to bake or fry, 6-inch diam	1 tortilla	104	3	18	153	1	2.3	0.6	0	19%
flour, ready to bake or fry	1 oz	92	2	16	136	1	2.0	0.5	0	19%
(Azteca)										
corn	1 tortilla	45	1	9	10	0	0.0	0.0	0	0%
flour, 7-inch diam	1 tortilla	80	2	14	110	0	2.0	0.0	0	22%
flour, 9-inch diam	1 tortilla	130	3	23	180	0	3.0	0.0	0	21%
(Fry's) flour, fajita style, extra soft	1 tortilla	100	2	17	160	0	2.0	0.0	0	19%

Food Name	Serving Size	Calories	Prot. gms	Carbs gms	Sod. mgs	Fiber gms	Fat gms	Sat. Fat gms	Chol. mgs	% Fat Cal.
(Garcia's)										
flour, burrito style	1 tortilla	220	5	37	220	2	5.0	1.5	0	21%
flour, fajita style	1 tortilla	100	2	17	220	1	2.5	0.5	0	23%
wheat, 8-inch diam	1 tortilla	160	4	24	360	2	5.0	1.5	0	29%
(LA LA'S) flour	1 tortilla	160	4	28	350	1	3.0	0.5	0	17%
(La Tortilla)										
flour, burrito sized, 99% fat free	1 tortilla	120	4	25	350	10	0.5	0.3	0	4%
flour, fat free	1 tortilla	60	2	13	180	6	0.0	0.0	0	0%
whole wheat, 99% fat free	1 tortilla	60	2	12	180	9	0.0	0.0	0	0%
(Mission)										
flour, burrito size 'Premium'	1 tortilla	230	6	40	395	0	6.0	0.0	0	23%
flour, light	1 tortilla	70	2	16	280	4	1.0	0.5	0	11%
flour, soft, taco size, 8-inch diam	1 tortilla	146	4	25	249	na	3.1	0.7	na	19%
(Old El Paso)										
corn	1 tortilla	60	1	10	170	0	1.0	0.0	0	17%
flour	1 tortilla	150	4	27	360	0	3.0	0.0	0	18%
(Tyson)										
flour, burrito style	1 tortilla	173	5	29	40	0	4.0	0.0	0	21%
flour, burrito style, large, heat pressed	1 tortilla	182	5	33	90	0	4.0	0.0	0	19%
flour, burrito style, small, hand stretched	1 tortilla	106	3	19	50	0	2.0	0.0	0	17%
flour, fajita style	1 tortilla	84	3	18	20	0	2.0	0.0	0	18%
flour, soft, taco size	1 tortilla	121	4	20	30	0	3.0	0.0	0	22%
TORTILLA CHIPS. See also CORN CHIPS AND SNACKS.										
(Bachman)										
	1 oz	140	2	19	140	0	6.0	0.0	0	39%
nacho cheese	1 oz	140	2	18	210	0	6.0	0.0	0	40%
no salt	1 oz	140	2	19	0	0	6.0	0.0	0	39%
(Barbara's Bakery)										
yellow corn, no salt added, organic	1 oz	140	2	18	15	0	7.0	0.0	0	44%
yellow corn, regular, organic	1 oz	140	2	18	120	0	7.0	0.0	0	44%
(Bearitos)										
blue corn, organic	1 oz	146	3	17	29	1	7.0	0.0	0	44%
blue corn, organic, unsalted'	1 oz	137	3	17	3	1	6.5	0.0	0	43%
no salt added	1 oz	140	2	16	5	2	7.0	1.3	1	47%
yellow corn, no salt added, organic	1 oz	148	2	17	2	1	7.2	0.0	0	46%
yellow corn, organic	1 oz	143	2	18	58	1	6.4	0.0	0	42%
(Bravos)										
nacho cheese flavored, round	1 oz	150	2	18	180	0	8.0	0.0	0	47%
nacho cheese flavored, strips	1 oz	140	2	18	220	0	7.0	0.0	0	44%
nacho cheese and jalapeño	1 oz	150	2	19	170	0	7.0	0.0	0	43%
(Buenitos)										
no salt added	1 oz	150	2	18	1	4	8.0	0.0	0	47%
'Tortilla Chips'	1 oz	150	2	18	80	4	8.0	0.0	0	47%
(Doritos)										
approx 18 chips	1 oz	140	2	19	230	0	6.0	0.0	0	39%
cool ranch	1 oz	140	2	18	160	1	7.0	1.5	0	44%
cool ranch, approx 16 chips	1 oz	140	2	18	170	2	7.0	0.0	0	44%
cool ranch, light	1 oz	120	2	21	240	0	4.0	0.0	0	28%
'Jumpin' Jack' approx 16 chips	1 oz	140	2	18	220	2	7.0	0.0	0	44%
nacho, spicy	1 oz	140	2	18	210	1	7.0	1.5	0	44%
nacho cheese, approx 15 chips	1 oz	140	2	18	240	0	7.0	0.0	0	44%
nacho cheese 'Light'	1 oz	120	2	21	290	0	4.0	0.0	0	28%
'Nacho Cheesier'	1 oz	140	2	17	190	1	7.0	1.5	0	45%
salsa and cheese, 'Thins'	1 oz	150	2	17	180	0	8.0	0.0	0	49%

Food Name	Serving Size	Calories	Prot. gms	Carbs gms	Sod. mgs	Fiber gms	Fat gms	Sat. Fat gms	Chol. mgs	% Fat Cal.
'Salsa Rio' approx 16 chips	1 oz	140	2	18	190	2	7.0	0.0	0	44%
salsa verde	1 oz	150	2	20	210	1	7.0	1.5	0	42%
taco, approx 16 chips	1 oz	140	2	18	250	2	7.0	0.0	0	44%
'Taco Bell'	1 oz	150	2	21	170	1	7.0	1.5	0	41%
toasted corn, approx 16 chips	1 oz	140	2	19	80	2	7.0	0.0	0	43%
toasted	1 oz	140	2	18	120	1	7.0	1.5	0	44%
white corn, lightly salted, 'Thins'	1 oz	140	2	19	135	0	7.0	0.0	0	43%
(Eagle) ranch	1 oz	140	2	17	190	0	8.0	0.0	1	49%
(Featherweight)										
low-salt, round	1 oz	150	2	18	10	0	8.0	0.0	0	47%
nacho cheese, low-salt	1 oz	150	2	18	45	0	8.0	0.0	0	47%
(Garden of Eden)										
black bean, organic	10 chips	150	3	18	55	1	7.0	0.5	0	43%
blue corn and sunflower seed, organic	10 chips	160	3	16	70	1	8.0	1.0	0	49%
blue corn, hot and spicy, organic	10 chips	140	2	3	80	2	7.0	1.0	0	76%
blue corn, organic, no salt added	10 chips	150	2	18	0	1	7.0	0.5	0	44%
blue corn, salted, organic	10 chips	150	2	18	55	1	7.0	0.5	0	44%
chipotle, hot and smoky, organic	10 chips	120	2	23	80	1	2.0	0.0	0	15%
unsalted, no oil added, organic	10 chips	110	2	23	10	1	1.0	0.0	0	8%
w/jalapeño, organic	10 chips	140	2	18	80	2	7.0	0.5	0	44%
yogurt and green onion, organic	10 chips	120	2	23	70	1	2.0	0.0	0	15%
(Guiltless Gourmet)										
baked, original	1 oz	110	2	22	160	2	1.0	0.0	0	9%
blue corn	1 oz	110	3	22	140	2	1.0	0.0	0	8%
chili lime	1 oz	110	2	22	200	2	1.0	0.0	0	9%
nacho, baked	1 oz	110	3	22	200	2	1.0	0.0	0	8%
original, no salt added	1 oz	110	2	22	26	2	1.0	0.0	0	9%
ranch	1 oz	110	3	22	200	2	1.0	0.0	0	8%
white corn	1 oz	110	3	22	140	2	1.0	0.0	0	8%
yellow corn, baked, no salt added, approx 24 chips	1 oz	110	3	22	26	3	1.0	0.0	0	8%
yellow corn, baked, w/salt, approx 24 chips	1 oz	110	3	22	160	3	1.0	0.0	0	8%
(Hain)										
sesame	1 oz	140	2	19	190	0	7.0	0.0	0	43%
sesame, cheese	1 oz	160	2	20	270	0	8.0	0.0	5	45%
sesame, no salt added	1 oz	140	2	19	0	0	7.0	0.0	5	43%
taco	1 oz	160	2	15	320	0	11.0	0.0	5	59%
(Keebler)										
cinnamon crispana, flour, 'Chacho's'	1 oz	140	2	19	70	0	7.0	1.0	0	43%
original, restaurant style 'Chacho's'	1 oz	140	3	18	180	0	7.0	1.0	5	43%
(Kettle Tias)										
blue corn, lightly salted	1 oz	140	3	18	80	2	6.0	0.5	0	39%
blue corn, no salt added	1 oz	140	3	18	2	2	6.0	0.5	0	39%
yellow corn, lightly salted	1 oz	140	2	19	80	2	7.0	0.5	0	43%
yellow corn, no salt added	1 oz	140	2	19	3	2	7.0	0.5	0	43%
(La Famous)										
no salt added	1 oz	140	2	18	5	0	7.0	0.0	0	44%
regular	1 oz	140	2	18	180	0	7.0	0.0	0	44%
(Laura Scudder's)										
nacho cheese, jalapeño, 'Strips'	1 oz	150	2	19	170	0	7.0	0.0	0	43%
nacho cheese, 'Triangles'	1 oz	140	2	18	220	0	7.0	0.0	0	44%
picante, 'Restaurant Style Strips'	1 oz	150	2	19	190	0	7.0	0.0	0	43%
restaurant style, lightly salted	1 oz	140	2	18	90	0	7.0	0.0	0	44%
(Louise's) 95% nonfat	1 oz	120	2	23	170	1	1.5	0.3	0	12%
(Mexi-Snax)										
hot	12 chips	140	2	21	70	0	5.0	0.0	0	33%

Food Name	Serving Size	Calories	Prot. gms	Carbs gms	Sod. mgs	Fiber gms	Fat gms	Sat. Fat gms	Chol. mgs	% Fat Cal.
no salt added	12 chips	140	2	21	0	0	6.0	0.0	0	37%
vegetable medley	12 chips	140	2	21	114	0	5.0	0.0	0	33%
(Mi Ranchito)										
jalapeño cheddar	10 chips	140	2	20	170	1	7.0	1.0	0	42%
spicy red chili, 'Rojo's'	10 chips	140	2	20	100	1	7.0	1.0	0	42%
(Michael Season's)										
white corn, lightly salted	1 oz	135	3	17	120	na	6.0	0.5	0	40%
yellow corn, lightly salted, organic	1 oz	135	2	19	120	na	5.0	0.5	0	35%
yellow corn, organic	1 oz	135	2	19	80	na	5.0	0.5	0	35%
(Old El Paso)										
crispy, approx 16 chips	1 oz	150	2	17	105	1	8.0	0.0	0	49%
'NaChips' approx 9 chips	1 oz	150	2	18	80	2	7.0	0.0	0	44%
white corn, low-sodium, round, 'NaChips'	1 oz	160	2	17	5	0	9.0	0.0	0	52%
(Planters)										
nacho cheese	1 oz	150	2	18	160	0	8.0	2.0	0	47%
traditional	1 oz	150	2	18	150	0	8.0	2.0	0	47%
(Santitas)										
food service product, 'Restaurant Strips'	1 oz	140	2	19	60	1	6.0	1.0	0	39%
100% white corn	1 oz	140	2	19	80	1	6.0	1.0	0	39%
restaurant style	1 oz	140	2	19	50	1	6.0	1.0	0	39%
(Slimchips) nonfat, approx 10 chips	0.4 oz	44	1	10	60	1	0.5	0.0	0	9%
(Tio Sancho) 'Microwave Snacks'	4 oz	567	9	74	590	4	26.1	0.0	0	41%
(Tostitos)										
approx 11 chips	1 oz	140	2	18	170	0	8.0	0.0	0	47%
baked	1 oz	110	2	24	200	2	1.0	0.0	0	8%
bite-size	1 oz	140	2	17	110	1	8.0	1.0	0	49%
lime and chile	1 oz	150	2	17	180	1	7.0	1.0	0	45%
nacho cheese, sharp, approx 11 chips	1 oz	150	2	17	200	0	8.0	0.0	0	49%
restaurant style	1 oz	140	2	19	110	1	6.0	1.0	0	39%
rounds	1 oz	150	1	18	85	1	8.0	1.0	0	49%
unsalted	1 oz	110	3	24	0	2	1.0	0.0	0	8%
white corn, baked, 'Cool Ranch'	1 oz	130	2	21	170	0	3.0	0.0	0	23%
(Vera Cruz)										
tortilla rounds, baked	1 oz	120	2	22	78	2	1.5	0.0	0	12%
tortilla rounds, baked, unsalted	1 oz	120	2	22	0	2	1.5	0.0	0	12%
(Wise) nacho cheese flavored, crispy, round	1 oz	150	2	18	180	0	8.0	0.0	0	47%
TORULA YEAST. See under YEAST.										
TOSTACO SHELL *(Old El Paso)*	1 shell	100	1	11	10	1	5.0	0.0	0	48%
TOSTADA CHIPS										
(Michael Season's) yellow corn, lightly salted, bite-sized	1 oz	135	2	19	120	na	5.0	0.5	0	35%
TOSTADA SHELL										
(Bearitos) yellow corn	1 shell	140	2	17	0	2	7.0	1.1	0	45%
(Lawry's)	1 shell	73	1	10	147	0	3.5	0.0	0	42%
(Ortega)	1 shell	50	0	8	5	0	2.0	0.0	0	36%
(Pancho Villa)	1 shell	55	1	6	65	0	3.0	0.0	0	49%
(Rosarita)										
	1 shell	63	1	9	10	0	2.4	0.5	18	36%
1-oz shell	2 shells	138	2	17	88	4	7.6	2.1	0	47%
(Tio Sancho)	1 shell	67	1	8	1	1	3.2	0.0	0	43%
TOWELGOURD. See GOURD, DISHCLOTH.										
TRAIL MIX SNACK										
(Harmony)										
'Deluxe Super'	1/4 cup	150	3	23	35	3	7.0	2.5	0	38%
nut and berry mix	1/4 cup	160	5	21	0	3	8.0	1.0	0	41%

Food Name	Serving Size	Calories	Prot. gms	Carbs gms	Sod. mgs	Fiber gms	Fat gms	Sat. Fat gms	Chol. mgs	% Fat Cal.
(Maranatha Natural)										
'Deluxe'	1/4 cup	150	5	13	5	3	9.0	1.5	0	53%
'Mountain Delight'	1/4 cup	140	5	15	30	3	8.0	2.0	0	47%
'Nature Trail'	1/4 cup	150	4	15	0	2	9.0	1.5	0	52%
'Snack Attack'	1/4 cup	140	2	16	0	2	8.0	3.0	0	50%
(Pacific Shores) all fruit	1/4 cup	110	0	21	20	2	2.0	1.5	0	18%
(Pilgram Joe's) cranberry	1/4 cup	150	5	12	5	3	9.0	1.5	0	54%
(Trader Joe's)										
'Muir Trail Mix'	1/4 cup	180	7	11	0	2	13.0	2.5	0	62%
w/carob chips, 'Mt. Baldy Mix'	1/4 cup	190	0	15	5	3	14.0	2.0	0	68%
TREE FERN										
cooked, chopped	1/2 cup	28	0	8	4	3	0.1	0.0	0	1%
cooked, whole, 6.5-inch long	1 frond	12	0	3	2	1	0.0	0.0	0	1%
TREE MUSHROOM. See MUSHROOM, OYSTER.										
TRITICALE	1 cup	645	25	138	10	na	4.0	0.7	0	5%
TROUT										
MIXED SPECIES										
baked, broiled, grilled, or microwaved	3 oz	162	23	0	57	0	7.2	1.3	63	40%
raw	3 oz	126	18	0	44	0	5.6	1.0	49	40%
RAINBOW										
farmed, baked, broiled, grilled, or microwaved	3 oz	144	21	0	36	0	6.1	1.8	58	38%
farmed, raw	3 oz	117	18	0	30	0	4.6	1.3	50	35%
wild, baked, broiled, grilled, or microwaved	3 oz	128	19	0	48	0	4.9	1.4	59	35%
wild, raw	3 oz	101	17	0	26	0	2.9	0.6	50	26%
SEA										
mixed species, baked, broiled, grilled, or microwaved	3 oz	113	18	0	63	0	3.9	1.1	90	31%
mixed species, raw	3 oz	88	14	0	49	0	3.1	0.9	71	31%
TUNA										
Canned										
in oil, drained	3 oz	158	23	0	337	0	6.9	1.4	26	39%
in water, drained	3 oz	99	22	0	287	0	0.7	0.2	26	6%
in water, no salt added, drained	3 oz	99	22	0	43	0	0.7	0.2	26	6%
solid, in olive oil *(Progresso)*	1/4 cup	160	0	0	250	0	12.0	2.0	30	100%
very low sodium *(Chicken of the Sea)*	2 oz	60	13	0	35	0	0.5	0.1	25	8%
Frozen, steak, w/o seasoning mix *(SeaPak)*	6 oz pkg	180	40	0	65	0	2.0	0.0	75	10%
ALBACORE										
Canned										
solid white, in soybean oil, drained *(Bumble Bee)*	2 oz	100	14	0	310	0	8.0	2.0	30	56%
solid white, in soybean oil, drained *(Finast)*	2 oz	145	14	1	320	0	10.0	0.0	0	60%
solid white, in soybean oil, drained *(S&W)*	2 oz	160	13	0	450	0	12.0	0.0	0	68%
solid white, in soybean oil, drained *(Star-Kist)*	2 oz	140	14	1	310	0	10.0	1.0	25	60%
solid white, in spring water, fancy *(Chicken of the Sea)*	2 oz	60	14	1	250	0	1.0	0.0	0	13%
solid white, in water, drained *(A&P)*	2 oz	70	15	1	310	0	1.0	0.0	0	12%
solid white, in water, drained *(Bumble Bee)*	2 oz	60	14	0	310	0	2.0	1.0	30	24%
solid white, in water, drained *(Finast)*	2 oz	70	15	1	310	0	1.0	0.0	0	12%
solid white, in water, drained *(Pathmark)*	2 oz	70	15	0	310	0	2.0	0.0	0	23%
solid white, in water, drained *(Star-Kist)*	2 oz	70	15	1	310	0	1.0	0.2	25	12%
solid white, in water, drained *(Weight Watchers)*	2 oz	70	15	1	210	0	1.0	0.2	25	12%
Frozen										
steak, white, boneless/skinless, raw *(Peter Pan Seafoods)*	3.5 oz	102	19	0	51	0	4.9	0.0	54	37%
BLUEFIN										
Fresh										
baked, broiled, grilled, or microwaved	3 oz	156	25	0	43	0	5.3	1.4	42	31%
raw	3 oz	122	20	0	33	0	4.2	1.1	32	31%

Food Name	Serving Size	Calories	Prot. gms	Carbs gms	Sod. mgs	Fiber gms	Fat gms	Sat. Fat gms	Chol. mgs	% Fat Cal.
CHUNK LIGHT										
Canned										
in Canola oil *(Chicken of the Sea)*	2 oz	110	13	0	250	0	6.0	0.3	30	51%
in oil *(S&W)*	3 oz	167	21	0	349	0	9.1	1.5	46	49%
in vegetable oil, w/liquid *(Chicken of the Sea)*	2 oz	160	12	1	250	0	12.0	0.0	0	68%
in soybean oil, drained *(Bumble Bee)*	2 oz	110	12	0	310	0	12.0	3.0	30	69%
in soybean oil, drained *(Finast)*	2 oz	150	13	1	310	0	13.0	0.0	0	68%
in soybean oil, drained *(Star-Kist)*	2 oz	150	13	1	310	0	13.0	1.0	25	68%
in soybean oil, drained, 'Fancy' *(S&W)*	2 oz	140	13	0	450	0	10.0	0.0	0	63%
in water *(Captains Choice)*	3 oz	90	18	0	465	0	2.0	0.0	0	20%
in water *(Chicken of the Sea)*	2 oz	60	13	0	250	0	0.5	0.2	30	8%
in water *(S&W)*	3 oz	106	23	0	349	0	0.8	0.0	53	7%
in water, diet, drained *(Star-Kist)*	2 oz	65	14	1	35	0	1.0	0.2	25	13%
in water, drained *(Bumble Bee)*	2 oz	50	12	0	310	0	1.0	0.5	30	16%
in water, drained *(Featherweight)*	2 oz	60	13	0	30	0	1.0	0.0	30	15%
in water, drained *(Finast)*	2 oz	60	13	1	310	0	1.0	0.0	0	14%
in water, drained *(Pathmark)*	2 oz	70	15	0	310	0	2.0	0.0	0	23%
in water, drained *(Star-Kist)*	2 oz	60	13	1	310	0	1.0	0.2	25	14%
in water, drained, 'Fancy' *(S&W)*	2 oz	60	13	0	500	0	1.0	0.0	0	15%
in water, low-sodium *(Chicken of the Sea)*	2 oz	60	14	0	90	0	0.5	0.1	30	7%
in water, no salt added, drained *(Weight Watchers)*	2 oz	60	14	1	210	0	1.0	0.2	25	13%
in water, 60% less salt, drained *(Star-Kist)*	2 oz	65	14	1	120	0	1.0	0.2	25	13%
CHUNK WHITE										
Canned										
in soybean oil, drained *(Bumble Bee)*	2 oz	110	12	0	310	0	12.0	3.0	30	69%
in water *(Chicken of the Sea)*	2 oz	60	13	0	250	0	1.0	0.1	25	15%
in water, diet, drained *(Star-Kist)*	2 oz	70	15	1	30	0	1.0	0.2	25	12%
in water, drained *(A&P)*	2 oz	100	12	1	310	0	5.0	0.0	0	46%
in water, drained *(Bumble Bee)*	2 oz	60	12	0	310	0	2.0	1.0	30	27%
in water, 60% less salt, drained *(Star-Kist)*	2 oz	70	15	1	120	0	1.0	0.2	25	12%
LIGHT										
Canned										
in oil, drained	3 oz	168	25	0	301	0	7.0	1.3	15	37%
in oil, no salt added, drained	3 oz	168	25	0	43	0	7.0	1.3	15	37%
in soybean oil, drained *(A&P)*	2 oz	150	13	1	310	0	13.0	0.0	0	68%
in water, drained *(A&P)*	2 oz	60	13	1	310	0	1.0	0.0	0	14%
in water, drained *(Empress)*	2 oz	60	12	0	310	0	1.0	0.0	0	16%
SKIPJACK / aku / katsuo / oceanic bonito										
Fresh										
baked, broiled, grilled, or microwaved	3 oz	112	24	0	40	0	1.1	0.4	51	9%
raw	3 oz	88	19	0	31	0	0.9	0.3	40	9%
SOLID LIGHT										
Canned										
in Canola oil *(Chicken of the Sea)*	2 oz	90	14	0	250	0	3.0	0.3	25	33%
in oil *(S&W)*	3 oz	121	26	0	349	0	2.3	0.0	30	17%
in soybean oil, drained *(Star-Kist)*	2 oz	150	13	1	310	0	13.0	1.0	25	68%
in soybean oil, drained, solid *(Progresso)*	1/3 cup	150	13	1	400	0	13.0	0.0	0	68%
in water *(Chicken of the Sea)*	2 oz	70	15	0	250	0	1.0	0.1	25	13%
in water, drained *(Star-Kist)*	2 oz	60	14	1	310	0	1.0	0.2	25	13%
in water, drained, 'Prime Catch' *(Star-Kist)*	2 oz	60	14	1	310	0	1.0	0.2	25	13%
SOLID WHITE										
Canned										
in soybean oil, drained *(Star-Kist)*	2 oz	140	14	1	310	0	10.0	1.0	25	60%
in water *(Captains Choice)*	2 oz	70	15	0	250	0	1.0	0.0	25	13%

Food Name	Serving Size	Calories	Prot. gms	Carbs gms	Sod. mgs	Fiber gms	Fat gms	Sat. Fat gms	Chol. mgs	% Fat Cal.
WHITE										
Canned										
in oil, no salt added, drained	3 oz	158	23	0	43	0	6.9	1.4	26	39%
in soybean oil, drained (A&P)	2 oz	150	13	1	310	0	10.0	0.0	0	62%
in water, drained	3 oz	109	20	0	320	0	2.5	0.7	36	21%
in water, no salt added, drained	3 oz	109	20	0	43	0	2.5	0.7	36	21%
YELLOWFIN / ahi										
Fresh										
baked, broiled, grilled, or microwaved	3 oz	118	25	0	40	0	1.0	0.3	49	8%
raw	3 oz	92	20	0	31	0	0.8	0.2	38	8%
raw boneless	1 oz	31	7	0	10	0	0.3	0.1	13	8%
Frozen										
steak, boneless, skinless, raw (Peter Pan Seafoods)	3.5 oz	131	23	0	61	0	4.1	0.0	45	28%
TUNA DISH/ENTRÉE										
(Banquet) pie, frozen	7 oz	540	17	44	810	0	33.0	0.0	30	55%
(Marie Callender's) chunky tuna and noodles	12 oz	960	18	43	1570	6	35.0	18.0	55	56%
(Stouffer's)										
tuna-noodle casserole	1 entrée	320	20	37	1130	0	10.0	3.5	40	28%
tuna-noodle casserole, frozen, food service product	1 oz	35	2	3	126	0	1.9	0.3	4	50%
(Weight Watchers) tuna-noodle casserole	1 entrée	270	13	39	590	4	7.0	3.5	35	23%
TUNA DISH/ENTRÉE MIX										
(Tuna Helper)										
au gratin meal, mix only	1/2 cup	190	6	34	730	1	3.5	1.0	3	16%
au gratin meal, prepared	1 cup	300	13	37	890	1	11.0	3.0	20	33%
buttery rice, prepared	1/5 pkg	160	4	32	830	1	2.0	0.0	0	11%
cheesy pasta meal, mix only	3/4 cup	170	5	29	710	1	3.0	1.0	3	17%
cheesy pasta meal, prepared	1 cup	280	14	32	890	1	11.0	3.0	20	35%
creamy broccoli, prepared	1/5 pkg	200	6	35	800	0	4.0	0.0	0	18%
creamy mushroom, prepared	1/5 pkg	140	5	28	580	0	1.0	0.0	0	6%
creamy pasta meal, mix only	3/4 cup	190	5	29	730	1	6.0	1.5	3	28%
creamy pasta meal, prepared	1 cup	300	14	31	910	1	13.0	3.5	20	39%
fettuccine Alfredo meal, mix only	3/4 cup	170	5	30	730	1	3.5	1.5	0	18%
fettuccine Alfredo meal, prepared	1 cup	310	14	32	950	1	14.0	3.5	15	41%
pasta salad, prepared	1/5 pkg	140	5	28	580	0	1.0	0.0	0	6%
pot pie, prepared	1/2 cup	340	5	35	920	1	20.0	5.0	0	53%
pot pie, prepared	1/6 pkg	290	4	31	730	0	17.0	0.0	0	52%
Romanoff meal, mix only	2/3 cup	210	7	38	650	1	3.0	1.0	5	13%
Romanoff meal, prepared	1 cup	280	15	38	800	1	8.0	1.5	20	25%
tetrazzini meal, mix only	2/3 cup	180	7	32	790	1	3.0	1.5	5	15%
tetrazzini meal, prepared	1 cup	310	17	33	1010	1	12.0	3.0	20	35%
TUNA SALAD SPREAD (Libby's) 'Spreadables'	1/3 cup	130	7	6	370	3	8.0	1.0	15	58%
TUNA SUBSTITUTE										
(Natural Touch) vegetarian, 'Tuno'	1/3 cup drained	60	7	2	360	1	2.0	0.5	0	30.0%
(Worthington)										
vegetarian, 'Tuno' 12-oz can	1/3 cup drained	80	7	4	380	1	4.0	0.5	0	45.0%
vegetarian, 'Tuno' 12-oz roll	1/2 cup drained	80	6	2	290	1	6.0	1.0	0	67.5%
TUNKA. See GOURD, WHITE.										
TURBOT, EUROPEAN										
baked, broiled, grilled, or microwaved	3 oz	104	17	0	163	0	3.2	na	53	28%
raw	3 oz	81	14	0	128	0	2.5	0.6	41	28%
TURKEY										
BACK										
Fresh										
all classes, meat and skin, raw	1 lb	896	81.6	0.0	304	0	59.2	16.0	336	62%

Food Name	Serving Size	Calories	Prot. gms	Carbs gms	Sod. mgs	Fiber gms	Fat gms	Sat. Fat gms	Chol. mgs	% Fat Cal.
all classes, meat and skin, raw	1 oz	56	5.1	0.0	19	0	3.7	1.0	21	62%
all classes, meat and skin, roasted	4 oz	276	30.2	0.0	83	0	16.3	4.7	103	55%
fryer/roaster, meat and skin, raw	4 oz	173	22.5	0	69	0	8.3	2.4	98	43%
fryer/roaster, meat and skin, roasted	4 oz	233	30.0	0	80	0	11.7	3.4	123	45%
fryer/roaster, meat only, raw	4 oz	137	23.6	0	75	0	4.0	1.4	85	26%
fryer/roaster, meat only, roasted	4 oz	194	32.0	0	83	0	6.5	2.2	109	30%
young hen, meat and skin, raw	4 oz	252	20.1	0	71	0	18.4	0.4	79	66%
young hen, meat and skin, roasted	4 oz	290	30.0	0	79	0	17.9	5.2	97	56%
young tom, meat and skin, raw	4 oz	205	21.2	0	81	0	12.7	3.6	90	56%
young tom, meat and skin, roasted	4 oz	272	30.7	0	88	0	15.6	4.5	107	52%
BREAST										
Fresh										
all classes, meat and skin, raw	1 lb	720	99.2	0.0	272	0	32.0	8.0	288	42%
all classes, meat and skin, raw	1 oz	45	32.6	0.0	71	0	8.4	2.4	84	37%
all classes, meat and skin, roasted	4 oz	214	32.6	0.0	71	0	8.4	2.4	84	37%
fryer/roaster, meat and skin, raw	4 oz	152	27.2	0	55	0	3.0	0.8	80	19%
fryer/roaster, meat and skin, roasted	4 oz	175	33.2	0	60	0	3.7	1.0	103	19%
fryer/roaster, meat and skin, pre-basted, roasted	4 oz	114	25.7	0	454	0	4.0	1.1	48	25%
young hen, meat and skin, raw	4 oz	191	24.7	0	63	0	9.5	2.6	71	45%
young hen, meat and skin, roasted	4 oz	222	33.0	0	66	0	9.0	2.6	82	37%
young tom, meat and skin, raw	4 oz	173	25.1	0	72	0	7.2	2.0	77	38%
young tom, meat and skin, roasted	4 oz	216	32.7	0	77	0	8.4	2.3	86	35%
Frozen or refrigerated										
barbecue, quartered *(Mr. Turkey)*	3.5 oz	95	21	1	901	0	0.8	0.2	35	7%
cooked *(Land O'Lakes)*	3 oz	100	20	0	55	0	1.0	1.0	50	10%
cooked *(Louis Rich)*	1 oz	47	8	0	21	0	1.5	0.6	21	29%
cooked, 'Cook-N-Bag' *(Longacre)*	1 oz	38	8	1	85	0	1.0	0.0	15	20%
cooked, 'Fresh Turkey Cuts' *(Louis Rich)*	1 oz	45	8	1	20	0	2.0	0.0	20	33%
8% self-basting solution *(Jennie-O)*	4 oz	160	22	0	200	0	8.0	2.0	65	45%
hen, cooked, w/o wings *(Louis Rich)*	1 oz	50	8	0	19	0	2.0	0.4	19	36%
hickory smoked, cooked *(Louis Rich)*	1 oz	33	5	1	346	0	1.0	0.3	13	27%
honey roasted, cooked *(Louis Rich)*	1 oz	33	5	1	318	0	0.8	0.3	12	22%
oven-roasted, cooked *(Louis Rich)*	1 oz	31	5	0	296	0	0.9	0.2	13	26%
raw, 'Cook-N-Bag' *(Longacre)*	1 oz	27	6	1	120	0	1.0	0.0	10	24%
raw, 'Ready-to-Cook' *(Longacre)*	1 oz	39	8	0	150	0	1.0	0.0	0	22%
raw, 'Tasti-Lean Tenders' *(Norbest)*	4 oz	135	28	0	81	0	2.0	0.0	0	14%
roast, cooked *(Louis Rich)*	1 oz	42	8	0	20	0	0.8	0.3	19	17%
roast, cooked, 'Fresh Turkey Cuts' *(Louis Rich)*	1 oz	40	8	1	20	0	1.0	0.0	20	20%
slices, cooked *(Louis Rich)*	1 oz	39	8	0	24	0	0.5	0.1	17	12%
smoked, cooked *(Louis Rich)*	1 oz	33	6	0	268	0	1.0	0.4	11	28%
smoked, cooked, no bone *(Norbest)*	1 oz	42	6	0	218	0	1.6	0.0	0	35%
steaks, cooked *(Louis Rich)*	1 oz	39	8	0	24	0	0.5	0.1	17	12%
steaks, cooked, 'Fresh Turkey Cuts' *(Louis Rich)*	1 oz	40	8	1	25	0	1.0	0.0	20	20%
steaks, cubed, raw *(Norbest)*	4 oz	135	28	0	81	0	2.0	0.0	0	14%
strips and tips, raw, 'Tasti-Lean' *(Norbest)*	4 oz	135	28	0	81	0	2.0	0.0	0	14%
tenderloins, cooked *(Louis Rich)*	1 oz	39	9	0	24	0	0.5	0.2	18	11%
tenderloins, cooked, 'Fresh Turkey Cuts' *(Louis Rich)*	1 oz	40	8	1	25	0	1.0	0.0	20	20%
COMPOSITE CUTS										
Canned										
chunk *(Hormel)*	6-3/4 oz	230	37	0	1278	0	10.0	0.0	0	38%
chunk *(Swanson)*	1 cup	360	64	16	880	4	8.0	2.0	140	18%
in broth, drained	5-oz can	231	34	0	663	0	9.7	2.8	94	38%
puréed *(Bryan Foods)*	1/3 cup	160	13	0	45	na	11.0	3.0	50	66%

Food Name	Serving Size	Calories	Prot. gms	Carbs gms	Sod. mgs	Fiber gms	Fat gms	Sat. Fat gms	Chol. mgs	% Fat Cal.
CUTLET										
Frozen or refrigerated, raw, 'Tasti-Lean' (Norbest)	4 oz	135	28	0	81	0	2.0	0.0	0	14%
DARK MEAT										
Fresh										
all classes, meat and skin, raw	1 lb	720	86.4	0.0	320	0	40.0	11.2	320	51%
all classes, meat and skin, raw	1 oz	45	5.4	0.0	20	0	2.5	0.7	20	51%
all classes, meat and skin, roasted	1 4 oz	251	31.2	0.0	86	0	13.1	4.0	101	49%
all classes, meat only, raw	1 lb	560	91.2	0.0	352	0	19.2	6.4	320	32%
all classes, meat only, raw	1 oz	35	5.7	0.0	22	0	1.2	0.4	20	32%
all classes, meat only, roasted	4 oz	212	32.4	0.0	90	0	8.2	2.7	96	36%
all classes, meat only, roasted, chopped or diced	1 cup	262	40.0	0.0	111	0	10.1	3.4	119	36%
fryer/roaster, meat and skin, raw	4 oz	147	23.0	0	75	0	5.5	1.6	99	33%
fryer/roaster, meat and skin, roasted	4 oz	208	31.8	0	87	0	8.1	2.4	134	35%
fryer/roaster, meat only, raw	4 oz	114	23.4	0	79	0	3.1	1.0	93	22%
fryer/roaster, meat only, roasted	4 oz	184	32.7	0	90	0	5.0	1.6	128	24%
fryer/roaster, meat only, roasted, chopped or diced	1 cup	227	40.0	0	111	0	6.0	2.0	157	24%
young hen, meat and skin, raw	4 oz	196	21.1	0	77	0	11.7	3.4	74	54%
young hen, meat and skin, roasted	4 oz	265	31.3	0	82	0	14.6	4.4	96	50%
young hen, meat only, raw	4 oz	149	22.9	0	84	0	5.5	1.8	71	34%
young hen, meat only, roasted	4 oz	220	22.9	0	62	0	6.3	2.1	65	37%
young hen, meat only, roasted, chopped or diced	1 cup	269	40.0	0	105	0	10.9	3.7	112	37%
young tom, meat and skin, raw	4 oz	174	21.8	0	86	0	9.0	2.6	88	47%
young tom, meat and skin, roasted	4 oz	235	31.0	0	91	0	12.4	3.8	104	45%
young tom, meat only, raw	4 oz	141	23.2	0	91	0	4.7	1.5	86	30%
young tom, meat only, roasted	4 oz	212	33.0	0	94	0	8.0	2.7	100	34%
GIBLETS										
Fresh										
all classes, raw	4 oz	150	22	2.4	101	0	4.8	1.5	328	29%
all classes, raw	1/2 oz	21	3	0	14	0	0.7	0.2	45	29%
all classes, w/fat, simmered	0.35 oz	17	3	0	6	0	0.5	0.2	42	27%
all classes, w/fat, simmered, chopped or diced	1 cup	242	39	3	86	0	7.4	2.2	606	27%
GIZZARD										
Fresh										
all classes, raw	1 med gizzard	132	22	1	90	0	4.2	1.2	179	29%
all classes, raw	1/4 oz	8	1	0	6	0	0.3	0.1	11	29%
all classes, simmered	0.14 oz	7	1	0	2	0	0.2	0.0	9	21%
all classes, simmered, chopped or diced	1 cup	236	43	1	78	0	5.6	1.6	336	21%
GROUND										
Fresh										
all classes, breaded, battered, fried	3.33-oz patty	266	13	15	752	0	16.9	4.4	58	57%
all classes, breaded, battered, fried	2.25-oz patty	181	9	10	512	0	11.5	3.0	40	57%
all classes, cooked	4-oz patty	193	22	0	88	0	10.8	2.8	84	50%
all classes, raw	4-oz patty	170	20	0	107	0	9.4	2.6	90	50%
Frozen or refrigerated										
(Louis Rich)	4 oz	190	20	0	140	0	12.0	3.5	90	57%
(Mr. Turkey)	1 oz	54	5	0	27	0	4.0	0.0	20	67%
burger patty (Shelton's)	1 serving	170	20	0	110	0	10.0	3.0	90	53%
cooked (Hudson)	1 oz	55	5	0	35	0	3.7	0.0	0	62%
cooked (Longacre)	1 oz	60	5	0	20	0	4.0	0.0	30	64%
extra lean, 97% fat-free (Turkey Store)	4 oz	120	27	0	75	0	1.5	0.5	55	11%
lean, 7% fat, w/natural flavorings (Turkey Store)	4 oz	160	23	0	80	0	8.0	2.0	70	44%
raw (Norbest)	1 oz	45	5	0	34	0	2.6	0.0	0	52%
w/natural flavoring (Louis Rich)	1 oz	50	8	0	33	0	2.2	0.7	24	40%

Food Name	Serving Size	Calories	Prot. gms	Carbs gms	Sod. mgs	Fiber gms	Fat gms	Sat. Fat gms	Chol. mgs	% Fat Cal.
HEART										
Fresh										
all classes, raw	1 med heart	41	5	0	25	0	2.0	0.6	33	44%
all classes, simmered, chopped or diced	1 cup	257	39	3	80	0	8.8	2.5	328	31%
HINDQUARTER										
Frozen or refrigerated, roast (Land O'Lakes)	3 oz	140	17	0	80	0	8.0	3.0	0	51%
LEG										
Fresh										
all classes, meat and skin, raw	1 lb	656	88.0	0.0	336	0	30.4	9.6	320	44%
all classes, meat and skin, raw	1 oz	41	5.5	0.0	21	0	1.9	0.6	320	44%
all classes, meat and skin, roasted	4 oz	236	31.6	0.0	87	0	11.1	3.5	96	44%
fryer/roaster, meat and skin, raw	4 oz	135	23	0	78	0	4.0	1.3	99	27%
fryer/roaster, meat and skin, roasted	4 oz	194	32.7	0	91	0	6.2	2.0	80	29%
fryer/roaster, meat only, raw	4 oz	123	23.3	0	81	0	2.7	0.9	96	20%
fryer/roaster, meat only, roasted	4 oz	182	33.2	0	92	0	4.3	1.4	136	21%
young hen, meat and skin, raw	4 oz	173	21.8	0	81	0	8.6	2.6	72	45%
young hen, meat and skin, roasted	4 oz	235	32.7	0	91	0	11.0	3.4	103	42%
Frozen or refrigerated										
(Land O'Lakes)	3 oz	120	17	0	85	0	5.0	2.0	0	40%
cooked (Louis Rich)	1 oz	56	8	0	22	0	2.6	0.9	27	42%
cooked, 'Fresh Turkey Cuts' (Louis Rich)	1 oz	55	8	1	25	0	3.0	0.0	30	43%
LIGHT MEAT										
Canned										
chunk white, in water, 97% fat-free (Valley Fresh)	2 oz	80	16	0	150	0	1.5	0.5	55	17%
white meat (Swanson)	2.5 oz	80	17	1	260	0	1.0	0.0	0	11%
Fresh										
all classes, meat and skin, raw	1 lb	720	97.6	0.0	272	0	33.6	9.6	288	44%
all classes, meat and skin, raw	1 oz	45	6.1	0.0	17	0	2.1	0.6	18	44%
all classes, meat and skin, roasted	4 oz	223	32.4	0.0	71	0	9.4	2.7	86	40%
all classes, meat only, raw	1 lb	528	107.2	0.0	288	0	6.4	1.6	272	12%
all classes, meat only, raw	1 oz	33	6.7	0.0	18	0	0.4	0.1	17	12%
all classes, meat only, roasted	4 oz	178	33.9	0.0	73	0	3.7	1.2	78	20%
all classes, meat only, roasted, chopped or diced	1 cup	220	41.9	0.0	90	0	4.5	1.4	97	20%
fryer/roaster, meat and skin, raw	4 oz	152	26.5	0	57	0	4.4	1.2	87	26%
fryer/roaster, meat and skin, roasted	4 oz	188	33	0	65	0	5.2	1.4	109	25%
fryer/roaster, meat only, raw	4 oz	123	27.6	0	59	0	0.6	0.2	75	4%
fryer/roaster, meat only, roasted	4 oz	160	34.1	0	64	0	1.3	0.4	98	8%
fryer/roaster, meat only, roasted, chopped or diced	1 cup	196	42	0	78	0	1.7	0.5	120	8%
young hen, meat and skin, raw	4 oz	189	24.8	0	63	0	9.3	2.5	71	44%
young hen, meat and skin, roasted	4 oz	237	32.5	0	66	0	10.8	3.0	84	41%
young hen, meat only, raw	4 oz	133	27.2	0	68	0	1.9	0.6	66	13%
young hen, meat only, raw	4 oz	184	34.6	0	68	0	4.3	1.3	78	21%
young hen, meat only, roasted, chopped or diced	1 cup	225	42.0	0	84	0	5.2	1.7	95	21%
young tom, meat and skin, raw	4 oz	179	25.0	0	72	0	8.0	2.2	77	41%
young tom, meat and skin, roasted	4 oz	218	32.8	0	76	0	8.8	2.4	86	36%
young tom, meat only, raw	4 oz	131	26.7	0	76	0	1.8	0.6	71	12%
young tom, meat only, roasted	4 oz	176	34.1	0	78	0	3.3	1.1	79	17%
LIVER										
Fresh										
all classes, raw	3.5 oz	140	20	4	98	0	4.0	1.3	475	26%
all classes, raw	0.25 oz	10	1	0	7	0	0.3	0.1	33	26%
all classes, simmered	0.18 oz	8	1	0	3	0	0.3	0.1	31	32%
all classes, simmered, chopped or diced	1 cup	237	34	5	90	0	8.3	2.6	876	32%

Food Name	Serving Size	Calories	Prot. gms	Carbs gms	Sod. mgs	Fiber gms	Fat gms	Sat. Fat gms	Chol. mgs	% Fat Cal.
NECK										
Fresh										
all classes, raw	1 lb	608	91.2	0.0	416	0	24.0	8.0	352	37%
all classes, raw	1 oz	38	5.7	0.0	26	0	1.5	0.5	22	37%
all classes, simmered	4 oz	204	30.4	0.0	64	0	8.2	2.8	138	38%
PATTY										
Frozen or refrigerated, kosher (Empire Kosher)	1 patty	200	13	14	280	1	10.0	2.0	5	45%
SKIN										
Fresh										
all classes, raw	1 lb	1760	57.6	0.0	160	0	168.0	43.2	576	87%
all classes, raw	1 oz	110	3.6	0.0	10	0	10.5	2.7	26	87%
all classes, roasted	1 oz	125	5.6	0.0	15	0	11.2	2.9	32	82%
fryer/roaster, raw	4 oz	325	18.0	0	39	0	26.8	6.9	159	75%
fryer/roaster, roasted	4 oz	343	23.5	0	71	0	26.6	7.1	165	70%
young hen, raw	4 oz	476	13.5	0	37	0	46.4	12.1	93	88%
young hen, roasted	4 oz	551	21.6	0	50	0	50.8	13.2	121	83%
young tom, raw	4 oz	421	15.7	0	45	0	39.4	10.3	108	85%
young tom, roasted	4 oz	482	21.4	0	68	0	42.5	11.1	132	80%
THIGH										
Frozen or refrigerated										
(Land O'Lakes)	3 oz	150	17	0	75	0	10.0	4.0	0	57%
cooked (Louis Rich)	1 oz	64	8	0	20	0	3.7	1.0	27	52%
cooked, 'Fresh Turkey Cuts' (Louis Rich)	1 oz	65	7	1	20	0	4.0	0.0	30	53%
WHOLE										
Frozen or refrigerated										
barbecue, kosher (Empire Kosher)	5 oz	250	35	0	320	0	12.0	3.5	100	44%
cooked, excluding giblets, 'Fresh Whole Turkey' (Louis Rich)	1 oz	50	8	1	25	0	2.0	0.0	25	33%
cooked, no bone (Norbest)	1 oz	42	6	0	105	0	1.5	0.0	0	34%
cooked, w/o giblets (Louis Rich)	1 oz	52	8	0	23	0	2.3	0.7	22	40%
young (Land O'Lakes) frozen/refrig., young	3 oz	130	17	1	55	0	7.0	2.0	65	47%
young, butter-basted (Land O'Lakes)	3 oz	140	17	1	135	0	8.0	3.0	85	50%
young, self-basting, broth (Land O'Lakes)	3 oz	120	18	1	145	0	5.0	2.0	77	37%
young, 3% self-basting solution, 'Natural Choice' (Jennie-O)	4 oz	170	22	0	120	0	8.0	2.5	85	45%
WING										
Fresh										
all classes, meat and skin, raw	1 lb	896	91.2	0.0	256	0	56.0	14.4	320	58%
all classes, meat and skin, raw	1 oz	56	5.7	0.0	16	0	3.5	0.9	20	58%
all classes, meat and skin, roasted	4 oz	260	31.0	0.0	69	0	14.1	3.8	92	51%
fryer/roaster, meat and skin, raw	3 oz	136	19.0	0	48	0	6.7	1.7	83	44%
fryer/roaster, meat and skin, roasted	3 oz	178	24	0	62	0	8.6	2.4	99	43%
fryer/roaster, meat only, raw	3 oz	92	19.8	0	56	0	1.0	0.3	69	10%
fryer/roaster, meat only, roasted	3 oz	141	25.2	0	66	0	3.0	1.0	9	19%
young hen, meat and skin, raw	3 oz	181	16.7	0	43	0	11.9	3.1	55	59%
young hen, meat and skin, roasted	3 oz	205	24.5	0	49	0	11.6	3.1	67	51%
young tom, meat and skin, raw	3 oz	160	17.1	0	51	0	9.7	2.6	63	54%
young tom, meat and skin, roasted	3 oz	188	24.5	0	57	0	9.8	2.9	69	47%
Frozen or refrigerated										
(Land O'Lakes)	3 oz	120	18	0	65	0	5.0	2.0	0	38%
cooked (Louis Rich)	1 oz	54	7	0	20	0	2.7	0.8	31	45%
cooked, 'Drumettes' (Louis Rich)	1 oz	51	8	0	20	0	2.2	0.7	29	39%
cooked, 'Fresh Turkey Cuts' (Louis Rich)	1 oz	55	7	1	20	0	3.0	0.0	30	46%
portions, cooked (Louis Rich)	1 oz	54	7	0	17	0	2.9	0.7	29	48%

Food Name	Serving Size	Calories	Prot. gms	Carbs gms	Sod. mgs	Fiber gms	Fat gms	Sat. Fat gms	Chol. mgs	% Fat Cal.
TURKEY DINNER/ENTRÉE										
(Armour) w/dressing and gravy, frozen, 'Classics'	11.5 oz	320	19	34	1280	0	12.0	0.0	50	34%
(Banquet)										
pie, frozen	7 oz	510	16	39	860	0	31.0	0.0	40	56%
pie, frozen, 'Supreme Microwave'	7 oz	430	15	30	740	0	27.0	0.0	35	57%
sliced, w/gravy, frozen, 'Cookin' Bags'	5 oz	100	7	5	0	0	6.0	0.0	0	53%
sliced, w/gravy, frozen, 'Family Entrées'	8 oz	150	12	8	0	0	8.0	0.0	0	47%
turkey entrée, frozen	1 entrée	280	14	34	1060	3	10.0	2.5	55	32%
turkey entrée, frozen	10.5 oz	390	18	35	1110	0	20.0	0.0	40	46%
turkey entrée, frozen, 'Extra Helping'	19 oz	750	29	68	1980	0	42.0	0.0	65	49%
w/dressing, potatoes, corn, in sauce	1 entrée	280	14	34	1061	3	9.9	2.5	52	32%
w/gravy and dressing, frozen, 'Healthy Balance'	11.25 oz	270	16	41	750	0	5.0	2.0	40	16%
w/mashed potatoes and corn, in seasoned sauce	1 serving	280	14	34	1061	3	9.9	2.5	52	32%
(Budget Gourmet)										
breast, Dijon, frozen	11.2 oz	340	20	37	860	0	12.0	0.0	65	32%
breast, sliced, frozen	11.1 oz	290	16	36	1200	0	9.0	0.0	45	28%
turkey à la king, w/rice, frozen	10 oz	390	20	36	740	0	18.0	0.0	75	42%
turkey entrée, glazed, frozen, 'Light'	1 entrée	250	15	38	730	2	4.0	2.0	30	15%
w/escalloped noodles 'Special Selections'	1 entrée	440	19	44	840	2	20.0	10.0	115	42%
(Butterball)										
breast, hickory-smoked, no skin, 99% fat-free	3 oz	80	17	1	710	0	1.0	0.0	35	11%
breast, roasted, no skin, 99% fat-free	3 oz	80	16	2	750	0	1.0	0.0	30	11%
breast, roasted, w/honey, no skin, 99% fat-free	3 oz	90	16	3	690	0	1.0	0.0	35	11%
(Dinty Moore)										
w/dressing and gravy, 'Micro Meal'	1 bowl	280	23	32	1120	4	7.0	2.0	35	22%
w/dressing and gravy, packaged, 'American Classics'	10 oz	290	28	33	910	0	5.0	1.0	40	16%
(Empire Kosher) pie, kosher	1 pie	470	21	46	820	11	23.0	5.0	25	44%
(Freezer Queen)										
croquettes, breaded, w/gravy, frozen	7 oz	250	13	19	940	0	13.0	0.0	0	48%
sliced, frozen	10 oz	280	16	36	1210	0	8.0	0.0	0	26%
sliced, w/gravy and dressing, frozen, 'Single Serve'	9 oz	230	17	32	1130	0	5.0	0.0	0	19%
sliced, w/gravy, frozen, 'Cook-In-Pouch'	5 oz	70	7	6	880	0	2.0	0.0	0	26%
sliced, w/gravy, frozen, 'Family Suppers'	7 oz	110	9	8	1160	0	5.0	0.0	0	40%
w/gravy and dressing, frozen, 'Deluxe Family'	7 oz	160	12	18	1130	0	5.0	0.0	0	27%
(Healthy Choice)										
breast medallions and vegetables, frozen, 'Classics'	12.5 oz	350	29	45	480	0	6.0	3.0	60	15%
breast, 'Traditional'	1 entrée	290	22	40	460	5	4.5	2.0	45	14%
breast, sliced, w/gravy and dressing, frozen	10 oz	270	27	30	530	0	4.0	2.0	50	14%
breast, traditional, frozen	1 meal	280	22	40	460	7	3.0	1.0	45	10%
'Country Inn Roast'	1 entrée	250	20	28	530	4	6.0	2.0	40	22%
country roast, w/mushrooms, gravy, rice	1 entrée	223	19	28	437	3	3.9	1.2	26	16%
roasted, w/mushrooms and gravy, frozen	8.5 oz	200	18	26	380	0	3.0	1.0	40	13%
tetrazzini, frozen	12.6 oz	340	23	49	490	0	6.0	3.0	40	16%
turkey and vegetables, 'Hearty Handfuls'	1 entrée	320	18	51	590	5	5.0	1.5	20	14%
w/mushrooms, 'Country Roast'	1 entrée	230	19	26	440	2	5.0	1.5	45	20%
w/vegetables, lowfat, frozen, 'Homestyle'	9.5 oz	230	24	28	470	0	3.0	1.0	35	11%
(Hormel) w/vegetable, microwave, 'Health Selections'	7.25 oz	220	15	35	420	0	2.0	1.0	20	8%
(Hudson) sliced, extra lean	1 slice	30	5	0	280	0	0.5	0.0	10	18%
(Hungry Man)										
pot pie	1 pie	650	21	65	1510	5	34.0	13.0	45	47%
turkey entrée, mostly white meat, frozen	1 entrée	510	29	64	1620	9	15.0	4.0	55	27%
(Jennie-O)										
white and dark meat, roasted, w/gravy	4 oz	150	19	3	780	0	7.0	1.5	70	42%

Food Name	Serving Size	Calories	Prot. gms	Carbs gms	Sod. mgs	Fiber gms	Fat gms	Sat. Fat gms	Chol. mgs	% Fat Cal.
white meat, roasted, w/gravy........................	4 oz	150	19	3	780	0	7.0	1.5	55	42%
(Le Menu)										
breast, sliced, w/mushroom gravy, frozen..............	10.5 oz	300	22	38	1020	0	7.0	0.0	0	21%
glazed, frozen, 'LightStyle'.........................	8.25 oz	260	18	34	720	0	6.0	0.0	35	21%
sliced, frozen, 'LightStyle'.........................	10 oz	210	21	21	540	0	5.0	0.0	30	21%
turkey divan, frozen, 'LightStyle'...................	10 oz	260	25	23	420	0	7.0	0.0	60	25%
white meat, w/gravy and stuffing, frozen..............	8 oz	200	19	19	610	0	5.0	1.0	25	23%
(Lean Cuisine)										
breast, sliced, in mushroom sauce w/rice, frozen........	8 oz	230	17	24	540	0	7.0	2.0	35	28%
breast, sliced, w/dressing, frozen....................	7 7/8 oz	200	16	23	590	0	5.0	1.0	25	22%
Dijon, frozen...................................	9.5 oz	210	20	20	590	0	6.0	2.0	45	25%
homestyle......................................	1 entrée	230	18	26	590	3	6.0	1.5	50	23%
homestyle, w/vegetables and pasta, frozen............	9 3/8 oz	230	21	25	550	0	5.0	2.0	50	20%
pot pie..	1 entrée	300	20	34	590	3	9.0	2.0	50	27%
tenderloins, glazed..............................	1 entrée	240	14	37	590	5	5.0	1.0	30	18%
(Libby's) w/gravy and dressing, microwave, 'Diner'.......	7 oz	170	11	15	830	1	7.0	2.0	35	38%
(Louis Rich)										
breast, roasted, 99 fat-free.......................	2 oz	50	11	1	620	0	0.5	0.0	25	9%
breast, roasted, dinner slices, 99% fat-free...........	1 slice	70	16	1	910	0	1.0	0.0	35	12%
nuggets/sticks, breaded..........................	1 serving	235	12	13	577	0	14.9	2.9	34	57%
nuggets/sticks, breaded..........................	1 piece	77	4	4	190	0	4.9	0.9	11	57%
patty, white meat, breaded........................	1 serving	220	12	13	550	0	13.0	2.5	35	54%
(Marie Callender's)										
grilled breast and rice pilaf.......................	11.7 oz	320	22	34	940	4	10.0	3.5	35	29%
pot pie..	1 pie	610	15	57	1070	3	36.0	9.0	15	53%
turkey w/gravy and dressing, frozen.................	14 oz	500	31	52	2040	4	19.0	9.0	80	34%
w/gravy and dressing, w/broccoli...................	1 entrée	504	31	52	2037	na	19.0	9.1	79	34%
(Morton) turkey entrée, frozen.....................	10 oz	230	15	28	1300	0	6.0	0.0	45	24%
(Mountain House) tetrazzini, freeze-dried, prepared.......	1 cup	200	13	20	0	0	8.0	0.0	0	35%
(Mrs. Paterson's)										
pie, w/broccoli, hand held, frozen, 'Aussie Pie'.........	5.5 oz	460	16	42	790	0	26.0	10.0	95	50%
(Norbest)										
breast, w/gravy, raw.............................	4 oz	115	21	1	492	0	2.4	0.0	0	20%
w/gravy, raw...................................	4 oz	115	20	1	600	0	2.7	0.0	0	22%
(Pierre)										
nuggets, product 1936...........................	1 piece	70	4	2	103	0	5.2	1.1	11	67%
nuggets, product 1937...........................	1 piece	49	3	1	81	0	3.7	0.7	8	67%
patty, breaded, flame-broiled, product 1939............	1 piece	287	15	8	453	0	21.3	4.5	42	67%
patty, flame-broiled, frozen, product 9719.............	1 piece	86	12	0	362	0	3.9	1.2	47	41%
patty, flame-broiled, frozen, product 9721.............	1 piece	105	15	0	446	0	4.8	1.5	58	41%
patty, strip-shaped, frozen, product 1938.............	1 piece	94	5	3	153	0	7.0	1.4	15	67%
(Pillsbury) casserole, frozen, 'Microwave Classic'.........	1 pkg	430	20	31	880	0	25.0	0.0	0	52%
(Right Course)										
sliced, in mild curry sauce, w/rice pilaf, frozen..........	8.75 oz	320	23	40	570	0	8.0	2.0	50	22%
(Shelton's)										
pot pie, white flour crust.........................	1 serving	220	15	18	360	1	10.0	5.0	50	41%
pot pie, whole wheat crust........................	1 serving	220	16	18	360	3	10.0	5.0	50	40%
(Stouffer's)										
breast, roasted, w/gravy and stuffing, frozen..........	7 7/8 oz	270	19	27	920	0	9.0	0.0	0	31%
pot pie..	1 entrée	530	21	36	1040	3	33.0	9.0	65	57%
roasted, w/stuffing, 'Homestyle'....................	1 entrée	280	19	25	950	1	11.0	3.0	40	36%
tetrazzini......................................	1 entrée	360	19	33	1060	1	17.0	7.0	55	42%
tetrazzini, frozen, food service product...............	1 oz	36	2	3	99	0	2.0	0.7	7	50%

Food Name	Serving Size	Calories	Prot. gms	Carbs gms	Sod. mgs	Fiber gms	Fat gms	Sat. Fat gms	Chol. mgs	% Fat Cal.
(Sunday House)										
young turkey, w/broth and caramel color	3 oz	110	16	0	560	0	5.0	1.5	60	41%
(Swanson)										
breast, w/pasta, frozen	11.25 oz	310	22	36	670	0	9.0	0.0	35	26%
pot pie	1 pie	400	10	42	700	3	21.0	8.0	25	48%
turkey and dressing, mostly white meat, w/gravy	1 entrée	240	13	30	830	2	9.0	2.0	20	32%
turkey entrée, frozen	11.5 oz	350	21	42	1090	0	11.0	0.0	0	28%
turkey entrée, frozen, 'Hungry Man'	17 oz	550	36	61	1810	0	18.0	0.0	0	29%
turkey entrée, mostly white meat, frozen	1 entrée	320	20	42	1030	4	8.0	3.0	35	23%
(Turkey By George)										
hickory barbecue, packaged	5 oz	190	28	8	840	0	5.0	0.0	65	24%
Italian parmesan, packaged	5 oz	170	28	3	860	0	5.0	0.0	70	27%
lemon pepper, packaged	5 oz	160	28	4	830	0	4.0	1.0	60	22%
mustard tarragon, packaged	5 oz	180	29	3	830	0	6.0	0.0	80	30%
(Tyson)										
pie, frozen	9 oz	370	13	39	981	0	18.0	0.0	34	44%
turkey entrée, frozen, 'Gourmet Selection'	11.5 oz	380	19	51	1350	0	11.0	0.0	0	26%
w/dressing, frozen, 'Elmer Fudd'	6.55 oz	260	10	40	510	0	7.0	0.0	18	24%
w/gravy, frozen, 'Gourmet Selections'	9.5 oz	320	19	34	900	0	12.0	0.0	35	34%
(Ultra Slim Fast)										
glazed, w/dressing, frozen	10.5 oz	340	28	49	570	0	5.0	0.0	50	13%
medallions, in herb sauce, frozen	12 oz	280	23	33	950	0	6.0	0.0	40	19%
(Weight Watchers)										
breast, stuffed	1 entrée	230	17	28	680	6	5.0	1.0	15	20%
medallions, roasted, w/mushroom sauce, frozen, 'Smart Ones'	8.5 oz	200	13	35	440	0	1.0	1.0	25	4%
medallions, 'Smart Ones'	1 entrée	190	10	34	530	4	2.0	0.5	20	9%
w/mushroom, rice, vegetable, 'Smart Ones'	1 entrée	214	15	35	504	3	1.7	0.4	24	7%
(Wonderbites)										
fajita, flame-broiled, product 2196, 'Dippers'	1 piece	34	5	1	132	0	1.3	0.4	14	34%
TURKEY FAT										
	1 cup	1846	0	0	0	0	204.6	60.3	209	98%
	1 tbsp	115	0	0	0	0	12.8	3.8	13	98%
	1 tsp	39	0	0	0	0	4.3	1.3	4	98%
TURKEY JERKY *(Shelton's)*	1/2 oz	50	9	1	125	0	0.5	0.0	25	10%
TURKEY SEASONING. See under SEASONING MIX.										
TURKEY SNACK STICKS										
(Turkey Store)										
breast meat, cheese, 'Gobble Stix'	1 stick	30	6	1	0	0	0.8	0.4	10	22%
breast meat, smoked, 'Gobble Stix'	1 stick	25	5	0	0	0	0.2	0.0	10	8%
TURKEY SPREAD										
(Libby's) turkey salad, 'Spreadables'	1/3 cup	150	7	7	310	2	10.0	1.5	25	62%
(Underwood) chunky 'Light'	2 1/8 oz	75	11	2	330	0	2.0	1.0	25	26%
TURKEY SUBSTITUTE										
(Worthington)										
canned, drained	2 slices	120	8	3	0	0	8.0	0.0	0	62%
slices	3 slices	193	13	3	580	2	14.0	2.4	2	65%
smoked, roll, frozen	4 slices	180	13	5	820	0	12.0	0.0	0	60%
vegetarian, 'Meatless Smoked Turkey'	3 slices	140	10	3	620	2	10.0	2.0	0	64.3%
vegetarian, 'Turkee Slices'	3 slices	170	13	3	580	2	12.0	1.5	0	63.5%
TURMERIC										
dried *(McCormick/Schilling)*	1 tsp	8	0	2	0	0	0.0	0.0	0	0%
ground	1 tbsp	24	1	4	3	1	0.7	0.2	0	23%

Food Name	Serving Size	Calories	Prot. gms	Carbs gms	Sod. mgs	Fiber gms	Fat gms	Sat. Fat gms	Chol. mgs	% Fat Cal.
ground............................	1 tsp	8	0	1	1	0	0.2	0.1	0	23%
ground (Durkee)...................	1 tsp	9	0	0	0	0	0.0	0.0	0	0%
ground (Laurel Leaf)...............	1 tsp	9	0	0	0	0	0.0	0.0	0	0%
ground (Spice Islands).............	1 tsp	7	0	1	1	0	0.2	0.0	0	23%
TURNIP. See also RUTABAGA.										
Canned										
(Stokely)........................	1/2 cup	20	2	3	350	0	0.0	0.0	0	0%
diced (Allens)....................	1/2 cup	16	2	2	25	0	1.0	0.0	0	36%
Fresh										
boiled, drained, cubed............	1 cup	33	1	8	78	3	0.1	0.0	0	3%
boiled, drained, mashed...........	1 cup	48	2	11	115	5	0.2	0.0	0	3%
raw, cubed.......................	1 cup	35	1	8	87	2	0.1	0.0	0	3%
Frozen										
cubes, boiled, drained............	1 cup	33	1	8	446	3	0.1	0.0	0	3%
diced (Southern)..................	3.5 oz	17	1	3	50	0	0.2	0.0	0	10%
mashed, boiled, drained...........	1 cup	48	2	11	658	5	0.2	0.0	0	3%
mashed, unprepared...............	10-oz pkg	45	3	8	71	5	0.5	0.0	0	8%
w/greens, boiled, drained.........	1 cup	28	3	5	24	3	0.3	0.0	0	8%
w/greens, unprepared.............	10-oz pkg	60	7	10	51	7	0.5	0.1	0	8%
TURNIP, CABBAGE. See KOHLRABI.										
TURNIP-ROOTED PARSLEY. See PARSLEY ROOT.										
TURNIP GREENS										
Canned										
chopped (Allens).................	1/2 cup	21	2	3	15	0	1.0	0.0	0	31%
chopped (Bush's Best)............	1/2 cup	20	2	3	310	0	0.0	0.0	0	0%
chopped, w/diced turnips (Allens)...	1/2 cup	19	2	1	15	0	1.0	0.0	0	43%
seasoned w/pork (Luck's)..........	1 cup	35	1	5	240	2	1.5	0.0	0	36%
w/diced turnips (Bush's Best)......	1/2 cup	25	1	4	370	2	0.0	0.0	0	0%
w/diced turnips (Stokely).........	1/2 cup	20	2	0	340	0	0.0	0.0	0	0%
w/liquid........................	1/2 cup	16	2	3	324	2	0.4	0.1	0	18%
Fresh										
boiled, drained, chopped..........	4 oz	23	1.3	4.9	33	3.5	0.3	0.1	0	10%
boiled, drained, chopped..........	1/2 cup	14	0.8	3.1	21	2.2	0.2	0.0	0	10%
raw, chopped....................	1 cup	15	1	3	22	2	0.2	0.0	0	9%
Frozen										
boiled, drained...................	10-oz pkg	66	7	11	33	7	0.9	0.2	0	12%
chopped (Flav-R-Pac).............	1/3 cup	30	2	2	20	2	0.0	0.0	0	0%
chopped (Frosty Acres)...........	3.3 oz	20	2	4	10	1	0.0	0.0	0	0%
chopped (Seabrook)..............	3.3 oz	20	2	4	11	1	0.0	0.0	0	0%
chopped (Southern)..............	3.5 oz	25	3	4	70	0	0.3	0.0	0	10%
chopped, boiled, drained..........	1 cup	29	2	6	42	5	0.3	0.1	0	10%
chopped, unprepared.............	10-oz pkg	62	7	10	34	7	0.9	0.2	0	12%
chopped, w/diced turnips (Flav-R-Pac).............	1/3 cup	30	2	2	20	2	0.0	0.0	0	0%
chopped or diced, unprepared......	1/2 cup	18	2	3	10	2	0.3	0.1	0	12%
w/diced turnips (Seabrook).......	3.3 oz	20	3	3	0	0	0.0	0.0	0	0%
TURNOVER. See under PASTRY.										
TUSCAN PEPPER. See PEPPER, TUSCAN.										
TURTLE, GREEN										
canned...........................	3.5 oz	106	23.4	0.0	68	0	0.7	0.0	50	6%
raw..............................	3.5 oz	89	19.8	0.0	68	0	0.5	0.0	50	5%
TUSK. See CUSK.										

U

Food Name	Serving Size	Calories	Prot. gms	Carbs gms	Sod. mgs	Fiber gms	Fat gms	Sat. Fat gms	Chol. mgs	% Fat Cal.
UCUHUBA BUTTER OIL										
....	1 cup	1927	0	0	0	0	218.0	185.7	0	100%
....	1 tbsp	120	0	0	0	0	13.6	11.6	0	100%
UDON. See under NOODLE, JAPANESE.										
UMEBOSHI / Japanese plum										
peeled and seeded	1 oz	13	0.1	3.4	<1	0.1	0.1	<0.1	0	6%
raw, approx 0.6 oz...........................	1 medium	5	<0.1	1.2	tr	0.1	<0.1	tr	0	6%
untrimmed...................................	1 lb	132	1.2	34.1	3	1.4	0.6	0.1	0	6%

V

Food Name	Serving Size	Calories	Prot. gms	Carbs gms	Sod. mgs	Fiber gms	Fat gms	Sat. Fat gms	Chol. mgs	% Fat Cal.
VANILLA EXTRACT										
....	1 cup	599	0	26	19	0	0.1	0.0	0	0%
....	1 tbsp	37	0	2	1	0	0.0	0.0	0	0%
....	1 tsp	12	0	1	0	0	0.0	0.0	0	0%
pure *(Virginia Dare)*........................	1 tsp	10	0	0	0	0	0.0	0.0	0	0%
VANILLA EXTRACT SUBSTITUTE										
imitation....................................	1 tbsp	7	0	2	0	0	0.0	0.0	0	0%
imitation....................................	1 tsp	2	0	1	0	0	0.0	0.0	0	0%
imitation, w/alcohol	1 tbsp	31	0	0	1	0	0.0	na	0	0%
imitation, w/alcohol	1 tsp	10	0	0	0	0	0.0	na	0	0%
VANILLA, BAKING chips, vanilla milk *(Hershey's)*	1/4 cup	240	3	25	65	0	14.0	0.0	0	53%
VEAL										
(NOTE: TRIMMED = Lean; separable fat removed after cooking. UNTRIMMED = Separable fat not removed.)										
BRAIN										
braised	3 oz	116	10	0	133	0	8.2	1.9	2635	64%
pan-fried	3 oz	181	12	0	150	0	14.2	3.4	1802	71%
raw	4 oz	134	12	0	144	0	9.3	2.2	1803	63%
BREAST										
Trimmed, whole, boneless, braised	3 oz	185	26	0	58	na	8.3	3.2	99	41%
Untrimmed										
plate half, boneless, braised	3 oz	240	22	0	54	na	16.1	6.3	95	61%
point half, boneless, braised	3 oz	211	24	0	56	na	12.0	4.7	97	52%
whole, boneless, braised.........................	3 oz	226	23	0	55	na	14.3	5.6	96	57%
GROUND										
broiled......................................	3 oz	146	21	0	71	0	6.4	2.6	88	40%
raw	4 oz	163	22	0	93	0	7.7	3.2	93	42%
HEART										
braised	3 oz	158	25	0	49	0	5.7	1.5	150	33%
raw	4 oz	125	19	0	87	0	4.5	1.2	118	33%
KIDNEY										
braised	3 oz	139	22	0	94	0	4.8	1.5	672	31%
raw	4 oz	112	18	1	202	0	3.5	1.1	413	28%
LEG										
Trimmed										
top round, braised.............................	3 oz	173	31	0	57	0	4.3	1.6	115	23%
top round, breaded, pan-fried	3 oz	175	24	8	387	0	5.3	1.4	96	27%

Food Name	Serving Size	Calories	Prot. gms	Carbs gms	Sod. mgs	Fiber gms	Fat gms	Sat. Fat gms	Chol. mgs	% Fat Cal.
top round, pan-fried	3 oz	156	28	0	65	0	3.9	1.1	91	23%
top round, raw	1 oz	30	6	0	18	0	0.5	0.1	22	15%
top round, roasted	3 oz	128	24	0	58	0	2.9	1.0	88	20%
Untrimmed										
top round, braised	3 oz	179	31	0	57	0	5.4	2.1	114	27%
top round, breaded, pan-fried	3 oz	194	23	8	386	0	7.8	2.6	95	36%
top round, pan-fried	3 oz	179	27	0	65	0	7.1	2.7	89	36%
top round, raw	1 oz	33	6	0	18	0	0.9	0.3	22	24%
top round, roasted	3 oz	136	24	0	58	0	4.0	1.6	88	26%
LEG AND SHOULDER										
Trimmed										
cubed for stew, braised	3 oz	160	30	0	79	0	3.7	1.1	123	21%
cubed for stew, raw	1 oz	31	6	0	24	0	0.7	0.2	24	21%
LIVER										
braised	3 oz	140	18	2	45	0	5.9	2.2	477	38%
pan-fried	3 oz	208	25	3	112	0	9.7	3.6	281	42%
raw	4 oz	152	20	5	70	0	5.0	1.8	350	29%
LOIN										
Trimmed										
braised	3 oz	192	29	0	71	0	7.8	2.2	106	37%
raw	1 oz	33	6	0	26	0	0.9	0.3	23	26%
roasted	3 oz	149	22	0	82	0	5.9	2.2	90	36%
Untrimmed										
braised	3 oz	241	26	0	68	0	14.6	5.7	100	55%
raw	1 oz	46	5	0	24	0	2.6	1.1	22	51%
roasted	3 oz	184	21	0	79	0	10.5	4.5	88	51%
LUNGS										
braised	3 oz	88	16	0	48	0	2.2	0.8	224	23%
raw	4 oz	102	18	0	122	0	2.6	0.9	260	23%
PANCREAS										
braised	3 oz	218	25	0	58	0	12.4	4.3	na	51%
raw	4 oz	206	17	0	76	0	14.9	5.1	196	65%
RIB										
Trimmed										
braised	3 oz	185	29	0	84	0	6.6	2.2	122	32%
raw	1 oz	34	6	0	27	0	1.1	0.3	24	29%
roasted	3 oz	150	22	0	82	0	6.3	1.8	98	38%
Untrimmed										
braised	3 oz	213	28	0	81	0	10.7	4.2	118	45%
raw	1 oz	46	5	0	25	0	2.6	1.1	23	50%
roasted	3 oz	194	20	0	78	0	11.9	4.6	94	55%
SHANK										
Trimmed										
fore and hind, braised	3 oz	150	27	0	80	0	3.7	1.0	107	22%
fore and hind, raw	1 oz	31	5	0	24	na	0.8	0.2	21	24%
Untrimmed										
fore and hind, braised	3 oz	162	27	0	79	na	5.3	1.8	105	29%
fore and hind, raw	1 oz	32	5	0	24	na	1.0	0.3	21	28%
SHOULDER										
Trimmed										
arm, braised	3 oz	171	30	0	77	0	4.5	1.3	132	24%
arm, raw	1 oz	30	6	0	24	0	0.6	0.2	24	19%
arm, roasted	3 oz	139	22	0	77	0	4.9	2.0	93	32%
blade, braised	3 oz	168	28	0	86	0	5.5	1.5	134	30%

Food Name	Serving Size	Calories	Prot. gms	Carbs gms	Sod. mgs	Fiber gms	Fat gms	Sat. Fat gms	Chol. mgs	% Fat Cal.
blade, raw	1 oz	32	6	0	28	0	0.9	0.3	26	26%
blade, roasted	3 oz	145	22	0	87	0	5.8	2.2	101	36%
whole, arm and blade, braised	3 oz	169	29	0	82	0	5.2	1.4	111	28%
whole, arm and blade, raw	1 oz	32	6	0	26	0	0.9	0.3	24	24%
whole, arm and blade, roasted	3 oz	145	22	0	82	0	5.6	2.1	97	35%
Untrimmed										
arm, braised	3 oz	201	29	0	74	0	8.7	3.4	126	39%
arm, raw	1 oz	37	5	0	24	0	1.5	0.6	23	37%
arm, roasted	3 oz	156	22	0	77	0	7.0	3.0	92	41%
blade, braised	3 oz	191	27	0	83	0	8.6	3.1	130	40%
blade, raw	1 oz	37	5	0	27	0	1.5	0.6	26	36%
blade, roasted	3 oz	158	21	0	85	0	7.4	2.9	99	42%
whole, arm and blade, braised	3 oz	194	27	0	81	0	8.6	3.2	107	40%
whole, arm and blade, raw	1 oz	37	5	0	26	0	1.5	0.6	25	37%
whole, arm and blade, roasted	3 oz	156	22	0	82	0	7.2	2.9	96	41%
SIRLOIN										
Trimmed										
braised	3 oz	173	29	0	69	0	5.5	1.5	96	29%
raw	1 oz	31	6	0	23	0	0.7	0.2	22	21%
roasted	3 oz	143	22	0	72	0	5.3	2.0	88	33%
Untrimmed										
braised	3 oz	214	27	0	67	0	11.2	4.4	92	47%
raw	1 oz	43	5	0	22	0	2.2	0.9	22	46%
roasted	3 oz	172	21	0	71	0	8.9	3.8	87	47%
SPLEEN										
braised	3 oz	110	20	0	49	0	2.5	0.8	380	20%
raw	4 oz	111	21	0	110	0	2.5	0.8	386	20%
THYMUS										
braised	3 oz	148	27	0	56	0	3.6	1.3	399	22%
raw	4 oz	112	20	0	94	0	2.8	1.0	304	22%
TONGUE										
braised	3 oz	172	22	0	54	0	8.6	3.7	202	45%
raw	4 oz	149	19	2	93	0	6.2	2.7	70	38%
VEAL DINNER/ENTRÉE										
(Armour) Parmigiana, frozen, 'Classics'	11.25 oz	400	18	34	1320	0	22.0	0.0	55	49%
(Banquet)										
Parmigiana	1 entrée	360	13	35	960	7	19.0	6.0	25	47%
Parmigiana, breaded patty, frozen, 'Cookin' Bags'	4 oz	230	10	20	0	0	11.0	0.0	0	45%
Parmigiana, w/tomato sauce, potato. peas in sauce	1 entrée	362	13	35	964	7	19.0	6.2	26	47%
(Contadina) Parmigiana, frozen	1 oz	42	3	3	165	na	2.3	na	8	49%
(Freezer Queen)										
Parmigiana, breaded, frozen, 'Cook-In-Pouch'	5 oz	220	11	17	560	0	12.0	0.0	0	49%
Parmigiana, breaded, frozen, 'Deluxe Family Suppers'	7 oz	300	17	22	820	0	15.0	0.0	0	46%
Parmigiana, platter, frozen	10 oz	400	22	32	870	0	20.0	0.0	0	45%
(Hormel)										
steak, breaded, frozen	4 oz	240	17	13	0	0	13.0	0.0	0	49%
steak, frozen	4 oz	130	22	2	0	0	4.0	0.0	0	27%
(Le Menu)										
Marsala, frozen, 'LightStyle'	10 oz	230	22	28	700	0	3.0	0.0	75	12%
Parmigiana, frozen	11.5 oz	390	24	36	840	0	17.0	0.0	0	39%
(Morton) Parmigiana, frozen	10 oz	260	10	35	1510	0	8.0	0.0	35	29%
(Pierre) veal and beef patty, Italian, frozen, product 1905	1 piece	279	14	12	591	1	19.6	7.9	36	63%
(Stouffer's) Parmigiana, w/spaghetti, 'Homestyle'	1 entrée	420	20	43	1200	6	19.0	4.0	75	40%

Food Name	Serving Size	Calories	Prot. gms	Carbs gms	Sod. mgs	Fiber gms	Fat gms	Sat. Fat gms	Chol. mgs	% Fat Cal.
(Swanson)										
Parmigiana	1 entrée	390	19	40	1060	5	18.0	8.0	85	41%
Parmigiana, 'Hungry Man'	1 entrée	640	34	74	1990	6	23.0	11.0	70	32%
Parmigiana, frozen, 'Homestyle Recipe'	10 oz	330	19	33	960	0	13.0	0.0	0	36%
(Weight Watchers)										
Parmigiana, breaded patty, frozen, 'Ultimate 200'	8.2 oz	150	22	5	550	0	4.0	1.0	50	25%
VEGETABLE CHIPS										
(Eden Foods)	1-oz bag	130	1	22	200	0	4.0	0.0	0	28%
sea vegetable *(Eden Foods)*	1-oz bag	130	1	22	200	0	5.0	0.0	0	33%
VEGETABLE DISH/ENTRÉE. See also individual listings.										
(Amy's Kitchen)										
pot pie	1 serving	360	7	44	540	4	18.0	11.0	45	44%
shepherd's pie	1 serving	160	5	27	490	5	4.0	0.0	0	22%
(Budget Gourmet)										
w/chicken, Chinese style, frozen	10 oz	280	11	47	590	0	7.0	1.0	10	21%
w/chicken, Italian style, frozen	10.25 oz	310	14	50	690	0	8.0	2.0	30	22%
(Dinty Moore) stew, canned	8 oz	155	5	20	850	0	6.0	2.0	14	35%
(Flav-R-Pac)										
stir-fry w/asparagus, frozen	1 cup	25	1	4	25	2	0.0	0.0	0	0%
stir-fry w/noodles, frozen	1 cup	50	2	9	25	2	0.0	0.0	0	0%
stir-fry w/rice, frozen	1 cup	80	3	18	15	2	0.0	0.0	0	0%
succotash, frozen	2/3 cup	100	4	22	50	2	1.0	0.0	0	8%
vegetarian dinner blend	3/4 cup	25	1	4	20	2	0.0	0.0	0	0%
(Frosty Acres) succotash, frozen	3.3 oz	100	4	19	47	1	0.0	0.0	0	0%
(Gardenburger)										
vegetable patty, vegetarian, roasted, 'Gourmet'	2.5 oz	120	7	17	270	2	2.8	1.5	10	21%
(Green Giant)										
broccoli, cauliflower, carrots, in cheese sauce	2/3 cup	80	3	11	560	2	2.5	1.5	5	29%
four vegetables in butter sauce w/pasta *(Green Giant)*	3/4 cup	70	3	11	280	2	2.0	1.5	5	24%
w/sauce, 'Garden Gourmet Fettuccine Primavera'	9.5 oz serving	307	13	34	734	2	13.3	4.4	14	39%
(Hanover) rice and vegetables w/soy sauce, 'Stir Fry 2'	1 cup	130	5	27	636	2	0.4	na	na	3%
(La Choy)										
chow mein, contains no meat	3/4 cup	35	2	6	820	2	0.4	0.0	0	10%
chow mein, meatless, canned	1 cup	55	3	10	854	1	0.7	0.0	0	11%
chow mein, vegetable, frozen, food service product	1 cup	108	2	20	1135	5	2.3	0.4	0	19%
(Morningstar Farms)										
vegetarian, 'Garden Grille'	1 patty	120	6	18	280	4	2.5	1.0	<5	18.8%
vegetarian, 'Garden Veggie Patties'	1 patty	100	10	3	350	4	2.5	0.5	0.0	22.5%
(Morton)										
w/beef, frozen	7 oz	430	11	27	740	0	31.0	0.0	30	65%
w/chicken, frozen	7 oz	420	14	27	740	0	28.0	0.0	35	61%
w/turkey, frozen	7 oz	420	14	27	740	0	28.0	0.0	40	61%
(Mountain House) stew, w/beef, freeze-dried, prepared	1 cup	230	11	27	77	0	7.0	0.0	0	29%
(Natural Touch)										
vegetarian, 'Dinner Entrée'	1 pattie	220	19	2	380	2	15.0	2.5	0	61.3%
vegetarian, 'Garden Veggie Pattie'	1 pattie	100	10	8	280	3	2.5	0.5	0	22.5%
vegetarian, 'Okara Patties'	1 pattie	110	11	4	360	3	5.0	1.0	0	40.9%
(S&W) succotash, canned, 'Country Style'	1/2 cup	80	4	16	250	0	1.0	0.0	0	10%
(Seabrook) succotash, frozen	3.3 oz	100	4	19	47	1	0.0	0.0	0	0%
(Shanghai) stir-fry, frozen	5.1 oz	75	6	11	510	0	1.0	0.0	0	12%
(Stokely) succotash, canned	1/2 cup	90	3	20	300	0	0.0	0.0	0	0%
(Stouffer's)										
chow mein, frozen, food service product	1 oz	14	0	2	156	0	0.7	0.1	0	44%
lasagna, frozen, food service product	1 oz	45	2	4	114	na	2.6	na	3	51%
(Tofu Classics) chow mein, Mandarin, prepared w/tofu	1/2 cup	110	8	14	390	0	6.0	0.0	0	38%

Food Name	Serving Size	Calories	Prot. gms	Carbs gms	Sod. mgs	Fiber gms	Fat gms	Sat. Fat gms	Chol. mgs	% Fat Cal.
(Ultra Slim Fast) and beef tips, country style	12 oz	230	21	26	960	0	5.0	0.0	45	19%
(Worthington)										
vegetarian, 'Multigrain Cutlets' 50-oz can	1 slice	80	12	4	300	3	1.5	0.5	0	16.9%
vegetarian, 'Multigrain Cutlets' 20-oz can	2 slices	100	15	5	390	4	2.0	0.5	0	18.0%
vegetarian, 'Vegetarian Cutlets'	1 slice	70	11	3	340	2	1.0	0.0	0	12.8%
VEGETABLE FLAKES (French's) dehydrated	1 tbsp	12	0	3	20	0	0.0	0.0	0	0%
VEGETABLE JUICE DRINK										
(Biotta)										
'Breuss Juice'	6 fl oz	67	2	13	147	0	0.1	0.0	0	1%
'Cocktail'	6 fl oz	50	2	10	497	0	0.1	0.0	0	2%
(Knudsen)										
'Very Veggie' blend, low-salt	8 fl oz	50	3	10	32	na	1.0	0.0	0	15%
'Very Veggie' fruit juice sweetened	8 fl oz	50	3	10	32	2	1.0	0.0	0	15%
'Very Veggie' low-sodium	8 fl oz	40	2	8	32	0	0.0	0.0	0	0%
'Very Veggie' organic	8 fl oz	40	2	8	0	0	0.0	0.0	0	0%
'Very Veggie' original	8 fl oz	40	2	8	560	0	0.0	0.0	0	0%
'Very Veggie' spicy	8 fl oz	40	2	8	560	0	0.0	0.0	0	0%
(Sacramento)	8 fl oz	30	3	9	850	2	0.0	0.0	0	0%
(Smucker's)										
hearty	8 fl oz	58	1	13	714	0	0.1	0.0	0	2%
hot and spicy	8 fl oz	58	1	13	650	0	0.1	0.0	0	2%
(V8)										
low-salt	8 fl oz	60	2	11	140	2	0.0	0.0	0	0%
100% juice	8 fl oz	50	1	10	620	1	0.0	0.0	0	0%
100% juice, lightly tangy	8 fl oz	60	2	11	340	1	0.0	0.0	0	0%
picante	11.5 fl oz	70	2	14	990	2	0.0	0.0	0	0%
spicy hot	8 fl oz	50	2	10	780	1	0.0	0.0	0	0%
(Veryfine) '100%'	6 fl oz	32	2	6	600	0	0.0	0.0	0	0%
VEGETABLE OIL. See also individual listings.										
salad or cooking	1 cup	1927	0	0	0	0	218.0	27.7	0	100%
salad or cooking	1 tbsp	120	0	0	0	0	13.6	1.7	0	100%
(Blue Plate)	1 tbsp	130	0	0	0	na	14.0	2.0	na	100%
(Crisco) Canola and corn oil blend	1 tbsp	120	0	0	0	0	14.0	1.5	0	100%
(Finast)	1 tbsp	120	0	0	0	0	14.0	2.0	0	100%
(Hain)										
'All Blend'	1 tbsp	120	0	0	0	0	14.0	2.0	0	100%
w/garlic, 'Garlic & Oil'	1 tbsp	120	0	0	0	0	14.0	3.0	0	100%
(Kroger)	1 tbsp	122	0	0	0	0	13.6	2.1	0	100%
(Mazola) Canola and corn oil blend, 'Right Blend'	1 tbsp	120	0	0	0	0	14.0	1.0	0	100%
(Pathmark)										
. . . .	1 tbsp	120	0	0	0	0	14.0	2.0	0	100%
'No Frills'	1 tbsp	130	0	0	0	0	14.0	2.0	0	100%
(Puritan)	1 tbsp	120	0	0	0	0	14.0	1.0	0	100%
(Wesson)										
. . . .	1 tbsp	122	0	0	0	0	13.6	2.0	0	100%
butter flavor	1 tbsp	122	0	0	0	0	13.6	2.0	0	100%
Canola and vegetable oil blend, 'Best Blend'	1 tbsp	120	0	0	0	0	14.0	1.0	0	100%
VEGETABLE OIL SPREAD. See MARGARINE; MARGARINE SPREAD; MARGARINE SUBSTITUTE.										
VEGETABLE OYSTER. See SALSIFY.										
VEGETABLE SPONGE. See GOURD, DISHCLOTH.										
VEGETABLES, MIXED										
Canned										
(A&P)										
'Eastern'	1/2 cup	45	2	8	330	0	1.0	0.0	0	18%

Food Name	Serving Size	Calories	Prot. gms	Carbs gms	Sod. mgs	Fiber gms	Fat gms	Sat. Fat gms	Chol. mgs	% Fat Cal.
no salt added.	1/2 cup	40	1	9	20	0	1.0	0.0	0	18%
'Western'	1/2 cup	40	1	9	380	0	1.0	0.0	0	18%
(Bush's Best) greens, mixed	1/2 cup	20	2	3	300	0	0.0	0.0	0	0%
(Chun King) chow mein	1/2 cup	10	1	2	15	1	0.0	0.0	0	0%
(Featherweight)	1/2 cup	40	2	8	25	0	0.0	0.0	0	0%
(Finast)										
	1/2 cup	40	1	8	390	0	0.0	0.0	0	0%
no salt added.	1/2 cup	40	2	8	25	0	0.0	0.0	0	0%
(Freshlike)										
water packed, no salt added	1/2 cup	35	2	8	25	0	0.0	0.0	0	0%
water packed, no sugar or salt added	1/2 cup	35	2	8	25	0	0.0	0.0	0	0%
(Green Giant)										
	1/2 cup	60	2	12	460	2	0.0	0.0	0	0%
'Garden Medley'	1/2 cup	35	1	9	350	1	0.0	0.0	0	0%
'Pantry Express'	1/2 cup	35	1	8	300	1	1.0	0.0	0	20%
(La Choy)										
Chinese.	1/2 cup	12	1	2	30	1	0.1	0.0	0	7%
Chinese, food service product.	2/3 cup	15	1	3	32	1	0.1	0.0	0	5%
chop suey	1/2 cup	9	1	2	330	1	0.1	0.0	0	8%
chop suey vegetables	1/2 cup	14	1	3	323	1	0.1	0.0	0	4%
chop suey vegetables, food service product	1/2 cup	11	1	2	439	1	0.4	0.0	0	21%
fancy	2/3 cup	9	1	1	32	1	0.1	0.0	0	8%
(P&Q)										
'Chunky Eastern'	1/2 cup	40	2	8	330	0	1.0	0.0	0	18%
'Chunky Western'	1/2 cup	40	2	9	380	0	1.0	0.0	0	18%
(Pathmark)										
	1/2 cup	35	2	8	320	0	0.0	0.0	0	0%
no salt added.	1/2 cup	35	2	7	25	0	0.0	0.0	0	0%
(S&W) 'Old Fashioned Harvest'	1/2 cup	35	1	6	380	0	0.0	0.0	0	0%
(Stokely)										
	1/2 cup	40	2	8	300	0	0.0	0.0	0	0%
no salt or sugar added	1/2 cup	40	2	8	25	0	0.0	0.0	0	0%
(Veg-All)										
large cut, 'Homestyle'	1/2 cup	35	2	9	380	0	0.0	0.0	0	0%
lite	1/2 cup	35	2	8	25	0	0.0	0.0	0	0%
original.	1/2 cup	35	2	8	320	0	0.0	0.0	0	0%
Frozen										
(A&P)										
	3.3 oz	65	3	13	55	0	1.0	0.0	0	12%
California blend	3.3 oz	25	2	5	25	0	1.0	0.0	0	24%
Italian style blend	3.3 oz	40	2	8	35	0	1.0	0.0	0	18%
Oriental style blend	3.3 oz	25	2	5	15	0	1.0	0.0	0	24%
winter blend	3.3 oz	24	2	6	190	0	1.0	0.0	0	22%
(Birds Eye)										
	3.3 oz	60	3	13	40	2	0.0	0.0	0	0%
broccoli, cauliflower, carrots, 'Farm Fresh'	4 oz	35	2	7	40	3	0.0	0.0	0	0%
broccoli, cauliflower, red peppers, 'Farm Fresh'	4 oz	30	3	5	25	3	0.0	0.0	0	0%
broccoli, corn, red peppers, 'Farm Fresh'	4 oz	60	3	14	15	3	1.0	0.0	0	12%
broccoli, green beans, pearl onions, red peppers	4 oz	35	2	7	15	3	0.0	0.0	0	0%
broccoli, red peppers, bamboo shoots, mushrooms	4 oz	30	3	5	20	3	0.0	0.0	0	0%
Brussels sprouts, cauliflower, carrots	4 oz	40	3	8	30	4	0.0	0.0	0	0%
cauliflower, baby carrots, snow pea pods	4 oz	40	2	8	35	3	0.0	0.0	0	0%
cauliflower, whole baby carrots, snow pea pods	4 oz	40	2	8	35	3	0.0	0.0	0	0%
cauliflower, zucchini, carrots, red peppers	4 oz	30	2	6	25	2	0.0	0.0	0	0%

Food Name	Serving Size	Calories	Prot. gms	Carbs gms	Sod. mgs	Fiber gms	Fat gms	Sat. Fat gms	Chol. mgs	% Fat Cal.
Chinese style, 'Stir-Fry'	3.3 oz	35	2	8	540	2	0.0	0.0	0	0%
Italian style, 'International Recipes'	3.3 oz	100	2	11	490	2	5.0	0.0	0	46%
Japanese style, 'International Recipes'	3.3 oz	90	2	10	420	2	5.0	0.0	0	48%
Japanese style, 'Stir-Fry'	3.3 oz	30	2	7	510	2	0.0	0.0	0	0%
New England style, 'International Recipes'	3.3 oz	130	3	14	430	2	7.0	0.0	0	48%
Oriental style, 'International Recipes'	3.3 oz	70	2	8	300	1	4.0	0.0	0	47%
pepper stir-fry, 'Farm Fresh Mixtures'	1 cup	25	1	5	15	2	0.0	0.0	0	0%
San Francisco style, 'International Recipes'	3.3 oz	100	2	11	400	1	5.0	0.0	0	46%
sugar snap peas, baby carrots, water chestnuts	3.2 oz	50	2	11	20	4	0.0	0.0	0	0%
(C&W)										
corn, broccoli, red peppers, 'Vegetable Stand'	2/3 cup	60	2	14	10	1	0.5	0.0	0	7%
peas, corn, green beans, baby carrots	3/4 cup	60	3	11	45	2	0.0	0.0	0	0%
petite peas and baby carrots, 'Early Harvest'	3.3 oz	60	4	12	95	0	0.0	0.0	0	0%
red, green, and yellow bell pepper strips	1/2 cup	20	1	4	10	2	0.0	0.0	0	0%
(Flav-R-Pac)										
Capri	3/4 cup	25	1	4	25	1	0.0	0.0	0	0%
fajita blend	3/4 cup	20	1	5	10	1	0.0	0.0	0	0%
fiesta	2/3 cup	60	4	10	131	6	0.0	0.0	0	0%
five vegetables	2/3 cup	60	3	12	50	2	0.5	0.0	0	7%
four vegetables	2/3 cup	50	2	9	45	2	0.0	0.0	0	0%
Italian, frozen	2/3 cup	30	1	5	30	2	0.0	0.0	0	0%
Italian, w/buttery sauce	1/2 cup	50	2	8	410	3	2.0	0.0	0	31%
Mexicali	2/3 cup	80	3	18	75	3	0.5	0.0	0	5%
omelette blend	3/4 cup	25	1	5	15	2	0.0	0.0	0	0%
Oriental	3/4 cup	25	1	4	15	2	0.0	0.0	0	0%
Scandinavian	3/4 cup	40	2	7	45	2	0.0	0.0	0	0%
stew vegetables	2/3 cup	40	1	9	45	1	0.0	0.0	0	0%
stew/soup vegetables	2/3 cup	40	1	9	45	1	0.0	0.0	0	0%
stir-fry blend, frozen	3/4 cup	25	1	5	20	2	0.0	0.0	0	0%
stir-fry blend, frozen, deluxe	3/4 cup	30	1	5	20	2	0.0	0.0	0	0%
w/buttery sauce, frozen	1/2 cup	90	4	16	540	4	2.5	0.0	0	22%
winter	1 cup	25	2	4	25	2	0.0	0.0	0	0%
(Freshlike)										
	3.3 oz	70	3	13	45	0	0.0	0.0	0	0%
'California Blend'	3.3 oz	30	2	6	20	0	0.0	0.0	0	0%
'Chuckwagon Blend'	3.3 oz	70	2	16	5	0	1.0	0.0	0	11%
'Country Blend'	3.3 oz	50	2	12	15	0	0.0	0.0	0	0%
for soup	3.3 oz	50	2	11	40	0	0.0	0.0	0	0%
for stew, 4-ways	3.3 oz	50	1	11	40	0	0.0	0.0	0	0%
for stew, 5-ways	3.3 oz	50	1	12	40	0	0.0	0.0	0	0%
'Italian Blend' food service product	3.3 oz	25	1	5	20	0	0.0	0.0	0	0%
'Italian Blend'	3.3 oz	30	2	7	20	0	0.0	0.0	0	0%
'Midwestern Blend'	3.3 oz	40	2	8	30	0	0.0	0.0	0	0%
'Oriental Blend'	3.3 oz	25	3	5	10	0	0.0	0.0	0	0%
'Scandinavian Blend'	3.3 oz	45	2	9	30	0	0.0	0.0	0	0%
'Winter Blend'	3.3 oz	25	3	5	25	0	0.0	0.0	0	0%
(Frosty Acres)										
	3.3 oz	65	3	13	50	1	0.0	0.0	0	0%
Dutch style	3.2 oz	30	2	5	30	0	0.0	0.0	0	0%
Italian style	3.2 oz	40	3	8	20	0	0.0	0.0	0	0%
Oriental style	3.2 oz	25	2	5	15	0	0.0	0.0	0	0%
(Green Giant)										
	1/2 cup	40	2	9	40	2	0.0	0.0	0	0%
broccoli, cauliflower, carrots 'One Serving'	1 pkg	30	3	7	40	3	0.0	0.0	0	0%

Food Name	Serving Size	Calories	Prot. gms	Carbs gms	Sod. mgs	Fiber gms	Fat gms	Sat. Fat gms	Chol. mgs	% Fat Cal.
California style, 'American Mixtures'	1/2 cup	25	2	6	40	2	0.0	0.0	0	0%
five vegetables in butter sauce	3/4 cup	60	2	8	300	2	2.0	1.5	5	31%
heartland style, 'American Mixtures'	1 cup	30	2	6	35	3	0.0	0.0	0	0%
LeSueur style, 'Valley Combinations'	1/2 cup	70	4	12	400	2	2.0	0.0	0	22%
Manhattan style, 'American Mixtures'	1 cup	25	2	4	15	2	0.0	0.0	0	0%
New England style, 'American Mixtures'	2/3 cup	70	2	13	70	3	1.5	0.0	0	18%
'Plain Polybag'	1/2 cup	40	2	9	40	2	0.0	0.0	0	0%
'Portion Pack'	3 oz	50	2	12	35	2	0.0	0.0	0	0%
San Francisco style, 'American Mixtures'	3/4 cup	30	1	6	20	2	0.0	0.0	0	0%
Santa Fe style, 'American Mixtures'	3/4 cup	60	2	13	10	2	0.0	0.0	0	0%
Seattle style, 'American Mixtures'	3/4 cup	25	1	5	15	2	0.0	0.0	0	0%
Western style, 'American Mixtures'	3/4 cup	50	1	9	10	2	1.5	0.0	0	25%
(Health Valley)	1/2 cup	68	3	14	39	2	0.0	0.0	0	0%
(La Choy) stir-fry vegetables, food service product	1/2 cup	34	3	6	2	1	0.1	0.0	0	1%
(Pictsweet)										
'California'	3/4 cup	20	1	4	25	1	0.0	0.0	0	0%
'Cantonese'	3.2 oz	35	2	7	25	0	0.0	0.0	0	0%
'Chinese Stir-Fry'	3/4 cup	30	1	5	200	2	0.0	0.0	0	0%
'Del Sol'	3.2 oz	30	2	6	25	0	0.0	0.0	0	0%
'Grande'	3/4 cup	45	2	10	15	2	0.5	0.0	0	9%
'Japanese'	3.2 oz	15	2	5	10	0	1.0	0.0	0	24%
low-sodium, vitamins A and C	3.2 oz	60	3	12	40	0	0.0	0.0	0	0%
'Oriental Stir-Fry'	3/4 cup	30	1	5	310	1	0.0	0.0	0	0%
peas, carrots	2/3 cup	50	3	9	75	3	0.0	0.0	0	0%
(Seabrook)	3.3 oz	65	3	13	50	1	0.0	0.0	0	0%
(Southern)	3.5 oz	69	3	14	60	0	0.0	0.0	0	0%
(Stokely)										
broccoli, cauliflower, baby carrots 'Singles'	3 oz	25	2	5	25	0	1.0	0.0	0	24%
'Singles'	3 oz	60	3	12	40	0	1.0	0.0	0	13%
(Trader Joe's) red, yellow, and green pepper strips, 'Melange a Trois'	1/3 cup	20	0	4	10	2	0.0	0.0	0	0%
(Veg-All)										
	3.3 oz	70	3	13	45	0	0.0	0.0	0	0%
'California Blend'	3.3 oz	30	2	6	20	0	0.0	0.0	0	0%
'Chuckwagon Blend'	3.3 oz	70	2	16	5	0	1.0	0.0	0	11%
'Country Blend'	3.3 oz	50	2	12	15	0	0.0	0.0	0	0%
for soup	3.3 oz	50	2	11	40	0	0.0	0.0	0	0%
for stew, 4-ways	3.3 oz	50	1	11	40	0	0.0	0.0	0	0%
for stew, 5-ways	3.3 oz	50	1	12	40	0	0.0	0.0	0	0%
'Italian Blend' food service product	3.3 oz	25	1	5	20	0	0.0	0.0	0	0%
'Italian Blend'	3.3 oz	30	2	7	20	0	0.0	0.0	0	0%
large cut	1/2 cup	45	1	9	350	2	0.0	0.0	0	0%
'Midwestern Blend'	3.3 oz	40	2	8	30	0	0.0	0.0	0	0%
'Oriental Blend'	3.3 oz	25	3	5	10	0	0.0	0.0	0	0%
'Scandinavian Blend'	3.3 oz	45	2	9	30	0	0.0	0.0	0	0%
'Winter Blend'	3.3 oz	25	3	5	25	0	0.0	0.0	0	0%

VEGETARIAN FOODS. See individual listings.
VEGGIE BURGER. See under BEEF SUBSTITUTE DINNER/ENTRÉE.
VENISON. See CARIBOU; DEER; ELK; MOOSE.
VERMOUTH
(Gallo)

Food Name	Serving Size	Calories	Prot. gms	Carbs gms	Sod. mgs	Fiber gms	Fat gms	Sat. Fat gms	Chol. mgs	% Fat Cal.
dry	2 fl oz	56	0	1	0	0	0.0	0.0	0	0%
sweet	2 fl oz	90	0	9	0	0	0.0	0.0	0	0%

Food Name	Serving Size	Calories	Prot. gms	Carbs gms	Sod. mgs	Fiber gms	Fat gms	Sat. Fat gms	Chol. mgs	% Fat Cal.
(Gambarelli & Davitto)										
dry	2 fl oz	64	0	2	4	0	0.0	0.0	0	0%
sweet	2 fl oz	77	0	8	4	0	0.0	0.0	0	0%
(Lejon)										
dry	2 fl oz	64	0	2	4	0	0.0	0.0	0	0%
sweet	2 fl oz	77	0	8	4	0	0.0	0.0	0	0%

VICHY WATER. See under SOFT DRINKS AND MIXERS.
VIENNA SAUSAGE. See under SAUSAGE.
VINE SPINACH. See SPINACH, VINE.
VINEGAR
APPLE CIDER

Food Name	Serving Size	Calories	Prot. gms	Carbs gms	Sod. mgs	Fiber gms	Fat gms	Sat. Fat gms	Chol. mgs	% Fat Cal.
	1 cup	34	0	14	2	0	0.0	0.0	0	0%
	1 tbsp	2	0	1	0	0	0.0	0.0	0	0%
(Hain)	1 tbsp	2	0	4	1	0	0.0	0.0	0	0%
(Heinz)	0.51 oz	2	0	0	1	0	0.0	0.0	0	0%
(Indian Summer)	1 cup	40	1	14	5	0	1.0	0.0	0	13%
(Lucky Leaf) pure	1 oz	4	0	2	0	0	0.0	0.0	0	0%
(Musselman's) pure	1 oz	4	0	2	0	0	0.0	0.0	0	0%
(S&W)	1 tbsp	0	0	0	0	0	0.0	0.0	0	0%
(White House) distilled, colored or white, distilled	1 oz	4	0	2	5	0	0.0	0.0	0	0%
MALT										
(Heinz) gourmet, 'Decanter'	0.51 oz	4	0	0	5	0	0.0	0.0	0	0%
(S&W) malt ale, 'International'	1 tbsp	0	0	0	0	0	0.0	0.0	0	0%
FLAVORED										
(Great Impressions)										
basil wine	1 tbsp	7	0	1	1	0	0.0	0.0	0	0%
garlic wine	1 tbsp	7	0	1	1	0	0.0	0.0	0	0%
hot paprika wine	1 tbsp	6	0	1	1	0	0.0	0.0	0	0%
raspberry wine	1 tbsp	7	0	1	1	0	0.0	0.0	0	0%
red wine	1 tbsp	6	0	1	1	0	0.0	0.0	0	0%
(Heinz)										
garlic wine, gourmet, 'Decanter'	0.51 oz	4	0	0	0	0	0.0	0.0	0	0%
tarragon, gourmet, 'Decanter'	0.51 oz	2	0	0	0	0	0.0	0.0	0	0%
(S&W)										
garlic wine, 'International'	1 tbsp	0	0	0	0	0	0.0	0.0	0	0%
Italian herb, 'International'	1 tbsp	0	0	0	0	0	0.0	0.0	0	0%
tarragon, 'International'	1 tbsp	0	0	0	0	0	0.0	0.0	0	0%
SALAD *(Heinz)* gourmet, 'Decanter'	0.51 oz	2	0	0	0	0	0.0	0.0	0	0%
WHITE										
(Heinz) white, distilled	1 tbsp	2	0	0	1	0	0.0	0.0	0	0%
(Indian Summer) white, distilled	1 cup	30	1	12	5	0	1.0	0.0	0	15%
(Lucky Leaf) white, distilled	1 oz	4	0	2	0	0	0.0	0.0	0	0%
(Musselman's) white, distilled	1 oz	4	0	2	0	0	0.0	0.0	0	0%
(S&W) white, distilled	1 tbsp	0	0	0	0	0	0.0	0.0	0	0%
WINE										
(Heinz) gourmet wine 'Decanter'	0.51 oz	4	0	0	0	0	0.0	0.0	0	0%
(Lucky Leaf) red	1 oz	0	0	0	0	0	0.0	0.0	0	0%
(Musselman's) red	1 oz	0	0	0	0	0	0.0	0.0	0	0%
(Regina)										
all varieties	1 oz	4	0	0	0	0	0.0	0.0	0	0%
red	1 oz	4	0	0	0	0	0.0	0.0	0	0%
(S&W) red, 'International'	1 tbsp	0	0	0	0	0	0.0	0.0	0	0%
VODKA										
80 proof	1 fl oz	64	0	0	0	0	0.0	0.0	0	0%

Food Name	Serving Size	Calories	Prot. gms	Carbs gms	Sod. mgs	Fiber gms	Fat gms	Sat. Fat gms	Chol. mgs	% Fat Cal.
86 proof	1 fl oz	70	0	0	0	0	0.0	0.0	0	0%
90 proof	1 fl oz	73	0	0	0	0	0.0	0.0	0	0%
94 proof	1 fl oz	76	0	0	0	0	0.0	0.0	0	0%
100 proof	1 fl oz	82	0	0	0	0	0.0	0.0	0	0%

W

Food Name	Serving Size	Calories	Prot. gms	Carbs gms	Sod. mgs	Fiber gms	Fat gms	Sat. Fat gms	Chol. mgs	% Fat Cal.
WAFFLE										
(Aunt Jemima)										
apple cinnamon, frozen	1 waffle	176	5	29	616	2	5.6	1.3	6	27%
buttermilk, frozen	1 waffle	179	4	29	615	1	5.8	1.4	7	28%
low-fat, frozen	2 waffles	160	5	32	540	1	1.5	0.5	0	8%
oat bran, frozen	2.5 oz	154	6	29	676	3	2.8	0.0	0	15%
original, frozen, 2.5 oz	1 waffle	173	4	28	591	2	5.6	1.4	6	28%
Quaker Oats, original, frozen	1 serving	197	5	30	563	na	6.0	1.6	12	28%
whole-grain wheat, frozen	5 oz waffle	154	6	29	676	3	2.8	0.0	0	15%
(Downyflake)										
apple and cinnamon, frozen 'Crisp & Healthy'	1 waffle	80	2	16	180	1	1.0	0.0	0	11%
butter, frozen, 'Hot-N-Buttery'	2 waffles	180	4	27	620	0	6.0	0.0	0	30%
buttermilk, frozen	2 waffles	190	5	32	750	0	5.0	0.0	0	23%
buttermilk, frozen, 'Jumbo'	2 waffles	170	4	30	630	0	4.0	1.0	0	21%
frozen, 'Jumbo'	2 waffles	170	4	30	570	0	4.0	1.0	0	21%
frozen, blueberry, frozen	2 waffles	180	4	32	570	0	4.0	0.0	0	20%
multigrain, frozen	2 waffles	250	6	28	500	4	4.0	0.0	0	21%
oat bran, frozen	2 waffles	260	6	30	650	3	13.0	0.0	0	45%
plain, frozen, 'Crisp & Healthy'	1 waffle	80	2	16	180	1	1.0	0.0	0	11%
regular, frozen	2 waffles	120	3	20	420	0	3.0	1.0	0	23%
rice bran, frozen	2 waffles	210	5	25	230	4	11.0	0.0	0	45%
(Eggo)										
apple, 'Fruit Top'	3.1 oz	190	3	32	250	0	6.0	1.0	0	28%
apple cinnamon	1 waffle	130	3	18	250	0	5.0	0.0	0	35%
banana bread, 'Kellogg's Nutri-Grain'	1 serving	212	5	32	280	2	7.4	1.3	0	31%
blueberry, frozen	1 waffle	130	3	18	250	0	5.0	0.0	0	35%
blueberry, frozen, 'Fruit Top'	3.1 oz	190	3	32	250	0	6.0	1.0	0	28%
blueberry, low-fat, 'Kellogg's Nutri-Grain'	1 serving	146	4	30	414	2	2.0	0.3	0	12%
blueberry, low-fat, round, 'Kellogg's Nutri-Grain'	1 waffle	73	2	15	207	1	1.0	0.1	0	12%
buttermilk, frozen	1 waffle	120	3	16	250	0	5.0	0.0	10	37%
cinnamon toast, mini, sets of four	3 sets	280	5	45	470	0	9.0	2.0	25	29%
golden oat	1 serving	139	5	26	270	2	2.3	0.4	1	15%
golden oat, round	1 serving	69	2	13	135	1	1.1	0.2	0	15%
homestyle	1 waffle	120	3	16	250	0	5.0	0.0	10	37%
homestyle, low-fat	1 serving	165	5	31	309	1	2.5	0.6	18	14%
homestyle, mini, frozen, sets of four	3 sets	240	6	34	520	0	8.0	1.5	25	31%
homestyle, round	1 waffle	83	2	15	155	0	1.2	0.3	9	14%
'Kellogg's Nutri-Grain'	1 waffle	130	3	18	250	2	5.0	0.0	0	35%
low-fat, 'Kellogg's Nutri-Grain'	1 serving	142	4	28	430	3	2.2	0.3	0	14%
low-fat, round, 'Kellogg's Nutri-Grain'	1 waffle	71	2	14	215	1	1.1	0.2	0	14%
multi-bran, 'Kellogg's Nutri-Grain'	2 waffles	180	5	32	400	6	6.0	1.0	0	27%
nonfat, 'Kellogg's Special K'	2 waffles	140	6	29	250	0	0.0	0.0	0	0%
nut and honey, frozen	2 waffles	240	6	32	430	0	10.0	2.0	25	37%

Food Name	Serving Size	Calories	Prot. gms	Carbs gms	Sod. mgs	Fiber gms	Fat gms	Sat. Fat gms	Chol. mgs	% Fat Cal.
oat bran, 'Common Sense'	1 waffle	110	3	16	220	2	4.0	0.0	0	32%
oat bran, w/fruit and nut, 'Common Sense'	1 waffle	120	3	17	220	2	5.0	0.0	0	36%
peach, 'Fruit Top'	3.1 oz	190	3	30	240	0	6.0	1.0	0	29%
raisin and bran, 'Kellogg's Nutri-Grain'	1 waffle	130	3	18	250	2	5.0	0.0	0	35%
strawberry	1 waffle	130	3	18	250	0	5.0	0.0	0	35%
strawberry, 'Fruit Top'	1 waffle	190	3	31	230	0	6.0	1.0	0	28%
wheat, whole grain, 'Kellogg's Nutri-Grain'	2 waffles	190	5	30	430	4	6.0	1.0	0	28%
(Krusteaz)										
blueberry, frozen	1 waffle	110	3	19	210	2	3.0	0.6	3	23%
buttermilk, frozen	1 waffle	100	3	16	190	2	2.0	0.0	4	19%
buttermilk, frozen	1 waffle	100	3	16	190	2	2.0	0.0	4	19%
golden, frozen	1 waffle	100	2	16	190	2	2.0	0.0	3	20%
(Med Diet) Belgian, low-protein	1 serving	237	0	46	14	0	7.0	2.0	0	26%
(Roman Meal) frozen	2 waffles	280	5	33	680	3	14.0	0.0	4	45%
(Van's)										
apple cinnamon, frozen	1 waffle	75	3	8	68	3	2.0	0.0	0	29%
Belgian, 7-grain, frozen	1 waffle	88	3	10	81	0	2.0	0.0	0	25%
Belgian, oat bran, frozen	1 waffle	89	3	11	124	0	2.0	0.0	0	24%
Belgian, original, frozen	1 waffle	86	3	14	54	0	2.0	0.0	0	21%
honey almond, frozen	1 waffle	75	3	8	68	3	2.0	0.0	0	29%
multigrain, frozen	1 waffle	75	3	8	68	3	2.0	0.0	0	29%
WAFFLE DISH/MEAL										
(Swanson)										
Belgian, w/sausage, frozen, 'Great Starts'	2.85 oz	280	7	21	420	0	19.0	0.0	0	60%
Belgian, w/sausage and strawberries, frozen	3.5 oz	210	3	31	240	0	8.0	0.0	0	35%
w/bacon, frozen, 'Great Starts'	2.2 oz	230	7	19	710	0	14.0	0.0	0	55%
WAFFLE MIX. See also PANCAKE/WAFFLE MIX.										
(Krusteaz) Belgian, prepared, 4-inch diam.	1 waffle	170	5	22	350	0	7.0	0.0	45	37%
WAKAME. See under SEA VEGETABLE.										
WALLEYE. See under PIKE; POLLACK										
WALNUT										
ALL TYPES										
chopped, natural, unsalted (Flanigan Farms)	1 oz	180	4	4	na	na	19.0	na	0	84%
halves and pieces (Azar)	2 oz	360	8	10	5	3	35.0	3.0	0	81%
halves and pieces, natural, unsalted (Flanigan Farms)	1/4 cup	180	7	5	0	2	18.0	1.5	0	77%
BLACK										
Dried										
	1 oz	172	7	3	0	1	16.0	1.0	0	78%
	1 tbsp	47	2	1	0	0	4.4	0.3	0	78%
(Planters)	1 oz	180	7	3	0	0	17.0	1.0	0	79%
chopped	1 cup	759	30	15	1	6	70.7	4.5	0	78%
shelled (Fisher)	1 oz	170	7	3	0	0	16.0	1.0	0	78%
Raw (Planters)	1 oz	180	7	3	0	0	17.0	1.0	0	79%
ENGLISH										
Dried										
in shell, whole, 7 med nuts	1 cup	183	4	4	1	2	18.3	1.7	0	83%
shelled (Diamond)	1 oz	192	5	4	0	0	19.0	0.0	0	83%
shelled, chopped (Fisher)	1 oz	180	4	5	0	0	18.0	2.0	0	82%
shelled, chopped	1 cup	785	18	16	2	8	78.3	7.4	0	83%
shelled, ground	1 cup	523	12	11	2	5	52.2	4.9	0	83%
shelled, ground (Fisher)	1 oz	180	4	5	0	0	18.0	2.0	0	82%
shelled, halved (Planters)	1 oz	190	4	3	0	0	20.0	2.0	0	87%
shelled, halved, 50 halves	1 cup	654	15	14	2	7	65.2	6.1	0	83%

Food Name	Serving Size	Calories	Prot. gms	Carbs gms	Sod. mgs	Fiber gms	Fat gms	Sat. Fat gms	Chol. mgs	% Fat Cal.
shelled, pieces (Planters)	1 oz	190	4	3	0	0	20.0	2.0	0	87%
shelled, pieces or chips	1 cup	785	18	16	2	8	78.3	7.4	0	83%
shelled, whole (Planters)	1 oz	190	4	3	0	0	20.0	2.0	0	87%
Raw (Fisher)	1 oz	180	4	5	0	0	18.0	2.0	0	82%
PERSIAN										
Dried										
shelled (Diamond)	1 oz	192	5	4	0	0	19.0	0.0	0	83%
shelled, halves (Planters)	1 oz	190	4	3	0	0	20.0	2.0	0	87%
shelled, pieces (Planters)	1 oz	190	4	3	0	0	20.0	2.0	0	87%
shelled, whole (Planters)	1 oz	190	4	3	0	0	20.0	2.0	0	87%
WALNUT OIL										
	1 cup	1927	0	0	0	0	218.0	19.8	0	100%
	1 tbsp	120	0	0	0	0	13.6	1.2	0	100%
(Hain)	1 tbsp	120	0	0	0	0	14.0	2.0	0	100%
(International Collection)	1 tbsp	120	0	0	0	0	14.0	1.0	0	100%
California, 100% pure (Loriva')	1 tbsp	125	0	0	0	0	14.0	1.0	0	100%
pure pressed, organic (Spectrum)	1 tbsp	120	0	0	0	0	14.0	1.0	0	100%
WASABI CHIPS										
(Eden Foods)										
	1-oz bag	130	1	22	200	0	4.0	0.0	0	28%
hot and spicy	1 oz bag	130	1	22	200	0	4.0	0.0	0	28%
WASABI ROOT / Japanese horseradish										
raw, sliced	1 cup	142	6	31	22	10	0.8	na	0	5%
raw, whole	1 med root	184	8	40	29	13	1.1	na	0	5%
WATER										
FLAVORED. See also under SOFT DRINKS AND MIXERS.										
(Cascadia)										
cherry blackberry, sparkling, w/juice	6 fl oz	2	0	0	0	0	0.0	0.0	0	0%
grapefruit, sparkling, w/juice	6 fl oz	2	0	0	0	0	0.0	0.0	0	0%
guava berry, sparkling, w/juice	6 fl oz	2	0	0	0	0	0.0	0.0	0	0%
lemonade, sparkling, w/juice	6 fl oz	2	0	0	0	0	0.0	0.0	0	0%
(Clearly Canadian)										
sparkling, 'Coastal Cranberry'	6 fl oz	70	0	16	10	0	0.0	0.0	0	0%
sparkling, 'Country Raspberry' sparkling	6 fl oz	70	0	16	10	0	0.0	0.0	0	0%
sparkling, 'Mountain Blackberry'	6 fl oz	70	0	16	10	0	0.0	0.0	0	0%
sparkling, 'Orchard Peach'	6 fl oz	70	0	16	10	0	0.0	0.0	0	0%
sparkling, 'Western Loganberry'	6 fl oz	70	0	16	10	0	0.0	0.0	0	0%
sparkling, 'Wild Cherry'	6 fl oz	70	0	16	10	0	0.0	0.0	0	0%
(H2OH!)										
lemon-lime, sparkling	6 fl oz	0	0	0	0	0	0.0	0.0	0	0%
natural berry, sparkling	6 fl oz	0	0	0	0	0	0.0	0.0	0	0%
(Quest)										
black cherry, sparkling, 'Refresher'	8 fl oz	2	0	0	35	0	0.0	0.0	0	0%
peach citrus, sparkling, 'Refresher'	8 fl oz	2	0	0	35	0	0.0	0.0	0	0%
raspberry, sparkling, 'Refresher'	8 fl oz	2	0	0	35	0	0.0	0.0	0	0%
red raspberry, sparkling, 'Refresher'	8 fl oz	2	0	0	35	0	0.0	0.0	0	0%
strawberry-kiwi, sparkling, 'Refresher'	8 fl oz	2	0	0	35	0	0.0	0.0	0	0%
tangerine lime, sparkling, 'Refresher'	8 fl oz	2	0	0	35	0	0.0	0.0	0	0%
UNFLAVORED										
(Perrier)	8 fl oz	0	0	0	2	0	0.0	0.0	0	0%
(Poland Spring)	8 fl oz	0	0	0	2	0	0.0	0.0	0	0%
distilled (Arrowhead)	1 liter	0	0	0	0	0	0.0	0.0	0	0%
drinking (Arrowhead)	1 liter	0	0	0	16	0	0.0	0.0	0	0%
fluoridated (Arrowhead)	1 liter	0	0	0	16	0	0.0	0.0	0	0%

Food Name	Serving Size	Calories	Prot. gms	Carbs gms	Sod. mgs	Fiber gms	Fat gms	Sat. Fat gms	Chol. mgs	% Fat Cal.
mineral *(Perrier)*	1 liter	0	0	0	19	0	0.0	0.0	0	0%
municipal	8 fl oz	0	0	0	7	0	0.0	0.0	0	0%
sparkling, natural *(Clearly Canadian)*	6 fl oz	0	0	0	3	0	0.0	0.0	0	0%
spring *(Arrowhead)*	1 liter	0	0	0	9	0	0.0	0.0	0	0%
spring, 'Arizona Tule' *(Arrowhead)*	1 liter	0	0	0	7	0	0.0	0.0	0	0%
Vichy *(Schweppes)*	6 fl oz	0	0	0	76	0	0.0	0.0	0	0%
WATER BUFFALO										
raw	1 oz	28	6	0	15	0	0.4	0.1	13	12%
roasted	3 oz	111	23	0	48	0	1.5	0.5	52	12%
roasted, diced	1 cup	183	37.6	0.0	78	0	2.5	0.8	85	13%
WATER CHESTNUT										
Canned										
Chinese *(LaChoy)*	1.28 oz	18	0	5	3	0	0.1	0.0	0	4%
Chinese, sliced, w/liquid	1/2 cup	35	1	9	6	2	0.0	0.0	0	1%
Chinese, whole, w/liquid	4 medium	14	0	3	2	1	0.0	0.0	0	1%
chopped *(LaChoy)*	0.63 oz	9	0	2	2	1	0.1	0.0	0	9%
sliced *(China Boy)*	1/2 cup	45	1	11	10	4	0.0	0.0	0	0%
sliced *(Chun King)*	1 oz	12	1	2	5	0	1.0	0.0	0	43%
sliced *(La Choy)*	2 tbsp	11	0	3	3	1	0.1	0.0	0	6%
sliced, food service product *(La Choy)*	2 tbsp	11	0	3	3	1	0.1	0.0	0	6%
whole *(La Choy)*	2 medium	10	0	2	2	1	0.1	0.0	0	6%
whole, food service product *(La Choy)*	2 medium	10	0	2	2	1	0.1	0.0	0	6%
Fresh										
Chinese, matai, raw, sliced	1/2 cup	60	1	15	9	2	0.1	0.0	0	1%
Chinese, matai, raw, whole	4 medium	35	1	9	5	1	0.0	0.0	0	1%
WATER CONVOLVULUS. See CABBAGE, SKUNK.										
WATERCRESS										
Fresh										
raw, chopped	1 cup	4	1	0	14	1	0.0	0.0	0	8%
raw, whole sprigs	10 medium	3	1	0	10	0	0.0	0.0	0	8%
raw, whole sprigs	1 medium	0	0	0	1	0	0.0	0.0	0	9%
WATERMELON										
raw, balls	1 cup	49	1	11	3	1	0.7	0.1	0	11%
raw, balls	10 balls	39	1	9	2	1	0.5	0.1	0	11%
raw, diced	1 cup	49	1	11	3	1	0.7	0.1	0	11%
raw, sliced, 1/16 of 10-inch diam melon	1 slice	92	2	21	6	1	1.2	0.1	0	11%
WATERMELON SEED										
dried, kernels	1 cup	602	31	17	107	na	51.2	10.6	0	71%
dried, kernels	1 oz	158	8	4	28	na	13.4	2.8	0	71%
WAX BEAN. See BEAN, WAX.										
WAX GOURD. See GOURD, WAX.										
WELSH RAREBIT. See under CHEESE DISH/ENTRÉE.										
WEST INDIAN CHERRY. See ACEROLA.										
WESTERN ENTRÉE										
(Banquet) frozen	11 oz	630	28	40	720	0	41.0	0.0	90	58%
(Morton) frozen	10 oz	290	14	29	1450	0	14.0	0.0	35	42%
(Swanson) frozen	11.5 oz	430	22	43	1060	0	19.0	0.0	0	40%
WHEAT										
BULGAR, gluten-free, 'Old World' *(Ener-G Foods)*	1/4 cup	181	5	39	2	8	0.6	0.0	0	3%
DURUM	1 cup	651	26	137	4	na	4.7	0.9	0	6%
HARD RED										
spring	1 cup	632	30	131	4	23	3.7	0.6	0	5%
spring or winter, whole grain *(Arrowhead Mills)*	2 oz	190	8	41	1	8	1.0	0.0	0	4%
winter	1 cup	628	24	137	4	23	3.0	0.5	0	4%

Food Name	Serving Size	Calories	Prot. gms	Carbs gms	Sod. mgs	Fiber gms	Fat gms	Sat. Fat gms	Chol. mgs	% Fat Cal.
HARD WHITE.	1 cup	657	22	146	4	na	3.3	0.5	0	4%
SOFT RED										
whole grain, for pastry (Arrowhead Mills)	2 oz	190	8	41	1	8	1.0	0.0	0	4%
winter.	1 cup	556	17	125	3	21	2.6	0.5	0	4%
SOFT WHITE	1 cup	571	18	127	3	21	3.3	0.6	0	5%
SPROUTED	1 cup	214	8	46	17	1	1.4	0.2	0	5%
WHEAT BRAN										
crude.	1 cup	125	9	37	1	25	2.5	0.4	0	16%
crude (Arrowhead Mills)	2 oz	50	10	30	3	24	2.0	0.0	0	10%
unprocessed (Quaker)	2 tbsp	8	1	4	0	3	0.2	0.0	0	9%
unprocessed, miller's bran, dry (Hodgson Mill).	1/4 cup	30	2	10	0	7	0.0	0.0	0	0%
unprocessed, natural (Miller's)	6 tbsp	70	4	17	2	12	1.0	0.0	0	10%
WHEAT CAKE (Quaker) lightly salted	1 cake	35	1	7	45	1	0.0	0.0	0	0%
WHEAT FLOUR. See under FLOUR.										
WHEAT GERM										
crude	1 cup	414	27	60	14	15	11.2	1.9	0	23%
toasted, plain, ready to eat	1 cup	432	33	56	5	15	12.1	2.1	0	23%
toasted, plain, ready to eat	1 oz	108	8	14	1	4	3.0	0.5	0	23%
(Arrowhead Mills) raw	2 oz	210	15	26	1	7	6.0	0.0	0	25%
(Hodgson Mill) untoasted, 25% protein, dry.	2 tbsp	55	4	7	0	4	1.0	0.0	0	17%
(Kretschmer)										
. . . .	2 tbsp	50	4	6	0	2	1.0	0.0	0	18%
honey crunch.	1 2/3 tbsp	52	4	8	2	1	1.1	0.2	0	19%
honey crunch, sodium-free, cholesterol-free.	1 oz	110	8	15	0	3	3.0	0.0	0	23%
sodium-free, cholesterol-free	2 tbsp	50	4	6	0	2	1.0	0.0	0	18%
WHEAT GERM NUTS (Anacon Foods)	1/2 oz	100	2	2	13	1	9.3	1.4	0	83%
WHEAT GERM OIL										
. . . .	1 cup	1927	0	0	0	0	218.0	41.0	0	100%
. . . .	1 tbsp	120	0	0	0	0	13.6	2.6	0	100%
WHEAT GLUTEN										
(Arrowhead Mills) Vita 1	1 oz	100	15	9	1	1	1.0	0.0	0	9%
(Hodgson Mill) Vital w/Vit-C.	1 tbsp	30	6	2	0	1	0.0	0.0	0	0%
WHEAT SNACKS										
wheat nuts, flavored, no salt added, all flavors										
except macadamia	1 oz	183	4	6	26	1	17.7	2.7	0	81%
wheat nuts, formulated, unflavored, salted	1 oz	176	4	7	143	1	16.4	2.5	0	78%
(Ralston)										
'Delicious'	16 crackers	140	2	23	220	1	4.0	0.5	na	26%
full fat, 'Delicious'.	16 crackers	140	3	20	120	2	6.0	1.0	0	37%
full fat, 'Grand Union'.	16 crackers	140	3	20	120	2	6.0	1.0	0	37%
full fat, 'Stop & Shop'.	16 crackers	140	3	20	120	2	6.0	1.0	0	37%
full fat, unsalted, 'Stop & Shop'	16 crackers	140	3	20	80	2	6.0	1.0	na	37%
'Grand Union'	16 crackers	140	2	23	220	1	4.0	0.5	na	26%
less fat.	16 crackers	140	2	23	220	1	4.0	0.5	0	26%
unsalted tops, 'Stop & Shop'	16 crackers	140	2	23	85	1	4.0	0.5	na	26%
WHEATGRASS										
powder (Pines)	1 tsp	13	1	2	1	1	0.0	0.0	0	0%
tablets (Pines).	7 tablets	13	1	2	1	1	0.0	0.0	0	0%
WHELK										
boiled, poached, or steamed.	3 oz	234	41	13	350	0	0.7	0.1	111	3%
raw	3 oz	116	20	7	175	0	0.3	0.0	55	3%
WHEY										
acid, dried	1 cup	193	7	42	552	0	0.3	0.2	2	1%
acid, dried	1 tbsp	10	0	2	28	0	0.0	0.0	0	1%

Food Name	Serving Size	Calories	Prot. gms	Carbs gms	Sod. mgs	Fiber gms	Fat gms	Sat. Fat gms	Chol. mgs	% Fat Cal.
acid, fluid.	1 quart	235	7	50	473	0	0.9	0.6	5	3%
acid, fluid.	1 cup	59	2	13	118	0	0.2	0.1	1	3%
sweet, dried.	1 cup	512	19	108	1565	0	1.6	1.0	9	3%
sweet, dried.	1 tbsp	26	1	6	81	0	0.1	0.1	0	3%
sweet, fluid.	1 quart	263	8	51	526	0	3.5	2.3	20	12%
sweet, fluid.	1 cup	66	2	13	132	0	0.9	0.6	5	12%
WHIPPED TOPPING. See CREAM TOPPING.										
WHISKEY										
80 proof.	1 fl oz	64	0	0	0	0	0.0	0.0	0	0%
86 proof.	1 fl oz	70	0	0	0	0	0.0	0.0	0	0%
90 proof.	1 fl oz	73	0	0	0	0	0.0	0.0	0	0%
94 proof.	1 fl oz	76	0	0	0	0	0.0	0.0	0	0%
100 proof.	1 fl oz	82	0	0	0	0	0.0	0.0	0	0%
WHISKEY SOUR. See under COCKTAIL; COCKTAIL MIX.										
WHITE ACRE PEAS, canned, fresh *(Allens)*.	1/2 cup	90	7	14	440	0	1.0	0.0	0	10%
WHITE BEAN. See BEAN, WHITE.										
WHITE CURRANT. See under CURRANT.										
WHITE GOURD. See CHINESE WATERMELON.										
WHITE MUSHROOM. See MUSHROOM, WHITE.										
WHITE PEPPER. See under PEPPER, GROUND.										
WHITE RICE. See under RICE.										
WHITE SUCKER. See SUCKER, WHITE.										
WHITEFISH										
mixed species, baked, broiled, grilled, or microwaved	3 oz	146	21	0	55	0	6.4	1.0	65	39%
mixed species, raw.	3 oz	114	16	0	43	0	5.0	0.8	51	39%
mixed species, smoked.	3 oz	92	20	0	866	0	0.8	0.2	28	8%
mixed species, smoked, flaked.	1 cup	147	32	0	1386	0	1.3	0.3	45	8%
WHITE-FLOWERED GOURD. See GOURD, BOTTLE.										
WHITING / silver hake										
Fresh										
mixed species, baked, broiled, grilled, or microwaved	3 oz	99	20	0	112	0	1.4	0.3	71	13%
mixed species, raw.	3 oz	77	16	0	61	0	1.1	0.2	57	13%
Frozen, 'Individually Wrapped' *(Booth).*	4 oz	80	19	0	85	0	1.0	0.0	0	11%
WILD RICE. See RICE, WILD.										
WINE. See also SHERRY; VERMOUTH; WINE, COOKING; WINE COOLER.										
(Mission Bell)										
'Arriba'.	2 fl oz	95	0	7	4	0	0.0	0.0	0	0%
'Diamond Red'.	2 fl oz	95	0	7	4	0	0.0	0.0	0	0%
'Silver Satin'.	2 fl oz	83	0	5	4	0	0.0	0.0	0	0%
'Silver Satin Bitter Lemon'.	2 fl oz	83	0	6	4	0	0.0	0.0	0	0%
'Swiss Up'.	2 fl oz	84	0	6	4	0	0.0	0.0	0	0%
BARBERA, white *(Colony)*.	4 fl oz	91	0	4	4	0	0.0	0.0	0	0%
BURGUNDY										
(Bravo) red.	4 fl oz	91	0	2	4	0	0.0	0.0	0	0%
(Carlo Rossi) red.	4 fl oz	92	0	2	0	0	0.0	0.0	0	0%
(Colony)										
red 'Classic'.	4 fl oz	90	0	1	4	0	0.0	0.0	0	0%
white, 'Classic'.	4 fl oz	80	0	1	4	0	0.0	0.0	0	0%
(Gallo)										
red.	4 fl oz	88	0	1	0	0	0.0	0.0	0	0%
red, 'Hearty'.	4 fl oz	92	0	2	0	0	0.0	0.0	0	0%
(Gambarelli & Davitto) red 'Parma'.	4 fl oz	91	0	2	4	0	0.0	0.0	0	0%
(Petri) red.	4 fl oz	91	0	2	4	0	0.0	0.0	0	0%

Food Name	Serving Size	Calories	Prot. gms	Carbs gms	Sod. mgs	Fiber gms	Fat gms	Sat. Fat gms	Chol. mgs	% Fat Cal.
CABERNET SAUVIGNON										
(Colony)	4 fl oz	88	0	1	4	0	0.0	0.0	0	0%
(Gallo)	4 fl oz	88	0	0	0	0	0.0	0.0	0	0%
CARBONATED										
(Jacques Bonet)										
almond	4 fl oz	104	0	8	4	0	0.0	0.0	0	0%
apricot	4 fl oz	111	0	10	4	0	0.0	0.0	0	0%
cherry	4 fl oz	106	0	8	4	0	0.0	0.0	0	0%
(Carlo Rossi) 'Paisano'	4 fl oz	92	0	2	0	0	0.0	0.0	0	0%
(Jacques Bonet)										
peach	4 fl oz	111	0	10	4	0	0.0	0.0	0	0%
raspberry	4 fl oz	106	0	8	4	0	0.0	0.0	0	0%
CHABLIS										
(Bravo)	4 fl oz	86	0	2	0	0	0.0	0.0	0	0%
(Carlo Rossi)										
pink	4 fl oz	92	0	4	0	0	0.0	0.0	0	0%
white	4 fl oz	84	0	2	0	0	0.0	0.0	0	0%
(Colony)										
	4 fl oz	98	0	5	4	0	0.0	0.0	0	0%
'Classic'	4 fl oz	84	0	2	4	0	0.0	0.0	0	0%
emerald	4 fl oz	102	0	5	4	0	0.0	0.0	0	0%
gold	4 fl oz	97	0	4	4	0	0.0	0.0	0	0%
ruby	4 fl oz	104	0	6	4	0	0.0	0.0	0	0%
(Gallo)										
	4 fl oz	80	0	4	0	0	0.0	0.0	0	0%
'Blanc'	4 fl oz	80	0	1	0	0	0.0	0.0	0	0%
(Petri)										
	4 fl oz	98	0	5	4	0	0.0	0.0	0	0%
'Chablis Blanc'	4 fl oz	86	0	2	4	0	0.0	0.0	0	0%
(Gambarelli & Davitto) 'Parma'	4 fl oz	86	0	2	4	0	0.0	0.0	0	0%
CHAMPAGNE										
(Jacques Bonet)										
brut	4 fl oz	92	0	2	4	0	0.0	0.0	0	0%
extra dry	4 fl oz	97	0	3	4	0	0.0	0.0	0	0%
pink	4 fl oz	98	0	4	4	0	0.0	0.0	0	0%
(Lejon)										
brut	4 fl oz	92	0	3	4	0	0.0	0.0	0	0%
extra dry	4 fl oz	97	0	2	4	0	0.0	0.0	0	0%
pink	4 fl oz	98	0	4	4	0	0.0	0.0	0	0%
CHENIN BLANC										
(Colony)	4 fl oz	86	0	2	4	0	0.0	0.0	0	0%
(Gallo)	4 fl oz	88	0	2	0	0	0.0	0.0	0	0%
CHIANTI										
(Carlo Rossi) 'Light'	4 fl oz	92	0	2	0	0	0.0	0.0	0	0%
(Petri)	4 fl oz	91	0	2	4	0	0.0	0.0	0	0%
COLD DUCK										
(Jacques Bonet)	4 fl oz	108	0	6	4	0	0.0	0.0	0	0%
(Lejon)	4 fl oz	108	0	6	4	0	0.0	0.0	0	0%
FRENCH COLOMBARD										
(Colony)	4 fl oz	84	0	2	4	0	0.0	0.0	0	0%
(Gallo)	4 fl oz	88	0	2	0	0	0.0	0.0	0	0%
GEWÜRZTRAMINER (Gallo)	4 fl oz	88	0	2	0	0	0.0	0.0	0	0%
MARSALA (Gambarelli & Davitto)	4 fl oz	77	0	4	4	0	0.0	0.0	0	0%

Food Name	Serving Size	Calories	Prot. gms	Carbs gms	Sod. mgs	Fiber gms	Fat gms	Sat. Fat gms	Chol. mgs	% Fat Cal.
MOSELLE *(Colony)* 'Rhineskeller'	4 fl oz	97	0	4	4	0	0.0	0.0	0	0%
MUSCATEL *(Italian Swiss Colony)*	2 fl oz	122	0	6	4	0	0.0	0.0	0	0%
PASTOSO *(Petri)*	4 fl oz	92	0	2	4	0	0.0	0.0	0	0%
PORT										
(Gallo)										
. . . .	2 fl oz	64	0	2	0	0	0.0	0.0	0	0%
tawny, 'Livingston Cellars'	2 fl oz	86	0	6	0	0	0.0	0.0	0	0%
white	2 fl oz	86	0	6	0	0	0.0	0.0	0	0%
(Italian Swiss Colony)										
. . . .	2 fl oz	85	0	6	4	0	0.0	0.0	0	0%
white	2 fl oz	86	0	6	4	0	0.0	0.0	0	0%
RED TABLE	3.5 fl oz	74	0	2	5	0	0.0	0.0	0	0%
RHINE										
(Bravo)	4 fl oz	97	0	4	4	0	0.0	0.0	0	0%
(Carlo Rossi)	4 fl oz	84	0	4	0	0	0.0	0.0	0	0%
(Colony) 'Classic'	4 fl oz	89	0	4	4	0	0.0	0.0	0	0%
(Gallo)	4 fl oz	80	0	4	0	0	0.0	0.0	0	0%
(Gambarelli & Davitto) 'Parma'	4 fl oz	92	0	1	4	0	0.0	0.0	0	0%
(Petri)	4 fl oz	97	0	4	4	0	0.0	0.0	0	0%
RIESLING *(Gallo)* 'Johannisberg'	4 fl oz	84	0	2	0	0	0.0	0.0	0	0%
ROSÉ										
(Bravo)	4 fl oz	92	0	3	4	0	0.0	0.0	0	0%
(Carlo Rossi) 'Vin Rose'	4 fl oz	88	0	3	0	0	0.0	0.0	0	0%
(Colony) 'Classic'	4 fl oz	89	0	3	4	0	0.0	0.0	0	0%
(Gallo)										
'Grenache'	4 fl oz	88	0	2	0	0	0.0	0.0	0	0%
'Red Rose'	4 fl oz	112	0	6	0	0	0.0	0.0	0	0%
'Vin Rose'	4 fl oz	88	0	3	0	0	0.0	0.0	0	0%
(Gambarelli & Davitto) 'Parma'	4 fl oz	92	0	3	4	0	0.0	0.0	0	0%
(Petri)	4 fl oz	92	0	3	4	0	0.0	0.0	0	0%
SAUVIGNON BLANC *(Gallo)*	4 fl oz	80	0	1	0	0	0.0	0.0	0	0%
TOKAY *(Italian Swiss Colony)*	2 fl oz	82	0	5	4	0	0.0	0.0	0	0%
WHITE TABLE	3.5 fl oz	70	0	1	5	0	0.0	0.0	0	0%
WINE, COOKING										
(Holland House)										
Marsala	1 fl oz	9	0	2	186	0	0.0	0.0	0	0%
red	1 fl oz	6	0	2	186	0	0.0	0.0	0	0%
sherry	1 fl oz	5	0	1	186	0	0.0	0.0	0	0%
vermouth	1 fl oz	2	0	1	186	0	0.0	0.0	0	0%
white	1 fl oz	2	0	1	186	0	0.0	0.0	0	0%
(Regina)										
Burgundy	1/4 cup	2	1	1	365	0	1.0	0.0	0	53%
Sauternes	1/4 cup	2	1	1	365	0	1.0	0.0	0	53%
sherry	1/4 cup	20	1	5	70	0	1.0	0.0	0	27%
WINE COOLER										
(Bartles & Jaymes)										
berry cooler, 'Light'	12 fl oz	150	0	32	0	0	0.0	0.0	0	0%
black cherry cooler, 'Light'	12 fl oz	139	0	30	0	0	0.0	0.0	0	0%
citrus cooler, 'Light'	6 fl oz	67	1	12	0	0	1.0	0.0	0	15%
tropical cooler, 'Light'	12 fl oz	151	0	32	0	0	0.0	0.0	0	0%

WINGED BEAN. See BEAN, WINGED.

WINTER RADISH. See under RADISH.

WINTER SQUASH. See SQUASH, WINTER.

Food Name	Serving Size	Calories	Prot. gms	Carbs gms	Sod. mgs	Fiber gms	Fat gms	Sat. Fat gms	Chol. mgs	% Fat Cal.
WOLF FISH / ocean catfish										
Fresh										
Atlantic, baked, broiled, or grilled	3 oz	105	19	0	93	0	2.6	0.4	50	22%
Atlantic, raw.	3 oz	82	15	0	72	0	2.0	0.3	39	22%
Frozen *(Booth)*.	4 oz	115	20	0	85	0	20.0	0.0	0	69%
WONTON WRAPPER										
including egg roll wrappers	1 oz	82	3	16	162	1	0.4	0.1	3	5%
including egg roll wrappers, 7-inch square	1 wrapper	93	3	19	183	1	0.5	0.1	3	5%
including egg roll wrappers, 3.5-inch square.	1 wrapper	23	1	5	46	0	0.1	0.0	1	5%
(Nasoya)	1 wrapper	23	1	5	19	0	0.0	0.0	0	0%

Y

Food Name	Serving Size	Calories	Prot. gms	Carbs gms	Sod. mgs	Fiber gms	Fat gms	Sat. Fat gms	Chol. mgs	% Fat Cal.
YAM										
Fresh										
boiled, drained, cubed.	1 cup	158	2	38	11	5	0.2	0.0	0	1%
boiled, drained, cubed.	1/2 cup	79	1	19	5	3	0.1	0.0	0	1%
raw, cubed.	1 cup	177	2	42	14	6	0.3	0.1	0	1%
Canned										
(Bush's Best)	1/2 cup	120	1	28	20	0	0.0	0.0	0	0%
cut, in light syrup *(Princella)*	2/3 cup	160	0	40	35	3	0.5	0.0	0	3%
orange pineapple *(Royal Prince)*.	1/2 cup	210	1	43	30	3	0.5	0.0	0	2%
CHINESE. See JICAMA.										
MOUNTAIN/HAWAIIAN										
Fresh										
raw, whole.	1 medium	281	6	69	55	na	0.4	0.1	0	1%
raw, cubed.	1/2 cup	46	1	11	9	na	0.1	0.0	0	1%
steamed, cubed.	1 cup	119	3	29	17	na	0.1	0.0	0	1%
YAM DISH										
(Flav-R-Pac) yam patties	2 pieces	150	1	33	200	3	1.0	0.0	0	6%
(Stouffer's) yam and apples, frozen, food service product. . .	1 oz	37	0	8	26	0	0.7	0.1	0	17%
YAMBEAN TUBER. See JICAMA.										
YARDLONG BEAN. See BEAN, YARDLONG.										
YAUTIA / tannia										
Fresh										
raw, sliced.	1 cup	132	2	32	28	2	0.5	0.1	0	3%
raw, whole.	1 med root	299	4	72	64	5	1.2	0.3	0	3%
YEAST										
BAKER'S										
active, dry	1 tbsp	35	5	5	6	3	0.6	0.1	0	13%
active, dry	1 tsp	12	2	2	2	1	0.2	0.0	0	13%
active dry *(Red Star)*.	0.25 oz	15	2	2	5	0	0.0	0.0	0	0%
active dry, 'RapidRise' *(Fleischmann's)*.	0.25 oz	20	3	3	10	0	0.0	0.0	0	0%
compressed.	0.6-oz cake	18	1	3	5	1	0.3	0.0	0	15%
BREWER'S										
debittered	1 oz	79	10.9	10.8	34	>0.5	0.3	0.0	0	3%
debittered	1 tbsp	23	3.1	3.1	10	>0.1	0.1	0.0	0	4%
torula.	1 oz	78	10.8	10.4	4	>0.9	0.3	0.0	0	3%
YELLOW BEAN. See BEAN, YELLOW.										
YELLOW MOMBIN. See JOBO.										
YELLOW PEPPER. See PEPPER, BANANA; PEPPER, BELL.										

Food Name	Serving Size	Calories	Prot. gms	Carbs gms	Sod. mgs	Fiber gms	Fat gms	Sat. Fat gms	Chol. mgs	% Fat Cal.
YELLOW SQUASH. See under SQUASH.										
YELLOW-EYE BEANS. See under BAKED BEANS, CANNED.										
YELLOWFIN TUNA. See under TUNA.										
YELLOWTAIL										
mixed species, baked, broiled, grilled, or microwaved	3 oz	159	25	0	43	0	5.7	na	60	32%
mixed species, raw	3 oz	124	20	0	33	0	4.5	1.1	47	32%
YOGURT										
(Crowley) all flavors, 'Swiss Style'	1 cup	240	8	48	150	0	2.0	0.0	10	7%
(Light n' Lively) all flavors except strawberry,										
nonfat, 'Free'............................	4.4 oz	50	4	8	60	0	0.0	0.0	0	0%
(Ripple) all flavors, fat-free, '70'	6 oz	70	5	13	85	0	0.0	0.0	5	0%
(Yoplait)										
all fruit flavors, custard style	6 oz	190	7	32	100	0	3.5	2.0	15	17%
all fruit flavors, light	6 oz	90	5	16	75	0	0.0	0.0	0	0%
all fruit flavors, nonfat	6 oz	90	5	16	75	0	0.0	0.0	0	0%
all fruit flavors, original, 99% fat-free..............	6 oz	180	6	34	80	0	1.5	1.0	10	8%
APPLE CINNAMON *(Dannon)* low-fat	1 container	240	9	46	140	1	3.0	1.5	15	11%
APPLE CRISP *(New Country)* low-fat	6 oz	150	5	30	85	0	2.0	0.0	0	11%
BANANA										
(Yoplait) custard style........................	6 oz	180	7	30	105	0	3.0	0.0	0	15%
(Dannon) lowfat, 'Sprinkl'ins'	4.1 oz	140	5	24	80	0	2.0	0.0	5	13%
BANANA BERRY										
(Light n' Lively) berry, low-fat, 1% milk fat, cultured	4.4 oz	130	5	24	75	0	1.0	0.0	10	7%
BERRY *(Yoplait)* w/wheat, raisins, walnuts, 'Breakfast'	6 oz	200	8	39	125	0	2.0	0.0	0	9%
BLACK CHERRY										
(Alta Dena)										
blended	8 oz	190	8	38	140	0	1.0	0.0	0	5%
fruit on the bottom........................	1 cup	240	12	40	150	0	4.0	0.0	0	15%
(Breyers) low-fat........................	8 oz	260	9	49	120	0	3.0	1.0	10	10%
(Knudsen) nonfat, 'Cal 70'	6 oz	70	5	12	75	0	0.0	0.0	5	0%
(Light n' Lively)										
....	8 oz	230	9	44	125	0	2.0	1.0	15	8%
nonfat, '100'....................	8 oz	100	8	17	100	0	0.0	0.0	0	0%
(Mountain High) natural, 'Honey Light'....................	8 oz	190	9	35	140	0	1.0	0.0	5	5%
BLUEBERRY										
(Alta Dena) fruit on the bottom, 'Maya'....................	1 cup	280	11	39	170	0	9.0	0.0	0	29%
(Breyers) low-fat....................	8 oz	250	9	48	120	0	2.0	1.0	10	7%
(Dannon)										
low-fat....................	1 container	240	9	46	140	1	3.0	1.5	15	11%
nonfat, blended	3/4 cup	160	7	33	105	0	0.0	0.0	5	0%
nonfat, light	8 oz	100	9	19	135	0	0.0	0.0	5	0%
(Knudsen) nonfat, 'Cal 70'	6 oz	70	6	11	80	0	0.0	0.0	5	0%
(Light n' Lively)										
....	8 oz	240	8	46	130	0	2.0	1.0	10	8%
nonfat, 'Free'	4.4 oz	50	4	8	60	0	0.0	0.0	0	0%
nonfat, '100'....................	8 oz	90	8	15	110	0	0.0	0.0	0	0%
(Mountain High) natural, 'Honey Light'....................	8 oz	190	9	35	140	0	1.0	0.0	5	5%
(New Country) 'Supreme'....................	6 oz	150	5	31	90	0	2.0	0.0	0	11%
(White Wave) nondairy....................	1 serving	150	5	31	55	1	1.0	0.0	0	6%
(Yoplait)										
fruit on the bottom....................	6 oz	170	7	35	105	0	0.0	0.0	5	0%
light	6 oz	90	5	16	70	0	0.0	0.0	5	0%
99% fat-free, original....................	6 oz	180	8	32	130	0	2.0	0.0	0	10%

Food Name	Serving Size	Calories	Prot. gms	Carbs gms	Sod. mgs	Fiber gms	Fat gms	Sat. Fat gms	Chol. mgs	% Fat Cal.
BLUEBERRIES AND CREAM										
(Weight Watchers) 'Ultimate 90'	1 cup	90	8	14	140	3	0.0	0.0	0	0%
BLUEBERRY AND VANILLA (Yoplait) parfait style	6 oz	200	8	34	120	0	3.0	0.0	0	14%
BLUEBERRY CHEESECAKE (Yogi) w/gelatin, 'Sundae'	5.6 oz	50	6	14	75	0	1.0	0.0	4	10%
BOYSENBERRY										
(Dannon) low-fat	1 container	240	9	45	150	1	3.0	1.5	15	11%
(Yoplait) 99% fat-free, original	6 oz	180	8	32	130	0	2.0	0.0	0	10%
CAPPUCCINO										
(Dannon) light	8 oz	100	9	16	135	0	0.0	0.0	5	0%
(Weight Watchers) 'Ultimate 90'	1 cup	90	8	14	140	0	0.0	0.0	0	0%
CHERRIES JUBILEE (Weight Watchers) 'Ultimate 90'	1 cup	90	8	14	140	0	0.0	0.0	0	0%
CHERRY										
(Dannon)										
low-fat	1 container	240	9	45	140	1	3.0	1.5	15	11%
low-fat, 'Sprinkl'ins'	4.1 oz	140	5	24	80	0	2.0	0.0	5	13%
(Light n' Lively)	4.4 oz	140	5	27	70	0	1.0	1.0	5	7%
(New Country) 'Supreme'	6 oz	150	5	32	90	0	2.0	0.0	0	11%
(Yoplait)										
custard style	6 oz	180	7	30	95	0	4.0	0.0	20	20%
light	6 oz	90	5	16	70	0	0.0	0.0	5	0%
99% fat-free, original	6 oz	180	8	32	130	0	2.0	0.0	0	10%
triple cherry, 'Trix'	6 oz	190	9	31	120	0	3.0	0.0	0	14%
w/almonds, 'Breakfast'	6 oz	200	8	38	90	2	3.0	2.0	10	13%
CHERRY VANILLA										
(Dannon)										
'Light'	8 oz	100	9	18	135	0	0.0	0.0	5	0%
low-fat, 'Sprinkl'ins'	4.1 oz	140	5	24	95	0	2.0	0.0	5	13%
nonfat, light	8 oz	100	9	18	135	0	0.0	0.0	5	0%
(Lite-Line) 1% fat, 'Swiss Style'	1 cup	240	10	45	150	0	2.0	0.0	0	8%
(Yogi) w/gelatin, 'Sundae'	5.6 oz	50	6	14	75	0	1.0	0.0	4	10%
(Yoplait)										
light, custard style	6 oz	90	6	17	85	0	0.0	0.0	5	0%
parfait style	6 oz	200	8	34	120	0	3.0	0.0	0	14%
COFFEE										
(Bison) low-fat	1 cup	210	11	33	160	0	4.0	0.0	10	17%
(Dannon)	8 oz	200	10	34	140	0	3.0	0.0	10	13%
(Friendship) low-fat	1 cup	210	11	35	170	0	3.0	0.0	14	13%
CRANBERRY RASPBERRY										
(Weight Watchers) 'Ultimate 90'	1 cup	90	8	14	140	0	0.0	0.0	0	0%
FRUIT CRUNCH (New Country) low-fat	6 oz	150	5	30	90	0	2.0	0.0	0	11%
GRAPE										
(Dannon) lowfat, 'Sprinkl'ins'	4.1 oz	140	5	24	110	0	2.0	0.0	5	13%
(Light n' Lively)	4.4 oz	130	6	24	70	0	1.0	1.0	10	7%
LEMON										
(Alta Dena) fruit on the bottom	1 cup	240	12	40	150	0	4.0	0.0	0	15%
(Bison) low-fat	1 cup	210	11	33	160	0	4.0	0.0	10	17%
(Dannon)										
	8 oz	200	10	34	140	0	3.0	0.0	10	13%
low-fat	1 container	210	10	36	160	0	3.0	2.0	15	13%
(Knudsen) nonfat, 'Cal 70'	6 oz	70	6	12	125	0	0.0	0.0	0	0%
(Light n' Lively) nonfat, '100'	8 oz	100	9	16	150	0	0.0	0.0	5	0%
(Mountain High) natural	8 oz	220	10	31	140	0	6.0	0.0	0	25%
(New Country) 'Supreme'	6 oz	150	5	31	90	0	2.0	0.0	0	11%
(Yoplait) 99% fat-free, original	6 oz	180	8	32	130	0	2.0	0.0	0	10%

Food Name	Serving Size	Calories	Prot. gms	Carbs gms	Sod. mgs	Fiber gms	Fat gms	Sat. Fat gms	Chol. mgs	% Fat Cal.
LEMON CHIFFON										
(Dannon)										
blended	6 oz	150	8	30	110	0	0.0	0.0	5	0%
'Light'	8 oz	100	9	15	135	0	0.0	0.0	5	0%
(Weight Watchers) 'Ultimate 90'	1 cup	90	8	14	140	1	0.0	0.0	0	0%
(Yogi) w/gelatin, 'Sundae'	5.6 oz	50	6	14	75	0	1.0	0.0	4	10%
MIXED BERRIES										
(Alta Dena) blended	8 oz	190	8	39	140	0	1.0	0.0	0	5%
(Breyers) low-fat	8 oz	250	9	48	120	0	2.0	1.0	10	7%
(New Country) low-fat	6 oz	150	5	31	85	0	2.0	0.0	0	11%
(Yoplait) custard style	6 oz	180	7	30	95	0	4.0	0.0	20	20%
ORANGE										
(Dannon) low-fat	1 container	240	9	45	135	0	3.0	1.5	15	11%
(New Country) 'Supreme'	6 oz	150	5	31	90	0	2.0	0.0	0	11%
ORANGE-PINEAPPLE *(Yogi)* w/gelatin, 'Sundae'	5.6 oz	50	6	14	75	0	1.0	0.0	4	10%
PEACH										
(Alta Dena) fruit on the bottom	1 cup	240	12	40	150	0	4.0	0.0	0	15%
(Breyers) low-fat	8 oz	250	9	48	120	0	2.0	1.0	10	7%
(Carnation) fruit on the bottom, 'Smooth'n Creamy'	8 oz	250	8	47	130	0	3.0	0.0	0	11%
(Dannon)										
low-fat	1 container	240	9	45	140	1	3.0	1.5	15	11%
nonfat, light	8 oz	100	9	17	135	0	0.0	0.0	5	0%
(Knudsen) nonfat, 'Cal 70'	6 oz	70	6	11	95	0	0.0	0.0	0	0%
(Light n' Lively)										
. . . .	8 oz	240	9	46	120	0	2.0	1.0	15	8%
nonfat, '100'	8 oz	100	9	16	115	0	0.0	0.0	5	0%
(Lite-Line) 1% fat, 'Swiss Style'	1 cup	230	10	42	150	0	2.0	0.0	0	8%
(Mountain High) natural	8 oz	220	10	31	140	0	6.0	0.0	0	25%
(Weight Watchers) 'Ultimate 90'	1 cup	90	8	14	140	0	0.0	0.0	0	0%
(Yogi) peachy, w/gelatin, 'Sundae'	5.6 oz	50	6	14	75	0	1.0	0.0	4	10%
(Yoplait)										
99% fat-free, original	6 oz	180	8	32	130	0	2.0	0.0	0	10%
nonfat, light, custard style	6 oz	90	6	17	85	0	0.0	0.0	5	0%
nonfat, fruit on the bottom	6 oz	170	7	35	105	0	0.0	0.0	5	0%
nonfat, w/granola, 'Crunch 'N Yogurt'	7 oz	220	8	43	125	0	2.0	0.0	5	8%
PEACH AND VANILLA *(Yoplait)* parfait style	6 oz	200	8	34	120	0	3.0	0.0	0	14%
PEACHES AND CREAM *(New Country)* low-fat	6 oz	150	5	31	90	0	2.0	0.0	0	11%
PIÑA COLADA *(Yoplait)* 99% fat-free, original	6 oz	180	8	32	130	0	2.0	0.0	0	10%
PINEAPPLE										
(Breyers) low-fat	8 oz	250	9	50	120	0	2.0	1.0	10	7%
(Knudsen) nonfat, 'Cal 70'	6 oz	70	6	12	125	0	0.0	0.0	0	0%
(Light n' Lively)	8 oz	230	9	47	120	0	2.0	1.0	10	7%
(Yoplait) 99% fat-free, original	6 oz	180	8	32	130	0	2.0	0.0	0	10%
PLAIN										
(Alta Dena)	1 cup	100	13	13	160	0	1.0	0.0	0	8%
(Bison)										
low-fat	1 cup	150	12	17	180	0	4.0	0.0	10	24%
nonfat	1 cup	120	12	16	170	0	0.0	0.0	0	0%
(Breyers) low-fat	8 oz	140	12	16	170	0	3.0	2.0	20	19%
(Crowley)										
. . . .	1 cup	160	10	14	150	0	8.0	0.0	30	43%
low-fat	1 cup	140	12	17	180	0	2.0	0.0	10	13%
nonfat	1 cup	120	13	17	180	0	1.0	0.0	1	7%
(Dannon)										

Food Name	Serving Size	Calories	Prot. gms	Carbs gms	Sod. mgs	Fiber gms	Fat gms	Sat. Fat gms	Chol. mgs	% Fat Cal.
low-fat	8 oz	140	10	16	160	0	4.0	0.0	15	26%
nonfat	8 oz	110	11	16	160	0	0.0	0.0	5	0%
(Friendship) low-fat, 1.5% fat	1 cup	150	12	17	190	0	3.0	0.0	14	19%
(Knudsen)										
	8 oz	200	12	16	170	0	9.0	5.0	35	42%
low-fat	8 oz	160	12	17	180	0	5.0	1.0	25	28%
(Lite-Line) 1.5% fat, 'Swiss Style'	1 cup	140	12	18	150	0	2.0	0.0	0	13%
(Meadow Gold) low-fat, 2% milk fat	1 cup	160	12	16	160	0	5.0	0.0	0	29%
(Mountain High) plain	1 cup	200	12	16	140	0	9.0	0.0	0	42%
(Weight Watchers) 'Ultimate 90'	1 cup	90	8	14	150	0	0.0	0.0	0	0%
(White Wave) nondairy	1 serving	180	12	18	70	5	7.0	1.5	0	34%
(Yoplait)										
98% fat-free, original	6 oz	120	10	15	150	0	2.0	0.0	15	15%
nonfat	8 oz	120	13	18	160	0	0.0	0.0	5	0%
RAINBOW PUNCH (Yoplait) 'Trix'	6 oz	190	9	31	120	0	3.0	0.0	0	14%
RASPBERRIES AND CREAM										
(Weight Watchers) 'Ultimate 90'	1 cup	90	8	14	140	0	0.0	0.0	0	0%
RASPBERRY										
(Alta Dena)										
blended	8 oz	180	8	37	140	0	1.0	0.0	0	5%
fruit on the bottom	1 cup	240	12	40	150	0	4.0	0.0	0	15%
(Breyers) low-fat	8 oz	250	9	48	120	0	2.0	1.0	10	7%
(Dannon)										
low-fat	1 container	240	9	45	150	1	3.0	1.5	15	11%
nonfat, blended	6 oz	150	8	30	110	0	0.0	0.0	5	0%
nonfat, 'Light'	8 oz	100	9	18	135	0	0.0	0.0	5	0%
(Knudsen) nonfat, 'Cal 70'	6 oz	70	6	11	80	0	0.0	0.0	5	0%
(Light n' Lively)										
nonfat, '100'	8 oz	90	8	15	105	0	0.0	0.0	0	0%
red	8 oz	230	9	43	130	0	2.0	1.0	10	8%
red, nonfat, 'Free'	4.4 oz	50	4	8	60	0	0.0	0.0	0	0%
(Meadow Gold)										
low-fat, natural, 'Sundae Style'	1 cup	250	10	42	160	0	4.0	0.0	0	15%
red, low-fat, 1.5% milk fat	1 cup	250	10	42	160	0	4.0	0.0	0	15%
(Mountain High) natural, 'Honey Light'	8 oz	190	9	35	140	0	1.0	0.0	5	5%
(New Country) red, 'Supreme'	6 oz	150	5	31	90	0	2.0	0.0	0	11%
(Yoplait)										
light	6 oz	90	5	16	70	0	0.0	0.0	5	0%
99% fat-free, original	6 oz	180	8	32	130	0	2.0	0.0	0	10%
nonfat, fruit on the bottom	6 oz	170	7	35	105	0	0.0	0.0	5	0%
STRAWBERRY										
(Alta Dena)										
blended	8 oz	180	8	37	140	0	1.0	0.0	0	5%
fruit on the bottom	1 cup	240	12	40	150	0	4.0	0.0	0	15%
fruit on the bottom, 'Maya'	1 cup	280	11	39	170	0	9.0	0.0	0	29%
(Breyers)										
	8 oz	218	9	41	118	0	1.8	1.1	20	8%
low-fat	8 oz	250	9	48	120	0	2.0	1.0	10	7%
nonfat, w/aspartame and fructose sweeteners	8 oz container	125	8	22	102	0	0.5	0.2	11	3%
'Smooth & Creamy'	8 oz	232	9	45	125	1	2.0	1.1	20	8%
(Carnation) 'Smooth 'n Creamy'	8 oz	230	8	44	115	0	3.0	0.0	0	11%
(Crowley) nonfat	1 cup	190	12	35	190	0	1.0	0.0	1	5%
(Dannon)										
low-fat	1 container	240	9	46	135	1	3.0	1.5	15	11%

Food Name	Serving Size	Calories	Prot. gms	Carbs gms	Sod. mgs	Fiber gms	Fat gms	Sat. Fat gms	Chol. mgs	% Fat Cal.
low-fat, 'Sprinkl'ins'	4.1 oz	140	5	24	95	0	2.0	0.0	5	13%
nonfat, blended	6 oz	150	8	30	110	0	0.0	0.0	5	0%
nonfat, light	8 oz	100	9	17	135	0	0.0	0.0	5	0%
(Knudsen)										
low-fat	8 oz	250	10	45	135	0	4.0	2.0	15	14%
nonfat, 'Cal 70'	6 oz	70	6	11	85	0	0.0	0.0	0	0%
(Light n' Lively)										
	8 oz	240	9	45	130	0	2.0	2.0	15	8%
	4.4 oz	135	4	27	56	0	1.0	0.6	11	7%
nonfat	4.4 oz	70	4	12	55	0	0.0	0.0	0	0%
nonfat, '100'	8 oz	90	8	15	105	0	0.0	0.0	5	0%
(Lite-Line) low-fat, 1% fat	1 cup	240	10	46	150	0	2.0	0.0	0	7%
(Mountain High) natural, 'Honey Light'	8 oz	190	9	35	140	0	1.0	0.0	5	5%
(New Country) 'Supreme'	6 oz	150	5	30	90	0	2.0	0.0	0	11%
(Sara Lee) 'Free & Light'	1/10 pkg	120	2	26	90	0	1.0	0.0	0	7%
(Weight Watchers) 'Ultimate 90'	1 cup	90	8	14	140	2	0.0	0.0	0	0%
(White Wave) nondairy	1 serving	150	5	30	40	3	1.0	0.0	0	6%
(Yoplait) custard style	6 oz	180	7	30	105	0	3.0	0.0	0	15%
99% fat-free, original	6 oz	180	8	32	130	0	2.0	0.0	0	10%
nonfat, fruit on the bottom	6 oz	170	7	35	105	0	0.0	0.0	5	0%
nonfat, light	6 oz	90	5	16	70	0	0.0	0.0	5	0%
nonfat, light, custard style	6 oz	90	6	17	85	0	0.0	0.0	5	0%
STRAWBERRY AND VANILLA *(Yoplait)* parfait style	6 oz	200	8	34	120	0	3.0	0.0	0	14%
STRAWBERRY CHEESECAKE										
(Yogi) w/gelatin, 'Sundae'	5.6 oz	50	6	14	75	0	1.0	0.0	4	10%
STRAWBERRY FRUIT BASKET										
(Knudsen) nonfat, 'Cal 70'	6 oz	70	6	11	75	0	0.0	0.0	5	0%
STRAWBERRY FRUIT CUP										
(Dannon) light	8 oz	100	9	17	135	0	0.0	0.0	5	0%
(Light n' Lively)										
	8 oz	240	9	47	120	0	2.0	1.0	15	7%
nonfat, 'Free'	4.4 oz	50	4	8	55	0	0.0	0.0	0	0%
'100'	8 oz	90	8	15	100	0	0.0	0.0	0	0%
(New Country) low-fat	6 oz	150	5	30	85	0	2.0	0.0	0	11%
STRAWBERRY-ALMOND *(Yoplait)* 'Breakfast Yogurt'	6 oz	200	8	38	90	2	3.0	2.0	10	13%
STRAWBERRY-BANANA										
(Alta Dena) fruit on the bottom	1 cup	180	12	35	128	0	1.0	0.0	0	5%
(Breyers) low-fat	8 oz	250	9	50	120	0	2.0	1.0	10	7%
(Carnation) 'Smooth 'n Creamy'	8 oz	240	9	42	125	0	4.0	0.0	0	15%
(Dannon)										
light	8 oz	100	9	17	135	0	0.0	0.0	5	0%
low-fat	1 container	240	9	43	140	1	3.0	1.5	15	11%
low-fat, 'Sprinkl'ins'	4.1 oz	140	5	24	95	0	2.0	0.0	5	13%
(Knudsen) nonfat, 'Cal 70'	6 oz	70	6	12	80	0	0.0	0.0	0	0%
(Light n' Lively)										
	8 oz	260	9	52	120	0	2.0	1.0	10	7%
nonfat, 'Free'	4.4 oz	50	4	8	60	0	0.0	0.0	0	0%
(Mountain High) natural, 'Honey Light'	8 oz	190	9	35	140	0	1.0	0.0	5	5%
(New Country)	6 oz	150	5	31	85	0	2.0	0.0	0	11%
(Weight Watchers) 'Ultimate 90'	1 cup	90	8	14	140	2	0.0	0.0	0	0%
(Yoplait)										
bash, 'Trix'	6 oz	190	9	31	120	0	3.0	0.0	0	14%
fruit on the bottom	6 oz	170	7	35	105	0	0.0	0.0	5	0%
light	6 oz	90	5	16	70	0	0.0	0.0	5	0%

Food Name	Serving Size	Calories	Prot. gms	Carbs gms	Sod. mgs	Fiber gms	Fat gms	Sat. Fat gms	Chol. mgs	% Fat Cal.
99% fat-free, original	6 oz	180	8	32	130	0	2.0	0.0	0	10%
w/wheat and walnuts, 'Breakfast'	6 oz	200	8	40	110	0	2.0	0.0	0	9%
STRAWBERRY-RHUBARB (Yoplait)	6 oz	190	8	32	110	0	3.0	0.0	10	14%
TROPICAL FRUIT										
(Dannon) nonfat, light	8 oz	100	9	18	135	0	0.0	0.0	5	0%
(Weight Watchers) nonfat, 'Ultimate 90'	1 cup	90	10	13	120	0	0.0	0.0	5	0%
(Yoplait) w/wheat, raisin, nuts, 'Breakfast'	6 oz	200	8	41	110	0	3.0	0.0	0	12%
VANILLA										
(Bison) low-fat	1 cup	210	11	33	160	0	4.0	0.0	10	17%
(Breyers) low-fat	8 oz	230	11	41	150	0	3.0	2.0	20	11%
(Crowley) low-fat	1 cup	200	12	33	170	0	2.0	0.0	10	9%
(Dannon)										
French, fat-free, blended	3/4 cup	150	7	31	100	0	0.0	0.0	5	0%
low-fat	1 container	210	10	36	160	0	3.0	2.0	15	13%
nonfat, light	8 oz	100	9	16	135	0	0.0	0.0	5	0%
w/wheat, 'Hearty Nuts & Raisins'	8 oz	270	9	48	120	0	5.0	0.0	10	16%
(Friendship) low-fat	1 cup	210	11	35	170	0	3.0	0.0	14	13%
(Knudsen)										
low-fat	8 oz	240	11	43	135	0	4.0	2.0	15	14%
nonfat, 'Cal 70'	6 oz	70	6	11	90	0	0.0	0.0	0	0%
(New Country) French, low-fat	6 oz	150	5	31	90	0	2.0	0.0	0	11%
(Weight Watchers) 'Ultimate 90'	1 cup	90	8	14	140	0	0.0	0.0	0	0%
(White Wave) nondairy	1 serving	140	6	23	45	1	2.5	0.0	0	16%
(Yoplait)										
	6 oz	180	9	29	120	0	3.0	0.0	15	15%
custard style	6 oz	180	7	30	110	0	4.0	0.0	20	20%
fat-free	6 oz	150	8	28	110	0	0.0	0.0	5	0%
nonfat, light, custard style	6 oz	90	6	17	85	0	0.0	0.0	5	0%
nonfat, w/granola, 'Crunch 'N Yogurt'	7 oz	220	8	43	125	0	2.0	0.0	5	8%
WILD BERRY										
(Light n' Lively) low-fat, 1% milk fat, cultured	4.4 oz	140	5	28	70	0	1.0	1.0	5	6%
YOGURT, FROZEN										
(Alta Dena) apricot mango	4 oz	90	3	20	210	0	0.0	0.1	0	0%
(Ben & Jerry's)										
black raspberry swirl	1/2 cup	150	4	32	65	0	0.0	0.0	0	0%
cappuccino	1/2 cup	140	4	30	75	0	0.0	0.0	0	0%
chocolate	1/2 cup	130	3	29	50	1	0.0	0.0	0	0%
vanilla fudge swirl	1/2 cup	140	5	31	75	1	0.0	0.0	0	0%
(Bison) chocolate	3.5 oz	94	3	18	50	0	2.0	0.0	5	18%
(Breyers)										
black cherry	1/2 cup	120	3	24	50	0	1.0	0.0	10	8%
chocolate	1/2 cup	120	3	24	65	0	1.0	0.0	10	8%
peach	1/2 cup	110	3	22	50	0	1.0	0.0	10	8%
red raspberry	1/2 cup	120	3	23	50	0	1.0	0.0	10	8%
strawberry	1/2 cup	110	3	22	45	0	1.0	0.0	10	8%
strawberry-banana	1/2 cup	110	3	22	45	0	1.0	0.0	10	8%
vanilla	1/2 cup	120	3	23	55	0	1.0	0.0	15	8%
(Cascadian Farm)										
chocolate, organic	1/2 cup	105	4	20	54	1	2.0	1.0	7	16%
strawberry, organic	1/2 cup	102	4	19	57	1	1.0	0.0	6	9%
vanilla, organic	1/2 cup	109	4	20	65	0	2.0	1.0	7	16%
(Crowley)										
banana, soft-serve, 'Peaks of Perfection'	1/2 cup	100	3	19	50	0	2.0	0.0	5	17%
cherry	3 oz	80	2	16	40	0	1.0	0.0	5	11%

Food Name	Serving Size	Calories	Prot. gms	Carbs gms	Sod. mgs	Fiber gms	Fat gms	Sat. Fat gms	Chol. mgs	% Fat Cal.
chocolate	3 oz	80	2	15	40	0	2.0	0.0	10	21%
chocolate, soft-serve, 'Peaks of Perfection'	1/2 cup	100	4	19	60	0	2.0	0.0	5	16%
lemon, soft-serve, 'Peaks of Perfection'	1/2 cup	100	3	19	50	0	2.0	0.0	5	17%
peach	3 oz	80	2	16	40	0	1.0	0.0	5	11%
plain, 'Peaks of Perfection'	1/2 cup	90	2	20	40	0	1.0	0.0	5	9%
raspberry	3 oz	80	2	16	40	0	1.0	0.0	5	11%
raspberry, soft-serve, 'Peaks of Perfection'	1/2 cup	100	3	19	50	0	2.0	0.0	5	17%
strawberry	3 oz	80	2	16	40	0	1.0	0.0	5	11%
strawberry, soft-serve, 'Peaks of Perfection'	1/2 cup	100	3	19	50	0	2.0	0.0	5	17%
vanilla	3 oz	80	2	15	40	0	2.0	0.0	10	21%
vanilla, soft-serve, 'Peaks of Perfection'	3.5 oz	100	3	19	50	0	2.0	0.0	5	17%
(Dannon)										
blueberry, soft-serve	1/2 cup	100	3	18	50	0	2.0	0.0	5	18%
butter pecan, soft-serve	1/2 cup	100	3	18	55	0	2.0	0.0	5	18%
cappuccino, light	4 oz	80	4	19	70	0	0.0	0.0	0	0%
cappuccino, soft-serve	1/2 cup	100	3	18	55	0	2.0	0.0	5	18%
caramel pecan, 'Pure Indulgence'	4 oz	180	4	22	70	0	8.0	0.0	20	41%
cheesecake, soft-serve	1/2 cup	100	4	18	55	0	2.0	0.0	5	17%
chocolate, light	4 oz	80	4	19	70	0	1.0	0.0	0	9%
chocolate, 'Pure Indulgence'	3 oz	130	5	24	75	0	3.0	0.0	10	19%
chocolate, soft-serve	1/2 cup	120	5	23	65	0	2.0	0.0	5	14%
chocolate nut, chunky, 'Pure Indulgence'	4 oz	190	5	24	60	0	9.0	0.0	20	41%
cookies and cream, 'Pure Indulgence'	4 oz	180	4	18	95	0	7.0	0.0	20	42%
Heath Bar crunch, 'Pure Indulgence'	4 oz	170	4	25	100	0	7.0	0.0	25	35%
lemon meringue, soft-serve	1/2 cup	100	4	18	55	0	2.0	0.0	5	17%
mixed berry, low-fat	1 container	240	9	45	150	1	3.0	1.5	15	11%
peach, light	4 oz	80	4	19	70	0	0.0	0.0	0	0%
peach, soft-serve	1/2 cup	100	4	18	55	0	2.0	0.0	5	17%
piña colada, soft-serve	1/2 cup	100	4	18	55	0	2.0	0.0	5	17%
raspberry soft-serve	1/2 cup	100	3	18	50	0	2.0	0.0	5	18%
red raspberry	4 oz	90	3	21	65	0	0.0	0.0	0	0%
red raspberry, soft-serve, nonfat	1/2 cup	90	3	21	65	0	0.0	0.0	0	0%
strawberry, light	4 oz	80	4	19	70	0	0.0	0.0	0	0%
strawberry-banana	1/2 cup	100	3	18	50	0	2.0	0.0	5	18%
vanilla, 'Pure Indulgence'	3 oz	130	5	25	50	0	3.0	0.0	10	18%
vanilla, light	4 oz	80	4	20	70	0	0.0	0.0	0	0%
(Dreyers)										
blueberry, 'Inspirations'	3 oz	80	2	15	40	0	1.0	0.0	5	12%
cherry, 'Inspirations'	3 oz	80	2	15	40	0	1.0	0.0	5	12%
cherry vanilla, fat-free	1/2 cup	90	3	19	45	na	0.0	0.0	0	0%
cherry vanilla, nonfat, 'Inspirations'	4 oz	90	4	19	80	0	0.0	0.0	0	0%
chocolate, 'Inspirations'	3 oz	80	2	15	40	0	1.0	0.0	5	12%
(Dreyers) chocolate fudge, fat-free	1/2 cup	100	3	22	75	na	0.0	0.0	0	0%
'Perfectly Peach' 'Inspirations'	3 oz	80	2	15	40	0	1.0	0.0	5	12%
raspberry, 'Inspirations'	3 oz	80	2	15	40	0	1.0	0.0	5	12%
strawberry, 'Inspirations'	3 oz	80	2	15	40	0	1.0	0.0	5	12%
strawberry-banana, 'Inspirations'	3 oz	80	2	15	40	0	1.0	0.0	5	12%
vanilla, fat-free	1/2 cup	80	3	18	45	na	0.0	0.0	0	0%
vanilla and chocolate, fat-free	1/2 cup	80	3	18	65	na	0.0	0.0	0	0%
vanilla chocolate swirl, 'Inspirations'	4 oz	90	4	19	85	0	0.0	0.0	0	0%
vanilla raspberry swirl, 'Inspirations'	3 oz	80	2	15	45	0	1.0	0.0	5	12%
(Edys)										
cherry vanilla	1/2 cup	90	3	19	45	na	0.0	0.0	0	0%
chocolate fudge	1/2 cup	100	3	22	75	na	0.0	0.0	0	0%

Food Name	Serving Size	Calories	Prot. gms	Carbs gms	Sod. mgs	Fiber gms	Fat gms	Sat. Fat gms	Chol. mgs	% Fat Cal.
vanilla	1/2 cup	80	3	18	45	na	0.0	0.0	0	0%
vanilla and chocolate	1/2 cup	80	3	18	65	na	0.0	0.0	0	0%
(Elan) chocolate almond	1/2 cup	160	5	23	65	0	7.0	0.0	0	36%
(Haagen-Dazs)										
banana, soft-serve, nonfat	1 oz	25	1	5	15	0	0.0	0.0	0	0%
chocolate, soft-serve	1 oz	30	1	4	13	0	1.0	0.0	3	31%
chocolate, soft-serve, nonfat	1 oz	30	1	6	20	0	0.0	0.0	0	0%
peach	3 oz	120	4	20	30	0	3.0	1.5	31	22%
'Praline Pandemonium' 'Extras'	4 oz	240	7	33	115	0	9.0	4.0	45	34%
raspberry, soft-serve	1 oz	30	1	5	15	0	1.0	0.0	3	27%
strawberry	3 oz	120	4	21	30	0	3.0	1.6	29	21%
strawberry, soft-serve	1 oz	25	1	5	10	0	0.0	0.0	0	0%
strawberry, soft-serve, nonfat	1 oz	25	1	5	10	0	0.0	0.0	0	0%
'Strawberry Cheesecake Craze' 'Extras'	4 oz	210	7	31	100	0	7.0	3.0	50	29%
vanilla almond crunch	3 oz	150	5	22	65	0	5.0	1.5	33	29%
(Sealtest)										
black cherry, nonfat, 'Free'	1/2 cup	110	2	24	50	0	0.0	0.0	0	0%
chocolate, nonfat, 'Free'	1/2 cup	110	3	24	55	0	0.0	0.0	0	0%
peach, nonfat, 'Free'	1/2 cup	100	2	23	35	0	0.0	0.0	0	0%
red raspberry, nonfat, 'Free'	1/2 cup	100	2	23	40	0	0.0	0.0	0	0%
strawberry, nonfat, 'Free'	1/2 cup	100	2	22	35	0	0.0	0.0	0	0%
(Stars)										
butter pecan	1/2 cup	210	5	18	110	0	14.0	6.0	30	58%
cappuccino fudge, fruit-sweetened	1/2 cup	110	4	22	65	0	0.0	0.0	0	0%
carob-peppermint, nonfat, fruit-sweetened	1/2 cup	110	4	22	65	0	0.0	0.0	0	0%
chocolate	1/2 cup	170	5	20	70	0	8.0	5.0	30	42%
dark chocolate, nonfat, fruit sweetened	1/2 cup	110	4	23	55	0	0.0	0.0	0	0%
espresso almond fudge	1/2 cup	200	5	23	110	1	10.0	5.0	30	45%
fruit, nonfat, fruit-sweetened, 'Black Leopard'	1/2 cup	100	4	20	60	0	0.0	0.0	0	0%
mango raspberry, nonfat, fruit sweetened	1/2 cup	100	4	23	55	0	0.0	0.0	0	0%
mint chip	1/2 cup	210	5	18	110	0	14.0	6.0	30	58%
peanut butter cup	1/2 cup	200	5	23	110	1	10.0	5.0	30	45%
'Vanilla Bean'	1/2 cup	170	5	20	70	0	8.0	5.0	30	42%
'Very Berry Blueberry' nonfat,	1/2 cup	110	4	23	55	0	0.0	0.0	0	0%
(Stonyfield Farm)										
apricot mango, nonfat, natural	4 oz	110	5	22	70	0	0.0	0.0	5	0%
(Stonyfield Farm)										
chocolate mint chip	4 oz	140	6	24	75	5	3.0	3.0	5	18%
chocolate peanut butter swirl	4 oz	210	9	20	70	1	10.0	2.0	5	44%
chocolate walnut amaretto	4 oz	150	7	21	80	1	5.0	1.0	5	29%
coffee, French roast, decaffeinated	4 oz	100	6	20	85	0	0.0	0.0	5	0%
coffee hazelnut fudge	4 oz	150	6	23	80	1	4.0	0.0	5	24%
'Double Raspberry'	4 oz	120	5	25	65	0	0.0	0.0	0	0%
'Double Strawberry'	4 oz	100	5	21	65	0	0.0	0.0	5	0%
Dutch chocolate, nonfat	4 oz	110	6	21	80	0	0.0	0.0	5	0%
mocha fudge, nonfat	4 oz	120	5	24	85	0	0.0	0.0	5	0%
'Very Vanilla'	4 oz	100	6	20	80	0	0.0	0.0	5	0%
(TCBY Treats)										
all flavors, regular	1/2 cup	140	4	23	60	0	3.0	2.0	15	20%
all flavors, hand-dipped, 96% nonfat	1/2 cup	110	3	22	65	1	2.5	1.0	5	18%
all flavors, hand-dipped, nonfat	1/2 cup	100	3	22	55	1	0.0	0.0	0	0%
all flavors, nonfat, no sugar added	1/2 cup	80	4	20	35	0	0.0	0.0	0	0%
all flavors, soft-serve, nonfat	1/2 cup	110	4	23	60	0	0.0	0.0	0	0%

Food Name	Serving Size	Calories	Prot. gms	Carbs gms	Sod. mgs	Fiber gms	Fat gms	Sat. Fat gms	Chol. mgs	% Fat Cal.
(Yoplait)										
caramel turtle fudge	1/2 cup	120	2	24	105	0	2.0	1.0	5	15%
chocolate fudge brownie	1/2 cup	110	3	24	75	1	1.5	0.5	5	11%
mixed berry	6 oz	180	8	32	130	0	2.0	0.0	0	10%
vanilla	1/2 cup	100	3	20	70	0	1.5	1.0	5	13%
YOGURT BAR, FROZEN										
(Cascadian Farm)										
blackberry, organic	1 bar	80	3	14	45	1	1.0	0.5	5	12%
chocolate, organic	1 bar	80	3	15	40	1	1.5	1.0	5	16%
vanilla, organic	1 bar	80	3	15	50	0	1.0	0.5	5	11%
(Dole)										
cherry, 'Fruit & Yogurt'	1 bar	80	2	17	22	0	1.0	0.0	0	11%
raspberry, 'Fruit & Yogurt'	1 bar	70	1	17	18	0	1.0	0.0	0	11%
strawberry, 'Fruit & Yogurt'	1 bar	70	1	17	16	0	1.0	0.0	0	11%
(Haagen-Dazs)										
peach	1 bar	100	2	18	20	0	1.0	1.0	15	10%
'Strawberry Daiquiri'	1 bar	100	2	20	20	0	1.0	1.0	20	9%
'Tropical Orange Passion'	1 bar	100	2	21	30	0	1.0	1.0	20	9%
(Yoplait)										
'Vanilla Orange Creme', lowfat	1 bar	30	1	8	25	0	0.5	0.0	0	11%
vanilla/chocolate/strawberry, w/dark chocolate coating	1 bar	110	2	11	35	0	6.0	5.0	5	51%
YOGURT DRINK. See under SPORTS AND DIET/NUTRITION DRINKS.										
YOKAN	1 oz	74	0.9	17.2	24	0	(tr)	0.0		0%
YUCA. See CASSAVA.										

Z

Food Name	Serving Size	Calories	Prot. gms	Carbs gms	Sod. mgs	Fiber gms	Fat gms	Sat. Fat gms	Chol. mgs	% Fat Cal.
ZANTE CURRANT. See under CURRANT.										
ZITI. See under PASTA.										
ZITI DISH/ENTRÉE. See under PASTA DISH/ENTRÉE.										
ZUCCHINI										
Canned, Italian style *(Progresso)*	1/2 cup	50	1	8	540	2	2.0	1.0	1	33%
Fresh										
baby, raw, whole	1 large	3	0	0	0	0	0.1	0.0	0	16%
baby, raw, whole	1 medium	2	0	0	0	0	0.0	0.0	0	16%
w/skin, boiled, drained, mashed	1/2 cup	19	1	5	4	2	0.1	0.0	0	3%
w/skin, boiled, drained, sliced	1 cup	29	1	7	5	3	0.1	0.0	0	3%
w/skin, raw, chopped	1 cup	17	1	4	4	1	0.2	0.0	0	8%
w/skin, raw, sliced	1 cup	16	1	3	3	1	0.2	0.0	0	8%
w/skin, raw, whole	1 large	45	4	9	10	4	0.5	0.1	0	8%
w/skin, raw, whole	1 medium	27	2	6	6	2	0.3	0.1	0	8%
w/skin, raw, whole	1 small	17	1	3	4	1	0.2	0.0	0	8%
Frozen										
(Seabrook)	3.3 oz	16	1	3	2	1	0.0	0.0	0	0%
(Southern)	3.5 oz	18	1	4	20	0	0.1	0.0	0	4%
breaded, kosher *(Empire Kosher)*	1 piece	100	5	18	280	1	0.0	0.0	0	0%
breaded, 'Quick Krisp' *(Stilwell)*	3.3 oz	200	4	24	410	0	10.0	0.0	15	45%
sliced *(Flav-R-Pac)*	2/3 cup	15	1	2	15	1	0.0	0.0	0	0%
w/skin, boiled, drained	1 cup	38	3	8	4	3	0.3	0.1	0	6%
w/skin, unprepared	3-lb pkg	231	16	49	27	18	1.8	0.4	0	6%
w/skin, unprepared	10-oz pkg	48	3	10	6	4	0.4	0.1	0	6%

PART TWO

VITAMIN AND MINERAL VALUES

Vitamin A • Thiamine • Riboflavin • Niacin •
Vitamin B_6 • Folic Acid • Vitamin B_{12} • Vitamin C •
Calcium • Iron • Magnesium • Potassium • Zinc •

A

Food Name	Serving Size	A I.U.	Thi mg	Rib mg	Nia mg	B₆ mg	Fol mcg	B₁₂ mcg	C mg	Calc mg	Iron mg	Mag mg	Pot mg	Zn mg
ABALONE														
mixed species, fried	3 oz	4	0.19	0.11	1.60	0.13	11.9	0.59	1.5	31.4	3.2	47.6	241	0.8
mixed species, raw	3 oz	4	0.16	0.01	1.30	0.13	4.3	0.62	1.7	26.4	2.7	40.8	213	0.7
ABALONE MUSHROOM. See MUSHROOM, OYSTER.														
ACEROLA, RAW / Barbados cherry / Puerto Rican cherry / West Indian cherry														
raw, trimmed	1 fruit	37	0.00	0.00	0.00	0.00	0.67	0.00	80.5	0.6	0.0	0.9	7	0.0
raw, untrimmed	1 cup	752	0.00	0.01	0.39	0.00	13.7	0.00	1644.0	11.8	0.2	17.6	143	0.1
ACEROLA JUICE														
	1 cup	1232	0.01	0.14	0.97	0.00	33.9	0.00	3872.0	24.2	1.2	29.0	235	0.2
	1 fl oz	154	0.00	0.00	0.12	0.00	4.2	0.00	483.0	3.0	0.2	3.6	29	0.0
ACORN														
dried	1 oz	0	0.00	0.00	0.68	0.20	32.5	0.00	0.0	15.3	0.3	23.2	201	0.2
raw	1 oz	11	0.00	0.00	0.52	0.15	24.7	0.00	0.0	11.6	0.2	17.6	153	0.1
ACORN FLOUR. See under FLOUR.														
ACORN SQUASH. See SQUASH, ACORN.														
ADZUKI BEAN. See BEAN, ADZUKI.														
AGAR. See under SEA VEGETABLE.														
AHI. See under TUNA.														
AKU. See under TUNA.														
ALASKA KING CRAB. See under CRAB.														
ALCOHOLIC BEVERAGES. See BEER AND MALT LIQUOR; COCKTAIL; COCKTAIL MIXER; LIQUEUR; and individual listings.														
ALFALFA SEEDS														
sprouted, raw	1 cup	51	0.00	0.00	0.16	0.00	11.9	0.00	2.7	10.6	0.3	8.9	26	0.3
sprouted, raw	1 tbsp	5	0.00	0.00	0.00	0.00	1.1	0.00	0.3	1.0	0.0	0.8	2	<0.1
ALGAE, spirulina, dried	1 cup	86	0.36	0.55	1.90	0.01	14.1	0.00	1.5	18.0	4.3	29.3	204	0.3
ALLSPICE														
ground	1 tbsp	32	0.00	0.00	0.17	0.00	2.2	0.00	2.4	39.6	0.4	8.1	62	<0.1
ground	1 tsp	10	0.00	0.00	0.01	0.00	0.7	0.00	0.8	12.6	0.1	2.6	20	<0.1
ALMOND														
ground	1 cup	10	0.23	0.77	3.70	0.12	27.6	0.00	0.0	236.0	4.1	261.0	692	3.2
whole kernels	1 almond	<1	0.00	0.00	0.01	0.00	0.4	0.00	0.0	3.0	<1.0	3.3	9	<0.1
whole kernels, approx 24	1 oz	3	0.01	0.23	1.10	0.00	8.2	0.00	0.0	70.3	1.2	78.0	206	1.0
Blanched														
	1 oz	2	0.01	0.16	1.00	0.00	8.5	0.00	0.0	61.2	1.1	78.0	195	0.9
	1 tbsp	<1	0.00	0.01	0.33	0.00	2.7	0.00	0.0	19.7	0.3	25.0	63	0.3
whole kernels	1 cup	10	0.29	0.81	5.30	0.17	43.5	0.00	0.0	313.0	5.4	399.0	996	4.5
Dry-roasted														
whole kernels, salted	1 cup	1	0.10	1.20	5.30	0.17	45.5	0.00	0.0	367.0	6.2	395.0	1029	4.9
whole kernels, salted, approx 22	1 oz	<1	0.00	0.24	1.10	0.00	9.4	0.00	0.0	75.4	1.3	81.1	211	1.0
whole kernels, unsalted	1 cup	1	0.10	1.20	5.30	0.17	45.5	0.00	0.0	367.0	6.2	395.0	1029	4.9
whole kernels, unsalted, approx 22	1 oz	<1	0.00	0.24	1.10	0.00	9.4	0.00	0.0	75.4	1.3	81.1	211	1.0
Honey-roasted														
unblanched	1 oz	0	0.00	0.27	0.80	0.00	9.1	0.00	0.2	74.6	0.8	68.0	159	0.7
unblanched, whole kernels	1 cup	0	0.16	1.40	4.10	0.12	46.1	0.00	1.0	379.0	4.1	346.0	806	3.7
Oil-roasted w/salt														
whole kernels, salted	1 cup	2	0.14	1.20	5.80	0.19	42.4	0.00	0.0	457.0	5.8	430.0	1097	4.8
whole kernels, salted, approx 22	1 oz	<1	0.00	0.22	1.00	0.00	7.7	0.00	0.0	82.5	1.0	77.7	198	0.9
whole kernels, unsalted	1 cup	2	0.14	1.20	5.80	0.19	42.4	0.00	0.0	457.0	5.8	430.0	1097	4.8
whole kernels, unsalted, approx 22	1 oz	<1	0.00	0.22	1.00	0.00	7.7	0.00	0.0	82.5	1.0	77.7	198	0.9

Food Name	Serving Size	A I.U.	Thi mg	Rib mg	Nia mg	B_6 mg	Fol mcg	B_{12} mcg	C mg	Calc mg	Iron mg	Mag mg	Pot mg	Zn mg
Unblanched														
sliced	1 cup	10	0.23	0.77	3.70	0.12	27.6	0.00	0.0	236.0	4.1	261.0	692	3.2
slivered	1 cup	11	0.26	0.88	4.20	0.14	31.3	0.00	0.0	268.0	4.6	297.0	786	3.6
whole	1 cup	14	0.34	1.20	5.60	0.19	41.2	0.00	0.0	352.0	6.1	391.0	1034	4.8
ALMOND BUTTER														
plain, salted	1 cup	0	0.33	1.50	7.20	0.19	163.0	0.00	1.8	675.0	9.3	758.0	1895	7.6
plain, salted	1 tbsp	0	0.00	0.10	0.46	0.00	10.4	0.00	0.1	43.2	0.6	48.5	121	0.5
plain, unsalted	1 cup	0	0.33	1.50	7.20	0.19	163.0	0.00	1.8	675.0	9.3	758.0	1895	7.6
plain, unsalted	1 tbsp	0	0.00	0.10	0.46	0.00	10.4	0.00	0.1	43.2	0.6	48.5	121	0.5
ALMOND OIL														
	1 cup	0	0.00	0.00	0.00	0.00	0.0	0.00	0.00	0.0	0.0	0.0	0	0.0
	1 tbsp	0	0.00	0.00	0.00	0.00	0.0	0.00	0.00	0.0	0.0	0.0	0	0.0
ALMOND PASTE														
	1 oz	<1	0.00	0.12	0.40	0.00	20.7	0.00	0.00	48.8	0.5	36.9	89	0.4
firmly packed	1 cup	5	0.19	0.94	3.20	0.01	166.0	0.00	0.2	390.0	3.6	295.0	713	3.4
AMARANTH	1 cup	0	0.16	0.41	2.50	0.44	95.5	0.00	8.2	298.0	14.8	519.0	714	6.2
AMARANTH LEAVES														
boiled, drained	1 cup	3656	0.00	0.18	0.74	0.23	75.0	0.00	54.3	276.0	3.0	72.6	846	1.2
raw	1 cup	817	0.00	0.00	0.18	0.01	23.9	0.00	12.1	60.2	0.7	15.4	171	0.3
	1 med leaf	408	0.00	0.00	0.01	0.00	11.9	0.00	6.1	30.1	0.3	7.7	86	0.1
AMERICAN BUFFALO. See BISON.														
ANCHO PEPPER. See PEPPER, ANCHO.														
ANCHOVY														
Canned														
European, in oil, boneless, drained	1 oz	20	0.00	0.10	5.60	0.01	3.5	0.25	0.0	65.8	1.3	19.6	154	0.7
European, in oil, drained	2 oz	32	0.00	0.16	9.00	0.01	5.6	0.40	0.0	104.0	2.1	31.1	245	1.1
European, in oil, drained	5 medium	14	0.00	0.01	4.00	0.00	2.5	0.18	0.0	46.4	0.9	13.8	109	0.5
European, in oil, drained	1 medium	3	0.00	0.00	0.80	0.00	0.5	0.00	0.0	9.3	0.2	2.8	22	0.1
Fresh, European, raw	3 oz	43	0.01	0.22	11.90	0.12	7.5	0.53	0.0	125.0	2.8	34.9	326	1.5
ANGLER FISH. See MONKFISH.														
ANISE SEED														
	1 tbsp	21	0.00	0.00	0.20	0.00	0.7	0.00	1.4	43.3	2.5	11.4	97	0.4
	1 tsp	7	0.00	0.00	0.01	0.00	0.2	0.00	0.4	13.6	0.8	3.6	30	0.1
ANTELOPE														
raw	1 oz	0	0.01	0.16	na	na	na	na	0.0	0.9	0.9	7.7	100	0.4
roasted	3 oz	0	0.22	0.62	na	na	na	na	0.0	3.4	3.6	23.8	316	1.4
roasted, boneless, yield from 1 lb raw	11.9 oz	0	0.88	2.50	na	na	na	na	0.0	13.6	14.3	95.2	1265	5.7
APPLE														
Canned, sweetened slices, drained	1 cup	104	0.00	0.00	0.15	0.01	0.6	0.00	0.8	8.2	0.5	4.1	139	<0.1
Dehydrated, sulfured														
low moisture, stewed	1 cup	37	0.00	0.01	0.27	0.10	0.2	0.00	1.2	7.7	0.8	9.7	262	0.1
low moisture, uncooked	1 cup	49	0.00	0.01	0.41	0.17	0.6	0.00	1.3	11.4	1.2	13.2	384	0.2
rings, uncooked	1 ring	0	0.00	0.00	0.01	0.00	0.0	0.00	0.3	0.9	<0.1	1.0	29	0.0
stewed	1 cup	43	0.00	0.01	0.33	0.13	0.0	0.00	2.5	7.7	0.8	10.2	268	0.1
uncooked	1 cup	0	0.00	0.14	0.80	0.11	0.0	0.00	3.4	12.0	1.2	13.8	387	0.2
Fresh														
boiled, peeled, sliced	1 cup	75	0.00	0.00	0.16	0.01	1.0	0.00	0.3	8.6	0.3	5.1	150	<0.1
microwaved, peeled, sliced	1 cup	68	0.00	0.00	0.10	0.01	1.0	0.00	0.5	8.5	0.3	5.1	158	<0.1
raw, peeled, quartered or chopped	1 cup	66	0.00	0.00	0.10	0.01	3.5	0.00	7.1	8.8	0.2	6.3	144	<0.1
raw, peeled, sliced	1 cup	48	0.00	0.00	0.10	0.01	0.4	0.00	4.4	4.4	<0.1	3.3	124	0.0
raw, peeled, whole, medium, approx														
3 per lb	1 apple	56	0.00	0.00	0.12	0.01	0.5	0.00	5.1	5.1	<0.1	3.8	145	<0.1
raw, unpeeled, sliced	1 cup	58	0.00	0.00	0.01	0.01	3.1	0.00	6.3	7.7	0.2	5.5	127	0.0

Food Name	Serving Size	A I.U.	Thi mg	Rib mg	Nia mg	B_6 mg	Fol mcg	B_{12} mcg	C mg	Calc mg	Iron mg	Mag mg	Pot mg	Zn mg
raw, unpeeled, whole, large, approx 2 per lb	1 large	112	0.00	0.00	0.16	0.10	5.9	0.00	12.1	14.8	0.4	10.6	244	<0.1
raw, unpeeled, whole, medium, approx 3 per lb	1 medium	73	0.00	0.00	0.11	0.01	3.9	0.00	7.9	9.7	0.3	6.9	159	<0.1
raw, unpeeled, whole, small, approx 4 per lb	1 small	56	0.00	0.00	0.01	0.01	3.0	0.00	6.0	7.4	0.2	5.3	122	0.0
Frozen, unsweetened	1 cup	59	0.00	0.00	0.01	0.01	1.2	0.00	0.2	6.9	0.3	5.2	133	<0.1
APPLE BUTTER														
	1 cup	333	0.01	0.01	0.32	0.14	2.8	0.00	2.0	39.5	0.9	14.1	257	0.2
	1 tbsp	20	0.00	0.00	0.00	0.00	0.2	0.00	0.1	2.4	<0.1	0.9	16	0.0
APPLE JUICE														
Canned, bottled or boxed														
unsweetened	8.45 fl oz	3	0.01	0.01	0.26	0.01	0.3	0.00	2.4	18.3	1.0	7.9	312	<0.1
unsweetened	1 cup	3	0.01	0.00	0.25	0.01	0.3	0.00	2.2	17.4	0.9	7.4	295	<0.1
unsweetened	1 fl oz	<1	0.00	0.00	0.00	0.00	0.0	0.00	0.3	2.2	0.1	0.9	37	0.0
unsweetened, w/added vitamin C	1 cup	3	0.01	0.00	na	0.01	0.3	0.00	103.0	17.4	0.9	7.4	295	<0.1
unsweetened, w/added vitamin C	1 fl oz	<1	0.00	0.00	na	0.00	0.0	0.00	12.9	2.2	0.1	0.9	37	0.0
Chilled or frozen														
concentrate, prepared	1 cup	0	0.00	0.00	0.01	0.01	0.7	0.00	1.4	14.3	0.6	11.9	301	0.1
concentrate, prepared	1 fl oz	0	0.00	0.00	0.00	0.00	<0.1	0.00	0.2	1.8	<0.1	1.5	38	0.0
concentrate, wadded vitamin C, prepared	1 cup	0	0.00	0.00	0.01	0.01	0.7	0.00	59.8	14.3	0.6	11.9	301	0.1
concentrate, w/added vitamin C, prepared	1 fl oz	0	0.00	0.00	0.00	0.00	<0.1	0.00	7.5	1.8	<0.1	1.5	38	0.0
concentrate, w/added vitamin C, undiluted	6 fl oz	0	0.00	0.11	0.28	0.25	2.1	0.00	188.0	42.2	1.9	35.9	945	0.3
APRICOT														
Canned														
halves, peeled, in extra light syrup, w/liquid	1 cup	3139	0.01	0.01	1.50	0.13	4.2	0.00	9.9	24.7	0.7	14.8	346	0.2
halves, peeled, in heavy syrup, w/liquid	1 cup	3173	0.01	0.01	0.97	0.14	4.4	0.00	8.0	23.2	0.8	18.1	361	0.3
halves, unpeeled, in heavy syrup, w/liquid	1/2 apricot	492	0.00	0.00	0.15	0.00	0.7	0.00	1.2	3.6	0.1	2.8	56	0.0
halves, unpeeled, in juice, w/liquid	1 cup	4126	0.00	0.01	0.84	0.13	4.1	0.00	12.0	29.3	0.7	24.4	403	0.3
halves, unpeeled, in juice, w/liquid	1/2 apricot	609	0.00	0.00	0.12	0.00	0.6	0.00	1.8	4.3	0.1	3.6	59	0.0
halves, unpeeled, in light syrup, w/liquid	1 cup	3345	0.00	0.01	0.77	0.14	4.3	0.00	6.8	27.8	1.0	20.2	349	0.3
halves, unpeeled, in light syrup, w/liquids	1/2 apricot	529	0.00	0.00	0.12	0.00	0.7	0.00	1.1	4.4	0.2	3.2	55	0.0
halves, unpeeled, in water, w/liquid	1 cup	3142	0.01	0.01	0.96	0.13	4.1	0.00	8.3	19.4	0.8	17.0	467	0.3
halves, unpeeled, in water, w/liquid	1/2 apricot	465	0.00	0.00	0.14	0.00	0.6	0.00	1.2	2.9	0.1	2.5	69	0.0
whole, peeled, in extra heavy syrup, w/liquid	1 cup	3619	0.00	0.01	0.84	0.13	3.9	0.00	5.9	19.7	1.5	19.7	310	0.3
whole, peeled, pitted, in heavy syrup, w/liquid	1 cup	3199	0.01	0.01	1.10	0.14	4.4	0.00	7.2	23.2	1.1	20.6	346	0.3
whole, peeled, pitted, in water, w/liquid	1 cup	4109	0.01	0.01	0.99	0.12	3.9	0.00	4.1	18.2	1.2	20.4	350	0.3
whole, unpeeled, in heavy syrup, w/liquid	1 cup	2952	0.01	0.01	0.90	0.13	4.1	0.00	7.4	21.6	0.7	16.8	336	0.3
Dehydrated, sulfured														
halves, stewed	1 cup	5908	0.00	0.01	2.40	0.28	0.0	0.00	4.0	40.0	4.2	42.5	1223	0.7
halves, uncooked	1 cup	9412	0.00	0.20	3.90	0.20	13.4	0.00	3.1	58.5	6.1	61.1	1791	1.0
low moisture, stewed	1 cup	10973	0.00	0.17	4.10	0.40	3.7	0.00	17.7	59.8	6.2	62.3	1813	1.0
low moisture, uncooked	1 cup	15076	0.01	0.18	4.30	0.62	5.2	0.00	11.3	72.6	7.5	75.0	2202	1.2
sweetened, halves, stewed	1 cup	5775	0.00	0.01	2.30	0.28	0.0	0.00	3.8	40.5	4.1	40.5	1196	0.7

Food Name	Serving Size	A I.U.	Thi mg	Rib mg	Nia mg	B₆ mg	Fol mcg	B₁₂ mcg	C mg	Calc mg	Iron mg	Mag mg	Pot mg	Zn mg
uncooked	1 half	253	0.00	0.00	0.11	0.00	0.4	0.00	<0.1	1.6	0.2	1.6	48	0.0
Fresh														
raw, whole	1 apricot	914	0.00	0.00	0.21	0.00	3.0	0.00	3.5	4.9	0.2	2.8	104	<0.1
raw, halves	1 cup	4049	0.01	0.01	0.93	0.01	13.3	0.00	15.5	21.7	0.8	12.4	459	0.4
raw, sliced	1 cup	4310	0.01	0.01	0.99	0.01	14.2	0.00	16.5	23.1	0.9	13.2	488	0.4
Frozen, sweetened	1 cup	4066	0.01	0.10	1.90	0.14	4.1	0.00	21.8	24.2	2.2	21.8	554	0.2
APRICOT KERNEL OIL														
	1 cup	0	0.00	0.00	0.00	0.00	0.0	0.00	0.0	0.0	0.0	0.0	0	0.0
	1 tbsp	0	0.00	0.00	0.00	0.00	0.0	0.00	0.0	0.0	0.0	0.0	0	0.0
ARROWHEAD														
boiled, drained	1 medium	0	0.00	0.00	0.14	0.00	1.1	0.00	0.0	0.8	0.1	5.9	106	0.0
raw	1 large	0	0.00	0.00	0.41	0.01	3.5	0.00	0.3	2.5	0.6	12.8	231	<0.1
raw	1 medium	0	0.00	0.00	0.20	0.00	1.7	0.00	0.1	1.2	0.3	6.1	111	0.0
ARROWROOT FLOUR. See under FLOUR.														
ARROWROOT														
raw, sliced	1 cup	23	0.17	0.01	2.00	0.32	406.0	0.00	2.3	7.2	2.7	30.0	545	0.8
raw, whole	1 med root	6	0.01	0.00	0.56	0.01	112.0	0.00	0.6	2.0	0.7	8.3	150	0.2
ARTICHOKE. See also ARTICHOKE, JERUSALEM.														
Fresh														
globe or French, boiled, drained	1 medium	212	0.01	0.01	1.20	0.13	61.2	0.00	12.0	54.0	1.5	72.0	425	0.6
globe or French, hearts, boiled, drained	1/2 cup	149	0.01	0.01	0.84	0.01	42.8	0.00	8.4	37.8	1.1	50.4	297	0.4
globe or French, raw	1 large	300	0.12	0.11	1.70	0.19	110.0	0.00	19.0	71.3	2.1	97.2	599	0.8
globe or French, raw	1 medium	237	0.01	0.01	1.30	0.15	87.0	0.00	15.0	56.3	1.6	76.8	474	0.6
Frozen														
globe or French, unprepared	9-oz pkg	393	0.15	0.36	2.20	0.21	320.0	0.00	13.5	48.5	1.3	68.8	632	0.8
globe or French, drained	9-oz pkg	394	0.15	0.38	2.20	0.21	285.0	0.00	12.0	50.4	1.3	74.4	634	0.9
globe or French, drained	1 cup	276	0.10	0.27	1.50	0.15	200.0	0.00	8.4	35.3	0.9	52.1	444	0.6
globe or French, no salt added, drained	1 cup	276	0.10	0.27	1.50	0.15	200.0	0.00	8.4	35.3	0.9	52.1	444	0.6
globe or French, no salt added, drained	9-oz pkg	394	0.15	0.38	2.20	0.21	285.0	0.00	12.0	50.4	1.3	74.4	634	0.9
ARTICHOKE, JERUSALEM / sunchoke														
raw, sliced	1 cup	30	0.30	0.01	1.90	0.12	20.1	0.00	6.0	21.0	5.1	25.5	644	0.2
ARUGULA / rucola / rugula														
raw	1/2 cup	237	0.00	0.00	0.00	0.00	9.7	0.00	1.5	16.0	0.2	4.7	37	<0.1
raw	1 leaf	48	0.00	0.00	0.00	0.00	1.9	0.00	0.3	3.2	0.0	0.9	7	0
ASIAN PEAR / Chinese pear / sand pear														
raw, whole, approx 2.25 x 2.5 inch diam	1 fruit	0	0.00	0.00	0.27	0.00	9.8	0.00	4.6	4.9	0.0	9.8	148	0
raw, whole, approx 3-3/8 x 3 inch diam	1 fruit	0	0.00	0.00	0.60	0.01	22.0	0.00	10.4	11.0	0.0	22.0	333	<0.1
ASPARAGUS														
Canned														
cuts, drained	1 cup	1285	0.15	0.24	2.30	0.27	231.0	0.00	44.5	38.7	4.4	24.2	416	1.0
cuts, no salt added, w\liquid	1/2 cup	642	0.01	0.11	1.00	0.12	104.0	0.00	20.1	18.3	0.7	11.0	210	0.6
cuts, w/liquid	1/2 cup	642	0.01	0.11	1.00	0.12	104.0	0.00	20.1	18.3	0.7	11.0	210	0.6
spears, drained, approx 5-inch long	1 spear	96	0.00	0.00	0.17	0.00	17.2	0.00	3.3	2.9	0.3	1.8	31	<0.1
Fresh														
cuts, boiled, drained, chopped	1/2 cup	485	0.11	0.11	0.97	0.11	131.0	0.00	9.7	18.0	0.7	9.0	144	0.4
cuts, raw	1 cup	781	0.19	0.17	1.60	0.18	172.0	0.00	17.7	28.1	1.2	24.1	366	0.6
spear tips, raw, 2 inches long or less	1 tip	20	0.00	0.00	0.00	0.00	4.5	0.00	0.5	0.7	0.0	0.6	10	0.0
spears, boiled, drained, 1/2-inch diam	4 spears	323	0.01	0.01	0.65	0.01	87.6	0.00	6.5	12.0	0.4	6.0	96	0.3
spears, raw, extra large, 8.75 to 10 inches	1 spear	140	0.00	0.00	0.28	0.00	30.7	0.00	3.2	5.0	0.2	4.3	66	0.1
spears, raw, large, 7.25 to 8.5 inches	1 spear	117	0.00	0.00	0.23	0.00	25.6	0.00	2.6	4.2	0.2	3.6	55	<0.1
spears, raw, medium, 5.25 to 7 inches	1 spear	93	0.00	0.00	0.19	0.00	20.5	0.00	2.1	3.4	0.1	2.9	44	<0.1
spears, raw, small, 5 inches long or less	1 spear	70	0.00	0.00	0.14	0.00	15.4	0.00	1.6	2.5	0.1	2.2	33	<0.1

Food Name	Serving Size	A I.U.	Thi mg	Rib mg	Nia mg	B$_6$ mg	Fol mcg	B$_{12}$ mcg	C mg	Calc mg	Iron mg	Mag mg	Pot mg	Zn mg
Frozen														
cuts, boiled, drained	1 cup	1472	0.12	0.19	1.90	0.00	242.0	0.00	43.9	41.4	1.2	23.4	392	1.0
cuts, no salt added, boiled, drained	1 cup	1472	0.12	0.19	1.90	0.00	242.0	0.00	43.9	41.4	1.2	23.4	392	1.0
cuts, unprepared	10-oz pkg	2692	0.34	0.37	3.40	0.32	542.0	0.00	90.3	71.0	2.1	39.8	719	1.7
spears, boiled, drained	10-oz pkg	2397	0.19	0.30	3.00	0.01	395.0	0.00	71.5	67.4	1.9	38.1	639	1.6
spears, boiled, drained	4 spears	491	0.00	0.01	0.62	0.00	80.8	0.00	14.6	13.8	0.4	7.8	131	0.3
spears, no salt added, boiled, drained	10-oz pkg	2397	0.19	0.30	3.00	0.01	395.0	0.00	71.5	67.4	1.9	38.1	639	1.6
spears, no salt added, boiled, drained	4 spears	491	0.00	0.01	0.62	0.00	80.8	0.00	14.6	13.8	0.4	7.8	131	0.3
spears, unprepared	4 spears	550	0.01	0.01	0.70	0.01	111.0	0.00	18.4	14.5	0.4	8.1	147	0.3
ATLANTIC COD. See under COD.														
ATLANTIC MACKEREL. See under MACKEREL.														
ATLANTIC OCEAN PERCH. See OCEAN PERCH.														
ATLANTIC POLLACK. See POLLACK.														
ATLANTIC SALMON. See under SALMON.														
ATLANTIC SARDINE. See under SARDINE.														
AUBERGINE. See EGGPLANT.														
AVOCADO														
ALL COMMERCIAL VARIETIES														
raw, cubed	1 cup	918	0.16	0.18	2.90	0.42	92.8	0.00	11.8	16.5	1.5	58.5	899	0.6
raw, puréed	1 cup	1408	0.25	0.28	4.40	0.64	142.0	0.00	18.2	25.3	2.3	89.7	1378	1.0
raw, sliced	1 cup	894	0.16	0.18	2.80	0.41	90.4	0.00	11.5	16.1	1.5	56.9	875	0.6
raw, whole	1 medium	1230	0.22	0.25	3.90	0.56	124.0	0.00	15.9	22.1	2.0	78.4	1204	0.8
CALIFORNIA														
raw, puréed	1 cup	1408	0.25	0.28	4.40	0.64	151.0	0.00	18.2	25.3	2.7	94.3	1458	1.0
raw, whole, peeled and pitted	1 medium	1059	0.19	0.21	3.30	0.48	113.0	0.00	13.7	19.0	2.0	70.9	1097	0.7
FLORIDA														
raw, puréed	1 cup	1408	0.25	0.28	4.40	0.64	123.0	0.00	18.2	25.3	1.2	78.2	1122	1.0
raw, whole, peeled and pitted	1 medium	1860	0.33	0.37	5.80	0.85	162.0	0.00	24.0	33.4	1.6	103.0	1484	1.3
AVOCADO OIL														
	1 cup	0	0.00	0.00	0.00	0.00	0.0	0.00	0.0	0.0	0.0	0.0	0	0.0
	1 tbsp	0	0.00	0.00	0.00	0.00	0.0	0.00	0.0	0.0	0.0	0.0	0	0.0
AWA / milkfish														
baked, broiled, grilled, or microwaved	3 oz	93	0.00	0.01	7.00	0.41	15.3	2.80	0.0	55.3	0.4	32.3	318	0.9
raw	3 oz	85	0.00	0.01	5.50	0.36	13.6	2.90	0.0	43.4	0.3	25.5	248	0.7

B

Food Name	Serving Size	A I.U.	Thi mg	Rib mg	Nia mg	B$_6$ mg	Fol mcg	B$_{12}$ mcg	C mg	Calc mg	Iron mg	Mag mg	Pot mg	Zn mg
BABASSU OIL. See PALM KERNEL OIL.														
BABY FOOD														
CEREAL														
Barley														
dry	1 tbsp	<1	0.07	0.07	0.86	0.01	0.7	0.00	0.2	19.1	1.1	2.8	10	0.08
dry	1/2 oz	2	0.41	0.41	5.40	0.06	4.3	0.00	0.3	119.0	7.1	17.3	59	0.47
prepared w/whole milk	1 oz	30	0.14	0.16	1.70	0.03	2.5	0.09	na	65.2	3.5	8.5	54	0.24
Cereal w/egg yolks														
junior	1 jar	245	0.01	0.08	0.08	0.03	5.6	0.10	1.2	40.8	0.9	5.1	60	0.49
junior	1 oz	41	0.00	0.01	0.01	0.01	0.9	0.02	0.2	6.8	0.1	0.9	10	0.08
strained	1 jar	159	0.01	0.05	0.06	0.02	3.7	0.08	0.9	27.1	0.5	3.4	44	0.32
strained	1 oz	40	0.00	0.01	0.01	0.01	0.9	0.02	0.2	6.8	0.1	0.9	11	0.08
w/eggs, strained	1 jar	182	0.01	0.06	0.06	0.03	10.6	0.09	0.9	30.5	0.6	3.4	50	0.37
w/eggs, strained	1 oz	46	0.00	0.01	0.02	0.01	2.7	0.02	0.2	7.7	0.2	0.9	13	0.09

Food Name	Serving Size	A I.U.	Thi mg	Rib mg	Nia mg	B_6 mg	Fol mcg	B_{12} mcg	C mg	Calc mg	Iron mg	Mag mg	Pot mg	Zn mg
Egg yolks and bacon														
junior	1 jar	160	0.09	0.13	0.45	0.04	7.0	0.15	1.5	47.6	0.8	8.5	60	0.46
junior	1 oz	27	0.01	0.02	0.08	0.01	1.2	0.03	0.4	7.9	0.1	1.4	10	0.08
High-protein														
dry	1/2 oz	2	0.40	0.41	5.10	0.07	28.5	0.00	0.3	109.0	7.1	34.2	203	0.66
dry	1 tbsp	<1	0.06	0.07	0.82	0.01	4.6	0.00	0.2	17.4	1.1	5.5	33	0.11
prepared w/whole milk	1 oz	30	0.13	0.16	1.60	0.03	10.0	0.09	na	61.8	3.4	13.6	99	0.30
w/apple and orange, dry	1/2 oz	8	0.54	0.61	3.40	0.05	27.0	0.04	0.4	107.0	6.7	22.6	189	0.38
w/apple and orange, dry	1 tbsp	1	0.09	0.10	0.57	0.01	4.6	0.01	0.1	18.0	1.1	3.8	32	0.07
w/apple and orange, prepared w/whole milk	1 oz	na	0.19	0.24	1.10	0.03	7.8	0.10	na	63.2	4.1	10.5	98	0.22
Mixed														
dry	1/2 oz	3	0.37	0.41	5.20	0.03	6.4	0.00	0.3	110.0	7.1	15.0	66	0.36
dry	1 tbsp	1	0.06	0.07	0.87	0.01	1.1	0.00	0.1	18.3	1.2	2.5	11	0.06
prepared w/whole milk	1 oz	30	0.12	0.17	1.60	0.02	3.2	0.09	0.3	62.4	3.0	7.7	56	0.20
prepared w/whole milk	1 oz	31	0.19	0.20	0.98	0.03	2.0	0.10	0.4	60.7	3.2	7.4	67	0.16
w/applesauce and bananas, junior	1 jar	32	0.48	0.60	6.90	0.24	6.3	0.00	15.5	6.8	9.5	11.9	54	0.37
w/applesauce and bananas, junior	1 oz	5	0.08	0.10	1.10	0.04	1.0	0.00	2.6	1.1	1.6	2.0	9	0.06
w/applesauce and bananas, strained	1 jar	20	0.32	0.40	4.50	0.16	4.1	0.00	28.8	6.8	7.5	9.0	46	0.22
w/applesauce and bananas, strained	1 oz	5	0.08	0.10	1.10	0.04	1.0	0.00	7.2	1.7	1.9	2.3	12	0.05
w/banana, dry	1/2 oz	19	0.57	0.53	3.10	0.06	2.6	0.04	0.54	104.0	7.1	13.5	100	0.21
w/banana, dry	1 tbsp	3	0.10	0.09	0.51	0.01	0.4	0.01	0.1	17.4	1.2	2.3	17	0.04
Oatmeal														
dry	1/2 oz	2	0.43	0.39	5.40	0.02	5.3	0.00	0.5	110.0	7.1	21.8	71	0.55
dry	1 tbsp	<1	0.07	0.07	0.90	0.00	0.9	0.00	0.1	18.3	1.2	3.6	12	0.09
prepared w/whole milk	1 oz	30	0.14	0.16	1.70	0.02	2.8	0.09	0.4	62.4	3.4	9.9	58	0.26
w/applesauce and bananas, junior	1 jar	48	0.41	0.82	5.70	0.41	6.0	0.00	32.5	10.2	9.4	18.7	82	0.56
w/applesauce and bananas, junior	1 oz	8	0.07	0.14	0.95	0.07	1.0	0.00	5.4	1.7	1.6	3.1	13	0.09
w/applesauce and bananas, strained	1 jar	34	0.47	0.41	5.70	0.23	4.0	0.00	24.6	10.2	6.4	12.4	53	0.40
w/applesauce and bananas, strained	1 oz	9	0.12	0.10	1.40	0.06	1.0	0.00	6.2	2.6	1.6	3.1	13	0.10
w/bananas, dry	1/2 oz	10	0.54	0.56	3.00	0.06	2.8	0.03	0.7	97.7	7.1	17.7	110	0.28
w/bananas, dry	1 tbsp	2	0.09	0.09	0.50	0.01	0.5	0.01	0.1	16.3	1.2	3.0	18	0.05
w/bananas, prepared w/whole milk	1 oz	28	0.18	0.21	0.96	0.03	2.1	0.09	0.5	58.4	3.2	8.5	70	0.18
w/fruit, instant, toddler, dry	1 tbsp	5	0.04	0.05	0.51	0.02	1.0	0.00	0.1	15.2	0.8	5.7	18	0.30
w/honey, dry	1/2 oz	3	0.39	0.40	5.20	0.00	5.0	0.00	0.0	164	9.5	20.7	37	0.53
w/honey, dry	1 tbsp	<1	0.07	0.07	0.87	0.00	0.9	0.00	0.0	27.7	1.6	3.5	6	0.09
w/honey, prepared w/whole milk	1 oz	na	0.14	0.17	1.70	0.02	2.8	0.09	na	81.9	3.1	9.9	48	0.26
Rice														
dry	1/2 oz	2	0.40	0.33	4.70	0.07	3.7	0.00	0.4	128.0	7.1	30.9	58	0.30
dry	1 tbsp	<1	0.07	0.06	0.78	0.01	0.6	0.00	0.1	21.3	1.2	5.2	10	0.05
prepared w/whole milk	1 oz	30	0.13	0.14	1.50	0.03	2.3	0.09	0.3	67.8	3.5	12.8	54	0.18
w/applesauce and bananas, strained	1 jar	24	0.29	0.48	4.50	0.26	2.8	0.00	35.7	19.2	7.6	3.4	32	0.09
w/applesauce and bananas, strained	1 oz	6	0.07	0.12	1.10	0.07	0.7	0.00	9.0	4.8	1.9	0.9	8	0.02
w/applesauce and bananas, strained	1 tbsp	3	0.04	0.07	0.64	0.04	0.4	0.00	5.1	2.7	1.1	0.5	5	0.01
w/applesauce and bananas, strained, 'Strained 2' (Heinz)	4.25-oz jar	25	0.31	0.51	4.80	0.28	3.0	0.00	37.9	20.4	8.1	3.6	34	0.10
w/applesauce and bananas, strained, 'Second Foods' (Gerber)	4-oz jar	24	0.29	0.48	4.50	0.26	2.8	0.00	35.7	19.2	7.6	3.4	32	0.09
w/banana, dry	1/2 oz	4	0.60	0.57	3.50	0.10	1.8	0.03	0.3	104.0	7.1	21.1	115	0.2
w/banana, dry	1 tbsp	1	0.10	0.10	0.58	0.02	0.3	0.01	0.1	17.3	1.2	3.5	19	>0.1
w/banana, prepared w/whole milk	1 oz	8	0.19	0.22	1.10	0.04	1.8	0.09	0.3	60.4	3.1	9.6	72	0.2
w/honey, prepared w/whole milk	1 oz	26	0.14	0.17	1.70	0.03	2.4	0.09	0.0	82.5	3.1	12.8	40	0.2
w/mixed fruit, junior	1 oz	4	0.04	0.05	0.60	0.03	0.3	0.01	2.6	4.5	0.7	1.4	14	>0.1
w/mixed fruit, junior	1 tbsp	2	0.02	0.02	0.32	0.02	0.2	0.00	1.4	2.4	0.4	0.8	8	>0.1

Food Name	Serving Size	A I.U.	Thi mg	Rib mg	Nia mg	B$_6$ mg	Fol mcg	B$_{12}$ mcg	C mg	Calc mg	Iron mg	Mag mg	Pot mg	Zn mg
w/mixed fruit, 'Third Foods' (Gerber)	6-oz jar	26	0.22	0.27	3.60	0.19	1.7	0.03	15.8	27.2	4.4	8.5	85	0.2
DESSERTS AND SNACKS														
Cookies and crackers														
arrowroot cookie	1 cookie	0	0.03	0.02	0.29	0.00	1.8	0.00	0.3	1.6	0.2	1.1	8	>0.1
arrowroot cookie	1 oz	0	0.14	0.12	1.60	0.01	9.9	0.02	1.6	9.1	0.9	6.2	44	0.2
pretzel	1 oz	2	0.13	0.10	1.00	0.02	24.1	0.00	1.1	7.1	1.1	7.9	39	0.2
pretzel	1 pretzel	<1	0.03	0.02	0.21	0.01	5.1	0.00	0.2	1.5	0.2	1.7	8	>0.1
teething biscuit	1 biscuit	13	0.03	0.06	0.48	0.01	5.4	0.01	1.0	28.9	0.4	3.9	36	0.1
teething biscuit	1 oz	33	0.07	0.15	1.20	0.03	13.9	0.02	2.6	74.6	1.0	9.9	92	0.3
zwieback	1 oz	16	0.06	0.07	0.37	0.02	24.7	0.00	1.5	5.7	0.2	4.0	87	0.2
zwieback	1 piece	4	0.02	0.02	0.09	0.01	6.1	0.00	0.4	1.4	<0.1	1.0	21	>0.1
zwieback toast (Gerber)	1 cracker	4	0.02	0.02	0.09	0.01	6.1	0.00	0.4	1.4	<0.1	1.0	21	>0.1
Cottage cheese														
Custard/pudding														
cherry-vanilla pudding, junior	1 oz	57	0.00	0.00	0.01	0.00	0.1	0.00	0.3	1.4	0.1	0.6	9	>0.1
cherry-vanilla pudding, strained	1 oz	57	0.00	0.00	0.01	0.00	0.1	0.00	0.3	1.4	0.1	0.6	10	>0.1
orange pudding, strained	1 oz	33	0.01	0.02	0.03	0.01	2.2	0.00	2.6	9.1	<0.1	1.4	24	>0.1
pineapple pudding, junior	1 oz	11	0.01	0.01	0.04	0.01	1.6	0.02	7.6	9.6	0.1	2.6	26	>0.1
pineapple pudding, junior	1 tbsp	6	0.01	0.01	0.02	0.01	0.8	0.01	4.0	5.1	<0.1	1.4	14	>0.1
pineapple pudding, junior, 'Third Foods' (Gerber)	6-oz jar	63	0.07	0.08	0.21	0.07	9.5	0.10	45.4	57.8	0.3	15.3	153	0.3
pineapple pudding, strained	1 oz	11	0.01	0.01	0.03	0.01	1.5	0.02	7.7	8.8	0.1	2.6	23	>0.1
pineapple pudding, strained	1 tbsp	6	0.01	0.01	0.02	0.01	0.8	0.01	4.1	4.7	<0.1	1.4	12	>0.1
pineapple pudding, strained, 'Second Foods' (Gerber)	4-oz jar	45	0.04	0.05	0.12	0.05	5.9	0.07	30.7	35.0	0.2	10.2	92	0.2
vanilla custard, junior	1 cup	108	0.03	0.12	0.17	0.07	13.7	0.53	0.9	124.0	0.5	11.4	156	0.7
vanilla custard, junior	1 oz	13	0.00	0.02	0.02	0.01	1.7	0.07	0.1	15.3	0.1	1.4	19	0.1
vanilla custard, junior	1 tbsp	7	0.00	0.01	0.01	0.01	0.8	0.03	0.1	7.6	<0.1	0.7	10	>0.1
vanilla custard, junior, 'Junior 3' (Heinz)	6-oz jar	80	0.02	0.09	0.13	0.05	10.2	0.39	0.7	91.8	0.4	8.5	116	0.5
vanilla custard, junior, 'Stages 3' (Beech-Nut)	6-oz jar	80	0.02	0.09	0.13	0.05	10.2	0.39	0.7	91.8	0.4	8.5	116	0.5
vanilla custard, junior, 'Third Foods' (Gerber)	6-oz jar	80	0.02	0.09	0.13	0.05	10.2	0.39	0.7	91.8	0.4	8.5	116	0.5
vanilla custard, strained	1 cup	147	0.03	0.18	0.09	0.05	13.7	0.02	1.8	126.0	0.6	11.4	151	0.6
vanilla custard, strained	1 oz	18	0.00	0.02	0.01	0.01	1.7	0.00	0.2	15.6	0.1	1.4	19	>0.1
vanilla custard, strained	1 tbsp	9	0.00	0.01	0.01	0.00	0.8	0.00	0.1	7.7	<0.1	0.7	9	>0.1
vanilla custard, strained, 'Strained 2' (Heinz)	4-oz jar	72	0.01	0.09	0.05	0.02	6.8	0.01	0.9	62.1	0.3	5.7	75	0.3
vanilla custard, strained 'Stages 2' (Beech-Nut)	4-oz jar	72	0.01	0.09	0.05	0.02	6.8	0.01	0.9	62.1	0.3	5.7	75	0.3
vanilla custard, strained 'Second Foods' (Gerber)	4-oz jar	72	0.01	0.09	0.05	0.02	6.8	0.01	0.9	62.1	0.3	5.7	75	0.3
Dutch apple dessert														
junior	1 oz	5	0.00	0.00	0.01	0.01	0.0	0.00	5.1	0.85	<0.1	1.1	19	>0.1
strained	1 oz	14	0.00	0.00	0.01	0.01	0.2	0.00	6.1	1.4	0.1	0.6	9	0.0
Fruit dessert														
junior	1 oz	68	0.01	0.00	0.04	0.01	1.0	0.00	0.9	2.6	0.1	1.4	27	>0.1
junior	1 tbsp	36	0.00	0.00	0.02	0.01	0.5	0.00	0.5	1.4	<0.1	0.8	14	>0.1
junior, 'Junior 3' (Heinz)	6-oz jar	406	0.04	0.02	0.25	0.06	6.0	0.00	5.1	15.3	0.4	8.5	162	>0.1
junior, 'Third Foods' (Gerber)	6-oz jar	406	0.04	0.02	0.25	0.06	6.0	0.00	5.1	15.3	0.4	8.5	162	>0.1
strained	1 oz	71	0.01	0.00	0.04	0.01	0.9	0.00	0.7	2.6	0.1	1.4	27	>0.1
strained	1 tbsp	38	0.00	0.00	0.02	0.01	0.5	0.00	0.4	1.4	<0.1	0.8	14	>0.1
strained, 'Strained 2' (Heinz)	4.25-oz jar	301	0.02	0.01	0.17	0.04	4.0	0.00	3.0	10.8	0.3	6.0	113	>0.1

Food Name	Serving Size	A I.U.	Thi mg	Rib mg	Nia mg	B$_6$ mg	Fol mcg	B$_{12}$ mcg	C mg	Calc mg	Iron mg	Mag mg	Pot mg	Zn mg
strained, 'Second Foods' (Gerber)	4-oz jar	284	0.02	0.01	0.16	0.04	3.7	0.00	2.8	10.2	0.3	5.7	106	>0.1
Peach cobbler														
junior.	1 oz	40	0.00	0.00	0.07	0.00	0.3	0.00	5.8	1.1	<0.1	0.6	16	>0.1
junior.	1 tbsp	21	0.00	0.00	0.04	0.00	0.2	0.00	3.1	0.6	<0.1	0.3	8	>0.1
junior, 'Third Foods' (Gerber)	6-oz jar	241	0.02	0.03	0.44	0.01	1.9	0.00	34.9	6.8	0.2	3.4	95	>0.1
strained.	1 oz	40	0.00	0.00	0.07	0.00	0.3	0.00	5.8	1.1	<0.1	0.6	15	>0.1
strained.	1 tbsp	21	0.00	0.00	0.04	0.00	0.2	0.00	3.1	0.6	<0.1	0.3	8	>0.1
strained, 'Strained 2' (Heinz).	4-oz jar	160	0.01	0.02	0.29	0.01	1.2	0.00	23.2	4.5	0.1	2.3	61	0.3
strained, 'Second Foods' (Gerber)	4-oz jar	160	0.01	0.02	0.29	0.01	1.2	0.00	23.2	4.5	0.1	2.3	61	0.3
DINNERS AND MAIN DISHES														
Apple and chicken dinner														
strained.	1 oz	9	0.01	0.02	0.16	0.02	0.3	0.01	0.1	5.1	0.1	1.7	27	0.1
strained, 'Strained 2' (Heinz). . . . . : . . .	4-oz jar	34	0.02	0.06	0.65	0.09	1.1	0.02	0.2	20.3	0.4	6.8	107	0.4
strained, 'Stages 2' (Beech-Nut).	4-oz jar	34	0.02	0.06	0.65	0.09	1.1	0.02	0.2	20.3	0.4	6.8	107	0.4
strained, 'Second Foods' (Gerber)	4-oz jar	34	0.02	0.06	0.65	0.09	1.1	0.02	0.2	20.3	0.4	6.8	107	0.4
Apple and ham dinner														
strained.	1 tbsp	<1	0.01	0.01	0.11	0.01	0.3	0.00	<0.1	0.6	0.1	1.1	18	>0.1
strained, 'Second Foods' (Gerber)	4-oz jar	7	0.07	0.07	0.82	0.08	2.3	0.02	0.1	4.5	0.3	7.9	136	0.5
Apple and turkey dinner														
strained.	1 tbsp	1	0.00	0.01	0.11	0.01	0.3	0.03	<0.1	0.8	0.1	1.1	18	>0.1
strained, 'Second Foods' (Gerber)	4-oz jar	10	0.02	0.09	0.86	0.08	2.3	0.20	0.1	5.7	0.6	7.9	136	0.6
Beef and rice dinner, toddler	1 oz	142	0.01	0.02	0.38	0.04	1.7	0.14	1.1	3.1	0.2	2.3	34	0.3
Beef lasagna dinner, toddler	1 oz	330	0.02	0.03	0.38	0.02	1.7	0.14	0.5	5.1	0.3	3.1	35	0.2
Beef noodle dinner														
junior.	1 oz	186	0.01	0.01	0.17	0.01	3.4	0.03	0.4	2.3	0.1	2.0	13	0.1
junior.	1 tbsp	105	0.00	0.01	0.09	0.01	1.9	0.02	0.2	1.3	0.1	1.1	7	>0.1
junior, 'Junior 3' (Heinz).	6-oz jar	1115	0.05	0.06	0.99	0.05	20.4	0.17	2.4	13.6	0.7	11.9	78	0.7
junior, 'Stages 3' (Beech-Nut).	6-oz jar	1115	0.05	0.06	0.99	0.05	20.4	0.17	2.4	13.6	0.7	11.9	78	0.7
junior, 'Third Foods' (Gerber)	6-oz jar	1115	0.05	0.06	0.99	0.05	20.4	0.17	2.4	13.6	0.7	11.9	78	0.7
strained.	1 oz	203	0.01	0.01	0.17	0.01	2.3	0.05	<0.1	2.8	0.1	2.8	25	0.2
strained.	1 tbsp	115	0.01	0.01	0.10	0.01	1.3	0.03	<0.1	1.6	0.1	1.6	14	0.1
strained, 'Second Foods' (Gerber)	4-oz jar	809	0.04	0.04	0.70	0.04	9.0	0.22	0.1	11.3	0.5	11.3	98	0.7
strained, 'Stages 2' (Beech-Nut).	4-oz jar	809	0.04	0.04	0.70	0.04	9.0	0.22	0.1	11.3	0.5	11.3	98	0.7
strained, 'Strained 2' (Heinz).	4-oz jar	809	0.04	0.04	0.70	0.04	9.0	0.22	0.1	11.3	0.5	11.3	98	0.7
Beef stew														
toddler. . . . . · 1 oz	1 oz	467	0.00	0.02	0.37	0.02	1.7	0.14	0.9	2.6	0.2	3.1	40	0.3
toddler, 'Table Time' (Beech-Nut)	6 oz	2803	0.02	0.11	2.20	0.13	10.2	0.87	5.1	15.3	1.2	18.7	241	1.5
Broccoli and chicken dinner														
strained.	1 oz	129	0.01	0.02	0.22	0.03	12.8	0.00	5.4	11.6	0.2	3.4	48	0.2
strained, 'Second Foods' (Gerber)	4-oz jar	514	0.02	0.10	0.88	0.10	50.9	0.01	21.5	46.3	0.6	13.6	191	0.7
strained, 'Strained 2' (Heinz).	4-oz jar	514	0.02	0.10	0.88	0.10	50.9	0.01	21.5	46.3	0.6	13.6	191	0.7
Carrot and beef dinner														
strained.	1 tbsp	2168	0.00	0.01	0.14	0.02	2.5	0.05	0.1	3.3	0.1	1.9	34	0.1
strained, 'Second Foods' (Gerber)	4-oz jar	16331	0.02	0.07	1.10	0.11	19.2	0.34	0.9	24.9	0.6	14.7	255	0.9
Chicken noodle dinner														
junior.	1 oz	490	0.01	0.01	0.20	0.02	2.0	0.00	<0.1	6.0	0.1	2.0	11	0.1
junior.	1 tbsp	277	0.01	0.01	0.11	0.01	1.1	0.00	<0.1	3.4	0.1	1.1	6	>0.1
junior, 'Junior 3' (Heinz).	6-oz jar	2939	0.05	0.07	1.20	0.09	11.9	0.02	0.2	35.7	0.7	11.9	66	0.7
junior, 'Stages 3' (Beech-Nut).	6-oz jar	2939	0.05	0.07	1.20	0.09	11.9	0.02	0.2	35.7	0.7	11.9	66	0.7
junior, 'Third Foods' (Gerber)	6-oz jar	2939	0.05	0.07	1.20	0.09	11.9	0.02	0.2	35.7	0.7	11.9	66	0.7
strained.	1 oz	619	0.01	0.02	0.20	0.02	3.1	0.01	<0.1	7.7	0.2	4.0	39	0.2
strained.	1 tbsp	349	0.01	0.01	0.12	0.01	1.8	0.00	<0.1	4.3	0.1	2.2	22	>0.1
strained, 'Second Foods' (Gerber)	4-oz jar	2466	0.05	0.07	0.82	0.07	12.4	0.02	0.1	30.5	0.7	15.8	157	0.6
strained, 'Stages 2' (Beech-Nut).	4-oz jar	2466	0.05	0.07	0.82	0.07	12.4	0.02	0.1	30.5	0.7	15.8	157	0.6

Food Name	Serving Size	A I.U.	Thi mg	Rib mg	Nia mg	B_6 mg	Fol mcg	B_{12} mcg	C mg	Calc mg	Iron mg	Mag mg	Pot mg	Zn mg
strained, 'Strained 2' (Heinz)	4-oz jar	2466	0.05	0.07	0.82	0.07	12.4	0.02	0.1	30.5	0.7	15.8	157	0.6
Chicken stew														
strained	1 cup	3169	0.04	0.07	0.67	0.09	11.9	0.28	2.3	84.7	0.6	11.4	151	0.5
strained	1 oz	392	0.01	0.01	0.08	0.01	1.5	0.03	0.3	10.5	0.1	1.4	19	>0.1
strained	1 tbsp	221	0.00	0.01	0.05	0.01	0.8	0.02	0.2	5.9	<0.1	0.8	11	>0.1
strained, 'Stages 2' (Beech-Nut)	4-oz jar	1564	0.02	0.04	0.33	0.04	5.9	0.14	1.1	41.8	0.3	5.7	75	0.3
strained, 'Strained 2' (Heinz)	4-oz jar	1564	0.02	0.04	0.33	0.04	5.9	0.14	1.1	41.8	0.3	5.7	75	0.3
toddler	6.25-oz jar	1788	0.06	0.13	2.00	0.08	28.3	0.25	3.4	63.7	1.2	17.7	163	0.7
toddler	1 oz	286	0.01	0.02	0.33	0.01	4.5	0.04	0.5	10.2	0.2	2.8	26	0.1
toddler	1 tbsp	162	0.01	0.01	0.18	0.01	2.6	0.02	0.3	5.8	0.1	1.6	15	>0.1
Green bean and turkey dinner														
strained	1 jar	410	0.03	0.11	1.20	0.08	27.1	0.05	1.9	41.8	0.9	23.7	189	0.7
strained	1 oz	103	0.01	0.03	0.29	0.02	6.8	0.01	0.5	10.5	0.2	6.0	47	0.2
strained, 'Second Foods' (Gerber)	4-oz jar	410	0.03	0.11	1.20	0.08	27.1	0.05	1.9	41.8	0.9	23.7	189	0.7
strained, 'Strained 2' (Heinz)	4-oz jar	410	0.03	0.11	1.20	0.08	27.1	0.05	1.9	41.8	0.9	23.7	189	0.7
Macaroni and cheese														
junior	1 oz	4	0.02	0.02	0.16	0.01	3.1	0.01	0.4	14.5	0.1	2.0	13	>0.1
strained	1 oz	24	0.01	0.02	0.15	0.01	3.1	0.04	<0.1	18.7	0.1	2.3	19	0.1
Macaroni, tomato, and beef dinner														
junior	1 jar	1175	0.08	0.09	1.30	0.08	15.3	0.41	2.5	23.8	0.6	11.9	122	0.6
junior	1 oz	196	0.01	0.02	0.21	0.01	2.6	0.07	0.4	4.0	0.1	2.0	20	0.1
junior	1 tbsp	111	0.01	0.01	0.12	0.01	1.4	0.04	0.2	2.2	0.1	1.1	12	>0.1
junior, 'Stages 3' (Beech-Nut)	6-oz jar	1175	0.08	0.09	1.30	0.08	15.3	0.41	2.5	23.8	0.6	11.9	122	0.6
junior, 'Third Foods' (Gerber)	6-oz jar	1175	0.08	0.09	1.30	0.08	15.3	0.41	2.5	23.8	0.6	11.9	122	0.6
strained	1 jar	992	0.04	0.05	0.81	0.06	10.2	0.17	0.3	19.2	0.5	13.6	127	0.6
strained	1 oz	249	0.01	0.01	0.20	0.02	2.6	0.04	0.1	4.8	0.1	3.4	32	0.2
strained	1 tbsp	140	0.01	0.01	0.11	0.01	1.4	0.02	0.1	2.7	0.1	1.9	18	>0.1
strained, 'Second Foods' (Gerber)	4-oz jar	992	0.04	0.05	0.81	0.06	10.2	0.17	0.3	19.2	0.5	13.6	127	0.6
strained, 'Stages 2' (Beech-Nut)	4-oz jar	992	0.04	0.05	0.81	0.06	10.2	0.17	0.3	19.2	0.5	13.6	127	0.6
strained, 'Strained 2' (Heinz)	4-oz jar	992	0.04	0.05	0.81	0.06	10.2	0.17	0.3	19.2	0.5	13.6	127	0.6
Mixed vegetable														
junior	1 oz	693	0.00	0.01	0.12	0.02	1.9	0.00	0.9	4.8	0.1	2.8	32	>0.1
strained	1 oz	773	0.00	0.01	0.14	0.02	2.3	0.00	0.8	6.2	0.1	3.1	34	>0.1
Pasta and vegetable dinner (Gerber)	4-oz jar	627	0.07	0.06	0.63	0.12	10.2	0.00	3.3	15.8	0.6	27.1	150	0.5
Spaghetti, tomato, and meat dinner														
junior	1 jar	2134	0.08	0.12	1.60	0.11	45.9	0.05	0.3	25.5	0.9	18.7	207	0.9
junior	1 oz	356	0.01	0.02	0.27	0.02	7.7	0.01	0.1	4.3	0.2	3.1	35	0.2
junior	1 tbsp	201	0.01	0.01	0.16	0.01	4.3	0.01	<0.1	2.4	0.1	1.8	20	>0.1
junior, 'Stages 3' (Beech-Nut)	6-oz jar	2134	0.08	0.12	1.60	0.11	45.9	0.05	0.3	25.5	0.9	18.7	207	0.9
junior, 'Third Foods' (Gerber)	6-oz jar	2134	0.08	0.12	1.60	0.11	45.9	0.05	0.3	25.5	0.9	18.7	207	0.9
toddler	1 jar	753	0.11	0.17	2.60	0.14	54.4	0.39	7.0	37.4	1.5	25.5	277	0.8
toddler	1 oz	126	0.02	0.03	0.44	0.02	9.1	0.07	1.2	6.2	0.3	4.3	46	0.1
toddler (Heinz)	6-oz jar	2134	0.08	0.12	1.60	0.11	45.9	0.05	0.3	25.5	0.9	18.7	207	0.9
Sweet potato and chicken dinner														
strained	1 tbsp	691	0.00	0.01	0.17	0.02	1.0	0.01	0.0	4.8	0.1	2.1	32	>0.1
strained, 'Stages 2' (Beech-Nut)	4-oz jar	4879	0.02	0.05	1.20	0.16	6.8	0.06	0.0	33.9	0.5	14.7	226	0.4
Turkey and barley dinner (Gerber)	4-oz jar	4240	0.03	0.07	1.10	0.09	18.1	0.02	3.1	23.7	0.6	14.7	157	0.6
Turkey and rice dinner														
junior	1 oz	535	0.01	0.01	0.20	0.02	2.3	0.01	0.1	6.8	0.1	2.6	24	0.1
junior	1 tbsp	302	0.01	0.01	0.11	0.01	1.3	0.00	0.1	3.8	0.1	1.4	14	>0.1
junior, 'Junior 3' (Heinz)	6-oz jar	3206	0.06	0.08	1.20	0.09	13.6	0.03	0.5	40.8	0.7	15.3	146	0.8
junior, 'Stages 3' (Beech-Nut) dinner	6-oz jar	3206	0.06	0.08	1.20	0.09	13.6	0.03	0.5	40.8	0.7	15.3	146	0.8
junior, 'Third Foods' (Gerber)	6-oz jar	3206	0.06	0.08	1.20	0.09	13.6	0.03	0.5	40.8	0.7	15.3	146	0.8
strained	1 oz	460	0.01	0.01	0.18	0.02	1.1	0.01	0.1	5.1	0.1	2.3	26	0.1

Food Name	Serving Size	A I.U.	Thi mg	Rib mg	Nia mg	B_6 mg	Fol mcg	B_{12} mcg	C mg	Calc mg	Iron mg	Mag mg	Pot mg	Zn mg
strained...............	1 tbsp	260	0.00	0.01	0.10	0.01	0.6	0.00	<0.1	2.9	0.1	1.3	15	>0.1
strained, 'Second Foods' (Gerber).........	4-oz jar	1833	0.03	0.05	0.73	0.06	4.5	0.02	0.2	20.3	0.3	9.0	103	0.5
strained, 'Stages 2' (Beech-Nut)..........	4-oz jar	1833	0.03	0.05	0.73	0.06	4.5	0.02	0.2	20.3	0.3	9.0	103	0.5
strained, 'Strained 2' (Heinz).............	4-oz jar	1833	0.03	0.05	0.73	0.06	4.5	0.02	0.2	20.3	0.3	9.0	103	0.5
Turkey stew														
Vegetable, dumpling, and beef dinner														
junior...............	1 oz	187	0.01	0.01	0.14	0.01	2.1	0.03	0.2	4.0	0.1	2.0	13	>0.1
strained...............	1 oz	118	0.01	0.01	0.16	0.01	2.0	0.03	0.2	4.0	0.1	1.7	13	0.1
Vegetable and bacon dinner														
junior...............	1 cup	4035	0.13	0.08	1.40	0.16	23.0	0.26	2.8	28.2	1.1	20.5	220	0.7
junior...............	1 oz	447	0.01	0.01	0.16	0.02	2.6	0.03	0.3	3.1	0.1	2.3	24	>0.1
junior...............	1 tbsp	252	0.01	0.01	0.09	0.01	1.4	0.02	0.2	1.8	0.1	1.3	14	>0.1
junior, 'Junior 3' (Heinz).................	6-oz jar	2679	0.09	0.05	0.93	0.11	15.3	0.17	1.9	18.7	0.7	13.6	146	0.5
junior, 'Third Foods' (Gerber).............	6-oz jar	2679	0.09	0.05	0.93	0.11	15.3	0.17	1.9	18.7	0.7	13.6	146	0.5
strained...............	1 cup	5847	0.08	0.10	1.20	0.15	7.7	0.15	0.8	35.8	0.8	25.6	297	0.8
strained...............	1 oz	648	0.01	0.01	0.13	0.02	0.9	0.02	0.1	4.0	0.1	2.8	33	>0.1
strained...............	1 tbsp	365	0.01	0.01	0.08	0.01	0.5	0.01	0.1	2.2	0.1	1.6	19	>0.1
strained, 'Second Foods' (Gerber).........	4-oz jar	2581	0.04	0.04	0.54	0.07	3.4	0.07	0.3	15.8	0.3	11.3	131	0.3
strained, 'Strained 2' (Heinz).............	4-oz jar	2581	0.04	0.04	0.54	0.07	3.4	0.07	0.3	15.8	0.3	11.3	131	0.3
Vegetable and beef dinner														
junior...............	1 cup	6513	0.07	0.11	1.60	0.18	10.2	0.44	0.8	30.7	0.0	28.2	312	1.3
junior...............	1 oz	721	0.01	0.01	0.17	0.02	1.1	0.05	0.1	3.4	0.1	3.1	35	0.1
junior...............	1 tbsp	407	0.00	0.01	0.10	0.01	0.6	0.03	0.1	1.9	0.1	1.8	20	>0.1
junior, 'Junior 3' (Heinz).................	6-oz jar	4325	0.05	0.07	1.00	0.12	6.8	0.29	0.5	20.4	0.7	18.7	207	0.9
junior, 'Stages 3' (Beech-Nut) dinner.......	6-oz jar	4325	0.05	0.07	1.00	0.12	6.8	0.29	0.5	20.4	0.7	18.7	207	0.9
junior, 'Third Foods' (Gerber).............	6-oz jar	4325	0.05	0.07	1.00	0.12	6.8	0.29	0.5	20.4	0.7	18.7	207	0.9
strained...............	1 cup	7478	0.09	0.12	2.10	0.18	20.5	0.46	0.5	43.5	1.5	38.4	404	1.4
strained...............	1 oz	828	0.01	0.01	0.23	0.02	2.3	0.05	0.1	4.8	0.2	4.3	45	0.2
strained...............	1 tbsp	467	0.01	0.01	0.13	0.01	1.3	0.03	<0.1	2.7	0.1	2.4	25	>0.1
strained (Earth's Best)	4.5-oz jar	3739	0.04	0.06	1.10	0.09	10.2	0.23	0.3	21.8	0.7	19.2	202	0.7
strained, 'Second Foods' (Gerber).........	4-oz jar	3301	0.04	0.05	0.94	0.08	9.0	0.20	0.2	19.2	0.7	16.9	179	0.6
strained, 'Stages 2' (Beech-Nut)..........	4-oz jar	3301	0.04	0.05	0.94	0.08	9.0	0.20	0.2	19.2	0.7	16.9	179	0.6
strained, 'Strained 2' (Heinz).............	4-oz jar	3301	0.04	0.05	0.94	0.08	9.0	0.20	0.2	19.2	0.7	16.9	179	0.6
Vegetable and chicken dinner														
junior...............	1 cup	6687	0.06	0.12	1.60	0.12	7.7	0.05	0.5	69.1	0.8	20.5	212	0.8
junior...............	1 oz	741	0.01	0.01	0.18	0.01	0.9	0.01	0.1	7.7	0.1	2.3	24	>0.1
junior...............	1 tbsp	418	0.00	0.01	0.10	0.01	0.5	0.00	<0.1	4.3	0.1	1.3	13	>0.1
junior, 'Stages 3' (Beech-Nut) dinner.......	6-oz jar	4440	0.04	0.08	1.10	0.08	5.1	0.03	0.3	45.9	0.6	13.6	141	0.5
junior, 'Third Foods' (Gerber).............	6-oz jar	4440	0.04	0.08	1.10	0.08	5.1	0.03	0.3	45.9	0.6	13.6	141	0.5
strained...............	1 cup	10578	0.08	0.13	1.80	0.18	12.8	0.03	0.3	69.1	1.4	35.8	404	1.2
strained...............	1 oz	1171	0.01	0.02	0.20	0.02	1.4	0.00	<0.1	7.7	0.2	4.0	45	0.1
strained...............	1 tbsp	661	0.01	0.01	0.12	0.01	0.8	0.00	<0.1	4.3	0.1	2.2	25	>0.1
strained, 'Second Foods' (Gerber).........	4-oz jar	4669	0.04	0.06	0.81	0.08	5.7	0.01	0.1	30.5	0.6	15.8	179	0.5
strained, 'Stages 2' (Beech-Nut)..........	4-oz jar	4669	0.04	0.06	0.81	0.08	5.7	0.01	0.1	30.5	0.6	15.8	179	0.5
strained, 'Strained 2' (Heinz).............	4-oz jar	4669	0.04	0.06	0.81	0.08	5.7	0.01	0.1	30.5	0.6	15.8	179	0.5
Vegetable and dumpling dinner														
Vegetable and ham dinner														
junior...............	1 cup	3628	0.08	0.10	1.30	0.12	20.5	0.08	2.8	35.8	0.6	20.5	248	0.8
junior...............	1 oz	402	0.01	0.01	0.14	0.01	2.3	0.01	0.3	4.0	0.1	2.3	28	>0.1
junior...............	1 tbsp	227	0.01	0.01	0.08	0.01	1.3	0.01	0.2	2.2	<0.1	1.3	16	>0.1
junior, 'Junior 3' (Heinz).................	6-oz jar	2409	0.05	0.07	0.87	0.08	13.6	0.05	1.9	23.8	0.4	13.6	165	0.5
junior, 'Third Foods' (Gerber).............	6-oz jar	2409	0.05	0.07	0.87	0.08	13.6	0.05	1.9	23.8	0.4	13.6	165	0.5
strained...............	1 cup	7352	0.09	0.14	1.70	0.18	7.7	0.15	4.1	41.0	1.1	30.7	361	0.8
strained...............	1 oz	814	0.01	0.02	0.19	0.02	0.9	0.02	0.5	4.5	0.1	3.4	40	>0.1

Food Name	Serving Size	A I.U.	Thi mg	Rib mg	Nia mg	B_6 mg	Fol mcg	B_{12} mcg	C mg	Calc mg	Iron mg	Mag mg	Pot mg	Zn mg
strained	1 tbsp	460	0.01	0.01	0.11	0.01	0.5	0.01	0.3	2.6	0.1	1.9	23	>0.1
strained, 'Second Foods' (Gerber)	4-oz jar	3245	0.04	0.06	0.76	0.08	3.4	0.07	1.8	18.1	0.5	13.6	159	0.4
strained, 'Stages 2' (Beech-Nut)	4-oz jar	3245	0.04	0.06	0.76	0.08	3.4	0.07	1.8	18.1	0.5	13.6	159	0.4
strained, 'Strained 2' (Heinz)	4-oz jar	3245	0.04	0.06	0.76	0.08	3.4	0.07	1.8	18.1	0.5	13.6	159	0.4
Vegetable and lamb dinner														
junior	1 oz	420	0.01	0.01	0.16	0.01	1.0	0.05	0.5	3.7	0.1	2.0	27	>0.1
strained	1 cup	5107	0.05	0.09	1.40	0.12	9.2	0.41	3.1	30.7	0.9	17.9	241	0.6
strained	1 oz	566	0.01	0.01	0.15	0.01	1.0	0.05	0.3	3.4	0.1	2.0	27	>0.1
strained	1 tbsp	319	0.00	0.01	0.09	0.01	0.6	0.03	0.2	1.9	0.1	1.1	15	>0.1
strained, 'Stages 2' (Beech-Nut)	4-oz jar	2254	0.02	0.04	0.60	0.05	4.1	0.18	1.4	13.6	0.4	7.9	106	0.2
strained, 'Strained 2' (Heinz)	4-oz jar	2254	0.02	0.04	0.60	0.05	4.1	0.18	1.4	13.6	0.4	7.9	106	0.2
Vegetable and noodle dinner														
Vegetable and turkey dinner														
junior	1 cup	4209	0.06	0.08	1.40	0.13	17.9	0.03	1.0	41.0	0.9	23.0	251	0.8
junior	1 oz	466	0.01	0.01	0.15	0.02	2.0	0.00	0.1	4.5	0.1	2.6	28	>0.1
junior	1 tbsp	263	0.00	0.01	0.09	0.01	1.1	0.00	0.1	2.6	0.1	1.4	16	>0.1
junior, 'Third Foods' (Gerber)	6-oz jar	2795	0.04	0.05	0.92	0.09	11.9	0.02	0.7	27.2	0.6	15.3	167	0.5
strained	1 cup	11254	0.05	0.06	1.20	0.11	25.6	0.05	1.8	69.1	1.0	33.3	261	1.8
strained	1 oz	1246	0.01	0.01	0.13	0.01	2.8	0.01	0.2	7.7	0.1	3.7	29	0.2
strained	1 tbsp	703	0.00	0.00	0.08	0.01	1.6	0.00	0.1	4.3	0.1	2.1	16	0.1
strained (Earth's Best)	4.5-oz jar	4967	0.02	0.03	0.53	0.05	11.3	0.02	0.8	30.5	0.4	14.7	115	0.8
strained, 'Second Foods' (Gerber)	4-oz jar	4967	0.02	0.03	0.53	0.05	11.3	0.02	0.8	30.5	0.4	14.7	115	0.8
toddler	1 oz	595	0.01	0.03	0.17	0.02	0.9	0.13	0.8	13.0	0.2	4.5	47	>0.1
Vegetable, noodle, and chicken dinner														
junior	1 oz	298	0.01	0.01	0.19	0.01	1.0	0.03	0.2	7.4	0.1	3.1	17	>0.1
strained	1 oz	402	0.01	0.01	0.12	0.01	0.9	0.02	0.2	7.9	0.1	2.8	16	>0.1
Vegetable, noodle, and turkey dinner														
junior	1 oz	282	0.01	0.01	0.09	0.01	0.8	0.03	0.2	9.1	0.1	2.6	21	>0.1
strained	1 oz	281	0.01	0.01	0.07	0.01	0.7	0.03	0.2	9.1	0.1	2.3	18	>0.1
FORMULA														
Infant formula, mix														
Liquid concentrate														
low-iron (Gerber)	1 fl oz	121	0.03	0.06	0.40	0.02	6.5	0.12	4.9	31.4	0.3	3.4	44	0.4
low-iron, 'Enfamil' (Mead Johnson)	1 fl oz	124	0.03	0.06	0.41	0.03	6.6	0.12	5.0	32.0	0.3	3.5	45	0.4
low-iron, 'Similac' (Ross)	1 fl oz	120	0.04	0.06	0.42	0.02	6.0	0.10	3.6	31.1	0.1	2.5	42	0.3
low-iron, 'SMA' (Wyeth-Ayerst)	1 fl oz	122	0.04	0.06	0.31	0.03	3.1	0.08	3.5	25.7	0.1	2.8	34	0.3
w/iron (Gerber)	1 fl oz	121	0.03	0.06	0.40	0.02	6.5	0.12	4.9	31.4	0.7	3.4	44	0.4
w/iron (Good Start)	1 fl oz	119	0.03	0.05	0.30	0.03	3.5	0.09	3.1	25.7	0.6	2.5	39	0.3
w/iron, 'Enfamil' (Mead Johnson)	1 fl oz	124	0.03	0.06	0.41	0.03	6.6	0.12	5.0	32.0	0.7	3.5	45	0.4
w/iron, 'Follow-Up' (Carnation)	1 fl oz	103	0.03	0.04	0.53	0.03	6.6	0.13	3.3	55.6	0.8	3.5	56	0.3
w/iron, 'Isomil SF' (Ross)	1 fl oz	120	0.02	0.06	0.54	0.02	6.0	0.18	3.6	42.1	0.7	3.1	43	0.3
w/iron, 'Isomil' (Ross)	1 fl oz	120	0.02	0.06	0.54	0.02	6.0	0.18	3.6	42.1	0.7	3.1	43	0.3
w/iron, 'I-Soyalac' (Carnation)	1 fl oz	129	0.04	0.04	0.52	0.04	6.3	0.13	4.9	41.4	0.8	4.4	48	0.3
w/iron, 'Nursoy' (Wyeth-Ayerst)	1 fl oz	124	0.04	0.06	0.31	0.03	3.1	0.13	3.4	37.1	0.7	4.4	43	0.3
w/iron, 'Nutramigen' (Mead Johnson)	1 fl oz	124	0.03	0.04	0.41	0.03	6.6	0.12	5.0	38.7	0.7	4.4	45	0.4
w/iron, 'Prosobee' (Mead Johnson)	1 fl oz	121	0.03	0.04	0.40	0.02	6.5	0.12	4.9	42.4	0.7	4.3	49	0.5
w/iron, 'Similac' (Ross)	1 fl oz	120	0.04	0.06	0.42	0.02	6.0	0.10	3.6	31.1	0.7	2.5	42	0.3
w/iron, 'SMA' (Wyeth-Ayerst)	1 fl oz	124	0.04	0.06	0.31	0.03	3.1	0.08	3.5	26.1	0.7	2.8	34	0.3
w/iron, 'Soyalac' (Carnation)	1 fl oz	129	0.03	0.04	0.52	0.04	6.3	0.13	5.0	42.1	0.8	5.0	49	0.3
Powder														
low-iron (Gerber)	1 scoop	133	0.04	0.06	0.44	0.03	7.1	0.13	5.3	34.9	0.3	3.6	48	0.4
low-iron, 'Enfamil' (Mead Johnson)	1 scoop	129	0.03	0.06	0.43	0.03	6.9	0.13	5.1	33.2	0.3	3.4	47	0.4
low-iron, 'Similac' (Ross)	1 scoop	137	0.05	0.07	0.48	0.03	6.9	0.11	4.1	35.6	0.1	2.7	48	0.3
low-iron, 'Similac PM 60/40' (Ross)	1 scoop	138	0.05	0.07	0.48	0.03	6.9	0.12	4.2	25.8	0.1	2.8	40	0.4

Food Name	Serving Size	A I.U.	Thi mg	Rib mg	Nia mg	B6 mg	Fol mcg	B12 mcg	C mg	Calc mg	Iron mg	Mag mg	Pot mg	Zn mg
low-iron, 'SMA' (Wyeth-Ayerst)	1 scoop	132	0.05	0.07	0.33	0.03	3.3	0.09	3.6	27.8	0.1	3.0	37	0.3
w/iron (Good Start)	1 scoop	134	0.03	0.06	0.33	0.04	4.0	0.10	3.7	28.7	0.7	3.0	44	0.3
w/iron, 'Enfamil' (Mead Johnson)	1 scoop	129	0.03	0.06	0.43	0.03	6.9	0.13	5.1	33.2	0.8	3.4	47	0.4
w/iron, 'Follow-Up' (Carnation)	1 scoop	111	0.04	0.04	0.57	0.03	7.0	0.14	3.5	59.8	0.8	3.8	60	0.3
w/iron, 'Gerber' (Mead Johnson)	1 scoop	133	0.04	0.06	0.44	0.03	7.1	0.13	5.3	34.9	0.8	3.6	48	0.4
w/iron, 'Isomil' (Ross)	1 scoop	135	0.03	0.04	0.61	0.03	6.7	0.20	4.0	47.2	0.8	3.4	49	0.3
w/iron, 'I-Soyalac' (Carnation)	1 scoop	68	0.02	0.02	0.27	0.02	3.4	0.07	2.6	22.0	0.4	2.3	26	0.2
w/iron, 'Lofenalac' (Mead Johnson)	1 scoop	137	0.04	0.04	0.56	0.03	6.9	0.14	3.6	41.3	0.8	4.8	45	0.4
w/iron, 'Nursoy' (Wyeth-Ayerst)	1 scoop	131	0.04	0.07	0.33	0.03	3.3	0.13	3.7	39.4	0.8	4.4	46	0.4
w/iron, 'Nutramigen' (Mead Johnson)	1 scoop	142	0.04	0.04	0.47	0.03	7.6	0.14	5.7	44.2	0.8	5.2	52	0.5
w/iron, 'Portagen' (Mead Johnson)	1 scoop	348	0.07	0.08	0.93	0.09	7.0	0.28	3.6	41.4	0.8	8.8	56	0.4
w/iron, 'Pregestimil' (Mead Johnson)	1 scoop	167	0.03	0.04	0.55	0.03	6.9	0.14	5.2	41.4	0.8	4.8	48	0.4
w/iron, 'Prosobee' (Mead Johnson)	1 scoop	133	0.04	0.04	0.45	0.03	7.1	0.13	5.3	46.4	0.8	4.9	53	0.5
w/iron, 'SAM' (Wyeth-Ayerst)	1 scoop	132	0.05	0.07	0.33	0.03	3.3	0.09	3.6	27.8	0.8	3.0	37	0.3
w/iron, 'Similac' (Ross)	1 scoop	137	0.05	0.07	0.48	0.03	6.9	0.11	4.1	35.6	0.8	2.7	48	0.3
w/iron, 'Soylac' (Carnation)	1 scoop	68	0.02	0.02	0.27	0.02	3.4	0.07	2.6	20.7	0.4	2.7	26	0.2
w/iron, prepared 'Lofenalac' (Mead Johnson)	1 fl oz	62	0.02	0.02	0.25	0.01	3.1	0.06	1.6	18.8	0.4	2.2	20	0.2
w/iron, prepared 'Portagen' (Mead Johnson)	1 fl oz	156	0.03	0.04	0.42	0.04	3.1	0.13	1.6	18.9	0.4	4.0	24	0.2
w/iron, prepared 'Pregestimil' (Mead Johnson)	1 fl oz	76	0.02	0.02	0.25	0.01	3.1	0.06	2.3	18.8	0.4	2.2	21	0.2
Infant formula, ready to use														
low-iron (Gerber)	1 fl oz	60	0.02	0.03	0.20	0.01	3.4	0.06	2.4	15.6	0.1	1.5	22	0.2
low-iron, 'Alimentum' (Ross)	1 fl oz	60	0.01	0.02	0.27	0.01	3.0	0.09	1.8	21.0	0.4	1.5	24	0.2
low-iron, 'Enfamil' (Mead Johnson)	1 fl oz	60	0.02	0.03	0.20	0.01	3.4	0.06	2.4	15.6	0.1	1.5	22	0.2
low-iron, 'Similac' (Ross)	1 fl oz	61	0.02	0.03	0.21	0.01	3.1	0.05	1.8	16.1	<0.1	1.2	21	0.2
low-iron, 'Similac Natural Care' (Ross)	1 fl oz	296	0.06	0.15	1.20	0.06	8.8	0.13	8.8	49.7	0.1	2.7	31	0.4
low-iron, 'Similac PM 60/40' (Mead Johnson)	1 fl oz	60	0.02	0.03	0.21	0.01	3.0	0.05	1.8	11.2	<0.1	1.2	20	0.2
low-iron, 'SMA' (Wyeth-Ayerst)	1 fl oz	60	0.02	0.03	0.15	0.01	1.5	0.04	1.7	12.5	<0.1	1.5	17	0.2
w/iron (Gerber)	1 fl oz	60	0.02	0.03	0.20	0.01	3.4	0.06	2.4	15.6	0.4	1.5	22	0.2
w/iron (Good Start)	1 fl oz	61	0.01	0.03	0.15	0.02	1.8	0.04	1.6	12.8	0.3	1.2	20	0.2
w/iron, 'Enfamil' (Mead Johnson)	1 fl oz	60	0.02	0.03	0.20	0.01	3.0	0.06	2.4	15.6	0.4	1.5	22	0.2
w/iron, 'Follow-Up' (Carnation)	1 fl oz	49	0.02	0.02	0.26	0.01	3.0	0.06	1.6	26.8	0.4	1.8	27	0.1
w/iron, 'Isomil' (Ross)	1 fl oz	60	0.01	0.02	0.27	0.01	3.0	0.09	1.8	21.0	0.4	1.5	22	0.2
w/iron, 'Isomil SF' (Ross)	1 fl oz	60	0.01	0.02	0.27	0.01	3.0	0.09	1.8	21.0	0.4	1.5	22	0.2
w/iron, 'I-Soyalac' (Carnation)	1 fl oz	63	0.02	0.02	0.25	0.02	3.0	0.06	2.4	20.1	0.4	2.1	24	0.2
w/iron, 'Nutramigen' (Mead Johnson)	1 fl oz	61	0.02	0.02	0.20	0.01	3.1	0.06	2.4	19.1	0.4	2.2	22	0.2
w/iron, 'Nutrsoy' (Wyeth-Ayerst)	1 fl oz	60	0.02	0.03	0.15	0.01	1.5	0.06	1.6	17.9	0.4	2.1	21	0.2
w/iron, 'Prosobee' (Mead Johnson)	1 fl oz	60	0.02	0.02	0.20	0.01	3.4	0.06	2.4	21.0	0.4	2.1	24	0.2
w/iron, 'Similac' (Ross)	1 fl oz	60	0.02	0.03	0.21	0.01	3.0	0.05	1.8	15.8	0.4	1.2	21	0.2
w/iron, 'Similac Special Care 24' (Ross)	1 fl oz	298	0.06	0.15	1.20	0.06	8.9	0.13	8.8	43.1	0.4	2.8	31	0.4
w/iron, 'SMA' (Wyeth-Ayerst)	1 fl oz	60	0.02	0.03	0.15	0.01	1.5	0.04	1.7	12.5	0.4	1.5	17	0.2
w/iron, 'Soyalac' (Carnation)	1 fl oz	63	0.02	0.02	0.25	0.02	3.0	0.06	2.4	18.9	0.4	2.4	24	0.2
Toddler formula, mix														
Liquid concentrate, soy, prepared, 'Next Step' (Mead Johnson)	1 fl oz	60	0.02	0.02	0.20	0.01	3.0	0.06	2.4	21.0	0.4	2.1	24	0.2
Powder, soy, prepared 'Next Step' (Mead Johnson)	1 fl oz	60	0.02	0.02	0.20	0.02	3.0	0.06	2.4	23.2	0.4	1.5	30	0.2
Toddler formula, ready to use, w/iron, 'Pediasure' (Ross)	1 fl oz	76	0.08	0.06	0.50	0.08	10.8	0.18	2.9	28.8	0.4	5.9	39	0.4

Food Name	Serving Size	A I.U.	Thi mg	Rib mg	Nia mg	B$_6$ mg	Fol mcg	B$_{12}$ mcg	C mg	Calc mg	Iron mg	Mag mg	Pot mg	Zn mg
FRUIT														
Apple and blueberry														
junior	1 oz	12	0.01	0.01	0.03	0.01	1.0	0.00	3.9	1.4	0.1	0.9	18	>0.1
strained	1 oz	6	0.01	0.01	0.03	0.01	1.0	0.00	7.9	1.1	0.1	0.9	20	>0.1
Apple and raspberry														
w/sugar, junior	1 oz	9	0.00	0.01	0.03	0.01	0.9	0.00	8.2	1.4	0.1	1.1	20	>0.1
w/sugar, strained	1 oz	6	0.00	0.01	0.03	0.01	1.0	0.00	7.6	1.4	0.1	1.1	23	>0.1
Apple and sweet potato (Gerber)	4-oz jar	2317	0.01	0.02	0.11	0.06	2.3	0.00	7.2	9.0	0.2	6.8	168	0.1
Applesauce														
junior	1 oz	3	0.00	0.01	0.02	0.01	0.5	0.00	10.7	1.4	0.1	0.9	22	>0.1
junior	1 tbsp	1	0.00	0.0	0.01	0.01	0.3	0.00	6.0	0.8	<0.1	0.5	12	>0.1
junior, 'Junior 3' (Heinz)	6-oz jar	15	0.02	0.05	0.11	0.05	2.9	0.00	64.3	8.5	0.4	5.1	131	>0.1
junior, 'Stages 3' (Beech-Nut)	6-oz jar	15	0.02	0.05	0.11	0.05	2.9	0.00	64.3	8.5	0.4	5.1	131	>0.1
junior, 'Third Foods' (Gerber)	6-oz jar	15	0.02	0.05	0.11	0.05	2.9	0.00	64.3	8.5	0.4	5.1	131	>0.1
strained	1 oz	5	0.00	0.01	0.02	0.01	0.5	0.00	10.9	1.1	0.1	0.9	20	>0.1
strained	1 tbsp	3	0.00	0.00	0.01	0.01	0.3	0.00	6.1	0.6	<0.1	0.5	11	0.00
strained (Earth's Best)	4.5-oz jar	22	0.02	0.04	0.08	0.04	2.4	0.00	49.0	5.1	0.3	3.8	91	>0.1
strained, 'Baby's First' (Beech-Nut)	2.5-oz jar	12	0.01	0.02	0.04	0.02	1.3	0.00	27.2	2.8	0.2	2.1	50	>0.1
strained, 'Beginner 1' (Heinz)	2.5-oz jar	12	0.01	0.02	0.04	0.02	1.3	0.00	27.2	2.8	0.2	2.1	50	>0.1
strained, 'First Foods' (Gerber)	2.5-oz jar	12	0.01	0.02	0.04	0.02	1.3	0.00	27.2	2.8	0.2	2.1	50	>0.1
strained, 'Second Foods' (Gerber)	4-oz jar	19	0.01	0.03	0.07	0.04	2.1	0.00	43.3	4.5	0.3	3.4	80	>0.1
strained, 'Stages 1' (Beech-Nut)	4-oz jar	19	0.01	0.03	0.07	0.04	2.1	0.00	43.3	4.5	0.3	3.4	80	>0.1
strained, 'Strained 2' (Heinz)	4-oz jar	19	0.01	0.03	0.07	0.04	2.1	0.00	43.3	4.5	0.3	3.4	80	>0.1
w/apricot, junior	1 oz	96	0.00	0.01	0.04	0.01	0.4	0.00	5.1	1.7	0.1	1.1	31	>0.1
w/apricot, junior	1 tbsp	54	0.00	0.01	0.02	0.01	0.2	0.00	2.9	1.0	<0.1	0.6	17	>0.1
w/apricot, junior, 'Junior 3' (Heinz)	6-oz jar	576	0.02	0.05	0.25	0.05	2.4	0.00	30.4	10.2	0.4	6.8	185	>0.1
w/apricot, strained	1 oz	110	0.00	0.01	0.04	0.01	0.4	0.00	5.4	1.7	0.1	1.1	34	>0.1
w/apricot, strained	1 tbsp	62	0.00	0.01	0.02	0.01	0.2	0.00	3.0	1.0	<0.1	0.6	19	>0.1
w/apricot, strained (Earth's Best)	4.5-oz jar	495	0.02	0.04	0.18	0.04	1.7	0.00	24.2	7.7	0.3	5.1	154	>0.1
w/apricot, strained, 'Second Foods' (Gerber)	4-oz jar	437	0.02	0.03	0.16	0.03	1.5	0.00	21.4	6.8	0.3	4.5	136	>0.1
w/apricot, strained, 'Stages 2' (Beech-Nut)	4-oz jar	437	0.02	0.03	0.16	0.03	1.5	0.00	21.4	6.8	0.3	4.5	136	>0.1
w/apricot, strained, 'Strained 2' (Heinz)	4-oz jar	437	0.02	0.03	0.16	0.03	1.5	0.00	21.4	6.8	0.3	4.5	136	>0.1
w/banana, junior	1 tbsp	3	0.00	0.01	0.03	0.02	0.5	0.00	2.8	0.8	<0.1	1.4	21	>0.1
w/banana, junior, 'Stages 3' (Beech-Nut)	6-oz jar	31	0.02	0.05	0.28	0.17	5.1	0.00	29.4	8.5	0.4	15.3	223	>0.1
w/cherry, junior	1 oz	13	0.00	0.01	0.04	0.01	0.1	0.00	12.1	0.3	0.1	1.1	37	>0.1
w/cherry, strained	1 oz	13	0.00	0.01	0.04	0.01	0.1	0.00	12.1	0.3	0.1	1.1	37	>0.1
w/pineapple, strained	1 oz	6	0.01	0.01	0.02	0.01	0.5	0.00	8.0	1.1	<0.1	0.9	22	0.0
w/pineapple, junior	1 oz	6	0.01	0.01	0.02	0.01	0.6	0.00	7.6	1.1	<0.1	1.1	22	>0.1
w/tapioca, junior	1 oz	205	0.00	0.00	0.06	0.01	0.5	0.00	5.1	2.3	0.1	1.1	35	>0.1
w/tapioca, junior	1 tbsp	108	0.00	0.00	0.03	0.00	0.2	0.00	2.7	1.2	<0.1	0.6	19	>0.1
w/tapioca, junior, 'Junior 3' (Heinz)	6-oz jar	1229	0.01	0.02	0.33	0.05	2.7	0.00	30.4	13.6	0.5	6.8	213	>0.1
w/tapioca, junior, 'Third Foods' (Gerber)	6-oz jar	1229	0.01	0.02	0.33	0.05	2.7	0.00	30.4	13.6	0.5	6.8	213	>0.1
w/tapioca, strained	1 oz	206	0.00	0.00	0.06	0.01	0.4	0.00	6.1	2.6	0.1	1.1	34	>0.1
w/tapioca, strained	1 tbsp	109	0.00	0.00	0.03	0.01	0.2	0.00	3.2	1.4	0.1	0.6	18	>0.1
w/tapioca, strained, 'Second Foods' (Gerber)	4-oz jar	819	0.01	0.02	0.22	0.03	1.7	0.00	24.4	10.2	0.3	4.5	137	<0.1
w/tapioca, strained, 'Strained 2' (Heinz)	4.25-oz jar	870	0.01	0.02	0.23	0.04	1.8	0.00	25.9	10.8	0.4	4.8	145	<0.1
Banana														
w/tapioca, junior	1 jar	75	0.03	0.03	0.37	0.24	10.9	0.00	43.7	13.6	0.5	20.4	184	0.1

Food Name	Serving Size	A I.U.	Thi mg	Rib mg	Nia mg	B$_6$ mg	Fol mcg	B$_{12}$ mcg	C mg	Calc mg	Iron mg	Mag mg	Pot mg	Zn mg
w/tapioca, junior	1 oz	13	0.00	0.01	0.06	0.04	1.8	0.00	7.3	2.3	0.1	3.4	31	<0.1
w/tapioca, junior	1 tbsp	7	0.00	0.00	0.03	0.02	1.0	0.00	3.9	1.2	0.1	1.8	16	<0.1
w/tapioca, junior, 'Junior 3' (Heinz)	6-oz jar	75	0.03	0.03	0.37	0.24	10.9	0.00	43.7	13.6	0.5	20.4	184	0.1
w/tapioca, junior, 'Third Foods' (Gerber)	6-oz jar	75	0.03	0.03	0.37	0.24	10.9	0.00	43.7	13.6	0.5	20.4	184	0.1
w/tapioca, strained	1 jar	49	0.01	0.04	0.21	0.13	6.2	0.00	18.9	5.7	0.2	11.3	99	<0.1
w/tapioca, strained	1 oz	12	0.00	0.01	0.05	0.03	1.6	0.00	4.7	1.4	0.1	2.8	25	<0.1
w/tapioca, strained	1 tbsp	7	0.00	0.01	0.03	0.02	0.8	0.00	2.5	0.8	<0.1	1.5	13	<0.1
w/tapioca, strained, 'Second Foods' (Gerber)	4-oz jar	49	0.01	0.04	0.21	0.13	6.2	0.00	18.9	5.7	0.2	11.3	99	<0.1
w/tapioca, strained, 'Strained 2' (Heinz)	4.25-oz jar	52	0.01	0.04	0.22	0.14	6.6	0.00	20.0	6.0	0.2	12.0	106	<0.1
Banana and pineapple														
w/tapioca, junior	1 jar	68	0.03	0.03	0.31	0.16	9.3	0.00	36.0	11.9	0.2	10.2	133	<0.1
w/tapioca, junior	1 oz	11	0.00	0.01	0.05	0.03	1.6	0.00	6.0	2.0	<0.1	1.7	22	<0.1
w/tapioca, junior	1 tbsp	6	0.00	0.00	0.03	0.01	0.8	0.00	3.2	1.1	<0.1	0.9	12	<0.1
w/tapioca, junior, 'Junior 3' (Heinz)	6-oz jar	68	0.03	0.03	0.31	0.16	9.3	0.00	36.0	11.9	0.2	10.2	133	<0.1
w/tapioca, junior, 'Third Foods' (Gerber)	6-oz jar	68	0.03	0.03	0.31	0.16	9.3	0.00	36.0	11.9	0.2	10.2	133	<0.1
w/tapioca, strained	1 jar	46	0.02	0.02	0.19	0.09	6.1	0.00	21.7	7.9	0.3	6.8	77	<0.1
w/tapioca, strained	1 oz	12	0.01	0.01	0.05	0.02	1.5	0.00	5.4	2.0	0.1	1.7	19	<0.1
w/tapioca, strained	1 tbsp	6	0.00	0.00	0.03	0.01	0.8	0.00	2.9	1.1	<0.1	0.9	10	<0.1
w/tapioca, strained, 'Second Foods' (Gerber)	4-oz jar	46	0.02	0.02	0.19	0.09	6.1	0.00	21.7	7.9	0.3	6.8	77	<0.1
w/tapioca, strained, 'Strained 2' (Heinz)	4.25-oz jar	49	0.02	0.02	0.20	0.10	6.5	0.00	23.0	8.4	0.3	7.2	82	<0.1
Guava and papaya														
w/tapioca, strained	1 oz	52	0.00	0.01	0.08	0.01	0.6	0.00	22.9	2.0	0.1	1.4	21	<0.1
w/tapioca, strained	1 oz	85	0.00	0.02	0.11	0.01	0.6	0.00	21.4	2.0	0.1	0.6	21	<0.1
Mango														
w/tapioca, strained	1 oz	189	0.01	0.01	0.07	0.03	0.6	0.00	35.3	1.1	<0.1	1.1	17	<0.1
w/tapioca, strained	1 tbsp	100	0.00	0.00	0.04	0.02	0.3	0.00	18.7	0.6	<0.1	0.6	9	<0.1
w/tapioca, strained (Gerber)	4-oz jar	751	0.03	0.03	0.29	0.13	2.3	0.00	141	4.5	0.1	4.5	67	<0.1
Papaya and applesauce														
w/tapioca, strained	1 oz	21.5	0.00	0.01	0.03	0.01	0.6	0.00	32.1	2.0	0.1	1.4	22	<0.1
Peach														
w/sugar, junior	1 jar	303	0.02	0.05	1.10	0.03	6.6	0.00	32.1	8.5	0.5	8.5	264	0.1
w/sugar, junior	1 oz	51	0.00	0.01	0.18	0.01	1.1	0.00	5.4	1.4	0.1	1.4	44	<0.1
w/sugar, junior	1 tbsp	29	0.00	0.01	0.10	0.00	0.6	0.00	3.0	0.8	<0.1	0.8	25	<0.1
w/sugar, junior, 'Junior 3' (Heinz)	6-oz jar	303	0.02	0.05	1.10	0.03	6.6	0.00	32.1	8.5	0.5	8.5	264	0.1
w/sugar, junior, 'Stages 3' (Beech-Nut)	6-oz jar	303	0.02	0.05	1.10	0.03	6.6	0.00	32.1	8.5	0.5	8.5	264	0.1
w/sugar, junior, 'Third Foods' (Gerber)	6-oz jar	303	0.02	0.05	1.10	0.03	6.6	0.00	32.1	8.5	0.5	8.5	264	0.1
w/sugar, strained	1 jar	182	0.01	0.04	0.69	0.02	4.4	0.00	35.5	6.8	0.3	6.8	183	0.1
w/sugar, strained	1 oz	46	0.00	0.01	0.17	0.00	1.1	0.00	8.9	1.7	0.1	1.7	46	<0.1
w/sugar, strained	1 tbsp	26	0.00	0.01	0.10	0.00	0.6	0.00	5.0	1.0	<0.1	1.0	26	<0.1
w/sugar, strained, 'Baby's First' (Beech-Nut)	2.5-oz jar	114	0.01	0.02	0.43	0.01	2.8	0.00	22.3	4.3	0.2	4.3	115	<0.1
w/sugar, strained, 'Beginner 1' (Heinz)	2.5-oz jar	114	0.01	0.02	0.43	0.01	2.8	0.00	22.3	4.3	0.2	4.3	115	<0.1
w/sugar, strained, 'First Foods' (Gerber)	2.5-oz jar	114	0.01	0.02	0.43	0.01	2.8	0.00	22.3	4.3	0.2	4.3	115	<0.1
w/sugar, strained, 'Second Foods' (Gerber)	4-oz jar	182	0.01	0.04	0.69	0.02	4.4	0.00	35.5	6.8	0.3	6.8	183	0.1
w/sugar, strained, 'Stages 1' (Beech-Nut)	4-oz jar	182	0.01	0.04	0.69	0.02	4.4	0.00	35.5	6.8	0.3	6.8	183	0.1

Food Name	Serving Size	A I.U.	Thi mg	Rib mg	Nia mg	B$_6$ mg	Fol mcg	B$_{12}$ mcg	C mg	Calc mg	Iron mg	Mag mg	Pot mg	Zn mg
w/sugar, strained, 'Strained 2' (Heinz)	4-oz jar	182	0.01	0.04	0.69	0.02	4.4	0.00	35.5	6.8	0.3	6.8	183	0.1
Pear														
junior	1 oz	10	0.00	0.01	0.05	0.00	1.1	0.00	6.2	2.3	0.1	2.6	33	<0.1
junior	1 tbsp	5	0.00	0.01	0.03	0.00	0.6	0.00	3.5	1.3	<0.1	1.4	18	<0.1
junior, 'Junior 3' (Heinz)	6-oz jar	58	0.02	0.05	0.32	0.02	6.5	0.00	37.4	13.6	0.4	15.3	196	0.1
junior, 'Stages 3' (Beech-Nut)	6-oz jar	58	0.02	0.05	0.32	0.02	6.5	0.00	37.4	13.6	0.4	15.3	196	0.1
junior, 'Third Foods' (Gerber)	6-oz jar	58	0.02	0.05	0.32	0.02	6.5	0.00	37.4	13.6	0.4	15.3	196	0.1
strained	1 oz	9	0.00	0.01	0.05	0.00	1.0	0.00	6.9	2.3	0.1	2.3	37	<0.1
strained	1 tbsp	5	0.00	0.00	0.03	0.00	0.6	0.00	3.9	1.3	<0.1	1.3	21	<0.1
strained (Earth's Best)	4.5-oz jar	37	0.02	0.03	0.21	0.01	4.1	0.00	27.7	9.0	0.3	9.0	147	<0.1
strained, 'Baby's First' (Beech-Nut)	2.5-oz jar	23	0.01	0.02	0.13	0.01	2.6	0.00	17.4	5.7	0.2	5.7	92	<0.1
strained, 'Beginner 1' (Heinz)	2.5-oz jar	23	0.01	0.02	0.13	0.01	2.6	0.00	17.4	5.7	0.2	5.7	92	<0.1
strained, 'First Foods' (Gerber)	2.5-oz jar	23	0.01	0.02	0.13	0.01	2.6	0.00	17.4	5.7	0.2	5.7	92	<0.1
strained, 'Second Foods' (Gerber)	4-oz jar	37	0.02	0.03	0.21	0.01	4.1	0.00	27.7	9.0	0.3	9.0	147	<0.1
strained, 'Stages 1' (Beech-Nut)	4-oz jar	37	0.02	0.03	0.21	0.01	4.1	0.00	27.7	9.0	0.3	9.0	147	<0.1
strained, 'Strained 2' (Heinz)	4-oz jar	37	0.02	0.03	0.21	0.01	4.1	0.00	27.7	9.0	0.3	9.0	147	<0.1
Pear and pineapple														
junior	1 oz	9	0.01	0.01	0.05	0.00	0.8	0.00	4.8	2.8	0.1	2.0	34	<0.1
junior	1 tbsp	5	0.00	0.00	0.03	0.00	0.5	0.00	2.7	1.6	<0.1	1.1	19	<0.1
junior, 'Third Foods' (Gerber)	6-oz jar	54	0.04	0.04	0.31	0.02	4.9	0.00	28.6	17.0	0.4	11.9	201	0.2
strained	1 oz	8	0.01	0.01	0.06	0.01	0.8	0.00	7.8	2.8	0.1	2.0	33	<0.1
strained	1 tbsp	5	0.00	0.00	0.03	0.00	0.5	0.00	4.4	1.6	<0.1	1.1	19	<0.1
strained, 'Second Foods' (Gerber)	4-oz jar	33	0.02	0.03	0.23	0.02	3.2	0.00	31.1	11.3	0.3	7.9	131	<0.1
strained, 'Stages 2' (Beech-Nut)	4-oz jar	33	0.02	0.03	0.23	0.02	3.2	0.00	31.1	11.3	0.3	7.9	131	<0.1
strained, 'Strained 2' (Heinz)	4-oz jar	33	0.02	0.03	0.23	0.02	3.2	0.00	31.1	11.3	0.3	7.9	131	<0.1
Plum														
w/tapioca, junior	1 oz	27	0.00	0.01	0.06	0.01	0.3	0.00	0.2	1.7	0.1	1.1	24	<0.1
w/tapioca, junior	1 tbsp	14	0.00	0.01	0.03	0.00	0.1	0.00	0.1	0.9	<0.1	0.6	12	<0.1
w/tapioca, junior, 'Third Foods' (Gerber)	6-oz jar	160	0.01	0.05	0.35	0.05	1.5	0.00	1.4	10.2	0.4	6.8	141	0.1
w/tapioca, strained	1 oz	27	0.00	0.01	0.06	0.01	0.3	0.00	0.3	1.7	0.1	1.1	24	<0.1
w/tapioca, strained	1 tbsp	14	0.00	0.00	0.03	0.00	0.1	0.00	0.2	0.9	<0.1	0.6	13	<0.1
w/tapioca, strained, 'Second Foods' (Gerber)	4-oz jar	107	0.01	0.03	0.24	0.03	1.0	0.00	1.2	6.8	0.2	4.5	96	<0.1
w/tapioca, strained, 'Strained 2' (Heinz)	4-oz jar	107	0.01	0.03	0.24	0.03	1.0	0.00	1.2	6.8	0.2	4.5	96	<0.1
Prune														
w/tapioca, junior	1 oz	115	0.01	0.02	0.15	0.02	<0.1	0.00	0.2	4.3	0.1	2.8	46	<0.1
w/tapioca, strained	1 oz	128	0.01	0.02	0.15	0.02	<0.1	0.00	0.2	4.3	0.1	2.8	50	<0.1
w/tapioca, strained	1 tbsp	68	0.00	0.01	0.08	0.01	<0.1	0.00	0.1	2.3	0.1	1.5	27	<0.1
w/tapioca, strained, 'Second Foods' (Gerber)	4-oz jar	512	0.03	0.09	0.59	0.09	0.2	0.00	0.9	16.9	0.4	11.3	200	0.1
w/tapioca, strained, 'Strained 2' (Heinz)	4.25-oz jar	544	0.03	0.09	0.63	0.10	0.2	0.00	1.0	18.0	0.4	12.0	212	0.1
Tropical fruit, junior	1 oz	6	0.00	0.01	0.02	0.01	0.9	0.00	5.3	2.8	0.1	1.4	16	<0.1
JUICE														
Apple														
	1 fl oz	6	0.00	0.01	0.03	0.01	<0.1	0.00	18.4	1.3	0.2	1.0	29	<0.1
(Earth's Best)	4.2 fl oz	24	0.01	0.02	0.11	0.04	0.1	0.00	75.8	5.2	0.8	3.9	119	<0.1
'First Foods' (Gerber)	4 fl oz	23	0.01	0.02	0.10	0.04	0.1	0.00	72.4	5.0	0.7	3.8	114	<0.1
'Stages 1' (Beech-Nut)	4 fl oz	23	0.01	0.02	0.10	0.04	0.1	0.00	72.4	5.0	0.7	3.8	114	<0.1
'Strained 2' (Heinz)	4 fl oz	23	0.01	0.02	0.10	0.04	0.1	0.00	72.4	5.0	0.7	3.8	114	<0.1
Apple-banana														
	1 fl oz	3	0.00	0.00	0.04	0.02	0.3	0.00	8.7	2.2	0.1	1.9	38	<0.1

Food Name	Serving Size	A I.U.	Thi mg	Rib mg	Nia mg	B$_6$ mg	Fol mcg	B$_{12}$ mcg	C mg	Calc mg	Iron mg	Mag mg	Pot mg	Zn mg
(Earth's Best)	4.2 fl oz	12	0.01	0.01	0.18	0.08	1.3	0.00	36.5	9.2	0.3	7.9	161	<0.1
'Second Foods' (Gerber)	4 fl oz	11	0.01	0.01	0.17	0.08	1.3	0.00	34.9	8.8	0.3	7.5	154	<0.1
'Stages 2' (Beech-Nut)	4 fl oz	11	0.01	0.01	0.17	0.08	1.3	0.00	34.9	8.8	0.3	7.5	154	<0.1
'Strained 2' (Heinz)	4 fl oz	11	0.01	0.01	0.17	0.08	1.3	0.00	34.9	8.8	0.3	7.5	154	<0.1
Apple-cherry	1 fl oz	2	0.00	0.01	0.03	0.01	0.1	0.00	18.2	1.6	0.2	0.9	31	<0.1
Apple-grape														
	1 fl oz	2	0.00	0.01	0.03	0.01	0.1	0.00	16.7	1.9	0.1	0.9	28	<0.1
(Earth's Best)	4.2 fl oz	8	0.01	0.03	0.14	0.05	0.4	0.00	70.2	7.9	0.5	3.9	118	<0.1
'Second Foods' (Gerber)	4 fl oz	8	0.01	0.03	0.14	0.04	0.4	0.00	67.0	7.5	0.5	3.8	113	<0.1
'Stages 2' (Beech-Nut)	4 fl oz	8	0.01	0.03	0.14	0.04	0.4	0.00	67.0	7.5	0.5	3.8	113	<0.1
'Strained 2' (Heinz)	4 fl oz	8	0.01	0.03	0.14	0.04	0.4	0.00	67.0	7.5	0.5	3.8	113	<0.1
w/calcium, 'Graduates' (Gerber)	6 fl oz	6	0.02	0.04	0.19	0.10	1.5	0.00	40.1	240.0	0.6	127.0	163	<0.1
Apple-peach	1 fl oz	20	0.00	0.00	0.07	0.01	0.4	0.00	18.3	0.9	0.2	0.9	30	<0.1
Apple-pineapple														
Apple-plum	1 fl oz	13	0.01	0.01	0.06	0.01	<0.1	0.00	18.2	1.6	0.2	0.9	32	<0.1
Apple-prune														
	4 fl oz	20	0.01	0.00	0.38	0.04	0.1	0.00	84.4	11.3	1.2	8.8	185	<0.1
	1 fl oz	5	0.00	0.00	0.09	0.01	<0.1	0.00	21.1	2.8	0.3	2.2	46	<0.1
Fruit punch														
w/calcium, 'Graduates' (Gerber)	6 fl oz	6	0.02	0.04	0.19	0.10	1.5	0.00	40.1	121.0	0.6	13.2	163	<0.1
Mixed fruit														
	4 fl oz	53	0.03	0.02	0.15	0.05	8.4	0.00	79.5	10.0	0.4	6.3	126	<0.1
	1 fl oz	13	0.01	0.00	0.04	0.01	2.1	0.00	19.8	2.5	0.1	1.6	32	<0.1
Orange														
	1 fl oz	17	0.01	0.01	0.08	0.02	8.2	0.00	19.5	3.7	0.1	2.8	57	<0.1
'Second Foods' (Gerber)	4 fl oz	69	0.06	0.04	0.30	0.07	33.0	0.00	78.1	15.0	0.2	11.3	230	<0.1
'Stages 3' (Beech-Nut)	4 fl oz	69	0.06	0.04	0.30	0.07	33.0	0.00	78.1	15.0	0.2	11.3	230	<0.1
'Strained 2' (Heinz)	4 fl oz	69	0.06	0.04	0.30	0.07	33.0	0.00	78.1	15.0	0.2	11.3	230	<0.1
Orange-apple	1 fl oz	23	0.01	0.01	0.06	0.01	3.8	0.00	24.0	3.1	0.1	1.6	43	<0.1
Orange-apple-banana														
	1 fl oz	8	0.01	0.01	0.08	0.02	3.0	0.00	10.0	1.6	0.1	1.9	42	<0.1
'Strained 2' (Heinz)	4 fl oz	34	0.05	0.03	0.33	0.08	12.1	0.00	40.1	6.3	0.4	7.5	168	<0.1
Orange-apricot	1 fl oz	67	0.02	0.01	0.08	0.02	6.2	0.00	26.8	1.9	0.1	2.2	62	<0.1
Orange-banana	1 fl oz	14	0.02	0.01	0.06	0.02	7.6	0.00	10.6	5.3	<0.1	4.4	62	<0.1
Orange-pineapple	1 fl oz	10	0.02	0.01	0.06	0.02	5.8	0.00	16.7	2.5	0.1	2.8	44	<0.1
Prune-orange	1 fl oz	41	0.01	0.04	0.12	0.02	4.1	0.00	19.9	3.7	0.3	2.5	57	<0.1
MEAT														
Beef														
junior	1 oz	17	0.00	0.05	0.93	0.03	1.6	0.42	0.5	2.3	0.5	2.6	54	0.6
junior	1 tbsp	9	0.00	0.02	0.49	0.02	0.9	0.22	0.3	1.2	0.3	1.4	29	0.3
junior, 'Junior 3' (Heinz)	2.5-oz jar	42	0.01	0.11	2.30	0.09	4.0	1.00	1.3	5.7	1.2	6.4	135	1.4
junior, 'Third Foods' (Gerber)	2.5-oz jar	42	0.01	0.11	2.30	0.09	4.0	1.00	1.3	5.7	1.2	6.4	135	1.4
strained	1 oz	19	0.00	0.04	0.81	0.04	1.6	0.40	0.6	2.0	0.4	4.8	62	0.7
strained	1 tbsp	10	0.00	0.02	0.43	0.02	0.8	0.21	0.3	1.1	0.2	2.5	33	0.4
strained, 'Second Foods' (Gerber)	2.5-oz jar	48	0.01	0.10	2.00	0.10	3.9	1.00	1.5	5.0	1.0	12.1	156	1.7
strained, 'Stages 1' (Beech-Nut)	2.5-oz jar	48	0.01	0.10	2.00	0.10	3.9	1.00	1.5	5.0	1.0	12.1	156	1.7
strained, 'Strained 2' (Heinz)	2.5-oz jar	48	0.01	0.10	2.00	0.10	3.9	1.00	1.5	5.0	1.0	12.1	156	1.7
Chicken														
junior	1 oz	11	0.00	0.05	0.97	0.05	3.1	0.11	0.4	15.6	0.3	3.1	35	0.3
junior	1 tbsp	6	0.00	0.02	0.51	0.03	1.7	0.06	0.2	8.3	0.2	1.6	18	0.2
junior, 'Junior 3' (Heinz)	2.5-oz jar	28	0.01	0.12	2.40	0.13	7.9	0.28	1.1	39.0	0.7	7.8	87	0.7
junior, 'Third Foods' (Gerber)	2.5-oz jar	28	0.01	0.12	2.40	0.13	7.9	0.28	1.1	39.0	0.7	7.8	87	0.7
strained	1 oz	15	0.00	0.04	0.92	0.06	2.9	0.11	0.5	18.1	0.4	3.7	40	0.3
strained	1 tbsp	8	0.00	0.02	0.49	0.03	1.6	0.06	0.3	9.6	0.2	1.9	21	0.2

Food Name	Serving Size	A I.U.	Thi mg	Rib mg	Nia mg	B_6 mg	Fol mcg	B_{12} mcg	C mg	Calc mg	Iron mg	Mag mg	Pot mg	Zn mg
strained, 'Second Foods' (Gerber)	2.5-oz jar	38	0.01	0.11	2.30	0.14	7.4	0.28	1.2	45.4	1.0	9.2	100	0.9
strained, 'Stages 1' (Beech-Nut)	2.5-oz jar	38	0.01	0.11	2.30	0.14	7.4	0.28	1.2	45.4	1.0	9.2	100	0.9
strained, 'Strained 2' (Heinz)	2.5-oz jar	38	0.01	0.11	2.30	0.14	7.4	0.28	1.2	45.4	1.0	9.2	100	0.9
Chicken stick														
	1 stick	1	0.00	0.02	0.20	0.01	1.1	0.04	0.2	7.3	0.2	1.4	11	0.1
'Graduates' (Gerber)	2.5-oz jar	8	0.01	0.14	1.40	0.07	7.9	0.28	1.2	51.8	1.1	9.9	75	0.7
Ham														
junior	1 oz	9	0.04	0.06	0.81	0.06	0.6	0.03	0.6	1.4	0.3	3.1	60	0.5
strained	1 oz	11	0.04	0.04	0.75	0.07	0.6	0.03	0.6	1.7	0.3	3.7	58	0.6
strained	1 tbsp	6	0.02	0.02	0.40	0.04	0.3	0.02	0.3	0.9	0.2	1.9	31	0.3
strained, 'Second Foods' (Gerber)	2.5-oz jar	27	0.10	0.11	1.90	0.18	1.4	0.07	1.5	4.3	0.7	9.2	145	1.6
Lamb														
junior	1 oz	8	0.01	0.05	0.91	0.05	0.6	0.64	0.5	2.0	0.5	2.8	60	0.7
strained	1 oz	9	0.01	0.06	0.83	0.04	0.7	0.62	0.3	2.0	0.4	3.7	58	0.8
strained	1 tbsp	5	0.00	0.03	0.44	0.02	0.3	0.33	0.2	1.1	0.2	1.9	31	0.4
strained, 'Second Foods' (Gerber)	2.5-oz jar	23	0.01	0.14	2.10	0.11	1.6	1.60	0.9	5.0	1.1	9.2	146	2.0
strained, 'Stages 1' (Beech-Nut)	2.5-oz jar	23	0.01	0.14	2.10	0.11	1.6	1.60	0.9	5.0	1.1	9.2	146	2.0
strained, 'Strained 2' (Heinz)	2.5-oz jar	23	0.01	0.14	2.10	0.11	1.6	1.60	0.9	5.0	1.1	9.2	146	2.0
Meat stick														
	1 jar	49	0.04	0.12	1.10	0.06	6.3	0.21	1.7	24.1	1.0	7.8	81	1.3
	1 stick	7	0.01	0.02	0.15	0.01	0.9	0.03	0.2	3.4	0.1	1.1	11	0.2
(Gerber) 'Graduates'	2.5-oz jar	49	0.04	0.12	1.10	0.06	6.3	0.21	1.7	24.1	1.0	7.8	81	1.3
Pork, strained	1 oz	11	0.04	0.06	0.64	0.06	0.5	0.28	0.5	1.4	0.3	2.8	63	0.6
Turkey														
junior	1 oz	9	0.01	0.07	0.99	0.05	3.4	0.30	0.7	7.9	0.4	3.4	51	0.5
junior	1 tbsp	5	0.00	0.04	0.52	0.03	1.8	0.16	0.4	4.2	0.2	1.8	27	0.3
junior, 'Third Foods' (Gerber)	2.5-oz jar	23	0.01	0.18	2.50	0.12	8.6	0.76	1.7	19.9	1.0	8.5	128	1.3
strained	1 oz	13	0.01	0.06	1.00	0.05	3.2	0.28	0.6	6.5	0.3	4.0	66	0.5
strained	1 tbsp	7	0.00	0.03	0.55	0.03	1.7	0.15	0.3	3.5	0.2	2.1	35	0.3
strained, 'Second Foods' (Gerber)	2.5-oz jar	33	0.01	0.15	2.60	0.13	8.0	0.71	1.6	16.3	0.9	9.9	164	1.3
strained, 'Stages 1' (Beech-Nut)	2.5-oz jar	33	0.01	0.15	2.60	0.13	8.0	0.71	1.6	16.3	0.9	9.9	164	1.3
strained, 'Strained 2' (Heinz)	2.5-oz jar	33	0.01	0.15	2.60	0.13	8.0	0.71	1.6	16.3	0.9	9.9	164	1.3
Turkey stick														
	1 jar	14	0.01	0.11	1.20	0.05	8.0	0.71	1.1	51.1	0.9	11.4	65	1.3
	1 stick	2	0.00	0.02	0.17	0.01	1.1	0.10	0.2	7.2	0.1	1.6	9	0.1
(Gerber) 'Graduates'	2.5-oz jar	14	0.01	0.11	1.20	0.05	8.0	0.71	1.1	51.1	0.9	11.4	65	1.3
Veal														
junior	1 oz	14	0.01	0.05	1.10	0.03	1.9	0.37	0.6	1.7	0.4	3.1	70	0.7
strained	1 oz	13	0.01	0.05	1.00	0.04	1.7	0.37	0.7	2.0	0.4	3.4	61	0.6
strained	1 tbsp	7	0.00	0.02	0.53	0.02	0.9	0.20	0.3	1.1	0.2	1.8	32	0.3
strained, 'Second Foods' (Gerber)	2.5-oz jar	33	0.01	0.11	2.50	0.11	4.2	0.92	1.6	5.0	0.9	8.5	153	1.4
strained, 'Stages 1' (Beech-Nut)	2.5-oz jar	33	0.01	0.11	2.50	0.11	4.2	0.92	1.6	5.0	0.9	8.5	153	1.4
strained, 'Strained 2' (Heinz)	2.5-oz jar	33	0.01	0.11	2.50	0.11	4.2	0.92	1.6	5.0	0.9	8.5	153	1.4
VEGETABLES														
Beets														
strained	1 cup	74	0.03	0.10	0.30	0.05	69.0	0.00	5.4	31.4	0.7	31.4	408	0.3
strained	1 oz	9	0.00	0.01	0.04	0.01	8.7	0.00	0.7	4.0	0.1	4.0	52	<0.1
strained	1 tbsp	5	0.00	0.01	0.02	0.00	4.3	0.00	0.3	2.0	0.1	2.0	26	<0.1
strained, 'Second Foods' (Gerber)	4-oz jar	37	0.01	0.05	0.15	0.03	34.8	0.00	2.7	15.8	0.4	15.8	206	0.1
strained, 'Strained 2' (Heinz)	4-oz jar	37	0.01	0.05	0.15	0.03	34.8	0.00	2.7	15.8	0.4	15.8	206	0.1
Carrots														
junior	1 cup	26454	0.05	0.09	1.10	0.18	38.8	0.00	12.3	51.5	0.9	24.6	452	0.4
junior	1 oz	3348	0.01	0.01	0.14	0.02	4.9	0.00	1.6	6.5	0.1	3.1	57	<0.1
junior	1 tbsp	1653	0.00	0.01	0.07	0.01	2.4	0.00	0.8	3.2	0.1	1.5	28	<0.1

Food Name	Serving Size	A I.U.	Thi mg	Rib mg	Nia mg	B$_6$ mg	Fol mcg	B$_{12}$ mcg	C mg	Calc mg	Iron mg	Mag mg	Pot mg	Zn mg
junior, 'Junior 3' (Heinz)	6-oz jar	20077	0.04	0.07	0.84	0.14	29.4	0.00	9.3	39.1	0.7	18.7	343	0.3
junior, 'Stages 3' (Beech-Nut)	6-oz jar	20077	0.04	0.07	0.84	0.14	29.4	0.00	9.3	39.1	0.7	18.7	343	0.3
junior, 'Third Foods' (Gerber)	6-oz jar	20077	0.04	0.07	0.84	0.14	29.4	0.00	9.3	39.1	0.7	18.7	343	0.3
strained	1 cup	25673	0.05	0.09	1.00	0.16	33.4	0.00	12.8	49.3	0.8	20.2	439	0.3
strained	1 oz	3249	0.01	0.01	0.13	0.02	4.2	0.00	1.6	6.2	0.1	2.6	56	<0.1
strained (Earth's Best)	4.5-oz jar	14670	0.03	0.05	0.59	0.09	19.1	0.00	7.3	28.2	0.5	11.5	251	0.2
strained (Earth's Best)	1 tbsp	1605	0.00	0.01	0.07	0.01	2.1	0.00	0.8	3.1	0.1	1.3	27	<0.1
strained, 'Baby's First (Beech-Nut)'	2.5-oz jar	8137	0.02	0.03	0.33	0.05	10.6	0.00	4.0	15.6	0.3	6.4	139	0.1
strained, 'Beginner 1' (Heinz)	2.5-oz jar	8137	0.02	0.03	0.33	0.05	10.6	0.00	4.0	15.6	0.3	6.4	139	0.1
strained, 'First Foods' (Gerber)	2.5-oz jar	8137	0.02	0.03	0.33	0.05	10.6	0.00	4.0	15.6	0.3	6.4	139	0.1
strained, 'Second Foods' (Gerber)	4-oz jar	12951	0.03	0.05	0.52	0.08	16.8	0.00	6.4	24.9	0.4	10.2	221	0.2
strained, 'Stages 1' (Beech-Nut)	4-oz jar	12951	0.03	0.05	0.52	0.08	16.8	0.00	6.4	24.9	0.4	10.2	221	0.2
strained, 'Strained 2' (Heinz)	4-oz jar	12951	0.03	0.05	0.52	0.08	16.8	0.00	6.4	24.9	0.4	10.2	221	0.2
Corn														
creamed, junior	1 cup	185	0.03	0.12	1.20	0.10	30.5	0.05	5.3	43.2	0.7	19.2	194	0.6
creamed, junior	1 oz	22	0.00	0.01	0.14	0.01	3.6	0.01	0.6	5.1	0.1	2.3	23	<0.1
creamed, junior	1 tbsp	12	0.00	0.01	0.08	0.01	1.9	0.00	0.3	2.7	<0.1	1.2	12	<0.1
creamed, junior, 'Junior 3' (Heinz)	6-oz jar	131	0.02	0.08	0.86	0.07	21.6	0.03	3.7	30.6	0.5	13.6	138	0.4
creamed, strained	1 cup	180	0.03	0.11	1.20	0.10	27.1	0.05	5.0	48.0	0.7	19.2	216	0.5
creamed, strained	1 oz	21	0.00	0.01	0.14	0.01	3.2	0.01	0.6	5.7	0.1	2.3	26	<0.1
creamed, strained	1 tbsp	11	0.00	0.01	0.08	0.01	1.7	0.00	0.3	3.0	<0.1	1.2	14	<0.1
creamed, strained, 'Second Foods' (Gerber)	4-oz jar	85	0.02	0.05	0.58	0.05	12.8	0.02	2.4	22.6	0.3	9.0	102	0.2
creamed, strained, 'Stages 2' (Beech-Nut)	4-oz jar	85	0.02	0.05	0.58	0.05	12.8	0.02	2.4	22.6	0.3	9.0	102	0.2
creamed, strained, 'Strained 2' (Heinz)	4-oz jar	85	0.02	0.05	0.58	0.05	12.8	0.02	2.4	22.6	0.3	9.0	102	0.2
Beans, green														
creamed, junior	1 cup	360	0.06	0.13	0.56	0.03	95.3	0.12	6.5	76.8	0.6	16.8	156	0.4
creamed, junior	1 oz	43	0.01	0.02	0.07	0.00	11.3	0.01	0.8	9.1	0.1	2.0	18	<0.1
creamed, junior	1 tbsp	23	0.0	0.01	0.04	0.00	6.0	0.01	0.4	4.8	<0.1	1.1	10	<0.1
creamed, junior, 'Junior 3' (Heinz)	6-oz jar	255	0.04	0.09	0.40	0.02	67.5	0.09	4.6	54.4	0.4	11.9	111	0.3
creamed, junior, 'Third Foods' (Gerber)	6-oz jar	255	0.04	0.09	0.40	0.02	67.5	0.09	4.6	54.4	0.4	11.9	111	0.3
junior	1 cup	1039	0.05	0.25	0.77	0.08	78.5	0.00	20.2	156.0	2.6	52.8	307	0.5
junior	1 oz	123	0.01	0.03	0.09	0.01	9.3	0.00	2.4	18.4	0.3	6.2	36	<0.1
junior	1 tbsp	65	0.00	0.02	0.05	0.01	4.9	0.00	1.3	9.8	0.2	3.3	19	<0.1
junior, 'Stages 3' (Beech-Nut) dinner	6-oz jar	736	0.04	0.17	0.55	0.06	55.6	0.00	14.3	111.0	1.8	37.4	218	0.3
strained	1 cup	1075	0.06	0.20	0.83	0.09	83.0	0.00	12.5	93.6	1.8	57.6	379	0.5
strained	1 oz	127	0.01	0.02	0.10	0.01	9.8	0.00	1.5	11.1	0.2	6.8	45	<0.1
strained	1 tbsp	67	0.00	0.01	0.05	0.01	5.2	0.00	0.8	5.8	0.1	3.6	24	<0.1
strained, 'Beginner 1' (Heinz)	2.5-oz jar	318	0.02	0.06	0.25	0.03	24.6	0.00	3.7	27.7	0.5	17.0	112	0.2
strained, 'First Foods' (Gerber)	2.5-oz jar	318	0.02	0.06	0.25	0.03	24.6	0.00	3.7	27.7	0.5	17.0	112	0.2
strained, 'Second Foods' (Gerber)	4-oz jar	506	0.03	0.10	0.39	0.04	39.1	0.00	5.9	44.1	0.9	27.1	179	0.2
strained, 'Stages 1' (Beech-Nut)	4-oz jar	506	0.03	0.10	0.39	0.04	39.1	0.00	5.9	44.1	0.9	27.1	179	0.2
strained, 'Strained 2' (Heinz)	4-oz jar	506	0.03	0.10	0.39	0.04	39.1	0.00	5.9	44.1	0.9	27.1	179	0.2
w/potatoes (Gerber)	4-oz jar	96	0.05	0.12	0.52	0.09	11.3	0.17	1.2	67.8	0.6	22.6	167	0.3
Garden vegetables, strained	1 oz	1720	0.02	0.02	0.22	0.03	11.4	0.00	1.6	7.9	0.2	6.0	48	<0.1
Mixed vegetables														
junior	1 cup	10068	0.07	0.08	1.60	0.19	9.8	0.00	6.0	26.4	1.0	26.4	408	0.7
junior	1 oz	1189	0.01	0.01	0.19	0.02	1.2	0.00	0.7	3.1	0.1	3.1	48	<0.1
junior	1 tbsp	629	0.00	0.01	0.10	0.01	0.6	0.00	0.4	1.6	0.1	1.6	26	<0.1
strained	1 jar	4510	0.03	0.03	0.37	0.06	4.4	0.00	1.9	14.7	0.4	11.3	144	0.2
strained	1 oz	1131	0.01	0.01	0.09	0.02	1.1	0.00	0.5	3.7	0.1	2.8	36	<0.1

Food Name	Serving Size	A I.U.	Thi mg	Rib mg	Nia mg	B₆ mg	Fol mcg	B₁₂ mcg	C mg	Calc mg	Iron mg	Mag mg	Pot mg	Zn mg
Peas														
creamed, strained	1 cup	206	0.21	0.13	1.90	0.11	54.5	0.19	3.8	31.2	1.3	38.4	211	0.9
creamed, strained	1 oz	24	0.03	0.02	0.23	0.01	6.4	0.02	0.5	3.7	0.2	4.5	25	0.1
creamed, strained	1 tbsp	13	0.01	0.01	0.12	0.01	3.4	0.01	0.2	1.9	0.1	2.4	13	<0.1
creamed, strained, 'Strained 2' (Heinz)	4-oz jar	97	0.10	0.06	0.92	0.05	25.7	0.09	1.8	14.7	0.6	18.1	99	0.4
strained	1 cup	1356	0.19	0.15	2.40	0.17	62.2	0.00	16.6	48.0	2.3	36.0	269	0.8
strained	1 oz	160	0.02	0.02	0.29	0.02	7.3	0.00	2.0	5.7	0.3	4.3	32	0.1
strained	1 tbsp	85	0.01	0.01	0.15	0.01	3.9	0.00	1.0	3.0	0.1	2.3	17	<0.1
strained, 'Baby's First' (Beech-Nut)	2.5-oz jar	401	0.06	0.04	0.72	0.05	18.4	0.00	4.9	14.2	0.7	10.7	80	0.3
strained, 'Beginner 1' (Heinz)	2.5-oz jar	401	0.06	0.04	0.72	0.05	18.4	0.00	4.9	14.2	0.7	10.7	80	0.3
strained, 'First Foods' (Gerber)	2.5-oz jar	401	0.06	0.04	0.72	0.05	18.4	0.00	4.9	14.2	0.7	10.7	80	0.3
strained, 'Second Foods' (Gerber)	4-oz jar	638	0.09	0.07	1.10	0.08	29.3	0.00	7.8	22.6	1.1	16.9	127	0.4
strained, 'Stages 1' (Beech-Nut)	4-oz jar	638	0.09	0.07	1.10	0.08	29.3	0.00	7.8	22.6	1.1	16.9	127	0.4
strained, 'Strained 2' (Heinz)	4-oz jar	638	0.09	0.07	1.10	0.08	29.3	0.00	7.8	22.6	1.1	16.9	127	0.4
Potato														
toddler	1 cup	0	0.03	0.02	0.57	0.11	9.8	0.00	17.1	6.5	0.3	24.4	179	0.3
toddler	1 tbsp	0	0.00	0.00	0.04	0.01	0.6	0.00	1.1	0.4	<0.1	1.5	11	<0.1
toddler, 'Graduates' (Gerber)	4.5 oz	0	0.01	0.01	0.25	0.05	4.3	0.00	7.5	2.8	0.1	10.7	78	0.1
Spinach														
creamed, strained	1 cup	10008	0.04	0.25	0.52	0.18	146.0	0.14	20.9	214.0	1.5	132	458	0.7
creamed, strained	1 oz	1182	0.00	0.03	0.06	0.02	17.2	0.02	2.5	25.2	0.2	15.6	54	<0.1
creamed, strained	1 tbsp	626	0.00	0.02	0.03	0.01	9.1	0.01	1.3	13.3	0.1	8.3	29	<0.1
creamed, strained, 'Second Foods' (Gerber)	4-oz jar	4712	0.02	0.12	0.24	0.09	68.7	0.07	9.8	101.0	0.7	62.1	216	0.4
Squash														
butternut, and corn (Gerber)	4-oz jar	3156	0.07	0.07	0.63	0.12	26.0	0.00	5.5	36.2	0.5	29.4	398	0.3
junior	1 cup	4511	0.03	0.15	0.85	0.16	34.5	0.00	17.5	53.8	0.8	26.9	414	0.2
junior	1 oz	571	0.00	0.02	0.11	0.02	4.4	0.00	2.2	6.8	0.1	3.4	52	<0.1
junior	1 tbsp	282	0.00	0.01	0.05	0.01	2.2	0.00	1.1	3.4	0.1	1.7	26	<0.1
junior, 'Third Foods' (Gerber)	6-oz jar	3424	0.02	0.11	0.64	0.12	26.2	0.00	13.3	40.8	0.6	20.4	315	0.1
strained	1 cup	4532	0.03	0.13	0.79	0.14	34.5	0.00	17.2	53.8	0.7	26.9	401	0.3
strained	1 oz	574	0.00	0.02	0.10	0.02	4.4	0.00	2.2	6.8	0.1	3.4	51	<0.1
strained (Earth's Best)	4.5-oz jar	2589	0.01	0.07	0.45	0.08	19.7	0.00	9.9	30.7	0.4	15.4	229	0.2
strained (Earth's Best)	1 tbsp	283	0.00	0.01	0.05	0.01	2.2	0.00	1.1	3.4	<0.1	1.7	25	<0.1
strained, 'Baby's First' (Beech-Nut)	2.5-oz jar	1436	0.01	0.04	0.25	0.05	10.9	0.00	5.5	17.0	0.2	8.5	127	0.1
strained, 'Beginner 1' (Heinz)	2.5-oz jar	1436	0.01	0.04	0.25	0.05	10.9	0.00	5.5	17.0	0.2	8.5	127	0.1
strained, 'First Foods' (Gerber)	2.5-oz jar	1436	0.01	0.04	0.25	0.05	10.9	0.00	5.5	17.0	0.2	8.5	127	0.1
strained, 'Second Foods' (Gerber)	4-oz jar	2286	0.01	0.06	0.40	0.07	17.4	0.00	8.7	27.1	0.3	13.6	202	0.1
strained, 'Stages 1' (Beech-Nut)	4-oz jar	2286	0.01	0.06	0.40	0.07	17.4	0.00	8.7	27.1	0.3	13.6	202	0.1
strained, 'Strained 2' (Heinz)	4-oz jar	2286	0.01	0.06	0.40	0.07	17.4	0.00	8.7	27.1	0.3	13.6	202	0.1
Sweet potato														
junior	1 cup	14865	0.06	0.08	0.86	0.25	23.1	0.00	21.5	35.8	0.9	26.9	544	0.3
junior	1 oz	1881	0.01	0.01	0.11	0.03	2.9	0.00	2.7	4.5	0.1	3.4	69	<0.1
junior	1 tbsp	929	0.00	0.01	0.05	0.02	1.4	0.00	1.3	2.2	0.1	1.7	34	<0.1
junior, 'Junior 3' (Heinz)	6-oz jar	11281	0.04	0.06	0.65	0.19	17.5	0.00	16.3	27.2	0.7	20.4	413	0.2
junior, 'Stages 3' (Beech-Nut)	6-oz jar	11281	0.04	0.06	0.65	0.19	17.5	0.00	16.3	27.2	0.7	20.4	413	0.2
junior, 'Third Foods' (Gerber)	6-oz jar	11281	0.04	0.06	0.65	0.19	17.5	0.00	16.3	27.2	0.7	20.4	413	0.2
strained	1 cup	14421	0.06	0.07	0.80	0.21	22.0	0.00	22.2	35.8	0.8	29.1	589	0.5
strained	1 oz	1825	0.01	0.01	0.10	0.03	2.8	0.00	2.8	4.5	0.1	3.7	75	<0.1
strained (Earth's Best)	4.5-oz jar	8241	0.04	0.04	0.46	0.12	12.5	0.00	12.7	20.5	0.5	16.6	337	0.3
strained (Earth's Best)	1 tbsp	901	0.00	0.01	0.05	0.01	1.4	0.00	1.4	2.2	0.1	1.8	37	<0.1
strained, 'Baby's First' (Beech-Nut)	2.5-oz jar	4571	0.02	0.02	0.25	0.07	7.0	0.00	7.0	11.4	0.3	9.2	187	0.2
strained, 'Beginner 1' (Heinz)	2.5-oz jar	4571	0.02	0.02	0.25	0.07	7.0	0.00	7.0	11.4	0.3	9.2	187	0.2
strained, 'First Foods' (Gerber)	2.5-oz jar	4571	0.02	0.02	0.25	0.07	7.0	0.00	7.0	11.4	0.3	9.2	187	0.2

Food Name	Serving Size	A I.U.	Thi mg	Rib mg	Nia mg	B$_6$ mg	Fol mcg	B$_{12}$ mcg	C mg	Calc mg	Iron mg	Mag mg	Pot mg	Zn mg
strained, 'Second Foods' (Gerber)	4-oz jar	7275	0.03	0.04	0.41	0.11	11.1	0.00	11.2	18.1	0.4	14.7	297	0.2
strained, 'Stages 1' (Beech-Nut).	4-oz jar	7275	0.03	0.04	0.41	0.11	11.1	0.00	11.2	18.1	0.4	14.7	297	0.2
strained, 'Strained 2' (Heinz).	4-oz jar	7275	0.03	0.04	0.41	0.11	11.1	0.00	11.2	18.1	0.4	14.7	297	0.2
BACON, COOKED														
cured, approx 12 slices per lb, raw	1 slice	0	0.14	0.04	1.10	0.05	0.8	0.35	0.0	2.7	0.2	3.4	58	0.4
cured, approx 20 slices per lb, raw	3 slices	0	0.25	0.07	1.90	0.10	1.4	0.63	0.0	4.8	0.4	6.1	104	0.8
cured, broiled, pan-fried or roasted	3 med slices	0	0.13	0.05	1.40	0.05	1.0	0.33	0.0	2.3	0.3	4.6	92	0.6
BACON, CANADIAN STYLE														
cured, 6 slices per 6-oz pkg, grilled	1 pkg	0	1.10	0.27	9.60	0.63	5.6	1.10	0.0	13.9	1.1	29.2	542	2.4
cured, 6 slices per 6-oz pkg, grilled	2 slices	0	0.38	0.09	3.20	0.21	1.9	0.36	0.0	4.7	0.4	9.8	181	0.8
cured, 6 slices per 6-oz pkg, unheated.	2 slices	0	0.43	0.10	3.50	0.22	2.3	0.38	0.0	4.5	0.4	9.6	195	0.8
cured, unheated	6-oz pkg	0	1.3	0.29	10.60	0.66	6.8	1.10	0.0	13.6	1.2	28.9	585	2.4
(Hormel)	1 serving	0	na	na	na	na	na	na	0.8	3.6	0.5	10.5	156	1.0
BACON SUBSTITUTE														
breakfast strips, beef, cured, cooked	3 slices	0	0.03	0.09	2.20	0.11	2.7	1.20	0.0	3.1	1.1	9.2	140	2.2
breakfast strips, beef, cured, uncooked	3 slices	0	0.04	0.08	2.00	0.12	3.4	1.10	16.3	2.7	0.8	7.5	104	2.6
breakfast strips, pork, cured, cooked	3 slices	0	0.25	0.13	2.60	0.12	1.4	0.60	0.0	4.8	0.7	8.8	158	1.3
breakfast strips, pork, cured, raw	3 slices	0	0.32	0.12	2.50	0.14	2.0	0.67	18.5	5.4	0.6	8.2	139	1.1
vegetarian, meatless	1 cup	127	6.30	0.69	10.9	0.69	59.8	0.00	0.0	33.1	3.5	27.4	245	0.6
vegetarian, meatless	1 strip	4	0.22	0.02	0.38	0.02	2.1	0.00	0.0	1.1	0.1	1.0	9	<0.1
(Louis Rich) turkey	1 serving	0	na	na	na	na	na	na	0.0	5.6	0.2	2.7	29	0.4
BAGEL														
BLUEBERRY														
(Lender's)														
4-inch diam, frozen, 'Bagel Shop'	1 bagel	0	0.27	0.20	4.10	0.06	75.5	0.00	0.0	57.1	1.8	na	158	na
frozen, 'Big'n Crusty'	1 serving	0	0.46	0.26	3.40	0.05	59.5	0.00	0.0	11.1	3.1	na	73	na
3-inch diam, refrigerated, 'Premium'	1 bagel	0	0.21	0.14	1.60	0.05	59.9	0.00	0.0	12.2	1.6	na	131	na
CINNAMON-RAISIN														
4.5-inch diam	1 bagel	86	0.45	0.33	3.60	0.07	106	0.00	0.8	22.4	4.5	33.0	175	1.3
3.5-inch diam	1 bagel	52	0.27	0.20	2.20	0.04	63.9	0.00	0.5	13.5	2.7	19.9	105	0.8
2.5-inch diam	1 bagel	19	0.10	0.07	0.80	0.02	23.4	0.00	0.2	4.9	1.0	7.3	39	0.3
EGG														
4.5-inch diam	1 bagel	120	0.59	0.26	3.80	0.10	96.8	0.18	0.7	14.3	4.4	27.5	75	0.9
3.5-inch diam	1 bagel	77	0.38	0.17	2.40	0.06	62.5	0.11	0.4	9.2	2.8	17.8	48	0.6
2.5-inch diam	1 bagel	28	0.14	0.06	0.90	0.02	22.9	0.04	0.2	3.4	1.0	6.5	18	0.2
OAT BRAN														
4.5-inch diam	1 bagel	4	0.36	0.37	3.30	0.05	89.1	0.00	0.2	13.2	3.4	34.1	127	1.0
3.5-inch diam	1 bagel	3	0.23	0.24	2.10	0.03	57.5	0.00	0.1	8.5	2.2	22.0	82	0.6
2.5-inch diam	1 bagel	1	0.09	0.09	0.77	0.01	21.1	0.00	0.1	3.1	0.8	8.1	30	0.2
PLAIN														
enriched, 4.5-inch diam	1 bagel	0	0.59	0.35	5.00	0.06	96.8	0.00	0.0	81.4	3.9	31.9	111	1.0
enriched, 4-inch diam	1 bagel	0	0.48	0.28	4.10	0.05	78.3	0.00	0.0	65.9	3.2	25.8	90	0.8
enriched, 3.5-inch diam	1 bagel	0	0.38	0.22	3.20	0.04	62.5	0.00	0.0	52.5	2.5	20.6	72	0.6
enriched, 3-inch diam	1 bagel	0	0.31	0.18	2.60	0.03	50.2	0.00	0.0	42.2	2.0	16.5	58	0.5
enriched, 2.5-inch diam	1 bagel	0	0.14	0.08	1.20	0.01	22.9	0.00	0.0	19.2	0.9	7.5	26	0.2
unenriched, 4.5-inch diam	1 bagel	0	0.18	0.06	1.90	0.06	24.2	0.00	0.0	81.4	1.5	31.9	111	1.0
unenriched, 4-inch diam	1 bagel	0	0.14	0.05	1.60	0.05	19.6	0.00	0.0	16.0	1.2	25.8	90	0.8
unenriched, 3.5-inch diam	1 bagel	0	0.12	0.04	1.20	0.04	15.6	0.00	0.0	12.8	1.0	20.6	72	0.6
unenriched, 3-inch diam	1 bagel	0	0.09	0.03	1.00	0.03	12.5	0.00	0.0	10.3	0.8	16.5	58	0.5
unenriched, 2.5-inch diam	1 bagel	0	0.04	0.01	0.46	0.01	5.7	0.00	0.0	4.7	0.4	7.5	26	0.2
BAKED BEANS, CANNED														
w/beef	1 cup	567	0.14	0.12	2.50	0.24	115	0.00	4.8	120.0	4.3	66.5	851	3.2
w/franfurters	1 cup	399	0.15	0.14	2.30	0.12	77.7	0.00	6.0	124.0	4.5	72.5	609	4.8
plain or vegetarian	1 cup	434	0.39	0.15	1.10	0.34	60.7	0.00	7.9	127.0	0.7	81.3	752	3.6

Food Name	Serving Size	A I.U.	Thi mg	Rib mg	Nia mg	B$_6$ mg	Fol mcg	B$_{12}$ mcg	C mg	Calc mg	Iron mg	Mag mg	Pot mg	Zn mg
w/pork	1 cup	450	0.13	0.10	1.10	0.16	91.8	0.00	5.1	134.0	4.3	86.0	782	3.7
w/pork, sweet sauce	1 cup	288	0.12	0.15	0.89	0.22	94.6	0.00	7.6	154.0	4.2	86.0	673	3.8
w/pork, tomato sauce	1 cup	314	0.13	0.12	1.30	0.17	56.9	0.00	7.8	142.0	8.3	88.5	759	14.8
w/pork, tomato sauce	1 tbsp	20	0.01	0.01	0.08	0.01	3.6	0.00	0.5	8.8	0.5	5.5	47	0.9

BAKING CHOCOLATE. See CHOCOLATE, BAKING.

BAKING POWDER
Double-acting

Food Name	Serving Size	A I.U.	Thi mg	Rib mg	Nia mg	B$_6$ mg	Fol mcg	B$_{12}$ mcg	C mg	Calc mg	Iron mg	Mag mg	Pot mg	Zn mg
sodium aluminum sulfate	1 tsp	0	0.00	0.00	0.00	0.00	0.0	0.00	0.0	270.0	0.5	1.2	1	0.0
sodium aluminum sulfate	1/2 tsp	0	0.00	0.00	0.00	0.00	0.0	0.00	0.0	135.0	0.3	0.6	<1	0.0
straight phosphate	1 tsp	0	0.00	0.00	0.00	0.00	0.0	0.00	0.0	339.0	0.5	1.8	<1	0.0
straight phosphate	1/2 tsp	0	0.00	0.00	0.00	0.00	0.0	0.00	0.0	169.0	0.3	0.9	<1	0.0
Low-sodium														
low-salt	1 tsp	0	0.00	0.00	0.00	0.00	0.0	0.00	0.0	217.0	0.4	1.4	505	<0.1
low-salt	1/2 tsp	0	0.00	0.00	0.00	0.00	0.0	0.00	0.0	108.0	0.2	0.7	253	<0.1
Regular														
	1 tsp	0	0.00	0.00	0.00	0.00	0.0	0.00	0.0	0.0	0.0	0.0	0	0.0
	1/2 tsp	0	0.00	0.00	0.00	0.00	0.0	0.00	0.0	0.0	0.0	0.0	0	0.0

BALSAM PEAR / bitter gourd
Leafy tips

Food Name	Serving Size	A I.U.	Thi mg	Rib mg	Nia mg	B$_6$ mg	Fol mcg	B$_{12}$ mcg	C mg	Calc mg	Iron mg	Mag mg	Pot mg	Zn mg
boiled, drained	1 cup	1005	0.09	0.16	0.58	0.44	50.8	0.00	32.2	24.4	0.6	54.5	349	0.2
raw	1 med leaf	69	0.01	0.01	0.04	0.03	5.1	0.00	3.5	3.4	0.1	3.4	24	<0.1
raw	1/2 cup	416	0.04	0.09	0.27	0.19	30.7	0.00	21.1	20.2	0.5	20.4	146	<0.1
Pods														
boiled, drained, 1/2-inch pieces	1 cup	140	0.06	0.07	0.35	0.05	63.4	0.00	40.9	11.2	0.5	19.8	396	1.0
boiled, drained, 1/2-inch pieces	1/2 cup	70.1	0.03	0.03	0.17	0.03	31.7	0.00	20.5	5.6	0.2	9.9	198	0.5
pods, raw, 1/2-inch pieces	1 cup	353	0.04	0.04	0.37	0.04	67.0	0.00	78.1	17.7	0.4	15.8	275	0.7
pods, raw, whole	1 medium	471	0.05	0.05	0.50	0.05	89.3	0.00	104.0	23.6	0.5	21.1	367	1.0

BAMBOO SHOOTS

Food Name	Serving Size	A I.U.	Thi mg	Rib mg	Nia mg	B$_6$ mg	Fol mcg	B$_{12}$ mcg	C mg	Calc mg	Iron mg	Mag mg	Pot mg	Zn mg
Canned, drained, 1/8-inch slices	1 cup	10.5	0.03	0.03	0.18	0.18	4.2	0.00	1.4	10.5	0.4	5.2	105	0.9
Fresh														
boiled, drained, 1/2-inch slices	1 cup	0	0.02	0.06	0.36	0.12	2.8	0.00	0.0	14.4	0.3	3.6	640	0.6
boiled, drained, whole	1 medium	0	0.03	0.07	0.43	0.14	3.3	0.00	0.0	17.3	0.4	4.3	768	0.7
raw, 1/2-inch pieces	1/2 cup	15	0.11	0.05	0.46	0.18	5.4	0.00	3.0	9.9	0.4	2.3	405	0.8
raw, 1/2-inch slices	1 cup	30	0.23	0.11	0.91	0.36	10.7	0.00	6.0	19.6	0.8	4.5	805	1.7

BANANA, DEHYDRATED
Dehydrated or powdered

Food Name	Serving Size	A I.U.	Thi mg	Rib mg	Nia mg	B$_6$ mg	Fol mcg	B$_{12}$ mcg	C mg	Calc mg	Iron mg	Mag mg	Pot mg	Zn mg
	1 cup	305	0.18	0.24	2.80	0.44	14.0	0.00	7.0	22.0	1.1	108.0	1491	0.6
	1 tbsp	19	0.01	0.02	0.17	0.03	0.9	0.00	0.4	1.4	0.1	6.7	92	<0.1
Fresh, raw														
mashed	1 cup	182	0.10	0.23	1.20	1.30	43.0	0.00	20.5	13.5	0.7	65.3	891	0.4
sliced	1 cup	122	0.07	0.15	0.81	0.87	28.6	0.00	13.7	9.0	0.5	43.5	594	0.2
whole, extra large, 9 inches long and up	1 banana	123	0.07	0.15	0.82	0.88	29.0	0.00	13.8	9.1	0.5	44.1	602	0.2
whole, extra small, up to 6 inches long	1 banana	66	0.04	0.08	0.44	0.47	15.5	0.00	7.4	4.9	0.3	23.5	321	0.1
whole, large, 8 to 8-7/8 inches long	1 banana	110	0.06	0.14	0.73	0.79	26.0	0.00	12.4	8.2	0.4	39.4	539	0.2
whole, medium, 7 to 7-7/8 inches long	1 banana	96	0.05	0.12	0.64	0.68	22.5	0.00	10.7	7.1	0.4	34.2	467	0.2
whole, small, 6 to 6-7/8 inches long	1 banana	82	0.05	0.10	0.55	0.58	19.3	0.00	9.2	6.1	0.3	29.3	400	0.2

BANANA CHIP

Food Name	Serving Size	A I.U.	Thi mg	Rib mg	Nia mg	B$_6$ mg	Fol mcg	B$_{12}$ mcg	C mg	Calc mg	Iron mg	Mag mg	Pot mg	Zn mg
	3 oz	71	0.07	0.01	0.60	0.22	11.9	0.00	5.4	15.3	1.1	64.6	456	0.6
	1.5 oz	35	0.04	0.01	0.30	0.11	5.9	0.00	2.6	7.6	0.5	31.9	225	0.3
	1 oz	24	0.02	0.01	0.20	0.07	4.0	0.00	1.8	5.1	0.4	21.5	152	0.2

BANANA PEPPER. See PEPPER, BANANA.

BARLEY

Food Name	Serving Size	A I.U.	Thi mg	Rib mg	Nia mg	B$_6$ mg	Fol mcg	B$_{12}$ mcg	C mg	Calc mg	Iron mg	Mag mg	Pot mg	Zn mg
	1 cup	41	1.20	0.52	8.50	0.58	35.0	0.00	0.0	60.7	6.6	245.0	832	5.1

Food Name	Serving Size	A I.U.	Thi mg	Rib mg	Nia mg	B$_6$ mg	Fol mcg	B$_{12}$ mcg	C mg	Calc mg	Iron mg	Mag mg	Pot mg	Zn mg
pearled, cooked	1 cup	11	0.13	0.10	3.20	0.18	25.1	0.00	0.0	17.3	2.1	34.5	146	1.3
pearled, raw	1 cup	44	0.38	0.23	9.20	0.52	46.0	0.00	0.0	58.0	5.0	158.0	560	4.3
BARLEY FLOUR. See under FLOUR.														
BARLEY MALT FLOUR. See under FLOUR.														
BASIL														
Fresh														
....	2 tbsp	205	0.00	0.00	0.05	0.01	3.4	0.00	1.0	8.2	0.2	4.3	25.5	<0.1
....	5 leaves	97	0.00	0.00	0.02	0.00	1.6	0.00	0.5	3.9	0.1	2.0	12	<0.1
Ground														
....	1 tbsp	422	0.01	0.01	0.31	0.05	12.3	0.00	2.8	95.1	1.9	19.0	154	0.3
....	1 tsp	131	0.00	0.00	0.10	0.02	3.8	0.00	0.9	29.6	0.6	5.9	48	<0.1
BASS, CALICO. See SUNFISH.														
BASS, FRESHWATER														
mixed species, baked, broiled, grilled,														
or microwaved	3 oz	98	0.07	0.08	1.30	0.12	14.4	2.00	1.8	87.5	1.6	32.3	388	0.7
mixed species, raw	3 oz	85	0.06	0.06	1.10	0.10	12.8	1.70	1.7	68.0	1.3	25.5	303	0.6
BASS, SEA														
mixed species, baked, broiled, grilled,														
or microwaved	3 oz	181	0.11	0.13	1.60	0.39	4.9	0.26	0.0	11.1	0.3	45.0	279	0.4
mixed species, raw	3 oz	156	0.09	0.10	1.40	0.34	4.3	0.26	0.0	8.5	0.3	34.9	218	0.3
BASS, STRIPED														
baked, broiled, grilled, or microwaved	3 oz	88.4	0.10	0.03	2.2	0.29	8.5	3.7	0	16.1	0.92	43.4	279	0.43
raw	3 oz	76.5	0.09	0.03	1.8	0.26	7.7	3.2	0	12.8	0.71	34.0	218	0.34
BAY LEAF														
crumbled........................	1 tbsp	111	0.00	0.01	0.04	0.02	3.2	0.00	0.8	15.0	0.8	2.2	10	0.0
crumbled........................	1 tsp	37	0.00	0.00	0.01	0.01	1.1	0.00	0.3	5.0	0.3	0.7	3	0.0
BEAN, ADZUKI														
Canned, mature seeds, sweetened..........	1 cup	15	0.30	0.17	1.90	0.25	316.0	0.00	0.0	65.1	3.3	91.8	352	4.6
Fresh														
mature seeds, boiled	1 cup	14	0.27	0.15	1.60	0.22	279.0	0.00	0.0	64.4	4.6	120.0	1224	4.1
mature seeds, raw	1 cup	34	0.90	0.43	5.20	0.69	1225.0	0.00	0.0	130.0	9.8	250.0	2470	9.9
BEAN, BLACK / black turtle bean														
Canned, mature seeds	1 cup	10	0.34	0.29	1.50	0.13	146.0	0.00	6.5	84.0	4.6	84.0	739	1.3
Dried														
mature seeds, boiled	1 cup	10	0.42	0.10	0.87	0.12	256.0	0.00	0.0	46.4	3.6	120.0	611	1.9
mature seeds, raw	1 cup	33	1.70	0.37	3.80	0.56	862.0	0.00	0.0	239.0	9.7	332.0	2877	7.1
mature seeds, raw	1 tbsp	2	0.11	0.02	0.24	0.04	53.8	0.00	0.0	14.9	0.6	20.7	179	0.4
BEAN, BLACK TURTLE. See BEAN, BLACK.														
BEAN, BROAD. See BEAN, FAVA.														
BEAN, CRANBERRY / borlotti / Roman bean / rose coco bean														
Canned, mature seeds	1 cup	0	0.10	0.10	1.30	0.14	201.0	0.00	2.1	88.4	4.0	83.2	676	2.2
Dried														
mature seeds, boiled	1 cup	0	0.37	0.12	0.91	0.14	366.0	0.00	0.0	88.5	3.7	88.5	685	2.0
mature seeds, raw	1 cup	4	1.50	0.41	2.80	0.60	1179.0	0.00	0.0	248.0	9.8	304.0	2597	7.1
BEAN, FAVA / broad bean / horse bean / jack bean														
Canned														
mature seeds	1 cup	26	0.05	0.13	2.50	0.12	83.7	0.00	4.6	66.6	2.6	81.9	620	1.6
Fresh														
immature seeds, raw	1 bean	28	0.01	0.01	0.12	0.00	7.7	0.00	2.6	1.8	0.2	3.0	20	<0.1
immature seeds, raw	1 cup	382	0.19	0.12	1.60	0.04	105.0	0.00	36.0	24.0	2.1	41.4	273	0.6
mature seeds, boiled	1 cup	26	0.17	0.15	1.20	0.12	177.0	0.00	0.5	61.2	2.5	73.1	456	1.7
mature seeds, raw	1 cup	80	0.83	0.50	4.20	0.55	634.0	0.00	2.1	155.0	10.1	288.0	1593	4.7
mature seeds, raw	1 tbsp	5	0.05	0.03	0.27	0.03	39.8	0.00	0.1	9.7	0.6	18.0	100	0.3
raw, in pod	1 cup	420	0.17	0.36	2.80	0.13	186.0	0.00	4.7	46.6	2.0	41.6	418	1.3

Food Name	Serving Size	A I.U.	Thi mg	Rib mg	Nia mg	B₆ mg	Fol mcg	B₁₂ mcg	C mg	Calc mg	Iron mg	Mag mg	Pot mg	Zn mg
raw, in pod	1 med pod	20	0.01	0.02	0.14	0.01	9.0	0.00	0.2	2.3	0.1	2.0	20	<0.1
BEAN, FRENCH / haricots. See also BEAN, GREEN.														
Fresh														
mature seeds, boiled	1 cup	5	0.23	0.11	0.97	0.19	132.0	0.00	2.1	112.0	1.9	99.1	655	1.1
mature seeds, raw	1 cup	15	0.98	0.41	3.80	0.74	733.0	0.00	8.5	342.0	6.3	346.0	2421	3.5
BEAN, GARBANZO. See CHICKPEA.														
BEAN, GOA. See BEAN, WINGED.														
BEAN, GREAT NORTHERN														
Canned, mature seeds	1 cup	3	0.38	0.16	1.20	0.28	213.0	0.00	3.4	139.0	4.1	134.0	920	1.7
Dried														
mature seeds, boiled	1 cup	2	0.28	0.10	1.20	0.21	181.0	0.00	2.3	120.0	3.8	88.5	692	1.6
mature seeds, raw	1 cup	6	1.20	0.43	3.60	0.82	882.0	0.00	9.7	320.0	10.0	346.0	2538	4.2
BEAN, GREEN / string bean / snap bean. See also BEAN, FRENCH.														
Canned														
drained	1 cup	471	0.02	0.08	0.27	0.05	42.9	0.00	6.5	35.1	1.2	17.6	147	0.4
drained	10 beans	216	0.01	0.04	0.13	0.02	19.7	0.00	3.0	16.1	0.6	8.1	68	0.2
no salt added, drained	1 cup	471	0.02	0.08	0.27	0.05	42.9	0.00	6.5	35.1	1.2	17.6	147	0.4
no salt added, drained	10 beans	216	0.01	0.04	0.13	0.02	19.7	0.00	3.0	16.1	0.6	8.1	68	0.2
no salt added, w/liquid	1/2 cup	385	0.03	0.06	0.24	0.04	21.8	0.00	4.1	28.8	1.1	15.6	110	0.2
seasoned, w/liquid	1/2 cup	599	0.03	0.06	0.27	0.05	20.2	0.00	3.5	25.1	0.5	14.8	106	0.2
w/liquid	1/2 cup	385	0.03	0.06	0.24	0.04	21.8	0.00	4.1	28.8	1.1	15.6	110	0.2
Freeze-Dried														
Fresh														
boiled, drained	1 cup	833	0.09	0.12	0.77	0.07	41.6	0.00	12.1	57.5	1.6	31.3	374	0.5
raw	1 cup	735	0.09	0.12	0.83	0.08	40.1	0.00	17.9	40.7	1.1	27.5	230	0.3
raw, whole, approx 4-inch long	10 beans	367	0.05	0.06	0.41	0.04	20.1	0.00	9.0	20.4	0.6	13.8	115	0.1
Frozen														
drained	1 cup	541	0.05	0.12	0.52	0.08	31.1	0.00	5.5	66.2	1.2	32.4	170	0.7
no salt added, drained	1 cup	541	0.05	0.12	0.52	0.08	31.1	0.00	5.5	66.2	1.2	32.4	170	0.7
unprepared	10-oz pkg	1363	0.28	0.26	1.40	0.12	41.7	0.00	36.6	119.0	2.4	62.5	528	0.7
unprepared	1 cup	595	0.12	0.11	0.62	0.05	18.2	0.00	16.0	52.1	1.1	27.3	231	0.3
BEAN, HORSE. See BEAN, FAVA.														
BEAN, HYACINTH														
immature seeds, boiled, drained	1 cup	124	0.05	0.08	0.42	0.02	40.5	0.00	4.4	35.7	0.7	36.5	228	0.3
immature seeds, raw	1 cup	87	0.06	0.07	0.42	0.02	49.2	0.00	10.3	40.0	0.6	32.0	202	0.3
mature seeds, boiled	1 cup	0	0.52	0.07	0.80	0.07	7.4	0.00	0.0	77.6	8.9	159.0	654	5.5
mature seeds, raw	1 cup	0	2.40	0.29	3.40	0.33	47.3	0.00	0.0	273	10.7	594.0	2594	19.5
BEAN, JACK. See BEAN, FAVA.														
BEAN, KIDNEY														
ALL TYPES														
Canned														
mature seeds	1 cup	0	0.28	0.18	1.30	0.18	126.0	0.00	3.1	69.1	3.1	79.4	658	1.4
Dried														
mature seeds, boiled	1 cup	0	0.28	0.10	1.00	0.21	229.0	0.00	2.1	49.6	5.2	79.7	713	1.9
mature seeds, boiled	1 tbsp	0	0.02	0.01	0.06	0.01	14.3	0.00	0.1	3.1	0.3	5.0	44.3	0.1
mature seeds, raw	1 cup	15	0.97	0.40	3.80	0.73	725.0	0.00	8.3	263.0	15.1	258.0	2587	5.1
Frozen, immature seeds, drained	10-oz pkg	519	0.22	0.17	2.40	0.36	48.2	0.00	18.0	87.1	6.1	174.0	1278	1.7
Sprouted														
immature seeds, frozen, drained	1/2 cup	150	0.06	0.05	0.69	0.10	13.9	0.00	5.2	25.2	1.8	50.4	370	0.5
mature seeds, raw	1 cup	4	0.68	0.46	5.40	0.16	108.0	0.00	71.2	31.3	1.5	38.6	344	0.7
CALIFORNIA RED														
Dried														
mature seeds, boiled	1 cup	5	0.23	0.11	0.96	0.18	131.0	0.00	2.1	117.0	5.3	85.0	742	1.5
mature seeds, raw	1 cup	15	0.97	0.40	3.80	0.73	725.0	0.00	8.3	359.0	17.2	294.0	2742	4.7

Food Name	Serving Size	A I.U.	Thi mg	Rib mg	Nia mg	B$_6$ mg	Fol mcg	B$_{12}$ mcg	C mg	Calc mg	Iron mg	Mag mg	Pot mg	Zn mg
RED														
Canned														
mature seeds	1 cup	0	0.27	0.23	1.20	0.06	130.0	0.00	2.8	61.4	3.2	71.7	658	1.4
mature seeds	1 tbsp	0	0.02	0.01	0.07	0.00	8.1	0.00	0.2	3.8	0.2	4.5	41	<0.1
Dried														
mature seeds, boiled	1 cup	0	0.28	0.10	1.00	0.21	229.0	0.00	2.1	49.6	5.2	79.7	713	1.9
mature seeds, boiled	1 tbsp	0	0.02	0.01	0.06	0.01	14.3	0.00	0.1	3.1	0.3	5.0	44	0.1
mature seeds, raw	1 cup	15	1.10	0.40	3.90	0.73	725.0	0.00	8.3	153.0	12.3	254.0	2501	5.1
mature seeds, raw	1 tbsp	1	0.07	0.03	0.26	0.05	48.1	0.00	0.6	10.1	0.8	16.8	166	0.3
ROYAL RED														
Dried														
mature seeds, boiled	1 cup	5	0.17	0.12	0.98	0.18	130.0	0.00	2.1	77.9	4.9	74.3	669	1.6
mature seeds, raw	1 cup	15	0.72	0.44	3.90	0.73	724.0	0.00	8.3	241.0	16.0	254.0	2477	4.9
BEAN, LIMA / butterbean														
Canned														
immature seeds, no salt added, w/liquid	1/2 cup	186	0.04	0.05	0.66	0.08	19.8	0.00	10.8	34.7	2.0	42.2	353	0.8
immature seeds, w/liquid	1/2 cup	186	0.04	0.05	0.66	0.08	19.8	0.00	9.1	34.7	2.0	42.2	353	0.8
large, mature seeds	1 cup	0	0.13	0.08	0.63	0.22	121.0	0.00		50.6	4.4	94.0	530	1.6
Dried														
baby, mature seeds, boiled, drained	1 cup	0	0.29	0.10	1.20	0.14	273.0	0.00	0.0	52.8	4.4	96.5	730	1.9
baby, mature seeds, raw	1 cup	10	1.20	0.44	3.50	0.66	808.0	0.00	0.0	164.0	12.5	380.0	2834	5.3
immature seeds, boiled, drained	1 cup	629	0.24	0.16	1.80	0.33	44.7	0.00	17.2	54.4	4.2	126.0	969	1.3
immature seeds, raw	1 cup	473	0.34	0.16	2.30	0.32	53.0	0.00	36.5	53.0	4.9	90.5	729	1.2
large, mature seeds, boiled, drained	1 cup	0	0.30	0.10	0.79	0.30	156.0	0.00	0.0	32.0	4.5	80.8	955	1.8
large, mature seeds, boiled, drained	1 tbsp	0	0.02	0.01	0.05	0.02	9.7	0.00	0.0	2.0	0.3	5.0	59	0.1
mature seeds, raw	1 cup	0	0.90	0.36	2.70	0.91	703.0	0.00	0.0	144.0	13.4	399.0	3069	5.0
mature seeds, raw	1 tbsp	0	0.06	0.02	0.17	0.06	43.9	0.00	0.0	9.0	0.8	24.9	191	0.3
Frozen														
baby, drained	10-oz pkg	519	0.22	0.17	2.40	0.36	48.2	0.00	18.0	87.1	6.1	174.0	1278	1.7
baby, drained	1/2 cup	150	0.06	0.05	0.69	0.10	13.9	0.00	5.2	25.2	1.8	50.4	370	0.5
baby, unprepared	10-oz pkg	537	0.32	0.21	2.90	0.45	78.4	0.00	23.6	99.4	6.3	142.0	1284	1.8
baby, unprepared	1/2 cup	155	0.09	0.06	0.84	0.13	22.6	0.00	6.8	28.7	1.8	41.0	371	0.5
Fordhook, immature seeds, no salt added, boiled, drained	1/2 cup	162	0.06	0.05	0.91	0.10	18.0	0.00	10.9	18.7	1.2	28.9	347	0.4
Fordhook, immature seeds, no salt added, boiled, drained	10-oz pkg	591	0.23	0.19	3.30	0.38	65.9	0.00	39.8	68.4	4.2	106.0	1269	1.4
Fordhook, immature seeds, unprepared	10-oz pkg	633	0.26	0.19	3.40	0.39	90.6	0.00	54.8	68.2	4.3	108.0	1358	1.4
Fordhook, immature seeds, unprepared	1/2 cup	178	0.07	0.05	0.95	0.11	25.5	0.00	15.4	19.2	1.2	30.4	382	0.4
BEAN, MOTH														
mature seeds, boiled, drained	1 cup	18	0.22	0.04	1.20	0.17	254.0	0.00	1.8	5.3	5.6	184.0	538	1.0
mature seeds, raw	1 cup	63	1.10	0.18	5.50	0.72	1272.0	0.00	7.8	294.0	21.3	747.0	2334	3.8
BEAN, MUNG														
Canned, mature seeds, sprouted, drained	1 cup	29	0.04	0.09	0.28	0.04	12.1	0.00	0.4	17.5	0.5	11.3	33.8	0.4
Dried														
mature seeds, boiled, drained	1 cup	49	0.33	0.12	1.20	0.14	321.0	0.00	2.0	54.5	2.8	97.0	537	1.7
mature seeds, raw	1 cup	236	1.30	0.48	4.70	0.79	1294.0	0.00	9.9	273.0	14.0	391.0	2579	5.5
mature seeds, raw	1 tbsp	15	0.08	0.03	0.29	0.05	81.2	0.00	0.6	17.2	0.9	24.6	162	<0.4
Sprouted														
mature seeds, boiled, drained	1 cup	17	0.06	0.13	1.00	0.07	36.3	0.00	14.1	14.9	0.8	17.4	125	0.6
mature seeds, raw	12-oz pkg	71	0.29	0.42	2.50	0.30	207.0	0.00	44.9	44.2	3.1	71.4	507	1.4
mature seeds, raw	1 cup	22	0.09	0.13	0.78	0.09	63.2	0.00	13.7	13.5	1.0	21.8	155	0.4
mature seeds, stir-fried	1 cup	38	0.17	0.22	1.50	0.16	86.3	0.00	19.8	16.1	2.4	40.9	272	1.1
BEAN, MUNGO														
mature seeds, boiled, drained	1 cup	56	0.27	0.14	2.70	0.10	170.0	0.00	1.8	95.4	3.1	113.0	416	1.5

Food Name	Serving Size	A I.U.	Thi mg	Rib mg	Nia mg	B$_6$ mg	Fol mcg	B$_{12}$ mcg	C mg	Calc mg	Iron mg	Mag mg	Pot mg	Zn mg
mature seeds, raw	1 cup	48	0.56	0.53	3.00	0.58	447.0	0.00	0.0	286.0	15.7	553.0	2035	6.9
BEAN, NAVY														
Canned, mature seeds	1 cup	3	0.37	0.14	1.30	0.27	163	0.00	1.8	123.0	4.8	123.0	755	2.0
Dried														
mature seeds, boiled, drained	1 cup	4	0.37	0.11	0.97	0.30	255.0	0.00	1.6	127.0	4.5	107.0	670	1.9
mature seeds, raw	1 cup	8	1.30	0.48	4.30	0.91	769.0	0.00	6.2	322.0	13.4	360.0	2371	5.3
Sprouted, mature seeds	1 cup	4	0.41	0.22	1.30	0.20	137.0	0.00	19.6	15.6	2.0	105.0	319	0.9
BEAN, PINK														
mature seeds, boiled, drained	1 cup	0	0.43	0.11	0.96	0.30	284.0	0.00	0.0	87.9	3.9	110.0	859	1.6
mature seeds, raw	1 cup	0	1.6	0.40	4.00	1.10	973.0	0.00	0.0	273.0	14.2	382.0	3074	5.4
BEAN, PINTO														
Canned, mature seeds	1 cup	58	0.24	0.15	0.70	0.18	144.0	0.00	2.2	103.0	3.5	64.8	583	1.7
Dried														
mature seeds, boiled, drained	1 cup	3	0.32	0.16	0.68	0.27	294.0	0.00	3.6	82.1	4.5	94.0	800	1.8
mature seeds, boiled, drained	1 tbsp	<1	0.02	0.01	0.04	0.02	18.2	0.00	0.2	5.1	0.3	5.8	49.6	0.1
mature seeds, raw	1 cup	10	1.10	0.46	2.80	0.85	977.0	0.00	14.1	234.0	11.3	307.0	2563	4.9
mature seeds, raw	1 tbsp	1	0.07	0.03	0.17	0.05	60.8	0.00	0.9	14.5	0.7	19.1	159	0.3
Frozen														
immature seeds, drained	10-oz pkg	0	0.78	0.31	1.80	0.55	95.1	0.00	2.0	148.0	7.7	153.0	1835	2.0
immature seeds, drained	3.3 oz	0	0.26	0.10	0.59	0.18	31.5	0.00	0.7	48.9	2.5	50.8	607	0.7
immature seeds, no salt added, drained	10-oz pkg	0	0.78	0.31	1.80	0.55	95.1	0.00	2.0	148.0	7.7	153.0	1835	2.0
immature seeds, no salt added, drained	3.3 oz	0	0.26	0.10	0.59	0.18	31.5	0.00	0.7	48.9	2.5	50.8	607	0.7
immature seeds, unprepared	10-oz pkg	0	0.97	0.34	2.00	0.61	143.0	0.00	2.8	165.0	8.5	170.0	2147	2.2
immature seeds, unprepared	3.3 oz	0	0.32	0.11	0.66	0.20	47.4	0.00	0.9	54.5	2.8	56.4	711	0.7
BEAN, ROMAN. See BEAN, CRANBERRY.														
BEAN, ROSE COCO. See BEAN, CRANBERRY.														
BEAN, SHELLY, canned, w/liquid	1 cup	559	0.08	0.13	0.50	0.12	44.1	0.00	7.6	71.0	2.4	36.8	267	0.7
BEAN, SNAP. See BEAN, GREEN; BEAN, WAX.														
BEAN, SOYA. See SOYBEAN.														
BEAN, STRING. See BEAN, GREEN; BEAN, WAX.														
BEAN, WAX / yellow snap bean														
Canned														
drained	1 cup	142	0.02	0.08	0.27	0.05	42.9	0.00	6.5	35.1	1.2	17.6	147	0.4
drained	10 beans	65	0.01	0.04	0.13	0.02	19.7	0.00	3.0	16.1	0.6	8.1	68	0.2
no salt added, drained	1/2 cup	71	0.01	0.04	0.14	0.03	21.6	0.00	3.3	17.7	0.6	8.8	74	0.2
no salt added, w/liquid	1/2 cup	76	0.03	0.06	0.24	0.04	21.8	0.00	4.8	28.8	1.1	15.6	118	0.2
w/liquid	1/2 cup	76	0.03	0.06	0.24	0.04	21.8	0.00	4.1	28.8	1.1	15.6	118	0.2
Fresh														
boiled, drained	1 cup	101	0.09	0.12	0.77	0.07	41.6	0.00	12.1	57.5	1.6	31.3	374	0.5
raw	1 cup	119	0.09	0.12	0.83	0.08	40.1	0.00	17.9	40.7	1.1	27.5	230	0.3
Frozen														
no salt added, drained	1 cup	151	0.05	0.12	0.52	0.08	31.1	0.00	5.5	66.2	1.2	32.4	170	0.7
unprepared	10-oz pkg	364	0.28	0.26	1.40	0.12	41.7	0.00	36.6	119.0	2.4	62.5	528	0.7
unprepared	1 cup	159	0.12	0.11	0.62	0.05	18.2	0.00	16.0	52.1	1.1	27.3	231	0.3
BEAN, WHITE														
Dried														
mature seeds, boiled	1 cup	0	0.21	0.08	0.25	0.17	144.0	0.00	0.0	161.0	6.6	113.0	1004	2.5
mature seeds, boiled	1 tbsp	0	0.01	0.01	0.02	0.01	9.0	0.00	0.0	10.1	0.4	7.1	63	0.2
mature seeds, raw	1 cup	0	0.88	0.29	0.97	0.64	783.0	0.00	0.0	485.0	21.1	384.0	3626	7.4
mature seeds, raw	1 tbsp	0	0.06	0.02	0.06	0.04	48.9	0.00	0.0	30.2	1.3	23.9	226	0.5
small, mature seeds, boiled	1 cup	0	0.42	0.11	0.49	0.23	245.0	0.00	0.0	131.0	5.1	122.0	829	2.0
small, mature seeds, raw	1 cup	0	1.60	0.45	2.90	0.94	830.0	0.00	0.0	372.0	16.6	393.0	3315	6.0
Canned, mature seeds	1 cup	0	0.25	0.10	0.30	0.20	171.0	0.00	0.0	191.0	7.8	134.0	1189	2.9

Food Name	Serving Size	A I.U.	Thi mg	Rib mg	Nia mg	B_6 mg	Fol mcg	B_{12} mcg	C mg	Calc mg	Iron mg	Mag mg	Pot mg	Zn mg
BEAN, WINGED / goa bean														
immature seeds, boiled, drained..........	1 cup	55	0.05	0.05	0.40	0.05	21.8	0.00	6.1	37.8	0.7	18.6	170	0.2
immature seeds, raw, sliced..............	1 cup	56	0.06	0.04	0.40	0.05	28.9	0.00	8.1	37.0	0.7	15.0	98	0.2
immature seeds, raw, whole.............	1 pod	21	0.02	0.02	0.14	0.02	10.5	0.00	2.9	13.4	0.2	5.4	36	0.0
mature seeds, boiled, drained	1 cup	4	0.33	0.18	1.30	0.23	143.0	0.00	3.2	110.0	4.4	131.0	575	1.9
mature seeds, raw	1 cup	0	1.90	0.82	5.60	0.32	81.2	0.00	0.0	801.0	24.5	326.0	1778	8.2
BEAN, YARDLONG														
boiled, drained, sliced.................	1 cup	468	0.09	0.10	0.66	0.03	46.3	0.00	16.8	45.8	1.0	43.7	302	0.4
boiled, drained, whole..................	1 pod	63	0.01	0.01	0.09	0.00	6.2	0.00	2.3	6.2	0.1	5.9	41	<0.1
mature seeds, boiled, drained	1 cup	27	0.36	0.11	0.94	0.16	249.0	0.00	0.68	71.8	4.5	168.0	539	1.8
mature seeds, raw	1 cup	87	1.50	0.39	3.60	0.62	1099.0	0.00	2.7	230.0	14.4	564.0	1932	5.8
raw, sliced...........................	1 cup	787	0.10	0.10	0.37	0.02	56.1	0.00	17.1	45.5	0.4	40.0	218	0.3
raw, whole...........................	1 pod	104	0.01	0.01	0.05	0.00	7.4	0.00	2.3	6.2	0.1	5.3	28.8	0.0
BEAN, YELLOW, mature seeds, raw..........	1 cup	12	1.40	0.65	4.80	0.87	762.0	0.00	0.0	325.0	13.7	435.0	2042	5.5
BEAR														
raw	1 oz	0	0.05	0.19	0.91	na	na	na	0.0	0.85	1.9	na	na	na
simmered	3 oz	0	0.09	0.70	2.80	0.25	5.1	2.10	0.0	4.3	9.1	19.6	224	9.7
simmered, yield from 1 lb raw,														
boneless.................	7.9 oz	0	0.28	2.30	9.30	0.80	16.6	6.80	0.0	13.8	29.7	63.7	729	28.4
BEAVER														
raw	1 oz	0	0.02	0.06	0.54	na	na	na	0.6	4.3	2.0	7.1	99	na
roasted	3 oz	0	0.04	0.26	1.90	0.40	9.3	7.10	2.5	18.7	8.5	24.6	343	2.9
roasted, yield from 1 lb raw, boneless	11 oz	0	0.16	0.97	6.90	1.50	34.4	26.00	9.4	68.9	31.3	90.8	1261	7.1
BEECHNUT, dried	1 oz	0	0.09	0.11	0.25	0.19	31.9	0.00	4.4	0.3	0.7	0.0	288	0.1
BEEF. See also under LUNCHEON MEAT.														
(NOTE: TRIMMED = Lean; separable fat removed after cooking. UNTRIMMED = Separable fat not removed.)														
BRAIN														
pan-fried............................	3 oz	0	0.11	0.22	3.20	0.33	5.1	12.90	2.8	7.7	1.9	12.8	301	1.1
raw	4 oz	0	0.17	0.31	5.20	0.29	4.5	12.30	18.8	9.0	2.4	14.7	363	1.4
raw	1 oz	0	0.04	0.08	1.30	0.07	1.1	3.10	4.7	2.3	0.6	3.7	91	0.4
simmered	3 oz	0	0.07	0.14	1.90	0.20	6.0	7.30	0.9	7.7	1.9	11.9	204	1.1
BRISKET, FLAT HALF														
Trimmed														
all grades, 0-inch fat, braised.............	3 oz	0	0.06	0.19	3.30	0.26	6.8	2.20	0.0	4.3	2.4	21.3	253	5.4
all grades, 1/4-inch fat, braised.............	3 oz	0	0.06	0.19	3.30	0.26	6.8	2.20	0.0	4.3	2.4	21.3	253	5.4
all grades, 1/4-inch fat, raw................	1 oz	0	0.03	0.05	1.20	0.13	2.0	0.69	0.0	1.4	0.5	6.8	99	1.0
Untrimmed														
all grades, 0-inch fat, braised	3 oz	0	0.06	0.18	3.20	0.26	6.8	2.20	0.0	4.3	2.3	20.4	246	5.2
all grades, 1/8-inch fat, braised............	3 oz	0	0.05	0.16	2.90	0.24	6.0	2.10	0.0	6.0	2.1	17.9	224	4.6
all grades, 1/8-inch fat, raw...............	4 oz	0	0.10	0.18	4.40	0.45	6.8	2.60	0.0	6.8	1.9	23.7	340	3.5
all grades, 1/4-inch fat, braised............	3 oz	0	0.05	0.15	2.70	0.22	5.1	2.00	0.0	6.8	1.9	16.1	207	4.1
all grades, 1/4-inch fat, raw...............	4 oz	0	0.10	0.17	4.00	0.42	6.8	2.40	0.0	6.8	1.8	20.3	307	3.2
BRISKET, POINT HALF														
Trimmed														
all grades, 0-inch fat, braised	3 oz	0	0.06	0.20	3.00	0.24	6.8	2.20	0.0	5.1	2.4	18.7	232	6.3
all grades, 1/4-inch fat, braised............	3 oz	0	0.06	0.20	3.00	0.24	6.8	2.20	0.0	5.1	2.4	18.7	232	6.3
all grades, 1/4-inch fat, raw...............	1 oz	0	0.03	0.05	1.00	0.12	2.0	0.69	0.0	1.4	0.6	6.2	88.7	1.4
Untrimmed														
all grades, 0-inch fat, braised	3 oz	0	0.05	0.16	2.60	0.20	6.0	2.00	0.0	6.8	2.0	15.3	198	5.0
all grades, 1/8-inch fat, braised............	3 oz	0	0.05	0.17	2.70	0.21	6.0	2.00	0.0	6.8	2.1	16.1	205	5.2
all grades, 1/8-inch fat, raw...............	1 oz	0	0.02	0.04	0.89	0.10	1.7	0.64	0.0	1.7	0.5	5.1	75	1.2
all grades, 1/4-inch fat, braised............	3 oz	0	0.05	0.15	2.40	0.20	5.1	1.90	0.0	7.7	1.9	14.4	188	4.5
all grades, 1/4-inch fat, raw...............	1 oz	0	0.02	0.04	0.81	0.09	1.7	0.60	0.0	2.0	0.4	4.5	66	1.1

Food Name	Serving Size	A I.U.	Thi mg	Rib mg	Nia mg	B_6 mg	Fol mcg	B_{12} mcg	C mg	Calc mg	Iron mg	Mag mg	Pot mg	Zn mg
BRISKET, WHOLE														
Trimmed														
all grades, 0-inch fat, braised,.............	3 oz	0	0.06	0.19	3.20	0.25	6.8	2.20	0.0	5.1	2.4	19.6	242	5.9
all grades, 1/4-inch fat, braised.............	3 oz	0	0.06	0.19	3.20	0.25	6.8	2.20	0.0	5.1	2.4	19.6	242	5.9
all grades, raw	1 oz	0	0.03	0.05	1.10	0.12	2.0	0.69	0.0	1.4	0.5	6.5	94	1.2
Untrimmed														
all grades, 0-inch fat, braised	3 oz	0	0.06	0.17	2.90	0.23	6.0	2.10	0.0	6.0	2.1	17.9	220	5.1
all grades, 1/8-inch fat, braised.............	3 oz	0	0.05	0.17	2.80	0.22	6.0	2.00	0.0	6.0	2.1	17.0	213	4.9
all grades, 1/8-inch fat, raw.............	1 oz	0	0.03	0.04	0.99	0.11	1.7	0.64	0.0	1.7	0.5	5.4	80	1.1
all grades, 1/4-inch fat, braised.............	3 oz	0	0.05	0.15	2.50	0.20	5.1	1.90	0.0	6.8	1.9	15.3	196	4.3
all grades, 1/4-inch fat, raw.............	1 oz	0	0.02	0.04	0.90	0.10	1.7	0.60	0.0	2.0	0.5	4.8	71	0.9
CHUCK, ARM POT ROAST														
Trimmed														
all grades, 0-inch fat, braised.............	3 oz	0	0.07	0.25	3.20	0.28	9.3	2.90	0.0	7.7	3.2	20.4	246	7.4
all grades, 1/4-inch fat, braised.............	3 oz	0	0.07	0.25	3.20	0.28	9.3	2.90	0.0	7.7	3.2	20.4	246	7.4
all grades, 1/4-inch fat, raw.............	1 oz	0	0.04	0.06	1.10	0.13	2.3	0.99	0.0	1.7	0.7	6.8	105	1.4
choice, 0-inch fat, braised.............	3 oz	0	0.07	0.25	3.20	0.28	9.3	2.90	0.0	7.7	3.2	20.4	246	7.4
choice, 1/4-inch fat, braised	3 oz	0	0.07	0.25	3.20	0.28	9.3	2.90	0.0	7.7	3.2	20.4	246	7.4
choice, 1/4-inch fat, raw	1 oz	0	0.04	0.06	1.10	0.13	2.3	0.99	0.0	1.7	0.7	6.8	105	1.4
prime, 1/2-inch fat, braised.............	3 oz	0	0.07	0.25	3.20	0.28	9.3	2.90	0.0	7.7	3.2	20.4	246	7.4
prime, 1/2-inch fat, raw.............	1 oz	0	0.04	0.06	1.10	0.13	2.3	0.99	0.0	1.7	0.7	6.8	105	1.4
select, 0-inch fat, braised	3 oz	0	0.07	0.25	3.20	0.28	9.3	2.90	0.0	7.7	3.2	20.4	246	7.4
select, 1/4-inch fat, braised.............	3 oz	0	0.07	0.25	3.20	0.28	9.3	2.90	0.0	7.7	3.2	20.4	246	7.4
select, 1/4-inch fat, raw.............	1 oz	0	0.04	0.06	1.10	0.13	2.3	0.99	0.0	1.7	0.7	6.8	105	1.4
Untrimmed														
all grades, 0-inch fat, braised	3 oz	0	0.06	0.22	2.90	0.26	8.5	2.70	0.0	8.5	2.9	17.9	224	6.4
all grades, 1/8-inch fat, braised.............	3 oz	0	0.06	0.21	2.80	0.25	7.7	2.60	0.0	8.5	2.8	17.0	217	6.1
all grades, 1/8-inch fat, raw.............	1 oz	0	0.03	0.05	0.93	0.11	2.0	0.88	0.0	2.0	0.6	5.7	89	1.2
all grades, 1/4-inch fat, braised.............	3 oz	0	0.06	0.20	2.70	0.24	7.7	2.50	0.0	8.5	2.6	16.1	209	5.8
all grades, 1/4-inch fat, raw.............	1 oz	0	0.03	0.05	0.92	0.11	2.0	0.87	0.0	2.0	0.6	5.7	87	1.1
choice, 1/4-inch fat, braised	3 oz	0	0.06	0.20	2.70	0.24	7.7	2.50	0.0	8.5	2.6	16.1	207	5.7
choice, 1/4-inch fat, raw	1 oz	0	0.03	0.05	0.91	0.11	2.0	0.86	0.0	2.0	0.6	5.4	87	1.1
prime, 1/2-inch fat, braised.............	3 oz	0	0.06	0.19	2.60	0.23	7.7	2.40	0.0	8.5	2.5	16.1	201	5.5
prime, 1/2-inch fat, raw.............	1 oz	0	0.03	0.05	0.88	0.10	2.0	0.83	0.0	2.0	0.6	5.1	82	1.1
select, 1/8-inch fat, raw.............	1 oz	0	0.03	0.05	0.94	0.11	2.0	0.89	0.0	2.0	0.6	5.7	90	1.2
select, 1/4-inch fat, braised.............	3 oz	0	0.06	0.20	2.70	0.25	7.7	2.50	0.0	8.5	2.7	17.0	213	5.9
select, 1/4-inch fat, raw.............	1 oz	0	0.03	0.05	0.93	0.11	2.0	0.87	0.0	2.0	0.6	5.7	88	1.2
CHUCK, BLADE ROAST														
Trimmed														
all grades, 0-inch fat, braised	3 oz	0	0.07	0.24	2.30	0.25	5.1	2.10	0.0	11.1	3.1	19.6	224	8.7
all grades, 1/4-inch fat, braised.............	3 oz	0	0.07	0.24	2.30	0.25	5.1	2.10	0.0	11.1	3.1	19.6	224	8.7
all grades, 1/4-inch fat, raw.............	1 oz	0	0.03	0.05	0.67	0.11	1.7	1.10	0.0	2.8	0.7	5.7	90	1.7
choice, 0-inch fat, braised.............	3 oz	0	0.07	0.24	2.30	0.25	5.1	2.10	0.0	11.1	3.1	19.6	224	8.7
choice, 1/4-inch fat, braised.............	3 oz	0	0.07	0.24	2.30	0.25	5.1	2.10	0.0	11.1	3.1	19.6	224	8.7
choice, 1/4-inch fat, raw	1 oz	0	0.03	0.05	0.67	0.11	1.7	1.10	0.0	2.8	0.7	5.7	90	1.7
prime, 1/2-inch fat, braised.............	3 oz	0	0.07	0.24	2.30	0.25	5.1	2.10	0.0	11.1	3.1	19.6	224	8.7
prime, 1/2-inch fat, raw.............	1 oz	0	0.03	0.05	0.67	0.11	1.7	1.10	0.0	2.8	0.7	5.7	90	1.7
select, 0-inch fat, braised	3 oz	0	0.07	0.24	2.30	0.25	5.1	2.10	0.0	11.1	3.1	19.6	224	8.7
select, 1/4-inch fat, braised.............	3 oz	0	0.07	0.24	2.30	0.25	5.1	2.10	0.0	11.1	3.1	19.6	224	8.7
select, 1/4-inch fat, raw.............	1 oz	0	0.03	0.05	0.67	0.11	1.7	1.10	0.0	2.8	0.7	5.7	90	1.7
Untrimmed														
all grades, 0-inch fat, braised	3 oz	0	0.06	0.21	2.10	0.22	4.3	2.00	0.0	11.1	2.7	17.0	201	7.3
all grades, 1/8-inch fat, braised.............	3 oz	0	0.06	0.20	2.10	0.22	4.3	1.90	0.0	11.1	2.7	16.1	198	7.1
all grades, 1/8-inch fat, raw.............	1 oz	0	0.03	0.05	0.62	0.10	1.4	0.96	0.0	2.8	0.6	4.8	77	1.4

Food Name	Serving Size	A I.U.	Thi mg	Rib mg	Nia mg	B$_6$ mg	Fol mcg	B$_{12}$ mcg	C mg	Calc mg	Iron mg	Mag mg	Pot mg	Zn mg
all grades, 1/4-inch fat, braised............	3 oz	0	0.06	0.20	2.10	0.22	4.3	1.90	0.0	11.1	2.6	16.1	196	7.1
all grades, 1/4-inch fat, raw..............	1 oz	0	0.03	0.05	0.61	0.10	1.4	0.95	0.0	2.8	0.6	4.8	76	1.4
choice, 1/8-inch fat, braised.............	3 oz	0	0.06	0.20	2.00	0.22	4.3	1.90	0.0	11.1	2.6	16.1	196	7.0
choice, 1/8-inch fat, raw	1 oz	0	0.03	0.05	0.61	0.10	1.4	0.95	0.0	2.8	0.6	4.8	76	1.4
choice, 1/4-inch fat, braised.............	3 oz	0	0.06	0.20	2.00	0.21	4.3	1.90	0.0	11.1	2.6	16.1	194	6.9
choice, 1/4-inch fat, raw	1 oz	0	0.03	0.05	0.61	0.10	1.4	0.94	0.0	2.8	0.6	4.5	75	1.4
prime, 1/2-inch fat, braised..............	3 oz	0	0.06	0.20	2.00	0.21	4.3	1.90	0.0	11.1	2.5	15.3	190	6.7
prime, 1/2-inch fat, raw..............	1 oz	0	0.03	0.05	0.60	0.10	1.4	0.91	0.0	2.8	0.5	4.5	71	1.3
select, 1/8-inch fat, braised..............	3 oz	0	0.06	0.21	2.10	0.22	4.3	2.00	0.0	11.1	2.7	17.0	201	7.4
select, 1/8-inch fat, raw..............	1 oz	0	0.03	0.05	0.62	0.10	1.4	0.97	0.0	2.8	0.6	4.8	78	1.4
select, 1/4-inch fat, braised.............	3 oz	0	0.06	0.21	2.10	0.22	4.3	2.00	0.0	11.1	2.7	17.0	199	7.2
select, 1/4-inch fat, raw..............	1 oz	0	0.03	0.05	0.62	0.10	1.4	0.97	0.0	2.8	0.6	4.8	77	1.4
FLANK														
Trimmed														
choice, 0-inch fat, braised..............	3 oz	0	0.12	0.16	3.90	0.31	7.7	2.90	0.0	5.1	3.0	20.4	298	5.1
choice, 0-inch fat, broiled..............	3 oz	0	0.09	0.16	4.30	0.29	6.8	2.80	0.0	6.0	2.2	20.4	352	4.1
choice, 0-inch fat, raw..............	1 oz	0	0.03	0.04	1.30	0.12	2.0	0.86	0.0	1.4	0.6	6.0	103	1.0
Untrimmed														
choice, 0-inch fat, braised..............	3 oz	0	0.12	0.15	3.80	0.30	7.7	2.80	0.0	5.1	2.8	19.6	286	4.9
choice, 0-inch fat, broiled..............	3 oz	0	0.09	0.15	4.20	0.29	6.8	2.70	0.0	6.0	2.1	19.6	342	4.0
choice, 0-inch fat, raw..............	4 oz	0	0.12	0.17	5.10	0.47	7.9	3.40	0.0	5.7	2.2	22.6	396	3.9
GROUND														
Extra lean, 17% fat														
baked, medium.....................	3 oz	0	0.03	0.20	3.50	0.19	7.7	1.50	0.0	6.0	1.9	14.4	190	4.5
baked, well done....................	3 oz	0	0.04	0.26	4.60	0.25	9.3	1.60	0.0	7.7	2.5	18.7	247	5.9
broiled, medium....................	3 oz	0	0.05	0.23	4.20	0.23	7.7	1.80	0.0	6.0	2.0	17.9	266	4.6
broiled, well done..................	3 oz	0	0.06	0.27	5.00	0.27	9.3	2.20	0.0	7.7	2.4	21.3	314	5.5
pan-fried, medium..................	3 oz	0	0.05	0.22	4.00	0.23	7.7	1.70	0.0	6.0	2.0	17.9	265	4.6
pan-fried, well done................	3 oz	0	0.06	0.26	4.60	0.26	8.5	2.00	0.0	6.8	2.3	20.4	306	5.3
raw	4 oz	0	0.07	0.28	5.10	0.29	9.0	2.30	0.0	7.9	2.2	22.6	321	4.7
raw	1 oz	0	0.02	0.07	1.30	0.07	2.3	0.58	0.0	2.0	0.6	5.7	81	1.2
Lean, 21% fat														
baked, medium.....................	3 oz	0	0.04	0.16	3.60	0.17	7.7	1.50	0.0	7.7	1.8	14.4	190	4.3
baked, well done....................	3 oz	0	0.06	0.20	4.60	0.22	10.2	1.90	0.0	10.2	2.3	17.9	243	5.5
broiled, medium	3 oz	0	0.04	0.18	4.40	0.22	7.7	2.00	0.0	9.3	1.8	17.9	256	4.6
broiled, well done	3 oz	0	0.05	0.20	5.10	0.26	9.3	2.30	0.0	10.2	2.1	20.4	297	5.3
pan-fried, medium..................	3 oz	0	0.04	0.19	4.10	0.24	7.7	1.90	0.0	8.5	1.9	17.0	254	4.4
pan-fried, well done	3 oz	0	0.05	0.20	4.60	0.27	8.5	2.20	0.0	9.3	2.1	19.6	289	5.0
raw	4 oz	0	0.06	0.24	5.10	0.28	9.0	2.60	0.0	9.0	2.0	20.3	295	4.4
raw	1 oz	0	0.01	0.06	1.30	0.07	2.3	0.66	0.0	2.3	0.5	5.1	74	1.1
Regular, 27% fat														
baked, medium.....................	3 oz	0	0.03	0.14	4.00	0.20	7.7	2.00	0.0	8.5	2.0	12.8	188	4.2
baked, well done....................	3 oz	0	0.03	0.17	5.00	0.25	9.3	2.50	0.0	10.2	2.5	16.1	233	5.2
broiled, medium....................	3 oz	0	0.03	0.16	4.90	0.23	7.7	2.50	0.0	9.3	2.1	17.0	248	4.4
broiled, well done	3 oz	0	0.03	0.18	5.50	0.26	8.5	2.80	0.0	10.2	2.3	18.7	278	4.9
pan-fried, medium..................	3 oz	0	0.03	0.17	5.00	0.20	7.7	2.30	0.0	9.3	2.1	17.0	255	4.3
pan-fried, well done	3 oz	0	0.03	0.18	5.50	0.23	8.5	2.50	0.0	11.1	2.3	18.7	282	4.8
raw	4 oz	0	0.04	0.17	5.10	0.27	7.9	3.00	0.0	9.0	2.0	18.1	258	4.0
raw	1 oz	0	0.01	0.04	1.30	0.07	2.0	0.75	0.0	2.3	0.5	4.5	65	1.0
HEART														
raw	4 oz	0	0.22	1.20	10.70	0.49	2.3	15.40	7.1	2.3	5.2	26.0	301	2.7
simmered	3 oz	0	0.12	1.30	3.50	0.18	1.7	12.20	1.3	5.1	6.4	21.3	198	2.7
KIDNEY														
raw	1 oz	249	0.11	0.72	2.30	0.14	22.7	7.70	2.5	1.7	2.1	4.8	73	0.5

Food Name	Serving Size	A I.U.	Thi mg	Rib mg	Nia mg	B_6 mg	Fol mcg	B_{12} mcg	C mg	Calc mg	Iron mg	Mag mg	Pot mg	Zn mg
simmered	3 oz	1055	0.16	3.50	5.10	0.44	83.3	43.60	0.7	14.4	6.2	15.3	152	3.6
LIVER														
braised	3 oz	30327	0.17	3.50	9.10	0.77	184.0	60.40	19.6	6.0	5.8	17.0	200	5.2
pan-fried	3 oz	30689	0.18	3.50	12.30	1.20	187.0	95.00	19.6	9.3	5.3	19.6	309	4.6
raw	4 oz	39941	0.29	3.10	14.40	1.10	280.0	78.20	24.9	6.8	7.7	21.5	365	4.4
LOIN, TOP														
Trimmed														
all grades, 0-inch fat, broiled	3 oz	0	0.08	0.17	4.50	0.36	6.8	1.70	0.0	6.8	2.1	22.9	337	4.4
all grades, 1/4-inch fat, broiled	3 oz	0	0.08	0.17	4.50	0.36	6.8	1.70	0.0	6.8	2.1	22.9	337	4.4
all grades, 1/4-inch fat, raw	1 oz	0	0.03	0.04	1.30	0.13	2.0	0.86	0.0	1.4	0.5	6.2	99	1.0
choice, 0-inch fat, broiled	3 oz	0	0.08	0.17	4.50	0.36	6.8	1.70	0.0	6.8	2.1	22.9	337	4.4
choice, 1/4-inch fat, broiled	3 oz	0	0.08	0.17	4.50	0.36	6.8	1.70	0.0	6.8	2.1	22.9	337	4.4
choice, 1/4-inch fat, raw	1 oz	0	0.03	0.04	1.30	0.13	2.0	0.86	0.0	1.4	0.5	6.2	99	1.0
prime, 1/4-inch fat, broiled	3 oz	0	0.08	0.17	4.50	0.36	6.8	1.70	0.0	6.8	2.1	22.9	337	4.4
prime, 1/4-inch fat, raw	1 oz	0	0.03	0.04	1.30	0.13	2.0	0.86	0.0	1.4	0.5	6.2	99	1.0
prime, 1/2-inch fat, raw	3 oz	0	0.08	0.17	4.50	0.36	6.8	1.70	0.0	6.8	2.1	22.9	337	4.4
select, 0-inch fat, broiled	3 oz	0	0.08	0.17	4.50	0.36	6.8	1.70	0.0	6.8	2.1	22.9	337	4.4
select, 1/4-inch fat, broiled	3 oz	0	0.08	0.17	4.50	0.36	6.8	1.70	0.0	6.8	2.1	22.9	337	4.4
select, 1/4-inch fat, raw	1 oz	0	0.03	0.04	1.30	0.13	2.0	0.86	0.0	1.4	0.5	6.2	99	1.0
Untrimmed														
all grades, 0-inch fat, broiled	3 oz	0	0.08	0.16	4.40	0.35	6.8	1.70	0.0	6.8	2.1	22.1	330	4.3
all grades, 1/8-inch fat, broiled	3 oz	0	0.07	0.15	4.10	0.32	6.0	1.70	0.0	7.7	1.9	20.4	306	4.0
all grades, 1/4-inch fat, broiled	3 oz	0	0.07	0.15	4.00	0.32	6.0	1.60	0.0	7.7	1.9	19.6	297	3.9
choice, 0-inch fat, broiled	3 oz	0	0.08	0.16	4.40	0.35	6.8	1.70	0.0	6.8	2.0	22.1	327	4.3
choice, 1/8-inch fat, broiled	3 oz	0	0.07	0.15	4.10	0.32	6.0	1.60	0.0	7.7	1.9	20.4	301	4.0
choice, 1/4-inch fat, broiled	3 oz	0	0.07	0.15	4.00	0.32	6.0	1.60	0.0	7.7	1.9	19.6	294	3.9
prime, 1/8-inch fat, broiled	3 oz	0	0.07	0.15	4.10	0.32	6.0	1.60	0.0	7.7	1.9	20.4	301	4.0
prime, 1/4-inch fat, broiled	3 oz	0	0.07	0.15	4.00	0.32	6.0	1.60	0.0	7.7	1.9	19.6	294	3.9
prime, 1/2-inch fat, broiled	3 oz	0	0.07	0.15	3.80	0.31	6.0	1.60	0.0	7.7	1.8	19.6	286	3.7
select, 0-inch fat, broiled	3 oz	0	0.08	0.16	4.40	0.35	6.8	1.70	0.0	6.8	2.1	22.1	330	4.3
select, 1/8-inch fat, broiled	3 oz	0	0.07	0.15	4.10	0.33	6.0	1.70	0.0	7.7	2.0	20.4	308	4.0
select, 1/4-inch fat, broiled	3 oz	0	0.07	0.15	4.10	0.32	6.0	1.60	0.0	7.7	1.9	20.4	301	4.0
LUNGS														
braised	3 oz	33	0.03	0.12	2.10	0.02	6.8	2.20	27.8	9.3	4.6	8.5	147	1.4
raw	4 oz	52	0.05	0.26	4.50	0.05	12.4	4.30	43.5	11.3	9.0	15.8	384	1.8
PANCREAS														
braised	3 oz	0	0.15	0.41	3.40	0.15	2.5	14.10	17.3	13.6	2.2	17.9	209	3.9
raw	4 oz	0	0.16	0.50	5.00	0.23	3.4	15.80	15.5	10.2	2.5	20.3	312	2.9
PORTERHOUSE														
Trimmed														
all grades, 0-inch fat, broiled	3 oz	0	0.09	0.21	3.90	0.34	6.8	1.90	0.0	6.0	2.6	22.9	312	4.5
all grades, 1/4-inch fat, broiled	3 oz	0	0.09	0.21	3.90	0.34	6.8	1.90	0.0	6.0	2.6	22.9	312	4.5
all grades, 1/4-inch fat, raw	1 oz	0	0.03	0.05	1.10	0.12	2.0	0.85	0.0	1.4	0.6	6.5	99	1.0
choice, 0-inch fat, broiled	3 oz	0	0.09	0.21	3.90	0.34	6.8	1.90	0.0	6.0	2.6	22.9	312	4.5
choice, 1/4-inch fat, broiled	3 oz	0	0.09	0.21	3.90	0.34	6.8	1.90	0.0	6.0	2.6	22.9	312	4.5
choice, 1/4-inch fat, raw	1 oz	0	0.03	0.05	1.10	0.12	2.0	0.85	0.0	1.4	0.6	6.5	99	1.0
select, 0-inch fat, broiled	3 oz	0	0.09	0.21	3.90	0.34	6.8	1.90	0.0	6.0	2.6	22.9	312	4.5
select, 1/4-inch fat, broiled	3 oz	0	0.09	0.21	3.90	0.34	6.8	1.90	0.0	6.0	2.6	22.9	312	4.5
select, 1/4-inch fat, raw	1 oz	0	0.03	0.05	1.10	0.12	2.0	0.85	0.0	1.4	0.6	6.5	99	1.0
Untrimmed														
all grades, 0-inch fat, broiled	3 oz	0	0.09	0.19	3.60	0.31	6.0	1.90	0.0	6.8	2.4	20.4	283	4.0
all grades, 1/8-inch fat, broiled	3 oz	0	0.09	0.19	3.50	0.30	6.0	1.80	0.0	6.8	2.3	19.6	273	3.9
all grades, 1/8-inch fat, raw	1 oz	0	0.03	0.05	1.00	0.11	1.7	0.77	0.0	1.7	0.6	5.4	85	0.9
all grades, 1/4-inch fat, broiled	3 oz	0	0.08	0.18	3.30	0.29	6.0	1.80	0.0	6.8	2.2	18.7	263	3.7

Food Name	Serving Size	A I.U.	Thi mg	Rib mg	Nia mg	B$_6$ mg	Fol mcg	B$_{12}$ mcg	C mg	Calc mg	Iron mg	Mag mg	Pot mg	Zn mg
all grades, 1/4-inch fat, raw	1 oz	0	0.03	0.05	0.99	0.11	1.7	0.76	0.0	1.7	0.5	5.4	85	0.9
choice, 1/8-inch fat, broiled	3 oz	0	0.09	0.19	3.50	0.30	6.0	1.80	0.0	6.8	2.3	19.6	274	3.9
choice, 1/8-inch fat, raw	1 oz	0	0.03	0.05	0.00	0.11	1.7	0.77	0.0	1.7	0.6	5.4	84	0.9
choice, 1/4-inch fat, broiled	3 oz	0	0.08	0.18	3.30	0.29	6.0	1.80	0.0	6.8	2.2	18.7	261	3.7
choice, 1/4-inch fat, raw	1 oz	0	0.03	0.05	0.00	0.11	1.7	0.77	0.0	1.7	0.6	5.4	84	0.9
select, 0-inch fat, broiled	3 oz	0	0.09	0.19	3.50	0.31	6.0	1.80	0.0	6.8	2.4	20.4	280	4.0
select, 1/8-inch fat, broiled	3 oz	0	0.09	0.19	3.40	0.30	6.0	1.80	0.0	6.8	2.3	19.6	272	3.9
select, 1/8-inch fat, raw	1 oz	0	0.03	0.05	1.00	0.11	1.7	0.79	0.0	1.7	0.6	5.7	88	0.9
select, 1/4-inch fat, broiled	3 oz	0	0.08	0.18	3.40	0.29	6.0	1.80	0.0	6.8	2.3	19.6	265	3.8
select, 1/4-inch fat, raw	1 oz	0	0.03	0.05	1.00	0.11	1.7	0.79	0.0	1.7	0.6	5.7	88	0.9
RIB, LARGE END														
Trimmed														
all grades, ribs 6-9, 0-inch fat, roasted	1 oz	0	0.03	0.05	0.88	0.10	1.7	0.92	0.0	2.0	0.6	6.0	97	1.4
all grades, ribs 6-9, 1/4-inch fat, broiled	3 oz	0	0.07	0.16	2.70	0.22	6.0	2.80	0.0	7.7	2.2	19.6	316	5.3
all grades, ribs 6-9, 1/4-inch fat, raw	1 oz	0	0.03	0.05	0.88	0.10	1.7	0.92	0.0	2.0	0.6	6.0	97	1.4
all grades, ribs 6-9, 1/4-inch fat, roasted	3 oz	0	0.08	0.19	3.80	0.22	7.7	2.20	0.0	6.8	2.4	21.3	303	6.3
choice, ribs 6-9, 0-inch fat, roasted	3 oz	0	0.08	0.19	3.80	0.22	7.7	2.20	0.0	6.8	2.4	21.3	303	6.3
choice, ribs 6-9, 1/4-inch fat, broiled	3 oz	0	0.07	0.16	2.70	0.22	6.0	2.80	0.0	7.7	2.2	19.6	316	5.3
choice, ribs 6-9, 1/4-inch fat, raw	1 oz	0	0.03	0.05	0.88	0.10	1.7	0.92	0.0	2.0	0.6	6.0	97	1.4
choice, ribs 6-9, 1/4-inch fat, roasted	3 oz	0	0.08	0.19	3.80	0.22	7.7	2.20	0.0	6.8	2.4	21.3	303	6.3
prime, ribs 6-9, 1/4-inch fat, broiled	3 oz	0	0.08	0.17	2.60	0.27	6.0	2.80	0.0	6.8	2.1	20.4	314	5.3
prime, ribs 6-9, 1/4-inch fat, raw	1 oz	0	0.03	0.05	0.88	0.10	1.7	0.92	0.0	2.0	0.6	6.0	97	1.4
prime, ribs 6-9, 1/4-inch fat, roasted	3 oz	0	0.08	0.19	3.80	0.22	7.7	2.20	0.0	6.8	2.4	21.3	303	6.3
prime, ribs 6-9, 1/2-inch fat, broiled	3 oz	0	0.07	0.17	2.60	0.27	6.0	2.80	0.0	6.8	2.1	20.4	31	5.3
prime, ribs 6-9, 1/2-inch fat, roasted	3 oz	0	0.07	0.19	3.80	0.22	7.7	2.20	0.0	6.8	2.4	21.3	303	6.3
select, ribs 6-9, 0-inch fat, roasted	3 oz	0	0.08	0.19	3.80	0.22	7.7	2.20	0.0	6.8	2.4	21.3	303	6.3
select, ribs 6-9, 1/4-inch fat, broiled	3 oz	0	0.07	0.16	2.70	0.22	6.0	2.80	0.0	7.7	2.2	19.6	316	5.3
select, ribs 6-9, 1/4-inch fat, raw	1 oz	0	0.03	0.05	0.88	0.10	1.7	0.92	0.0	2.0	0.6	6.0	97	1.4
select, ribs 6-9, 1/4-inch fat, roasted	3 oz	0	0.08	0.19	3.80	0.22	7.7	2.20	0.0	6.8	2.4	21.3	303	6.3
Untrimmed														
all grades, ribs 6-9, 0-inch fat, roasted	3 oz	0	0.06	0.16	3.10	0.20	6.0	2.00	0.0	8.5	2.0	17.0	251	5.0
all grades, ribs 6-9, 1/8-inch fat, raw	1 oz	0	0.02	0.04	0.74	0.08	1.4	0.77	0.0	2.3	0.5	4.5	74	1.1
all grades, ribs 6-9, 1/8-inch fat, roasted	3 oz	0	0.06	0.16	3.10	0.20	6.0	2.0	0.0	8.5	2.0	17.0	249	5.0
all grades, ribs 6-9, 1/4-inch fat, raw	1 oz	0	0.02	0.04	0.73	0.08	1.4	0.76	0.0	2.3	0.5	4.3	73	1.0
all grades, ribs 6-9, 1/4-inch fat, roasted	3 oz	0	0.06	0.15	3.10	0.20	6.0	2.00	0.0	8.5	2.0	16.1	245	4.8
choice, ribs 6-9, 0-inch fat, roasted	3 oz	0	0.06	0.16	3.10	0.20	6.0	2.00	0.0	8.5	2.0	17.0	247	4.9
choice, ribs 6-9, 1/8-inch fat, raw	1 oz	0	0.02	0.04	0.73	0.08	1.4	0.76	0.0	2.3	0.5	4.3	72	1.0
choice, ribs 6-9, 1/8-inch fat, roasted	3 oz	0	0.06	0.15	3.10	0.19	6.0	2.00	0.0	8.5	2.0	16.1	243	4.8
choice, ribs 6-9, 1/4-inch fat, raw	1 oz	0	0.02	0.04	0.72	0.08	1.4	0.75	0.0	2.3	0.5	4.3	70	1.0
choice, ribs 6-9, 1/4-inch fat, roasted	3 oz	0	0.06	0.15	3.00	0.19	6.0	2.00	0.0	8.5	1.9	16.1	241	4.7
prime, ribs 6-9, 1/8-inch fat, raw	1 oz	0	0.02	0.04	0.72	0.08	1.4	0.75	0.0	2.3	0.5	4.3	70	1.0
prime, ribs 6-9, 1/4-inch fat, raw	1 oz	0	0.02	0.04	0.71	0.08	1.4	0.73	0.0	2.3	0.5	4.3	69	1.0
prime, ribs 6-9, 1/4-inch fat, roasted	3 oz	0	0.06	0.15	3.00	0.19	6.0	2.00	0.0	8.5	1.9	16.1	243	4.8
prime, ribs 6-9, 1/2-inch fat, raw	1 oz	0	0.02	0.04	0.70	0.08	1.4	0.73	0.0	2.3	0.5	4.0	68	1.0
prime, ribs 6-9, 1/2-inch fat, roasted	3 oz	0	0.06	0.15	3.00	0.19	6.0	2.00	0.0	8.5	1.9	16.1	240	4.7
select, ribs 6-9, 1/8-inch fat, raw	1 oz	0	0.02	0.04	0.75	0.08	1.4	0.78	0.0	2.3	0.5	4.5	75	1.1
select, ribs 6-9, 1/8-inch fat, roasted	3 oz	0	0.06	0.16	3.20	0.20	6.8	2.00	0.0	7.7	2.0	17.0	254	5.1
select, ribs 6-9, 1/4-inch fat, raw	1 oz	0	0.02	0.04	0.74	0.08	1.4	0.77	0.0	2.3	0.5	4.5	74	1.1
select, ribs 6-9, 1/4-inch fat, roasted	3 oz	0	0.06	0.16	3.10	0.20	6.0	2.00	0.0	8.5	2.0	17.0	251	5.0
RIB, SHORTRIB														
Trimmed														
choice, braised	3 oz	0	0.06	0.17	2.70	0.24	6.0	2.90	0.0	9.3	2.9	18.7	266	6.6

Food Name	Serving Size	A I.U.	Thi mg	Rib mg	Nia mg	B6 mg	Fol mcg	*B12 mcg	C mg	Calc mg	Iron mg	Mag mg	Pot mg	Zn mg
choice, raw	3 oz	0	0.06	0.17	2.70	0.24	6.0	2.90	0.0	9.3	2.9	18.7	266	6.6
Untrimmed														
choice, braised	3 oz	0	0.04	0.13	2.10	0.19	4.3	2.20	0.0	10.2	2.0	12.8	190	4.1
choice, raw	1 oz	0	0.02	0.03	0.72	0.09	1.4	0.73	0.0	2.6	0.4	4.0	66	0.9
RIB, SMALL END														
Trimmed														
all grades, ribs 10-12, 0-inch fat, broiled	3 oz	0	0.09	0.19	4.10	0.34	6.8	2.80	0.0	11.1	2.2	22.9	335	5.9
all grades, ribs 10-12, 1/4-inch fat, broiled	3 oz	0	0.09	0.19	4.10	0.34	6.8	2.80	0.0	11.1	2.2	22.9	335	5.9
all grades, ribs 10-12, 1/4-inch fat, raw	1 oz	0	0.03	0.04	1.10	0.12	1.7	1.00	0.0	2.8	0.6	6.2	106	1.3
all grades, ribs 10-12, 1/4-inch fat, roasted	3 oz	0	0.06	0.16	3.20	0.24	6.8	2.80	0.0	10.2	2.5	21.3	338	5.3
choice, ribs 10-12, 0-inch fat, broiled	3 oz	0	0.09	0.19	4.10	0.34	6.8	2.80	0.0	11.1	2.2	22.9	335	5.9
choice, ribs 10-12, 0-inch fat, raw	1 oz	0	0.03	0.04	1.10	0.12	1.7	1.00	0.0	2.8	0.6	6.2	106	1.3
choice, ribs 10-12, 1/4-inch fat, broiled	3 oz	0	0.09	0.19	4.10	0.34	6.8	2.80	0.0	11.1	2.2	22.9	335	5.9
choice, ribs 10-12, 1/4-inch fat, raw	1 oz	0	0.03	0.04	1.10	0.12	1.7	1.00	0.0	2.8	0.6	6.2	106	1.3
choice, ribs 10-12, 1/4-inch fat, roasted	3 oz	0	0.06	0.16	3.20	0.24	6.8	2.80	0.0	10.2	2.5	21.3	338	5.3
prime, ribs 10-12, 1/4-inch fat, broiled	3 oz	0	0.09	0.19	4.10	0.34	6.8	2.80	0.0	11.1	2.2	22.9	335	5.9
prime, ribs 10-12, 1/4-inch fat, raw	1 oz	0	0.03	0.04	1.10	0.12	1.7	1.00	0.0	2.8	0.6	6.2	106	1.3
prime, ribs 10-12, 1/4-inch fat, roasted	3 oz	0	0.07	0.16	3.10	0.32	6.8	2.90	0.0	11.1	2.0	21.3	343	5.3
prime, ribs 10-12, 1/2-inch fat, broiled	3 oz	0	0.09	0.18	4.10	0.34	6.8	2.80	0.0	11.1	2.2	22.9	335	5.9
prime, ribs 10-12, 1/2-inch fat, roasted	3 oz	0	0.07	0.17	3.10	0.32	6.8	2.90	0.0	11.1	2.0	21.3	343	5.3
select, ribs 10-12, 0-inch fat, broiled	3 oz	0	0.09	0.19	4.10	0.34	6.8	2.80	0.0	11.1	2.2	22.9	335	5.9
select, ribs 10-12, 1/4-inch fat, broiled	3 oz	0	0.09	0.19	4.10	0.34	6.8	2.80	0.0	11.1	2.2	22.9	335	5.9
select, ribs 10-12, 1/4-inch fat, raw	1 oz	0	0.03	0.04	1.10	0.12	1.7	1.00	0.0	2.8	0.6	6.2	106	1.3
select, ribs 10-12, 1/4-inch fat, roasted	3 oz	0	0.06	0.16	3.20	0.24	6.8	2.80	0.0	10.2	2.5	21.3	338	5.3
Untrimmed														
all grades, ribs 10-12, 0-inch fat, broiled	3 oz	0	0.08	0.16	3.60	0.30	6.0	2.60	0.0	11.1	2.0	19.6	292	5.1
all grades, ribs 10-12, 1/8-inch fat, broiled	3 oz	0	0.08	0.16	3.40	0.29	6.0	2.50	0.0	11.1	1.9	18.7	280	4.8
all grades, ribs 10-12, 1/8-inch fat, raw	1 oz	0	0.02	0.04	0.89	0.10	1.4	0.85	0.0	2.8	0.5	4.8	83	1.0
all grades, ribs 10-12, 1/8-inch fat, roasted	3 oz	0	0.05	0.14	2.70	0.20	5.1	2.40	0.0	11.1	2.1	17.0	275	4.2
all grades, ribs 10-12, 1/4-inch fat, broiled	3 oz	0	0.08	0.15	3.40	0.28	6.0	2.50	0.0	11.1	1.9	18.7	276	4.8
all grades, ribs 10-12, 1/4-inch fat, raw	1 oz	0	0.02	0.04	0.88	0.10	1.4	0.84	0.0	2.8	0.5	4.8	81	1.0
all grades, ribs 10-12, 1/4-inch fat, roasted	3 oz	0	0.05	0.14	2.70	0.20	5.1	2.40	0.0	11.1	2.0	17.0	272	4.1
choice, ribs 10-12, 0-inch fat, broiled	3 oz	0	0.08	0.16	3.60	0.30	6.0	2.60	0.0	11.1	2.0	19.6	292	5.1
choice, ribs 10-12, 0-inch fat, raw	1 oz	0	0.02	0.04	0.92	0.10	1.4	0.88	0.0	2.8	0.5	5.1	87	1.1
choice, ribs 10-12, 1/8-inch fat, broiled	3 oz	0	0.08	0.16	3.40	0.29	6.0	2.50	0.0	11.1	1.9	18.7	277	4.8
choice, ribs 10-12, 1/8-inch fat, raw	1 oz	0	0.02	0.04	0.93	0.11	1.4	0.89	0.0	2.8	0.5	5.1	89	1.1
choice, ribs 10-12, 1/8-inch fat, roasted	3 oz	0	0.05	0.14	2.70	0.20	5.1	2.40	0.0	11.1	2.0	17.0	271	4.1
choice, ribs 10-12, 1/4-inch fat, broiled	3 oz	0	0.08	0.15	3.40	0.28	6.0	2.40	0.0	11.1	1.9	18.7	274	4.7
choice, ribs 10-12, 1/4-inch fat, raw	1 oz	0	0.02	0.03	0.86	0.10	1.4	0.83	0.0	2.8	0.5	4.5	80	1.0
choice, ribs 10-12, 1/4-inch fat, roasted	3 oz	0	0.05	0.14	2.6	0.20	5.1	2.40	0.0	11.1	2.0	16.1	267	4.1
prime, ribs 10-12, 1/8-inch fat, broiled	3 oz	0	0.08	0.16	3.50	0.29	6.0	2.50	0.0	11.1	1.9	18.7	282	4.9
prime, ribs 10-12, 1/8-inch fat, raw	1 oz	0	0.02	0.04	0.87	0.10	1.4	0.84	0.0	2.8	0.5	4.8	81	1.0
prime, ribs 10-12, 1/8-inch fat, roasted	3 oz	0	0.05	0.14	2.60	0.26	6.0	2.40	0.0	11.1	1.7	17.0	275	4.1
prime, ribs 10-12, 1/4-inch fat, broiled	3 oz	0	0.08	0.16	3.40	0.29	6.0	2.50	0.0	11.1	1.9	18.7	279	4.8
prime, ribs 10-12, 1/4-inch fat, raw	1 oz	0	0.02	0.03	0.86	0.10	1.4	0.83	0.0	2.8	0.5	4.5	80	1.0
prime, ribs 10-12, 1/4-inch fat, roasted	3 oz	0	0.05	0.14	2.60	0.26	5.1	2.40	0.0	11.1	1.6	16.1	270	4.0
prime, ribs 10-12, 1/2-inch fat, broiled	3 oz	0	0.07	0.16	3.40	0.29	6.0	2.50	0.0	11.1	1.9	18.7	277	4.8

Food Name	Serving Size	A I.U.	Thi mg	Rib mg	Nia mg	B_6 mg	Fol mcg	B_{12} mcg	C mg	Calc mg	Iron mg	Mag mg	Pot mg	Zn mg
prime, ribs 10-12, 1/2-inch fat, raw..........	1 oz	0	0.02	0.04	0.85	0.10	1.4	0.82	0.0	2.8	0.5	4.5	78	0.0
prime, ribs 10-12, 1/2-inch fat, roasted......	3 oz	0	0.05	0.14	2.50	0.26	6.0	2.40	0.0	11.1	1.6	16.1	269	4.0
select, ribs 10-12, 1/8-inch fat, broiled......	3 oz	0	0.08	0.16	3.50	0.29	6.0	2.50	0.0	11.1	1.9	18.7	281	4.9
select, ribs 10-12, 1/8-inch fat, raw..........	1 oz	0	0.02	0.04	0.90	0.10	1.4	0.86	0.0	2.8	0.5	4.8	84	1.1
select, ribs 10-12, 1/8-inch fat, roasted.....	3 oz	0	0.05	0.14	2.70	0.20	5.1	2.50	0.0	11.1	2.1	17.0	279	4.3
select, ribs 10-12, 1/4-inch fat, broiled......	3 oz	0	0.08	0.16	3.40	0.29	6.0	2.50	0.0	11.1	1.9	18.7	279	4.8
select, ribs 10-12, 1/4-inch fat, raw..........	1 oz	0	0.02	0.04	0.88	0.10	1.4	0.85	0.0	2.8	0.5	4.8	82	1.0
select, ribs 10-12, 1/4-inch fat, roasted.....	3 oz	0	0.05	0.14	2.70	0.20	5.1	2.40	0.0	11.1	2.0	17.0	275	4.2
RIB, WHOLE														
Trimmed														
all grades, ribs 6-12, 1/4-inch fat, broiled	3 oz	0	0.08	0.17	3.30	0.27	6.0	2.80	0.0	9.3	2.2	21.3	324	5.6
all grades, ribs 6-12, 1/4-inch fat, raw.......	1 oz	0	0.03	0.05	0.95	0.11	1.7	0.95	0.0	2.3	0.6	6.0	100	1.4
all grades, ribs 6-12, 1/4-inch fat, roasted...........................	3 oz	0	0.07	0.18	3.50	0.23	6.8	2.50	0.0	8.5	2.4	21.3	318	5.9
choice, ribs 6-12, 1/4-inch fat, broiled.......	3 oz	0	0.08	0.17	3.30	0.27	6.0	2.80	0.0	9.3	2.2	21.3	324	5.6
choice, ribs 6-12, 1/4-inch fat, raw	1 oz	0	0.03	0.05	0.95	0.11	1.7	0.95	0.0	2.3	0.6	6.0	100	1.4
choice, ribs 6-12, 1/4-inch fat, roasted	3 oz	0	0.07	0.18	3.50	0.23	6.8	2.50	0.0	8.5	2.4	21.3	318	5.9
prime, ribs 6-12, 1/4-inch fat, broiled	3 oz	0	0.08	0.18	3.20	0.30	6.0	2.80	0.0	8.5	2.1	21.3	322	5.6
prime, ribs 6-12, 1/4-inch fat, raw...........	1 oz	0	0.03	0.05	0.95	0.11	1.7	0.95	0.0	2.3	0.6	6.0	100	1.4
prime, ribs 6-12, 1/4-inch fat, roasted.......	3 oz	0	0.07	0.18	3.50	0.26	7.7	2.50	0.0	8.5	2.2	21.3	320	5.9
prime, ribs 6-12, 1/2-inch fat, broiled	3 oz	0	0.08	0.17	3.20	0.30	6.8	2.80	0.0	8.5	2.1	21.3	322	5.6
prime, ribs 6-12, 1/2-inch fat, roasted.......	3 oz	0	0.07	0.18	3.50	0.26	6.8	2.50	0.0	8.5	2.2	21.3	320	5.9
select, ribs 6-12, 1/4-inch fat, broiled	3 oz	0	0.08	0.17	3.30	0.27	6.0	2.80	0.0	9.3	2.2	21.3	324	5.6
select, ribs 6-12, 1/4-inch fat, raw...........	1 oz	0	0.03	0.05	0.95	0.11	1.7	0.95	0.0	2.3	0.6	6.0	100	1.4
select, ribs 6-12, 1/4-inch fat, roasted	3 oz	0	0.07	0.18	3.50	0.23	6.8	2.50	0.0	8.5	2.4	21.3	318	5.9
Untrimmed														
all grades, ribs 6-12, 1/8-inch fat, broiled	3 oz	0	0.07	0.14	2.80	0.23	5.1	2.50	0.0	9.3	1.9	17.0	268	4.5
all grades, ribs 6-12, 1/8-inch fat, raw.......	1 oz	0	0.02	0.04	0.79	0.09	1.4	0.79	0.0	2.6	0.5	4.5	76	1.0
all grades, ribs 6-12, 1/8-inch fat, roasted...........................	3 oz	0	0.06	0.15	2.90	0.20	6.0	2.20	0.0	9.3	2.0	17.0	259	4.6
all grades, ribs 6-12, 1/4-inch fat, broiled	3 oz	0	0.07	0.14	2.80	0.23	5.1	2.40	0.0	10.2	1.8	17.0	265	4.4
all grades, ribs 6-12, 1/4-inch fat, raw.......	1 oz	0	0.02	0.04	0.79	0.09	1.4	0.80	0.0	2.6	0.5	4.5	77	1.1
all grades, ribs 6-12, 1/4-inch fat, roasted..........................	3 oz	0	0.06	0.14	2.90	0.20	6.0	2.20	0.0	9.3	2.0	17.0	256	4.5
choice, ribs 6-12, 1/8-inch fat, broiled.......	3 oz	0	0.07	0.14	2.80	0.23	5.1	2.40	0.0	9.3	1.9	17.0	266	4.4
choice, ribs 6-12, 1/8-inch fat, raw	1 oz	0	0.02	0.04	0.79	0.09	1.4	0.79	0.0	2.6	0.5	4.5	76	1.0
choice, ribs 6-12, 1/8-inch fat, roasted	3 oz	0	0.06	0.14	2.90	0.20	6.0	2.20	0.0	9.3	2.0	17.0	257	4.6
choice, ribs 6-12, 1/4-inch fat, broiled.......	3 oz	0	0.07	0.14	2.70	0.23	5.1	2.40	0.0	10.2	1.8	16.1	262	4.4
choice, ribs 6-12, 1/4-inch fat, raw	1 oz	0	0.02	0.04	0.77	0.09	1.4	0.78	0.0	2.6	0.5	4.3	74	1.0
choice, ribs 6-12, 1/4-inch fat, roasted	3 oz	0	0.06	0.14	2.90	0.20	6.0	2.10	0.0	9.3	2.0	16.1	252	4.5
prime, ribs 6-12, 1/8-inch fat, broiled	3 oz	0	0.07	0.15	2.70	0.26	5.1	2.40	0.0	9.3	1.8	17.0	264	4.4
prime, ribs 6-12, 1/8-inch fat, raw...........	1 oz	0	0.02	0.04	0.78	0.09	1.4	0.78	0.0	2.6	0.5	4.5	75	1.0
prime, ribs 6-12, 1/8-inch fat, roasted.......	3 oz	0	0.06	0.15	2.90	0.22	6.0	2.20	0.0	9.3	1.8	17.0	258	4.6
prime, ribs 6-12, 1/4-inch fat, broiled	3 oz	0	0.07	0.14	2.70	0.26	5.1	2.40	0.0	9.3	1.8	17.0	260	4.3
prime, ribs 6-12, 1/4-inch fat, raw...........	1 oz	0	0.02	0.04	0.77	0.09	1.4	0.77	0.0	2.6	0.5	4.3	73	0.0
prime, ribs 6-12, 1/4-inch fat, roasted.......	3 oz	0	0.06	0.14	2.80	0.22	6.0	2.10	0.0	9.3	1.8	16.1	254	4.5
prime, ribs 6-12, 1/2-inch fat, broiled	3 oz	0	0.06	0.14	2.60	0.25	5.1	2.30	0.0	10.2	1.7	16.1	252	4.2
prime, ribs 6-12, 1/2-inch fat, raw...........	1 oz	0	0.02	0.04	0.76	0.09	1.4	0.77	0.0	2.6	0.5	4.3	72	1.0
prime, ribs 6-12, 1/2-inch fat, roasted.......	3 oz	0	0.06	0.14	2.80	0.21	6.0	2.10	0.0	9.3	1.8	15.3	245	4.3
select, ribs 6-12, 1/8-inch fat, broiled	3 oz	0	0.07	0.14	2.80	0.24	5.1	2.50	0.0	9.3	1.9	17.0	273	4.6
select, ribs 6-12, 1/8-inch fat, raw..........	1 oz	0	0.02	0.04	0.81	0.09	1.4	0.81	0.0	2.6	0.5	4.8	79	1.1

Food Name	Serving Size	A I.U.	Thi mg	Rib mg	Nia mg	B_6 mg	Fol mcg	B_{12} mcg	C mg	Calc mg	Iron mg	Mag mg	Pot mg	Zn mg
select, ribs 6-12, 1/8-inch fat, roasted	3 oz	0	0.06	0.15	3.00	0.20	6.0	2.20	0.0	9.3	2.0	17.0	264	4.7
select, ribs 6-12, 1/4-inch fat, broiled	3 oz	0	0.07	0.14	2.80	0.23	5.1	2.50	0.0	9.3	1.9	17.0	269	4.5
select, ribs 6-12, 1/4-inch fat, raw	1 oz	0	0.02	0.04	0.80	0.09	1.4	0.80	0.0	2.6	0.5	4.5	77	1.1
select, ribs 6-12, 1/4-inch fat, roasted	3 oz	0	0.06	0.15	3.00	0.20	6.0	2.20	0.0	9.3	2.0	17.0	260	4.7

ROUND, BOTTOM

Trimmed

Food Name	Serving Size	A I.U.	Thi mg	Rib mg	Nia mg	B_6 mg	Fol mcg	B_{12} mcg	C mg	Calc mg	Iron mg	Mag mg	Pot mg	Zn mg
all grades, 0-inch fat, braised	3 oz	0	0.06	0.22	3.50	0.31	9.3	2.10	0.0	4.3	2.9	21.3	262	4.7
all grades, 0-inch fat, roasted	3 oz	0	0.07	0.20	3.50	0.32	10.2	2.30	0.0	4.3	2.7	23.8	332	3.9
all grades, 1/4-inch fat, braised	3 oz	0	0.06	0.22	3.50	0.31	9.3	2.10	0.0	4.3	2.9	21.3	262	4.7
all grades, 1/4-inch fat, raw	1 oz	0	0.03	0.06	1.20	0.16	2.8	0.83	0.0	1.1	0.7	7.1	105	0.0
all grades, 1/4-inch fat, roasted	3 oz	0	0.07	0.20	3.50	0.32	10.2	2.30	0.0	4.3	2.7	23.8	332	3.9
choice, 0-inch fat, braised	3 oz	0	0.06	0.22	3.50	0.31	9.3	2.10	0.0	4.3	2.9	21.3	262	4.7
choice, 0-inch fat, roasted	3 oz	0	0.07	0.20	3.50	0.32	10.2	2.30	0.0	4.3	2.7	23.8	332	3.9
choice, 1/4-inch fat, braised	3 oz	0	0.06	0.22	3.50	0.31	9.3	2.10	0.0	4.3	2.9	21.3	262	4.7
choice, 1/4-inch fat, raw	1 oz	0	0.03	0.06	1.20	0.16	2.8	0.83	0.0	1.1	0.7	7.1	105	0.0
choice, 1/4-inch fat, roasted	3 oz	0	0.07	0.20	3.50	0.32	10.2	2.30	0.0	4.3	2.7	23.8	332	3.9
prime, 1/2-inch fat, broiled	3 oz	0	0.06	0.22	3.50	0.31	9.3	2.10	0.0	4.3	2.9	21.3	262	4.7
prime, 1/2-inch fat, raw	1 oz	0	0.03	0.06	1.20	0.16	2.8	0.83	0.0	1.1	0.7	7.1	105	0.0
select, 0-inch fat, braised	3 oz	0	0.06	0.22	3.50	0.31	9.3	2.10	0.0	4.3	2.9	21.3	262	4.7
select, 0-inch fat, roasted	3 oz	0	0.07	0.20	3.50	0.32	10.2	2.30	0.0	4.3	2.7	23.8	332	3.9
select, 1/4-inch fat, braised	3 oz	0	0.06	0.22	3.50	0.31	9.3	2.10	0.0	4.3	2.9	21.3	262	4.7
select, 1/4-inch fat, raw	1 oz	0	0.03	0.06	1.20	0.16	2.8	0.83	0.0	1.1	0.7	7.1	105	0.0
select, 1/4-inch fat, roasted	3 oz	0	0.07	0.20	3.50	0.32	10.2	2.30	0.0	4.3	2.7	23.8	332	3.9

Untrimmed

Food Name	Serving Size	A I.U.	Thi mg	Rib mg	Nia mg	B_6 mg	Fol mcg	B_{12} mcg	C mg	Calc mg	Iron mg	Mag mg	Pot mg	Zn mg
all grades, 0-inch fat, braised	3 oz	0	0.06	0.22	3.40	0.31	9.3	2.10	0.0	4.3	2.9	21.3	258	4.6
all grades, 0-inch fat, roasted	3 oz	0	0.07	0.20	3.40	0.32	10.2	2.30	0.0	4.3	2.6	23.8	330	3.9
all grades, 1/8-inch fat, braised	3 oz	0	0.06	0.20	3.30	0.29	8.5	2.00	0.0	5.1	2.7	19.6	246	4.3
all grades, 1/8-inch fat, raw	1 oz	0	0.03	0.05	1.10	0.15	2.6	0.79	0.0	1.4	0.6	6.5	98	0.9
all grades, 1/8-inch fat, roasted	3 oz	0	0.07	0.20	3.30	0.31	10.2	2.20	0.0	4.3	2.5	22.1	313	3.7
all grades, 1/4-inch fat, braised	3 oz	0	0.06	0.20	3.20	0.28	8.5	2.00	0.0	5.1	2.7	18.7	240	4.2
all grades, 1/4-inch fat, raw	1 oz	0	0.03	0.05	1.10	0.15	2.6	0.78	0.0	1.4	0.6	6.2	95	0.9
all grades, 1/4-inch fat, roasted	3 oz	0	0.07	0.20	3.20	0.30	9.3	2.20	0.0	5.1	2.4	21.3	304	3.6
choice, 0-inch fat, braised	3 oz	0	0.06	0.21	3.40	0.30	9.3	2.10	0.0	4.3	2.9	20.4	257	4.6
choice, 0-inch fat, roasted	3 oz	0	0.07	0.20	3.40	0.32	10.2	2.30	0.0	4.3	2.6	23.8	327	3.9
choice, 1/8-inch fat, braised	3 oz	0	0.06	0.20	3.20	0.29	8.5	2.00	0.0	5.1	2.7	19.6	245	4.3
choice, 1/8-inch fat, raw	1 oz	0	0.03	0.05	1.10	0.15	2.6	0.79	0.0	1.4	0.6	6.5	97	0.9
choice, 1/8-inch fat, roasted	3 oz	0	0.07	0.20	3.30	0.30	10.2	2.20	0.0	5.1	2.5	22.1	311	3.7
choice, 1/4-inch fat, braised	3 oz	0	0.06	0.20	3.20	0.28	8.5	2.00	0.0	5.1	2.7	18.7	240	4.2
choice, 1/4-inch fat, raw	1 oz	0	0.03	0.05	1.10	0.15	2.6	0.78	0.0	1.4	0.6	6.2	94	0.9
choice, 1/4-inch fat, roasted	3 oz	0	0.07	0.19	3.20	0.29	9.3	2.20	0.0	5.1	2.4	21.3	302	3.6
prime, 1/2-inch fat, braised	3 oz	0	0.06	0.20	3.20	0.29	8.5	2.00	0.0	5.1	2.7	19.6	244	4.3
prime, 1/2-inch fat, raw	1 oz	0	0.03	0.05	1.10	0.15	2.6	0.78	0.0	1.4	0.6	6.2	94	0.9
select, 0-inch fat, braised	3 oz	0	0.06	0.22	3.40	0.31	9.3	2.10	0.0	4.3	2.9	21.3	258	4.6
select, 0-inch fat, roasted	3 oz	0	0.07	0.20	3.40	0.32	10.2	2.30	0.0	4.3	2.6	23.8	330	3.9
select, 1/8-inch fat, braised	3 oz	0	0.06	0.20	3.30	0.29	8.5	2.00	0.0	5.1	2.7	19.6	246	4.3
select, 1/8-inch fat, raw	1 oz	0	0.03	0.05	1.10	0.15	2.6	0.80	0.0	1.4	0.6	6.5	98	0.9
select, 1/8-inch fat, roasted	3 oz	0	0.07	0.20	3.30	0.31	10.2	2.20	0.0	4.3	2.5	22.1	314	3.7
select, 1/4-inch fat, braised	3 oz	0	0.06	0.20	3.20	0.28	8.5	2.00	0.0	5.1	2.7	19.6	241	4.2
select, 1/4-inch fat, raw	1 oz	0	0.03	0.05	1.10	0.15	2.6	0.79	0.0	1.4	0.6	6.5	96	0.9
select, 1/4-inch fat, roasted	3 oz	0	0.07	0.20	3.20	0.30	9.3	2.20	0.0	5.1	2.5	22.1	307	3.6

ROUND, EYE OF

Trimmed

Food Name	Serving Size	A I.U.	Thi mg	Rib mg	Nia mg	B_6 mg	Fol mcg	B_{12} mcg	C mg	Calc mg	Iron mg	Mag mg	Pot mg	Zn mg
all grades, 0-inch fat, roasted	3 oz	0	0.08	0.14	3.20	0.32	6.0	1.80	0.0	4.3	1.7	22.9	336	4.0
all grades, 1/4-inch fat, raw	1 oz	0	0.03	0.04	1.10	0.13	2.0	0.91	0.0	1.1	0.4	6.5	109	0.8

Food Name	Serving Size	A I.U.	Thi mg	Rib mg	Nia mg	B6 mg	Fol mcg	B12 mcg	C mg	Calc mg	Iron mg	Mag mg	Pot mg	Zn mg
all grades, 1/4-inch fat, roasted	3 oz	0	0.08	0.14	3.20	0.32	6.0	1.80	0.0	4.3	1.7	22.9	336	4.0
choice, 0-inch fat, roasted................	3 oz	0	0.08	0.14	3.20	0.32	6.0	1.80	0.0	4.3	1.7	22.9	336	4.0
choice, 1/4-inch fat, raw	1 oz	0	0.03	0.04	1.10	0.13	2.0	0.91	0.0	1.1	0.4	6.5	109	0.8
choice, 1/4-inch fat, roasted	3 oz	0	0.08	0.14	3.20	0.32	6.0	1.80	0.0	4.3	1.7	22.9	336	4.0
prime, 1/2-inch fat, raw..................	1 oz	0	0.03	0.04	1.10	0.13	2.0	0.91	0.0	1.1	0.4	6.5	109	0.8
prime, 1/2-inch fat, roasted..............	3 oz	0	0.07	0.14	3.20	0.32	6.0	1.80	0.0	4.3	1.7	22.9	336	4.0
select, 0-inch fat, roasted	3 oz	0	0.08	0.14	3.20	0.32	6.0	1.80	0.0	4.3	1.7	22.9	336	4.0
select, 1/4-inch fat, raw.................	1 oz	0	0.03	0.04	1.10	0.13	2.0	0.91	0.0	1.1	0.4	6.5	109	0.8
select, 1/4-inch fat, roasted.............	3 oz	0	0.08	0.14	3.20	0.32	6.0	1.80	0.0	4.3	1.7	22.9	336	4.0
Untrimmed														
all grades, 0-inch fat, roasted	3 oz	0	0.08	0.14	3.20	0.32	6.0	1.80	0.0	4.3	1.6	22.9	333	4.0
all grades, 1/8-inch fat, raw..........	1 oz	0	0.03	0.04	1.00	0.12	2.0	0.88	0.0	1.1	0.4	6.2	103	0.8
all grades, 1/8-inch fat, roasted	3 oz	0	0.07	0.14	3.10	0.32	6.0	1.80	0.0	4.3	1.6	22.1	324	3.9
all grades, 1/4-inch fat, raw...........	1 oz	0	0.03	0.04	0.95	0.12	1.7	0.83	0.0	1.4	0.4	5.7	95	0.8
all grades, 1/4-inch fat, roasted	3 oz	0	0.07	0.14	3.00	0.30	6.0	1.80	0.0	5.1	1.6	20.4	308	3.7
choice, 0-inch fat, roasted.............	3 oz	0	0.08	0.14	3.20	0.32	6.0	1.80	0.0	4.3	1.6	22.9	333	4.0
choice, 1/8-inch fat, raw	1 oz	0	0.03	0.04	1.00	0.12	2.0	0.87	0.0	1.1	0.4	6.2	103	0.8
choice, 1/8-inch fat, roasted	3 oz	0	0.07	0.14	3.10	0.32	6.0	1.80	0.0	4.3	1.6	22.1	324	3.9
choice, 1/4-inch fat, raw	1 oz	0	0.03	0.04	0.95	0.12	1.7	0.83	0.0	1.4	0.4	5.7	95	0.8
choice, 1/4-inch fat, roasted	3 oz	0	0.07	0.14	3.00	0.30	5.1	1.80	0.0	5.1	1.6	20.4	305	3.7
select, 1/8-inch fat, raw.............	1 oz	0	0.03	0.04	1.00	0.12	2.0	0.88	0.0	1.1	0.4	6.2	103	0.8
select, 1/8-inch fat, roasted..........	3 oz	0	0.07	0.14	3.10	0.32	6.0	1.80	0.0	4.3	1.6	22.1	324	3.9
select, 1/4-inch fat, raw.............	1 oz	0	0.03	0.04	0.96	0.12	1.7	0.84	0.0	1.4	0.4	5.7	96	0.8
select, 1/4-inch fat, roasted...........	3 oz	0	0.07	0.14	3.00	0.30	6.0	1.80	0.0	5.1	1.6	21.3	310	3.7
prime, 1/2-inch fat, raw.............	1 oz	0	0.03	0.04	0.96	0.12	1.7	0.84	0.0	1.4	0.4	6.0	96	0.8
prime, 1/2-inch fat, roasted...........	3 oz	0	0.07	0.14	3.00	0.30	6.0	1.80	0.0	5.1	1.6	21.3	311	3.7
ROUND, FULL CUT														
Trimmed														
choice, 1/4-inch fat, broiled...........	3 oz	0	0.09	0.19	3.60	0.34	8.5	2.70	0.0	4.3	2.3	23.8	359	3.9
choice, 1/4-inch fat, raw	1 oz	0	0.03	0.05	1.10	0.14	2.6	0.84	0.0	1.1	0.6	7.1	106	0.0
select, 1/4-inch fat, broiled	3 oz	0	0.09	0.19	3.60	0.35	8.5	2.70	0.0	4.3	2.3	23.8	360	4.0
select, 1/4-inch fat, raw................	1 oz	0	0.03	0.05	1.10	0.14	2.6	0.84	0.0	1.1	0.6	7.1	106	0.0
Untrimmed														
choice, 1/8-inch fat, broiled...........	3 oz	0	0.08	0.18	3.40	0.32	7.7	2.60	0.0	5.1	2.2	22.1	336	3.7
choice, 1/8-inch fat, raw	1 oz	0	0.03	0.05	1.10	0.13	2.3	0.80	0.0	1.1	0.6	6.2	97	0.9
choice, 1/4-inch fat, broiled...........	3 oz	0	0.08	0.18	3.40	0.32	7.7	2.60	0.0	5.1	2.1	21.3	333	3.7
choice, 1/4-inch fat, raw	1 oz	0	0.03	0.05	1.10	0.13	2.3	0.79	0.0	1.1	0.6	6.2	96	0.9
select, 1/8-inch fat, broiled	3 oz	0	0.09	0.18	3.40	0.32	7.7	2.60	0.0	5.1	2.2	22.1	336	3.7
select, 1/8-inch fat, raw.............	1 oz	0	0.03	0.05	1.10	0.13	2.3	0.80	0.0	1.1	0.6	6.2	97	0.9
select, 1/4-inch fat, broiled	3 oz	0	0.08	0.18	3.40	0.32	7.7	2.60	0.0	5.1	2.2	22.1	333	3.7
select, 1/4-inch fat, raw.............	1 oz	0	0.03	0.05	1.10	0.13	2.3	0.79	0.0	1.1	0.6	6.2	96	0.9
ROUND, TOP														
Trimmed														
all grades, 0-inch fat, braised	3 oz	0	0.06	0.21	3.20	0.24	7.7	2.30	0.0	3.4	2.8	22.1	284	3.9
all grades, 1/4-inch fat, braised..........	3 oz	0	0.06	0.21	3.20	0.24	7.7	2.30	0.0	3.4	2.8	22.1	284	3.9
all grades, 1/4-inch fat, broiled	3 oz	0	0.10	0.23	5.10	0.48	10.2	2.10	0.0	5.1	2.4	26.4	376	4.7
all grades, 1/4-inch fat, raw...............	1 oz	0	0.03	0.05	1.20	0.14	2.6	0.81	0.0	0.9	0.6	7.1	109	0.8
choice, 0-inch fat, braised................	3 oz	0	0.06	0.21	3.20	0.24	7.7	2.30	0.0	3.4	2.8	22.1	284	3.9
choice, 1/4-inch fat, braised	3 oz	0	0.06	0.21	3.20	0.24	7.7	2.30	0.0	3.4	2.8	22.1	284	3.9
choice, 1/4-inch fat, broiled.............	3 oz	0	0.10	0.23	5.10	0.48	10.2	2.10	0.0	5.1	2.4	26.4	376	4.7
choice, 1/4-inch fat, pan-fried...........	3 oz	0	0.09	0.24	4.70	0.52	11.1	2.90	0.0	4.3	2.7	29.8	436	3.9
choice, 1/4-inch fat, raw	1 oz	0	0.03	0.05	1.20	0.14	2.6	0.81	0.0	0.9	0.6	7.1	109	0.8
prime, 1/2-inch fat, broiled	3 oz	0	0.10	0.23	5.10	0.48	10.2	2.10	0.0	5.1	2.4	26.4	376	4.7
prime, 1/4-inch fat, broiled	3 oz	0	0.10	0.23	5.10	0.48	10.2	2.10	0.0	5.1	2.4	26.4	376	4.7

Food Name	Serving Size	A I.U.	Thi mg	Rib mg	Nia mg	B_6 mg	Fol mcg	B_{12} mcg	C mg	Calc mg	Iron mg	Mag mg	Pot mg	Zn mg
prime, 1/4-inch fat, raw	1 oz	0	0.03	0.05	1.20	0.14	2.6	0.81	0.0	0.9	0.6	7.1	109	0.8
select, 0-inch fat, braised	3 oz	0	0.06	0.21	3.20	0.24	7.7	2.30	0.0	3.4	2.8	22.1	284	3.9
select, 1/4-inch fat, braised	3 oz	0	0.06	0.21	3.20	0.24	7.7	2.30	0.0	3.4	2.8	22.1	284	3.9
select, 1/4-inch fat, broiled	3 oz	0	0.10	0.23	5.10	0.48	10.2	2.10	0.0	5.1	2.4	26.4	376	4.7
select, 1/4-inch fat, raw	1 oz	0	0.03	0.05	1.20	0.14	2.6	0.81	0.0	0.9	0.6	7.1	109	0.8
Untrimmed														
all grades, 0-inch fat, braised	3 oz	0	0.06	0.21	3.20	0.24	7.7	2.30	0.0	3.4	2.8	21.3	281	3.8
all grades, 1/8-inch fat, braised	3 oz	0	0.06	0.20	3.10	0.23	7.7	2.20	0.0	4.3	2.7	20.4	271	3.7
all grades, 1/8-inch fat, broiled	3 oz	0	0.09	0.22	4.90	0.46	10.2	2.10	0.0	5.1	2.4	25.5	360	4.5
all grades, 1/8-inch fat, raw	1 oz	0	0.03	0.05	1.20	0.14	2.6	0.78	0.0	0.9	0.6	6.8	103	0.8
all grades, 1/4-inch fat, braised	3 oz	0	0.06	0.20	3.10	0.23	7.7	2.20	0.0	4.3	2.7	20.4	268	3.6
all grades, 1/4-inch fat, broiled	3 oz	0	0.09	0.22	4.90	0.45	9.3	2.10	0.0	6.0	2.3	24.6	356	4.5
all grades, 1/4-inch fat, raw	1 oz	0	0.03	0.05	1.20	0.14	2.3	0.77	0.0	1.1	0.6	6.5	100	0.8
choice, 0-inch fat, braised	3 oz	0	0.06	0.21	3.20	0.24	7.7	2.30	0.0	3.4	2.8	21.3	281	3.8
choice, 1/8-inch fat, braised	3 oz	0	0.06	0.20	3.10	0.23	7.7	2.20	0.0	4.3	2.7	20.4	269	3.7
choice, 1/8-inch fat, broiled	3 oz	0	0.09	0.22	4.90	0.46	10.2	2.10	0.0	5.1	2.4	25.5	360	4.5
choice, 1/8-inch fat, pan-fried	3 oz	0	0.09	0.22	4.40	0.48	10.2	2.80	0.0	5.1	2.5	28.1	408	3.7
choice, 1/8-inch fat, raw	1 oz	0	0.03	0.05	1.20	0.14	2.6	0.78	0.0	0.9	0.6	6.8	103	0.8
choice, 1/4-inch fat, braised	3 oz	0	0.06	0.20	3.00	0.23	7.7	2.20	0.0	4.3	2.6	20.4	265	3.6
choice, 1/4-inch fat, broiled	3 oz	0	0.09	0.22	4.90	0.45	9.3	2.10	0.0	6.0	2.3	24.6	356	4.5
choice, 1/4-inch fat, pan-fried	3 oz	0	0.09	0.22	4.30	0.48	10.2	2.70	0.0	5.1	2.5	27.2	400	3.6
choice, 1/4-inch fat, raw	1 oz	0	0.03	0.05	1.20	0.14	2.3	0.77	0.0	1.1	0.6	6.5	100	0.8
prime, 1/2-inch fat, broiled	3 oz	0	0.10	0.22	5.00	0.46	9.3	2.10	0.0	5.1	2.4	25.5	363	4.4
prime, 1/2-inch fat, raw	1 oz	0	0.03	0.05	1.20	0.14	2.6	0.78	0.0	1.1	0.6	6.5	103	0.8
prime, 1/8-inch fat, broiled	3 oz	0	0.10	0.22	5.10	0.47	10.2	2.10	0.0	5.1	2.4	25.5	371	4.7
prime, 1/8-inch fat, raw	1 oz	0	0.03	0.05	1.20	0.14	2.6	0.79	0.0	0.9	0.6	6.8	105	0.8
prime, 1/4-inch fat, broiled	3 oz	0	0.10	0.22	5.00	0.47	10.2	2.10	0.0	5.1	2.4	25.5	367	4.6
prime, 1/4-inch fat, raw	1 oz	0	0.03	0.05	1.20	0.14	2.6	0.79	0.0	0.9	0.6	6.8	104	0.8
select, 0-inch fat, braised	3 oz	0	0.06	0.21	3.20	0.24	7.7	2.30	0.0	3.4	2.8	21.3	281	3.8
select, 1/8-inch fat, braised	3 oz	0	0.06	0.20	3.10	0.23	7.7	2.20	0.0	3.4	2.7	21.3	273	3.7
select, 1/8-inch fat, broiled	3 oz	0	0.09	0.22	4.90	0.46	10.2	2.10	0.0	5.1	2.4	25.5	361	4.5
select, 1/8-inch fat, raw	1 oz	0	0.03	0.05	1.20	0.14	2.6	0.78	0.0	0.9	0.6	6.8	103	0.8
select, 1/4-inch fat, braised	3 oz	0	0.06	0.20	3.10	0.23	7.7	2.20	0.0	4.3	2.7	20.4	269	3.7
select, 1/4-inch fat, broiled	3 oz	0	0.09	0.22	4.90	0.45	9.3	2.10	0.0	6.0	2.3	24.6	356	4.5
select, 1/4-inch fat, raw	1 oz	0	0.03	0.05	1.20	0.14	2.6	0.77	0.0	1.1	0.6	6.5	101	0.8
ROUND TIP														
Trimmed														
all grades, 0-inch fat, roasted	3 oz	0	0.09	0.23	3.20	0.34	6.8	2.50	0.0	4.3	2.5	22.9	328	6.0
all grades, 1/4-inch fat, raw	1 oz	0	0.03	0.06	0.96	0.13	2.3	0.91	0.0	1.1	0.6	6.8	103	1.4
all grades, 1/4-inch fat, roasted	3 oz	0	0.09	0.23	3.20	0.34	6.8	2.50	0.0	4.3	2.5	22.9	328	6.0
choice, 0-inch fat, roasted	3 oz	0	0.09	0.23	3.20	0.34	6.8	2.50	0.0	4.3	2.5	22.9	328	6.0
choice, 1/4-inch fat, raw	1 oz	0	0.03	0.06	0.96	0.13	2.3	0.91	0.0	1.1	0.6	6.8	103	1.4
choice, 1/4-inch fat, roasted	3 oz	0	0.09	0.23	3.20	0.34	6.8	2.50	0.0	4.3	2.5	22.9	328	6.0
prime, 1/4-inch fat, raw	1 oz	0	0.03	0.06	0.96	0.13	2.3	0.91	0.0	1.1	0.6	6.8	103	1.4
prime, 1/2-inch fat, roasted	3 oz	0	0.08	0.23	3.20	0.34	6.8	2.50	0.0	4.3	2.5	22.9	328	6.0
prime, 1/4-inch fat, roasted	3 oz	0	0.09	0.23	3.20	0.34	6.8	2.50	0.0	4.3	2.5	22.9	328	6.0
select, 0-inch fat, roasted	3 oz	0	0.09	0.23	3.20	0.34	6.8	2.50	0.0	4.3	2.5	22.9	328	6.0
select, 1/4-inch fat, raw	1 oz	0	0.03	0.06	0.96	0.13	2.3	0.91	0.0	1.1	0.6	6.8	103	1.4
select, 1/4-inch fat, roasted	3 oz	0	0.09	0.23	3.20	0.34	6.8	2.50	0.0	4.3	2.5	22.9	328	6.0
Untrimmed														
all grades, 0-inch fat, roasted	3 oz	0	0.09	0.22	3.10	0.33	6.8	2.40	0.0	4.3	2.4	22.1	321	5.9
all grades, 1/8-inch fat, raw	1 oz	0	0.03	0.05	0.90	0.12	2.0	0.85	0.0	1.4	0.6	6.2	93	1.3
all grades, 1/8-inch fat, roasted	3 oz	0	0.08	0.22	3.10	0.32	6.8	2.40	0.0	5.1	2.4	22.1	312	5.7
all grades, 1/4-inch fat, raw	1 oz	0	0.03	0.05	0.88	0.11	2.0	0.84	0.0	1.4	0.6	6.0	91	1.2

Food Name	Serving Size	A I.U.	Thi mg	Rib mg	Nia mg	B_6 mg	Fol mcg	B_{12} mcg	C mg	Calc mg	Iron mg	Mag mg	Pot mg	Zn mg
all grades, 1/4-inch fat, roasted	3 oz	0	0.08	0.21	3.00	0.32	6.0	2.30	0.0	5.1	2.3	21.3	305	5.5
choice, 0-inch fat, roasted.	3 oz	0	0.09	0.22	3.10	0.33	6.8	2.40	0.0	4.3	2.4	22.1	321	5.9
choice, 1/8-inch fat, raw	1 oz	0	0.03	0.05	0.89	0.12	2.0	0.85	0.0	1.4	0.6	6.0	92	1.2
choice, 1/8-inch fat, roasted	3 oz	0	0.08	0.21	3.00	0.32	6.8	2.40	0.0	5.1	2.4	21.3	310	5.6
choice, 1/4-inch fat, raw	1 oz	0	0.03	0.05	0.88	0.11	2.0	0.84	0.0	1.4	0.6	6.0	90	1.2
choice, 1/4-inch fat, roasted	3 oz	0	0.08	0.21	3.00	0.32	6.0	2.30	0.0	5.1	2.3	20.4	301	5.4
prime, 1/4-inch fat, raw.	1 oz	0	0.03	0.05	0.89	0.11	2.0	0.85	0.0	1.4	0.6	6.0	92	1.2
prime, 1/4-inch fat, roasted.	3 oz	0	0.08	0.20	2.90	0.32	6.0	2.30	0.0	5.1	2.3	20.4	298	5.4
prime, 1/2-inch fat, raw	1 oz	0	0.03	0.05	0.88	0.11	2.0	0.84	0.0	1.4	0.6	5.7	90	1.2
prime, 1/2-inch fat, roasted	3 oz	0	0.08	0.20	2.90	0.31	6.0	2.30	0.0	6.0	2.3	20.4	294	5.3
select, 1/8-inch fat, raw.	1 oz	0	0.03	0.05	0.90	0.12	2.0	0.86	0.0	1.4	0.6	6.2	94	1.3
select, 1/8-inch fat, roasted.	3 oz	0	0.08	0.22	3.10	0.32	6.8	2.40	0.0	5.1	2.4	22.1	315	5.7
select, 1/4-inch fat, raw	1 oz	0	0.03	0.05	0.89	0.12	2.0	0.85	0.0	1.4	0.6	6.0	93	1.2
select, 1/4-inch fat, roasted.	3 oz	0	0.08	0.21	3.00	0.32	6.8	2.40	0.0	5.1	2.4	21.3	308	5.6
SHANK CROSSCUTS														
Trimmed														
choice, 1/4-inch fat, raw	1 oz	0	0.03	0.06	1.60	0.13	2.3	0.94	0.0	5.7	0.7	4.0	110	2.0
choice, 1/4-inch fat, simmered	3 oz	0	0.12	0.18	5.00	0.32	8.5	3.20	0.0	27.2	3.3	25.5	380	8.9
Untrimmed														
choice, 1/4-inch fat, raw	3 oz	0	0.09	0.17	4.50	0.37	6.8	2.70	0.0	16.1	1.9	11.1	304	5.4
choice, 1/4-inch fat, simmered	3 oz	0	0.10	0.17	4.50	0.29	7.7	3.00	0.0	25.5	3.0	22.9	343	7.9
SIRLOIN, TOP														
Trimmed														
all grades, 0-inch fat, broiled.	3 oz	0	0.11	0.25	3.60	0.38	8.5	2.40	0.0	9.3	2.9	27.2	343	5.5
all grades, 1/4-inch fat, broiled	3 oz	0	0.11	0.25	3.60	0.38	8.5	2.40	0.0	9.3	2.9	27.2	343	5.5
all grades, 1/4-inch fat, raw.	1 oz	0	0.04	0.07	1.00	0.13	2.3	0.90	0.0	2.0	0.8	6.8	102	1.2
choice, 0-inch fat, broiled	3 oz	0	0.11	0.25	3.60	0.38	8.5	2.40	0.0	9.3	2.9	27.2	343	5.5
choice, 1/4-inch fat, broiled.	3 oz	0	0.11	0.25	3.60	0.38	8.5	2.40	0.0	9.3	2.9	27.2	343	5.5
choice, 1/4-inch fat, pan-fried	3 oz	0	0.12	0.28	3.70	0.42	8.5	3.10	0.0	9.3	3.3	28.1	395	5.4
choice, 1/4-inch fat, raw	1 oz	0	0.04	0.07	1.00	0.13	2.3	0.90	0.0	2.0	0.8	6.8	102	1.2
select, 0-inch fat, broiled.	3 oz	0	0.11	0.25	3.60	0.38	8.5	2.40	0.0	9.3	2.9	27.2	343	5.5
select, 1/4-inch fat, broiled	3 oz	0	0.11	0.25	3.60	0.38	8.5	2.40	0.0	9.3	2.9	27.2	343	5.5
select, 1/4-inch fat, raw.	1 oz	0	0.04	0.07	1.00	0.13	2.3	0.90	0.0	2.0	0.8	6.8	102	1.2
Untrimmed														
all grades, 0-inch fat, broiled.	3 oz	0	0.10	0.24	3.50	0.36	8.5	2.40	0.0	9.3	2.8	26.4	331	5.3
all grades, 1/8-inch fat, broiled	3 oz	0	0.10	0.23	3.40	0.36	7.7	2.30	0.0	9.3	2.6	24.6	316	5.1
all grades, 1/8-inch fat, raw.	1 oz	0	0.03	0.06	0.93	0.11	2.0	0.83	0.0	2.0	0.7	6.0	91	1.1
all grades, 1/4-inch fat, broiled	3 oz	0	0.09	0.23	3.30	0.35	7.7	2.30	0.0	9.3	2.6	24.6	311	5.0
all grades, 1/4-inch fat, raw.	1 oz	0	0.03	0.06	0.91	0.11	2.0	0.82	0.0	2.0	0.7	6.0	89	1.0
choice, 0-inch fat, broiled	3 oz	0	0.10	0.24	3.50	0.36	8.5	2.40	0.0	9.3	2.7	25.5	328	5.3
choice, 1/8-inch fat, broiled.	3 oz	0	0.09	0.23	3.40	0.35	7.7	2.30	0.0	9.3	2.6	24.6	314	5.0
choice, 1/8-inch fat, pan-fried	3 oz	0	0.10	0.25	3.30	0.37	7.7	2.80	0.0	10.2	2.9	23.8	345	4.7
choice, 1/8-inch fat, raw	1 oz	0	0.03	0.06	0.92	0.11	2.0	0.83	0.0	2.0	0.7	6.0	90	1.0
choice, 1/4-inch fat, broiled.	3 oz	0	0.09	0.23	3.30	0.35	7.7	2.30	0.0	9.3	2.6	23.8	309	4.9
choice, 1/4-inch fat, pan-fried	3 oz	0	0.10	0.24	3.20	0.36	7.7	2.80	0.0	10.2	2.8	23.8	337	4.6
choice, 1/4-inch fat, raw	1 oz	0	0.03	0.06	0.91	0.11	2.0	0.82	0.0	2.3	0.7	5.7	88	1.0
select, 0-inch fat, broiled.	3 oz	0	0.10	0.25	3.60	0.87	8.5	2.40	0.0	9.3	2.8	26.4	334	5.4
select, 1/8-inch fat, broiled	3 oz	0	0.10	0.23	3.40	0.36	7.7	2.30	0.0	9.3	2.6	24.6	316	5.1
select, 1/8-inch fat, raw.	1 oz	0	0.03	0.06	0.93	0.12	2.0	0.84	0.0	2.0	0.7	6.0	92	1.1
select, 1/4-inch fat, broiled	3 oz	0	0.09	0.23	3.40	0.35	7.7	2.30	0.0	9.3	2.6	24.6	314	5.0
select, 1/4-inch fat, raw.	1 oz	0	0.03	0.06	0.92	0.11	2.0	0.82	0.0	2.0	0.7	6.0	90	1.0
SPLEEN														
braised	3 oz	0	0.04	0.26	4.70	0.03	3.4	4.30	42.8	10.2	33.5	16.1	241	2.4
raw	4 oz	0	0.06	0.42	9.50	0.08	4.5	6.40	51.4	10.2	50.3	24.9	485	2.4

Food Name	Serving Size	A I.U.	Thi mg	Rib mg	Nia mg	B_6 mg	Fol mcg	B_{12} mcg	C mg	Calc mg	Iron mg	Mag mg	Pot mg	Zn mg
T-BONE														
Trimmed														
all grades, 0-inch fat, broiled	3 oz	0	0.09	0.21	3.90	0.33	6.8	1.90	0.0	5.1	2.7	23.8	321	4.5
all grades, 1/4-inch fat, broiled	3 oz	0	0.09	0.21	3.90	0.33	6.8	1.90	0.0	5.1	2.7	23.8	321	4.5
all grades, 1/4-inch fat, raw	1 oz	0	0.03	0.05	1.10	0.12	2.0	0.85	0.0	1.4	0.7	6.5	100	1.0
choice, 0-inch fat, broiled	3 oz	0	0.09	0.21	3.90	0.33	6.8	1.90	0.0	5.1	2.7	23.8	321	4.5
choice, 1/4-inch fat, broiled	3 oz	0	0.09	0.21	3.90	0.33	6.8	1.90	0.0	5.1	2.7	23.8	321	4.5
choice, 1/4-inch fat, raw	1 oz	0	0.03	0.05	1.10	0.12	2.0	0.85	0.0	1.4	0.7	6.5	100	1.0
select, 0-inch fat, broiled	3 oz	0	0.09	0.21	3.90	0.33	6.8	1.90	0.0	5.1	2.7	23.8	321	4.5
select, 1/4-inch fat, broiled	3 oz	0	0.09	0.21	3.90	0.33	6.8	1.90	0.0	5.1	2.7	23.8	321	4.5
select, 1/4-inch fat, raw	1 oz	0	0.03	0.05	1.10	0.12	2.0	0.85	0.0	1.4	0.7	6.5	100	1.0
Untrimmed														
all grades, 0-inch fat, broiled	3 oz	0	0.09	0.20	3.60	0.31	6.0	1.90	0.0	6.0	2.5	21.3	296	4.1
all grades, 1/8-inch fat, broiled	3 oz	0	0.09	0.19	3.50	0.30	6.0	1.80	0.0	6.8	2.4	20.4	286	4.0
all grades, 1/8-inch fat, raw	1 oz	0	0.03	0.05	1.00	0.11	1.7	0.79	0.0	1.7	0.6	5.7	88	0.9
all grades, 1/4-inch fat, broiled	3 oz	0	0.08	0.18	3.40	0.29	6.0	1.80	0.0	6.8	2.3	19.6	276	3.8
all grades, 1/4-inch fat, raw	1 oz	0	0.03	0.05	1.00	0.11	1.7	0.78	0.0	1.7	0.6	5.7	88	0.9
choice, 0-inch fat, broiled	3 oz	0	0.09	0.20	3.60	0.31	6.0	1.90	0.0	6.0	2.5	21.3	295	4.1
choice, 1/8-inch fat, broiled	3 oz	0	0.09	0.19	3.50	0.30	6.0	1.80	0.0	6.8	2.4	20.4	284	3.9
choice, 1/8-inch fat, raw	1 oz	0	0.03	0.05	1.00	0.11	1.7	0.78	0.0	1.7	0.6	5.7	87	0.9
choice, 1/4-inch fat, broiled	3 oz	0	0.08	0.18	3.40	0.28	6.0	1.80	0.0	6.8	2.3	19.6	273	3.8
choice, 1/4-inch fat, raw	1 oz	0	0.03	0.05	1.00	0.11	1.7	0.78	0.0	1.7	0.6	5.4	87	0.9
select, 0-inch fat, broiled	3 oz	0	0.09	0.20	3.70	0.31	6.0	1.90	0.0	6.0	2.5	22.1	299	4.2
select, 1/8-inch fat, broiled	3 oz	0	0.09	0.19	3.60	0.30	6.0	1.90	0.0	6.8	2.4	21.3	291	4.0
select, 1/8-inch fat, raw	1 oz	0	0.03	0.05	1.10	0.11	2.0	0.80	0.0	1.7	0.6	5.7	90	1.0
select, 1/4-inch fat, broiled	3 oz	0	0.09	0.19	3.50	0.30	6.0	1.80	0.0	6.8	2.4	20.4	284	3.9
select, 1/4-inch fat, raw	1 oz	0	0.03	0.05	1.00	0.11	2.0	0.80	0.0	1.7	0.6	5.7	90	0.9
TENDERLOIN														
Trimmed														
all grades, 0-inch fat, broiled	3 oz	0	0.11	0.26	3.30	0.37	6.0	2.20	0.0	6.0	3.0	25.5	356	4.8
all grades, 1/4-inch fat, broiled	3 oz	0	0.11	0.26	3.30	0.37	6.0	2.20	0.0	6.0	3.0	25.5	356	4.8
all grades, 1/4-inch fat, raw	1 oz	0	0.04	0.07	0.97	0.12	2.0	0.82	0.0	1.7	0.8	6.8	104	1.0
all grades, 1/4-inch fat, roasted	3 oz	0	0.09	0.26	2.90	0.25	7.7	2.30	0.0	6.0	3.1	22.9	332	4.1
choice, 0-inch fat, broiled	3 oz	0	0.11	0.26	3.30	0.37	6.0	2.20	0.0	6.0	3.0	25.5	356	4.8
choice, 1/4-inch fat, broiled	3 oz	0	0.11	0.26	3.30	0.37	6.0	2.20	0.0	6.0	3.0	25.5	356	4.8
choice, 1/4-inch fat, raw	1 oz	0	0.04	0.07	0.97	0.12	2.0	0.82	0.0	1.7	0.8	6.8	104	1.0
choice, 1/4-inch fat, roasted	3 oz	0	0.15	0.28	3.90	0.48	7.7	3.30	0.0	6.8	3.1	27.2	416	4.1
prime, 1/4-inch fat, broiled	3 oz	0	0.11	0.26	3.30	0.37	6.0	2.20	0.0	6.0	3.0	25.5	356	4.8
prime, 1/4-inch fat, raw	1 oz	0	0.04	0.07	0.97	0.12	2.0	0.82	0.0	1.7	0.8	6.8	104	1.0
prime, 1/4-inch fat, roasted	3 oz	0	0.09	0.27	2.90	0.32	6.8	2.40	0.0	6.0	3.1	22.9	334	4.4
prime, short loin, 1/2-inch fat, broiled	3 oz	0	0.11	0.25	3.30	0.37	6.0	2.20	0.0	6.0	3.0	25.5	356	4.8
prime, short loin, 1/2-inch fat, roasted	3 oz	0	0.09	0.27	2.90	0.32	6.8	2.40	0.0	6.0	3.1	22.9	334	4.4
select, 0-inch fat, broiled	3 oz	0	0.11	0.26	3.30	0.37	6.0	2.20	0.0	6.0	3.0	25.5	356	4.8
select, 1/4-inch fat, broiled	3 oz	0	0.11	0.26	3.30	0.37	6.0	2.20	0.0	6.0	3.0	25.5	356	4.8
select, 1/4-inch fat, raw	1 oz	0	0.04	0.07	0.97	0.12	2.0	0.82	0.0	1.7	0.8	6.8	104	1.0
select, 1/4-inch fat, roasted	3 oz	0	0.09	0.26	2.90	0.25	7.7	2.30	0.0	6.0	3.1	22.9	332	4.1
Untrimmed														
all grades, 0-inch fat, broiled	3 oz	0	0.10	0.25	3.20	0.36	6.0	2.10	0.0	6.0	2.9	24.6	341	4.5
all grades, 1/8-inch fat, raw	1 oz	0	0.03	0.06	0.84	0.11	1.7	0.73	0.0	2.0	0.7	5.4	85	0.9
all grades, 1/8-inch fat, roasted	3 oz	0	0.10	0.23	3.00	0.33	5.1	2.10	0.0	6.8	2.7	22.1	318	4.2
all grades, 1/4-inch fat, broiled	3 oz	0	0.09	0.22	3.00	0.33	5.1	2.00	0.0	6.8	2.7	22.1	313	4.1
all grades, 1/4-inch fat, raw	1 oz	0	0.03	0.06	0.83	0.11	1.7	0.72	0.0	2.0	0.7	5.4	84	0.8
all grades, 1/4-inch fat, roasted	3 oz	0	0.07	0.22	2.50	0.21	6.0	2.10	0.0	7.7	2.6	18.7	277	3.4
choice, 0-inch fat, broiled	3 oz	0	0.10	0.24	3.20	0.36	6.0	2.10	0.0	6.0	2.9	23.8	338	4.5

Food Name	Serving Size	A I.U.	Thi mg	Rib mg	Nia mg	B_6 mg	Fol mcg	B_{12} mcg	C mg	Calc mg	Iron mg	Mag mg	Pot mg	Zn mg
choice, 1/8-inch fat, broiled	3 oz	0	0.09	0.22	3.00	0.33	5.1	2.10	0.0	6.8	2.7	22.1	315	4.2
choice, 1/8-inch fat, raw	1 oz	0	0.03	0.06	0.84	0.11	1.7	0.73	0.0	2.0	0.7	5.4	85	0.9
choice, 1/8-inch fat, roasted	3 oz	0	0.13	0.23	3.30	0.41	6.8	2.90	0.0	7.7	2.6	22.1	346	3.4
choice, 1/4-inch fat, broiled	3 oz	0	0.09	0.22	3.00	0.33	5.1	2.00	0.0	6.8	2.7	22.1	310	4.1
choice, 1/4-inch fat, raw	1 oz	0	0.03	0.06	0.83	0.11	1.7	0.72	0.0	2.0	0.7	5.4	84	0.8
choice, 1/4-inch fat, roasted	3 oz	0	0.13	0.23	3.30	0.40	6.8	2.80	0.0	7.7	2.6	22.1	340	3.4
prime, 1/8-inch fat, broiled	3 oz	0	0.09	0.22	3.00	0.33	5.1	2.00	0.0	6.8	2.7	22.1	313	4.1
prime, 1/8-inch fat, raw	1 oz	0	0.03	0.06	0.85	0.11	1.7	0.74	0.0	2.0	0.7	5.7	86	0.9
prime, 1/8-inch fat, roasted	3 oz	0	0.08	0.23	2.60	0.28	6.0	2.10	0.0	6.8	2.7	19.6	286	3.7
prime, 1/4-inch fat, broiled	3 oz	0	0.09	0.22	3.00	0.32	5.1	2.00	0.0	6.8	2.6	21.3	308	4.1
prime, 1/4-inch fat, raw	1 oz	0	0.03	0.06	0.84	0.11	1.7	0.73	0.0	2.0	0.7	5.4	85	0.9
prime, 1/4-inch fat, roasted	3 oz	0	0.08	0.23	2.50	0.28	6.0	2.10	0.0	7.7	2.6	18.7	281	3.7
prime, short loin, 1/2-inch fat, broiled	3 oz	0	0.09	0.22	2.90	0.32	6.0	2.00	0.0	6.8	2.6	22.1	308	4.1
prime, short loin, 1/2-inch fat, roasted	3 oz	0	0.07	0.22	2.50	0.27	6.0	2.10	0.0	7.7	2.6	18.7	277	3.6
select, 0-inch fat, broiled	3 oz	0	0.10	0.25	3.20	0.36	6.0	2.10	0.0	6.0	2.9	24.6	341	4.5
select, 1/8-inch fat, broiled	3 oz	0	0.10	0.23	3.10	0.34	5.1	2.10	0.0	6.8	2.7	22.9	320	4.3
select, 1/8-inch fat, raw	1 oz	0	0.03	0.06	0.84	0.11	1.7	0.73	0.0	2.0	0.7	5.4	85	0.9
select, 1/8-inch fat, roasted	3 oz	0	0.08	0.22	2.50	0.21	6.8	2.10	0.0	7.7	2.6	18.7	281	3.4
select, 1/4-inch fat, broiled	3 oz	0	0.10	0.23	3.00	0.33	5.1	2.10	0.0	6.8	2.7	22.1	318	4.2
select, 1/4-inch fat, raw	1 oz	0	0.03	0.06	0.83	0.11	1.7	0.72	0.0	2.0	0.7	5.4	84	0.8
select, 1/4-inch fat, roasted	3 oz	0	0.07	0.22	2.50	0.21	6.0	2.10	0.0	7.7	2.6	18.7	277	3.4
THYMUS														
braised	3 oz	0	0.07	0.19	1.60	0.07	0.9	1.30	25.7	8.5	1.3	8.5	368	1.9
raw	4 oz	0	0.12	0.39	3.90	0.18	2.3	2.40	38.4	7.9	2.4	15.8	407	2.3
TONGUE														
raw	4 oz	0	0.14	0.38	4.80	0.35	7.9	4.30	3.5	6.8	3.3	18.1	356	3.2
simmered	3 oz	0	0.03	0.30	1.80	0.14	4.3	5.00	0.4	6.0	2.9	14.4	153	4.1
TRIPE														
raw	4 oz	0	0.01	0.19	0.07	0.05	2.3	1.70	3.8	10.2	2.2	9.0	305	2.8
raw	1 oz	0	0.00	0.05	0.02	0.01	0.6	0.44	1.0	2.6	0.6	2.3	77	0.7
BEEF, CORNED. See also under HASH.														
Canned														
cured	1 oz	0	0.01	0.04	0.69	0.04	2.6	0.46	0.0	3.4	0.6	4.0	39	1.0
cured, sliced, 0.75-oz slices	1 slice	0	0.00	0.03	0.51	0.03	1.9	0.34	0.0	2.5	0.4	2.9	29	0.8
Fresh														
brisket, cured, cooked	3 oz	0	0.02	0.14	2.60	0.20	5.1	1.40	0.0	6.8	1.6	10.2	123	3.9
brisket, cured, raw	1 oz	0	0.01	0.05	1.00	0.08	1.4	0.51	7.7	2.0	0.5	4.0	84	0.8
BEEF DINNER/ENTRÉE. See also BEEF, CORNED; CHILI; MEAT LOAF DINNER/ENTRÉE; SANDWICH.														
(Banquet)														
Salisbury steak, w/gravy, potatoes, corn, in sauce	1 pkg	0	na	na	na	na	na	na	na	na	2.1	1127.0	na	na
Salisbury steak, w/gravy, potatoes, corn, in sauce	1 serving	0	na	na	na	na	na	na	na	na	2.1	1127.0	na	na
Salisbury steak, w/gravy, potatoes, corn, in sauce, 'Extra Helping'	1 pkg	na	na	na	na	na	na	na	0.0	112.0	1.9	na	na	na
Salisbury steak, w/gravy, potatoes, corn, in sauce, 'Extra Helping'	1 serving	na	na	na	na	na	na	na	0.0	112.0	1.9	na	na	na
(Castleberry Premium)														
stew	1 pkg	2604	na	na	na	na	na	na	na	na	na	na	na	na
stew	1 serving	938	na	na	na	na	na	na	na	na	na	na	na	na
(Dinty Moore)														
stew, canned	1 pkg yield	7183	na	na	na	na	na	na	4.7	34.0	3.0	42.5	714	4.7
stew, canned	1 cup	3988	na	na	na	na	na	na	2.6	18.9	1.7	23.6	396	2.6

Food Name	Serving Size	A I.U.	Thi mg	Rib mg	Nia mg	B$_6$ mg	Fol mcg	B$_{12}$ mcg	C mg	Calc mg	Iron mg	Mag mg	Pot mg	Zn mg
(Healthy Choice)														
Salisbury steak, w/mushroom gravy, mashed potato, corn, frozen	1 pkg	1014	na	na	na	na	na	na	11.7	42.4	2.2	na	na	na
steak, w/mushroom gravy, mashed potato, corn, frozen	1 serving	1014	na	na	na	na	na	na	11.7	42.4	2.2	na	na	na
(Lean Cuisine)														
Oriental, w/vegetables, rice	1 pkg	2550	na	na	na	na	na	na	26.5	na	na	na	na	na
Oriental, w/vegetables, rice	1 serving	2550	na	na	na	na	na	na	26.5	na	na	na	na	na
(Lean Magic 30)														
and turkey barbecue, flame-broiled, product 9126	1 piece	156	0.14	0.09	2.40	0.26	1.7	1.40	1.3	33.1	1.9	26.4	245	3.2
and turkey patty, flame-broiled, w/tangy glaze	1 piece	52.7	0.14	0.10	2.40	0.25	1.7	1.10	0.0	26.4	1.8	28.1	252	3.7
and turkey patty, flame-broiled, w/teriyaki sauce	1 piece	12.4	0.03	0.02	0.56	0.06	0.4	0.26	0.0	6.2	0.4	6.6	59	0.9
(Lean Magic)														
barbecue, flame-broiled, product 3732	1 piece	101	0.14	0.11	2.70	0.27	2.7	1.40	1.2	25.2	1.7	28.6	275	4.0
patty, flame-broiled	1 piece	52	0.16	0.16	3.10	0.29	3.5	1.70	0.0	24.9	2.3	31.9	296	5.4
patty, flame-broiled, w/onion.	1 piece	45	0.14	0.15	2.90	0.28	5.2	1.60	0.52	23.7	2.2	28.9	283	5.0
patty, mesquite, flame-broiled. . . . . : .	1 piece	52	0.16	0.16	3.10	0.29	3.5	1.70	0.0	25.6	2.3	31.9	296	5.4
rib, barbecue, flame-broiled, 'Rib-B-Q' product 3733	1 piece	80	0.10	0.11	2.40	0.25	3.4	1.30	1.2	17.7	1.5	22.4	252	3.4
rib, barbecue, flame-broiled, 'Rib-B-Q' product 3832	1 piece	101	0.14	0.14	2.70	0.26	3.4	1.50	1.2	26.5	2.0	27.9	260	4.7
rib, barbecue, flame-broiled, 'Rib-B-Q' product 3833	1 piece	80	0.10	0.14	2.50	0.23	4.1	1.60	1.2	19.0	1.9	21.8	233	4.3
rib, barbecue, flame-broiled, 'Rib-B-Q' product 4150	1 piece	221	0.13	0.10	2.30	0.22	1.9	1.20	2.6	23.7	1.6	23.7	226	3.2
Salisbury steak, flame-broiled	1 piece	152	0.11	0.16	2.50	0.24	7.4	1.60	2.1	25.9	2.1	23.7	245	4.4
(Nestlé)														
stew, canned, 'Chef Mate'.	1 cup	3107	0.18	0.25	3.10	0.30	na	0.55	2.5	63.0	1.6	35.3	388	2.5
stew, canned, 'Chef Mate'.	1 pkg	37397	2.20	3.00	37.40	3.60	na	6.70	30.3	758	19.1	425.0	4671	30.0
(Pierre)														
and onion, breaded, flame-broiled, 'Two-Fers' product 9681.	1 piece	19	0.05	0.05	1.00	0.10	1.6	0.60	0.22	10.5	0.7	10.5	99	1.7
finger, country-fried, product 3714	1 piece	<1	0.05	0.05	0.86	0.04	8.6	0.35	0.0	3.1	0.6	3.1	52	0.7
finger, country-fried, product 3813	1 piece	13	0.08	0.06	1.10	0.07	9.4	0.39	0.0	8.3	0.8	7.0	72	1.2
finger, country-fried, product 3814	1 piece	<1	0.06	0.07	1.00	0.06	10.4	0.43	0.0	4.2	0.8	3.9	61	1.0
flame-broiled, product 9600	1 piece	99	0.14	0.15	2.70	0.26	6.1	1.70	1.6	31.2	2.1	27.4	268	4.6
flame-broiled, 'Two-Fers' product 9684.	1 piece	23	0.06	0.06	1.20	0.11	1.2	0.67	0.0	11.5	0.8	12.4	111	1.9
nugget, country-fried, product 1910	1 piece	<1	0.03	0.03	0.54	0.02	5.4	0.22	0.0	2.1	0.4	1.8	31	0.5
nugget, country-fried, product 1935	1 piece	16	0.04	0.04	0.56	0.04	6.1	0.25	0.0	5.5	0.5	3.8	39	0.6
nugget, country-fried, product 3811	1 piece	<1	0.04	0.04	0.64	0.03	6.4	0.27	0.0	2.6	0.5	2.4	37	0.6
patty, country-fried, product 1840.	1 piece	52	0.33	0.26	4.40	0.27	38.9	1.60	0.0	34.6	3.2	29.2	294	4.8
patty, country-fried, product 1845.	1 piece	98	0.26	0.24	3.40	0.21	36.5	1.50	0.0	33.1	2.7	22.9	235	3.7
patty, country-fried, product 3712	1 piece	29	0.27	0.24	4.10	0.22	38.1	1.50	0.0	25.1	2.9	21.8	263	3.9
patty, country-fried, product 3713	1 piece	32	0.29	0.27	4.50	0.24	41.4	1.70	0.0	27.3	3.2	24.0	288	4.3
patty, country-fried, product 3812.	1 piece	47	0.30	0.24	4.10	0.25	36.0	1.50	0.0	31.6	3.2	27.3	274	4.5
patty, flame-broiled, deluxe, product 9100.	1 piece	57	0.16	0.15	3.00	0.29	3.1	1.70	0.0	27.7	2.2	31.6	289	5.1
patty, flame-broiled, deluxe, product 9110.	1 piece	42	0.12	0.11	2.30	0.22	2.3	1.30	0.0	20.5	1.6	23.4	214	3.8
patty, flame-broiled, product 3771	1 piece	30	0.11	0.11	2.60	0.26	3.5	1.40	0.0	16.6	1.5	24.1	268	3.6

Food Name	Serving Size	A I.U.	Thi mg	Rib mg	Nia mg	B$_6$ mg	Fol mcg	B$_{12}$ mcg	C mg	Calc mg	Iron mg	Mag mg	Pot mg	Zn mg
patty, flame-broiled, product 3774	1 piece	42	0.15	0.16	3.60	0.36	4.8	2.00	0.0	21.9	2.1	33.3	371	5.0
patty, flame-broiled, product 3781	1 piece	31	0.11	0.12	2.60	0.27	3.5	1.40	0.0	16.7	1.5	24.3	270	3.7
patty, flame-broiled, w/onion, deluxe, product 9680	1 piece	93	0.26	0.25	5.00	0.49	7.7	3.00	1.1	52.0	3.7	52.0	490	8.2
patty, flame-broiled, w/onion, product 3879.	1 piece	46	0.14	0.14	2.80	0.27	4.4	1.60	0.5	24.4	2.1	28.1	272	4.8
patty, flame-broiled, w/onion, product 9675.	1 piece	46	0.14	0.14	2.70	0.26	4.4	1.60	0.5	25.2	2.0	27.4	265	4.6
patty, flame-broiled, w/onions, product 3779.	1 piece	30	0.11	0.11	2.50	0.26	4.4	1.40	0.5	17.0	1.5	23.7	270	3.5
patty, frozen, flame-broiled, product 3871.	1 piece	50	0.15	0.15	2.90	0.28	3.5	1.60	0.0	24.1	2.1	29.7	276	5.0
patty, frozen, flame-broiled, product 3874.	1 piece	69	0.20	0.20	4.00	0.38	4.8	2.20	0.0	33.3	2.9	40.9	380	6.8
patty, frozen, flame-broiled, product 3881.	1 piece	51	0.15	0.15	2.90	0.28	3.5	1.60	0.0	24.3	2.1	29.9	278	5.0
patty, frozen, flame-broiled, product 9220.	1 piece	63	0.16	0.11	2.40	0.24	1.8	1.30	0.0	28.8	1.7	28.8	234	4.0
patty, frozen, flame-broiled, product 9230.	1 piece	78	0.20	0.13	3.00	0.29	2.2	1.50	0.0	35.5	2.1	35.5	289	5.0
patty, jalapeño, flame-broiled, product 3778.	1 piece	118	0.10	0.11	2.50	0.26	3.5	1.40	2.0	16.7	1.5	22.9	262	3.5
patty, jalapeño, flame-broiled, product 3878.	1 piece	141	0.15	0.15	2.90	0.28	3.5	1.60	2.0	26.9	2.2	29.7	277	5.0
patty, less fat, flame-broiled, product 3772.	1 piece	52	0.15	0.12	2.90	0.29	2.8	1.50	0.0	24.1	1.8	31.2	300	4.3
patty, mesquite, flame-broiled, product 3770.	1 piece	30	0.11	0.11	2.60	0.26	3.5	1.40	0.0	16.6	1.5	24.1	268	3.6
patty, mesquite, flame-broiled, product 3773.	1 piece	52	0.15	0.12	2.90	0.29	2.8	1.50	0.0	24.9	1.7	31.2	300	4.3
patty, mesquite, flame-broiled, product 3780.	1 piece	31	0.11	0.11	2.60	0.27	3.5	1.40	0.0	16.7	1.5	24.3	270	3.7
patty, mesquite, flame-broiled, product 3870.	1 piece	50	0.15	0.15	2.90	0.28	3.5	1.60	0.0	24.8	2.1	29.7	276	5.0
patty, mesquite, flame-broiled, product 3880.	1 piece	51	0.15	0.15	2.90	0.28	3.5	1.60	0.0	25.0	2.1	29.9	278	5.0
patty, mesquite, flame-broiled, product 9103.	1 piece	57	0.16	0.12	2.90	0.29	3.1	1.50	0.0	27.7	1.8	31.6	295	4.3
patty, New York strip, flame-broiled, product 3777	1 piece	23	0.10	0.11	2.50	0.26	3.5	1.40	0.0	13.2	1.4	22.2	261	3.4
patty, New York strip, flame-broiled, product 3877	1 piece	42	0.14	0.15	2.80	0.27	3.5	1.60	0.0	21.4	2.0	27.6	265	4.8
Salisbury steak, flame-broiled, less fat, product 3721	1 piece	93	0.13	0.12	2.60	0.27	5.9	1.40	1.6	28.9	1.7	27.4	279	3.8
Salisbury steak, flame-broiled, product 3720.	1 piece	68	0.09	0.11	2.30	0.24	6.5	1.40	1.5	19.4	1.4	20.2	248	3.1
Salisbury steak, flame-broiled, product 3820.	1 piece	91	0.13	0.15	2.60	0.25	5.8	1.60	1.5	28.8	2.0	25.9	259	4.5
steak, country-fried, frozen, product 1610.	1 piece	1	0.21	0.23	3.80	0.16	37.8	1.50	0.0	15.1	2.7	13.0	217	3.4
steak, country-fried, frozen, product 3710.	1 piece	1	0.21	0.23	3.70	0.17	37.8	1.50	0.0	14.0	2.7	14.0	224	3.2
steak, country-fried, frozen, product 3810.	1 piece	2	0.25	0.28	4.30	0.23	43.2	1.80	0.0	17.3	3.2	16.2	252	4.2

Food Name	Serving Size	A I.U.	Thi mg	Rib mg	Nia mg	B6 mg	Fol mcg	B12 mcg	C mg	Calc mg	Iron mg	Mag mg	Pot mg	Zn mg
steak, flame-broiled, product 3760	1 piece	0	0.05	0.10	2.10	0.21	3.9	1.30	0.0	4.5	1.2	14.9	219	2.6
steak, flame-broiled, product 3765	1 piece	0	0.05	0.10	2.10	0.21	3.9	1.30	0.0	4.5	1.2	14.9	219	2.6
steak, frozen, flame-broiled, product 3860	1 piece	0	0.05	0.14	2.20	0.20	4.5	1.60	0.0	5.8	1.7	14.3	198	3.7
steak, frozen, flame-broiled, product 9010	1 piece	0	0.05	0.14	2.40	0.21	4.4	1.70	0.0	7.4	1.8	14.8	209	3.8
steak, frozen, flame-broiled, product 9017	1 piece	0	0.05	0.15	2.40	0.21	5.2	1.70	0.0	8.1	1.8	14.8	212	3.9
steak, frozen, flame-broiled, product 9503	1 piece	0	0.05	0.13	2.10	0.19	4.3	1.50	0.0	5.5	1.6	13.4	185	3.5
steak, mesquite, flame-broiled, product 3763	1 piece	0	0.05	0.10	2.20	0.22	4.0	1.40	0.0	5.4	1.2	14.7	224	2.7
steak, mesquite, frozen, flame-broiled, product 3863	1 piece	0	0.05	0.14	2.30	0.20	4.7	1.60	0.0	6.7	1.7	14.7	202	3.8
(Stouffer's)														
creamed chipped beef	1 pkg	0	na	na	na	na	na	na	na	473.0	2.3	na	na	na
creamed chipped beef	1 serving	0	na	na	na	na	na	na	na	190.0	0.9	na	na	na
Salisbury steak, w/gravy, macaroni and cheese, 'Homestyle'	1 pkg	0	na	na	na	na	na	na	na	196.0	2.3	na	na	na
Salisbury steak, w/gravy, macaroni and cheese, 'Homestyle'	1 serving	0	na	na	na	na	na	na	na	196.0	2.3	na	na	na
BEEF JERKY														
chopped and formed.	1 oz	0	0.04	0.04	0.49	0.05	38.0	0.28	0.0	5.7	1.5	14.5	169	2.3
cured, dried.	1 oz	0	0.02	0.06	1.50	0.10	3.1	0.75	0.0	1.7	1.3	9.1	126	1.5
BEEF STEW. See under BEEF DINNER/ENTRÉE.														
BEEF SUBSTITUTE														
(Morningstar Farms)														
ground beef substitute, vegetarian, 'Burger Style Recipe Crumbles'.	1 cup	0	9.90	0.35	3.00	0.54	na	4.40	0.0	79.2	6.4	2.2	178	1.6
BEEF SUBSTITUTE DINNER/ENTRÉE														
(Green Giant)														
burger, vegetable protein, vegetarian, original, 'Harvest Burger'	1 pkg	0	1.30	0.80	25.30	1.60	86.9	0.00	0.0	409.0	15.5	282.0	1738	32.5
burger, vegetable protein, vegetarian, original, 'Harvest Burger'	1 patty	0	0.32	0.20	6.30	0.39	21.6	0.00	0.0	102.0	3.9	70.2	432	8.1
(Morningstar Farms)														
burger, vegetarian, 'Better'N Burgers'.	1 pkg	0	12.3	26.6	198.00	9.50	11797.0	0.00	0.0	4164.0	139.0	776.0	20818	35.9
burger, vegetarian, 'Better'N Burgers'.	1 patty	0	0.26	0.55	4.10	0.20	246.0	0.00	0.0	86.7	2.9	16.1	434	0.8
burger, vegetarian, 'Garden Veggie Patties'.	1 pkg	36290	306.00	4.80	0.00	0.00	1365.0	0.00	0.0	2286.0	57.5	1397	8509	27.3
burger, vegetarian, 'Garden Veggie Patties'.	1 cup	2880	24.30	0.38	0.00	0.00	108.0	0.00	0.0	181.0	4.6	111.0	675	2.2
burger, vegetarian, 'Garden Veggie Patties'.	1 patty	766	6.50	0.10	0.00	0.00	28.8	0.00	0.0	48.2	1.2	29.5	180	0.6
burger, vegetarian, spicy black bean	1 pkg	7946	461.00	8.00	0.00	12.10	na	4.00	0.0	3214	105.0	2500.0	15401	53.1
burger, vegetarian, spicy black bean	1 patty	139	8.10	0.14	0.00	0.21	na	0.07	0.0	56.2	1.8	43.7	269	0.9
(Natural Touch)														
burger, vegetarian, 'Garden Veggie Patties'.	1 pkg	36290	306.00	4.80	0.00	0.00	na	0.00	0.0	2286.0	57.5	1397.0	8509	27.3
burger, vegetarian, 'Garden Veggie Patties'.	1 cup	2880	24.30	0.38	0.00	0.00	na	0.00	0.0	181.0	4.6	111.0	675	2.2
burger, vegetarian, 'Garden Veggie Patties'.	1 patty	766	6.50	0.10	0.00	0.00	na	0.00	0.0	48.2	1.2	29.5	180	0.6
burger, vegetarian, 'Vegan Burger'	1 patty	0	0.26	0.55	4.10	0.20	246.0	0.00	0.0	86.7	2.9	16.1	434	0.8

Food Name	Serving Size	A I.U.	Thi mg	Rib mg	Nia mg	B_6 mg	Fol mcg	B_12 mcg	C mg	Calc mg	Iron mg	Mag mg	Pot mg	Zn mg
burger, vegetarian, 'Vegan Burger'	1 pkg	0	12.30	26.6	198.00	9.50	11797.0	0.00	0.0	4164.0	139.0	776.0	20818	35.9
BEEF TALLOW	1 cup	0	0.00	0.00	0.00	0.00	0.0	0.00	0.0	0.0	0.0	0.0	<1	0.0
BEEFALO														
composite of cuts, raw	1 oz	0	0.01	0.03	1.30	na	4.3	0.69	2.0	5.1	0.7	na	124	1.4
composite of cuts, roasted	3 oz	0	0.03	0.09	4.20	na	15.3	2.20	7.7	20.4	2.6	na	390	5.4
BEER AND MALT LIQUOR														
beer, light	12 fl oz	0.0	0.03	0.11	1.40	0.12	14.5	0.04	0.0	17.7	0.1	17.7	64	0.1
beer, regular . . . . '. .	12 fl oz	0.0	0.02	0.09	1.60	0.18	21.4	0.07	0.0	17.8	0.1	21.4	89	<0.1
malt beverage	8 fl oz	5	0.04	0.11	2.60	0.06	33.2	0.05	1.2	11.8	0.1	16.6	19	<0.1
BEET														
Canned														
diced, drained	1 cup	17	0.02	0.06	0.25	0.09	47.4	0.00	6.4	23.6	2.9	26.7	232	0.3
Harvard, sliced, w/liquids	1 cup	27	0.03	0.12	0.21	0.14	71.3	0.00	5.9	27.1	0.9	46.7	403	0.6
no salt added, w/liquid	1 cup	64	0.03	0.09	0.37	0.14	71.3	0.00	6.9	32.0	1.6	39.4	349	0.6
pickled, sliced, w/liquid	1 cup	25	0.02	0.11	0.57	0.11	60.2	0.00	5.2	25.0	0.9	34.0	336	0.6
regular pack, w/liquid	1 cup	64	0.03	0.09	0.37	0.14	71.3	0.00	6.9	32.0	1.6	39.4	325	0.6
shredded, drained.	1 cup	21	0.02	0.08	0.31	0.11	58.9	0.00	8.0	29.3	3.5	33.1	289	0.4
sliced, drained	1 cup	19	0.02	0.07	0.27	0.10	51.3	0.00	7.0	25.5	3.1	28.9	252	0.4
sliced, drained	1 slice	1	0.00	0.00	0.01	0.01	2.4	0.00	0.3	1.2	0.2	1.4	12	<0.1
whole, drained	1 cup	18	0.02	0.07	0.26	0.09	49.2	0.00	6.7	24.4	3.0	27.7	241	0.3
whole, drained	1 medium	3	0.00	0.01	0.04	0.01	7.2	0.00	1.0	3.6	0.4	4.1	36	0.0
Fresh														
boiled, drained, sliced.	1/2 cup	30	0.02	0.03	0.28	0.06	68.0	0.00	3.1	13.6	0.7	19.6	259	0.3
boiled, drained, whole, 2-inch diam	2 beets	35	0.03	0.04	0.33	0.07	80.0	0.00	3.6	16.0	0.8	23.0	305	0.3
raw, sliced.	1 cup	52	0.04	0.05	0.45	0.09	148	0.00	6.7	21.8	1.1	31.3	442	0.5
raw, whole, 2-inch diam	1 beet	31	0.03	0.03	0.27	0.06	89.4	0.00	4.0	13.1	0.7	18.9	267	0.3
BEET GREENS														
boiled, drained, 1-inch pieces.	1 cup	7344	0.17	0.42	0.72	0:19	20.6	0.00	35.9	164.0	2.7	97.9	1309	0.7
boiled, drained, 1-inch pieces.	1/2 cup	3672	0.08	0.21	0.36	0.10	10.3	0.00	17.9	82.1	1.4	49.0	654	0.4
raw . . . . : . . .	1 cup	2318	0.04	0.08	0.15	0.04	5.6	0.00	11.4	45.2	1.3	27.4	208	0.1
raw	1 med leaf	1952	0.03	0.07	0.13	0.03	4.7	0.00	9.6	38.1	1.1	23.0	175	0.1
raw, 1-inch pieces.	1/2 cup	1159	0.02	0.04	0.08	0.02	2.8	0.00	5.7	22.6	0.6	13.7	104	<0.1
BELLYFISH. See MONKFISH.														
BERRIES. See individual listings.														
BISON / American buffalo														
raw	1 oz	0	na	0.03	0.54	na	na	na	0.0	1.7	0.7	7.1	97	0.8
ribeye, trimmed to 0-inch fat, raw	4 oz	3	0.05	0.10	2.10	0.28	na	2.50	0.0	6.8	3.2	27.1	389	3.6
ribeye, trimmed to 0-inch fat, raw	1 oz	1	0.01	0.03	0.52	0.07	na	0.62	0.0	1.7	0.8	6.8	98	0.9
roasted	3 oz	0	0.09	0.23	3.20	0.34	6.8	2.40	0.0	6.8	2.9	22.1	307	3.1
roasted, boneless, yield from 1 lb raw	11.9 oz	0	0.34	0.92	12.6	1.40	27.2	9.70	0.0	27.2	11.6	88.4	1227	12.5
shoulder, trimmed to 0-inch fat, raw	4 oz	2	0.05	0.11	2.10	0.25	na	2.50	0.0	4.5	3.4	27.1	364	5.7
shoulder, trimmed to 0-inch fat, raw	1 oz	1	0.01	0.03	0.53	0.06	na	0.62	0.0	1.1	0.9	6.8	91	1.4
top round, trimmed to 0-inch fat, raw	4 oz	3	0.05	0.10	2.20	0.32	na	2.10	0.0	5.7	3.3	28.3	390	4.0
top round, trimmed to 0-inch fat, raw	1 oz	1	0.01	0.03	0.57	0.07	na	0.65	0.0	1.4	0.9	6.8	95	1.0
BITTER GOURD. See BALSAM PEAR.														
BLACK BEAN. See BEAN, BLACK.														
BLACK CURRANT. See under CURRANT.														
BLACK PEPPER. See PEPPER, BLACK.														
BLACK TURTLE BEAN. See BEAN, BLACK.														
BLACKBERRY														
Canned, in heavy syrup, w/liquid	1 cup	561	0.07	0.10	0.73	0.09	67.8	0.00	7.2	53.8	1.7	43.5	253	0.5
Fresh, raw	1 cup	238	0.04	0.06	0.58	0.08	49.0	0.00	30.2	46.1	0.8	28.8	282	0.4
Frozen														
unsweetened	1 cup	172	0.04	0.07	1.80	0.09	51.3	0.00	4.7	43.8	1.2	33.2	211	0.4

Food Name	Serving Size	A I.U.	Thi mg	Rib mg	Nia mg	B$_6$ mg	Fol mcg	B$_{12}$ mcg	C mg	Calc mg	Iron mg	Mag mg	Pot mg	Zn mg
unsweetened	18-oz pkg	581	0.15	0.23	6.20	0.31	173.0	0.00	15.8	148.0	4.1	112.0	714	1.3
BLACK-EYED PEAS / cowpeas														
Canned														
Crowder, Southern, mature seeds, boiled, drained	1 cup	26	0.35	0.10	0.85	0.17	358.0	0.00	0.7	41.3	4.3	91.2	478	2.2
Crowder, Southern, mature seeds, w/pork	1 cup	0	0.15	0.12	1.00	0.11	122.0	0.00	0.5	40.8	3.4	103.0	427	2.5
Dried														
Catjang, mature seeds, boiled, drained	1 cup	17	0.28	0.08	1.20	0.16	242.0	0.00	0.7	44.5	5.2	164.0	641	3.2
Catjang, mature seeds, uncooked	1 cup	55	1.10	0.28	4.70	0.60	1067.0	0.00	2.5	142	16.6	556.0	2296	10.2
Crowder, Southern, mature seeds, uncooked	1 cup	84	1.40	0.38	3.50	0.60	1056.0	0.00	2.5	184	13.8	307.0	1857	5.6
Crowder, Southern, mature seeds, uncooked	1 tbsp	5	0.09	0.02	0.22	0.04	66.4	0.00	0.2	11.6	0.9	19.3	117	0.4
immature seeds, boiled, drained	1 cup	1305	0.17	0.24	2.30	0.11	210.0	0.00	3.6	211	1.8	85.8	690	1.7
immature seeds, uncooked	1 cup	1185	0.16	0.21	2.10	0.10	244.0	0.00	3.6	183	1.6	74.0	625	1.5
Fresh														
leafy tips, boiled, drained, chopped	1 cup	305	0.14	0.08	0.53	0.07	32.0	0.00	9.8	36.6	0.6	32.9	186	0.1
leafy tips, raw, chopped	1 cup	256	0.13	0.06	0.40	0.06	36.5	0.00	13.0	22.7	0.7	15.5	164	0.1
leafy tips, raw, whole	1 med leaf	21	0.01	0.01	0.03	0.01	3.0	0.00	1.1	1.9	0.1	1.3	14	<0.1
young pods w/seeds, boiled, drained	1 cup	1330	0.09	0.09	0.76	0.12	24.3	0.00	16.1	52.3	0.7	39.0	186	0.2
young pods w/seeds, raw, chopped	1 cup	1504	0.14	0.13	1.10	0.16	49.4	0.00	31.0	61.1	0.9	54.5	202	0.3
young pods w/seeds, raw, whole	1 med pod	192	0.02	0.02	0.14	0.02	6.3	0.00	4.0	7.8	0.1	7.0	26	0.0
Frozen														
immature seeds, drained	1 cup	128	0.44	0.11	1.20	0.16	240.0	0.00	4.4	39.1	3.6	85.0	638	2.4
immature seeds, unprepared	10-oz pkg	239	0.70	0.20	2.30	0.30	531.0	0.00	11.4	73.8	6.7	156.0	1252	4.5
immature seeds, unprepared	1 cup	134	0.39	0.11	1.30	0.17	299.0	0.00	6.4	41.6	3.8	88.0	706	2.5
BLUE CRAB. See under CRAB.														
BLUEBERRIES														
Canned														
in heavy syrup, w/liquids	1 cup	164	0.09	0.14	0.29	0.09	4.1	0.00	2.8	12.8	0.8	10.2	102	0.2
Fresh														
raw	1 pint	402	0.19	0.20	1.40	0.14	25.7	0.00	52.3	24.1	0.7	20.1	358	0.4
raw	50 berries	68	0.03	0.03	0.24	0.02	4.4	0.00	8.8	4.1	0.1	3.4	61	<0.1
Frozen														
unthawed	1 cup	145	0.07	0.07	0.52	0.05	9.3	0.00	18.9	8.7	0.3	7.3	129	0.2
sweetened	10-oz pkg	125	0.06	0.15	0.72	0.17	19.0	0.00	2.8	17.0	1.1	5.7	170	0.2
sweetened, thawed	1 cup	101	0.05	0.12	0.58	0.14	15.4	0.00	2.3	13.8	0.9	4.6	138	0.1
unsweetened	20-oz pkg	459	0.18	0.21	2.90	0.34	38.0	0.00	14.2	45.4	1.0	28.4	306	0.4
unsweetened, unthawed	1 cup	126	0.05	0.06	0.81	0.09	10.4	0.00	3.9	12.4	0.3	7.8	84	0.1
BLUEFIN TUNA. See under TUNA.														
BLUEFISH														
baked, broiled, grilled, or microwaved	3 oz	390	0.06	0.08	6.20	0.39	1.7	5.30	0.0	7.7	0.5	35.7	405	0.9
raw	3 oz	338	0.05	0.07	5.10	0.34	1.4	4.60	0.0	6.0	0.4	28.1	316	0.7
BOAR, WILD														
raw	1 oz	0	0.11	0.03	1.10	na	na	na	0.0	3.4	na	na	na	na
roasted	3 oz	0	0.26	0.12	3.60	0.35	5.1	0.59	0.0	13.6	1.0	22.9	337	2.6
roasted, boneless, yield from 1 lb raw	11.9 oz	0	1.10	0.48	14.30	1.40	20.4	2.40	0.0	54.4	3.8	91.8	1346	10.2
BOBWHITE. See QUAIL.														
BOK CHOY / Chinese cabbage / napa cabbage / pak-choi / pe-tsai														
boiled, drained	1 med leaf	135	0.01	0.01	0.07	0.03	7.5	0.00	2.2	4.5	<0.1	1.4	32	<0.1
boiled, drained, shredded	1 cup	4366	0.05	0.11	0.73	0.28	69.0	0.00	44.2	158.0	1.8	18.7	631	0.3
raw, head, whole	1 medium	25200	0.34	0.59	4.20	1.60	552	0.00	378.0	882.0	6.7	160.0	2117	1.6
raw, leaf, whole	1 medium	420	0.01	0.01	0.07	0.03	9.2	0.00	6.3	14.7	0.1	2.7	35.3	<0.1

Food Name	Serving Size	A I.U.	Thi mg	Rib mg	Nia mg	B₆ mg	Fol mcg	B₁₂ mcg	C mg	Calc mg	Iron mg	Mag mg	Pot mg	Zn mg
raw, shredded	1 cup	2100	0.03	0.05	0.35	0.14	46.0	0.00	31.5	73.5	0.6	13.3	176	0.1
BONITO, OCEANIC. See under TUNA.														
BORAGE, fresh, raw, 1-inch pieces	1 cup	3738	0.05	0.13	0.80	0.08	11.7	0.00	31.1	82.8	2.9	46.3	418	0.2
BORECOLE. See KALE.														
BORLOTTI. See BEAN, CRANBERRY.														
BOTTLE GOURD. See GOURD, BOTTLE.														
BOYSENBERRIES														
Canned, in heavy syrup . . . . . :	1 cup	102	0.07	0.07	0.59	0.10	88.1	0.00	15.9	46.1	1.1	28.2	230	0.5
Frozen														
unsweetened	1 cup	88	0.07	0.05	1.00	0.07	83.6	0.00	4.1	35.6	1.1	21.1	183	0.3
unsweetened	10-oz pkg	190	0.15	0.11	2.20	0.16	180.0	0.00	8.8	76.7	2.4	45.4	395	0.6
BRAMBLE. See RASPBERRY.														
BRATWURST. See under SAUSAGE.														
BRAZIL NUT / paranut														
BRAZIL NUT, DRIED														
dried, unblanched, approx 6–8 kernels	1 oz	0	0.28	0.04	0.46	0.07	1.1	0.00	0.2	49.9	1.0	63.8	170	1.3
dried, unblanched, shelled, approx														
32 kernels	1 cup	0	1.40	0.17	2.30	0.35	5.6	0.00	1.0	246.0	4.8	315.0	840	6.4
BREAD														
BROWN														
canned	1 slice	39	0.01	0.05	0.50	0.04	5.0	0.01	0.0	31.5	0.9	28.4	143	0.2
canned . . . . : .	1 oz	25	0.00	0.03	0.32	0.02	3.1	0.00	0.0	19.8	0.6	17.9	90	0.1
EGG, 5x3x1/2-inch slices	1 slice	30	0.17	0.17	1.90	0.03	42.0	0.04	0.0	37.2	1.2	7.6	46	0.3
FRENCH														
large slices, approx 5 x 2-1/2 x 1 inch	1 slice	0	0.18	0.12	1.70	0.02	33.3	0.00	0.0	26.3	0.9	9.4	40	0.3
medium slices, approx 4-3/4 x 4 x 1/2 inch . . .	0	.0.13	0.08	1.20	0.01	23.8	0.00	0.0	18.8	0.6	6.8	28	0.2	
small slices, approx 2-1/2 x 2 x 1/2 inch	1 slice	0	0.08	0.05	0.71	0.01	14.3	0.00	0.0	11.3	0.4	4.0	17	0.1
INDIAN FRY														
Navajo, 10.5-inch diam	1 serving	0	0.69	0.49	5.80	0.04	118.0	0.00	0.0	373.0	5.8	25.6	118	0.8
Navajo, 5-inch diam	1 serving	0	0.39	0.27	3.30	0.02	66.6	0.00	0.0	210.0	3.2	14.4	67	0.5
ITALIAN														
large slices, approx 4-1/2 x 3-1/4 x 3/4														
inch	1 slice	0	0.14	0.09	1.30	0.01	28.5	0.00	0.0	23.4	0.9	8.1	33	0.3
medium slices	1 slice	0	0.10	0.06	0.88	0.01	19.0	0.00	0.0	15.6	0.6	5.4	22	0.2
small slices, approx 3-1/4 x 2-1/2 x														
1/2 inch	1 slice	0	0.05	0.03	0.44	0.01	9.5	0.00	0.0	7.8	0.3	2.7	11	<0.1
MIXED GRAIN														
7-grain, w/whole grain, large slices	1 slice	0	0.13	0.11	1.40	0.11	25.6	0.02	0.1	29.1	1.1	17.0	65	0.4
7-grain, w/whole-grain, medium slices	1 slice	0	0.11	0.09	1.10	0.09	20.8	0.02	0.1	23.7	0.9	13.8	53	0.3
OAT BRAN														
. . . .	1 slice	2	0.15	0.10	1.40	0.02	24.3	0.00	0.0	19.5	0.9	10.5	44	0.3
lower calorie	1 slice	<1	0.08	0.05	0.86	0.02	15.2	0.00	0.0	13.1	0.7	12.7	24	0.2
OATMEAL														
. . . .	1 slice	4	0.11	0.07	0.85	0.02	16.7	0.01	0.0	17.8	0.7	10.0	38	0.3
lower calorie	1 slice	1	0.08	0.06	0.70	0.01	12.7	0.02	0.1	26.4	0.5	5.5	29	0.2
PITA														
white, enriched, large, 6.5-inch diam	1 pita	0	0.36	0.20	2.80	0.02	57.0	0.00	0.0	51.6	1.6	15.6	72	0.5
white, enriched, small, 4-inch diam	1 pita	0	0.17	0.09	1.30	0.01	26.6	0.00	0.0	24.1	0.7	7.3	34	0.2
white, unenriched, large, 6.5-inch diam	1 pita	0	0.16	0.06	1.30	0.02	14.4	0.00	0.0	51.6	0.8	15.6	72	0.5
PROTEIN, w/gluten	1 slice	<1	0.07	0.08	0.81	0.01	19.6	0.00	0.0	23.6	0.8	12.3	61	0.4
PUMPERNICKEL														
regular slices	1 slice	0	0.09	0.08	0.80	0.03	20.8	0.00	0.0	17.7	0.8	14.0	54	0.4
snack size	1 slice	0	0.02	0.02	0.22	0.01	5.6	0.00	0.0	4.8	0.2	3.8	15	0.1
thick slices, approx 5x4x3/8 inch	1 slice	0	0.11	0.10	0.99	0.04	25.6	0.00	0.0	21.8	0.9	17.3	67	0.5

Food Name	Serving Size	A I.U.	Thi mg	Rib mg	Nia mg	B6 mg	Fol mcg	B12 mcg	C mg	Calc mg	Iron mg	Mag mg	Pot mg	Zn mg
thin slices	1 slice	0	0.07	0.06	0.62	0.03	16.0	0.00	0.0	13.6	0.6	10.8	42	0.3
RAISIN														
enriched, large slices	1 slice	0	0.11	0.13	1.10	0.02	27.8	0.00	<0.1	21.1	0.9	8.3	73	0.2
enriched, medium slices	1 slice	0	0.09	0.10	0.90	0.02	22.6	0.00	<0.1	17.2	0.8	6.8	59	0.2
enriched, thin slices	1 slice	0	0.08	0.09	0.80	0.02	20.0	0.00	<0.1	15.2	0.7	6.0	52	0.2
unenriched, large slices	1 slice	0	0.06	0.06	0.48	0.02	10.9	0.00	<0.1	21.1	0.6	8.3	73	0.2
unenriched, medium slices	1 slice	0	0.05	0.05	0.39	0.02	8.8	0.00	<0.1	17.2	0.5	6.8	59	0.2
unenriched, thin slices	1 slice	0	0.04	0.04	0.34	0.02	7.8	0.00	<0.1	15.2	0.4	6.0	52	0.2
RICE BRAN	1 slice	1	0.18	0.08	1.80	0.07	17.6	0.00	0.0	18.6	1.0	21.6	58	0.4
RYE														
lower calorie, medium slices	1 slice	1	0.08	0.06	0.58	0.02	11.0	0.01	0.1	17.5	0.7	5.1	23	0.2
lower calorie, thick slices	1 slice	1	0.12	0.08	0.81	0.03	15.4	0.01	0.1	24.3	1.0	7.0	31	0.2
lower calorie, thin slices	1 slice	1	0.07	0.05	0.51	0.02	9.6	0.01	0.1	15.2	0.6	4.4	20	0.1
regular, medium slices	1 slice	2	0.14	0.11	1.20	0.02	27.5	0.00	0.1	23.4	0.9	12.8	53	0.4
regular, snack size	1 slice	<1	0.03	0.02	0.27	0.01	6.0	0.00	<0.1	5.1	0.2	2.8	12	<0.1
regular, thin slices	1 slice	1	0.09	0.07	0.76	0.02	17.2	0.00	0.1	14.6	0.6	8.0	33	0.2
WHEAT														
	1 slice	0	0.11	0.07	1.00	0.02	19.3	0.00	0.0	26.3	0.8	11.5	50	0.3
cracked wheat, large or thick sliced	1 slice	0	0.11	0.07	1.10	0.09	18.3	0.01	0.0	12.9	0.8	15.6	53	0.2
cracked wheat, regular	1 slice	0	0.09	0.06	0.92	0.08	15.3	0.01	0.0	10.8	0.7	13.0	44	0.3
cracked wheat, regular, crust removed	1 slice	0	0.04	0.03	0.45	0.04	7.4	0.00	0.0	5.2	0.3	6.3	22	0.2
cracked wheat, thin sliced	1 slice	0	0.07	0.05	0.73	0.06	12.2	0.00	0.0	8.6	0.6	10.4	35	0.3
cracked wheat, thin sliced, crust removed	1 slice	0	0.03	0.02	0.34	0.03	5.7	0.00	0.0	4.0	0.3	4.9	17	0.1
lower calorie	1 slice	0	0.10	0.07	0.89	0.03	16.3	0.00	<0.1	18.4	0.7	9.0	28	0.3
WHEAT BERRY														
	1 slice	0	0.11	0.07	1.00	0.02	19.3	0.00	0.0	26.3	0.8	11.5	50	0.3
lower calorie	1 slice	0	0.10	0.07	0.89	0.03	16.3	0.00	<0.1	18.4	0.7	9.0	28	0.3
WHEAT BRAN	1 slice	0	0.14	0.10	1.60	0.06	24.8	0.00	0.0	26.6	1.1	29.2	82	0.5
WHEAT GERM	1 slice	<1	0.10	0.11	1.30	0.02	26.3	0.02	0.1	24.9	1.0	7.8	71	0.3
WHITE														
lower calorie, medium slices	1 slice	1	0.09	0.07	0.84	0.01	21.9	0.06	0.1	21.6	0.7	5.3	18	0.3
low-salt, medium slices	1 slice	0	0.12	0.09	0.99	0.02	23.8	0.01	0.0	27.0	0.8	6.0	30	0.2
low-salt, thick slices	1 slice	0	0.14	0.10	1.20	0.02	28.5	0.01	0.0	32.4	0.9	7.2	36	0.2
low-salt, thin slices	1 slice	0	0.09	0.07	0.79	0.01	19.0	0.01	0.0	21.6	0.6	4.8	24	0.1
regular, medium slices	1 slice	0	0.12	0.09	0.99	0.02	23.8	0.01	0.0	27.0	0.8	6.0	30	0.1
regular, medium slices, crust removed	1 slice	0	0.06	0.04	0.48	0.01	11.4	0.00	0.0	13.0	0.4	2.9	14	<0.1
regular, thick slices	1 slice	0	0.14	0.10	1.20	0.02	28.5	0.01	0.0	32.4	0.9	7.2	36	0.2
regular, thin slices	1 slice	0	0.09	0.07	0.79	0.01	19.0	0.01	0.0	21.6	0.6	4.8	24	0.1
regular, very thin slices	1 slice	0	0.07	0.05	0.59	0.01	14.3	0.01	0.0	16.2	0.5	3.6	18	<0.1
WHOLE WHEAT	1 slice	0	0.10	0.06	1.10	0.05	14.0	0.00	0.0	20.2	0.9	24.1	71	0.5
BREAD, QUICK														
BANANA, made w/margarine	1 oz	132	0.05	0.06	0.41	0.04	9.4	0.03	0.5	6.0	0.4	4.0	38	0.1
CORNBREAD, made w/2% milk	1 oz	79	0.08	0.08	0.64	0.03	18.1	0.04	0.1	70.6	0.7	7.1	42	0.2
IRISH SODA, 3.75x3x1/2-inch slices	1 slice	116	0.18	0.16	1.40	0.05	28.2	0.03	0.5	48.6	1.6	13.8	160	0.3
BREAD, QUICK, MIX														
BANANA *(Keebler Elfin Loaf)* prepared w/margarine	1 loaf	264	0.10	0.11	0.82	0.09	18.8	0.06	1.0	12.0	0.8	8.0	76	0.2
CORNBREAD														
unenriched	1 oz	33	0.01	0.01	0.27	0.04	3.1	0.03	<0.1	16.2	0.2	6.8	32	0.2
enriched	1 oz	33	0.12	0.08	0.95	0.04	29.8	0.03	<0.1	16.2	0.7	6.8	32	0.2
unenriched, prepared	1 oz	58	0.07	0.08	0.58	0.03	15.6	0.05	<0.1	20.7	0.5	5.7	36	0.2
BREAD CRUMBS														
plain, dry, grated	1 cup	1	0.83	0.47	7.40	0.11	118.0	0.02	0.0	245.0	6.6	49.7	239	1.3

Food Name	Serving Size	A I.U.	Thi mg	Rib mg	Nia mg	B₆ mg	Fol mcg	B₁₂ mcg	C mg	Calc mg	Iron mg	Mag mg	Pot mg	Zn mg
plain, dry, grated	1 oz	<1	0.22	0.12	1.90	0.03	30.9	0.01	0.0	64.4	1.7	13.0	63	0.4
seasoned, dry, grated	1 cup	16	0.19	0.20	3.30	0.18	131.0	0.05	0.5	119.0	3.8	45.6	324	1.1
seasoned, dry, grated	1 oz	4	0.05	0.05	0.77	0.04	30.9	0.01	0.1	28.1	0.9	10.8	77	0.3
BREADFRUIT, RAW														
Fresh, raw, whole, small fruit	1/4 fruit	38	0.11	0.03	0.86	0.10	13.4	0.00	27.8	16.3	0.5	24.0	470	0.1
Frozen, unthawed	1 cup	88	0.24	0.07	2.00	0.22	30.8	0.00	63.8	37.4	1.2	55.0	1078	0.3
BREADFRUIT SEEDS														
boiled	1 oz	68	0.08	0.05	1.50	0.08	13.9	0.00	1.7	17.3	0.2	14.2	248	0.2
raw	1 oz	73	0.14	0.09	0.12	0.09	15.0	0.00	1.9	10.2	1.0	15.3	267	0.3
roasted	1 oz	83	0.12	0.07	2.10	0.12	16.8	0.00	2.2	24.4	0.3	17.6	307	0.3
BREADNUT TREE SEEDS														
dried	1 cup	346	0.05	0.22	3.40	1.10	181.0	0.00	74.6	150.0	7.4	184.0	3228	3.1
dried	1 oz	61	0.01	0.04	0.59	0.19	32.0	0.00	13.2	26.6	1.3	32.6	570	0.5
raw, 8–14 seeds	1 oz	70	0.02	0.02	0.25	0.11	18.8	0.00	7.8	27.8	0.6	19.3	335	0.3
BREADSTICKS														
plain, pieces	1 cup	0	0.27	0.25	2.40	0.03	56.1	0.00	0.0	10.1	2.0	14.7	57	0.4
plain, 7-5/8 x 5/8 inch	1 breadstick	0	0.06	0.06	0.53	0.01	12.2	0.00	0.0	2.2	0.4	3.2	12	<0.1
plain, 9-1/4 x 3/8 inch	1 breadstick	0	0.04	0.03	0.32	0.00	7.3	0.00	0.0	1.3	0.3	1.9	7	<0.1
plain, small, 4.25-inch long	1 breadstick	0	0.03	0.03	0.26	0.00	6.1	0.00	0.0	1.1	0.2	1.6	6	<0.1
BREAKFAST DRINK MIX														
(Carnation)														
regular, prepared w/8 fl oz 2% milk	9 oz	2250	0.40	0.50	5.20	0.50	92.0	1.50	30.0	550.0	4.6	110.0	627	4.0
sugarless, prepared w/8 fl oz 2% milk	9 oz	2250	0.40	0.50	5.20	0.50	92.0	1.50	30.0	550.0	4.6	110.0	627	4.0
BREAKFAST SANDWICH														
(Pierre)														
ham and cheese, wrapped, 'Ham n Go'														
product 1295	1 piece	386	0.00	0.02	0.01	0.00	40.5	0.05	0.0	68.1	1.3	1.8	8	0.2
ham, w/cheese, 'Ham-n-Go'														
product 1293	1 piece	323	na	na	na	na	40.9	na	0.0	30.4	1.5	na	1.0	na
wrapped, 'Link-N-Dog'														
'Dine'n w/Pierre'	1 piece	34	0.07	0.07	1.40	0.13	31.9	0.80	0.2	31.9	1.6	13.5	134	2.3
wrapped, 'Saus-A-Rage'														
'Dine'n w/Pierre'	1 piece	354	0.07	0.07	1.40	0.13	42.7	0.79	0.1	40.9	1.8	13.3	134	2.3
(Sunny Fresh)														
egg and cheese biscuit, precooked,														
frozen	1 pkg	24647	28.5	36.60	243.00	4.40	na	32.10	0.0	12145.0	270.0	357.0	4763	35.7
egg and cheese biscuit, precooked, .0														
frozen	1 serving	205	0.24	0.30	2.00	0.04	na	0.27	0.0	101.0	2.3	3.0	40	0.3
egg and cheese pocket sandwich, pre-														
cooked, frozen, 'Breakfast Stuff-Its'	1 pkg	26331	14.5	23.70	175.00	3.40	na	25.30	0.0	7501.0	113.0	306.0	3674	27.6
egg and cheese pocket sandwich,														
pre-cooked, frozen, 'Breakfast Stuff-Its'	1 serving	219	0.12	0.20	1.50	0.03	na	0.21	0.0	62.5	0.94	2.6	31	0.2
ham, w/cheese, precooked, frozen	1 pkg	25592	28.6	37.60	243.00	4.60	na	34.70	14.5	12723.0	294.0	434.0	5639	39.0
ham, w/cheese, precooked, frozen	1 serving	213	0.24	0.31	2.00	0.04	na	0.29	0.1	106	2.4	3.6	47	0.3
BREAKFAST STRIP. See under BACON SUBSTITUTE.														
BROAD BEAN. See BEAN, FAVA.														
BROCCOLI														
Fresh														
boiled, drained, chopped	1/2 cup	1083	0.04	0.09	0.45	0.11	39.0	0.00	58.2	35.9	0.7	18.7	228	0.3
boiled, drained, spears, large, 11-12														
inches long	1 spear	3886	0.15	0.32	1.60	0.40	140.0	0.00	209.0	129.0	2.4	67.2	818	1.0
boiled, drained, spears, medium,														
7.5-8 inches long	1 spear	2498	0.10	0.20	1.00	0.26	90.0	0.00	134.0	82.8	1.5	43.2	526	0.7

Food Name	Serving Size	A I.U.	Thi mg	Rib mg	Nia mg	B6 mg	Fol mcg	B12 mcg	C mg	Calc mg	Iron mg	Mag mg	Pot mg	Zn mg
boiled, drained, spears, small, 5 inches														
long	1 spear	1943	0.08	0.16	0.80	0.20	70.0	0.00	104.0	64.4	1.2	33.6	409	0.5
raw, bunch	1 medium	9375	0.40	0.72	3.90	0.97	432	0.00	567.0	292.0	5.3	152.0	1976	2.4
raw, chopped	1 cup	1357	0.06	0.11	0.56	0.14	62.5	0.00	82.0	42.2	0.8	22.0	286	0.4
raw, chopped or diced	1/2 cup	678	0.03	0.05	0.28	0.07	31.2	0.00	41.0	21.1	0.4	11.0	143	0.2
raw, florets	1 cup	2130	0.05	0.08	0.45	0.11	50.4	0.00	66.2	34.1	0.6	17.8	231	0.3
raw, florets	1 medium	330	0.01	0.01	0.07	0.02	7.8	0.00	10.3	5.3	0.1	2.8	36	<0.1
raw, spears, medium, 7-5/8 inches long	1 spear	2328	0.10	0.18	0.96	0.24	107.0	0.00	141.0	72.5	1.3	37.8	491	0.6
raw, spears, small, 5 inches long, raw	1 spear	478	0.02	0.04	0.20	0.05	22.0	0.00	28.9	14.9	0.3	7.8	101	0.1
Frozen														
chopped, no salt added, drained	1 cup	3481	0.10	0.15	0.84	0.24	104.0	0.00	73.8	93.8	1.1	36.8	331	0.5
chopped, unprepared	1 cup	3223	0.08	0.15	0.73	0.20	105.0	0.00	88.0	87.4	1.3	28.1	331	0.7
chopped, unprepared	10-oz pkg	5867	0.15	0.27	1.30	0.37	190.0	0.00	160.0	159.0	2.3	51.1	602	1.4
chopped, drained	1 cup	3481	0.10	0.15	0.84	0.24	104.0	0.00	73.8	93.8	1.1	36.8	331	0.6
spears, no salt added, drained	1/2 cup	1741	0.05	0.08	0.42	0.12	27.6	0.00	36.9	46.9	0.6	18.4	166	0.3
spears, no salt added, drained	10-oz pkg	4730	0.14	0.20	1.10	0.33	75.0	0.00	100.0	128.0	1.5	50.0	450	0.8
unprepared	10-oz pkg	4058	0.20	0.32	1.30	0.50	268.0	0.00	194.0	116.0	2.0	45.4	710	1.0
unprepared	2-lb pkg	12961	0.65	1.00	4.20	1.60	855.0	0.00	619.0	372.0	6.5	145.0	2268	3.1
drained	1/2 cup	1741	0.05	0.08	0.42	0.12	27.6	0.00	36.9	46.9	0.6	18.4	166	0.3
drained	10-oz pkg	4730	0.14	0.20	1.10	0.33	75.0	0.00	100.0	128.0	1.5	50.0	450	0.8
BROCCOLI, CHINESE, cooked	1 cup	1441	0.08	0.13	0.39	0.06	87.1	0.00	24.8	88.0	0.5	15.8	230	0.3
BROTH. See under SOUP.														
BROWN RICE. See under RICE.														
BROWNIE. See under CAKE, SNACK.														
BROWN RICE FLOUR. See under FLOUR.														
BRUSSELS SPROUTS														
Fresh														
boiled, drained	1/2 cup	561	0.08	0.06	0.47	0.14	46.8	0.00	48.4	28.1	0.9	15.6	247	0.3
boiled, drained, whole	1 medium	151	0.02	0.02	0.13	0.04	12.6	0.00	13.0	7.6	0.3	4.2	67	<0.1
raw	1 cup	777	0.12	0.08	0.66	0.19	53.8	0.00	74.8	37.0	1.2	20.2	342	0.4
raw	1 medium	168	0.03	0.02	0.14	0.04	11.6	0.00	16.1	8.0	0.3	4.4	74	<0.1
Frozen														
drained	1 cup	913	0.16	0.17	0.83	0.45	157.0	0.00	70.8	37.2	1.1	37.2	504	0.6
no salt added, drained	1 cup	913	0.16	0.17	0.83	0.45	157.0	0.00	70.8	37.2	1.1	37.2	504	0.6
unprepared	2-lb pkg	7392	0.95	1.10	5.80	1.80	1119.0	0.00	672.0	236	8.4	181.0	3356	2.8
unprepared	10-oz pkg	2315	0.30	0.35	1.80	0.57	350.0	0.00	210.0	73.8	2.6	56.8	1051	0.9
BUCKWHEAT	1 cup	0	0.17	0.72	11.90	0.36	51.0	0.00	0.0	30.6	3.7	393.0	782	4.1
BUCKWHEAT FLOUR. See under FLOUR.														
BUCKWHEAT GROATS, ROASTED / kasha														
cooked	1 cup	0	0.07	0.07	1.60	0.13	23.5	0.00	0.0	11.8	1.3	85.7	148	1.0
dry	1 cup	0	0.37	0.44	8.40	0.58	68.9	0.00	0.0	27.9	4.1	362.0	525	4.0
BUFFALO, AMERICAN. See BISON.														
BULGUR														
cooked	1 cup	0	0.10	0.05	1.80	0.15	32.8	0.00	0.0	18.2	1.7	58.2	124	1.0
cooked	1 tbsp	0	0.01	0.00	0.08	0.01	1.5	0.00	0.0	0.84	0.1	2.7	6	<0.1
dry	1 cup	0	0.33	0.16	7.20	0.48	37.8	0.00	0.0	49.0	3.4	230.0	574	2.7
BUN. See BUN, FRANKFURTER; BUN, HAMBURGER; BUN, SWEET; ENGLISH MUFFIN; ROLL.														
BUN, FRANKFURTER														
foot-long, brown-and-serve	1 bun	0	0.42	0.27	3.50	0.05	81.7	0.05	0.1	102.0	2.7	19.8	114	0.7
lower calorie	1 bun	<1	0.17	0.08	2.10	0.02	40.9	0.04	0.1	25.4	1.3	8.6	34	0.3
lower calorie	1 oz	<1	0.11	0.05	1.40	0.01	26.9	0.03	0.1	16.7	0.9	5.7	22	0.2
mixed grain	1 bun	<1	0.20	0.13	1.90	0.04	40.9	0.00	0.0	40.9	1.7	18.9	69	0.5
mixed grain	1 oz	<1	0.13	0.09	1.30	0.03	26.9	0.00	0.0	26.9	1.1	12.5	45	0.3
plain	1 bun	0	0.21	0.13	1.70	0.02	40.9	0.03	<0.1	59.8	1.4	8.6	61	0.3

Food Name	Serving Size	A I.U.	Thi mg	Rib mg	Nia mg	B$_6$ mg	Fol mcg	B$_{12}$ mcg	C mg	Calc mg	Iron mg	Mag mg	Pot mg	Zn mg
plain	1 oz	0	0.14	0.09	1.10	0.01	26.9	0.02	<0.1	39.4	0.9	5.7	40	0.2
BUN, HAMBURGER														
lower calorie	1 bun	<1	0.17	0.08	2.10	0.02	40.9	0.04	0.1	25.4	1.3	8.6	34	0.3
lower calorie	1 oz	<1	0.11	0.05	1.40	0.01	26.9	0.03	0.1	16.7	0.9	5.7	22	0.2
mixed grain	1 bun	<1	0.20	0.13	1.90	0.04	40.9	0.00	0	40.9	1.7	18.9	69	0.5
mixed grain	1 oz	<1	0.13	0.09	1.30	0.03	26.9	0.00	0	26.9	1.1	12.5	45	0.3
plain	1 bun	0	0.21	0.13	1.70	0.02	40.9	0.03	<0.1	59.8	1.4	8.6	61	0.3
plain	1 oz	0	0.14	0.09	1.10	0.01	26.9	0.02	<0.1	39.4	0.9	5.7	40	0.2
BUN, SWEET. See also PASTRY.														
HONEYBUN														
glazed, yeast-leavened, 4x3-inch oval	1 bun	9	0.24	0.14	1.90	0.04	27.9	0.06	0.1	27.9	1.3	14.3	70	0.5
glazed, yeast-leavened, 4.5x3.5-inch oval	1 bun	11	0.28	0.17	2.20	0.04	33.5	0.07	0.1	33.5	1.6	17.2	84	0.6
glazed, yeast-leavened, 5x3.5-inch oval	1 bun	12	0.31	0.18	2.40	0.05	36.5	0.08	0.1	36.5	1.7	18.7	92	0.7
BURBOT														
baked, broiled, grilled, or microwaved	3 oz	14	0.36	0.15	1.70	0.29	0.9	0.78	0.0	54.4	1.0	34.9	440	0.8
raw	3 oz	13	0.32	0.12	1.40	0.26	0.9	0.68	0.0	42.5	0.8	27.2	343	0.7
BURDOCK ROOT / gobo														
boiled, drained, sliced, 1-inch pieces	1 cup	0	0.05	0.07	0.40	0.35	24.4	0.00	3.3	61.3	1.0	48.8	450	0.5
boiled, drained, whole	1 med root	0	0.07	0.10	0.53	0.46	32.4	0.00	4.3	81.3	1.3	64.7	598	0.6
raw, sliced, 1-inch pieces	1 cup	0	0.01	0.04	0.35	0.28	26.9	0.00	3.5	48.4	0.9	44.8	363	0.4
raw, whole	1 med root	0	0.02	0.05	0.47	0.37	35.6	0.00	4.7	64.0	1.2	59.3	480	0.5
BURGER. See under BEEF DINNER/ENTRÉE; BEEF SUBSTITUTE DINNER/ENTRÉE; and individual ground meat listings.														
BUSH NUT. See MACADAMIA NUT.														
BUTTER														
salted	1 cup	6942	0.01	0.08	0.10	0.01	6.8	0.28	0.0	54.5	0.4	4.5	59	0.1
salted	1 stick	3468	0.01	0.04	0.05	0.00	3.4	0.14	0.0	27.2	0.2	2.3	30	<0.1
salted	1 tbsp	434	0.00	0.01	0.01	0.00	0.4	0.02	0.0	3.4	<0.1	0.4	4	<0.1
salted, 1-inch square, 1/3-inch high	1 pat	153	0.00	0.00	0.00	0.00	0.2	0.01	0.0	1.2	<0.1	0.1	1	0.0
unsalted	1 cup	6942	0.01	0.08	0.10	0.01	6.4	0.29	0.0	53.3	0.4	4.5	59	0.1
unsalted	1 stick	3468	0.01	0.04	0.05	0.00	3.2	0.15	0.0	26.6	0.2	2.3	30	<0.1
unsalted	1 tbsp	434	0.00	0.01	0.01	0.00	0.4	0.02	0.0	3.3	<0.1	0.4	4	<0.1
unsalted, 1-inch square, 1/3-inch high	1 pat	153	0.00	0.00	0.00	0.00	0.1	0.01	0.0	1.2	<0.1	0.1	1	0.0
whipped, salted	1 cup	4618	0.01	0.05	0.06	0.01	4.2	0.19	0.0	35.5	0.2	3.3	39	<0.1
whipped, salted	1 stick	2312	0.00	0.03	0.03	0.00	2.1	0.09	0.0	17.8	0.1	1.6	20	<0.1
whipped, salted	1 tbsp	287	0.00	0.00	0.00	0.00	0.3	0.01	0.0	2.2	<0.1	0.2	2	<0.1
whipped, salted, 1-inch square, 1/3-inch high	1 pat	116	0.00	0.00	0.00	0.00	0.1	0.01	0.0	0.9	<0.1	0.1	1.0	0.0
BUTTER OIL														
anhydrous	1 cup	7688	0.00	0.01	0.01	0.00	0.4	0.03	0.0	8.0	0.0	0.9	10	<0.1
anhydrous	1 tbsp	480	0.00	0.00	0.00	0.00	<0.1	0.00	0.0	0.5	0.0	0.1	<1	0.0
BUTTERBEAN. See BEAN, LIMA.														
BUTTERBUR / fuki														
Canned														
chopped	1 cup	0	0.01	0.01	0.17	0.04	3.2	0.00	14.8	42.2	0.8	2.5	15	<0.1
stalks, whole	3 medium	0	0.00	0.00	0.06	0.02	1.2	0.00	5.4	15.3	0.3	0.9	5	<0.1
Fresh														
raw, chopped	1 cup	47.0	0.02	0.02	0.19	0.09	9.8	0.00	29.6	96.8	0.1	13.2	616	0.2
raw, petioles, whole	1 medium	3	0.00	0.00	0.01	0.01	0.5	0.00	1.6	5.2	<0.1	0.7	33	<0.1
BUTTERFISH														
baked, broiled, grilled, or microwaved	3 oz	93	0.12	0.16	4.90	0.29	14.4	1.60	0.0	23.8	0.5	27.2	409	0.8
raw	3 oz	85	0.10	0.13	3.80	0.26	12.8	1.60	0.0	18.7	0.4	21.3	319	0.7
BUTTERHEAD LETTUCE. See under LETTUCE.														

Food Name	Serving Size	A I.U.	Thi mg	Rib mg	Nia mg	B$_6$ mg	Fol mcg	B$_{12}$ mcg	C mg	Calc mg	Iron mg	Mag mg	Pot mg	Zn mg
BUTTERMILK														
cultured, low-fat	1 quart	323	0.33	1.50	0.57	0.33	49.0	2.10	9.6	1141.0	0.5	107.0	1483	4.1
cultured, low-fat	1 cup	80.8	0.08	0.38	0.14	0.08	12.3	0.54	2.4	285.0	0.1	26.8	371	1.0
cultured, low-fat	1 fl oz	10	0.01	0.05	0.02	0.01	1.5	0.07	0.3	35.6	<0.1	3.4	46	0.1
dry	1 cup	262	0.47	1.90	1.10	0.41	56.9	4.60	6.8	1421.0	0.4	131.0	1910	4.8
dry	1 tbsp	14	0.03	0.10	0.06	0.02	3.1	0.25	0.4	77.0	<0.1	7.1	103	0.3
BUTTERNUT, DRIED														
dried	1 cup	149	0.46	0.18	1.30	0.67	79.4	0.00	3.8	63.6	4.8	284.0	505	3.8
dried	1 oz	35	0.11	0.04	0.30	0.16	18.8	0.00	0.9	15.0	1.1	67.2	119	0.9
dried	1 nutmeat	4	0.01	0.00	0.03	0.02	2.0	0.00	0.1	1.6	0.1	7.1	13	<0.1
BUTTERNUT SQUASH. See under SQUASH.														
BUTTERSCOTCH. See under CANDY COATING.														
BUTTERSCOTCH TOPPING	2 tbsp	37	0.01	0.04	0.02	0.01	0.8	0.04	0.1	21.7	0.1	2.9	34	<0.1
BUTTON MUSHROOM. See MUSHROOM, WHITE.														

C

Food Name	Serving Size	A I.U.	Thi mg	Rib mg	Nia mg	B$_6$ mg	Fol mcg	B$_{12}$ mcg	C mg	Calc mg	Iron mg	Mag mg	Pot mg	Zn mg
CABBAGE, CHINESE. See BOK CHOY.														
CABBAGE, COMMON														
boiled, drained, shredded	1/2 cup	99	0.04	0.04	0.21	0.09	15.0	0.00	15.1	23.3	0.1	6.0	73	<0.1
boiled, drained, whole, medium, approx 5.75-inch diam	1 head	1666	0.72	0.69	3.60	1.40	252.0	0.00	254.0	391.0	2.1	101.0	1224	1.1
raw, chopped	1 cup	118	0.05	0.04	0.27	0.09	38.3	0.00	28.7	41.8	0.5	13.3	219	0.2
raw, leaf, large leaf	1 leaf	44	0.02	0.01	0.10	0.03	14.2	0.00	10.6	15.5	0.2	5.0	81	<0.1
raw, leaf, medium leaf	1 leaf	31	0.01	0.01	0.07	0.02	9.9	0.00	7.4	10.8	0.1	3.5	57	<0.1
raw, leaf, small leaf	1 leaf	20	0.01	0.01	0.05	0.01	6.5	0.00	4.8	7.0	0.1	2.3	37	<0.1
raw, shredded	1 cup	93	0.04	0.03	0.21	0.07	30.1	0.00	22.5	32.9	0.4	10.5	172	0.1
raw, whole, large, approx 7-inch diam	1 head	1660	0.62	0.50	3.70	1.20	537.0	0.00	402.0	587.0	7.4	187.0	3070	2.2
raw, whole, medium head, approx 5.75-inch diam	1 head	1208	0.45	0.36	2.70	0.87	390.0	0.00	292.0	427.0	5.4	136.0	2234	1.6
raw, whole, small head, approx 4.5-inch diam	1 head	950	0.36	0.29	2.10	0.69	307.0	0.00	230.0	336.0	4.2	107.0	1756	1.3
CABBAGE, DANISH														
raw, shredded	1/2 cup	44	0.02	0.01	0.11	0.03	19.8	0.00	17.9	16.4	0.2	5.3	86	<0.1
raw, whole, medium	1 head	1144	0.45	0.27	2.70	0.86	515.0	0.00	381.0	427.0	5.1	136.0	2234	1.6
CABBAGE, NAPA. See BOK CHOY.														
CABBAGE, RED														
boiled, drained, leaf	1 leaf	6	0.01	0.00	0.04	0.03	2.8	0.00	7.6	8.1	0.1	2.4	32	<0.1
boiled, drained, shredded	1/2 cup	20	0.03	0.02	0.15	0.11	9.4	0.00	25.8	27.8	0.3	8.3	105	0.1
raw, chopped	1 cup	36	0.05	0.03	0.27	0.19	18.4	0.00	50.7	45.4	0.4	13.3	183	0.2
raw, leaf, medium	1 leaf	9	0.01	0.01	0.07	0.05	4.8	0.00	13.1	11.7	0.1	3.5	47	<0.1
raw, shredded	1 cup	28	0.04	0.02	0.21	0.15	14.5	0.00	39.9	35.7	0.3	10.5	144	0.25
raw, whole, large, approx 5.5-inch diam	1 head	454	0.57	0.34	3.40	2.40	235.0	0.00	646.0	578.0	5.6	170.0	2336	2.4
raw, whole, medium, approx 5-inch diam	1 head	336	0.42	0.25	2.50	1.80	174.0	0.00	478.0	428.0	4.1	126.0	1728	1.8
raw, whole, small, approx 4-inch diam	1 head	227	0.28	0.17	1.70	1.20	117.0	0.00	323.0	289.0	2.8	85.0	1168	1.2
CABBAGE, SAVOY														
boiled, drained, shredded	1 cup	1289	0.07	0.03	0.04	0.22	67.1	0.00	24.6	43.5	0.6	34.8	267	0.3
raw, shredded	1 cup	700	0.05	0.02	0.21	0.13	56.1	0.00	21.7	24.5	0.3	19.6	161	0.2

Food Name	Serving Size	A I.U.	Thi mg	Rib mg	Nia mg	B₆ mg	Fol mcg	B₁₂ mcg	C mg	Calc mg	Iron mg	Mag mg	Pot mg	Zn mg
CABBAGE, SKUNK / swamp cabbage / water convolvulus														
boiled, drained, chopped	1 cup	5096	0.05	0.08	0.49	0.08	34.1	0.00	15.7	52.9	1.3	29.4	278	0.2
raw, shredded.	1 cup	3528	0.02	0.06	0.50	0.05	32.0	0.00	30.8	43.1	0.9	39.8	175	0.1
CABBAGE DISH/ENTRÉE														
(Lean Cuisine) stuffed, w/meat and														
tomato sauce, potato	1 serving	0	na	na	na	na	na	na	53.0	105	na	na	na	na
CABBAGE TURNIP. See KOHLRABI.														
CALABASH GOURD. See GOURD, BOTTLE.														
CALAMARI. See SQUID.														
CALICO BASS. See SUNFISH.														
CANADIAN BACON. See BACON, CANADIAN STYLE.														
CANDY. See also CANDY COATING.														
(Nestlé) 'Butterfinger' round 'BBs'	10 pieces	0	0.02	0.02	0.65	0.02	7.0	0.00	0.0	7.0	0.2	20.5	99	0.3
CANDY BAR														
(Hershey's)														
'Caramello' 5-oz bar	1 bar	na	na	na	na	na	na	na	na	261.0	1.0	na	na	na
'Caramello' 1.6-oz bar.	1 bar	na	na	na	na	na	na	na	na	82.8	0.3	na	na	na
'5th Avenue' 2-oz bar	1 bar	32	0.08	0.07	2.00	0.05	21.7	0.07	0.1	42.2	0.7	36.5	169	0.7
'5th Avenue' snack size, 0.6 oz	1 bar	9	0.02	0.02	0.55	0.01	6.1	0.02	<0.1	11.8	0.2	10.2	48	0.2
'Kit Kat' 3.375-oz bar	1 bar	156	0.17	0.52	2.40	0.12	136.0	0.15	0.7	158.0	0.9	37.4	279	1.2
'Kit Kat' 2.8-oz bar	1 bar	127	0.14	0.42	2.00	0.10	111.0	0.13	0.65	129.0	0.7	30.4	227	1.0
'Kit Kat' 1.62-oz bar	1 bar	75	0.08	0.25	1.20	0.06	65.3	0.07	0.3	75.9	0.4	17.9	134	0.6
'Kit Kat' 1.5-oz bar	1 bar	69	0.07	0.23	1.10	0.05	59.6	0.07	0.3	69.3	0.4	16.4	122	0.5
'Kit Kat' mini, 0.35-oz bar	1 bar	16	0.02	0.05	0.26	0.01	14.2	0.02	0.1	16.5	0.1	3.9	29	0.1
'Mounds' 1.9-oz bar	1 bar	3	0.02	0.03	0.15	0.05	1.6	0.00	0.2	8.0	1.1	29.7	131	0.5
'Mounds' snack size, 0.7-oz bar	1 bar	1	0.01	0.01	0.05	0.02	0.6	0.00	0.1	2.9	0.4	10.6	47	0.2
'Mr. Goodbar' 2.6-oz bar	1 bar	104	0.12	0.19	2.40	0.07	28.5	0.22	0.2	78.8	1.0	62.8	326	1.3
'Mr. Goodbar' 1.75-oz bar	1 bar	70	0.08	0.13	1.60	0.04	19.1	0.15	0.2	52.9	0.6	42.1	219	0.9
'Special Dark' extra large, 8 oz	1 bar	80	0.07	0.16	0.91	0.08	4.5	0.00	0.0	61.3	5.4	252.0	679	3.3
'Special Dark' large, 4-oz bar	1 bar	40	0.03	0.08	0.45	0.04	2.3	0.00	0.0	30.5	2.7	125.0	338	1.6
'Special Dark' 2.8-oz bar	1 bar	28	0.02	0.06	0.32	0.03	1.6	0.00	0.0	21.3	1.9	87.7	236	1.1
'Special Dark' 2.2-oz bar.	1 bar	22	0.02	0.04	0.25	0.02	1.2	0.00	0.0	16.7	1.5	68.6	185	0.9
'Special Dark' 1.45-oz bar.	1 bar	14	0.01	0.03	0.16	0.01	0.8	0.00	0.0	11.1	1.0	45.5	123	0.6
'Whatchamacallit' 1.7-oz bar.	1 bar	34	0.22	0.29	3.50	0.27	4.8	0.16	0.1	54.7	0.3	28.8	148	0.6
(M&M Mars)														
'Mars' almond, 1.76-oz bar	1 bar	94	0.02	0.16	0.47	0.03	9.5	0.18	0.4	84.0	0.6	36.0	163	0.6
'Milky Way' 2.15-oz bar	1 bar	66	0.02	0.14	0.21	0.03	6.1	0.20	0.6	79.3	0.5	20.7	147	0.4
'Milky Way' 2.1-oz bar	1 bar	65	0.02	0.13	0.21	0.03	6.0	0.19	0.6	78.0	0.5	20.4	145	0.4
'Milky Way' 2.05-oz bar	1 bar	63	0.02	0.13	0.20	0.03	5.8	0.19	0.6	75.4	0.4	19.7	140	0.4
'Milky Way' 1.9-oz bar	1 bar	58	0.02	0.12	0.19	0.03	5.4	0.17	0.5	70.2	0.4	18.4	130	0.4
'Milky Way' 0.8-oz bar	1 bar	25	0.01	0.05	0.08	0.01	2.3	0.07	0.2	29.9	0.2	7.8	55	0.2
'Milky Way' fun size	1 bar	19	0.01	0.04	0.06	0.01	1.8	0.06	0.2	23.4	0.1	6.1	43	0.1
'Snickers' king size, 4-oz bar.	1 bar	172	0.11	0.17	4.70	0.10	45.2	0.17	0.7	106.0	0.9	81.4	366	2.7
'Snickers' 2-oz bar	1 bar	87	0.06	0.09	2.40	0.05	22.8	0.09	0.3	53.6	0.4	41.0	185	1.3
'Snickers' fun size	1 bar	23	0.02	0.02	0.63	0.01	6.0	0.02	0.1	14.1	0.1	10.8	49	0.4
'3 Musketeers' 2.13-oz bar	1 bar	48	0.02	0.08	0.14	0.01	0.0	0.10	0.2	50.4	0.4	17.4	80	0.3
'3 Musketeers' 1.813-oz bar	1 bar	41	0.02	0.07	0.12	0.01	0.0	0.09	0.2	42.8	0.4	14.8	68	0.3
'3 Musketeers' 0.8-oz bar	1 bar	18	0.01	0.03	0.05	0.00	0.0	0.04	0.1	19.3	0.2	6.7	31	0.1
'3 Musketeers' fun size	1 bar	13	0.01	0.02	0.04	0.00	0.0	0.03	0.1	13.9	0.1	4.8	22	0.1
'Twix' 11-oz pkg.	1 pkg	296	0.50	0.71	3.70	0.08	74.9	0.56	1.2	281.0	2.5	99.8	630	2.4
'Twix' 3.35-oz bar	4 bars	90	0.15	0.22	1.10	0.03	22.8	0.17	0.4	85.5	0.8	30.4	192	0.7
'Twix' 2.06-oz bar	2 bars	55	0.09	0.13	0.69	0.02	13.9	0.10	0.2	52.2	0.5	18.6	117	0.5
'Twix' 2-oz pkg.	1 pkg	54	0.09	0.13	0.68	0.02	13.7	0.10	0.2	51.3	0.5	18.2	115	0.5
'Twix' peanut, 9.43-oz pkg.	1 pkg	192	0.26	0.40	10.8	0.38	66.8	0.35	1.6	206.0	2.4	198.0	951	3.7

Food Name	Serving Size	A I.U.	Thi mg	Rib mg	Nia mg	B6 mg	Fol mcg	B12 mcg	C mg	Calc mg	Iron mg	Mag mg	Pot mg	Zn mg
'Twix' peanut, 2.06-oz pkg.	1 pkg	42	0.06	0.09	2.30	0.08	14.5	0.08	0.4	44.7	0.5	42.9	206	0.8
'Twix' peanut, 1.89-oz pkg.	1 pkg	39	0.05	0.08	2.20	0.08	13.5	0.07	0.3	41.6	0.5	40.0	192	0.8
'Twix' peanut, 1.77-oz pkg.	1 pkg	36	0.05	0.08	2.00	0.07	12.5	0.07	0.3	38.5	0.5	37.0	178	0.7
(Nestlé)														
'100 Grand' 1.5-oz bar	1 bar	35	0.12	0.19	1.40	0.14	30.1	0.11	0.2	49.0	0.1	16.3	97	0.4
'100 Grand' miniature	1 bar	17	0.06	0.09	0.69	0.07	14.7	0.05	0.1	23.9	0.1	8.0	48	0.2
'Baby Ruth' 2.28-oz bar	1 bar	0	0.06	0.06	1.80	0.04	20.1	0.03	0.0	26.6	0.1	52.0	257	0.8
'Baby Ruth' 2.1-oz bar	1 bar	0	0.06	0.06	1.70	0.04	18.6	0.03	0.0	24.6	0.1	48.0	238	0.8
'Baby Ruth' 1.2-oz bar	1 bar	0	0.03	0.03	0.94	0.02	10.5	0.02	0.0	13.9	0.1	27.2	135	0.4
'Baby Ruth' miniature	1 bar	0	0.02	0.02	0.58	0.01	6.5	0.01	0.0	8.6	<0.1	16.8	83	0.3
'Baby Ruth' fun size	1 bar	0	0.01	0.01	0.39	0.01	4.3	0.01	0.0	5.7	<0.1	11.2	55	0.2
'Butterfinger' king size	1 bar	0	0.09	0.08	2.70	0.08	29.2	0.01	0.0	29.2	0.8	85.3	411	1.3
'Butterfinger' 2.16-oz bar	1 bar	0	0.05	0.04	1.50	0.04	16.5	0.01	0.0	16.5	0.5	48.2	232	0.7
'Butterfinger' 1.6-oz bar	1 bar	0	0.04	0.03	1.10	0.03	12.2	0.01	0.0	12.2	<0.1	35.5	171	0.5
'Butterfinger' fun size	1 bar	0	0.02	0.02	0.52	0.01	5.7	0.00	0.0	5.7	0.2	16.6	80	0.3
'Butterfinger' bite size	1 bar	0	0.01	0.01	0.17	0.01	1.9	0.00	0.0	1.9	0.1	5.5	27	0.1
'Chunky' 1.4-oz bar	1 bar	25	0.04	0.16	0.76	0.05	8.8	0.15	0.1	57.2	0.5	29.2	214	0.7
'Chunky' 1.25-oz bar	1 bar	22	0.03	0.14	0.67	0.04	7.7	0.13	0.1	50.0	0.4	25.6	187	0.6
'Crunch' 1.55-oz bar	1 bar	30	0.15	0.25	1.70	0.17	34.8	0.16	0.1	74.4	0.2	25.5	151	0.6
'Crunch' 1.4-oz bar	1 bar	28	0.14	0.23	1.60	0.16	31.6	0.15	0.1	67.6	0.2	23.2	138	0.6
'Crunch' miniature	1 bar	7	0.03	0.06	0.40	0.04	7.9	0.04	<0.1	16.9	0.1	5.8	34	0.1
'Oh Henry!' 2-oz bar	1 bar	27	0.01	0.09	1.60	0.04	17.1	0.12	0.1	62.1	0.3	35.2	185	0.7
CARAMEL														
(Hershey's)														
in milk chocolate, 1.91-oz pkg 'Rolo'	1 pkg	77	0.03	0.12	0.11	0.02	2.6	0.15	0.2	81.1	0.3	20.7	131	0.5
in milk chocolate, 1.74-oz roll 'Rolo'	1 roll	72	0.03	0.11	0.11	0.02	2.5	0.14	0.2	75.0	0.3	19.1	122	0.5
in milk chocolate, 0.2-oz pieces 'Rolo'	1 piece	4	0.00	0.01	0.01	0.00	0.2	0.01	<0.1	4.6	<0.1	1.2	7	<0.1
CHOCOLATE														
(M&M Mars)														
'M&M's' mini, 5-oz pkg	1 pkg	318	0.09	0.33	0.35	0.05	7.1	0.41	0.9	165.0	1.7	65.3	416	1.5
'M&Ms' plain	1 cup	422	0.11	0.44	0.47	0.06	12.5	0.56	1.0	218.0	2.3	85.3	553	2.0
'M&Ms' plain	10 pieces	14	0.00	0.02	0.02	0.00	0.4	0.02	<0.1	7.3	0.1	2.9	19	<0.1
'M&Ms' plain, 1.69-oz pkg.	1 pkg	97	0.03	0.10	0.11	0.01	2.9	0.13	0.2	50.4	0.5	19.7	128	<0.1
'M&Ms' plain, 1.48-oz box.	1 box	85	0.02	0.09	0.09	0.01	2.5	0.11	0.2	44.1	0.5	17.2	112	<0.1
FRUIT														
(M&M Mars)														
'Skittles' original, bite size	1 cup	0	0.00	0.04	0.04	0.01	0.0	0.00	137.0	0.0	<0.1	2.0	10	<0.1
'Skittles' original, bite size, 4-oz pkg	1 pkg	0	0.00	0.02	0.02	0.01	0.0	0.00	75.6	0.0	<0.1	1.1	6	<0.1
'Skittles' original, bite size, 2.3-oz pkg	1 pkg	0	0.00	0.01	0.01	0.00	0.0	0.00	43.5	0.0	<0.1	0.7	3	<0.1
'Skittles' original, bite size, 2.17-oz pkg	1 pkg	0	0.00	0.01	0.01	0.00	0.0	0.00	41.5	0.0	<0.1	0.6	3	<0.1
'Skittles' original, bite size, 2-oz pkg	1 pkg	0	0.00	0.01	0.01	0.00	0.0	0.00	38.1	0.0	<0.1	0.6	3	<0.1
'Skittles' original, bite size	10 pieces	0	0.00	0.00	0.00	0.00	0.0	0.00	7.2	0.0	0.0	0.1	<1	0.0
chews, 'Starburst'	48 pieces	0	0.00	0.00	0.00	0.00	0.0	0.00	21.2	1.6	0.1	0.4	<1	0.0
chews, 'Starburst'	1 piece	0	0.00	0.00	0.00	0.00	0.0	0.00	2.6	0.2	<0.1	0.1	<1	0.0
chews, 'Starburst' 16-oz pkg	1 pkg	0	0.01	0.01	0.02	0.00	0.0	0.00	240.0	18.2	0.6	4.5	9	0.0
chews, 'Starburst' 2.07-oz pkg	1 pkg	0	0.00	0.00	0.00	0.00	0.0	0.00	31.2	2.4	0.1	0.6	1.2	0.0
chews, 'Starburst' fun size.	1 pkg	0	0.00	0.00	0.00	0.00	0.0	0.00	22.2	1.7	0.1	0.4	<1	0.0
GUM (Chiclets)	10 pieces	0	0.00	0.00	0.00	0.00	0.0	0.00	0.0	0.0	0.0	0.0	0	0.0
GUMDROP														
1-inch diam.	1 gumdrop	0	0.00	0.00	0.00	0.00	0.0	0.00	0.0	0.4	1.0	0.1	<1	0.0
3/4-inch diam	1 gumdrop	0	0.00	0.00	0.00	0.00	0.0	0.00	0.0	0.1	<0.1	<0.1	<1	0.0
1/2-inch diam	1 gumdrop	0	0.00	0.00	0.00	0.00	0.0	0.00	0.0	0.1	<0.1	<0.1	<1	0.0

Food Name	Serving Size	A I.U.	Thi mg	Rib mg	Nia mg	B₆ mg	Fol mcg	B₁₂ mcg	C mg	Calc mg	Iron mg	Mag mg	Pot mg	Zn mg
JELLIED AND GUMMED														
gummy bears	10 pieces	0	0.00	0.00	0.00	0.00	0.0	0.00	0.0	0.7	0.1	0.2	1	0.0
gummy fish	10 pieces	0	0.00	0.00	0.00	0.00	0.0	0.00	0.0	1.5	0.2	0.5	3	0.0
gummy worms	10 pieces	0	0.00	0.00	0.00	0.00	0.0	0.00	0.0	2.2	0.3	0.7	4	0.0
jelly ring, 1 1/4 inch diam	1 ring	0	0.00	0.00	0.00	0.00	0.0	0.00	0.0	0.3	<0.1	0.1	<1	0.0
jellybeans, large, 10 pieces	1 oz	0	0.00	0.00	0.00	0.00	0.0	0.00	0.0	0.9	0.3	0.6	11	<0.1
jellybeans, small	10 pieces	0	0.00	0.00	0.00	0.00	0.0	0.00	0.0	0.3	0.1	0.2	4	<0.1
MARSHMALLOW														
miniature	1 cup	<1	0.00	0.00	0.04	0.00	0.5	0.00	0.0	1.5	0.1	1.0	3	<0.1
miniature	10 pieces	<1	0.00	0.00	0.01	0.00	0.1	0.00	0.0	0.2	<0.1	0.1	<1	0.0
regular size	1 piece	<1	0.00	0.00	0.01	0.00	0.1	0.00	0.0	0.2	<0.1	0.1	<1	0.0
MINT														
(Nestlé)														
'After Eight'	5 pieces	8	0.02	0.02	0.12	0.01	0.4	0.00	0.0	9.4	0.6	18.4	69	0.2
'After Eight'	1 piece	2	0.00	0.00	0.03	0.00	0.1	0.00	0.0	1.9	0.1	3.7	14	<0.1
PEANUT														
(M&M Mars)														
chocolate, candy-coated, 'M&Ms'	1 cup	158	0.17	0.29	6.40	0.14	59.5	0.31	0.9	172.0	2.0	126.0	588	3.9
chocolate, candy-coated, 'M&Ms' 1.74-oz pkg	1 pkg	46	0.05	0.08	1.80	0.04	17.1	0.09	0.3	49.5	0.6	36.3	170	1.1
chocolate, candy-coated, 'M&Ms' 1.67-oz pkg	1 pkg	44	0.05	0.08	1.80	0.04	16.4	0.09	0.2	47.5	0.5	34.8	163	1.1
chocolate, candy-coated, 'M&Ms' fun size pkg	1 pkg	20	0.02	0.04	0.79	0.02	7.3	0.04	0.1	21.2	0.2	15.5	73	0.5
chocolate, candy-coated, 'M&Ms'	10 pieces	19	0.02	0.03	0.75	0.02	7.0	0.04	0.1	20.2	0.2	14.8	69	0.5
(Nestlé)														
chocolate-covered, 'Goobers' 7-oz pkg.	1 pkg	0	0.24	0.42	10.3	0.42	15.8	0.57	0.0	251.0	2.7	236.0	994	4.3
chocolate-covered, 'Goobers'	1/4 cup	0	0.05	0.09	2.10	0.09	3.3	0.12	0.0	52.1	0.6	48.8	206	0.9
chocolate-covered, 'Goobers' 1.375-oz pkg . .		0	0.05	0.08	2.00	0.08	3.1	0.11	0.0	49.5	0.5	46.4	196	0.9
chocolate-covered, 'Goobers'	10 pieces	0	0.01	0.02	0.52	0.02	0.8	0.03	0.0	12.7	0.1	11.9	50	0.2
PEANUT BUTTER														
(Hershey's)														
'Reese's Peanut Butter Cup' individual, 0.6 oz	1 piece	12	0.04	0.03	0.79	0.03	9.3	0.03	<0.1	13.3	0.2	15.1	60	0.3
'Reese's Peanut Butter Cup' miniature	5 pieces	29	0.10	0.07	1.80	0.06	21.4	0.06	0.1	30.4	0.5	34.7	137	0.7
'Reese's Peanut Butter Cup' miniature	1 piece	5	0.02	0.01	0.32	0.01	3.9	0.01	<0.1	5.5	0.1	6.2	25	0.1
'Reese's Peanut Butter Cup' 2-pack, 1.6 oz . .		33	0.11	0.08	2.10	0.07	24.8	0.07	0.1	35.1	0.5	40.0	158	0.8
'Reese's Pieces'	1/4 cup	1	0.05	0.07	1.30	0.03	13.2	0.10	0.2	38.5	0.4	20.7	108	0.4
'Reese's Pieces'	1.6-oz pkg	1	0.04	0.07	1.30	0.03	12.9	0.10	0.2	37.7	0.4	20.2	106	0.4
'Reese's Pieces'	50 pieces	<1	0.04	0.06	1.10	0.03	10.9	0.08	0.2	32.0	0.3	17.2	90	0.3
'Reese's Pieces'	10 pieces	<1	0.01	0.01	0.23	0.01	2.2	0.02	<0.1	6.6	0.1	3.5	19	<0.1
PECAN														
(Demet's)														
turtles	1 piece	28	0.03	0.04	0.06	0.01	1.7	0.07	0.1	26.9	0.2	8.9	52	0.3
turtles, 6-oz pkg	1 pkg	277	0.26	0.41	0.58	0.09	17.0	0.68	1.2	269.0	2.3	89.1	524	2.4
RAISIN														
(Nestlé)														
chocolate-covered, 'Raisinets' 1.58-oz pkg	1 pkg	17	0.04	0.10	0.18	0.05	2.3	0.10	0.1	48.6	0.5	20.3	231	0.4
chocolate-covered, 'Raisinets'	10 pieces	4	0.01	0.02	0.04	0.01	0.5	0.02	<0.1	10.8	0.1	4.5	51	<0.1
CANDY COATING														
bars, butterscotch, confectioner's coating	1 oz	0	0.02	0.00	0.02	0.00	0.3	0.03	<0.1	9.6	<0.1	1.4	53.0	0.0
bars, white, confectioner's coating	3 oz	29.8	0.05	0.24	0.63	0.05	14.4	0.52	0.42	169	0.2	10.2	243	0.6

Food Name	Serving Size	A I.U.	Thi mg	Rib mg	Nia mg	B$_6$ mg	Fol mcg	B$_{12}$ mcg	C mg	Calc mg	Iron mg	Mag mg	Pot mg	Zn mg
chips, butterscotch, confectioner's														
coating	1 cup	0	0.14	0.00	0.12	0.03	1:7	0.17	0.2	57.8	0.1	8.5	318	0.2
chip, white, confectioner's coating	1 cup	59.5	0.11	0.48	1.30	0.10	28.9	1.00	0.9	338.0	0.4	20.4	486	1.3
CANOLA OIL														
	1 cup	0	0.00	0.00	0.00	0.00	0.0	0.00	0.0	0.0	0.0	0.0	0	0.0
	1 tbsp	0	0.00	0.00	0.00	0.00	0.0	0.00	0.0	0.0	0.0	0.0	0	0.0
CANTALOUPE. See MELON, CANTALOUPE.														
CAPE GOOSEBERRY / ground cherry / poha														
raw	1 cup	1008	0.15	0.06	3.9	na	na	0	15.4	12.6	1.4	na	na	na
CAPERS, canned, drained	1 tbsp	12.0	0.00	0.01	0.06	0.00	2.0	0.00	0.4	3.4	0.1	2.8	3.4	<0.1
CARAMBOLA. See STAR FRUIT.														
CARAWAY SEED														
	1 tbsp	24.3	0.03	0.03	0.24	0.02	0.67	0.00	1.4	46.2	1.	17.3	91	0.4
	1 tsp	7.6	0.01	0.01	0.08	0.01	0.21	0.00	0.4	14.5	0.3	5.4	28	0.1
CARDAMOM														
ground	1 tbsp	0	0.01	0.01	0.06	na	na	0.00	1.2	22.2	0.8	13.3	65	0.4
ground	1 tsp	0	0.00	0.00	0.02	na	na	0.00	0.4	7.7	0.3	4.6	22	0.2
CARDONI. See CARDOON.														
CARDOON / cardoni														
raw, shredded	1 cup	214	0.04	0.05	0.53	0.08	50.4	0.00	3.6	125.0	1.2	74.8	712	0.3
CARIBOU														
raw	1 oz	0	0.09	0.20	1.60	0.11	1.1	1.80	0.0	4.8	1.3	7.4	84	1.1
roasted	3 oz	0	0.21	0.77	4.90	0.27	4.3	5.60	2.5	18.7	5.2	22.9	264	4.5
roasted, yield from 1 lb raw, boneless	11.9 oz	0	0.85	3.10	19.7	1.10	17.0	22.60	10.2	74.8	21.0	91.8	1054	17.9
CARISSA / Natal plum														
Fresh														
raw, sliced	1 cup	60	0.06	0.09	0.30	na	na	0.00	57.0	16.5	2.0	24.0	390	na
raw, whole, peeled and seeded	1 fruit	8	0.01	0.01	0.04	na	na	0.00	7.6	2.2	0.3	3.2	52	na
CAROB FLAVOR DRINK MIX														
powder, mix only	1 tbsp	0	0.00	0.00	0.09	0.02	0.0	0.00	0.0	3.8	0.6	0.6	12.5	<0.1
powder, prepared w/milk	8 fl oz	307	0.10	0.39	0.30	0.12	12.3	0.87	2.3	292.0	0.7	33.3	369	<0.1
CAROB FLOUR. See under FLOUR.														
CARP														
baked, broiled, grilled, or microwaved	3 oz	27	0.12	0.06	1.80	0.19	14.7	1.30	1.4	44.2	1.4	32.3	363	1.6
raw	3 oz	25	0.10	0.05	1.40	0.16	12.8	1.30	1.4	34.9	1.1	24.6	283	1.3
CARROT														
Canned														
regular pack, mashed, drained	1 cup	31405	0.04	0.07	1.30	0.26	21.0	0.00	6.2	57.0	1.5	18.2	408	0.6
regular pack, sliced, drained	1 cup	20110	0.03	0.04	0.81	0.16	13.4	0.00	3.9	36.5	0.9	11.7	261	0.4
regular pack, sliced, drained	1 slice	386	0.00	0.00	0.02	0.00	0.3	0.00	<0.1	0.7	<0.1	0.2	5	<0.1
regular pack, sliced, w//liquid	1/2 cup	11894	0.02	0.03	0.52	0.14	10.0	0.00	2.5	38.1	0.6	11.1	213	0.4
sliced, no salt added, drained	1 cup	20110	0.03	0.04	0.81	0.16	13.4	0.00	3.9	36.5	0.9	11.7	261	0.4
sliced, no salt added, drained	1 slice	386	0.00	0.00	0.02	0.00	0.3	0.00	<0.1	0.7	<0.1	0.2	5	<0.1
sliced, no salt added, mashed	1 cup	31405	0.04	0.07	1.30	0.26	21.0	0.00	6.2	57.0	1.5	18.2	408	0.6
sliced, no salt added, w/liquid	1/2 cup	11894	0.02	0.03	0.52	0.14	10.0	0.00	2.5	38.1	0.6	11.1	194	0.4
Fresh														
baby, raw, large	1 carrot	2252	0.01	0.01	0.13	0.01	5.0	0.00	1.3	3.5	0.1	1.8	42	<0.1
baby, raw, medium	1 carrot	1501	0.00	0.01	0.09	0.01	3.3	0.00	<0.1	2.3	<0.1	1.2	28	<0.1
boiled, drained, sliced	1/2 cup	19152	0.03	0.04	0.40	0.19	10.8	0.00	1.8	24.2	0.5	10.1	177	0.2
boiled, drained, whole, medium	1 carrot	11295	0.02	0.03	0.23	0.11	6.4	0.00	1.1	14.3	0.3	6.0	104	0.1
raw, chopped	1 cup	36005	0.12	0.08	1.20	0.19	17.9	0.00	11.9	34.6	0.6	19.2	413	0.3
raw, cut, strips or slices	1 cup	34317	0.12	0.07	1.10	0.18	17.1	0.00	11.3	32.9	0.6	18.3	394	0.2
raw, cut, 3-inch strips	1 strip	1969	0.01	0.00	0.07	0.01	1.0	0.00	0.7	1.9	<0.1	1.1	23	<0.1
raw, grated	1 cup	30942	0.11	0.07	1.00	0.16	15.4	0.00	10.2	29.7	0.6	16.5	355	0.2

Food Name	Serving Size	A I.U.	Thi mg	Rib mg	Nia mg	B$_6$ mg	Fol mcg	B$_{12}$ mcg	C mg	Calc mg	Iron mg	Mag mg	Pot mg	Zn mg
raw, whole, large, 7.25–8.5-inch														
long	1 carrot	20253	0.07	0.04	0.67	0.11	10.1	0.00	6.7	19.4	0.4	10.8	233	0.1
raw, whole, medium, 5.5–7.25-inch														
long	1 carrot	17159	0.06	0.04	0.57	0.09	8.5	0.00	5.7	16.5	0.3	9.2	197	0.1
raw, whole, small, 5.5-inch long	1 carrot	14065	0.05	0.03	0.46	0.07	7.0	0.00	4.7	13.5	0.3	7.5	162	0.1
Frozen														
sliced, drained	1 cup	25845	0.04	0.05	0.64	0.19	15.8	0.00	4.1	40.9	0.7	14.6	231	0.4
sliced, no salt, drained	1 cup	25845	0.04	0.05	0.64	0.19	15.8	0.00	4.1	40.9	0.7	14.6	231	0.4
sliced, unprepared	10-oz pkg	60441	0.11	0.13	1.80	0.51	27.3	0.00	12.2	90.9	1.7	31.2	514	0.7
sliced, unprepared	1/2 cup	13620	0.03	0.03	0.40	0.12	6.1	0.00	2.8	20.5	0.4	7.0	116	0.2
CARROT JUICE														
canned	1 cup	25833	0.22	0.13	0.91	0.51	9.0	0.00	20.1	56.6	1.1	33.0	689	0.4
canned	1 fl oz	3229	0.03	0.02	0.11	0.06	1.1	0.00	2.5	7.1	0.1	4.1	86	<0.1
CASABA MELON. See MELON, CASABA.														
CASHEW / heart nut														
Dry roasted														
halves and whole, salted	1 cup	0	0.27	0.27	1.90	0.35	94.8	0.00	0.0	61.6	8.2	356.0	774	7.7
halves and whole, unsalted	1 cup	0	0.27	0.27	1.90	0.35	94.8	0.00	0.0	61.6	8.2	356.0	774	7.7
salted	1 oz	0	0.06	0.06	0.40	0.07	19.6	0.00	0.0	12.8	1.7	73.7	160	1.6
unsalted	1 oz	0	0.06	0.06	0.40	0.07	19.6	0.00	0.0	12.8	1.7	73.7	160	1.6
unsalted	1 tbsp	0	0.02	0.02	0.12	0.02	6.0	0.00	0.0	3.9	0.5	22.4	49	0.5
Oil roasted														
halves and whole, salted	1 cup	0	0.55	0.23	2.30	0.33	88.0	0.00	0.0	53.3	5.3	332.0	689	6.2
halves and whole, unsalted	1 cup	0	0.55	0.23	2.30	0.33	88.0	0.00	0.0	53.3	5.3	332.0	689	6.2
salted, approx 18 kernels	1 oz	0	0.12	0.05	0.51	0.07	19.2	0.00	0.0	11.6	1.2	72.3	150	1.3
unsalted, approx 18 kernels	1 oz	0	0.12	0.05	0.51	0.07	19.2	0.00	0.0	11.6	1.2	72.3	150	1.3
CASHEW BUTTER														
salted	1 oz	0	0.09	0.05	0.45	0.07	19.4	0.00	0.0	12.2	1.4	73.1	155	1.5
salted	1 tbsp	0	0.05	0.03	0.26	0.04	10.9	0.00	0.0	6.9	0.8	41.3	87	0.8
unsalted	1 oz	0	0.09	0.05	0.45	0.07	19.4	0.00	0.0	12.2	1.4	73.1	155	1.5
unsalted	1 tbsp	0	0.05	0.03	0.26	0.04	10.9	0.00	0.0	6.9	0.8	41.3	87	0.8
CASSAVA / manioc / yuca														
raw, chopped or sliced	1 cup	52	0.18	0.10	1.80	0.18	55.6	0.00	42.4	33.0	0.6	43.3	558	0.7
raw, whole	1 root	102	0.35	0.20	3.50	0.36	110.0	0.00	84.0	65.3	1.1	85.7	1106	1.4
CATFISH, CHANNEL														
breaded, fried	3 oz	24	0.06	0.11	1.90	0.16	25.5	1.60	0.0	37.4	1.2	22.9	289	0.7
farmed, baked, broiled, grilled, or														
microwaved	3 oz	43	0.36	0.06	2.10	0.14	6.0	2.40	0.7	7.7	0.7	22.1	273	0.9
farmed, raw	3 oz	43	0.31	0.06	2.00	0.16	8.5	2.10	0.5	7.7	0.4	19.6	254	0.6
wild, baked, broiled, grilled, or														
microwaved	3 oz	43	0.19	0.06	2.00	0.09	8.5	2.50	0.7	9.3	0.3	23.8	356	0.5
wild, raw	3 oz	43	0.18	0.06	1.60	0.10	8.5	1.90	0.6	11.9	0.3	19.6	304	0.4
CATFISH, OCEAN. See WOLF FISH.														
CATSUP / ketchup														
	1 cup	2438	0.21	0.17	3.30	0.42	36.0	0.00	36.2	45.6	1.7	52.8	1154	0.6
	1 tbsp	152	0.01	0.01	0.20	0.03	2.3	0.00	2.3	2.9	0.1	3.3	72	<0.1
	1 pkt	61	0.01	0.00	0.08	0.01	0.9	0.00	0.9	1.1	<0.1	1.3	28	<0.1
low-salt	1 cup	2438	0.21	0.17	3.30	0.42	36.0	0.00	36.2	45.6	1.7	52.8	1154	0.6
low-salt	1 tbsp	152	0.01	0.01	0.20	0.03	2.3	0.00	2.3	2.9	0.1	3.3	72	<0.1
low-salt	1 pkt	61	0.01	0.00	0.08	0.01	0.9	0.00	0.9	1.1	<0.1	1.3	29	<0.1
CAULIFLOWER														
Fresh														
green, cooked	1/5 head	127	0.06	0.09	0.61	0.19	36.9	0.00	65.3	28.8	0.7	17.1	250	0.6
green, raw, chopped	1 cup	97	0.05	0.07	0.47	0.14	36.5	0.00	56.4	21.1	0.5	12.8	192	0.4

Food Name	Serving Size	A I.U.	Thi mg	Rib mg	Nia mg	B6 mg	Fol mcg	B12 mcg	C mg	Calc mg	Iron mg	Mag mg	Pot mg	Zn mg
green, raw, florets	1 floret	38	0.02	0.03	0.18	0.06	14.3	0.00	22.0	8.3	0.2	5.0	75	0.2
green, raw, whole, large, approx 6–7-inch diam	1 head	777	0.41	0.52	3.80	1.10	291.0	0.00	450.0	169.0	3.7	102.0	1533	3.3
green, raw, whole, medium, approx 5–6-inch diam	1 head	655	0.34	0.44	3.20	0.96	246.0	0.00	380.0	142.0	3.1	86.2	1293	2.8
green, raw, whole, small, approx 4-inch diam	1 head	494	0.26	0.33	2.40	0.72	185.0	0.00	286.0	107.0	2.4	65.0	975	2.1
white, boiled, drained, 1-inch pieces	1/2 cup	11	0.03	0.03	0.25	0.11	27.3	0.00	27.5	9.9	0.2	5.6	88	0.1
white, boiled, drained, florets	3 florets	9	0.02	0.03	0.22	0.09	23.8	0.00	23.9	8.6	0.2	4.9	77	0.1
white, raw, chopped	1 cup	19	0.06	0.06	0.53	0.22	57.0	0.00	46.4	22.0	0.4	15.0	303	<0.1
white, raw, florets	1 floret	3	0.01	0.01	0.07	0.03	7.4	0.00	6.0	2.9	>0.1	1.9	39	<0.1
white, raw, whole, large, approx 6–7-inch diam	1 head	160	0.48	0.53	4.40	1.90	479.0	0.00	390.0	185.0	3.7	126.0	2545	2.4
white, raw, whole, medium, approx 5–6-inch diam	1 head	109	0.33	0.36	3.00	1.30	328.0	0.00	267.0	127.0	2.5	86.3	1742	1.6
white, raw, whole, small, approx 4-inch diam	1 head	50	0.15	0.17	1.40	0.59	151.0	0.00	123.0	58.3	1.2	39.8	803	0.7
Frozen														
drained, 1-inch pieces	1 cup	40	0.07	0.10	0.56	0.16	73.8	0.00	56.3	30.6	0.7	16.2	250	0.2
no salt added, drained, 1-inch pieces	1 cup	40	0.07	0.10	0.56	0.16	73.8	0.00	56.3	30.6	0.7	16.2	250	0.2
unprepared	10-oz pkg	88	0.14	0.20	1.20	0.35	181.0	0.00	139.0	62.5	1.5	34.1	548	0.6
unprepared, 1-inch pieces	1/2 cup	21	0.03	0.05	0.28	0.08	42.2	0.00	32.2	14.5	0.4	7.9	127	0.1
CAVIAR														
black or red, granular	1 oz	530	0.05	0.18	0.03	0.09	14.2	5.70	0.0	78.0	3.4	85.0	51	0.3
black or red, granular	1 tbsp	299	0.03	0.10	0.02	0.05	8.0	3.20	0.0	44.0	1.9	48.0	29	0.2
CAYENNE. See under PEPPER, GROUND.														
CECI. CECI. See CHICKPEA.														
CELERIAC														
boiled, drained, chopped	1 cup	0	0.04	0.06	0.66	0.16	5.3	0.00	5.6	40.3	0.7	18.6	268	0.31
raw	1 cup	0	0.08	0.09	1.10	0.26	11.9	0.00	12.5	67.1	1.1	31.2	468	0.5
CELERY														
boiled, drained, diced	1 cup	99	0.03	0.04	0.24	0.07	16.5	0.00	4.6	31.5	0.3	9.0	213	0.1
boiled, drained, whole	2 stalks	198	0.07	0.07	0.48	0.13	33.0	0.00	9.2	63.0	0.6	18.0	426	0.2
raw, cut, approx 4-inch strips	1 cup	5	0.00	0.00	0.01	0.00	1.1	0.00	0.3	1.6	<0.1	0.4	12	0.0
raw, cut, approx 4-inch strips	1 strip	161	0.06	0.05	0.39	0.10	33.6	0.00	8.4	48.0	0.5	13.2	344	0.2
raw, diced	1 cup	166	0.06	0.06	0.40	0.11	34.7	0.00	8.7	49.6	0.5	13.6	356	0.2
raw, diced	1 tbsp	10	0.00	0.00	0.02	0.01	2.1	0.00	0.5	3.0	<0.1	0.8	22	<0.1
raw, whole, large, 11–12 inch long	1 stalk	86	0.03	0.03	0.21	0.06	17.9	0.00	4.5	25.6	0.3	7.0	184	<0.1
raw, whole, medium, 7.5–8-inch long	1 stalk	54	0.02	0.02	0.13	0.04	11.2	0.00	2.8	16.0	0.2	4.4	115	<0.1
raw, whole, small, approx 5-inch long	1 stalk	23	0.01	0.01	0.06	0.02	4.8	0.00	1.2	6.8	<0.1	1.9	49	<0.1
CELERY SEED														
	1 tbsp	3	0.02	0.02	0.20	0.02	0.7	0.00	1.1	115	2.9	28.6	91	0.5
	1 tsp	1	0.01	0.01	0.06	0.01	0.2	0.00	0.3	35.3	0.9	8.8	28	0.1
CELLOPHANE NOODLES. See under NOODLE.														
CELTUCE, fresh, raw	1 med leaf	280	0.00	0.01	0.04	0.04	3.6	0.00	1.6	3.1	<0.1	2.2	26	<0.1
CEREAL, HOT														
FARINA														
enriched, cooked w/water	1 cup	0	0.19	0.12	1.30	0.02	53.6	0.00	0.0	4.7	1.2	4.7	30	0.2
enriched, cooked w/water	3/4 cup	0	0.14	0.09	0.96	0.02	40.3	0.00	0.0	3.5	0.9	3.5	23	0.1
enriched, cooked w/water	1 tbsp	0	0.01	0.01	0.08	0.00	3.4	0.00	0.0	0.3	<0.1	0.3	2	<0.1
enriched, cooked w/water, salt	1 cup	0	0.19	0.12	1.30	0.02	53.6	0.00	0.0	4.7	1.2	4.7	30	0.2
enriched, cooked w/water, salt	3/4 cup	0	0.14	0.09	0.96	0.02	40.3	0.00	0.0	3.5	0.9	3.5	23	0.1
enriched, unprepared	1 cup	0	1.00	0.63	7.10	0.10	304.0	0.00	0.0	24.6	6.5	22.9	165	0.9
enriched, unprepared	1 tbsp	0	0.06	0.04	0.44	0.01	18.9	0.00	0.0	1.5	0.4	1.4	10	<0.1

Food Name	Serving Size	A I.U.	Thi mg	Rib mg	Nia mg	B$_6$ mg	Fol mcg	B$_{12}$ mcg	C mg	Calc mg	Iron mg	Mag mg	Pot mg	Zn mg
unenriched, cooked w/water	1 cup	0	0.02	0.02	0.23	0.02	4.7	0.00	0.0	4.7	<0.1	4.7	30	0.2
unenriched, cooked w/water	3/4 cup	0	0.02	0.02	0.17	0.02	3.5	0.00	0.0	3.5	<0.1	3.5	23	0.1
unenriched, cooked w/water, salt	1 cup	0	0.02	0.02	0.23	0.02	4.7	0.00	0.0	4.7	<0.1	4.7	30	0.2
unenriched, cooked w/water, salt	3/4 cup	0	0.02	0.02	0.17	0.02	3.5	0.00	0.0	3.5	<0.1	3.5	23	0.1
unenriched, unprepared	1 cup	0	0.11	0.18	1.20	0.10	42.2	0.00	0.0	24.6	2.6	22.9	165	0.9
unenriched, unprepared	1 tbsp	0	0.01	0.01	0.08	0.01	2.6	0.00	0.0	1.5	0.2	1.4	10	<0.1
(Quaker)	1/4 cup	0	0.19	0.11	1.50	0.02	67.8	0.00	0.0	5.3	13.2	7.5	43	0.3
GRITS. See GRITS.														
MULTIGRAIN														
(Quaker) unprepared	1/2 cup	3	0.12	0.05	1.40	0.10	10.4	0.00	0.0	13.6	1.2	46.0	164	1.3
(Roman Meal)														
oats, wheat, and other grains, prepared w/water, salt	1 cup	22	0.31	0.22	3.30	0.38	24.0	0.00	0.0	26.4	1.4	74.4	257	2.9
oats, wheat, and other grains, prepared w/water, salt	3/4 cup	16	0.23	0.16	2.40	0.28	18.0	0.00	0.0	19.8	1.0	55.8	193	1.5
oats, wheat, and other grains, prepared w/water, salt	1 cup	22	0.31	0.22	3.30	0.38	24.0	0.00	0.0	26.4	1.4	74.4	257	1.9
oats, wheat, and other grains, prepared w/water, salt	3/4 cup	16	0.23	0.16	2.40	0.28	18.0	0.00	0.0	19.8	1.0	55.8	193	1.5
oats, wheat, and other grains, unprepared	1 cup	42	0.62	0.44	6.50	0.76	70.0	0.00	0.0	55.0	2.8	150.0	513	3.9
oats, wheat, and other grains, unprepared	1/4 cup	11	0.16	0.11	1.60	0.19	17.5	0.00	0.0	13.8	0.7	37.5	128	1.0
wheat w/other grains, plain, prepared w/water	1 cup	0	0.24	0.12	3.10	0.11	24.1	0.00	0.0	28.9	2.1	108.0	301	1.8
wheat w/other grains, plain, prepared w/water	1 cup	0	0.18	0.09	2.30	0.09	18.1	0.00	0.0	21.7	1.6	81.5	226	1.3
wheat w/other grains, plain, prepared w/water, salt	3/4 cup	0	0.18	0.09	2.30	0.09	18.1	0.00	0.0	21.7	1.6	81.5	226	1.3
wheat w/other grains, plain, prepared w/water, salt	3/4 cup	0	0.18	0.09	2.30	0.09	18.1	0.00	0.0	21.7	1.6	81.5	226	1.3
wheat w/other grains, plain, unprepared	1 cup	0	0.47	0.23	6.30	0.23	65.1	0.00	0.0	60.5	4.3	220.0	614	3.6
wheat w/other grains, plain, unprepared	1/3 cup	0	0.16	0.08	2.10	0.08	21.7	0.00	0.0	20.1	1.4	73.5	205	1.2
wheat w/other grains, plain, unprepared	1 tbsp	0	0.03	0.02	0.39	0.02	4.1	0.00	0.0	3.8	0.3	13.7	38	0.2
OAT BRAN														
(Quaker) 'Mother's' unprepared	1/2 cup	40	0.39	0.12	0.32	0.04	15.2	0.00	0.0	31.6	3.2	96.4	232	1.7
OATMEAL AND OATS														
regular, quick, or instant, not fortified, unprepared	1 cup	82	0.59	0.11	0.63	0.10	25.9	0.00	0.0	42.1	3.4	120.0	284	2.5
regular, quick, or instant, not fortified, unprepared	1/3 cup	27	0.20	0.04	0.21	0.03	8.6	0.00	0.0	14.0	1.1	40.0	95	0.8
(Maypo)														
oat, w/other grains, prepared w/water	1 cup	2338	0.72	0.72	9.40	0.96	9.6	2.90	28.8	125.0	8.4	50.4	211	1.5
oat, w/other grains, prepared w/water	3/4 cup	1753	0.54	0.54	7.00	0.72	7.2	2.20	21.6	93.6	6.3	37.8	158	1.1
oat, w/other grains, prepared w/water	1 tbsp	146	0.05	0.05	0.58	0.06	0.6	0.18	1.8	7.8	0.5	3.1	13	<0.1
oat, w/other grains, prepared w/water, salt	1 cup	2338	0.72	0.72	9.40	0.96	9.6	2.90	28.8	125.0	8.4	50.4	211	1.5
oat, w/other grains, prepared w/water, salt	3/4 cup	1753	0.54	0.54	7.00	0.72	7.2	2.20	21.6	93.6	6.3	37.8	158	1.1
oat, w/other grains, unprepared	1 cup	4974	1.50	1.70	19.9	2.00	25.4	5.90	60.2	265.0	17.9	108.0	449	3.1
oat, w/other grains, unprepared	3/4 cup	2487	0.75	0.85	10.0	0.99	12.7	3.00	30.1	133.0	8.9	54.0	225	1.6
(Quaker)														
apple spice, microwave, 'Quick 'n Hearty'	1 pkt	1050	0.31	0.36	4.20	0.42	84.2	0.00	0.5	108.0	4.0	36.5	138	0.8

Food Name	Serving Size	A I.U.	Thi mg	Rib mg	Nia mg	B$_6$ mg	Fol mcg	B$_{12}$ mcg	C mg	Calc mg	Iron mg	Mag mg	Pot mg	Zn mg
brown sugar cinnamon, microwave, 'Quick 'n Hearty'	1 pkt	1050	0.31	0.36	4.20	0.42	84.0	0.00	<0.1	108.0	4.0	40.3	125	0.9
cinnamon double raisin, microwave, 'Quick 'n Hearty'	1 pkt	1050	0.31	0.36	4.20	0.42	84.1	na	0.5	108.0	4.0	39.5	188	0.8
'Cinnamagic' instant, unprepared	1 pkt	1275	0.36	0.23	3.80	0.42	103.0	0.00	0.1	178.0	6.3	37.2	118	0.9
fruit punch flavor, instant, 'Power Rangers' unprepared	1 pkt	1273	0.35	0.22	3.80	0.42	108.0	0.00	0.0	176.0	6.2	34.8	99	0.8
fruit and cream, instant, unprepared	1 pkt	1050	0.31	0.36	4.20	0.42	84.0	0.01	0.1	106.0	4.0	27.6	97	0.6
honey bran, microwave, 'Quick 'n Hearty'	1 pkt	1050	0.31	0.36	4.20	0.42	84.0	0.00	0.0	108.0	4.0	41.4	118	0.9
low-salt, instant, unprepared	1 pkt	1050	0.31	0.36	4.20	0.42	84.3	0.00	0.0	107.0	8.2	37.5	105	0.8
maple and brown sugar, instant, prepared w/water	1 pkt	1008	0.30	0.34	4.00	0.40	80.6	0.00	0.0	105.0	3.9	38.8	112	0.9
maple and brown sugar, instant, unprepared	1 pkt	1050	0.31	0.36	4.20	0.42	83.8	0.00	0.0	108.0	4.0	40.0	117	0.9
regular flavor, microwave, 'Quick 'n Hearty'	1 pkt	1050	0.31	0.36	4.20	0.42	84.1	0.00	0.0	108.0	8.5	38.6	110	0.9
w/apples and cinnamon, instant, prepared w/water	1 pkt	1019	0.30	0.35	4.10	0.41	93.9	0.00	0.3	104.0	3.9	29.8	106	0.7
w/apples and cinnamon, instant, unprepared	1 pkt	1050	0.31	0.36	4.20	0.42	84.0	0.00	0.3	106.0	4.0	30.1	109	0.7
(Ralston)														
prepared w/water, salt	1 cup	0	0.20	0.18	2.00	0.11	17.7	0.11	0.0	12.7	1.6	58.2	154	1.4
prepared w/water, salt	3/4 cup	0	0.15	0.13	1.50	0.09	13.3	0.08	0.0	9.5	1.2	43.7	116	1.1
(Under Cover Bears)														
plain, instant, prepared w/water	1 pkt	1032	0.36	0.19	3.70	0.51	66.5	0.00	0.0	111.0	4.3	29.0	68	0.6
RICE														
(Cream of Rice)														
cream of, prepared w/water, no salt	1 cup	0	0.00	0.00	0.98	0.07	7.3	0.00	0.0	7.3	0.5	7.3	49	0.4
cream of, prepared w/water, no salt	3/4 cup	0	0.00	0.00	0.73	0.05	5.5	0.00	0.0	5.5	0.4	5.5	37	0.3
cream of, prepared w/water, no salt	1 tbsp	0	0.00	0.00	0.06	0.00	0.5	0.00	0.0	0.5	<0.1	0.5	3	<0.1
cream of, prepared w/water, salt	1 cup	0	0.00	0.00	0.98	0.07	7.3	0.00	0.0	7.3	0.5	7.3	49	0.4
cream of, prepared w/water, salt	3/4 cup	0	0.00	0.00	0.73	0.05	5.5	0.00	0.0	5.5	0.4	5.5	37	0.3
cream of, unprepared	1 cup	0	0.35	0.17	5.20	0.34	50.2	0.00	0.0	41.5	2.2	39.8	247	1.9
cream of, unprepared	1 tbsp	0	0.02	0.01	0.31	0.02	3.0	0.00	0.0	2.4	0.1	2.3	15	0.1
WHEAT														
(Cream of Wheat)														
cream of, apple, banana and maple flavored, 'Mix 'N Eat' prepared	1 pkt	1251	0.45	0.30	5.00	0.45	101.0	0.00	0.0	40.5	8.1	9.0	56	0.2
cream of, apple, banana and maple flavored, 'Mix 'N Eat' unprepared	1 pkt	1250	0.39	0.25	5.00	0.50	99.8	0.00	0.0	40.0	8.1	9.2	55	0.2
cream of, instant, prepared w/water	1 cup	0	0.24	0.00	1.70	0.03	149.0	0.00	0.0	60.3	12.1	14.5	48	0.4
cream of, instant, prepared w/water	3/4 cup	0	0.18	0.00	1.30	0.02	112.0	0.00	0.0	45.3	9.1	10.9	36	0.3
cream of, instant, prepared w/water, salt	1 cup	0	0.24	0.00	1.70	0.03	149.0	0.00	0.0	60.3	12.1	14.5	48	0.4
cream of, instant, prepared w/water, salt	3/4 cup	0	0.18	0.00	1.30	0.02	112.0	0.00	0.0	45.3	9.1	10.9	36	0.3
cream of, instant, prepared w/water, salt	1 tbsp	0	0.02	0.00	0.11	0.00	9.4	0.00	0.0	3.8	0.8	0.91	3	<0.1
cream of, plain, 'Mix 'N Eat' prepared	1 pkt	1252	0.43	0.28	5.00	0.57	101.0	0.00	0.0	19.9	8.1	7.1	38	0.2
cream of, plain, 'Mix 'N Eat' unprepared	1 pkt	1250	0.37	0.26	5.00	0.51	100.0	0.00	0.0	20.1	8.1	7.7	38	0.2
cream of, quick, prepared w/water	1 cup	0	0.24	0.00	1.40	0.03	108.0	0.00	0.0	50.2	10.3	11.9	45	0.3

Food Name	Serving Size	A I.U.	Thi mg	Rib mg	Nia mg	B$_6$ mg	Fol mcg	B$_{12}$ mcg	C mg	Calc mg	Iron mg	Mag mg	Pot mg	Zn mg
cream of, quick, prepared w/water	3/4 cup	0	0.18	0.00	1.10	0.02	80.5	0.00	0.0	37.6	7.7	8.9	34	0.2
cream of, quick, prepared w/water	1 tbsp	0	0.02	0.00	0.09	0.00	6.7	0.00	0.0	3.1	0.6	0.8	3	<0.1
cream of, quick, prepared w/water, salt	1 cup	0	0.24	0.00	1.40	0.03	108.0	0.00	0.0	50.2	10.3	11.9	45	0.3
cream of, quick, prepared w/water, salt	3/4 cup	0	0.18	0.00	1.10	0.02	80.5	0.00	0.0	37.6	7.7	8.9	34	0.2
cream of, quick, unprepared	1 cup	0	0.88	0.35	7.40	0.16	213.0	0.00	0.0	248.0	50.3	58.1	229	1.7
cream of, quick, unprepared	1 tbsp	0	0.06	0.02	0.46	0.01	13.3	0.00	0.0	15.5	3.1	3.6	14	0.1
cream of, regular, prepared w/water	1 cup	0	0.25	0.00	1.50	0.04	45.2	0.00	0.0	50.2	10.3	10.0	43	0.3
cream of, regular, prepared w/water	3/4 cup	0	0.19	0.00	1.10	0.03	33.8	0.00	0.0	37.6	7.7	7.5	32	0.2
cream of, regular, prepared w/water	1 tbsp	0	0.02	0.00	0.09	0.00	2.8	0.00	0.0	3.1	0.6	0.6	23	<0.1
cream of, regular, prepared w/water, salt	1 cup	0	0.25	0.00	1.50	0.04	45.2	0.00	0.0	50.2	10.3	10.0	43	0.3
cream of, regular, prepared w/water, salt	3/4 cup	0	0.19	0.00	1.10	0.03	33.8	0.00	0.0	37.6	7.7	7.5	32	0.2
cream of, regular, unprepared	1 cup	0	0.89	0.36	7.50	0.16	635.0	0.00	0.0	251.0	50.9	60.5	205	1.7
cream of, regular, unprepared	1 tbsp	0	0.06	0.02	0.48	0.01	41.1	0.00	0.0	16.2	3.3	3.9	13	0.1
(Malt-O-Meal)														
and barley, plain or chocolate, prepared w/water	1 cup	0	0.48	0.24	5.80	0.02	4.8	0.00	0.0	4.8	9.6	4.8	31	0.2
and barley, plain or chocolate, prepared w/water	3/4 cup	0	0.36	0.18	4.30	0.01	3.6	0.00	0.0	3.6	7.2	3.6	23	0.1
and barley, plain or chocolate, prepared w/water	1 tbsp	0	0.03	0.02	0.36	0.00	0.3	0.00	0.0	0.3	0.6	0.3	2	<0.1
and barley, plain or chocolate, prepared w/water, salt	1 cup	0	0.48	0.24	5.80	0.02	4.8	0.00	0.0	4.8	9.6	4.8	31	0.2
and barley, plain or chocolate, prepared w/water, salt	3/4 cup	0	0.36	0.18	4.30	0.01	3.6	0.00	0.0	3.6	7.2	3.6	23	0.1
and barley, plain, unprepared	1 cup	0	2.10	1.50	29.0	0.10	39.6	0.00	0.0	23.1	47.2	21.4	155	0.9
and barley, plain, unprepared	1 tbsp	0	0.13	0.09	1.80	0.01	2.5	0.00	0.0	1.4	2.9	1.3	10	<0.1
(Maltex)														
'Maltex' prepared w/water	1 cup	0	0.25	0.10	2.40	0.08	22.4	0.00	0.0	17.4	1.8	57.3	266	1.9
'Maltex' prepared w/water	3/4 cup	0	0.19	0.08	1.80	0.06	16.8	0.00	0.0	13.1	1.3	43.0	200	1.4
'Maltex' prepared w/water	1 tbsp	0	0.02	0.01	0.15	0.01	1.4	0.00	0.0	1.1	0.1	3.6	17	0.1
'Maltex' prepared w/water, salt	1 cup	0	0.25	0.10	2.40	0.08	22.4	0.00	0.0	17.4	1.8	57.3	266	1.9
'Maltex' prepared w/water, salt	3/4 cup	0	0.19	0.08	1.80	0.06	16.8	0.00	0.0	13.1	1.3	43.0	200	1.4
'Maltex' unprepared	1 cup	0	0.79	0.30	7.00	0.23	86.1	0.00	0.0	54.4	5.3	168.0	787	5.5
'Maltex' unprepared	1/4 cup	0	0.20	0.08	1.80	0.06	21.7	0.00	0.0	13.7	1.3	42.2	198	1.4
(Ralston)														
'Ralston' prepared w/water	1 cup	0	0.20	0.18	2.00	0.11	17.7	0.11	0.0	12.7	1.6	58.2	154	1.4
'Ralston' prepared w/water	3/4 cup	0	0.15	0.13	1.50	0.09	13.3	0.08	0.0	9.5	1.2	43.7	116	1.1
'Ralston' prepared w/water	1 tbsp	0	0.01	0.01	0.13	0.01	1.1	0.01	0.0	0.8	0.1	3.6	10	<0.1
'Ralston' unprepared	1 cup	0	0.64	0.57	6.20	0.34	70.8	0.33	0.0	41.3	5.0	179.0	463	4.2
'Ralston' unprepared	1/4 cup	0	0.16	0.14	1.60	0.09	18.0	0.08	0.0	10.5	1.3	45.6	118	1.1
(Wheatena)														
'Wheatena' prepared w/water	1 cup	0	0.02	0.05	1.30	0.05	17.0	0.00	0.0	9.7	1.4	48.6	187	1.7
'Wheatena' prepared w/water	3/4 cup	0	0.02	0.04	1.00	0.04	12.7	0.00	0.0	7.3	1.0	36.4	140	1.3
'Wheatena' prepared w/water, salt	1 cup	0	0.02	0.05	1.30	0.05	17.0	0.00	0.0	9.7	1.4	48.6	187	1.7
'Wheatena' prepared w/water, salt	3/4 cup	0	0.02	0.04	1.00	0.04	12.7	0.00	0.0	7.3	1.0	36.4	140	1.3
'Wheatena' unprepared	1 cup	0	0.10	0.20	5.00	0.17	83.2	0.00	0.0	39.5	5.0	183.0	694	6.2
'Wheatena' unprepared	1/4 cup	0	0.03	0.05	1.20	0.04	20.6	0.00	0.0	9.8	1.2	45.5	172	1.5
CEREAL, READY-TO-EAT														
(Chex) See under *(General Mills)*.														
(General Mills)														
'Basic 4'	1 cup	1250	0.37	0.42	5.00	0.50	99.5	0.00	15.0	310.0	4.5	40.1	162	3.8
'Berry Berry Kix'	3/4 cup	750	0.38	0.43	5.00	0.50	99.9	0.00	15.0	66.0	4.5	5.7	24	3.8

Food Name	Serving Size	A I.U.	Thi mg	Rib mg	Nia mg	B_6 mg	Fol mcg	B_{12} mcg	C mg	Calc mg	Iron mg	Mag mg	Pot mg	Zn mg
'Body Buddies'	1 cup	750	0.38	0.43	5.00	0.50	99.9	1.50	15.0	49.5	8.1	6.6	26	3.8
'Boo Berry'	1 cup	0	0.38	0.43	5.00	0.50	99.9	0.00	15.0	20.4	4.5	2.7	18	3.8
'Cheerios'	1 cup	1250	0.38	0.43	5.00	0.50	99.9	0.00	15.0	55.2	8.1	32.7	89	3.8
'Cheerios' apple cinnamon	3/4 cup	750	0.38	0.43	5.00	0.50	99.9	0.00	15.0	35.4	4.5	20.1	60	3.8
'Cheerios' honey nut	1 cup	750	0.38	0.43	5.00	0.50	99.9	0.00	15.0	20.4	4.5	29.4	85	3.8
'Cheerios' multigrain	1 cup	750	0.38	0.43	5.00	0.50	99.9	0.00	15.0	57.0	8.1	29.7	97	3.8
'Cheerios Plus' multigrain	1 cup	500	1.50	1.70	20.0	2.00	400.0	6.00	15.0	100.0	18.0	27.9	88	15.0
'Chex' bran	1 cup	107	0.64	0.27	8.60	0.88	173.0	2.60	26.0	29.4	14.0	69.1	216	6.5
'Chex' corn	1 cup	0	0.38	0.00	5.00	0.50	99.9	1.50	6.0	100.0	9.0	8.4	32	0.4
'Chex' honey nut	3/4 cup	0	0.38	0.44	5.00	0.51	100.0	1.50	6.0	102.0	9.0	0.0	27	0
'Chex' multi-bran	1 cup	0	0.32	0.00	4.40	0.44	88.2	1.30	5.1	95.1	13.7	59.8	191	3.2
'Chex' rice	1.25 cup	0	0.38	0.02	5.00	0.50	99.8	1.50	6.0	104.0	9.0	9.3	36	0
'Chex' wheat	1 cup	0	0.23	0.04	3.00	0.30	60.0	0.90	3.6	60.0	9.0	33.6	116	0.8
'Cinnamon Streusel' Betty Crocker	3/4 cup	750	0.38	0.43	5.00	0.50	99.9	0.00	15.0	33.9	4.5	14.4	58	3.8
'Cinnamon Toast Crunch'	3/4 cup	750	0.38	0.43	5.00	0.50	99.9	0.00	15.0	42.3	4.5	13.5	44	3.8
'Cocoa Puffs'	1 cup	0	0.38	0.43	5.00	0.50	99.9	0.00	15.0	33.0	4.5	6.6	52	3.8
'Cookie-Crisp'	1 cup	0	0.39	0.27	5.30	0.54	106.0	1.60	0.0	5.7	4.8	8.4	29	3.2
'Corn Flakes'	1 cup	96	0.13	0.03	1.10	0.02	1.8	0.00	0.0	1.8	0.6	2.8	22	<0.1
'Count Chocula'	1 cup	0	0.38	0.43	5.00	0.50	99.9	0.00	15.0	28.5	4.5	9.3	63	3.8
'Country Corn Flakes'	1 cup	750	0.38	0.48	5.00	0.50	99.9	0.00	15.0	53.4	8.1	7.2	40	3.8
'Crispy Wheats 'N Raisins'	1 cup	1250	0.37	0.42	5.00	0.50	99.5	0.00	0.0	69.3	4.5	42.4	230	1.1
'Crunchy Bran'	3/4 cup	38	0.08	0.42	5.00	0.50	100.0	0.00	0.0	20.5	7.6	14.3	56	3.8
'Dutch Apple' Betty Crocker	1 cup	750	0.37	0.42	5.00	0.50	99.5	0.00	15.0	57.2	4.5	24.2	101	4.9
'Fiber One'	1/2 cup	0	0.38	0.43	5.00	0.50	99.9	0.00	9.0	58.5	4.5	68.1	217	1.2
'40% Bran Flakes'	1 cup	2160	0.64	0.73	8.60	0.88	173.0	2.60	26.0	22.5	7.8	118.0	286	2.0
'40% Bran Flakes'	1 oz	1250	0.37	0.42	5.00	0.51	100.0	1.50	15.0	13.0	4.5	68.0	166	1.2
'Frankenberry'	1 cup	0	0.38	0.43	5.00	0.50	99.9	0.00	15.0	24.6	4.5	2.7	16	3.8
'Golden Grahams'	3/4 cup	750	0.38	0.43	5.00	0.50	99.9	0.00	15.0	14.4	4.5	9.3	53	3.8
'Honey Frosted Wheaties'	3/4 cup	750	0.38	0.43	5.00	0.50	99.9	0.00	15.0	7.8	4.5	10.8	56	3.8
'Honey Nut Clusters'	1 cup	0	0.37	0.42	5.00	0.50	100.0	0.00	9.0	71.5	4.5	51.7	171	1.0
'Kaboom'	1.25 cup	750	0.38	0.43	5.00	0.50	99.9	0.00	15.0	50.4	8.1	18.9	60	3.8
'Kix'	1 1/3 cup	1250	0.38	0.43	5.00	0.50	99.9	0.00	15.0	43.5	8.1	9.3	41	3.8
'Lucky Charms'	1 cup	750	0.38	0.43	5.00	0.50	99.9	0.00	15.0	32.4	4.5	19.5	54	3.8
'Nature Valley Granola' cinnamon and raisin	3/4 cup	0	0.18	0.04	0.56	0.08	8.3	0.00	0.0	42.9	1.3	55.0	189	0.9
'Nature Valley Granola' fruit, low-fat	2/3 cup	0	0.09	0.05	0.95	0.06	7.2	0.00	0.0	39.6	1.4	18.7	162	0.9
'Nature Valley Granola' fruit and nut	2/3 cup	0	0.19	0.09	0.64	0.07	9.9	0.00	0.0	45.6	1.7	55.5	194	1.1
'Nature Valley Granola' toasted oats	3/4 cup	0	0.17	0.06	0.61	0.08	8.3	0.00	0.0	41.3	1.7	52.3	183	1.1
'Oatmeal Crisp w/Almonds'	1 cup	0	0.37	0.42	5.00	0.50	99.5	0.00	9.0	35.8	4.5	57.2	185	3.8
'Oatmeal Crisp w/Apples'	1 cup	0	0.37	0.42	5.00	0.50	99.5	0.00	9.0	23.1	4.5	45.1	160	3.8
'Oatmeal Raisin Crisp'	1 cup	750	0.37	0.42	5.00	0.50	100.0	0.00	0.0	38.0	4.5	44.5	212	3.8
'Raisin Bran'	1 cup	1852	0.56	0.62	7.40	0.73	148.0	2.20	1.7	26.9	27.3	84.6	287	1.7
'Raisin Bran'	1-1/3 oz	1250	0.38	0.42	5.00	0.49	100.0	1.50	1.1	18.1	18.4	57.1	194	1.1
'Raisin Nut Bran'	1 cup	0	0.37	0.42	5.00	0.50	99.5	0.00	0.0	73.7	4.5	53.9	218	1.1
'Reese's Peanut Butter Puffs'	3/4 cup	750	0.38	0.43	5.00	0.50	99.9	0.00	15.0	21.0	4.5	15.9	62	3.8
'S'Mores Grahams'	3/4 cup	750	0.38	0.43	5.00	0.50	99.9	0.00	15.0	14.4	4.5	10.8	48	3.8
'Sugar Frosted Flakes'	1 cup	1675	0.49	0.57	6.70	0.68	2.7	2.00	20.1	4.2	1.0	2.7	24	0.8
'Sun Crunchers'	1 cup	750	0.37	0.42	5.00	0.50	99.5	0.00	15.0	85.3	4.5	43.5	130	0.8
'Team Cheerios'	1 cup	500	0.38	0.43	5.00	0.50	203.0	1.50	6.0	106.0	4.5	21.6	70	3.8
'Total'	3/4 cup	1250	1.50	1.70	20.10	2.00	400.0	7.70	60.0	258.0	18.0	32.1	97	15.0
'Total Corn Flakes'	1 1/3 cup	1250	1.50	1.70	20.10	2.00	400.0	8.10	60.0	237.0	18.0	7.8	34	15.0
'Total Raisin Bran'	1 cup	1250	1.50	1.70	20.00	2.00	400.0	6.40	0.0	238.0	18.0	44.5	287	15.0
'Triples'	1 cup	1250	0.38	0.43	5.00	0.50	99.9	0.00	15.0	41.1	8.1	6.9	31	3.8
'Trix'	1 cup	750	0.38	0.43	5.00	0.50	99.9	0.00	15.0	32.1	4.5	3.6	18	3.8

Food Name	Serving Size	A I.U.	Thi mg	Rib mg	Nia mg	B$_6$ mg	Fol mcg	B$_{12}$ mcg	C mg	Calc mg	Iron mg	Mag mg	Pot mg	Zn mg
'Wheaties'	1 cup	750	0.38	0.43	5.00	0.50	99.9	0.00	15.0	54.6	8.1	31.8	104	0.7
(Heartland)														
'Heartland Natural' plain	1 cup	65	0.36	0.16	1.60	0.19	64.4	0.00	1.1	74.8	4.3	147.0	385	3.0
'Heartland Natural, plain	1 oz	15.9	0.09	0.04	0.40	0.05	15.9	0.00	0.3	18.4	1.1	36.3	95	0.8
'Heartland Natural' w/coconut	1 cup	57	0.35	0.15	1.80	0.17	56.7	0.00	1.1	66.2	5.4	138.0	384	2.7
'Heartland Natural' w/coconut	1 oz	15	0.09	0.04	0.48	0.05	15.3	0.00	0.3	17.9	1.5	37.1	104	0.7
'Heartland Natural' w/raisins	1 cup	63	0.32	0.14	1.50	0.20	44.0	0.00	1.1	66.0	4.0	141.0	415	2.8
(Honeybran)														
'Honeybran'	1 cup	1543	0.46	0.53	6.20	0.63	23.4	1.90	18.6	16.1	5.6	45.9	151	0.9
'Honeybran'	1 oz	1250	0.37	0.42	5.00	0.51	19.0	1.50	15.0	13.0	4.5	37.1	122	0.7
(Kellogg's)														
'All-Bran'	1/2 cup	750	0.39	0.42	5.00	0.51	90.0	1.50	15.0	106.0	4.5	129.0	342	3.8
'All-Bran Bran Buds'	1/3 cup	750	0.39	0.42	5.00	0.51	90.0	0.00	15.0	20.1	4.5	83.4	270	6.5
'All-Bran' w/extra fiber	1/2 cup	866	0.42	0.48	5.80	0.57	120.0	1.70	17.3	116.0	5.2	120.0	300	4.3
'Apple Jacks'	1 cup	750	0.39	0.42	5.00	0.51	106.0	0.00	15.0	3.3	4.5	8.7	32	3.8
'Apple Raisin Crisp'	1 cup	778	0.39	0.44	5.20	0.50	110.0	1.50	0.0	14.8	1.9	9.9	85	1.5
'Bran Flakes'	3/4 cup	1208	0.38	0.44	5.00	0.49	102.0	1.40	15.0	13.9	8.1	60.0	175	3.8
'Cinnamon Mini Buns'	3/4 cup	750	0.39	0.42	5.00	0.51	90.0	0.00	15.0	3.9	4.5	11.1	37	3.8
'Cocoa Frosted Flakes'	3/4 cup	750	0.37	0.43	5.00	0.50	93.0	1.50	15.0	0.6	4.5	3.1	19	<0.1
'Cocoa Krispies'	3/4 cup	750	0.37	0.43	5.00	0.50	93.0	0.00	15.0	4.0	1.8	11.5	60	1.5
'Common Sense Oat Bran Flakes'	3/4 cup	750	0.39	0.42	5.00	0.51	90.0	1.50	0.0	14.7	8.4	47.7	120	3.8
'Corn Flakes'	1 cup	700	0.36	0.39	4.70	0.48	98.8	0.00	14.0	1.1	8.7	3.4	26	0.2
'Corn Pops'	1 cup	775	0.40	0.43	5.20	0.53	109.0	0.00	15.5	2.5	1.9	2.5	23	1.6
'Cracklin' Oat Bran'	3/4 cup	842	0.42	0.48	5.60	0.56	153.0	0.00	16.8	24.8	2.0	76.5	255	1.6
'Crispix'	1 cup	750	0.38	0.44	5.00	0.49	87.0	0.00	15.0	3.5	1.8	7.0	35	1.5
'Double Dip Crunch'	3/4 cup	776	0.39	0.45	5.20	0.51	90.0	0.00	15.5	2.1	1.9	5.1	21	1.6
'Froot Loops'	1 cup	703	0.39	0.42	5.00	0.51	90.0	0.00	14.1	3.3	4.2	8.7	32	3.8
'Frosted Bran'	3/4 cup	726	0.36	0.42	4.80	0.48	90.0	1.40	14.5	9.3	4.3	37.8	122	3.6
'Frosted Flakes'	3/4 cup	750	0.37	0.43	5.00	0.50	93.0	0.00	15.0	0.6	4.5	2.8	21	0.2
'Frosted Krispies'	3/4 cup	866	0.42	0.48	5.80	0.57	120.0	0.00	17.3	2.1	2.1	7.2	23	0.4
'Frosted Mini-Wheats' bite size	1 cup	0	0.33	0.39	4.70	0.44	110.0	1.40	0.0	0.0	15.4	55.5	186	1.4
'Frosted Mini-Wheats' regular	1 cup	0	0.36	0.41	5.00	0.46	102.0	1.50	0.0	18.4	14.3	51.5	170	1.5
'Fruity Marshmallow Krispies'	3/4 cup	804	0.39	0.45	5.40	0.54	120.0	0.00	16.1	1.5	1.9	6.3	18	0.3
granola, w/o raisins, low-fat	1/2 cup	842	0.44	0.50	5.60	0.55	110.0	1.70	1.6	22.6	2.0	46.8	138	4.2
granola, w/raisins, low-fat	2/3 cup	688	0.33	0.39	4.60	0.44	110.0	1.40	1.6	24.2	1.9	45.6	156	3.5
'Healthy Choice Almond Crunch with Raisins'	1 cup	474	0.50	0.55	6.70	0.66	110.0	2.00	0.0	26.9	6.0	49.0	198	1.4
'Healthy Choice Multigrain' flakes	1 cup	500	0.54	0.60	7.00	0.69	90.0	2.10	0.0	8.7	6.3	29.1	100	1.5
'Healthy Choice Toasted Brown Sugar Squares'	1.25 cup	509	0.55	0.60	7.20	0.71	110.0	2.10	0.0	18.7	6.4	59.4	214	1.5
'Honey Crunch Corn Flakes'	3/4 cup	750	0.39	0.42	5.00	0.51	90.0	0.00	15.0	4.2	1.8	7.2	31	0.2
'Just Right' fruit and nut	1 cup	1146	0.33	0.39	4.60	0.44	110.0	1.40	0.0	0.0	14.8	33.0	156	1.0
'Just Right' w/crunchy nuggets	1 cup	1250	0.39	0.44	5.00	0.50	102.0	1.50	0.0	14.3	16.2	34.1	121	0.9
'Mini-Wheats' apple cinnamon	3/4 cup	0	0.39	0.44	5.00	0.50	110.0	1.50	0.0	20.9	16.2	48.4	166	1.5
'Mini-Wheats' blueberry	3/4 cup	0	0.39	0.44	5.10	0.50	110.0	1.50	0.0	19.3	16.5	51.1	183	1.5
'Mini-Wheats' raisin	3/4 cup	0	0.39	0.44	5.20	0.50	110.0	1.50	0.0	18.7	16.8	47.9	260	1.5
'Mini-Wheats' strawberry	1 cup	0	0.44	0.50	5.50	0.55	110.0	1.60	0.0	22.0	17.8	66.0	187	1.6
'Mueslix' apple and orange crunch	3/4 cup	778	0.39	0.44	5.20	0.50	110.0	1.30	0.0	33.5	4.7	62.7	209	3.1
'Mueslix' raisin and almond crunch, w/dates	2/3 cup	200	0.39	0.44	5.00	0.00	110.0	1.50	0.0	19.8	4.5	46.8	230	3.7
'Nut & Honey Crunch'	1.25 cup	750	0.39	0.44	5.00	0.50	110.0	0.00	15.0	5.5	4.5	5.0	60	0.4
'Nutri-Grain Wheat'	3/4 cup	0	0.39	0.42	5.00	0.51	90.0	1.50	15.0	9.6	1.0	24.3	110	3.8
'Pop-Tarts Crunch' strawberry, frosted	3/4 cup	682	0.33	0.39	4.60	0.45	90.0	0.00	13.8	2.4	4.1	9.6	27	3.4
'Product 19'	1 cup	750	1.50	1.70	20.0	2.00	390.0	6.00	60.0	2.7	18.0	12.3	41	15.0

Food Name	Serving Size	A I.U.	Thi mg	Rib mg	Nia mg	B6 mg	Fol mcg	B12 mcg	C mg	Calc mg	Iron mg	Mag mg	Pot mg	Zn mg
'Raisin Bran'	1 cup	832	0.43	0.49	5.60	0.55	122.0	1.60	0.0	35.4	5.0	89.1	437	4.1
'Razzle Dazzle Rice Krispies'	3/4 cup	500	0.36	0.42	5.00	0.50	112.0	1.50	15.0	2.0	1.8	8.1	27	0.6
'Rice Krispies'	1.25 cup	825	0.43	0.46	5.50	0.56	116.0	0.00	16.5	3.3	2.0	15.8	42	0.6
'Rice Krispies' apple cinnamon	3/4 cup	776	0.39	0.45	5.20	0.51	90.0	1.50	15.5	2.1	1.9	7.8	31	0.3
'Rice Krispies Treats'	3/4 cup	750	0.39	0.42	5.00	0.51	90.0	1.50	15.0	1.8	1.8	6.3	19	0.3
'Smacks'	3/4 cup	750	0.38	0.43	5.00	0.51	99.9	0.00	15.1	3.0	1.8	15.9	42	0.4
'Smart Start'	1 cup	750	1.50	1.70	20.0	2.00	400.0	6.00	15.0	10.5	18.0	29.5	102	15.0
'Special K'	1 cup	750	0.53	0.59	7.00	0.71	93.0	0.00	15.0	4.7	8.7	17.7	55	3.8
'Temptations' French vanilla almond	3/4 cup	866	0.42	0.48	5.80	0.57	120.0	0.00	17.3	10.8	5.2	6.9	41	0.2
'Temptations' honey roasted pecan	1 cup	776	0.39	0.45	5.20	0.51	90.0	0.00	15.5	0.6	4.7	2.7	29	0.1
(Malt-O-Meal)														
'Berry Colossal Crunch'	3/4 cup	0	0.38	0.43	5.00	0.50	99.9	0.00	0.0	2.4	4.5	5.7	40	3.8
'Colossal Crunch'	3/4 cup	0	0.38	0.43	5.00	0.50	99.9	0.00	0.0	3.0	4.5	15.0	40	3.8
'Corn Bursts'	1 cup	750	0.75	0.85	10.00	0.00	99.8	1.50	15.0	11.2	1.8	1.2	16	1.5
'Crispy Rice'	1 cup	750	0.45	0.51	6.00	0.50	120.0	1.80	15.0	0.0	1.8	7.9	46	0.6
'Marchmallow Mateys'	1 cup	500	0.38	0.43	5.00	0.50	200.0	1.50	6.0	99.9	5.7	18.0	62	4.2
'Toasty O's'	1 cup	1250	0.38	0.43	5.00	0.50	99.9	0.00	15.0	39.9	8.1	32.1	93	3.8
'Tootie Fruities'	1 cup	750	0.37	0.43	5.00	0.50	99.8	1.50	15.0	99.8	4.5	8.0	39	3.8
(Nature Valley) See under (General Mills).														
(Post)														
'Alpha-Bits' w/marshmallows	1 cup	750	0.37	0.43	5.00	0.50	100.0	1.50	0.0	4.1	2.7	11.9	29	1.5
'Banana Nut Crunch'	1 cup	750	0.38	0.42	5.00	0.50	99.7	1.50	0.1	21.2	16.2	48.4	171	1.5
'Blueberry Morning'	1.25 cup	750	0.37	0.42	5.00	0.50	100.0	1.50	0.0	14.8	1.8	23.6	91	0.9
'Bran Flakes'	3/4 cup	750	0.38	0.43	5.00	0.50	99.9	1.50	0.0	16.8	8.1	64.2	185	1.5
'Cocoa Pebbles'	3/4 cup	750	0.37	0.43	5.00	0.50	100.0	1.50	0.0	3.5	1.8	10.7	42	1.5
'Frosted Alpha-Bits'	1 cup	750	0.37	0.43	5.00	0.50	99.8	1.50	0.0	9.6	2.7	25.0	62	1.5
'Frosted Shredded Wheat' bite size	1 cup	0	0.37	0.43	5.00	0.50	99.8	1.50	0.0	6.8	1.8	48.4	170	1.5
'Fruit & Fibre' w/dates, raisins and walnuts	1 cup	750	0.37	0.42	5.00	0.50	100.0	1.50	0.0	23.6	5.4	66.0	244	1.5
'Fruity Pebbles'	3/4 cup	750	0.38	0.42	5.00	0.50	99.9	1.50	0.0	1.4	1.8	5.1	30	1.5
'Golden Crisp'	3/4 cup	750	0.38	0.42	5.00	0.50	99.9	1.50	0.0	4.0	1.8	16.5	34	1.5
'Grape-Nuts'	1/2 cup	750	0.38	0.42	5.00	0.50	99.8	1.50	0.0	19.7	16.2	58.0	178	1.2
'Grape-Nuts Flakes'	3/4 cup	750	0.37	0.43	5.00	0.50	100.0	1.50	0.0	11.3	8.1	29.9	99	1.2
'Great Grains' crunchy pecan	2/3 cup	750	0.38	0.45	5.00	0.50	100.0	1.50	0.1	14.8	2.7	46.1	170	1.2
'Great Grains' raisin, date, and pecan	2/3 cup	750	0.38	0.43	5.00	0.50	99.9	1.50	<0.1	16.7	3.6	45.4	176	1.2
'Honey Bunches Of Oats'	3/4 cup	750	0.38	0.43	5.00	0.50	99.9	1.50	0.0	6.3	8.1	16.5	52	0.3
'Honey Bunches Of Oats' w/almonds	3/4 cup	750	0.38	0.42	5.00	0.50	100.0	1.50	<0.1	11.5	8.1	21.4	70	0.3
'Honeycomb'	1 1/3 cup	750	0.37	0.43	5.00	0.50	100.0	1.50	0.0	4.9	2.7	10.7	35	1.5
'100% Bran'	1/3 cup	750	0.37	0.43	5.00	0.50	100.0	1.50	0.0	22.0	8.1	80.6	275	3.8
'Oreo O's'	3/4 cup	750	0.38	0.42	5.00	0.50	99.9	1.50	0.0	5.1	1.8	14.8	49	1.5
'Raisin Bran'	1 cup	750	0.38	0.42	5.00	0.50	99.7	1.50	0.0	26.6	10.8	88.5	357	2.2
'Shredded Wheat' original	2 biscuits	0	0.12	0.05	2.60	0.18	19.8	0.00	0.0	20.2	1.4	54.3	196	1.3
'Shredded Wheat' spoon size	1 cup	0	0.13	0.06	2.70	0.20	20.6	0.00	0.0	21.1	1.6	56.8	203	1.3
'Shredded Wheat N Bran' original	1.25 cup	0	0.15	0.07	3.70	0.20	27.1	0.00	0.0	26.6	2.5	80.8	248	1.9
'Toasties' corn flakes	1 cup	750	0.38	0.43	5.00	0.50	100.0	1.50	0.0	0.8	5.4	4.5	33	0.1
'Waffle Crisp'	1 cup	750	0.38	0.43	5.00	0.50	100.0	1.50	0.0	5.9	1.8	11.7	34	1.5
(Quaker)														
'Apple Zaps'	3/4 cup	1002	0.38	0.43	5.00	0.50	100.0	0.00	12.0	2.7	4.5	15.0	53	3.8
'Cap'n Crunch'	3/4 cup	36	0.38	0.42	5.00	0.50	100.0	0.00	0.0	5.4	4.5	9.4	35	3.8
'Cap'n Crunch's Crunchberries'	3/4 cup	33	0.37	0.42	5.00	0.50	100.0	0.01	<0.1	6.5	4.5	9.9	37	4.0
'Cap'n Crunch's Peanut Butter Crunch'	3/4 cup	37	0.38	0.42	5.00	0.50	100.0	0.00	0.0	2.7	4.5	18.6	62	3.8
'Cinnamon Life'	1 cup	16	0.63	0.71	8.40	0.83	168.0	0.00	0.1	135.0	7.5	41.5	113	6.3
'Cinnamon Oatmeal Squares'	1 cup	548	0.41	0.46	5.50	0.55	110.0	0.00	6.6	41.4	14.6	70.2	250	4.1
'Cocoa Blasts'	1 cup	1100	0.41	0.47	5.50	0.55	110.0	0.00	13.2	8.9	5.0	18.5	71	4.1

Food Name	Serving Size	A I.U.	Thi mg	Rib mg	Nia mg	B₆ mg	Fol mcg	B₁₂ mcg	C mg	Calc mg	Iron mg	Mag mg	Pot mg	Zn mg
'Corn Blasts'	1 cup	1100	0.41	0.47	5.50	0.55	110.0	0.00	13.2	10.9	5.0	17.5	64	4.1
'Frosted Flakers'	3/4 cup	750	0.38	0.42	5.00	0.50	100.0	0.00	15.0	0.9	4.7	8.4	34	0.2
'Fruitangy Oh!s'	1 cup	1034	0.39	0.44	5.20	0.52	104.0	0.00	12.4	2.8	4.7	18.0	59	3.9
'Honey Graham Oh!'	3/4 cup	1004	0.38	0.43	5.00	0.50	100.0	0.00	12.0	12.4	4.5	12.7	45	3.8
'King Vitaman'	1.25 cup	1044	0.39	0.44	5.20	0.52	104.0	1.60	12.4	3.7	8.7	26.0	86	3.9
'Kretschmer Honey Crunch Wheat Germ'	1 2/3 tbsp	13	0.19	0.10	0.66	0.07	46.6	0.00	0.0	7.0	1.1	38.1	135	1.9
'Marshmallow Safari'	3/4 cup	1000	0.38	0.42	5.00	0.50	99.9	0.00	12.0	26.1	4.5	16.8	42	3.8
'Oat Bran'	1.25 cup	519	0.39	0.44	5.20	0.52	104.0	0.00	6.2	30.2	16.0	99.2	257	3.9
'Oat Life, Plain'	3/4 cup	12	0.40	0.45	5.30	0.53	107.0	0.00	0.0	97.6	9.0	31.0	79	4.0
'Oatmeal Squares'	1 cup	563	0.42	0.48	5.60	0.56	113.0	0.00	6.8	35.8	15.7	70.0	228	4.2
'100% Natural,' oats, honey, and raisins	1/2 cup	4	0.14	0.09	0.77	0.08	11.7	0.05	0.3	38.8	1.7	47.9	214	1.1
'100% Natural,' oats and honey'	1/2 cup	3	0.17	0.08	0.85	0.09	12.0	0.05	0.1	46.1	1.4	50.4	211	1.2
'100% Natural,' whole grain w/raisins, lowfat	1/2 cup	9	0.14	0.06	0.91	0.07	11.5	0.00	0.4	30.0	1.3	39.5	169	0.9
'Puffed Rice'	1 cup	0	0.06	0.01	0.88	0.00	1.4	0.00	0.0	1.3	0.4	4.2	16	0.2
'Puffed Wheat'	1.25 cup	2	0.06	0.04	1.80	0.02	5.1	0.06	0.0	3.6	0.7	19.9	55	0.5
'Quisp'	1 cup	34	0.38	0.43	5.10	0.51	102.0	0.00	0.0	5.1	4.6	13.8	36	3.8
'Sun Country Granola' w/almonds'	1/2 cup	0	0.18	0.10	0.54	0.07	19.4	0.04	<0.1	49.0	2.5	51.9	221	1.1
'Sun Country Granola' w/raisins and dates	1/2 cup	0	0.09	0.07	0.26	0.04	9.6	0.06	0.1	23.9	1.3	26.0	133	0.5
'Toasted Oatmeal' honey nut	1 cup	500	0.37	0.42	5.00	0.50	100.0	0.02	6.0	26.9	4.5	53.4	185	3.9
(Rice Krinkles)														
'Frosted Rice Krinkles'	1 cup	1984	0.58	0.68	7.90	0.81	159.0	2.40	0.0	6.3	2.8	12.2	23	2.4
'Frosted Rice Krinkles' single serving box		939	0.28	0.32	3.70	0.38	75.2	1.10	0.0	3.0	1.3	5.8	11	1.1

CHARD. See SWISS CHARD.

CHAYOTE

Food Name	Serving Size	A I.U.	Thi mg	Rib mg	Nia mg	B₆ mg	Fol mcg	B₁₂ mcg	C mg	Calc mg	Iron mg	Mag mg	Pot mg	Zn mg
boiled, drained, chopped, 1-inch pieces	1 cup	75	0.04	0.06	0.67	0.19	29.0	0.00	12.8	20.8	0.4	19.2	277	0.5
raw, chopped, 1-inch pieces	1 cup	74	0.03	0.04	0.62	0.10	123.0	0.00	10.2	22.4	0.5	15.8	165	1.0
raw, whole, 5.75-inches	1 chayote	114	0.05	0.06	0.95	0.15	189.0	0.00	15.6	34.5	0.7	24.4	254	1.5

CHEESE. See also CHEESE FOOD; CHEESE PRODUCT; CHEESE SPREAD; CHEESE SUBSTITUTE.

AMERICAN

Food Name	Serving Size	A I.U.	Thi mg	Rib mg	Nia mg	B₆ mg	Fol mcg	B₁₂ mcg	C mg	Calc mg	Iron mg	Mag mg	Pot mg	Zn mg
pasteurized, process	1 oz	343	0.01	0.10	0.02	0.02	2.2	0.20	0.0	174.0	0.1	6.3	46	0.9
pasteurized, process, diced	1 cup	1693	0.04	0.49	0.10	0.10	10.9	0.97	0.0	862.0	0.6	31.1	227	4.2
pasteurized, process, w/disodium phosphate added	1 oz	343	0.01	0.10	0.02	0.02	2.2	0.20	0.0	174.0	0.1	6.3	46	0.9
pasteurized process w/disodium phosphate added, melted	1 cup	2951	0.07	0.86	0.17	0.17	19.0	1.70	0.0	1502.0	1.0	54.3	395	7.3
pasteurized process w/ disodium phosphate added, shredded	1 cup	1367	0.03	0.40	0.08	0.08	8.8	0.79	0.0	696.0	0.4	25.1	183	3.4

BLUE

Food Name	Serving Size	A I.U.	Thi mg	Rib mg	Nia mg	B₆ mg	Fol mcg	B₁₂ mcg	C mg	Calc mg	Iron mg	Mag mg	Pot mg	Zn mg
	1 oz	204	0.01	0.11	0.29	0.05	10.3	0.34	0.0	150.0	<0.1	6.5	73	0.8
crumbled	1 cup	973	0.04	0.52	1.40	0.22	49.1	1.60	0.0	712.0	0.4	31.0	346	3.6

BRICK

Food Name	Serving Size	A I.U.	Thi mg	Rib mg	Nia mg	B₆ mg	Fol mcg	B₁₂ mcg	C mg	Calc mg	Iron mg	Mag mg	Pot mg	Zn mg
	1 oz	307	0.00	0.10	0.03	0.02	5.8	0.36	0.0	191.0	0.1	6.9	39	0.7
diced	1 cup	1430	0.02	0.46	0.16	0.09	26.8	1.70	0.0	889.0	0.6	32.1	179	3.4
shredded	1 cup	1224	0.02	0.40	0.13	0.07	22.9	1.40	0.0	761.0	0.5	27.5	153	2.9

BRIE

Food Name	Serving Size	A I.U.	Thi mg	Rib mg	Nia mg	B₆ mg	Fol mcg	B₁₂ mcg	C mg	Calc mg	Iron mg	Mag mg	Pot mg	Zn mg
	1 oz	189	0.02	0.15	0.11	0.07	18.4	0.47	0.0	52.2	0.1	5.7	43	0.7
melted	1 cup	1601	0.17	1.20	0.91	0.56	156.0	4.00	0.0	442.0	1.2	48.0	365	5.7
sliced	1 cup	960	0.10	0.75	0.55	0.34	93.6	2.40	0.0	265.0	0.7	28.8	219	3.4

CAMEMBERT

Food Name	Serving Size	A I.U.	Thi mg	Rib mg	Nia mg	B₆ mg	Fol mcg	B₁₂ mcg	C mg	Calc mg	Iron mg	Mag mg	Pot mg	Zn mg
	1 cup	2271	0.07	1.20	1.60	0.56	153.0	3.20	0.0	953.0	0.8	49.1	459	5.9
	1 oz	262	0.01	0.14	0.18	0.06	17.6	0.37	0.0	110.0	<0.1	5.7	53	0.7

Food Name	Serving Size	A I.U.	Thi mg	Rib mg	Nia mg	B$_6$ mg	Fol mcg	B$_{12}$ mcg	C mg	Calc mg	Iron mg	Mag mg	Pot mg	Zn mg
CARAWAY	1 oz	299	0.01	0.13	0.05	0.02	5.2	0.08	0.0	191.0	0.2	6.3	26	0.8
CHEDDAR														
low-fat	1 oz	66	0.00	0.06	0.01	0.01	3.1	0.14	0.0	118.0	0.1	4.5	19	0.5
low-fat, diced	1 cup	308	0.02	0.29	0.07	0.06	14.5	0.65	0.0	548.0	0.6	21.1	87	2.4
low-fat, shredded	1 cup	263	0.01	0.25	0.06	0.05	12.4	0.55	0.0	469.0	0.5	18.1	75	2.1
low-salt	1 oz	297	0.01	0.11	0.02	0.02	5.1	0.23	0.0	199.0	0.2	7.7	32	0.9
low-salt, diced	1 cup	1382	0.03	0.50	0.11	0.10	23.8	1.10	0.0	928.0	1.0	35.6	1	4.1
low-salt, shredded	1 cup	1183	0.02	0.42	0.10	0.09	20.3	0.94	0.0	794.0	0.8	30.5	127	3.5
regular	1 oz	300	0.01	0.11	0.02	0.02	5.2	0.23	0.0	204.0	0.2	7.9	28	0.9
regular, diced	1 cup	1398	0.04	0.50	0.11	0.10	24.0	1.10	0.0	952.0	0.9	36.7	130	4.1
regular, melted	1 cup	2584	0.07	0.92	0.20	0.18	44.4	2.00	0.0	1760.0	1.7	67.8	240	8.6
regular, shredded	1 cup	1197	0.03	0.42	0.09	0.08	20.6	0.94	0.0	815.0	0.8	31.4	111	3.5
CHESHIRE	1 oz	279	0.01	0.08	0.02	0.02	5.2	0.23	0.0	182.0	<0.1	5.9	27	0.8
COLBY														
low-fat	1 oz	66	0.00	0.06	0.01	0.01	3.1	0.14	0.0	118.0	0.1	4.5	19	0.5
low-fat, diced	1 cup	308	0.02	0.29	0.07	0.06	14.5	0.65	0.0	548.0	0.6	21.1	87	2.4
low-fat, shredded	1 cup	263	0.01	0.25	0.06	0.05	12.4	0.55	0.0	469.0	0.4	18.1	75	2.1
low-salt	1 oz	297	0.01	0.11	0.02	0.02	5.1	0.23	0.0	199.0	0.2	7.7	32	0.9
low-salt, diced	1 cup	1382	0.03	0.50	0.11	0.10	23.8	1.10	0.0	928.0	1.0	35.6	148	4.1
low-salt, shredded	1 cup	1183	0.02	0.42	0.10	0.09	20.3	0.94	0.0	794.0	0.8	30.5	127	3.5
regular	1 oz	293	0.00	0.11	0.03	0.02	5.2	0.23	0.0	194.0	0.2	7.3	36	0.9
regular, diced	1 cup	1365	0.02	0.50	0.12	0.10	24.0	1.10	0.0	904.0	1.0	34.1	167	4.1
regular, shredded	1 cup	1168	0.02	0.42	0.11	0.09	20.6	0.93	0.0	774.0	0.9	29.2	143	3.5
COTTAGE CHEESE														
creamed, large curd, creamed	1 cup	342	0.04	0.34	0.27	0.14	25.6	1.30	0.0	126.0	0.3	11.0	177	0.8
creamed, large or small curd	4 oz	184	0.02	0.18	0.14	0.08	13.8	0.70	0.0	67.8	0.2	5.9	95	0.4
nonfat, dry, large or small curd	4 oz	34	0.03	0.16	0.17	0.09	16.7	0.93	0.0	35.8	0.3	4.5	37	0.5
nonfat, dry, large or small curd, not packed	1 cup	44	0.04	0.21	0.23	0.12	21.5	1.20	0.0	46.0	0.3	5.7	47	0.7
1% fat	4 oz	42	0.02	0.19	0.14	0.08	14.0	0.71	0.0	68.8	0.1	6.0	97	0.4
1% fat, not packed	1 cup	84	0.05	0.37	0.29	0.15	28.0	1.40	0.0	138.0	0.3	12.1	193	0.9
2% fat	4 oz	79	0.03	0.21	0.16	0.09	14.8	0.81	0.0	77.4	0.2	6.8	109	0.5
2% fat, not packed	1 cup	158	0.05	0.42	0.33	0.17	29.6	1.60	0.0	155.0	0.4	13.6	217	1.0
CREAM CHEESE														
	1 cup	3311	0.04	0.46	0.23	0.11	30.6	0.98	0.0	185.0	2.8	14.9	277	1.3
	3 oz pkg	1213	0.01	0.17	0.09	0.04	11.2	0.36	0.0	67.9	1.0	5.5	101	0.5
	1 oz	405	0.01	0.06	0.03	0.01	3.7	0.12	0.0	22.7	0.3	1.8	34	0.2
	1 tbsp	207	0.00	0.03	0.02	0.01	1.9	0.06	0.0	11.6	0.2	0.93	17	<0.1
whipped	1 tbsp	143	0.00	0.02	0.01	0.01	1.3	0.04	0.0	8.0	0.1	0.64	12	<0.1
EDAM														
	7-oz pkg	1814	0.07	0.77	0.16	0.15	32.1	3.00	0.0	1447.0	0.9	58.9	372	7.4
	1 oz	260	0.01	0.11	0.02	0.02	4.6	0.44	0.0	207.0	0.1	8.4	53	1.1
FETA														
	1 oz	127	0.04	0.24	0.28	0.12	9.1	0.48	0.0	140.0	0.2	5.4	18	0.8
crumbled	1 cup	671	0.23	1.30	1.50	0.64	48.0	2.50	0.0	739.0	1.0	28.8	93	4.3
FONTINA														
	8-oz pkg	2665	0.05	0.46	0.34	0.19	13.6	3.80	0.0	1249.0	0.5	31.8	144	7.9
	1 oz	333	0.01	0.06	0.04	0.02	1.7	0.47	0.0	156.0	0.0	4.0	18	1.0
diced	1 cup	1550	0.03	0.27	0.20	0.11	7.9	2.20	0.0	726.0	0.3	18.5	84	4.6
shredded	1 cup	1268	0.02	0.22	0.16	0.09	6.5	1.80	0.0	594.0	0.3	15.1	69	3.8
GJETOST														
	8-oz pkg	2527	0.71	3.10	1.80	0.61	10.4	5.50	0.0	908.0	1.2	159.0	3198	2.6
	1 oz	316	0.09	0.39	0.23	0.08	1.3	0.69	0.0	113.0	0.2	19.8	399	0.3
GOAT														
hard	1 oz	451	0.04	0.34	0.68	0.02	1.1	0.03	0.0	254.0	0.5	15.3	14	0.5

Food Name	Serving Size	A I.U.	Thi mg	Rib mg	Nia mg	B$_6$ mg	Fol mcg	B$_{12}$ mcg	C mg	Calc mg	Iron mg	Mag mg	Pot mg	Zn mg
semisoft	1 oz	378	0.02	0.19	0.33	0.02	0.6	0.06	0.0	84.5	0.5	8.2	45	0.2
soft	1 oz	267	0.02	0.11	0.12	0.07	3.4	0.05	0.0	39.7	0.5	4.5	7	0.3
GOUDA														
	7-oz pkg	1275	0.06	0.66	0.13	0.16	41.4	3.00	0.0	1386.0	0.5	57.4	239	7.7
	1 oz	183	0.01	0.10	0.02	0.02	5.9	0.44	0.0	198.0	<0.1	8.2	34	1.1
GRUYERE														
	6-oz pkg	2072	0.10	0.47	0.18	0.14	17.7	2.70	0.0	1719.0	0.3	61.0	138	6.6
	1 oz	346	0.02	0.08	0.03	0.02	2.9	0.45	0.0	287.0	<0.1	10.2	23	1.1
diced	1 cup	1609	0.08	0.37	0.14	0.11	13.7	2.10	0.0	1335.0	0.2	47.4	107	5.1
shredded	1 cup	1317	0.07	0.30	0.11	0.09	11.2	1.70	0.0	1092.0	0.2	38.8	88	4.2
JACK. See MONTEREY JACK.														
LIMBURGER														
	8-oz pkg	2908	0.18	1.10	0.36	0.20	131.0	2.40	0.0	1128.0	0.3	47.7	291	4.8
	1 cup	1717	0.11	0.67	0.21	0.12	77.0	1.40	0.0	666.0	0.2	28.1	172	2.8
	1 oz	363	0.02	0.14	0.05	0.02	16.3	0.29	0.0	141.0	<0.1	6.0	36	0.6
MONTEREY JACK														
	1 oz	269	0.00	0.11	0.03	0.02	5.2	0.23	0.0	212.0	0.2	7.7	23	0.9
	6-oz pkg	1615	0.03	0.66	0.16	0.13	30.9	1.40	0.0	1269.0	1.2	45.9	137	5.1
diced	1 cup	1254	0.02	0.52	0.12	0.10	24.0	1.10	0.0	985.0	1.0	35.7	107	4.0
shredded	1 cup	1074	0.02	0.44	0.11	0.09	20.6	0.93	0.0	843.0	0.8	30.5	91	3.4
MOZZARELLA														
part skim	1 oz	166	0.01	0.09	0.03	0.02	2.5	0.23	0.0	183.0	<0.1	6.6	24	0.8
part skim, low-moisture	1 oz	199	0.01	0.10	0.03	0.02	2.8	0.26	0.0	207.0	<0.1	7.4	27	0.9
part skim, low-moisture, diced	1 cup	928	0.03	0.45	0.16	0.10	13.1	1.20	0.0	965.0	0.3	34.7	125	4.1
part skim, low moisture, shredded	1 cup	794	0.02	0.39	0.13	0.09	11.2	1.00	0.0	826.0	0.3	29.7	107	3.5
whole milk	1 oz	225	0.00	0.07	0.02	0.02	2.0	0.19	0.0	147.0	<0.1	5.3	19	0.6
whole milk, low moisture	1 oz	256	0.01	0.08	0.03	0.02	2.2	0.21	0.0	163.0	<0.1	5.9	21	0.7
whole milk, low-moisture, shredded	1 cup	887	0.02	0.27	0.09	0.06	7.8	0.73	0.0	579.0	0.2	20.8	75	2.5
MUENSTER														
	6-oz pkg	1904	0.02	0.54	0.17	0.10	20.6	2.50	0.0	1219.0	0.7	46.5	228	4.8
	1 oz	318	0.00	0.09	0.03	0.02	3.4	0.42	0.0	203.0	0.1	7.8	38	0.8
diced	1 cup	1478	0.02	0.42	0.14	0.07	16.0	1.90	0.0	947.0	0.5	36.1	177	3.7
shredded	1 cup	1266	0.02	0.36	0.12	0.06	13.7	1.70	0.0	811.0	0.5	30.9	152	3.2
NEUFCHATEL														
	3-oz pkg	964	0.01	0.17	0.11	0.04	9.6	0.22	0.0	64.0	0.2	6.5	97	0.4
	1 oz	321	0.00	0.06	0.04	0.01	3.2	0.08	0.0	21.3	<0.1	2.2	32	0.2
PARMESAN														
grated	1 cup	701	0.05	0.39	0.32	0.11	8.0	1.40	0.0	1376.0	1.0	50.8	107	3.2
grated	1 oz	199	0.01	0.11	0.09	0.03	2.3	0.40	0.0	390.0	0.3	14.4	30	0.9
grated	1 tbsp	35	0.00	0.02	0.02	0.01	0.4	0.07	0.0	68.8	<0.1	2.5	5	0.2
hard	1 oz	171	0.01	0.09	0.08	0.03	2.0	0.34	0.0	336.0	0.2	12.4	26	0.8
shredded	1 tbsp	32	0.00	0.02	0.01	0.01	0.4	0.07	0.0	62.6	<0.1	2.5	5	0.2
PIMIENTO														
pasteurized, process	1 oz	358	0.01	0.10	0.02	0.02	2.2	0.20	0.6	174.0	0.1	6.3	46	0.8
pasteurized, process, diced	1 cup	1767	0.04	0.50	0.11	0.10	10.9	0.97	3.1	860.0	0.6	31.1	226	4.2
pasteurized, process, melted	1 cup	3079	0.07	0.86	0.19	0.17	19.0	1.70	5.5	1499.0	1.0	54.2	395	7.3
pasteurized, process, shredded	1 cup	1426	0.03	0.40	0.09	0.08	8.8	0.79	2.5	694.0	0.5	25.1	183	3.4
PORT DU SALUT														
	6-oz pkg	2266	0.02	0.41	0.10	na	30.9	2.50	0.0	1105.0	0.7	41.3	231	4.4
	1 oz	378	0.00	0.07	0.02	na	5.2	0.42	0.0	184.0	0.1	6.9	39	0.7
diced	1 cup	1760	0.02	0.32	0.08	na	24.0	2.00	0.0	858.0	0.6	32.1	179	3.4
shredded	1 cup	1506	0.02	0.27	0.07	na	20.6	1.70	0.0	734.0	0.5	27.5	153	2.9
PROVOLONE														
	6-oz pkg	1386	0.03	0.55	0.27	0.12	17.7	2.50	0.0	1285.0	0.9	46.9	235	5.5
	1 oz	231	0.01	0.09	0.04	0.02	2.9	0.41	0.0	214.0	0.2	7.8	40	0.9

Food Name	Serving Size	A I.U.	Thi mg	Rib mg	Nia mg	B$_6$ mg	Fol mcg	B$_{12}$ mcg	C mg	Calc mg	Iron mg	Mag mg	Pot mg	Zn mg
diced........................	1 cup	1076	0.03	0.42	0.21	0.10	13.7	1.90	0.0	998.0	0.7	36.4	183	4.3
QUESO ANEJO														
Mexican	1 oz	63	0.01	0.06	0.01	0.01	0.3	0.39	0.0	193.0	0.1	7.9	25	0.8
Mexican, crumbled	1 cup	292	0.03	0.28	0.04	0.06	1.3	1.80	0.0	898.0	0.6	37.0	115	3.9
QUESO ASEDERO														
Mexican	1 oz	63	0.01	0.06	0.05	0.02	2.3	0.28	0.0	187.0	0.1	7.4	24	0.9
Mexican, diced	1 cup	294	0.03	0.29	0.24	0.07	10.6	1.30	0.0	873.0	0.7	34.3	114	4.0
Mexican, shredded............	1 cup	252	0.02	0.25	0.20	0.06	9.0	1.10	0.0	747.0	0.6	29.4	97	3.4
QUESO CHIHUAHUA														
Mexican	1 oz	64	0.01	0.06	0.04	0.02	0.6	0.29	0.0	185.0	0.1	6.5	15	1.0
Mexican, diced	1 cup	300	0.02	0.30	0.20	0.07	2.6	1.40	0.0	859.0	0.6	30.4	69	4.6
Mexican, shredded............	1 cup	257	0.02	0.25	0.17	0.06	2.3	1.20	0.0	736.0	0.5	26.0	59	4.0
RICOTTA														
part skim...................	1 cup	1063	0.05	0.46	0.19	0.05	32.2	0.72	0.0	669.0	1.1	36.3	308	3.3
part skim...................	1/2 cup	536	0.03	0.23	0.10	0.03	16.2	0.36	0.0	337.0	0.6	18.3	155	1.7
part skim...................	1 oz	122	0.01	0.05	0.02	0.01	3.7	0.08	0.0	77.1	0.1	4.2	35	0.4
whole milk..................	1 cup	1205	0.03	0.48	0.26	0.11	30.0	0.83	0.0	509.0	0.9	27.8	257	2.9
whole milk..................	1/2 cup	608	0.02	0.24	0.13	0.05	15.1	0.42	0.0	257.0	0.5	14.0	130	1.4
ROMANO														
....	5 oz pkg	811	0.05	0.53	0.11	0.12	9.7	1.60	0.0	1511.0	1.1	58.1	123	3.7
....	1 oz	162	0.01	0.11	0.02	0.02	1.9	0.32	0.0	302.0	0.2	11.6	25	0.7
ROQUEFORT														
....	1 oz	297	0.01	0.17	0.21	0.04	13.9	0.18	0.0	188.0	0.1	8.4	26	0.6
....	3-oz pkg	890	0.03	0.50	0.62	0.11	41.6	0.55	0.0	563.0	0.5	25.1	77	1.8
SWISS														
....	1 oz	240	0.01	0.10	0.03	0.02	1.8	0.47	0.0	272.0	<0.1	10.2	31	1.1
diced.......................	1 cup	1115	0.03	0.48	0.12	0.11	8.4	2.20	0.0	1268.0	0.2	47.4	146	5.1
melted......................	1 cup	2062	0.05	0.89	0.22	0.20	15.6	4.10	0.0	2345.0	0.4	87.6	270	9.5
shredded....................	1 cup	913	0.02	0.39	0.10	0.09	6.9	1.80	0.0	1038.0	0.2	38.8	120	4.2
TILSIT														
....	6-oz pkg	1777	0.10	0.61	0.35	0.11	34.0	3.60	0.0	1190.0	0.4	22.1	110	6.0
....	1 oz	296	0.02	0.10	0.06	0.02	5.7	0.59	0.0	198.0	<0.1	3.7	18	1.0
CHEESE FOOD. See also CHEESE PRODUCT.														
AMERICAN														
cold pack	8-oz pkg	1600	0.07	1.00	0.17	0.32	12.3	2.90	0.0	1129.0	1.9	67.4	824	6.8
cold pack	1 oz	200	0.01	0.13	0.02	0.04	1.5	0.36	0.0	141.0	0.2	8.4	103	0.9
pasteurized, process	8-oz pkg	2073	0.07	1.00	0.32	0.32	16.6	2.50	0.0	1303.0	1.9	69.3	633	6.8
pasteurized, process	1 oz	259	0.01	0.13	0.04	0.04	2.1	0.32	0.0	163.0	0.2	8.7	79	0.9
pasteurized, process, diced	1 cup	1032	0.03	0.50	0.16	0.16	8.2	1.30	0.0	649.0	1.0	34.5	315	3.4
pasteurized, process, w/disodium phosphate added................	8-oz pkg	2073	0.07	1.00	0.32	0.32	16.6	2.50	0.0	1303.0	1.9	69.3	633	6.8
pasteurized, process, w/disodium phosphate added................	1 oz	259	0.01	0.13	0.04	0.04	2.1	0.32	0.0	163.0	0.2	8.7	79	0.9
SWISS														
pasteurized process	8-oz pkg	1943	0.03	0.91	0.24	0.08	13.2	5.20	0.0	1642.0	1.4	63.6	645	8.1
pasteurized process	1 oz	243	0.00	0.11	0.03	0.01	1.6	0.65	0.0	205.0	0.2	7.9	81	1.0
pasteurized, process, diced	1 cup	1131	0.02	0.39	0.05	0.05	8.3	1.70	0.0	1081.0	0.9	40.8	302	5.1
pasteurized, process, w/disodium phosphate added.................	1 oz	229	0.00	0.08	0.01	0.01	1.7	0.35	0.0	219.0	0.2	8.3	61	1.0
pasteurized, process, w/disodium phosphate added, diced.........	1 cup	913	0.02	0.31	0.04	0.04	6.7	1.40	0.0	872.0	0.7	32.9	244	4.1
CHEESE PRODUCT														
(Kraft)														
American, pasteurized process	1 slice	455	na	0.06	na	na	na	na	<0.1	150.0	<0.1	na	49.6	0.5

Food Name	Serving Size	A I.U.	Thi mg	Rib mg	Nia mg	B$_6$ mg	Fol mcg	B$_{12}$ mcg	C mg	Calc mg	Iron mg	Mag mg	Pot mg	Zn mg
'Cheez Whiz' light, pasteurized process	2 tbsp	220	na	0.12	na	na	na	na	0.1	146.0	<0.1	na	104	0.8
'Cheez Whiz' pasteurized process	2 tbsp	214	na	0.08	na	na	na	na	0.1	118.0	<0.1	na	79	0.5
'Velveeta' less fat, pasteurized process	1 oz	275	na	0.18	na	na	na	na	<0.1	161.0	<0.1	na	97	0.7
CHEESE SAUCE. See under SAUCE.														
CHEESE SOUP. See under SOUP.														
CHEESE SPREAD														
AMERICAN														
pasteurized, process	1 cup	1923	0.12	1.10	0.32	0.28	17.1	0.98	0.0	1371.0	0.8	69.6	590	6.3
pasteurized, process	1 oz	223	0.01	0.12	0.04	0.03	2.0	0.11	0.0	159.0	<0.1	8.1	69	0.7
pasteurized, process, diced	1 cup	1103	0.07	0.60	0.18	0.16	9.8	0.56	0.0	787.0	0.5	39.9	339	3.6
pasteurized, process, w/disodium phosphate added	1 oz	223	0.01	0.12	0.04	0.03	2.0	0.11	0.0	159.0	<0.1	8.1	69	0.7
(Kraft) 'Velveeta' pasteurized, process	1 oz	310	na	0.10	na	na	na	na	<0.1	130.0	<0.1	na	94	0.5
CHEESE SUBSTITUTE														
MOZZARELLA														
	3 oz	1238	0.02	0.38	0.27	0.04	9.3	0.69	<0.1	519.0	0.3	34.9	387	1.6
	1 oz	413	0.01	0.13	0.09	0.01	3.1	0.23	<0.1	173.0	0.1	11.6	129	0.5
shredded	1 cup	1645	0.03	0.50	0.36	0.06	12.4	0.92	0.1	689.0	0.5	46.3	514	2.2
CHERIMOYA. See CUSTARD APPLE.														
CHERRY														
SOUR														
Canned														
red, in extra heavy syrup, w/liquid	1 cup	1817	0.04	0.10	0.42	0.12	19.3	0.00	5.0	26.1	3.3	13.1	238	0.2
red, in heavy syrup, w/liquid	1 cup	1828	0.04	0.10	0.43	0.11	19.5	0.00	5.1	25.6	3.3	15.4	238	0.2
red, in light syrup, w/liquid	1 cup	1830	0.04	0.10	0.43	0.11	19.4	0.00	5.0	25.2	3.3	15.1	239	0.2
red, in water, w/liquid	1 cup	1840	0.04	0.10	0.43	0.11	19.5	0.00	5.1	26.8	3.3	14.6	239	0.2
Fresh														
red, raw	1 cup	1989	0.05	0.06	0.62	0.07	11.6	0.00	15.5	24.8	0.5	13.9	268	0.2
red, raw, pitted	1 cup	1321	0.03	0.04	0.41	0.05	7.7	0.00	10.3	16.5	0.3	9.3	178	0.1
Frozen														
red, unsweetened	18-oz pkg	4437	0.22	0.17	0.70	0.34	22.9	0.00	8.7	66.3	2.7	45.9	632	0.5
red, unsweetened, unthawed	1 cup	1349	0.07	0.05	0.21	0.10	7.0	0.00	2.6	20.1	0.8	13.9	192	0.2
SWEET														
Canned														
pitted, in extra heavy syrup w/liquid	1 cup	394	0.06	0.10	1.00	0.08	11.0	0.00	9.4	23.5	0.9	20.9	371	0.3
pitted, in heavy syrup, w/liquid	1 cup	390	0.05	0.10	1.00	0.08	10.6	0.00	9.1	22.8	0.9	22.8	367	0.3
pitted, in juice, w/liquid	1 cup	313	0.05	0.06	1.00	0.08	10.5	0.00	6.3	35.0	1.4	30.0	328	0.3
pitted, in light syrup, w/liquid	1 cup	396	0.05	0.10	1.00	0.08	10.6	0.00	9.3	22.7	0.9	22.7	373	0.3
pitted, in water, w/liquid	1 cup	397	0.06	0.10	1.00	0.07	10.4	0.00	5.5	27.3	0.9	22.3	325	0.2
Fresh														
raw	1 cup	250	0.06	0.07	0.47	0.04	4.9	0.00	8.2	17.6	0.5	12.9	262	<0.1
raw, medium	1 cherry	15	0.00	0.00	0.03	0.00	0.3	0.00	0.5	1.0	<0.1	0.8	15	0.0
raw, pitted	1 cup	310	0.07	0.09	0.58	0.05	6.1	0.00	10.2	21.8	0.6	15.9	325	0.0
Frozen														
sweetened	10-oz pkg	537	0.08	0.13	0.50	0.10	11.9	0.00	2.8	34.1	1.0	28.4	565	0.1
sweetened, thawed	1 cup	490	0.07	0.12	0.46	0.09	10.9	0.00	2.6	31.1	0.9	25.9	515	0.1
CHERRY, SURINAM. See PITANGA.														
CHERVIL														
dried	1 tbsp	111	0.01	0.01	0.10	0.02	5.2	0.00	1.0	25.6	0.6	2.5	90	0.2
dried	1 tsp	35	0.00	0.00	0.03	0.01	1.6	0.00	0.3	8.1	0.2	0.8	28	<0.1
CHESTNUT, CHINESE														
boiled or steamed	1 oz	39	0.03	0.04	0.16	0.08	13.2	0.00	7.0	3.4	0.3	16.4	87	0.2
dried	1 oz	93	0.07	0.08	0.37	0.19	31.2	0.00	16.6	8.2	0.7	38.8	206	0.4

Food Name	Serving Size	A I.U.	Thi mg	Rib mg	Nia mg	B6 mg	Fol mcg	B12 mcg	C mg	Calc mg	Iron mg	Mag mg	Pot mg	Zn mg
raw	1 oz	57	0.05	0.05	0.23	0.12	19.2	0.00	10.2	5.1	0.4	23.8	127	0.3
roasted	1 oz	1	0.04	0.03	0.42	0.12	20.5	0.00	10.9	5.4	0.4	25.5	135	0.3
CHESTNUT, EUROPEAN / Italian chestnut / sweet chestnut														
boiled or steamed	1 oz	5	0.04	0.03	0.21	0.07	10.9	0.00	7.6	13.0	0.5	15.3	203	<0.1
dried, peeled	1 oz	0	0.10	0.02	0.24	0.19	31.2	0.00	4.3	18.1	0.7	21.0	281	0.1
dried, unpeeled	1 oz	0	0.08	0.10	0.24	0.19	31.0	0.00	4.3	19.0	0.7	21.0	280	0.1
raw, peeled	1 oz	7	0.04	0.01	0.31	0.10	16.4	0.00	11.4	5.4	0.3	8.5	137	0.1
raw, unpeeled	1 cup	41	0.34	0.24	1.70	0.55	89.9	0.00	62.4	39.1	1.5	46.4	751	0.8
raw, unpeeled	1 oz	8	0.07	0.05	0.33	0.11	17.6	0.00	12.2	7.7	0.3	9.1	147	0.2
roasted	1 cup	34	0.35	0.25	1.90	0.71	100.0	0.00	37.2	41.5	1.3	47.2	847	0.8
roasted, approx 3 kernels	1 oz	7	0.07	0.05	0.38	0.14	19.8	0.00	7.4	8.2	0.3	9.4	168	0.2
roasted	10 kernels	20	0.20	0.15	1.10	0.42	58.8	0.00	21.8	24.4	0.8	27.7	497	0.5
CHESTNUT, ITALIAN. See CHESTNUT, EUROPEAN.														
CHESTNUT, JAPANESE														
boiled or steamed	1 oz	4	0.04	0.02	0.15	0.03	4.8	0.00	2.7	3.1	0.2	5.1	34	0.1
dried	1 oz	25	0.23	0.11	0.99	0.19	30.8	0.00	17.4	20.4	1.0	32.6	218	0.7
dried	1 cup	133	1.20	0.59	5.40	1.00	168.0	0.00	95.0	112.0	5.2	178.0	1190	4.0
raw	1 oz	11	0.10	0.05	0.42	0.08	13.2	0.00	7.5	8.8	0.4	13.9	93	0.3
roasted	1 oz	21	0.13	na	0.20	0.12	16.7	0.00	7.9	9.9	0.6	18.1	121	0.4
CHESTNUT, SWEET. See CHESTNUT, EUROPEAN.														
CHEWING GUM. See under CANDY, GUM.														
CHIA SEEDS, dried	1 oz	10.2	0.25	0.05	1.6	0.20	32.4	0	4.5	150	2.8	21.8	292	1.5
CHICKEN														
AVERAGE OF ALL PARTS														
Fresh														
broiler/fryer, meat and skin, batter-dipped, fried	4 oz	102	0.09	0.22	10.27	0.47	10.3	0.35	0.0	19.5	1.6	28.6	267	2.3
broiler/fryer, meat and skin, flour-coated, fried	4 oz	102	0.10	0.22	10.26	0.47	10.3	0.35	0.0	19.3	1.6	28.6	268	2.3
broiler/fryer, meat and skin, raw	4 oz	160	0.07	0.14	7.78	0.39	6.9	0.35	1.8	12.6	1.0	22.9	216	1.5
broiler/fryer, meat and skin, roasted	4 oz	184	0.07	0.19	9.71	0.46	5.7	0.34	0.0	17.2	1.5	26.3	255	2.2
broiler/fryer, meat and skin, roasted, chopped or diced	1 cup	225	0.09	0.23	11.90	0.56	7.0	0.42	0.0	21.0	1.8	32.2	312	2.7
broiler/fryer, meat and skin, stewed	4 oz	167	0.05	0.17	6.39	0.25	5.7	0.23	0.0	14.9	1.3	21.7	190	2.0
broiler/fryer, meat and skin, stewed, chopped or diced	1 cup	204	0.06	0.21	7.80	0.31	7.0	0.28	0.00	18.2	1.6	26.6	232	2.5
broiler/fryer, meat only, fried	4 oz	67	0.10	0.23	11.06	0.55	7.9	0.39	0.0	19.5	1.5	30.9	293	2.6
broiler/fryer, meat only, fried, chopped or diced	1 cup	83	0.12	0.28	13.50	0.67	9.8	0.48	0.0	23.8	1.9	37.8	360	3.1
broiler/fryer, meat only, raw	4 oz	59	0.08	0.16	9.39	0.49	8.0	0.42	2.6	13.7	1.0	28.6	262	1.7
broiler/fryer, meat only, roasted	4 oz	61	0.08	0.20	10.5	0.54	6.9	0.38	0.0	17.1	1.4	28.6	278	2.4
broiler/fryer, meat only, roasted, chopped or diced	1 cup	74.2	0.10	0.25	12.8	0.66	8.4	0.46	0	21.0	1.7	35.0	340	2.9
broiler/fryer, meat only, stewed	4 oz	57	0.06	0.17	6.98	0.29	6.8	0.25	0.0	16.0	1.3	24.0	206	2.3
broiler/fryer, meat only, stewed, chopped or diced	1 cup	70	0.07	0.23	8.60	0.36	8.4	0.31	0.0	19.6	1.6	29.4	252	2.8
capon, meat and skin, raw	4 oz	147	0.07	0.14	8.31	0.41	6.9	0.4	1.9	12.6	1.2	23.9	248	1.3
capon, meat and skin, roasted	4 oz	78	0.08	0.19	10.20	0.49	6.9	0.38	0.0	15.9	1.7	27.4	292	2.0
roaster, meat and skin, raw	4 oz	150	0.07	0.13	7.51	0.36	6.9	0.36	1.7	11.4	1.1	21.7	224	1.2
roaster, meat and skin, roasted	4 oz	95	<0.01	0.16	8.48	0.40	5.7	0.31	0.0	13.7	1.4	22.9	241	1.6
roaster, meat only, raw	4 oz	51	0.07	0.15	9.02	0.48	8.0	0.41	2.4	11.4	1.2	26.3	272	1.4
roaster, meat only, roasted	4 oz	47	0.07	0.17	9.02	0.47	5.7	0.33	0.0	13.7	1.4	24.0	262	1.7
roaster, meat only, roasted, chopped or diced	1 cup	57.4	0.09	0.21	11.0	0.57	7.0	0.41	0.0	16.8	1.7	29.4	321	2.1

Food Name	Serving Size	A I.U.	Thi mg	Rib mg	Nia mg	B_6 mg	Fol mcg	B_{12} mcg	C mg	Calc mg	Iron mg	Mag mg	Pot mg	Zn mg
stewing, meat and skin, raw	4 oz	203	0.13	0.19	7.17	0.38	6.9	0.37	0.4	11.4	1.2	22.9	233	1.3
stewing, meat and skin, stewed	4 oz	150	0.11	0.27	6.61	0.29	5.7	0.26	0.0	14.8	1.5	22.9	208	2.1
stewing, meat only, raw	4 oz	120	0.17	0.24	8.54	0.50	8.0	0.44	3.8	11.4	1.2	27.5	287	1.6
stewing, meat only, stewed	4 oz	44	0.13	0.32	7.34	0.35	6.8	0.30	0.0	14.8	1.7	25.1	231	2.3
stewing, meat only, stewed, chopped or diced	1 cup	157	0.16	0.39	9.00	0.43	8.4	0.36	0.0	18.2	2.0	30.8	283	2.9
BACK														
Fresh														
broiler/fryer, meat and skin, batter-dipped, fried	4 oz	136	0.13	0.25	6.67	0.27	22.9	0.30	0.0	29.7	1.7	21.7	206	1.3
broiler/fryer, meat and skin, flour-coated, fried	141		0.13	0.27	8.41	0.35	17.1	0.32	0.0	27.5	1.9	26.3	259	2.9
broiler/fryer, meat and skin, raw	4 oz	286	0.06	0.14	5.54	0.22	6.8	0.29	1.8	14.9	1.1	17.1	165	1.4
broiler/fryer, meat and skin, roasted	4 oz	397	0.06	0.22	7.76	0.30	6.9	0.30	0.0	23.9	1.6	22.9	123	2.6
broiler/fryer, meat and skin, stewed, chopped or diced	1 cup	493	0.07	0.24	6.9	0.24	8.0	0.29	0.0	28.8	2.0	25.6	232	3.1
broiler/fryer, meat only, fried	4 oz	112	0.12	0.30	8.87	0.39	10.2	0.35	0.0	29.8	1.9	28.6	288	2.1
broiler/fryer, meat only, raw	4 oz	113	0.09	0.18	7.61	0.38	10.3	0.40	3.6	19.5	1.2	25.1	233	2.1
broiler/fryer, meat only, roasted	4 oz	109	0.09	0.26	7.99	0.40	8.0	0.34	0.0	27.4	1.6	15.1	271	3.1
broiler/fryer, meat only, stewed	4 oz	103	0.05	0.19	5.17	0.22	7.9	0.24	0.0	23.9	1.4	19.3	181	2.7
BREAST														
Fresh														
broiler/fryer, meat and skin, batter-dipped, fried	4 oz	77	0.13	0.16	12.00	0.49	17.1	0.34	0.0	22.9	1.5	27.4	229	1.1
broiler/fryer, meat and skin, flour-coated, fried	4 oz	57	0.09	0.15	15.74	0.66	6.9	0.38	0.0	18.3	1.4	34.3	296	1.3
broiler/fryer, meat and skin, raw	4 oz	95	0.07	0.09	11.35	0.61	4.6	0.39	1.1	12.5	0.9	28.6	251	0.9
broiler/fryer, meat and skin, roasted	4 oz	106	0.08	0.14	14.58	0.64	4.5	0.36	0.0	16.0	1.2	30.9	280	1.2
broiler/fryer, meat and skin, roasted, chopped or diced	1 cup	130	0.09	0.17	17.8	0.78	5.6	0.45	0.0	19.6	1.5	37.8	343	1.4
broiler/fryer, meat and skin, stewed	4 oz	94	0.05	0.14	8.94	0.33	3.4	0.24	0.0	14.9	1.0	25.1	204	1.1
broiler/fryer, meat and skin, stewed, chopped or diced	1 cup	115	0.06	0.16	10.9	0.41	4.2	0.29	0.0	18.2	1.3	30.8	249	1.4
broiler/fryer, meat only, fried	4 oz	26	0.09	0.15	16.88	0.73	4.5	0.4	0.0	18.3	1.3	35.5	315	1.2
broiler/fryer, meat only, raw	4 oz	24	0.08	0.11	12.78	0.63	4.6	0.44	1.4	12.6	0.82	32.0	292	0.9
broiler/fryer, meat only, roasted	4 oz	24	0.08	0.13	15.68	0.69	4.5	0.39	0.0	17.1	1.2	33.1	292	1.1
broiler/fryer, meat only, roasted, chopped or diced	1 cup	29.4	0.10	0.16	19.2	0.84	5.6	0.48	0.0	21.0	1.5	40.6	358	1.4
broiler/fryer, meat only, stewed	4 oz	22	0.05	0.13	9.62	0.37	3.5	0.26	0.0	14.8	1.0	27.4	214	<0.1
broiler/fryer, meat only, stewed, chopped or diced	1 cup	26.6	0.06	0.17	11.9	0.46	4.2	0.32	0.0	18.2	1.2	33.6	262	1.4
DARK MEAT														
Fresh														
broiler/fryer, meat and skin, batter-dipped, fried	4 oz	118	0.14	0.25	6.41	0.28	20.6	0.31	0.0	24.0	1.6	22.9	211	2.4
broiler/fryer, meat and skin, flour-coated, fried	4 oz	119	0.11	0.27	7.83	0.37	12.5	0.34	0.0	19.4	1.7	27.5	263	3.0
broiler/fryer, meat and skin, raw	4 oz	194	0.07	0.17	5.97	0.29	8.0	0.33	2.4	12.6	1.1	2.2	203	1.8
broiler/fryer, meat and skin, roasted	4 oz	230	0.08	0.24	7.25	0.36	8.0	0.33	0.0	17.2	1.6	25.1	251	2.9
broiler/fryer, meat and skin, stewed	4 oz	212	0.06	0.20	5.16	0.19	6.8	0.23	0.0	16.0	1.5	20.6	189	2.6
broiler/fryer, meat only, fried	4 oz	90	0.11	0.29	8.04	0.43	10.3	0.38	0.0	20.6	1.8	28.6	289	3.3
broiler/fryer, meat only, fried, chopped or diced	1 cup	111	0.13	0.35	9.90	0.52	12.6	0.46	0.0	25.2	2.1	35.0	354	4.1
broiler/fryer, meat only, raw	4 oz	82	0.08	0.21	7.13	0.38	11.4	0.41	3.6	13.7	1.2	26.3	254	2.3

Food Name	Serving Size	A I.U.	Thi mg	Rib mg	Nia mg	B_6 mg	Fol mcg	B_{12} mcg	C mg	Calc mg	Iron mcg	Mag mg	Pot mg	Zn mg
broiler/fryer, meat only, roasted	4 oz	82	0.08	0.25	7.48	0.41	0.4	0.37	0.0	17.2	1.6	26.2	274	3.2
broiler/fryer, meat only, roasted, chopped or diced	1 cup	101	0.10	0.32	9.20	0.50	11.2	0.45	0.0	21.0	1.9	32.2	336	3.9
broiler/fryer, meat only, stewed	4 oz	79	0.07	0.26	5.45	0.24	8.0	0.25	0.0	15.9	1.6	22.9	207	3.1
broiler/fryer, meat only, stewed, chopped or diced	1 cup	97	0.08	0.28	6.60	0.29	9.8	0.31	0.0	19.6	1.9	28.0	253	3.7
roaster, meat only, raw	4 oz	69	0.08	0.20	6.68	0.36	10.3	0.38	3.4	10.3	1.3	23.9	260	1.9
roaster, meat only, roasted	4 oz	62	0.07	0.22	6.57	0.35	8.0	0.30	0.0	12.5	1.6	22.9	257	2.4
roaster, meat only, roasted, chopped or diced	1 cup	76	0.09	0.27	8.00	0.43	9.8	0.38	0.0	15.4	1.9	28.0	314	3.0
stewing, meat only, raw	4 oz	155	0.19	0.32	6.20	0.39	11.4	0.42	5.2	11.4	1.4	26.2	276	2.4
stewing, meat only, stewed	4 oz	166	0.14	0.39	5.17	0.27	9.1	0.28	0.0	13.8	1.9	25.2	233	3.6
stewing, meat only, stewed, chopped or diced	1 cup	203	0.18	0.49	6.40	0.34	11.2	0.35	0.0	16.8	2.3	30.8	286	4.4
DRUMSTICK														
Fresh														
broiler/fryer, meat and skin, batter-dipped, fried	4 oz	90	0.13	0.24	5.85	0.32	20.5	0.22	0.0	19.4	1.5	22.9	213	2.7
broiler/fryer, meat and skin, flour-coated, fried	4 oz	96	0.08	0.28	7.09	0.39	11.4	0.35	0.0	13.8	15.7	26.4	262	3.3
broiler/fryer, meat and skin, fried	4 oz	70	0.09	0.27	6.86	0.46	10.5	0.41	0.0	13.7	1.5	27.4	285	3.7
broiler/fryer, meat and skin, roasted, chopped or diced	1 cup	140	0.10	0.30	8.40	0.48	11.20	0.45	0.0	16.8	1.9	32.2	321	4.0
broiler/fryer, meat and skin, stewed, chopped or diced	1 cup	127	0.07	0.27	5.90	0.27	9.8	0.31	0.0	15.4	1.9	28.0	258	3.7
broiler/fryer, meat only, raw	4 oz	65	0.09	0.22	6.49	0.40	11.4	0.43	3.7	12.7	1.2	26.3	258	2.5
broiler/fryer, meat only, roasted	4 oz	69	0.09	0.26	7.03	0.44	10.1	0.40	0.0	13.6	1.49	27.3	281	3.6
broiler/fryer, meat only, roasted, chopped or diced	1 cup	84	0.11	0.33	8.50	0.55	12.6	0.48	0.0	16.8	1.8	33.6	344	4.5
broiler/fryer, meat only, stewed	4 oz	65	0.08	0.24	4.89	0.24	8.9	0.29	0.0	12.7	1.6	24.1	227	3.5
broiler/fryer, meat only, stewed, chopped or diced	1 cup	91	0.09	0.34	6.90	0.37	12.8	0.38	0.0	17.6	2.2	33.6	318	4.8
GIBLETS														
Fresh														
broiler/fryer, fried	1 oz	3409	0.02	0.44	3.08	0.18	108.4	3.74	2.4	5.1	2.9	7.3	94	1.8
broiler/fryer, fried, chopped or diced	1 cup	17297	0.14	2.20	15.90	0.88	550.0	19.30	12.6	26.1	15.0	36.3	479	9.1
broiler/fryer, raw	1 oz	2528	0.02	0.29	1.86	0.12	98.5	3.23	4.6	2.9	1.6	5.1	65	0.9
broiler/fryer, simmered	1 oz	2122	0.02	0.27	1.16	0.10	107.3	2.86	2.2	3.5	1.8	5.7	45	1.3
broiler/fryer, simmered, chopped or diced	1 cup	10775	0.13	1.40	5.90	0.49	545.0	14.70	11.6	17.4	9.3	29.0	229	6.6
capon, raw	1 oz	4162	0.03	0.31	2.06	0.14	112.5	3.65	5.2	2.9	1.7	5.1	65	0.9
capon, simmered	1 oz	3790	0.03	0.31	1.17	0.10	118.2	0.34	2.6	3.6	1.9	5.7	44	1.3
capon, simmered, chopped or diced	1 cup	19236	0.14	1.50	6.00	0.55	600.0	1.70	13.1	18.9	9.9	29.0	222	6.8
roaster, raw	1 oz	2741	0.02	0.23	1.83	0.10	78.9	2.74	3.8	2.9	1.6	4.9	65	0.9
roaster, simmered, chopped or diced	1 cup	11797	0.11	1.20	5.80	0.44	439.0	12.30	9.4	17.4	8.8	29.0	232	6.7
roaster, simmered	1 oz	2324	0.02	0.23	1.14	0.09	86.7	2.48	1.8	3.4	1.7	5.7	46	1.3
stewing, raw	1 oz	2999	0.03	0.32	2.45	0.15	99.9	3.06	3.3	2.9	1.7	5.1	65	0.9
stewing, simmered	1 oz	2724	0.03	0.30	1.41	0.12	104.9	2.69	1.6	3.7	1.8	5.7	44	1.2
stewing, simmered, chopped or diced	1 cup	13827	0.13	1.50	7.20	0.59	532.0	13.70	8.0	18.9	9.3	29.0	223	6.2
GIZZARD														
Fresh														
all classes, raw	1 oz	62	0.00	0.05	1.35	0.05	14.8	0.59	0.9	2.3	1.0	4.7	68	0.9
all classes, simmered	1 oz	54	0.00	0.08	1.14	0.04	15.1	0.57	0.4	2.9	1.2	5.7	51	1.3
all classes, simmered, chopped or diced	1 cup	273	0.04	0.35	5.80	0.17	76.8	2.80	2.3	14.5	6.0	29.0	260	6.4

Food Name	Serving Size	A I.U.	Thi mg	Rib mg	Nia mg	B_6 mg	Fol mcg	B_{12} mcg	C mg	Calc mg	Iron mg	Mag mg	Pot mg	Zn mg
HEART														
Fresh														
all classes, simmered, chopped or diced	1 cup	41	0.10	1.10	4.10	0.46	116.0	10.60	2.6	27.6	13.1	29.0	191	10.6
all classes, raw	1 medium	2	0.01	0.04	0.30	0.02	4.4	0.45	0.2	0.7	0.4	0.9	11	0.4
LEG														
Fresh														
broiler/fryer, meat and skin, batter-dipped, fried	4 oz	104	0.13	0.25	6.26	0.31	20.6	0.32	0.0	20.6	1.6	22.9	217	2.5
broiler/fryer, meat and skin, flour-coated, fried	4 oz	105	0.10	0.27	7.51	0.39	12.6	0.36	0.0	14.8	1.6	27.5	266	3.1
broiler/fryer, meat and skin, roasted	4 oz	154	0.08	0.25	7.12	0.38	7.9	0.35	0.0	13.7	1.5	26.3	240	2.9
broiler/fryer, meat and skin, roasted, chopped or diced	1 cup	189	0.10	0.30	8.70	0.46	9.8	0.42	0.0	16.8	1.9	32.2	315	3.6
broiler/fryer, meat and skin, stewed	4 oz	142	0.06	0.21	5.18	0.21	6.9	0.23	0.0	12.6	1.5	22.9	201	2.7
broiler/fryer, meat and skin, stewed, chopped or diced	1 cup	174	0.08	0.27	6.40	0.25	8.4	0.28	0.0	15.4	1.9	28.0	246	3.4
broiler/fryer, meat only, fried	4 oz	76	0.10	0.29	7.55	0.45	10.2	0.39	0.0	14.9	1.6	28.6	290	3.5
broiler/fryer, meat only, boneless/skinless	4 oz	75	0.10	0.28	7.66	0.45	10.3	0.39	0.0	14.8	1.6	28.6	291	3.4
broiler/fryer, meat only, raw	4 oz	140	0.08	0.19	6.22	0.33	12.6	0.36	2.8	11.4	1.1	23.9	226	2.1
broiler/fryer, meat only, raw, boneless/skinless	4 oz	70	0.09	0.22	6.95	0.38	11.4	0.41	3.7	12.6	1.1	26.3	262	2.4
broiler/fryer, meat only, roasted	4 oz	72	0.08	0.26	7.21	0.42	9.2	0.36	0.0	13.6	1.5	27.5	276	3.2
broiler/fryer, meat only, roasted, boneless/skinless	4 oz	72	0.08	0.26	7.22	0.42	9.1	0.36	0.0	13.7	1.4	27.4	277	3.2
broiler/fryer, meat only, roasted, chopped or diced	1 cup	88	0.11	0.33	8.80	0.52	11.2	0.45	0.0	16.8	1.8	33.6	339	4.0
broiler/fryer, meat only, stewed	4 oz	69	0.08	0.25	5.52	0.25	9.1	0.27	0.0	12.6	1.60	30.0	217	3.2
broiler/fryer, meat only, stewed, boneless/skinless	4 oz	69	0.07	0.25	5.43	0.24	9.2	0.26	0.0	12.6	1.6	24.0	217	3.2
broiler/fryer, meat only, stewed, chopped or diced	1 cup	96	0.09	0.35	7.70	0.34	12.8	0.37	0.0	17.6	2.2	33.6	304	4.4
LIGHT MEAT														
Fresh														
broiler/fryer, meat and skin, batter-dipped, fried	4 oz	118	0.14	0.25	6.43	0.29	20.6	0.31	0.0	24.0	1.6	22.9	211	2.4
broiler/fryer, meat and skin, flour-coated, fried	4 oz	90	0.13	0.17	10.40	0.45	18.3	0.32	0.0	22.9	1.4	25.2	211	1.2
broiler/fryer, meat and skin, raw	4 oz	113	0.07	0.10	10.15	0.55	4.5	0.38	1.0	12.6	0.91	26.3	233	1.1
broiler/fryer, meat and skin, roasted	4 oz	126	0.07	0.14	12.70	0.60	3.5	0.36	0.0	17.1	1.3	28.6	260	1.4
broiler/fryer, meat and skin, stewed	4 oz	110	0.05	0.13	7.92	0.31	3.4	0.23	0.0	14.9	1.1	22.9	191	1.3
broiler/fryer, meat only, fried	4 oz	34	0.09	0.14	15.36	0.71	4.6	0.41	0.0	18.2	1.3	33.2	299	1.4
broiler/fryer, meat only, fried, chopped or diced	1 cup	42	0.10	0.18	18.70	0.88	5.6	0.50	0.0	22.4	1.6	40.6	368	1.8
broiler/fryer, meat only, raw	4 oz	32	0.08	0.10	12.08	0.61	4.5	0.43	1.4	13.8	0.8	30.9	273	1.1
broiler/fryer, meat only, roasted	4 oz	33	0.07	0.12	14.10	0.68	4.6	0.39	0.0	17.1	1.21	30.9	282	1.4
broiler/fryer, meat only, roasted, chopped or diced	1 cup	41	0.09	0.16	17.40	0.84	5.6	0.48	0.0	21.0	1.5	37.8	346	1.7
broiler/fryer, meat only, stewed	4 oz	31	0.05	0.13	8.85	0.37	3.4	0.26	0.0	14.8	1.1	25.1	206	1.4
broiler/fryer, meat only, stewed, chopped or diced	1 cup	38	0.06	0.16	10.90	0.46	4.2	0.32	0.0	18.2	1.3	30.8	252	1.7
roaster, meat only, raw	4 oz	31	0.08	0.10	11.66	0.63	4.6	0.45	1.4	12.6	1.0	28.6	287	0.75
roaster, meat only, roasted	4 oz	29	0.07	0.10	12.00	0.62	3.4	0.35	0.0	14.8	1.2	26.2	270	0.9

Food Name	Serving Size	A I.U.	Thi mg	Rib mg	Nia mg	B_6 mg	Fol mcg	B_{12} mcg	C mg	Calc mg	Iron mg	Mag mg	Pot mg	Zn mg
roaster, meat only, roasted, chopped or diced	1 cup	35	0.09	0.13	14.70	0.76	4.2	0.43	0.0	18.2	1.5	32.2	330	1.1
stewing, meat only, raw	4 oz	80	0.15	0.14	11.30	0.65	4.6	0.46	2.1	12.6	1.1	29.7	298	0.7
stewing, meat only, stewed	4 oz	83	0.11	0.23	9.82	0.45	4.6	0.30	0.0	16.1	1.4	26.2	227	0.9
stewing, meat only, stewed, chopped or diced	1 cup	102	0.13	0.27	12.00	0.55	5.6	0.38	0.0	19.6	1.7	32.2	279	1.2
LIVER														
Fresh														
all classes, raw	1 oz	5871	0.03	0.57	2.66	0.23	210.9	6.6	9.7	3.1	2.5	5.7	65	0.9
all classes, simmered	1 oz	4680	0.05	0.52	1.29	0.19	220.0	5.71	4.5	3.9	2.4	6.2	40	1.2
all classes, simmered, chopped or diced	1 cup	22925	0.21	2.40	6.20	0.81	1078.0	27.10	22.1	19.6	11.9	29.4	196	6.1
NECK														
Fresh														
broiler/fryer, meat and skin, batter-dipped, fried	1 oz	49	0.04	0.07	1.29	0.05	4.3	0.07	0.0	8.9	0.6	46	43.2	0.7
broiler/fryer, meat and skin, flour-coated, fried	1 oz	54	0.03	0.08	1.53	0.08	3.1	0.08	0.0	8.8	0.7	5.5	51	0.9
broiler/fryer, meat and skin, raw	1 oz	62	0.01	0.06	1.03	0.06	1.4	0.08	0.3	5.1	0.5	3.6	39	0.5
broiler/fryer, meat and skin, simmered	1 oz	46	0.00	0.08	0.94	0.03	0.9	0.05	0.0	7.8	0.6	3.6	31	0.8
broiler/fryer, meat only, fried	1 oz	46	0.04	0.08	1.43	0.12	2.3	0.08	0.0	11.8	0.86	5.7	61	1.2
broiler/fryer, meat only, raw	1 oz	42	0.00	0.05	1.19	0.10	2.3	0.10	0.8	7.6	0.6	4.8	50	0.8
broiler/fryer, meat only, simmered	1 oz	34	0.00	0.06	1.14	0.06	1.7	0.06	0.0	12.6	0.7	4.6	40	1.1
SKIN														
Fresh														
broiler/fryer, batter-dipped, fried	1 oz	31	0.04	0.04	0.75	0.01	9.0	0.04	0.0	5.9	0.3	2.7	17	0.2
broiler/fryer, flour-coated, fried	1 oz	66	0.03	0.05	1.68	0.03	9.4	0.05	0.0	4.0	0.4	4.8	36	0.3
broiler/fryer, raw	1 oz	75	0.01	0.02	1.12	0.03	0.9	0.07	0.0	3.1	0.3	3.7	29	0.3
broiler/fryer, roasted	1 oz	75	0.01	0.04	1.58	0.03	0.6	0.06	0.0	3.9	0.4	4.3	39	0.4
broiler/fryer, stewed	1 oz	57	<0.01	0.03	1.07	0.02	0.6	0.03	0.0	3.4	0.3	3.7	33	0.3
THIGH														
Fresh														
broiler/fryer, meat and skin, batter-dipped, fried	4 oz	109	0.13	0.27	6.51	0.29	21.7	0.32	0.0	20.6	1.6	24.1	219	2.4
broiler/fryer, meat and skin, flour-coated, fried	4 oz	112	0.11	0.28	7.92	0.37	13.6	0.35	0.0	16.0	1.7	28.6	271	2.9
broiler/fryer, meat and skin, raw	4 oz	165	0.07	0.17	6.20	0.29	8.0	0.34	2.7	11.4	1.1	22.9	219	1.8
broiler/fryer, meat and skin, roasted	4 oz	188	0.07	0.24	7.19	0.35	7.9	0.33	0.0	13.6	1.5	25.1	254	2.8
broiler/fryer, meat and skin, roasted, chopped or diced	1 cup	231	0.09	0.30	8.90	0.43	9.8	0.41	0.0	16.8	1.9	30.8	311	3.3
broiler/fryer, meat and skin, stewed	4 oz													
broiler/fryer, meat only, fried	4 oz	80	0.11	0.29	8.13	0.44	10.3	0.37	0.0	14.9	1.7	29.7	297	3.3
broiler/fryer, meat only, raw	4 oz	74	0.08	0.22	7.29	0.38	11.4	0.39	3.5	11.4	1.2	27.5	263	2.2
broiler/fryer, meat only, roasted	4 oz	74	0.09	0.26	7.47	0.40	9.2	0.35	0.0	13.6	1.4	27.5	273	2.9
broiler/fryer, meat only, roasted, chopped or diced	1 cup	91	0.10	0.32	9.10	0.49	11.2	0.43	0.0	16.8	1.8	33.6	333	3.6
broiler/fryer, meat only, simmered	4 oz	71	0.08	0.25	6.02	0.25	8.1	0.25	0.0	12.5	1.6	24.1	210	2.9
broiler/fryer, meat only, simmered, chopped or diced	1 cup	86	0.09	0.30	7.30	0.29	9.8	0.29	0.0	15.4	2.0	29.4	256	3.6
broiler/fryer, meat and skin, stewed	4 oz	173	0.07	0.22	5.55	0.20	6.9	0.22	0.0	12.6	1.6	21.7	195	2.5
WING														
Fresh														
broiler/fryer, meat and skin, batter-dipped, fried	4 oz	129	0.12	0.16	5.91	0.35	20.5	0.28	0.0	22.9	1.5	18.1	158	1.6

Food Name	Serving Size	A I.U.	Thi mg	Rib mg	Nia mg	B$_6$ mg	Fol mcg	B$_{12}$ mcg	C mg	Calc mg	Iron mg	Mag mg	Pot mg	Zn mg
broiler/fryer, meat and skin, flour-coated, fried	4 oz	143	0.06	0.18	7.82	0.48	6.6	0.30	0.0	17.4	1.4	21.7	202	2.0
broiler/fryer, meat and skin, fried	4 oz	70	0.09	0.19	8.29	0.67	4.6	0.38	0.0	17.1	1.3	23.8	238	2.4
broiler/fryer, meat and skin, raw	4 oz	168	0.04	0.12	6.69	0.39	4.7	0.35	0.8	13.8	1.1	20.5	178	1.5
broiler/fryer, meat and skin, roasted	4 oz	181	0.05	0.16	7.62	0.49	3.4	0.33	0.0	16.9	1.47	21.8	210	2.1
broiler/fryer, meat and skin, roasted, chopped or diced	1 cup	221	0.06	0.18	9.30	0.59	4.2	0.41	0.0	21.0	1.8	26.6	258	2.5
broiler/fryer, meat and skin, stewed	4 oz	152	0.05	0.14	5.24	0.24	3.4	0.19	0.0	13.8	1.3	18.1	159	1.9
broiler/fryer, meat and skin, stewed, chopped or diced	1 cup	186	0.06	0.14	6.50	0.31	4.2	0.25	0.0	16.8	1.6	22.4	195	2.3
CHICKEN DINNER/ENTRÉE. See also CHILI; ENCHILADA; FAJITA MIX; SANDWICH.														
(Banquet)														
fried chicken, w/mashed potatoes and corn, in seasoned sauce	1 serving	0	na	na	na	na	na	na	1.4	38.8	1.4	na	na	na
pot pie, frozen	1 serving	1142	na	na	na	na	na	na	0.0	27.7	1.1	na	na	na
(Barber Foods)														
cordon bleu, w/cheese and ham, frozen	1 pkg	435	na	na	na	na	na	na	292.0	na	na	na	na	na
cordon bleu, w/cheese and ham, frozen	1 serving	215	na	na	na	na	na	na	144.0	na	na	na	na	na
w/broccoli and cheese stuffing, frozen	1 pkg	170	na	na	na	na	na	na	27.2	238.0	na	na	na	na
w/broccoli and cheese stuffing, frozen	1 serving	84	na	na	na	na	na	na	13.4	118.0	na	na	na	na
(Budget Gourmet) French, light, w/vegetables, potato, sauce	1 serving	2295	na	na	na	na	na	na	na	na	na	na	na	na
(Chun King)														
sweet and sour, w/vegetables, fruit, sauce, canned	1 pkg	0	na	na	na	na	na	na	147.0	na	na	na	na	na
sweet and sour, w/vegetables, fruit, sauce, canned	1 serving	0	na	na	na	na	na	na	30.2	na	na	na	na	na
(Healthy Choice)														
cacciatore, in sauce, w/vegetables	1 entrée	266	na	na	na	na	na	na	na	53.1	2.2	na	750	na
teriyaki, w/rice, vegetable, apple cherry compote	1 entrée	1182	na	na	na	na	na	na	12.2	37.4	1.1	na	424	na
(Kid Cuisine) nuggets, w/macaroni and cheese, corn, pudding, 'Cosmic'	1 serving	0	na	na	na	na	na	na	na	206.0	2.9	na	na	na
(Lunch Express)														
Alfredo	1 entrée	2426	na	na	na	na	na	na	24.2	147.0	na	na	na	na
stir-fry, w/rice and vegetables, frozen	1 entrée	5271	na	na	na	na	na	na	23.7	na	na	na	na	na
(Marie Callender's) pot pie, frozen	1 serving	1133	na	na	na	na	na	na	0.0	37.4	na	na	na	na
(Mrs. Paterson's) pie, hand held pie, frozen, Aussie Pie'	1 serving	363	na	na	na	na	na	na	na	na	3.0	na	na	na
(Pierre)														
barbecue, frozen, 'Chix-B-Q' product 9845	1 piece	127	0.12	0.11	4.50	0.27	5.4	0.35	0.0	23.8	1.3	19.7	186	2.9
breaded, frozen, 'Two-Fers' product 1870	1 piece	25	0.08	0.06	1.90	0.08	0.6	0.11	0.0	8.2	0.6	6.2	55.3	0.6
breast, breaded, frozen, cooked, product 1881	1 piece	17	0.06	0.05	2.40	0.08	6.7	0.05	0.0	5.3	0.4	4.2	42	0.2
breast patty, fillet-shaped, flame-broiled, 'Caboose' product 9863	1 piece	73	0.12	0.08	6.00	0.33	1.8	0.49	0.0	22.2	1.1	25.2	204	2.1
breast patty, fillet-shaped, flame-broiled, product 9820	1 piece	37	0.05	0.07	7.30	0.34	6.0	0.19	0.0	25.5	1.3	27.2	225	0.8
breast patty, fillet-shaped, flame-broiled, product 9916	1 piece	84	0.14	0.10	7.80	0.42	2.3	0.58	0.0	27.3	1.4	32.0	252	2.6
breast patty, mesquite, fillet-shaped, flame-broiled, product 9816	1 piece	44	0.04	0.07	6.40	0.27	5.2	0.16	0.0	23.7	1.1	22.9	189	0.7
nuggets, breaded, frozen, product 3800	1 piece	20	0.04	0.04	0.89	0.04	4.1	0.10	0.0	5.1	0.3	3.4	30	0.4

Food Name	Serving Size	A I.U.	Thi mg	Rib mg	Nia mg	B₆ mg	Fol mcg	B₁₂ mcg	C mg	Calc mg	Iron mg	Mag mg	Pot mg	Zn mg
patty, breaded, frozen, product 1915	1 piece	51	0.16	0.12	3.80	0.15	1.1	0.23	0.0	16.5	1.1	12.5	111	1.2
patty, cutlet-shaped, flame-broiled, frozen, product 9835	1 piece	87	0.14	0.13	6.00	0.36	3.0	0.58	0.0	25.9	1.3	28.9	246	2.9
patty, cutlet-shaped, honey mustard, flame-broiled, frozen, product 9852	1 piece	91	0.14	0.13	5.90	0.35	3.4	0.57	0.59	25.5	1.5	28.9	243	2.9
patty, cutlet-shaped, mesquite, flame-broiled, frozen, product 9805	1 piece	100	0.14	0.13	6.30	0.34	6.7	0.41	0.0	25.2	1.4	22.9	224	3.2
patty, cutlet-shaped, rotisserie style, flame-broiled, frozen, product 9878	1 piece	93	0.17	0.12	7.10	0.39	na	0.68	0.0	30.8	1.5	33.8	269	3.2
patty, cutlet-shaped, teriyaki sauce, flame-broiled, frozen, product 9829	1 piece	89	0.14	0.13	5.90	0.35	3.4	0.57	0.0	26.4	1.3	28.9	243	2.9
patty, fillet-shaped, flame-broiled, frozen, product 9840	1 piece	92	0.12	0.11	4.50	0.28	5.4	0.36	0.0	20.4	1.2	19.8	187	2.9
(Stouffer's)														
parmigiana, w/pasta Alfredo, homestyle, frozen.	9 7/8 oz	2426	na	na	na	na	na	na	24.2	147.0	na	na	na	na
pie, frozen.	1 entrée	4670	na	na	na	na	na	na	na	102.0	3.0	na	na	na
(Tyson)														
mesquite, w/barbecue sauce, corn, potato.	1 entrée	474	na	na	na	na	na	na	0.0	na	na	na	na	na
roasted, w/garlic sauce, pasta, vegetable	1 entrée	na	na	na	na	na	na	na	na	na	1.6	na	na	na
(Wonderbites)														
barbecue, flame-broiled, frozen, 'Dippers'.	1 piece	38	0.04	0.03	1.50	0.09	0.8	0.14	0.2	7.3	0.4	7.1	60	0.7
breast, flame-broiled, frozen, 'Dippers'	1 piece	22	0.03	0.02	1.90	0.10	1.3	0.09	0.0	5.2	0.3	5.6	52	0.6
Buffalo flavored, flame-broiled, frozen, 'Dippers'.	1 piece	70	0.04	0.03	1.50	0.09	0.8	0.16	0.4	7.4	0.4	7.8	64	0.8
chili salsa, breaded, frozen, 'Dippers'	1 piece	60	0.06	0.05	1.30	0.06	6.7	0.17	1.1	8.0	0.5	5.3	47	0.5
flame-broiled, frozen, 'Dippers'	1 piece	21	0.03	0.03	1.50	0.09	0.7	0.14	0.0	6.3	0.3	7.0	60	0.7
honey mustard, flame-broiled, frozen, 'Dippers'.	1 piece	23	0.03	0.03	1.50	0.09	1.5	0.09	0.2	5.3	0.4	5.5	53	0.7
Italian, flame-broiled, frozen, 'Dippers'	1 piece	28	0.04	0.03	1.50	0.09	0.8	0.16	0.2	7.8	0.4	8.0	65	0.8
teriyaki, flame broiled, frozen, 'Dippers' product 3727	1 piece	6.4	0.03	0.03	0.64	0.07	9.0	0.36	0	4.2	0.39	6.0	70.4	0.88
teriyaki, flame broiled, frozen, 'Dippers' product 3827	1 piece	12.8	0.04	0.04	0.73	0.07	0.80	0.41	0	6.8	0.55	7.8	73.8	1.3
teriyaki, flame broiled, frozen, 'Dippers' product 9879	1 piece	22.1	0.04	0.03	1.5	0.09	0.84	0.14	0	6.5	0.33	7.1	60.1	0.71
CHICKEN FAT														
. . . .	1 cup	0	0.00	0.00	0.00	0.00	0.0	0.00	0.0	0.0	0.0	0.0	0	0.0
. . . .	1 tbsp	0	0.00	0.00	0.00	0.00	0.0	0.00	0.0	0.0	0.0	0.0	0	0.0
CHICKPEA FLOUR. See under FLOUR.														
CHICKPEA / ceci / garbanzo														
Canned, mature seed	1 cup	58	0.07	0.08	0.33	1.10	160.0	0.00	9.1	76.8	3.2	69.6	413	2.5
Fresh														
mature seed, boiled	1 cup	44	0.19	0.10	0.86	0.23	282.0	0.00	2.1	80.4	4.7	78.7	477	2.5
mature seed, raw	1 cup	134	0.95	0.42	3.10	1.10	1113.0	0.00	8.0	210.0	12.5	230.0	1750	6.9
mature seed, raw	1 tbsp	8	0.06	0.03	0.19	0.07	69.6	0.00	0.5	13.1	0.8	14.4	109	0.4
CHICORY, raw, trimmed, chopped.	1/2 cup	7200	0.11	0.18	0.90	0.19	197	0	43.2	180	1.6	54.0	756	0.76
CHICORY, WITLOOF														
raw	1/2 cup	13.1	0.03	0.01	0.07	0.02	16.6	0	1.3	8.6	0.11	4.5	95.0	0.07
raw, medium, approx 2.1 oz	1 head	15.4	0.03	0.01	0.09	0.02	19.6	0	1.5	10.1	0.13	5.3	112	0.09
CHICORY ROOT														
raw, medium, approx 2.6 oz	1 root	3.6	0.02	0.02	0.24	0.14	13.7	0	3.0	24.6	0.48	13.2	174	0.20

Food Name	Serving Size	A I.U.	Thi mg	Rib mg	Nia mg	B$_6$ mg	Fol mcg	B$_{12}$ mcg	C mg	Calc mg	Iron mg	Mag mg	Pot mg	Zn mg
raw, 1-inch pieces.	1/2 cup	2.7	0.02	0.01	0.18	0.11	10.3	0	2.3	18.4	0.36	9.9	131	0.15
CHILI														
(El Rio)														
con carne, w/o beans, canned	1 pkg	778	na	na	na	na	na	na	na	na	7.2	na	na	na
con carne, w/o beans, canned	1 serving	478	na	na	na	na	na	na	na	na	4.4	na	na	na
(Hormel)														
turkey, w/beans, canned.	1 cup	1650	na	na	na	na	na	na	1.5	116	3.5	69.2	682	2.7
vegetarian, w/beans, canned	1 cup	1941	na	na	na	na	na	na	1.2	96.3	3.5	81.5	803	1.7
w/beans, canned	1 cup	968	na	na	na	na	na	na	0.5	69.2	3.2	59.3	662	2.7
w/o beans, canned	1 cup	2384	na	na	na	na	na	na	0.0	49.6	2.6	37.8	349	2.6
(Nalley's) con carne, w/beans, canned	1 serving	0	na	na	na	na	na	na	na	na	4.6	na	na	na
(Nestlé)														
spicy, w/beans, canned, 'Chef Mate'	1 cup	2004	0.15	0.15	3.0	0.26	na	0.86	1.3	83.5	5.4	53.1	648	2.8
w/beans, canned 'Chef Mate'	1 cup	3013	0.11	0.20	3.5	0.23	na	1.4	0.76	88.5	4.8	45.5	511	3.9
w/o beans, canned, 'Chef Mate'	1 cup	2900	0.14	0.27	4.8	0.34	na	1.8	1.8	67.5	4.5	45.0	530	4.5
(Open Range)														
w/beans, canned	1 pkg	0	na	na	na	na	na	na	na	na	5.0	na	na	na
w/beans, canned	1 serving	0	na	na	na	na	na	na	na	na	2.7	na	na	na
(Stagg)														
w/beans, canned, 'Classic'	1 cup	1161	na	na	na	na	na	na	2.5	91.4	4.0	64.2	785	2.7
w/beans, canned, 'Country'	1 cup	514	na	na	na	na	na	na	1.7	56.8	3.5	51.9	558	2.5
w/beans, canned, 'Dynamite'	1 cup	1252	na	na	na	na	na	na	3.0	104	4.4	69.2	778	2.7
w/beans, canned, 'Ranchhouse'.	1 cup	1082	na	na	na	na	na	na	5.2	114	4.2	81.5	867	2.0
w/beans, canned, 'Silverado'	1 cup	1247	na	na	na	na	na	na	5.2	88.9	3.7	71.6	815	2.7
CHILI PEPPER. See PEPPER, CHILI.														
CHILI POWDER. See under SEASONING MIX.														
CHINESE APPLE. See POMEGRANATE.														
CHINESE BROCCOLI. See BROCCOLI, CHINESE.														
CHINESE CABBAGE. See BOK CHOY.														
CHINESE FUNGUS / Jew's ear / pepeao														
dried	1 cup	0	0.20	0.08	0.72	0.23	38.5	0.00	0.3	27.1	1.5	35.0	170	1.8
raw, approx 0.2 oz	1 piece	0	0.01	0.01	0.00	0.01	1.1	0.00	<0.1	<0.1	<0.1	1.5	3	<0.1
raw, sliced	1 cup	0	0.08	0.20	0.07	0.09	18.9	0.00	0.6	15.8	0.6	24.8	43	0.7
CHINESE GOOSEBERRY. See KIWI FRUIT.														
CHINESE NOODLE. See under PASTA.														
CHINESE PARSLEY. See CORIANDER.														
CHINESE PARSLEY LEAF. See CORIANDER LEAF.														
CHINESE PARSLEY SEED. See CORIANDER SEED; PEAS, SNOW.														
CHINESE PEAR. See ASIAN PEAR.														
CHINESE RADISH. See DAIKON.														
CHINESE YAM. See JICAMA.														
CHINOOK SALMON. See under SALMON.														
CHIVES														
Fresh														
raw, chopped	1 tbsp	131	0.00	0.00	0.02	0.00	3.1	0.00	1.7	2.8	<0.1	1.3	9	<0.1
raw, chopped	1 tsp	44	0.00	0.00	0.01	0.00	1.1	0.00	0.6	0.9	<0.1	0.4	3	<0.1
Freeze-dried														
. . . .	1/4 cup	546	0.01	0.01	0.05	0.02	0.9	0.00	5.3	6.5	0.2	5.1	24	<0.1
. . . .	1 tbsp	137	0.00	0.00	0.01	0.00	0.2	0.00	1.3	1.6	<0.1	1.3	6	<0.1
CHOCOLATE. See CHOCOLATE, BAKING. See also under CANDY.														
CHOCOLATE, BAKING														
Bits														
milk chocolate, 'Mini Baking Bits'														
(M&M Mars).	1 pkg	25402	6.80	26.20	27.90	3.60	567.0	34.0	68.0	13154.0	139.0	5216.0	33226	120

Food Name	Serving Size	A I.U.	Thi mg	Rib mg	Nia mg	B₆ mg	Fol mcg	B₁₂ mcg	C mg	Calc mg	Iron mg	Mag mg	Pot mg	Zn mg
milk chocolate, 'Mini Baking Bits'														
(M&M Mars)............	1 serving	32	0.01	0.03	0.04	0.01	0.7	0.04	<0.1	16.5	0.2	6.5	42	0.2
semisweet, 'Mini Baking Bits'														
(M&M Mars) Mini Baking Bits...........	12-oz pkg	248	0.17	0.29	1.30	0.16	95.2	0.00	0.0	116.0	10.0	360.0	1142	5.1
semisweet, 'Mini Baking Bits'														
(M&M Mars) Mini Baking Bits...........	1 tbsp	10	0.01	0.01	0.06	0.01	3.9	0.00	0.0	4.8	0.4	14.8	47	0.2
Liquid............	1 oz	3	0.01	0.08	0.59	0.02	5.4	0.00	0.0	15.3	1.2	75.1	331	1.0
Squares														
Mexican............	1 square	4	0.01	0.02	0.37	0.01	0.4	0.00	<0.1	6.8	0.4	19.0	79	0.3
unsweetened............	1-oz square	28	0.02	0.05	0.32	0.03	2.0	0.00	0.0	21.0	1.8	87.9	236	1.1
unsweetened, grated............	1 cup	129	0.11	0.22	1.50	0.13	9.2	0.00	0.0	97.7	8.3	409.0	1100	5.3
CHOCOLATE MILK														
1% fat............	1 quart	2000	0.38	1.70	1.30	0.41	48.0	3.40	9.3	1147.0	2.4	133.0	1702	4.1
1% fat............	1 cup	500	0.10	0.41	0.32	0.10	12.0	0.85	2.3	287.0	0.6	33.3	426	1.0
2% fat............	1 quart	2000	0.37	1.60	1.30	0.41	48.0	3.40	9.2	1136.0	2.4	132.0	1688	4.1
2% fat............	1 cup	500	0.09	0.41	0.32	0.10	12.0	0.85	2.3	284.0	0.6	33.0	422	1.0
2% fat............	1 fl oz	62	0.01	0.05	0.04	0.01	1.5	0.11	0.3	35.4	<0.1	4.1	53	0.1
whole............	1 quart	1210	0.37	1.60	1.30	0.40	47.0	3.30	9.1	1121.0	2.4	130.0	1669	4.1
whole............	1 cup	303	0.09	0.41	0.31	0.10	11.8	0.83	2.3	280.0	0.6	32.6	417	1.0
whole............	1 fl oz	37.8	0.01	0.05	0.04	0.01	1.5	0.10	0.3	35.0	<0.1	4.1	52	0.1
CHORIZO. See under SAUSAGE.														
CHRYSANTEMUM LEAVES														
raw, whole............	1 med leaf	337	0.02	0.03	0.10	0.03	31.9	0.00	0.3	21.1	0.4	5.8	102	0.1
raw, chopped............	1 cup	954	0.07	0.07	0.27	0.09	90.3	0.00	0.7	59.7	1.2	16.3	289	0.4
CHRYSANTHEMUM GARLAND														
boiled, drained, 1-inch pieces............	1 cup	5050	0.02	0.16	0.72	0.12	50.2	0.00	23.9	69.0	3.7	18.0	569	0.2
raw, 1-inch pieces............	1 cup	3669	0.01	0.06	0.22	0.03	19.1	0.00	9.3	14.0	0.8	4.3	143	<0.1
raw, whole, approx 8.75-inch long.........	1 stem	2055	0.00	0.03	0.12	0.02	10.7	0.00	5.2	7.8	0.4	2.4	80	<0.1
CHUB / cisco														
raw............	3 oz	85	0.08	0.09	2.10	0.26	12.8	0.85	0.0	10.2	0.3	14.4	301	0.3
smoked............	1 oz	267	0.01	0.05	0.66	0.08	0.6	1.20	0.0	7.4	0.1	4.8	83	<0.1
smoked............	3 oz	802	0.04	0.14	2.00	0.23	1.8	3.60	0.0	22.1	0.4	14.4	249	0.3
CHUM SALMON. See under SALMON.														
CILANTRO LEAF														
raw, chopped............	1 cup	2820	0.03	0.08	0.60	0.06	28.5	0.00	16.2	30.8	0.8	12.0	235	<0.1
raw, minced............	1 tsp	98	0.00	0.00	0.02	0.00	0.99	0.00	0.6	1.1	<0.1	0.4	8	0.0
CINNAMON														
ground............	1 tbsp	18	0.01	0.01	0.09	0.02	2.0	0.00	1.9	83.5	2.6	3.8	34	0.1
ground............	1 tsp	6	0.00	0.00	0.03	0.01	0.7	0.00	0.7	28.3	0.9	1.3	12	<0.1
CISCO. See CHUB.														
CITRONELLA. See LEMONGRASS.														
CLAM														
Canned														
mixed species, drained............	1 cup	912	0.24	0.68	5.40	0.18	46.1	158.00	35.4	147.0	44.7	28.8	1005	4.4
mixed species, drained............	3 oz	485	0.13	0.36	2.90	0.09	24.5	84.10	18.8	78.2	23.8	15.3	534	2.3
mixed species, w/liquid............	1 cup	72	0.02	0.05	0.43	0.02	4.8	12.00	2.4	31.2	0.7	26.4	358	0.2
mixed species, w/liquid............	3 oz	26	0.01	0.02	0.15	0.01	1.7	4.30	0.9	11.1	0.3	9.3	127	<0.1
Fresh														
mixed species, boiled or steamed............	3 oz	485	0.13	0.36	2.90	0.09	24.5	84.10	18.8	78.2	23.8	15.3	534	2.3
mixed species, boiled or steamed, small....	20 clams	1083	0.28	0.81	6.40	0.21	54.7	188.00	42.0	175.0	53.1	34.2	1193	5.2
mixed species, breaded, fried............	3 oz	257	0.09	0.21	1.80	0.05	30.6	34.20	8.5	53.5	11.8	11.9	277	1.2
mixed species, breaded, fried, small........	20 clams	568	0.19	0.46	3.90	0.11	67.7	75.70	18.8	118.0	26.2	26.3	613	2.7
mixed species, raw............	3 oz	255	0.07	0.18	1.50	0.05	13.6	42.00	11.1	39.1	11.9	7.7	267	1.2

Food Name	Serving Size	A I.U.	Thi mg	Rib mg	Nia mg	B_6 mg	Fol mcg	B_{12} mcg	C mg	Calc mg	Iron mg	Mag mg	Pot mg	Zn mg
mixed species, raw, large	9 clams	540	0.14	0.38	3.20	0.11	28.8	89.00	23.4	82.8	25.2	16.2	565	2.5
mixed species, raw, large	1 clam	60	0.02	0.04	0.35	0.01	3.2	9.90	2.6	9.2	2.8	1.8	63	0.3
mixed species, raw, medium	1 clam	44	0.01	0.03	0.26	0.01	2.3	7.20	1.9	6.7	2.0	1.3	45.5	0.2
mixed species, raw, small	1 clam	27	0.01	0.02	0.16	0.01	1.4	4.50	1.2	4.1	1.3	0.8	28.3	0.1
CLAM-TOMATO JUICE														
canned	5.5 fl oz	357	0.07	0.05	0.32	0.14	26.4	50.8	6.8	19.9	0	36.5	149	1.8
canned	1 fl oz	64.9	0.01	0.01	0.06	0.03	4.8	9.2	1.2	3.6	0.18	6.6	27.2	0.33
CLOUD EAR FUNGI														
dried	1 cup	0	0.00	0.24	1.80	0.03	10.6	0.00	0.0	44.5	1.6	23.2	211.0	0.4
dried, whole	1 medium	0	0.00	0.04	0.28	0.01	1.7	0.00	0.0	7.2	0.3	3.7	33.9	<0.1
CLOVES														
ground	1 tbsp	35	0.01	0.02	0.10	0.09	6.1	0.00	5.3	42.6	0.6	17.4	73	<0.1
ground	1 tsp	11	0.00	0.01	0.03	0.03	2.0	0.00	1.7	13.6	0.2	5.5	23	<0.1
COATING MIX. See SEASONING AND COATING MIX.														
COBNUT. See HAZELNUT.														
COCKTAIL. See also COCKTAIL MIX; LIQUEUR.														
DAIQUIRI														
canned	6.8 fl oz	4	0.00	0.00	0.03	0.01	1.7	0.00	2.7	0.0	>0.1	2.1	23	>0.1
canned	1 fl oz	<1	0.00	0.00	0.00	0.00	0.2	0.00	0.4	0.0	0.0	0.3	3	>0.1
PIÑA COLADA														
canned	6.8 fl oz	53	0.04	0.01	0.23	0.04	13.3	0.00	3.3	2.2	>0.1	13.3	184	0.4
canned	1 fl oz	8	0.01	0.00	0.03	0.01	2.0	0.00	0.5	0.3	>0.1	2.0	27	>0.1
TEQUILA SUNRISE														
canned	6.8 fl oz	205	0.08	0.03	0.40	0.11	22.4	0.00	40.7	0.0	>0.1	14.8	21	1.3
canned	1 fl oz	30	0.01	0.01	0.06	0.02	3.3	0.00	6.0	0.0	>0.1	2.2	3	0.2
WHISKEY SOUR														
canned	6.8 fl oz	27	0.02	0.01	0.04	0.00	0.0	0.00	3.3	0.0	>0.1	2.1	23	0.1
canned	1 fl oz	4	0.00	0.00	0.01	0.00	0.0	0.00	0.5	0.0	0.0	0.3	3	>0.1
COCKTAIL MIX														
WHISKEY SOUR														
bottled	1 fl oz	7	0.00	0.00	0.00	0.00	0.0	0.00	0.8	0.6	>0.1	0.3	97	>0.1
bottled, w/added potassium and sodium	1 fl oz	7	0.00	0.00	0.00	0.00	0.0	0.00	0.9	0.7	>0.1	0.3	2	>0.1
instant, dry	1 pkt	5	0.00	0.00	0.00	0.00	0.0	0.00	0.5	45.4	>0.1	3.2	3	>0.1
COCOA														
unsweetened	1 cup	17	0.07	0.21	1.90	0.10	27.5	0.00	0.0	110.0	11.9	429.0	1311	5.9
unsweetened	1 tbsp	1	0.00	0.01	0.12	0.01	1.7	0.00	0.0	6.9	0.8	26.9	82	0.4
unsweetened, European style (Hershey's)	1 cup	na	na	na	na	na	na	na	na	129	36.0	na	4365	na
unsweetened, European style (Hershey's)	1 tbsp	na	na	na	na	na	na	na	na	7.5	2.1	na	254	na
unsweetened, processed w/alkali	1 cup	17	0.10	0.40	2.10	0.10	27.5	0.00	0.0	95.5	13.3	409.0	2158	5.5
unsweetened, processed w/alkali	1 tbsp	1	0.01	0.03	0.13	0.01	1.7	0.00	0.0	6.0	0.8	25.7	135	0.3
COCOA, HOT, MIX														
(Alba 66)														
w/aspartame, mix only	1 pkt	6	0.05	0.27	0.21	0.06	2.8	0.37	0.0	110.0	0.9	39.7	516	0.7
(Carnation)														
rich, mix only	1 pkt	0	0.03	0.12	0.16	0.03	2.0	0.10	0.0	40.0	0.3	27.4	194	0.4
sugarless, mix only	1 pkt	0	0.06	0.22	0.18	0.05	5.8	0.45	0.4	123.0	0.4	27.0	288	0.6
w/marshmallows, mix only	1 pkt	0	0.03	0.12	0.10	0.03	1.1	0.12	0.0	41.2	0.2	16.2	142	0.2
(Swiss Miss)														
w/aspartame, w/added calcium or phosphorus, w/o added salt or vitamin A, mix only	1 pkt	240	0.04	0.21	0.16	0.05	2.2	0.29	0.0	216.0	0.7	31.2	405	0.5

Food Name	Serving Size	A I.U.	Thi mg	Rib mg	Nia mg	B_6 mg	Fol mcg	B_{12} mcg	C mg	Calc mg	Iron mg	Mag mg	Pot mg	Zn mg
w/aspartame, w/added salt and vitamin A, w/o added calcium or phosphorus, mix only	1 pkt	5	0.04	0.21	0.16	0.05	2.2	0.29	0.0	86.4	0.7	31.2	405	0.5
COCOA BUTTER OIL														
	1 cup	0	0.00	0.00	0.00	0.00	0.0	0.00	0.0	0.0	0.0	0.0	0	0.0
	1 tbsp	0	0.00	0.00	0.00	0.00	0.0	0.00	0.0	0.0	0.0	0.0	0	0.0
COCONUT														
Dried														
meat, creamed	1 oz	0	0.02	0.03	0.17	0.09	2.6	0.00	0.4	7.4	0.9	26.1	156	0.6
meat, sweetened, flaked, canned	1 cup	0	0.02	0.02	0.23	0.18	5.5	0.00	0.0	10.8	1.4	37.7	249	1.2
meat, sweetened, flaked, canned	4 oz	0	0.03	0.02	0.35	0.27	8.1	0.00	0.0	16.0	2.1	55.9	369	1.8
meat, sweetened, flaked, packaged	1 cup	0	0.02	0.02	0.22	0.19	5.8	0.00	0.0	10.4	1.3	35.5	234	1.3
meat, sweetened, flaked, packaged	1 oz	0	0.01	0.01	0.09	0.07	2.2	0.00	0.0	4.0	0.5	13.6	90	0.5
meat, sweetened, shredded	1 cup	0	0.03	0.02	0.44	0.25	7.5	0.00	0.7	13.9	1.8	46.5	313	1.7
meat, sweetened, shredded	7-oz pkg	0	0.06	0.04	0.94	0.54	16.1	0.00	1.4	29.9	3.8	99.5	671	3.6
meat, sweetened, toasted	1 oz	0	0.02	0.03	0.17	0.09	2.6	0.00	0.4	7.7	0.9	26.1	157	0.6
meat, unsweetened	1 oz	0	0.02	0.03	0.17	0.09	2.6	0.00	0.4	7.4	0.9	25.5	154	0.6
Fresh														
meat, raw, shredded	1 cup	0	0.05	0.02	0.43	0.04	21.1	0.00	2.6	11.2	1.9	25.6	285	0.9
meat, raw, 2x2x1/2-inch pieces	1 piece	0	0.03	0.01	0.24	0.02	11.9	0.00	1.5	6.3	1.1	14.4	160	0.5
meat, raw, whole	1 medium	0	0.26	0.08	2.1	0.21	105	0.00	13.1	55.6	9.6	127.0	1413	4.4
COCONUT CREAM														
Canned														
liquid expressed from grated meat	1 cup	0	0.07	0.12	0.11	0.09	42.3	0.00	5.3	3.0	1.5	50.3	299	1.8
liquid expressed from grated meat	1 tbsp	0	0.00	0.01	0.01	0.01	2.7	0.00	0.3	0.2	0.1	3.2	19	0.1
Fresh														
liquid expressed from grated meat, raw	1 cup	0	0.07	0.00	2.10	0.11	55.2	0.00	6.7	26.4	5.5	67.2	780	2.3
liquid expressed from grated meat, raw	1 tbsp	0	0.01	0.00	0.13	0.01	3.5	0.00	0.4	1.6	0.3	4.2	49	0.1
COCONUT MILK														
Canned														
liquid expressed from grated meat and water	1 cup	0	0.05	0.00	1.40	0.06	30.5	0.00	2.3	40.7	7.5	104.0	497	1.3
liquid expressed from grated meat and water	1 tbsp	0	0.00	0.00	0.10	0.00	2.0	0.00	0.2	2.7	0.5	6.9	33	<0.1
Fresh														
liquid expressed from grated meat and water, raw	1 cup	0	0.06	0.00	1.80	0.08	38.6	0.00	6.7	38.4	3.9	88.8	631	1.6
liquid expressed from grated meat and water, raw	1 tbsp	0	0.00	0.00	0.11	0.01	2.4	0.00	0.4	2.4	0.3	5.5	40	0.1
Frozen														
liquid expressed from grated meat and water	1 cup	0	0.06	0.00	1.60	0.07	34.1	0.00	2.6	9.6	1.9	76.8	557	1.4
liquid expressed from grated meat and water	1 tbsp	0	0.00	0.00	0.10	0.01	2.1	0.00	0.2	0.6	0.1	4.8	35	<0.1
COCONUT OIL														
	1 cup	0	0.00	0.00	0.00	0.00	0.0	0.00	0.0	0.0	<0.1	0.0	0	0.0
	1 tbsp	0	0.00	0.00	0.00	0.00	0.0	0.00	0.0	0.0	<0.1	0.0	0	0.0
COCONUT WATER														
liquid from coconuts	1 cup	0	0.07	0.14	0.19	0.08	6.0	0.00	5.8	57.6	0.7	60.0	600	0.2
liquid from coconuts	1 tbsp	0	0.01	0.01	0.01	0.01	0.4	0.00	0.4	3.6	<0.1	3.8	38	<0.1
COD														
ALASKAN / sablefish / skil														
baked, broiled, grilled, or microwaved	3 oz	287	0.10	0.10	4.40	0.29	14.4	1.20	0.0	38.3	1.4	60.4	390	0.4
raw	3 oz	264	0.09	0.08	3.40	0.26	12.8	1.30	0.0	29.8	1.1	46.8	304	0.3

Food Name	Serving Size	A I.U.	Thi mg	Rib mg	Nia mg	B_6 mg	Fol mcg	B_{12} mcg	C mg	Calc mg	Iron mg	Mag mg	Pot mg	Zn mg
smoked	3 oz	347	0.11	0.10	4.50	0.33	16.7	1.70	0.0	42.5	1.4	62.9	400	0.4
ATLANTIC														
Canned														
w/liquid	3 oz	39	0.07	0.07	2.10	0.24	6.9	0.89	0.9	17.9	0.42	34.9	449	0.5
Dried and salted														
	3 oz	120	0.23	0.20	6.40	0.73	21.0	8.50	3.0	136.0	2.1	113.0	1239	1.4
5.5x1.5x1/2-inch pieces	1 piece	113	0.21	0.19	6.00	0.69	19.8	8.00	2.8	128.0	2.0	106.0	1166	1.3
	1 oz	40	0.08	0.07	2.10	0.25	7.0	2.80	1.0	45.4	0.7	37.7	413	0.5
Fresh														
baked, broiled, grilled, or microwaved	3 oz	39	0.08	0.07	2.10	0.24	6.9	0.89	0.9	11.9	0.4	35.7	207	0.5
raw	3 oz	34	0.07	0.06	1.80	0.21	6.0	0.77	0.9	13.6	0.3	27.2	351	0.4
PACIFIC														
baked, broiled, grilled, or microwaved	3 oz	27.2	0.02	0.04	2.1	0.39	6.8	0.88	2.5	7.7	0.28	26.4	439	0.43
raw	3 oz	23.8	0.02	0.04	1.7	0.34	5.6	0.77	2.5	6.0	0.22	20.4	343	0.34
COD LIVER OIL. See under FISH OIL.														
COFFEE														
Brewed														
decaffeinated, prepared w/tap water	6 fl oz	0	0.00	0.00	0.40	0.00	0.0	0.00	0.0	3.6	<0.1	8.9	96	<0.1
regular, prepared w/distilled water	6 fl oz	0	0.00	0.00	0.40	0.00	0.2	0.00	0.0	3.6	<0.1	10.7	123	<0.1
regular, prepared w/tap water	6 fl oz	0	0.00	0.00	0.40	0.00	0.2	0.00	0.0	3.6	<0.1	8.9	96	<0.1
Instant														
regular, powder, mix only	1 tsp	0	0.00	0.00	0.25	0.00	0.0	0.00	0.0	1.3	<0.1	2.9	32	0.0
regular, powder, mix only	1 rounded tsp	0	0.00	0.02	0.51	0.00	0.0	0.00	0.0	2.5	<0.1	5.6	63	0.0
regular, powder, prepared	6 fl oz	0	0.00	0.03	0.51	0.00	0.0	0.00	0.0	5.4	<0.1	7.2	63	<0.1
w/chicory, powder, mix only	1 rounded tsp	0	0.00	0.01	0.39	0.00	0.0	0.00	0.0	1.9	<0.1	3.8	61	<0.1
w/chicory, powder, prepared	6 fl oz	0	0.00	0.01	0.39	0.00	0.0	0.00	0.0	5.4	<0.1	5.4	61	<0.1
FLAVORED														
Instant														
(General Foods)														
café Francais, 'International Coffees' mix only	1-1/3 tbsp	0	na	na	na	na	na	na	0	3.1	<0.1	na	129	na
French vanilla, 'International Coffees' mix only	1-1/3 tbsp	0	na	na	na	na	na	na	0	1.7	<0.1	na	76	na
French vanilla, sugarless, 'International Coffees' mix only	1-1/3 tbsp	0	na	na	na	na	na	na	0	4.3	<0.1	na	72	na
Suisse mocha, 'International Coffees' mix only	1-1/3 tbsp	0	na	na	na	na	na	na	0	2.3	0.3	na	117	na
Suisse mocha, sugar-free, 'International Coffees' mix only	1-1/3 tbsp	0	na	na	na	na	na	na	0	5.3	0.3	na	112	na
COFFEE SUBSTITUTE														
cereal grain beverage, mix only	1 tsp	0	0.02	0.00	0.39	0.02	0.6	0.00	0.0	1.2	0.1	5.6	42	<0.1
cereal grain beverage, prepared w/milk	6 fl oz	229	0.07	0.30	0.54	0.08	9.1	0.65	1.7	220.0	0.2	29.6	318	0.7
cereal grain beverage, prepared w/water	6 fl oz	0	0.01	0.00	0.39	0.02	0.5	0.00	0.0	5.4	0.1	7.2	43	<0.1
COHO SALMON. See under SALMON.														
COLE. See KALE.														
COLESLAW														
fresh	1/2 cup	381	0.04	0.04	0.16	0.08	15.9	0.00	19.6	27.0	0.4	6.0	109	0.1
fresh	1 tbsp	51	0.01	0.01	0.02	0.01	2.1	0.00	2.6	3.6	<0.1	0.8	15	<0.1
COLEWORT. See KALE.														
COLLARDS														
Fresh														
boiled, drained, chopped	1 cup	5945	0.08	0.20	1.10	0.24	177.0	0.00	34.6	226.0	0.87	32.3	494	0.8

Food Name	Serving Size	A I.U.	Thi mg	Rib mg	Nia mg	B₆ mg	Fol mcg	B₁₂ mcg	C mg	Calc mg	Iron mg	Mag mg	Pot mg	Zn mg
raw, chopped	1 cup	1377	0.02	0.05	0.27	0.06	59.8	0.00	12.7	52.2	0.07	3.2	61	<0.1
Frozen														
chopped, unprepared	3-lb pkg	77754	0.68	1.50	8.70	1.60	995.0	0.00	544.0	2736.0	14.6	395.0	3443	3.5
chopped, unprepared	10-oz pkg	16225	0.14	0.31	1.80	0.33	208.0	0.00	114.0	571.0	3.0	82.4	719	0.7
no salt added, chopped, drained	1 cup	10168	0.08	0.20	1.10	0.19	129.0	0.00	44.9	357.0	1.9	51.0	427	0.5
COLORADO PINYON. See PINE NUT.														
CONVOLVULUS, WATER. See CABBAGE, SKUNK.														
COOKIE														
(Archway)														
'Aunt Bea's Pound Cake' 'Home Style'	1 serving	22	0.07	0.06	0.50	na	na	na	0.0	9.6	0.5	na	21	na
hermits, 'Home Style'	1 serving	9	0.07	0.06	0.58	na	na	na	0.0	13.3	0.7	na	37	na
windmill, old fashioned, 'Home Style'	1 serving	3	0.07	0.05	0.58	na	na	na	0.0	7.2	0.7	na	20	na
ANIMAL CRACKER	1 cracker	0	0.01	0.01	0.09	0.00	2.1	0.00	0.0	1.1	<0.1	0.5	3	<0.1
APPLE CINNAMON														
(Archway) 'Home Style'	1 serving	<1	0.07	0.06	0.57	na	17.2	na	0.0	8.3	0.6	na	23	na
APPLE RAISIN														
(Archway) gourmet, 'Home Style'	1 serving	8	0.07	0.04	0.36	na	na	na	0.0	7.3	0.6	na	57	na
APRICOT														
(Archway) filled, 'Home Style'	1 serving	14	0.06	0.05	0.49	na	na	na	0.0	5.3	0.5	na	32	na
BLACK WALNUT														
(Archway) icebox, 'Home Style'	1 serving	15	0.07	0.06	0.55	na	17.5	na	0.0	5.0	0.7	na	20	na
CARAMEL														
(Snackwell's) 'Caramel Delights'	1 serving	<1	0.01	0.02	0.09	0.01	9.5	0.02	<0.1	8.5	0.1	4.7	22	0.1
CARROT														
(Archway) cake, gourmet, 'Home Style'.......	1 serving	251	0.06	0.05	0.41	na	na	na	0.0	11.2	0.7	na	11	na
CHERRY														
(Archway) filled, 'Home Style'	1 serving	22	0.07	0.05	0.48	na	na	na	0.0	6.0	0.5	na	30	na
CHOCOLATE														
wafer..................................	1 oz	3	0.06	0.08	0.81	0.01	14.2	0.03	0.0	8.8	1.1	15.0	60	0.3
wafer..................................	1 wafer	<1	0.01	0.02	0.17	0.00	3.0	0.01	0.0	1.9	0.2	3.2	13	<0.1
(Archway)														
devil's food, nonfat, 'Home Style'	1 serving	0	0.06	0.04	0.44	na	13.0	na	0.0	2.0	0.5	na	54	na
Dutch cocoa, 'Home Style'	1 serving	5	0.06	0.04	0.47	na	na	na	0.0	2.9	0.6	na	46	na
mud pie, 'Home Style'..................	1 serving	8	0.05	0.05	0.45	na	12.3	na	0.0	7.3	0.7	na	67	na
(Snackwell's) devil's food cake, nonfat	1 serving	<1	0.01	0.03	0.22	0.00	3.0	0.01	<0.1	4.8	0.5	4.0	18	<0.1
CHOCOLATE CHIP														
(Archway)														
and toffee, gourmet, 'Home Style'..........	1 serving	20	0.07	0.05	0.57	na	na	na	0.0	3.9	0.6	na	21	na
drop, 'Home Style'.....................	1 serving	21	0.06	0.06	0.50	na	na	na	0.0	9.5	0.6	na	27	na
ice box, 'Home Style'	1 serving	12	0.06	0.05	0.46	na	na	na	0.0	4.8	0.6	na	27	na
no sugar, 'Home Style'	1 serving	5	0.06	0.05	0.44	na	na	na	0.0	61.9	0.5	na	19	na
rocky road, gourmet, 'Home Style'	1 serving	22	0.06	0.06	0.51	na	na	na	0.0	5.3	0.8	na	54	na
rocky road, sugarless, 'Home Style'	1 serving	3	0.06	0.05	0.45	na	na	na	0.0	40.3	0.7	na	58	na
(Keebler)														
regular, enriched, 'Rich, 'n Chips'	1 large	<1	0.03	0.04	0.38	0.01	5.9	0.00	0.0	3.5	0.4	4.3	19	<0.1
(Nabisco)														
'Chips Ahoy'	1 cookie	<1	0.03	0.04	0.39	0.01	6.0	0.00	0.0	3.5	0.4	4.4	19	<0.1
mini, 'Chips Ahoy!'	1 cookie	<1	0.01	0.01	0.06	0.00	0.9	0.00	0.0	0.6	<0.1	0.7	3	<0.1
pecan, 'Selections' 'Chips Ahoy!'	1 cookie	<1	0.03	0.03	0.33	0.01	5.0	0.00	0.0	3.0	0.3	3.7	16	<0.1
CINNAMON *(Archway)* honey hearts,														
nonfat, 'Home Style'	1 serving	0	0.10	0.06	0.78	na	23.4	na	0.0	6.3	0.8	na	20	na
COCONUT														
(Archway) macaroon, 'Home Style'	1 serving	0	0.01	0.01	0.07	na	1.1	na	0.0	3.3	0.4	na	57	na

Food Name	Serving Size	A I.U.	Thi mg	Rib mg	Nia mg	B₆ mg	Fol mcg	B₁₂ mcg	C mg	Calc mg	Iron mg	Mag mg	Pot mg	Zn mg
FIG														
(Figaroo) bar	1 cookie	14	0.07	0.09	0.81	0.03	11.6	0.04	0.1	27.5	1.2	11.6	89	0.2
FORTUNE														
	1 cookie	<1	0.02	0.01	0.15	0.00	4.4	0.00	0.0	0.9	0.1	0.6	3	<0.1
	1 oz	<1	0.05	0.04	0.52	0.00	15.6	0.00	0.0	3.4	0.4	2.0	12	<0.1
GINGER														
snap, large 3.5–4-inch diam	1 cookie	<1	0.06	0.09	1.00	0.03	23.0	0.00	0.0	24.6	2.0	15.7	111	0.2
snap, medium	1 cookie	<1	0.01	0.02	0.23	0.01	5.0	0.00	0.0	5.4	0.5	3.4	24	<0.1
(Archway)														
snap, iced, 'Home Style'	1 serving	0	0.10	0.07	0.91	na	24.8	na	0.0	7.8	1.3	na	25	na
snap, less fat, 'Home Style'	1 serving	0	0.11	0.07	0.92	na	24.3	na	0.0	9.0	1.4	na	47	na
GRAHAM														
(Keebler) chocolate, 'Selects'	1 serving	na	na	na	na	na	na	na	na	na	na	na	na	na
(Nabisco)	1 serving	0	0.06	0.07	1.10	0.03	12.9	na	0.0	22.1	1.2	16.5	50	0.5
LEMON														
(Archway)														
drop, 'Home Style'	1 serving	14	0.07	0.06	0.54	na	na	na	0.0	8.9	0.5	na	20	na
frosty, 'Home Style'	1 serving	0	0.06	0.05	0.51	na	15.3	na	0.0	10.7	0.4	na	24	na
nuggets, nonfat, 'Home Style'	1 serving	0	0.10	0.06	0.77	na	23.0	na	0.0	4.5	0.7	na	20	na
snap, 'Home Style'	1 serving	11	0.10	0.07	0.74	na	23.3	na	0.0	9.3	0.7	na	24	na
MINT														
(Snackwell's) creme	1 serving	<1	0.02	0.03	0.31	0.01	5.0	0.00	0.0	5.0	0.6	10.0	37	0.2
MOLASSES														
(Archway)														
	1 serving	12	0.07	0.06	0.66	na	na	na	0.0	8.6	1.1	na	29	na
dark, 'Home Style'	1 serving	0	0.08	0.06	0.75	na	19.0	na	0.0	13.4	1.2	na	96	na
iced, 'Home Style'	1 serving	5	0.07	0.04	0.44	na	na	na	0.0	8.1	0.6	na	45	na
old fashioned, 'Home Style'	1 serving	12	0.08	0.06	0.69	na	na	na	0.0	9.1	1.2	na	29	na
(Little Debbie)	1 cookie	0	0.07	0.05	0.61	0.02	14.8	0.00	0.0	14.8	1.3	10.4	69	<0.1
OATMEAL														
(Archway)														
apple-filled	1 piece	3	0.07	0.04	0.44	na	13.3	na	0.0	7.3	0.7	na	46	na
date-filled, 'Home Style'	1 serving	6	0.07	0.04	0.45	na	na	na	0.0	8.5	0.5	na	52	na
golden, gourmet, 'Ruth's' 'Home Style'	1 serving	8	0.08	0.05	0.52	na	na	na	0.0	7.6	0.6	na	59	na
'Home Style'	1 serving	7	0.07	0.04	0.47	na	na	na	0.0	7.8	0.6	na	46	na
pecan, gourmet, 'Home Style'	1 serving	9	0.07	0.04	0.40	na	na	na	0.0	5.9	0.8	na	43	na
raisin, 'Home Style'	1 serving	7	0.07	0.04	0.45	na	na	na	0.0	8.1	0.6	na	60	na
raisin, nonfat, 'Home Style'	1 serving	<1	0.08	0.04	0.51	na	14.6	na	0.0	11.5	1.0	na	87	na
raspberry, nonfat, 'Home Style'	1 serving	<1	0.08	0.04	0.51	na	14.6	na	0.0	11.8	0.0	na	89	na
'Ruth's'	1 serving	9	0.07	0.04	0.44	na	na	na	0.0	8.1	0.7	na	48	na
sugar-free, 'Home Style'	1 serving	<1	0.07	0.04	0.43	na	13.9	na	0.0	4.8	0.5	na	21	na
ORANGE														
(Archway) frosty, 'Home Style'	1 serving	0	0.06	0.05	0.48	na	15.1	na	0.0	11.2	0.4	na	24	na
PEANUT														
(Archway) jumble, 'Home Style'	1 serving	8	0.06	0.04	1.10	na	na	na	0.0	7.4	1.0	na	59	na
PEANUT BUTTER														
(Archway)														
gourmet, old fashioned, 'Home Style'	1 serving	15	0.06	0.05	1.20	na	na	na	0.0	6.0	0.7	na	52	na
'Home Style'	1 serving	13	0.05	0.04	0.92	na	na	na	0.0	7.3	0.6	na	44	na
(Little Debbie) wafer, w/peanut butter, chocolate covered	1 serving	na	na	na	na	na	na	na	1.1	na	na	na	na	na
PECAN														
(Archway) iced, 'Home Style'	1 serving	9	0.07	0.05	0.56	na	na	na	0.0	4.1	0.5	na	17	na

Food Name	Serving Size	A I.U.	Thi mg	Rib mg	Nia mg	B_6 mg	Fol mcg	B_{12} mcg	C mg	Calc mg	Iron mg	Mag mg	Pot mg	Zn mg
RASPBERRY														
(Archway) filled, 'Home Style'	1 serving	11	0.08	0.05	0.48	na	na	na	0.0	6.0	0.5	na	31	na
SANDWICH														
chocolate, w/creme filling	1 cookie	<1	0.01	0.02	0.21	0.00	4.3	0.00	0.0	2.6	0.4	4.5	18	<0.1
chocolate, w/creme filling, chocolate-coated	1 cookie	<1	0.02	0.04	0.23	0.01	3.1	0.01	0.0	6.0	0.5	6.6	41	0.1
chocolate, w/extra creme filling	1 cookie	0	0.01	0.02	0.20	0.00	5.6	0.00	0.0	3.1	0.4	4.4	16	<0.1
SHORTBREAD														
(Archway) sugarless, 'Home Style'	1 serving	na	0.06	0.05	0.51	na	15.4	na	0.0	2.2	0.4	na	14	na
STRAWBERRY														
(Archway) filled, 'Home Style'	1 serving	11	0.07	0.05	0.48	na	na	na	0.0	6.3	0.6	na	34	na
SUGAR														
(Archway)														
'Home Style'	1 serving	8	0.07	0.06	0.59	na	na	na	0.0	7.2	0.5	na	20	na
nonfat, 'Home Style'	1 serving	0	0.06	0.04	0.50	na	15.2	na	0.0	2.6	0.4	na	12	na
VANILLA														
(Keebler)														
wafer, 'Keebler Golden'	1 serving	na	na	na	na	na	na	na	na	na	na	na	na	na
COOKIE CRUMB TOPPING														
(Nabisco) 'Oreo Crunchies'	1 serving	<1	0.01	0.02	0.20	0.00	3.3	0.00	na	2.6	0.5	5.3	21	0.1
COOKIE CRUMBS														
chocolate wafer crumbs	1 cup	15	0.23	0.30	3.20	0.06	56.0	0.10	0.0	34.7	4.5	59.4	235	1.2
COOKIE DOUGH														
(Pillsbury) chocolate chip, refrigerated	1 serving	na	na	na	na	na	na	na	na	na	na	na	na	na
COOKING OIL. See individual listings.														
CORIANDER / Chinese parsley														
CORIANDER, RAW														
CORIANDER LEAF/ Chinese parsley leaf														
dried	1 tbsp	105	0.02	0.03	0.19	0.02	4.9	0	10.2	22.4	0.76	12.5	80.4	0.09
dried	1 tsp	35.1	0.01	0.01	0.06	0.01	1.6	0	3.4	7.5	0.26	4.2	26.8	0.03
fresh, raw, chopped	1/4 cup	111	0	0.01	0.03	0	0.41	0	0.42	3.9	0.08	1.0	21.7	0.02
fresh, raw, whole, med plants	9 plants	553	0.02	0.02	0.15	0.02	2.1	0	2.1	19.6	0.39	5.2	108	0.09
CORIANDER SEED/ Chinese parsley seed														
	1 tbsp	0	0.01	0.02	0.11	na	0	0	1.1	35.4	0.82	16.5	63.4	0.23
	1 tsp	0	0	0.01	0.04	na	0	0	0.38	12.8	0.29	5.9	22.8	0.09
CORN														
WHITE														
Canned														
kernels, sweet, drained	1 cup	0	0.05	0.13	2.00	0.08	79.7	0.00	13.9	8.2	1.4	32.8	320	0.6
kernels, sweet, no salt added, w/liquid	1/2 cup	0	0.03	0.08	1.20	0.05	48.8	0.00	7.0	5.1	0.5	20.5	210	0.5
kernels, sweet, vacuum-packed	1/2 cup	0	0.04	0.08	1.20	0.06	51.8	0.00	8.5	5.3	0.4	24.1	195	0.5
kernels, sweet, w/liquid	1/2 cup	0	0.03	0.08	1.20	0.05	48.8	0.00	7.0	5.1	0.5	20.5	210	0.5
sweet, vacuum packed, no salt added	1/2 cup	0	0.04	0.08	1.20	0.06	51.8	0.00	8.5	5.3	0.4	24.1	195	0.5
Fresh														
kernels, sweet, boiled, drained	1/2 cup	0	0.07	0.06	1.10	0.11	25.4	0.00	2.5	3.3	0.3	15.6	121	0.3
kernels, sweet, raw	1 cup	0	0.31	0.09	2.60	0.09	70.5	0.00	10.5	3.1	0.8	57.0	416	0.7
on the cob, sweet, large ears, 7.75 to 9 inches	1 ear	0	0.29	0.09	2.40	0.08	65.5	0.00	9.7	2.9	0.7	52.9	386	0.6
on the cob, sweet, med ears, 6.75 to 7.5 inches	1 ear	0	0.18	0.05	1.50	0.05	41.2	0.00	6.1	1.8	0.4	33.3	243	0.4
on the cob, sweet, small ears, 5.5 to 6.5 inches	1 ear	0	0.15	0.04	1.20	0.04	33.4	0.00	5.0	1.5	0.4	27.0	197	0.3
Frozen														
kernels, sweet, boiled, drained	10-oz pkg	0	0.24	0.20	3.70	0.37	88.0	0.00	8.8	11.4	1.0	54.0	417	1.1

Food Name	Serving Size	A I.U.	Thi mg	Rib mg	Nia mg	B_6 mg	Fol mcg	B_{12} mcg	C mg	Calc mg	Iron mg	Mag mg	Pot mg	Zn mg
kernels, sweet, boiled, drained	1/2 cup	0	0.14	0.06	1.20	0.18	25.0	0.00	3.9	2.5	0.5	23.8	206	0.5
kernels, sweet, no salt added, boiled, drained	1/2 cup	0	0.14	0.06	1.20	0.18	25.0	0.00	3.9	2.5	0.5	23.8	206	0.5
YELLOW														
Canned														
brine pack, w/liquid	1/2 cup	195	0.03	0.08	1.20	0.05	48.8	0.00	7.0	5.1	0.5	20.5	210	0.5
kernels, sweet, drained	1 cup	256	0.05	0.13	2.00	0.08	79.7	0.00	13.9	8.2	1.4	32.8	320	0.6
kernels, sweet, w/liquid	1/2 cup	195	0.03	0.08	1.20	0.05	48.8	0.00	7.0	5.1	0.5	20.5	210	0.5
sweet, no salt added, vacuum-packed	1/2 cup	253	0.04	0.08	1.20	0.06	51.8	0.00	8.5	5.3	0.4	24.1	195	0.5
sweet, vacuum-packed	1/2 cup	253	0.04	0.08	1.20	0.06	51.8	0.00	8.5	5.3	0.4	24.1	195	0.5
Fresh														
baby, sweet, whole, boiled, drained	1 ear	17	0.02	0.01	0.13	0.01	3.7	0.00	0.5	0.2	<0.1	2.6	20	<0.1
kernels, sweet, boiled, drained	1/2 cup	178	0.18	0.06	1.30	0.05	38.0	0.00	5.1	1.6	0.5	26.2	204	0.4
kernels, sweet, raw	1 cup	433	0.31	0.09	2.60	0.09	70.5	0.00	10.5	3.1	0.8	57.0	416	0.7
on the cob, large ears, 7.75 to 9 inches	1 ear	402	0.29	0.09	2.40	0.08	65.5	0.00	9.7	2.9	0.7	52.9	386	0.6
on the cob, medium ears, 6.75 to 7.5 inches.	1 ear	253	0.18	0.05	1.50	0.05	41.2	0.00	6.1	1.8	0.5	33.3	243	0.4
on the cob, small ears, 5.5 to 6.5 inches	1 ear	205	0.15	0.04	1.20	0.04	33.4	0.00	5.0	1.5	0.4	27.0	197	0.3
Frozen														
kernels, sweet, boiled, drained	10-oz pkg	625	0.24	0.20	3.70	0.37	88.0	0.00	8.8	11.4	1.0	54.0	417	1.1
kernels, sweet, boiled, drained	1/2 cup	173	0.14	0.06	1.20	0.18	25.0	0.00	3.9	2.5	0.5	23.8	206	0.5
kernels, sweet, no salt added, boiled, drained.	1/2 cup	173	0.14	0.06	1.20	0.18	25.0	0.00	3.9	2.5	0.5	23.8	206	0.5
kernels, sweet, unprepared	10-oz pkg	369	0.24	0.20	4.90	0.51	101.0	0.00	18.2	11.4	1.2	51.1	596	1.1
kernels, sweet, unprepared	1/2 cup	107	0.07	0.06	1.40	0.15	29.3	0.00	5.2	3.3	0.3	14.8	172	0.3
CORN BRAN, crude	1 cup	54	0.01	0.08	2.10	0.12	3.0	0.00	0.0	31.9	2.1	48.6	33	1.2
CORN CHIPS AND SNACKS.														
(Cornuts)														
nuggets, toasted, barbecue	1 oz	96	0.10	0.04	0.43	0.05	0.0	0.00	0.1	4.8	0.5	30.9	81	0.5
nuggets, toasted, nacho	1 oz	11	0.10	0.02	0.34	0.06	4.3	0.00	4.4	9.9	0.5	30.9	88	0.5
nuggets, toasted, plain	1 oz	0	0.01	0.04	0.48	0.07	0.0	0.00	0.0	2.6	0.5	32.0	79	0.5
CORN FLOUR. See under FLOUR. See also CORNMEAL.														
CORN SYRUP														
dark.	1 cup	0	0.04	0.03	0.07	0.03	0.0	0.00	0.0	59.0	1.2	26.2	144	0.1
dark.	1 tbsp	0	<0.01	<0.01	<0.01	<0.01	0.0	0.00	0.0	3.6	<0.1	1.6	9	<0.1
high-fructose.	1 cup	0	0.00	0.06	0.00	0.00	0.0	0.00	0.0	0.0	<0.1	0.0	0	0.1
high-fructose.	1 tbsp	0	0.00	<0.01	0.00	0.00	0.0	0.00	0.0	0.0	<0.1	0.0	0	<0.1
light.	1 cup	0	0.04	0.03	0.07	0.03	0.0	0.00	0.0	9.8	0.2	6.6	13	<0.1
light.	1 tbsp	0	<0.01	<0.01	<0.01	<0.01	0.0	0.00	0.0	0.6	<0.1	0.4	<1	<0.1
table blend, w/sugar	1 cup	0	0.02	0.15	0.06	0.03	9.5	0.00	0.0	72.7	2.3	28.4	199	0.1
table blend, w/sugar	1 tbsp	0	<0.01	0.01	<0.01	<0.01	0.6	0.00	0.0	4.6	0.2	1.8	13	<0.1
CORNED BEEF HASH. See under HASH.														
CORNISH GAME HEN														
meat and skin, raw	1/2 medium	181	0.12	0.29	9.50	0.50	5.0	0.55	0.8	18.5	1.3	30.2	396	1.9
meat and skin, roasted	1/2 medium	137	0.09	0.26	7.60	0.40	2.6	0.36	0.7	16.8	1.2	23.2	316	1.9
meat only, raw.	1/2 medium	90	0.11	0.26	8.10	0.46	3.6	0.48	0.7	14.4	0.9	25.2	323	1.6
meat only, roasted	1/2 medium	71	0.08	0.25	6.90	0.39	2.2	0.33	0.7	14.3	0.9	20.9	275	1.7
CORNMEAL														
WHITE														
Regular														
enriched, degermed	1 cup	0	0.99	0.56	6.90	0.35	258.0	0.00	0.0	6.9	5.7	55.2	224	1.0
unenriched, degermed	1 cup	0	0.19	0.07	1.40	0.35	66.2	0.00	0.0	6.9	1.5	55.2	224	1.0
whole-grain.	1 cup	0	0.47	0.25	4.40	0.37	31.0	0.00	0.0	7.3	4.2	155.0	350	2.2
Self-rising														
bolted, plain, enriched	1 cup	0	0.81	0.49	6.50	0.66	228.0	0.00	0.0	440.0	7.0	105.0	311	2.4

Food Name	Serving Size	A I.U.	Thi mg	Rib mg	Nia mg	B₆ mg	Fol mcg	B₁₂ mcg	C mg	Calc mg	Iron mg	Mag mg	Pot mg	Zn mg
bolted, w/wheat flour added, enriched	1 cup	0	1.20	0.74	8.80	0.65	313.0	0.00	0.0	508.0	8.4	91.8	352	2.4
enriched, degermed	1 cup	0	0.94	0.53	6.30	0.54	258.0	0.00	0.0	483.0	6.5	67.6	235	1.4
YELLOW														
Regular														
enriched, degermed	1 cup	570	0.99	0.56	6.90	0.35	258.0	0.00	0.0	6.9	5.7	55.2	224	1.0
unenriched, degermed	1 cup	570	0.19	0.07	1.40	0.35	66.2	0.00	0.0	6.9	1.5	55.2	224	1.0
whole-grain	1 cup	572	0.47	0.25	4.40	0.37	31.0	0.00	0.0	7.3	4.2	155.0	350	2.2
Self-rising														
bolted, plain, enriched	1 cup	572	0.81	0.49	6.50	0.66	228.0	0.00	0.0	440.0	7.0	105.0	311	2.4
bolted, w/wheat flour added, enriched	1 cup	488	1.20	0.74	8.80	0.65	313.0	0.00	0.0	508.0	8.4	91.8	352	2.4
enriched, degermed	1 cup	570	0.94	0.53	6.30	0.54	258.0	0.00	0.0	483.0	6.5	67.6	235	1.4
CORNSTARCH	1 cup	0	0.00	0.00	0.00	0.00	0.0	0.00	0.0	2.6	0.6	3.8	4	<0.1
COTTAGE CHEESE. See under CHEESE.														
COTTONSEED FLOUR. See under FLOUR.														
COTTONSEED KERNELS														
roasted	1 cup	659	1.10	0.38	4.50	1.20	348.0	0.00	13.4	149.0	8.0	656.0	2012	8.9
roasted	1 tbsp	44	0.08	0.03	0.30	0.08	23.3	0.00	0.9	10.0	0.5	44.0	135	0.6
COTTONSEED MEAL, partially defatted	1 oz	130	0.63	0.12	1.20	0.23	68.5	0.00	0.7	143.0	3.8	215.0	530	3.5
COTTONSEED OIL														
. . . .	1 cup	0	0.00	0.00	0.00	0.00	0.0	0.00	0.0	0.0	0.0	0.0	0	0.0
. . . .	1 tbsp	0	0.00	0.00	0.00	0.00	0.0	0.00	0.0	0.0	0.0	0.0	0	0.0
COUSCOUS														
cooked	1 cup	0	0.10	0.04	1.5	0.08	23.6	0	0	12.6	0.60	12.6	91.1	0.41
uncooked	1 cup	0	0.33	0.14	5.2	0.27	79.2	0	0	42.2	2.0	42.2	306	1.4
uncooked	1 oz	0	0.05	0.02	0.84	0.04	12.9	0	0	6.9	0.33	6.9	49.9	0.22
COWPEAS. See BLACK-EYED PEAS.														
CRAB														
ALASKA KING														
boiled, poached, or steamed	1 med leg	39	0.07	0.07	1.80	0.24	68.3	15.40	10.2	79.1	1.0	84.4	351	10.2
boiled, poached, or steamed	3 oz	25	0.05	0.05	1.10	0.15	43.4	9.80	6.5	50.1	0.7	53.5	223	6.5
raw	1 med leg	41	0.07	0.07	1.90	0.26	75.7	15.50	12.0	79.1	1.0	84.3	351	10.2
raw	3 oz	20	0.04	0.04	0.94	0.13	37.4	7.70	6.0	39.1	0.5	41.6	173	5.1
BLUE														
Canned														
. . . .	1 cup	7	0.11	0.11	1.90	0.20	57.4	0.62	3.6	136.0	1.1	52.6	505	5.4
. . . .	1 oz	1	0.02	0.02	0.39	0.04	12.0	0.13	0.8	28.6	0.2	11.1	106	1.1
. . . .	3 oz	4	0.07	0.07	1.20	0.13	36.1	0.39	2.3	85.8	0.7	33.1	318	3.4
drained	6.5-oz can	6	0.10	0.11	1.70	0.19	53.1	0.57	3.4	126.0	1.1	48.8	468	5.0
Fresh														
boiled, poached, or steamed	3 oz	5	0.09	0.04	2.80	0.15	43.2	6.20	2.8	88.4	0.8	28.1	275	3.6
boiled, poached, or steamed, flakes														
and pieces	1 cup	7	0.12	0.06	3.90	0.21	59.9	8.60	3.9	123.0	1.1	38.9	382	5.0
boiled, poached, or steamed, pieces	1 cup	8	0.14	0.07	4.50	0.24	68.6	9.90	4.5	140.0	1.2	44.5	437	5.7
boiled, poached, or steamed, w/o shell	1 oz	2	0.03	0.01	0.94	0.05	14.4	2.10	0.9	29.5	0.3	9.4	92	1.2
raw	1 med crab	1	0.02	0.01	0.57	0.03	9.2	1.90	0.6	18.7	0.2	7.1	69	0.7
raw	3 oz	4	0.07	0.03	2.30	0.13	37.4	7.70	2.5	75.7	0.6	28.9	280	3.0
DUNGENESS														
boiled, poached, or steamed	1 med crab	132	0.07	0.26	4.60	0.22	53.3	13.20	4.6	74.9	0.6	73.7	518	6.9
boiled, poached, or steamed	3 oz	88	0.05	0.17	3.10	0.15	35.7	8.80	3.1	50.1	0.4	49.3	347	4.6
raw	1 med crab	147	0.08	0.27	5.10	0.25	71.7	14.70	5.7	75.0	0.6	73.3	577	7.0
raw	3 oz	77	0.04	0.14	2.70	0.13	37.4	7.70	3.0	39.1	0.3	38.3	301	3.6
QUEEN														
boiled, poached, or steamed	3 oz	147	0.08	0.21	2.50	0.15	35.7	8.80	6.1	28.1	2.4	53.5	170	3.1
raw	3 oz	128	0.07	0.17	2.10	0.13	37.4	7.70	6.0	22.1	2.1	41.6	147	2.4
CRAB SUBSTITUTE														
Alaska king style, made from surimi	3 oz	56	0.03	0.02	0.15	0.03	1.4	1.40	0.0	11.1	0.3	36.5	77	0.3

Food Name	Serving Size	A I.U.	Thi mg	Rib mg	Nia mg	B$_6$ mg	Fol mcg	B$_{12}$ mcg	C mg	Calc mg	Iron mg	Mag mg	Pot mg	Zn mg
made from surimi	1 oz	19	0.01	0.01	0.06	0.01	0.5	0.45	0.0	2.6	<0.1	12.2	32	<0.1
made from surimi	3 oz	56	0.02	0.02	0.19	0.03	1.4	1.40	0.0	7.7	0.2	36.5	95	0.3
CRABAPPLE, raw, sliced	1 cup	44	0.03	0.02	0.11	na	na	0.00	8.8	19.8	0.4	7.7	213	na
CRACKER														
matzo, egg	1/2 oz	6	0.11	0.09	0.72	0.01	16.6	0.03	<0.1	5.7	0.4	3.4	21	0.1
matzo, egg and onion	1/2 oz	3	0.08	0.06	0.69	0.02	22.4	0.03	<0.1	5.1	0.6	4.3	12	0.1
matzo, plain	1/2 oz	0	0.06	0.04	0.55	0.02	16.6	0.00	0.0	1.8	0.5	3.5	16	0.1
matzo, whole wheat	1/2 oz	0	0.05	0.04	0.77	0.02	5.0	0.00	0.0	3.3	0.7	19.0	45	0.4
melba toast, plain	1/2 oz	0	0.06	0.04	0.58	0.01	17.6	0.00	0.0	13.2	0.5	8.4	29	0.3
melba toast, plain, no salt added	1/2 oz	0	0.06	0.04	0.58	0.01	17.6	0.00	0.0	13.2	0.5	8.4	29	0.3
melba toast, plain, no salt added, rounds	1 piece	0	0.01	0.01	0.12	0.00	3.7	0.00	0.0	2.8	0.1	1.8	6	<0.1
melba toast, plain, rounds	1 piece	0	0.01	0.01	0.12	0.00	3.7	0.00	0.0	2.8	0.1	1.8	6	<0.1
melba toast, rye	1/2 oz	0	0.07	0.04	0.67	0.01	12.1	0.00	0.0	11.1	0.5	5.5	27	0.2
melba toast, wheat	1/2 oz	0	0.06	0.04	0.72	0.02	18.7	0.00	0.0	6.1	0.6	7.9	21	0.2
oyster	1/2 oz	0	0.08	0.07	0.74	0.01	17.6	0.00	0.0	16.9	0.8	3.8	18	0.1
oyster, low-salt	1/2 oz	0	0.08	0.07	0.74	0.01	17.6	0.00	0.0	16.9	0.8	3.8	103	0.1
saltine	1/2 oz	0	0.08	0.07	0.74	0.01	17.6	0.00	0.0	16.9	0.8	3.8	18	0.1
saltine, low-salt	1/2 oz	0	0.08	0.07	0.74	0.01	17.6	0.00	0.0	16.9	0.8	3.8	103	0.1
saltine, unsalted tops	1/2 oz	0	0.08	0.07	0.74	0.01	17.6	0.00	0.0	16.9	0.8	3.8	18	0.1
(Cheez-It) cheese flavor	1 cup	100	0.35	0.27	2.90	0.34	49.6	0.28	0.0	93.6	3.0	22.3	66	0.7
(Euphrates)														
wheat	1 cracker	0	0.02	0.01	0.20	0.01	1.8	0.00	0.0	2.0	0.2	2.5	7.3	<0.1
wheat, low-salt	1 cracker	0	0.02	0.01	0.20	0.01	1.8	0.00	0.0	2.0	0.2	2.5	8.1	<0.1
(Keebler)														
'Wheatables'	1 cracker	0	0.01	0	0.05	0	0.44	0	0.0	0.49	0.04	0.62	1.8	0.02
'Wheatables' low-salt	1 cracker	0	0.01	0.00	0.05	0.00	0.4	0.00	0.0	0.5	<0.1	0.6	2	<0.1
(Nabisco)														
'Harvest Wheat'	1 cracker	0	0.02	0.01	0.15	0.00	1.3	0.00	0.0	1.5	0.1	1.9	6	<0.1
'Harvest Wheat' low-salt	1 cracker	0	0.02	0.01	0.15	0.00	1.3	0.00	0.0	1.5	0.1	1.9	6	<0.1
'Premium' saltine, original	1 serving	0	0.05	0.06	0.61	0.01	11.8	na	0.0	27.0	0.7	2.9	14	na
'Ritz'	1 serving	0	0.04	0.05	0.61	0.01	9.6	0.00	0.0	23.5	0.7	3.2	15	0.2
'Ritz' wheat	1 cracker	0	0.02	0.01	0.15	0.00	1.3	0.00	0.0	1.5	0.1	1.9	6	<0.1
'Ritz' wheat, low salt	1 cracker	0	0.02	0.01	0.15	0.00	1.3	0.00	0.0	1.5	0.1	1.9	6	<0.1
'Triscuit' wheat	10 bits	0	0.02	0.01	0.45	0.02	2.8	0.00	0.0	5.0	0.3	9.9	30	0.2
'Twigs' cheese	1 cracker	3.2	0.01	0.01	0.09	0.01	1.6	0.01	0.0	3.0	0.1	0.7	3	<0.1
'Wheat Thins'	1 cracker	0	0.02	0.01	0.15	0.00	1.3	0.00	0.0	1.5	0.1	1.9	6	<0.1
'Wheat Thins' low-salt	1 cracker	0	0.02	0.01	0.15	0.00	1.3	0.00	0.0	1.5	0.1	1.9	6	<0.1
'Wheatsworth'	1 cracker	0	0.02	0.01	0.15	0.00	1.3	0.00	0.0	1.5	0.1	1.9	6	<0.1
'Wheatsworth' low-salt	1 cracker	0	0.02	0.01	0.15	0.00	1.3	0.00	0.0	1.5	0.1	1.9	6	<0.1
(RyKrisp) crispbread, rye, triple cracker	1 wafer	0	0.06	0.04	0.26	0.05	11.8	0.00	0.0	7.8	0.6	19.5	80	0.6
(Snackwell's)														
cheese, zesty	1 serving	47.7	0.07	0.10	1.10	0.03	17.1	0.02	0.2	12.9	0.9	9.9	47	0.5
cracked pepper	7 crackers	0.28	0.04	0.05	0.75	0.01	11.5	0.00	<0.1	23.8	0.5	3.8	16	0.1
French onion	1 serving	6.6	0.07	0.09	1.10	0.03	17.1	0.02	0.2	11.7	0.9	9.6	44	0.5
Italian ranch	1 serving	11.4	0.07	0.09	1.10	0.02	21.9	0.02	0.2	12.3	0.9	6.6	42	0.3
salsa, snack	1 serving	14.1	0.07	0.09	1.10	0.03	21.9	0.01	0.2	12.6	0.9	9.6	41	0.5
wheat	1 serving	0	0.04	0.06	na	na	na	na	0.0	22.4	0.6	6.9	29	0.3
wheat thins, baked	1 serving	0	0.09	0.09	1.20	0.03	12.2	na	0.0	23.2	1.1	15.1	56	na
(Sunshine)														
wheat, heart-shaped	1 cracker	0	0.01	0.01	0.10	0.00	0.9	0.00	0.0	1.0	<0.1	1.2	4	<0.1
wheat, heart-shaped, low-salt	1 cracker	0	0.01	0.01	0.10	0.00	0.9	0.00	0.0	1.0	<0.1	1.2	4	<0.1
(Wasa) crispbread, rye	1 crispbread	0	0.02	0.02	0.10	0.02	4.7	0.00	0.0	3.1	0.2	7.8	32	0.2
CRACKER MEAL														
	1 cup	0	0.80	0.54	6.60	0.05	132.0	0.00	0.0	26.4	5.3	27.6	132	0.8
	1 oz	0	0.20	0.13	1.60	0.01	32.6	0.00	0.0	6.5	1.3	6.8	33	0.2

Food Name	Serving Size	A I.U.	Thi mg	Rib mg	Nia mg	B_6 mg	Fol mcg	B_12 mcg	C mg	Calc mg	Iron mg	Mag mg	Pot mg	Zn mg
CRANBERRY, RAW														
Fresh														
raw, chopped	1 cup	51	0.03	0.02	0.11	0.07	1.9	0.00	14.8	7.7	0.2	5.5	78	0.1
raw, whole	1 cup	44	0.03	0.02	0.10	0.06	1.6	0.00	12.8	6.7	0.2	4.8	68	0.1
CRANBERRY BEAN. See BEAN, CRANBERRY.														
CRANBERRY JUICE COCKTAIL. See under FRUIT JUICE DRINK.														
CRANBERRY SAUCE														
canned, sweetened	1 cup	55	0.04	0.06	0.28	0.04	2.8	0.00	5.5	11.1	0.6	8.3	72	0.1
canned, sweetened, 1/2-inch slices	1 slice	11	0.01	0.01	0.06	0.01	0.6	0.00	1.1	2.3	0.1	1.7	15	<0.1
CRAPPIE. See SUNFISH.														
CRAYFISH														
mixed species, farmed, cooked	3 oz	43	0.04	0.07	1.40	0.11	9.3	2.60	0.4	43.4	0.9	28.1	202	1.3
mixed species, farmed, raw	3 oz	43	0.04	0.03	1.60	0.07	25.5	1.80	0.4	21.3	0.5	25.5	222	0.9
mixed species, wild, cooked	3 oz	43	0.04	0.07	1.90	0.07	37.4	1.80	0.8	51.0	0.7	28.1	252	1.5
mixed species, wild, raw	3 oz	44	0.06	0.03	1.90	0.09	31.4	1.70	1.0	22.9	0.7	22.9	257	1.1
CREAM														
half and half	1 cup	1050	0.09	0.36	0.19	0.09	6.0	0.80	2.1	254.0	0.2	24.6	314	1.2
half and half	1 fl oz	131	0.01	0.05	0.02	0.01	0.8	0.10	0.3	31.7	<0.1	3.1	39	0.2
half and half	1 tbsp	65	0.01	0.02	0.01	0.01	0.4	0.05	0.1	15.7	<0.1	1.5	19	<0.1
heavy, whipping	1 cup	3499	0.05	0.26	0.09	0.06	8.8	0.43	1.4	154.0	<0.1	16.7	179	0.6
heavy, whipping	1 fl oz	438	0.01	0.03	0.01	0.01	1.1	0.05	0.2	19.3	<0.1	2.1	23	<0.1
heavy, whipping	1 tbsp	221	0.00	0.02	0.01	0.00	0.6	0.03	<0.1	9.7	<0.1	1.1	11	<0.1
heavy, whipping, whipped	1 cup	1757	0.03	0.13	0.05	0.03	4.4	0.22	0.7	77.2	<0.1	8.4	90	0.3
light	1 cup	1519	0.08	0.35	0.14	0.08	5.5	0.53	1.8	231.0	0.1	20.8	292	0.7
light	1 fl oz	190	0.01	0.04	0.02	0.01	0.7	0.07	0.2	28.9	<0.1	2.6	37	<0.1
light	1 tbsp	95	0.01	0.02	0.01	0.01	0.3	0.03	0.1	14.4	<0.1	1.3	18	<0.1
light, whipping	1 cup	2694	0.06	0.30	0.10	0.07	8.8	0.47	1.5	166.0	<0.1	17.3	231	0.6
light, whipping	1 tbsp	169	0.00	0.02	0.01	0.00	0.6	0.03	<0.1	10.4	<0.1	1.1	15	<0.1
light, whipping, whipped	1 cup	1352	0.03	0.15	0.05	0.03	4.4	0.23	0.7	83.3	<0.1	8.7	116	0.3
CREAM CHEESE. See under CHEESE.														
CREAM OF TARTAR														
	1 tsp	0	0.00	0.00	0.00	0.00	0.0	0.00	0.0	0.2	0.1	<0.1	495	<0.1
	1/2 tsp	0	0.00	0.00	0.00	0.00	0.0	0.00	0.0	0.1	<0.1	<0.1	248	<0.1
CRIMINI MUSHROOM. See MUSHROOM, CRIMINI.														
CROAKER, ATLANTIC														
breaded, fried	3 oz	64	0.08	0.11	3.70	0.22	28.9	1.80	0.0	27.2	0.7	35.7	289	0.4
raw	3 oz	51	0.06	0.08	3.60	0.26	12.8	2.10	0.0	12.8	0.3	34.0	293	0.4
CROUTONS														
seasoned	1 cup	16	0.20	0.17	1.90	0.03	35.2	0.06	0.0	38.4	1.1	16.8	72	0.4
seasoned	4 cubes	<1	0.01	0.00	0.05	0.00	0.9	0.00	0.0	0.9	<0.1	0.4	2	<0.1
CROWDER PEAS. See under BLACK-EYED PEAS.														
CUCUMBER														
Fresh														
peeled, raw, chopped	1 cup	98	0.03	0.02	0.14	0.10	18.6	0.00	3.7	18.6	0.2	16.0	197	0.2
peeled, raw, sliced	1 cup	88	0.03	0.01	0.12	0.09	16.7	0.00	3.3	16.7	0.2	14.3	176	0.2
peeled, raw, sticks, 4-inches	1 stick	7	0.00	0.00	0.01	0.01	1.3	0.00	0.3	1.3	<0.1	1.1	13	<0.1
peeled, raw, whole, large, 8.25 inches	1 cucumber	207	0.06	0.03	0.29	0.20	39.2	0.00	7.8	39.2	0.5	33.6	414	0.4
peeled, raw, whole, small 6-3/8 inches	1 cucumber	117	0.03	0.02	0.16	0.11	22.1	0.00	4.4	22.1	0.3	19.0	234	0.2
w/peel, raw, whole, large, 8.25 inches	1 cucumber	647	0.07	0.07	0.67	0.13	39.1	0.00	16.0	42.1	0.8	33.1	433	0.6
w/peel, raw, sliced	1/2 cup	112	0.01	0.01	0.12	0.02	6.8	0.00	2.8	7.3	0.1	5.7	75	0.1
CUMIN SEED														
whole	1 tbsp	76	0.04	0.02	0.28	0.02	0.6	0.00	0.5	55.8	4.0	21.9	107	0.3
whole	1 tsp	27	0.01	0.01	0.10	0.01	0.2	0.00	0.2	19.5	1.4	7.7	38	0.1
CUPU ASSU OIL														
	1 cup	0	0.00	0.00	0.00	0.00	0.0	0.00	0.0	0.0	na	0.0	0	0.0
	1 tbsp	0	0.00	0.00	0.00	0.00	0.0	0.00	0.0	0.0	na	0.0	0	0.0

Food Name	Serving Size	A I.U.	Thi mg	Rib mg	Nia mg	B$_6$ mg	Fol mcg	B$_{12}$ mcg	C mg	Calc mg	Iron mg	Mag mg	Pot mg	Zn mg
CURRANT														
BLACK / European currant, raw..............	1 cup	258	0.06	0.06	0.34	0.07	na	0.00	203.0	61.6	1.7	26.9	361	0.3
RED OR WHITE, raw.....................	1 cup	134	0.05	0.06	0.11	0.08	9.0	0.00	45.9	37.0	1.1	14.6	308	0.3
ZANTE, dried......................	1 cup	105	0.23	0.20	2.30	0.43	14.7	0.00	6.8	124.0	4.7	59.0	1284	0.9
CURRY POWDER. See under SEASONING MIX.														
CUSK / torsk / tusk														
baked, broiled, grilled, or microwaved	3 oz	59	0.04	0.14	2.80	0.38	1.7	1.00	0.0	11.1	0.9	34.0	428	0.4
raw...........................	3 oz	51	0.04	0.11	2.30	0.33	1.7	0.89	0.0	8.5	0.7	26.4	333	0.3
CUSTARD APPLE / cherimoya														
raw, whole, peeled and seeded	1 fruit	55	0.55	0.60	7.10	na	na	0.00	49.2	126.0	2.7	na	na	na
CUTTLEFISH														
mixed species, cooked	3 oz	574	0.01	1.50	1.90	0.23	20.4	4.60	7.2	153.0	9.2	51.0	541	2.9
mixed species, raw.....................	3 oz	319	0.01	0.77	1.00	0.13	13.6	2.50	4.5	76.5	5.1	25.5	301	1.5

D

Food Name	Serving Size	A I.U.	Thi mg	Rib mg	Nia mg	B$_6$ mg	Fol mcg	B$_{12}$ mcg	C mg	Calc mg	Iron mg	Mag mg	Pot mg	Zn mg
DAIKON / Chinese radish / Oriental radish														
boiled, drained, sliced..................	1 cup	0	0.00	0.03	0.22	0.06	25.6	0.00	22.2	25.0	0.2	13.2	419	0.2
dried	1 cup	0	0.31	0.79	3.90	0.72	342.0	0.00	0.0	730.0	7.8	197.0	4053	2.5
raw, untrimmed........................	1 lb	0	0.07	0.07	0.68	0.16	95.3	0.00	74.4	91.3	1.4	54.1	767	0.5
DAIQUIRI. See under COCKTAIL.														
DANDELION GREENS														
boiled, drained, chopped	1 cup	12285	0.14	0.18	0.54	0.17	13.1	0.00	18.9	147.0	1.9	25.2	244	0.3
raw, chopped	1 cup	7700	0.11	0.14	0.44	0.14	15.0	0.00	19.3	103.0	1.7	19.8	218	0.2
DANISH CABBAGE. See CABBAGE, DANISH.														
DANISH PASTRY. See under PASTRY; PASTRY, TOASTER.														
DATE														
Domestic, natural and dry														
pitted, chopped........................	1 cup	89	0.16	0.18	3.90	0.34	22.4	0.00	0.0	57.0	2.0	62.3	1161	0.5
whole	1 medium	4	0.01	0.01	0.18	0.02	1.0	0.00	0.0	2.7	0.1	2.9	54	<0.1
DATE, INDIAN. See TAMARIND.														
DEER														
raw..............................	1 oz	0	0.06	0.14	1.80	0.11	1.1	1.8	0.0	1.4	1.0	6.5	90	0.6
roasted	3 oz	0	0.15	0.51	5.70	na	na	na	0.0	6.0	3.8	20.4	285	2.3
DESSERT TOPPING														
(Nestlé)														
'Butterfinger'..........................	1 cup	0	0.15	0.12	4.30	0.12	47.0	0.02	0.0	47.0	1.3	137.0	663	2.0
'Butterfinger'..........................	2 tbsp	0	0.02	0.02	0.62	0.02	6.8	0.00	0.0	6.8	0.2	19.8	95	0.3
'Crunch'	2 tbsp	17	0.08	0.14	0.95	0.10	19.0	0.09	<0.1	40.6	0.1	13.9	83	0.3
crunchy, 'Buncha Crunch'..............	2-lb pkg	816	5.20	6.60	75.0	6.2	1351.0	2.80	5.4	1170.0	5.4	644.0	3156	15.5
crunchy, 'Buncha Crunch'..............	2 tbsp	18	0.12	0.15	1.70	0.14	29.8	0.06	0.1	25.8	0.1	14.2	70	0.3
'Rainbow Morsel'......................	3-lb pkg	68	0.49	0.84	3.80	0.45	27.2	0.00	9.5	422.0	21.9	1034.0	3266	14.7
'Rainbow Morsel'......................	1 pkt	<1	0.01	0.01	0.04	0.01	0.3	0.00	0.1	4.3	0.2	10.6	34	0.2
DILL SEED														
....	1 tbsp	4	0.03	0.02	0.19	0.02	0.7	0.00	1.4	100.0	1.1	16.9	78	0.3
....	1 tsp	1	0.01	0.01	0.06	0.01	0.2	0.00	0.4	31.8	0.3	5.4	25	0.1
DILL WEED														
dried..........................	1 tbsp	181	0.01	0.01	0.09	0.05	na	0.00	1.6	55.3	1.5	14.0	103	0.1
dried..........................	1 tsp	59	0.00	0.00	0.03	0.02	na	0.00	0.5	17.8	0.5	4.5	33	<0.1
DILL WEED														
fresh, sprigs	1 cup	687	0.01	0.03	0.14	0.02	13.3	0.00	7.6	18.5	0.6	4.9	66	<0.1
fresh, sprigs, medium..................	5 sprigs	77	0.00	0.00	0.02	0.00	1.5	0.00	0.9	2.1	<0.1	0.6	7	<0.1

Food Name	Serving Size	A I.U.	Thi mg	Rib mg	Nia mg	B$_6$ mg	Fol mcg	B$_{12}$ mcg	C mg	Calc mg	Iron mg	Mag mg	Pot mg	Zn mg
DINNER ROLL. See under ROLL.														
DISHCLOTH GOURD. See GOURD, DISHCLOTH.														
DOCK, raw, chopped	1 cup	5320	0.05	0.13	0.67	0.16	17.6	0.00	63.8	58.5	3.2	137.0	519	0.3
DOLPHIN FISH. See MAHI MAHI.														
DRAGON'S EYE. See LONGAN.														
DRESSING. See SALAD DRESSING; STUFFING MIX.														
DRUM, FRESHWATER														
baked, broiled, grilled, or microwaved	3 oz	167	0.07	0.18	2.40	0.29	14.4	2.00	0.9	65.5	1.0	32.3	300	0.7
raw	3 oz	145	0.06	0.14	2.00	0.26	12.8	1.70	0.9	51.0	0.8	25.5	234	0.6
DUCK														
AVERAGE OF ALL PARTS														
Domestic														
meat and skin, raw	3 oz	144	0.17	0.18	3.37	0.16	11.1	0.22	2.4	9.4	2.1	12.8	179	1.2
meat and skin, roasted	3 oz	180	0.15	0.23	4.11	0.15	5.2	0.26	0.0	9.4	2.3	13.7	175	1.6
meat and skin, roasted, chopped														
or diced	1 cup	294	0.24	0.38	6.80	0.25	8.4	0.42	0.0	15.4	3.8	22.4	286	2.6
meat only, raw.	3 oz	68	0.31	0.39	4.57	0.29	21.5	0.34	4.9	9.4	2.1	16.3	232	1.6
meat only, roasted, chopped or diced	1 cup	108	0.36	0.66	7.1	0.35	14.0	0.56	0	16.8	3.8	28.0	353	3.6
Wild, meat and skin, raw	3 oz	75	0.30	0.23	2.83	0.47	18.0	0.57	4.4	4.3	3.6	17.1	213	0.6
BREAST														
Domestic														
meat and skin, roasted	3 oz	na	na	na	6.7	na	na	na	2.4	6.8	2.8	na	na	na
meat only, broiled	3 oz	na	na	na	8.8	na	na	na	2.7	7.7	3.8	na	na	na
meat only, broiled, chopped or diced	1 cup	na	na	na	18.0	na	na	na	5.6	15.7	7.8	na	na	na
Wild, meat only, raw	3 oz	45	0.35	0.27	2.99	0.54	21.4	0.65	5.3	2.6	3.8	18.9	230	0.6
LEG														
Domestic														
meat and skin, roasted	3 oz	na	na	na	4.9	na	na	na	1.3	8.5	1.8	na	na	na
meat only, braised.	3 oz	na	na	na	4.5	na	na	na	2.0	8.5	2.0	na	na	na
meat only, braised, chopped or diced	1 cup	na	na	na	9.3	na	na	na	4.0	17.4	4.1	na	na	na
LIVER, domestic, raw.	1 oz	1140	0.17	0.26	1.86	0.23	210.9	15.43	1.3	3.1	8.9	6.9	66	0.9
DUCK FAT														
. . . .	1 cup	0	0.00	0.00	0.00	0.00	0.0	0.00	0.0	0.0	0.0	0.0	0	0.0
. . . .	1 tbsp	0	0.00	0.00	0.00	0.00	0.0	0.00	0.0	0.0	0.0	0.0	0	0.0
DUNGENESS CRAB. See under CRAB.														
DURIAN														
raw or frozen, chopped or diced	1 cup	109	0.91	0.49	2.60	0.77	na	0.00	47.9	14.6	1.0	72.9	1059	0.7
raw or frozen, whole	1 medium	271	2.30	1.20	6.50	1.90	na	0.00	119.0	36.1	2.6	181.0	2625	1.7

E

Food Name	Serving Size	A I.U.	Thi mg	Rib mg	Nia mg	B$_6$ mg	Fol mcg	B$_{12}$ mcg	C mg	Calc mg	Iron mg	Mag mg	Pot mg	Zn mg
ÉCLAIR. See under PASTRY.														
EEL														
mixed species, baked, broiled, grilled,														
or microwaved	3 oz	3219	0.16	0.04	3.80	0.07	14.7	2.50	1.5	22.1	0.5	22.1	297	1.8
mixed species, baked, broiled, grilled,														
or microwaved, 1-inch cubes	1 piece	644	0.03	0.01	0.76	0.01	2.9	0.49	0.3	4.4	0.1	4.4	59	0.4
mixed species, raw	3 oz	2954	0.13	0.03	3.00	0.06	12.8	2.50	1.5	17.0	0.4	17.0	231	1.4
EGG														
CHICKEN														
Dried														
white, flakes, glucose-reduced	1/2 lb	0	0.08	4.90	1.50	0.05	203.0	1.10	0.0	189.0	0.5	152.0	2364	0.3

Food Name	Serving Size	A I.U.	Thi mg	Rib mg	Nia mg	B_6 mg	Fol mcg	B_{12} mcg	C mg	Calc mg	Iron mg	Mag mg	Pot mg	Zn mg
white, powder, glucose-reduced	1 tbsp	0	0.01	0.32	0.10	0.00	13.4	0.07	0.0	12.5	<0.1	10.1	156	<0.1
white, powder, glucose-reduced, sifted.	1 cup	0	0.04	2.50	0.77	0.03	102.0	0.56	0.0	95.7	0.3	76.9	1194	0.2
whole	1 tbsp	45	0.01	0.08	0.02	0.02	8.6	0.20	0.0	11.6	0.3	2.1	25	0.3
whole, sifted	1 cup	765	0.17	1.30	0.26	0.33	145.0	3.40	0.0	196	5.8	35.7	419	4.5
whole, stabilized, glucose-reduced.	1 tbsp	103	0.02	0.06	0.01	0.02	9.7	0.53	0.0	11.1	0.4	2.4	26	0.3
whole, stabilized, glucose-reduced, sifted	1 cup	1743	0.28	1.00	0.22	0.36	164.0	8.90	0.0	189.0	7.0	41.4	438	4.9
yolk, powdered	1 tbsp	53	0.01	0.08	0.00	0.03	9.8	0.21	0.0	11.4	0.2	0.5	10	0.2
yolk, powdered, sifted	1 cup	881	0.19	1.30	0.06	0.44	163.0	3.60	0.0	190.0	3.6	8.7	163	3.3
Fresh														
white, raw	1 cup	0	0.02	1.10	0.22	0.01	7.3	0.49	0.0	14.6	<0.1	26.7	347	<0.1
white, raw, large	1 white	0	0.00	0.15	0.03	0.00	1.0	0.07	0.0	2.0	<0.1	3.7	48	0.1
whole, cooked, omelet-style	1 tbsp	99	0.01	0.06	0.01	0.02	4.4	0.11	0.0	6.4	0.2	1.4	15	0.1
whole, cooked, omelet-style, large	1 egg	399	0.03	0.24	0.04	0.07	17.7	0.43	0.0	25.6	0.7	5.5	62	0.6
whole, fried, large	1 egg	394	0.03	0.24	0.04	0.07	17.5	0.42	0.0	25.3	0.7	5.1	61	0.6
whole, hard-boiled	1 tbsp	48	0.01	0.04	0.01	0.01	3.7	0.09	0.0	4.3	0.1	0.9	11	<0.1
whole, hard-boiled, chopped	1 cup	762	0.09	0.70	0.09	0.17	59.8	1.50	0.0	68.0	1.6	13.6	171	1.4
whole, hard-boiled, large	1 egg	280	0.03	0.26	0.03	0.06	22.0	0.56	0.0	25.0	0.6	5.0	63	0.5
whole, poached, large	1 egg	316	0.03	0.22	0.03	0.06	17.5	0.40	0.0	24.5	0.7	5.0	60	0.6
whole, raw.	1 cup	1543	0.15	1.20	0.18	0.34	114.0	2.40	0.0	119.0	3.5	24.3	294	2.7
whole, raw, extra large	1 egg	368	0.04	0.29	0.04	0.08	27.3	0.58	0.0	28.4	0.8	5.8	70	0.6
whole, raw, jumbo	1 egg	413	0.04	0.33	0.05	0.09	30.6	0.65	0.0	31.9	0.9	6.5	79	0.7
whole, raw, large	1 egg	318	0.03	0.25	0.04	0.07	23.5	0.50	0.0	24.5	0.7	5.0	61	0.6
whole, raw, medium	1 egg	279	0.03	0.22	0.03	0.06	20.7	0.44	0.0	21.6	0.6	4.4	53	0.5
whole, raw, small	1 egg	235	0.02	0.19	0.03	0.05	17.4	0.37	0.0	18.1	0.5	3.7	45	0.4
whole, scrambled	1 cup	1500	0.11	0.96	0.17	0.26	66.0	1.70	0.4	156.0	2.6	26.4	304	2.2
whole, scrambled	1 tbsp	93	0.01	0.06	0.01	0.02	4.1	0.11	<0.1	9.7	0.2	1.6	18.9	0.1
whole, scrambled, large	1 egg	416	0.03	0.27	0.05	0.07	18.3	0.47	0.1	43.3	0.7	7.3	84	0.6
yolk, raw	1 cup	4726	0.41	1.60	0.04	0.95	355.0	7.60	0.0	333.0	8.6	21.9	228	7.6
yolk, raw	1 yolk	323	0.03	0.11	0.00	0.07	24.2	0.52	0.0	22.7	0.6	1.5	16	0.5
Frozen														
whole	1/2 lb	3201	0.35	1.20	0.10	0.78	263.0	4.10	0.0	313.0	7.6	20.4	268	6.5
whole, raw, sugared	1/2 lb	2985	0.31	1.20	0.05	0.65	316.0	4.00	0.0	279.0	7.1	22.7	234	6.4
DUCK, fresh, whole, raw, medium	1 egg	930	0.11	0.28	0.14	0.17	56.0	3.80	0.0	44.6	2.7	11.6	156	1.0
GOOSE, fresh, whole, raw, medium	1 egg	1843	0.21	0.55	0.27	0.34	109.0	7.30	0.0	86.7	5.2	22.5	302	1.9
QUAIL, fresh, whole, raw, medium.	1 egg	27	0.01	0.07	0.01	0.01	6.0	0.14	0.0	5.8	0.3	1.1	12	0.1
TURKEY, fresh, whole, raw, medium	1 egg	438	0.09	0.37	0.02	0.10	56.2	1.30	0.0	78.2	3.2	10.6	112	1.2
EGG NOODLE. See under NOODLE.														
EGGPLANT / aubergine														
raw, cubed	1 cup	69	0.04	0.03	0.49	0.07	15.6	0.00	1.4	5.7	0.2	11.5	178	0.12
raw, whole, approx 1.25 lb, peeled	1 eggplant	385	0.24	0.16	2.70	0.39	87.0	0.00	7.8	32.1	1.2	64.1	994	0.6
raw, whole, approx 1.25 lb, unpeeled	1 eggplant	460	0.28	0.19	3.30	0.46	104.0	0.00	9.3	38.4	1.5	76.7	1189	0.8
ELDERBERRY, fresh, raw	1 cup	870	0.10	0.09	0.72	0.33	8.7	0.00	52.2	55.1	2.3	7.3	406	0.2
ELK														
raw	1 oz	0	na	na	na	na	na	na	0.0	1.1	0.8	6.5	89	0.7
roasted	3 oz	0	na	na	na	na	na	na	0.0	4.3	3.1	20.4	279	2.7
ENCHILADA/ENCHILADA ENTRÉE														
(Healthy Choice)														
chicken, suprema, w/green sauce, rice, corn, apple raspberry	1 serving	768	na	na	na	na	na	na	18.2	134.0	0.8	na	384	na
(Lean Cuisine)														
chicken enchilada Suiza, w/sour cream sauce, rice	1 serving	0	na	na	na	na	na	na	na	184.0	na	na	na	na

FIG 755

Food Name	Serving Size	A I.U.	Thi mg	Rib mg	Nia mg	B_6 mg	Fol mcg	B_{12} mcg	C mg	Calc mg	Iron mg	Mag mg	Pot mg	Zn mg
(Stouffer's)														
chicken enchilada, w/Mexican rice, Monterey Jack sauce	1 serving	756	na	na	na	na	na	na	15.3	255.0	na	na	na	na
(Weight Watchers)														
chicken enchilada Suiza, w/sour cream sauce and cheese	1 serving	0	na	na	na	na	na	na	na	250	na	na	na	na
ENCHILADA SAUCE. See under SAUCE.														
ENDIVE														
raw, chopped	1/2 cup	513	0.02	0.02	0.10	0.01	35.5	0.00	1.6	13.0	0.2	3.8	79	0.2
raw, whole, approx 1.3 lb	1 head	10517	0.41	0.39	2.10	0.10	728.0	0.00	33.3	267.0	4.3	77.0	1611	4.1
ENGLISH MUFFIN														
(Thomas') plain	1 muffin	0	na	na	na	na	82.7	0.20	0.06	76.4	1.7	na	na	na
ENOKI. See MUSHROOM, ENOKI.														
ENSURE. See under MEDICAL NUTRITIONALS.														
EPAZOTE														
fresh, raw, chopped	1 tbsp	<1	0.00	0.00	0.01	0.00	1.7	0.00	<0.1	2.2	<0.1	1.0	5	<0.1
fresh, raw, whole sprigs	1 medium	1	0.00	0.01	0.01	0.00	4.3	0.00	<0.1	5.5	<0.1	2.4	13	<0.1
EPPAW, raw	1 cup	0	0.11	0.12	0.30	0.18	24.3	0.00	13.0	110.0	1.1	32.0	340	1.1
EUROPEAN CHESTNUT. See CHESTNUT, EUROPEAN.														
EUROPEAN CURRANT. See under CURRANT.														

F

Food Name	Serving Size	A I.U.	Thi mg	Rib mg	Nia mg	B_6 mg	Fol mcg	B_{12} mcg	C mg	Calc mg	Iron mg	Mag mg	Pot mg	Zn mg
FAJITA/FAJITA ENTRÉE														
(Wonderbites)														
beef, flame-broiled, 'Dippers'	1 piece	12	0.04	0.04	0.69	0.07	0.9	0.38	<0.1	6.3	0.53	7.2	68	1.2
beef, flame-broiled, product 9971	1 piece	13	0.04	0.03	0.69	0.07	0.7	0.39	0.0	6.8	0.52	7.4	67	1.2
turkey, flame-broiled, 'Dippers'	1 piece	50	0.03	0.04	0.88	0.08	3.4	0.22	<0.1	6.8	0.43	5.4	58	0.8
FAJITA MIX														
(Tyson)														
chicken, kit, frozen	1 pkg	386	na	na	na	na	na	na	73.3	na	na	na	na	na
chicken, kit, frozen	1 serving	55	na	na	na	na	na	na	10.4	na	na	na	na	na
FARINA. See under CEREAL, HOT.														
FATHEAD. See SHEEPSHEAD.														
FAVA BEAN. See BEAN, FAVA.														
FEIJOA, RAW														
raw, puréed	1 cup	0	0.02	0.08	0.70	0.12	92.3	0.00	49.3	41.3	0.19	21.9	377	0.1
raw, whole, trimmed	1 medium	0	0.00	0.02	0.14	0.03	19.0	0.00	10.2	8.5	0.04	4.5	78	<0.1
FENNEL / finnochio														
fresh, raw, sliced	1 cup	117	0.01	0.03	0.56	0.04	23.5	0.00	10.4	42.6	0.6	14.8	360	0.2
fresh, raw, whole, bulb	1 medium	314	0.02	0.08	1.50	0.11	63.2	0.00	28.1	115.0	1.7	39.8	969	0.5
FENNEL SEED														
whole	1 tbsp	8	0.02	0.02	0.35	na	na	0.00	1.2	69.4	1.1	22.3	98	0.2
whole	1 tsp	3	0.01	0.01	0.12	na	na	0.00	0.4	23.9	0.4	7.7	34	<0.1
FENUGREEK SEED														
whole	1 tbsp	7	0.04	0.04	0.18	na	6.3	0.00	0.3	19.5	3.7	21.2	85	0.3
whole	1 tsp	2	0.01	0.01	0.06	na	2.1	0.00	0.1	6.5	1.2	7.1	29	<0.1
FIG														
Canned														
in extra heavy syrup, w//liquid	1 cup	94	0.06	0.09	1.10	na	na	0.00	2.6	67.9	0.7	26.1	253	0.3
in heavy syrup, w/liquid	1 cup	96	0.06	0.10	1.10	0.18	5.2	0.00	2.6	69.9	0.7	25.9	256	0.3

Food Name	Serving Size	A I.U.	Thi mg	Rib mg	Nia mg	B₆ mg	Fol mcg	B₁₂ mcg	C mg	Calc mg	Iron mg	Mag mg	Pot mg	Zn mg
in heavy syrup, w/liquid.	1 medium	10	0.01	0.01	0.12	0.02	0.6	0.00	0.3	7.6	<0.1	2.8	28	<0.1
in light syrup, w/liquid	1 cup	93	0.06	0.10	1.10	0.18	5.0	0.00	2.5	68.0	0.7	25.2	257	0.3
in light syrup, w/liquid	1 medium	10	0.01	0.01	0.12	0.02	0.6	0.00	0.3	7.6	<0.1	2.8	29	<0.1
in water, w/liquid.	1 cup	94	0.06	0.09	1.10	0.17	5.0	0.00	2.5	69.4	0.7	24.8	255	0.3
in water, w/liquids	1 medium	10	0.01	0.01	0.12	0.02	0.5	0.00	0.3	7.6	<0.1	2.7	28	<0.1
Dried														
raw, chopped	1 cup	265	0.14	0.17	1.40	0.45	14.9	0.00	1.6	287.0	4.4	117	1427	1.0
raw, whole.	1 medium	25	0.01	0.02	0.13	0.04	1.4	0.00	0.2	27.4	0.4	11.2	135	0.1
stewed	1 cup	412	0.03	0.28	1.70	0.34	2.6	0.00	11.4	158.0	2.4	64.8	780	0.5
Fresh														
raw, large, approx 2.5-inch diam.	1 fig	91	0.04	0.03	0.26	0.07	3.8	0.00	1.3	22.4	0.2	10.9	148	0.1
raw, medium, approx 2.25-inch diam	1 fig	71	0.03	0.03	0.20	0.06	3.0	0.00	1.0	17.5	0.2	8.5	116	<0.1
raw, small, approx 1.5-inch diam	1 fig	57	0.02	0.02	0.16	0.05	2.4	0.00	0.8	14.0	0.2	6.8	93	<0.1
FILBERT. See HAZELNUT.														
FILO DOUGH. See PHYLLO DOUGH.														
FINNOCHIO. See FENNEL.														
FIREWEED LEAVES														
raw, chopped	1 cup	828	0.01	0.03	1.10	0.14	25.8	0.00	0.5	98.7	0.6	35.9	114	0.6
raw, whole.	1 plant	792	0.01	0.03	1.00	0.14	24.6	0.00	0.5	94.4	0.5	34.3	109	0.6
FISH. See individual listings.														
FISH OIL														
COD LIVER														
. . . .	1 cup	218000	na	0.00	0.00	0.00	0.0	0.00	0.0	0.0	0.0	0.0	0	0
. . . .	1 tbsp	13600	na	0.00	0.00	0.00	0.0	0.00	0.0	0.0	0.0	0.0	0	0
HERRING														
. . . .	1 cup	0	0.00	0.00	0.00	0.00	0.0	0.00	0.0	0.0	0.0	0.0	0	0
. . . .	1 tbsp	0	0.00	0.00	0.00	0.00	0.0	0.00	0.0	0.0	0.0	0.0	0	0
MENHADEN														
. . . .	1 cup	0	0.00	0.00	0.00	0.00	0.0	0.00	0.0	0.0	0.0	0.0	0	0
. . . .	1 tbsp	0	0.00	0.00	0.00	0.00	0.0	0.00	0.0	0.0	0.0	0.0	0	0
fully hydrogenated	1 cup	0	0.00	0.00	0.00	0.00	0.0	0.00	0.0	0.0	0.0	0.0	0	0
fully hydrogenated	1 tbsp	0	0.00	0.00	0.00	0.00	0.0	0.00	0.0	0.0	0.0	0.0	0	0
SALMON														
. . . .	1 cup	0	0.00	0.00	0.00	0.00	0.0	0.00	0.0	0.0	0.0	0.0	0	0
. . . .	1 tbsp	0	0.00	0.00	0.00	0.00	0.0	0.00	0.0	0.0	0.0	0.0	0	0
SARDINE														
. . . .	1 cup	0	0.00	0.00	0.00	0.00	0.0	0.00	0.0	0.0	0.0	0.0	0	0
. . . .	1 tbsp	0	0.00	0.00	0.00	0.00	0.0	0.00	0.0	0.0	0.0	0.0	0	0
FLATFISH. See FLOUNDER; HALIBUT; SOLE.														
FLAXSEED														
. . . .	1 cup	0	0.26	0.25	2.20	1.40	431.0	0.00	2.0	308.0	9.6	561	1056	6.5
. . . .	1 tbsp	0	0.02	0.02	0.17	0.11	33.4	0.00	0.2	23.9	0.8	43.4	82	0.5
FLOUNDER														
baked, broiled, grilled, or microwaved	3 oz	32	0.07	0.10	1.90	0.20	7.8	2.10	0.0	15.3	0.3	49.3	292	0.5
raw	3 oz	28	0.08	0.07	2.50	0.18	6.8	1.30	1.4	15.3	0.3	26.4	307	0.4
raw, boneless	1 oz	9	0.03	0.02	0.82	0.06	2.3	0.43	0.5	5.1	0.1	8.8	102	0.1
FLORIDA POMPANO. See POMPANO, FLORIDA.														
FLOUR. See also individual listings.														
ACORN, full fat.	1 oz	15	0.04	0.04	0.68	0.20	32.2	0.00	0.0	12.2	0.3	31.2	202	0.2
ARROWROOT	1 cup	0	0.00	0.00	0.00	0.01	9.0	0.00	0.0	51.2	0.4	3.8	14	<0.1
BARLEY.	1 cup	0	0.55	0.17	9.30	0.59	11.8	0.00	0.0	47.4	4.0	142.0	457	3.0
BARLEY MALT.	1 cup	31	0.50	0.50	9.10	1.10	61.6	0.00	0.9	59.9	7.6	157.0	363	3.3
BUCKWHEAT, whole groat	1 cup	0	0.50	0.23	7.40	0.70	64.8	0.00	0.0	49.2	4.9	301.0	692	3.7

Food Name	Serving Size	A I.U.	Thi mg	Rib mg	Nia mg	B$_6$ mg	Fol mcg	B$_{12}$ mcg	C mg	Calc mg	Iron mg	Mag mg	Pot mg	Zn mg
CAROB														
....	1 cup	14	0.06	0.47	2.00	0.38	29.9	0.00	0.2	358.0	3.0	55.6	852	<0.1
....	1 tbsp	1	0.00	0.04	0.15	0.03	2.3	0.00	<0.1	27.8	0.2	4.3	66	<0.1
CHICKPEA, besan..................	1 cup	38	0.45	0.10	1.60	0.45	402.0	0.00	0.0	41.4	4.5	153.0	778	2.6
CORN. See also CORNMEAL.														
masa, enriched.............	1 cup	0	1.60	0.86	11.20	0.42	213.0	0.00	0.0	161.0	8.2	125.0	340	2.0
white, whole grain............	1 cup	0	0.29	0.09	2.20	0.43	29.3	0.00	0.0	8.2	2.8	109.0	369	2.0
yellow, degermed, unenriched	1 cup	64	0.09	0.07	3.30	0.12	60.5	0.00	0.0	2.5	1.1	22.7	113	0.5
yellow, enriched	1 cup	535	1.60	0.86	11.20	0.42	213.0	0.00	0.0	161.0	8.2	125.0	340	2.0
yellow, whole grain	1 cup	549	0.29	0.09	2.20	0.43	29.3	0.00	0.0	8.2	2.8	109.0	369	2.0
COTTONSEED														
low-fat	1 oz	122	0.59	0.11	1.10	0.22	64.6	0.00	0.7	134.0	3.6	203.0	499	3.3
partially defatted	1 cup	408	2.00	0.38	3.80	0.72	216.0	0.00	2.3	449.0	11.9	678.0	1666	11.0
partially defatted	1 tbsp	22	0.11	0.02	0.20	0.04	11.5	0.00	0.1	23.9	0.6	36.0	89	0.6
PEANUT														
defatted.................	1 cup	0	0.42	0.29	16.20	0.30	149.0	0.00	0.0	84.0	1.3	222	774	3.1
defatted.................	1 oz	0	0.20	0.14	7.70	0.14	70.4	0.00	0.0	39.7	0.6	105	366	1.4
low-fat.................	1 cup	0	0.27	0.10	6.90	0.18	80.0	0.00	0.0	78.0	2.8	28.8	815	3.6
low-fat.................	1 oz	0	0.13	0.05	3.30	0.09	37.8	0.00	0.0	36.9	1.3	13.6	385	1.7
POTATO	1 cup	0	0.36	0.08	5.60	1.2	40.0	0.00	6.1	104.0	2.2	104	1602	0.9
RICE, brown....................	1 cup	0	0.70	0.13	10.0	1.20	25.3	0.00	0.0	17.4	3.1	177.0	457	3.9
RICE, white	1 cup	0	0.22	0.03	4.10	0.69	6.3	0.00	0.0	15.8	0.6	55.3	120	1.3
SESAME														
high-fat.................	1 oz	20	0.76	0.08	3.80	0.04	8.7	0.00	0.0	45.1	4.3	102	120	3.0
low-fat.................	1 oz	18	0.71	0.08	3.60	0.04	8.2	0.00	0.0	42.2	4.0	95.8	113	2.8
partially defatted	1 oz	20	0.72	0.08	3.60	0.04	8.2	0.00	0.0	42.5	4.1	103	120	3.0
SOY														
defatted.................	1 tbsp	3	0.04	0.02	0.16	0.04	18.9	0.00	0.0	14.9	0.6	18.0	148	0.2
defatted, stirred.............	1 cup	40	0.70	0.25	2.60	0.57	305.0	0.00	0.0	241.0	9.2	290	2384	2.5
full-fat.................	1 tbsp	6.2	0.03	0.06	0.23	0.02	17.9	0.00	0.0	10.7	0.3	22.3	131	0.2
full-fat, roasted, stirred	1 cup	94	0.35	0.80	2.80	0.30	193.0	0.00	0.0	160.0	4.9	314	1735	3.0
full-fat, stirred	1 cup	101	0.49	0.97	3.60	0.39	290.0	0.00	0.0	173.0	5.4	360	2113	3.3
low-fat.................	1 tbsp	2	0.02	0.02	0.12	0.03	22.6	0.00	0.0	10.3	0.3	12.6	141	<0.1
low-fat, stirred	1 cup	35	0.33	0.25	1.90	0.46	361.0	0.00	0.0	165.0	5.3	202	2262	1.0
SUNFLOWER SEED														
partially defatted	1 cup	31	2.00	0.17	4.70	0.48	142.0	0.00	0.8	73.0	4.2	221	43	3.2
partially defatted	1 tbsp	2	0.13	0.01	0.29	0.03	8.9	0.00	<0.1	4.6	0.3	13.8	3	0.2
TRITICALE, whole-grain	1 cup	0	0.49	0.17	3.70	0.52	96.2	0.00	0.0	45.5	3.4	199	606	3.5
WHEAT														
White														
bread, enriched..........	1 cup	0	1.10	0.70	10.30	0.05	211.0	0.00	0.0	20.6	6.0	34.3	137	1.2
cake, enriched	1 cup	0	1.20	0.59	9.30	0.05	211.0	0.00	0.0	19.2	10.0	21.9	144	0.9
enriched, bleached	1 cup	0	0.98	0.62	7.40	0.06	193.0	0.00	0.0	18.8	5.8	27.5	134	0.9
enriched, calcium-fortified.............	1 cup	0	0.98	0.62	7.40	0.06	193.0	0.00	0.0	315.0	5.8	27.5	134	0.9
enriched, self-rising	1 cup	0	0.84	0.52	7.30	0.06	193.0	0.00	0.0	423.0	5.8	23.8	155	0.8
enriched, unbleached	1 cup	0	0.98	0.62	7.40	0.06	193.0	0.00	0.0	18.8	5.8	27.5	134	0.9
tortilla, enriched	1 cup	0	0.82	0.55	6.50	0.04	151.0	0.00	0.0	228.0	7.8	23.3	111	0.7
unenriched	1 cup	0	0.15	0.05	1.60	0.06	32.5	0.00	0.0	18.8	1.5	27.5	134	0.9
Whole wheat	1 cup	0	0.54	0.26	7.60	0.41	52.8	0.00	0.0	40.8	4.7	166	486	3.5
FRANKFURTER														
(Butcher Boy Meats) turkey..............	1 serving	166	0.03	0.08	1.20	0.12	3.9	0.14	0.5	82.9	1.0	7.8	106	1.6
(Hormel) beef, 'Wrangler'	1 frank	7	na	na	na	na	na	na	11.1	7.8	1.0	7.9	96	1.3
(Louis Rich)														
turkey and chicken	1 serving	0	na	na	na	na	na	na	0.0	59.0	1.0	10.3	72	0.8
turkey and chicken, w/cheese............	1 serving	0	na	na	na	na	na	na	0.0	109.0	0.9	9.9	71	0.8

Food Name	Serving Size	A I.U.	Thi mg	Rib mg	Nia mg	B$_6$ mg	Fol mcg	B$_{12}$ mcg	C mg	Calc mg	Iron mg	Mag mg	Pot mg	Zn mg
(Loma Linda)														
vegetarian, canned, 'Big Franks'	1 pkg	na	3.10	7.50	64.30	7.50	na	32.70	na	113.0	11.0	na	675	13.3
vegetarian, canned, 'Big Franks'	1 link	na	0.28	0.68	5.80	0.67	na	2.90	na	10.2	1.0	na	62	1.2
(Morningstar Farms)														
vegetarian, 'Deli Franks'	1 pkg	0	14.50	2.30	0.00	1.20	na	0.91	0.0	1724.0	61.2	363.0	5035	38.1
vegetarian, 'Deli Franks'	1 serving	0	0.14	0.02	0.00	0.01	na	0.01	0.0	17.1	0.6	3.6	50	0.38
(Oscar Mayer)														
beef	1 frank	na	0.02	0.05	0.98	0.05	6.8	0.51	0.0	5.0	0.5	5.8	77	0.9
beef, bun-length	1 frank	0	na	na	na	na	na	na	0.0	7.4	0.9	8.6	90	1.3
beef, fat-free	1 frank	0	na	na	na	na	na	na	0.0	10.0	0.9	9.5	234	1.2
beef light	1 frank	0	na	na	na	na	na	na	0.0	12.0	0.9	10.3	229	1.2
fat-free	1 frank	0	na	na	na	na	na	na	0.0	7.5	0.5	10.5	236	0.6
pork and turkey	1 frank	0	na	na	na	na	na	na	0.0	27.0	0.5	7.7	73	0.8
pork, turkey, and beef, light	1 frank	0	na	na	na	na	na	na	0.0	21.7	0.7	9.7	226	1.0
turkey, w/cheese	1 frank	0	na	na	na	na	na	na	0.0	73.8	0.7	11.3	59	0.8
FRENCH ARTICHOKE. See under ARTICHOKE.														
FRENCH BEAN. See BEAN, FRENCH.														
FRENCH TOAST														
(French Toast Boat) cinnamon	1 piece	22	0.27	0.18	1.90	0.00	na	0.01	0.07	36.4	1.9	0.65	85	<0.1
(Pierre) cinnamon, wedge, product 1847	1 piece	20	0.09	0.04	0.69	0.00	na	0.01	0.0	49.4	0.6	0	8	<0.1
(Sunny Fresh)														
bagel, w/maple syrup, frozen	1 pkg	14629	2.20	12.10	11.7	3.30	na	28.40	0.0	3175.0	54.4	284	5443	27.8
bagel, w/maple syrup, frozen	1 serving	183	0.03	0.15	0.15	0.04	na	0.35	0.0	39.7	0.7	3.5	68	0.4
cinnamon swirl	1 pkg	0	na	na	na	na	na	na	na	na	2.5	na	na	na
cinnamon swirl	1 serving	0	na	na	na	na	na	na	na	na	2.5	na	na	na
FRESHWATER BASS. See BASS, FRESHWATER.														
FROGFISH. See MONKFISH.														
FRUIT DRINK														
(Kool-Aid)														
grape-berry, 'Kool-Aid Splash'	1 serving	0	na	na	na	na	na	na	0.0	0.0	<0.1	na	13	na
tropical, 'Kool-Aid Burst'	1 serving	0	na	na	na	na	na	na	0.0	0.0	<0.1	na	8	na
FRUIT DRINK MIX														
(Country Time)														
lemonade, pink, sugar-free, w/vitamin C,														
mix only	1/8 cap/tub	na	na	na	na	na	na	na	6.6	na	na	na	na	na
lemonade, w/vitamin C, mix only	1/8 cap/tub	na	na	na	na	na	na	na	6.8	na	na	na	na	na
(Crystal Light) lemonade drink,														
w/NutraSweet, prepared	8 fl oz	0.02	na	na	na	na	na	na	<0.1	0.1	0.0	na	63	na
(Kool-Aid)														
tropical punch, sugar-sweetened,														
powder	1 serving	0	na	na	na	na	na	na	6.0	27.9	<0.1	na	<1	na
tropical punch, unsweetened, ...	1 serving	0	na	na	na	na	na	na	6.0	6.6	0.0	na	0	na
(Tang)														
orange flavored, mix only	2 tbsp	500	0.00	0.17	2.00	0.20	0.0	0.00	60.0	92.3	<0.1	0.0	48	0.01
orange flavored, prepared	8 fl oz	500	0.00	0.17	2.00	0.20	0.0	0.00	60.0	92.3	<0.1	0.0	48	0.01
orange flavored, sugarless, prepared	8 fl oz	500	0.00	0.17	2.00	0.20	0.0	0.00	60.0	34.5	0.0	6.9	78	0
FRUIT JUICE BLEND														
ORANGE-GRAPEFRUIT														
unsweetened, canned	1 cup	294	0.14	0.07	0.83	0.06	35.3	0.00	71.9	19.8	1.1	24.7	390	0.17
unsweetened, canned	1 fl oz	36.8	0.02	0.01	0.10	0.01	4.4	0.00	9.0	2.5	0.1	3.1	49	0.02
PINEAPPLE-GRAPEFRUIT JUICE														
canned	1 cup	87.5	0.08	0.04	0.67	0.11	26.3	0.00	115	17.5	0.8	15.0	153	.15
canned	1 fl oz	11.0	0.01	0.01	0.08	0.01	3.3	0.00	14.4	2.2	0.1	1.9	19	.02

Food Name	Serving Size	A I.U.	Thi mg	Rib mg	Nia mg	B_6 mg	Fol mcg	B_{12} mcg	C mg	Calc mg	Iron mg	Mag mg	Pot mg	Zn mg
PINEAPPLE-ORANGE														
canned	1 cup	1328	0.08	0.05	0.52	0.12	27.3	0.00	56.3	12.5	0.7	15.0	115	0.15
canned	1 fl oz	166	0.01	0.01	0.07	0.02	3.4	0.00	7.0	1.6	<0.1	1.9	14	0.02
FRUIT JUICE DRINK														
cranberry juice cocktail	8 fl oz	10	0.02	0.02	0.09	0.05	0.5	0.00	89.6	7.6	0.4	5.1	46	0.2
cranberry juice cocktail, diet	8 fl oz	10	0.02	0.02	0.08	0.05	0.5	0.00	76.3	21.3	0.1	4.7	52	<0.1
(Capri Sun)														
fruit punch, all natural, ready-to-drink	1 serving	8.4	na	na	na	na	na	na	2.7	2.1	<0.1	na	25	na
FRUIT SNACK														
(Farley) w/vitamins A, C, and E	1 pouch	1413	na	na	na	na	na	na	23.5	na	na	na	na	na
(Sunkist) strawberry roll, w/vitamins A, C, and E	1 roll	175	na	na	na	na	na	na	17.1	na	na	na	na	na
FRUIT SPREAD														
(Polaner) strawberry, 'All Fruit Spreadable Fruit'	1 tbsp	na	na	na	na	na	na	na	na	na	na	na	na	na
FUKI. See BUTTERBUR.														

G

Food Name	Serving Size	A I.U.	Thi mg	Rib mg	Nia mg	B_6 mg	Fol mcg	B_{12} mcg	C mg	Calc mg	Iron mg	Mag mg	Pot mg	Zn mg
GARBANZO. See CHICKPEA.														
GARDEN CRESS														
boiled, drained	1 cup	10395	0.08	0.22	1.10	0.21	50.0	0.00	31.1	82.3	1.1	35.1	477	0.20
boiled, drained	1/2 cup	5236	0.04	0.11	0.54	0.11	25.2	0.00	15.6	41.5	0.5	17.7	240	0.10
raw	1 cup	4650	0.04	0.13	0.50	0.12	40.2	0.00	34.5	40.5	0.7	19.0	303	0.12
GARLIC														
raw, chopped	1 cup	0	0.27	0.15	0.95	1.70	4.2	0.00	42.4	246.0	2.3	34.0	545	1.6
raw, chopped	1 tsp	0	0.01	0.00	0.02	0.04	<0.1	0.00	0.9	5.1	<0.1	0.7	11.2	0.03
raw, whole	1 med clove	0	0.01	0.00	0.02	0.04	<0.1	0.00	0.9	5.4	<0.1	0.8	12.0	0.04
raw, whole	3 med cloves	0	0.02	0.01	0.06	0.11	0.3	0.00	2.8	16.3	0.2	2.3	36.1	0.10
GARLIC POWDER														
	1 tbsp	0	0.04	0.01	0.06	0.23	0.2	0.00	1.5	6.7	0.2	4.9	92.5	0.22
	1 tsp	0	0.01	0.00	0.02	0.08	<0.1	0.00	0.5	2.2	<0.1	1.6	30.8	0.07
GELATIN DESSERT														
(Jell-O) strawberry, sugar-free	1 snack	0	na	na	na	na	na	na	0.0	0.0	<0.1	na	2.8	na
GELATIN DESSERT MIX														
(Jell-O) strawberry, sugar-free, prepared	1/2 cup	0	na	na	na	na	na	na	0.0	0.5	<0.1	na	0.45	na
GELATIN DRINK														
(Knox) orange flavor, diet	1 envelope	0	0	0.02	0.01	na	na	na	29.7	7.4	0.1	1.8	1.4	0.01
GIN														
80 proof	1 fl oz	0	0.00	0.00	0.00	0.00	0.0	0.00	0.0	0.0	<0.1	0.0	0.56	0.01
86 proof	1 fl oz	0	0.00	0.00	0.00	0.00	0.0	0.00	0.0	0.0	<0.1	0.0	0.56	0.01
90 proof	1 fl oz	0	0.00	0.00	0.00	0.00	0.0	0.00	0.0	0.0	<0.1	0.0	0.56	0.01
94 proof	1 fl oz	0	0.00	0.00	0.00	0.00	0.0	0.00	0.0	0.0	<0.1	0.0	0.56	0.01
100 proof	1 fl oz	0	0.00	0.00	0.00	0.00	0.0	0.00	0.0	0.0	<0.1	0.0	0.56	0.01
GINGER														
Dried														
ground	1 tbsp	8	0.00	0.01	0.28	0.06	2.1	0.00	0.4	6.3	0.6	9.9	72.5	0.26
ground	1 tsp	3	0.00	0.00	0.09	0.02	0.7	0.00	0.1	2.1	0.2	3.3	24.2	0.09
Fresh														
raw, minced	1 tsp	0	0.00	0.00	0.01	0.00	0.2	0.00	0.1	0.4	<0.1	0.9	8.3	0.01
raw, sliced, 1-inch diam.	1/4 cup	0	0.01	0.01	0.17	0.04	2.7	0.00	1.2	4.3	0.1	10.3	99.6	0.08

Food Name	Serving Size	A I.U.	Thi mg	Rib mg	Nia mg	B₆ mg	Fol mcg	B₁₂ mcg	C mg	Calc mg	Iron mg	Mag mg	Pot mg	Zn mg
GINKGO NUT														
Canned														
approx 78 kernels	1 cup	522	0.21	0.08	5.6	0.31	50.7	0.00	14.1	6.2	0.5	24.8	279	0.33
approx 14 kernels	1 oz	96	0.04	0.02	1.0	0.06	9.3	0.00	2.6	1.1	<0.1	4.5	51.0	0.06
Dried	1 oz	309	0.12	0.05	3.3	0.18	30.0	0.00	8.3	5.7	0.5	15.0	283	0.19
Fresh, raw	1 oz	158	0.06	0.03	1.70	0.09	15.3	0.00	4.3	0.6	0.3	7.7	145	0.10
GLOBE ARTICHOKE. See under ARTICHOKE.														
GLUTINOUS RICE. See under RICE.														
GOA BEAN. See BEAN, WINGED.														
GOAT														
raw	1 oz	0	0.03	0.14	1.10	na	1.4	0.32	0	3.7	0.8	na	109	1.1
roasted	3 oz	0	0.08	0.52	3.40	0.00	4.3	1.00	0	14.4	3.2	0.0	344	4.5
GOAT'S MILK. See under MILK.														
GOBO. See BURDOCK ROOT.														
GOOSE.														
AVERAGE OF ALL PARTS														
meat and skin, raw	4 oz	63	0.10	0.28	4.11	0.43	4.6	0.39	4.8	13.7	2.9	20.6	352	1.9
meat and skin, roasted	4 oz	80	0.09	0.37	4.74	0.43	2.3	0.47	0.0	14.8	3.2	25.2	376	2.9
meat and skin, roasted, chopped or diced . . .	1 cup	98	0.11	0.45	5.80	0.52	2.8	0.57	0.0	18.2	4.0	30.8	461	3.7
meat only, roasted	4 oz	46	0.10	0.45	4.64	0.54	13.7	0.56	0.0	16.0	3.3	28.6	444	3.6
LIVER. See also PÂTÉ, CANNED.														
raw	1 oz	8857	0.16	0.26	1.84	0.21	210.9	15.32	1.3	12.2	8.8	6.8	66	0.9
GOOSE FAT														
. . . .	1 cup	0	0.00	0.00	0.00	0.00	0.0	0.00	0.0	0.0	0.0	0.0	0	0
. . . .	1 tbsp	0	0.00	0.00	0.00	0.00	0.0	0.00	0.0	0.0	0.0	0.0	0	0
GOOSEBERRY														
Canned, in light syrup, w/liquids	1 cup	348	0.05	0.13	0.39	0.03	8.1	0.00	25.2	40.3	0.8	15.1	194	0.28
Fresh, raw	1 cup	435	0.06	0.05	0.45	0.12	9.0	0.00	41.5	37.5	0.5	15.0	297	0.18
GOOSEFISH. See MONKFISH.														
GOURD, BOTTLE / calabash gourd / white-flowered gourd														
boiled, drained, cubed	1 cup	0	0.04	0.03	0.57	0.06	6.3	0.00	12.4	35.0	0.4	16.1	248	1.0
raw, cubed	1/2 cup	9	0.02	0.01	0.19	0.02	3.4	0.00	5.9	15.1	0.1	6.4	87.0	0.41
raw, whole, medium	1 gourd	123	0.22	0.17	2.50	0.31	45.5	0.00	77.9	200.0	1.5	84.8	1157	5.4
GOURD, CALABASH. See GOURD, BOTTLE.														
GOURD, DISHCLOTH / loofah gourd / rag gourd / sponge gourd / towelgourd / vegetable sponge														
boiled, drained, cubed	1 cup	463	0.08	0.08	0.46	0.18	21.4	0.00	10.1	16.0	0.6	35.6	806	0.30
boiled, drained, sliced	1/2 cup	231	0.04	0.04	0.23	0.09	10.7	0.00	5.1	8.0	0.3	17.8	403	0.15
raw, cubed	1 cup	390	0.05	0.06	0.38	0.04	6.4	0.00	11.4	19.0	0.3	13.3	132	0.07
raw, whole, medium	1 gourd	730	0.09	0.11	0.71	0.08	11.9	0.00	21.4	35.6	0.6	24.9	247	0.13
GOURD, LOOFAH. See GOURD, DISHCLOTH.														
GOURD, RAG. See GOURD, DISHCLOTH.														
GOURD, SPONGE. See GOURD, DISHCLOTH.														
GOURD, WAX														
boiled, drained, cubed	1 cup	0	0.06	0.00	0.67	0.06	6.5	0.00	18.4	31.5	0.7	17.5	8.8	1.0
raw, cubed	1 cup	0	0.05	0.14	0.53	0.05	6.9	0.00	17.2	25.1	0.5	13.2	7.9	0.81
raw, whole, medium	1 gourd	0	2.30	6.30	22.80	2.00	296.0	0.00	741.0	1083.0	22.8	570.0	342	34.8
GOURD, WHITE-FLOWERED. See GOURD, BOTTLE.														
GRAHAM CRACKER. See under COOKIE.														
GRANADILLA. See PASSIONFRUIT.														
GRAPE														
AMERICAN (Concord, Delaware, Niagara)														
Fresh														
slipskin	1 medium	2	0.00	0.00	0.01	0.00	<0.1	0.00	0.10	0.3	<0.1	0.1	4.6	0
slipskin	1 cup	92	0.09	0.05	0.28	0.10	3.6	0.00	3.7	12.9	0.3	4.6	176	0.04

Food Name	Serving Size	A I.U.	Thi mg	Rib mg	Nia mg	B_6 mg	Fol mcg	B_{12} mcg	C mg	Calc mg	Iron mg	Mag mg	Pot mg	Zn mg
EUROPEAN (Muskat, Tokay, Thompson)														
Canned														
Thompson, seedless, in heavy syrup, w/liquid	1 cup	164	0.08	0.06	0.32	0.17	6.7	0.00	2.6	25.6	2.4	15.4	264	0.13
Thompson, seedless, in water, w/liquid	1 cup	162	0.08	0.06	0.32	0.16	6.4	0.00	2.5	24.5	2.4	14.7	262	0.12
Fresh														
red or green	1 medium	4	0.01	0.00	0.02	0.01	0.2	0.00	0.6	0.6	<0.1	0.3	10.7	0
red or green, seedless	1 cup	112	0.14	0.09	0.46	0.17	6.0	0.00	16.6	16.9	0.4	9.2	285	0.08
red or green, seedless	1 medium	4	0.01	0.00	0.02	0.01	0.2	0.00	0.5	0.6	<0.1	0.3	9.3	0
GRAPE JUICE														
unsweetened	1 cup	20.2	0.07	0.09	0.66	0.16	6.6	0.00	0.3	22.8	0.6	25.3	334	0.13
unsweetened	1 fl oz	3	0.01	0.01	0.08	0.02	0.8	0.00	<0.1	2.8	<0.1	3.2	41.7	0.02
GRAPE LEAVES														
raw	1 cup	3779	0.01	0.05	0.33	0.06	11.6	0.00	1.6	50.8	0.4	13.3	38.1	0.09
raw	1 medium	810	0.00	0.01	0.07	0.01	2.5	0.00	0.3	10.9	<0.1	2.9	8.2	0.02
GRAPEFRUIT														
PINK														
Fresh														
Arizona, sections, w/juice	1 cup	596	0.08	0.05	0.44	0.10	28.1	0.00	87.6	25.3	0.2	20.7	338	0.16
Arizona, whole, approx 3.75-inch diam	1/2 fruit	319	0.04	0.03	0.23	0.05	15.0	0.00	46.9	13.5	0.1	11.1	181	0.09
California, sections, w/juice	1 cup	596	0.08	0.05	0.44	0.10	28.1	0.00	87.6	25.3	0.2	20.7	338	0.16
California, whole, approx 3.75-inch diam	1/2 fruit	319	0.04	0.03	0.23	0.05	15.0	0.00	46.9	13.5	0.1	11.1	181	0.09
Florida, sections, w/juice	1 cup	596	0.09	0.05	0.46	0.10	21.6	0.00	85.1	34.5	0.3	18.4	292	0.16
Florida, whole, approx 3.75-inch diam	1/2 fruit	319	0.05	0.03	0.25	0.05	11.6	0.00	45.5	18.4	0.2	9.8	156	0.09
sections, w/juice	1 cup	285	0.08	0.05	0.57	0.10	23.5	0.00	79.1	27.6	0.2	18.4	320	0.16
whole, approx 4.5-inch diam	1/2 fruit	206	0.06	0.03	0.41	0.07	16.9	0.00	57.1	19.9	0.2	13.3	231	0.12
whole, approx 4-inch diam	1/2 fruit	159	0.05	0.03	0.32	0.05	13.1	0.00	44.0	15.4	0.1	10.2	178	0.09
whole, approx 3.75-inch diam	1/2 fruit	319	0.04	0.03	0.23	0.05	15.0	0.00	46.9	13.5	0.2	9.8	159	0.09
whole, approx 3.5-inch diam	1/2 fruit	124	0.04	0.02	0.25	0.04	10.2	0.00	34.4	12.0	<0.1	8.0	139	0.07
RED														
Fresh														
Arizona, sections, w/juice	1 cup	596	0.08	0.05	0.44	0.10	28.1	0.00	87.6	25.3	0.2	20.7	338	0.16
Arizona, whole, approx 3.75-inch diam	1/2 fruit	319	0.04	0.03	0.23	0.05	15.0	0.00	46.9	13.5	0.1	11.1	181	0.09
California, sections, w/juice	1 cup	596	0.08	0.05	0.44	0.10	28.1	0.00	87.6	25.3	0.2	20.7	338	0.16
California, whole, approx 3.75-inch diam	1/2 fruit	319	0.04	0.03	0.23	0.05	15.0	0.00	46.9	13.5	0.1	11.1	181	0.09
Florida, sections, w/juice	1 cup	596	0.09	0.05	0.46	0.10	21.6	0.00	85.1	34.5	0.3	18.4	292	0.16
Florida, whole, approx 3.75-inch diam	1/2 fruit	319	0.05	0.03	0.25	0.05	11.6	0.00	45.5	18.4	0.2	9.8	156	0.09
sections, w/juice	1 cup	285	0.08	0.05	0.57	0.10	23.5	0.00	79.1	27.6	0.2	18.4	320	0.16
whole, approx 4.5-inch diam	1/2 fruit	206	0.06	0.03	0.41	0.07	16.9	0.00	57.1	19.9	0.2	13.3	231	0.12
whole, approx 4-inch diam	1/2 fruit	159	0.05	0.03	0.32	0.05	13.1	0.00	44.0	15.4	0.1	10.2	178	0.09
whole, approx 3.75-inch diam	1/2 fruit	319	0.04	0.03	0.23	0.05	15.0	0.00	46.9	13.5	0.2	9.8	159	0.09
whole, approx 3.5-inch diam	1/2 fruit	124	0.04	0.02	0.25	0.04	10.2	0.00	34.4	12.0	<0.1	8.0	139	0.07
WHITE														
Canned														
sections, in juice, w/liquid	1 cup	0	0.07	0.05	0.62	0.05	21.9	0.00	84.4	37.4	0.5	27.4	421	0.20
sections, in light syrup, w/liquid	1 cup	0	0.10	0.05	0.62	0.05	21.6	0.00	54.1	35.6	1.0	25.4	328	0.20
sections, in water, w/liquid	1 cup	0	0.10	0.05	0.61	0.05	21.5	0.00	53.2	36.6	1.0	24.4	322	0.22
Fresh														
California, sections, w/juice	1 cup	23	0.09	0.05	0.62	0.10	27.1	0.00	76.6	27.6	0.2	20.7	329	0.16
California, whole, approx 3.75-inch diam	1/2 fruit	12	0.04	0.02	0.32	0.05	13.9	0.00	39.3	14.2	<0.1	10.6	169	0.08
Florida, sections, w/juice	1 cup	23	0.09	0.05	0.46	0.10	21.6	0.00	85.1	34.5	0.1	20.7	345	0.16

Food Name	Serving Size	A I.U.	Thi mg	Rib mg	Nia mg	B6 mg	Fol mcg	B12 mcg	C mg	Calc mg	Iron mg	Mag mg	Pot mg	Zn mg
Florida, whole, approx 3.75-inch diam	1/2 fruit	12	0.05	0.02	0.24	0.05	11.1	0.00	43.7	17.7	<0.1	10.6	177	0.08
sections, w/juice	1 cup	285	0.08	0.05	0.57	0.10	23.5	0.00	79.1	27.6	0.2	18.4	320	0.16
whole, approx 3.5-inch diam.	1/2 fruit	124	0.04	0.02	0.25	0.04	10.2	0.00	34.4	12.0	<0.1	8.0	139	0.07
whole, approx 3.75-inch diam.	1/2 fruit	12	0.04	0.02	0.32	0.05	11.8	0.00	39.3	14.2	<0.1	10.6	175	0.08
whole, approx 4-inch diam	1/2 fruit	159	0.05	0.03	0.32	0.05	13.1	0.00	44.0	15.4	0.1	10.2	178	0.09
whole, approx 4.5-inch diam.	1/2 fruit	206	0.06	0.03	0.41	0.07	16.9	0.00	57.1	19.9	0.2	13.3	231	0.12
GRAPEFRUIT JUICE														
canned, unsweetened.	1 cup	17	0.10	0.05	0.57	0.05	25.7	0.00	72.1	17.3	0.5	24.7	378	0.22
fresh-squeezed, pink, unsweetened.	1 cup	1087	0.10	0.05	0.49	0.11	25.2	0.00	93.9	22.2	0.5	29.6	400	0.12
fresh-squeezed, white, unsweetened	1 cup	25	0.10	0.05	0.49	0.11	25.2	0.00	93.9	22.2	0.5	29.6	400	0.12
frozen concentrate, unsweetened.	6 fl oz	64	0.30	0.16	1.60	0.32	26.5	0.00	248	55.9	1.0	78.7	1002	0.37
frozen concentrate, unsweetened, prepared.	1 cup	22	0.10	0.05	0.54	0.11	8.9	0.00	83.2	19.8	0.4	27.2	336	0.12
GRAPESEED OIL														
. . . .	1 cup	0	0.00	0.00	0.00	0.00	0.0	0.00	0.0	0.0	0.0	0.0	0	0
. . . .	1 tbsp	0	0.00	0.00	0.00	0.00	0.0	0.00	0.0	0.0	0.0	0.0	0	0
GRAVY														
BEEF														
(Pepperidge Farm)														
hearty	1 jar	0	na	na	na	na	na	na	na	na	na	na	na	na
hearty	1 serving	0	na	na	na	na	na	na	na	na	na	na	na	na
BROWN *(Heinz)* savory, 'HomeStyle'.	1/4 cup	na	na	na	na	na	na	na	na	na	na	na	na	na
SAUSAGE														
(Nestlé)														
country, 'Chef-Mate'	1 pkg	0	4.70	1.80	31.20	1.90	29.8	10.10	3.0	179.0	16.4	149.0	2292	16.4
country, 'Chef-Mate'	1/4 cup	0	0.10	0.04	0.65	0.04	0.6	0.21	<0.1	3.7	0.34	3.1	47.7	0.34
GRAVY MIX														
AU JUS														
(Custom Foods)														
base, 'Red Label' mix only	16-oz pkg	222	0.41	0.21	3.10	1.20	222.0	1.40	2.3	7541.0	13.4	114.0	835	6.6
base, 'Red Label' mix only	1 serving	5	0.01	0.01	0.07	0.03	4.9	0.03	<0.1	166.0	0.30	2.5	18.4	0.14
instant, 'Superb' mix only	4-oz pkg	44	1.4	0.62	6.70	0.47	na	0.28	4.5	172.0	32.5	32.8	299	2.2
instant, 'Superb' mix only	1 serving	3	0.09	0.04	0.40	0.03	na	0.02	0.3	10.2	1.9	1.9	17.8	0.13
(Nestlé)														
'Trio' mix only	7-oz pkg	0	0.00	0.00	0.01	0.00	0.0	0.00	0.0	204.0	5.5	2.0	7.9	0.10
'Trio' mix only	1 tsp	0	0.00	0.00	0.00	0.00	0.0	0.00	0.0	3.1	<0.1	<0.1	0.12	0
BEEF														
(Custom Foods)														
instant, 'Superb' mix only	16-oz pkg	182	0.85	2.30	4.90	0.63	45.4	2.80	4.1	640.0	28.5	186.0	2043	3.5
instant, 'Superb' mix only	1 serving	3	0.01	0.03	0.07	0.01	0.7	0.04	<0.1	9.4	0.4	2.7	30.1	0.05
BISCUIT														
(Custom Foods)														
old-fashioned, 'Superb' mix only	1 pkg	3196	1.30	1.40	9.20	0.20	224.0	1.60	2.0	252.0	41.1	81.6	4223	3.5
old-fashioned, 'Superb' mix only	1 serving	46	0.02	0.02	0.13	0.00	3.2	0.02	<0.1	3.6	0.6	1.2	60.2	0.05
peppered, 'Superb'	1 pkg	2924	2.40	2.00	17.1	0.27	224.0	1.50	5.4	238.0	1.9	109.0	952	3.7
peppered, 'Superb'	1 serving	42	0.03	0.03	0.25	0.00	3.2	0.02	<0.1	3.4	<0.1	1.6	13.6	0.05
BROWN														
(Custom Foods)														
instant, 'Superb' mix only	1 pkg	177	1.10	2.10	10.30	1.30	454.0	1.50	8.6	527.0	33.6	145.0	1666	4.4
instant, 'Superb' mix only	1 serving	3	0.02	0.03	0.15	0.02	6.7	0.02	0.1	7.8	0.5	2.1	24.6	0.06
(Nestlé)														
'Trio' mix only	16-oz pkg	0	0.11	0.07	0.95	0.06	118.0	0.00	0.0	163.0	8.2	36.2	63.4	2.9
'Trio' mix only	1 tbsp	0	0.00	0.00	0.01	0.00	1.6	0.00	0.0	2.2	0.1	0.5	0.84	0.04
'Trio Supreme' mix only.	16-oz pkg	227	1.80	3.10	25.9	1.90	1258.0	0.00	0.0	386.0	0.0	213	2515	7.1

Food Name	Serving Size	A I.U.	Thi mg	Rib mg	Nia mg	B$_6$ mg	Fol mcg	B$_{12}$ mcg	C mg	Calc mg	Iron mg	Mag mg	Pot mg	Zn mg
'Trio Supreme' mix only	1 tbsp	3	0.02	0.04	0.34	0.03	16.6	0.01	0.0	5.1	0.0	2.8	33.2	0.09
CHICKEN														
(Custom Foods)														
instant, 'Superb' mix only	16-oz pkg	363	1.30	2.60	17.9	0.91	232.0	1.90	4.1	486.0	24.4	173.0	1884	5.7
instant, 'Superb' mix only	1 serving	5	0.02	0.04	0.26	0.01	3.4	0.03	<0.1	7.2	0.4	2.5	27.8	0.08
(Nestlé)														
'Trio' mix only	1 pkg	1333	0.52	1.80	11.0	0.86	103.0	2.50	7.7	1026.0	8.3	167.0	1744	7.6
'Trio' mix only	1 tbsp	17	0.01	0.02	0.14	0.01	1.3	0.03	0.1	12.8	0.1	2.1	21.8	0.10
'Trio Supreme' mix only	1 pkg	2739	2.50	6.80	38.0	2.10	2007.0	2.30	0.0	737.0	0.0	295.0	3788	8.3
'Trio Supreme' mix only	1 tbsp	39	0.04	0.10	0.54	0.03	28.3	0.03	0.0	10.4	0.0	4.2	53.4	0.12
COUNTRY														
(Custom Foods)														
(Nestlé)														
'Trio' mix only	1 pkg	0	0.77	1.20	7.80	0.24	62.4	0.56	0.0	406.0	8.1	87.4	867	4.0
'Trio' mix only	1 tbsp	0	0.01	0.02	0.10	0.00	0.8	0.01	0.0	5.2	0.1	1.1	11.1	0.05
PORK														
(Custom Foods)														
instant, 'Superb' mix only	16-oz pkg	531	0.54	1.10	3.80	0.33	81.7	1.50	6.4	531.0	17.9	99.9	944	3.3
instant, 'Superb' mix only	1 serving	8	0.01	0.02	0.06	0.01	1.2	0.02	<0.1	7.8	0.3	1.5	13.9	0.05
SOUTHERN														
(Nestlé)														
'Trio' mix only	1 pkg	898	0.11	0.40	0.36	0.13	11.0	0.85	2.6	276.0	2.3	51.5	508	1.2
'Trio' mix only	1 serving	24	0.00	0.01	0.01	0.00	0.3	0.02	<0.1	7.5	<0.1	1.4	13.8	0.03
TURKEY														
(Custom Foods)														
instant, 'Superb' mix only	16-oz pkg	636	0.59	1.20	5.40	0.93	114.0	1.70	4.1	522.0	43.4	136.0	1389	5.1
instant, 'Superb' mix only	1 serving	9	0.01	0.02	0.08	0.01	1.7	0.03	<0.1	7.7	0.6	2.0	20.5	0.08
(Nestlé)														
'Trio' mix only	1 pkg	0	1.70	5.40	19.40	1.70	902.0	3.90	0.0	680.0	6.8	323.0	4065	7.1
'Trio' mix only	1 serving	0	0.02	0.08	0.27	0.03	12.7	0.05	0.0	9.6	0.1	4.6	57.4	0.10

GREAT NORTHERN BEAN. See BEAN, GREAT NORTHERN.

GREEN BEAN. See BEAN, GREEN; BEAN, FRENCH.

GREEN ONION. See SCALLION.

GREEN PEAS. See PEAS, GREEN.

GREEN PEPPER. See PEPPER, BELL.

GREENLAND HALIBUT. See under HALIBUT.

GRITS

CORN

Instant

(Quaker)

Food Name	Serving Size	A I.U.	Thi mg	Rib mg	Nia mg	B$_6$ mg	Fol mcg	B$_{12}$ mcg	C mg	Calc mg	Iron mg	Mag mg	Pot mg	Zn mg
butter flavor, dry	1 pkt	54	0.18	0.20	2.40	0.03	47.0	0.00	0.0	2.0	8.1	7.6	54	0.1
cheddar cheese flavor, dry	1 pkt	4	0.17	0.19	2.20	0.05	43.7	0.06	0.0	12.9	8.1	10.4	48	0.2
plain, dry	1 pkt	0	0.19	0.21	2.50	0.06	49.6	0.00	0.0	5.9	8.5	10.1	41	0.2
w/imitation bacon bits, dry	1 pkt	0	0.18	0.20	2.30	0.06	46.8	0.00	0.0	10.6	8.1	9.5	71	0.2
w/imitation ham bits, dry	1 pkt	0	0.17	0.20	2.30	0.06	46.5	0.06	0.0	14.6	8.1	14.0	50	0.2
Quick-cooking														
white, enriched, dry	1 cup	0	0.00	0.59	7.70	0.23	292.0	0.00	0.0	3.1	6.1	42.1	214	0.6
white, enriched, dry	1 tbsp	0	0.06	0.04	0.48	0.01	18.1	0.00	0.0	0.2	0.4	2.6	13	<0.1
white, unenriched, dry	1 cup	0	0.20	0.06	1.90	0.23	7.8	0.00	0.0	3.1	1.6	42.1	214	0.6
white, unenriched, dry	1 tbsp	0	0.01	0.00	0.12	0.01	0.5	0.00	0.0	0.2	0.1	2.6	13	<0.1
white, enriched, cooked w/water, w/o salt	1 cup	0	0.24	0.14	2.00	0.06	75.0	0.00	0.0	0.0	1.5	9.7	53	0.1
white, enriched, cooked w/water, w/o salt	3/4 cup	0	0.18	0.11	1.50	0.04	56.4	0.00	0.0	0.0	1.2	7.3	40	0.1

Food Name	Serving Size	A I.U.	Thi mg	Rib mg	Nia mg	B6 mg	Fol mcg	B12 mcg	C mg	Calc mg	Iron mg	Mag mg	Pot mg	Zn mg
white, unenriched, cooked w/water, w/o salt	1 cup	0	0.05	0.02	0.48	0.06	2.4	0.00	0.0	0.0	0.5	9.7	53	0.1
white, unenriched, cooked w/water, w/o salt	3/4 cup	0	0.04	0.02	0.36	0.04	1.8	0.00	0.0	0.0	0.4	7.3	40	0.1
yellow, unenriched, dry	1 cup	686	0.20	0.06	1.90	0.23	7.8	0.00	0.0	3.1	1.6	42.1	214	0.6
yellow, unenriched, dry	1 tbsp	43	0.01	0.00	0.12	0.01	0.5	0.00	0.0	0.2	0.1	2.6	13	0.0
yellow, enriched, dry	1 cup	686	0.00	0.59	7.70	0.23	292.0	0.00	0.0	3.1	6.1	42.1	214	0.6
yellow, enriched, dry	1 tbsp	43	0.06	0.04	0.48	0.01	18.1	0.00	0.0	0.2	0.4	2.6	13	<0.1
yellow, enriched, cooked w/water, w/o salt	1 cup	145	0.24	0.14	2.00	0.06	75.0	0.00	0.0	0.0	1.5	9.7	53	0.2
yellow, enriched, cooked w/water, w/o salt	3/4 cup	109	0.18	0.11	1.50	0.04	56.4	0.00	0.0	0.0	1.2	7.3	40	0.1
yellow, unenriched, cooked w/water, w/o salt	1 cup	145	0.05	0.02	0.48	0.06	2.4	0.00	0.0	0.0	0.5	9.7	53	0.2
yellow, unenriched, cooked w/water, w/o salt	3/4 cup	109	0.04	0.02	0.36	0.04	1.8	0.00	0.0	0.0	0.4	7.3	40	0.1
HOMINY														
Canned														
white	1 cup	0	0.01	0.01	0.05	0.01	1.6	0.00	0.0	16.5	1.0	26.4	15	1.7
yellow	1 cup	176	0.01	0.01	0.05	0.01	1.6	0.00	0.0	16.0	1.0	25.6	14	1.7
GROUND CHERRY. See CAPE GOOSEBERRY.														
GROUND HUSK TOMATO. See TOMATILLO.														
GROUPER														
mixed species, baked, broiled, grilled, or microwaved	3 oz	140	0.07	0.01	0.32	0.30	8.7	0.59	0.0	17.9	0.9	31.4	404	0.4
raw	3 oz	122	0.06	0.00	0.27	0.26	7.5	0.51	0.0	22.9	0.8	26.4	411	0.4
GUANABANA / soursop														
pulp	1 cup	5	0.16	0.11	2.00	0.13	31.5	0.00	46.4	31.5	1.4	47.3	626	0.2
raw, whole, approx 2.1 lb	1 medium	13	0.44	0.31	5.60	0.37	87.5	0.00	129.0	87.5	3.8	131.0	1738	0.6
GUAVA														
raw, chopped	1 cup	1307	0.08	0.08	2.00	0.24	23.1	0.00	303.0	33.0	0.5	16.5	469	0.4
raw, whole, trimmed	1 medium	713	0.05	0.05	1.10	0.13	12.6	0.00	165.0	18.0	0.3	9.0	256	0.2
GUAVA, STRAWBERRY														
raw, chopped	1 cup	220	0.07	0.07	1.50	na	na	0.00	90.3	51.2	0.5	41.5	712	na
raw, whole, trimmed	1 medium	5	0.00	0.00	0.04	na	na	0.00	2.2	1.3	<0.1	1.0	17.5	na
GUINEA HEN														
meat and skin, raw	4 oz	105	0.07	0.18	8.75	0.45	5.7	0.38	1.5	12.6	0.9	25.1	221	1.3
meat only, raw	4 oz	47	0.07	0.13	10.06	0.54	6.9	0.42	1.9	12.6	0.9	27.4	251	1.4
GUM. See under CANDY.														

H

Food Name	Serving Size	A I.U.	Thi mg	Rib mg	Nia mg	B6 mg	Fol mcg	B12 mcg	C mg	Calc mg	Iron mg	Mag mg	Pot mg	Zn mg
HADDOCK														
Fresh														
baked, broiled, grilled, or microwaved	3 oz	54	0.03	0.04	3.90	0.29	11.3	1.20	0.0	35.7	1.1	42.5	339	0.4
raw	3 oz	47	0.03	0.03	3.20	0.26	9.8	1.00	0.0	28.1	0.9	33.1	264	0.3
Smoked														
fillet	3 oz	62	0.04	0.04	4.30	0.34	13.0	1.40	0.0	41.6	1.2	45.9	353	0.4
fillet, boneless	1 oz	21	0.01	0.01	1.40	0.11	4.3	0.45	0.0	13.9	0.4	15.3	118	0.1
HADDOCK, NORWAY. See OCEAN PERCH.														
HAKE, SILVER. See WHITING.														

Food Name	Serving Size	A I.U.	Thi mg	Rib mg	Nia mg	B$_6$ mg	Fol mcg	B$_{12}$ mcg	C mg	Calc mg	Iron mg	Mag mg	Pot mg	Zn mg
HALIBUT														
ATLANTIC														
baked, broiled, grilled, or microwaved	3 oz	152	0.06	0.08	6.10	0.34	11.7	1.20	0.0	51.0	0.9	91.0	490	0.5
raw	3 oz	132	0.05	0.06	5.00	0.29	10.2	1.00	0.0	40.0	0.7	70.5	383	0.4
GREENLAND														
baked, broiled, grilled, or microwaved	3 oz	51	0.06	0.09	1.60	0.41	0.9	0.82	0.0	3.4	0.7	28.1	292	0.4
raw	3 oz	47	0.05	0.07	1.30	0.36	0.9	0.85	0.0	2.5	0.6	22.1	228	0.3
PACIFIC														
baked, broiled, grilled, or microwaved	3 oz	152	0.06	0.08	6.10	0.34	11.7	1.20	0.0	51.0	0.9	91.0	490	0.5
raw	3 oz	132	0.05	0.06	5.00	0.29	10.2	1.00	0.0	40.0	0.7	70.5	383	0.4
HAM. See also PORK. Also see under LUNCHEON MEAT.														
(NOTE: TRIMMED = Lean; separable fat removed. UNTRIMMED = Separable fat not removed.)														
Bone in, whole														
trimmed, fully cooked, baked	3 oz	0	0.58	0.22	4.30	0.40	3.4	0.59	0.0	6.0	0.8	18.7	269	2.2
trimmed, fully cooked, baked, chopped	1 cup	0	0.95	0.36	7.00	0.66	5.6	0.98	0.0	9.8	1.3	30.8	442	3.6
trimmed, fully cooked, unheated	1 oz	0	0.26	0.06	1.50	0.15	1.1	0.25	0.0	2.0	0.2	5.1	105	0.6
trimmed, fully cooked, unheated, chopped	1 cup	0	1.30	0.32	7.40	0.74	5.6	1.20	0.0	9.8	1.1	25.2	519	2.9
untrimmed, fully cooked, unheated, chopped	1 cup	0	1.10	0.27	6.20	0.57	5.6	1.00	48.9	9.8	1.0	21.0	434	2.5
untrimmed, fully cooked, heated, chopped	1 cup	0	0.84	0.31	6.20	0.53	4.2	0.90	0.0	9.8	1.2	26.6	400	3.2
Boneless														
center slice, country-style, trimmed, unheated	4 oz	0	0.64	0.27	4.40	0.47	5.7	0.99	0.0	11.3	1.3	28.3	576	3.2
center slice, country style, untrimmed, unheated	4 oz	0	0.95	0.23	5.40	0.53	4.5	0.90	0.0	7.9	0.9	18.1	381	2.1
extra lean, approx 5% fat, baked	3 oz	0	0.64	0.17	3.40	0.34	2.5	0.55	0.0	6.8	1.3	11.9	244	2.4
extra lean, approx 5% fat, baked, chopped	1 cup	0	1.10	0.28	5.60	0.56	4.2	0.91	0.0	11.2	2.1	19.6	402	4.0
extra lean and regular, baked	3 oz	0	0.63	0.24	4.50	0.30	2.5	0.58	0.0	6.8	1.2	16.1	308	2.2
extra lean and regular, baked, chopped	1 cup	0	1.00	0.39	7.50	0.49	4.2	0.95	0.0	11.2	2.0	26.6	507	3.7
extra lean and regular, unheated, chopped	1 cup	0	1.20	0.34	7.10	0.53	4.2	1.10	0.0	9.8	1.3	25.2	416	2.9
regular, approx 11% fat, baked	3 oz	0	0.62	0.28	5.20	0.26	2.5	0.59	0.0	6.8	1.1	18.7	348	2.1
regular, approx 11% fat, baked, chopped	1 cup	0	1.00	0.46	8.60	0.43	4.2	0.98	0.0	11.2	1.9	30.8	573	3.5
steak, unheated	1 oz	0	0.23	0.06	1.40	0.11	1.1	0.22	9.2	1.1	0.3	5.4	92	0.6
Patty, cured, unheated	1 oz	0	0.13	0.04	0.85	0.05	0.9	0.31	0.0	2.3	0.3	2.8	68	0.5
HAMBURGER. See under BEEF; BEEF DISH/ENTRÉE.														
HAMBURGER BUN. See BUN, HAMBURGER.														
HAMBURGER RELISH. See under RELISH.														
HAMBURGER SUBSTITUTE. See under BEEF SUBSTITUTE DISH/ENTRÉE.														
HARD ROLL. See under ROLL.														
HARICOTS. See BEAN, FRENCH.														
HASH														
CORNED BEEF														
(Armour)														
canned	1 pkg	0	na	na	na	na	na	na	na	na	4.0	na	na	na
canned	1 serving	0	na	na	na	na	na	na	na	na	2.2	na	na	na
(Hormel) canned	1 cup	0	na	na	na	na	na	na	2.1	44.8	2.4	30.7	406	3.3
(Nestlé)														
'Chef Mate'	1 pkg	0	0.22	0.30	6.30	0.58	na	2.50	1.5	45.5	3.0	38.0	536	7.5
'Chef Mate'	1 cup	0	2.60	3.50	75.70	6.90	na	29.40	18.2	546.0	35.8	455.0	6430	90.1

Food Name	Serving Size	A I.U.	Thi mg	Rib mg	Nia mg	B$_6$ mg	Fol mcg	B$_{12}$ mcg	C mg	Calc mg	Iron mg	Mag mg	Pot mg	Zn mg
HAZELNUT / cob nut / filbert														
dried	1 oz	11	0.18	0.03	0.51	0.16	32.0	0.00	1.8	32.3	1.3	46.2	193	0.7
dried	10 medium	6	0.09	0.02	0.25	0.08	15.8	0.00	0.9	16.0	0.7	22.8	95	0.3
dried, blanched	1 oz	11	0.14	0.03	0.44	0.17	22.1	0.00	0.6	42.2	0.9	45.4	187	0.6
dried, chopped	1 cup	46	0.74	0.13	2.10	0.65	130.0	0.00	7.1	131.0	5.4	187.0	782	2.8
dried, ground	1 cup	30	0.48	0.08	1.40	0.42	84.8	0.00	4.7	85.5	3.5	122.0	510	1.8
dried, whole	1 cup	54	0.87	0.15	2.40	0.76	153.0	0.00	8.4	154.0	6.3	220.0	918	3.3
dry-roasted, no salt added	1 oz	17	0.10	0.04	0.58	0.18	24.9	0.00	1.1	34.6	1.2	49.0	214	0.7
HAZELNUT OIL														
	1 cup	0	0.00	0.00	0.00	0.00	0.0	0.00	0.0	0.0	0.0	0.0	0	0
	1 tbsp	0	0.00	0.00	0.00	0.00	0.0	0.00	0.0	0.0	0.0	0.0	0	0
HEART NUT. See CASHEW.														
HEARTS OF PALM. See under PALM.														
HERRING														
ATLANTIC														
fillet, baked, broiled, grilled, or microwaved	3 oz	87	0.10	0.25	3.50	0.30	9.8	11.20	0.6	62.9	1.2	34.9	356	1.1
fillet, kippered, small, approx 2-3/8 x 1-3/8 x 1/4 inch	1 fillet	26	0.03	0.06	0.88	0.08	2.7	3.70	0.2	16.8	0.3	9.2	89	0.3
fillet, kippered, medium, approx 5 x 1.75 x 1/4 inch	1 fillet	52	0.05	0.13	1.80	0.17	5.5	7.50	0.4	33.6	0.6	18.4	179	0.5
fillet, kippered, large, approx 7 x 2.25 x 1/4 inch	1 fillet	83	0.08	0.21	2.90	0.27	8.9	12.20	0.7	54.6	1.0	29.9	291	0.9
fillet, kippered, boneless	1 oz	36	0.04	0.09	1.20	0.12	3.9	5.30	0.3	23.8	0.4	13.0	127	0.4
pickled	1 cup	1205	0.05	0.20	4.60	0.24	3.4	6.00	0.0	108.0	1.7	11.2	97	0.7
pickled, approx 1.75 x 7/8 x 1/2 inch	1 piece	129	0.01	0.02	0.50	0.03	0.4	0.64	0.0	11.6	0.2	1.2	10	<0.1
pickled, boneless	1 oz	244	0.01	0.04	0.94	0.05	0.7	1.20	0.0	21.8	0.4	2.3	20	0.2
raw	3 oz	80	0.08	0.20	2.70	0.26	8.5	11.60	0.6	48.5	0.9	27.2	278	0.8
raw, boneless	1 oz	27	0.03	0.07	0.91	0.09	2.8	3.90	0.2	16.2	0.3	9.1	93	0.3
PACIFIC														
baked, broiled, grilled, or miocrowaved	3 oz	99	0.06	0.22	2.40	0.44	5.1	8.20	0.0	90.1	1.2	34.9	461	0.6
raw	3 oz	90	0.05	0.17	1.90	0.38	4.3	8.50	0.0	70.5	0.9	27.2	360	0.5
HERRING OIL. See under FISH OIL.														
HICKORY NUT, DRIED														
	1 cup	157	1.00	0.16	1.10	0.23	48.0	0.00	2.4	73.2	2.5	208.0	523	5.2
	1 oz	37	0.25	0.04	0.26	0.05	11.3	0.00	0.6	17.3	0.6	49.0	124	1.2
	1 medium	3.9	0.03	0.00	0.03	0.01	1.2	0.00	<0.1	1.8	<0.1	5.2	13	0.1
HIRITAKE. See MUSHROOM, OYSTER.														
HOMINY. See under GRITS.														
HONEY														
strained or extracted	1 cup	0	0.00	0.13	0.41	0.08	6.8	0.00	1.7	20.3	1.4	6.8	176	0.8
strained or extracted	1 tbsp	0	0.00	0.01	0.03	0.01	0.4	0.00	0.1	1.3	<0.1	0.42	11	<0.1
HONEYDEW MELON. See MELON, HONEYDEW.														
HORSE														
raw	1 oz	0	0.04	0.03	1.30	0.11	na	0.85	0.3	1.7	1.1	6.8	102	0.8
roasted	3 oz	0	0.09	0.10	4.10	0.28	na	2.70	1.7	6.8	4.3	21.3	322	3.2
HORSE BEAN. See BEAN, FAVA.														
HORSERADISH														
prepared	1 tbsp	<1	0.00	0.00	0.06	0.01	8.6	0.00	3.7	8.4	<0.1	4.0	37	0.1
prepared	1 tsp	<1	0.00	0.00	0.02	0.00	2.9	0.00	1.2	2.8	<0.1	1.4	12	<0.1
HORSERADISH, JAPANESE. See WASABI ROOT.														
HORSERADISH TREE														
leafy tips, boiled, drained, chopped	1 cup	2945	0.09	0.21	0.84	0.39	9.4	0.00	13.0	63.4	0.9	63.4	144	0.2
leafy tips, raw, chopped	1 cup	1588	0.05	0.14	0.47	0.25	8.4	0.00	10.9	38.9	0.8	30.9	71	0.1
pods, boiled, drained, sliced	1 cup	83	0.05	0.08	0.70	0.13	35.9	0.00	114.0	23.6	0.5	49.6	539	0.5

Food Name	Serving Size	A I.U.	Thi mg	Rib mg	Nia mg	B₆ mg	Fol mcg	B₁₂ mcg	C mg	Calc mg	Iron mg	Mag mg	Pot mg	Zn mg
pods, raw, sliced....................	1 cup	74	0.05	0.07	0.62	0.12	44.3	0.00	141.0	30.0	0.4	45.0	461	0.
pods, raw, whole, approx 15 1/3 inch long	1 pod	8	0.01	0.01	0.07	0.01	4.9	0.00	15.5	3.3	<0.1	5.0	51	<0.1

HOT COCOA. See COCOA, HOT, MIX.
HOT DOG. See FRANKFURTER.
HOT DOG BUN. See BUN, FRANKFURTER.
HUBBARD SQUASH. See SQUASH, HUBBARD.
HUMPBACK SALMON. See under SALMON.
HUNGARIAN PEPPER. See PEPPER, HUNGARIAN.
HYACINTH BEAN. See BEAN, HYACINTH.

I

Food Name	Serving Size	A I.U.	Thi mg	Rib mg	Nia mg	B₆ mg	Fol mcg	B₁₂ mcg	C mg	Calc mg	Iron mg	Mag mg	Pot mg	Zn mg
ICE CREAM.														
(Healthy Choice) praline and caramel, low-fat...................	1/2 cup	199	na	na	na	na	na	na	0	99.4	0.08	na	na	na

ICEBERG LETTUCE. See LETTUCE, ICEBERG.
ICED TEA. See TEA.
INDIAN DATE. See TAMARIND.
INDIAN FRY BREAD. See under BREAD.
INFANT FORMULA. See under BABY FOOD.
IRISH MOSS. See under SEA VEGETABLE.
ITALIAN CHESTNUT. See CHESTNUT, EUROPEAN.
ITALIAN MUSHROOM. See MUSHROOM, CRIMINI.
ITALIAN STONE PINE NUT. See PINE NUT.

J

Food Name	Serving Size	A I.U.	Thi mg	Rib mg	Nia mg	B₆ mg	Fol mcg	B₁₂ mcg	C mg	Calc mg	Iron mg	Mag mg	Pot mg	Zn mg
JACK BEAN. See BEAN, FAVA.														
JACK MACKEREL. See under MACKEREL.														
JACKFRUIT														
Fresh, raw, sliced........................	1 cup	490	0.05	0.18	0.66	0.18	23.1	0.00	11.1	56.1	1.0	61.0	500	0.7
Canned, in syrup, drained..........	1 cup	4	0.06	0.06	1.20	0.08	24.9	0.00	0.9	78.3	0.5	17.8	171	0.2
JALAPEÑO. See PEPPER, JALAPEÑO.														
JAMBOLAN. See JAVA PLUM.														
JAPANESE HORSERADISH. See WASABI ROOT.														
JAPANESE MEDLAR. See LOQUAT.														
JAVA PLUM / jambolan														
cut up	1 cup	4	0.01	0.02	0.35	0.05	na	0.00	19.3	25.6	0.3	20.3	107	na
whole	3 fruits	<1	0.00	0.00	0.02	0.00	na	0.00	1.3	1.7	<0.1	1.4	7	na
JEW'S EAR. See CHINESE FUNGUS.														
JELLYBEAN. See under CANDY.														
JERUSALEM ARTICHOKE. See ARTICHOKE, JERUSALEM.														
JICAMA / Chinese yam / Mexican potato / sicama / yambean tuber														
raw, sliced.................	1 cup	27	0.03	0.04	0.26	0.06	15.6	0.00	26.3	15.6	0.8	15.6	195	0.2
raw, whole.................	1 medium	138	0.13	0.19	1.30	0.28	79.1	0.00	133.0	79.1	4.0	79.1	989	1.1
JUTE POTHERB														
boiled, drained	1 cup	4511	0.08	0.17	0.77	0.50	90.3	0.00	28.7	184.0	2.7	53.9	479	0.7
raw	1 cup	1557	0.04	0.15	0.35	0.17	34.4	0.00	10.4	58.2	1.3	17.9	157	0.2

K

Food Name	Serving Size	A I.U.	Thi mg	Rib mg	Nia mg	B$_6$ mg	Fol mcg	B$_{12}$ mcg	C mg	Calc mg	Iron mg	Mag mg	Pot mg	Zn mg
KAISER ROLL. See under ROLL.														
KALE / cole / colewort														
Fresh														
boiled, drained, chopped	1 cup	9620	0.07	0.09	0.65	0.18	17.3	0.00	53.3	93.6	1.2	23.4	296	0.3
raw, chopped	1 cup	5963	0.07	0.09	0.67	0.18	19.6	0.00	80.4	90.5	1.1	22.8	299	0.3
Frozen														
boiled, drained, chopped	1 cup	8260	0.06	0.15	0.87	0.11	18.6	0.00	32.8	179.0	1.2	23.4	417	0.2
boiled, drained, chopped or diced	1/2 cup	4130	0.03	0.07	0.44	0.06	9.3	0.00	16.4	89.7	0.6	11.7	209	0.1
unprepared	10-oz pkg	17759	0.16	0.32	2.00	0.26	47.4	0.00	112.0	386.0	2.6	51.1	946	0.5
unprepared	3.3 oz	5878	0.05	0.11	0.66	0.09	15.7	0.00	36.9	128.0	0.9	16.9	313	0.2
KALE, SCOTCH														
boiled, drained, chopped	1 cup	2592	0.05	0.05	1.00	0.18	17.3	0.00	68.6	172.0	2.5	74.1	356	0.3
raw, chopped	1 cup	2077	0.05	0.04	0.87	0.15	18.8	0.00	87.1	137.0	2.0	59.0	302	0.3
KANPYO / dried gourd strips	1/2 cup	0	0.00	0.01	0.78	0.14	16.5	0.00	<0.1	75.6	1.4	33.8	427	1.6
KATSUO. See under TUNA.														
KATURAY / sesbania flower														
flowers, raw, whole	1 cup	0	0.02	0.02	0.09	na	20.4	0.00	14.6	3.8	0.2	2.4	37	na
flowers, raw, whole	1 medium	0	0.00	0.00	0.01	na	3.1	0.00	2.2	0.6	<0.1	0.4	5.5	na
flowers, steamed	1 cup	0	0.05	0.05	0.26	na	59.2	0.00	38.5	22.9	0.6	12.5	111	na
KELP. See under SEA VEGETABLE.														
KETA SALMON. See under SALMON.														
KETCHUP. See CATSUP.														
KIDNEY BEAN. See BEAN, KIDNEY.														
KING CRAB. See under CRAB.														
KING MACKEREL. See under MACKEREL.														
KING SALMON. See under SALMON.														
KIWI FRUIT / Chinese gooseberry														
Fresh														
raw, cut up	1 cup	310	0.04	0.09	0.89	0.16	67.3	0.00	173.0	46.0	0.7	53.1	588	0.3
raw, peeled	1 large	159	0.02	0.05	0.46	na	na	0.00	68.3	23.7	0.4	27.3	302	na
raw, peeled	1 medium	133	0.02	0.04	0.38	na	na	0.00	57.0	19.8	0.3	22.8	252	na
KOHLRABI / cabbage turnip														
boiled, drained, sliced	1 cup	58	0.07	0.03	0.64	0.25	20.0	0.00	89.1	41.3	0.7	31.4	561	0.5
raw, sliced	1 cup	49	0.07	0.03	0.54	0.20	21.7	0.00	83.7	32.4	0.5	25.6	473	<0.1
KUMQUAT, raw, trimmed	1 medium	57	0.02	0.02	0.10	0.01	3.0	0.00	7.1	8.4	<0.1	2.5	37	<0.1

L

Food Name	Serving Size	A I.U.	Thi mg	Rib mg	Nia mg	B$_6$ mg	Fol mcg	B$_{12}$ mcg	C mg	Calc mg	Iron mg	Mag mg	Pot mg	Zn mg
LAMB, AUSTRALIAN														
(NOTE: All USDA choice grade. TRIMMED = Lean; separable fat removed. UNTRIMMED = Separable fat not removed.)														
COMPOSITE CUTS														
Trimmed														
cooked	3 oz	na	0.11	0.31	4.90	0.34	na	2.60	na	13.6	1.7	20.4	270	4.4
raw	3 oz	na	0.13	0.25	4.80	0.33	na	2.40	na	10.2	1.4	18.7	272	3.6
Untrimmed														
cooked	3 oz	na	0.11	0.28	4.60	0.31	na	2.40	na	14.4	1.6	18.7	256	4.0

Food Name	Serving Size	A I.U.	Thi mg	Rib mg	Nia mg	B₆ mg	Fol mcg	B₁₂ mcg	C mg	Calc mg	Iron mg	Mag mg	Pot mg	Zn mg
raw	3 oz	na	0.11	0.22	4.20	0.29	na	2.10	na	11.1	1.2	17.0	241	3.1
LEG / CENTER SLICE														
Trimmed														
center slice, broiled	3 oz	na	0.12	0.36	4.90	0.39	na	2.70	na	11.1	2.1	22.1	301	4.4
center slice, raw	1 oz	na	0.04	0.09	1.60	0.12	na	0.85	na	2.6	0.6	7.1	97	1.0
Untrimmed														
center slice, broiled	3 oz	na	0.11	0.34	4.70	0.37	na	2.60	na	11.9	2.0	21.3	291	4.2
center slice, raw	3 oz	na	0.12	0.25	4.42	0.33	na	2.41	na	8.6	1.5	19.7	273	2.8
LEG / FORESHANK														
Trimmed														
braised	3 oz	na	0.08	0.24	4.6	0.22	na	2.70	na	11.9	1.6	18.7	217	6.7
raw	3 oz	na	0.09	0.20	4.9	0.25	na	2.30	na	9.3	1.3	17.0	251	5.2
Untrimmed														
braised	3 oz	na	0.07	0.22	4.3	0.21	na	2.50	na	13.6	1.5	17.9	207	5.9
raw	3 oz	na	0.08	0.19	4.5	0.22	na	2.10	na	10.2	1.2	16.1	230	4.6
LEG / SHANK														
Trimmed														
raw	3 oz	na	0.13	0.27	4.7	0.34	na	2.60	na	6.0	1.4	18.7	280	3.8
roasted	3 oz	na	0.12	0.36	4.9	0.39	na	2.70	na	6.8	1.8	21.3	280	4.1
Untrimmed														
raw	3 oz	na	0.12	0.25	4.3	0.31	na	2.30	na	7.7	1.3	17.0	256	3.4
roasted	3 oz	na	0.11	0.33	4.6	0.36	na	2.60	na	8.5	1.7	19.6	266	3.8
LEG / SIRLOIN														
Trimmed														
raw	3 oz	na	0.13	0.27	4.7	0.34	na	2.60	na	8.5	1.5	19.6	279	3.0
roasted	3 oz	na	0.12	0.36	4.9	0.39	na	2.70	na	11.1	1.9	21.3	270	4.0
Untrimmed														
raw	3 oz	na	0.11	0.23	4.00	0.29	na	2.20	na	10.2	1.3	17.0	237	2.5
roasted	3 oz	na	0.11	0.32	4.50	0.35	na	2.50	na	12.8	1.8	19.6	252	3.6
LEG /WHOLE														
Trimmed														
raw	3 oz	na	0.13	0.27	4.70	0.34	na	2.60	na	6.8	1.4	19.6	280	3.6
roasted	3 oz	na	0.12	0.36	4.90	0.39	na	2.70	na	7.7	1.8	21.3	277	4.1
Untrimmed														
raw	3 oz	na	0.12	0.24	4.20	0.30	na	2.30	na	8.5	1.3	17.0	251	3.2
roasted	3 oz	na	0.11	0.33	4.60	0.36	na	2.60	na	9.3	1.7	19.6	263	3.8
LOIN														
Trimmed														
broiled	3 oz	na	0.15	0.28	6.90	0.44	na	1.70	na	17.9	1.9	22.1	289	3.0
raw	3 oz	na	0.16	0.27	6.20	0.41	na	1.60	na	12.8	1.5	20.4	278	2.3
Untrimmed														
broiled	3 oz	na	0.15	0.27	6.70	0.42	na	1.70	na	17.9	1.8	21.3	281	2.9
raw	3 oz	na	0.14	0.25	5.70	0.38	na	1.50	na	12.8	1.4	18.7	257	2.1
RIB														
Trimmed														
raw	3 oz	na	0.15	0.23	5.40	0.37	na	1.50	na	8.5	1.4	18.7	259	2.6
roasted	3 oz	na	0.12	0.25	5.10	0.36	na	1.70	na	12.8	1.5	19.6	257	3.1
Untrimmed														
raw	3 oz	na	0.12	0.20	4.30	0.29	na	1.40	na	11.1	1.1	15.3	216	2.1
roasted	3 oz	na	0.11	0.23	4.70	0.33	na	1.60	na	14.4	1.4	17.9	240	2.8
SHOULDER / ARM														
Trimmed														
braised	3 oz	na	0.08	0.22	3.70	0.17	na	2.80	na	22.9	2.1	19.6	228	5.6
raw	3 oz	na	0.10	0.20	3.90	0.25	na	2.60	na	12.8	1.3	18.7	276	3.5

Food Name	Serving Size	A I.U.	Thi mg	Rib mg	Nia mg	B$_6$ mg	Fol mcg	B$_{12}$ mcg	C mg	Calc mg	Iron mg	Mag mg	Pot mg	Zn mg
Untrimmed, raw....................	3 oz	na	0.09	0.18	3.40	0.22	na	2.20	na	13.6	1.1	16.1	239	3.0
SHOULDER / BLADE														
Trimmed														
broiled............................	3 oz	na	0.09	0.25	4.00	0.18	na	3.00	na	23.8	1.4	17.9	268	5.4
raw	3 oz	na	0.10	0.20	3.90	0.25	na	2.60	na	16.1	1.2	17.0	253	4.4
Untrimmed														
broiled............................	3 oz	na	0.08	0.23	3.80	0.17	na	2.80	na	23.8	1.3	17.0	251	4.8
raw	3 oz	na	0.09	0.18	3.40	0.22	na	2.20	na	16.1	1.0	14.4	221	3.7
SHOULDER / WHOLE														
Trimmed														
cooked	3 oz	na	0.09	0.25	4.00	0.18	na	3.00	na	23.8	1.6	18.7	262	5.7
raw	3 oz	na	0.10	0.20	3.90	0.25	na	2.60	na	15.3	1.2	17.9	260	4.1
Untrimmed														
cooked	3 oz	na	0.08	0.23	3.80	0.17	na	2.80	na	23.8	1.5	17.9	245	5.0
raw	3 oz	na	0.09	0.18	3.40	0.22	na	2.20	na	15.3	1.1	15.3	227	3.5
SIRLOIN CHOP														
Trimmed														
broiled............................	3 oz	na	0.12	0.36	4.90	0.39	na	2.70	na	11.1	2.1	22.1	301	4.4
raw	1 oz	na	0.04	0.09	1.60	0.12	na	0.85	na	2.6	0.6	7.1	97	1.0
Untrimmed														
broiled............................	3 oz	na	0.11	0.33	4.60	0.36	na	2.60	na	11.9	2.0	21.3	286	4.1
raw	1 oz	na	0.04	0.08	1.40	0.10	na	0.77	na	3.1	0.5	6.2	87	0.9
LAMB, NEW ZEALAND														
COMPOSITE CUTS														
Trimmed														
cooked	3 oz	0	0.11	0.42	6.50	0.12	0.0	2.50	0.0	11.1	2.0	18.7	160	3.7
raw	1 oz	0	0.04	0.11	1.90	0.04	0.0	0.77	0.0	2.3	0.5	5.4	49	0.9
Untrimmed														
cooked	3 oz	0	0.09	0.35	6.20	0.09	0.9	2.30	0.0	12.8	1.8	16.1	137	3.1
raw	1 oz	0	0.04	0.09	1.90	0.03	0.3	0.69	0.0	3.7	0.4	4.3	39	0.7
LEG/FORESHANK														
Trimmed														
braised	3 oz	0	0.06	0.31	4.80	0.08	0.9	2.10	0.0	8.5	1.9	13.6	106	4.8
raw	1 oz	0	0.04	0.11	1.80	0.04	0.3	0.77	0.0	2.0	0.5	4.8	43	1.1
Untrimmed														
braised	3 oz	0	0.06	0.28	5.20	0.07	0.9	2.10	0.0	11.9	1.8	12.8	100	4.1
raw	1 oz	0	0.04	0.10	1.80	0.03	0.3	0.72	0.0	2.8	0.4	4.3	37	0.9
LEG/WHOLE														
Trimmed														
raw	1 oz	0	0.04	0.12	2.00	0.04	0.0	0.74	0.0	1.1	0.5	5.7	51	0.9
roasted	3 oz	0	0.10	0.42	6.40	0.12	0.0	2.20	0.0	6.0	1.9	17.9	156	3.4
Untrimmed														
raw	1 oz	0	0.04	0.11	1.90	0.04	0.3	0.70	0.0	2.0	0.5	5.1	45	0.8
roasted	3 oz	0	0.10	0.39	6.40	0.11	0.9	2.20	0.0	7.7	1.8	17.0	145	3.1
LOIN														
Trimmed														
broiled............................	3 oz	0	0.11	0.36	6.70	0.12	0.0	2.20	0.0	17.9	2.0	18.7	161	2.8
raw	1 oz	0	0.05	0.10	2.00	0.04	0.0	0.65	0.0	4.3	0.5	5.4	45	0.7
Untrimmed														
broiled............................	3 oz	0	0.10	0.31	6.70	0.09	0.9	2.10	0.0	19.6	1.7	16.1	135	2.3
raw	1 oz	0	0.04	0.08	1.90	0.03	0.3	0.59	0.0	4.8	0.4	4.3	34	0.5
RIB														
Trimmed														
raw	1 oz	0	0.04	0.09	1.70	0.03	0.0	0.70	0.0	3.1	0.5	4.8	44	0.8

Food Name	Serving Size	A I.U.	Thi mg	Rib mg	Nia mg	B_6 mg	Fol mcg	B_{12} mcg	C mg	Calc mg	Iron mg	Mag mg	Pot mg	Zn mg
roasted	3 oz	0	0.09	0.28	5.20	0.09	0.0	1.90	0.0	11.9	1.6	13.6	124	2.9
Untrimmed														
raw	1 oz	0	0.03	0.07	1.80	0.03	0.3	0.63	0.0	4.3	0.4	3.7	34	0.6
roasted	3 oz	0	0.08	0.23	5.80	0.07	0.9	2.00	0.0	16.1	1.5	11.9	105	2.2
SHOULDER / WHOLE														
Trimmed														
braised	3 oz	0	0.07	0.31	5.00	0.07	0.0	3.20	0.0	22.9	2.0	17.0	141	4.8
raw	1 oz	0	0.04	0.10	1.50	0.03	0.0	1.00	0.0	4.3	0.4	5.1	46	1.0
Untrimmed														
braised	3 oz	0	0.07	0.28	5.30	0.06	0.9	3.00	0.0	22.9	1.8	15.3	128	4.0
raw	1 lb	0	0.03	0.09	1.50	0.02	0.3	0.89	0.0	4.8	0.4	4.3	39	0.8
LAMB, U.S.														

(NOTE: All USDA choice grade. TRIMMED = Lean; separable fat removed. UNTRIMMED = Separable fat not removed.)

Food Name	Serving Size	A I.U.	Thi mg	Rib mg	Nia mg	B_6 mg	Fol mcg	B_{12} mcg	C mg	Calc mg	Iron mg	Mag mg	Pot mg	Zn mg
BRAIN														
braised	3 oz	0	0.09	0.20	2.10	0.09	4.3	7.90	10.2	10.2	1.4	11.9	174	1.2
pan-fried	3 oz	0	0.14	0.32	3.90	0.20	6.0	20.50	19.6	17.9	1.7	18.7	304	1.7
raw	4 oz	0	0.15	0.34	4.40	0.33	3.4	12.80	18.1	10.2	2.0	13.6	336	1.3
COMPOSITE CUTS														
Trimmed														
cooked	3 oz	0	0.09	0.24	5.40	0.14	19.6	2.20	0.0	12.8	1.7	22.1	292	4.5
raw	1 oz	0	0.04	0.07	1.70	0.05	6.5	0.74	0.0	2.8	0.5	7.4	79.4	1.2
Untrimmed														
cooked	3 oz	0	0.09	0.21	5.70	0.11	15.3	2.20	0.0	14.4	1.6	19.6	264	3.8
raw	1 oz	0	0.03	0.06	1.70	0.04	5.1	0.68	0.0	3.4	0.5	6.2	65	0.9
GROUND														
broiled	3 oz	0	0.09	0.21	5.70	0.12	16.1	2.20	0.0	18.7	1.5	20.4	288	4.0
raw	4 oz	0	0.12	0.24	6.70	0.15	20.3	2.60	0.0	18.1	1.8	23.7	251	3.9
HEART														
braised	3 oz	0	0.14	1.00	3.70	0.26	1.7	9.50	6.0	11.9	4.7	20.4	160	3.1
raw	4 oz	0	0.42	1.10	7.00	0.44	2.3	11.60	5.7	6.8	5.2	19.3	358	2.1
KIDNEYS														
braised	3 oz	387	0.30	1.80	5.10	0.10	68.8	67.10	10.2	15.3	10.5	17.0	151	3.2
raw	4 oz	358	0.70	2.50	8.50	0.25	31.8	59.40	12.5	14.7	7.2	19.3	314	2.5
LEG/FORESHANK														
Trimmed														
braised	3 oz	0	0.03	0.16	4.30	0.09	16.1	1.90	0.0	17.0	1.9	19.6	227	7.4
raw	1 oz	0	0.03	0.06	1.50	0.05	6.2	0.69	0.0	2.6	0.5	7.1	67	1.7
Untrimmed														
braised	3 oz	0	0.07	0.28	8.10	0.15	25.2	3.40	0.0	29.6	3.2	32.6	380	11.4
raw	1 oz	0	0.03	0.05	1.60	0.04	5.4	0.66	0.0	3.1	0.5	6.2	61	1.5
LEG/SHANK														
Trimmed														
raw	1 oz	0	0.04	0.07	1.80	0.05	6.5	0.75	0.0	1.7	0.5	7.7	82	1.1
roasted	3 oz	0	0.09	0.24	5.40	0.14	20.4	2.30	0.0	6.8	1.8	22.1	291	4.3
Untrimmed														
raw	1 oz	0	0.04	0.07	1.80	0.04	5.7	0.71	0.0	2.3	0.5	6.8	74	1.0
roasted	3 oz	0	0.09	0.23	5.60	0.14	18.7	2.30	0.0	8.5	1.7	21.3	277	4.0
LEG/SIRLOIN														
Trimmed														
raw	1 oz	0	0.04	0.07	1.80	0.05	6.8	0.78	0.0	2.0	0.5	7.7	81	1.1
roasted	3 oz	0	0.10	0.26	5.30	0.14	17.9	2.20	0.0	6.8	1.9	21.3	283	4.1
Untrimmed														
raw	1 oz	0	0.03	0.07	1.80	0.04	5.1	0.70	0.0	2.8	0.5	6.2	66	0.9
roasted	3 oz	0	0.09	0.24	5.60	0.12	14.4	2.10	0.0	9.3	1.7	18.7	256	3.5

Food Name	Serving Size	A I.U.	Thi mg	Rib mg	Nia mg	B$_6$ mg	Fol mcg	B$_{12}$ mcg	C mg	Calc mg	Iron mg	Mag mg	Pot mg	Zn mg
LEG/WHOLE														
Trimmed														
raw	1 oz	0	0.04	0.07	1.80	0.05	6.5	0.77	0.0	1.7	0.5	7.7	82	1.1
roasted	3 oz	0	0.09	0.25	5.40	0.14	19.6	2.20	0.0	6.8	1.8	22.1	287	4.2
Untrimmed														
raw	1 oz	0	0.04	0.07	1.80	0.04	5.4	0.71	0.0	2.6	0.5	6.5	71	0.9
roasted	3 oz	0	0.09	0.23	5.60	0.13	17.0	2.20	0.0	9.3	1.7	20.4	266	3.7
LEG AND SHOULDER														
Trimmed														
braised	3 oz	0	0.06	0.20	5.10	0.10	17.9	2.30	0.0	12.8	2.4	23.8	221	5.6
broiled	3 oz	0	0.09	0.26	5.60	0.12	19.6	2.60	0.0	11.1	2.0	26.4	285	4.9
raw	1 oz	0	0.04	0.07	1.70	0.05	6.5	0.77	0.0	2.6	0.5	7.4	81	1.2
LIVER														
braised	3 oz	21203	0.20	3.40	10.30	0.42	62.0	65.00	3.4	6.8	7.0	18.7	188	6.7
pan-fried	3 oz	22098	0.30	3.90	14.20	0.81	340.0	72.80	11.1	7.7	8.7	19.6	299	4.8
raw	4 oz	27910	0.39	4.10	18.30	1.00	261.0	102.00	4.5	7.9	8.4	21.5	355	5.3
LOIN														
Trimmed														
broiled	3 oz	0	0.09	0.24	5.80	0.14	20.4	2.10	0.0	16.1	1.7	23.8	320	3.5
raw	1 oz	0	0.04	0.07	1.80	0.05	6.8	0.63	0.0	3.4	0.5	7.7	78	0.9
roasted	3 oz	0	0.09	0.23	5.80	0.14	21.3	1.80	0.0	14.4	2.1	22.9	227	3.5
Untrimmed														
broiled	3 oz	0	0.09	0.21	6.00	0.11	15.3	2.10	0.0	17.0	1.5	20.4	278	3.0
raw	1 oz	0	0.03	0.06	1.80	0.04	4.8	0.58	0.0	4.3	0.5	6.0	61	0.7
roasted	3 oz	0	0.09	0.20	6.00	0.09	16.1	1.90	0.0	15.3	1.8	19.6	209	2.9
LUNGS														
braised	3 oz	90	0.03	0.12	2.10	0.05	6.8	2.10	23.8	10.2	3.9	9.3	108	1.6
raw	4 oz	101	0.05	0.27	4.70	0.13	13.6	4.50	35.2	11.3	7.3	15.9	270	2.0
PANCREAS														
braised	3 oz	0	0.02	0.18	2.20	0.04	11.1	4.70	17.0	10.2	1.8	16.1	247	2.3
raw	4 oz	0	0.03	0.28	4.20	0.08	14.7	6.80	20.4	9.1	2.6	23.8	476	2.2
RIB														
Trimmed														
broiled	3 oz	0	0.09	0.21	5.60	0.13	17.9	2.20	0.0	13.6	1.9	24.6	266	4.5
raw	1 oz	0	0.03	0.06	1.70	0.05	6.0	0.68	0.0	3.4	0.5	7.1	75	1.1
roasted	3 oz	0	0.08	0.20	5.20	0.13	18.7	1.80	0.0	17.9	1.5	19.6	268	3.8
Untrimmed														
broiled	3 oz	0	0.08	0.19	6.00	0.09	11.9	2.20	0.0	16.1	1.6	19.6	230	3.4
raw	1 oz	0	0.03	0.05	1.70	0.03	4.0	0.59	0.0	4.3	0.4	5.1	53.9	0.8
roasted	3 oz	0	0.08	0.18	5.70	0.09	12.8	1.90	0.0	18.7	1.4	17.0	230	3.0
SHOULDER / ARM														
Trimmed														
braised	3 oz	0	0.06	0.23	5.40	0.11	18.7	2.30	0.0	22.1	2.3	24.6	287	6.2
broiled	3 oz	0	0.09	0.25	5.80	0.12	19.6	2.50	0.0	14.4	2.0	25.5	289	4.9
raw	1 oz	0	0.03	0.07	1.70	0.04	6.8	0.76	0.0	3.4	0.5	7.1	81	1.2
roasted	3 oz	0	0.09	0.23	5.40	0.12	21.3	2.20	0.0	13.6	1.9	22.1	235	4.5
Untrimmed														
braised	3 oz	0	0.06	0.21	5.70	0.09	15.3	2.20	0.0	21.3	2.0	22.1	260	5.2
broiled	3 oz	0	0.09	0.23	6.00	0.10	15.3	2.40	0.0	15.3	1.8	22.1	263	4.2
raw	1 oz	0	0.03	0.06	1.70	0.04	5.4	0.69	0.0	4.0	0.4	6.0	68	0.9
roasted	3 oz	0	0.08	0.21	5.70	0.10	17.0	2.20	0.0	15.3	1.7	19.6	220	3.8
SHOULDER / BLADE														
Trimmed														
braised	3 oz	0	0.05	0.19	4.80	0.10	17.9	2.50	0.0	23.8	2.2	22.1	216	6.9

Food Name	Serving Size	A I.U.	Thi mg	Rib mg	Nia mg	B$_6$ mg	Fol mcg	B$_{12}$ mcg	C mg	Calc mg	Iron mg	Mag mg	Pot mg	Zn mg
broiled.	3 oz	0	0.09	0.22	5.20	0.14	17.9	2.40	0.0	20.4	1.5	22.1	313	5.5
raw	1 oz	0	0.03	0.06	1.50	0.05	6.5	0.80	0.0	4.5	0.5	6.8	76	1.4
roasted	3 oz	0	0.08	0.21	4.60	0.13	21.3	2.30	0.0	17.9	1.8	21.3	219	5.5
Untrimmed														
braised	3 oz	0	0.05	0.18	5.10	0.09	15.3	2.40	0.0	22.9	2.0	20.4	207	5.8
broiled.	3 oz	0	0.08	0.21	5.40	0.13	15.3	2.30	0.0	20.4	1.5	20.4	286	4.8
raw	1 oz	0	0.03	0.06	1.50	0.04	5.4	0.73	0.0	4.8	0.4	6.0	65	1.2
roasted	3 oz	0	0.08	0.20	5.00	0.09	17.9	2.30	0.0	17.9	1.6	18.7	209	4.7
SHOULDER / WHOLE														
Trimmed														
braised	3 oz	0	0.05	0.20	5.10	0.10	17.9	2.50	0.0	22.1	2.3	22.9	222	6.4
broiled.	3 oz	0	0.09	0.24	5.20	0.12	19.6	2.60	0.0	17.9	1.9	24.6	275	5.6
raw	1 oz	0	0.03	0.06	1.50	0.05	6.5	0.79	0.0	4.3	0.5	6.8	78	1.4
roasted	3 oz	0	0.08	0.22	4.90	0.13	21.3	2.30	0.0	16.1	1.8	21.3	225	5.1
Untrimmed														
braised	3 oz	0	0.06	0.19	5.40	0.09	14.4	2.40	0.0	21.3	2.0	20.4	211	5.4
broiled.	3 oz	0	0.08	0.22	5.50	0.10	16.1	2.50	0.0	17.9	1.7	22.1	256	4.9
raw	1 oz	0	0.03	0.06	1.60	0.04	5.4	0.72	0.0	4.5	0.4	6.0	65	1.1
roasted	3 oz	0	0.08	0.20	5.20	0.11	17.9	2.20	0.0	17.0	1.7	19.6	213	4.4
SPLEEN														
braised	3 oz	0	0.04	0.27	5.00	0.07	3.4	4.50	22.1	11.1	32.9	17.9	211	3.3
raw	4 oz	0	0.05	0.40	9.00	0.13	4.5	6.10	26.1	10.2	47.5	23.8	406	3.2
TONGUE														
braised	3 oz	0	0.07	0.36	3.10	0.14	2.5	5.40	6.0	8.5	2.2	13.6	134	2.5
raw	4 oz	0	0.17	0.43	5.30	0.20	4.5	8.20	6.8	10.2	3.0	23.8	291	2.6
LAMB'S QUARTERS														
fresh, boiled, drained, chopped	1 cup	17460	0.18	0.47	1.60	0.31	24.5	0.00	66.6	464.0	1.3	41.4	518	0.5
LARD														
. . . .	1 cup	0	0.00	0.00	0.00	0.00	0.0	0.00	0.0	0.1	0.0	<0.1	<1	0.2
. . . .	1 tbsp	0	0.00	0.00	0.00	0.00	0.0	0.00	0.0	<0.1	0.0	0	0	<0.1
LASAGNA/LASAGNA ENTRÉE														
(Budget Gourmet)														
w/Italian Sausage	1 entrée	2161	na	na	na	na	na	na	na	316.0	2.7	na	na	na
(Stouffer's)														
w/meat, sauce	1 pkg	0	na	na	na	na	na	na	na	637.0	na	na	na	na
w/meat, sauce	1 serving	0	na	na	na	na	na	na	na	230.0	na	na	na	na
LAVER. See under SEA VEGETABLE.														
LEEK														
Fresh														
boiled, drained, chopped	1/4 cup	12	0.01	0.01	0.05	0.03	6.3	0.00	1.1	7.8	0.3	3.6	23	<0.1
boiled, drained, whole.	1 medium	57	0.03	0.03	0.25	0.14	30.1	0.00	5.2	37.2	1.4	17.4	108	<0.1
raw, chopped	1 cup	85	0.05	0.03	0.36	0.21	57.0	0.00	10.7	52.5	1.9	24.9	160	0.1
raw, whole.	1 medium	85	0.05	0.03	0.36	0.21	57.0	0.00	10.7	52.5	1.9	24.9	160	0.1
Freeze-dried														
bulb/lower leaf portion	1/4 cup	2	0.01	0.00	0.03	0.01	2.9	0.00	0.9	2.9	<0.1	1.3	19	<0.1
bulb/lower leaf portion	1 tbsp	<1	0.00	0.00	0.01	0.00	0.7	0.00	0.2	0.7	<0.1	0.3	4.8	0.0
LEMON														
Fresh														
raw, sectioned, w/o peel	1 cup	61.5	0.09	0.04	0.21	0.17	22.5	0	112	55.1	1.3	17.0	293	0.13
raw, sliced, w/o peel, 1/8 of 2-1/8-inch														
diam lemon	1 wedge	2.0	0	0	0.01	0.01	0.74	0	3.7	1.8	0.04	0.56	9.7	0
raw, whole, w/o peel, 2-1/8-inch diam.	1 lemon	16.8	0.02	0.01	0.06	0.05	6.1	0	30.7	15.1	0.35	4.6	80.0	0.04
raw, w/peel, w/o seeds, 2-3/8-inch diam.	1 lemon	24.4	0.03	0.02	0.08	0.07	8.9	0	44.5	21.8	0.50	6.7	116	0.05

Food Name	Serving Size	A I.U.	Thi mg	Rib mg	Nia mg	B_6 mg	Fol mcg	B_{12} mcg	C mg	Calc mg	Iron mg	Mag mg	Pot mg	Zn mg
LEMON JUICE														
Canned or bottled														
....	1 cup	37	0.10	0.02	0.48	0.11	24.6	0.00	60.5	26.8	0.3	19.5	249	0.2
....	1 fl oz	5	0.01	0.00	0.06	0.01	3.1	0.00	7.6	3.4	<0.1	2.4	31	<0.1
....	1 tbsp	3	0.01	0.00	0.03	0.01	1.5	0.00	3.8	1.7	<0.1	1.2	16	<0.1
unsweetened, single strength...........	1 cup	32	0.14	0.03	0.33	0.15	23.2	0.00	76.9	19.5	0.3	19.5	217	0.1
unsweetened, single strength...........	1 fl oz	4	0.02	0.00	0.04	0.02	2.9	0.00	9.6	2.4	<0.1	2.4	27	<0.1
Fresh														
....	1 cup	49	0.07	0.02	0.24	0.12	31.5	0.00	112	17.1	<0.1	14.6	303	0.1
....	1 fl oz	6	0.01	0.00	0.03	0.02	3.9	0.00	14.0	2.1	<0.1	1.8	38	<0.1
juice of 1/8 of 2 1/8 inch-diam lemon	0.2 oz	9	0.01	0.01	0.05	0.02	6.1	0.00	21.6	3.3	<0.1	2.8	58	<0.1
juice of 2 1/8 inch-diam lemon	1.6 oz	1	0.00	0.00	0.01	0.00	0.8	0.00	2.7	0.4	0.0	0.4	7	0.0
LEMON PEEL														
raw, grated	1 tbsp	3	0.00	0.01	0.02	0.01	0.8	0.00	7.7	8.0	<0.1	0.9	10	<0.1
raw, grated	1 tsp	1	0.00	0.00	0.01	0.00	0.3	0.00	2.6	2.7	<0.1	0.3	3	<0.1
LEMONADE. See under FRUIT DRINK MIX.														
LEMONGRASS / citronella														
raw	1 cup	7	0.04	0.09	0.74	0.05	50.3	0.00	1.7	43.5	5.5	40.2	484	1.5
raw	1 tbsp	<1	0.00	0.01	0.05	0.00	3.6	0.00	0.1	3.1	0.4	2.9	35	0.1
LENTIL														
Dried														
mature seeds, boiled	1 cup	15.8	0.34	0.14	2.1	0.35	358	0	3.0	37.6	6.6	71.3	731	2.5
mature seeds, boiled	1 tbsp	0.98	0.02	0.01	0.13	0.02	22.2	0	0.19	2.3	0.41	4.4	45.4	0.16
mature seeds, raw	1 cup	74.9	0.91	0.47	5.0	1.0	831	0	11.9	97.9	17.3	205	1738	6.9
mature seeds, raw	1 tbsp	4.7	0.06	0.03	0.32	0.06	51.9	0	0.74	6.1	1.1	12.8	109	0.43
pink, raw	1 cup	111	0.98	0.20	2.9	0.77	392	0	3.3	78.7	14.5	138	1110	7.5
Sprouted, raw	1 cup	34.6	0.18	0.10	0.87	0.15	76.9	0	12.7	19.3	2.5	28.5	248	1.2
LETTUCE														
BIBB, BOSTON, OR BUTTERHEAD														
leaf, large	1 leaf	146	0.01	0.01	0.05	0.01	11.0	0	1.2	4.8	0.05	1.9	38.5	0.03
leaf, medium...........	1 leaf	72.8	0.01	0.01	0.02	0	5.5	0	0.60	2.4	0.02	0.97	19.3	0.01
leaf, small	1 leaf	48.5	0	0	0.02	0	3.7	0	0.40	1.6	0.02	0.65	12.8	0.01
shredded...........	1 cup	534	0.03	0.03	0.17	0.03	40.3	0	4.4	17.6	0.17	7.2	141	0.09
whole, approx 5-inch diam	1 head	1581	0.10	0.10	0.49	0.08	119	0	13.0	52.2	0.49	21.2	419	0.28
COS														
inner leaf, whole...........	1 med leaf	260	0.01	0.01	0.05	0.01	13.6	0	2.4	3.6	0.11	0.60	29.0	0.03
shredded...........	1/2 cup	728	0.03	0.03	0.14	0.01	38.0	0	6.7	10.1	0.31	1.7	81.2	0.07
ICEBERG														
leaf, large	1 leaf	49.5	0.01	0.01	0.03	0.01	8.4	0	0.58	2.9	0.08	1.4	23.7	0.03
leaf, medium...........	1 leaf	26.4	0	0	0.02	0	4.5	0	0.31	1.5	0.04	0.72	12.6	0.02
leaf, small	1 leaf	16.5	0	0	0.01	0	2.8	0	0.20	0.95	0.03	0.45	7.9	0.01
shredded or chopped	1 cup	182	0.03	0.02	0.10	0.02	30.8	0	2.1	10.4	0.28	5.0	86.9	0.12
whole, approx 6-inch diam	1 head	1779	0.25	0.16	1.0	0.22	302	0	21.0	102	2.7	48.5	852	1.2
LOOSELEAF														
leaf, medium...........	1 leaf	190	0.01	0.01	0.04	0.01	5.0	0	1.8	6.8	0.14	1.1	26.4	0.03
shredded...........	1/2 cup	532	0.01	0.02	0.11	0.02	13.9	0	5.0	19.0	0.39	3.1	73.9	0.08
ROMAINE														
inner leaf, whole...........	1 med leaf	260	0.01	0.01	0.05	0.01	13.6	0	2.4	3.6	0.11	0.60	29.0	0.03
shredded...........	1/2 cup	728	0.03	0.03	0.14	0.01	38.0	0	6.7	10.1	0.31	1.7	81.2	0.07
LIMA BEAN. See BEAN, LIMA.														
LIME														
fresh, raw, whole, approx 2-inch dia	1 lime	6.7	0.02	0.01	0.13	0.03	5.5	0	19.5	22.1	0.40	4.0	68.3	0.07
LIME JUICE														
Canned or bottled														
unsweetened	1 cup	39.4	0.08	0.01	0.40	0.07	19.4	0	15.7	29.5	0.57	17.2	185	0.15

Food Name	Serving Size	A I.U.	Thi mg	Rib mg	Nia mg	B_6 mg	Fol mcg	B_{12} mcg	C mg	Calc mg	Iron mg	Mag mg	Pot mg	Zn mg
unsweetened	1 fl oz	4.9	0.01	0	0.05	0.01	2.4	0	2.0	3.7	0.07	2.2	23.1	0.02
Fresh														
	1 cup	24.6	0.05	0.03	0.25	0.11	20.2	0	72.1	22.1	0.07	14.8	268	0.15
	1 fl oz	3.1	0.01	0	0.03	0.01	2.5	0	9.0	2.8	0.01	1.8	33.6	0.02
juice of 2 1/8 inch-diam lime	1.3 oz	3.8	0.01	0	0.04	0.02	3.1	0	11.1	3.4	0.01	2.3	41.4	0.02
juice of 1/8 of 2 1/8 inch-diam lime	0.2 oz	0.50	0	0	0.01	0	0.41	0	1.5	0.45	0	0.30	5.5	0
LING														
baked, broiled, grilled, or microwaved	3 oz	97.8	0.11	0.20	2.4	0.30	6.8	0.55	0	37.4	0.71	68.8	413	0.85
raw	3 oz	85.0	0.09	0.16	2.0	0.26	6.0	0.48	0	28.9	0.55	53.5	322	0.66
LINGCOD														
baked, broiled, grilled, or microwaved	3 oz	49.3	0.03	0.12	2.0	0.29	8.5	3.5	0	15.3	0.35	28.1	476	0.49
raw	3 oz	42.5	0.03	0.10	1.6	0.26	7.7	3.1	0	11.9	0.27	22.1	371	0.38
LIQUEUR														
COFFEE														
w/cream, 34 proof	1 fl oz	54.1	0.0	0.02	0.02	0.01	0.0	0.04	0.0	5.0	0.04	0.62	10.0	0.05
53 proof	1 fl oz	0.0	0	0.0	0.05	0.0	0	0.0	0	0.35	0.02	1.0	10.4	0.01
63 proof	1 fl oz	0.0	0	0.0	0.05	0.0	0	0.0	0	0.35	0.02	1.0	10.4	0.01
CRÈME DE MENTHE, 72 proof	1 fl oz	0.0	0	0.0	0.0	0.0	0	0.0	0	0.0	0.02	0.0	0	0.01
LIQUOR. See individual listings.														
LITCHI / lychee														
dried	1 medium	0	0	0.01	0.08	0	0.30	0	4.6	0.82	0.04	1.1	27.8	0.01
raw	1 cup	0	0.02	0.12	1.1	0.19	26.6	0	136	9.5	0.59	19.0	325	0.13
raw, trimmed, approx 0.6 oz	1 medium	0	0	0.01	0.06	0.01	1.3	0	6.9	0.48	0.03	0.96	16.4	0.01
LIVER. See under individual meat listings. Also see PÂTÉ, CANNED.														
LIVERWURST. See under LUNCHEON MEAT.														
LOBSTER														
NORTHERN														
boiled, poached, or steamed	1 cup	126	0.01	0.10	1.6	0.11	16.1	4.5	0	88.5	0.57	50.8	510	4.2
boiled, poached or steamed	3 oz	74.0	0.01	0.06	0.91	0.07	9.4	2.6	0	51.9	0.33	29.8	299	2.5
raw	3 oz	60.4	0.01	0.04	1.2	0.05	7.7	0.79	0	40.8	0.26	22.9	234	2.6
SPINY, MIXED SPECIES														
boiled, poached or steamed	3 oz	17.0	0.01	0.05	4.2	0.15	0.85	3.4	1.8	53.5	1.2	43.4	177	6.2
raw	3 oz	14.4	0.01	0.04	3.6	0.13	0.51	3.0	1.7	41.6	1.0	34.0	153	4.8
LOGANBERRY, frozen	1 cup	51.5	0.07	0.05	1.2	0.10	37.8	0	22.5	38.2	0.94	30.9	213	0.50
LONGAN / dragon's eye														
raw, trimmed	1 fruit	na	0	0	0.01	na	na	0	2.7	0.03	0	0.32	8.5	0
LOOFAH GOURD. See GOURD, DISHCLOTH.														
LOQUAT / Japanese medlar														
raw, cubed	1 cup	2277	0.03	0.04	0.27	0.15	20.9	0	1.5	23.8	0.42	19.4	396	0.08
raw, whole	1 medium	244	0	0	0.03	0.02	2.2	0	0.16	2.6	0.05	2.1	42.6	0.01
LOTTE. See MONKFISH.														
LOTUS ROOT														
boiled, drained, sliced	1/2 cup	0	0.08	0.01	0.18	0.13	4.7	0	16.4	15.6	0.54	13.2	218	0.20
raw, whole, 9.5-inch long	1 root	0	0.18	0.25	0.46	0.30	14.6	0	50.6	51.8	1.3	26.4	639	0.45
LOTUS SEED														
dried	1 cup	16.0	0.20	0.05	0.51	0.20	33.2	0	0	52.2	1.1	67.2	438	0.34
dried, whole, approx 42 kernels	1 oz	14.2	0.18	0.04	0.45	0.18	29.4	0	0	46.2	1.0	59.5	388	0.30
raw	1 oz	3.7	0.05	0.01	0.12	0.05	7.9	0	0	12.5	0.27	15.9	104	0.08
LOX. See under SALMON.														
LUNCHEON MEAT														
BEEF														
(Carl Budding)														
smoked, sliced	1 pkg	na	0.06	0.17	2.70	na	na	na	na	9.9	1.6	na	239	na
smoked, sliced	2 oz	na	0.05	0.14	2.20	na	na	na	na	7.9	1.3	na	191	na

Food Name	Serving Size	A I.U.	Thi mg	Rib mg	Nia mg	B$_6$ mg	Fol mcg	B$_{12}$ mcg	C mg	Calc mg	Iron mg	Mag mg	Pot mg	Zn mg
BOLOGNA														
beef	1 oz	0	0.01	0.03	0.68	0.04	1.4	0.40	0.0	3.4	0.5	3.4	45	0.6
beef, 4-inch diam, 1/8-inch slices	1 slice	0	0.01	0.03	0.55	0.04	1.1	0.33	0.0	2.8	0.4	2.8	36	0.5
beef, Lebanon	1 oz	0	0.02	0.05	1.20	0.07	0.9	0.72	0.0	3.7	0.7	4.5	85	1.1
beef and pork	1 oz	0	0.05	0.04	0.73	0.05	1.4	0.38	0.0	3.4	0.4	3.1	51	0.6
beef and pork, 4-inch diam, 1/8-inch slices	1 slice	0	0.04	0.03	0.59	0.04	1.1	0.31	0.0	2.8	0.4	2.5	41	0.5
pork	1 oz	0	0.15	0.05	1.10	0.08	1.4	0.26	0.0	3.1	0.2	4.0	80	0.6
pork, 4-inch diam, 1/8inch slices	1 slice	0	0.12	0.04	0.90	0.06	1.1	0.21	0.0	2.5	0.2	3.2	65	0.5
pork and beef, Lebanon, 4-inch diam, 1/8-inch slices	1 slice	0	0.01	0.04	1.00	0.06	0.7	0.59	0.0	3.0	0.6	3.7	69	0.9
turkey	1 oz	0	0.02	0.05	1.00	0.06	2.0	0.08	0.0	23.8	0.4	4.0	56	0.5
(Louis Rich) turkey	1 serving	0	na	na	na	na	na	na	0.0	34.7	0.5	6.2	43	0.5
(Oscar Mayer)														
beef	1 slice	0	0.01	0.03	0.68	0.05	3.6	0.40	0.0	3.4	0.4	3.9	47	0.6
beef, light	1 slice	0	na	na	na	na	na	na	0.0	3.6	0.3	3.9	44	0.5
chicken, pork, and beef	1 slice	0	na	na	na	na	na	na	0.0	19.3	0.5	5.9	43.1	0.40
fat-free	1 slice	0	na	na	na	na	na	na	0.0	4.2	0.3	6.2	43.7	0.32
pork, chicken, and beef, light	1 slice	0	na	na	na	na	na	na	0.0	14.0	0.4	5.6	45.6	0.45
Wisconsin made ring	1 slice	0	0.16	0.08	1.50	0.08	na	0.71	0.0	8.4	0.7	8.4	77.8	1.0
CHICKEN BREAST														
(Carl Budding)														
smoked, w/dark meat, sliced	1 pkg	na	0.05	0.18	4.80	na	na	na	na	88.0	1.1	na	182	na
smoked, w/dark meat, sliced	2 oz	na	0.04	0.14	3.80	na	na	na	na	70.3	0.9	na	145	na
(Louis Rich)														
baked, 'Classic Baked Grill'	1 slice	0	na	na	na	na	na	na	0.0	1.8	0.3	7.0	64	0.2
roasted, 'Cold Cuts'	1 slice	0	na	na	na	na	na	na	0.0	4.8	0.4	6.7	85	0.3
roasted, deluxe, 'Cold Cuts'	1 slice	0	na	na	na	na	na	na	0.0	2.0	0.3	6.7	74	0.2
(Oscar Mayer)														
honey-glazed	1 slice	0	na	na	na	na	na	na	0.0	1.3	0.2	4.7	43	<0.1
roasted	1 slice	0	na	na	na	na	na	na	0.0	1.6	0.2	4.7	41	<0.1
CORNED BEEF LOAF														
(Carl Budding)														
chopped, pressed	1 pkg	na	0.06	0.17	3.00	na	na	na	na	12.1	1.7	na	250	na
chopped, pressed	2 oz	na	0.05	0.14	2.40	na	na	na	na	9.6	1.4	na	200	na
HAM														
(Carl Budding)														
smoked, sliced	1 pkg	na	0.53	0.25	3.70	na	na	na	na	11.4	1.4	na	241	na
smoked, sliced	2 oz	na	0.42	0.20	2.90	na	na	na	na	9.1	1.2	na	193	na
(Hormel) 'Cure 81'	1 serving	0	na	na	na	na	na	na	1.3	3.3	0.7	16.5	268	1.7
(Louis Rich) turkey, 10% water added	1 serving	0	na	na	na	na	na	na	0.0	1.4	0.4	6.2	81	0.7
(Oscar Mayer)														
chopped, w/natural juice	1 serviing	0	na	na	na	na	na	na	0.0	2.5	0.4	6.4	73	0.6
smoked, 40% ham/water product	1 slice	0	na	na	na	na	na	na	0.0	1.8	0.2	4.3	37	0.3
smoked, 40% ham/water product	1 serving	0	na	na	na	na	na	na	0.0	5.2	0.4	12.7	110	0.7
water added, boiled	1 serving	0	na	na	na	na	na	na	0.0	6.3	0.9	19.5	178	1.2
water added, boiled	1 slice	0	na	na	na	na	na	na	0.0	2.1	0.3	6.5	59	0.4
water added, baked, 96% fat free	1 serving	0	na	na	na	na	na	na	0.0	6.3	0.8	19.5	169	1.1
water added, baked, 96% fat free	1 slice	0	na	na	na	na	na	na	0.0	2.1	0.3	6.5	56	0.4
water added, smoked, cooked	1 serving	0	na	na	na	na	na	na	0.0	6.3	0.8	19.5	169	1.1
water added, smoked, cooked	1 slice	0	na	na	na	na	na	na	0.0	2.1	0.3	6.5	56	0.4
HEAD CHEESE (Oscar Mayer)	1 serving	28	0.01	0.05	0.27	0.04	0.3	0.27	0.0	5.9	0.5	3.1	8	0.3
HAM AND CHEESE LOAF (Oscar Mayer)	1 serving	31	0.16	0.05	0.97	0.07	0.8	0.21	0.0	18.8	0.2	5.3	74	0.5
HONEY LOAF (Oscar Mayer)	1 serving	0	0.19	0.08	1.00	0.11	2.2	0.26	0.0	6.2	0.4	5.9	101	0.7

Food Name	Serving Size	A I.U.	Thi mg	Rib mg	Nia mg	B_6 mg	Fol mcg	B_{12} mcg	C mg	Calc mg	Iron mg	Mag mg	Pot mg	Zn mg
LIVER CHEESE														
(Oscar Mayer) pork fat wrapped	1 serving	8590	0.08	0.84	4.60	0.17	42.9	9.20	1.1	3.4	4.5	5.3	82	1.5
LIVERWURST														
(Oscar Mayer)														
Braunschweiger, sliced.	1 serving	4404	0.06	0.45	2.60	0.09	13.2	5.30	2.5	2.5	2.7	3.9	57	0.9
Braunschweiger, tube.	1 serving	9335	0.13	0.87	4.60	0.19	34.2	10.4	5.0	5.0	5.5	6.7	103	1.8
LOAF														
(Hormel)														
pork w/chicken, light, 'Spam'.	2 oz	0	na	na	na	na	na	na	21.6	21.6	0.8	10.1	258	1.2
pork w/ham, 'Spam'	2 oz	0	na	na	na	na	na	na	0.5	8.0	0.5	7.7	128	1.0
OLD FASHIONED LOAF (Oscar Mayer)	1 serving	0	na	na	na	na	na	na	0.0	31.6	0.4	6.4	82	0.5
OLIVE LOAF														
(Oscar Mayer) chicken, pork, turkey	1 serving	0	na	na	na	na	na	na	0.0	31.1	0.5	7.6	52	0.3
PASTRAMI														
(Carl Budding)														
beef, smoked, chopped, pressed	1 pkg	na	0.06	0.16	2.90	na	na	na	na	12.1	1.7	na	259	na
beef, smoked, chopped, pressed	2 oz	na	0.05	0.13	2.30	na	na	na	na	9.6	1.4	na	207	na
PICKLE AND PIMIENTO LOAF														
(Oscar Mayer)														
. . . .	1 slice													
w/chicken	1 serving	0	na	na	na	na	na	na	0.0	30.8	0.6	8.1	49	0.3
SALAMI														
(Louis Rich)														
cotto, turkey	1 serving	na	na	na	na	na	na	na	0.0	8.7	0.5	5.9	62	0.7
turkey	1 serving	0	na	na	na	na	na	na	0.0	11.2	0.4	6.2	61	0.7
(Oscar Mayer)														
beer	1 slice	0	na	na	na	na	na	na	0.0	2.1	0.3	4.1	49	0.5
cotto, beef.	1 slice	na	na	na	na	na	na	na	0.0	1.6	0.6	3.9	48	0.5
cotto, beef, pork, and chicken.	1 slice	0	na	na	na	na	na	na	0.0	17.3	0.7	6.7	50	0.5
Genoa.	1 slice	0	0.06	0.03	0.38	0.03	na	0.12	0.0	1.8	0.2	2.1	30	0.3
hard	1 slice	na	0.05	0.02	0.45	0.04	0.3	0.17	0.0	1.1	0.2	1.9	32	0.3
SPICE LOAF (Oscar Mayer)	1 serving	0	na	na	na	na	na	na	0.0	30.5	0.4	6.7	76	0.6
TURKEY BREAST														
(Carl Budding)														
and dark meat, smoked, sliced.	1 pkg	na	0.13	0.22	4.20	na	na	na	na	42.6	1.3	na	234	na
and dark meat, smoked, sliced.	2 oz	na	0.10	0.18	3.30	na	na	na	na	34.0	1.0	na	187	na
(Louis Rich)														
and white meat, roasted	1 serving	0	na	na	na	na	na	na	0.0	1.7	0.3	6.2	62	0.3
and white meat, smoked.	1 serving	0	na	na	na	na	na	na	0.0	2.5	0.2	9.8	73	0.3
honey-roasted, fat-free	1 serving	0	na	na	na	na	na	na	0.0	8.4	0.6	15.7	147	0.6
roasted, fat-free	1 slice	0	na	na	na	na	na	na	0.0	3.1	0.3	7.6	57	0.2
roasted, fat-free	1 serving	0	na	na	na	na	na	na	0.0	9.5	0.6	16.2	150	0.5
smoked, 'Carving Board'.	1 slice	0	na	na	na	na	na	na	0.0	3.3	0.3	6.8	69	0.2
smoked, 'Carving Board'.	1 serving	0	na	na	na	na	na	na	0.0	6.8	0.7	13.9	140	0.4
smoked, fat-free	1 serving	0	na	na	na	na	na	na	0.0	9.0	0.6	15.1	161	0.5
(Oscar Mayer)														
smoked	1 serving	0	na	na	na	na	na	na	0.0	5.2	0.4	15.6	113	0.4
smoked.	1 slice	0	na	na	na	na	na	na	0.0	1.3	0.1	3.9	28	0.1
TURKEY HAM. See under LUNCHEON MEAT, HAM.														
LUPIN														
mature seeds, boiled	1 cup	11.6	0.22	0.09	0.82	0.02	98.4	0	1.8	84.7	2.0	89.6	407	2.3
mature seeds, raw	1 cup	41.4	1.2	0.40	3.9	0.64	639	0	8.6	317	7.8	356	1823	8.6

LYCHEE. See LITCHI.

M

Food Name	Serving Size	A I.U.	Thi mg	Rib mg	Nia mg	B$_6$ mg	Fol mcg	B$_{12}$ mcg	C mg	Calc mg	Iron mg	Mag mg	Pot mg	Zn mg
MACADAMIA NUT / bush nut														
dried, whole, 10–12 kernels	1 oz	0	0.34	0.05	0.70	0.08	3.1	0.00	0.3	24.1	1.0	36.9	104	0.4
dried, whole or halves	1 cup	0	1.60	0.22	3.30	0.37	14.7	0.00	1.6	114	4.9	174.0	493	1.7
dry-roasted, salted, whole, 10-12 kernels	1 oz	0	0.20	0.03	0.65	0.10	2.8	0.00	0.2	19.8	0.8	33.5	103	0.4
dry-roasted, salted, whole or halves	1 cup	0	0.95	0.12	3.00	0.48	13.4	0.00	0.9	93.8	3.6	158.0	486	1.7
dry-roasted, unsalted, whole, 10-12 kernels	1 oz	0	0.20	0.03	0.65	0.10	2.8	0.00	0.2	19.8	0.8	33.5	103	0.4
dry-roasted, unsalted, whole or halves	1 cup	0	0.95	0.12	3.00	0.48	13.4	0.00	0.9	93.8	3.6	158.0	486	1.7
MACARONI. See under PASTA.														
MACARONI DISH/ENTRÉE. See under PASTA DISH ENTRÉE.														
MACE														
ground	1 tbsp	42	0.02	0.02	0.07	0.02	4.0	0.00	1.1	13.4	0.7	8.6	25	0.1
ground	1 tsp	14	0.01	0.01	0.02	0.01	1.3	0.00	0.4	4.3	0.2	2.8	8	<0.1
MACKEREL														
ATLANTIC														
baked, broiled, grilled, or microwaved	3 oz	153	0.14	0.35	5.80	0.39	1.3	16.10	0.3	12.8	1.3	82.5	341	0.8
raw	3 oz	140	0.15	0.27	7.70	0.34	1.1	7.40	0.3	10.2	1.4	64.6	267	0.5
JACK, mixed species														
Canned, drained	1 cup	825	0.08	0.40	11.70	0.40	9.5	13.20	1.7	458	3.9	70.3	369	1.9
Fresh														
baked, broiled, grilled, or microwaved	3 oz	40	0.12	0.46	9.10	0.32	1.7	3.60	1.8	24.6	1.3	30.6	443	0.7
raw	3 oz	37	0.09	0.36	7.10	0.28	1.7	3.70	1.7	19.6	1.0	23.8	345	0.6
KING														
baked, broiled, grilled, or microwaved	3 oz	713	0.10	0.49	8.90	0.43	7.7	15.30	1.4	34.0	1.9	34.9	474	0.6
raw	3 oz	618	0.09	0.41	7.30	0.38	6.5	13.30	1.4	26.4	1.5	27.2	370	0.5
PACIFIC, mixed species														
baked, broiled, grilled, or microwaved	3 oz	40	0.12	0.46	9.10	0.32	1.7	3.60	1.8	24.6	1.3	30.6	443	0.7
raw	3 oz	37	0.09	0.36	7.10	0.28	1.7	3.70	1.7	19.6	1.0	23.8	345	0.6
SPANISH														
baked, broiled, grilled, or microwaved	3 oz	93	0.11	0.18	4.30	0.39	1.0	6.00	1.4	11.1	0.6	32.3	471	0.5
raw	3 oz	85	0.11	0.14	2.00	0.34	0.9	2.00	1.4	9.3	0.4	28.1	379	0.4
MAHI MAHI / dolphin fish														
baked, broiled, grilled, or microwaved	3 oz	177	0.02	0.07	6.30	0.39	5.1	0.59	0.0	16.1	1.2	32.3	453	0.5
raw	3 oz	153	0.02	0.06	5.20	0.34	4.3	0.51	0.0	12.8	0.9	25.5	354	0.4
MALABAR SPINACH. See SPINACH, MALABAR.														
MALABAR LIQUOR. See under BEER AND MALT LIQUOR.														
MALT SYRUP. See under SYRUP.														
MALTED MILK FLAVOR DRINK MIX														
CHOCOLATE FLAVOR														
w/added nutrients, powder, mix only	1 cup	10216	2.40	3.20	39.70	3.40	72.6	0.16	117.0	346	13.6	74.9	931	0.8
w/added nutrients, powder, prepared w/milk	8 fl oz	3058	0.73	1.30	10.90	1.00	31.8	0.88	33.9	384	3.8	53.0	620	1.2
w/o added nutrients, powder, mix only	1 envelope	19	0.04	0.04	0.42	0.03	4.2	0.04	0.3	12.6	0.5	14.7	130	0.2
w/o added nutrients, powder, prepared w/milk	8 fl oz	326	0.13	0.44	0.63	0.14	16.4	0.93	2.6	305	0.6	47.7	498	1.1
NATURAL FLAVOR														
w/added nutrients, powder, prepared	8 fl oz	2531	0.71	1.10	10.40	0.87	21.7	1.00	29.4	371	3.6	47.7	572	1.1
w/o added nutrients, powder, prepared	8 fl oz	368	0.20	0.59	1.30	0.19	21.7	1.00	2.9	355	0.3	53.0	530	1.1
MAMMY APPLE														
raw, trimmed, whole, approx 3.1 lb	1 medium	1946	0.17	0.34	3.40	0.85	118.0	0.00	118.0	93.1	5.9	135.0	398	0.9

Food Name	Serving Size	A I.U.	Thi mg	Rib mg	Nia mg	B_6 mg	Fol mcg	B_{12} mcg	C mg	Calc mg	Iron mg	Mag mg	Pot mg	Zn mg
MANDARIN ORANGE. See also TANGERINE.														
Canned														
in juice	1 cup	2121	0.20	0.07	1.10	0.11	11.5	0.00	85.2	27.4	0.7	27.4	331	1.3
in light syrup	1 cup	2117	0.13	0.11	1.10	0.11	11.6	0.00	49.9	17.6	0.9	20.2	197	0.6
MANGO														
raw, sliced	1 cup	6425	0.10	0.09	0.96	0.22	23.1	0.00	45.7	16.5	0.2	14.8	257	<0.1
raw, trimmed, whole, medium, approx 10.6 oz	1 mango	8061	0.12	0.12	1.20	0.28	29.0	0.00	57.3	20.7	0.3	18.6	323	<0.1
MANGOSTEEN														
Canned														
in syrup	1 cup	na	0.12	0.12	0.62	0.04	67.0	0.00	6.3	25.9	0.7	28.1	104	0.5
in syrup, drained	1 cup	na	0.11	0.11	0.56	0.04	60.8	0.00	5.7	23.5	0.6	25.5	94	0.4
MANIOC. See CASSAVA.														
MAPLE SYRUP. See under SYRUP.														
MARGARINE														
coconut, hydrogenated and regular, w/safflower and hydrogenated palm	1 stick	4050	0.01	0.04	0.03	0.01	1.3	0.11	0.2	33.9	0.0	2.9	48	na
coconut, hydrogenated and regular, w/safflower and hydrogenated palm	1 tsp	168	0.00	0.00	0.00	0.00	<0.1	0.00	<0.1	1.4	0.0	0.1	2.0	na
corn, hydrogenated	1 stick	4050	0.01	0.04	0.03	0.01	1.3	0.11	0.2	33.9	0.0	2.9	48	na
corn, hydrogenated	1 tsp	168	0.00	0.00	0.00	0.00	<0.1	0.00	<0.1	1.4	0.0	0.1	2	na
corn, hydrogenated and regular	1 stick	4050	0.01	0.04	0.03	0.01	1.3	0.11	0.2	33.9	0.0	2.9	48	0.0
corn, hydrogenated and regular	1 tsp	168	0.00	0.00	0.00	0.00	<0.1	0.00	<0.1	1.4	0.0	0.1	2	0.0
corn, hydrogenated and regular, soft	1 cup	8106	0.02	0.07	0.05	0.02	2.4	0.19	0.3	60.2	0.0	5.2	86	0.0
corn, hydrogenated and regular, soft	1 tsp	168	0.00	0.00	0.00	0.00	<0.1	0.00	<0.1	1.2	0.0	0.1	2	0.0
corn, w/hydrogenated soybean and cottonseed	1 stick	4050	0.01	0.04	0.03	0.01	1.3	0.11	0.2	33.9	0.0	2.9	48	0.0
corn, w/hydrogenated soybean and cottonseed	1 tsp	168	0.00	0.00	0.00	0.00	<0.1	0.00	<0.1	1.4	0.0	0.1	2	0.0
corn, w/hydrogenated soybean and cottonseed, unsalted	1 stick	4050	0.01	0.02	0.02	0.01	0.8	0.06	0.1	19.7	0.0	1.7	28	0.0
corn, w/ hydrogenated soybean and cottonseed, unsalted	1 tsp	168	0.00	0.00	0.00	0.00	<0.1	0.00	0.0	0.82	0.0	<0.1	1	0.0
lard, hydrogenated	1 stick	0	0.00	0.00	0.00	0.00	0.0	0.00	0.0	0	0.0	0.0	48	0.0
lard, hydrogenated	1 tsp	0	0.00	0.00	0.00	0.00	0.0	0.00	0.0	0	0.0	0.0	2	0.0
safflower, w/hydrogenated cottonseed and peanut, soft	1 cup	8106	0.02	0.07	0.05	0.02	2.4	0.19	0.3	60.2	0.0	5.2	86	0.0
safflower, w/hydrogenated cottonseed and peanut, soft	1 tsp	168	0.00	0.00	0.00	0.00	<0.1	0.00	<0.1	1.2	0.0	0.1	2	0.0
safflower, w/hydrogenated soybean	1 stick	4050	0.01	0.04	0.03	0.01	1.3	0.11	0.2	33.9	0.0	2.9	48	0.0
safflower, w/hydrogenated soybean	1 tsp	168	0.00	0.00	0.00	0.00	<0.1	0.00	<0.1	1.4	0.0	0.1	2	0.0
safflower, w/hydrogenated soybean and cottonseed	1 stick	4050	0.01	0.04	0.03	0.01	1.3	0.11	0.2	33.9	0.0	2.9	48	0.0
safflower, w/hydrogenated soybean and cottonseed	1 tsp	168	0.00	0.00	0.00	0.00	<0.1	0.00	<0.1	1.4	0.0	0.1	2	0.0
soybean, hydrogenated	1 stick	4035	0.01	0.04	0.03	0.01	1.3	0.11	0.2	33.8	0.0	2.9	48	0.0
soybean, hydrogenated	1 tsp	168	0.00	0.00	0.00	0.00	<0.1	0.00	<0.1	1.4	0.0	0.1	2	0.0
soybean, hydrogenated and regular	1 stick	4050	0.01	0.04	0.03	0.01	1.3	0.11	0.2	33.9	0.0	2.9	48	na
soybean, hydrogenated and regular	1 tsp	168	0.00	0.00	0.00	0.00	<0.1	0.00	<0.1	1.4	0.0	0.1	2	na
soybean, hydrogenated and regular, and cottonseed, liquid	1 cup	8106	0.05	0.18	0.11	0.04	6.0	0.48	0.8	150	0.0	13.1	214	0.0
soybean hydrogenated and regular, and cottonseed, liquid	1 tsp	168	0.00	0.00	0.00	0.00	0.1	0.01	<0.1	3.1	0.0	0.3	4	0.0

Food Name	Serving Size	A I.U.	Thi mg	Rib mg	Nia mg	B6 mg	Fol mcg	B12 mcg	C mg	Calc mg	Iron mg	Mag mg	Pot mg	Zn mg
soybean, hydrogenated and regular, soft, salted	1 cup	8106	0.02	0.07	0.05	0.02	2.4	0.19	0.3	60.2	0.0	5.2	86	0.0
soybean, hydrogenated and regular, soft, salted	1 tsp	168	0.00	0.00	0.00	0.00	<0.1	0.00	<0.1	1.2	0.0	0.1	2	0.0
soybean, hydrogenated and regular, soft, unsalted	1 cup	8106	0.02	0.07	0.05	0.02	2.4	0.19	0.3	60.2	0.0	5.2	86	0.0
soybean, hydrogenated and regular, soft, unsalted	1 tsp	168	0.00	0.00	0.00	0.00	<0.1	0.00	<0.1	1.2	0.0	0.1	2	0.0
soybean, hydrogenated, w/corn and hydrogenated cottonseed	1 stick	4050	0.01	0.04	0.03	0.01	1.3	0.11	0.2	33.9	0.0	2.9	48	0.0
soybean, hydrogenated, w/corn and hydrogenated cottonseed	1 tsp	168	0.00	0.00	0.00	0.00	<0.1	0.00	<0.1	1.4	0.0	0.1	2	0.0
soybean, hydrogenated, w/cottonseed	1 stick	4050	0.01	0.04	0.03	0.01	1.3	0.11	0.2	33.9	0.0	2.9	48	0.0
soybean, hydrogenated, w/cottonseed	1 tsp	168	0.00	0.00	0.00	0.00	<0.1	0.00	<0.1	1.4	0.0	0.1	2	0.0
soybean, hydrogenated, w/cottonseed, soft	1 cup	8106	0.02	0.07	0.05	0.02	2.4	0.19	0.3	60.2	0.0	5.2	86	0.0
soybean, hydrogenated, w/cottonseed, soft	1 tsp	168	0.00	0.00	0.00	0.00	<0.1	0.00	<0.1	1.2	0.0	0.1	2	0.0
soybean, hydrogenated, w/hydrogenated and regular palm, soft	1 cup	8106	0.02	0.07	0.05	0.02	2.4	0.19	0.3	60.2	0.0	5.2	86	0.0
soybean, hydrogenated, w/hydrogenated and regular palm, soft	1 tsp	168	0.00	0.00	0.00	0.00	<0.1	0.00	<0.1	1.2	0.0	0.1	2	0.0
soybean, hydrogenated, w/safflower, soft	1 cup	8106	0.02	0.07	0.05	0.02	2.4	0.19	0.3	60.2	0.0	5.2	86	0.0
soybean, hydrogenated, w/safflower, soft	1 tsp	168	0.00	0.00	0.00	0.00	<0.1	0.00	<0.1	1.2	0.0	0.1	2	0.0
soybean and cottonseed, hydrogenated, soft	1 cup	8106	0.02	0.07	0.05	0.02	2.4	0.19	0.3	60.2	0.0	5.2	86	0.0
soybean and cottonseed, hydrogenated, soft	1 tsp	168	0.00	0.00	0.00	0.00	<0.1	0.00	<0.1	1.2	0.0	0.1	2	0.0
soybean and cottonseed, hydrogenated, soft, unsalted	1 cup	8106	0.02	0.07	0.05	0.02	2.4	0.19	0.3	60.2	0.0	5.2	86	0.0
soybean and cottonseed, hydrogenated, soft, unsalted	1 tsp	168	0.00	0.00	0.00	0.00	<0.1	0.00	<0.1	1.2	0.0	0.1	2	0.0
sunflower, w/hydrogenated cottonseed and peanut, soft	1 cup	8106	0.02	0.07	0.05	0.02	2.4	0.19	0.3	60.2	0.0	5.2	86	0.0
sunflower, w/hydrogenated cottonseed and peanut, soft	1 tsp	168	0.00	0.00	0.00	0.00	<0.1	0.00	<0.1	1.2	0.0	0.1	2	0.0
sunflower, w/hydrogenated soybean and cottonseed	1 stick	4050	0.01	0.04	0.03	0.01	1.3	0.11	0.2	33.9	0.0	2.9	48	0.0
sunflower, w/hydrogenated soybean and cottonseed	1 tsp	168	0.00	0.00	0.00	0.00	<0.1	0.00	<0.1	1.4	0.0	0.1	2	0.0
MARGARINE SPREAD														
margarine-butter blend, 60% corn oil margarine, 40% butter	1 stick	4035	0.01	0.04	0.04	0.01	2.3	0.07	0.1	31.6	<0.1	2.3	41	<0.1
margarine-butter blend, 60% corn oil margarine, 40% butter	1 tsp	179	0.00	0.00	0.00	0.00	0.1	0.00	<0.1	1.4	0.0	0.1	2	0.0
MARGARINE SUBSTITUTE														
corn, hydrogenated and regular, 40% fat	1 cup	8285	0.01	0.05	0.03	0.01	1.6	0.13	0.2	41.3	0.0	3.6	59	0.0
corn, hydrogenated and regular, 40% fat	1 tsp	171	0.00	0.00	0.00	0.00	<0.1	0.00	<0.1	0.85	0.0	<0.1	1	0.0
soybean, hydrogenated, 40% fat	1 cup	8285	0.01	0.05	0.03	0.01	1.6	0.13	0.2	41.3	0.0	3.6	59	0.0
soybean, hydrogenated, 40% fat	1 tsp	171	0.00	0.00	0.00	0.00	<0.1	0.00	<0.1	0.85	0.0	<0.1	1	0.0

Food Name	Serving Size	A I.U.	Thi mg	Rib mg	Nia mg	B_6 mg	Fol mcg	B_{12} mcg	C mg	Calc mg	Iron mg	Mag mg	Pot mg	Zn mg
soybean, hydrogenated, w/cottonseed, 40% fat	1 cup	8285	0.01	0.05	0.03	0.01	1.6	0.13	0.2	41.3	0.0	3.6	59	0.0
soybean, hydrogenated, w/cottonseed, 40% fat	1 tsp	171	0.00	0.00	0.00	0.00	<0.1	0.00	<0.1	0.85	0.0	<0.1	1	0.0
soybean, hydrogenated, w/hydrogenated and regular palm, 40% fat	1 cup	8285	0.01	0.05	0.03	0.01	1.6	0.13	0.2	41.3	0.0	3.6	59	0.0
soybean, hydrogenated/ w.hydrogenated and regular palm, 40% fat	1 tsp	171	0.00	0.00	0.00	0.00	<0.1	0.00	<0.1	0.85	0.0	<0.1	1	0.0
soybean, hydrogenated, w/hydrogenated and regular palm, 60% fat, tub	1 cup	8178	0.02	0.06	0.04	0.01	1.9	0.15	0.3	47.9	0.0	4.2	68	0.0
soybean, hydrogenated, w/hydrogenated and regular palm, 60% fat, tub	1 tsp	171	0.00	0.00	0.00	0.00	<0.1	0.00	<0.1	1.0	0.0	<0.1	1	0.0
soybean and cottonseed, hydrogenated, 40% fat	1 cup	8285	0.01	0.05	0.03	0.01	1.6	0.13	0.2	41.3	0.0	3.6	59	0.0
soybean and cottonseed, hydrogenated, 40% fat	1 tsp	171	0.00	0.00	0.00	0.00	<0.1	0.00	<0.1	0.85	0.0	<0.1	1	0.0
soybean and cottonseed, hydrogenated, 60% fat, tub	1 cup	8178	0.02	0.06	0.04	0.01	1.9	0.15	0.3	47.9	0.0	4.2	68	0.0
soybean and cottonseed, hydrogenated, 60% fat, tub	1 tsp	171	0.00	0.00	0.00	0.00	<0.1	0.00	<0.1	1.0	0.0	<0.1	1	0.0
soybean and palm, hydrogenated, 60% fat, stick	1 cup	8178	0.02	0.06	0.04	0.01	1.9	0.15	0.3	47.9	0.0	4.2	68	0.0
soybean and palm, hydrogenated, 60% fat, stick	1 tsp	171	0.00	0.00	0.00	0.00	<0.1	0.00	<0.1	1.0	0.0	<0.1	1	0.0
MARJORAM														
dried	1 tbsp	137	0.01	0.01	0.07	0.02	4.7	0.00	0.9	33.8	1.4	5.9	26	<0.1
dried	1 tsp	48	0.00	0.00	0.03	0.01	1.6	0.00	0.3	11.9	0.5	2.1	9	<0.1
MARSHMALLOW. See under CANDY.														
MATAI. See under WATER CHESTNUT.														
MATZO. See under CRACKER.														
MAYONNAISE														
(Kraft)														
light	1 tbsp	28	na	na	na	na	na	na	<0.1	<0.1	<0.1	na	8	na
nonfat	1 tbsp	16	na	na	na	na	na	na	0.0	<0.1	<0.1	na	8	na
MEAT LOAF DINNER/ENTRÉE														
(Banquet) w/tomato sauce, potatoes, carrots in sauce, 'Extra Helping'	1 pkg	2088	na	na	na	na	na	na	7.7	77.0	3.9	na	na	na
(Healthy Choice) traditional, w/potato, vegetable, apple praline	1 pkg	745	na	na	na	na	na	na	55.4	47.6	2.2	na	na	na
(Lean Magic) flame broiled	1 piece	152	0.11	0.16	2.50	0.24	7.4	1.60	2.1	25.9	2.1	23.7	245	4.4
(Lean Magic 30) flame broiled	1 piece	158	0.09	0.11	1.90	0.19	6.8	1.10	2.2	27.8	1.9	19.5	200	2.7
(Pierre)														
flame-broiled, product 3724	1 piece	110	0.09	0.11	2.30	0.24	5.9	1.40	1.6	20.0	1.4	20.7	249	3.1
flame-broiled, product 3725	1 piece	124	0.12	0.12	2.50	0.26	5.9	1.40	1.7	25.2	1.6	25.2	262	3.6
flame-broiled, product 3824	1 piece	126	0.12	0.14	2.60	0.24	5.9	1.60	1.6	26.6	2.0	24.4	249	4.3
MEATBALL DINNER/ENTRÉ														
(Lean Cuisine) Swedish, w/pasta, frozen	1 entrée	0	na	na	na	na	na	na	na	na	2.1	na	na	na
MEDICAL NUTRITIONALS														
CRITICAL CARE SUPPORT														
(Nestlé Clinical Nutrition)														
'Crucial' for tube feeding, lactose- and gluten-free, low-residue, ready to use	1000 ml	6000	3.00	2.40	28.00	4.00	540.0	8.00	1000.0	1000	18.0	400.0	1872	36.0

Food Name	Serving Size	A I.U.	Thi mg	Rib mg	Nia mg	B6 mg	Fol mcg	B12 mcg	C mg	Calc mg	Iron mg	Mag mg	Pot mg	Zn mg
'Crucial' for tube feeding, lactose- and gluten-free, low-residue, ready to use	250 ml	1500	0.75	0.60	7.00	1.00	135.0	2.00	250.0	250	4.5	100.0	468	9.0
(Novartis [Sandoz])														
'Impact' ready to use.	1000 ml	6700	2.00	1.70	20.00	1.50	400.0	8.00	80.0	800	12.0	270.0	1400	15.0
'Impact' ready to use, 1 can, ...	250 ml	1670	0.50	0.43	5.00	0.37	100.0	2.00	20.0	200	3.0	66.7	350	3.8
'Impact 1.5' for fluid restriction or high caloric needs, ready to use, ...	1000 ml	8000	2.40	2.10	24.00	1.80	480.0	9.60	96.0	960	14.0	320.0	1680	18.0
'Impact 1.5' for fluid restriction or high caloric needs, ready to use, 1 can	250 ml	2000	0.60	0.51	6.00	0.44	120.0	2.40	24.0	240	3.6	80.0	420	4.5
'Impact with Fiber' ready to use	1000 ml	700	2.00	1.70	20.00	1.50	400.0	8.00	80.0	800	12.0	270.0	1400	15.0
'Impact with Fiber' ready to use, 1 can, ...	250 ml	1670	0.50	0.43	5.00	0.37	100.0	2.00	20.0	200	3.0	66.7	350	3.8
(Ross)														
'Perative' for tube feeding (not parenteral use), kosher, gluten- and lactose-free, low-residue, ready to use, ...	1 liter	8666	1.90	2.30	26.00	2.60	520.0	7.80	260.0	867	15.6	347.0	1730	19.5
'Perative' for tube feeding (not parenteral use), kosher, gluten- and lactose-free, low-residue, ready to use	8 fl oz	2053	0.48	0.53	6.20	0.62	124.0	1.90	62.0	206	3.7	82.2	410	4.6
DIABETES/GLUCOSE INTOLERANCE SUPPORT														
(Mead Johnson Nutritionals)														
'Choice DM' for oral or tube feeding, ready to use	1000 ml	5300	1.60	1.80	21.00	2.10	420.0	6.40	250.0	1060	19.0	420.0	1820	21.0
'Choice DM' for oral or tube feeding, ready to use	8 fl oz	1250	0.38	0.43	5.00	0.50	100.0	1.50	60.0	250	4.5	100.0	430	5.0
(Nestlé Clinical Nutrition)														
'Glytrol with Fiber' for oral or tube feeding, kosher, sucrose-, lactose-, and gluten-free, ready to use	1000 ml	4000	2.00	2.40	28.00	4.00	400.0	8.00	140.0	720	12.8	286.0	1400	15.0
'Glytrol with Fiber' for oral or tube feeding, kosher, sucrose-, lactose-, and gluten-free, ready to use	250 ml	1000	0.50	0.60	7.00	1.00	100.0	2.00	35.0	180	3.2	71.5	350	3.8
(Novartis [Sandoz])														
'Diabetisource with Fiber' ready to use.	1000 ml	6700	1.50	1.70	20.00	2.00	400.0	6.00	200.0	670	12.0	270.0	1400	15.0
'Diabetisource with Fiber' ready to use.	250 ml	1670	0.38	0.43	5.00	0.50	100.0	1.50	50.0	167	3.0	66.7	350	3.8
'Resource Diabetic with Fiber' for oral or tube feeding, ready to use	1000 ml	5300	1.60	1.80	21.00	2.10	220.0	6.30	160.0	930	9.5	110.0	1100	12.0
'Resource Diabetic with Fiber' for oral or tube feeding, ready to use	237 ml	1250	0.38	0.43	5.00	0.50	100.0	1.50	37.5	220	2.3	25.0	270	2.8
(Ross)														
'Glucerna with Fiber' for oral or tube feeding (not parenteral use), kosher, gluten- and lactose-free, low-residue, ready to use	1 liter	6320	1.60	1.80	21.10	2.10	422.0	6.30	211.0	704	12.7	282.0	1570	15.9
'Glucerna with Fiber' for oral or tube feeding (not parenteral use), kosher, gluten- and lactose-free, low-residue, ready to use	8 fl oz	1500	0.38	0.43	5.00	0.50	100.0	1.50	50.0	167	3.0	66.7	370	3.8
ELEMENTAL DIET														
(B. Braun/McGaw)														
'Immun-Aid' for oral or tube feeding, high-nitrogen, powder, prepared	2000 ml	5330	1.50	1.70	20.00	20.00	400.0	6.00	120.0	1000	18.0	400.0	2110	50.0
'Immun-Aid' for oral or tube feeding, high-nitrogen, powder, prepared	500 ml	1333	0.38	0.43	5.00	5.00	100.0	1.50	30.0	250	4.5	100.0	530	13.0

Food Name	Serving Size	A I.U.	Thi mg	Rib mg	Nia mg	B$_6$ mg	Fol mcg	B$_{12}$ mcg	C mg	Calc mg	Iron mg	Mag mg	Pot mg	Zn mg
(Mead Johnson Nutritionals)														
'Criticare HN' high-nitrogen, ready to use....	1000 ml	2600	2.00	2.30	26.00	2.60	210.0	7.90	159.0	530	9.5	210.0	1320	10.6
'Criticare HN' high-nitrogen, ready to use....	8 fl oz	630	0.48	0.54	6.30	0.63	50.0	1.90	38.0	125	2.3	50.0	310	2.5
(Nestlé Clinical Nutrition)														
'Peptamen' for tube feeding, isotonic, lactose- and gluten-free, low-residue, ready to use........................	1000 ml	3333	2.00	2.40	28.00	4.00	540.0	8.00	340.0	800	18.0	300.0	1500	24.0
'Peptamen' for tube feeding, isotonic, lactose- and gluten-free, low-residue, ready to use........................	250 ml	833	0.50	0.60	7.00	1.00	135.0	2.00	85.0	200	4.5	75.0	375	6.0
'Peptamen Oral' oral, lactose- and gluten-free, low-residue, ready to use.....	1000 ml	3333	2.00	2.40	28.00	4.00	540.0	8.00	340.0	800	18.0	300.0	1500	24.0
'Peptamen Oral' oral, lactose- and gluten-free, low-residue, ready to use.....	250 ml	833	0.50	0.60	7.00	1.00	135.0	2.00	85.0	200	4.5	75.0	375	6.0
'Peptamen VHP' for tube feeding, very high protein, isotonic, lactose- and gluten-free, low-residue, ready to use.....	1000 ml	3333	2.00	2.40	28.00	4.00	540.0	8.00	340.0	800	18.0	300.0	1500	24.0
'Peptamen VHP' for tube feeding, very high protein, isotonic, lactose- and gluten-free, low-residue, ready to use.....	250 ml	833	0.50	0.60	7.00	1.00	135.0	2.00	85.0	200	4.5	75.0	375	6.0
'Peptamen VHP' oral, very high protein, lactose- and gluten-free, low-residue, ready to use........................	1000 ml	3333	2.00	2.40	28.00	4.00	540.0	8.00	340.0	800	18.0	300.0	1500	24.0
'Peptamen VHP' oral, very high protein, lactose- and gluten-free, low-residue, ready to use........................	250 ml	833	0.50	0.60	7.00	1.00	135.0	2.00	85.0	200	4.5	75.0	375	6.0
'Reabilan' for tube feeding, lactose and gluten-free, low-residue, ready to use.....	1000 ml	2660	1.50	1.50	20.00	2.00	250.0	3.00	100.0	500	10.0	250.0	1250	10.0
'Reabilan' for tube feeding, lactose and gluten-free, low-residue, ready to use.....	375 ml	1000	0.56	0.56	7.50	0.75	94.0	1.10	37.5	187	3.8	94.0	469	3.8
'Reabilan HN' for tube feeding, high-nitrogen, lactose- and gluten-free, low-residue, ready to use..............	1000 ml	3538	2.00	2.00	26.60	2.70	332.0	4.00	133.0	665	13.3	332.0	1662	13.3
'Reabilan HN' for tube feeding, high-nitrogen, lactose- and gluten-free, low-residue, ready to use..............	375 ml	1328	0.75	0.75	10.00	1.00	125.0	1.50	50.0	250	5.0	125.0	623	5.0
(Novartis [Sandoz])														
'Tolerex' powder, prepared	1000 ml	2800	0.83	0.94	11.00	1.10	220.0	3.30	33.0	560	10.0	220.0	1200	8.3
'Tolerex' powder, prepared, 1 packet	300 ml	833	0.25	0.28	3.30	0.33	67.0	1.00	10.0	167	3.0	66.7	350	2.5
'Vivonex Plus' high-nitrogen, powder, prepared..........................	1000 ml	4200	1.70	1.90	22.00	2.20	440.0	6.70	67.0	560	10.0	220.0	1100	13.0
'Vivonex Plus' high-nitrogen, powder, prepared..........................	300 ml	1250	0.50	0.57	6.70	0.67	133.0	2.00	20.0	167	3.0	66.7	317	3.8
'Vivonex T.E.N' for gastrointestinal impairment, powder, prepared...........	1000 ml	2500	1.50	1.70	20.00	2.00	400.0	6.00	60.0	500	9.0	200.0	780	10.0
'Vivonex T.E.N' for gastrointestinal impairment, powder, prepared, 1 packet	300 ml	750	0.45	0.51	6.00	0.60	120.0	1.80	18.0	150	2.7	60.0	235	3.0
FAT MALABSORPTION SUPPORT														
(Mead Johnson Nutritionals)														
'Lipisorb' lactose-free, low-residue, powder, 2 calories per ml, prepared.......	8 fl oz	1800	0.56	0.63	7.20	0.72	144.0	2.20	22.0	330	4.4	96.0	600	4.8
'Lipisorb' lactose-free, low-residue, powder, 1 calorie per ml, prepared	8 fl oz	900	0.28	0.31	3.60	0.36	72.0	1.10	10.8	168	2.2	48.0	300	2.4

Food Name	Serving Size	A I.U.	Thi mg	Rib mg	Nia mg	B$_6$ mg	Fol mcg	B$_{12}$ mcg	C mg	Calc mg	Iron mg	Mag mg	Pot mg	Zn mg
'Lipisorb' lactose-free, low-residue, ready to use	1000 ml	6300	1.90	2.20	25.00	2.50	510.0	7.60	76.0	850	15.2	340.0	1690	16.9
'Lipisorb' lactose-free, low-residue, ready to use	8 fl oz	1500	0.46	0.52	6.00	0.60	120.0	1.80	18.0	200	3.6	80.0	400	4.0
GASTROINTESTINAL SUPPORT														
(Nestlé Clinical Nutrition)														
'Elementra' for oral or tube feeding, elemental protein, powder, 2 scoops	6.6 gm	na	na	na	na	na	na	na	na	60.0	na	4.9	85	na
(Novartis [Sandoz])														
'Sandosource Peptide' semi-elemental, low-fat, ready to use	1000 ml	5700	1.70	1.90	23.00	2.30	460.0	6.90	170.0	570	10.0	230.0	1600	13.0
'Sandosource Peptide' semi-elemental, low-fat, ready to use	250 ml	1430	0.43	0.49	5.70	0.57	114.0	1.70	42.9	143	2.6	57.1	400	3.3
(Ross)														
'Alitraq' for oral or tube feeding (not parenteral use), kosher, gluten-free, low-residue, powder, prepared	1 liter	3998	2.00	2.30	27.00	2.70	267.0	8.00	200.0	733	15.0	3.4	1200	20.0
'Alitraq' for oral or tube feeding (not parenteral use), kosher, gluten-free, low-residue, powder, prepared	300 ml	1200	0.60	0.68	8.00	0.80	80.0	2.40	60.0	220	4.4	1.0	360	6.0
'Vital High Nitrogen' for oral or tube feeding (not parenteral use), kosher, gluten- and lactose-free, low-residue, powder, prepared	1 liter	3332	2.00	2.30	26.70	2.70	533.0	8.00	200.0	667	12.0	3.4	1400	15.0
'Vital High Nitrogen' for oral or tube feeding (not parenteral use), kosher, gluten- and lactose-free, low-residue, powder, prepared	300 ml	1000	0.60	0.68	8.00	0.80	160.0	2.40	60.0	200	3.6	1.0	420	4.5
GENERAL PURPOSE														
(Mead Johnson Nutritionals)														
'Boost' oral, milk-based, cholesterol- and lactose-free	8 fl oz	1250	0.38	0.43	5.00	0.70	140.0	2.10	60.0	300	3.6	100	400	4.5
'Sustacal' oral, milk-based, lactose-free, cholesterol-free, powder, prepared	8 fl oz	1290	0.40	0.20	6.80	0.55	133.0	1.00	20.0	290	6.0	105	560	4.0
'Sustacal' oral, milk-based, moderate protein, fiber-free, lactose-free, low-residue, ready to use	8 fl oz	1010	0.33	0.40	4.70	0.47	89.0	1.30	13.3	240	4.0	90.0	490	3.3
'Sustacal Pudding' lactose-free, fiber-free	8 fl oz	750	0.23	0.26	3.00	0.30	60.0	0.90	9.0	225	2.7	60.0	320	2.3
'Sustacal with Fiber' oral, milk-based, w/fiber, lactose-free, ready to use	8 fl oz	830	0.37	0.43	5.00	0.50	100.0	1.50	30.0	200	3.0	67.0	330	3.3
(Novartis [Sandoz])														
'Resource' fruit beverage, low-electrolyte, fat-free	1000 ml	2600	1.60	1.80	21.00	2.10	210.0	6.30	160.0	570	9.5	210	63	16.0
'Resource' fruit beverage, low-electrolyte, fat-free, 1 Brik Pak	237 ml	625	0.38	0.43	5.00	0.50	50.0	1.50	37.5	135	2.3	50.0	15	3.8
(Ross)														
'Ensure' for oral or tube feeding (not parenteral use), kosher, gluten- and lactose-free, low-residue, powder, prepared	1 liter	2650	1.60	1.90	21.20	2.20	424.0	6.40	159.0	530	9.6	212.0	1564	12.0
'Ensure' for oral or tube feeding (not parenteral use), kosher, gluten- and lactose-free, low-residue, powder, prepared	8 fl oz	625	0.38	0.43	5.00	0.50	100.0	1.50	37.5	125	2.3	50.0	370	2.8

Food Name	Serving Size	A I.U.	Thi mg	Rib mg	Nia mg	B_6 mg	Fol mcg	B_{12} mcg	C mg	Calc mg	Iron mg	Mag mg	Pot mg	Zn mg
'Ensure' for oral or tube feeding (not parenteral use), kosher, gluten- and lactose-free, low-residue, ready to use	1 liter	5284	1.60	1.90	21.20	2.20	423.0	6.40	127.0	1268	19.0	5.3	1564	16.1
'Ensure' for oral or tube feeding (not parenteral use), kosher, gluten- and lactose-free, low-residue, ready to use	8 fl oz	1250	0.38	0.43	5.00	0.50	100.0	1.50	30.0	300	4.5	1.3	370	3.8
'Ensure Pudding' oral, patients w/swallowing impairments, kosher, gluten-free, 9.2 g lactose/serving	5-oz can	850	0.26	0.29	3.40	0.34	68.0	1.10	15.4	200	3.1	68.0	330	3.8
'Ensure with Fiber' for oral or tube feeding (not parenteral use), fiber-fortified, kosher, gluten- and lactose-free, low-residue, ready to use	1 liter	3595	1.70	1.90	21.60	2.20	432.0	1.90	216.0	719	13.0	288.0	1693	16.2
'Ensure with Fiber' for oral or tube feeding (not parenteral use), fiber-fortified, kosher, gluten- and lactose-free, low-residue, ready to use	8 fl oz	850	0.39	0.44	5.10	0.51	102.0	0.44	51.0	170	3.1	68.0	400	3.8
GERIATRIC														
(Nestlé Clinical Nutrition)														
'Probalance with Fiber' for oral or tube feeding, high-fiber, kosher, lactose- and gluten-free, ready to use	1000 ml	4000	2.30	2.50	40.00	4.00	1200.0	12.00	240.0	1250	18.0	400.0	1560	24.0
'Probalance with Fiber' for oral or tube feeding, high-fiber, kosher, lactose- and gluten-free, ready to use	250 ml	1000	0.56	0.64	10.00	1.00	300.0	3.00	60.0	312	4.5	100.0	390	6.0
HEALING SUPPORT														
(Mead Johnson Nutritionals)														
'Protain XL' for tube feeding, high-protein, w/fiber, ready to use	1000 ml	7000	2.40	2.70	32.0	3.20	480.0	15.00	240.0	800	18.0	320.0	1760	30.0
'Protain XL' for tube feeding, high-protein, w/fiber, ready to use	8 fl oz	1660	0.57	0.64	7.60	0.76	114.0	3.50	57.0	189	4.3	76.0	420	7.1
'Traumacal' for oral or tube feeding, high-calorie, high-nitrogen	1000 ml	2500	1.90	2.20	25.00	2.50	200.0	7.50	148.0	750	8.9	200.0	1390	14.8
'Traumacal' for oral or tube feeding, high-calorie, high-nitrogen	8 fl oz	590	0.45	0.51	5.90	0.59	47.0	1.80	35.0	177	2.1	47.0	330	3.5
(Nestlé Clinical Nutrition)														
'Replete' isotonic, kosher, lactose- and gluten-free, low-residue, ready to use	1000 ml	4000	3.00	2.40	28.00	4.00	540.0	8.00	340.0	1000	18.0	400.0	1500	24.0
'Replete' isotonic, kosher, lactose- and gluten-free, low-residue, ready to use	250 ml	1000	0.75	0.60	7.00	1.00	135.0	2.00	85.0	250	4.5	100.0	375	6.0
'Replete with Fiber' for oral or tube feeding, isotonic, high-fiber, kosher, lactose- and gluten-free, ready to use	1000 ml	4000	3.00	2.40	28.00	4.00	540.0	8.00	340.0	1000	18.0	400.0	1500	24.0
'Replete with Fiber' for oral or tube feeding, isotonic, high-fiber, kosher, lactose- and gluten-free, ready to use	250 ml	1000	0.75	0.60	7.00	1.00	135.0	2.00	85.0	250	4.5	100.0	375	6.0
(Ross)														
'Promote' for oral or tube feeding, high-protein, kosher, gluten- and lactose-free, low-residue, ready to use	1 liter	7250	2.30	2.50	30.0	3.00	600.0	9.00	340.0	1200	18.0	400.0	1980	24.0
'Promote' for oral or tube feeding, high-protein, kosher, gluten- and lactose-free, low-residue, ready to use	8 fl oz	1720	0.54	0.61	7.10	0.72	143.0	2.20	80.6	285	4.3	94.9	470	5.7

Food Name	Serving Size	A I.U.	Thi mg	Rib mg	Nia mg	B$_6$ mg	Fol mcg	B$_{12}$ mcg	C mg	Calc mg	Iron mg	Mag mg	Pot mg	Zn mg
'Promote with Fiber' for oral or tube feeding, high-protein, kosher, gluten- and lactose-free, low-residue, ready to use	1 liter	7250	2.30	2.50	30.00	3.00	600.0	9.00	340.0	1200	18.0	400.0	1980	24.0
'Promote with Fiber' for oral or tube feeding, high-protein, kosher, gluten- and lactose-free, low-residue, ready to use	8 fl oz	1720	0.54	0.61	7.10	0.72	143.0	0.61	80.6	285	4.3	94.9	470	5.7
HEPATIC SUPPORT														
(B. Braun/McGaw)														
'Hepatic-Aid II' for oral or tube feeding, amino acid and calories, powder, prepared	340 ml	na	na	na	na	na	na	na	na	na	na	na	na	na
(Nestlé Clinical Nutrition)														
'Nutrihep' for oral or tube feeding, kosher, lactose- and gluten-free, ready to use	1000 ml	5000	1.50	1.70	20.00	2.00	400.0	6.00	96.0	100	18.0	400.0	1320	15.2
'Nutrihep' for oral or tube feeding, kosher, lactose- and gluten-free, ready to use	250 ml	1250	0.38	0.43	5.00	0.50	100.0	1.50	24.0	250	4.5	100.0	330	3.8
HIV/AIDS SUPPORT														
(Ross)														
'Advera with Fiber' for oral or tube feeding (not parenteral use), kosher, gluten- and lactose-free, ready to use	1 liter	10778	3.20	2.90	25.40	3.40	507.0	50.70	381.0	10788	19.1	338.0	2532	15.9
'Advera with Fiber' for oral or tube feeding (not parenteral use), kosher, gluten- and lactose-free, ready to use	8 fl oz	2550	0.75	0.68	6.00	0.80	120.0	12.00	90.0	260	4.5	80.0	600	3.8
HYDRATION SUPPORT														
(Ross)														
'Equalyte' enteral rehydration solution	8 fl oz	0	0.00	0.00	0.00	na	0.0	na	0.0	0.0	0.0	0.0	210	0.0
'Equalyte' rehydration solution, for oral or tube feeding (not parenteral use), kosher, gluten- and lactose-free, ready to use	1 liter	na	na	na	na	na	na	na	na	na	na	na	875	na
'Introlite' rehydration solution, for tube feeding (not parenteral use), low calorie, kosher, gluten- and lactose-free, low-residue, ready to use	1 liter	3788	1.70	1.90	22.80	2.30	455.0	1.90	228.0	758.0	13.7	304.0	1570	17.1
'Pedialyte' for children	8 fl oz	0	0.00	0.00	0.00	na	0.0	na	0.0	0.0	0.0	na	183	na
INTACT PROTEIN DIET														
(Mead Johnson Nutritionals)														
'Comply' for tube feeding, high-calorie, lactose-free, ready to use	1000 ml	6000	1.80	2.00	24.00	3.40	600.0	18.00	180.0	1200.0	22.0	480.0	1850	24.0
'Comply' for tube feeding, high-calorie, lactose-free, ready to use	8 fl oz	1420	0.43	0.48	5.70	0.80	142.0	4.30	43.0	280.0	5.1	114.0	440	5.7
'Isocal' for tube feeding, lactose-free, low-residue, ready to use	1000 ml	2600	2.00	2.30	26.00	2.60	210.0	7.90	159.0	630.0	9.5	210.0	1320	10.6
'Isocal' for tube feeding, lactose-free, low-residue, ready to use	8 fl oz	630	0.48	0.54	6.30	0.63	50.0	1.90	38.0	150.0	2.2	50.0	310	2.5
'Isocal HN' for tube feeding, high-nitrogen, isotonic, low-residue, ready to use	1000 ml	4200	3.20	3.60	42.00	4.20	340.0	12.70	250.0	850.0	15.2	340.0	1610	16.9

Food Name	Serving Size	A I.U.	Thi mg	Rib mg	Nia mg	B_6 mg	Fol mcg	B_{12} mcg	C mg	Calc mg	Iron mg	Mag mg	Pot mg	Zn mg
'Isocal HN' for tube feeding, high-nitrogen, isotonic, low-residue, ready to use	8 fl oz	1000	0.75	0.85	10.00	1.00	80.0	3.00	60.0	200.0	3.6	80.0	380	4.0
'Ultracal with Fiber' for tube feeding, high-nitrogen, w/fiber, ready to use	1000 ml	4200	3.20	3.60	42.00	4.20	340.0	12.70	250.0	850.0	15.2	340.0	1610	16.9
'Ultracal with Fiber' for tube feeding, high-nitrogen, w/fiber, ready to use	8 fl oz	1000	0.75	0.85	10.00	1.00	80.0	3.00	60.0	200.0	3.6	80.0	380	4.0
(Nestlé Clinical Nutrition)														
'Nubasics' oral, low-sodium, kosher, lactose-, gluten-, and cholesterol-free, low-residue, ready to use	250 ml	750	0.40	0.45	5.20	0.75	100.0	1.50	26.0	125.0	2.3	50.0	312	2.6
'Nubasics Complete Nutrition Bar' oral, low-sodium, kosher, lactose- and gluten-free	1 bar	375	0.20	0.25	2.60	0.35	50.0	0.75	13.0	100.0	1.1	40.0	220	1.3
'Nubasics Complete Nutrition Soup' oral, low-cholesterol, lactose- and gluten-free, low-residue, 1 envelope	56 g	750	0.40	0.45	5.20	0.75	100.0	1.50	26.0	165.0	2.3	50.0	310	2.6
'Nubasics Decaffeinated Coffee Beverage' oral, kosher, lactose-, gluten-, and cholesterol-free, powder	2 scoops	375	0.20	0.23	2.60	0.37	50.0	0.75	20.0	110.0	1.3	32.0	310	1.3
'Nubasics Juice Drink' oral, kosher, lactose-, gluten-, and cholesterol-free; low-residue	163 ml	400	0.20	0.25	2.60	0.35	50.0	1.30	20.0	83.0	1.5	33.3	50.0	1.6
'Nubasics Plus' oral, high-calorie, low-sodium, kosher, lactose-, gluten-, and cholesterol-free, low-residue, ready to use	250 ml	1125	0.60	0.70	7.80	1.10	150.0	2.20	39.0	187.0	3.4	75.0	467	3.9
'Nubasics 2.0' oral, very high calorie; kosher, lactose- and gluten-free, low-residue, ready to use	250 ml	2000	1.00	1.20	14.00	2.00	270.0	4.00	70.0	335.0	6.0	134.0	480	7.0
'Nubasics VHP' oral, high-protein, low-sodium, kosher, lactose-, gluten-, and cholesterol-free, ready to use	250 ml	750	0.40	0.45	5.20	0.75	100.0	1.50	26.0	145.0	2.3	50.0	312	2.6
'Nubasics with Fiber' oral, high-protein with fiber, low-sodium, kosher, lactose-, gluten-, and cholesterol-free, low-residue, ready to use	250 ml	750	0.40	0.45	5.20	0.75	100.0	1.50	26.0	125.0	2.3	50.0	312	2.6
'Nutren 1.0' for oral or tube feeding, kosher, lactose- and gluten-free, low-residue, ready to use	1000 ml	4000	2.00	2.40	28.00	4.00	540.0	8.00	140.0	668.0	12.0	268.0	1248	14.0
'Nutren 1.0' for oral or tube feeding, kosher, lactose- and gluten-free, low-residue, ready to use	250 ml	1000	0.50	0.60	7.00	1.00	135.0	2.00	35.0	167.0	3.0	67.0	312	3.5
'Nutren 1.0 with Fiber' for oral or tube feeding, high-fiber, kosher, lactose- and gluten-free, ready to use	1000 ml	4000	2.00	2.40	28.00	4.00	540.0	8.00	140.0	668.0	12.0	268	1248	14.0
'Nutren 1.0 with Fiber' for oral or tube feeding, high-fiber, kosher, lactose- and gluten-free, ready to use	250 ml	1000	0.50	0.60	7.00	1.00	135.0	2.00	35.0	167.0	3.0	67.0	312	3.5
'Nutren 1.5' for oral or tube feeding, high-calorie, kosher, lactose- and gluten-free, low-residue, ready to use	1000 ml	6000	3.00	3.60	42.00	6.00	800.0	12.00	212.0	1000.0	18.0	400	1872	20.0

Food Name	Serving Size	A I.U.	Thi mg	Rib mg	Nia mg	B_6 mg	Fol mcg	B_{12} mcg	C mg	Calc mg	Iron mg	Mag mg	Pot mg	Zn mg
'Nutren 1.5' for oral or tube feeding, high-calorie, kosher, lactose- and gluten-free, low-residue, ready to use	250 ml	1500	0.75	0.90	10.50	1.50	200.0	3.00	53.0	250.0	4.5	100	468	5.0
'Nutren 2.0' for oral or tube feeding, very high calorie, kosher, lactose- and gluten-free, low-residue, ready to use	1000 ml	8000	4.00	4.80	56.00	8.00	1080.0	16.00	280.0	1340.0	24.0	536.0	1920	28.0
'Nutren 2.0' for oral or tube feeding, very high calorie, kosher, lactose- and gluten-free, low-residue, ready to use	250 ml	2000	1.00	1.20	14.00	2.00	270.0	4.00	70.0	335.0	6.0	134.0	480	7.0
(Novartis [Sandoz])														
'Citrotein' fruit-flavored, lactose-free, low-residue, powder, prepared.	100 ml	5200	3.10	3.60	42.00	4.30	830.0	13.00	240.0	1100.0	38.0	420.0	550	16.0
'Citrotein' fruit-flavored, lactose-free, low-residue, powder, prepared.	254 ml	1330	0.80	0.91	10.70	1.10	210.0	3.20	60.0	270.0	9.6	107.0	140	4.0
'Compleat' for tube feeding, blenderized, ready to use	1000 ml	3300	1.50	1.70	20.00	2.00	270.0	6.00	60.0	670.0	13.0	270.0	1400	15.0
'Compleat' for tube feeding, blenderized, ready to use, 1 can	250 ml	833	0.38	0.43	5.00	0.50	66.7	1.50	15.0	167.0	3.0	66.7	350	3.8
'Compleat Modified with Fiber' for tube feeding, blenderized, lactose-free, isotonic, ready to use.	1000 ml	3300	1.50	1.70	20.00	2.00	270.0	6.00	60.0	670.0	12.0	270.0	1400	15.0
'Compleat Modified with Fiber' for tube feeding, blenderized, lactose-free, isotonic, ready to use, 1 can	250 ml	833	0.38	0.43	5.00	0.50	66.7	1.50	15.0	167.0	3.0	66.7	350	3.8
'Fibersource HN' for oral or tube feeding, high-fiber, high-nitrogen, lactose- and gluten-free, ready to use	1000 ml	3300	2.00	2.30	27.00	2.70	270.0	8.00	200.0	670.0	12.0	270.0	1800	17.0
'Fibersource HN' for oral or tube feeding, high-fiber, high-nitrogen, lactose- and gluten-free, ready to use	250 ml	833	0.50	0.57	6.70	0.67	66.7	2.00	50.0	167.0	3.0	66.7	450	4.2
'Fibersource' for oral or tube feeding, high-fiber, lactose- and gluten-free, ready to use	1000 ml	3300	2.00	2.30	27.00	2.70	270.0	8.00	200.0	670.0	12.0	270.0	1800	17.0
'Fibersource' for oral or tube feeding, high-fiber, lactose- and gluten-free, ready to use, 1 can	250 ml	833	0.50	0.57	6.70	0.67	66.7	2.00	50.0	167.0	3.0	66.7	450	4.2
'Isosource HN' for oral or tube feeding, protein maintenance, lactose-, gluten-, and fiber-free, ready to use	1000 ml	3300	2.00	2.30	27.00	2.70	270.0	8.00	200.0	670.0	12.0	270.0	1700	17.0
'Isosource HN' for oral or tube feeding, protein maintenance, lactose-, gluten-, and fiber-free, ready to use	250 ml	833	0.50	0.57	6.70	0.67	66.7	2.00	50.0	167.0	3.0	66.7	417	4.2
'Isosource 1.5 with Fiber' high-calorie, high-nitrogen, ready to use	1000 ml	11000	3.20	3.60	43.00	4.30	640.0	13.00	320.0	1100.0	19.0	430.0	2100	32.0
'Isosource 1.5 with Fiber' high-calorie, high-nitrogen, ready to use, 1 can	250 ml	2680	0.80	0.91	10.70	1.10	161.0	3.20	80.4	268.0	4.8	107.0	536	8.0
'Isosource Standard' for oral or tube feeding, protein maintenance, lactose-, gluten-, and fiber-free, ready to use.	1000 ml	3300	2.00	2.30	27.00	270.0	270.0	8.00	200.0	670.0	12.0	270.0	1700	17.0
'Isosource Standard' for oral or tube feeding, protein maintenance, lactose-, gluten-, and fiber-free, ready to use.	250 ml	833	0.50	0.57	6.70	0.67	66.7	2.00	50.0	167.0	3.0	66.7	417	4.2
'Isosource VHN with Fiber' for oral or tube feeding, w/fiber, ready to use.	1000 ml	8000	2.40	2.70	32.00	3.20	480.0	9.60	240.0	800.0	14.0	320.0	1600	24.0

Food Name	Serving Size	A I.U.	Thi mg	Rib mg	Nia mg	B_6 mg	Fol mcg	B_{12} mcg	C mg	Calc mg	Iron mg	Mag mg	Pot mg	Zn mg
'Isosource VHN with Fiber' for oral or tube feeding, w/fiber, ready to use........ (Ross)	250 ml	2000	0.60	0.68	8.00	0.80	120.0	2.40	60.0	200.0	3.6	80.0	400	6.0
'Ensure High Protein' oral (not parenteral use), kosher, gluten- and lactose-free, low-residue, ready to use	8 fl oz	1250	0.38	0.43	5.00	0.50	100.0	1.50	30.0	250.0	4.5	100.0	500	5.6
'Ensure Plus' for oral or tube feeding (not parenteral use), high-calorie, kosher, gluten- and lactose-free, low-residue, ready to use.............	1 liter	3522	2.10	2.40	28.20	2.80	564.0	8.50	212.0	705.0	12.7	282.0	1940	15.9
'Ensure Plus' for oral or tube feeding (not parenteral use), high-calorie, kosher, gluten- and lactose-free, low-residue, ready to use..............	8 fl oz	834	0.50	0.57	6.70	0.67	134.0	2.00	50.0	167.0	3.0	67.0	460	3.8
'Ensure Plus HN' for oral or tube feeding (not parenteral use), high calorie, kosher, gluten- and lactose-free, low-residue, ready to use..............	1 liter	5280	3.20	3.60	42.30	4.20	845.0	12.70	317.0	1056.0	19.1	423.0	1820	23.8
'Ensure Plus HN' for oral or tube feeding (not parenteral use), high calorie, kosher, gluten- and lactose-free, low-residue, ready to use..............	8 fl oz	1250	0.75	0.85	10.00	1.00	200.0	3.00	75.0	250.0	4.5	100.0	430	5.6
'Jevity with Fiber' for tube feeding (not parenteral use), fiber-fortified, isotonic, kosher, gluten-and lactose-free, low-residue, ready to use..............	1 liter	3788	1.70	1.90	22.80	2.30	455.0	6.80	228.0	909.0	13.7	304.0	1570	13.7
'Jevity with Fiber' for tube feeding (not parenteral use), fiber-fortified, isotonic, kosher, gluten-and lactose-free, low-residue, ready to use..............	8 fl oz	893	0.41	0.46	5.40	0.54	108.0	1.70	53.6	215.0	3.2	71.5	370	3.2
'Jevity Plus with Fiber' for tube feeding (not parenteral use), high-nitrogen, kosher, gluten- and lactose-free, ready to use......................	1 liter	5000	2.30	2.50	30.00	3.00	600.0	9.00	300.0	1200.0	18.0	400.0	1850	22.5
'Jevity Plus with Fiber' for tube feeding (not parenteral use), high-nitrogen, kosher, gluten- and lactose-free, ready to use............................	8 fl oz	1190	0.54	0.61	7.10	0.72	143.0	2.20	71.3	285.0	4.3	95.0	380	5.3
'Osmolite' for oral or tube feeding (not parenteral use), high-nitrogen, isotonic, kosher, gluten- and lactose-free, low-residue, ready to use..............	1 liter	2650	1.60	1.80	21.20	2.10	424.0	6.40	159.0	530.0	9.5	212.0	1020	12.0
'Osmolite' for oral or tube feeding (not parenteral use), high-nitrogen, isotonic, kosher, gluten- and lactose-free, low-residue, ready to use..............	8 fl oz	625	0.38	0.43	5.00	0.50	100.0	1.50	37.5	125.0	2.3	50.0	240	2.8
'Osmolite HN' for tube feeding (not parenteral use), high-nitrogen, kosher, gluten- and lactose-free, low-residue, ready to use......................	1 liter	3788	1.70	1.90	22.80	2.30	455.0	6.80	228.0	758.0	13.7	304.0	1570	17.1
'Osmolite HN' for tube feeding (not parenteral use), high-nitrogen, kosher, gluten- and lactose-free, low-residue, ready to use......................	8 fl oz	893	0.41	0.46	5.40	0.54	108.0	1.70	53.6	179.0	3.2	71.5	370	4.0

Food Name	Serving Size	A I.U.	Thi mg	Rib mg	Nia mg	B_6 mg	Fol mcg	B_{12} mcg	C mg	Calc mg	Iron mg	Mag mg	Pot mg	Zn mg
'Osmolite HN Plus' for tube feeding (not parenteral use), high-calorie, high-nitrogen, kosher, gluten- and lactose-free, low-residue, ready to use	1 liter	5000	2.30	2.50	30.00	3.00	600.0	2.50	300.0	1200.0	18.0	400.0	1940	22.5
'Osmolite HN Plus' for tube feeding (not parenteral use), high-calorie, high-nitrogen, kosher, gluten- and lactose-free, low-residue, ready to use	8 fl oz	1190	0.54	0.61	7.10	0.72	143.0	0.61	71.3	285.0	4.3	95.0	460	5.3
'Twocal HN' for oral or tube feeding (not parenteral use), high-calorie, high-protein, kosher, gluten- and lactose-free, low-residue, ready to use	1 liter	5263	2.60	2.90	33.70	3.40	674.0	10.10	316.0	1052.0	19.0	421.0	2456	23.7
'Twocal HN' for oral or tube feeding (not parenteral use), high-calorie, high-protein, kosher, gluten- and lactose-free, low-residue, ready to use	8 fl oz	1250	0.60	0.68	8.00	0.80	160.0	2.40	75.0	250.0	4.5	100.0	580	5.6
PEDIATRIC														
(Mead Johnson Nutritionals)														
'Kindercal with Fiber' for oral or tube feeding, lactose-free, isotonic, ready to use.........................	1000 ml	4100	1.70	2.10	21.00	2.10	161.0	5.90	250.0	850.0	10.6	210.0	1310	12.7
'Kindercal with Fiber' for oral or tube feeding, lactose-free, isotonic, ready to use	8 fl oz	970	0.40	0.50	4.90	25.00	38.0	1.40	58.0	200.0	2.5	50.0	310	3.0
'Portagen' for GI disorders, children under 2 years, powder, prepared.........	5 fl oz	780	156.00	188.00	2.10	0.21	15.6	0.63	8.1	94.0	1.9	20.0	125	0.9
(Nestlé Clinical Nutrition)														
'Nutren Junior' for oral or tube feeding, children 1–10 years, kosher, lactose- and gluten-free, low-residue, ready to use.........................	1000 ml	2400	2.40	2.00	20.00	2.40	400.0	6.00	100.0	1000.0	15.0	200.0	1320	15.0
'Nutren Junior' for oral or tube feeding, children 1–10 years, kosher, lactose- and gluten-free, low-residue, ready to use............................	250 ml	600	0.60	0.50	5.00	0.60	100.0	1.50	25.0	250.0	3.8	50.0	330	3.8
'Nutren Junior with Fiber' for oral or tube feeding, children 1–10 years, kosher, lactose- and gluten-free, low-residue, ready to use..............	1000 ml	2400	2.40	2.00	20.00	2.40	400.0	6.00	100.0	1000.0	15.0	200.0	1320	15.0
'Nutren Junior with Fiber' for oral or tube feeding, children 1–10 years, kosher, lactose- and gluten-free, low-residue, ready to use..............	250 ml	600	0.60	0.50	5.00	0.60	100.0	1.50	25.0	250.0	3.8	50.0	330	3.8
'Peptamen Junior' for tube feeding, GI patients, children 1-10 years, lactose- and gluten-free, low-residue, ready to use	1000 ml	2400	2.40	2.00	20.00	2.40	400.0	6.00	100.0	1000.0	14.0	200.0	1320	15.0
'Peptamen Junior' for tube feeding, GI patients, children 1-10 years, lactose- and gluten-free, low-residue, ready to use	250 ml	600	0.60	0.50	5.00	0.60	100.0	1.50	25.0	250.0	3.5	50.0	330	3.8
'Peptamen Junior Oral' oral, for children 1-10 years, lactose- and gluten-free, low-residue, ready to use	1000 ml	2400	2.40	2.00	20.00	2.40	400.0	6.00	100.0	1000.0	14.0	200.0	1320	15.0
'Peptamen Junior Oral' oral, for children 1-10 years, lactose- and gluten-free, low-residue, ready to use	250 ml	600	0.60	0.50	5.00	0.60	100.0	1.50	25.0	250.0	3.5	50.0	330	3.8

Food Name	Serving Size	A I.U.	Thi mg	Rib mg	Nia mg	B$_6$ mg	Fol mcg	B$_{12}$ mcg	C mg	Calc mg	Iron mg	Mag mg	Pot mg	Zn mg
(Novartis [Sandoz])														
'Vivonex Pediatric' for oral or tube feeding, children 1–10 years, powder, prepared........................	1000 ml	2500	1.50	1.80	20.00	2.00	200.0	3.00	100.0	970.0	10.0	200.0	1200	12.0
'Vivonex Pediatric' for oral or tube feeding, children 1–10 years, powder, prepared........................	250 ml	625	0.38	0.45	5.00	0.50	50.0	0.75	25.0	243.0	2.5	50.0	300	3.0
(Ross)														
'Pediasure' for oral or tube feeding (not parenteral use) kosher, gluten- and lactose-free, low-residue, not for children with galactosemia.........	1 liter	2570	2.70	2.10	17.00	2.60	370.0	2.10	100.0	970.0	14.0	200.0	1310	12.0
'Pediasure' for oral or tube feeding (not parenteral use) kosher, gluten- and lactose-free, low-residue, not for children with galactosemia.............	8 fl oz	610	0.64	0.50	4.00	0.62	88.0	0.50	24.0	230.0	3.3	47.0	310	2.8
'Pediasure with Fiber' for oral or tube feeding (not parenteral use), kosher, gluten- and lactose-free, ready to use, not for children with galactosemia........	1 liter	2570	2.70	2.10	17.00	2.60	370.0	2.10	100.0	970.0	14.0	200.0	1310	12.0
'Pediasure with Fiber' for oral or tube feeding (not parenteral use), kosher, gluten- and lactose-free, ready to use, not for children with galactosemia........	8 fl oz	610	0.64	0.50	4.00	0.62	88.0	0.50	24.0	230.0	3.3	47.0	310	2.8
PROTEIN SUPPLEMENT														
(Mead Johnson Nutritionals) 'Casec'.........	100 gm	na	na	na	na	na	na	na	na	1400.0	na	na	10	na
(Novartis [Sandoz])														
'Meritene' oral, powder, prepared..........	1000 ml	4800	1.40	2.60	19.00	1.90	400.0	6.90	58.0	2200.0	17.0	380.0	2800	14.0
'Meritene' oral, powder, prepared..........	275 ml	1250	0.38	0.68	5.00	0.50	100.0	1.80	15.0	570.0	4.5	100.0	730	3.8
(Ross)														
'Promod' for oral or tube feeding (not parenteral use), powder, gluten-free, low-residue, kosher, 2 scoops...........	6.6 gm	na	na	na	na	na	na	na	na	44.0	na	na	65	na
PULMONARY SUPPORT														
(Mead Johnson Nutritionals)														
'Respalor' for oral or tube feeding, high-nitrogen, high-calorie, ready to use...........................	1000 ml	3500	2.70	3.00	35.00	3.50	280.0	10.60	210.0	710.0	12.7	280.0	1480	13.9
'Respalor' for oral or tube feeding, high-nitrogen, high-calorie, ready to use...........................	8 fl oz	830	0.62	0.72	8.30	0.83	67.0	2.50	50.0	167.0	3.0	67.0	350	3.3
(Nestlé Clinical Nutrition)														
'Nutrivent' for tube feeding, kosher, lactose- and gluten-free, low-residue, ready to use......................	1000 ml	6000	3.00	3.60	42.00	6.00	812.0	12.00	210.0	1200.0	18.0	480.0	1872	21.2
'Nutrivent' for tube feeding, kosher, lactose- and gluten-free, low-residue, ready to use......................	250 ml	1500	0.75	0.90	10.50	1.50	203.0	3.00	53.0	300.0	4.5	120.0	468	5.3
(Ross)														
'Pulmocare' for oral or tube feeding (not parenteral use), kosher, gluten- and lactose-free, low-residue, ready to use......................	1 liter	11740	3.20	3.60	42.30	4.20	845.0	12.70	317.0	1056.0	19.1	423.0	1730	23.8

Food Name	Serving Size	A I.U.	Thi mg	Rib mg	Nia mg	B6 mg	Fol mcg	B12 mcg	C mg	Calc mg	Iron mg	Mag mg	Pot mg	Zn mg
'Pulmocare' for oral or tube feeding (not parenteral use), kosher, gluten- and lactose-free, low-residue, ready to use	8 fl oz	2752	0.75	0.85	10.00	1.00	200.0	3.00	75.0	250.0	4.5	100.0	410	5.6
RENAL SUPPORT														
(Mead Johnson Nutritionals)														
'Magnacal' for oral or tube feeding, high-calorie, ready to use..............	1000 ml	5000	3.80	4.30	50.00	10.00	800.0	14.80	101.0	1010.0	18.2	200.0	1270	20.0
'Magnacal' for oral or tube feeding, high-calorie, ready to use..............	8 fl oz	1180	0.90	1.00	11.80	2.40	189.0	3.50	24.0	240.0	4.3	47.0	300	4.7
(Nestlé Clinical Nutrition)														
'Renalcal Diet' for oral or tube feeding, patients w/renal failure, high-calorie, kosher, lactose- and gluten-free, low-residue, ready to use..............	1000 ml	na	1.50	1.70	20.00	7.00	600.0	6.00	60.0	na	na	na	na	14.0
'Renalcal Diet' for oral or tube feeding, patients w/renal failure, high-calorie, kosher, lactose- and gluten-free, low-residue, ready to use..............	250 ml	na	0.38	0.43	5.00	1.80	150.0	1.50	15.0	na	na	na	na	3.5
(Ross)														
'Nepro' for oral or tube feeding (not parenteral use), dialzed patients, kosher, gluten- and lactose-free, low-residue, ready to use..............	1 liter	4210	2.50	2.90	33.70	8.80	1053.0	10.10	105.0	1368.0	18.9	211.0	1057	23.6
'Nepro' for oral or tube feeding (not parenteral use), dialzed patients, kosher, gluten- and lactose-free, low-residue, ready to use..........................	8 fl oz	1000	0.60	0.68	8.00	2.10	250.0	2.40	25.0	325.0	4.5	50.0	250	5.6
'Suplena' for oral or tube feeding (not parenteral use), predialyzed patients, kosher, gluten- and lactose-free, low-residue, ready to use..............	1 liter	1053	2.50	2.90	33.70	8.60	1053.0	10.10	105.0	1385	18.9	211.0	1116	23.6
'Suplena' for oral or tube feeding (not parenteral use), predialyzed patients, kosher, gluten- and lactose-free, low-residue, ready to use..............	8 fl oz	250	0.60	0.68	8.00	2.00	250.0	2.40	25.0	329.0	4.5	50.0	265	5.6
MEDLAR, JAPANESE. See LOQUAT.														
MELBA TOAST. See under CRACKER.														
MELON, CANTALOUPE / muskmelon														
balls	1 cup	5706	0.06	0.04	1.00	0.20	30.1	0.00	74.7	19.5	0.4	19.5	547	0.3
balls	10 balls	4449	0.05	0.03	0.79	0.16	23.5	0.00	58.2	15.2	0.3	15.2	426	0.2
cubed	1 cup	5158	0.06	0.03	0.92	0.18	27.2	0.00	67.5	17.6	0.3	17.6	494	0.3
diced	1 cup	5029	0.06	0.03	0.90	0.18	26.5	0.00	65.8	17.2	0.3	17.2	482	0.3
wedges, 1/8 of large melon..............	1 wedge	3288	0.04	0.02	0.58	0.12	17.3	0.00	43.0	11.2	0.2	11.2	315	0.2
1/8 of medium melon	1 wedge	2225	0.03	0.01	0.40	0.08	11.7	0.00	29.1	7.6	0.1	7.6	213	0.1
1/8 of small melon	1 wedge	1773	0.02	0.01	0.32	0.06	9.3	0.00	23.2	6.0	0.1	6.0	170	<0.1
whole, large, approx 6-1/2-inch diam	1 melon	26243	0.29	0.17	4.70	0.94	138	0.00	344.0	89.5	1.7	89.5	2515	1.3
whole, medium, approx 5-inch diam........	1 melon	17796	0.20	0.12	3.20	0.64	93.8	0.00	233.0	60.7	1.2	60.7	1706	0.9
whole, small, approx 4 1/4 inch diam	1 melon	14218	0.16	0.09	2.50	0.51	75.0	0.00	186.0	48.5	0.9	48.5	1363	0.7
MELON, CASABA														
cubed	1 cup	51	0.10	0.03	0.68	0.20	28.9	0.00	27.2	8.5	0.7	13.6	357	0.3
sliced, medium	1/10 melon	49	0.10	0.03	0.66	0.20	27.9	0.00	26.2	8.2	0.7	13.1	344	0.3
whole, medium	1 melon	492	0.98	0.33	6.60	2.00	279.0	0.00	262.0	82.0	6.6	131.0	3444	2.6
MELON, HONEYDEW														
balls	1 cup	71	0.14	0.03	1.10	0.10	10.6	0.00	43.9	10.6	0.1	12.4	480	0.1

Food Name	Serving Size	A I.U.	Thi mg	Rib mg	Nia mg	B₆ mg	Fol mcg	B₁₂ mcg	C mg	Calc mg	Iron mg	Mag mg	Pot mg	Zn mg
balls	10 balls	55	0.11	0.03	0.83	0.08	8.3	0.00	34.2	8.3	0.1	9.7	374	0.1
diced	1 cup	68	0.13	0.03	1.00	0.10	10.2	0.00	42.2	10.2	0.1	11.9	461	0.1
wedges, 1/8 of 5.25-inch diam melon	1 wedge	50	0.10	0.02	0.75	0.07	7.5	0.00	31.0	7.5	<0.1	8.8	339	<0.1
wedges, 1/8 of 6- to 7-inch diam melon	1 wedge	64	0.12	0.03	0.96	0.09	9.6	0.00	39.7	9.6	0.1	11.2	434	0.1
whole, approx 5.25-inch diam	1 melon	400	0.77	0.18	6.00	0.59	60.0	0.00	248.0	60.0	0.7	70.0	2710	0.7
whole, 6- to 7-inch diam	1 melon	512	0.99	0.23	7.70	0.76	76.8	0.00	317.0	76.8	0.9	89.6	3469	0.9

MENHADEN OIL. See under FISH OIL.

MEXICAN STYLE DINNER/ENTRÉE. See also individual listings.

(Patio)

w/tamale, beef enchilada, beans, rice	1 serving	628	na	na	na	na	na	na	4.9	241.0	2.9	na	na	na

MEXICAN POTATO. See JICAMA.

MILK

COW

Condensed

sweetened, canned	1 cup	1004	0.28	1.30	0.64	0.16	34.3	1.40	8.0	868.0	0.6	78.5	1136	2.9
sweetened, canned	1 fl oz	125	0.03	0.16	0.08	0.02	4.3	0.17	1.0	108.0	<0.1	9.8	142	0.4

Evaporated

Nonfat/skim

	1 cup	1004	0.12	0.79	0.45	0.14	22.0	0.61	3.2	741.0	0.7	69.1	849	2.3
	1/2 cup	502	0.06	0.40	0.22	0.07	11.0	0.31	1.6	371.0	0.4	34.6	424	1.2
	1 fl oz	125	0.01	0.10	0.06	0.02	2.7	0.08	0.4	92.3	<0.1	8.6	106	0.3

Whole

	1/2 cup	500	0.06	0.40	0.24	0.06	10.0	0.20	2.4	329.0	0.2	30.5	382	0.9
	1 fl oz	125	0.02	0.10	0.06	0.02	2.5	0.05	0.6	82.2	<0.1	7.6	96	0.2

Dry

Nonfat/skim

calcium-reduced	1/4 lb	9	0.18	1.90	0.75	0.34	55.9	4.50	7.5	316.0	0.4	67.8	768	4.6
calcium-reduced	1 oz	2	0.05	0.47	0.19	0.08	14.0	1.10	1.9	79.4	<0.1	17.0	193	1.1
instant	1 cup	1612	0.28	1.20	0.61	0.23	33.9	2.70	3.8	837.0	0.2	79.6	1160	3.0
instant	1/3 cup	545	0.10	0.40	0.20	0.08	11.5	0.92	1.3	283.0	<0.1	26.9	392	1.0
regular	1 cup	43	0.50	1.90	1.10	0.43	60.1	4.80	8.1	1508.0	0.4	132.0	2153	4.9
regular	1/4 cup	11	0.13	0.47	0.28	0.11	15.0	1.20	2.0	377.0	0.1	33.0	538	1.2
vitamin A	1 cup	2638	0.50	1.9	1.10	0.43	60.0	4.80	8.1	1508.0	0.4	132.0	2153	4.9
vitamin A	1/4 cup	659	0.13	0.47	0.28	0.11	15.0	1.20	2.0	377.0	0.1	33.0	538	1.2

Whole

	1 cup	1180	0.36	1.50	0.83	0.39	47.4	4.20	11.1	1168.0	0.6	108.0	1702	4.3
	1/4 cup	295	0.09	0.39	0.21	0.10	11.8	1.00	2.8	292.0	0.2	27.0	426	1.1

Fresh

Low-fat, 1% fat

vitamin A	1 quart	2001	0.38	1.60	0.85	0.42	49.8	3.60	9.5	1200.0	0.5	135.0	1524	3.8
vitamin A	1 cup	500	0.10	0.41	0.21	0.11	12.4	0.90	2.4	300.0	0.1	33.7	381	0.9
vitamin A, protein-fortified	1 quart	1998	0.44	1.90	0.98	0.49	58.1	4.20	11.3	1397.0	0.6	157.0	1774	4.4
vitamin A, protein-fortified	1 cup	499	0.11	0.47	0.25	0.12	14.5	1.00	2.8	349.0	0.2	39.3	444	1.1
vitamin A, school milk carton	1/2 pint	500	0.10	0.41	0.21	0.11	12.4	0.90	2.4	300.0	0.1	33.7	381	0.9
vitamin A, w/added nonfat milk solids	1 quart	1999	0.39	1.70	0.88	0.44	51.9	3.70	9.8	1251.0	0.5	141.0	1589	3.9
vitamin A, w/added nonfat milk solids	1 cup	500	0.10	0.42	0.22	0.11	13.0	0.94	2.5	313.0	0.1	35.2	397	0.9

Low-fat, 2% fat

vitamin A	1 quart	2001	0.38	1.60	0.84	0.42	49.8	3.60	9.3	1187.0	0.5	133.0	1507	3.8
vitamin A	1 cup	500	0.10	0.40	0.21	0.11	12.4	0.89	2.3	297.0	0.1	33.4	377	0.9
vitamin A, protein-fortified	1 quart	1998	0.44	1.90	0.99	0.50	59.0	4.20	11.0	1408.0	0.6	158.0	1788	4.4
vitamin A, protein-fortified	1 cup	499	0.11	0.48	0.25	0.13	14.8	1.10	2.8	352.0	0.2	39.6	447	1.1
vitamin A, school milk carton	1/2 pint	500	0.10	0.40	0.21	0.11	12.4	0.89	2.3	297.0	0.1	33.4	377	0.9
vitamin A, w/added nonfat milk solids	1 quart	1999	0.39	1.70	0.88	0.44	51.9	3.70	9.8	1251.0	0.5	141.0	1589	3.9

Food Name	Serving Size	A I.U.	Thi mg	Rib mg	Nia mg	B$_6$ mg	Fol mcg	B$_{12}$ mcg	C mg	Calc mg	Iron mg	Mag mg	Pot mg	Zn mg
vitamin A, w/added nonfat milk solids.......	1 cup	500	0.10	0.42	0.22	0.11	13.0	0.94	2.5	313.0	0.1	35.2	397	0.9
w/added nonfat milk solids..............	1 quart	735	0.44	1.90	0.99	0.45	52.9	3.80	11.0	1402.0	0.6	142.0	1781	4.0
w/added nonfat milk solids..............	1 cup	184	0.11	0.47	0.25	0.11	13.2	0.95	2.7	351.0	0.2	35.5	445	1.0
Nonfat/skim														
....	1 quart	69	0.35	1.40	0.86	0.39	49.0	3.70	9.6	1205.0	0.4	108.0	1627	3.9
....	1 cup	17	0.09	0.34	0.22	0.10	12.3	0.93	2.4	301.0	0.1	26.9	407	0.9
vitamin A..........................	1 quart	1999	0.35	1.40	0.86	0.39	51.0	3.70	9.6	1209.0	0.4	111.0	1623	3.9
vitamin A..........................	1 cup	500	0.09	0.34	0.22	0.10	12.7	0.93	2.4	302.0	0.1	27.8	406	0.9
vitamin A, protein-fortified.............	1 quart	1998	0.44	1.90	0.99	0.49	59.0	4.20	11.0	1407.0	0.6	158.0	1786	4.4
vitamin A, protein-fortified.............	1 cup	499	0.11	0.48	0.25	0.12	14.8	1.10	2.8	352.0	0.2	39.5	446	1.1
vitamin A, w/added nonfat milk solids.......	1 quart	1999	0.40	1.70	0.89	0.45	52.9	3.80	9.9	1265.0	0.5	142.0	1673	4.0
vitamin A, w/added nonfat milk solids.......	1 cup	500	0.10	0.43	0.22	0.11	13.2	0.95	2.5	316.0	0.1	35.5	418	1.0
Whole														
low-salt...........................	1 quart	1269	0.20	1.00	0.42	0.33	48.8	3.50	9.2	984.0	0.5	48.8	2467	3.7
low-salt...........................	1 cup	317	0.05	0.26	0.11	0.08	12.2	0.88	2.3	246.0	0.1	12.2	617	0.9
regular, 3.7% fat.....................	1 quart	1347	0.37	1.60	0.82	0.41	48.8	3.50	14.3	1161.0	0.5	131.0	1474	3.7
regular, 3.7% fat.....................	1 cup	337	0.09	0.39	0.20	0.10	12.2	0.87	3.6	290.0	0.1	32.7	368	0.9
regular, 3.25% fat....................	1 quart	1230	0.37	1.60	0.82	0.41	48.8	3.50	9.2	1165.0	0.5	131.0	1479	3.7
regular, 3.25% fat....................	1 cup	307	0.09	0.40	0.20	0.10	12.2	0.87	2.3	291.0	0.1	32.8	370	0.9
regular, 3.25% fat....................	1 tbsp	19	0.01	0.03	0.01	0.01	0.8	0.05	0.1	18.1	<0.1	2.0	23	<0.1
regular, 3.25% fat, school milk carton.......	1/2 pint	307	0.09	0.40	0.20	0.10	12.2	0.87	2.3	291.0	0.1	32.8	370	0.9
GOAT														
....	1 quart	1806	0.47	1.30	2.70	0.45	5.9	0.63	12.6	1303.0	0.5	136.0	1995	2.9
....	1 cup	451	0.12	0.34	0.68	0.11	1.5	0.16	3.1	326.0	0.1	34.1	499	0.7
....	1 fl oz	56	0.02	0.04	0.08	0.01	0.2	0.02	0.4	40.7	<0.1	4.3	62	<0.1
INDIAN BUFFALO														
....	1 quart	1737	0.51	1.30	0.89	0.22	54.7	3.50	22.0	1649.0	1.2	304.0	1734	2.1
....	1 cup	434	0.13	0.33	0.22	0.06	13.7	0.89	5.5	412.0	0.3	75.9	434	0.5
HUMAN														
....	1 cup	593	0.03	0.09	0.44	0.03	12.8	0.11	12.3	79.2	<0.1	8.4	126	0.4
....	1 fl oz	74	0.00	0.01	0.06	0.00	1.6	0.01	1.5	9.9	<0.1	1.0	16	<0.1
SHEEP														
....	1 quart	1441	0.64	3.50	4.10	0.59	68.6	7.00	40.8	1895.0	0.9	180.0	1338	5.3
....	1 cup	360	0.16	0.87	1.00	0.15	17.1	1.70	10.2	474.0	0.3	45.0	334	1.3
MILK SUBSTITUTE														
w/lauric acid oil, fluid....................	1 quart	0	0.12	0.86	0.00	0.00	0.0	0.00	0.0	317	3.8	62.3	1116	11.5
w/lauric acid oil, fluid....................	1 cup	0	0.03	0.22	0.00	0.00	0.0	0.00	0.0	79.3	0.9	15.6	279	2.9
w/hydrogenated vegetable oils, fluid........	1 quart	0	0.12	0.86	0.00	0.00	0.0	0.00	0.0	317	3.8	62.3	1116	11.5
w/hydrogenated vegetable oils, fluid........	1 cup	0	0.03	0.22	0.00	0.00	0.0	0.00	0.0	79.3	0.9	15.6	279	2.9
w/hydrogenated vegetable oils, fluid........	1 fl oz	0	0.00	0.03	0.00	0.00	0.0	0.00	0.0	9.9	0.12	1.9	35	0.4
MILKFISH. See AWA.														
MILLET														
cooked	1 cup	0	0.18	0.14	2.30	0.19	33.1	0.00	0.0	5.2	1.1	76.6	108	1.6
raw................................	1 cup	0	0.84	0.58	9.40	0.77	170.0	0.00	0.0	16.0	6.0	228.0	390	3.4
MISO....................	1 cup	239	0.27	0.69	2.40	0.59	90.8	0.00	0.0	182.0	7.5	116.0	451	9.1
MOLASSES														
....	1 cup	0	0.13	0.01	3.00	2.20	0.0	0.00	0.0	672.0	15.5	794	4802	0.9
....	1 tbsp	0	0.01	0.00	0.19	0.13	0.0	0.00	0.0	41.0	0.9	48.4	293	<0.1
blackstrap.........................	1 cup	0	0.11	0.17	3.50	2.30	3.3	0.00	0.0	2821.0	57.4	705.0	8174	3.3
blackstrap.........................	1 tbsp	0	0.01	0.01	0.22	0.14	0.2	0.00	0.0	172.0	3.5	43.0	498	0.2
MONKFISH / angler fish / bellyfish / frogfish / goosefish / sea devil														
baked, broiled, grilled, or microwaved	3 oz	39	0.03	0.06	2.2	0.23	6.8	0.88	0.9	8.5	0.4	22.9	436	0.5
raw................................	3 oz	34	0.02	0.05	1.80	0.20	6.0	0.77	0.9	6.8	0.3	17.9	340	0.4

Food Name	Serving Size	A I.U.	Thi mg	Rib mg	Nia mg	B_6 mg	Fol mcg	B_{12} mcg	C mg	Calc mg	Iron mg	Mag mg	Pot mg	Zn mg
MOOSE														
raw	3 oz	0	0.04	0.30	4.51	na	na	na	4.3	5.1	3.6	20.6	286	3.2
roasted	3 oz	0	0.04	0.29	4.50	0.32	3.4	5.40	4.3	5.1	3.6	20.4	284	3.1
MOTH BEAN. See BEAN, MOTH.														
MOUNTAIN YAM. See under YAM.														
MOUSSE MIX (Alsa) dark chocolate	2.5 tbsp	na	na	na	na	na	na	na	na	na	na	na	na	na
MULBERRY														
fresh, raw	1 cup	35	0.04	0.14	0.87	0.07	8.4	0.00	51.0	54.6	2.6	25.2	272	0.2
fresh, raw	10 medium	4	0.00	0.02	0.09	0.01	0.9	0.00	5.5	5.8	0.3	2.7	29	<0.1
MULLET, STRIPED														
baked, broiled, grilled, or microwaved	3 oz	120	0.09	0.09	5.4	0.42	8.3	0.21	1.0	26.4	1.2	28.1	389	0.75
raw	3 oz	104	0.08	0.07	4.4	0.36	7.2	0.19	1.0	34.9	0.87	24.6	303	0.44
MUNG BEAN. See BEAN, MUNG.														
MUNGO BEAN. See BEAN, MUNGO.														
MUSHROOM, BUTTON. See MUSHROOM, WHITE.														
MUSHROOM, CRIMINI														
brown, Italian, fresh, raw	1 piece	0	0.01	0.07	0.53	0.02	2.0	0.01	0.0	2.5	<0.1	1.3	63	0.2
MUSHROOM, ENOKI														
Fresh														
raw, whole	1 large	<1	0.00	0.01	0.18	0.00	1.5	0.00	0.6	<0.1	<0.1	0.8	19	<0.1
raw, whole	1 medium	<1	0.00	0.00	0.11	0.00	0.9	0.00	0.4	<0.1	<0.1	0.5	11	<0.1
MUSHROOM, OYSTER / abalone / hiritake / shimeji / tree mushroom														
raw	1 large	71	0.08	0.53	5.30	0.18	69.6	0.00	0.0	8.9	2.6	29.6	764	1.2
raw	1 small	7	0.01	0.05	0.54	0.02	7.0	0.00	0.0	0.9	0.3	3.0	77	0.1
MUSHROOM, SHIITAKE														
Dried														
whole	4 medium	0	0.05	0.19	2.10	0.14	24.5	0.00	0.5	1.6	0.3	19.8	230	1.1
whole	1 medium	0	0.01	0.05	0.51	0.04	5.9	0.00	0.1	0.4	<0.1	4.8	55	0.3
Fresh														
cooked, pieces	1 cup	0	0.05	0.25	2.20	0.23	30.3	0.00	0.4	4.3	0.6	20.3	170	1.9
cooked, whole	4 medium	0	0.03	0.12	1.10	0.11	15.0	0.00	0.2	2.2	0.3	10.1	84	0.9
MUSHROOM, STRAW														
Canned														
pieces, drained	1 cup	0	0.02	0.13	0.41	0.03	69.2	0.00	0.0	18.2	2.6	12.7	142	1.2
pieces, drained	1 med piece	0	0.00	0.00	0.01	0.00	2.1	0.00	0.0	0.6	<0.1	0.4	4	<0.1
MUSHROOM, TREE. See MUSHROOM, OYSTER.														
MUSHROOM, WHITE / button mushroom														
Canned														
caps, drained	8 caps	0	0.04	0.01	0.75	0.03	5.8	0.00	0.0	5.2	0.4	7.0	61	0.3
pieces, drained	1 cup	0	0.13	0.03	2.50	0.10	19.2	0.00	0.0	17.2	1.2	23.4	201	1.1
pieces, drained	1/2 cup	0	0.07	0.02	1.20	0.05	9.6	0.00	0.0	8.6	0.6	11.7	101	0.6
slices, drained	10 slices	0	0.03	0.01	0.64	0.02	4.9	0.00	0.0	4.4	0.3	6.0	52	0.3
whole, drained, large	1 mushroom	0	0.01	0.00	0.26	0.01	2.0	0.00	0.0	1.8	0.1	2.4	21	0.1
whole, drained, medium	1 mushroom	0	0.01	0.00	0.19	0.01	1.5	0.00	0.0	1.3	0.1	1.8	16	<0.1
whole, drained, small	1 mushroom	0	0.01	0.00	0.11	0.00	0.9	0.00	0.0	0.8	<0.1	1.1	9	<0.1
Fresh														
boiled drained, sliced	1 cup	0	0.11	0.47	7.00	0.15	28.4	0.00	6.2	9.4	2.7	18.7	555	1.4
boiled, drained, chopped	1 tbsp	0	0.01	0.03	0.44	0.01	1.8	0.00	0.4	0.6	0.2	1.2	35	<0.1
boiled, drained, sliced	1/2 cup	0	0.06	0.23	3.50	0.07	14.2	0.00	3.1	4.7	1.4	9.4	278	0.7
boiled, drained, whole, medium	1 mushroom	0	0.01	0.04	0.54	0.01	2.2	0.00	0.5	0.7	0.2	1.4	43	0.1
raw, pieces or slices	1 cup	0	0.06	0.30	2.80	0.07	8.4	0.03	1.6	3.5	0.7	7.0	259	0.5
raw, sliced	1/2 cup	0	0.03	0.15	1.40	0.04	4.2	0.01	0.8	1.8	0.4	3.5	130	0.3
raw, whole	1 cup	0	0.09	0.41	3.90	0.10	11.5	0.04	2.2	4.8	0.0	9.6	355	0.7

Food Name	Serving Size	A I.U.	Thi mg	Rib mg	Nia mg	B$_6$ mg	Fol mcg	B$_{12}$ mcg	C mg	Calc mg	Iron mg	Mag mg	Pot mg	Zn mg
raw, whole, large	1 mushroom	0	0.02	0.10	0.93	0.02	2.8	0.01	0.5	1.1	0.2	2.3	85	0.2
raw, whole, medium	1 mushroom	0	0.02	0.08	0.73	0.02	2.2	0.01	0.4	0.9	0.2	1.8	67	0.1
raw, whole, small	1 mushroom	0	0.01	0.04	0.40	0.01	1.2	0.00	0.2	0.5	0.1	1.0	37	<0.1
MUSKMELON. See MELON, CANTALOUPE.														
MUSKRAT, RAW														
raw	1 oz	0	0.03	0.15	1.80	na	na	na	1.4	7.1	na	6.2	78	na
roasted	3 oz	0	0.07	0.60	6.10	0.40	9.3	7.10	6.0	30.6	6.0	22.1	272	1.9
MUSSEL, BLUE														
boiled, poached, or steamed	3 oz	258	0.26	0.36	2.50	0.09	64.3	20.40	11.6	28.1	5.7	31.4	228	2.3
raw	1 cup	240	0.24	0.32	2.40	0.08	63.0	18.00	12.0	39.0	5.9	51.0	480	2.4
raw	3 oz	136	0.14	0.18	1.40	0.04	35.7	10.20	6.8	22.1	3.4	28.9	272	1.4
raw, large	1 mussel	32	0.03	0.04	0.32	0.01	8.4	2.40	1.6	5.2	0.8	6.8	64	0.3
raw, medium	1 mussel	26	0.03	0.03	0.26	0.01	6.7	1.90	1.3	4.2	0.6	5.4	51	0.3
raw, small	1 mussel	16	0.02	0.02	0.16	0.01	4.2	1.20	0.8	2.6	0.4	3.4	32	0.2
raw, w/o shell	1 oz	45	0.05	0.06	0.45	0.01	11.9	3.40	2.3	7.4	1.1	9.6	91	0.5
MUSTARD, PREPARED														
yellow	1 cup	330	0.13	0.06	1.10	0.18	20.0	0.00	7.3	200.0	4.6	95.0	378	1.5
yellow	1 tsp	7	0.00	0.00	0.02	0.00	0.4	0.00	0.1	4.0	<0.1	1.9	8	<0.1
MUSTARD GREENS														
Fresh														
boiled, drained, chopped	1 cup	4243	0.06	0.09	0.61	0.14	103.0	0.00	35.4	104.0	0.9	21.0	283	0.2
raw, chopped	1 cup	2968	0.05	0.06	0.45	0.10	105.0	0.00	39.2	57.7	0.8	17.9	198	0.1
Frozen														
boiled, drained	10-oz pkg	9476	0.09	0.11	0.55	0.23	147.0	0.00	29.3	214.0	2.4	27.6	295	0.4
boiled, drained, chopped, no salt added	1 cup	6705	0.06	0.08	0.39	0.16	104.0	0.00	20.7	152.0	1.7	19.5	209	0.3
boiled, drained, chopped or diced	1/2 cup	3353	0.03	0.04	0.19	0.08	52.1	0.00	10.3	75.8	0.8	9.8	104	0.2
boiled, drained, no salt added	10-oz pkg	9476	0.09	0.11	0.55	0.23	147.0	0.00	29.3	214.0	2.4	27.6	295	0.4
chopped, unprepared	1 cup	7526	0.07	0.09	0.46	0.19	202.0	0.00	36.9	169.0	1.9	21.9	248	0.3
unprepared	10-oz pkg	14640	0.14	0.17	0.89	0.37	393.0	0.00	71.9	329.0	3.7	42.6	483	0.7
MUSTARD OIL														
	1 cup	0	0.00	0.00	0.00	0.00	0.0	0.00	0.0	0.0	0.0	0.0	0	0.0
	1 tbsp	0	0.00	0.00	0.00	0.00	0.0	0.00	0.0	0.0	0.0	0.0	0	0.0
MUSTARD SEED														
yellow	1 tbsp	7	0.06	0.04	0.88	0.03	8.5	0.00	0.3	58.4	1.1	33.4	76	0.6
yellow	1 tsp	2	0.02	0.01	0.26	0.01	2.5	0.00	0.1	17.2	0.3	9.8	23	0.2
MUSTARD SPINACH / tendergreen														
boiled, drained, chopped	1 cup	14760	0.07	0.11	0.77	0.17	131.0	0.00	117.0	284.0	1.4	12.6	513	0.2
raw, chopped	1 cup	14850	0.10	0.14	1.00	0.23	238.0	0.00	195.0	315.0	2.3	16.5	674	0.3
MUTTON TALLOW														
	1 cup	0	0.00	0.00	0.00	0.00	0.0	0.00	0.0	0.0	0.0	0.0	0	0.0
	1 tbsp	0	0.00	0.00	0.00	0.00	0.0	0.00	0.0	0.0	0.0	0.0	0	0.0
MUTTONFISH. See OCEAN POUT.														

N

Food Name	Serving Size	A I.U.	Thi mg	Rib mg	Nia mg	B$_6$ mg	Fol mcg	B$_{12}$ mcg	C mg	Calc mg	Iron mg	Mag mg	Pot mg	Zn mg
NAPA. See BOK CHOY.														
NAPOLES														
cooked	1 cup	684	0.02	0.06	0.44	0.10	4.5	0.00	7.9	244.0	0.8	70.0	291	0.3
cooked	1 pad	133	0.00	0.01	0.09	0.02	0.9	0.00	1.5	47.6	0.1	13.6	57	<0.1
raw, sliced	1 cup	357	0.01	0.04	0.45	0.06	2.6	0.00	11.5	140.0	0.6	49.9	274	0.3

Food Name	Serving Size	A I.U.	Thi mg	Rib mg	Nia mg	B$_6$ mg	Fol mcg	B$_{12}$ mcg	C mg	Calc mg	Iron mg	Mag mg	Pot mg	Zn mg
NATAL PLUM. See CARISSA.														
NATTO	1 cup	0	0.28	0.33	0.00	0.23	14.0	0.00	22.8	380.0	15.1	201.0	1276	5.3
NAVY BEAN. See BEAN, NAVY.														
NECTARINE														
raw, sliced	1 cup	1016	0.02	0.06	1.40	0.04	5.1	0.00	7.5	6.9	0.2	11.0	293	0.1
raw, trimmed, whole, approx 2.5 inch diam	1 nectarine	1001	0.02	0.06	1.30	0.03	5.0	0.00	7.3	6.8	0.2	10.9	288	0.1
NEW ZEALAND SPINACH. See SPINACH, NEW ZEALAND.														
NOODLE. See also PASTA.														
CELLOPHANE. See under CHINESE.														
CHINESE														
cellophane/long rice, mung bean, dry	1 cup	0	0.21	0.00	0.28	0.07	2.8	0.00	0.0	35.0	3.0	4.2	14	0.6
chow mein	1 cup	38	0.26	0.19	2.70	0.05	40.5	0.00	0.0	9.0	2.1	23.4	54	0.6
chow mein	1.5 oz	37	0.25	0.18	2.60	0.05	38.7	0.00	0.0	8.6	2.0	22.4	52	0.6
rice, cooked	1 cup	0	0.03	0.01	0.13	0.01	5.3	0.00	0.0	7.0	0.3	5.3	7	0.4
EGG														
enriched, cooked	1 cup	32	0.30	0.13	2.40	0.06	102	0.14	0.0	19.2	2.5	30.4	45	1.0
enriched, dry	2 oz	35	0.60	0.27	4.60	0.07	132	0.23	0.0	17.7	2.6	34.2	133	0.9
enriched, dry	1 cup	24	0.40	0.18	3.10	0.05	87.8	0.15	0.0	11.8	1.7	22.8	89	0.6
spinach, enriched, cooked	1 cup	165	0.39	0.20	2.40	0.18	102	0.22	0.0	30.4	1.7	38.4	59	1.0
spinach, enriched, dry	2 oz	180	0.62	0.27	3.70	0.23	132	0.23	0.0	31.9	2.4	46.7	202	1.0
spinach, enriched, dry	1 cup	120	0.41	0.18	2.50	0.16	87.8	0.15	0.0	21.3	1.6	31.2	135	0.7
unenriched, cooked	1 cup	32	0.05	0.03	0.64	0.06	11.2	0.14	0.0	19.2	0.9	30.4	45	1.0
unenriched, dry	1 cup	24	0.07	0.03	0.80	0.05	11.0	0.15	0.0	11.8	0.7	22.8	89	0.6
JAPANESE														
soba, cooked	1 cup	0	0.11	0.03	0.58	0.05	8.0	0.00	0.0	4.6	0.6	10.3	40	0.1
soba, dry	2 oz	0	0.27	0.07	1.80	0.14	34.2	0.00	0.0	19.9	1.5	54.1	144	0.9
somen, cooked	1 cup	0	0.04	0.06	0.17	0.02	3.5	0.00	0.0	14.1	0.9	3.5	51	0.4
somen, dry	2 oz	0	0.06	0.02	0.50	0.03	8.0	0.00	0.0	13.1	0.8	16.0	94	0.3
RICE. See under CHINESE.														
SOBA. See under JAPANESE.														
UDON. See under JAPANESE.														
NORTHERN PIKE. See under PIKE.														
NORWAY HADDOCK. See OCEAN PERCH, ATLANTIC.														
NUTMEG BUTTER OIL														
. . . .	1 cup	0	0.00	0.00	0.00	0.00	0.0	0.00	0.0	0.0	0.0	0.0	0	0.0
. . . .	1 tbsp	0	0.00	0.00	0.00	0.00	0.0	0.00	0.0	0.0	0.0	0.0	0	0.0
NUTMEG														
ground	1 tbsp	7	0.02	0.00	0.09	0.02	5.3	0.00	0.2	12.9	0.2	12.8	25	0.2
ground	1 tsp	2	0.01	0.00	0.03	0.01	1.7	0.00	<0.1	4.1	<0.1	4.0	8	<0.1
NUTS, MIXED														
Dry-roasted														
w/peanuts, salted	1 cup	21	0.27	0.27	6.40	0.41	69.0	0.00	0.6	95.9	5.1	308.0	818	5.2
w/peanuts, salted	1 oz	4	0.06	0.06	1.30	0.08	14.3	0.00	0.1	19.8	1.0	63.8	169	1.1
w/peanuts, unsalted	1 cup	21	0.27	0.27	6.40	0.41	69.0	0.00	0.6	95.9	5.1	308.0	818	5.2
w/peanuts, unsalted	1 oz	4	0.06	0.06	1.30	0.08	14.3	0.00	0.1	19.8	1.0	63.8	169	1.1
Oil-roasted														
w/peanuts, salted	1 cup	29	0.73	0.70	2.80	0.26	81.2	0.00	0.7	153.0	3.7	361.0	783	6.7
w/peanuts, salted	1 oz	6	0.14	0.14	0.56	0.05	16.0	0.00	0.1	30.1	0.7	71.2	154	1.3
w/peanuts, unsalted	1 cup	27	0.71	0.32	7.20	0.34	118	0.00	0.7	153.0	4.6	334.0	825	7.2
w/peanuts, unsalted	1 oz	5	0.14	0.06	1.40	0.07	23.5	0.00	0.1	30.6	0.9	66.6	165	1.4
w/o peanuts, unsalted	1 cup	29	0.73	0.70	2.80	0.26	81.2	0.00	0.7	153.0	3.7	361.0	783	6.7
w/o peanuts, unsalted	1 oz	6	0.14	0.14	0.56	0.05	16.0	0.00	0.1	30.1	0.7	71.2	154	1.3

O

Food Name	Serving Size	A I.U.	Thi mg	Rib mg	Nia mg	B₆ mg	Fol mcg	B₁₂ mcg	C mg	Calc mg	Iron mg	Mag mg	Pot mg	Zn mg
OAT. See also under CEREAL, HOT.														
. . . .	1 cup	0	1.20	0.22	1.50	0.19	87.4	0.00	0.0	84.2	7.4	276.0	669	6.2
OAT BRAN														
cooked	1 cup	0	0.35	0.07	0.32	0.06	13.1	0.00	0.0	21.9	1.9	87.6	201	1.2
raw	1 cup	0	1.10	0.21	0.88	0.16	48.9	0.00	0.0	54.5	5.1	221.0	532	2.9
OAT VEGETABLE OIL														
. . . .	1 cup	0	0.00	0.00	0.00	0.00	0.0	0.00	0.0	0.0	0.0	0.0	0	0.0
. . . .	1 tbsp	0	0.00	0.00	0.00	0.00	0.0	0.00	0.0	0.0	0.0	0.0	0	0.0
OCEAN CATFISH. See WOLF FISH.														
OCEAN PERCH, ATLANTIC / Norway haddock / red perch / rose perch														
baked, broiled, grilled, or microwaved	3 oz	39	0.11	0.11	2.10	0.23	8.8	0.98	0.7	116.0	1.0	33.1	298	0.5
raw	3 oz	34	0.09	0.09	1.70	0.20	7.7	0.85	0.7	91.0	0.8	25.5	232	0.4
raw, boneless	1 oz	11	0.03	0.03	0.57	0.07	2.6	0.28	0.2	30.3	0.3	8.5	77.4	0.1
OCEAN POUT / muttonfish														
baked, broiled, grilled, or microwaved	3 oz	39	0.08	0.06	2.20	0.23	6.8	0.88	0.0	11.1	0.3	14.4	436	1.1
raw	3 oz	34	0.07	0.05	1.80	0.20	6.0	0.77	0.0	8.5	0.2	11.1	340	0.9
OCEANIC BONITO. See under TUNA.														
OCTOPUS														
common, boiled, poached, or steamed	3 oz	230	0.05	0.07	3.20	0.55	20.4	30.60	6.8	90.1	8.1	51.0	536	2.9
common, raw	3 oz	128	0.03	0.03	1.80	0.31	13.6	17.00	4.3	45.0	4.5	25.5	298	1.4
OHELOBERRY														
raw	1 cup	1162	0.02	0.05	0.38	na	na	0.00	8.4	9.8	0.1	8.4	53	na
raw	10 medium	91	0.00	0.00	0.03	na	na	0.00	0.7	0.8	<0.1	0.7	4	na
OKRA														
Fresh														
boiled, drained, sliced	1/2 cup	473	0.09	0.11	0.72	0.04	134.0	0.00	11	88.3	0.6	46.9	215	0.6
boiled, drained, whole, approx 3-inch														
long	8 pods	489	0.11	0.05	0.74	0.16	38.8	0.00	14	53.5	0.4	48.5	274	0.5
raw, sliced	1 cup	660	0.20	0.06	1.00	0.22	87.8	0.00	21	81.0	0.8	57.0	303	0.6
raw, whole, approx 3-inch long	8 pods	627	0.19	0.06	0.95	0.20	83.4	0.00	20	77.0	0.8	54.1	288	0.6
Frozen														
boiled, drained	10-oz pkg	1311	0.25	0.31	2.00	0.12	371.0	0.00	31	245.0	1.7	130.0	597	1.6
boiled, drained, no salt added	10-oz pkg	1311	0.25	0.31	2.00	0.12	371.0	0.00	31	245.0	1.7	130.0	597	1.6
unprepared	10-oz pkg	1315	0.25	0.30	2.00	0.12	419.0	0.00	35	230.0	1.6	122.0	599	1.5
unprepared	3-lb pkg	6301	1.20	1.40	9.60	0.57	2009.0	0.00	169	1102.0	7.8	585.0	2872	7.2
OLIVE														
chopped	1 tbsp	34	0.00	0.00	0.00	0.00	0.0	0.00	<0.1	7.4	0.3	0.3	<1	<0.1
whole, jumbo	1 olive	29	0.00	0.00	0.00	0.00	0.0	0.00	0.1	7.8	0.3	0.3	<1	<0.1
whole, large	1 olive	18	0.00	0.00	0.00	0.00	0.0	0.00	<0.1	3.9	0.1	0.2	<1	<0.1
whole, small	1 olive	13	0.00	0.00	0.00	0.00	0.0	0.00	<0.1	2.8	0.1	0.1	<1	<0.1
whole, super colossal	1 olive	53	0.00	0.00	0.00	0.00	0.0	0.00	0.2	14.3	0.5	0.6	1	<0.1
OLIVE OIL														
salad or cooking	1 cup	0	0.00	0.00	0.00	0.00	0.0	0.00	0.0	0.4	0.8	<0.1	0	0.1
salad or cooking	1 tbsp	0	0.00	0.00	0.00	0.00	0.0	0.00	0.0	<0.1	<0.1	0.0	0	<0.1
ONION														
GREEN. See SCALLION.														
RED, WHITE, OR YELLOW														
Canned														
chopped or diced, w/liquid	1/2 cup	0	0.04	0.01	0.07	0.15	10.9	0.00	4.8	50.4	0.2	6.7	124	0.3
whole, w/liquid	1 medium	0	0.02	0.00	0.04	0.09	6.1	0.00	2.7	28.4	<0.1	3.8	70	0.2

Food Name	Serving Size	A I.U.	Thi mg	Rib mg	Nia mg	B6 mg	Fol mcg	B12 mcg	C mg	Calc mg	Iron mg	Mag mg	Pot mg	Zn mg
Fresh														
boiled, drained, chopped	1 cup	0	0.09	0.05	0.35	0.27	31.5	0.00	10.9	46.2	0.5	23.1	349	0.4
boiled, drained, chopped	1 tbsp	0	0.01	0.00	0.03	0.02	2.3	0.00	0.8	3.3	<0.1	1.6	25	<0.1
boiled, drained, chopped or diced	1/2 cup	36	0.02	0.03	0.15	0.07	14.1	0.00	2.7	16.8	0.3	6.3	113	<0.1
boiled, drained, chopped or diced	1 tbsp	5	0.00	0.00	0.02	0.01	2.0	0.00	0.4	2.4	<0.1	0.9	16	<0.1
boiled, drained, sliced, medium, 1/8 inch thick	1 slice	0	0.01	0.00	0.02	0.02	1.8	0.00	0.6	2.6	<0.1	1.3	20	<0.1
boiled, drained, whole.	1 cup	44	0.03	0.04	0.28	0.15	28.1	0.00	10.7	56.7	0.7	16.8	212	0.2
boiled, drained, whole, medium, approx 2.5-inch diam	1 onion	0	0.04	0.02	0.16	0.12	14.1	0.00	4.9	20.7	0.2	10.3	156	0.2
raw, chopped	1 cup	0	0.07	0.03	0.24	0.19	30.4	0.00	10.2	32.0	0.4	16.0	251	0.3
raw, chopped	1 tbsp	0	0.00	0.00	0.02	0.01	1.9	0.00	0.6	2.0	<0.1	1.0	16	<0.1
raw, sliced.	1 cup	0	0.05	0.02	0.17	0.13	21.9	0.00	7.4	23.0	0.3	11.5	181	0.2
raw, sliced, medium, 1/8-inch thick	1 slice	0	0.01	0.00	0.02	0.02	2.7	0.00	0.9	2.8	<0.1	1.4	22	<0.1
raw, whole, medium, approx 2.5-inch diam	1 onion	0	0.05	0.02	0.16	0.13	20.9	0.00	7.0	22.0	0.2	11.0	173	0.2
Frozen														
chopped, unprepared	10-oz pkg	99	0.09	0.08	0.43	0.21	49.1	0.00	9.4	48.3	0.94	19.9	352	0.20
whole, unprepared	10-oz pkg	74	0.07	0.07	0.50	0.26	60.2	0.00	22.7	102	1.3	28.4	403	0.34
ONION FLAKES														
dehydrated	1 tbsp	0	0.03	0.01	0.05	0.08	8.3	0.00	3.8	12.8	0.08	4.6	81.1	0.10
dehydrated	1/4 cup	0	0.07	0.01	0.14	0.22	23.2	0.00	10.5	36.0	0.22	12.9	227	0.27
ONION POWDER														
. . . .	1 tbsp	0	0.03	0.00	0.04	0.10	10.8	0.00	0.95	23.6	0.17	7.9	61.3	0.15
. . . .	1 tsp	0	0.01	0.00	0.01	0.03	3.5	0.00	0.31	7.6	0.05	2.6	19.8	0.05
OPOSSUM, roasted.	3 oz	0	0.09	0.32	7.20	0.40	8.5	7.10	0	14.4	3.9	28.9	372	1.9
ORANGE														
ALL VARIETIES														
raw, peeled, sections	1 cup	369	0.16	0.07	0.51	0.11	54.5	0.00	95.8	72.0	0.18	18.0	326	0.13
raw, peeled, whole, large, approx 3 1/16 inch diam.	1 orange	377	0.16	0.07	0.52	0.11	55.8	0.00	97.9	73.6	0.18	18.4	333	0.13
raw, peeled, whole, medium, approx 2 5/8 inch diam.	1 orange	269	0.11	0.05	0.37	0.08	39.7	0.00	69.7	52.4	0.13	13.1	237	0.09
raw, peeled, whole, small, approx 2 3/8 inch diam.	1 orange	197	0.08	0.04	0.27	0.06	29.1	0.00	51.1	38.4	0.10	9.6	174	0.07
raw, w/peel	1 cup	425	0.17	0.09	0.85	0.16	51.0	0.00	121	119	1.4	23.8	333	0.19
raw, medium, w/peel, w/o seeds.	1 orange	398	0.16	0.08	0.80	0.15	47.7	0.00	113	111	1.3	22.3	312	0.17
CALIFORNIA														
Navel														
peeled, raw, sections, w/o membranes	1 cup	302	0.14	0.07	0.48	0.11	55.6	0.00	94.5	66.0	0.20	16.5	294	0.10
peeled, raw, whole, medium, approx 2 7/8 inch diam.	1 orange	256	0.12	0.06	0.41	0.10	47.2	0.00	80.2	56.0	0.17	14.0	249	0.08
Valencia														
peeled, raw, sections, w/o membranes.	1 cup	414	0.16	0.07	0.49	0.11	69.5	0.00	87.3	72.0	0.16	18.0	322	0.11
peeled, raw, whole, medium, approx 2 5/8 inch diam.	1 orange	278	0.11	0.05	0.33	0.08	46.7	0.00	58.7	48.4	0.11	12.1	217	0.07
FLORIDA														
raw, whole, peeled, medium, approx 2 11/16 inch diam.	1 orange	302	0.15	0.06	0.60	0.08	26.1	0.00	68.0	64.9	0.14	15.1	255	0.12
raw, whole, peeled, medium, approx 2 5/8 inch diam.	1 orange	282	0.14	0.06	0.56	0.07	24.4	0.00	63.5	60.6	0.13	14.1	238	0.11
raw, sections, peeled, w/o membranes	1 cup	370	0.19	0.07	0.74	0.09	32.0	0.00	83.3	79.5	0.17	18.5	313	0.15

ORANGE DRINK. See under FRUIT DRINK MIX.

Food Name	Serving Size	A I.U.	Thi mg	Rib mg	Nia mg	B$_6$ mg	Fol mcg	B$_{12}$ mcg	C mg	Calc mg	Iron mg	Mag mg	Pot mg	Zn mg
ORANGE JUICE														
California, refrigerated....................	1 cup	364	0.28	0.05	0.70	0.13	72.2	0.00	106	24.9	0.42	27.4	473	0.10
California, refrigerated	1 fl oz	45	0.04	0.01	0.09	0.02	9.0	0.00	13.3	3.1	0.05	3.4	59.1	0.01
fresh-squeezed..........................	1 cup	496	0.22	0.07	0.99	0.10	75.1	0.00	124	27.3	0.50	27.3	496	0.12
fresh-squeezed..........................	1 fl oz	62	0.03	0.01	0.12	0.01	9.4	0.00	15.5	3.4	0.06	3.4	62.0	0.02
fresh-squeezed, juice from 1 medium	3 oz	172	0.08	0.03	0.34	0.03	26.1	0.00	43.0	9.5	0.17	9.5	172	0.04
frozen concentrate, prepared	1 cup	194	0.20	0.05	0.50	0.11	109.0	0.00	96.9	22.4	0.25	24.9	473	0.13
frozen concentrate, prepared	1 fl oz	24	0.03	0.01	0.06	0.01	13.6	0.00	12.1	2.8	0.03	3.1	59.1	0.02
frozen concentrate, undiluted	1 cup	784	0.80	0.18	2.00	0.44	441.0	0.00	392	90.9	0.99	96.6	1914	0.51
frozen concentrate, undiluted............	6 fl oz	588	0.60	0.14	1.50	0.33	331.0	0.00	294	68.2	0.75	72.4	1436	0.38
frozen concentrate, undiluted............	1 fl oz	98	0.10	0.02	0.25	0.06	55.1	0.00	49.0	11.4	0.12	12.1	239	0.06
refrigerated.	1 cup	194	0.28	0.05	0.70	0.13	45.1	0.00	81.9	24.9	0.42	27.4	473	0.10
refrigerated.	1 fl oz	24	0.04	0.01	0.09	0.02	5.6	0.00	10.2	3.1	0.05	3.4	59.1	0.01
unsweetened, canned.	1 cup	436	0.15	0.07	0.78	0.22	45.1	0.00	85.7	19.9	1.1	27.4	436	0.17
unsweetened, canned.	1 fl oz	54	0.02	0.01	0.10	0.03	5.6	0.00	10.7	2.5	0.14	3.4	54.4	0.02
unsweetened, juice box	8.45 fl oz	460	0.16	0.07	0.83	0.23	47.6	0.00	90.5	21.0	1.2	28.9	460	0.18
ORANGE JUICE BLEND. See under FRUIT JUICE BLEND.														
ORANGE PEEL														
grated, raw	1 tbsp	25	0.01	0.01	0.05	0.01	1.8	0.00	8.2	9.7	0.05	1.3	12.7	0.02
grated, raw	1 tsp	8	0.00	0.00	0.02	0.00	0.6	0.00	2.7	3.2	0.02	0.44	4.2	0.01
ORANGE ROUGHY / slimehead														
baked, broiled, grilled, or microwaved	3 oz	69	0.10	0.16	3.10	0.29	6.8	2.00	0	32.3	0.20	32.3	327	0.82
raw	3 oz	59	0.09	0.13	2.50	0.26	6.0	1.70	0	25.5	0.15	25.5	255	0.64
OREGANO														
ground	1 tbsp	311	0.02	0.01	0.28	0.05	12.3	0.00	2.3	70.9	2.0	12.2	75.1	0.20
ground	1 tsp	104	0.01	0.01	0.09	0.02	4.1	0.00	0.75	23.6	0.66	4.0	25.0	0.07
ORIENTAL RADISH. See DAIKON.														
OYSTER														
EASTERN														
Canned														
....	3 oz	255	0.13	0.14	1.10	0.08	7.6	16.30	4.3	38.3	5.7	45.9	195	77.3
....	1 medium	24	0.01	0.01	0.10	0.01	0.7	1.50	0.4	3.6	0.5	4.3	18	7.3
drained	1 oz	69	0.04	0.04	0.29	0.02	2.0	4.40	1.1	10.3	1.5	12.4	53	20.9
drained	1 cup	486	0.24	0.27	2.00	0.15	14.4	31.00	8.1	72.9	10.9	87.5	371	147.0
w/liquid	12 oz	816	0.41	0.45	3.40	0.26	24.2	52.00	13.6	122.0	18.2	147.0	623	247.0
w/liquid	1 cup	744	0.37	0.41	3.10	0.24	22.1	47.50	12.4	112.0	16.6	134.0	568	226.0
Fresh														
breaded and fried	3 oz	257	0.13	0.17	1.40	0.05	26.4	13.30	3.2	52.7	5.9	49.3	207	74.1
breaded and fried	6 medium	266	0.13	0.18	1.50	0.06	27.3	13.80	3.3	54.6	6.1	51.0	215	76.7
farmed, cooked......................	3 oz	54	0.11	0.05	1.50	0.07	20.4	20.70	5.1	47.6	6.6	28.1	129	38.4
farmed, cooked......................	6 medium	37	0.08	0.03	1.10	0.05	14.2	14.30	3.5	33.0	4.6	19.5	90	26.6
farmed, raw.........................	3 oz	21	0.09	0.06	1.10	0.05	15.3	13.80	4.0	37.4	4.9	28.1	105	32.2
farmed, raw.........................	6 medium	21	0.09	0.06	1.10	0.05	15.1	13.60	3.9	37.0	4.9	27.7	104	31.9
wild, cooked, dry heat.................	3 oz	0	0.07	0.07	1.40	0.08	15.3	23.60	3.5	38.3	3.7	39.1	143	62.6
wild, cooked, dry heat.................	6 medium	0	0.05	0.05	0.99	0.05	10.6	16.40	2.4	26.6	2.6	27.1	99	43.4
wild, cooked, moist heat...............	3 oz	153	0.16	0.15	2.10	0.10	11.9	38.00	5.1	76.5	10.2	80.8	239	154.0
wild, cooked, moist heat...............	6 medium	76	0.08	0.08	1.00	0.05	5.9	14.70	2.5	37.8	5.0	39.9	118	76.3
wild, raw............................	1 cup	248	0.25	0.24	3.40	0.15	24.8	48.30	9.2	112.0	16.5	117.0	387	225.0
wild, raw............................	6 medium	84	0.08	0.08	1.20	0.05	8.4	16.30	3.1	37.8	5.6	39.5	131	76.3
PACIFIC														
cooked	3 oz	413	0.11	0.38	3.10	0.08	12.8	24.50	10.9	13.6	7.8	37.4	257	28.3
cooked	1 medium	122	0.03	0.11	0.90	0.02	3.8	7.20	3.2	4.0	2.3	11.0	76	8.3
raw	3 oz	230	0.06	0.20	1.70	0.04	8.5	13.60	6.8	6.8	4.3	18.7	143	14.1
raw	1 medium	135	0.03	0.12	1.00	0.03	5.0	8.00	4.0	4.0	2.6	11.0	84	8.3

Food Name	Serving Size	A I.U.	Thi mg	Rib mg	Nia mg	B₆ mg	Fol mcg	B₁₂ mcg	C mg	Calc mg	Iron mg	Mag mg	Pot mg	Zn mg

OYSTER MUSHROOM. See MUSHROOM, OYSTER.
OYSTER PLANT. See SALSIFY.

P

Food Name	Serving Size	A I.U.	Thi mg	Rib mg	Nia mg	B₆ mg	Fol mcg	B₁₂ mcg	C mg	Calc mg	Iron mg	Mag mg	Pot mg	Zn mg
PACIFIC COD. See under COD.														
PACIFIC MACKEREL. See under MACKEREL.														
PACIFIC MACKEREL. See ROCKFISH, PACIFIC.														
PAK-CHOI. See BOK CHOY.														
PALM, HEARTS OF														
Canned														
....	1 cup	0	0.02	0.08	0.64	0.03	56.9	0.00	11.5	84.7	4.6	55.5	258	1.7
....	1 piece	0	0.00	0.02	0.14	0.01	12.9	0.00	2.6	19.1	1.0	12.5	58	0.4
PALM KERNEL OIL / babassu oil														
....	1 cup	0	0.00	0.00	0.00	0.00	0.0	0.00	0.0	0.0	0.0	0.0	0	0.0
....	1 tbsp	0	0.00	0.00	0.00	0.00	0.0	0.00	0.0	0.0	0.0	0.0	0	0.0
....	2 tbsp	0	0.00	0.00	0.00	0.00	0.0	0.00	0.0	0.0	0.0	0.0	0	0.0
PALM OIL														
....	1 cup	0	0.00	0.00	0.00	0.00	0.0	0.00	0.0	0.0	<0.1	0.0	0	0.0
....	1 tbsp	0	0.00	0.00	0.00	0.00	0.0	0.00	0.0	0.0	0.0	0.0	0	0.0
PANCAKE, buttermilk *(Krusteaz)* mini,														
frozen, microwave	1 serving	3002	na	na	na	na	na	na	na	na	1.5	na	na	na
PAPAYA														
raw, cubed	1 cup	398	0.04	0.05	0.47	0.03	53.2	0.00	86.5	33.6	0.1	14.0	360	0.1
raw, mashed	1 cup	653	0.06	0.07	0.78	0.04	87.4	0.00	142.0	55.2	0.2	23.0	591	0.2
raw, whole, large, 5.75 inch long,														
3.25 inch diam..	1 papaya	1079	0.10	0.12	1.30	0.07	144.0	0.00	235.0	91.2	0.4	38.0	977	0.3
raw, whole, medium, 5 1/8 inch long,														
3 inch diam..	1 papaya	863	0.08	0.10	1.00	0.06	116.0	0.00	188.0	73.0	0.3	30.4	781	0.2
raw, whole, small, 4.5 inch long, 2.75														
inch diam..	1 papaya	432	0.04	0.05	0.51	0.03	57.8	0.00	93.9	36.5	0.2	15.2	391	0.1
PAPRIKA														
ground	1 tbsp	4182	0.05	0.12	1.10	0.14	7.3	0.00	4.9	12.2	1.6	12.7	162	0.3
ground	1 tsp	1273	0.01	0.04	0.32	0.04	2.2	0.00	1.5	3.7	0.5	3.9	49	<0.1
PARSLEY														
dried	1 tbsp	303	0.00	0.02	0.10	0.01	2.3	0.00	1.6	19.1	1.3	3.2	50	<0.1
dried	1 tsp	70	0.00	0.00	0.02	0.00	0.5	0.00	0.4	4.4	0.3	0.8	11	<0.1
dried (McCormick/Schilling)	1 tsp													
freeze-dried	1/4 cup	885	0.02	0.03	0.15	0.02	21.5	0.00	2.1	2.5	0.8	5.2	88	<0.1
freeze-dried	1 tbsp	253	0.00	0.01	0.04	0.01	6.1	0.00	0.6	0.7	0.2	1.5	25	<0.1
fresh, raw	1 cup	3120	0.05	0.06	0.79	0.05	91.2	0.00	79.8	82.8	3.7	30.0	332	0.6
fresh, raw	10 sprigs	520	0.01	0.01	0.13	0.01	15.2	0.00	13.3	13.8	0.6	5.0	55	0.1
fresh, raw	1 tbsp	198	0.00	0.00	0.05	0.00	5.8	0.00	5.1	5.2	0.2	1.9	21	<0.1
PARSLEY, CHINESE. See CORIANDER.														
PARSNIP														
boiled, drained, sliced..........	1/2 cup	0	0.07	0.04	0.56	0.07	45.4	0.00	10.1	28.9	0.5	22.6	286	0.2
boiled, drained, whole, approx 9 inch														
long	1 parsnip	0	0.13	0.08	1.20	0.15	93.1	0.00	20.8	59.2	0.9	46.4	587	0.4
raw, sliced	1 cup	0	0.12	0.07	0.93	0.12	88.8	0.00	22.6	47.9	0.8	38.6	499	0.8
PASSION FRUIT / granadilla														
purple, raw, sliced..........	1 cup	1652	0.00	0.31	3.50	0.24	33.0	0.00	70.8	28.3	3.8	68.4	821	0.2
purple, raw, whole, trimmed	1 medium	126	0.00	0.02	0.27	0.02	2.5	0.00	5.4	2.2	0.3	5.2	63	<0.1

Food Name	Serving Size	A I.U.	Thi mg	Rib mg	Nia mg	B6 mg	Fol mcg	B12 mcg	C mg	Calc mg	Iron mg	Mag mg	Pot mg	Zn mg
PASSION-FRUIT JUICE														
purple, raw	1 cup	1771	0.00	0.32	3.60	0.12	17.3	0.00	73.6	9.9	0.6	42.0	687	0.1
purple, raw	1 fl oz	222	0.00	0.04	0.45	0.02	2.2	0.00	9.2	1.2	<0.1	5.3	86	<0.1
yellow, raw	1 cup	5953	0.00	0.25	5.50	0.15	19.8	0.00	45.0	9.9	0.9	42.0	687	0.2
yellow, raw	1 fl oz	745	0.00	0.03	0.69	0.02	2.5	0.00	5.6	1.2	0.1	5.3	86	<0.1
PASTA. See also NOODLE.														
(NOTE: 2 ounces uncooked pasta = approximately 1 cup cooked.)														
CORN														
cooked	1 cup	79.8	0.07	0.03	0.78	0.08	8.4	0.00	0.0	1.4	0.4	50.4	43	0.9
cry	2 oz	96.9	0.13	0.05	1.40	0.12	14.3	0.00	0.0	2.3	0.5	67.8	168	1.0
dry	1 cup	179	0.24	0.09	2.60	0.22	26.3	0.00	0.0	4.2	0.9	125.0	309	1.9
MACARONI														
elbows, enriched, cooked	1 cup	0	0.29	0.14	2.30	0.05	98.0	0.00	0.0	9.8	2.0	25.2	43	0.7
elbows, protein-fortified, dry	1 cup	0	1.10	0.44	7.10	0.17	215.0	0.00	0.0	36.3	3.9	60.5	187	1.7
elbows, unenriched, cooked	1 cup	0	0.03	0.03	0.56	0.05	9.8	0.00	0.0	9.8	0.7	25.2	43	0.7
elbows, unenriched, dry	1 cup	0	0.10	0.06	1.80	0.11	18.9	0.00	0.0	18.9	1.4	50.4	170	1.3
elbows, whole wheat, cooked	1 cup	0	0.15	0.06	0.99	0.11	7.0	0.00	0.0	21.0	1.5	42.0	62	1.1
elbows, whole wheat, dry	1 cup	0	0.28	0.08	2.90	0.13	32.5	0.00	0.0	22.8	2.1	81.5	123	1.4
small shells, enriched, dry	1 cup	0	0.96	0.41	7.00	0.10	215.0	0.00	0.0	16.7	3.6	44.6	151	1.1
small shells, enriched, cooked	1 cup	0	0.23	0.11	1.90	0.04	80.5	0.00	0.0	8.1	1.6	20.7	36	0.6
small shells, protein-fortified, cooked	1 cup	0	0.34	0.19	2.10	0.07	94.3	0.00	0.0	11.5	0.8	34.5	48	0.6
small shells, protein-fortified, dry	1 cup	0	1.10	0.44	7.10	0.17	215.0	0.00	0.0	36.3	3.9	60.5	187	1.7
spirals, enriched, cooked	1 cup	0	0.27	0.13	2.20	0.05	93.8	0.00	0.0	9.4	1.9	24.1	42	0.7
spirals, enriched, dry	1 cup	0	0.86	0.37	6.30	0.09	194.0	0.00	0.0	15.1	3.2	40.3	136	1.0
spirals, vegetable, enriched, dry	1 cup	91.2	0.59	0.30	4.20	0.07	132.0	0.00	0.0	19.4	2.4	26.2	162	0.4
spirals, whole wheat, dry	1 cup	0	0.51	0.15	5.40	0.23	59.9	0.00	0.0	42.0	3.8	150.0	226	2.5
vegetable, enriched, cooked	1 cup	71.0	0.15	0.08	1.40	0.03	87.1	0.00	0.0	14.7	0.7	25.5	42	0.6
vegetable, enriched, dry	1 cup	134	0.87	0.44	6.20	0.11	194.0	0.00	0.0	28.6	3.6	38.6	239	0.6
SPAGHETTI														
enriched, cooked	1 cup	0	0.29	0.14	2.30	0.05	98.0	0.00	0.0	9.8	2.0	25.2	43	0.7
enriched, dry	2 oz	0	0.59	0.25	4.30	0.06	132.0	0.00	0.0	10.3	2.2	27.4	92	0.7
protein-fortified, cooked	1 cup	0	0.42	0.23	2.60	0.09	115.0	0.00	0.0	14.0	1.0	42.0	59	0.7
spinach, cooked	1 cup	213	0.14	0.14	2.10	0.13	16.8	0.00	0.0	42.0	1.5	86.8	81	1.5
spinach, dry	2 oz	263	0.21	0.11	2.60	0.18	27.4	0.00	0.0	33.1	1.2	99.2	214	1.6
unenriched, cooked	1 cup	0	0.03	0.03	0.56	0.05	9.8	0.00	0.0	9.8	0.7	25.2	43	0.7
unenriched, dry	2 oz	0	0.05	0.03	0.97	0.06	10.3	0.00	0.0	10.3	0.7	27.4	92	0.7
whole wheat, cooked	1 cup	0	0.15	0.06	0.99	0.11	7.0	0.00	0.0	21.0	1.5	42.0	62	1.1
whole wheat, dry	2 oz	0	0.28	0.08	2.90	0.13	32.5	0.00	0.0	22.8	2.1	81.5	123	1.4
PASTA DISH/ENTRÉE														
(Chef Boyardee) macaroni and mini meatballs, canned, 'Teenage Mutant Ninja Turtles'	1 serving	278	na	na	na	na	na	na	0.4	21.2	0.9	na	na	na
spaghetti and meatballs, in tomato sauce, canned	1 pkg	608	na	na	na	na	na	na	1.7	29.8	3.1	na	na	na
spaghetti and meatballs, in tomato sauce, canned	1 serving	343	na	na	na	na	na	na	0.9	16.8	1.8	na	na	na
(Healthy Choice)														
beef macaroni, frozen	1 serving	514	0.28	0.16	3.10	0.19	106.0	0.12	58.1	45.6	2.7	36.0	365	1.2
spaghetti Bolognese, frozen	1 serving	492	0.34	3.8	0.50	0.20	130.0	0.17	15.3	50.9	3.5	42.5	408	1.4
(Lean Cuisine)														
spaghetti w/meat sauce, frozen	1 serving	544	na	na	na	na	na	na	34.9	na	2.1	na	na	na
spaghetti w/meatballs, w/sauce, frozen	1 serving	0	na	na	na	na	na	na	na	94.2	2.4	na	na	na
(Michelinas)														
spaghetti and meatballs, w/Pomodoro sauce, low-fat, frozen	1 serving	520	na	na	na	na	na	na	8.8	na	2.9	na	na	na

Food Name	Serving Size	A I.U.	Thi mg	Rib mg	Nia mg	B_6 mg	Fol mcg	B_{12} mcg	C mg	Calc mg	Iron mg	Mag mg	Pot mg	Zn mg
(Nestlé)														
macaroni and cheese, canned, 'Chef Mate'.	1 pkg	2517	3.8	4.0	30.00	0.85	na	2.40	0.0	2426.0	23.1	394	1820	18.8
macaroni and cheese, canned, 'Chef Mate'.	1 cup	210	0.32	0.33	2.50	0.07	na	0.20	0.0	202.0	1.9	32.9	152	1.6
PASTA DISH/ENTRÉE MIX														
(Kraft) macaroni and cheese, original, unprepared.	1 serving	50	0.67	0.41	4.50	na	65.1	na	0.4	92.4	2.6	na	296	na
PASTA SAUCE. See under SAUCE.														
PASTRY. See also PASTRY, TOASTER.														
APPLE														
(Pepperidge Farm)														
turnover, frozen, ready to bake.	1 serving	na	na	na	na	na	na	na	na	na	1.2	na	na	na
ÉCLAIR														
(Tasty-Klair) custard-filled, prepared.	1 éclair	811	0.13	0.30	0.90	0.07	31.6	0.38	0.3	71.2	1.3	16.9	132	0.7
(Weight Watchers) chocolate, frozen.	1 éclair	na	na	na	na	na	na	na	na	na	na	na	na	na
PASTRY, TOASTER														
APPLE														
(Kellogg's)														
cinnamon, frosted, low-fat, 'Pop Tarts'	1 pastry	500	0.16	0.16	2.0	0.21	52.0	0	0	5.7	1.8	4.7	28.1	0.16
cinnamon, 'Pop Tarts'	1 pastry	500	0.15	0.17	2.0	0.20	41.6	0	0	12.0	1.8	5.7	47.3	0.34
BERRY														
(Kellogg's) wild, frosted, 'Pop Tarts'	1 pastry	500	0.16	0.16	2.0	0.22	54.0	0	0	11.3	1.8	5.4	44.3	0.16
BLUEBERRY														
(Kellogg's)														
frosted, 'Pop Tarts'	1 pastry	500	0.15	0.17	2.0	0.20	41.6	0	0	12.5	1.8	8.3	49.4	0.64
low-fat, 'Pop Tarts'	1 pastry	500	0.16	0.16	2.0	0.21	52.0	0	0	5.7	1.8	4.7	29.6	0.16
plain, 'Pop Tarts'	1 pastry	500	0.15	0.17	2.0	0.20	41.6	0	0	12.5	1.8	8.3	49.4	0.66
BROWN SUGAR CINNAMON														
(Kellogg's)														
frosted, 'Pop Tarts'	1 pastry	500	0.15	0.17	2.0	0.20	40.0	0	0	14.5	1.8	7.5	55.5	1.2
frosted w/cinnamon, low-fat, 'Pop Tarts'	1 pastry	500	0.15	0.15	2.0	0.20	50.0	0	0	7.0	1.8	5.0	30.5	0.15
plain, 'Pop Tarts'	1 pastry	500	0.15	0.17	2.0	0.20	40.0	0	0	15.5	1.8	8.0	67.5	0.61
CHERRY														
(Kellogg's)														
low-fat, 'Pop Tarts'	1 pastry	500	0.16	0.16	2.0	0.21	52.0	0	0	5.7	1.8	4.7	29.6	0.16
plain, 'Pop Tarts'	1 pastry	500	0.15	0.17	2.0	0.20	41.6	0	0	14.6	1.8	8.3	59.3	0.64
CHOCOLATE FUDGE														
(Kellogg's)														
fudge, frosted, 'Pop Tarts'	1 pastry	500	0.16	0.16	2.0	0.21	52.0	0	0	19.8	1.8	15.1	82.2	0.26
fudge, frosted, low-fat, 'Pop Tarts'	1 pastry	500	0.16	0.16	2.0	0.21	52.0	0	0	13.5	1.8	14.6	61.9	0.26
milk chocolate, 'Pop Tarts' *(Kellogg's)*	1 pastry	500	0.16	0.16	2.0	0.21	52.0	0	0	19.8	1.8	12.0	81.6	0.21
vanilla creme, frosted, 'Pop Tarts'	1 pastry	500	0.15	0.17	2.0	0.21	52.0	0	0	15.6	1.8	11.4	62.4	0.62
CINNAMON														
(Pillsbury)														
'Danish' 'Toaster Strudel' enriched	1 pastry	6.4	0.16	0.14	1.50	0.02	32.9	0.05	<0.1	37.6	1.0	10.1	66	0.4
'Danish' 'Toaster Strudel' unenriched	1 pastry	6.4	0.10	0.05	0.58	0.02	17.5	0.05	0.1	37.6	0.4	10.1	66	0.4
FRUIT														
(Pillsbury)														
'Danish' 'Toaster Strudel' enriched	1 pastry	39.2	0.14	0.12	1.10	0.02	17.5	0.05	2.1	24.4	0.9	8.0	44	0.3
'Danish' 'Toaster Strudel' unenriched	1 pastry	39.2	0.03	0.05	0.41	0.02	8.5	0.07	2.1	24.4	0.4	8.0	44	0.3
GRAPE *(Kellogg's)* frosted, 'Pop Tarts'	1 pastry	500	0.15	0.17	2.0	0.21	52.0	0	0	12.0	1.8	10.9	59.8	0.68
RASPBERRY														
(Kellogg's) frosted, 'Pop Tarts'	1 pastry	500	0.15	0.17	2.0	0.21	52.0	0	0	11.4	1.8	8.3	44.2	0.63

Food Name	Serving Size	A I.U.	Thi mg	Rib mg	Nia mg	B$_6$ mg	Fol mcg	B$_{12}$ mcg	C mg	Calc mg	Iron mg	Mag mg	Pot mg	Zn mg
S'MORES *(Kellogg's)* 'Pop Tarts'	1 pastry	500	0.16	0.16	2.0	0.21	52.0	0	0	15.1	1.8	10.9	65.0	0.21
STRAWBERRY														
(Kellogg's)														
frosted, 'Pop Tarts'	1 pastry	500	0.16	0.16	2.0	0.21	52.0	0	0	11.4	1.8	5.2	44.2	0.16
frosted, low-fat, 'Pop Tarts'	1 pastry	500	0.16	0.16	2.0	0.21	52.0	0	0	5.2	1.8	4.2	25.5	0.16
low-fat, 'Pop Tarts'	1 pastry	500	0.16	0.16	2.0	0.21	52.0	0	0	5.7	1.8	4.7	28.1	0.16
'Pastry Swirls' 'Pop Tarts'	1 pastry	0	na	na	na	na	na	na	0	19.8	1.1	na	na	na
'Pop Tarts'	1 pastry	500	0.16	0.16	2.0	0.21	52.0	0	0	12.5	1.8	5.7	48.4	0.16
PÂTÉ, CANNED														
chicken liver	1 oz	205	0.02	0.40	2.10	0.07	91.0	2.30	2.8	2.8	2.6	3.7	27	0.6
chicken liver	1 tbsp	94	0.01	0.18	0.98	0.03	41.7	1.00	1.3	1.3	1.2	1.7	12	0.3
goose liver, de foie gras, smoked	1 oz	945	0.03	0.09	0.71	0.02	17.0	2.70	0.6	19.8	1.6	3.7	39	0.3
goose liver, de foie gras, smoked	1 tbsp	433	0.01	0.04	0.33	0.01	7.8	1.20	0.3	9.1	0.7	1.7	18	0.1
PATTYPAN SQUASH. See SQUASH, SCALLOP.														
PEACH														
Canned														
extra light, halves or slices, w/liquid	1 cup	667	0.05	0.05	2.00	0.05	8.2	0.00	7.4	12.3	0.7	12.3	183	0.2
in extra heavy syrup, halves or slices,														
w/liquid	1 cup	343	0.03	0.06	1.40	0.05	8.1	0.00	3.1	7.9	0.8	13.1	217	0.2
in heavy syrup, halves, w/liquid	1/2 med fruit	325	0.01	0.02	0.60	0.02	3.1	0.00	2.7	2.9	0.3	4.9	90	<0.1
in heavy syrup, slices, w/liquid	1 cup	870	0.03	0.06	1.60	0.05	8.4	0.00	7.3	7.9	0.7	13.1	241	0.2
in heavy syrup, whole, w/liquid	1 cup	767	0.03	0.09	1.30	0.05	7.7	0.00	12.8	14.5	0.7	16.9	206	0.2
in juice, halves, w/liquid	1/2 fruit	373	0.01	0.02	0.57	0.02	3.3	0.00	3.5	5.9	0.3	6.9	125	0.1
in juice, whole, w/liquid	1 cup	953	0.02	0.04	1.50	0.05	8.5	0.00	9.0	15.0	0.7	17.5	320	0.3
in juice, halves or slices, w/liquid	1 cup	945	0.02	0.04	1.40	0.05	8.4	0.00	8.9	14.9	0.7	17.4	317	0.3
in light syrup, halves, w/liquid	1/2 fruit	347	0.01	0.03	0.58	0.02	3.2	0.00	2.4	2.9	0.4	4.9	95	<0.1
in light syrup, halves or slices, w/liquid	1 cup	889	0.02	0.06	1.50	0.05	8.3	0.00	6.0	7.5	0.9	12.6	243	0.2
in water, halves, w/liquid	1/2 fruit	521	0.01	0.02	0.51	0.02	3.3	0.00	2.8	2.0	0.3	4.9	97	<0.1
in water, halves or slices, w/liquid	1 cup	1298	0.02	0.05	1.30	0.05	8.3	0.00	7.1	4.9	0.8	12.2	242	0.2
Dried														
sulfured, stewed	1 cup	958	0.02	0.14	4.90	0.13	6.8	0.00	16.5	38.7	5.5	55.7	1341	0.8
sulfured, uncooked	1 cup	1644	0.05	0.13	5.60	0.18	7.7	0.00	12.3	44.1	6.4	66.1	1567	0.9
sulfured, uncooked, halves	1 cup	3461	0.00	0.34	7.00	0.11	0.5	0.00	7.7	44.8	6.5	67.2	1594	0.9
sulfured, uncooked, halves	1/2 medium	281	0.00	0.03	0.57	0.01	<0.1	0.00	0.6	3.6	0.5	5.5	129	<0.1
Fresh														
raw, sliced	1 cup	910	0.03	0.07	1.70	0.03	5.8	0.00	11.2	8.5	0.2	11.9	335	0.2
raw, whole, large, 2.75 inch diam,														
2.5 per lb	1 peach	840	0.03	0.06	1.60	0.03	5.3	0.00	10.4	7.8	0.2	11.0	309	0.2
raw, whole, medium, 2.5 inch diam,														
4 per lb	1 peach	524	0.02	0.04	0.97	0.02	3.3	0.00	6.50	4.9	<1	6.9	193	0.1
raw, whole, small, 2 inch diam, 5 per lb	1 peach	423	0.01	0.03	0.78	0.01	2.7	0.00	5.20	4.0	<0.1	5.5	156	0.1
Frozen														
sliced, thawed	1 cup	710	0.03	0.09	1.60	0.05	8.0	0.00	236.0	7.5	0.9	12.5	325	0.1
sweetened, sliced	10-oz pkg	807	0.04	0.10	1.90	0.05	9.1	0.00	268.0	8.5	1.1	14.2	369	0.1
sweetened, sliced	10 med slices	440	0.02	0.05	1.00	0.03	5.0	0.00	146.0	4.7	0.6	7.8	202	<0.1
PEANUT														
ALL TYPES														
Dry roasted														
salted	1 oz	0	0.12	0.03	3.80	0.07	41.2	0.00	0.0	15.3	0.6	49.9	187	0.9
salted	1 medium	0	0.00	0.00	0.14	0.00	1.5	0.00	0.0	0.5	<0.1	1.8	7	<0.1
unsalted	1 cup	0	0.64	0.14	19.7	0.37	212.0	0.00	0.0	78.8	3.3	257	961	4.8
unsalted	1 oz	0	0.12	0.03	3.80	0.07	41.2	0.00	0.0	15.3	0.6	49.9	187	0.9

Food Name	Serving Size	A I.U.	Thi mg	Rib mg	Nia mg	B_6 mg	Fol mcg	B_{12} mcg	C mg	Calc mg	Iron mg	Mag mg	Pot mg	Zn mg
unsalted	1 medium	0	0.00	0.00	0.14	0.00	1.5	0.00	0.0	0.5	<0.1	1.8	7	<0.1
Oil roasted														
salted	1 medium	0	0.00	0.00	0.13	0.00	1.1	0.00	0.0	0.8	<0.1	1.7	6	<0.1
salted, chopped	1 cup	0	0.36	0.16	20.60	0.37	181.0	0.00	0.0	127.0	2.6	266.0	982	9.5
salted, halves and whole	1 cup	0	0.36	0.16	20.60	0.37	181.0	0.00	0.0	127.0	2.6	266.0	982	9.5
unsalted, shelled	1 oz	0	0.07	0.03	4.00	0.07	35.6	0.00	0.0	24.9	0.5	52.4	193	1.9
unsalted, chopped	1 cup	0	0.34	0.14	19.00	0.34	167.0	0.00	0.0	117.0	2.4	246.0	907	8.8
Raw														
	1 cup	0	0.93	0.20	17.60	0.51	350.0	0.00	0.0	134.0	6.7	245.0	1029	4.8
	1 oz	0	0.18	0.04	3.40	0.10	68.0	0.00	0.0	26.1	1.3	47.6	200	0.9
SPANISH														
Oil roasted														
salted	1 cup	0	0.47	0.13	22.00	0.38	185.0	0.00	0.0	147.0	3.4	247.0	1141	2.9
salted	1 oz	0	0.09	0.02	4.20	0.07	35.7	0.00	0.0	28.4	0.7	47.6	220	0.6
unsalted	1 cup	0	0.47	0.13	22.00	0.38	185.0	0.00	0.0	147.0	3.4	247.0	1141	2.9
unsalted	1 oz	0	0.09	0.02	4.20	0.07	35.7	0.00	0.0	28.4	0.7	47.6	220	0.6
Raw														
	1 cup	0	0.99	0.20	23.30	0.51	350.0	0.00	0.0	155.0	5.7	274.0	1086	3.1
	1 oz	0	0.19	0.04	4.50	0.10	68.0	0.00	0.0	30.1	1.1	53.3	211	0.6
VALENCIA														
Oil roasted														
salted	1 cup	0	0.13	0.22	20.60	0.35	181.0	0.00	0.0	77.8	2.4	230.0	881	4.4
salted	1 oz	0	0.03	0.04	4.10	0.07	35.6	0.00	0.0	15.3	0.5	45.4	174	0.9
unsalted	1 cup	0	0.13	0.22	20.60	0.35	181.0	0.00	0.0	77.8	2.4	230.0	881	4.4
unsalted	1 oz	0	0.03	0.04	4.10	0.07	35.6	0.00	0.0	15.3	0.5	45.4	174	0.9
Raw														
unsalted	1 cup	0	0.93	0.44	18.80	0.50	358.0	0.00	0.0	90.5	3.1	269.0	485	4.9
unsalted	1 oz	0	0.18	0.09	3.60	0.10	69.6	0.00	0.0	17.6	0.6	52.2	94	0.9
VIRGINIA														
Oil roasted														
salted	1 cup	0	0.40	0.16	21.0	0.36	179.0	0.00	0.0	123.0	2.4	269.0	932	9.5
salted	1 oz	0	0.08	0.03	4.20	0.07	35.6	0.00	0.0	24.4	0.5	53.3	185	1.9
unsalted	1 cup	0	0.40	0.16	21.00	0.36	179.0	0.00	0.0	123.0	2.4	269.0	932	9.5
unsalted	1 oz	0	0.08	0.03	4.20	0.07	35.6	0.00	0.0	24.4	0.5	53.3	185	1.9
Raw														
unsalted	1 cup	0	0.95	0.19	18.10	0.51	349	0.00	0.0	130.0	3.7	250.0	1007	6.5
unsalted	1 oz	0	0.19	0.04	3.50	0.10	67.7	0.00	0.0	25.2	0.7	48.5	196	1.3
PEANUT BUTTER														
chunky	1 cup	0	0.32	0.29	35.30	1.20	237.0	0.00	0.0	106.0	4.9	410.0	1927	7.2
chunky	2 tbsp	0	0.04	0.04	4.40	0.14	29.4	0.00	0.0	13.1	0.6	50.9	239	0.9
chunky, no salt added	1 cup	0	0.32	0.29	35.30	1.20	237.0	0.00	0.0	106.0	4.9	410.0	1927	7.2
chunky, no salt added	2 tbsp	0	0.04	0.04	4.40	0.14	29.4	0.00	0.0	13.1	0.6	50.9	239	0.9
smooth	1 cup	0	0.21	0.27	34.60	1.20	191.0	0.00	0.0	98.0	4.7	410.0	1726	7.5
smooth	2 tbsp	0	0.03	0.03	4.30	0.14	23.7	0.00	0.0	12.2	0.6	50.9	214	0.9
smooth, no salt added	1 cup	0	0.21	0.27	34.60	1.20	191.0	0.00	0.0	98.0	4.7	410.0	1726	7.5
smooth, no salt added	2 tbsp	0	0.03	0.03	4.30	0.14	23.7	0.00	0.0	12.2	0.6	50.9	214	0.9
PEANUT FLOUR. See under FLOUR.														
PEANUT OIL														
	1 cup	0	0.00	0.00	0.00	0.00	0.0	0.00	0.0	0.2	<0.1	<0.1	<1	<0.1
	1 tbsp	0	0.00	0.00	0.00	0.00	0.0	0.00	0.0	<0.1	0.0	<0.1	0	0.0
PEAR														
Canned														
in extra heavy syrup, halves, w/liquid	1 cup	0	0.03	0.06	0.63	0.04	3.2	0.00	2.9	13.3	0.6	10.6	170	0.2

Food Name	Serving Size	A I.U.	Thi mg	Rib mg	Nia mg	B_6 mg	Fol mcg	B_{12} mcg	C mg	Calc mg	Iron mg	Mag mg	Pot mg	Zn mg
in extra heavy syrup, halves, w/1.75 tbsp liquid	1 med half	0	0.01	0.02	0.19	0.01	0.9	0.00	0.9	4.0	0.2	3.2	51	<0.1
in extra light syrup, halves, w/liquid	1 cup	0	0.03	0.05	0.99	0.04	3.0	0.00	4.9	17.3	0.5	12.3	111	0.2
in extra light syrup, halves, w/liquid	1 med half	0	0.01	0.02	0.30	0.01	0.9	0.00	1.5	5.3	0.2	3.8	34	<0.1
in heavy syrup, w/liquid	1 cup	0	0.03	0.06	0.64	0.04	3.2	0.00	2.9	13.3	0.6	10.6	173	0.2
in heavy syrup, w/liquid	1 med half	0	0.01	0.02	0.18	0.01	0.9	0.00	0.8	3.8	0.2	3.0	49	<0.1
in juice, halves, w/liquid	1 cup	15	0.03	0.03	0.50	0.04	3.0	0.00	4.0	22.3	0.7	17.4	238	0.2
in juice, halves, w/liquid	1 med half	5	0.01	0.01	0.15	0.01	0.9	0.00	1.2	6.8	0.2	5.3	73	<0.1
in light syrup, halves, w/liquid	1 cup	0	0.03	0.04	0.39	0.04	3.0	0.00	1.8	12.6	0.7	10.0	166	0.2
in light syrup, halves, w/liquid	1/2 fruit	0	0.01	0.01	0.12	0.01	0.9	0.00	0.5	3.8	0.2	3.0	50	<0.1
in water, halves, w/liquid	1 cup	0	0.02	0.02	0.13	0.03	2.9	0.00	2.4	9.8	0.5	9.8	129	0.2
in water, halves, w/liquid	1 med half	0	0.01	0.01	0.04	0.01	0.9	0.00	0.8	3.0	0.2	3.0	40	<0.1
Dried														
sulfured, stewed, halves	1 cup	107	0.01	0.05	0.90	0.09	0.0	0.00	10.2	40.8	2.6	40.8	658	0.5
sulfured, uncooked, halves	1 cup	5.4	0.01	0.26	2.50	0.13	0.0	0.00	12.6	61.2	3.8	59.4	959	0.7
sulfured, uncooked, halves	1 med half	<1	0.00	0.03	0.25	0.01	0.0	0.00	1.3	6.1	0.4	5.9	96	<0.1
Fresh														
sliced	1 cup	33.0	0.03	0.07	0.17	0.03	12.0	0.00	6.6	18.1	0.4	9.9	206	0.2
whole, large, 2 per lb	1 pear	41.8	0.04	0.08	0.21	0.04	15.3	0.00	8.4	23.0	0.5	12.5	261	0.2
whole, medium, 2.5 per lb	1 pear	33.2	0.03	0.07	0.17	0.03	12.1	0.00	6.6	18.3	0.4	10.0	208	0.2
whole, small, 3 per lb	1 pear	27.8	0.03	0.06	0.14	0.03	10.1	0.00	5.6	15.3	0.4	8.3	174	0.2
PEAS, BLACK-EYED. See BLACK-EYED PEAS.														
PEAS, CROWDER. See under BLACK-EYED PEAS.														
PEAS, GREEN														
Canned														
drained	1 cup	1306	0.21	0.13	1.20	0.11	75.3	0.00	16.3	34.0	1.6	28.9	294	1.2
no salt added, drained	1/2 cup	653	0.10	0.07	0.62	0.05	37.7	0.00	8.2	17.0	0.8	14.4	147	0.6
no salt added, w/liquid	1/2 cup	477	0.14	0.09	1.00	0.08	35.3	0.00	12.2	22.3	1.3	21.1	124	0.9
Fresh														
boiled, drained	1 cup	955	0.41	0.24	3.20	0.35	101	0.00	22.7	43.2	2.5	62.4	434	1.9
boiled, drained	1/2 cup	534	0.23	0.08	1.20	0.09	46.9	0.00	7.9	19.2	1.3	23.2	134	0.8
raw	1 cup	928	0.39	0.19	3.00	0.25	94.3	0.00	58.0	36.3	2.1	47.9	354	1.8
Frozen														
boiled, drained	10-oz pkg	1690	0.72	0.25	3.70	0.29	148.0	0.00	25.0	60.7	4.0	73.4	425	2.4
unprepared	10-oz pkg	2065	0.73	0.28	4.80	0.35	151.0	0.00	51.1	62.5	4.3	71.0	423	2.3
unprepared	1/2 cup	523	0.19	0.07	1.20	0.09	38.2	0.00	13.0	15.8	1.1	18.0	107	0.6
Sprouted, mature seeds, raw	1 cup	199	0.27	0.19	3.70	0.32	173.0	0.00	12.5	43.2	2.7	67.2	457	1.3
PEAS, PIGEON														
immature seeds, boiled, drained	1 cup	199	0.54	0.25	3.30	0.08	153.0	0.00	43.0	62.7	2.4	61.2	698	1.3
immature seeds, raw	1 cup	216	0.62	0.26	3.40	0.11	266.0	0.00	60.1	64.7	2.5	105.0	850	1.6
immature seeds, raw	10 seeds	6	0.02	0.01	0.09	0.00	6.9	0.00	1.6	1.7	<0.1	2.7	22	<0.1
red gram, mature seeds, boiled	1 cup	5	0.25	0.10	1.30	0.08	186.0	0.00	0.0	72.2	1.9	77.3	645	1.5
red gram, mature seeds, raw	1 cup	57	1.30	0.38	6.10	0.58	935.0	0.00	0.0	267.0	10.7	375.0	2854	5.7
PEAS, SNOW / Chinese pea pods														
Fresh														
edible-podded, boiled, drained	1 cup	210	0.20	0.12	0.86	0.23	46.6	0.00	76.6	67.2	3.2	41.6	384	0.6
edible-podded, raw, whole	10 pods	49	0.05	0.03	0.20	0.05	14.2	0.00	20.4	14.6	0.7	8.2	68	0.1
edible-podded, raw, chopped	1 cup	142	0.15	0.08	0.59	0.16	40.9	0.00	58.8	42.1	2.0	23.5	196	0.3
edible-podded, raw, whole	1 cup	91	0.10	0.05	0.38	0.10	26.3	0.00	37.8	27.1	1.3	15.1	126	0.2
Frozen														
edible-podded, boiled, drained	1 cup	267	0.10	0.19	0.90	0.28	56.3	0.00	35.2	94.4	3.8	44.8	347	0.8
edible-podded, boiled, drained	10-oz pkg	423	0.16	0.30	1.40	0.44	89.1	0.00	55.7	149.0	6.1	70.8	549	1.2
edible-podded, no salt added, boiled, drained	1 cup	267	0.10	0.19	0.90	0.28	56.3	0.00	35.2	94.4	3.8	44.8	347	0.8

Food Name	Serving Size	A I.U.	Thi mg	Rib mg	Nia mg	B_6 mg	Fol mcg	B_{12} mcg	C mg	Calc mg	Iron mg	Mag mg	Pot mg	Zn mg
edible-podded, no salt added, boiled, drained	10-oz pkg	423	0.16	0.30	1.40	0.44	89.1	0.00	55.7	149.0	6.1	70.8	549	1.2
edible-podded, unprepared	1/2 cup	101	0.04	0.07	0.36	0.11	28.9	0.00	15.8	36.0	1.4	16.6	138	0.3
edible-podded, unprepared	10-oz pkg	398	0.17	0.28	1.40	0.44	114.0	0.00	62.5	142.0	5.7	65.3	545	1.2
PEAS, SPLIT														
mature seeds, boiled	1 cup	14	0.37	0.11	1.70	0.09	127.0	0.00	0.8	27.4	2.5	70.6	710	2.0
mature seeds, boiled	1 tbsp	<1	0.02	0.01	0.11	0.01	7.9	0.00	<0.1	1.7	0.2	4.4	44	0.1
mature seeds, raw	1 cup	294	1.40	0.42	5.7	0.34	539.0	0.00	3.5	108	8.7	227.0	1933	5.9
PECAN														
Dried														
chopped	1 cup	92	0.79	0.16	1.40	0.25	26.2	0.00	1.3	83.3	3.0	144.0	488	5.4
halves	1 cup	83	0.71	0.14	1.30	0.23	23.8	0.00	1.2	75.6	2.7	131.0	443	4.9
halves, approx 20 pieces	1 oz	22	0.19	0.04	0.33	0.06	6.2	0.00	0.3	19.8	0.7	34.3	116	1.3
Dry roasted														
unsalted	1 oz	40	0.13	0.03	0.33	0.05	4.5	0.00	0.3	20.4	0.8	37.4	120	1.4
salted	1 oz	40	0.13	0.03	0.33	0.05	4.5	0.00	0.3	20.4	0.8	37.4	120	1.4
Oil roasted														
salted	1 cup	114	0.52	0.12	1.30	0.21	16.5	0.00	1.1	73.7	2.7	133.0	431	4.9
salted, halves, approx 15 pieces	1 oz	30	0.13	0.03	0.34	0.05	4.3	0.00	0.3	19.0	0.7	34.3	111	1.3
unsalted	1 cup	114	0.52	0.12	1.30	0.21	16.5	0.00	1.1	73.7	2.7	133.0	431	4.9
unsalted, halves, approx 15 pieces	1 oz	30	0.13	0.03	0.34	0.05	4.3	0.00	0.3	19.0	0.7	34.3	111	1.3
PECTIN MIX, unsweetened, dry	1.75 oz	2	0.00	0.03	0.00	0.01	0.50	0.00	0.0	3.5	1.4	0.5	3.5	0.2
PEPEAO. See CHINESE FUNGUS.														
PEPPER, ANCHO, dried, whole	1 medium	3474	0.03	0.38	1.10	0.60	11.7	0.00	0.3	10.4	1.9	19.2	410	0.2
PEPPER, BANANA														
raw, chopped	1 cup	422	0.10	0.07	1.50	0.44	36.0	0.00	103.0	17.4	0.6	21.1	317	0.3
raw, whole, small, approx 4-inch long	1 pepper	112	0.03	0.02	0.41	0.12	9.6	0.00	27.3	4.6	0.2	5.6	85	<0.1
raw, whole, medium, approx 4.5-inch long	1 pepper	156	0.04	0.03	0.57	0.16	13.3	0.00	38.0	6.4	0.2	7.8	118	0.1
raw, whole, large, approx 5-inch long	1 pepper	255	0.06	0.04	0.93	0.27	21.8	0.00	62.0	10.5	0.3	12.8	192	0.2
PEPPER, BELL / green pepper / red pepper / sweet pepper / yellow pepper														
Canned or jarred														
green, halves, w/liquid	1 cup	217	0.04	0.04	0.77	0.25	22.8	0.00	65.1	57.4	1.1	15.4	204	0.3
red, halves, w/liquid	1 cup	728	0.04	0.04	0.77	0.25	22.8	0.00	65.1	57.4	1.1	15.4	204	0.3
red, halves, w/liquid	1/2 cup	364	0.02	0.02	0.39	0.13	11.4	0.00	32.5	28.7	0.6	7.7	102	0.1
Freeze-Dried														
	1/4 cup	100	0.02	0.02	0.12	0.04	3.7	0.00	30.4	2.1	0.2	3.0	51	<0.1
	1 tbsp	25	0.01	0.01	0.03	0.01	0.9	0.00	7.6	0.5	<0.1	0.8	14	<0.1
red	1/4 cup	1236	0.02	0.02	0.12	0.04	3.7	0.00	30.4	2.1	0.2	3.0	51	<0.1
red	1 tbsp	309	0.01	0.01	0.03	0.01	0.9	0.00	7.6	0.5	<0.1	0.8	13	<0.1
Fresh														
green, boiled, drained, chopped	1/2 cup	403	0.04	0.02	0.32	0.16	10.9	0.00	50.6	6.1	0.3	6.8	113	<0.1
green, boiled, drained, minced	1 tbsp	69	0.01	0.00	0.06	0.03	1.9	0.00	8.6	1.0	<0.1	1.2	19	<0.1
green, boiled, drained, strips	1 cup	799	0.08	0.04	0.64	0.32	21.6	0.00	100.0	12.2	0.6	13.5	224	0.2
green, raw, chopped	1 cup	942	0.10	0.05	0.76	0.37	32.8	0.00	133.0	13.4	0.7	14.9	264	0.2
green, raw, minced	1 tbsp	59	0.01	0.00	0.05	0.02	2.0	0.00	8.3	0.8	<0.1	0.93	17	<0.1
green, raw, rings, 3-inch diam, 1/4-inch thick	1 ring	63	0.01	0.00	0.05	0.03	2.2	0.00	8.9	0.9	<0.1	1.0	18	<0.1
green, raw, sliced	1 cup	581	0.06	0.03	0.47	0.23	20.2	0.00	82.2	8.3	0.4	9.2	163	0.1
green, raw, strips	10 strips	171	0.02	0.01	0.14	0.07	5.9	0.00	24.1	2.4	0.1	2.7	48	<0.1
green, raw, whole, approx 2.75-inch long, 2.5-inch diam.	1 pepper	752	0.08	0.04	0.61	0.29	26.2	0.00	106.0	10.7	0.6	11.9	211	0.1
green, raw, whole, approx 3.75-inch long, 3-inch diam	1 pepper	1036	0.11	0.05	0.83	0.41	36.1	0.00	146.0	14.8	0.8	16.4	290	0.2

Food Name	Serving Size	A I.U.	Thi mg	Rib mg	Nia mg	B$_6$ mg	Fol mcg	B$_{12}$ mcg	C mg	Calc mg	Iron mg	Mag mg	Pot mg	Zn mg
red, boiled, drained, chopped	1/2 cup	2557	0.04	0.02	0.32	0.16	10.9	0.00	116.0	6.1	0.3	6.8	113	<0.1
red, boiled, drained, minced . . . . , .	1 tbsp	436	0.01	0.00	0.06	0.03	1.9	0.00	19.8	1.0	<0.1	1.2	19	<0.1
red, boiled, drained, strips	1 cup	5076	0.08	0.04	0.64	0.32	21.6	0.00	231.0	12.2	0.6	13.5	224	0.2
red, raw, chopped	1 cup	8493	0.10	0.05	0.76	0.37	32.8	0.00	283.0	13.4	0.7	14.9	264	0.2
red, raw, minced	1 tbsp	530	0.01	0.00	0.05	0.02	2.0	0.00	17.7	0.8	<0.1	0.9	16.5	<0.1
red, raw, rings, 3-inch diam, 1/4-inch thick	1 ring	570	0.01	0.00	0.05	0.03	2.2	0.00	19.0	0.9	<0.1	1.0	18	<0.1
red, raw, sliced	1 cup	5244	0.06	0.03	0.47	0.23	20.2	0.00	175.0	8.3	0.4	9.2	163	0.1
red, raw, whole, approx 2.75-inch long, 2.5-inch diam.	1 medium	6783	0.08	0.04	0.61	0.29	26.2	0.00	226.0	10.7	0.6	11.9	211	0.1
red, raw, whole, approx 3.75-inch long, 3-inch diam.	1 large	9348	0.11	0.05	0.83	0.41	36.1	0.00	312.0	14.8	0.8	16.4	290	0.2
yellow, raw, strips	10 strips	124	0.02	0.01	0.46	0.09	13.5	0.00	95.4	5.7	0.2	6.2	110	<0.1
yellow, whole, approx 3.75-inch long, 3-inch diam	1 pepper	443	0.05	0.05	1.70	0.31	48.4	0.00	341.0	20.5	0.9	22.3	394	0.3
Frozen														
green, chopped, unprepared	10-oz pkg	1042	0.20	0.11	3.90	0.39	40.0	0.00	167.0	25.6	1.8	22.7	258	0.2
red, chopped, unprepared	10-oz pkg	13524	0.20	0.11	3.90	0.39	40.0	0.00	167.0	25.6	1.8	22.7	258	0.2
red, chopped, unprepared	1 oz	1333	0.02	0.01	0.38	0.04	3.9	0.00	16.4	2.5	0.2	2.2	25.5	<0.1
PEPPER, CHILI / chile														
Canned or jarred														
green, chopped, no seeds, w/liquid	1/2 cup	415	0.01	0.03	0.54	0.10	6.8	0.00	46.2	4.8	0.3	9.5	127	0.1
green, whole, no seeds, w/liquid.	1 med	445	0.02	0.04	0.58	0.11	7.3	0.00	49.6	5.1	0.4	10.2	137	0.1
red, chopped, no seeds, w/liquid	1/2 cup	8087	0.01	0.03	0.54	0.10	6.8	0.00	46.2	4.8	0.3	9.5	127	0.1
red, whole, no seeds, w/liquid.	1 med	8681	0.02	0.04	0.58	0.11	7.3	0.00	49.6	5.1	0.4	10.2	137	0.1
Fresh														
green, chopped or diced.	1/2 cup	578	0.07	0.07	0.71	0.21	17.6	0.00	182.0	13.5	0.9	18.8	255	0.2
green, raw, whole	1 med	347	0.04	0.04	0.43	0.13	10.5	0.00	109.0	8.1	0.5	11.3	153	0.1
Sun-dried														
hot, chopped.	1 cup	9801	0.03	0.45	3.2	0.30	18.9	0.00	11.6	16.6	2.2	32.6	692	0.4
hot, whole.	1 med	143	0.00	0.01	0.05	0	0.3	0.00	0.2	0.2	<0.1	0.5	10	<0.1
PEPPER, GROUND														
BLACK														
. . . .	1 tbsp	12	0.01	0.02	0.07	0.02	0.6	0.00	1.3	27.9	1.8	12.4	81	<0.1
. . . .	1 tsp	4	0.00	0.01	0.02	0.01	0.2	0.00	0.4	9.2	0.6	4.1	26	<0.1
. . . .	1 dash	<1	0.00	0.00	0.00	0.00	<0.1	0.00	<0.1	0.4	<0.1	0.2	1	0.0
CAYENNE														
. . . .	1 tbsp	2205	0.02	0.05	0.46	0.11	5.6	0.00	4.1	7.9	0.4	8.1	107	0.1
. . . .	1 tsp	749	0.01	0.02	0.16	0.04	1.9	0.00	1.4	2.7	0.1	2.7	36	<0.1
RED														
. . . .	1 tbsp	2205	0.02	0.05	0.46	0.11	5.6	0.00	4.1	7.9	0.4	8.1	107	0.1
. . . .	1 tsp	749	0.01	0.02	0.16	0.04	1.9	0.00	1.4	2.7	0.1	2.7	36	<0.1
WHITE														
. . . .	1 tbsp	0	0.00	0.01	0.02	0.02	0.7	0.00	1.5	18.8	1.0	6.4	5	<0.1
. . . .	1 tsp	0	0.00	0.00	0.01	0.01	0.2	0.00	0.5	6.4	0.3	2.2	2	<0.1
PEPPER, HUNGARIAN, raw, whole	1 medium	38	0.02	0.02	0.29	0.14	14.3	0.00	25.1	3.2	0.1	4.3	55	<0.1
PEPPER, JALAPEÑO														
Canned or jarred														
chopped, w/liquid	1 cup	2312	0.06	0.05	0.55	0.26	19.0	0.00	13.6	31.3	2.6	20.4	262	0.5
sliced, w/liquid	1 cup	1768	0.05	0.04	0.42	0.20	14.6	0.00	10.4	23.9	2.0	15.6	201	0.3
whole, w/liquid	1 med	374	0.01	0.01	0.09	0.04	3.1	0.00	2.2	5.1	0.4	3.3	43	<0.1
Fresh														
raw, sliced.	1 cup	194	0.13	0.05	1.00	0.46	42.3	0.00	39.9	9.0	0.6	17.1	194	0.2
raw, whole.	1 pepper	30	0.02	0.01	0.16	0.07	6.6	0.00	6.2	1.4	0.1	2.7	30	<0.1

Food Name	Serving Size	A I.U.	Thi mg	Rib mg	Nia mg	B$_6$ mg	Fol mcg	B$_{12}$ mcg	C mg	Calc mg	Iron mg	Mag mg	Pot mg	Zn mg
PEPPER, PERSIL, dried	1 medium	2503	0.01	0.22	0.50	0.30	11.9	0.00	0.45	6.8	0.7	9.1	156	0.1
PEPPER, SERRANO														
raw, chopped	1 cup	984	0.06	0.09	1.60	0.53	24.1	0.00	47.1	11.6	0.9	23.1	320	0.3
raw, whole.	1 medium	57	0.00	0.01	0.09	0.03	1.4	0.00	2.7	0.67	<0.1	1.3	19	<0.1
PEPPER, SWEET. See PEPPER, BELL.														
PEPPER, YELLOW. See PEPPER, BANANA; PEPPER, BELL.														
PEPPER DISH/ENTRÉE														
(Stouffer's)														
stuffed, w/beef, in tomato sauce, frozen	1 pkg	0	na	na	na	na	na	na	173	na	na	na	na	na
stuffed, w/beef, in tomato sauce, frozen	1 serving	0	na	na	na	na	na	na	86.7	na	na	na	na	na
PEPPERMINT														
fresh, raw, chopped	2 tbsp	136	0.00	0.01	0.06	0.00	3.6	0.00	1.0	7.8	0.2	2.6	18	<0.1
fresh, raw, whole.	2 leaves	4.2	0.00	0.00	0.00	0.00	0.11	0.00	<0.1	0.2	<0.1	<0.1	<1	0.0
PERCH														
baked, broiled, grilled, or microwaved	3 oz	27	0.07	0.10	1.60	0.12	4.9	1.90	1.4	86.7	1.0	32.3	292	1.2
raw	3 oz	24	0.06	0.09	1.30	0.10	4.3	1.60	1.4	68.0	0.8	25.5	229	0.9
PERCH, RED. See OCEAN PERCH.														
PERCH, ROSE. See OCEAN PERCH.														
PERSIL PEPPER. See PEPPER, PERSIL.														
PERSIMMON														
Japanese, dried, trimmed, whole, approx 2.5 inch diam	1 fruit	190	na	0.01	0.06	na	na	0.00	0	8.5	0.3	10.5	273	0.1
Japanese, raw, whole, approx 2.5 inch diam	1 fruit	3641	0.05	0.03	0.17	0.17	12.6	0.00	12.6	13.4	0.3	15.1	270	0.2
native, raw, trimmed, approx 2.5 inch diam	1 fruit	na	na	na	na	na	na	0.00	16.5	6.8	0.6	na	77.5	na
PE-TSAI. See BOK CHOY.														
PHEASANT														
average of all parts, meat and skin.	3 oz	152	0.06	0.12	5.49	0.55	5.2	0.67	4.6	10.3	0.9	17.1	208	0.8
average of all parts, meat only	3 oz	141	0.07	0.13	5.78	0.63	5.2	0.71	5.2	11.1	0.9	17.1	225	0.8
breast, meat only, raw.	3 oz	126	0.07	0.10	7.35	0.61	3.4	0.71	5.1	2.6	0.7	17.9	207	0.5
leg, meat only, raw	3 oz	167	0.06	0.18	3.20	0.63	8.6	0.72	5.1	24.8	1.6	17.1	254	1.3
PHYLLO DOUGH	1 oz	0	0.15	0.10	1.20	0.01	21.0	0.00	0.0	3.1	0.9	4.3	21	0.1
PICKLE														
DILL														
low-salt, whole, approx 3.75 inch long	1 pickle	214	0.01	0.02	0.04	0.01	0.7	0.00	1.2	5.8	0.3	7.2	75	<0.1
regular, chopped or diced.	1 cup	470	0.02	0.04	0.09	0.02	1.4	0.00	2.7	12.9	0.8	15.7	166	0.2
regular, slices	1 cup	510	0.02	0.05	0.09	0.02	1.6	0.00	2.9	13.9	0.8	17.1	180	0.2
regular, spears	1 spear	99	0.00	0.01	0.02	0.00	0.3	0.00	0.6	2.7	0.2	3.3	35	<0.1
regular, whole, approx 4-inch long	1 pickle	444	0.02	0.04	0.08	0.02	1.4	0.00	2.6	12.2	0.7	14.8	157	0.2
regular, whole, approx 3.75 inch long.	1 pickle	214	0.01	0.02	0.04	0.01	0.7	0.00	1.2	5.8	0.3	7.2	75	<0.1
regular, whole, 3.5-inch long.	1 pickle	122	0.01	0.01	0.02	0.01	0.4	0.00	0.7	3.3	0.2	4.1	42.9	<0.1
SOUR														
low-salt, approx 3.75-inch long.	1 pickle	94	0.00	0.01	0.00	0.01	0.5	0.00	0.7	0.0	0.3	2.6	15	<0.1
low-salt, approx 4-inch long	1 pickle	196	0.00	0.01	0.00	0.01	0.9	0.00	1.4	0.0	0.5	5.4	31	<0.1
low-salt, chopped or diced	1 cup	207	0.00	0.01	0.00	0.01	1.0	0.00	1.4	0.0	0.6	5.7	33	<0.1
low-salt, slices	1 cup	225	0.00	0.02	0.00	0.01	1.1	0.00	1.6	0.0	0.6	6.2	36	<0.1
low-salt, spears.	1 spear	44	0.00	0.00	0.00	0.00	0.2	0.00	0.3	0.0	0.1	1.2	7	<0.1
low-salt, whole, approx 3.5-inch long	1 pickle	54	0.00	0.00	0.00	0.00	0.3	0.00	0.4	0.0	0.1	1.5	9	<0.1
regular, slices	1 cup	225	0.00	0.02	0.00	0.01	1.1	0.00	1.6	0.0	0.6	6.2	36	<0.1
regular, spears	1 spear	44	0.00	0.00	0.00	0.00	0.2	0.00	0.3	0.0	0.1	1.2	7	<0.1
regular, whole, approx 3.5-inch long.	1 pickle	54	0.00	0.00	0.00	0.00	0.3	0.00	0.4	0.0	0.2	1.5	9	<0.1
regular, whole, approx 3.75-inch long.	1 pickle	94	0.00	0.01	0.00	0.01	0.5	0.00	0.7	0.0	0.3	2.6	15	<0.1
regular, whole, approx 4-inch long	1 pickle	196	0.00	0.01	0.00	0.01	0.9	0.00	1.4	0.0	0.5	5.4	31	<0.1

Food Name	Serving Size	A I.U.	Thi mg	Rib mg	Nia mg	B$_6$ mg	Fol mcg	B$_{12}$ mcg	C mg	Calc mg	Iron mg	Mag mg	Pot mg	Zn mg
SWEET														
gherkin, whole, approx 2.5-inch long	1 pickle	19	0.00	0.01	0.03	0.00	0.2	0.00	0.18	0.6	<0.1	0.6	5	<0.1
gherkin, whole, approx 2.75-inch long	1 pickle	32	0.00	0.01	0.04	0.00	0.3	0.00	0.30	1.0	0.2	1.0	8	<0.1
gherkin, whole, approx 2 1/8 inch long	1 pickle	8	0.00	0.00	0.01	0.00	<0.1	0.00	<0.1	0.2	<0.1	0.2	2	<0.1
low-salt, chopped or diced	1 cup	202	0.01	0.05	0.28	0.02	1.6	0.00	1.9	6.4	0.9	6.4	51	0.1
low-salt, slices	1 cup	214	0.02	0.05	0.30	0.03	1.7	0.00	2.0	6.8	1.0	6.8	55	<0.1
low-salt, slices	1 slice	8	0.00	0.00	0.01	0.00	<0.1	0.00	<0.1	0.2	<0.1	0.2	2	<0.1
regular, chopped	1 cup	202	0.01	0.05	0.28	0.02	1.6	0.00	1.9	6.4	0.9	6.4	51	0.1
regular, sliced	1 cup	214	0.02	0.05	0.30	0.03	1.7	0.00	2.0	6.8	1.0	6.8	54	0.1
regular, whole, approx 3-inch long	1 pickle	44	0.00	0.01	0.06	0.01	0.4	0.00	0.4	1.4	0.2	1.4	11	<0.1
PICKLE RELISH. See under RELISH.														
PIE														
APPLE														
(Banquet)														
frozen, ready to bake	1 serving	0	na	na	na	na	na	na	0	10.1	0.3	na	na	na
PIE CRUST														
(Nabisco)														
vanilla wafer crumb, 'Nilla'	1 slice	3	0.05	0.05	0.70	0.01	8.4	0.03	na	11.5	0.5	2.2	19	<0.1
PIGEON. See SQUAB.														
PIGEON PEA. See PEAS, PIGEON.														
PIGNOLI NUT. See PINE NUT.														
PIG'S EAR. See under PORK.														
PIG'S FEET. See under PORK.														
PIG'S HEART. See under PORK.														
PIG'S JOWL. See under PORK.														
PIG'S TAIL. See under PORK.														
PIG'S TONGUE. See under PORK.														
PIKE														
NORTHERN														
baked, broiled, grilled, or microwaved	3 oz	69	0.06	0.07	2.40	0.12	14.7	2.00	3.2	62.0	0.6	34.0	281	0.7
raw	3 oz	60	0.05	0.05	2.00	0.10	12.8	1.70	3.2	48.5	0.5	26.4	220	0.6
WALLEYE														
baked, broiled, grilled, or microwaved	3 oz	69	0.27	0.17	2.40	0.12	14.4	2.00	0.0	120	1.4	32.3	424	0.7
raw	3 oz	60	0.23	0.14	2.00	0.10	12.8	1.70	0.0	93.5	1.1	25.5	331	0.5
PILI NUT, CANARY TREE														
dried	1 cup	49	1.10	0.11	0.62	0.14	71.6	0.00	0.7	174.0	4.2	362.0	608	3.6
dried, approx 15 kernels	1 oz	12	0.26	0.03	0.15	0.03	16.9	0.00	0.2	41.1	1.0	85.6	144	0.8
PIMIENTO, CANNED														
Canned or jarred														
	1 cup	5098	0.03	0.12	1.20	0.41	11.5	0.00	163.0	11.5	3.2	11.5	303	0.4
chopped	1 tbsp	319	0.00	0.01	0.07	0.03	0.72	0.00	10.2	0.7	0.2	0.7	19	<0.1
sliced	1 slice	27	0.00	0.00	0.01	0.00	0.06	0.00	0.9	<0.1	<0.1	<0.1	2	0.0
whole	1 medium	1752	0.01	0.04	0.41	0.14	4.0	0.00	56.0	4.0	1.1	4.0	104	0.1
PIÑA COLADA. See under COCKTAIL.														
PINE NUT / Colorado pinyon / Italian stone pine nut / pignoli / pinnochio /piñon														
dried	1 cup	39	1.1	0.26	4.90	0.15	77.9	0.00	2.6	35.4	12.5	317.0	815	5.8
dried	1 oz	8	0.23	0.05	1.00	0.03	16.2	0.00	0.5	7.4	2.6	66.1	170	1.2
dried	1 tbsp	3	0.07	0.02	0.31	0.01	4.9	0.00	0.2	2.2	0.8	20.0	52	0.4
dried	10 medium	<1	0.02	0.00	0.06	0.00	1.0	0.00	<0.1	0.5	0.2	4.2	11	<0.1
PINEAPPLE														
Canned														
chunks, in extra heavy syrup, w/liquid	1 cup	36	0.23	0.07	0.73	0.19	12.0	0.00	19.0	36.4	1.0	39.0	265	0.3
chunks, in heavy syrup, w/liquid	1 cup	36	0.23	0.06	0.73	0.19	11.7	0.00	18.8	35.6	0.9	40.6	264	0.3
chunks, in juice, w/liquid	1 cup	95	0.24	0.05	0.71	0.18	12.0	0.00	23.7	34.9	0.7	34.9	304	0.3

Food Name	Serving Size	A I.U.	Thi mg	Rib mg	Nia mg	B_6 mg	Fol mcg	B_{12} mcg	C mg	Calc mg	Iron mg	Mag mg	Pot mg	Zn mg
chunks, in light syrup, w/liquid	1 cup	38	0.23	0.06	0.74	0.19	11.8	0.00	18.9	35.3	0.9	40.3	265	0.3
chunks, in water, w/liquid	1 cup	37	0.23	0.06	0.73	0.18	11.8	0.00	18.9	36.9	0.9	44.3	312	0.3
crushed, in extra heavy syrup, w/liquid	1 cup	36	0.23	0.07	0.73	0.19	12.0	0.00	19.0	36.4	1.0	39.0	265	0.3
crushed, in heavy syrup, w/liquid	1 cup	36	0.23	0.06	0.73	0.19	11.7	0.00	18.8	35.6	0.9	40.6	264	0.3
crushed, in juice, w/liquid	1 cup	95	0.24	0.05	0.71	0.18	12.0	0.00	23.7	34.9	0.7	34.9	304	0.3
crushed, in light syrup, w/liquid	1 cup	38	0.23	0.06	0.74	0.19	11.8	0.00	18.9	35.3	0.9	40.3	265	0.3
crushed, in water, w/liquid	1 cup	37	0.23	0.06	0.73	0.18	11.8	0.00	18.9	36.9	0.9	44.3	312	0.3
rings, in heavy syrup, 3-inch diam, w/liquid	1 ring	7	0.04	0.01	0.14	0.04	2.3	0.00	3.6	6.9	0.2	7.8	51	<0.1
rings, in juice, 3-inch diam, w/liquid	1 ring	18	0.05	0.01	0.13	0.04	2.3	0.00	4.5	6.6	0.1	6.6	57	<0.1
rings, in light syrup, 3-inch diam, w/liquid	1 ring	7	0.04	0.01	0.14	0.04	2.3	0.00	3.6	6.7	0.2	7.7	50	<0.1
rings, in water, 3-inch diam, w/liquid	1 ring	7	0.04	0.01	0.14	0.04	2.3	0.00	3.6	7.0	0.2	8.5	60	<0.1
sliced, in extra heavy syrup, w/liquid	1 cup	36	0.23	0.07	0.73	0.19	12.0	0.00	19.0	36.4	1.0	39.0	265	0.3
sliced, in heavy syrup, w/liquid	1 cup	36	0.23	0.06	0.73	0.19	11.7	0.00	18.8	35.6	0.9	40.6	264	0.3
sliced, in juice, w/liquid	1 cup	95	0.24	0.05	0.71	0.18	12.0	0.00	23.7	34.9	0.7	34.9	304	0.3
sliced, in light syrup, w/liquid	1 cup	38	0.23	0.06	0.74	0.19	11.8	0.00	18.9	35.3	0.9	40.3	265	0.3
sliced, in water, w/liquid	1 cup	37	0.23	0.06	0.73	0.18	11.8	0.00	18.9	36.9	0.9	44.3	312	0.3
Fresh														
raw, diced	1 cup	36	0.14	0.06	0.65	0.14	16.4	0.00	23.9	10.8	0.6	21.7	175	0.1
raw, sliced, 3.5 inch diam, 3/4 inch thick	1 slice	19	0.08	0.03	0.35	0.07	8.9	0.00	12.9	5.9	0.3	11.8	94.9	<0.1
raw, sliced, 3.5 inch diam, 1/2 inch thick	1 slice	13	0.05	0.02	0.23	0.05	5.9	0.00	8.6	3.9	0.2	7.8	63.3	<0.1
raw, whole, trimmed	1 medium	109	0.43	0.17	2.00	0.41	50.0	0.00	72.7	33.0	1.7	66.1	533	0.4
Frozen														
chunks, sweetened	1 cup	74	0.25	0.07	0.73	0.18	26.0	0.00	19.6	22.1	0.9	24.5	245	0.3
PINEAPPLE JUICE														
Can, bottle, box, or carton														
unsweetened, w/added ascorbic acid	1 cup	13	0.14	0.06	0.64	0.24	57.8	0.00	60.0	42.5	0.7	32.5	335	0.3
unsweetened, w/o added ascorbic acid	1 cup	13	0.14	0.06	0.64	0.24	57.8	0.00	26.8	42.5	0.7	32.5	335	0.3
Frozen or chilled														
concentrate, prepared	1 cup	25	0.17	0.05	0.50	0.19	26.5	0.00	30.0	27.5	0.8	22.5	340	0.3
concentrate, unprepared	6 fl oz	108	0.50	0.13	1.90	0.55	79.5	0.00	90.7	84.2	1.9	75.6	1020	0.9
PINEAPPLE-GRAPEFRUIT JUICE. See under FRUIT JUICE BLEND.														
PINEAPPLE-ORANGE JUICE. See under FRUIT JUICE BLEND.														
PINK BEAN. See BEAN, PINK.														
PINK GRAPEFRUIT JUICE. See under GRAPEFRUIT JUICE.														
PINK SALMON. See under SALMON.														
PINNOCHIO. See PINE NUT.														
PIÑON. See PINE NUT.														
PINTO BEAN. See BEAN, PINTO.														
PINYON, COLORADO. See PINE NUT.														
PISTACHIO														
Dried														
raw	1 cup	708	1.10	0.20	1.70	2.20	65.3	0.00	6.4	137.0	5.5	155.0	1251	2.8
raw	30 nuts	99	0.16	0.03	0.23	0.31	9.2	0.00	0.9	19.3	0.8	21.8	176	0.4
raw, approx 47 kernels	1 oz	157	0.25	0.05	0.37	0.48	14.5	0.00	1.4	30.3	1.2	34.3	277	0.6
Dry roasted														
salted	1 cup	682	1.1	0.20	1.80	2.20	64.0	0.00	2.9	138.0	5.3	154.0	1322	2.9
salted, approx 47 kernels	1 oz	151	0.24	0.05	0.40	0.48	14.2	0.00	0.7	30.6	1.2	34.0	293	0.7
unsalted	1 cup	682	1.10	0.20	1.80	2.20	64.0	0.00	2.9	138.0	5.3	154.0	1322	2.9
unsalted, approx 47 kernels	1 oz	151	0.24	0.05	0.40	0.48	14.2	0.00	0.7	30.6	1.2	34.0	293	0.7
PITA. See under BREAD.														

Food Name	Serving Size	A I.U.	Thi mg	Rib mg	Nia mg	B$_6$ mg	Fol mcg	B$_{12}$ mcg	C mg	Calc mg	Iron mg	Mag mg	Pot mg	Zn mg
PITANGA / Surinam cherry														
raw	1 cup	2595	0.05	0.07	0.52	na	na	0.00	45.5	15.6	0.4	20.8	178	na
raw, trimmed, whole	1 fruit	105	0.00	0.00	0.02	na	na	0.00	1.8	0.6	<0.1	0.8	7.2	na
PLANTAIN														
cooked, mashed	1 cup	1818	0.09	0.10	1.50	0.48	52.0	0.00	21.8	4.0	1.2	64.0	930	0.3
cooked, sliced	1 cup	1400	0.07	0.08	1.20	0.37	40.0	0.00	16.8	3.1	0.9	49.3	716	0.2
raw, sliced	1 cup	1668	0.08	0.08	1.00	0.44	32.6	0.00	27.2	4.4	0.9	54.8	739	0.2
raw, whole	1 medium	2017	0.09	0.10	1.20	0.54	39.4	0.00	32.9	5.4	1.1	66.2	893	0.3
PLUM														
Canned														
purple, in heavy syrup, w/liquid	1 medium	119	0.01	0.02	0.13	0.01	1.1	0.00	0.2	4.1	0.4	2.3	42	<0.1
purple, in juice, w/liquid	1 medium	464	0.01	0.03	0.22	0.01	1.2	0.00	1.3	4.6	0.2	3.7	71	<0.1
purple, in light syrup, w/liquid	1 medium	121	0.01	0.02	0.14	0.01	1.2	0.00	0.2	4.1	0.4	2.3	43	<0.1
purple, in water, w/liquid	1 medium	420	0.01	0.02	0.17	0.01	1.2	0.00	1.2	3.2	<0.1	2.3	58	<0.1
purple, pitted, in extra heavy syrup, w/liquid	1 cup	663	0.04	0.10	0.74	0.07	6.5	0.00	1.0	23.5	2.1	13.1	232	0.2
purple, pitted, in heavy syrup, w/liquid	1 cup	668	0.04	0.10	0.75	0.07	6.5	0.00	1.0	23.2	2.2	12.9	235	0.2
purple, pitted, in juice, w/liquid	1 cup	2543	0.06	0.15	1.20	0.07	6.6	0.00	7.1	25.2	0.9	20.2	388	0.3
purple, pitted, in light syrup, w/liquid	1 cup	665	0.04	0.10	0.75	0.07	6.6	0.00	1.0	22.7	2.2	12.6	234	0.2
purple, pitted, in water, w/liquid	1 cup	2276	0.05	0.10	0.92	0.07	6.5	0.00	6.7	17.4	0.4	12.4	314	0.2
Fresh														
raw, sliced	1 cup	533	0.07	0.16	0.82	0.13	3.6	0.00	15.7	6.6	0.2	11.6	284	0.2
raw, whole, approx 2 1/8 inch diam	1 plum	213	0.03	0.06	0.33	0.05	1.5	0.00	6.3	2.6	<0.1	4.6	114	<0.1
POHA. See CAPE GOOSEBERRY.														
POI	1 cup	48	0.31	0.10	2.6	0.66	51.4	0.00	9.6	38.4	2.1	57.6	439	0.5
POKEBERRY SHOOT														
boiled, drained	1 cup	14355	0.12	0.41	1.80	0.18	14.4	0.00	135.0	87.5	2.0	23.1	304	0.3
boiled, drained	1 tbsp	870	0.01	0.03	0.11	0.01	0.87	0.00	8.2	5.3	0.1	1.4	18	<0.1
raw	1 cup	13920	0.13	0.53	1.90	0.23	25.3	0.00	218.0	84.8	2.7	28.8	387	0.4
POLISH SAUSAGE. See under SAUSAGE.														
POLLACK														
ATLANTIC														
baked, broiled, grilled, or microwaved	3 oz	34	0.05	0.19	3.40	0.28	2.5	3.10	0.0	65.5	0.5	73.1	388	0.5
raw	3 oz	30	0.04	0.16	2.80	0.24	2.5	2.70	0.0	51.0	0.4	57.0	303	0.4
WALLEYE														
baked, broiled, grilled, or microwaved	3 oz	65	0.06	0.07	1.40	0.06	3.1	3.60	0.0	5.1	0.2	62.0	329	0.5
raw	3 oz	56	0.06	0.05	1.10	0.05	2.6	2.60	0.0	4.3	0.2	48.5	277	0.4
POMEGRANATE / Chinese apple														
raw, whole, medium, approx 3-3/8 inch diam	1 pomegranate	0	0.05	0.05	0.46	0.16	9.2	0.00	9.4	4.6	0.5	4.6	399	0.2
POMELO / pummelo														
raw, sections	1 cup	0	0.07	0.05	0.42	0.07	na	0.00	116.0	7.6	0.2	11.4	410	0.2
raw, trimmed	1 medium	0	0.21	0.16	1.30	0.22	na	0.00	371.0	24.4	0.7	36.5	1315	0.5
POMPANO, FLORIDA														
baked, broiled, grilled, or microwaved	3 oz	102	0.58	0.13	3.20	0.20	14.7	1.00	0.0	36.5	0.6	26.4	541	0.6
raw	3 oz	94	0.48	0.10	2.50	0.17	12.8	1.10	0.0	18.7	0.5	22.9	324	0.6
raw, boneless	1 oz	31	0.16	0.03	0.85	0.06	4.3	0.37	0.0	6.2	0.2	7.7	108	0.2
POPCORN														
(NOTE: All popcorn is popped unless otherwise noted.)														
AIR-POPPED														
	1 cup	16	0.02	0.02	0.16	0.02	1.8	0.00	0.0	0.8	0.2	10.5	24	0.3
	1 oz	56	0.06	0.08	0.55	0.07	6.5	0.00	0.0	2.8	0.8	37.1	85	0.9
white	1 cup	2	0.02	0.02	0.16	0.02	1.8	0.00	0.0	0.8	0.2	10.5	24	0.3
white	1 oz	8	0.06	0.08	0.55	0.07	6.5	0.00	0.0	2.8	0.8	37.1	85	0.9

Food Name	Serving Size	A I.U.	Thi mg	Rib mg	Nia mg	B$_6$ mg	Fol mcg	B$_{12}$ mcg	C mg	Calc mg	Iron mg	Mag mg	Pot mg	Zn mg
OIL-POPPED														
....	1 cup	17	0.02	0.02	0.17	0.02	1.9	0.00	<0.1	1.1	0.3	11.9	25	0.3
....	1 oz	44	0.04	0.04	0.44	0.06	4.8	0.00	<0.1	2.8	0.8	30.6	634	0.8
white	1 cup	1	0.02	0.02	0.17	0.02	1.9	0.00	<0.1	1.1	0.3	11.9	25	0.3
white	1 oz	3	0.04	0.04	0.44	0.06	4.8	0.00	<0.1	2.8	0.8	30.6	64	0.8
POPPY SEED														
....	1 tbsp	0	0.08	0.02	0.09	0.04	5.1	0.00	0.3	127.0	0.8	29.2	67	0.9
....	1 tsp	0	0.02	0.01	0.03	0.01	1.6	0.00	<0.1	40.6	0.3	9.3	30	0.3
POPPY SEED FILLING (Solo) 'Sokal'	2 tbsp	na	na	na	na	na	na	na	na	116.0	na	na	na	na
POPPY SEED OIL														
....	1 cup	0	0.00	0.00	0.00	0.00	0.0	0.00	0.0	0.0	0.0	0.0	0	0.0
....	1 tbsp	0	0.00	0.00	0.00	0.00	0.0	0.00	0.0	0.0	0.0	0.0	0	0.0
PORK. See also HAM.														
(NOTE: TRIMMED = Lean; separable fat removed. UNTRIMMED = Separable fat not removed.)														
BACKFAT														
Fresh, wholesale cuts, raw	1 oz	4	0.02	0.01	0.28	0.01	0.28	0.05	<0.1	0.6	<0.1	0.6	18	0.1
BACKRIB														
Fresh														
Untrimmed														
raw	1 oz	3	0.17	0.07	1.30	0.11	1.1	0.23	<0.1	9.1	0.3	4.5	66	0.7
roasted	3 oz	8	0.36	0.17	3.00	0.26	2.5	0.54	0.3	38.3	1.2	17.9	268	2.9
BELLY														
Fresh, wholesale cuts, raw	1 oz	3	0.11	0.07	1.30	0.04	0.3	0.24	<0.1	1.4	0.2	1.1	52	0.3
BRAIN														
Fresh														
braised	3 oz	0	0.07	0.19	2.80	0.12	3.4	1.20	11.9	7.7	1.5	10.2	166	1.3
raw	4 oz	0	0.17	0.31	4.80	0.22	6.8	2.50	15.3	11.3	1.8	15.8	292	1.4
raw	1 oz	0	0.04	0.08	1.20	0.05	1.7	0.62	3.8	2.8	0.5	4.0	73	0.4
CENTER LOIN														
Fresh														
Trimmed														
chop, bone in, braised	3 oz	6	0.70	0.19	4.10	0.34	2.5	0.43	0.9	19.6	0.9	17.0	312	1.9
chop, bone in, broiled	3 oz	7	0.98	0.26	4.70	0.40	5.1	0.63	0.3	26.4	0.7	22.9	319	2.0
chop, bone in, pan fried	3 oz	7	1.10	0.28	5.10	0.44	5.1	0.65	1.0	19.6	0.8	27.2	382	2.1
chop or roast, bone-in, raw	3 oz	4	0.68	0.12	2.84	0.30	2.8	0.32	0.6	11.7	0.5	12.8	202	0.9
roast, bone in, roasted	3 oz	6	0.78	0.23	4.60	0.32	3.4	0.49	0.9	21.3	0.9	18.7	308	1.8
Untrimmed														
chop, bone in, braised	3 oz	7	0.65	0.18	3.90	0.32	2.5	0.42	0.8	22.1	0.9	16.1	300	1.8
chop, bone in, broiled	3 oz	8	0.91	0.25	4.50	0.36	5.1	0.62	0.3	28.1	0.7	21.3	304	1.9
chop, bone in, pan fried	3 oz	7	0.97	0.26	4.80	0.40	5.1	0.62	0.9	22.9	0.8	24.6	361	2.0
chop or roast, bone-in, raw	3 oz	4	0.68	0.13	3.01	0.31	3.2	0.35	0.6	15.3	0.5	13.3	211	0.9
roast, bone in, roasted	3 oz	6	0.73	0.22	4.40	0.30	3.4	0.48	0.8	22.9	0.8	17.0	299	1.7
CENTER RIB														
Fresh														
Trimmed														
chop, bone in, braised	3 oz	5	0.53	0.21	4.40	0.29	1.7	0.46	0.3	18.7	0.8	16.1	344	1.8
chop, bone in, broiled	3 oz	5	0.95	0.28	5.20	0.40	2.5	0.65	0.3	26.4	0.7	23.8	357	2.0
chop, bone in, pan-fried	3 oz	5	0.74	0.28	5.00	0.34	2.5	0.64	0.3	17.0	0.7	22.9	387	1.8
roast, bone in, roasted	3 oz	5	0.64	0.27	5.50	0.29	2.5	0.58	0.3	22.1	0.8	18.7	371	1.8
Untrimmed														
chop, bone in, braised	3 oz	6	0.50	0.20	4.20	0.27	1.7	0.45	0.3	21.3	0.8	15.3	329	1.7
chop, bone in, broiled	3 oz	6	0.88	0.26	4.90	0.37	2.5	0.62	0.3	28.1	0.7	22.1	341	1.9
chop, bone in, pan-fried	3 oz	6	0.68	0.26	4.70	0.31	2.5	0.60	0.3	20.4	0.6	21.3	366	1.7
roast, bone in, roasted	3 oz	5	0.61	0.26	5.20	0.28	2.5	0.56	0.3	23.8	0.8	17.9	358	1.8

Food Name	Serving Size	A I.U.	Thi mg	Rib mg	Nia mg	B_6 mg	Fol mcg	B_{12} mcg	C mg	Calc mg	Iron mg	Mag mg	Pot mg	Zn mg
CHITTERLINGS														
Fresh														
raw	1 oz	0	0.00	0.02	0.02	0.00	0.6	0.23	1.2	5.7	0.5	1.7	33	0.6
simmered	3 oz	0	0.00	0.07	0.09	0.01	2.5	0.88	0	22.9	3.1	8.5	7	4.3
CHOP														
Refrigerated or frozen														
center cut, 'Always Tender' (Hormel)	4 oz	0	na	na	na	na	na	na	1.9	15.5	0.7	23.0	344	1.7
center cut, 'Always Tender' (Hormel)	1 oz	0	na	na	na	na	na	na	0.5	3.9	0.2	5.8	87	0.4
COMPOSITE CUTS														
Fresh														
Trimmed														
loin and shoulder, cooked	3 oz	6	0.72	0.29	4.40	0.37	5.1	0.64	0.3	17.9	0.9	22.1	319	2.5
loin and shoulder, raw	1 oz	2	0.27	0.08	1.40	0.14	1.4	0.19	0.2	4.5	0.3	6.5	108	0.6
Untrimmed														
leg, loin, shoulder, spareribs, cooked	3 oz	7	0.65	0.28	4.20	0.34	5.1	0.65	0.3	21.3	0.9	20.4	301	2.5
leg, loin, shoulder, spareribs, raw	1 oz	2	0.23	0.07	1.30	0.12	1.7	0.19	0.2	4.3	0.3	5.7	92	0.6
loin and shoulder, cooked	3 oz	7	0.72	0.28	4.20	0.34	5.1	0.63	0.3	20.4	0.8	20.4	308	2.2
loin and shoulder, raw	1 oz	2	0.25	0.07	1.30	0.13	1.4	0.18	0.2	5.4	0.2	6.0	99	0.5
EAR														
Fresh														
raw	1 oz	0	0.02	0.03	0.22	0.01	0.0	0.02	0.0	6.0	0.7	2.0	16	<0.1
simmered	1 medium	0	0.02	0.08	0.62	0.01	0.0	0.04	0.0	20.0	1.7	7.8	44	0.2
FEET														
Fresh														
pickled, cured	1 oz	0	0.00	0.01	0.10	0.11	1.1	0.18	0.0	9.1	0.2	1.1	67	0.4
PORK FEET, RAW														
raw	1/2 medium	0	0.04	0.10	1.10	0.11	1.9	0.26	0.0	56.0	0.5	6.7	260	1.2
raw	1 oz	0	0.01	0.03	0.32	0.03	0.6	0.08	0.0	16.7	0.1	2.0	78	0.4
simmered	3 oz	0	0.01	0.05	0.44	0.08	0.9	0.15	0.0	38.3	0.4	4.3	124	0.9
GROUND														
Fresh														
cooked	3 oz	7	0.60	0.19	3.60	0.33	5.1	0.46	0.6	18.7	1.1	20.4	308	2.7
raw	4 oz	8	0.83	0.27	4.90	0.43	5.7	0.79	0.8	15.8	1.0	21.5	324	2.5
raw	1 oz	2	0.21	0.07	1.20	0.11	1.4	0.20	0.2	4.0	0.3	5.4	81	0.6
HEART														
Fresh														
braised	1 cup	32	0.81	2.5	8.80	0.57	5.8	5.50	2.9	10.2	8.5	34.8	299	4.5
braised	1 medium	28	0.72	2.2	7.80	0.50	5.2	4.90	2.6	9.0	7.5	31.0	266	4.0
raw	1 medium	57	1.40	2.7	15.3	0.88	9.0	8.60	12.0	11.3	10.6	42.9	664	6.3
raw	1 oz	7	0.17	0.34	1.90	0.11	1.1	1.10	1.5	1.4	1.3	5.4	83	0.8
JOWL														
Fresh														
raw	4 oz	10	0.44	0.27	5.10	0.10	1.1	0.93	0.0	4.5	0.5	3.4	167	0.9
raw	1 oz	3	0.11	0.07	1.30	0.03	0.3	0.23	0.0	1.1	0.1	0.85	42.0	0.2
KIDNEYS														
Fresh														
braised	1 cup	364	0.55	2.2	8.10	0.64	57.4	10.9	14.8	18.2	7.4	25.2	200	5.8
braised	3 oz	221	0.34	1.3	4.90	0.39	34.9	6.60	9.0	11.1	4.5	15.3	122	3.5
raw	1 oz	56	0.10	0.48	2.30	0.13	11.9	2.40	3.8	2.6	1.4	4.8	65	0.8
LEG, RUMP HALF														
Fresh														
Trimmed														
raw	1 oz	2	0.30	0.08	1.40	0.13	0.9	0.20	0.4	1.7	0.3	7.1	107	0.6
roasted	3 oz	8	0.68	0.30	4.20	0.29	2.5	0.64	0.2	6.0	0.9	24.6	332	2.6

Food Name	Serving Size	A I.U.	Thi mg	Rib mg	Nia mg	B_6 mg	Fol mcg	B_{12} mcg	C mg	Calc mg	Iron mg	Mag mg	Pot mg	Zn mg
roasted, diced	1 cup	12.2	1.10	0.48	6.60	0.46	4.0	1.00	0.3	9.4	1.5	39.1	528	4.1
Untrimmed														
raw	1 oz	2.0	0.26	0.07	1.20	0.11	0.9	0.18	0.3	1.4	0.22	6.0	94	0.5
roasted	3 oz	7.7	0.64	0.28	4.00	0.27	2.5	0.61	0.2	10.2	0.9	22.9	318	2.4
roasted, diced	1 cup	12	1.00	0.44	6.30	0.43	4.0	0.97	0.3	16.2	1.4	36.5	505	3.8
LEG, SHANK HALF														
Fresh														
Trimmed														
raw	1 oz	2	0.25	0.08	1.30	0.14	1.4	0.20	0.3	2.0	0.3	7.1	96	0.7
roasted	3 oz	7	0.54	0.29	4.10	0.39	5.1	0.60	0.3	6.0	0.9	21.3	306	2.9
roasted, diced	1 cup	11	0.85	0.46	6.60	0.62	8.1	0.96	0.5	9.4	1.5	33.8	486	4.7
Untrimmed														
raw	1 oz	2	0.21	0.07	1.10	0.11	1.1	0.17	0.2	1.7	0.2	5.4	81	0.5
roasted	3 oz	8	0.49	0.26	3.80	0.34	4.3	0.56	0.3	12.8	0.8	18.7	287	2.6
roasted, diced	1 cup	12	0.78	0.41	6.00	0.54	6.8	0.89	0.4	20.3	1.3	29.7	456	4.1
LEG, WHOLE														
Fresh														
Trimmed														
raw	1 oz	2	0.25	0.07	1.50	0.14	2.6	0.20	0.3	1.7	0.3	7.1	105	0.6
roasted	3 oz	8	0.59	0.30	4.20	0.38	10.2	0.61	0.3	6.0	0.9	21.3	317	2.8
roasted, diced	1 cup	12	0.93	0.47	6.70	0.61	16.2	0.97	0.5	9.4	1.5	33.8	504	4.4
Untrimmed														
raw	1 oz	2	0.21	0.06	1.30	0.11	2.0	0.18	0.2	1.4	0.3	5.7	89	0.6
roasted	3 oz	9	0.54	0.27	3.90	0.34	8.5	0.58	0.3	11.9	0.9	18.7	299	2.5
roasted, diced	1 cup	14	0.86	0.42	6.20	0.54	13.5	0.92	0.4	18.9	1.4	29.7	475	4.0
LIVER														
Fresh														
braised	3 oz	15297	0.22	1.90	7.20	0.48	139.0	15.90	20.1	8.5	15.2	11.9	128	5.7
raw	1 oz	6138	0.08	0.85	4.30	0.20	60.1	7.40	7.2	2.6	6.6	5.1	77	1.6
LOIN														
Fresh														
Trimmed														
blade, braised	3 oz	6	0.45	0.23	3.30	0.30	2.5	0.60	0.7	20.4	1.1	15.3	277	3.3
blade, broiled	3 oz	6	0.63	0.30	3.90	0.38	3.4	0.80	0.7	19.6	0.9	22.1	318	3.4
blade, pan-fried	3 oz	6	0.62	0.30	3.80	0.35	3.4	0.82	0.7	18.7	0.9	22.1	310	3.3
blade, roasted	3 oz	7	0.49	0.29	4.00	0.37	4.3	0.68	0.3	24.6	1.1	20.4	297	3.2
ribs, country-style, braised	3 oz	6	0.46	0.24	3.50	0.31	2.5	0.63	0.7	21.3	1.2	15.3	293	3.4
ribs, country-style, raw	1 oz	2	0.23	0.08	1.20	0.14	1.1	0.24	0.2	6.5	0.3	6.0	96	0.8
ribs, country-style, roasted	3 oz	7	0.49	0.29	4.00	0.37	4.3	0.68	0.3	24.6	1.1	20.4	297	3.2
whole, braised	3 oz	6	0.56	0.23	3.90	0.33	3.4	0.47	0.5	15.3	0.9	17.0	329	2.1
whole, broiled	3 oz	6	0.79	0.29	4.50	0.42	5.1	0.61	0.6	14.4	0.8	24.6	372	2.1
whole, roasted	3 oz	7	0.86	0.28	5.00	0.47	6.0	0.62	0.5	15.3	0.9	23.8	361	2.1
Untrimmed														
blade, braised	3 oz	7	0.41	0.20	3.10	0.25	1.7	0.55	0.5	26.4	0.9	12.8	258	2.8
blade, broiled	3 oz	7	0.55	0.25	3.50	0.32	3.4	0.71	0.6	24.6	0.8	18.7	292	2.9
blade, pan-fried	3 oz	7	0.53	0.25	3.40	0.29	3.4	0.71	0.5	25.5	0.8	17.9	282	2.7
blade, roasted	3 oz	8	0.45	0.25	3.60	0.32	3.4	0.62	0.2	28.9	0.9	17.0	277	2.8
ribs, country-style, braised	3 oz	7	0.43	0.22	3.30	0.28	2.5	0.59	0.6	24.6	1.0	14.4	279	3.0
ribs, country-style, raw	1 oz	2	0.20	0.07	1.10	0.12	1.1	0.21	0.2	7.7	0.3	5.1	86	0.7
ribs, country-style, roasted	3 oz	8	0.76	0.29	3.70	0.38	4.3	0.67	0.3	21.3	0.9	19.6	292	2.0
whole, braised	3 oz	6	0.54	0.22	3.80	0.31	2.5	0.46	0.5	17.9	0.9	16.1	318	2.0
whole, broiled	3 oz	6	0.75	0.27	4.30	0.39	4.3	0.59	0.5	16.1	0.7	23.8	360	2.0
whole, roasted	3 oz	8	0.84	0.27	4.70	0.44	5.1	0.60	0.5	16.1	0.8	22.1	347	2.0

Food Name	Serving Size	A I.U.	Thi mg	Rib mg	Nia mg	B$_6$ mg	Fol mcg	B$_{12}$ mcg	C mg	Calc mg	Iron mg	Mag mg	Pot mg	Zn mg
Refrigerated or frozen														
boneless, 'Always Tender' (Hormel)	1 oz	0	na	na	na	na	na	na	0.4	1.2	0.2	5.9	87	0.5
boneless, 'Always Tender' (Hormel)	4 oz	0	na	na	na	na	na	na	1.5	4.9	0.7	23.7	347	1.8
LUNGS														
Fresh														
braised	3 oz	0	0.07	0.27	1.20	0.07	1.7	1.70	6.7	6.8	13.9	10.2	128	2.1
raw	1 oz	0	0.02	0.12	0.95	0.03	0.9	0.78	3.5	2.0	5.4	4.0	86	0.6
PANCREAS														
Fresh														
braised	3 oz	0	0.08	0.56	2.70	0.37	4.3	14.5	4.8	13.6	2.3	19.6	143	3.6
raw	1 oz	0	0.03	0.13	0.98	0.13	0.9	4.60	4.3	3.1	0.6	4.8	56	0.7
SHOULDER														
Fresh														
Trimmed														
arm picnic, braised	3 oz	7	0.51	0.31	5.00	0.35	4.3	0.60	0.3	6.8	1.7	18.7	344	4.2
arm picnic, raw	1 oz	1	0.25	0.09	1.30	0.14	1.1	0.21	0.3	1.7	0.3	6.0	97	0.8
arm picnic, roasted	3 oz	6	0.49	0.30	3.70	0.35	4.3	0.66	0.3	7.7	1.2	17.0	298	3.5
Boston blade, braised	3 oz	8	0.61	0.34	3.60	0.25	1.7	0.83	0.3	24.6	1.7	17.0	350	4.7
Boston blade, broiled	3 oz	7	0.64	0.37	3.70	0.26	4.3	0.96	0.3	28.1	1.3	20.4	292	4.3
Boston blade, roasted	3 oz	8	0.95	0.34	4.20	0.37	6.8	0.99	0.9	22.9	1.3	22.1	363	3.6
whole, raw	1 oz	2	0.25	0.09	1.20	0.12	1.4	0.24	0.2	4.0	0.4	6.0	97	0.9
whole, roasted	3 oz	6	0.53	0.32	3.60	0.27	4.3	0.73	0.5	15.3	1.3	17.0	294	3.5
whole, roasted, diced	1 cup	9	0.85	0.50	5.80	0.43	6.8	1.20	0.8	24.3	2.0	27.0	467	5.6
Untrimmed														
arm picnic, braised	3 oz	8	0.46	0.26	4.40	0.30	3.4	0.55	0.3	15.3	1.4	16.1	314	3.6
arm picnic, braised, diced	1 cup	12	0.73	0.41	7.00	0.47	5.4	0.88	0.4	24.3	2.2	25.6	498	5.6
arm picnic, raw	1 oz	2	0.21	0.07	1.10	0.11	1.1	0.18	0.2	1.4	0.3	4.8	82	0.7
arm picnic, roasted	3 oz	7	0.44	0.26	3.30	0.30	3.4	0.60	0.2	16.1	1.0	14.4	276	2.9
arm picnic, roasted, diced	1 cup	11	0.70	0.41	5.30	0.47	5.4	0.96	0.3	25.6	1.6	22.9	439	4.7
Boston blade, braised	3 oz	9	0.57	0.31	3.40	0.23	1.7	0.77	0.3	27.2	1.6	15.3	331	4.3
Boston blade, broiled	3 oz	8	0.59	0.34	3.50	0.23	3.4	0.90	0.3	30.6	1.2	17.9	277	3.8
Boston blade, roasted	3 oz	6	0.54	0.30	3.50	0.20	4.3	0.75	0.6	23.8	1.2	15.3	282	3.4
whole, raw	1 oz	2	0.22	0.08	1.10	0.10	1.4	0.21	0.2	4.3	0.3	5.1	86	0.8
whole, roasted	3 oz	7	0.49	0.28	3.40	0.25	4.3	0.68	0.4	20.4	1.1	15.3	280	3.2
whole, roasted, diced	1 cup	11	0.78	0.44	5.40	0.39	6.8	1.10	0.7	32.4	1.8	24.3	444	5.0
SIRLOIN														
Fresh														
Trimmed														
chop, bone in, braised	3 oz	6	0.59	0.24	3.40	0.38	2.5	0.48	0.8	11.1	1.1	17.0	286	2.2
chop, bone in, broiled	3 oz	7	0.88	0.34	4.00	0.46	5.1	0.71	0.3	15.3	1.1	22.9	320	2.3
roast, bone in, roasted	3 oz	6	0.68	0.28	4.70	0.36	5.1	0.66	0.3	17.0	0.9	21.3	311	2.2
Untrimmed														
chop, bone in, braised	3 oz	6	0.56	0.22	3.20	0.35	2.5	0.48	0.7	15.3	1.0	16.1	276	2.1
chop, bone in, broiled	3 oz	7	0.81	0.29	3.80	0.46	4.3	0.64	0.8	14.4	0.8	24.6	326	2.2
roast, bone in, roasted	3 oz	7	0.64	0.27	4.50	0.33	5.1	0.65	0.3	19.6	0.9	20.4	298	2.1
SPARERIBS														
Fresh														
Untrimmed														
braised	3 oz	9	0.35	0.33	4.70	0.30	3.4	0.92	0.0	40.0	1.6	20.4	272	3.9
raw	1 oz	3	0.17	0.08	1.40	0.12	1.1	0.25	0.0	8.8	0.3	6.2	73	0.8
SPLEEN														
Fresh														
braised	3 oz	0	0.12	0.22	5.00	0.05	3.4	2.30	9.9	11.1	18.9	12.8	193	3.0
raw	1 oz	0	0.04	0.09	1.70	0.02	1.1	0.92	8.1	2.8	6.3	3.7	112	0.7

Food Name	Serving Size	A I.U.	Thi mg	Rib mg	Nia mg	B_6 mg	Fol mcg	B_{12} mcg	C mg	Calc mg	Iron mg	Mag mg	Pot mg	Zn mg
STOMACH														
Fresh														
raw	4 oz	0	0.10	0.13	5.00	0.05	2.3	1.10	0.0	11.3	2.5	10.2	227	2.3
raw	1 oz	0	0.02	0.03	1.30	0.01	0.6	0.28	0.0	2.8	0.6	2.6	57	0.6
TAIL														
Fresh														
raw	4 oz	0	0.24	0.12	2.30	0.42	5.7	0.99	0.0	20.3	1.1	9.0	394	2.6
raw	1 oz	0	0.06	0.03	0.58	0.11	1.4	0.25	0.0	5.1	0.3	2.3	99	0.7
simmered	3 oz	0	0.06	0.06	0.95	0.23	3.4	0.47	0.0	11.9	0.7	6.0	133	1.4
TENDERLOIN														
Fresh														
Trimmed														
broiled	3 oz	6	0.84	0.33	4.40	0.45	5.1	0.85	0.9	4.3	1.2	30.6	383	2.5
raw	1 oz	2	0.28	0.08	1.30	0.15	1.4	0.23	0.3	1.4	0.4	7.4	104	0.6
roasted	3 oz	6	0.80	0.33	4.00	0.36	5.1	0.47	0.3	5.1	1.3	23.8	371	2.2
Untrimmed														
broiled	3 oz	6	0.82	0.32	4.30	0.44	5.1	0.83	0.9	4.3	1.2	29.8	377	2.5
raw	1 oz	2	0.27	0.08	1.20	0.14	1.4	0.22	0.3	1.4	0.3	7.1	102	0.6
roasted	3 oz	6	0.79	0.33	4.00	0.35	5.1	0.47	0.3	5.1	1.2	22.9	368	2.2
TONGUE														
Fresh														
braised	3 oz	0	0.27	0.43	4.50	0.20	3.4	2.00	1.4	16.1	4.2	17.0	201	3.9
raw	4 oz	0	0.55	0.55	6.00	0.27	4.5	3.20	5.0	18.1	3.8	20.3	275	3.4
raw	1 oz	0	0.14	0.14	1.50	0.07	1.1	0.81	1.2	4.5	0.9	5.1	69	0.9
TOP LOIN														
Fresh														
Trimmed														
chop, boneless, braised	3 oz	5	0.48	0.23	4.00	0.29	4.3	0.39	0.3	19.6	0.9	17.0	358	1.9
chop, boneless, broiled	3 oz	5	0.76	0.28	4.40	0.34	7.7	0.59	0.3	26.4	0.7	23.8	357	2.0
chop, boneless, pan-fried	3 oz	5	0.71	0.32	4.80	0.36	6.8	0.57	0.3	18.7	0.7	25.5	425	1.9
roast, boneless, raw	1 oz	2	0.24	0.08	1.40	0.13	2.0	0.15	<0.1	6.0	0.2	6.5	119	0.5
roast, boneless, roasted	3 oz	7	0.54	0.27	4.60	0.34	7.7	0.47	0.3	4.3	0.9	21.3	301	2.0
Untrimmed														
chop, boneless, braised	3 oz	6	0.47	0.22	3.90	0.28	3.4	0.39	0.3	17.9	0.8	16.1	346	1.8
chop, boneless, broiled	3 oz	5	0.73	0.26	4.30	0.32	6.8	0.59	0.3	24.6	0.7	22.9	344	1.9
chop, boneless, pan-fried	3 oz	6	0.68	0.30	4.60	0.34	6.8	0.55	0.3	17.9	0.7	23.8	407	1.9
chop or roast, boneless, raw	1 oz	1	0.23	0.07	1.30	0.12	1.7	0.14	<0.1	5.4	0.2	6.0	111	0.4
roast, boneless, roasted	3 oz	7	0.52	0.25	4.40	0.32	6.8	0.47	0.3	4.3	0.7	19.6	291	1.9
PORK, SALT														
cured, raw	8 oz	0	0.49	0.14	3.70	0.18	2.3	0.66	0	13.6	0.0	15.9	150	2.0
cured, raw	1 oz	0	0.06	0.02	0.46	0.02	0.3	0.08	0	1.7	0.1	2.0	18	0.3
PORK DINNER/ENTRÉE														
(Hormel)														
loin fillet, lemon garlic, 'Always Tender'	1 oz	0	na	na	na	na	na	na	0.5	1.5	0.2	5.5	152	0.4
loin fillet, lemon garlic, 'Always Tender'	4 oz	0	na	na	na	na	na	na	1.9	6.2	0.7	22.2	607	1.5
tenderlion, peppercorn, 'Always Tender'	4 oz	0	na	na	na	na	na	na	1.6	15.9	1.2	23.6	657	1.6
tenderloin, teriyaki, 'Always Tender'	4 oz	0	na	na	na	na	na	na	3.0	7.7	1.1	24.3	601	1.7
(Pierre)														
nuggets, breaded, frozen, product 1921	1 piece	5	0.07	0.04	0.50	0.03	4.5	0.11	<0.1	4.7	0.3	3.1	39	0.5
patty, country fried, frozen, product 1920	1 piece	102	0.50	0.28	3.60	0.23	36.5	0.85	<0.1	38.3	2.3	23.8	264	2.6

Food Name	Serving Size	A I.U.	Thi mg	Rib mg	Nia mg	B6 mg	Fol mcg	B12 mcg	C mg	Calc mg	Iron mg	Mag mg	Pot mg	Zn mg
patty, country fried, frozen, product 3701	1 piece	97	0.45	0.28	3.60	0.19	35.2	0.93	0.3	38.7	2.3	22.0	242	3.2
patty, country fried, frozen, product 3801	1 piece	96	0.50	0.27	3.50	0.22	34.3	0.81	<0.1	35.2	2.2	22.9	258	2.6
steak, country fried, frozen, product 3700	1 piece	6	0.56	0.33	4.00	0.14	37.1	0.53	0.4	27.3	2.0	10.9	227	2.4
steak, country fried, frozen, product 3800	1 piece	8	0.73	0.35	4.60	0.24	41.4	0.36	0.2	24.0	2.1	15.3	291	1.6
(Wonderbites)														
and turkey, barbecue, flame broiled, product 9119, 'Lean Magic 30'	1 piece	158	0.37	0.15	2.60	0.25	1.7	0.62	1.4	34.9	1.9	27.2	252	3.0
barbecue, flame broiled, product 1830	1 piece	225	0.35	0.14	2.70	0.22	1.3	0.59	2.6	33.3	1.3	23.0	254	2.7
barbecue, flame broiled, product 3734	1 piece	84	0.50	0.20	2.90	0.26	2.7	0.52	1.3	21.8	1.2	23.1	281	2.5
barbecue, flame broiled, product 3735	1 piece	20	0.12	0.05	0.69	0.06	0.6	0.12	0.3	5.1	0.3	5.4	66	0.6
barbecue, flame broiled, product 3834	1 piece	104	0.46	0.18	3.00	0.28	2.0	0.67	1.3	30.6	1.4	28.6	294	3.1
barbecue, flame broiled, product 3835, 'Dippers'	1 piece	25	0.12	0.04	0.73	0.07	0.6	0.20	0.4	8.8	0.3	6.6	68	0.9
barbecue, flame broiled, product 9800	1 piece	195	0.47	0.19	3.60	0.31	2.2	0.81	2.1	37.0	1.5	30.3	306	3.6
barbecue, flame broiled, product 9966, 'Dippers'	1 piece	48	0.12	0.05	0.82	0.07	0.5	0.18	0.5	8.1	0.4	7.4	79	0.8
barbecue, flame broiled, w/100 serving trays, product 9968	1 piece	48	0.13	0.05	0.84	0.07	0.7	0.23	0.6	9.7	0.4	7.2	78	0.9
barbecue, less fat, flame broiled, product 3730	1 piece	26	0.12	0.05	0.77	0.07	0.5	0.17	0.3	7.3	0.4	7.1	75	0.8
barbecue, less fat, flame broiled, product 3731	1 piece	106	0.48	0.20	3.10	0.29	2.1	0.68	1.3	29.7	1.4	29.0	304	3.2
barbecue, ready to cook, product 1190	1 piece	259	0.40	0.14	2.90	0.26	1.5	0.72	3.2	35.5	1.4	25.2	251	2.9
barbecue, ready to cook, product 1330	1 piece	298	0.45	0.16	3.30	0.29	1.7	0.82	3.7	41.6	1.6	28.9	284	3.3
Oriental crunch, flame-broiled, frozen, 'Dippers'	1 piece	15	0.16	0.06	1.00	0.07	6.5	0.22	<0.1	11.9	0.6	7.1	86	0.9
Oriental crunch, product 3702	1 piece	7	0.12	0.07	0.85	0.04	6.2	0.16	0.1	8.4	0.5	3.9	66	0.7
rib, barbecue, flame broiled, frozen, product 3736	1 piece	39	0.12	0.05	0.78	0.07	0.6	0.17	0.3	8.6	0.4	7.2	76	0.8
rib, barbecue, flame broiled, product 1805, 'Lean Magic'	1 piece	268	0.53	0.17	3.90	0.30	1.7	0.73	2.9	40.3	1.7	28.6	305	3.2
rib, barbecue, flame broiled, product 1809, 'Lean Magic'	1 piece	41	0.15	0.05	0.85	0.08	0.8	0.24	0.4	10.7	0.4	7.6	79	1.0
rib, flame broiled, frozen, product 3831, 'Lean Magic'	1 piece	106	0.49	0.20	3.20	0.29	2.8	0.68	1.3	28.3	1.5	29.7	308	3.3
rib, barbecue, flame broiled, product 3830, 'Lean Magic'	1 piece	26	0.14	0.05	0.80	0.07	0.9	0.23	0.4	9.0	0.4	7.1	75	0.9
teriyaki, flame broiled, product 3759	1 piece	7	0.13	0.06	0.77	0.07	0.8	0.13	<0.1	5.4	0.3	6.2	78	0.6
PORK FAT														
leaf, raw	1 oz	0	0.03	0.02	0.35	0.01	0	0.07	0.0	0.3	<0.1	0.3	8.8	<0.1
leaf, fresh	4 oz	0	0.12	0.07	1.40	0.03	0	0.26	0.0	1.1	0.1	1.1	35	0.2
PORK SKINS														
barbecue	1 oz	428	0.02	0.12	0.95	0.04	8.8	0.04	0.4	12.2	0.3	0.0	51	0.2
barbecue	1/2 oz	214	0.01	0.06	0.48	0.02	4.4	0.02	0.2	6.1	0.2	0.0	26	0.1
plain	1 oz	37	0.03	0.08	0.44	0.01	0	0.18	0.1	8.5	0.3	3.1	36	0.2
plain	1/2 oz	19	0.01	0.04	0.22	0.00	0	0.09	<0.1	4.3	0.1	1.6	18	<0.1
POTATO														
Canned														
sliced, drained	1 cup	0	0.12	0.02	1.60	0.34	11.2	0.00	9.2	9.0	2.3	25.2	412	0.5

Food Name	Serving Size	A I.U.	Thi mg	Rib mg	Nia mg	B$_6$ mg	Fol mcg	B$_{12}$ mcg	C mg	Calc mg	Iron mg	Mag mg	Pot mg	Zn mg
whole, drained	1 medium	0	0.02	0.01	0.32	0.07	2.2	0.00	1.8	1.8	0.4	4.9	80	0.1
whole, w/liquid	1 cup	0	0.10	0.06	2.70	0.41	13.5	0.00	22.8	117	2.2	42.0	615	1.2
Fresh														
baked, flesh and skin, 2-1/3 x 4-3/4 inch	1 potato	0	0.22	0.07	3.30	0.70	22.2	0.00	26.1	20.2	2.7	54.5	844	0.7
baked, flesh only	1/2 cup	0	0.06	0.01	0.85	0.18	5.6	0.00	7.8	3.0	0.2	15.3	239	0.2
baked, flesh only, 2 1/3 x 4 3/4 inch	1 potato	0	0.16	0.03	2.20	0.47	14.2	0.00	20.0	7.8	0.6	39.0	610	0.5
boiled, cooked in skin, flesh only	1/2 cup	0	0.08	0.02	1.10	0.23	7.8	0.00	10.1	3.9	0.2	17.2	296	0.2
boiled, cooked in skin, flesh only, 2.5 inch diam	1 potato	0	0.14	0.03	2.00	0.41	13.6	0.00	17.7	6.8	0.4	29.9	515	0.4
boiled, cooked w/o skin, flesh only	1/2 cup	0	0.08	0.02	1.00	0.21	6.9	0.00	5.8	6.2	0.2	15.6	256	0.2
boiled, cooked w/o skin, flesh only, 2.5 inch diam	1 potato	0	0.13	0.03	1.80	0.36	12.0	0.00	10.0	10.8	0.4	27.0	443	0.4
microwaved, cooked in skin, flesh and skin, 2.5 inch diam	1 potato	0	0.24	0.07	3.50	0.69	24.2	0.00	30.5	22.2	2.5	54.5	903	0.7
microwaved, cooked in skin, flesh and skin	1/2 cup	0	0.10	0.02	1.30	0.25	9.7	0.00	11.8	3.9	0.3	19.5	321	0.3
microwaved, cooked in skin, flesh and skin, 2-1/3 x 4.75 inch	1 potato	0	0.20	0.04	2.50	0.50	19.3	0.00	23.6	7.8	0.6	39.0	641	0.5
raw, diced, flesh and skin	1/2 cup	0	0.07	0.03	1.10	0.20	9.6	0.00	14.8	5.3	0.6	15.8	407	0.3
raw, sliced	1 cup	0	0.28	0.06	3.10	0.47	22.9	0.00	25.8	14.6	1.8	23.7	630	0.6
raw, whole, large, 3–4.25 inch diam, flesh and skin	1 potato	0	0.16	0.06	2.70	0.48	23.6	0.00	36.2	12.9	1.4	38.6	999	0.7
raw, whole, long, 2 1/3 x 4 3/4 inch, flesh and skin	1 potato	0	0.18	0.07	3.00	0.53	25.9	0.00	39.8	14.1	1.5	42.4	1097	0.8
raw, whole, medium, 2.25–3 inch diam, flesh and skin	1 potato	0	0.11	0.04	1.80	0.32	15.6	0.00	24.0	8.5	0.9	25.6	662	0.5
raw, whole, small, 1.75–2.25 inch diam, flesh and skin	1 potato	0	0.08	0.03	1.40	0.24	11.8	0.00	18.1	6.4	0.7	19.3	500	0.4
skin, baked	1 skin	0	0.07	0.06	1.80	0.36	12.5	0.00	7.8	19.7	4.1	24.9	332	0.3
skin, boiled	1 skin	0	0.01	0.01	0.41	0.08	3.3	0.00	1.8	15.3	2.1	10.2	138	0.2
skin, microwaved	1 skin	0	0.04	0.04	1.30	0.28	9.6	0.00	8.9	26.7	3.4	21.5	377	0.3
skin, raw	1 skin	0	0.01	0.01	0.39	0.09	6.6	0.00	4.3	11.4	1.2	8.7	157	0.1
POTATO, MEXICAN. See JICAMA.														
POTATO FLOUR. See under FLOUR.														
POTATO DISH/ENTRÉE														
(Crispy Crowns) puffs, frozen, prepared	10 puffs	10	0.12	0.04	1.30	0.14	9.9	0.00	4.1	18.0	0.9	11.4	228	0.2
(Healthy Choice) cheddar broccoli, w/cheese sauce, frozen	1 pkg	331	na	na	na	na	na	na	28.9	241.0	1.1	na	na	na
PRETZEL														
twists, hard, salted	1 oz	0	0.13	0.18	1.50	0.03	48.5	0.00	0.0	10.2	1.2	9.9	41	0.2
twists, hard, salted	10 twists	0	0.28	0.37	3.20	0.07	103.0	0.00	0.0	21.6	2.6	21.0	88	0.5
twists, hard, unsalted	1 oz	0	0.05	0.03	0.54	0.03	23.5	0.00	0.0	10.2	0.5	9.9	41	0.2
twists, hard, unsalted	10 twists	0	0.11	0.06	1.20	0.07	49.8	0.00	0.0	21.6	1.0	21.0	88	0.5
whole wheat, hard	1 oz	0	0.13	0.08	1.90	0.08	15.3	0.00	0.3	7.9	0.8	8.5	122	0.2
(M&M Mars)														
w/cheddar, 'Combos'	1 oz	19	0.09	0.16	0.90	0.01	2.3	0.03	0	55.9	0.3	6.2	37	0.2
w/cheddar, 'Combos'	10 combos	20	0.09	0.17	0.95	0.01	2.4	0.04	0	59.1	0.3	6.6	39	0.2
PRICKLY PEAR														
raw, sliced	1 cup	76	0.02	0.09	0.69	0.09	8.9	0.00	20.9	83.4	0.5	127	328	0.2
raw, whole, trimmed	1 fruit	53	0.01	0.06	0.47	0.06	6.2	0.00	14.4	57.7	0.3	87.5	227	0.1
PRUNE														
Canned														
in heavy syrup, w/liquid	1 cup	1865	0.08	0.28	2.00	0.47	0.2	0.00	6.6	39.8	0.9	35.1	529	0.5

Food Name	Serving Size	A I.U.	Thi mg	Rib mg	Nia mg	B₆ mg	Fol mcg	B₁₂ mcg	C mg	Calc mg	Iron mg	Mag mg	Pot mg	Zn mg
in heavy syrup, w/liquid................	5 medium	685	0.03	0.11	0.75	0.17	<0.1	0.00	2.4	14.6	0.4	12.9	194	0.2
Dried														
low-moisture, stewed....................	1 cup	1464	0.13	0.08	2.80	0.54	0.6	0.00	0.0	67.2	3.3	58.8	988	0.7
low-moisture, uncooked..................	1 cup	2326	0.16	0.22	4.00	0.98	2.5	0.00	0.0	95.0	4.6	84.5	1397	1.0
pitted, stewed...........................	1 cup	759	0.06	0.25	1.80	0.54	0.3	0.00	7.2	57.0	2.8	49.6	828	0.6
pitted, uncooked........................	1 cup	3378	0.14	0.28	3.30	0.45	6.3	0.00	5.6	86.7	4.2	76.5	1267	0.9
uncooked...............................	1 medium	167	0.01	0.01	0.17	0.02	0.3	0.00	0.3	4.3	0.2	3.8	63	<0.1
PRUNE JUICE														
canned.................................	1 cup	8	0.04	0.18	2.00	0.56	1.0	0.00	10.5	30.7	3.0	35.8	707	0.5
canned.................................	1 fl oz	<1	0.01	0.02	0.25	0.07	0.1	0.00	1.3	3.8	0.4	4.5	88	<0.1
PUDDING. See also PUDDING/PIE FILLING MIX.														
CHOCOLATE (Jell-O) fat free.............	1 serving	174	na	na	na	na	na	na	0.3	89.3	0.6	na	235	na
VANILLA (Jell-O) fat free..................	1 serving	174	na	na	na	na	na	na	0.3	85.9	<0.1	na	123	na
PUDDING/PIE FILLING MIX														
CHOCOLATE														
(Jell-O)														
cook and serve, nonfat, lower calorie.......	1 serving	<1	na	na	na	na	na	na	0.0	5.3	0.7	na	88	na
cook and serve, sugar-free, prepared.......	1 serving	0	na	na	na	na	na	na	0.0	6.9	1.2	na	139	na
fat-free, sugar-free, prepared.............	1 serving	<1	na	na	na	na	na	na	0.1	13.9	0.8	na	122	na
instant, mix only........................	1 serving	0	na	na	na	na	na	na	0.0	4.5	0.6	na	81	na
VANILLA														
(Jell-O)														
cook and serve, nonfat, lower calorie.......	1 serving	0	na	na	na	na	na	na	0.0	2.3	<0.1	na	3	na
cook and serve, sugar-free, prepared.......	1 serving	0	na	na	na	na	na	na	0.0	11.8	<0.1	na	3	na
fat-free, sugar-free, prepared.............	1 serving	0	na	na	na	na	na	na	0.0	2.5	<0.1	na	2	na
instant, mix only........................	1 pkg	0	na	na	na	na	na	na	0.1	1.0	<0.1	na	1	na
PUERTO RICAN CHERRY. See ACEROLA.														
PUMMELO. See POMELO.														
PUMPKIN														
Fresh														
boiled, drained, mashed.................	1 cup	2651	0.08	0.19	1.00	0.11	20.8	0.00	11.5	36.8	1.4	22.1	564	0.6
raw, cubed, 1-inch cubes................	1 cup	1856	0.06	0.13	0.70	0.07	18.8	0.00	10.4	24.4	0.9	13.9	394	0.4
Canned														
....	1 cup	54037	0.06	0.13	0.90	0.14	30.1	0.00	10.3	63.7	3.4	56.4	505	0.4
no salt added..........................	1 cup	54037	0.06	0.13	0.90	0.14	30.1	0.00	10.3	63.7	3.4	56.4	505	0.4
PUMPKIN FLOWER														
boiled, drained.........................	1 cup	2324	0.02	0.04	0.41	0.07	54.7	0.00	6.7	49.6	1.2	33.5	142	0.1
raw....................................	1 cup	643	0.01	0.03	0.23	na	19.4	0.00	9.2	12.9	0.2	7.9	57	na
raw, whole.............................	1 medium	39	0.00	0.00	0.01	na	1.2	0.00	0.6	0.8	<0.1	0.48	4	na
PUMPKIN LEAF														
boiled, drained.........................	1 cup	1757	0.05	0.10	0.60	0.14	17.6	0.00	0.7	30.5	2.3	27.0	311	0.1
raw....................................	1 cup	757	0.04	0.05	0.36	0.08	14.1	0.00	4.3	15.2	0.9	14.8	170	<0.1
PUMPKIN SEED														
dried, kernels..........................	1 cup	524	0.29	0.44	2.40	0.31	79.3	0.00	2.6	59.3	20.7	738.0	1114	10.3
dried, kernels, hulled, approx 142 seeds....	1 oz	108	0.06	0.09	0.50	0.06	16.3	0.00	0.5	12.2	4.2	152.0	229	2.1
roasted, kernels........................	1 cup	863	0.48	0.72	4.00	0.20	130.0	0.00	4.1	97.6	33.9	1212.0	1830	16.9
roasted, kernels........................	1 oz	108	0.06	0.09	0.49	0.03	16.3	0.00	0.5	12.2	4.2	151.0	229	2.1
roasted, whole.........................	1 cup	40	0.02	0.03	0.18	0.02	5.8	0.00	0.3	35.2	2.1	168.0	588	6.6
roasted, whole, approx 85 seeds..........	1 oz	18	0.01	0.02	0.08	0.01	2.6	0.00	<0.1	15.6	0.9	74.3	261	2.9
PUMPKINFISH. See SUNFISH.														
PURSLANE / pussley														
boiled, drained.........................	1 cup	2130	0.04	0.10	0.53	0.08	9.8	0.00	12.1	89.7	0.9	77.0	561	0.2
raw....................................	1 cup	568	0.02	0.05	0.21	0.03	4.9	0.00	9.0	27.9	0.9	29.2	212	<0.1

Q

Food Name	Serving Size	A I.U.	Thi mg	Rib mg	Nia mg	B₆ mg	Fol mcg	B₁₂ mcg	C mg	Calc mg	Iron mg	Mag mg	Pot mg	Zn mg
QUAIL / bobwhite														
meat and skin, raw	3 oz	208	0.21	0.23	6.46	0.51	6.9	0.36	5.2	11.1	3.4	19.7	185	2.1
meat only, raw	3 oz	49	0.24	0.24	7.02	0.45	5.9	0.40	6.2	11.2	3.9	21.4	203	2.3
QUEEN CRAB. See under CRAB.														
QUINCE, raw, trimmed	1 medium	80	0.02	0.03	0.18	0.04	2.8	0.00	13.8	10.1	0.6	7.4	181	<0.1
QUINOA, uncooked	1 cup	0	0.34	0.67	5.0	0.38	83.3	0.00	0.0	102.0	15.7	357.0	1258	5.6

R

Food Name	Serving Size	A I.U.	Thi mg	Rib mg	Nia mg	B₆ mg	Fol mcg	B₁₂ mcg	C mg	Calc mg	Iron mg	Mag mg	Pot mg	Zn mg
RABBIT														
domesticated, composite cuts, raw	1 oz	0	0.03	0.04	2.10	0.14	2.3	2.00	0.0	3.7	0.5	5.4	94	0.5
domesticated, composite cuts, roasted	3 oz	0	0.08	0.18	7.20	0.40	9.3	7.10	0.0	16.1	1.9	17.9	326	1.9
domesticated, composite cuts, stewed	3 oz	0	0.05	0.14	6.10	0.29	7.7	5.50	0.0	17.0	2.0	17.0	255	2.0
wild, raw	1 oz	0	0.01	0.02	1.80	na	na	na	0.0	3.4	0.9	8.2	107	na
wild, stewed	3 oz	0	0.02	0.06	5.40	0.29	6.8	5.50	0.0	15.3	4.1	26.4	292	2.0
RACCOON, roasted	3 oz	0	0.50	0.44	4.00	0.40	9.3	7.10	0.0	11.9	6.0	25.5	338	1.9
RADICCHIO														
fresh, raw, leaf	1 med leaf	2	0.00	0.00	0.02	0.01	4.8	0.00	0.6	1.5	<0.1	1.0	24	<0.1
fresh, raw, shredded	1 cup	11	0.01	0.01	0.10	0.02	24.0	0.00	3.2	7.6	0.2	5.2	121	0.3
RADISH														
CHINESE. See DAIKON.														
ORIENTAL. See DAIKON.														
RED														
fresh, raw, sliced	1 cup	9	0.01	0.05	0.35	0.08	31.3	0.00	26.4	24.4	0.3	10.4	269	0.4
fresh, raw, sliced	1/2 cup	5	0.00	0.03	0.17	0.04	15.7	0.00	13.2	12.2	0.2	5.2	135	0.2
fresh, raw, whole, large, 1–1.25-inch diam	1 radish	<1	0.00	0.00	0.03	0.01	2.4	0.00	2.1	1.9	<0.1	0.8	21	<0.1
fresh, raw, whole, medium, 3/4–1-inch diam	1 radish	<1	0.00	0.00	0.01	0.00	1.2	0.00	1.0	0.9	<0.1	0.4	10	<0.1
fresh, raw, whole, small, under 3/4-inch diam	1 radish	<1	0.00	0.00	0.01	0.00	0.5	0.00	0.5	0.4	<0.1	0.2	5	<0.1
WHITE ICICLE														
raw, sliced	1/2 cup	0	0.02	0.01	0.15	0.04	7.0	0.00	14.5	13.5	0.4	4.5	140	<0.1
raw, whole, approx 7-inch long	1 medium	0	0.01	0.00	0.05	0.01	2.4	0.00	4.9	4.6	0.14	1.5	48	<0.1
RADISH SEED, sprouted, raw	1 cup	149	0.04	0.04	1.10	0.11	36.0	0.00	11.0	19.4	0.33	16.7	33	0.2
RAG GOURD. See GOURD, DISHCLOTH.														
RAINBOW SMELT. See SMELT, RAINBOW.														
RAINBOW TROUT. See under TROUT.														
RAISIN														
Golden														
seedless	1 cup packed	73	0.01	0.32	1.90	0.53	5.4	0.00	5.3	87.5	3.0	57.8	1231	0.5
seedless	1 cup	64	0.01	0.28	1.70	0.47	4.8	0.00	4.6	76.8	2.6	50.8	1082	0.5
Dark														
seeded	1 cup packed	0	0.19	0.30	1.80	0.31	5.4	0.00	8.9	46.2	4.3	49.5	1361	0.3
seeded	1 cup	0	0.16	0.26	1.60	0.27	4.8	0.00	7.8	40.6	3.8	43.5	1196	0.3
seedless, mini-box	0.5 oz	1	0.02	0.01	0.12	0.04	0.5	0.00	0.5	6.9	0.3	4.6	105	<0.1
seedless	1 cup packed	13	0.26	0.14	1.40	0.41	5.4	0.00	5.4	80.8	3.4	54.5	1239	0.5

Food Name	Serving Size	A I.U.	Thi mg	Rib mg	Nia mg	B_6 mg	Fol mcg	B_{12} mcg	C mg	Calc mg	Iron mg	Mag mg	Pot mg	Zn mg
seedless	1 cup	12	0.23	0.13	1.20	0.36	4.8	0.00	4.8	71.0	3.0	47.9	1089	0.4
seedless	50 medium	2	0.04	0.02	0.21	0.07	0.9	0.00	0.9	12.7	0.5	8.6	195	<0.1
RAMBUTAN														
canned, in syrup	1 cup	6	0.03	0.05	2.90	0.04	17.1	0.00	10.5	47.1	0.8	15.0	90	0.2
canned, in syrup	1 medium	<1	0.00	0.00	0.12	0.00	0.7	0.00	0.4	2.0	<0.1	0.6	4	<0.1
canned, in syrup, drained	1 cup	5	0.02	0.03	2.00	0.03	12.0	0.00	7.3	33.0	0.5	10.5	63	0.1
RASPBERRY / bramble														
Canned, in heavy syrup, w/liquid	1 cup	85	0.05	0.08	1.10	0.11	26.9	0.00	22.3	28.2	1.1	30.7	241	0.4
Fresh														
raw	1 pint	406	0.09	0.28	2.80	0.18	81.1	0.00	78.0	68.6	1.8	56.2	474	1.4
raw	1 cup	160	0.04	0.11	1.10	0.07	32.0	0.00	30.8	27.1	0.7	22.1	187	0.6
raw	10 medium	25	0.01	0.02	0.17	0.01	4.9	0.00	4.8	4.2	0.11	3.4	29	<0.1
Frozen														
red, sweetened	10-oz pkg	170	0.05	0.13	0.65	0.10	73.8	0.00	46.9	42.6	1.8	36.9	324	0.5
red, sweetened, unthawed	1 cup	150	0.05	0.11	0.57	0.09	65.0	0.00	41.3	37.5	1.6	32.5	285	0.5
RED CABBAGE. See CABBAGE, RED.														
RED CURRANT. See under CURRANT.														
RED PEPPER. See under PEPPER, BELL.														
RED PERCH. See OCEAN PERCH.														
RED SALMON. See under SALMON.														
RELISH														
HAMBURGER														
pickle	1/2 cup	326	0.02	0.05	0.75	0.02	1.2	0.00	2.8	4.9	1.4	8.5	93	0.1
pickle	1 tbsp	40	0.00	0.01	0.09	0.00	0.2	0.00	0.3	0.6	0.2	1.1	11	<0.1
HOT DOG														
pickle	1/2 cup	204	0.05	0.05	0.61	0.02	1.2	0.00	1.2	6.1	1.5	23.2	95	0.3
pickle	1 tbsp	25	0.01	0.01	0.08	0.00	0.2	0.00	0.2	0.8	0.2	2.9	12	<0.1
PICKLE														
sweet	1 cup	380	0.00	0.08	0.57	0.04	2.5	0.00	2.5	7.3	2.1	12.3	61	0.3
sweet	1 tbsp	23	0.00	0.01	0.04	0.00	0.2	0.00	0.2	0.5	0.1	0.8	4	<0.1
RENNIN, emzyme tablet, unsweetened	0.35 oz	0	0.00	0.00	0.00	0.00	0.0	0.00	0.0	370.0	0.7	1.8	29	0.6
RICE														
BROWN														
long grain, cooked	1 cup	0	0.19	0.05	3.00	0.28	7.8	0.00	0.0	19.5	0.8	83.8	84	1.2
long grain, raw	1 cup	0	0.74	0.17	9.40	0.94	37.0	0.00	0.0	42.5	2.7	265.0	413	3.7
medium grain, cooked	1 cup	0	0.20	0.02	2.60	0.29	7.8	0.00	0.0	19.5	1.0	85.8	154	1.2
medium grain, raw	1 cup	0	0.79	0.08	8.20	0.97	38.0	0.00	0.0	62.7	3.4	272.0	509	3.8
GLUTINOUS														
white, cooked	1 cup	0	0.04	0.02	0.51	0.05	1.7	0.00	0.0	3.5	0.2	8.7	17	0.7
white, raw	1 cup	0	0.33	0.10	4.00	0.20	12.9	0.00	0.0	20.4	3.0	42.5	142	2.2
WHITE														
long grain, cooked	1 cup	0	0.26	0.02	2.30	0.15	91.6	0.00	0.0	15.8	1.9	19.0	55	0.8
long grain, dry	1 cup	0	1.1	0.09	7.80	0.30	427.0	0.00	0.0	51.8	8.0	46.3	213	2.0
long grain, parboiled, cooked	1 cup	0	0.19	0.13	6.70	0.65	31.4	0.00	0.0	111.0	2.8	57.4	222	1.8
long grain, parboiled, dry	1 cup	0	1.1	0.13	6.70	0.65	427.0	0.00	0.0	111.0	6.6	57.4	222	1.8
long grain, precooked or instant, enriched, dry	1 cup	0	0.59	0.06	5.20	0.04	219.0	0.00	0.0	17.1	4.0	11.4	17	0.9
long grain, precooked or instant, enriched, prepared	1 cup	0	0.12	0.08	1.50	0.02	67.7	0.00	0.0	13.2	1.0	8.3	6.6	0.4
medium grain, cooked	1 cup	0	0.31	0.03	3.40	0.09	108.0	0.00	0.0	5.6	2.8	24.2	54	0.8
medium grain, dry	1 cup	na	0.14	0.09	3.10	0.28	17.6	0.00	0.0	17.6	1.6	68.3	168	2.3
short grain, cooked	1 cup	0	0.30	0.03	2.80	0.11	110.0	0.00	0.0	1.9	2.7	14.9	48	0.7
short grain, dry	1 cup	0	1.1	0.10	8.20	0.34	462.0	0.00	0.0	6.0	8.5	46.0	152	2.2

Food Name	Serving Size	A I.U.	Thi mg	Rib mg	Nia mg	B₆ mg	Fol mcg	B₁₂ mcg	C mg	Calc mg	Iron mg	Mag mg	Pot mg	Zn mg
RICE, WILD														
cooked	1 cup	0	0.09	0.14	2.10	0.22	42.6	0.00	0.0	4.9	0.9	52.5	166	2.2
raw	1 cup	30	0.18	0.42	10.80	0.63	152.0	0.00	0.0	33.6	3.1	283.0	683	9.5
RICE CAKE														
BROWN RICE														
	1 cake													
	1 cake	0	0.01	0.01	0.73	0.01	1.9	0.00	0.0	1.0	0.1	13.6	27	0.2
buckwheat	1 cake	0	0.01	0.01	0.73	0.01	1.9	0.00	0.0	1.0	0.1	13.6	27	0.2
buckwheat, unsalted	1 cake	0	0.01	0.01	0.58	0.01	1.7	0.00	0.0	0.8	0.1	10.3	25	0.2
corn	1 cake	0	0.01	0.02	0.59	0.01	1.8	0.00	0.0	1.9	0.2	12.3	27	0.2
multigrain	1 cake	0	0.01	0.02	0.59	0.01	1.8	0.00	0.0	1.9	0.2	12.3	27	0.2
multigrain, unsalted	1 cake	4	0.01	0.02	0.70	0.01	1.9	0.00	0.0	1.0	0.1	11.8	26	0.3
plain	1 cake	4	0.01	0.02	0.70	0.01	1.9	0.00	0.0	1.0	0.1	11.8	26	0.3
plain, unsalted	1 cake	<1	0.01	0.01	0.63	0.01	0.5	0.00	0.0	1.9	0.2	13.0	28	0.3
rye	1 cake	0	0.00	0.01	0.65	0.01	1.6	0.00	0.3	1.1	0.1	12.2	26	0.3
w/sesame seed	1 cake	0	0.00	0.01	0.65	0.01	1.6	0.00	0.3	1.1	0.1	12.2	26	0.3
w/sesame seed, unsalted	1 cake													
RICE FLOUR. See under FLOUR.														
ROCKFISH, PACIFIC														
baked, broiled, grilled, or microwaved	3 oz	186	0.04	0.07	3.30	0.23	8.8	1.00	0.0	10.2	0.5	28.9	442	0.5
mixed species, raw	3 oz	162	0.03	0.06	2.70	0.20	7.7	0.85	0.0	7.7	0.4	22.1	344	0.4
ROLL														
DINNER														
egg, 2.5-inch diam	1 roll	9	0.18	0.18	1.10	0.02	36.8	0.08	0.0	20.6	1.2	8.8	36	0.4
plain, 2x2x2 inches	1 roll	0	0.14	0.09	1.10	0.02	26.6	0.02	<0.1	33.3	0.9	6.4	37	0.2
rye, 2 3/8 inch diam	1 roll	2	0.11	0.08	1.10	0.02	24.4	0.00	0.0	8.5	0.8	15.3	51	0.3
whole wheat, 2.5-inch diam	1 roll	0	0.09	0.06	1.30	0.07	10.8	0.00	0.0	38.2	0.9	30.6	98	0.7
HARD, 3.5-inch diam	1 roll	0	0.27	0.19	2.40	0.02	54.1	0.00	0.0	54.1	1.9	15.4	62	0.5
KAISER, 3.5-inch diam	1 roll	0	0.27	0.19	2.40	0.02	54.1	0.00	0.0	54.1	1.9	15.4	62	0.5
ROLL, SWEET, DOUGH														
(Pillsbury)														
cinnamon, w/icing, refrigerated	1 serving	na	na	na	na	na	na	na	na	na	na	na	na	na
ROMAN BEAN. See BEAN, CRANBERRY.														
ROOT BEER. See under SOFT DRINKS AND MIXERES.														
ROSE COCO BEAN. See BEAN, CRANBERRY.														
ROSE PERCH. See OCEAN PERCH.														
ROUGHY, ORANGE. See ORANGE ROUGHY.														
RUCOLA. See ARUGULA.														
RUGULA. See ARUGULA.														
RUM														
80 proof	1 fl oz	0	0.00	0.00	0.00	0.00	0.0	0.00	0.0	0.0	<0.1	0.0	<1	<0.1
86 proof	1 fl oz	0	0.00	0.00	0.00	0.00	0.0	0.00	0.0	0.0	<0.1	0.0	<1	<0.1
90 proof	1 fl oz	0	0.00	0.00	0.00	0.00	0.0	0.00	0.0	0.0	<0.1	0.0	<1	<0.1
94 proof	1 fl oz	0	0.00	0.00	0.00	0.00	0.0	0.00	0.0	0.0	<0.1	0.0	<1	<0.1
100 proof	1 fl oz	0	0.00	0.00	0.00	0.00	0.0	0.00	0.0	0.0	<0.1	0.0	<1	<0.1

S

Food Name	Serving Size	A I.U.	Thi mg	Rib mg	Nia mg	B₆ mg	Fol mcg	B₁₂ mcg	C mg	Calc mg	Iron mg	Mag mg	Pot mg	Zn mg
SABLEFISH. See under COD.														
SAFFLOWER OIL														
over 70% oleic	1 cup	0	0.00	0.00	0.00	0.00	0.0	0.00	0.0	0.0	0.0	0.0	0	0.0
over 70% oleic	1 tbsp	0	0.00	0.00	0.00	0.00	0.0	0.00	0.0	0.0	0.0	0.0	0	0.0

Food Name	Serving Size	A I.U.	Thi mg	Rib mg	Nia mg	B$_6$ mg	Fol mcg	B$_{12}$ mcg	C mg	Calc mg	Iron mg	Mag mg	Pot mg	Zn mg
salad or cooking, over 70% linoleic	1 cup	0	0.00	0.00	0.00	0.00	0.0	0.00	0.0	0.0	0.0	0.0	0	0.0
salad or cooking, over 70% linoleic	1 tbsp	0	0.00	0.00	0.00	0.00	0.0	0.00	0.0	0.0	0.0	0.0	0	0.0
salad or cooking, over 70% oleic	1 cup	0	0.00	0.00	0.00	0.00	0.0	0.00	0.0	0.0	0.0	0.0	0	0.0
salad or cooking, over 70% oleic	1 tbsp	0	0.00	0.00	0.00	0.00	0.0	0.00	0.0	0.0	0.0	0.0	0	0.0
SAFFLOWER SEED, kernels, dried	1 oz	14	0.33	0.12	0.65	0.33	45.5	0.00	0.0	22.1	1.4	100.0	195	1.4
SAFFLOWER SEED MEAL														
partially defatted	1 oz	14	0.33	0.12	0.64	0.33	45.1	0.00	0.0	21.8	1.4	99.2	19	1.4
SAFFRON														
	1 tbsp	11	0.00	0.01	0.03	0.03	2.0	0.00	1.7	2.3	0.2	5.5	36	<0.1
	1 tsp	4	0.00	0.00	0.01	0.01	0.7	0.00	0.6	0.8	<0.1	1.8	12	<0.1
SAGE														
ground	1 tbsp	118	0.02	0.01	0.11	0.02	5.5	0.00	0.7	33.0	0.6	8.6	21	<0.1
ground	1 tsp	41	0.01	0.00	0.04	0.01	1.9	0.00	0.2	11.6	0.2	3.0	8	<0.1
SALAD DRESSING														
BLUE CHEESE														
regular	1 cup	515	0.03	0.25	0.25	0.09	19.8	0.67	4.9	198.0	0.5	0.0	91	0.7
regular	1 tbsp	32	0.00	0.02	0.02	0.01	1.2	0.04	0.3	12.4	<0.1	0.0	6	<0.1
no salt added	1 cup	515	0.03	0.25	0.25	na	na	na	4.9	198.0	0.5	na	91	na
no salt added	1 tbsp	32	0.00	0.02	0.02	na	na	na	0.3	12.4	<0.1	na	6	na
FRENCH														
low-fat, 5 calories per tsp	1 cup	3380	0.00	0.00	0.00	0.00	0.0	0.00	0.0	28.6	1.0	0	205	0.5
low-fat, 5 calories per tsp	1 tbsp	212	0.00	0.00	0.00	0.00	0.0	0.00	0.0	1.8	<0.1	0	12.9	<0.1
low-fat, 5 calories per teaspoon, no salt added	1 cup	52	0.00	0.00	0.00	na	na	na	0.0	28.6	1.0	na	205	na
low-fat, 5 calories per teaspoon, no salt added	1 tbsp	3	0.00	0.00	0.00	na	na	na	0.0	1.8	<0.1	na	13	na
regular	1 cup	3250	0.02	0.04	0.01	0.03	10.5	0.35	0.0	27.5	1.0	0.0	198	0.2
regular	1 tbsp	203	0.00	0.00	0.00	0.00	0.7	0.02	0.0	1.7	<0.1	0.0	12	<0.1
ITALIAN														
diet, 2 calories per tsp, no salt added	1 cup	0	0.00	0.00	0.00	na	na	na	0.0	4.8	0.5	na	36	na
diet, 2 calories per tsp, no salt added	1 tbsp	0	0.00	0.00	0.00	na	na	na	0.0	0.3	<0.1	na	2	na
no salt added	1 cup	183	0.05	0.01	0.44	na	na	na	<0.1	23.5	0.5	na	35	na
no salt added	1 tbsp	12	0.00	0.00	0.03	na	na	na	0.0	1.5	<0.1	na	2	na
regular	1 cup	183	0.02	0.05	0.01	0.03	11.5	0.38	0.0	23.5	0.5	1.5	35	0.3
regular	1 tbsp	12	0.00	0.00	0.00	0.00	0.7	0.02	0.0	1.5	<0.1	<0.1	2	<0.1
(Kraft)														
nonfat, 'Free'	2 tbsp	52	na	na	na	na	na	na	0.4	13.9	<0.1	na	38	na
zesty	2 tbsp	11	na	na	na	na	na	na	0.2	1.2	<0.1	na	9	na
MAYONNAISE TYPE														
(Kraft)														
'Miracle Whip Light'	1 tbsp	5	na	na	na	na	na	na	0.0	0.8	<0.1	na	4	na
nonfat, 'Miracle Whip-Free'	1 tbsp	11	na	na	na	na	na	na	0.0	0.9	<0.1	na	8	na
RANCH														
(Kraft)														
	2 tbsp	11	na	na	na	na	na	na	<0.1	8.4	<0.1	na	14	na
light, 'Light Done Right!'	2 tbsp	12	na	na	na	na	na	na	<0.1	7.8	<0.1	na	40	na
nonfat	2 tbsp	3	na	na	na	na	na	na	<0.1	9.1	<0.1	na	31	na
RUSSIAN														
diet	1 cup	146	0.02	0.03	0.01	0.02	9.1	0.30	15.6	49.4	1.6	1.2	408	0.3
diet	1 tbsp	9	0.00	0.00	0.00	0.00	0.6	0.02	0.9	3.1	0.1	<0.1	26	<0.1
regular	1 cup	1691	0.12	0.12	1.50	0.07	25.5	0.73	14.7	46.5	1.5	3.7	385	1.1
regular	1 tbsp	106	0.01	0.01	0.09	0.01	1.6	0.05	0.9	2.9	<0.1	0.2	24	<0.1
SESAME SEED														
	1 cup	1691	0.00	0.00	0.00	0.00	0.0	0.00	0.0	46.5	1.5	0.0	385	0.3
	1 tbsp	106	0.00	0.00	0.00	0.00	0.0	0.00	0.0	2.9	<0.1	0.0	24	<0.1

Food Name	Serving Size	A I.U.	Thi mg	Rib mg	Nia mg	B6 mg	Fol mcg	B12 mcg	C mg	Calc mg	Iron mg	Mag mg	Pot mg	Zn mg
SOUR CREAM TYPE														
non-butterfat, cultured..................	1 cup	24	0.09	0.38	0.17	0.04	27.7	0.77	2.2	266.0	<0.1	23.3	380	0.9
non-butterfat, cultured..................	1 tbsp	1	0.01	0.02	0.01	0.00	1.4	0.04	0.1	13.6	0.0	1.2	19	<0.1
THOUSAND ISLAND														
diet, 10 calories per teaspoon	1 cup	784	0.03	0.05	0.01	0.04	13.7	0.45	0.0	26.9	1.5	1.7	277	0.4
diet, 10 calories per teaspoon	1 tbsp	49	0.00	0.00	0.00	0.00	0.9	0.03	0.0	1.7	<0.1	0.1	17	<0.1
regular	1 cup	800	0.03	0.06	0.01	0.04	15.7	0.52	0.0	27.5	1.5	5.0	283	0.4
regular	1 tbsp	50	0.00	0.00	0.00	0.00	0.9	0.03	0.0	1.7	<0.1	0.3	18	<0.1
SALISBURY STEAK. See under BEEF DINNER/ENTRÉE.														
SALMON														
ATLANTIC														
Fresh														
farmed, baked, broiled, grilled, or														
microwaved	3 oz	43	0.29	0.12	6.80	0.55	28.9	2.40	3.1	12.8	0.3	25.5	326	0.4
farmed, raw...........................	3 oz	43	0.29	0.10	6.40	0.54	22.1	2.40	3.3	10.2	0.3	23.8	308	0.3
wild, baked, broiled, grilled, or														
microwaved	3 oz	37	0.23	0.41	8.60	0.80	24.6	2.60	0.0	12.8	0.9	31.4	534	0.7
wild, raw	3 oz	34	0.19	0.32	6.70	0.69	21.3	2.70	0.0	10.2	0.7	24.6	417	0.5
CHINOOK / king														
Fresh														
baked, broiled, grilled, or microwaved	3 oz	422	0.04	0.13	8.50	0.39	29.8	2.40	3.5	23.8	0.8	104	429	0.5
raw.................................	3 oz	387	0.03	0.10	6.70	0.34	25.5	2.50	3.4	18.7	0.6	80.8	335	0.4
Smoked														
....	3 oz	75	0.02	0.09	4.00	0.24	1.6	2.80	0.0	9.3	0.7	15.3	149	0.3
boneless	1 oz	25	0.01	0.03	1.30	0.08	0.5	0.92	0.0	3.1	0.2	5.1	50	<0.1
flaked	1 cup	120	0.03	0.14	6.40	0.38	2.6	4.40	0.0	15.0	1.2	24.5	238	0.4
lox.................................	3 oz	75	0.02	0.09	4.00	0.24	1.6	2.80	0.0	9.3	0.7	15.3	149	0.3
lox.................................	1 oz	25	0.01	0.03	1.30	0.08	0.5	0.92	0.0	3.1	0.2	5.1	50	<0.1
CHUM / keta														
Canned														
drained, w/bone	3 oz	52	0.02	0.14	6.00	0.32	17.0	3.70	0.0	212	0.6	25.5	255	0.9
drained, w/bone, no salt added...........	3 oz	52	0.02	0.14	6.00	0.32	17.0	3.70	0.0	212	0.6	25.5	255	0.9
Fresh														
baked, broiled, grilled, or microwaved	3 oz	97	0.08	0.19	7.20	0.39	4.3	2.90	0.0	11.9	0.6	23.8	468	0.5
raw.................................	3 oz	84	0.07	0.15	6.00	0.34	3.4	2.50	0.0	9.3	0.5	18.7	365	0.4
COHO / silver														
farmed, baked, broiled, grilled, or														
microwaved	3 oz	167	0.09	0.10	6.30	0.48	11.9	2.70	1.3	10.2	0.3	28.9	391	0.4
farmed, raw...........................	3 oz	160	0.08	0.09	5.80	0.56	11.1	2.30	0.9	10.2	0.3	26.4	383	0.4
wild, baked, broiled, grilled, or														
microwaved	3 oz	111	0.06	0.12	6.80	0.48	11.1	4.30	1.2	38.3	0.5	28.1	369	0.5
wild, boiled or poached.................	3 oz	92	0.10	0.14	6.60	0.47	7.7	3.80	0.9	39.1	0.6	29.8	387	0.4
wild, raw	3 oz	85	0.10	0.12	6.10	0.47	7.7	3.50	0.9	30.6	0.5	26.4	360	0.4
HUMPBACK. See PINK.														
KETA. See COHO.														
KING. See CHINOOK.														
PINK / humpback														
Canned														
w/bone and liquid	3 oz	47	0.02	0.16	5.60	0.26	13.1	3.70	0.0	181.0	0.7	28.9	277	0.8
w/bone and liquid, no salt added	3 oz	47	0.02	0.16	5.60	0.26	13.1	3.70	0.0	181.0	0.7	28.9	277	0.8
Fresh														
baked, broiled, grilled, or microwaved	3 oz	116	0.17	0.06	7.20	0.20	4.3	2.90	0.0	14.4	0.8	28.1	352	0.6
raw.................................	3 oz	100	0.14	0.05	6.00	0.17	3.4	2.50	0.0	11.1	0.7	22.1	275	0.5
RED. See SOCKEYE.														
SILVER. See COHO.														

Food Name	Serving Size	A I.U.	Thi mg	Rib mg	Nia mg	B$_6$ mg	Fol mcg	B$_{12}$ mcg	C mg	Calc mg	Iron mg	Mag mg	Pot mg	Zn mg
SOCKEYE / red														
Canned														
drained, w/bone	3 oz	150	0.01	0.16	4.70	0.26	8.3	0.26	0.0	203.0	0.9	24.6	320	0.9
drained, w/bone, no salt added	3 oz	150	0.01	0.16	4.70	0.26	8.3	0.26	0.0	203.0	0.9	24.6	320	0.9
Fresh														
baked, broiled, grilled, or microwaved	3 oz	178	0.18	0.14	5.70	0.19	4.3	4.90	0.0	6.0	0.5	26.4	319	0.4
raw	3 oz	163	0.17	0.13	4.90	0.16	3.4	4.30	0.0	5.1	0.4	20.4	332	0.5
SALMON OIL. See under FISH OIL.														
SALSA														
(La Victoria)														
'Brava'	1 tbsp	103	na	na	na	na	na	na	0.4	1.0	<0.1	na	na	na
chili dip, chunky	2 tbsp	63	na	na	na	na	na	na	3.1	4.2	<0.1	na	na	na
green chili, mild	2 tbsp	139	na	na	na	na	na	na	4.1	4.6	0.3	na	na	na
green jalapeño	2 tbsp	85	na	na	na	na	na	na	3.6	4.8	0.1	na	na	na
hot, thick and chunky	2 tbsp	159	na	na	na	na	na	na	1.6	3.4	<0.1	na	na	na
jalapeña, red	2 tbsp	755	na	na	na	na	na	na	9.8	6.4	<0.1	na	na	na
medium, thick and chunky	2 tbsp	175	na	na	na	na	na	na	4.4	5.8	<0.1	na	na	na
mild, thick and chunky	2 tbsp	231	na	na	na	na	na	na	4.3	5.4	<0.1	na	na	na
picante, medium	2 tbsp	140	na	na	na	na	na	na	2.5	4.2	<0.1	na	na	na
picante, mild	2 tbsp	126	na	na	na	na	na	na	1.9	4.6	<0.1	na	na	na
'Ranchera' hot	2 tbsp	362	na	na	na	na	na	na	1.3	4.9	<0.1	na	na	na
'Suprema' medium	2 tbsp	98	na	na	na	na	na	na	1.5	2.7	<0.1	na	na	na
'Suprema' mild	2 tbsp	185	na	na	na	na	na	na	4.4	4.6	<0.1	na	na	na
'Victoria' hot	2 tbsp	52	na	na	na	na	na	na	3.6	2.4	<0.1	na	na	na
SALSIFY / oyster plant / vegetable oyster														
boiled, drained, sliced	1 cup	0	0.08	0.23	0.53	0.29	20.5	0.00	6.2	63.5	0.7	24.3	382	0.4
raw, sliced	1 cup	0	0.11	0.29	0.67	0.37	35.0	0.00	10.6	79.8	0.93	30.6	505	0.5
SALT														
table	1 cup	0	0.00	0.00	0.00	0.00	0.0	0.00	0.0	70.1	0.9	2.9	23	0.3
table	1 dash	0	0.00	0.00	0.00	0.00	0.0	0.00	0.0	0.1	0.0	0.0	<1	<0.1
table	1 tbsp	0	0.00	0.00	0.00	0.00	0.0	0.00	0.0	4.3	<0.1	0.2	1	<0.1
table	1 tsp	0	0.00	0.00	0.00	0.00	0.0	0.00	0.0	1.4	<0.1	<0.1	<1	<0.1
SALT PORK. See PORK, SALT.														
SAND PEAR. See ASIAN PEAR.														
SANDWICH														
BEEF														
(Pierre)														
submarine, flame-broiled	1 piece	30	0.11	0.11	2.60	0.26	3.5	1.40	0.0	15.9	1.5	24.1	268	3.6
submarine, flame-broiled, 'Hot Diggity Sub'	1 piece	50	0.15	0.15	2.90	0.28	3.5	1.60	0.0	24.1	2.1	29.7	276	5.0
CHICKEN														
(Hot Pockets)														
w/broccoli, cheese, stuffed, 'Croissant Pockets'	1 pkg	678	na	na	na	na	na	na	12.5	na	7.6	na	na	na
w/broccoli, cheese, stuffed, 'Croissant Pockets'	1 serving	339	na	na	na	na	na	na	6.3	na	3.8	na	na	na
(Lean Pockets)														
supreme, glazed, frozen	1 pkg	1530	na	na	na	na	na	na	na	242.0	na	na	na	na
supreme, glazed, frozen	1 serving	768	na	na	na	na	na	na	na	122.0	na	na	na	na
(Weight Watchers)														
w/broccoli, cheese, pocket sandwich, 'On-The-Go'	1 pkg	235	na	na	na	na	na	na	na	91.7	na	na	na	na
HAM														
(Hot Pockets)														
and cheese, stuffed	1 pkg	0	na	na	na	na	na	na	na	502.0	5.2	na	na	na

Food Name	Serving Size	A I.U.	Thi mg	Rib mg	Nia mg	B_6 mg	Fol mcg	B_{12} mcg	C mg	Calc mg	Iron mg	Mag mg	Pot mg	Zn mg
and cheese, stuffed	1 serving	0	na	na	na	na	na	na	na	251.0	2.6	na	na	na
(Red Baron)														
and cheese, 'Premium Pockets'	1 pkg	0	na	na	na	na	na	na	na	385.0	na	na	na	na
and cheese, 'Premium Pockets'	1 serving	0	na	na	na	na	na	na	na	190.0	na	na	na	na
PIZZA														
(Hot Pockets)														
pepperoni, stuffed, frozen	1 pkg	899	na	na	na	na	na	na	na	561.0	6.3	na	na	na
pepperoni, stuffed, frozen	1 serving	449	na	na	na	na	na	na	na	280.0	3.2	na	na	na
SANDWICH SPREAD														
(Oscar Mayer) pork, chicken, and beef	1 serving	30	na	na	na	na	na	na	0.0	8.1	0.24	3.6	35	0.3
SAPODILLA														
fresh, raw, pulp	1 cup	145	0.00	0.05	0.48	0.09	33.7	0.00	35.4	50.6	1.9	28.9	465	0.2
fresh, raw, whole	1 medium	102	0.00	0.03	0.34	0.06	23.8	0.00	25.0	35.7	1.4	20.4	328	0.2
SAPOTE / marmalade plum														
raw, trimmed	1 medium	923	0.02	0.05	4.00	na	na	0.00	45.0	87.8	2.3	67.5	774	na
SARDINE														
ATLANTIC														
Canned														
in oil, drained, w/bone	1 oz	64	0.02	0.06	1.50	0.05	3.3	2.50	0.0	108.0	0.8	11.1	113	0.4
in oil, drained, w/bone	2 medium	54	0.02	0.05	1.30	0.04	2.8	2.10	0.0	91.7	0.7	9.4	95	0.3
in oil, drained, w/bone	1 cup	334	0.12	0.34	7.80	0.25	17.6	13.30	0.0	569.0	4.4	58.1	592	2.0
MIXED SPECIES														
Canned														
in tomato sauce, drained, w/bone	1 cup	325	0.04	0.21	3.70	0.11	21.6	8.00	0.9	214.0	2.0	30.3	303	1.2
in tomato sauce, drained, w/bone	1 medium	139	0.02	0.09	1.60	0.05	9.2	3.40	0.4	91.2	0.9	12.9	130	0.5
SARDINE OIL. See under FISH OIL.														
SAUCE														
BARBECUE														
(Bull's Eye) Ridge's	2 tbsp	na	na	na	na	na	na	na	na	na	na	na	na	na
(Kraft)														
hickory smoke	2 tbsp	114	na	na	na	na	na	na	<0.1	5.1	0.2	na	28	na
original	2 tbsp	114	na	na	na	na	na	na	<0.1	5.1	0.2	na	28	na
(Marzetti) original, 'Texas Best'	2 tbsp	na	na	na	na	na	na	na	na	na	na	na	na	na
CHEESE														
(La Victoria)														
cheddar	1/4 cup	112	na	na	na	na	na	na	0.0	60.0	0.5	na	na	na
nacho, w/jalapeno peppers	1/4 cup	39	na	na	na	na	na	na	1.1	63.7	0.9	na	na	na
(Nestlé)														
cheddar, 'Chef Mate'	1 cup	156	0.01	0.16	0.17	0.03	7.4	0.22	2.2	184.0	0.7	14.9	65	1.3
cheddar, 'Chef Mate'	1/4 cup	39	0.00	0.04	0.04	0.01	1.9	0.06	0.6	45.9	0.2	3.7	16	0.3
cheddar, sharp, 'Chef Mate'	1 cup	1210	0.02	0.31	0.07	0.05	12.6	0.38	0.3	544.0	0.5	25.2	81	2.6
cheddar, sharp, 'Chef Mate'	1/4 cup	302	0.00	0.08	0.02	0.01	3.1	0.10	<0.1	136.0	0.1	6.3	20	0.7
con queso, 'Que Bueno'	1 cup	688	0.01	0.16	0.17	0.03	7.6	0.23	0.0	471.0	0.0	15.1	66	1.3
con queso, 'Que Bueno'	1/4 cup	172	0.00	0.04	0.04	0.01	1.9	0.06	0.0	118.0	0.0	3.8	16	0.3
golden, 'Chef-Mate'	1 cup	799	0.02	0.31	0.07	0.05	12.6	0.38	0.0	643.0	0.6	25.2	81	2.6
golden, 'Chef-Mate'	1/4 cup	200	0.00	0.08	0.02	0.01	3.1	0.10	0.0	161.0	0.1	6.3	20	0.7
jalapeño, 'Que Bueno'	1 pkg	3396	0.12	2.00	2.00	0.39	90.2	2.70	24.0	2554.0	5.7	180.0	781	16.2
jalapeño, 'Que Bueno'	1/4 cup	71	0.00	0.04	0.04	0.01	1.9	0.06	0.5	53.5	0.1	3.8	16	0.3
nacho, mild, 'Que Bueno'	1 cup	512	0.02	0.31	0.07	0.05	12.6	0.38	0.3	471.0	0.8	25.2	81	2.6
nacho, mild, 'Que Bueno'	1/4 cup	128	0.00	0.08	0.02	0.01	3.1	0.10	<0.1	118.0	0.2	6.3	20	0.7
nacho, 'Que Bueno'	1 cup	1923	0.02	0.31	0.07	0.05	12.6	0.38	1.8	723.0	0.6	25.2	81	2.6
nacho, 'Que Bueno'	1/4 cup	481	0.00	0.08	0.02	0.01	3.1	0.10	0.4	181.0	0.2	6.3	20	0.7
CREOLE														
(Nestlé)														
'Chef Mate'	1 cup	935	0.13	0.10	2.10	0.28	34.7	0.00	0.0	139.0	1.2	34.7	749	0.4

Food Name	Serving Size	A I.U.	Thi mg	Rib mg	Nia mg	B_6 mg	Fol mcg	B_{12} mcg	C mg	Calc mg	Iron mg	Mag mg	Pot mg	Zn mg
'Chef Mate'	1/4 cup	234	0.03	0.03	0.53	0.07	8.7	0.00	0.0	34.7	0.3	8.7	187	0.1
ENCHILADA														
(La Victoria)	1/4 cup	1393	na	na	na	na	na	na	2.7	7.2	<0.1	na	na	na
(Nestlé)														
'Que Bueno'	1 pkg	15844	2.10	1.40	40.90	5.60	308.0	0.00	274.0	925.0	39.7	655.0	10717	7.3
'Que Bueno'	2 tbsp	123	0.02	0.01	0.32	0.04	2.4	0.00	2.1	7.2	0.3	5.1	83	<0.1
HOT DOG														
(Nestlé)														
chili, 'Chef-Mate'	1 pkg	20577	2.40	2.30	32.10	3.60	1072.0	6.40	3.1	949.0	47.5	612.0	7257	26.6
chili, 'Chef-Mate'	1/4 cup	423	0.05	0.05	0.66	0.07	22.1	0.13	<0.1	19.5	0.9	12.6	149	0.6
Coney Island, 'Chef-Mate	1 cup	2522	0.13	0.13	3.00	0.35	32.2	0.15	0.3	79.4	4.4	47.1	791	1.0
Coney Island, 'Chef-Mate	1/4 cup	631	0.03	0.03	0.76	0.09	8.1	0.04	<0.1	19.8	1.1	11.8	198	0.3
HOT SAUCE														
(Tabasco) pepper	1 tsp	77	0.00	0.00	0.01	0.01	<0.1	0.00	0.2	0.6	<0.1	0.6	6	<0.1
(Tabasco) pepper	1/4 tsp	20	0.00	0.00	0.00	0.00	<0.1	0.00	0.05	0.1	<0.1	0.1	2	0.0
ITALIAN														
(Nestlé) 'Chef-Mate'	1 cup	504	0.16	0.09	2.30	0.35	33.3	0.00	8.6	70.4	0.8	41.0	778	0.5
(Nestlé) 'Chef-Mate'	1/4 cup	244	0.08	0.05	1.10	0.17	16.1	0.00	4.2	34.1	0.4	19.8	377	0.3
LEMON														
(Nestlé) 'Chef-Mate'	1 pkg	0	0.15	0.11	0.74	0.17	21.3	0.00	183.0	85.0	8.1	42.5	425	0.9
(Nestlé) 'Chef-Mate'	2 tbsp	0	0.00	0.00	0.01	0.00	0.3	0.00	2.8	1.3	0.1	0.64	6	<0.1
MARINARA														
(Contadina)														
	1 cup	875	0.11	0.08	1.40	0.21	22.5	0.00	17.5	47.5	1.5	30.0	518	0.3
	1/2 cup	438	0.05	0.04	0.71	0.11	11.3	0.00	8.8	23.8	0.8	15.0	259	0.2
MOLE POBLANO (La Victoria)	2 oz	11742	na	na	na	na	na	na	0.0	58.1	1.6	na	na	na
PASTA / spaghetti. See also SAUCE, MARINARA.														
(Nestlé)														
spaghetti	1 cup	1000	0.16	0.12	3.90	0.36	25.0	0.00	22.3	62.5	2.1	55.0	958	0.5
spaghetti	1/2 cup	500	0.08	0.06	1.90	0.18	12.5	0.00	11.1	31.3	1.1	27.5	479	0.3
(Prego) spaghetti, traditional,														
'100% Natural'	2 tbsp	734	na	na	na	na	na	na	13.5	na	na	na	na	na
(Ragu) smooth, traditional 'Old World'	1/2 cup	646	na	na	na	na	na	na	na	na	1.0	na	na	na
PICANTE														
(Nestlé)														
'Que Bueno'	1 pkg	10717	2.00	1.60	37.20	4.80	386.0	0.00	73.2	1619.0	19.3	578.0	10331	6.6
'Que Bueno'	2 tbsp	83.4	0.02	0.01	0.29	0.04	3.0	0.00	0.6	12.6	0.2	4.5	80	<0.1
(Contadina) deluxe	1/4 cup	420	0.04	0.03	0.90	0.09	6.3	0.01	7.1	34.0	0.6	13.2	223	0.2
(Nestlé) deluxe	1 pkg	20043	1.80	1.60	42.70	4.10	301.0	0.60	340.0	1623.0	27.0	631.0	10638	7.5
SHOYU. See under Soy, below.														
SOY														
from hydrolyzed vegetable protein	1/4 cup	0	0.02	0.06	1.60	0.08	7.5	0.00	0.0	2.9	0.9	3.5	88	0.2
from hydrolyzed vegetable protein	1 tbsp	0	0.01	0.02	0.51	0.03	2.3	0.00	0.0	0.9	0.3	1.1	27	<0.1
from hydrolyzed vegetable protein	1 tsp	0	0.00	0.01	0.17	0.01	0.8	0.00	0.0	0.3	<0.1	0.4	9	<0.1
shoyu, from soy and wheat	1 cup	0	0.09	0.42	5.60	0.38	40.8	0.00	0.0	48.5	4.9	110.0	1017	1.3
shoyu, from soy and wheat	1 tbsp	0	0.01	0.03	0.35	0.02	2.6	0.00	0.0	3.0	0.3	6.9	64	<0.1
shoyu, from soy and wheat	1 tsp	0	0.00	0.01	0.12	0.01	0.9	0.00	0.0	1.0	0.1	2.3	21	<0.1
shoyu, from soy and wheat, low-sodium	1 cup	0	0.13	0.33	8.60	0.43	39.5	0.00	0.0	43.4	5.2	86.7	459	0.9
shoyu, from soy and wheat, low-sodium	1 tbsp	0	0.01	0.02	0.60	0.03	2.8	0.00	0.0	3.1	0.4	6.1	32	<0.1
shoyu, from soy and wheat, low-sodium	1 tsp	0	0.00	0.01	0.18	0.01	0.8	0.00	0.0	0.9	0.1	1.8	10	<0.1
tamari, from soy	1 tbsp	0	0.01	0.03	0.71	0.04	3.3	0.00	0.0	3.6	0.4	7.2	38	<0.1
tamari, from soy	1 tsp	0	0.00	0.01	0.24	0.01	1.1	0.00	0.0	1.2	0.1	2.4	13	<0.1

Food Name	Serving Size	A I.U.	Thi mg	Rib mg	Nia mg	B_6 mg	Fol mcg	B_{12} mcg	C mg	Calc mg	Iron mg	Mag mg	Pot mg	Zn mg
STIR-FRY														
(Nestlé)														
all-purpose, 'Chef-Mate'	1 pkg	503	0.28	0.77	18.30	0.93	80.5	0.00	94.6	201.0	15.3	201.0	1047	2.4
all-purpose, 'Chef-Mate'	1 tbsp	4	0.00	0.01	0.14	0.01	0.6	0.00	0.7	1.5	0.1	1.5	8	<0.1
(Nestlé) glaze, 'Chef-Mate'	2 tbsp	48	0.02	0.01	0.09	0.03	2.6	0.00	2.6	15.0	0.4	5.8	72	<0.1
SZECHUAN														
(Nestlé)														
Chef-Mate'	1 pkg	12772	0.29	0.70	12.50	1.00	82.8	15.30	33.1	228.0	15.5	207.0	1656	2.5
Chef-Mate'	2 tbsp	197	0.00	0.01	0.19	0.02	1.3	0.24	0.5	3.5	0.2	3.2	26	<0.1
TACO														
(La Victoria)														
green, medium	1 tbsp	12	na	na	na	na	na	na	0.7	1.2	<0.1	na	na	na
green, mild	1 tbsp	12	na	na	na	na	na	na	0.7	1.2	<0.1	na	na	na
red, medium	1 tbsp	251	na	na	na	na	na	na	2.8	3.3	<0.1	na	na	na
red, mild	1 tbsp	251	na	na	na	na	na	na	2.8	3.3	<0.1	na	na	na
TAMARI. See under Soy, above.														
TERIYAKI														
(Nestlé)														
'Chef-Mate'	1 pkg	0	0.21	0.56	12.20	0.64	62.1	0.00	0.0	166.0	11.6	166.0	1035	2.1
'Chef-Mate'	1 tbsp	0	0.00	0.00	0.09	0.01	0.5	0.00	0.0	1.3	<0.1	1.3	8	<0.1
SAUCE MIX														
ALFREDO														
(Knorr) CPC, mix only	2 tbsp	na	na	na	na	na	na	na	na	na	na	na	na	na
CHEESE														
(Custom Foods)														
cheddar, 'Superb' mix only	1 serving	57	0.03	0.10	0.34	0.03	19.0	0.07	0.1	40.5	<0.1	5.1	61	0.2
nacho, 'Superb' mix only	1 serving	43	0.03	0.10	0.34	0.03	19.0	0.07	0.2	43.3	0.1	5.1	61	0.2
(Nestlé)														
nacho, 'Trio' mix only	2 tbsp	22	0.03	0.08	0.29	0.02	16.1	0.06	0.3	20.0	<0.1	4.3	51	0.1
supreme, 'Trio' mix only	2 tbsp	18	0.03	0.08	0.29	0.02	16.1	0.06	0.0	24.0	0.0	4.3	51	0.1
'Trio' mix only	2 tbsp	21	0.03	0.08	0.29	0.02	16.1	0.06	0.0	22.0	<0.1	4.3	51	0.1
ITALIAN														
(Custom Foods) all purpose, 'Red Label'														
mix only	1 serving	3	0.01	0.00	0.03	0.02	2.5	0.00	<0.1	6.0	1.1	2.2	25	<0.1
SAUERKRAUT														
canned, drained	1 cup	43	0.05	0.05	0.34	0.31	55.9	0.00	34.7	70.8	3.5	30.7	401	0.5
canned, w/liquid	1 cup	26	0.03	0.03	0.20	0.19	33.7	0.00	20.9	42.6	2.1	18.5	241	0.37
SAUSAGE														
(Oscar Mayer) 'Smokie Links'	1 serving	0	na	na	na	na	na	na	0.0	4.3	0.5	7.3	77	0.9
BEEF *(Oscar Mayer)* 'Smokies'	1 serving	0	na	na	na	na	na	na	0.0	4.7	0.8	6.5	74	1.3
BEERWURST														
beef, 4-inch diam, 1/8 inch slice	1 slice	0	0.02	0.03	0.78	0.04	0.7	0.45	0.0	2.1	0.4	2.8	40	0.6
beef, 2.5-inch diam, 1/4-inch slice	1 slice	0	0.00	0.01	0.20	0.01	0.2	0.12	0.0	0.5	<0.1	0.7	10	0.2
pork, 4-inch diam, 1/8 inch slice	1 slice	0	0.13	0.04	0.75	0.08	0.7	0.20	0.0	1.8	0.2	3.0	58	0.4
pork, 2.5-inch diam, 1/4-inch slice	1 slice	0	0.03	0.01	0.20	0.02	0.2	0.05	0.0	0.5	<0.1	0.8	15	0.1
BOCKWURST														
pork, veal, milk, and egg, raw	1 oz	7	0.12	0.05	1.20	0.07	1.7	0.23	0.0	4.5	0.2	5.1	77	0.4
pork, veal, milk, egg, raw, 7 links per lb.	1 link	15	0.27	0.11	2.70	0.15	3.9	0.53	0.0	10.4	0.4	11.7	176	1.0
BRATWURST														
pork, cooked	1 oz	0	0.14	0.05	0.91	0.06	0.6	0.27	0.3	12.5	0.4	4.3	60	0.7
pork, cooked, 4 per 12 oz pkg	1 link	0	0.43	0.16	2.70	0.18	1.7	0.81	0.9	37.4	1.1	12.8	180	2.0
pork and beef, w/nonfat dry milk added	1 oz	0	0.07	0.06	0.94	0.04	1.4	0.58	0.0	13.6	0.3	4.5	80	0.6
BRAUNSCHWEIGER														
	1 oz	3983	0.07	0.43	2.40	0.09	12.5	5.70	0.0	2.6	2.7	3.1	56	0.8
2.5-inch diam, 1/4-inch slice	1 slice	2529	0.05	0.27	1.50	0.06	7.9	3.60	0.0	1.6	1.7	2.0	36	0.5

Food Name	Serving Size	A I.U.	Thi mg	Rib mg	Nia mg	B_6 mg	Fol mcg	B_{12} mcg	C mg	Calc mg	Iron mg	Mag mg	Pot mg	Zn mg
CERVELAT														
beef and pork	1 oz	0	0.04	0.09	1.20	0.07	0.6	1.60	0.0	3.7	0.7	4.0	77	0.7
beef and pork, 4-inch diam, 1/8-inch slice	1 slice	0	0.04	0.08	0.99	0.06	0.5	1.30	0.0	3.0	0.6	3.2	62	0.6
(Oscar Mayer)														
	1 serving	na	0.11	0.13	2.0	0.14	2.3	1.70	0.0	4.1	1.0	6.9	105	0.9
	1 slice	na	0.05	0.07	1.00	0.07	1.1	0.86	0.0	2.1	0.5	3.5	52	0.5
beef	1 serving	na	0.07	0.15	2.00	0.12	2.3	2.50	0.0	3.7	1.1	6.9	107	1.1
beef	1 slice	na	0.04	0.08	0.99	0.06	1.1	1.30	0.0	1.8	0.6	3.5	54	0.5
CHEESE (Oscar Mayer) 'Smokies'	1 serving	69	na	na	na	na	na	na	0.0	19.4	0.5	6.9	78	0.8
CHORIZO														
pork and beef	1 oz	0	0.18	0.09	1.50	0.15	0.6	0.57	0.0	2.3	0.5	5.1	113	0.9
pork and beef, 4-inch link	1 link	0	0.38	0.18	3.10	0.32	1.2	1.20	0.0	4.8	0.9	10.8	239	2.0
HONEY ROLL														
beef	1 oz	0	0.02	0.05	1.20	0.08	1.1	0.67	0.0	2.6	0.6	4.5	83	0.9
beef, 4-inch diam, 1/8-inch slice	1 slice	0	0.02	0.04	0.96	0.06	0.9	0.54	0.0	2.1	0.5	3.7	67	0.8
ITALIAN STYLE														
pork, cooked, 5 links per lb.	1 link	0	0.42	0.16	2.80	0.22	3.4	0.87	1.3	16.1	1.0	12.1	204	1.6
pork, cooked, 4 links per lb.	1 link	0	0.52	0.19	3.50	0.27	4.2	1.10	1.7	19.9	1.2	14.9	252	2.0
pork, raw, 7 links per lb.	1 link	0	0.52	0.15	3.00	0.27	7.3	0.83	1.8	16.4	1.1	12.7	230	1.6
pork, raw, 4 links per lb.	1 link	0	0.64	0.19	3.70	0.34	9.0	1.00	2.3	20.3	1.3	15.8	286	2.0
KIELBASA, pork and beef	1 oz	0	0.07	0.06	0.82	0.05	1.4	0.46	0.0	12.5	0.4	4.5	77	0.6
KNOCKWURST														
pork and beef	1 oz	0	0.10	0.04	0.78	0.05	0.6	0.34	0.0	3.1	0.3	3.1	56	0.5
pork and beef, 4-inch x 1 1/8 inch diam	1 link	0	0.23	0.10	1.90	0.12	1.4	0.80	0.0	7.5	0.6	7.5	135	1.1
LIVER. See SAUSAGE, BRAUNSCHWEIGER.														
LUNCHEON														
pork and beef	1 oz	0	0.06	0.06	1.00	0.06	0.9	0.56	0.0	3.7	0.4	4.0	70	0.7
pork and beef, 4-inch diam, 1/8-inch slice	1 slice	0	0.05	0.05	0.81	0.05	0.7	0.45	0.0	3.0	0.3	3.2	56	0.6
MORTADELLA														
beef and pork	1 oz	0	0.03	0.04	0.76	0.04	0.9	0.42	0.0	5.1	0.4	3.1	46	0.6
beef and pork, 15 per 8-oz pkg.	1 slice	0	0.02	0.02	0.40	0.02	0.5	0.22	0.0	2.7	0.2	1.6	24	0.3
NEW ENGLAND STYLE														
pork and beef	1 oz	0	0.18	0.07	0.99	0.10	2.0	0.38	0.0	2.0	0.3	4.5	91	0.8
pork and beef, 4-inch diam, 1/8-inch slice	1 slice	0	0.15	0.06	0.80	0.08	1.6	0.31	0.0	1.6	0.2	3.7	74	0.6
PEPPERONI														
pork and beef, 10 1/4 inch long x 1 3/8-inch diam	1 sausage	0	0.80	0.63	12.40	0.63	10.0	6.30	0.0	25.1	3.5	40.2	871	6.3
pork and beef, 1 3/8-inch diam, 1/8-inch slice	1 slice	0	0.02	0.01	0.27	0.01	0.2	0.14	0.0	0.6	<0.1	0.9	19.1	0.1
(Hormel) turkey, 'Pillow Pak'	1 serving	15	na	na	na	na	na	na	0.0	7.8	0.8	12.4	135	1.3
POLISH STYLE. See also KIELBASA.														
pork	1 oz	0	0.14	0.04	0.98	0.05	0.6	0.28	0.3	3.4	0.4	4.0	67	0.6
pork, 10-inch long x 1.25-inch diam	1 sausage	0	1.10	0.34	7.8	0.43	4.5	2.20	2.3	27.2	3.3	31.8	538	4.4
PORK														
link, 4-inch long x 1 1/8 inch diam	1 link	0	0.48	0.17	3.10	0.24	3.4	1.10	1.4	20.4	0.8	12.9	228	1.9
link, fresh, cooked, 4-inch long x 7/8-inch diam before cooking	1 link	0	0.10	0.03	0.59	0.04	0.3	0.23	0.3	4.2	0.2	2.2	47	0.3
link, fresh, raw, 7/8-inch diam x 4-inch long	1 link	0	0.15	0.05	0.79	0.07	1.1	0.32	0.6	5.0	0.3	3.1	57	0.5
link, 2-inch long x 3/4-inch diam	1 link	0	0.11	0.04	0.72	0.06	0.8	0.26	0.3	4.8	0.2	3.0	54	0.5
patty, fresh, cooked, 3 7/8 inch diam x 1/4-inch thick before cooking	1 patty	0	0.20	0.07	1.20	0.09	0.5	0.47	0.5	8.6	0.3	4.6	98	0.7
patty, fresh, raw 3 7/8 inch diam x 1/4-inch thick	1 patty	0	0.31	0.09	1.60	0.14	2.3	0.64	1.1	10.3	0.5	6.3	116	0.9

Food Name	Serving Size	A I.U.	Thi mg	Rib mg	Nia mg	B₆ mg	Fol mcg	B₁₂ mcg	C mg	Calc mg	Iron mg	Mag mg	Pot mg	Zn mg
(Oscar Mayer)														
link	2 links	0	na	na	na	na	na	na	0.0	7.7	0.8	8.6	114	1.2
link, cooked	1 link	0	na	na	na	na	na	na	0.0	3.8	0.4	4.3	57	0.6
PORK AND BEEF														
link, 4-inch long x 1 1/8 inch diam	1 link	0	0.18	0.12	2.2	0.12	1.4	1.00	0.0	6.8	1.0	8.2	129	1.4
link, fresh, cooked, 4-inch long x 7/8-inch diam before cooking	1 link	0	0.05	0.02	0.44	0.01	0.3	0.06	0.0	1.3	0.2	1.6	25	0.2
link, 2-inch long x 3/4-inch diam	1 link	0	0.04	0.03	0.52	0.03	0.3	0.24	0.0	1.6	0.2	1.9	30	0.3
patty, fresh, cooked, 3 7/8 inch diam x 1/4-inch thick before cooking	1 patty	0	0.10	0.04	0.91	0.01	0.5	0.12	0.0	2.7	0.3	3.2	51	0.5
PORK AND TURKEY														
(Oscar Mayer)														
little, 'Smokies'	1 link	0	na	na	na	na	na	na	0.0	1.0	0.1	1.5	16	0.2
w/cheese, little, 'Smokies'	1 link	0	na	na	na	na	na	na	0.0	6.0	0.1	1.9	14	0.2
SALAMI. See also under LUNCHEON MEAT.														
beef, cooked	1 oz	0	0.03	0.05	0.92	0.05	0.6	0.87	0.0	2.6	0.6	4.0	64	0.6
beef, cooked, 4-inch diam, 1/8-inch slice	1 slice	0	0.02	0.04	0.75	0.04	0.5	0.70	0.0	2.1	0.5	3.2	52	0.5
beef and pork, cooked	1 oz	0	0.07	0.11	1.00	0.06	0.6	1.00	0.0	3.7	0.8	4.3	56	0.6
beef and pork, cooked, 4-inch diam, 1/8-inch slice	1 slice	0	0.06	0.09	0.82	0.05	0.5	0.84	0.0	3.0	0.6	3.5	46	0.5
pork and beef, dry or hard, 3 1/8 inch, 1/16-inch slice	1 slice	0	0.06	0.03	0.49	0.05	0.2	0.19	0.0	0.8	0.2	1.7	38	0.3
pork, dry or hard, 3 1/8 inch, 1/16-inch slice	1 slice	0	0.09	0.03	0.56	0.06	0.2	0.28	0.0	1.3	0.1	2.2	38	0.4
TURKEY *(Louis Rich)* smoked	1 serving	0	na	na	na	na	na	na	0.0	14.6	0.8	11.8	113	1.2
VEGETARIAN														
(Morningstar Farms)														
'Breakfast Patties'	1 pkg	0	578.00	14.30	197.00	20.40	na	161.00	0.0	1959.0	206.0	122.0	10940	39.6
'Breakfast Patties'	1 patty	0	5.40	0.13	1.80	0.19	na	1.50	0.0	18.2	1.9	1.1	102	0.4
VIENNA, beef and pork, canned, 7/8-inch diam x 2-inch long	1 sausage	0	0.01	0.02	0.26	0.02	0.6	0.16	0.0	1.6	0.1	1.1	16	0.3
SAVORY, GROUND														
ground	1 tbsp	226	0.02	na	0.18	na	na	0.00	2.2	93.8	1.7	16.6	46	0.2
ground	1 tsp	72	0.01	na	0.06	na	na	0.00	0.7	29.8	0.5	5.3	15	<0.1
SAVOY CABBAGE. See CABBAGE, SAVOY.														
SCALLION														
raw, tops and bulb, chopped	1 cup	385	0.06	0.08	0.53	0.06	64.0	0.00	18.8	72.0	1.5	20.0	276	0.4
raw, tops and bulb, chopped	1 tbsp	23	0.00	0.01	0.03	0.00	3.8	0.00	1.1	4.3	<0.1	1.2	17	<0.1
raw, tops and bulb, whole, large, 5-1/4 inch long	1 scallion	96	0.01	0.02	0.13	0.02	16.0	0.00	4.7	18.0	0.4	5.0	69	0.1
raw, tops and bulb, whole, medium, 4-1/8-inch long	1 scallion	58	0.01	0.01	0.08	0.01	9.6	0.00	2.8	10.8	0.2	3.0	41	<0.1
raw, tops and bulb, whole, small, 3-inch long	1 scallion	19	0.00	0.00	0.03	0.00	3.2	0.00	0.9	3.6	<0.1	1.0	14	<0.1
SCALLOP														
mixed species, breaded and fried	2 large	23	0.01	0.03	0.47	0.04	11.5	0.41	0.7	13.0	0.3	18.3	103	0.3
mixed species, raw	2 large	15	0.00	0.02	0.34	0.05	4.8	0.46	0.9	7.2	<0.1	16.8	97	0.3
mixed species, raw	3 oz	43	0.01	0.06	0.98	0.13	13.6	1.30	2.5	20.4	0.3	47.6	274	0.8
SCALLOP SQUASH. See SQUASH, SCALLOP.														
SCALLOP SUBSTITUTE														
made from surimi	3 oz	56	0.01	0.01	0.26	0.03	1.4	1.40	0.0	6.8	0.3	36.5	88	0.3
SCOTCH KALE. See KALE, SCOTCH.														
SCUP / sea bream														
baked, broiled, grilled, or microwaved	3 oz	88	0.11	0.10	4.20	0.29	14.4	1.40	0.0	43.4	0.6	24.6	313	0.5

Food Name	Serving Size	A I.U.	Thi mg	Rib mg	Nia mg	B_6 mg	Fol mcg	B_{12} mcg	C mg	Calc mg	Iron mg	Mag mg	Pot mg	Zn mg
raw	1 cup	149	0.18	0.17	6.80	0.50	24.9	2.30	0.0	66.4	0.9	38.2	476	0.8
raw	3 oz	77	0.09	0.09	3.50	0.26	12.8	1.20	0.0	34.0	0.5	19.6	244	0.4
raw, boneless	1 oz	26	0.03	0.03	1.20	0.09	4.3	0.40	0.0	11.3	0.2	6.5	81	0.1
SEA BASS. See BASS, SEA.														
SEA BREAM. See SCUP.														
SEA DEVIL. See MONKFISH.														
SEA PERCH. See OCEAN PERCH, ATLANTIC.														
SEA TROUT. See under TROUT.														
SEA VEGETABLE														
AGAR, raw	2 tbsp	0	0.00	0.00	0.01	0.00	8.5	0.00	0	5.4	0.2	6.7	23	<0.1
IRISH MOSS, raw	2 tbsp	12	0.00	0.05	0.06	0.01	18.2	0.00	0.3	7.2	0.9	14.4	6	0.2
KELP, raw	2 tbsp	12	0.01	0.02	0.05	0.00	18.0	0.00	0.3	16.8	0.3	12.1	9	0.1
LAVER														
raw	10 sheets	1353	0.03	0.12	0.38	0.04	38.0	0.00	10.1	18.2	0.5	0.5	93	0.3
raw	2 tbsp	520	0.01	0.05	0.15	0.02	14.6	0.00	3.9	7.0	0.2	0.2	36	0.1
WAKAME, raw	2 tbsp	36	0.01	0.02	0.16	0.00	19.6	0.00	0.3	15.0	0.2	10.7	5.0	<0.1
SEASONING AND COATING MIX														
PORK														
(Shake 'N Bake) original recipe,	1 serving	na	na	na	na	na	na	na	na	na	na	na	na	na
SEASONING MIX														
CHILI POWDER														
	1 tbsp	2620	0.03	0.06	0.59	0.14	7.5	0.00	4.8	20.9	1.1	12.8	144	0.2
	1 tsp	908	0.01	0.02	0.20	0.05	2.6	0.00	1.7	7.2	0.4	4.4	50	<0.1
CURRY POWDER														
	1 tbsp	62	0.02	0.02	0.22	0.04	9.7	0.00	0.7	30.1	1.9	16.0	97	0.3
	1 tsp	20	0.01	0.01	0.07	0.01	3.1	0.00	0.2	9.6	0.6	5.1	31	<0.1
SEAWEED. See SEA VEGETABLE.														
SEMOLINA														
enriched	1 cup	0	1.40	0.95	10.00	0.17	257.0	0.00	0.0	28.4	7.3	78.5	311	1.8
unenriched	1 cup	0	0.47	0.13	5.50	0.17	120.0	0.00	0.0	28.4	2.1	78.5	311	1.8
SERRANO PEPPER. See PEPPER, SERRANO.														
SESAME BUTTER / tahini														
	1 tbsp	8	0.04	0.03	1.10	0.13	16.0	0.00	0.0	154.0	3.1	57.9	93	1.2
made from raw and stone ground kernels	1 oz	19	0.36	0.14	1.70	0.04	27.7	0.00	0.0	119.0	0.7	27.2	117	1.3
made from raw and stone ground kernels	1 tbsp	10	0.19	0.08	0.89	0.02	14.7	0.00	0.0	63.0	0.4	14.4	62	0.7
made from roasted and toasted kernels	1 oz	19	0.35	0.13	1.50	0.04	27.7	0.00	0.0	121.0	2.5	26.9	117	1.3
made from roasted and toasted kernels	1 tbsp	10	0.18	0.07	0.82	0.02	14.7	0.00	0.0	63.9	1.3	14.3	62	0.7
made from unroasted kernels, hulls removed	1 oz	19	0.45	0.03	1.60	0.04	27.7	0.00	0.0	40.0	1.8	100.0	130	3.0
made from unroasted kernels, hulls removed	1 tbsp	9	0.22	0.02	0.79	0.02	13.7	0.00	0.0	19.7	0.9	49.4	64	1.5
SESAME FLOUR. See under FLOUR.														
SESAME MEAL, partially defatted	1 oz	19	0.73	0.08	3.60	0.04	8.4	0.00	0.0	43.4	4.1	98.1	115	2.9
SESAME OIL														
	1 cup	0	0.00	0.00	0.00	0.00	0.0	0.00	0.0	0.0	0.0	0.0	0	0.0
	1 tbsp	0	0.00	0.00	0.00	0.00	0.0	0.00	0.0	0.0	0.0	0.0	0	0.0
SESAME SEED / sim sim														
Dried														
hulled	1 cup	99	1.10	0.13	7.00	0.22	144	0.00	0.0	197.0	11.7	521.0	611	15.4
hulled	1 tbsp	5	0.06	0.01	0.38	0.01	7.7	0.00	0.0	10.5	0.6	27.8	33	0.8
hulled	1 tsp	2	0.02	0.00	0.13	0.00	2.6	0.00	0.0	3.5	0.2	9.4	11	0.3

Food Name	Serving Size	A I.U.	Thi mg	Rib mg	Nia mg	B$_6$ mg	Fol mcg	B$_{12}$ mcg	C mg	Calc mg	Iron mg	Mag mg	Pot mg	Zn mg
whole	1 cup	13	1.10	0.36	6.50	1.10	139	0.00	0.0	1404.0	21.0	505.0	674	11.2
whole	1 tbsp	<1	0.07	0.02	0.41	0.07	8.7	0.00	0.0	87.8	1.3	31.6	42	0.7
Roasted and toasted, whole	1 oz	3	0.23	0.07	1.30	0.23	27.8	0.00	0.0	280.0	4.2	101.0	135	2.0
Toasted														
hulled, salted	1 cup	85	1.50	0.60	7.00	0.19	123.0	0.00	0.0	168.0	10.0	443.0	520	13.1
hulled, salted	1 oz	19	0.34	0.13	1.50	0.04	27.2	0.00	0.0	37.1	2.2	98.1	115	2.9
hulled, unsalted	1 cup	85	1.50	0.60	7.00	0.19	123.0	0.00	0.0	168.0	10.0	443.0	520	13.1
hulled, unsalted	1 oz	19	0.34	0.13	1.50	0.04	27.2	0.00	0.0	37.1	2.2	98.1	115	2.9
SESAME STICKS														
wheat-based, salted	2 oz	50	0.07	0.04	0.88	0.05	12.5	0.00	0.0	96.4	0.4	25.5	100	0.7
wheat-based, salted	1 oz	25	0.04	0.02	0.44	0.02	6.2	0.00	0.0	48.2	0.2	12.8	50	0.3
SESBANIA FLOWER. See KATURAY.														
SHAD, AMERICAN														
baked, broiled, grilled, or microwaved	3 oz	102	0.16	0.26	9.20	0.39	14.4	0.12	0.0	51.0	1.1	32.3	418	0.4
raw	3 oz	94	0.13	0.20	7.10	0.34	12.8	0.13	0.0	40.0	0.8	25.5	326	0.3
SHALLOT														
Freeze-dried														
chopped	1/4 cup	2020	0.01	0.00	0.04	0.06	4.2	0.00	1.4	6.6	0.2	3.7	59	<0.1
chopped	1 tbsp	505	0.00	0.00	0.01	0.02	1.0	0.00	0.4	1.6	<0.1	0.9	15	<0.1
Fresh, raw, chopped	1 tbsp	119	0.01	0.00	0.02	0.04	3.4	0.00	0.8	3.7	0.1	2.1	33	<0.1
SHARK														
mixed species, batter-dipped, fried	3 oz	153	0.06	0.08	2.40	0.26	12.8	1.00	0.0	42.5	0.9	36.5	132	0.4
SHEA NUT OIL														
	1 cup	0	0.00	0.00	0.00	0.00	0.0	0.00	0.0	0.0	0.0	0.0	0	0.0
	1 tbsp	0	0.00	0.00	0.00	0.00	0.0	0.00	0.0	0.0	0.0	0.0	0	0.0
SHEEPSHEAD / fathead														
baked, broiled, grilled, or microwaved	3 oz	98	0.01	0.04	1.50	0.30	14.7	2.00	0.0	31.4	0.6	29.8	435	0.54
raw	3 oz	85	0.01	0.03	1.30	0.26	12.8	1.70	0.0	17.9	0.4	27.2	343	0.33
SHELLIE BEAN. See BEAN, SHELLY.														
SHELLY BEAN. See BEAN, SHELLY.														
SHIITAKE. See MUSHROOM, SHIITAKE.														
SHIMEJI. See MUSHROOM, OYSTER.														
SHORTENING														
For baking														
hydrogenated soybean oil w/ palm and cottonseed oils	1 cup	0	0.00	0.00	0.00	0.00	0.0	0.00	0.0	0.0	0.0	0.0	0	0.0
hydrogenated soybean oil w/ palm and cottonseed oils	1 tbsp	0	0.00	0.00	0.00	0.00	0.0	0.00	0.0	0.0	0.0	0.0	0	0.0
For bread														
hydrogenated soybean oil w/cottonseed oil	1 cup	0	0.00	0.00	0.00	0.00	0.0	0.00	0.0	0.0	0.0	0.0	0	0.0
hydrogenated soybean oil w/cottonseed oil	1 tbsp	0	0.00	0.00	0.00	0.00	0.0	0.00	0.0	0.0	0.0	0.0	0	0.0
For cake and frosting														
hydrogenated soybean oil	1 cup	0	0.00	0.00	0.00	0.00	0.0	0.00	0.0	0.0	0.0	0.0	0	0.0
hydrogenated soybean oil	1 tbsp	0	0.00	0.00	0.00	0.00	0.0	0.00	0.0	0.0	0.0	0.0	0	0.0
For cake mix														
hydrogenated soybean and cottonseed oils	1 cup	0	0.00	0.00	0.00	0.00	0.0	0.00	0.0	0.0	0.0	0.0	0	0.0
hydrogenated soybean and cottonseed oils	1 tbsp	0	0.00	0.00	0.00	0.00	0.0	0.00	0.0	0.0	0.0	0.0	0	0.0
For confectionery														
fractionated palm oil	1 cup	0	0.00	0.00	0.00	0.00	0.0	0.00	0.0	0.0	0.0	0.0	0	0.0
fractionated palm oil	1 tbsp	0	0.00	0.00	0.00	0.00	0.0	0.00	0.0	0.0	0.0	0.0	0	0.0

Food Name	Serving Size	A I.U.	Thi mg	Rib mg	Nia mg	B_6 mg	Fol mcg	B_{12} mcg	C mg	Calc mg	Iron mg	Mag mg	Pot mg	Zn mg
hydrogenated coconut and/or palm kernel oil	1 cup	0	0.00	0.00	0.00	0.00	0.0	0.00	0.0	0.0	0.0	0.0	0	0.0
hydrogenated coconut and/or palm kernel oil	1 tbsp	0	0.00	0.00	0.00	0.00	0.0	0.00	0.0	0.0	0.0	0.0	0	0.0
For frying														
heavy-duty, beef tallow and cottonseed oil	1 cup	0	0.00	0.00	0.00	0.00	0.0	0.00	0.0	0.0	0.0	0.0	0	0.0
heavy-duty, beef tallow and cottonseed oil	1 tbsp	0	0.00	0.00	0.00	0.00	0.0	0.00	0.0	0.0	0.0	0.0	0	0.0
heavy-duty, hydrogenated palm oil	1 cup	0	0.00	0.00	0.00	0.00	0.0	0.00	0.0	0.0	0.0	0.0	0	0.0
heavy-duty, hydrogenated palm oil	1 tbsp	0	0.00	0.00	0.00	0.00	0.0	0.00	0.0	0.0	0.0	0.0	0	0.0
heavy-duty, hydrogenated soybean (under 1% linoleic)	1 cup	0	0.00	0.00	0.00	0.00	0.0	0.00	0.0	0.0	0.0	0.0	0	0.0
heavy-duty, hydrogenated soybean (under 1% linoleic)	1 tbsp	0	0.00	0.00	0.00	0.00	0.0	0.00	0.0	0.0	0.0	0.0	0	0.0
heavy-duty, hydrogenated soybean (30% linoleic), w/stabilizers	1 cup	0	0.00	0.00	0.00	0.00	0.0	0.00	0.0	0.0	0.0	0.0	0	0.0
heavy-duty, hydrogenated soybean (30% linoleic), w/stabilizers	1 tbsp	0	0.00	0.00	0.00	0.00	0.0	0.00	0.0	0.0	0.0	0.0	0	0.0
hydrogenated soybean and cottonseed oils	1 cup	0	0.00	0.00	0.00	0.00	0.0	0.00	0.0	0.0	0.0	0.0	0	0.0
hydrogenated soybean and cottonseed oils	1 tbsp	0	0.00	0.00	0.00	0.00	0.0	0.00	0.0	0.0	0.0	0.0	0	0.0
Household														
hydrogenated soybean and cottonseed oils	1 cup	0	0.00	0.00	0.00	0.00	0.0	0.00	0.0	0.0	0.0	0.0	0	0.0
hydrogenated soybean and cottonseed oils	1 tbsp	0	0.00	0.00	0.00	0.00	0.0	0.00	0.0	0.0	0.0	0.0	0	0.0
hydrogenated soybean oil w/ palm oil	1 cup	0	0.00	0.00	0.00	0.00	0.0	0.00	0.0	0.0	0.0	0.0	0	0.0
hydrogenated soybean oil w/ palm oil	1 tbsp	0	0.00	0.00	0.00	0.00	0.0	0.00	0.0	0.0	0.0	0.0	0	0.0
lard and vegetable oil	1 cup	0	0.00	0.00	0.00	0.00	0.0	0.00	0.0	0.0	0.0	0.0	0	0.0
lard and vegetable oil	1 tbsp	0	0.00	0.00	0.00	0.00	0.0	0.00	0.0	0.0	0.0	0.0	0	0.0
Industrial														
hydrogenated soybean oil w/cottonseed oil	1 cup	0	0.00	0.00	0.00	0.00	0.0	0.00	0.0	0.0	0.0	0.0	0	0.0
hydrogenated soybean oil w/cottonseed oil	1 tbsp	0	0.00	0.00	0.00	0.00	0.0	0.00	0.0	0.0	0.0	0.0	0	0.0
lard and vegetable oil	1 cup	0	0.00	0.00	0.00	0.00	0.0	0.00	0.0	0.0	0.0	0.0	0	0.0
lard and vegetable oil	1 tbsp	0	0.00	0.00	0.00	0.00	0.0	0.00	0.0	0.0	0.0	0.0	0	0.0
Multipurpose														
hydrogenated soybean and palm oils	1 cup	0	0.00	0.00	0.00	0.00	0.0	0.00	0.0	0.0	0.0	0.0	0	0.0
hydrogenated soybean and palm oils	1 tbsp	0	0.00	0.00	0.00	0.00	0.0	0.00	0.0	0.0	0.0	0.0	0	0.0

SHOYU. See under SAUCE.

SHRIMP

Food Name	Serving Size	A I.U.	Thi mg	Rib mg	Nia mg	B_6 mg	Fol mcg	B_{12} mcg	C mg	Calc mg	Iron mg	Mag mg	Pot mg	Zn mg
Canned														
mixed species	1 cup	77	0.04	0.05	3.50	0.14	2.3	1.40	2.9	75.5	3.5	52.5	269	1.6
mixed species	10 medium	19	0.01	0.01	0.88	0.04	0.6	0.36	0.7	18.9	0.9	13.1	67	0.4
mixed species	3 oz	51	0.02	0.03	2.30	0.09	1.5	0.95	2.0	50.1	2.3	34.9	179	1.1
mixed species, cooked	1 oz	17	0.01	0.01	0.78	0.03	0.5	0.32	0.7	16.7	0.8	11.6	60	0.4
Fresh														
mixed species, boiled, poached, or steamed	3 oz	186	0.03	0.03	2.20	0.11	3.0	1.30	1.9	33.1	2.6	28.9	155	1.3
mixed species, large, boiled, poached, or steamed	4 shrimp	48	0.01	0.01	0.57	0.03	0.8	0.33	0.5	8.6	0.7	7.5	40	0.3

Food Name	Serving Size	A I.U.	Thi mg	Rib mg	Nia mg	B$_6$ mg	Fol mcg	B$_{12}$ mcg	C mg	Calc mg	Iron mg	Mag mg	Pot mg	Zn mg
mixed species, raw	3 oz	153	0.02	0.03	2.20	0.09	2.5	0.99	1.7	44.2	2.0	31.4	157	0.9
mixed species, raw, large	4 shrimp	50	0.01	0.01	0.71	0.03	0.8	0.33	0.6	14.6	0.7	10.4	52	0.3
mixed species, raw, medium	1 shrimp	11	0.00	0.00	0.15	0.01	0.2	0.07	0.1	3.1	0.1	2.2	11	<0.1
mixed species, raw, small	1 shrimp	9	0.00	0.00	0.13	0.01	0.2	0.06	0.1	2.6	0.1	1.9	9	<0.1
SHRIMP SUBSTITUTE														
made from surimi	3 oz	56	0.02	0.03	0.14	0.03	1.4	1.40	0.0	16.1	0.5	36.5	767	0.3
SICAMA. See JICAMA.														
SILVER HAKE. See WHITING.														
SILVER SALMON. See under SALMON.														
SIM SIM. See SESAME SEED.														
SISYMBRIUM SEED														
dried, whole	1 cup	47	0.14	0.31	12.4	0.58	70.5	0.0	22.7	1208.0	<0.1	232.0	1576	0.2
dried, whole	1 oz	18	0.05	0.12	4.80	0.22	27.0	0.0	8.7	463.0	<0.1	89.0	604	<0.1
SKIL. See COD, ALASKAN.														
SKIPJACK. See under TUNA.														
SKUNK CABBAGE. See CABBAGE, SKUNK.														
SLIMEHEAD. See ORANGE ROUGHY.														
SMELT, RAINBOW														
baked, broiled, grilled, or microwaved	3 oz	49	0.01	0.12	1.50	0.14	3.90	3.4	0.0	65.5	0.9	32.3	316	1.8
raw	3 oz	43	0.01	0.10	1.20	0.13	3.40	2.9	0.0	51.0	0.8	25.5	247	1.4
SNACK MIX														
(General Mills)														
'Chex'	2/3 cup	41	0.44	0.14	4.80	0.44	0.0	3.50	13.5	9.9	7.0	17.9	76	0.6
'Chex'	2 oz	82	0.88	0.28	9.50	0.88	0.0	7.00	26.9	19.8	14.0	35.7	153	1.2
(Nabisco)														
original flavor, 'Doo Dads'	1 cup	86	0.20	0.15	3.00	0.12	22.7	0.01	<0.1	42.0	1.4	34.0	157	1.3
original flavor, 'Doo Dads'	1/2 cup	43	0.10	0.07	1.50	0.06	11.3	0.00	<0.1	21.0	0.7	17.0	79	0.6
SNAP BEAN. See BEAN, GREEN; BEAN, WAX.														
SNAPPER														
mixed species, baked, broiled, grilled, or microwaved	3 oz	98	0.05	0.00	0.29	0.39	4.9	3.00	1.4	34.0	0.2	31.4	444	0.4
mixed species, raw	3 oz	85	0.04	0.00	0.24	0.34	4.3	2.50	1.4	27.2	0.2	27.2	354	0.3
SOBA NOODLE. See under NOODLE.														
SOCKEYE SALMON. See under SALMON.														
SODA. See SOFT DRINKS AND MIXERS														
SOFT DRINKS AND MIXERS														
club soda	12 fl oz	0	0.00	0.00	0.00	0.00	0.0	0.00	0.0	17.8	<0.1	3.5	7	0.4
club soda	1 fl oz	0	0.00	0.00	0.00	0.00	0.0	0.00	0.0	1.5	0.0	0.3	<1	<0.1
cola	12 fl oz	0	0.00	0.00	0.00	0.00	0.0	0.00	0.0	11.1	0.1	3.7	4	<0.1
cola	1 fl oz	0	0.00	0.00	0.00	0.00	0.0	0.00	0.0	0.9	<0.1	0.3	<1	0.0
cola, caffeine-free	12 fl oz	0	0.00	0.00	0.00	0.00	0.0	0.00	0.0	11.1	0.1	3.7	4	<0.1
cola, caffeine-free	1 fl oz	0	0.00	0.00	0.00	0.00	0.0	0.00	0.0	0.9	<0.1	0.3	<.1	0.0
cola, diet, w/aspartame	12 fl oz	0	0.02	0.08	0.00	0.00	0.0	0.00	0.0	14.2	0.1	3.5	0	0.3
cola, diet, w/aspartame	1 fl oz	0	0.00	0.01	0.00	0.00	0.0	0.00	0.0	1.2	<0.1	0.3	0	<0.1
cola, diet, w/aspartame, caffeine-free	12 fl oz	0	0.02	0.08	0.00	0.00	0.0	0.00	0.0	14.2	0.1	3.5	0	0.3
cola, diet, w/aspartame, caffeine-free	1 fl oz	0	0.00	0.01	0.00	0.00	0.0	0.00	0.0	1.2	<0.1	0.3	0	<0.1
cola, diet, w/saccharin	12 fl oz	0	0.00	0.00	0.00	0.00	0.0	0.00	0.0	14.2	0.1	3.5	7	0.2
cola, diet, w/saccharin	1 fl oz	0	0.00	0.00	0.00	0.00	0.0	0.00	0.0	1.2	<0.1	0.3	<1	<0.1
cream soda	1 fl oz	0	0.00	0.00	0.00	0.00	0.0	0.00	0.0	1.5	<0.1	0.3	<1	<0.1
cream soda	12 fl oz	0	0.00	0.00	0.00	0.00	0.0	0.00	0.0	18.6	0.2	3.7	4	0.3
diet, all flavors except cola, w/aspartame	12 fl oz	0	0.00	0.00	0.00	0.00	0.0	0.00	0.0	14.2	0.1	3.5	7	0.0
diet, all flavors except cola, w/aspartame	1 fl oz	0	0.00	0.00	0.00	0.00	0.0	0.00	0.0	1.2	<0.1	0.3	<1	0.0
ginger ale	12 fl oz	0	0.00	0.00	0.00	0.00	0.0	0.00	0.0	11.0	0.7	3.7	4	0.2
ginger ale	1 fl oz	0	0.00	0.00	0.00	0.00	0.0	0.00	0.0	0.9	<0.1	0.3	<1	<0.1

Food Name	Serving Size	A I.U.	Thi mg	Rib mg	Nia mg	B_6 mg	Fol mcg	B_{12} mcg	C mg	Calc mg	Iron mg	Mag mg	Pot mg	Zn mg
grape soda	12 fl oz	0	0.00	0.00	0.00	0.00	0.0	0.00	0.0	11.2	0.3	3.7	4	0.3
grape soda	1 fl oz	0	0.00	0.00	0.00	0.00	0.0	0.00	0.0	0.9	<0.1	0.3	<1	<0.1
lemon-lime soda	12 fl oz	0	0.00	0.00	0.06	0.00	0.0	0.00	0.0	7.4	0.3	3.7	4	0.2
lemon-lime soda	1 fl oz	0	0.00	0.00	0.01	0.00	0.0	0.00	0.0	0.6	<0.1	0.3	<1	<0.1
lemon-lime soda, w/caffeine	12 fl oz	0	0.00	0.00	0.06	0.00	0.0	0.00	0.0	7.4	0.3	3.7	4	0.2
lemon-lime soda, w/caffeine	1 fl oz	0	0.00	0.00	0.01	0.00	0.0	0.00	0.0	0.6	<0.1	0.3	<1	<0.1
orange soda	12 fl oz	0	0.00	0.00	0.00	0.00	0.0	0.00	0.0	18.6	0.2	3.7	7	0.4
orange soda	1 fl oz	0	0.00	0.00	0.00	0.00	0.0	0.00	0.0	1.6	<0.1	0.3	<1	<0.1
root beer	12 fl oz	0	0.00	0.00	0.00	0.00	0.0	0.00	0.0	18.5	0.2	3.7	4	0.3
root beer	1 fl oz	0	0.00	0.00	0.00	0.00	0.0	0.00	0.0	1.5	<0.1	0.3	<1	<0.1
tonic water	12 fl oz	0	0.00	0.00	0.00	0.00	0.0	0.00	0.0	3.7	<0.1	0.0	0	0.4
tonic water	1 fl oz	0	0.00	0.00	0.00	0.00	0.0	0.00	0.0	0.3	0.0	0.0	0	<0.1
SOLE														
baked, broiled, grilled, or microwaved	3 oz	32	0.07	0.10	1.90	0.20	7.8	2.10	0.0	15.3	0.3	49.3	292	0.5
raw	3 oz	28	0.08	0.07	2.50	0.18	6.8	1.30	1.4	15.3	0.3	26.4	307	0.4
raw, boneless	1 oz	9	0.03	0.02	0.82	0.06	2.3	0.43	0.5	5.1	0.1	8.8	102	0.1
SOMEN. See under NOODLE.														
SORGHUM	1 cup	0	0.46	0.27	5.60	na	na	0.00	0.0	53.8	8.4	na	672	na
SORGHUM SYRUP. See under SYRUP.														
SOUP. See also SOUP MIX.														
ASPARAGUS, CREAM OF														
Canned, condensed														
prepared w/milk	1 cup	600	0.10	0.28	0.88	0.06	29.8	0.50	4.0	174.0	0.9	19.8	360	0.9
unprepared	10.75-oz can	1083	0.13	0.19	1.90	0.03	58.0	0.12	6.7	70.2	2.0	9.2	421	2.1
unprepared	1 cup	891	0.11	0.16	1.60	0.03	47.7	0.10	5.5	57.7	1.6	7.5	346	1.8
BEAN														
Canned, condensed														
w/frankfurter, prepared	1 cup	870	0.11	0.07	1.00	0.13	30.0	0.08	1.0	87.5	2.4	47.5	478	1.2
w/frankfurter, unprepared	1 cup	1741	0.22	0.13	2.10	0.26	63.1	0.16	1.8	174.0	4.7	97.3	955	2.4
w/pork, prepared	1 cup	888	0.09	0.03	0.57	0.04	31.9	0.05	1.5	81.0	2.0	45.5	402	1.0
w/pork, unprepared	11.5-oz can	2158	0.21	0.08	1.40	0.10	77.3	0.10	3.9	196.0	5.0	108	978	2.5
w/pork, unprepared	1 cup	1781	0.17	0.07	1.10	0.08	63.8	0.08	3.2	161.0	4.1	88.8	807	2.1
Canned, ready to use														
w/ham, chunky, commercial product	19.25-oz can	8878	0.33	0.33	3.80	0.27	65.5	0.16	9.8	175	7.3	104.0	956	2.4
w/ham, chunky, commercial product	1 cup	3951	0.15	0.15	1.70	0.12	29.2	0.07	4.4	77.8	3.2	46.2	425	1.1
BEEF														
Canned, ready to use														
chunky	19-oz can	5864	0.13	0.34	6.10	0.30	30.2	1.40	15.6	70.1	5.2	10.8	755	5.9
chunky	1 cup	2611	0.06	0.15	2.70	0.13	13.4	0.62	7.0	31.2	2.3	4.8	336	2.6
BEEF BARLEY														
Canned, ready to use														
(Progresso)														
	10.5-oz can	3776	na	na	na	na	na	na	na	na	2.9	na	na	na
low-fat, 'Healthy Classics'	1 cup	2338	0.13	0.13	2.90	0.19	24.1	0.36	3.6	28.9	1.9	31.3	366	1.5
BEEF BROTH/BOUILLON														
Canned, condensed														
prepared	1 cup	0	0.02	0.03	0.71	0.02	2.9	0.00	0.9	9.6	0.5	0.0	154	0.4
unprepared	10.5-oz can	0	0.05	0.07	1.70	0.06	7.2	0.00	2.1	20.9	1.3	0.0	373	0.9
unprepared	1 cup	0	0.04	0.06	1.40	0.05	5.9	0.00	1.7	17.2	1.1	0.0	308	0.7
Canned, ready to use														
	14-oz can	0	0.01	0.08	3.10	0.04	7.9	0.28	0.0	23.8	0.7	7.9	214	0.0
	10.5-oz can	0	0.01	0.12	4.60	0.06	11.7	0.41	0.0	35.2	0.0	11.7	316	0.0
	1 cup	0	0.01	0.05	1.90	0.02	4.8	0.17	0.0	14.4	0.4	4.8	130	0.0
and tomato juice	5.5-oz can	215	0.00	0.05	0.28	0.04	7.2	0.08	1.5	18.5	0.9	5.0	161	<0.1

Food Name	Serving Size	A I.U.	Thi mg	Rib mg	Nia mg	B_6 mg	Fol mcg	B_{12} mcg	C mg	Calc mg	Iron mg	Mag mg	Pot mg	Zn mg
and tomato juice	1 oz	39.0	0.00	0.01	0.05	0.01	1.3	0.02	0.3	3.4	0.2	0.92	29	<0.1
BEEF MUSHROOM														
Canned, condensed														
prepared	1 cup	0	0.04	0.06	0.95	0.05	9.8	0.20	4.6	4.9	0.9	9.8	154	1.5
unprepared	10.75-oz can	0	0.06	0.18	2.70	0.12	21.4	0.49	0.0	12.2	2.1	21.4	384	3.4
unprepared	1 cup	0	0.05	0.15	2.30	0.10	17.6	0.40	0.0	10.0	1.8	17.6	316	2.8
BEEF NOODLE														
Canned, condensed														
prepared	1 cup	630	0.07	0.06	1.10	0.04	19.5	0.20	0.2	14.6	1.1	4.9	100	1.5
unprepared	10.75-oz can	1531	0.17	0.14	2.60	0.09	45.8	0.49	0.9	36.6	2.7	15.3	241	3.7
unprepared	1 cup	1260	0.14	0.12	2.10	0.08	37.6	0.40	0.8	30.1	2.2	12.6	198	3.1
BEEF VEGETABLE														
Canned, ready to use														
country, chunky	1 cup	4374	na	na	na	na	na	na	na	na	2.2	na	na	na
w/barley, prepared	1 cup	720	na	na	na	na	na	na	na	na	na	na	na	na
BLACK BEAN														
Canned, condensed														
prepared	1 cup	506	0.08	0.05	0.53	0.09	24.7	0.03	0.7	44.5	2.1	42.0	274	1.4
unprepared	11-oz can	1388	0.13	0.12	1.30	0.22	62.4	0.00	0.6	109.0	4.7	103.0	780	3.4
unprepared	1 cup	1144	0.11	0.10	1.10	0.18	51.4	0.00	0.5	90.0	3.9	84.8	643	2.8
BROCCOLI CREAM OF														
Canned, ready to use														
(Progresso) 'Healthy Classics'	1 cup	293	0.03	0.06	0.32	0.07	29.3	0.00	5.9	41.5	1.2	14.6	161	0.3
CELERY, CREAM OF														
Canned, condensed														
prepared w/milk	1 cup	461	0.07	0.25	0.44	0.06	8.4	0.50	1.5	186.0	0.7	22.3	310	0.2
prepared w/water	1 cup	307	0.03	0.05	0.33	0.01	2.4	0.24	0.2	39.0	0.6	7.3	122	0.2
unprepared	10.75-oz can	744	0.07	0.12	0.81	0.03	5.8	0.12	0.6	97.6	1.5	15.3	299	0.4
unprepared	1 cup	612	0.06	0.10	0.67	0.03	4.8	0.10	0.5	80.3	1.3	12.6	246	0.3
CHEESE														
Canned, condensed														
prepared w/milk	1 cup	1242	0.06	0.33	0.50	0.08	10.0	0.43	1.3	289.0	0.8	20.1	341	0.7
prepared w/water	1 cup	1087	0.02	0.14	0.40	0.03	4.9	0.00	0.0	141.0	0.7	4.9	153	0.6
unprepared	11-oz can	2643	0.04	0.33	0.97	0.06	9.4	0.00	0.0	346.0	1.8	9.4	374	1.6
unprepared	1 cup	2177	0.03	0.27	0.80	0.05	7.7	0.00	0.0	285.0	1.5	7.7	308	1.3
CHICKEN														
Canned, condensed														
w/dumplings, prepared	1 cup	518	0.02	0.07	1.80	0.04	2.4	0.17	0.0	14.5	0.6	4.8	116	0.4
w/dumplings, unprepared	10.5-oz can	1261	0.04	0.18	4.30	0.09	6.0	0.39	0.0	35.8	1.5	8.9	283	0.9
w/dumplings, unprepared	1 cup	1041	0.03	0.14	3.50	0.07	4.9	0.32	0.0	29.5	1.3	7.4	234	0.7
Canned, ready to use														
chunky	19-oz can	2792	0.18	0.37	9.50	0.11	9.7	0.54	2.7	53.9	3.7	16.2	377	2.2
chunky	10.75-oz can	1580	0.10	0.21	5.40	0.06	5.5	0.30	1.5	30.5	2.1	9.2	214	1.2
chunky	1 cup	1243	0.08	0.17	4.20	0.05	4.3	0.24	1.2	24.0	1.7	7.2	168	0.9
CHICKEN, CREAM OF														
Canned, condensed														
prepared w/milk	1 cup	714	0.07	0.26	0.92	0.07	7.7	0.55	1.2	181	0.7	17.4	273	0.7
prepared w/water	1 cup	561	0.03	0.06	0.82	0.02	1.7	0.10	0.2	34.2	0.6	2.4	87.8	0.6
unprepared	10.75-oz can	1360	0.07	0.15	2.00	0.04	4.0	0.21	0.3	82.3	1.5	6.1	214	1.5
unprepared	1 cup	1119	0.06	0.12	1.60	0.03	3.3	0.18	0.3	67.8	1.2	5.0	176	1.3
CHICKEN BROTH/BOUILLON														
Canned, condensed														
prepared	1 cup	0	0.01	0.07	3.30	0.02	4.8	0.24	0.0	9.6	0.5	2.4	206	0.3
unprepared	10.75-oz can	0	0.02	0.14	6.80	0.06	12.2	0.61	0.0	18.3	1.3	6.1	519	0.6

Food Name	Serving Size	A I.U.	Thi mg	Rib mg	Nia mg	B6 mg	Fol mcg	B12 mcg	C mg	Calc mg	Iron mg	Mag mg	Pot mg	Zn mg
unprepared........................	1 cup	0	0.02	0.12	5.60	0.05	10.0	0.50	0.0	15.1	1.0	5.0	427	0.5
CHICKEN GUMBO														
Canned, condensed														
prepared........................	1 cup	137	0.02	0.05	0.66	0.06	4.9	0.02	4.9	24.4	0.9	4.9	76	0.4
unprepared......................	10.75-oz can	329	0.61	0.92	1.60	0.15	15.3	0.06	12.2	58.0	2.2	9.2	183	0.9
unprepared......................	1 cup	271	0.50	0.75	1.30	0.13	12.6	0.05	10.0	47.7	1.8	7.5	151	0.8
CHICKEN MUSHROOM														
Canned, condensed														
prepared........................	1 cup	1135	0.02	0.11	1.60	0.05	0.2	0.05	0.0	29.3	0.9	9.8	154	0.9
unprepared......................	10.75-oz can	2760	0.06	0.27	4.00	0.12	6.1	0.15	0.0	70.2	2.1	21.4	384	2.4
unprepared......................	1 cup	2272	0.05	0.23	3.30	0.10	5.0	0.13	0.0	57.7	1.8	17.6	316	2.0
CHICKEN NOODLE														
Canned, condensed														
prepared........................	1 cup	711	0.05	0.06	1.40	0.03	21.7	0.14	0.2	16.9	0.8	4.8	55	0.4
unprepared......................	10.5-oz can	1585	0.16	0.16	3.70	0.06	47.7	0.39	0.0	32.8	1.8	11.9	134	0.7
unprepared......................	1 cup	1309	0.13	0.13	3.00	0.05	39.4	0.32	0.0	27.1	1.5	9.8	111	0.6
(Campbell's)														
unprepared......................	10.75-oz can	680	0.19	0.14	3.70	0.12	42.7	0.21	0.0	33.5	1.8	18.3	137	0.7
Canned, ready to use														
chunky.........................	19-oz can	2744	0.16	0.38	9.70	0.11	86.2	0.70	0.0	53.9	3.2	21.6	243	2.2
chunky.........................	1 cup	1222	0.07	0.17	4.30	0.05	38.4	0.31	0.0	24.0	1.4	9.6	108	0.9
w/celery and carrots, homestyle...........	1 cup	662	na	na	na	na	na	na	na	na	1.5	na	na	na
w/meatballs, chunky.....................	20-oz can	5318	0.28	0.28	5.70	0.11	51.0	0.57	17.6	68.0	4.0	22.7	352	1.1
w/meatballs, chunky.....................	1 cup	2326	0.12	0.12	2.50	0.05	22.3	0.25	7.7	29.8	1.7	9.9	154	0.5
(Progresso) 'Healthy Classics'..............	1 cup	920	0.11	0.11	3.40	0.05	33.2	0.21	0.7	19.0	1.1	9.5	209	0.4
CHICKEN RICE														
Canned, condensed														
prepared........................	1 cup	660	0.02	0.02	1.10	0.02	0.9	0.14	0.2	16.9	0.8	0	101	0.3
unprepared......................	10.5-oz can	1606	0.04	0.06	2.70	0.06	2.7	0.39	0.3	41.7	1.8	0	244	0.6
unprepared......................	1 cup	1326	0.03	0.05	2.30	0.05	2.2	0.32	0.3	34.4	1.5	0	202	0.5
Canned, ready to use														
chunky.........................	19-oz can	13157	0.05	0.22	9.20	0.11	8.6	0.70	8.6	75.5	4.2	21.6	243	2.2
chunky.........................	1 cup	5858	0.02	0.10	4.10	0.05	3.8	0.31	3.8	33.6	1.9	9.6	108	0.9
(Progresso)														
wild rice, w/vegetables..................	1 cup	1315	na	na	na	na	na	na	na	na	na	na	na	na
w/vegetables, 'Healthy Classics'...........	1 cup	1644	0.12	0.07	2.60	0.07	35.9	0.10	0.7	23.9	1.2	23.9	275	0.4
CHICKEN VEGETABLE														
Canned, condensed														
prepared........................	1 cup	2656	0.04	0.06	1.20	0.05	4.8	0.12	0.9	16.9	0.9	7.2	154	0.4
unprepared......................	10.5-oz can	6461	0.11	0.14	3.00	0.12	11.9	0.30	2.4	41.7	2.1	14.9	375	0.9
unprepared......................	1 cup	5333	0.09	0.11	2.50	0.10	9.8	0.25	2.0	34.4	1.7	12.3	310	0.7
Canned, ready to use														
chunky.........................	19-oz can	13453	0.09	0.37	7.40	0.22	26.9	0.54	12.4	59.3	3.3	21.6	825	4.9
chunky.........................	1 cup	5990	0.04	0.17	3.30	0.10	12.0	0.24	5.5	26.4	1.5	9.6	367	2.2
CHILI BEEF														
Canned, condensed														
prepared........................	1 cup	1510	0.06	0.08	1.10	0.16	17.5	0.33	4.0	42.5	2.1	30.0	525	1.4
unprepared......................	11.25-oz can	3665	0.14	0.19	2.60	0.38	44.7	0.77	9.9	105	5.2	73.4	1276	3.4
unprepared......................	1 cup	3022	0.12	0.15	2.10	0.32	36.8	0.63	8.2	86.8	4.3	60.5	1052	2.8
CLAM CHOWDER														
Canned, condensed														
Manhattan, prepared..................	1 cup	964	0.03	0.04	0.82	0.10	9.8	4.00	3.9	26.8	1.6	12.2	188	0.9
Manhattan, unprepared................	10.75-oz can	2339	0.07	0.10	2.00	0.24	24.4	9.90	9.8	58.0	4.0	24.4	458	2.3
Manhattan, unprepared................	1 cup	1925	0.06	0.08	1.60	0.20	20.1	8.10	8.0	47.7	3.3	20.1	377	1.9

Food Name	Serving Size	A I.U.	Thi mg	Rib mg	Nia mg	B6 mg	Fol mcg	B12 mcg	C mg	Calc mg	Iron mg	Mag mg	Pot mg	Zn mg
New England, prepared w/milk	1 cup	164	0.07	0.24	1.00	0.13	9.7	10.20	3.5	186.0	1.5	22.3	300	0.8
New England, prepared w/water	1 cup	7.3	0.02	0.04	0.96	0.08	3.7	8.00	2.0	43.9	1.5	7.3	146	0.8
New England, unprepared	10.75-oz can	24.4	0.05	0.09	2.30	0.18	8.8	23.90	5.8	101.0	3.4	18.3	278	1.8
New England, unprepared	1 cup	20.1	0.04	0.08	1.90	0.15	7.3	19.60	4.8	82.8	2.8	15.1	228	1.5
Canned, ready to use														
Manhattan, chunky	19-oz can	7395	0.13	0.14	4.20	0.59	21.0	17.80	27.5	151.0	5.9	43.1	862	3.8
Manhattan, chunky	1 cup	3293	0.06	0.06	1.80	0.26	9.4	7.90	12.2	67.2	2.6	19.2	384	1.7
(Progresso)														
New England, 'Healthy Classics'	1 cup	244	0.05	0.09	0.86	0.09	29.3	6.20	5.1	17.1	0.9	12.2	283	0.4
CRAB														
Canned, ready to use														
....	13-oz can	764	0.29	0.11	2.00	0.19	22.1	0.29	0.0	99.6	1.8	22.1	494	2.2
....	1 cup	505	0.20	0.07	1.30	0.12	14.6	0.20	0.0	65.9	1.2	14.6	327	1.5
ESCAROLE														
Canned, ready to use														
....	19.5-oz can	4839	0.17	0.11	5.10	0.50	77.4	1.10	10.0	71.9	1.7	11.1	592	5.0
....	1 cup	2170	0.07	0.05	2.30	0.22	34.7	0.50	4.5	32.2	0.7	5.0	265	2.2
GARLIC AND PASTA														
Canned, ready to use														
(Progresso) 'Healthy Classics'	1 cup	3086	0.23	0.13	2.00	0.10	63.2	0.00	0.0	50.4	0.9	34.0	299	0.6
GAZPACHO														
Canned, ready to use														
....	13-oz can	3937	0.07	0.04	1.40	0.22	14.8	0.00	10.7	36.9	1.5	11.1	339	0.4
....	1 cup	2603	0.05	0.02	0.93	0.15	9.8	0.00	7.1	24.4	0.9	7.3	224	0.2
GREEN PEA														
Canned, condensed														
prepared w/milk	1 cup	356	0.16	0.27	1.30	0.10	7.9	0.43	2.8	173.0	2.0	55.9	376	1.8
prepared w/water	1 cup	203	0.11	0.07	1.20	0.05	1.8	0.00	1.8	27.5	1.9	40.0	190	1.7
unprepared	11.25-oz can	488	0.26	0.17	3.00	0.13	4.5	0.00	4.1	67.0	4.7	95.7	463	4.1
unprepared	1 cup	402	0.22	0.14	2.50	0.11	3.7	0.00	3.4	55.2	3.9	78.9	381	3.4
LENTIL														
Canned, ready to use														
w/ham	20-oz can	822	0.40	0.26	3.10	0.51	113.0	0.68	9.6	96.4	6.1	51.0	816	1.7
w/ham	1 cup	360	0.17	0.11	1.40	0.22	49.6	0.30	4.2	42.2	2.7	22.3	357	0.7
(Progresso) 'Healthy Classics'	1 cup	951	0.11	0.09	0.70	0.16	102.0	0.00	0.9	41.1	2.7	41.1	336	1.0
MINESTRONE														
Canned, condensed														
prepared	1 cup	2338	0.05	0.04	0.94	0.10	36.1	0.00	1.2	33.7	0.9	7.2	313	0.7
unprepared	10.5-oz can	5686	0.13	0.11	2.30	0.24	86.4	0.00	2.7	83.4	2.2	17.9	760	1.8
unprepared	1 cup	4694	0.11	0.09	1.90	0.20	71.3	0.00	2.2	68.9	1.8	14.8	627	1.5
Canned, ready to use														
chunky	19-oz can	9772	0.12	0.26	2.60	0.54	119.0	0.00	10.8	135	4.0	32.3	1374	3.2
chunky	1 cup	4351	0.06	0.12	1.20	0.24	52.8	0.00	4.8	60.0	1.8	14.4	612	1.4
(Progresso) 'Healthy Classics'	1 cup	1357	0.15	0.08	1.00	0.14	60.3	0.00	0.7	38.6	1.7	31.3	306	0.7
MUSHROOM														
Canned, condensed														
w/beef stock, prepared	1 cup	1254	0.03	0.10	1.20	0.04	9.3	0.00	0.9	9.8	0.8	9.8	159	1.4
w/beef stock, unprepared	10.75-oz can	3050	0.09	0.23	2.90	0.09	22.3	0.00	2.4	24.4	2.0	21.4	384	3.4
w/beef stock, unprepared	1 cup	2510	0.07	0.19	2.40	0.08	18.3	0.00	2.0	20.1	1.7	17.6	316	2.8
MUSHROOM, CREAM OF														
Canned, condensed														
prepared w/milk	1 cup	154	0.08	0.28	0.91	0.06	9.9	0.50	2.2	179	0.6	19.8	270	0.6
prepared w/water	1 cup	0	0.05	0.09	0.72	0.02	4.9	0.05	0.9	46.4	0.5	4.9	100	0.6
unprepared	10.75-oz can	0	0.07	0.20	2.00	0.03	9.2	0.30	2.7	79.3	1.3	12.2	204	1.4

Food Name	Serving Size	A I.U.	Thi mg	Rib mg	Nia mg	B_6 mg	Fol mcg	B_{12} mcg	C mg	Calc mg	Iron mg	Mag mg	Pot mg	Zn mg
unprepared	1 cup	0	0.06	0.17	1.60	0.03	7.5	0.25	2.3	65.3	1.1	10.0	168	1.2
MUSHROOM BARLEY														
Canned, condensed														
prepared	1 cup	198	0.02	0.09	0.88	0.17	4.9	0.00	0.0	12.2	0.5	9.8	93	0.5
unprepared	10.75-oz can	482	0.06	0.21	2.10	0.43	15.3	0.00	0.0	30.5	1.2	21.4	232	1.2
unprepared	1 cup	397	0.05	0.18	1.80	0.35	12.6	0.00	0.0	25.1	1.0	17.6	191	1.0
ONION														
Canned, condensed														
prepared	1 cup	0	0.03	0.02	0.60	0.05	15.2	0.00	1.2	26.5	0.7	2.4	68	0.6
unprepared	10.5-oz can	0	0.08	0.06	1.50	0.12	37.0	0.00	3.0	65.6	1.6	6.0	167	1.5
unprepared	1 cup	0	0.07	0.05	1.20	0.10	30.5	0.00	2.5	54.1	1.4	4.9	138	1.2
ONION, CREAM OF														
Canned, condensed														
prepared w/milk	1 cup	451	0.10	0.27	0.60	0.07	22.3	0.50	2.5	179	0.7	22.3	310	0.6
prepared w/water	1 cup	295	0.05	0.08	0.50	0.02	6.8	0.05	1.2	34.2	0.6	4.9	120	0.2
unprepared	10.75-oz can	720	0.12	0.18	1.20	0.06	17.4	0.12	3.0	82.3	1.5	15.3	299	0.4
unprepared	1 cup	592	0.10	0.15	1.00	0.05	14.3	0.10	2.5	67.8	1.3	12.6	246	0.3
OYSTER STEW														
Canned, condensed														
unprepared	10.5-oz can	173	0.05	0.09	0.57	0.03	6.0	5.30	7.7	53.6	2.4	11.9	119	25.0
unprepared	1 cup	143	0.04	0.07	0.47	0.03	4.9	4.40	6.4	44.3	2.0	9.8	98	20.7
prepared w/milk	1 cup	225	0.07	0.23	0.34	0.06	9.8	2.60	4.4	167.0	1.1	19.6	235	10.3
prepared w/water	1 cup	69.9	0.02	0.04	0.23	0.01	2.4	2.20	3.1	21.7	1.0	4.8	48	10.3
PEPPER POT														
Canned, condensed														
prepared	1 cup	865	0.05	0.05	1.20	0.06	9.6	0.17	1.4	24.1	0.9	4.8	152	1.2
unprepared	10.5-oz can	2104	0.13	0.12	3.00	0.15	23.8	0.42	3.3	56.6	2.2	11.9	370	3.0
unprepared	1 cup	1737	0.11	0.10	2.50	0.12	19.7	0.34	2.7	46.7	1.8	9.8	305	2.5
POTATO, CREAM OF														
Canned, condensed														
prepared w/milk	1 cup	444	0.08	0.24	0.64	0.09	9.2	0.50	1.2	166.0	0.6	17.4	322	0.7
prepared w/water	1 cup	288	0.03	0.04	0.54	0.04	2.9	0.05	0.0	19.5	0.5	2.4	137	0.6
unprepared	10.75-oz can	702	0.09	0.09	1.30	0.09	7.3	0.12	0.0	48.8	1.2	3.0	332	1.5
unprepared	1 cup	577	0.07	0.07	1.10	0.08	6.0	0.10	0.0	40.2	0.9	2.5	274	1.3
SCOTCH BROTH														
Canned, condensed														
prepared	1 cup	2179	0.02	0.05	1.20	0.07	9.6	0.27	0.9	14.5	0.8	4.8	159	1.6
unprepared	10.5-oz can	5301	0.05	0.11	2.80	0.18	23.8	0.66	2.1	35.8	2.0	8.9	387	3.9
unprepared	1 cup	4376	0.04	0.09	2.30	0.15	19.7	0.54	1.7	29.5	1.7	7.4	320	3.2
SHRIMP, CREAM OF														
Canned, condensed														
unprepared	10.75-oz can	384	0.05	0.07	1.00	0.09	9.2	1.40	0.0	42.7	1.3	21.4	143	1.8
unprepared	1 cup	316	0.04	0.06	0.85	0.08	7.5	1.20	0.0	35.1	1.1	17.6	118	1.5
prepared w/milk	1 cup	312	0.06	0.23	0.53	0.45	9.9	1.00	1.2	164	0.6	22.3	248	0.8
SPLIT PEA														
Canned, condensed														
w/ham, prepared w/water	1 cup	445	0.15	0.08	1.50	0.07	2.5	0.25	1.5	22.8	2.3	48.1	400	1.3
w/ham, unprepared	11.5-oz can	1079	0.36	0.18	3.60	0.16	6.2	0.65	3.6	52.2	5.5	117.0	968	3.2
w/ham, unprepared	1 cup	890	0.30	0.15	3.00	0.14	5.1	0.54	3.0	43.0	4.6	96.8	799	2.6
Canned, ready to use														
w/ham, chunky	19-oz can	10942	0.26	0.21	5.70	0.48	10.2	0.54	15.6	75.5	4.8	86.2	685	7.0
w/ham, chunky	1 cup	4872	0.12	0.09	2.50	0.22	4.6	0.24	7.0	33.6	2.1	38.4	305	3.1
(Progresso) 'Healthy Classics'	1 cup	1847	0.18	0.07	1.20	0.19	50.6	0.03	0.0	43.0	1.9	35.4	463	1.0

Food Name	Serving Size	A I.U.	Thi mg	Rib mg	Nia mg	B₆ mg	Fol mcg	B₁₂ mcg	C mg	Calc mg	Iron mg	Mag mg	Pot mg	Zn mg
STOCKPOT														
Canned, condensed														
prepared	1 cup	3979	0.04	0.05	1.20	0.09	9.9	0.00	2.0	22.2	0.9	4.9	237	1.2
unprepared	11-oz can	9672	0.11	0.13	3.00	0.22	25.0	0.00	5.0	53.0	2.1	9.4	577	2.8
unprepared	1 cup	7967	0.09	0.10	2.40	0.18	20.6	0.00	4.1	43.7	1.7	7.7	475	2.3
TOMATO														
Canned, condensed														
prepared w/milk	1 cup	848	0.13	0.25	1.50	0.16	20.8	0.45	67.7	159.0	1.8	22.3	449	0.3
prepared w/water	1 cup	688	0.09	0.05	1.40	0.11	14.6	0.00	66.4	12.2	1.8	7.3	264	0.2
unprepared	10.75-oz can	1693	0.21	0.12	3.40	0.27	35.7	0.00	162.0	33.5	4.3	18.3	641	0.6
unprepared	1 cup	1393	0.18	0.10	2.80	0.23	29.4	0.00	133.0	27.6	3.5	15.1	527	0.5
(Progresso)														
garden, 'Healthy Classics'	1 cup	1348	0.17	0.10	1.60	0.11	24.5	0.00	4.4	56.4	1.6	29.4	304	0.5
TOMATO BEEF														
Canned, condensed														
w/noodles, prepared	1 cup	534	0.08	0.09	1.90	0.09	19.5	0.20	0.0	17.1	1.1	7.3	220	0.8
w/noodles, unprepared	10.75-oz can	1296	0.20	0.22	4.50	0.21	45.8	0.46	0.0	42.7	2.7	18.3	537	1.8
w/noodles, unprepared	1 cup	1067	0.17	0.18	3.70	0.18	37.6	0.38	0.0	35.1	2.2	15.1	442	1.5
TOMATO BISQUE														
Canned, condensed														
prepared w/milk	1 cup	879	0.11	0.27	1.30	0.14	21.3	0.43	7.0	186.0	0.9	25.1	605	0.6
unprepared	11-oz can	1753	0.16	0.17	2.80	0.22	37.4	0.00	14.4	96.7	2.0	21.8	1014	1.4
unprepared	1 cup	1444	0.13	0.14	2.30	0.18	30.8	0.00	11.8	79.7	1.6	18.0	835	1.2
TOMATO RICE														
Canned, condensed														
prepared	1 cup	756	0.06	0.05	1.10	0.08	13.6	0.00	14.8	22.2	0.8	4.9	331	0.5
unprepared	11-oz can	1835	0.15	0.12	2.60	0.19	34.3	0.00	35.9	56.2	1.9	12.5	802	1.2
unprepared	1 cup	1511	0.12	0.10	2.10	0.15	28.3	0.00	29.6	46.3	1.6	10.3	660	1.0
TURKEY														
Canned, condensed														
prepared	1 cup	293	0.07	0.06	1.40	0.04	19.5	0.15	0.2	12.2	0.9	4.9	76	0.6
unprepared	10.75-oz can	711	0.18	0.16	3.40	0.09	45.8	0.40	0.3	27.4	2.3	12.2	183	1.4
unprepared	1 cup	585	0.15	0.13	2.80	0.08	37.6	0.33	0.3	22.6	1.9	10.0	151	1.2
Canned, ready to use														
chunky	18.75-oz can	16130	0.08	0.24	8.10	0.69	25.0	4.80	14.4	112	4.3	53.2	814	4.8
chunky	1 cup	7156	0.04	0.11	3.60	0.31	11.1	2.10	6.4	49.6	1.9	23.6	361	2.1
TURKEY VEGETABLE														
Canned, condensed														
prepared	1 cup	2444	0.03	0.04	1.00	0.05	4.8	0.17	0.0	16.9	0.8	4.8	176	0.6
unprepared	10.5-oz can	5948	0.07	0.10	2.40	0.12	11.9	0.42	0.0	41.7	1.8	8.9	426	1.5
unprepared	1 cup	4910	0.06	0.08	2.00	0.10	9.8	0.34	0.0	34.4	1.5	7.4	352	1.2
VEGETABLE														
Canned, ready to use														
chunky	19-oz can	13200	0.16	0.15	2.70	0.43	37.2	0.00	13.5	124.0	3.7	16.2	889	7.0
chunky	1 cup	5878	0.07	0.07	1.20	0.19	16.6	0.00	6.0	55.2	1.6	7.2	396	3.1
(Progresso) 'Healthy Classics'	1 cup	3196	0.08	0.07	1.80	0.07	28.6	0.07	1.4	30.9	1.5	21.4	290	0.4
VEGETABLE BEEF														
Canned, condensed														
broth, prepared	1 cup	2089	0.05	0.05	0.97	0.06	9.6	0.00	2.4	16.9	0.9	7.2	193	0.8
broth, unprepared	10.5-oz can	5087	0.13	0.11	2.40	0.14	25.3	0.00	5.7	41.7	2.4	14.9	468	1.9
broth, unprepared	1 cup	4199	0.10	0.09	1.90	0.11	20.9	0.00	4.7	34.4	1.9	12.3	386	1.6
prepared	1 cup	1891	0.04	0.05	1.00	0.08	10.5	0.32	2.4	17.1	1.1	4.9	173	1.5
unprepared	10.75-oz can	4599	0.09	0.12	2.50	0.18	25.6	0.76	5.8	39.6	2.7	15.3	421	3.8
unprepared	1 cup	3785	0.07	0.10	2.10	0.15	21.1	0.63	4.8	32.6	2.2	12.6	346	3.1

Food Name	Serving Size	A I.U.	Thi mg	Rib mg	Nia mg	B$_6$ mg	Fol mcg	B$_{12}$ mcg	C mg	Calc mg	Iron mg	Mag mg	Pot mg	Zn mg
SOUP MIX														
ASPARAGUS, CREAM OF, prepared	1 cup	271	0.05	0.05	0.50	0.01	7.5	0.03	0.8	22.6	0.5	2.5	133	0.7
BEAN, w/bacon, prepared	1 cup	53	0.05	0.27	0.40	0.03	7.9	0.03	1.1	55.6	1.3	29.1	326	0.7
BEEF														
broth, cubed, mix only	1 cube	2	0.01	0.01	0.12	0.01	1.2	0.04	0.0	2.2	<0.1	1.8	15	<0.1
broth, dried, prepared	1 cup	4	0.01	0.02	0.36	0.02	2.6	0.08	0.0	4.8	<0.1	4.1	36	0.0
BEEF NOODLE, prepared	1 cup	8	0.12	0.06	0.69	0.04	15.1	0.00	0.5	5.0	0.3	10.0	80	0.1
BROCCOLI														
(Lipton)														
and cheese, 'Cup-A-Soup' mix only	1 serving	47.2	0.00	0.01	0.06	na	3.7	na	3.0	46.4	0.2	na	na	na
CAULIFLOWER, prepared	1 cup	5	0.08	0.08	0.51	0.03	2.6	0.18	2.6	10.2	0.5	2.6	105	0.3
CELERY, prepared	1 cup	269	0.03	0.05	0.30	0.00	2.0	0.05	0.3	35.6	0.5	5.1	109	0.1
CHICKEN														
broth, cubed, mix only	1 cube	20	0.00	0.02	0.10	0.00	1.3	0.01	<0.1	7.5	<0.1	2.2	12	0.0
broth, dried, mix only	1 tsp	10	0.00	0.01	0.05	0.00	0.6	0.01	<0.1	3.7	<0.1	1.1	6	0.0
broth, dried, prepared	8 fl oz	40	0.01	0.03	0.20	0.01	2.6	0.02	<0.1	15.0	<0.1	4.5	25	<0.1
(Lipton)														
broth, 'Cup-A-Soup' mix only	1 serving	<1	0.00	0.00	0.17	na	0.0	na	<0.1	1.9	<0.1	na	na	na
w/pasta, fat-free, 'Cup-A-Soup' mix only	1 serving	1081	0.08	0.03	0.69	na	14.0	na	<0.1	2.9	0.4	na	na	na
w/pasta, beans, 'Kettle Creations' prepared	1 serving	465	0.20	0.14	1.60	na	29.4	na	1.7	37.5	1.1	na	na	na
hearty, supreme, 'Cup-A-Soup' mix only	1 serving	25	0.06	0.05	0.59	na	0.0	na	0.1	22.9	0.2	na	na	na
CHICKEN, CREAM OF														
prepared	1 cup	407	0.10	0.20	2.60	0.05	5.2	0.26	0.5	75.7	0.3	5.2	214	1.6
(Lipton)														
'Cup-A-Soup' mix only	1 envelope	25	0.06	0.05	0.60	na	0.0	na	0.1	18.9	<0.1	na	na	na
CHICKEN NOODLE														
prepared	1 cup	15	0.20	0.08	1.10	0.03	17.7	0.05	0	5.0	0.5	7.6	33	0.2
(Lipton)														
'Cup-A-Soup' mix only	1 serving	777	0.77	0.41	7.60	na	98.0	na	1.5	44.0	3.1	na	na	na
hearty, 'Cup-A-Soup' mix only	1 envelope	41	0.12	0.06	1.30	na	17.0	na	0.1	5.9	0.5	na	na	na
real chicken broth, 'Soup Secrets' mix only	1 serving	18	0.21	0.08	1.00	na	19.8	na	<0.1	3.4	0.5	na	na	na
'Soup Secrets' mix only	1 serving	23	0.24	0.09	1.60	na	0.0	na	<0.1	9.6	0.7	na	na	na
CHICKEN RICE, prepared w/water	1 cup	0	0.00	0.00	0.35	0.02	0.5	0.07	0	7.2	0.0	0.0	9	0.1
CHICKEN VEGETABLE														
prepared w/water	1 cup	15	0.07	0.05	0.69	0.09	2.5	0.10	1.3	15.0	0.6	22.6	68	0.2
CLAM CHOWDER														
Manhattan, prepared	1 cup	1015	0.03	0.04	0.86	0.11	10.0	4.30	4.2	25.1	1.7	10.6	198	0.9
New England, prepared	1 cup	9	0.02	0.16	0.84	0.07	3.3	8.90	2.0	76.5	1.3	6.8	205	0.7
CONSOMMÉ w/gelatin, prepared	1 cup	8	0.00	0.03	0.57	0.03	4.0	0.13	0.0	7.5	0.1	7.5	57	0.0
GREEN PEA														
prepared w/water	1 cup	49	0.22	0.15	1.30	0.05	42.0	0.27	0.0	21.7	1.0	46.1	238	0.6
(Lipton)														
'Cup-A-Soup' mix only	1 serving	0	0.01	0.02	0.21	na	0.0	na	<0.1	0.63	0.6	na	na	na
HERB														
(Lipton)														
Fiesta, 'Recipe Secrets' mix only	1 serving	149	0.04	0.04	0.29	na	2.1	na	1.5	9.5	0.3	na	na	na
savory, w/garlic 'Recipe Secrets' mix only	1 serving	44	0.03	0.03	0.30	na	0.0	na	1.7	6.9	0.2	na	na	na
LEEK, prepared	1 cup	5	0.05	0.03	0.25	0.03	7.6	0.03	2.5	30.5	0.5	10.2	89	0.2
LENTIL														
(Lipton)														
homestyle, 'Kettle Creations' prepared	1 serving	467	0.03	0.02	0.20	na	28.8	na	1.2	7.9	1.8	na	na	na

Food Name	Serving Size	A I.U.	Thi mg	Rib mg	Nia mg	B$_6$ mg	Fol mcg	B$_{12}$ mcg	C mg	Calc mg	Iron mg	Mag mg	Pot mg	Zn mg
MINESTRONE, prepared.................	1 cup	295	0.08	0.05	1.00	0.10	35.5	0.00	1.0	38.1	1.0	7.6	340	0.8
MUSHROOM														
prepared............................	1 cup	8	0.28	0.11	0.50	0.03	5.1	0.25	1.0	65.8	0.5	5.1	200	<0.1
(Lipton)														
beefy, 'Recipe Secrets' mix only	1 serving	<1	0.00	0.01	0.08	na	0.0	na	0.2	10.8	0.1	na	na	na
MUSHROOM, CREAM OF														
(Lipton) 'Cup-A-Soup' mix only	1 serving	<1	0.01	0.02	0.22	na	0.0	na	0.1	17.1	<0.1	na	na	na
NOODLE														
(Lipton)														
giggle noodle, 'Soup Secrets' mix only	1 serving	19	0.26	0.10	1.30	na	25.3	na	<0.1	3.6	0.7	na	na	na
ring noodle, 'Cup-A-Soup' mix only.........	1 serving	1861	0.11	0.05	0.81	na	16.8	na	0.2	4.2	0.4	na	na	na
ring noodle, 'Soup Secrets' mix only........	1 serving	18	0.23	0.09	1.10	na	21.8	na	<0.1	3.4	0.6	na	na	na
w/extra noodle, 'Soup Secrets'														
mix only	1 servingg	17	0.34	0.14	1.8	na	33.8	na	<0.1	3.5	0.9	na	na	na
(Top Ramen) Oriental, mix only.............	1 serving	na	na	na	na	na	na	na	na	na	1.8	na	na	na
Chicken flavor														
(Top Ramen)														
individual package, mix only..............	1 container	400	na	na	na	na	na	na	na	na	2.2	na	na	na
ONION														
prepared............................	1 cup	3	0.03	0.06	0.48	0.00	1.5	0.00	0.3	12.3	0.2	4.9	64	<0.1
(Lipton)														
'Recipe Secrets' mix only	1 serving	0	0.01	0.02	0.04	na	0.0	na	0.8	14.5	0.1	na	na	na
beefy, 'Recipe Secrets' mix only	1 serving	0	0.02	0.02	0.12	na	0.0	na	0.7	11.2	0.1	na	na	na
ONION MUSHROOM														
(Lipton) 'Recipe Secrets' mix only	1 serving	0	0.20	0.02	0.30	na	0.0	na	0.5	10.1	0.1	na	na	na
OXTAIL, prepared	1 cup	10	0.03	0.03	0.76	0.03	5.1	0.25	0.0	10.1	0.3	10.1	84	0.0
PASTA														
(Lipton) spirals, 'Soup Secrets' mix only	1 serving	17	0.23	0.09	1.20	na	24.5	na	<0.1	5.4	0.4	na	na	na
PASTA AND BEAN														
(Lipton)														
homestyle, 'Kettle Creations' mix only	1 serving	415	0.17	0.08	1.00	na	46.2	na	1.8	39.9	1.4	na	na	na
TOMATO														
prepared............................	1 cup	832	0.06	0.05	0.78	0.10	6.6	0.08	4.5	53.0	0.4	13.3	294	0.2
(Lipton) 'Cup-A-Soup' mix only	1 envelope	203	0.17	0.34	0.96	na	5.7	na	3.9	91.0	0.3	na	na	na
TOMATO VEGETABLE														
prepared............................	1 cup	190	0.06	0.05	0.79	0.05	10.1	0.00	6.1	7.6	0.6	20.2	104	0.2
(Lipton)														
'Cup-A-Soup' mix only	1 serving	2023	0.08	0.03	0.54	na	13.3	na	0.5	5.9	0.4	na	na	na
'Recipe Secrets' mix only	1 serving	20	0.02	0.02	0.13	na	0.0	na	8.4	19.6	0.3	na	na	na
spring, 'Cup-A-Soup' mix only............	1 envelope	1765	0.08	0.04	0.62	na	13.5	na	0.6	3.8	0.4	na	na	na
VEGETABLE, CREAM OF, prepared	1 cup	36	1.20	0.11	0.52	0.03	7.8	0.13	3.9	31.2	0.5	10.4	96	0.3
VEGETABLE BEEF, prepared	1 cup	238	0.03	0.04	0.46	0.05	7.6	0.25	1.3	12.7	0.9	22.8	76	0.3
SOUR CREAM														
cultured.............................	1 cup	1817	0.08	0.34	0.15	0.04	24.8	0.69	2.0	268.0	0.1	25.8	331	0.6
cultured.............................	1 tbsp	95	0.00	0.02	0.01	0.00	1.3	0.04	0.1	14.0	<0.1	1.3	17	<0.1
half and half, less fat, cultured	1 cup	1094	0.09	0.36	0.16	0.04	26.1	0.73	2.1	253.0	0.2	24.4	312	1.2
half and half, less fat, cultured	1 tbsp	68	0.01	0.02	0.01	0.00	1.6	0.05	0.1	15.7	<0.1	1.5	19	<0.1
(Breakstone's)														
less fat.............................	2 tbsp	326	na	na	na	na	na	na	0.3	49.9	<0.1	na	65	na
nonfat..............................	2 tbsp	217	na	na	na	na	na	na	0.4	45.1	<0.1	na	70	na
SOUR CREAM SUBSTITUTE														
cultured.............................	1 cup	0	0.00	0.00	0.00	0.00	0.0	0.00	0.0	5.8	0.9	14.7	369	2.7
cultured.............................	1 oz	0	0.00	0.00	0.00	0.00	0.0	0.00	0.0	0.7	0.1	1.8	46	0.3

SOURSOP. See GUANABANA.

Food Name	Serving Size	A I.U.	Thi mg	Rib mg	Nia mg	B_6 mg	Fol mcg	B_{12} mcg	C mg	Calc mg	Iron mg	Mag mg	Pot mg	Zn mg
SOY FLOUR. See under FLOUR.														
SOY MEAL														
defatted, raw............................	1 cup	49	0.84	0.31	3.20	0.69	369.0	0.00	0.0	298.0	16.7	373.0	3038	6.2
defatted, raw, crude protein basis														
Nx6.25	1 cup	49	0.84	0.31	3.20	0.69	369.0	0.00	0.0	298.0	16.7	373.0	3038	6.2
SOY PROTEIN CONCENTRATE														
produced by acid wash..................	1 oz	0	0.09	0.04	0.20	0.04	96.4	0.00	0.0	103.0	3.1	39.7	128	1.2
produced by acid wash, crude protein														
basis Nx6.25	1 oz	0	0.09	0.04	0.20	0.04	96.4	0.00	0.0	103.0	3.1	39.7	128	1.2
produced by alcohol extraction............	1 oz	0	0.09	0.04	0.20	0.04	96.4	0.00	0.0	103.0	3.1	89.3	624	1.2
SOY PROTEIN ISOLATE														
....	1 oz	0	0.05	0.03	0.41	0.03	49.9	0.00	0.0	50.5	4.1	11.1	23	1.1
K type.................................	1 oz	0	0.05	0.03	0.41	0.03	49.9	0.00	0.0	50.5	4.1	11.1	451	1.1
K type, crude protein basis..............	1 oz	0	0.05	0.03	0.41	0.03	49.9	0.00	0.0	50.5	4.1	11.1	451	1.1
(Protein Technologies)														
'ProPlus'	1 oz	527	0.74	0.28	10.2	0.74	56.7	2.80	0.0	56.7	5.1	na	454	17.0
'Supro'	1 oz	0	0.06	0.03	0.09	na	56.7	0.00	0.0	56.7	4.5	11.3	28	1.1
SOY SAUCE. See under SAUCE.														
SOYBEAN														
Dried														
mature, boiled..........................	1 cup	16	0.27	0.49	0.69	0.40	92.5	0.00	2.9	175.0	8.8	148.0	886	2.0
mature, boiled..........................	1 tbsp	1	0.02	0.03	0.04	0.03	5.8	0.00	0.2	10.9	0.6	9.2	55	0.1
mature, dry-roasted	1 cup	40	0.73	1.30	1.80	0.39	352.0	0.00	7.9	241.0	6.8	392.0	2346	8.2
mature, raw............................	1 cup	45	1.60	1.60	3.00	0.70	698.0	0.00	11.2	515.0	29.2	521.0	3342	9.1
mature, roasted	1 cup	344	0.17	0.25	2.40	0.36	363.0	0.00	3.8	237.0	6.7	249.0	2528	5.4
mature, sprouted, raw...................	1/2 cup	4	0.12	0.04	0.40	0.06	60.2	0.00	5.4	23.4	0.7	25.2	169	0.4
mature, sprouted, raw...................	10 sprouts	1	0.03	0.01	0.12	0.02	17.2	0.00	1.5	6.7	0.2	7.2	48	0.1
mature, sprouted, steamed...............	1 cup	10	0.19	0.05	1.00	0.10	75.2	0.00	7.8	55.5	1.2	56.4	334	0.9
Green														
boiled, drained	1 cup	281	0.47	0.28	2.30	0.11	200.0	0.00	30.6	261.0	4.5	108.0	970	1.6
raw	1 cup	461	1.10	0.45	4.20	0.17	422.0	0.00	74.2	504.0	9.1	166.0	1587	2.5
SOYBEAN OIL														
salad or cooking	1 cup	0	0.00	0.00	0.00	0.00	0.0	0.00	0.0	<0.1	<0.1	<0.1	0	0.0
salad or cooking	1 tbsp	0	0.00	0.00	0.00	0.00	0.0	0.00	0.0	<0.1	0.0	0.0	0	0.0
salad or cooking, hydrogenated	1 cup	0	0.00	0.00	0.00	0.00	0.0	0.00	0.0	0.0	0.0	0.0	0	0.0
salad or cooking, hydrogenated	1 tbsp	0	0.00	0.00	0.00	0.00	0.0	0.00	0.0	0.0	0.0	0.0	0	0.0
SOYBEAN-COTTONSEED OIL														
salad or cooking, hydrogenated	1 cup	0	0.00	0.00	0.00	0.00	0.0	0.00	0.0	0.0	0.0	0.0	0	0.0
salad or cooking, hydrogenated	1 tbsp	0	0.00	0.00	0.00	0.00	0.0	0.00	0.0	0.0	0.0	0.0	0	0.0
SOYBEAN-LECITHIN OIL														
....	1 cup	0	0.00	0.00	0.00	0.00	0.0	0.00	0.0	0.0	0.0	0.0	0	0.0
....	1 tbsp	0	0.00	0.00	0.00	0.00	0.0	0.00	0.0	0.0	0.0	0.0	0	0.0
SOYMILK														
....	1 cup	78	0.39	0.17	0.36	0.10	3.7	0.00	0.0	9.8	1.4	46.5	345	0.6
....	1 fl oz	10	0.05	0.02	0.05	0.01	0.5	0.00	0.0	1.2	0.2	5.8	43	<0.1
SPAGHETTI. See under PASTA														
SPAGHETTI DISH/ENTRÉE. See under PASTA DISH/ENTRÉE.														
SPAGHETTI SQUASH. See SQUASH, SPAGHETTI.														
SPANISH MACKEREL. See under MACKEREL.														
SPANISH PEANUT. See under PEANUT.														
SPEARMINT														
dried.................................	1 tbsp	169	0.01	0.02	0.11	0.04	8.5	0.00	0.0	23.8	1.4	9.6	31	<0.1
dried.................................	1 tsp	53	0.00	0.01	0.03	0.01	2.6	0.00	0.0	7.4	0.4	3.0	9	<0.1

Food Name	Serving Size	A I.U.	Thi mg	Rib mg	Nia mg	B$_6$ mg	Fol mcg	B$_{12}$ mcg	C mg	Calc mg	Iron mg	Mag mg	Pot mg	Zn mg
fresh	2 tbsp	462	0.01	0.02	0.11	0.02	12.0	0.00	1.5	22.7	1.4	7.2	52	0.1
SPINACH. See also SPINACH DISH/ENTRÉE.														
Canned														
drained	1 cup	18781	0.03	0.29	0.83	0.21	209.0	0.00	30.6	272.0	4.9	163.0	740	0.9
no salt, w/liquid	1 cup	15051	0.04	0.25	0.63	0.19	136.0	0.00	31.6	194.0	3.7	131.0	538	0.9
regular pack, w/liquid	1 cup	15051	0.04	0.25	0.63	0.19	136.0	0.00	31.6	194.0	3.7	131.0	538	0.9
Fresh														
boiled, drained	1 cup	14742	0.17	0.42	0.88	0.44	262.0	0.00	17.6	245.0	6.4	157.0	839	1.4
raw	1 cup	2015	0.02	0.06	0.22	0.06	58.3	0.00	8.4	29.7	0.8	23.7	167	0.2
raw	1 med leaf	672	0.01	0.02	0.07	0.02	19.4	0.00	2.8	9.9	0.3	7.9	56	<0.1
Frozen														
chopped or leaf, boiled, drained	10 oz pkg	17125	0.13	0.37	0.92	0.32	237.0	0.00	27.1	321.0	3.3	152.0	656	1.5
chopped or leaf, boiled, drained	1/2 cup	7395	0.06	0.16	0.40	0.14	102.0	0.00	11.7	139.0	1.4	65.5	283	0.7
chopped or leaf, no salt added, drained	10-oz pkg	17125	0.13	0.37	0.92	0.32	237.0	0.00	27.1	321.0	3.3	152.0	656	1.5
chopped or leaf, no salt added, drained	1/2 cup	7395	0.06	0.16	0.40	0.14	102.0	0.00	11.7	139.0	1.4	65.5	283	0.7
chopped or leaf, unprepared	10-oz pkg	22033	0.24	0.44	1.20	0.40	340.0	0.00	69.0	315.0	5.8	165.0	917	1.3
chopped or leaf, unprepared	1 cup	12102	0.13	0.24	0.68	0.22	187.0	0.00	37.9	173.0	3.2	90.5	504	0.7
SPINACH, MALABAR														
cooked	1 med bunch	197	0.02	0.02	0.13	0.02	19.4	0.00	1.0	21.1	0.3	8.2	44	<0.1
cooked	1 cup	510	0.05	0.06	0.35	0.04	50.2	0.00	2.6	54.6	0.7	21.1	113	0.1
SPINACH, NEW ZEALAND														
boiled, drained, chopped	1 cup	6520	0.05	0.19	0.70	0.43	14.9	0.00	28.8	86.4	1.2	57.6	184	0.6
raw, chopped	1 cup	2464	0.02	0.07	0.28	0.17	8.3	0.00	16.8	32.5	0.5	21.8	73	0.2
SPINACH DISH/ENTRÉE														
(Budget Gourmet) au gratin, frozen	1 pkg	7078	na	na	na	na	na	na	27.1	243	2.0	na	na	na
(Stouffer's)														
cream of, side dish	1/2 cup	4563	na	na	na	na	na	na	na	141	na	na	na	na
creamed	1 pkg	9127	na	na	na	na	na	na	na	283	na	na	na	na
SPINY LOBSTER. See under LOBSTER.														
SPIRULINA. See under ALGAE.														
SPLIT PEA. See PEAS, SPLIT.														
SPONGE GOURD. See GOURD, DISHCLOTH.														
SPOT														
baked, broiled, grilled, or microwaved	3 oz	98	0.16	0.23	7.20	0.39	5.1	2.90	0.0	15.3	0.4	45.9	541	0.6
raw	3 oz	85	0.14	0.19	6.00	0.34	4.3	2.50	0.0	11.9	0.3	35.7	422	0.4
SPRING ONION. See SCALLION.														
SQUAB														
average of all parts, meat and skin, raw	3 oz	208	0.18	0.19	5.19	0.35	5.1	0.35	4.4	10.3	3.0	18.8	171	1.9
average of all parts, meat only, raw	3 oz	81	0.24	0.24	5.87	0.44	6.0	0.41	6.2	11.1	3.9	21.4	203	2.3
light meat, meat only, raw	3 oz	58	0.24	0.25	7.40	0.54	4.0	0.47	5.2	10.1	2.3	28.3	263	2.7
SQUASH. See also ZUCCHINI.														
ACORN														
baked, cubed	1 cup	877	0.34	0.03	1.80	0.40	38.3	0.00	22.1	90.2	1.9	88.2	896	0.4
boiled, mashed	1 cup	632	0.25	0.02	1.30	0.29	27.7	0.00	15.9	63.7	1.4	63.7	644	0.3
raw, cubed	1 cup	476	0.20	0.01	0.98	0.22	23.4	0.00	15.4	46.2	0.9	44.8	486	0.2
raw, whole, 4-inch diam	1 squash	1465	0.60	0.04	3.00	0.66	72.0	0.00	47.4	142.0	3.0	138.0	1496	0.6
BUTTERNUT														
Fresh														
baked, cubed	1 cup	14352	0.15	0.04	2.00	0.25	39.4	0.00	31.0	84.0	1.2	59.5	582	0.3
raw, cubed	1 cup	10920	0.14	0.03	1.70	0.22	37.4	0.00	29.4	67.2	0.9	47.6	493	0.2
Frozen														
boiled, mashed	1 cup	8014	0.12	0.09	1.10	0.17	39.4	0.00	8.4	45.6	1.4	21.6	319	0.3
unprepared	4-lb pkg	86891	1.60	1.10	13.40	2.00	428.0	0.00	112.0	526.0	16.0	254.0	3846	3.1

Food Name	Serving Size	A I.U.	Thi mg	Rib mg	Nia mg	B₆ mg	Fol mcg	B₁₂ mcg	C mg	Calc mg	Iron mg	Mag mg	Pot mg	Zn mg
unprepared	12-oz pkg	16286	0.31	0.20	2.50	0.37	80.2	0.00	21.1	98.6	3.0	47.6	721	0.6
HUBBARD														
baked, cubed	1 cup	12372	0.15	0.10	1.10	0.35	33.2	0.00	19.5	34.9	0.9	45.1	734	0.3
boiled, mashed	1 cup	9452	0.10	0.07	0.79	0.24	22.9	0.00	15.3	23.6	0.7	30.7	505	0.2
raw, cubed	1 cup	6264	0.08	0.05	0.58	0.18	19.0	0.00	12.8	16.2	0.5	22.0	371	0.2
PATTYPAN. See SQUASH, SCALLOP.														
SCALLOP / pattypan squash														
boiled, mashed	1 cup	204	0.12	0.06	1.10	0.20	49.7	0.00	25.9	36.0	0.8	45.6	336	0.6
boiled, sliced	1 cup	153	0.09	0.05	0.83	0.15	37.3	0.00	19.4	27.0	0.6	34.2	252	0.4
raw, sliced	1 cup	143	0.09	0.04	0.78	0.14	39.1	0.00	23.4	24.7	0.5	29.9	237	0.4
SPAGHETTI														
boiled or baked, drained	1 cup	171	0.06	0.03	1.30	0.15	12.4	0.00	5.4	32.5	0.5	17.1	181	0.3
raw, cubed	1 cup	51	0.04	0.02	0.96	0.10	12.1	0.00	2.1	23.2	0.3	12.1	109	0.2
SUMMER. See also ZUCCHINI.														
Canned														
crookneck or straightneck, no salt added, mashed, drained	1 cup	290	0.04	0.07	1.00	0.10	25.0	0.00	6.5	28.8	1.7	31.2	230	0.7
crookneck or straightneck, no salt added, diced, drained	1 cup	254	0.03	0.06	0.88	0.09	21.8	0.00	5.7	25.2	1.5	27.3	202	0.6
crookneck or straightneck, no salt added, sliced, drained	1 cup	261	0.04	0.06	0.90	0.09	22.5	0.00	5.8	25.9	1.5	28.1	207	0.6
Fresh														
all varieties, boiled, drained, sliced	1 cup	517	0.08	0.07	0.92	0.12	36.2	0.00	9.9	48.6	0.7	43.2	346	0.7
all varieties, raw, sliced	1 cup	221	0.07	0.04	0.62	0.12	28.9	0.00	16.7	22.6	0.5	26.0	220	0.3
all varieties, raw, whole	1 large	633	0.21	0.12	1.80	0.35	82.7	0.00	47.8	64.6	1.5	74.3	630	0.8
all varieties, raw, whole	1 medium	384	0.13	0.07	1.10	0.21	50.2	0.00	29.0	39.2	0.9	45.1	382	0.5
all varieties, raw, whole	1 small	231	0.08	0.04	0.65	0.13	30.2	0.00	17.5	23.6	0.5	27.1	230	0.3
crookneck or straightneck, boiled, drained, sliced	1 cup	517	0.09	0.09	0.92	0.17	36.2	0.00	9.9	48.6	0.7	43.2	346	0.7
crookneck or straightneck, boiled, drained, sliced	1/2 cup	258	0.04	0.04	0.46	0.09	18.1	0.00	5.0	24.3	0.3	21.6	173	0.4
crookneck or straightneck, raw, sliced	1 cup	439	0.07	0.06	0.59	0.14	29.8	0.00	10.9	27.3	0.6	27.3	276	0.4
Frozen														
crookneck or straightneck, drained, sliced	1 cup	374	0.07	0.09	0.84	0.19	24.4	0.00	13.1	38.4	0.0	51.8	486	0.7
crookneck or straightneck, sliced, unprepared	1 cup	363	0.05	0.06	0.52	0.11	15.3	0.00	8.3	23.4	0.6	29.9	272	0.5
WINTER														
Fresh														
all varieties, baked, cubed	1 cup	7292	0.17	0.05	1.40	0.15	57.4	0.00	19.7	28.7	0.7	16.4	896	0.5
all varieties, raw, cubed	1 cup	4710	0.11	0.03	0.93	0.10	25.2	0.00	14.3	36.0	0.7	24.4	406	0.2
SQUID / calamari														
mixed species, fried	3 oz	30	0.05	0.39	2.20	0.05	11.9	1.00	3.6	33.1	0.9	32.3	237	1.5
mixed species, raw	3 oz	28	0.02	0.35	1.80	0.05	4.2	1.10	4.0	27.2	0.6	28.1	209	1.3
mixed species, raw, boneless	1 oz	9	0.01	0.12	0.62	0.02	1.4	0.37	1.3	9.1	0.2	9.4	70	0.4
SQUIRREL														
raw	1 oz	0	0.02	0.06	1.10	na	na	na	0.0	0.6	1.3	6.8	86	na
roasted	3 oz	0	0.05	0.25	3.90	0.32	7.7	5.50	0.0	2.5	5.8	23.8	299	1.5
STAR FRUIT / carambola														
raw, cubed	1 cup	675	0.04	0.04	0.56	0.14	19.2	0.00	29.0	5.5	0.4	12.3	223	0.2
raw, sliced	1 cup	532	0.03	0.03	0.44	0.11	15.1	0.00	22.9	4.3	0.3	9.7	176	0.1
raw, whole, large, approx 4.5-inch long	1 fruit	626	0.04	0.03	0.52	0.13	17.8	0.00	26.9	5.1	0.3	11.4	207	0.1
raw, whole, medium, approx 3 5/8 inch long	1 fruit	449	0.03	0.03	0.37	0.09	12.7	0.00	19.3	3.6	0.2	8.2	148	0.1

Food Name	Serving Size	A I.U.	Thi mg	Rib mg	Nia mg	B$_6$ mg	Fol mcg	B$_{12}$ mcg	C mg	Calc mg	Iron mg	Mag mg	Pot mg	Zn mg
raw, whole, small, approx 3-inch long.......	1 fruit	345	0.02	0.02	0.29	0.07	9.8	0.00	14.8	2.8	0.2	6.3	114	<0.1

STRAW MUSHROOM. See MUSHROOM, STRAW.

STRAWBERRY

Canned, in heavy syrup, w/liquid.............	1 cup	66	0.05	0.09	0.14	0.12	71.1	0.00	80.5	33.0	1.2	20.3	218	0.2

Fresh

raw, halved................	1 cup	41	0.03	0.10	0.35	0.09	26.9	0.00	86.2	21.3	0.6	15.2	252	0.2
raw, puréed................	1 cup	63	0.05	0.15	0.53	0.14	41.1	0.00	132.0	32.5	0.9	23.2	385	0.3
raw, sliced................	1 cup	45	0.03	0.11	0.38	0.10	29.4	0.00	94.1	23.2	0.6	16.6	276	0.2
raw, trimmed................	1 pint	96	0.07	0.24	0.82	0.21	63.2	0.00	202.0	50.0	1.4	35.7	593	0.5
raw, whole................	1 cup	39	0.03	0.10	0.33	0.09	25.5	0.00	81.6	20.2	0.6	14.4	239	0.2
raw, whole, extra large, approx 1 5/8 inch diam................	1 berry	7	0.01	0.02	0.06	0.02	4.8	0.00	15.3	3.8	0.1	2.7	44.8	<0.1
raw, whole, large, approx 1 3/8 inch diam................	1 berry	5	0.00	0.01	0.04	0.01	3.2	0.00	10.2	2.5	<0.1	1.8	29.9	<0.1
raw, whole, medium, approx 1 1/4 inch diam................	1 berry	3	0.00	0.01	0.03	0.01	2.1	0.00	6.8	1.7	<0.1	1.2	19.9	<0.1
raw, whole, small, approx 1 inch diam.......	1 berry	2	0.00	0.01	0.02	0.00	1.2	0.00	4.0	0.9	<0.1	0.7	11.6	<0.1

Frozen

sliced, sweetened................	10-oz pkg	68	0.05	0.14	1.10	0.09	42.3	0.00	118.0	31.2	1.7	19.9	278	0.2
sliced, sweetened, thawed................	1 cup	61	0.04	0.13	1.00	0.08	38.0	0.00	106.0	28.1	1.5	17.9	250	0.2
whole, sweetened................	10-oz pkg	77	0.04	0.22	0.83	0.08	10.8	0.00	112.0	31.2	1.3	17.0	278	0.1
whole, sweetened, thawed................	1 cup	69	0.04	0.20	0.75	0.07	9.7	0.00	101.0	28.1	1.2	15.3	250	0.1
whole, unsweetened................	1 med berry	5	0.00	0.00	0.05	0.00	1.8	0.00	4.4	1.7	<0.1	1.2	16	<0.1
whole, unsweetened................	20 oz pkg	255	0.13	0.21	2.60	0.16	95.3	0.00	234.0	90.7	4.3	62.4	839	0.7
whole, unsweetened, thawed.............	1 cup	99	0.05	0.08	1.00	0.06	37.1	0.00	91.1	35.4	1.7	24.3	327	0.3
whole, unsweetened, unthawed..........	1 cup	67	0.03	0.06	0.69	0.04	25.0	0.00	61.4	23.8	1.1	16.4	221	0.2

STRAWBERRY GUAVA. See GUAVA, STRAWBERRY.

STRING BEAN. See BEAN, GREEN.

STRIPED BASS. See BASS, STRIPED.

STRIPED MULLET. See MULLET, STRIPED.

STUFFING MIX

(Brownberry) sage and onion, mix only.......	1 serving	na	na	na	na	na	na	na	na	na	2.6	na	na	na
(Stove Top) chicken flavor.................	1 serving	30	0.11	0.08	1.10	na	22.4	na	0.9	17.6	1.2	na	75	na

STURGEON

mixed species, baked, broiled, grilled, or microwaved..................	3 oz	687	0.07	0.08	8.60	0.20	14.7	2.10	0.0	14.4	0.77	38.3	309	0.5
mixed species, baked, broiled, grilled, or microwaved, flaked.................	1 cup	1099	0.11	0.12	13.70	0.31	23.5	3.40	0.0	23.1	1.2	61.2	495	0.7
mixed species, raw.................	3 oz	595	0.06	0.06	7.10	0.17	12.8	1.90	0.0	11.1	0.6	29.8	241	0.4
mixed species, smoked.................	3 oz	793	0.08	0.08	9.40	0.23	17.0	2.50	0.0	14.4	0.8	40.0	322	0.5
mixed species, smoked.................	1 oz	265	0.03	0.03	3.10	0.08	5.7	0.82	0.0	4.8	0.3	13.3	107	0.2

SUCCOTASH. See under VEGETABLE DISH/ENTRÉE.

SUCKER, WHITE

baked, broiled, grilled, or microwaved.......	3 oz	167	0.01	0.07	1.2	0.20	14.4	2.00	0.0	76.5	1.4	32.3	414	0.8
raw.................	3 oz	145	0.01	0.06	1.0	0.17	12.8	1.70	0.0	59.5	1.1	25.5	323	0.6

SUET

beef, raw.................	4 oz	0	0.01	0.02	0.29	0.03	1.1	0.30	0.0	2.3	0.2	1.1	18	0.3
beef, raw.................	1 oz	0	0	0	0.07	0.01	0.3	0.08	0.0	0.6	<0.1	0.3	5	<0.1

SUGAR

CANE

Brown

granulated.................	1 tsp	0	0.00	0.00	0.00	0.00	<0.1	0.00	0.0	2.7	<0.1	0.9	11	<0.1
packed.................	1 cup	0	0.02	0.02	0.18	0.06	2.2	0.00	0.0	187.0	4.2	63.8	761	0.4

Food Name	Serving Size	A I.U.	Thi mg	Rib mg	Nia mg	B$_6$ mg	Fol mcg	B$_{12}$ mcg	C mg	Calc mg	Iron mg	Mag mg	Pot mg	Zn mg
packed	1 tsp	0	0.00	0.00	0.00	0.00	<0.1	0.00	0.0	3.9	<0.1	1.3	16	<0.1
unpacked	1 cup	0	0.01	0.01	0.12	0.04	1.4	0.00	0.0	123.0	2.8	42.0	502	0.3
unpacked	1 tsp	0	0.00	0.00	0.00	0.00	<0.1	0.00	0.0	2.5	<0.1	0.9	10	<0.1
White														
confectioner's/powdered	1 tsp	0	0.00	0.00	0.00	0.00	0.0	0.00	0.0	<0.1	0.0	0.0	<1	0.0
confectioner's/powdered, unsifted	1 cup	0	0.00	0.00	0.00	0.00	0.0	0.00	0.0	1.2	<0.1	0.0	2	<0.1
confectioner's/powdered, unsifted	1 tbsp	0	0.00	0.00	0.00	0.00	0.0	0.00	0.0	<0.1	<0.1	0.0	<1	0.0
cubes	1 cube	0	0.00	0.00	0.00	0.00	0.0	0.00	0.0	<0.1	0.0	0.0	<1	0.0
granulated	1 cup	0	0.00	0.04	0.00	0.00	0.0	0.00	0.0	2.0	0.1	0.0	4	<0.1
granulated	1 tsp	0	0.00	0.00	0.00	0.00	0.0	0.00	0.0	<0.1	0.0	0.0	<1	0.0
MAPLE														
	1 oz	7	0.00	0.00	0.01	0.00	0.0	0.00	0.0	25.5	0.5	5.4	78	1.7
	1 tsp	<1	0.00	0.00	0.00	0.00	0.0	0.00	0.0	2.7	<0.1	0.6	8	0.2
approx 1.75 x 1.25 x 1/2 inch pieces	1 piece	7	0.00	0.00	0.01	0.00	0.0	0.00	0.0	25.2	0.5	5.3	77	1.7
SUGAR APPLE / sweetsop														
raw, pulp	1 cup	15	0.28	0.28	2.20	0.50	35.0	0.00	90.8	60.0	1.5	52.5	618	0.25
raw, whole, approx 2 7/8 inch diam.	1 fruit	9	0.17	0.17	1.40	0.31	21.7	0.00	56.3	37.2	0.9	32.5	383	0.16
SUMMER SQUASH. See under SQUASH. See also ZUCCHINI.														
SUNCHOKE. See ARTICHOKE, JERUSALEM.														
SUNFISH / calico bass / crappie / pumpkinfish														
baked, broiled, grilled, or microwaved	3oz	49	0.08	0.07	1.20	0.12	14.4	2.00	0.9	87.5	1.3	32.3	382	1.7
raw	3 oz	42	0.07	0.06	1.00	0.10	12.8	1.70	0.9	68.0	1.0	25.5	298	1.3
SUNFLOWER BUTTER														
salted	1 oz	15	0.09	0.08	1.50	0.23	67.3	0.00	0.8	34.6	1.3	105.0	20	1.5
salted	1 tbsp	8	0.05	0.05	0.85	0.13	38.0	0.00	0.4	19.5	0.8	59.0	12	0.9
unsalted	1 oz	15	0.09	0.08	1.50	0.23	67.3	0.00	0.8	34.6	1.3	105.0	20	1.5
unsalted	1 tbsp	8	0.05	0.05	0.85	0.13	38.0	0.00	0.4	19.5	0.8	59.0	12	0.9
SUNFLOWER SEED														
Dried														
kernels	1 cup	72	3.30	0.36	6.50	1.1	327.0	0.00	2.0	167	9.7	510.0	992	7.3
kernels, in shell	1 cup	23	1.10	0.12	2.10	0.35	105.0	0.00	0.6	53.4	3.1	163.0	317	2.3
Oil-roasted														
kernels, salted	1 cup	69	0.43	0.38	5.60	1.1	316.0	0.00	1.9	75.6	9.0	171.0	652	7.0
kernels, salted	1 oz	15	0.09	0.08	1.20	0.23	66.3	0.00	0.4	15.9	1.9	36.0	137	1.5
kernels, shelled, salted	1 cup	69	0.43	0.38	5.60	1.1	316.0	0.00	1.9	75.6	9.0	171.0	652	7.0
kernels, unsalted	1 cup	69	0.43	0.38	5.60	1.1	316.0	0.00	1.9	75.6	9.0	171.0	652	7.0
kernels, unsalted	1 oz	15	0.09	0.08	1.20	0.23	66.3	0.00	0.4	15.9	1.9	36.0	137	1.5
Dry-roasted														
kernels, hulled, unsalted	1 cup	0	0.14	0.32	9.00	1.0	304.0	0.00	1.8	89.6	4.9	165.0	1088	6.8
kernels, salted	1 cup	0	0.14	0.32	9.00	1.0	304.0	0.00	1.8	89.6	4.9	165.0	1088	6.8
kernels, salted	1 oz	0	0.03	0.07	2.00	0.23	67.3	0.00	0.4	19.8	1.1	36.6	241	1.5
kernels, unsalted	1 oz	0	0.03	0.07	2.00	0.23	67.3	0.00	0.4	19.8	1.1	36.6	241	1.5
Toasted														
kernels, salted	1 cup	0	0.44	0.38	5.60	1.1	319.0	0.00	1.9	76.4	9.1	173.0	658	7.1
kernels, salted	1 oz	0	0.09	0.08	1.20	0.23	67.4	0.00	0.4	16.2	1.9	36.6	139	1.5
kernels, unsalted	1 cup	0	0.44	0.38	5.60	1.1	319.0	0.00	1.9	76.4	9.1	173.0	658	7.1
kernels, unsalted	1 oz	0	0.09	0.08	1.20	0.23	67.4	0.00	0.4	16.2	1.9	36.6	139	1.5
SUNFLOWER SEED FLOUR. See under FLOUR.														
SUNFLOWER SEED OIL														
at least 60% linoleic	1 cup	0	0.00	0.00	0.00	0.00	0.0	0.00	0.0	0	0	0.0	0	0.0
at least 60% linoleic	1 tbsp	0	0.00	0.00	0.00	0.00	0.0	0.00	0.0	0	0	0.0	0	0.0
less than 60% linoleic	1 cup	0	0.00	0.00	0.00	0.00	0.0	0.00	0.0	0.41	<0.1	0.4	0	0.0
less than 60% linoleic	1 tbsp	0	0.00	0.00	0.00	0.00	0.0	0.00	0.0	0.03	0	<0.1	0	0.0

Food Name	Serving Size	A I.U.	Thi mg	Rib mg	Nia mg	B6 mg	Fol mcg	B12 mcg	C mg	Calc mg	Iron mg	Mag mg	Pot mg	Zn mg
linoleic, hydrogenated..............	1 cup	0	0.00	0.00	0.00	0.00	0.0	0.00	0.0	0	0	0.0	0	0.0
linoleic, hydrogenated..............	1 tbsp	0	0.00	0.00	0.00	0.00	0.0	0.00	0.0	0	0	0.0	0	0.0

SURIMI. See under CRAB SUBSTITUTE; SCALLOP SUBSTITUTE; SHRIMP SUBSTITUTE.

SURIMI

	Serving Size	A I.U.	Thi mg	Rib mg	Nia mg	B6 mg	Fol mcg	B12 mcg	C mg	Calc mg	Iron mg	Mag mg	Pot mg	Zn mg
....	1 oz	19	0.01	0.01	0.06	0.01	0.5	0.45	0.0	2.6	<0.1	12.2	32	<0.1
....	3 oz	56	0.02	0.02	0.19	0.03	1.4	1.40	0.0	7.7	0.2	36.5	95	0.3

SURINAM CHERRY. See PITANGA.

SWAMP CABBAGE. See CABBAGE, SKUNK.

SWEET CHESTNUT. See CHESTNUT, EUROPEAN.

SWEET POTATO

Fresh

Food Name	Serving Size	A I.U.	Thi mg	Rib mg	Nia mg	B6 mg	Fol mcg	B12 mcg	C mg	Calc mg	Iron mg	Mag mg	Pot mg	Zn mg
baked in skin.........................	1 cup	43644	0.15	0.25	1.20	0.48	45.2	0.00	49.2	56.0	0.9	40.0	696	0.6
baked in skin.........................	1 large	39280	0.13	0.23	1.10	0.43	40.7	0.00	44.3	50.4	0.8	36.0	626	0.5
baked in skin.........................	1 medium	24877	0.08	0.14	0.69	0.28	25.8	0.00	28.0	31.9	0.5	22.8	397	0.3
baked in skin.........................	1 small	13093	0.04	0.08	0.36	0.14	13.6	0.00	14.8	16.8	0.3	12.0	209	0.2
boiled, w/o skin......................	1 medium	25752	0.08	0.21	0.97	0.37	16.8	0.00	25.8	31.7	0.9	15.1	278	0.4
boiled, w/o skin, mashed	1 cup	55937	0.17	0.46	2.10	0.80	36.4	0.00	56.1	68.9	1.8	32.8	604	0.9
raw, approx 5-inch long long...........	1 potato	26082	0.09	0.19	0.88	0.33	17.9	0.00	29.5	28.6	0.8	13.0	265	0.4
raw, cubed	1 cup	26684	0.09	0.20	0.90	0.34	18.4	0.00	30.2	29.3	0.8	13.3	271	0.4

Canned

Food Name	Serving Size	A I.U.	Thi mg	Rib mg	Nia mg	B6 mg	Fol mcg	B12 mcg	C mg	Calc mg	Iron mg	Mag mg	Pot mg	Zn mg
mashed............................	1 cup	38571	0.07	0.23	2.40	0.60	27.3	0.00	13.3	76.5	3.4	61.2	536	0.5
mashed, vacuum pack	1 cup	20357	0.09	0.14	1.90	0.48	42.3	0.00	67.3	56.1	2.3	56.1	796	0.5
pieces, vacuum pack	1 cup	15966	0.07	0.11	1.50	0.38	33.2	0.00	52.8	44.0	1.8	44.0	624	0.4
syrup pack, drained	1 cup	14028	0.05	0.07	0.67	0.12	15.5	0.00	21.2	33.3	1.9	23.5	378	0.3
syrup pack, w/liquid	1 cup	13039	0.06	0.11	1.00	0.12	14.8	0.00	23.9	34.2	1.8	29.6	422	0.4
Frozen, cubes	1 cup	32799	0.12	0.09	1.10	0.31	37.5	0.00	23.4	65.1	0.9	38.7	642	0.6

SWEET POTATO LEAF

Fresh

Food Name	Serving Size	A I.U.	Thi mg	Rib mg	Nia mg	B6 mg	Fol mcg	B12 mcg	C mg	Calc mg	Iron mg	Mag mg	Pot mg	Zn mg
raw, whole, 12.25-inch leaf..............	1 leaf	164	0.03	0.06	0.18	0.03	12.8	0.00	1.8	5.9	0.1	9.8	82.9	<0.1
raw, chopped	1 cup	360	0.06	0.12	0.40	0.07	28.0	0.00	3.9	12.9	0.4	21.4	181	0.1
steamed, chopped	1 cup	586	0.07	0.17	0.64	0.10	31.2	0.00	0.9	15.4	0.4	39.0	305	0.2

SWEETBREAD. See BEEF, PANCREAS; BEEF THYMUS, LAMB, PANCREAS; VEAL, PANCREAS; VEAL, THYMUS.

SWEETENER. See CORN SYRUP; HONEY; SUGAR, CANE; SUGAR, MAPLE; SYRUP.

SWEETSOP. See SUGAR APPLE.

SWISS CHARD / chard

Fresh

Food Name	Serving Size	A I.U.	Thi mg	Rib mg	Nia mg	B6 mg	Fol mcg	B12 mcg	C mg	Calc mg	Iron mg	Mag mg	Pot mg	Zn mg
boiled, drained, chopped	1 cup	5493	0.06	0.15	0.63	0.15	15.1	0.00	31.5	102	4.0	151.0	961	0.6
raw, chopped	1 cup	1188	0.01	0.03	0.14	0.04	5.0	0.00	10.8	18.4	0.7	29.2	136	0.1
raw, whole...........................	1 med leaf	1584	0.02	0.04	0.19	0.05	6.6	0.00	14.4	24.5	0.9	38.9	182	0.2

SWORDFISH

Food Name	Serving Size	A I.U.	Thi mg	Rib mg	Nia mg	B6 mg	Fol mcg	B12 mcg	C mg	Calc mg	Iron mg	Mag mg	Pot mg	Zn mg
baked, broiled, grilled, or microwaved	3 oz	116	0.04	0.10	10.0	0.32	2.0	1.70	0.9	5.1	0.9	28.9	314	1.3
raw	3 oz	101	0.03	0.08	8.20	0.28	1.7	1.50	0.9	3.4	0.7	22.9	245	0.9

SYRUP

MALT

	Serving Size	A I.U.	Thi mg	Rib mg	Nia mg	B6 mg	Fol mcg	B12 mcg	C mg	Calc mg	Iron mg	Mag mg	Pot mg	Zn mg
....	1 cup	0	0.04	1.50	31.20	1.90	46.1	0.00	0.0	234	3.7	276.0	1229	0.5
....	1 tbsp	0	0.00	0.09	1.900	0.12	2.9	0.00	0.0	14.6	0.2	17.3	76.8	<0.1

MAPLE

	Serving Size	A I.U.	Thi mg	Rib mg	Nia mg	B6 mg	Fol mcg	B12 mcg	C mg	Calc mg	Iron mg	Mag mg	Pot mg	Zn mg
....	1 cup	0	0.02	0.03	0.10	0.01	0.0	0.00	0.0	211	3.8	44.1	643	13.1
....	1 tbsp	0	0.00	0.00	0.01	0.00	0.0	0.00	0.0	13.4	0.2	2.8	40.8	0.8

SORGHUM

	Serving Size	A I.U.	Thi mg	Rib mg	Nia mg	B6 mg	Fol mcg	B12 mcg	C mg	Calc mg	Iron mg	Mag mg	Pot mg	Zn mg
....	1 cup	0	0.33	0.51	0.33	2.20	0.0	0.00	0.0	495	12.5	330.0	3300	1.4
....	1 tbsp	0	0.02	0.03	0.02	0.14	0.0	0.00	0.0	31.5	0.8	21.0	210	<0.1

T

Food Name	Serving Size	A I.U.	Thi mg	Rib mg	Nia mg	B_6 mg	Fol mcg	B_{12} mcg	C mg	Calc mg	Iron mg	Mag mg	Pot mg	Zn mg
TACO SHELL														
baked	1 oz	0	0.07	0.02	0.38	0.08	29.8	0.00	0.0	45.4	0.7	29.8	51	0.4
baked, large, 6.5-inch dia.	1 shell	0	0.05	0.01	0.28	0.06	22.1	0.00	0.0	33.6	0.5	22.1	38	0.3
baked, medium, 5-inch diam.	1 shell	0	0.03	0.01	0.18	0.04	14.0	0.00	0.0	21.3	0.3	14.0	24	0.2
baked, mini, 3-inch diam.	1 shell	0	0.01	0.00	0.07	0.02	5.30	0.00	0.0	8.0	0.1	5.3	9	<0.1
baked, no salt added	1 oz	0	0.07	0.02	0.38	0.08	29.8	0.00	0.0	45.4	0.7	29.8	51	0.4
baked, no salt added, medium, 5-inch diam	1 shell	0	0.03	0.01	0.18	0.04	13.7	0.00	0.0	20.8	0.3	13.7	23	0.2
baked, no salt added, mini, 3-inch diam	1 shell	0	0.01	0.00	0.07	0.02	5.30	0.00	0.0	8.0	0.1	5.3	9	<0.1
TAHINI. See SESAME BUTTER.														
TAMARIND / Indian date														
Fresh														
raw, pulp	1 cup	36	0.51	0.18	2.30	0.08	16.8	0.00	4.2	88.8	3.4	110.0	754	0.1
raw, whole, approx 1 x 3 inches	1 fruit	<1	0.01	0.00	0.04	0.00	0.3	0.00	<0.1	1.5	<0.1	1.8	13	0.0
TANGERINE. See also MANDARIN ORANGE.														
Fresh														
raw, sections	1 cup	1794	0.20	0.04	0.31	0.13	39.8	0.00	60.1	27.3	0.2	23.4	306	0.47
raw, whole, large, approx 2.5-inch diam	1 fruit	902	0.10	0.02	0.16	0.07	20.0	0.00	30.2	13.7	0.1	11.8	154	0.23
raw, whole, medium, approx 2 3/8 inch diam	1 fruit	773	0.09	0.02	0.13	0.06	17.1	0.00	25.9	11.8	<0.1	10.1	132	0.2
raw, whole, small, approx 2.25 inch diam	1 fruit	644	0.07	0.02	0.11	0.05	14.3	0.00	21.6	9.8	<0.1	8.4	110	0.2
TANGERINE JUICE														
canned, sweetened	1 cup	1046	0.15	0.05	0.25	0.08	11.5	0.00	54.8	44.8	0.5	19.9	443	<0.1
canned, sweetened	1 fl oz	131	0.02	0.01	0.03	0.01	1.4	0.00	6.8	5.6	<0.1	2.5	55	<0.1
fresh, raw	1 cup	1037	0.15	0.05	0.25	0.10	11.4	0.00	76.6	44.5	0.5	19.8	440	<0.1
fresh, raw	1 fl oz	130	0.02	0.01	0.03	0.01	1.4	0.00	9.6	5.6	<0.1	2.5	55	<0.1
frozen concentrate, diluted	1 cup	1381	0.13	0.05	0.22	0.10	11.1	0.00	58.3	19.3	0.2	19.3	272	<0.1
frozen concentrate, diluted	1 fl oz	172	0.02	0.01	0.03	0.01	1.4	0.00	7.3	2.4	<0.1	2.4	34	<0.1
frozen concentrate, undiluted	6 fl oz	4310	0.39	0.14	0.70	0.31	34.7	0.00	182.0	57.8	0.7	59.9	850	0.2
TANNIER. See YAUTIA.														
TAPIOCA, pearl, dry	1 cup	0	0.01	0.00	0.00	0.01	6.1	0.00	0.0	30.4	2.4	1.5	17	0.2
TARO														
cooked, sliced	1 cup	0	0.14	0.04	0.67	0.44	25.3	0.00	6.6	23.8	0.9	39.6	639	0.4
raw, sliced	1 cup	0	0.10	0.03	0.62	0.29	23.1	0.00	4.7	44.7	0.6	34.3	615	0.2
Tahitian, cooked, sliced	1 cup	2417	0.06	0.27	0.66	0.16	9.9	0.00	52.1	204.0	2.1	69.9	854	0.1
Tahitian, raw, sliced	1 cup	2556	0.08	0.30	1.20	0.14	11.4	0.00	120.0	161.0	1.6	58.8	758	0.1
TARO CHIPS														
	1 oz	0	0.05	0.01	0.15	0.12	5.7	0.00	1.4	17.0	0.3	23.8	214	0.1
	10 chips	0	0.04	0.01	0.12	0.10	4.6	0.00	1.1	13.8	0.3	19.3	174	<0.1
TARO LEAF														
raw, chopped	1 cup	1351	0.06	0.13	0.42	0.04	35.2	0.00	14.6	30.0	0.6	12.6	181	0.1
raw, whole, 11x6.5-inch leaf	1 leaf	483	0.02	0.05	0.15	0.02	12.6	0.00	5.2	10.7	0.2	4.5	65	<0.1
steamed, chopped	1 cup	6145	0.20	0.55	1.80	0.10	70.0	0.00	51.5	125	1.7	29.0	667	0.3
TARO SHOOT														
cooked, sliced	1 cup	71	0.05	0.07	1.10	0.16	3.6	0.00	26.5	19.6	0.6	11.2	482	0.8
raw, whole	1 med shoot	42	0.03	0.04	0.66	0.09	2.7	0.00	17.4	10.0	0.5	6.6	276	0.4
raw, sliced	1/2 cup	22	0.02	0.02	0.34	0.05	1.4	0.00	9.0	5.2	0.3	3.4	143	0.2
TARRAGON														
ground	1 tbsp	202	0.01	0.06	0.43	0.06	13.2	0.00	2.4	54.7	1.6	16.6	145	0.2
ground	1 tsp	67	0.00	0.02	0.14	0.02	4.4	0.00	0.8	18.2	0.5	5.5	48	<0.1

Food Name	Serving Size	A I.U.	Thi mg	Rib mg	Nia mg	B6 mg	Fol mcg	B12 mcg	C mg	Calc mg	Iron mg	Mag mg	Pot mg	Zn mg
TEA														
BLACK														
Brewed														
decaffeinated, prepared w/tap water	6 fl oz	0	0.00	0.03	0.00	0.00	8.9	0.00	0.0	0.0	<0.1	5.3	66	<0.1
decaffeinated, prepared w/tap water	8 fl oz	0	0.00	0.03	0.00	0.00	11.8	0.00	0.0	0.0	<0.1	7.1	88	<0.1
regular, prepared w/distilled water	6 fl oz	0	0.00	0.03	0.00	0.00	9.3	0.00	0.0	0.0	<0.1	1.8	37	<0.1
regular, prepared w/tap water	6 fl oz	0	0.00	0.03	0.00	0.00	9.3	0.00	0.0	0.0	<0.1	5.3	66	<0.1
regular, prepared w/tap water	8 fl oz	0	0.00	0.03	0.00	0.00	12.3	0.00	0.0	0.0	<0.1	7.1	88	<0.1
Instant														
powder, unsweetened	1 tsp	0	0.00	0.01	0.09	0.01	0.7	0.00	0.0	0.4	<0.1	2.5	46	<0.1
powder, unsweetened, prepared	8 fl oz	0	0.00	0.01	0.09	0.01	0.7	0.00	0.0	4.7	<0.1	4.7	47	<0.1
(Crystal Light)														
sugar-free, prepared	8 fl oz	0	na	na	na	na	na	na	0.0	0.2	<0.1	na	17	na
HERBAL/FLAVORED														
Brewed														
chamomile, brewed	6 fl oz	36	0.02	0.01	0.00	0.00	1.1	0.00	0.0	3.6	0.1	1.8	16	<0.1
chamomile, brewed	8 fl oz	47	0.02	0.01	0.00	0.00	1.4	0.00	0.0	4.7	0.2	2.4	21	0.1
herbal, all types, except chamomile	6 fl oz	0	0.02	0.01	0.00	0.00	1.1	0.00	0.0	3.6	0.1	1.8	16	<0.1
herbal, all types, except chamomile	8 fl oz	0	0.02	0.01	0.00	0.00	1.4	0.00	0.0	4.7	0.2	2.4	21	0.1
TEASEED OIL														
....	1 cup	0	0.00	0.00	0.00	0.00	0.0	0.00	0.0	0.0	0.0	0.0	0	0.0
....	1 tbsp	0	0.00	0.00	0.00	0.00	0.0	0.00	0.0	0.0	0.0	0.0	0	0.0
TEMPEH	1 cup	0	0.13	0.59	4.40	0.36	39.7	0.13	0.0	184.0	4.5	134.0	684	1.9
TENDERGREEN. See MUSTARD SPINACH.														
TEQUILA SUNRISE. See under COCKTAIL.														
THYME, FRESH														
fresh	1 tsp	38	0.00	0.00	0.02	0.00	0.4	0.00	1.3	3.2	0.1	1.3	5	<0.1
fresh	1/2 tsp	19	0.00	0.00	0.01	0.00	0.2	0.00	0.6	1.6	<0.1	0.6	2	<0.1
ground	1 tbsp	163	0.02	0.02	0.21	0.05	11.8	0.00	2.1	81.2	5.3	9.5	35	0.3
ground	1 tsp	53	0.01	0.01	0.07	0.02	3.8	0.00	0.7	26.5	1.7	3.1	11	<0.1
TILEFISH														
baked, broiled, grilled, or microwaved	3 oz	59	0.12	0.16	3.00	0.26	14.7	2.10	0.0	22.1	0.3	28.1	435	0.5
raw	3 oz	51	0.10	0.14	2.50	0.22	12.8	1.90	0.0	22.1	0.2	23.8	368	0.3
TOFU														
fried	1 oz	0	0.05	0.01	0.03	0.03	7.6	0.00	0.0	105.0	1.4	17.0	41	0.6
fuyu, salted and fermented	1 block	18	0.02	0.01	0.04	0.01	3.2	0.00	<0.1	5.1	0.2	5.7	8	0.2
fuyu, salted and fermented, prepared														
w/calcium sulfate	1 block	18	0.02	0.01	0.04	0.01	3.2	0.00	<0.1	135.0	0.2	6.4	8	0.2
okara	1 cup	0	0.02	0.02	0.12	0.14	32.2	0.00	0.0	97.6	1.6	31.7	260	0.7
EXTRA FIRM														
w/nigari	1/5 block	9	0.04	0.04	0.30	0.04	23.7	0.00	0.5	93.7	1.6	64.6	121	1.0
(Mori-Nu)														
silken	1 slice	0	0.07	0.03	0.20	0.01	na	0.00	0.0	26.0	1.0	22.7	129	0.5
silken, light	1 slice	0	0.03	0.02	0.09	0.00	na	0.00	0.0	36.1	0.7	8.4	48	0.2
FIRM														
nigan	1/2 cup	209	0.20	0.13	0.48	0.12	36.9	0.00	0.3	861.0	13.2	73.1	299	2.0
prepared w/calcium sulfate	1/2 cup	10	0.12	0.13	0.01	0.08	41.6	0.00	0.3	204.0	1.8	58.0	222	1.3
(Mori-Nu)														
silken	1 slice	0	0.09	0.03	0.21	0.01	na	0.00	0.0	26.9	0.9	22.7	163	0.5
HARD, w/nigari	1/4 block	na	0.05	0.09	0.78	0.05	26.8	0.00	0.4	421.0	3.4	64.7	178	2.0
REGULAR, prepared w/calcium sulfate	1/2 cup	105	0.10	0.06	0.24	0.06	18.6	0.00	0.1	434.0	6.6	37.2	150	<1.0
SOFT														
nigan	1 cubic-inch	1.2	0.01	0.01	0.09	0.01	7.7	0.00	<0.1	19.5	0.2	4.8	21	0.1
nigan, 1/2-inch pieces	1 cup	17	0.12	0.09	1.30	0.13	109.0	0.00	0.5	275.0	2.8	67.0	298	1.6

Food Name	Serving Size	A I.U.	Thi mg	Rib mg	Nia mg	B6 mg	Fol mcg	B12 mcg	C mg	Calc mg	Iron mg	Mag mg	Pot mg	Zn mg
(Mori-Nu)														
silken..............................	1 slice	0	0.08	0.03	0.25	0.01	na	0.00	0.0	26.0	0.7	24.4	151	0.4
TOMATILLO / ground husk tomato														
raw..................................	1 medium	39	0.02	0.01	0.63	0.02	2.4	0.00	4.0	2.4	0.2	6.8	91.1	0.08
raw, chopped or diced..............	1/2 cup	75	0.03	0.02	1.20	0.04	4.6	0.00	7.7	4.6	0.4	13.2	177	0.14
TOMATO														
Canned														
red, stewed.....................	1 cup	1380	0.12	0.09	1.80	0.04	13.8	0.00	29.1	84.2	1.9	30.6	607	0.4
red, w/green chilies..............	1 cup	940	0.08	0.05	1.50	0.25	21.9	0.00	14.9	48.2	0.6	26.5	258	0.3
red, wedges, in tomato juice.............	1 cup	1509	0.15	0.07	1.80	0.30	26.4	0.00	38.6	67.9	1.2	28.7	655	0.4
red, whole.....................	1 cup	1428	0.11	0.07	1.80	0.22	18.7	0.00	34.1	72.0	1.3	28.8	530	0.4
red, whole.....................	1 medium	660	0.05	0.03	0.82	0.10	8.70	0.00	15.8	33.3	0.6	13.3	245	0.2
red, whole, no salt added..............	1 cup	1428	0.11	0.07	1.80	0.22	18.7	0.00	34.1	72.0	1.3	28.8	545	0.4
red, whole, no salt added..............	1 medium	660	0.05	0.03	0.82	0.10	8.70	0.00	15.8	33.3	0.6	13.3	252	0.2
Fresh, raw, ripe														
cherry, red, ripe, June–October	1 cup	928	0.09	0.07	0.94	0.12	22.4	0.00	38.7	7.5	0.7	16.0	331	0.1
cherry, red, ripe, June–October, medium	1 tomato	106	0.01	0.01	0.11	0.01	2.50	0.00	4.4	0.9	<0.1	1.9	38	<0.1
cherry, red, ripe, November–May	1 cup	928	0.09	0.07	0.94	0.12	22.4	0.00	14.9	7.5	0.7	16.4	331	0.1
cherry, red, ripe, November–May, medium	1 tomato	106	0.01	0.01	0.11	0.01	2.50	0.00	1.7	0.9	<0.1	1.9	38	<0.1
cherry, red, ripe, year-round average	1 cup	928	0.09	0.07	0.94	0.12	22.4	0.00	28.5	7.5	0.7	16.4	331	0.1
cherry, red, ripe, year-round average, medium	1 tomato	106	0.01	0.01	0.11	0.01	2.5	0.00	3.2	0.9	<0.1	1.9	38	<0.1
green, raw, chopped.....................	1 cup	1156	0.11	0.07	0.90	0.15	15.8	0.00	42.1	23.4	0.9	18.0	367	0.1
green, raw, whole, large	1 tomato	1168	0.11	0.07	0.91	0.15	16.0	0.00	42.6	23.7	0.9	18.2	371	0.1
green, raw, whole, medium..............	1 tomato	790	0.07	0.05	0.61	0.10	10.8	0.00	28.8	16.0	0.6	12.3	251	<0.1
green, raw, whole, small	1 tomato	584	0.06	0.04	0.46	0.07	8.0	0.00	21.3	11.8	0.5	9.1	186	<0.1
orange, raw, chopped....................	1 cup	2364	0.07	0.05	0.94	0.10	45.8	0.00	25.3	7.9	0.7	12.6	335	0.2
orange, raw, whole, medium.............	1 tomato	1661	0.05	0.04	0.66	0.07	32.2	0.00	17.8	5.5	0.5	8.9	235	0.2
plum, red, ripe, raw, June–October, medium	1 tomato	386	0.04	0.03	0.39	0.05	9.3	0.00	16.1	3.1	0.3	6.8	138	<0.1
plum, red, ripe, raw, November–May, medium	1 tomato	386	0.04	0.03	0.39	0.05	9.3	0.00	6.2	3.1	0.3	6.8	138	<0.1
plum, red, ripe, raw, year-round average, whole, medium	1 tomato	386	0.04	0.03	0.39	0.05	9.3	0.00	11.8	3.1	0.3	6.8	138	<0.1
red, ripe, boiled........................	1 cup	1783	0.17	0.14	1.80	0.23	31.2	0.00	54.7	14.4	1.3	33.6	670	0.3
red, ripe, boiled, medium	2 tomatoes	1828	0.17	0.14	1.80	0.23	32.0	0.00	56.1	14.8	1.4	34.4	686	0.3
red, ripe, raw, June–October, medium	1 tomato	766	0.07	0.06	0.77	0.10	18.4	0.00	32.0	6.2	0.6	13.5	273	0.1
red, ripe, raw, June–October, 1/2-inch slices, medium....................	1 slice	168	0.02	0.01	0.17	0.02	4.0	0.00	7.0	1.4	0.1	3.0	60	<0.1
red, ripe, raw, June–October, 1/4-inch slices, medium....................	1 slice	125	0.01	0.01	0.13	0.02	3.0	0.00	5.2	1.0	<0.1	2.2	44	<0.1
red, ripe, raw, June–October, quartered, medium	1 wedge	193	0.02	0.02	0.20	0.03	4.7	0.00	8.1	1.6	0.1	3.4	69	<0.1
red, ripe, raw, June–October, whole, 3 inch diam........................	1 tomato	1134	0.11	0.09	1.10	0.15	27.3	0.00	47.3	9.1	0.8	20.0	404	0.2
red, ripe, raw, June–October, whole, 2-3/5 inch diam	1 tomato	766	0.07	0.06	0.77	0.10	18.4	0.00	32.0	6.2	0.6	13.5	273	0.1
red, ripe, raw, June–October, whole, 2-2/5 inch diam	1 tomato	567	0.05	0.04	0.57	0.07	13.7	0.00	23.7	4.5	0.4	10.0	202	<0.1
red, ripe, raw, November–May, chopped or sliced...........................	1 cup	1121	0.11	0.09	1.10	0.14	27.0	0.00	18.0	9.0	0.8	19.8	400	0.2
red, ripe, raw, November–May, medium, quartered....................	1 wedge	193	0.02	0.02	0.20	0.03	4.7	0.00	3.1	1.6	0.1	3.4	69	<0.1

Food Name	Serving Size	A I.U.	Thi mg	Rib mg	Nia mg	B$_6$ mg	Fol mcg	B$_{12}$ mcg	C mg	Calc mg	Iron mg	Mag mg	Pot mg	Zn mg
red, ripe, raw, November–May, medium, 1/2-inch slices	1 slice	168	0.02	0.01	0.17	0.02	4.0	0.00	2.7	1.4	0.1	3.0	60	<0.1
red, ripe, raw, November–May, medium, 1/4-inch slices	1 slice	125	0.01	0.01	0.13	0.02	3.0	0.00	2.0	1.0	<0.1	2.2	44	<0.1
red, ripe, raw, November–May, whole, 3 inch diam.	1 large	1134	0.11	0.09	1.10	0.15	27.3	0.00	18.2	9.1	0.8	20.0	404	0.2
red, ripe, raw, November–May, whole, 2 3/5 inch diam.	1 tomato	766	0.07	0.06	0.77	0.10	18.4	0.00	12.3	6.2	0.6	13.5	273	0.1
red, ripe, stewed	1 cup	673	0.11	0.08	1.10	0.09	11.1	0.00	18.4	26.3	1.1	15.2	249	0.2
year round average, chopped or sliced.	1 cup	1121	0.11	0.09	1.10	0.14	27.0	0.00	34.4	9.0	0.8	19.8	400	0.2
year round average, medium, 1/2-inch slices	1 slice	168	0.02	0.01	0.17	0.02	4.0	0.00	5.2	1.4	0.1	3.0	60	<0.1
year round average, medium, 1/4-inch slices	1 med slice	125	0.01	0.01	0.13	0.02	3.0	0.00	3.8	1.0	<0.1	2.2	44	<0.1
year round average, medium, quartered	1 wedge	193	0.02	0.02	0.20	0.03	4.7	0.00	5.9	1.6	0.1	3.4	69	<0.1
year round average, whole, 2-2/5-inch diam.	1 tomato	567	0.05	0.04	0.57	0.07	13.7	0.00	17.4	4.5	0.4	10.0	202	<0.1
year round average, whole, 2-3/5-inch diam.	1 tomato	766	0.07	0.06	0.77	0.10	18.4	0.00	23.5	6.2	0.6	13.5	273	0.1
year round average, whole, 3-inch diam.....	1 tomato	1134	0.11	0.09	1.10	0.15	27.3	0.00	34.8	9.1	0.8	20.0	404	0.2
yellow, raw, chopped.	1 cup	0	0.06	0.07	1.60	0.08	41.7	0.00	12.5	15.3	0.7	16.7	359	0.4
yellow, raw, whole, medium	1 tomato	0	0.09	0.10	2.50	0.12	63.6	0.00	19.1	23.3	1.0	25.4	547	0.6
Sun-dried														
	1 cup	472	0.28	0.26	4.90	0.18	36.7	0.00	21.2	59.4	4.9	105.0	1851	1.1
	1 piece	18	0.01	0.01	0.18	0.01	1.4	0.00	0.8	2.2	0.2	3.9	69	<0.1
packed in oil, drained	1 cup	1415	0.21	0.42	4.00	0.35	25.3	0.00	112.0	51.7	2.9	89.1	1722	0.9
packed in oil, drained	1 piece	39	0.01	0.01	0.11	0.01	0.7	0.00	3.1	1.4	<0.1	2.4	47	<0.1
TOMATO JUICE.														
canned	1 cup	1351	0.11	0.08	1.60	0.27	48.4	0.00	44.5	21.9	1.4	26.7	535	0.3
canned	6 fl oz	1012	0.09	0.06	1.20	0.20	36.2	0.00	33.3	16.4	1.1	20.0	400	0.3
canned, no salt added	1 cup	1351	0.11	0.08	1.60	0.27	48.4	0.00	44.5	21.9	1.4	26.7	535	0.3
canned, no salt added	6 fl oz	1012	0.09	0.06	1.20	0.20	36.2	0.00	33.3	16.4	1.1	20.0	400	0.3
canned, no salt added	1 fl oz	169	0.01	0.01	0.20	0.03	6.0	0.00	5.6	2.7	0.2	3.3	67	<0.1
TOMATO PASTE														
	6-oz can	4157	0.26	0.32	5.50	0.65	38.1	0.00	72.1	59.5	3.3	86.7	1593	1.4
	1/2 cup	3203	0.20	0.25	4.20	0.50	29.3	0.00	55.5	45.9	2.5	66.8	1227	1.0
no salt added	1 cup	6406	0.41	0.50	8.40	0.00	58.7	0.00	111.0	91.7	5.1	134.0	2455	2.1
no salt added	6-oz can	4157	0.26	0.32	5.50	0.65	38.1	0.00	72.1	59.5	3.3	86.7	1593	1.4
no salt added	1 tbsp	401	0.03	0.03	0.53	0.06	3.7	0.00	7.0	5.7	0.3	8.4	154	0.1
TOMATO PURÉE														
	1 cup	3188	0.18	0.14	4.30	0.38	27.5	0.00	26.0	42.5	3.1	60.0	1065	0.6
no salt added	1 cup	3188	0.18	0.14	4.30	0.38	27.5	0.00	26.0	42.5	3.1	60.0	1065	0.6
TOMATOSEED OIL														
	1 cup	0	0.00	0.00	0.00	0.00	0.0	0.00	0.0	0.0	0.0	0.0	0	0.0
	1 tbsp	0	0.00	0.00	0.00	0.00	0.0	0.00	0.0	0.0	0.0	0.0	0	0.0
TONIC WATER. See under SOFT DRINKS AND MIXERS.														
TORSK. See CUSK.														
TORTILLA														
corn, no salt added, ready to bake or fry	1 oz	0	0.03	0.02	0.42	0.06	32.3	0.00	0.0	49.6	0.4	18.4	44	0.3
corn, no salt added, ready-to-bake or fry, 6-inch diam	1 tortilla	0	0.03	0.02	0.39	0.06	29.6	0.00	0.0	45.5	0.4	16.9	40	0.2
corn, ready-to-bake or fry...............	1 oz	0	0.03	0.02	0.42	0.06	32.3	0.00	0.0	49.6	0.4	18.4	44	0.3
flour, ready to bake or fry, 12-inch diam	1 tortilla	0	0.62	0.34	4.20	0.06	144.0	0.00	0.0	45.6	3.9	30.4	153	0.8
flour, ready to bake or fry, 10-inch diam	1 tortilla	0	0.38	0.21	2.60	0.04	88.6	0.00	0.0	90.0	2.4	18.7	94	0.5

Food Name	Serving Size	A I.U.	Thi mg	Rib mg	Nia mg	B_6 mg	Fol mcg	B_{12} mcg	C mg	Calc mg	Iron mg	Mag mg	Pot mg	Zn mg
flour, ready to bake or fry, 7–8-inch diam	1 tortilla	0	0.26	0.14	1.80	0.03	60.3	0.00	0.0	19.1	1.6	12.7	64	0.4
corn, ready-to-bake or fry, 6-inch diam	1 tortilla	0	0.03	0.02	0.39	0.06	29.6	0.00	0.0	45.5	0.4	16.9	40	0.2
flour, ready to bake or fry	1 oz	0	0.15	0.08	1.00	0.01	34.9	0.00	0.0	35.4	0.9	7.4	37	0.2
TOWELGOURD. See GOURD, DISHCLOTH.														
TREE FERN														
cooked, chopped	1/2 cup	142	0.00	0.21	2.50	0.13	10.7	0.00	21.3	5.7	0.1	3.5	4	0.2
cooked, whole, 6.5-inch long	1 frond	62	0.00	0.09	1.10	0.06	4.7	0.00	9.3	2.5	<0.1	1.6	2	0.1
TREE MUSHROOM. See MUSHROOM, OYSTER.														
TRITICALE	1 cup	0	0.80	0.26	2.70	0.27	140.0	0.00	0.0	71.0	4.9	250.0	637	6.6
TRITICALE FLOUR. See under FLOUR.														
TROUT														
MIXED SPECIES														
baked, broiled, grilled, or microwaved	3 oz	54	0.36	0.36	4.90	0.20	12.8	6.40	0.4	46.8	1.6	23.8	394	0.7
raw	3 oz	49	0.30	0.28	3.80	0.17	11.3	6.60	0.4	36.5	1.3	18.7	307	0.6
RAINBOW														
farmed, baked, broiled, grilled, or microwaved	3 oz	244	0.20	0.07	7.50	0.34	20.4	4.20	2.8	73.1	0.3	27.2	375	0.4
farmed, raw	3 oz	236	0.17	0.06	7.00	0.53	9.3	3.20	2.5	57.0	0.2	27.2	383	0.4
wild, baked, broiled, grilled, or microwaved	3 oz	43	0.13	0.08	4.90	0.29	16.1	5.40	1.7	73.1	0.3	26.4	381	0.4
wild, raw	3 oz	53	0.11	0.09	4.60	0.34	10.2	3.80	2.0	57.0	0.6	26.4	409	0.9
SEA														
mixed species, baked, broiled, grilled, or microwaved	3 oz	98	0.06	0.18	2.50	0.39	5.1	2.90	0.0	18.7	0.3	34.0	371	0.5
mixed species, raw	3 oz	85	0.05	0.14	2.00	0.34	4.3	2.50	0.0	14.4	0.2	26.4	290	0.4
TUNA														
Canned														
in oil, drained	3 oz	68	0.01	0.07	9.90	0.36	3.9	1.90	0.0	3.4	0.6	28.9	283	0.4
in water, drained	3 oz	48	0.03	0.06	11.3	0.30	3.4	2.50	0.0	9.3	1.3	22.9	201	0.7
in water, no salt added, drained	3 oz	48	0.03	0.06	11.3	0.30	3.4	2.50	0.0	9.3	1.3	22.9	201	0.7
BLUEFIN														
Fresh														
baked, broiled, grilled, or microwaved	3 oz	2142	0.24	0.26	9.00	0.45	1.9	9.20	0.0	8.5	1.1	54.4	275	0.7
raw	3 oz	1856	0.20	0.21	7.40	0.39	1.6	8.00	0.0	6.8	0.9	42.5	214	0.5
LIGHT														
Canned														
in oil, drained	3 oz	66	0.03	0.10	10.5	0.09	4.5	1.90	0.0	11.1	1.2	26.4	176	0.8
in oil, no salt added, drained	3 oz	66	0.03	0.10	10.5	0.09	4.5	1.90	0.0	11.1	1.2	26.4	176	0.8
SKIPJACK / aku / katsuo / oceanic bonito														
baked, broiled, grilled, or microwaved	3 oz	51	0.03	0.10	15.9	0.83	8.5	1.90	0.9	31.4	1.4	37.4	444	0.9
raw	3 oz	44	0.03	0.09	13.1	0.72	7.7	1.60	0.9	24.6	1.1	28.9	346	0.7
WHITE														
Canned														
in oil, no salt added, drained	3 oz	68	0.01	0.07	9.90	0.36	3.9	1.90	0.0	3.4	0.6	28.9	283	0.4
in water, drained	3 oz	16	0.01	0.04	4.90	0.18	1.7	0.99	0.0	11.9	0.8	28.1	201	0.4
in water, no salt added, drained	3 oz	16	0.01	0.04	4.90	0.18	1.7	0.99	0.0	11.9	0.8	28.1	201	0.4
YELLOWFIN / ahi														
Fresh														
baked, broiled, grilled, or microwaved	3 oz	58	0.43	0.05	10.10	0.88	1.7	0.51	0.0	17.9	0.8	54.4	484	0.6
raw	3 oz	50	0.37	0.04	8.30	0.77	1.6	0.44	0.0	13.6	0.6	42.5	377	0.4
raw boneless	1 oz	17	0.12	0.01	2.80	0.26	0.5	0.15	0.3	4.5	0.2	14.2	126	0.2
TURBOT, EUROPEAN														
baked, broiled, grilled, or microwaved	3 oz	34	0.07	0.08	2.30	0.21	7.7	2.20	1.4	19.6	0.4	55.3	259	0.2

Food Name	Serving Size	A I.U.	Thi mg	Rib mg	Nia mg	B_6 mg	Fol mcg	B_{12} mcg	C mg	Calc mg	Iron mg	Mag mg	Pot mg	Zn mg
raw	3 oz	29	0.06	0.07	1.90	0.18	6.8	1.90	1.4	15.3	0.3	43.4	202	0.2
TURKEY														
BACK														
Fresh														
all classes, meat and skin, raw	4 oz	11	0.07	0.21	2.07	0.32	10.3	0.41	0.0	19.4	1.9	20.6	270	3.0
all classes, meat and skin, roasted	4 oz	0	0.06	0.26	3.93	0.34	9.2	0.39	0.0	37.7	2.5	25.1	297	4.5
all classes, meat and skin, roasted, chopped or diced	1 cup	0	0.08	0.31	4.8	0.42	11.2	0.48	0	46.2	3.1	30.8	364	5.5
fryer/roaster, meat and skin, raw	4 oz	7	0.05	0.18	3.75	0.37	11.4	0.44	0.0	21.7	1.6	21.7	233	2.2
fryer/roaster, meat and skin, roasted	4 oz	0	0.04	0.22	4.04	0.35	10.3	0.41	0.0	41.1	2.1	22.9	237	3.8
fryer/roaster, meat only, raw	4 oz	0	0.05	0.20	4.11	0.43	12.6	0.46	0.0	21.7	1.7	23.9	254	2.3
fryer/roaster, meat only, roasted	4 oz	0	0.06	0.23	4.39	0.46	11.4	0.47	0.0	41.1	2.1	25.2	248	4.4
young hen, meat and skin, raw	4 oz	9	0.07	0.20	2.72	0.31	10.3	0.38	0.0	20.6	2.0	20.6	264	2.0
young hen, meat and skin, roasted	4 oz	0	0.06	0.24	4.06	0.33	9.2	0.38	0.0	35.4	2.5	26.3	301	4.4
young tom, meat and skin, raw	4 oz	13	0.08	0.22	3.31	0.35	10.3	0.41	0.0	19.4	1.7	20.6	280	3.3
young tom, meat and skin, roasted	4 oz	0	0.06	0.27	3.82	0.36	9.1	0.39	0.0	39.9	2.5	25.1	302	4.6
BREAST														
Fresh														
all classes, meat and skin, raw	4 oz	7	0.06	0.13	5.95	0.55	7.9	0.48	0.0	14.8	1.3	27.5	314	1.8
all classes, meat and skin, roasted	4 oz	0	0.06	0.15	7.28	0.54	6.9	0.41	0.0	23.9	1.6	30.8	329	2.3
fryer/roaster, meat and skin, raw	4 oz	0	0.05	0.13	7.15	0.67	9.1	0.53	0.0	11.4	1.3	31.9	335	1.4
fryer/roaster, meat and skin, roasted	4 oz	0	0.05	0.15	8.55	0.63	6.9	0.45	0.0	13.7	1.8	33.1	334	1.9
fryer/roaster, meat and skin, pre-basted, roasted	4 oz	0	0.06	0.15	10.36	0.37	5.7	0.37	0.0	10.3	0.8	23.9	283	1.7
young hen, meat and skin, raw	4 oz	2	0.06	0.14	5.61	0.55	8.0	0.47	0.0	14.9	1.6	27.5	304	1.8
young hen, meat and skin, roasted	4 oz	0	0.06	0.15	7.63	0.53	6.9	0.39	0.0	25.1	1.5	29.7	330	2.2
young tom, meat and skin, raw	4 oz	8	0.07	0.12	4.43	0.55	7.9	0.48	0.0	14.9	1.2	27.4	322	1.8
young tom, meat and skin, roasted	4 oz	0	0.07	1.15	6.91	0.56	6.9	0.41	0.0	23.9	1.6	30.9	330	2.4
DARK MEAT														
Fresh														
all classes, meat and skin, raw	4 oz	6	0.08	0.23	3.23	0.37	11.4	0.44	0.0	19.4	1.9	22.9	298	3.4
all classes, meat and skin, roasted	4 oz	0	0.07	0.26	4.07	0.36	10.3	0.41	0.0	37.7	2.6	26.3	313	4.7
all classes, meat and skin, roasted, chopped or diced	1 cup	0	0.08	0.33	4.90	0.45	12.6	0.50	0.0	46.2	3.2	32.2	384	5.8
all classes, meat only, raw	4 oz	0	0.09	0.25	3.55	0.41	12.6	0.46	0.0	19.4	1.9	25.1	327	3.7
all classes, meat only, roasted	4 oz	0	0.08	0.29	4.14	0.41	10.3	0.43	0.0	36.5	2.6	27.4	332	5.1
all classes, meat only, roasted, chopped or diced	1 cup	0	0.09	0.35	5.10	0.50	12.6	0.52	0.0	44.8	3.3	33.6	406	6.2
fryer/roaster, meat and skin, raw	4 oz	3	0.05	0.21	3.25	0.39	11.4	0.45	0.0	15.9	1.8	22.9	265	2.9
fryer/roaster, meat and skin, roasted	4 oz	0	0.05	0.27	3.88	0.38	10.2	0.42	0.0	30.8	2.7	26.3	271	4.4
fryer/roaster, meat only, raw	4 oz	0	0.06	0.23	3.36	0.42	12.6	0.47	0.0	14.9	1.9	25.1	279	3.0
fryer/roaster, meat only, roasted	4 oz	0	0.06	0.29	4.02	0.44	11.4	0.44	0.0	29.8	2.8	27.4	281	4.8
fryer/roaster, meat only, roasted, chopped or diced	1 cup	0	0.07	0.35	4.90	0.53	14.0	0.55	0.0	36.4	3.4	33.6	344	5.8
young hen, meat and skin, raw	4 oz	5	0.08	0.23	3.01	0.37	11.4	0.44	0.0	20.6	2.1	22.9	296	3.2
young hen, meat and skin, roasted	4 oz	0	0.06	0.26	4.20	0.36	9.2	0.39	0.0	35.5	2.6	26.3	316	4.6
young hen, meat only, raw	4 oz	0	0.08	0.25	3.25	0.41	12.6	0.46	0.0	20.6	2.2	26.3	328	3.5
young hen, meat only, roasted	4 oz	0	0.07	0.27	4.30	0.39	10.3	0.42	0.0	34.3	2.7	28.6	334	5.0
young hen, meat only, roasted, chopped or diced	1 cup	0	0.08	0.33	5.30	0.48	12.6	0.50	0.0	42.0	3.3	35.0	409	6.1
young tom, meat and skin, raw	4 oz	7	0.09	0.23	3.53	0.38	11.4	0.44	0.0	19.4	1.8	22.9	303	3.5
young tom, meat and skin, roasted	4 oz	0	0.07	0.28	3.88	0.38	10.3	0.42	0.0	39.9	2.6	26.3	315	4.9
young tom, meat only, raw	4 oz	0	0.10	0.26	3.78	0.41	12.5	0.46	0.0	19.4	1.9	23.9	332	3.9
young tom, meat only, roasted	4 oz	0	0.08	0.29	4.06	0.42	11.4	0.43	0.0	39.9	2.7	26.3	335	5.2

Food Name	Serving Size	A I.U.	Thi mg	Rib mg	Nia mg	B$_6$ mg	Fol mcg	B$_{12}$ mcg	C mg	Calc mg	Iron mg	Mag mg	Pot mg	Zn mg
GIBLETS														
Fresh														
all classes, raw	1 oz	2189	0.02	0.32	1.79	0.12	97.7	8.04	1.1	2.3	1.9	5.4	90	0.7
all classes, w/fat, simmered	1 oz	1726	0.03	0.26	1.29	0.09	98.6	6.86	0.5	3.7	1.9	4.9	57	1.1
all classes, w/fat, simmered, chopped or diced	1 cup	8752	0.07	1.03	6.50	0.48	500.0	34.80	2.5	18.9	9.7	24.6	290	5.3
GIZZARD														
Fresh														
all classes, raw	1 medium	245	0.06	0.26	3.90	0.16	58.8	2.40	3.6	10.2	4.3	19.2	388	2.3
all classes, raw	1 oz	62	0.00	0.08	0.98	0.04	14.7	0.61	0.9	2.6	1.1	4.9	98	0.6
all classes, simmered	1 oz	53	0.00	0.07	0.86	0.07	14.9	0.57	0.4	4.3	1.6	5.4	60	1.2
all classes, simmered, chopped or diced	1 cup	268	0.05	0.47•	4.50	0.17	75.4	2.80	2.3	21.8	7.9	27.6	306	6.0
GROUND														
Fresh														
all classes, cooked	4-oz patty	0	0.04	0.14	4.00	0.32	5.7	0.27	0.00	20.5	1.6	19.7	221	2.3
all classes, raw	4-oz patty	6	0.06	0.15	4.00	0.40	8.0	0.39	0.0	14.8	1.4	21.7	266	2.2
HEART														
Fresh														
all classes, raw	1 medium	9	0.06	0.32	1.20	0.10	20.9	2.10	0.9	2.6	1.4	6.4	80	1.0
all classes, simmered, chopped or diced	1 cup	41	0.10	1.30	4.70	0.46	115.0	10.40	2.5	18.9	10.0	31.9	265	7.6
LEG														
Fresh														
all classes, meat and skin, raw	4 oz	3	0.09	0.24	3.37	0.39	11.4	0.45	0.0	19.5	1.9	24.1	312	3.5
all classes, meat and skin, roasted	4 oz	0	0.06	0.27	4.02	0.37	10.3	0.42	0.0	36.5	2.6	26.2	320	4.8
fryer/roaster, meat and skin, raw	4 oz	2	0.06	0.23	3.00	0.40	11.4	0.46	0.0	12.6	1.9	24.0	282	3.3
fryer/roaster, meat and skin, roasted	4 oz	0	0.07	0.29	3.76	0.39	10.3	0.42	0.0	26.3	2.9	27.4	287	4.7
fryer/roaster, meat only, raw	4 oz	0	0.06	0.25	3.07	0.42	12.5	0.47	0.0	11.4	1.9	25.2	290	3.4
fryer/roaster, meat only, roasted	4 oz	0	0.07	0.30	3.75	0.43	11.4	0.43	0.0	25.2	30.4	28.6	295	4.8
young hen, meat and skin, raw	4 oz	2	0.09	0.24	3.05	0.39	11.4	0.45	0.0	20.6	2.2	25.1	312	3.4
young hen, meat and skin, roasted	4 oz	0	0.06	0.26	4.18	0.37	10.3	0.40	0.0	34.3	2.6	27.4	322	4.8
LIGHT MEAT														
Fresh														
all classes, meat and skin, raw	4 oz	7	0.06	0.13	5.84	0.55	7.9	0.48	0.0	14.9	1.4	27.4	310	1.8
all classes, meat and skin, roasted	4 oz	0	0.07	0.15	7.23	0.54	6.9	0.40	0.0	24.0	1.6	29.7	326	2.4
all classes, meat and skin, roasted, chopped or diced	1 cup	0	0.08	0.19	8.80	0.66	8.4	0.49	0.0	29.4	2.0	36.4	399	2.9
all classes, meat only, raw	4 oz	0	0.08	0.14	6.70	0.64	9.1	0.52	0.0	13.7	1.4	30.9	349	1.8
all classes, meat only, roasted	4 oz	0	0.07	0.15	7.81	0.62	6.8	0.42	0.0	21.7	1.6	32.0	349	2.3
all classes, meat only, roasted, chopped or diced	1 cup	0	0.09	0.18	9.60	0.76	8.4	0.52	0.0	26.6	1.9	39.2	427	2.9
fryer/roaster, meat and skin, raw	4 oz	6	0.04	0.13	5.89	0.58	9.1	0.50	0.0	13.7	1.4	27.5	289	1.7
fryer/roaster, meat and skin, roasted	4 oz	0	0.05	0.16	7.15	0.56	6.9	0.41	0.0	20.5	1.9	29.7	299	2.4
fryer/roaster, meat only, raw	4 oz	0	0.04	0.13	6.55	0.66	9.2	0.53	0.0	11.4	1.4	29.7	315	1.6
fryer/roaster, meat only, roasted	4 oz	0	0.04	0.15	7.91	0.65	6.8	0.45	0.0	17.2	1.8	31.9	316	2.4
fryer/roaster, meat only, roasted, chopped or diced	1 cup	0	0.06	0.19	9.70	0.80	8.4	0.55	0.0	21.0	2.2	39.2	388	2.9
young hen, meat and skin, raw	4 oz	6	0.06	0.14	5.61	0.55	8.0	0.48	0.0	14.9	1.6	27.4	305	1.8
young hen, meat and skin, roasted	4 oz	0	0.06	0.15	7.51	0.53	6.8	0.39	0.0	26.3	1.6	29.7	327	2.3
young hen, meat only, raw	4 oz	0	0.07	0.15	6.45	0.64	9.2	0.51	0.0	13.7	1.6	30.9	342	1.8
young hen, meat only, roasted	4 oz	0	0.07	0.14	8.16	0.59	6.9	0.41	0.0	24.0	1.5	31.9	348	2.2
young hen, meat only, roasted, chopped or diced	1 cup	0	0.09	0.18	9.20	0.77	8.4	0.53	0.0	25.2	1.9	39.2	431	2.9
young tom, meat and skin, raw	4 oz	9	0.07	0.12	6.05	0.54	7.9	0.48	0.0	14.9	1.2	27.4	316	1.9
young tom, meat and skin, roasted	4 oz	0	0.07	0.15	6.89	0.55	6.9	0.41	0.0	24.0	1.6	30.8	328	2.4

Food Name	Serving Size	A I.U.	Thi mg	Rib mg	Nia mg	B$_6$ mg	Fol mcg	B$_{12}$ mcg	C mg	Calc mg	Iron mg	Mag mg	Pot mg	Zn mg
young tom, meat only, raw	4 oz	0	0.08	0.13	6.90	0.63	9.1	0.51	0.0	13.7	1.2	30.9	359	1.9
young tom, meat only, roasted	4 oz	0	0.08	0.15	7.52	0.63	6.8	0.44	0.0	20.6	1.6	32.0	352	2.4
LIVER														
Fresh														
all classes, raw	1 oz	5155	0.00	0.61	2.89	0.20	211.0	17.96	1.3	1.99	3.1	6.1	85	0.7
all classes, simmered	1 oz	3594	0.00	0.39	1.71	0.17	190.3	13.71	0.6	3.1	2.2	4.3	55	0.9
all classes, simmered, chopped or diced	1 cup	17613	0.07	2.00	8.30	0.73	932.0	66.50	2.7	15.4	10.9	21.0	272	4.3
NECK														
Fresh														
all classes, raw	1 oz	0	0.02	0.07	0.90	0.09	3.1	0.12	0.0	9.8	0.6	5.5	86	1.5
all classes, simmered	1 oz	0	0.00	0.06	0.49	0.06	2.3	0.06	0.0	10.6	0.7	4.3	43	2.0
SKIN														
Fresh														
all classes, raw	4 oz	43	0.02	0.09	1.70	0.09	4.5	0.27	0.0	20.6	1.5	9.2	117	1.5
all classes, roasted	4 oz	0	0.02	0.17	3.04	0.09	4.6	0.27	0.0	39.9	2.0	18.3	183	2.4
fryer/roaster, raw	4 oz	38	0.03	0.10	1.98	0.10	5.8	0.35	0.0	21.7	1.5	11.4	138	1.8
fryer/roaster, roasted	4 oz	0	0.03	0.18	3.02	0.09	4.5	0.26	0.0	40.0	2.2	19.5	207	2.4
young hen, raw	4 oz	31	0.02	0.09	1.57	0.07	4.5	0.25	0.0	21.7	1.7	9.2	122	1.4
young hen, roasted	4 oz	0	0.02	0.15	3.21	0.08	4.5	0.27	0.0	36.6	2.1	17.1	177	2.3
young tom, raw	4 oz	56	0.02	0.09	1.79	0.09	4.5	0.29	0.0	20.6	1.4	9.2	110	1.4
young tom, roasted	4 oz	0	0.02	0.18	2.90	0.09	4.6	0.29	0.0	42.2	2.0	19.4	184	2.4
WING														
Fresh														
all classes, meat and skin, raw	3 oz	9	0.05	0.10	3.89	0.36	5.9	0.34	0.0	11.9	1.1	17.9	206	1.3
all classes, meat and skin, roasted	3 oz	0	0.04	0.11	4.99	0.36	4.9	0.29	0.0	20.7	1.2	21.4	228	1.8
fryer/roaster, meat and skin, raw	3 oz	9	0.02	0.09	2.62	0.33	5.9	0.33	0.0	11.9	1.2	14.5	153	1.6
fryer/roaster, meat and skin, roasted	3 oz	0	0.03	0.14	3.12	0.38	1.5	5.14	0.0	25.0	1.5	17.1	343	2.8
fryer/roaster, meat only, raw	3 oz	0	0.03	0.09	3.07	0.46	5.9	0.36	0.0	10.2	1.2	18.1	172	1.7
fryer/roaster, meat only, roasted	3 oz	0	0.05	0.15	3.53	0.50	6.1	0.35	0.0	22.2	1.5	18.7	175	3.3
young hen, meat and skin, raw	3 oz	7	0.05	0.09	3.57	0.33	5.9	0.33	0.0	11.9	1.2	18.1	204	1.3
young hen, meat and skin, roasted	3 oz	0	0.03	0.12	5.20	0.37	4.3	0.28	0.0	20.5	1.2	21.4	230	1.7
young tom, meat and skin, raw	3 oz	12	0.06	0.08	3.99	0.34	5.9	0.34	0.0	11.1	0.9	17.9	214	1.3
young tom, meat and skin, roasted	3 oz	0	0.04	0.12	4.89	0.37	5.3	0.29	0.0	19.6	1.3	21.6	232	1.8
TURKEY DINNER/ENTRÉE														
(Banquet)														
w/dressing, potatoes, corn, in sauce	1 entrée	84	na	na	na	na	na	na	na	47.2	1.4	na	na	na
w/mashed potatoes and corn, in seasoned sauce	1 entrée	84	na	na	na	na	na	na	na	47.2	1.4	na	na	na
(Healthy Choice)														
country roast, w/mushrooms, gravy, rice	1 entrée	864	na	na	na	na	na	na	na	21.6	1.0	na	na	na
(Louis Rich)														
nuggets/sticks, breaded	1 serving	0	na	na	na	na	na	na	0.0	7.7	0.7	17.9	150	1.6
nuggets/sticks, breaded	1 piece	0	na	na	na	na	na	na	0.0	2.5	0.2	5.9	49	0.5
(Marie Callender's)														
w/gravy and dressing, w/broccoli	1 entrée	397	na	na	na	na	na	na	23.8	131.0	4.4	na	na	na
(Pierre)														
nuggets, product 1936	1 piece	5	0.04	0.04	0.84	0.04	4.8	0.06	0.0	5.8	0.4	3.0	36	0.4
nuggets, product 1937	1 piece	1	0.03	0.03	0.60	0.03	3.1	0.03	0.0	4.0	0.3	2.1	25	0.3
patty, breaded, flame-broiled, product 1939	1 piece	74	0.16	0.20	3.2	0.17	24.5	0.52	0.0	28.4	1.8	12.6	149	1.6
patty, flame-broiled, frozen, product 9719	1 piece	0	na	na	na	na	na	na	0.0	13.8	1.1	na	19	na
patty, flame-broiled, frozen, product 9721	1 piece	0	na	na	na	na	na	na	0.0	17.0	1.3	na	23	na

Food Name	Serving Size	A I.U.	Thi mg	Rib mg	Nia mg	B$_6$ mg	Fol mcg	B$_{12}$ mcg	C mg	Calc mg	Iron mg	Mag mg	Pot mg	Zn mg
patty, strip-shaped, frozen, product 1938	1 piece	2	0.05	0.06	1.10	0.06	5.9	0.06	0.0	7.6	0.5	4.0	48	0.5
TURKEY FAT														
....	1 cup	0	0.00	0.00	0.00	0.00	0.0	0.00	0.0	0.0	0.0	0.0	0	0.0
....	1 tbsp	0	0.00	0.00	0.00	0.00	0.0	0.00	0.0	0.0	0.0	0.0	0	0.0
....	1 tsp	0	0.00	0.00	0.00	0.00	0.0	0.00	0.0	0.0	0.0	0.0	0	0.0
TURMERIC														
ground	1 tbsp	0	0.01	0.02	0.35	0.12	2.7	0.00	1.8	12.4	2.8	13.1	172	0.3
ground	1 tsp	0	0.00	0.01	0.11	0.04	0.9	0.00	0.6	4.0	0.9	4.2	56	0.1
TURNIP														
Fresh														
boiled, drained, cubed	1 cup	0	0.04	0.04	0.47	0.11	14.4	0.00	18.1	34.3	0.3	12.5	211	0.3
boiled, drained, mashed	1 cup	0	0.06	0.05	0.69	0.15	21.2	0.00	26.7	50.6	0.5	18.4	311	0.5
raw, cubed	1 cup	0	0.05	0.04	0.52	0.12	18.9	0.00	27.3	39.0	0.4	14.3	248	0.4
raw, cubed	1/2 cup	0	0.03	0.02	0.26	0.06	9.4	0.00	13.7	19.5	0.2	7.2	124	0.2
Frozen														
cubes, boiled, drained.	1 cup	0	0.04	0.04	0.47	0.11	14.4	0.00	18.1	34.3	0.3	12.5	211	0.3
mashed, boiled, drained	1 cup	0	0.06	0.05	0.69	0.15	21.2	0.00	26.7	50.6	0.5	18.4	311	0.5
mashed, unprepared	10-oz pkg	74	0.09	0.06	1.10	0.14	21.9	0.00	12.5	65.3	2.0	28.4	389	0.4
w/greens, boiled, drained	1 cup	8412	0.05	0.11	0.48	0.10	35.0	0.00	15.3	148.0	2.2	19.6	101	0.2
w/greens, unprepared.	10-oz pkg	17347	0.13	0.25	1.10	0.21	115.0	0.00	73.3	324.0	4.6	51.1	233	0.5
TURNIP, CABBAGE. See KOHLRABI.														
TURNIP GREENS														
Canned, w/liquid	1/2 cup	4196	0.01	0.07	0.42	0.04	48.2	0.00	18.1	138.0	1.8	23.4	165	0.3
Fresh														
boiled, drained, chopped	1/2 cup	7917	0.07	0.10	0.59	0.26	170.0	0.00	39.5	197.0	1.2	31.7	292	0.2
raw, chopped	1 cup	4180	0.04	0.06	0.33	0.14	107.0	0.00	33.0	105.0	0.6	17.1	163	0.1
Frozen														
boiled, drained	10-oz pkg	17545	0.12	0.16	1.00	0.15	86.7	0.00	48.0	334.0	4.3	57.2	493	0.9
chopped, boiled, drained	1 cup	7917	0.07	0.10	0.59	0.26	170.0	0.00	39.5	197.0	1.2	31.7	292	0.2
chopped, unprepared	10-oz pkg	17563	0.13	0.26	1.10	0.28	209.0	0.00	76.1	335.0	4.3	76.7	523	0.5
chopped or diced, unprepared	1/2 cup	5071	0.04	0.08	0.31	0.08	60.4	0.00	22.0	96.8	1.2	22.1	151	0.1
TURNOVER. See under PASTRY.														
TUSK. See CUSK.														

U

Food Name	Serving Size	A I.U.	Thi mg	Rib mg	Nia mg	B$_6$ mg	Fol mcg	B$_{12}$ mcg	C mg	Calc mg	Iron mg	Mag mg	Pot mg	Zn mg
UCUHUBA BUTTER OIL														
....	1 cup	0	0.00	0.00	0.00	0.00	0.0	0.00	0.0	0.0	0.0	0.0	0	0.0
....	1 tbsp	0	0.00	0.00	0.00	0.00	0.0	0.00	0.0	0.0	0.0	0.0	0	0.0

V

Food Name	Serving Size	A I.U.	Thi mg	Rib mg	Nia mg	B$_6$ mg	Fol mcg	B$_{12}$ mcg	C mg	Calc mg	Iron mg	Mag mg	Pot mg	Zn mg
VANILLA EXTRACT														
....	1 cup	0	0.02	0.20	0.88	0.05	0.0	0.00	0.0	22.9	0.3	25.0	308	0.2
....	1 tbsp	0	0.00	0.01	0.06	0.00	0.0	0.00	0.0	1.4	<0.1	1.6	19	<0.1
....	1 tsp	0	0.00	0.00	0.02	0.00	0.0	0.00	0.0	0.5	<0.1	0.5	6	<0.1

Food Name	Serving Size	A I.U.	Thi mg	Rib mg	Nia mg	B_6 mg	Fol mcg	B_{12} mcg	C mg	Calc mg	Iron mg	Mag mg	Pot mg	Zn mg
VANILLA EXTRACT SUBSTITUTE														
imitation	1 tbsp	0	0.00	0.00	0.02	0.00	0.0	0.00	0.0	0.4	<0.1	0.1	0	0.0
imitation	1 tsp	0	0.00	0.00	0.01	0.00	0.0	0.00	0.0	0.1	0.0	<0.1	0	0.0
imitation, w/alcohol	1 tbsp	0	0.00	0.01	0.04	0.00	0.0	0.00	0.0	0.0	<0.1	0.7	13	<0.1
imitation, w/alcohol	1 tsp	0	0.00	0.00	0.01	0.00	0.0	0.00	0.0	0.0	<0.1	0.2	4	0.0
VEAL														
(NOTE: TRIMMED = Lean; separable fat removed after cooking. UNTRIMMED = Separable fat not removed.)														
BRAIN														
braised	3 oz	0	0.07	0.17	2.10	0.14	2.5	8.20	11.1	13.6	1.4	13.6	182	1.4
pan-fried	3 oz	0	0.13	0.31	4.80	0.28	5.1	18.10	12.8	8.5	0.9	15.3	401	1.5
raw	4 oz	0	0.15	0.29	4.90	0.32	3.4	13.80	15.9	11.3	2.4	15.9	357	1.3
BREAST														
Trimmed, whole, boneless, braised	3 oz	na	0.05	0.28	7.60	0.25	12.8	1.30	na	7.7	0.7	18.7	246	3.6
Untrimmed														
plate half, boneless, braised	3 oz	na	0.05	0.25	6.70	0.22	11.1	1.10	na	6.8	0.6	16.1	226	3.0
point half, boneless, braised	3 oz	na	0.05	0.26	7.10	0.23	11.9	1.20	na	7.7	0.7	17.9	236	3.3
whole, boneless, braised	3 oz	na	0.05	0.25	6.80	0.22	11.1	1.10	na	7.7	0.7	17.0	231	3.1
GROUND														
broiled	3 oz	0	0.06	0.23	6.80	0.33	9.3	1.10	0.0	14.4	0.8	20.4	286	3.3
raw	4 oz	na	0.09	0.30	8.50	0.46	14.7	1.50	0.0	16.9	0.9	27.1	356	3.5
HEART														
braised	3 oz	0	0.30	0.79	4.10	0.18	1.7	12.30	8.5	6.8	3.7	15.3	169	1.9
raw	4 oz	0	0.59	1.10	7.30	0.49	2.3	15.60	9.1	5.7	4.8	20.4	296	1.7
KIDNEY														
braised	3 oz	569	0.16	1.70	3.90	0.15	17.9	31.40	6.8	24.6	2.6	20.4	135	3.6
raw	4 oz	349	0.36	2.20	7.90	0.42	23.8	32.00	5.7	12.5	3.8	18.1	308	2.2
LEG														
Trimmed														
top round, braised	3 oz	0	0.05	0.31	9.10	0.32	15.3	1.00	0.0	7.7	1.1	25.5	329	3.4
top round, breaded, pan-fried	3 oz	29	0.14	0.31	9.20	0.36	23.8	1.10	0.0	33.1	1.4	27.2	326	2.4
top round, pan-fried	3 oz	0	0.06	0.32	10.70	0.43	13.6	1.30	0.0	6.0	0.7	27.2	376	2.9
top round, raw	1 oz	0	0.02	0.08	2.70	0.13	4.0	0.30	0.0	1.4	0.2	7.7	105	0.7
top round, roasted	3 oz	0	0.05	0.28	8.60	0.26	13.6	1.00	0.0	5.1	0.8	23.8	334	2.6
Untrimmed														
top round, braised	3 oz	0	0.05	0.30	9.00	0.31	15.3	0.99	0.0	6.8	1.1	24.6	326	3.4
top round, breaded, pan-fried	3 oz	29	0.14	0.30	8.80	0.34	22.9	1.10	0.0	33.1	1.4	26.4	315	2.3
top round, pan-fried	3 oz	0	0.06	0.30	10.20	0.42	12.8	1.20	0.0	5.1	0.8	26.4	361	2.7
top round, raw	1 oz	0	0.02	0.08	2.70	0.13	4.0	0.29	0.0	1.4	0.2	7.4	104	0.7
top round, roasted	3 oz	0	0.05	0.27	8.40	0.26	13.6	0.99	0.0	5.1	0.8	23.8	331	2.6
LEG AND SHOULDER														
Trimmed														
cubed for stew, braised	3 oz	0	0.06	0.34	7.10	0.32	13.6	1.40	0.0	24.6	1.2	23.8	291	5.1
cubed for stew, raw	1 oz	0	0.03	0.08	2.10	0.13	3.7	0.42	0.0	4.8	0.3	7.1	94	1.0
LIVER														
braised	3 oz	22851	0.11	1.60	7.20	0.42	645.0	31.00	26.4	6.0	2.2	16.1	174	8.1
pan-fried	3 oz	15978	0.21	2.90	14.40	0.73	272.0	54.40	18.7	10.2	4.4	22.1	372	6.7
raw	4 oz	16720	0.22	2.00	13.30	0.84	728.0	53.10	24.9	10.2	5.4	20.4	331	4.6
LOIN														
Trimmed														
braised	3 oz	0	0.04	0.29	8.50	0.24	12.8	1.10	0.0	27.2	0.9	22.9	252	3.5
raw	1 oz	0	0.02	0.07	2.60	0.16	4.0	0.34	0.0	4.8	0.2	7.1	92	0.7
roasted	3 oz	0	0.05	0.26	8.00	0.32	13.6	1.10	0.0	17.9	0.7	22.1	289	2.8
Untrimmed														
braised	3 oz	0	0.03	0.26	7.70	0.22	11.9	1.00	0.0	23.8	0.9	20.4	238	3.1

Food Name	Serving Size	A I.U.	Thi mg	Rib mg	Nia mg	B$_6$ mg	Fol mcg	B$_{12}$ mcg	C mg	Calc mg	Iron mg	Mag mg	Pot mg	Zn mg
raw	1 oz	0	0.02	0.07	2.40	0.15	3.7	0.32	0.0	4.5	0.2	6.5	86	0.7
roasted	3 oz	0	0.04	0.24	7.50	0.29	12.8	1.10	0.0	16.1	0.7	21.3	276	2.6
LUNGS														
braised	3 oz	0	0.03	0.11	1.90	0.05	6.8	2.00	28.9	6.0	3.1	6.8	121	1.0
raw	4 oz	0	0.05	0.26	4.60	0.13	12.5	4.30	44.2	7.9	5.9	13.6	311	1.3
PANCREAS														
braised	3 oz	0	0.16	0.43	3.50	0.16	2.5	14.70	5.1	15.3	2.0	20.4	236	4.4
raw	4 oz	0	0.15	0.48	4.80	0.22	3.4	15.20	18.1	21.5	2.4	20.4	315	2.9
RIB														
Trimmed														
braised	3 oz	0	0.05	0.26	6.70	0.29	13.6	1.30	0.0	20.4	1.2	22.1	270	5.1
raw	1 oz	0	0.02	0.07	2.00	0.13	3.7	0.39	0.0	4.0	0.3	6.5	87	0.9
roasted	3 oz	0	0.05	0.25	6.40	0.23	11.9	1.30	0.0	10.2	0.8	20.4	264	3.8
Untrimmed														
braised	3 oz	0	0.04	0.25	6.40	0.27	13.6	1.20	0.0	18.7	1.2	21.3	260	4.7
raw	1 oz	0	0.02	0.07	1.90	0.12	3.4	0.37	0.0	3.7	0.2	6.2	82	0.9
roasted	3 oz	0	0.04	0.23	5.90	0.21	11.1	1.20	0.0	9.3	0.8	18.7	251	3.5
SHANK														
Trimmed														
fore and hind, braised	3 oz	0	0.04	0.26	8.20	0.23	14.4	1.40	na	28.9	1.1	21.3	263	5.8
fore and hind, raw	1 oz	na	0.02	0.08	2.20	0.13	4.3	0.39	na	5.7	0.2	6.0	90	1.1
Untrimmed														
fore and hind, braised	3 oz	na	0.04	0.25	8.00	0.23	14.4	1.40	na	28.1	1.1	21.3	259	5.6
fore and hind, raw	1 oz	na	0.02	0.08	2.10	0.12	4.3	0.39	na	5.7	0.2	6.0	89	1.1
SHOULDER														
Trimmed														
arm, braised	3 oz	0	0.05	0.28	9.10	0.26	16.1	1.50	0.0	25.5	1.2	25.5	295	5.3
arm, raw	1 oz	0	0.02	0.08	2.20	0.13	4.5	0.40	0.0	6.2	0.3	7.4	96	0.9
arm, roasted	3 oz	0	0.06	0.28	7.00	0.26	14.4	1.30	0.0	22.9	1.0	22.9	303	3.7
blade, braised	3 oz	0	0.05	0.31	4.80	0.21	12.8	1.70	0.0	34.0	1.3	23.8	259	6.3
blade, raw	1 oz	0	0.03	0.09	1.60	0.11	2.8	0.53	0.0	6.5	0.3	6.5	84	1.3
blade, roasted	3 oz	0	0.06	0.31	4.90	0.20	9.3	1.80	0.0	23.8	0.9	20.4	264	4.9
whole, arm and blade, braised	3 oz	0	0.05	0.30	5.70	0.22	13.6	1.60	0.0	31.4	1.2	23.8	271	6.0
whole, arm and blade, raw	1 oz	0	0.03	0.08	1.70	0.11	3.1	0.48	0.0	6.2	0.3	6.8	88	1.2
whole, arm and blade, roasted	3 oz	0	0.06	0.29	5.50	0.22	11.1	1.60	0.0	22.9	0.9	21.3	278	4.5
Untrimmed														
arm, braised	3 oz	0	0.05	0.26	8.60	0.25	15.3	1.50	0.0	23.8	1.2	24.6	283	4.9
arm, raw	1 oz	0	0.02	0.08	2.20	0.13	4.3	0.39	0.0	6.0	0.3	7.1	93	0.9
arm, roasted	3 oz	0	0.05	0.27	6.80	0.25	14.4	1.30	0.0	22.1	0.9	22.1	296	3.6
blade, braised	3 oz	0	0.05	0.30	4.70	0.20	12.8	1.60	0.0	32.3	1.2	22.1	252	6.0
blade, raw	1 oz	0	0.03	0.09	1.50	0.11	2.8	0.52	0.0	6.5	0.3	6.5	82	1.2
blade, roasted	3 oz	0	0.06	0.30	4.90	0.20	9.3	1.70	0.0	23.8	0.9	20.4	260	4.7
whole, arm and blade, braised	3 oz	0	0.05	0.29	5.50	0.21	12.8	1.60	0.0	29.8	1.2	22.9	263	5.6
whole, arm and blade, raw	1 oz	0	0.03	0.08	1.80	0.11	3.4	0.47	0.0	6.2	0.3	6.5	86	1.1
whole, arm and blade, roasted	3 oz	0	0.06	0.29	5.40	0.22	10.2	1.50	0.0	22.9	0.9	21.3	274	4.4
SIRLOIN														
Trimmed														
braised	3 oz	0	0.05	0.32	6.00	0.32	13.6	1.40	0.0	16.1	1.0	24.6	288	4.0
raw	1 oz	0	0.02	0.09	2.50	0.15	4.0	0.38	0.0	3.1	0.2	7.4	99	0.8
roasted	3 oz	0	0.05	0.32	7.90	0.29	13.6	1.30	0.0	11.9	0.8	22.9	310	3.0
Untrimmed														
braised	3 oz	0	0.04	0.30	5.60	0.30	12.8	1.30	0.0	14.4	1.0	22.9	273	3.7
raw	1 oz	0	0.02	0.09	2.40	0.14	3.7	0.36	0.0	3.1	0.2	6.8	93	0.7

Food Name	Serving Size	A I.U.	Thi mg	Rib mg	Nia mg	B₆ mg	Fol mcg	B₁₂ mcg	C mg	Calc mg	Iron mg	Mag mg	Pot mg	Zn mg
roasted	3 oz	0	0.05	0.30	7.50	0.27	12.8	1.20	0.0	11.1	0.8	22.1	298	2.8
SPLEEN														
braised	3 oz	0	0.04	0.25	4.50	0.06	3.4	4.10	34.0	6.0	6.3	11.9	183	1.6
raw	4 oz	0	0.05	0.40	9.00	0.13	4.5	6.10	46.5	6.8	10.6	19.3	411	1.8
THYMUS														
braised	3 oz	0	0.05	0.14	1.70	0.08	0.9	1.90	62.9	2.5	1.7	14.4	291	2.6
raw	4 oz	0	0.09	0.19	2.90	0.13	3.4	3.60	63.5	2.3	2.2	18.1	491	3.5
TONGUE														
braised	3 oz	0	0.06	0.30	1.30	0.13	7.7	4.50	5.1	7.7	1.8	15.3	138	3.8
raw	4 oz	1	0.19	0.47	2.50	0.22	5.7	6.90	5.7	7.9	3.1	19.3	307	3.0
VEGETABLE DISH/ENTRÉE														
Canned														
succotash, drained	1 cup	564	0.32	0.18	2.50	0.22	63.0	0.00	15.7	32.6	2.9	102.0	787	1.2
succotash, no salt added, drained	1 cup	564	0.32	0.18	2.50	0.22	63.0	0.00	15.7	32.6	2.9	102.0	787	1.2
succotash, w/cream style corn, drained	1 cup	375	0.07	0.17	1.60	0.34	118.0	0.00	17.0	29.3	1.5	2.7	487	1.1
succotash, w/whole kernel corn, w/liquid	1 cup	372	0.07	0.15	1.60	0.13	80.8	0.00	11.7	28.1	1.4	48.5	416	1.3
Frozen														
succotash, boiled, drained	1 cup	393	0.13	0.12	2.20	0.16	56.4	0.00	10.0	25.5	1.5	39.1	451	0.8
succotash, no salt added, boiled, drained	1 cup	393	0.13	0.12	2.20	0.16	56.4	0.00	10.0	25.5	1.5	39.1	451	0.8
succotash, unprepared	10-oz pkg	730	0.25	0.20	3.90	0.28	118.0	0.00	24.1	45.4	2.7	68.2	838	1.3
succotash, unprepared	1 cup	401	0.14	0.11	2.10	0.16	64.9	0.00	13.3	25.0	1.5	37.4	460	0.73
(Banquet) Parmigiana, w/tomato sauce, potato, peas in sauce	1 entrée	252	na	na	na	na	na	na	27.8	66.3	2.3	na	na	na
(Pierre) veal and beef patty, Italian, frozen, product 1905	1 piece	54	0.29	0.22	3.90	0.22	3.4	1.20	0.2	36.5	2.4	25.5	249	3.8
VEGETABLE OIL. See also individual listings.														
salad or cooking	1 cup	0	0.00	0.00	0.00	0.00	0.0	0.00	0.0	0.0	0.0	0.0	0	0.0
salad or cooking	1 tbsp	0	0.00	0.00	0.00	0.00	0.0	0.00	0.0	0.0	0.0	0.0	0	0.0
VEGETABLE OYSTER. See SALSIFY.														
VEGETABLE SPONGE. See GOURD, DISHCLOTH.														
VEGETABLES, MIXED														
Canned														
drained	1 cup	18985	0.08	0.08	0.94	0.13	38.5	0.00	8.2	44.0	1.7	26.1	474	0.7
w/liquid	1 cup	12448	0.08	0.10	1.20	0.19	44.1	0.00	9.3	51.5	1.6	36.8	338	1.3
Frozen														
boiled, drained	10-oz pkg	11762	0.20	0.33	2.30	0.20	52.3	0.00	8.8	68.8	2.3	60.5	465	1.3
boiled, drained	1/2 cup	3892	0.07	0.11	0.77	0.07	17.3	0.00	2.9	22.8	0.8	20.0	154	0.5
no salt added, boiled, drained	10-oz pkg	11762	0.20	0.33	2.30	0.20	52.3	0.00	8.8	68.8	2.3	60.5	465	1.3
no salt added, boiled, drained	1/2 cup	3892	0.07	0.11	0.77	0.07	17.3	0.00	2.9	22.8	0.8	20.0	154	0.5
unprepared	10-oz pkg	14422	0.35	0.24	3.60	0.27	82.4	0.00	29.5	71.0	2.7	68.2	602	1.3
VINEGAR, APPLE CIDER														
	1 cup	0	0.00	0.00	0.00	0.00	0.0	0.00	0.0	14.4	1.4	52.8	240	0.0
	1 tbsp	0	0.00	0.00	0.00	0.00	0.0	0.00	0.0	0.9	<0.1	3.3	15	0.0
VODKA														
80 proof	1 fl oz	0	0.00	0.00	0.00	0.00	0.0	0.00	0.0	0.0	<0.1	0.0	<1	<0.1
86 proof	1 fl oz	0	0.00	0.00	0.00	0.00	0.0	0.00	0.0	0.0	<0.1	0.0	<1	<0.1
90 proof	1 fl oz	0	0.00	0.00	0.00	0.00	0.0	0.00	0.0	0.0	<0.1	0.0	<1	<0.1
94 proof	1 fl oz	0	0.00	0.00	0.00	0.00	0.0	0.00	0.0	0.0	<0.1	0.0	<1	<0.1
100 proof	1 fl oz	0	0.00	0.00	0.00	0.00	0.0	0.00	0.0	0.0	<0.1	0.0	<1	<0.1

W

Food Name	Serving Size	A I.U.	Thi mg	Rib mg	Nia mg	B₆ mg	Fol mcg	B₁₂ mcg	C mg	Calc mg	Iron mg	Mag mg	Pot mg	Zn mg
WAFFLE														
(Aunt Jemima)														
Quaker Oats, original, frozen	1 serving	na	na	na	na	na	na	na	na	na	5.2	na	na	na
(Eggo)														
banana bread, 'Kellogg's Nutri-Grain'	1 serving	1000	0.31	0.31	4.00	0.39	39.8	1.20	1.1	39.8	3.6	14.0	140	0.5
blueberry, low-fat, 'Kellogg's Nutri-Grain'.	1 serving	897	0.27	0.31	3.60	0.36	35.7	1.10	0.0	42.7	3.2	37.8	48	na
blueberry, low-fat, round, 'Kellogg's Nutri-Grain'.	1 waffle	449	0.13	0.15	1.80	0.18	17.9	0.54	0.0	21.4	1.6	18.9	24	na
golden oat.	1 serving	897	0.28	0.35	3.60	0.35	28.7	1.10	0.6	46.2	3.2	30.8	134	na
golden oat, round	1 waffle	449	0.14	0.17	1.80	0.17	14.3	0.53	0.3	23.1	1.6	15.4	67	na
homestyle, low-fat.	1 serving	1013	0.62	0.52	5.20	0.33	53.9	1.10	0.0	40.6	3.9	47.6	100	na
homestyle, round	1 waffle	506	0.31	0.26	2.60	0.16	26.9	0.55	0.0	20.3	1.9	23.8	50	na
low-fat, 'Kellogg's Nutri-Grain'.	1 serving	897	0.27	0.31	3.60	0.36	35.7	1.10	0.0	42.7	3.2	39.2	50	na
low-fat, round, 'Kellogg's Nutri-Grain'	1 waffle	449	0.13	0.15	1.80	0.18	17.9	0.54	0.0	21.4	1.6	19.6	25	na
WAKAME. See under SEA VEGETABLE.														
WALLEYE. See under PIKE; POLLACK.														
WALNUT														
BLACK														
Dried														
. . . .	1 oz	84	0.06	0.03	0.20	0.16	18.6	0.00	0.9	16.4	0.9	57.3	149	0.9
. . . .	1 tbsp	23	0.02	0.01	0.05	0.04	5.1	0.00	0.3	4.5	0.2	15.8	41	0.3
chopped	1 cup	370	0.27	0.14	0.86	0.69	81.9	0.00	4.0	72.5	3.8	253	655	4.3
ENGLISH														
Dried														
in shell, whole, 7 med nuts	1 cup	12	0.10	0.04	0.54	0.15	27.4	0.00	0.4	29.1	0.8	44.2	123	0.9
shelled, chopped	1 cup	49	0.41	0.18	2.30	0.64	118.0	0.00	1.6	125.0	3.5	190.0	529	3.7
shelled, ground	1 cup	33	0.27	0.12	1.50	0.43	78.4	0.00	1.0	83.2	2.3	126.0	353	2.5
shelled, halved, 50 halves	1 cup	41	0.34	0.15	1.90	0.54	98.0	0.00	1.3	104.0	2.9	158.0	441	3.1
shelled, pieces or chips	1 cup	49	0.41	0.18	2.30	0.64	118.0	0.00	1.6	125.0	3.5	190.0	529	3.7
WALNUT OIL														
. . . .	1 cup	0	0.00	0.00	0.00	0.00	0.0	0.00	0.0	0.0	0.0	0.0	0	0.0
. . . .	1 tbsp	0	0.00	0.00	0.00	0.00	0.0	0.00	0.0	0.0	0.0	0.0	0	0.0
WASABI ROOT / Japanese horseradish														
raw, sliced.	1 cup	60	0.17	0.15	0.97	0.36	23.4	0.00	54.5	166.0	1.3	89.7	738	2.1
raw, whole, medium	1 root	78	0.22	0.19	1.30	0.46	30.4	0.00	70.8	216.0	1.7	117.0	960	2.7
WATER														
UNFLAVORED														
(Perrier).	8 fl oz	0	0.00	0.00	0.00	0.00	0.0	0.00	0.0	33.2	0.0	0.0	0	0.0
(Poland Spring).	8 fl oz	0	0.00	0.00	0.00	0.00	0.0	0.00	0.0	2.4	<0.1	2.4	0	0.0
municipal	8 fl oz	0	0.00	0.00	0.00	0.00	0.0	0.00	0.0	4.7	<0.1	2.4	0	<0.1
WATER BUFFALO														
raw	1 oz	0	0.01	0.06	1.70	0.15	2.3	0.47	0.0	3.4	0.5	9.1	84	0.6
roasted	3 oz	0	0.03	0.21	5.30	0.39	7.7	1.50	0.0	12.8	1.8	28.1	266	2.2
WATER CHESTNUT														
Canned														
Chinese, sliced, w/liquid	1/2 cup	3	0.01	0.02	0.25	0.11	4.1	0.00	0.9	2.8	0.6	3.5	83	0.3
Chinese, whole, w/liquid	4 medium	1	0.00	0.01	0.10	0.05	1.6	0.00	0.4	1.1	0.2	1.4	33	0.1
Fresh														
Chinese, matai, raw, sliced	1/2 cup	0	0.09	0.12	0.62	0.20	10.0	0.00	2.5	6.8	<0.1	13.6	362	0.31
Chinese, matai, raw, whole.	4 medium	0	0.05	0.07	0.36	0.12	5.8	0.00	1.4	4.0	<0.1	7.9	210	0.18

Food Name	Serving Size	A I.U.	Thi mg	Rib mg	Nia mg	B6 mg	Fol mcg	B12 mcg	C mg	Calc mg	Iron mg	Mag mg	Pot mg	Zn mg
WATER CONVOLVULUS. See CABBAGE, SKUNK.														
WATERCRESS														
raw, chopped	1 cup	1598	0.03	0.04	0.07	0.04	3.1	0.00	14.6	40.8	<0.1	7.1	112	<0.1
raw, whole sprigs	10 medium	1175	0.02	0.03	0.05	0.03	2.3	0.00	10.8	30.0	<0.1	5.3	83	<0.1
raw, whole sprigs	1 medium	118	0.00	0.00	0.01	0.00	0.2	0.00	1.1	3.0	<0.1	0.5	8.3	0
WATERMELON														
raw, balls	1 cup	564	0.12	0.03	0.31	0.22	3.4	0.00	14.8	12.3	0.3	16.9	179	0.1
raw, balls	10 balls	447	0.10	0.02	0.24	0.18	2.7	0.00	11.7	9.8	0.2	13.4	142	<0.1
raw, diced	1 cup	556	0.12	0.03	0.30	0.22	3.3	0.00	14.6	12.2	0.3	16.7	176	0.1
raw, sliced, 1/16 of 10-inch diam melon	1 slice	1047	0.23	0.06	0.57	0.41	6.3	0.00	27.5	22.9	0.5	31.5	332	0.2
WATERMELON SEED														
dried, kernels	1 cup	0	0.20	0.16	3.80	0.10	62.5	0.00	0.0	58.3	7.9	556.0	700	11.1
dried, kernels	1 oz	0	0.05	0.04	1.00	0.03	16.4	0.00	0.0	15.3	2.1	146.0	184	2.9
WAX BEAN. See BEAN, WAX.														
WAX GOURD. See GOURD, WAX.														
WEST INDIAN CHERRY. See ACEROLA.														
WHEAT														
DURUM	1 cup	0	0.80	0.23	12.9	0.80	83.1	0.00	0.0	65.3	6.8	276.0	828	8.0
HARD RED														
spring	1 cup	0	0.97	0.21	11.0	0.65	82.6	0.00	0.0	48.0	6.9	238.0	653	5.3
winter	1 cup	0	0.73	0.22	10.5	0.58	73.0	0.00	0.0	55.7	6.1	242.0	697	5.1
HARD WHITE	1 cup	0	0.74	0.21	8.40	0.71	72.2	0.00	0.0	61.4	8.8	179.0	829	6.4
SOFT RED, winter	1 cup	0	0.66	0.16	8.10	0.46	68.9	0.00	0.0	45.4	5.4	212.0	667	4.4
SOFT WHITE	1 cup	0	0.69	0.18	8.00	0.64	68.2	0.00	0.0	57.1	9.0	151.0	731	5.8
SPROUTED	1 cup	0	0.24	0.17	3.30	0.29	41.0	0.00	2.8	30.2	2.3	88.6	183	1.8
WHEAT BRAN, crude	1 cup	0	0.30	0.34	7.90	0.76	45.8	0.00	0.0	42.3	6.1	354.0	686	4.2
WHEAT FLOUR. See under FLOUR.														
WHEAT GERM														
crude	1 cup	0	2.2	0.57	7.80	1.50	323	0.00	0.0	44.9	7.2	275.0	1026	14.1
toasted, plain, ready to eat	1 cup	0	1.90	0.93	6.30	1.10	398	0.00	6.8	50.9	10.3	362.0	1070	18.8
toasted, plain, ready to eat	1 oz	0	0.47	0.23	1.60	0.28	99.8	0.00	1.7	12.8	2.6	90.7	268	4.7
WHEAT GERM OIL														
	1 cup	0	0.00	0.00	0.00	0.00	0.0	0.00	0.0	0.0	0.0	0.0	0	0.0
	1 tbsp	0	0.00	0.00	0.00	0.00	0.0	0.00	0.0	0.0	0.0	0.0	0	0.0
WHEAT SNACKS														
wheat nuts, flavored, no salt added, all flavors except macadamia	1 oz	<1	0.06	0.06	0.28	0.07	26.6	0.00	<0.1	5.7	0.6	16.4	74	0.8
wheat nuts, formulated, unflavored, salted	1 oz	<1	0.09	0.09	0.42	0.11	40.3	0.00	<0.1	7.4	0.7	16.4	90	0.8
WHELK														
boiled, poached, or steamed	3 oz	138	0.04	0.18	1.70	0.55	9.7	15.40	5.8	96.0	8.6	146.0	590	2.8
raw	3 oz	72	0.02	0.09	0.89	0.29	5.4	7.70	3.4	48.5	4.3	73.1	295	1.4
WHEY														
acid, dried	1 cup	33	0.35	1.20	0.66	0.35	18.9	1.40	0.5	1171.0	0.7	113.0	1304	3.6
acid, dried	1 tbsp	2	0.02	0.06	0.03	0.02	0.9	0.07	<0.1	59.6	<0.1	5.8	66	0.2
acid, fluid	1 cup	17	0.10	0.34	0.19	0.10	5.4	0.44	0.2	253.0	0.2	24.0	352	1.1
acid, fluid	1 quart	69	0.41	1.40	0.78	0.41	21.6	1.80	0.6	1011.0	0.8	95.8	1408	4.2
sweet, dried	1 cup	64	0.75	3.20	1.80	0.85	16.8	3.40	2.2	1154.0	1.3	255.0	3016	2.9
sweet, dried	1 tbsp	3	0.04	0.17	0.09	0.04	0.9	0.18	0.1	59.7	<0.1	13.2	156	0.2
sweet, fluid	1 cup	39	0.09	0.39	0.18	0.08	2.0	0.68	0.3	115.0	0.2	20.3	396	0.3
sweet, fluid	1 quart	157	0.35	1.60	0.73	0.30	7.9	2.70	0.9	461.0	0.6	81.3	1584	1.3
WHISKEY														
80 proof	1 fl oz	0	0.00	0.00	0.00	0.00	0.0	0.00	0.0	0.0	<0.1	0.0	<1	<0.1
86 proof	1 fl oz	0	0.00	0.00	0.00	0.00	0.0	0.00	0.0	0.0	<0.1	0.0	<1	<0.1

Food Name	Serving Size	A I.U.	Thi mg	Rib mg	Nia mg	B6 mg	Fol mcg	B12 mcg	C mg	Calc mg	Iron mg	Mag mg	Pot mg	Zn mg
90 proof	1 fl oz	0	0.00	0.00	0.00	0.00	0.0	0.00	0.0	0.0	<0.1	0.0	<1	<0.1
94 proof	1 fl oz	0	0.00	0.00	0.00	0.00	0.0	0.00	0.0	0.0	<0.1	0.0	<1	<0.1
100 proof	1 fl oz	0	0.00	0.00	0.00	0.00	0.0	0.00	0.0	0.0	<0.1	0.0	<1	<0.1

WHISKEY SOUR. See under COCKTAIL; COCKTAIL MIX

WHITE BEAN. See BEAN, WHITE.

WHITE CURRANT. See under CURRANT.

WHITE FLOUR. See under FLOUR.

WHITE MUSHROOM. See MUSHROOM, WHITE.

WHITE-FLOWERED GOURD. See GOURD, BOTTLE.

WHITEFISH

Food Name	Serving Size	A I.U.	Thi mg	Rib mg	Nia mg	B6 mg	Fol mcg	B12 mcg	C mg	Calc mg	Iron mg	Mag mg	Pot mg	Zn mg
mixed species, baked, broiled, grilled, or microwaved	3 oz	111	0.14	0.13	3.30	0.29	14.4	0.82	0.0	28.1	0.4	35.7	345	1.1
mixed species, raw	3 oz	102	0.12	0.10	2.50	0.26	12.8	0.85	0.0	22.1	0.3	28.1	269	0.8
mixed species, smoked	3 oz	162	0.03	0.09	2.00	0.33	6.2	2.80	0.0	15.3	0.4	19.6	360	0.4
mixed species, smoked, flaked	1 cup	258	0.04	0.14	3.30	0.53	9.9	4.40	0.0	24.5	0.7	31.3	575	0.7

WHITING / silver hake

Food Name	Serving Size	A I.U.	Thi mg	Rib mg	Nia mg	B6 mg	Fol mcg	B12 mcg	C mg	Calc mg	Iron mg	Mag mg	Pot mg	Zn mg
mixed species, baked, broiled, grilled, or microwaved	3 oz	97	0.06	0.05	1.40	0.15	12.8	2.20	0.0	52.7	0.4	22.9	369	0.5
mixed species, raw	3 oz	84	0.05	0.04	1.10	0.13	11.1	2.00	0.0	40.8	0.3	17.9	212	0.8

WHOLE WHEAT FLOUR. See under FLOUR.

WILD RICE. See RICE, WILD.

WINGED BEAN. See BEAN, WINGED.

WINTER SQUASH. See under SQUASH.

WOLF FISH / ocean catfish

Food Name	Serving Size	A I.U.	Thi mg	Rib mg	Nia mg	B6 mg	Fol mcg	B12 mcg	C mg	Calc mg	Iron mg	Mag mg	Pot mg	Zn mg
Atlantic, baked, broiled, grilled, or microwaved	3 oz	368	0.18	0.08	2.20	0.39	5.1	2.00	0.0	6.8	0.1	32.3	327	0.9
Atlantic, raw	3 oz	319	0.15	0.07	1.80	0.34	4.3	1.70	0.0	5.1	<0.1	25.5	255	0.7

WONTON WRAPPER

Food Name	Serving Size	A I.U.	Thi mg	Rib mg	Nia mg	B6 mg	Fol mcg	B12 mcg	C mg	Calc mg	Iron mg	Mag mg	Pot mg	Zn mg
including egg roll wrappers	1 oz	4	0.15	0.11	1.50	0.01	24.4	0.01	0.0	13.3	0.9	5.7	23	0.2
including egg roll wrappers, 7-inch square	1 wrapper	5	0.17	0.12	1.70	0.01	27.5	0.01	0.0	15.0	1.1	6.4	26	0.2
including egg roll wrappers, 3.5-inch square	1 wrapper	1	0.04	0.03	0.43	0.00	6.9	0.00	0.0	3.8	0.3	1.6	7	<0.1

Y

Food Name	Serving Size	A I.U.	Thi mg	Rib mg	Nia mg	B6 mg	Fol mcg	B12 mcg	C mg	Calc mg	Iron mg	Mag mg	Pot mg	Zn mg

YAM

Fresh

Food Name	Serving Size	A I.U.	Thi mg	Rib mg	Nia mg	B6 mg	Fol mcg	B12 mcg	C mg	Calc mg	Iron mg	Mag mg	Pot mg	Zn mg
boiled, drained, cubed	1 cup	0	0.13	0.04	0.75	0.31	21.8	0.00	16.5	19.0	0.71	24.5	911	0.3
boiled, drained, cubed	1/2 cup	0	0.07	0.02	0.38	0.16	10.9	0.00	8.2	9.5	0.35	12.2	456	0.1
raw, cubed	1 cup	0	0.17	0.05	0.83	0.44	34.5	0.00	25.6	25.5	0.81	31.5	1224	0.4

CHINESE. See JICAMA.

MOUNTAIN/HAWAIIAN

Fresh

Food Name	Serving Size	A I.U.	Thi mg	Rib mg	Nia mg	B6 mg	Fol mcg	B12 mcg	C mg	Calc mg	Iron mg	Mag mg	Pot mg	Zn mg
raw, whole	1 medium	0	0.43	0.08	2.0	0.75	58.8	0.00	10.9	109.0	1.8	50.4	1756	1.1
raw, cubed	1/2 cup	0	0.07	0.01	0.33	0.12	9.5	0.00	1.8	17.7	0.3	8.2	284	0.2
steamed, cubed	1 cup	0	0.13	0.02	0.19	0.30	17.5	0.00	0.0	11.6	0.6	14.5	718	0.5

YAMBEAN TUBER. See JICAMA.

YARDLONG BEAN. See BEAN, YARDLONG.

YAUTIA / tannier

Food Name	Serving Size	A I.U.	Thi mg	Rib mg	Nia mg	B6 mg	Fol mcg	B12 mcg	C mg	Calc mg	Iron mg	Mag mg	Pot mg	Zn mg
raw, sliced	1 cup	15	0.13	0.05	0.90	0.32	22.9	0.00	7.0	12.2	1.3	32.4	807	0.7

Food Name	Serving Size	A I.U.	Thi mg	Rib mg	Nia mg	B$_6$ mg	Fol mcg	B$_{12}$ mcg	C mg	Calc mg	Iron mg	Mag mg	Pot mg	Zn mg
raw, whole..........................	1 med root	34	0.30	0.12	2.00	0.72	51.9	0.00	15.9	27.4	3.0	73.2	1824	1.5
YEAST														
baker's, active, dry	1 tbsp	<1	0.28	0.66	4.80	0.19	281.0	0.00	<0.1	7.7	2.0	11.8	240	0.8
baker's, active, dry	1 tsp	<1	0.09	0.22	1.60	0.06	93.6	0.00	<0.1	2.6	0.7	3.9	80	0.3
baker's, compressed...................	0.6-oz cake	0	0.32	0.19	2.10	0.07	133.0	0.00	<0.1	3.2	0.6	6.8	102	1.7
YELLOW BEAN. See BEAN, WAX; BEAN; YELLOW.														
YELLOW PEPPER. See under PEPPER.														
YELLOW SNAP BEAN. See BEAN, WAX.														
YELLOWFIN TUNA. See under TUNA.														
YELLOWTAIL														
baked, broiled, grilled, or microwaved	3 oz	88	0.15	0.04	7.40	0.16	3.4	1.10	2.5	24.6	0.5	32.3	457	0.6
raw	3 oz	81	0.12	0.03	5.80	0.14	3.1	1.10	2.4	19.6	0.4	25.5	357	0.4
YOGURT														
(Breyers)														
strawberry, low-fat.....................	8 oz	77	na	0.43	na	na	na	1.20	0.0	284.0	0.2	na	436	na
strawberry, nonfat, w/aspartame and														
fructose sweeteners...................	8 oz	9	na	0.32	na	na	na	0.93	1.4	216.0	0.3	na	331	na
strawberry, 'Smooth & Creamy'	8 oz	70	na	0.41	na	na	na	1.20	0.0	245.0	0.3	na	402	na
YOKAN	1 slice	<1	0.00	0.00	0.01	0.00	1.1	0.00	0.0	3.8	0.2	2.5	6.3	<0.1
YUCA. See CASSAVA.														

Z

Food Name	Serving Size	A I.U.	Thi mg	Rib mg	Nia mg	B$_6$ mg	Fol mcg	B$_{12}$ mcg	C mg	Calc mg	Iron mg	Mag mg	Pot mg	Zn mg
ZANTE CURRANT. See under CURRANT.														
ZUCCHINI														
Canned, Italian style	1 cup	1224	0.10	0.09	1.20	0.34	68.6	0.00	5.2	38.6	1.5	31.8	622	0.6
Fresh														
baby, raw............................	1 large	78	0.01	0.01	0.11	0.02	3.2	0.00	5.5	3.4	0.1	5.3	73	0.1
baby, raw............................	1 medium	54	0.01	0.00	0.08	0.02	2.2	0.00	3.8	2.3	<0.1	3.6	51	<0.1
w/skin, boiled, drained, mashed	1/2 cup	288	0.05	0.05	0.51	0.09	20.2	0.00	5.5	15.6	0.4	26.4	304	0.2
w/skin, boiled, drained, sliced.............	1 cup	432	0.07	0.07	0.77	0.14	30.2	0.00	8.3	23.4	0.6	39.6	455	0.3
w/skin, raw, whole.....................	1 large	1098	0.23	0.10	1.30	0.29	71.4	0.00	29.1	48.5	1.4	71.1	801	0.7
w/skin, raw, whole.....................	1 medium	666	0.14	0.06	0.78	0.17	43.3	0.00	17.6	29.4	0.8	43.1	486	0.4
w/skin, raw, whole.....................	1 small	401	0.08	0.04	0.47	0.11	26.1	0.00	10.6	17.7	0.5	26.0	293	0.2
w/skin, raw, chopped	1 cup	422	0.09	0.04	0.50	0.11	27.4	0.00	11.2	18.6	0.5	27.3	308	0.3
w/skin, raw, sliced.....................	1 cup	384	0.08	0.03	0.45	0.10	25.0	0.00	10.2	16.9	0.5	24.9	280	0.2
Frozen														
w/skin, boiled, drained	1 cup	963	0.09	0.09	0.86	0.10	17.4	0.00	8.3	37.9	1.1	29.0	433	0.5
w/skin, unprepared.....................	10-oz pkg	1375	0.14	0.12	1.20	0.14	28.1	0.00	15.1	51.1	1.4	36.9	619	0.6
w/skin, unprepared.....................	3-lb pkg	6587	0.65	0.57	5.90	0.68	135.0	0.00	72.1	245.0	6.9	177.0	2967	2.9

PART THREE

FAST-FOOD/CHAIN RESTAURANT VALUES

Calories • Protein • Carbohydrates • Sodium •

Fiber • Fat • Saturated Fat • Cholesterol •

Percentage of Calories from Fat

Food Name	Serving Size	Calories	Prot. gms	Carbs gms	Sod. mgs	Fiber gms	Fat gms	Sat. Fat gms	Chol. mgs	% Fat Cal.
ARBY'S										
BACON	2 strips	90	5	0	220	0	7.0	10.0	3	76%
BISCUIT										
w/margarine	2.8 oz	270	5	26	750	0	16.0	0.0	3	54%
CATSUP/KETCHUP	1 pkt	10	na	3	90	0	0.0	0.0	0	0%
CHEESE										
Swiss	1 slice	45	3	0	220	0	3.0	10.0	2	69%
CROISSANT										
	2.2 oz	260	6	28	300	0	16.0	20.0	10	51%
DRESSING										
Thousand Island	2.5 oz	350	0	11	580	0	33.0	15.0	5	87%
bleu cheese	2.5 oz	390	3	3	770	0	39.0	30.0	6	94%
buttermilk ranch	2.5 oz	210	0	2	600	0	49.0	5.0	7	98%
buttermilk ranch, reduced calorie	2 oz	50	0	12	710	0	0.0	0.0	0	0%
honey French	2.5 oz	350	0	24	530	0	27.0	0.0	4	72%
Italian, lower calorie	2.19 oz	20	0	4	1110	0	1.0	0.0	0	36%
EGG										
scrambled	1.8 oz	70	6	0	70	0	5.0	220.0	2	65%
FINGER MEAL										
chicken	10.7 oz	880	35	81	2240	0	47.0	60.0	8	48%
FINGER SNACK										
chicken	7.4 oz	610	20	62	1610	0	32.0	30.0	6	47%
jalapeño bites	3.9 oz	330	7	29	670	2	21.0	40.0	9	57%
mozzarella sticks	4.8 oz	470	18	34	1330	2	29.0	60.0	14	56%
onion petals	4 oz	410	4	43	300	2	24.0	0.0	3	53%
FRENCH FRIES										
cheddar curly	6 oz	450	8	52	1420	0	25.0	5.0	6	49%
curly, large	7 oz	600	8	75	1710	0	30.0	0.0	7	45%
curly, medium	4.5 oz	380	5	49	1100	0	19.0	0.0	5	44%
curly, small	3.8 oz	320	4	40	910	0	16.0	0.0	4	45%
homestyle, large	7.5 oz	630	8	86	1240	6	29.0	0.0	5	41%
homestyle, medium	5 oz	420	5	57	830	4	19.0	0.0	3	41%
homestyle, small	4 oz	340	4	46	660	3	15.0	0.0	3	40%
FRENCH TOASTIX, w/o powdered sugar or syrup	3 hotcakes	370	7	48	440	4	17.0	0.0	4	41%
HAM	1.5 oz	50	7	1	830	0	3.0	30.0	1	46%
HOT CHOCOLATE	8.6 oz	110	2	23	120	0	1.0	0.0	1	8%
MAPLE SYRUP	1.5 oz	220	0	54	50	0	0.0	0.0	0	0%
MUSTARD										
German	1 pkt	5	0	0	60	0	0.0	0.0	0	0%
honey	1 oz	130	0	5	170	0	12.0	10.0	2	84%
ORANGE JUICE	10 oz	140	1	34	0	0	0.0	0.0	0	0%
SAUCE										
Arby's	1 pkt	15	0	3	110	0	0.0	0.0	0	0%
barbecue dipping	1 oz	40	0	10	350	0	0.0	0.0	0	0%
beef stock aus jus	2 oz	10	0	0	440	0	0.0	0.0	0	0%
bronco berry	1.5 oz	90	0	23	35	0	0.0	0.0	0	0%
horsey	1 pkt	60	0	3	100	0	5.0	0.0	1	79%
marinara sauce	1.5 oz	35	1	4	260	0	1.5	0.0	0	40%
tangy Southwest	1.52 oz	250	0	3	280	0	25.0	30.0	4	95%
SANDWICH										
Arby-Q	6.6 oz	380	19	42	990	3	15.0	30.0	5	36%
Beef 'N Cheddar	7 oz	510	26	45	1250	3	28.0	50.0	9	47%
chicken, bacon 'n Swiss	7.8 oz	610	37	52	1620	5	30.0	75.0	9	43%
chicken breast fillet	7.6 oz	560	30	49	1080	6	28.0	55.0	6	44%

Food Name	Serving Size	Calories	Prot. gms	Carbs gms	Sod. mgs	Fiber gms	Fat gms	Sat. Fat gms	Chol. mgs	% Fat Cal.
chicken cordon bleu	8.9 oz	650	40	50	2120	5	34.0	90.0	9	46%
fish fillet sandwich	7.9 oz	540	23	51	880	2	27.0	40.0	7	45%
French dip sub	7.1 oz	490	30	43	1440	3	22.0	56.0	8	40%
grilled chicken deluxe	8.7 oz	420	30	42	930	3	16.0	60.0	4	33%
grilled chicken, lowfat	6.3 oz	280	30	33	920	4	5.0	50.0	2	15%
hot ham 'n Swiss sub	9.7 oz	570	30	47	2660	2	31.0	100.0	10	48%
Italian sub	10.3 oz	800	28	49	2610	2	54.0	85.0	16	61%
Philly beef 'n Swiss sub	11.1 oz	780	39	52	2140	4	48.0	90.0	16	54%
roast beef, big Montana	11 oz	720	50	44	2270	7	40.0	110.0	17	49%
roast beef, giant	8.1 oz	550	34	43	1560	5	28.0	70.0	11	45%
roast beef, junior	4.6 oz	340	18	36	790	3	16.0	30.0	6	40%
roast beef, regular	5.6 oz	400	23	36	1030	3	20.0	40.0	7	43%
roast beef, super	8.7 oz	530	24	50	1190	5	27.0	40.0	9	45%
roast beef melt w/cheddar	5.4 oz	380	19	38	960	3	19.0	30.0	7	43%
roast beef sub	10.7 oz	770	32	48	2170	3	49.0	70.0	15	58%
roast chicken club	8.4 oz	540	37	39	1590	3	29.0	70.0	8	46%
roast chicken deluxe, low-fat	7 oz	260	23	32	950	4	5.0	40.0	2	17%
roast turkey deluxe, lowfat	6.9 oz	230	19	33	870	4	5.0	25.0	2	18%
turkey sub	10.7 oz	670	29	49	2130	2	39.0	60.0	10	53%
POTATO, BAKED										
broccoli 'n cheddar	13.6 oz	550	14	71	730	7	25.0	50.0	13	40%
chicken broccoli	15.8 oz	830	35	68	970	7	47.0	60.0	8	51%
cool ranch	12.3 oz	500	8	67	150	6	23.0	25.0	7	41%
deluxe	12.3 oz	610	14	68	860	6	31.0	80.0	19	46%
jalapeño	14.6 oz	660	15	72	930	6	36.0	50.0	14	48%
Philly chicken	15.8 oz	880	32	75	1020	7	53.0	70.0	10	53%
w/butter and sour cream	11.3 oz	500	8	65	170	6	24.0	60.0	15	43%
POTATO CAKES	2 cakes	220	2	21	460	3	14.0	0.0	3	58%
SALAD										
garden, w/one crouton packet, 2 saltine crackers	10.2 oz	110	9	16	150	1	3.0	0.0	0	21%
grilled chicken, low-fat	14.2 oz	190	25	16	530	1	4.0	40.0	1	18%
roast chicken, lowfat	14.2 oz	200	25	16	800	1	5.0	40.0	1	22%
w/one crouton packet, 2 saltine crackers	5.4 oz	90	5	12	130	0	3.0	0.0	0	28%
SAUSAGE PATTY	1.4 oz	200	7	1	290	0	19.0	60.0	7	84%
SHAKE										
chocolate	10.3 oz	390	8	69	270	0	9.0	10.0	6	21%
jamocha	10.3 oz	380	8	66	300	0	9.0	10.0	6	21%
strawberry	10.3 oz	380	8	67	270	0	9.0	10.0	6	21%
vanilla	10.3 oz	380	8	67	270	0	9.0	12.0	6	21%
TURNOVER										
iced apple	3.4 oz	360	4	54	180	6	14.0	0.0	3	35%
iced cherry	3.5 oz	350	4	53	190	0	14.0	0.0	3	36%
ARTHUR TREACHER'S										
CHICKEN PATTIES										
	2 patties	369	27	17	495	0	21.6	65.0	4	53%
SANDWICH										
chicken	1 sandwich	413	16	44	708	0	19.2	32.0	3	42%
fish	1 sandwich	440	16	39	836	0	24.0	42.0	4	49%
COD FILLET, 'Bake'n Broil' tail shape	5 oz	245	20	10	144	0	14.2	0.0	0	52%
COLESLAW										
	3 oz	123	1	11	266	0	8.2	7.0	1	60%
DESSERT, Lemon Luv	1 serving	276	3	35	314	0	13.9	1.0	2	45%
FISH FILLET	5.2 oz	355	19	25	450	0	19.8	56.0	3	50%
FRENCH FRIES, chips	4 oz	276	4	35	39	0	13.2	5.0	2	43%

Food Name	Serving Size	Calories	Prot. gms	Carbs gms	Sod. mgs	Fiber gms	Fat gms	Sat. Fat gms	Chol. mgs	% Fat Cal.
HUSHPUPPY, 'Krunch Pup'	1 piece	203	5	12	446	0	14.8	25.0	4	66%
SHRIMP	7 pieces	381	13	27	538	0	24.4	93.0	3	58%
AU BON PAIN										
BAGEL										
cinnamon	1 bagel	395	14	86	605	4	2.0	0.0	1	4%
onion	1 bagel	390	16	81	665	4	2.0	0.0	1	4%
plain	1 bagel	380	15	79	665	3	2.0	0.0	1	5%
sesame	1 bagel	425	17	81	665	4	5.0	0.0	1	10%
BREAD										
baguette	1 loaf	810	27	166	1830	0	2.0	0.0	1	2%
cheese	1 loaf	1670	70	269	4140	0	29.0	75.0	9	16%
four-grain	1 loaf	1420	57	262	3050	0	11.0	1.0	1	7%
multigrain	2 slices	391	16	77	2040	0	3.0	1.0	1	7%
onion herb	1 loaf	1430	52	263	2390	0	13.0	0.0	1	9%
pita pocket	2 slices	80	3	18	0	0	1.0	0.0	0	10%
ponsienne	1 loaf	1490	49	166	3380	0	4.0	0.0	1	4%
rye	2 slices	374	14	73	2170	0	4.0	0.0	1	9%
CHICKEN POT PIE	1 serving	440	18	46	1109	0	21.0	45.0	7	43%
COOKIE										
chocolate chip	1 cookie	280	2	37	70	0	15.0	25.0	9	46%
chocolate chunk, w/pecan, 'Gourmet'	1 cookie	290	3	37	200	0	17.0	10.0	6	49%
cookie, oatmeal, oatmeal raisin, 'Gourmet'	1 cookie	250	4	41	230	0	9.0	10.0	0	31%
peanut butter, 'Gourmet'	1 cookie	290	7	33	250	0	15.0	10.0	6	46%
shortbread, 'Gourmet'	1 cookie	425	5	46	385	0	26.0	68.0	16	53%
white chocolate chunk, w/pecan, 'Gourmet'	1 cookie	300	3	37	200	0	17.0	10.0	6	49%
CROISSANT										
almond	1 croissant	420	8	41	250	0	25.0	95.0	12	53%
apple	1 croissant	250	4	38	150	0	10.0	25.0	6	35%
blueberry cheese	1 croissant	380	7	44	280	0	20.0	60.0	12	47%
chocolate	1 croissant	400	5	46	220	0	24.0	35.0	14	51%
cinnamon raisin	1 croissant	390	7	60	240	0	13.0	35.0	8	30%
coconut pecan	1 croissant	440	7	51	290	0	23.0	45.0	12	47%
hazelnut chocolate	1 croissant	480	6	56	220	0	28.0	35.0	14	50%
croissant, plain	1 croissant	220	5	29	240	0	10.0	25.0	6	40%
raspberry cheese	1 croissant	400	7	49	280	0	20.0	60.0	12	45%
strawberry cheese	1 croissant	400	7	49	280	0	20.0	60.0	12	45%
sweet cheese	1 croissant	420	8	45	310	0	23.0	70.0	14	49%
MUFFIN										
blueberry, gourmet	1 muffin	390	8	66	410	0	4.0	40.0	0	11%
bran, gourmet	1 muffin	390	7	73	940	0	11.0	20.0	0	24%
carrot, gourmet	1 muffin	450	7	58	610	0	22.0	15.0	5	43%
corn, gourmet	1 muffin	460	8	71	510	0	17.0	25.0	3	33%
cranberry walnut, gourmet	1 muffin	350	7	53	730	0	13.0	15.0	0	33%
oat bran apple gourmet	1 muffin	400	7	71	590	0	2.0	0.0	0	5%
pumpkin gourmet	1 muffin	410	6	63	500	0	16.0	20.0	2	34%
whole grain, gourmet	1 muffin	440	10	68	310	0	16.0	30.0	2	32%
PASTRY										
cheese Danish	1 Danish	390	8	43	530	2	22.0	78.0	12	49%
cherry Danish	1 Danish	335	7	42	480	2	16.0	50.0	8	42%
cherry dumpling Danish	1 Danish	360	5	59	255	1	13.0	0.0	2	31%
raspberry Danish	1 Danish	335	6	43	480	2	16.0	50.0	8	42%
ROLL										
'Alpine'	1 roll	220	8	43	810	0	3.0	0.0	0	12%
braided	1 roll	387	10	64	1540	0	11.0	34.0	3	25%

Food Name	Serving Size	Calories	Prot. gms	Carbs gms	Sod. mgs	Fiber gms	Fat gms	Sat. Fat gms	Chol. mgs	% Fat Cal.
country seed	1 roll	220	9	37	460	0	4.0	0.0	0	16%
croissant	1 roll	300	7	38	240	0	14.0	35.0	8	41%
French	1 roll	320	10	65	710	0	1.0	0.0	0	3%
hearth	1 roll	370	16	69	600	0	3.0	0.0	0	7%
'Petit Pain'	1 roll	220	7	44	490	0	1.0	0.0	0	4%
pumpernickel	1 roll	210	8	42	1005	0	2.0	0.0	0	8%
raisin	1 roll	250	8	46	480	0	4.0	0.0	0	14%
rye	1 roll	230	8	44	0	0	2.0	0.0	0	8%
soft	1 roll	310	8	50	410	0	8.0	0.0	0	24%
vegetable	1 roll	230	6	40	410	0	5.0	0.0	0	20%
SALAD										
garden, small	1 salad	20	5	5	10	0	1.0	0.0	0	18%
garden w/grilled chicken	1 salad	110	14	9	330	0	2.0	30.0	0	16%
garden w/shrimp	1 salad	102	11	8	193	0	2.0	105.0	0	19%
garden w/tuna	1 salad	350	21	11	480	0	25.0	40.0	4	64%
Italian, low-calorie	1 salad	68	0	3	360	0	6.0	5.0	0	82%
SANDWICH										
chicken, cracked pepper, on French roll	1 sandwich	440	33	66	1390	0	3.0	50.0	0	6%
chicken, cracked pepper, on hearth roll	1 sandwich	490	39	70	1280	0	5.0	50.0	0	9%
chicken, cracked pepper, on soft roll	1 sandwich	430	31	51	1090	0	10.0	50.0	0	22%
chicken, grilled, on French roll	1 sandwich	450	33	66	1320	0	5.0	60.0	0	10%
chicken, grilled, on hearth roll	1 sandwich	500	39	70	1210	0	7.0	60.0	0	13%
chicken, grilled, on soft roll	1 sandwich	440	31	51	1020	0	12.0	60.0	0	25%
chicken, tarragon, on French roll	1 sandwich	590	34	68	1014	0	16.0	70.0	0	26%
chicken, tarragon, on hearth roll	1 sandwich	640	40	72	904	0	18.0	70.0	0	27%
chicken, tarragon, on soft roll	1 sandwich	580	32	53	714	0	23.0	70.0	0	38%
ham, on French roll	1 sandwich	470	27	68	1680	0	8.0	115.0	0	16%
ham, on hearth roll	1 sandwich	520	33	72	1570	0	10.0	115.0	0	18%
ham, on soft roll	1 sandwich	460	25	53	1380	0	15.0	115.0	0	30%
ham and cheese croissant, hot, filled	1 sandwich	370	10	38	280	0	20.0	55.0	12	48%
roast beef, on French roll	1 sandwich	500	34	66	1020	0	9.0	60.0	0	17%
roast beef, on hearth roll	1 sandwich	550	40	70	910	0	11.0	60.0	0	18%
roast beef, on soft roll	1 sandwich	490	32	51	720	0	16.0	60.0	0	30%
spinach and cheese croissant, hot, filled	1 sandwich	290	9	29	310	0	16.0	45.0	10	49%
turkey and cheddar croissant, hot, filled	1 sandwich	410	16	38	680	0	22.0	70.0	13	48%
turkey and havarti croissant, hot, filled	1 sandwich	410	17	38	630	0	21.0	70.0	13	46%
turkey sandwich, smoked, on French roll	1 sandwich	420	32	65	1660	0	2.0	35.0	0	4%
turkey sandwich, smoked, on hearth roll	1 sandwich	470	38	69	1550	0	4.0	35.0	0	8%
turkey sandwich, smoked, on soft roll	1 sandwich	410	30	50	1360	0	9.0	35.0	0	20%
SANDWICH FILLING										
boursin cheese	1 serving	290	6	2	390	0	29.0	90.0	18	89%
brie cheese	1 serving	300	18	3	510	0	24.0	85.0	15	72%
provolone cheese	1 serving	155	10	1	180	0	12.6	36.0	7	72%
SOUP										
beef barley	1 bowl	112	9	15	901	0	3.0	18.0	0	22%
beef barley	1 cup	75	6	10	600	0	2.0	12.0	0	22%
broccoli, cream of	1 bowl	302	8	18	219	0	26.0	54.0	12	69%
broccoli, cream of	1 cup	201	5	12	146	0	17.0	36.0	8	69%
chicken, w/noodle	1 bowl	119	12	14	743	0	1.7	26.0	1	13%
chicken, w/noodle	1 cup	79	8	9	495	0	1.0	17.0	1	12%
chili, vegetarian	1 bowl	208	9	37	763	0	4.0	0.0	1	16%
chili, vegetarian	1 cup	139	6	24	508	0	3.0	0.0	1	18%
clam chowder	1 bowl	433	17	36	1029	0	27.0	90.0	15	53%
clam chowder	1 cup	289	11	24	687	0	18.0	60.0	9	54%

Food Name	Serving Size	Calories	Prot. gms	Carbs gms	Sod. mgs	Fiber gms	Fat gms	Sat. Fat gms	Chol. mgs	% Fat Cal.
minestrone	1 cup	105	5	20	265	0	2.0	1.0	0	15%
split pea	1 bowl	264	18	45	453	0	2.0	1.0	0	7%
split pea	1 cup	176	12	30	303	0	1.0	1.0	0	5%
tomato Florentine	1 bowl	92	4	15	221	0	1.7	0.0	1	17%
tomato Florentine	1 cup	61	3	10	147	0	1.0	0.0	1	15%
vegetarian, garden	1 bowl	44	2	9	92	0	1.0	0.0	1	17%
vegetarian, garden	1 cup	29	1	6	61	0	1.0	0.0	1	24%

BASKIN ROBBINS
ICE
grape	1/2 cup	100	0	27	10	0	0.0	0.0	0	0%
margarita	1/2 cup	110	0	28	10	0	0.0	0.0	0	0%

ICE CREAM
'Berries 'n Banana,' sugarless	1/2 cup	80	4	15	55	0	1.0	5.0	1	11%
'Call Me Nuts,' sugarless	1/2 cup	110	3	21	55	1	2.0	5.0	1	16%
'Cappuccino Blast,' w/whipped cream	1 serving	160	3	22	60	0	7.0	30.0	4	39%
'Caramel Banana Surprise,' nonfat	1/2 cup	110	3	24	95	0	0.0	0.0	0	0%
caramel praline, soft serve, nonfat	1/2 cup	120	4	25	85	0	0.0	0.0	0	0%
'Cherry Cordial,' sugarless	1/2 cup	100	3	18	55	0	2.0	5.0	2	18%
chocolate chip, 'Chillyburger'	1 serving	220	4	27	100	1	11.0	25.0	7	44%
chocolate chip, sugarless	1/2 cup	100	4	17	70	0	2.5	5.5	2	21%
chocolate chip, sugarless, 'Low, Lite 'n Luscious'	1 serving	100	3	20	0	0	2.0	4.0	0	16%
chocolate marshmallow, nonfat	1/2 cup	110	4	26	75	1	0.0	0.0	0	0%
chocolate vanilla twist, nonfat	1/2 cup	100	4	21	100	0	0.0	0.0	0	0%
'Chocolate Wonder,' nonfat	1/2 cup	90	4	20	70	1	0.0	0.0	0	0%
'Chunky Banana,' sugarless	1/2 cup	90	3	16	55	0	1.5	5.0	1	15%
coconut fudge, sugarless	1/2 cup	110	3	20	60	1	1.5	5.0	1	13%
'Double Raspberry,' light	1/2 cup	90	3	16	40	0	2.0	10.0	1	19%
espresso, light	1/2 cup	110	3	18	55	0	4.0	10.0	3	30%
'Jamoca Swirl,' nonfat	1/2 cup	110	3	23	105	0	0.0	0.0	0	0%
'Jamoca Swiss Almond,' sugarless	1/2 cup	100	3	16	65	0	2.5	5.0	2	23%
'Just Chocolate Vanilla' dairy, nonfat	1/2 cup	100	4	21	60	0	0.0	0.0	0	0%
'Just Peachy' dairy, nonfat	1/2 cup	100	3	22	60	0	0.0	0.0	0	0%
'Kookaberry Kiwi,' nonfat	1/2 cup	90	3	20	90	0	0.0	0.0	0	0%
'Mocha Cappuccino Blast,' nonfat	1 serving	120	3	26	75	0	0.0	0.0	0	0%
peach, nonfat	1/2 cup	100	3	22	90	0	0.0	0.0	0	0%
peanut butter cream, nonfat	1/2 cup	100	4	21	110	0	0.0	0.0	0	0%
pineapple cheesecake, nonfat	1/2 cup	110	3	24	100	0	0.0	0.0	0	0%
pineapple coconut, sugarless	1/2 cup	90	3	16	60	0	1.5	5.0	1	15%
'Pistachio Creme Chip,' light	1/2 cup	120	4	17	55	0	4.0	10.0	3	30%
'Pralines 'n Cream'	1 scoop	280	4	35	180	0	14.0	36.0	0	45%
praline, light	1/2 cup	120	3	18	65	0	4.0	10.0	2	30%
'Raspberry Revelation' sugarless	1/2 cup	100	3	20	55	1	1.0	5.0	1	9%
'Rocky Path,' light	1/2 cup	130	4	19	55	1	4.0	10.0	2	28%
strawberry, sugarless, 'Low, Lite 'n Luscious'	1 serving	80	2	17	70	0	1.0	3.0	0	11%
'Strawberry Royal,' light	1/2 cup	110	2	19	120	0	3.0	9.0	0	24%
vanilla, soft serve, nonfat	1/2 cup	120	5	25	85	0	0.0	0.0	0	0%
'Thin Mint,' sugarless	1/2 cup	100	3	16	65	0	2.5	5.0	2	23%
'Vanilla Bean,' nonfat	1/2 cup	100	4	20	110	0	0.0	0.0	0	0%
'Vanilla Swiss Almond,' sugarless	1/2 cup	110	3	20	60	1	2.0	5.0	2	16%

ICE CREAM BAR
'Cappuccino Blast'	1 bar	120	2	18	35	0	5.0	20.0	3	36%
'Sundae Bars' chocolate, caramel ribbon, light	1 bar	150	3	24	75	0	5.0	11.0	0	29%

ICE CREAM CONE
waffle, cone and cup, plain	1 cone	140	3	28	5	0	2.0	0.0	0	13%

Food Name	Serving Size	Calories	Prot. gms	Carbs gms	Sod. mgs	Fiber gms	Fat gms	Sat. Fat gms	Chol. mgs	% Fat Cal.
sugar, cone and cup, plain	1 cone	60	1	11	45	0	1.0	0.0	0	16%
SHERBET										
orange	1/2 cup	120	1	26	25	0	1.5	5.0	1	11%
rainbow	1/2 cup	120	1	26	25	0	1.5	5.0	1	11%
SORBET										
fruit whip, nonfat	1 serving	80	0	24	20	0	0.0	0.0	0	0%
raspberry cranberry	1/2 cup	110	0	29	10	0	0.0	0.0	0	0%
red raspberry	1/2 cup	120	0	30	10	0	0.0	0.0	0	0%
strawberry, soft-serve, nonfat	1 serving	100	0	20	20	0	0.0	0.0	0	0%
TOPPING										
butterscotch	1 oz	100	1	24	80	0	1.0	3.0	1	9%
hot fudge	1 oz	100	1	17	45	0	3.0	0.0	1	27%
hot fudge, nonfat, sugar-free	1 oz	90	2	20	96	1	0.0	0.0	0	0%
praline caramel	1 oz	90	0	19	105	0	0.0	0.0	0	0%
strawberry	1 oz	60	0	14	5	0	0.0	0.0	0	0%
YOGURT, FROZEN										
black cherry, nonfat	1/2 cup	110	3	24	50	0	0.0	0.0	0	0%
blueberry, lowfat	1/2 cup	120	4	24	70	0	1.5	5.0	1	11%
cheesecake, lowfat	1/2 cup	120	4	21	75	0	1.5	10.0	1	12%
chocolate, lowfat	1/2 cup	120	5	23	75	0	1.5	5.0	1	11%
chocolate, lowfat, large	9 oz	315	9	54	90	0	9.0	9.0	0	24%
chocolate, lowfat, medium	7 oz	246	7	42	70	0	7.0	7.0	0	24%
chocolate mint, nonfat	1/2 cup	100	4	23	60	1	0.0	0.0	0	0%
coconut, nonfat, large	9 oz	180	9	45	90	0	0.0	0.0	0	0%
coconut, nonfat, medium	7 oz	140	7	35	70	0	0.0	0.0	0	0%
coconut, nonfat, small	5 oz	100	5	25	50	0	0.0	0.0	0	0%
Dutch chocolate, nonfat	1/2 cup	100	4	23	60	1	0.0	0.0	0	0%
'For Heaven's Cake,' low-fat	1/2 cup	120	3	24	75	0	2.0	10.0	2	14%
'Have Your Cake,' low-fat	1/2 cup	110	4	22	100	0	1.0	4.0	1	8%
Kahlua frozen, nonfat	1/2 cup	100	3	21	55	0	0.0	0.0	0	0%
key lime nonfat	1/2 cup	100	3	22	55	0	0.0	0.0	0	0%
'Mango in Paradise,' nonfat	1/2 cup	130	4	28	70	1	0.0	0.0	0	0%
maple walnut, nonfat	1/2 cup	100	3	22	55	0	0.0	0.0	0	0%
peach, nonfat	1/2 cup	100	3	22	50	0	0.0	0.0	0	0%
'Peppermint Twist,' nonfat	1/2 cup	100	3	22	55	0	0.0	0.0	0	0%
pina colada, nonfat	1/2 cup	110	3	22	50	0	0.0	0.0	0	0%
raspberry, nonfat	1/2 cup	100	3	22	55	0	0.0	0.0	0	0%
raspberry, nonfat, large	9 oz	225	9	45	90	0	0.0	0.0	0	0%
raspberry, nonfat, medium	7 oz	164	7	35	70	0	0.0	0.0	0	0%
raspberry, nonfat, small	5 oz	125	5	25	50	0	0.0	0.0	0	0%
strawberry, low-fat, large	9 oz	270	9	54	90	0	9.0	9.0	0	24%
strawberry, low-fat, medium	7 oz	211	7	42	70	0	7.0	7.0	0	24%
strawberry, low-fat, small	5 oz	150	5	30	50	0	5.0	5.0	0	24%
strawberry, nonfat	1/2 cup	100	3	23	55	0	0.0	0.0	0	0%
strawberry, nonfat, large	9 oz	225	9	45	90	0	0.0	0.0	0	0%
strawberry, nonfat, medium	7 oz	176	7	35	70	0	0.0	0.0	0	0%
vanilla, low-fat, large	9 oz	270	9	54	90	0	9.0	9.0	0	24%
vanilla, low-fat, medium	7 oz	211	7	42	70	0	7.0	7.0	0	24%
vanilla, nonfat	1/2 cup	110	4	23	65	0	0.0	0.0	0	0%

BIG BOY RESTAURANT
DESSERT

Food Name	Serving Size	Calories	Prot. gms	Carbs gms	Sod. mgs	Fiber gms	Fat gms	Sat. Fat gms	Chol. mgs	% Fat Cal.
'No-no' frozen	1 serving	75	2	17	36	0	0.0	0.0	0	0%
yogurt, frozen, nonfat	1 serving	72	2	16	31	0	0.0	0.0	0	0%

Food Name	Serving Size	Calories	Prot. gms	Carbs gms	Sod. mgs	Fiber gms	Fat gms	Sat. Fat gms	Chol. mgs	% Fat Cal.
ENTRÉE										
chicken and vegetable stir-fry	1 serving	562	43	68	750	0	14.0	68.0	0	22%
chicken breast, w/salad, no dressing, oat bran bread	1 serving	349	38	20	342	0	13.0	65.0	0	34%
chicken breast, w/mozzarella, salad, no dressing, bread	1 serving	370	42	24	353	0	12.0	76.0	0	29%
chicken, Cajun, w/salad, no dressing, oat bran bread	1 serving	349	38	20	612	0	13.0	65.0	0	34%
cod, baked, w/salad, no dressing, oat bran bread	1 serving	364	43	20	371	0	12.0	68.0	0	30%
cod, Dijon, baked, w/salad, no dressing, bread	1 serving	427	44	21	567	0	18.0	68.0	0	38%
cod, broiled, w/salad, no dressing, oat bran bread	1 serving	364	43	20	371	0	12.0	68.0	0	30%
cod, Dijon, broiled, w/salad, no dressing, bread	1 serving	427	44	21	567	0	18.0	68.0	0	38%
cod, Cajun, w/salad, no dressing, oat bran bread	1 serving	364	43	20	461	0	12.0	68.0	0	30%
spaghetti marinara, w/salad, no dressing, oat bran bread	1 serving	450	15	87	761	0	6.0	8.0	0	12%
vegetable stir-fry	1 serving	408	9	74	703	0	10.0	0.0	0	21%
SALAD										
chicken breast, Dijon	1 salad	391	42	31	415	0	11.0	65.0	0	25%
dinner, no dressing	1 salad	19	1	4	11	0	0.0	0.0	0	0%
SALAD DRESSING, buttermilk	1 serving	36	0	4	151	0	2.0	10.0	0	53%
SANDWICH										
chicken w/mozzarella, on pita, 'Heart Smart'	1 sandwich	404	42	26	421	0	13.0	76.0	0	30%
turkey, on pita, 'Heart Smart'	1 sandwich	224	22	24	833	0	5.0	75.0	0	20%
SIDE DISH										
corn	1 serving	90	3	21	1	0	1.0	0.0	0	9%
mixed vegetables	1 serving	27	2	5	42	0	0.0	0.0	0	0%
potato, baked	1 serving	163	5	37	7	0	0.0	0.0	0	0%
rice	1 serving	114	3	25	633	0	0.0	0.0	0	0%
roll	1 roll	139	3	30	187	0	0.0	2.0	0	0%
SOUP										
cabbage	1 bowl	43	2	9	727	0	1.0	1.0	0	17%
cabbage	1 cup	37	2	8	623	0	0.0	1.0	0	0%
BOJANGLES										
BISCUIT	1 serving	239	4	30	588	0	11.0	1.0	0	42%
CHICKEN										
breast, no skin, 'Southern'	3.5 oz	239	25	10	766	0	11.5	91.7	0	43%
breast, no skin, 'Southern'	4 oz	271	28	11	869	0	13.0	104.0	0	43%
leg, no skin, 'Southern'	1.8 oz	128	7	5	312	0	12.0	54.0	0	69%
leg, no skin, 'Southern'	3.5 oz	251	14	10	611	0	23.5	105.8	0	69%
thigh, no skin, 'Southern'	3.5 oz	291	21	11	653	0	18.7	97.0	0	57%
thigh, no skin, 'Southern'	3.2 oz	264	19	10	592	0	17.0	88.0	0	57%
SANDWICH, chicken fillet, grilled, no mayo	1 sandwich	329	27	37	418	0	7.0	59.0	0	20%
SIDE DISH										
coleslaw	1 serving	105	1	19	406	0	4.0	0.0	0	31%
dirty rice	1 serving	167	5	21	397	0	7.0	12.0	0	38%
pinto bean, Cajun	1 serving	124	6	25	463	0	0.0	0.0	0	0%
BONANZA RESTAURANTS										
HALIBUT FILLET										
	6 oz	139	26	3	128	0	2.0	60.0	0	13%
	3.5 oz	82	15	2	75	0	1.2	35.3	0	13%
RIBEYE STEAK										
	5.5 oz	196	28	1	563	0	8.0	50.0	0	38%
	3.5 oz	126	18	1	361	0	5.1	32.1	0	38%
BOSTON MARKET										
CHICKEN										
drumstick, Tabasco barbecue	1 drumstick	130	14	4	190	0	6.0	50.0	2	43%

Food Name	Serving Size	Calories	Prot. gms	Carbs gms	Sod. mgs	Fiber gms	Fat gms	Sat. Fat gms	Chol. mgs	% Fat Cal.
1/4 chicken, dark meat, w/o skin	1/4 chicken	190	22	1	440	0	10.0	115.0	3	49%
1/4 chicken, dark meat, w/skin	1/4 chicken	320	30	2	500	0	21.0	155.0	6	60%
1/4 chicken, teriyaki, dark meat, w/skin	1/4 chicken	340	40	17	890	0	12.0	135.0	4	32%
1/4 chicken, teriyaki, dark meat, w/skin	1/4 chicken	380	30	17	870	0	21.0	155.0	6	50%
1/4 chicken, w/skin	1/4 chicken	590	70	4	1010	0	33.0	280.0	10	50%
1/4 chicken, w/wing, white meat, w/skin	1/4 chicken	280	0	2	510	0	12.0	135.0	4	93%
1/4 chicken, w/o wing, white meat, w/o skin	1/4 chicken	170	33	2	480	0	4.0	85.0	1	20%
Southwest, savory	1 portion	400	40	26	1670	4	15.0	100.0	5	34%
triple topped	1 portion	470	50	20	1350	1	22.0	155.0	12	41%
wing, Tabasco barbecue	1 wing	110	9	4	170	0	7.0	30.0	2	55%
CHICKEN POT PIE	1 pie	780	32	61	1480	4	46.0	135.0	13	53%
CORNBREAD	1 loaf	200	3	33	390	1	6.0	25.0	2	27%
DESSERT										
brownie	1 piece	450	6	47	190	3	27.0	80.0	7	53%
chocolate chip cookie	1 cookie	340	4	48	240	1	17.0	25.0	6	42%
cinnamon apple pie	1/5 pie	390	2	46	250	2	23.0	0.0	4	52%
GRAVY, chicken	1 oz	15	0	2	170	0	1.0	0.0	0	53%
HAM, Boston hearth, lean	5 oz	210	25	9	1490	0	9.0	75.0	4	37%
MEAT LOAF										
w/brown gravy	7 oz	390	30	19	1040	1	22.0	120.0	8	50%
w/chunky tomato sauce	8 oz	370	30	22	1170	2	18.0	120.0	8	44%
SALAD										
Caesar, entrée	10 oz	510	17	17	1130	3	42.0	35.0	11	74%
Caesar, side	4 oz	200	7	7	450	1	17.0	15.0	5	73%
Caesar, w/o dressing	8 oz	230	16	14	500	3	12.0	20.0	6	47%
chicken Caesar	13 oz	650	43	17	1580	3	45.0	105.0	12	63%
chicken, chunky	3/4 cup	370	28	3	800	1	27.0	120.0	5	66%
tossed, individual, w/Caesar dressing	1 salad	380	5	18	810	3	31.0	15.0	5	75%
tossed, individual, w/fat-free ranch dressing	1 salad	160	5	29	940	4	2.5	0.0	0	14%
tossed, individual, w/old Venice dressing	1 salad	340	4	20	1110	3	27.0	0.0	4	72%
SANDWICH										
barbecue chicken	1 sandwich	540	30	84	1690	3	9.0	75.0	3	15%
barbecue chicken pastry	1 sandwich	640	17	56	1260	1	39.0	60.0	12	55%
broccoli chicken cheddar pastry	1 sandwich	690	21	45	1050	2	47.0	85.0	13	62%
chicken, w/cheese and sauce sandwich	1 sandwich	750	41	72	1860	5	33.0	135.0	12	40%
chicken, w/o cheese and sauce	1 sandwich	430	34	62	910	4	4.5	65.0	1	10%
chicken salad	1 sandwich	680	39	63	1360	4	30.0	120.0	5	40%
ham, w/cheese and sauce	1 sandwich	750	38	72	1730	5	34.0	100.0	12	41%
ham and cheddar pastry	1 sandwich	640	19	47	1560	1	41.0	60.0	13	58%
ham sub, w/o cheese and sauce	1 sandwich	440	25	66	1450	4	8.0	45.0	3	17%
Italian chicken pastry	1 sandwich	630	21	43	910	2	41.0	60.0	12	59%
meatloaf, w/cheese	1 sandwich	860	46	95	2270	6	33.0	165.0	16	34%
meatloaf, w/o cheese	1 sandwich	690	40	86	1610	6	21.0	120.0	7	27%
turkey, open faced	1 sandwich	500	37	61	2170	3	12.0	80.0	2	22%
turkey, w/cheese and sauce	1 sandwich	710	45	68	1390	4	28.0	110.0	10	36%
turkey club	1 sandwich	650	39	64	1590	4	26.0	105.0	8	36%
turkey sub, w/o cheese and sauce	1 sandwich	400	45	61	1070	4	3.5	60.0	1	7%
SIDE DISH										
applesauce, cinnamon	3/4 cup	250	0	56	45	3	4.5	0.0	1	15%
applesauce, cinnamon, low-fat, chunky	3/4 cup	250	1	62	30	2	0.0	0.0	0	0%
barbecue baked beans	3/4 cup	270	8	48	540	12	5.0	0.0	2	17%
black rice and beans	1 cup	300	8	45	1050	5	10.0	0.0	2	30%
broccoli cauliflower au gratin	3/4 cup	200	9	14	600	3	11.0	20.0	7	52%
broccoli rice casserole	3/4 cup	240	5	26	800	2	12.0	40.0	8	47%
broccoli w/red peppers	3/4 cup	60	3	5	130	3	3.5	0.0	1	50%
butternut squash, low-fat	3/4 cup	160	2	25	580	3	6.0	15.0	4	33%

Food Name	Serving Size	Calories	Prot. gms	Carbs gms	Sod. mgs	Fiber gms	Fat gms	Sat. Fat gms	Chol. mgs	% Fat Cal.
carrots, honey glazed	3/4 cup	280	1	35	80	4	15.0	0.0	3	48%
chili, chicken	1 cup	220	18	21	1000	6	7.0	40.0	2	29%
coleslaw	3/4 cup	300	2	30	540	3	19.0	20.0	3	57%
corn, whole kernel	3/4 cup	180	5	30	170	2	4.0	0.0	1	20%
coyote bean salad	3/4 cup	190	4	24	210	9	9.0	0.0	1	42%
cranberry relish, low-fat	3/4 cup	370	2	84	5	5	5.0	0.0	1	12%
fruit salad	3/4 cup	70	1	15	10	1	0.5	0.0	0	7%
green beans	3/4 cup	80	1	5	200	3	6.0	0.0	0	69%
green bean casserole	3/4 cup	130	2	10	440	2	9.0	20.0	5	63%
macaroni and cheese	3/4 cup	280	13	32	830	1	11.0	30.0	6	35%
potato, baked, sweet low-fat	1 potato	460	6	94	510	10	7.0	0.0	1	14%
potato, mashed, homestyle	2/3 cup	190	3	24	570	1	9.0	25.0	6	43%
potato, mashed, homestyle, w/gravy	3/4 cup	210	4	26	740	1	10.0	25.0	6	43%
potato, new, low-fat	3/4 cup	130	3	25	150	2	2.5	0.0	0	17%
potato planks, oven-roasted, low-fat	5 planks	180	3	32	370	3	5.0	0.0	1	24%
potato salad, old-fashioned	3/4 cup	340	2	30	870	2	24.0	30.0	4	63%
red beans and rice, low-fat	1 cup	260	8	45	1050	4	5.0	5.0	0	18%
rice pilaf	2/3 cup	180	5	32	600	2	5.0	0.0	1	23%
spinach, creamed	3/4 cup	260	9	11	740	2	20.0	55.0	13	69%
squash casserole	3/4 cup	330	7	20	1110	3	24.0	70.0	13	67%
stuffing, savory	3/4 cup	310	6	44	1140	3	12.0	0.0	2	35%
sweet potato casserole	3/4 cup	280	3	39	190	2	18.0	10.0	5	49%
vegetables, steamed, low-fat	2/3 cup	35	2	7	35	3	0.5	0.0	0	11%
zucchini marinana, low-fat	3/4 cup	60	1	7	330	2	3.0	0.0	0	46%
SOUP										
chicken noodle	1 cup	130	11	12	1310	2	4.5	40.0	1	31%
chicken tortilla	1 cup	220	10	19	1410	2	11.0	35.0	4	46%
potato	1 cup	270	8	24	1020	2	16.0	40.0	8	53%
tomato bisque	1 cup	280	4	16	1280	2	23.0	50.0	10	72%
TURKEY, breast, rotisserie, skinless, low-fat	5 oz	170	36	1	850	0	1.0	100.0	1	6%

BRAUM'S

Food Name	Serving Size	Calories	Prot. gms	Carbs gms	Sod. mgs	Fiber gms	Fat gms	Sat. Fat gms	Chol. mgs	% Fat Cal.
	1 serving	180	3	16	35	0	3.0	0.0	0	26%
diet, sugarless, w/NutraSweet	1 serving	90	3	13	0	0	3.0	0.0	0	30%
nonfat	1 serving	90	4	20	55	0	0.0	0.0	0	0%
'Premium Light'	1 serving	102	3	15	0	56	3.0	0.0	0	27%

BRAZIER. See DAIRY QUEEN/BRAZIER.

BRESLER'S

Food Name	Serving Size	Calories	Prot. gms	Carbs gms	Sod. mgs	Fiber gms	Fat gms	Sat. Fat gms	Chol. mgs	% Fat Cal.
ICE CREAM, 'Royal Lites,' all flavors	1 serving	132	5	9	70	0	5.0	16.0	0	45%
SHERBET, all flavors	1 serving	160	1	34	0	0	2.0	6.0	0	11%
YOGURT, FROZEN										
gourmet, all flavors	1 serving	116	4	22	0	0	2.0	7.0	0	15%
nonfat, all flavors	1 serving	108	4	24	0	0	0.0	0.0	0	0%

BURGER CHEF
BREAKFAST

Food Name	Serving Size	Calories	Prot. gms	Carbs gms	Sod. mgs	Fiber gms	Fat gms	Sat. Fat gms	Chol. mgs	% Fat Cal.
sausage biscuit	1 serving	418	16	33	1313	0	25.0	45.0	0	53%
scrambled eggs and bacon platter	1 serving	567	21	50	1108	0	31.0	0.0	0	50%
scrambled eggs and sausage platter	1 serving	668	26	50	1411	0	40.0	479.0	0	54%
'Sunrise' w/bacon	1 serving	392	19	30	978	0	21.0	384.0	0	49%
'Sunrise' w/sausage	1 sandwich	526	26	30	1412	0	33.0	419.0	0	57%
CHEESEBURGER										
regular	1 serving	278	14	28	641	0	12.0	37.0	0	39%
double patty	1 serving	402	23	28	835	0	22.0	74.0	0	49%

Food Name	Serving Size	Calories	Prot. gms	Carbs gms	Sod. mgs	Fiber gms	Fat gms	Sat. Fat gms	Chol. mgs	% Fat Cal.
DESSERT, apple turnover	1 serving	237	2	38	0	0	9.0	0.0	0	34%
HAMBURGER										
'Big Chef'	1 serving	556	22	37	840	0	36.0	78.0	0	58%
mushroom, single patty	1 serving	520	28	34	744	0	29.0	92.0	0	51%
regular	1 serving	235	11	27	480	0	9.0	27.0	0	35%
'Super Chef'	1 serving	604	27	35	1088	0	39.0	99.0	0	59%
'Top Chef'	1 serving	541	30	29	1007	0	33.0	100.0	0	56%
HAMBURGER MEAL, 'Funmeal'	1 serving	514	14	85	513	0	19.0	27.0	0	30%
SANDWICH										
chicken club	1 sandwich	521	36	33	0	0	25.0	0.0	0	45%
'Fisherman's Fillet'	1 sandwich	534	26	41	0	0	32.0	0.0	0	52%
SIDE DISH										
french fries, large	1 serving	285	4	36	456	0	14.0	0.0	0	44%
french fries, regular	1 serving	204	3	26	327	0	10.0	0.0	0	44%
'Hash Rounds'	1 serving	235	3	26	349	0	14.0	0.0	0	52%
salad, lettuce	1 salad	11	1	3	8	0	0.0	0.0	0	0%
BURGER KING										
BEVERAGE										
chocolate shake, medium	1 serving	440	12	75	330	4	10.0	30.0	6	21%
chocolate shake, medium, syrup added	1 serving	570	14	105	520	3	10.0	30.0	6	16%
chocolate shake, small	1 serving	330	9	58	250	3	7.0	25.0	4	19%
chocolate shake, small, syrup added	1 serving	390	10	72	350	2	7.0	20.0	4	16%
'Coca-Cola Classic,' medium	22 fl oz	280	0	70	na	0	0.0	0.0	0	0%
coffee	12 fl oz	5	0	1	5	0	0.0	0.0	0	0%
'Diet Coke,' medium	22 fl oz	1	0	0	na	0	0.0	0.0	0	0%
orange juice,'Tropicana'	10 fl oz	140	2	33	0	0	0.0	0.0	0	0%
milk, 2%	8 fl oz	130	8	12	120	0	5.0	20.0	3	36%
'Sprite,' medium	22 fl oz	260	0	66	na	0	0.0	0.0	0	0%
strawberry shake, medium, syrup added	1 medium	550	13	104	350	2	9.0	30.0	5	15%
strawberry shake, small, syrup added	1 serving	390	10	72	260	1	7.0	20.0	4	16%
vanilla shake, medium	1 medium	430	13	73	330	2	9.0	30.0	5	19%
vanilla shake, small	1 small	330	10	56	250	1	7.0	20.0	4	19%
BREAKFAST										
bacon	3 pieces	40	3	0	170	na	3.0	10.0	1	69%
biscuit	1 serving	300	6	35	830	1	15.0	0.0	3	45%
biscuit w/egg	1 sandwich	380	11	37	1010	1	21.0	140.0	5	50%
biscuit w/sausage	1 sandwich	490	13	36	1240	1	33.0	35.0	10	60%
biscuit w/sausage, egg and cheese	1 sandwich	620	20	37	1650	1	43.0	185.0	14	63%
'Cini-Minis' w/vanilla icing	1 serving	110	0	20	40	na	3.0	0.0	0	25%
'Cini-Minis' w/o vanilla icing	4 rolls	440	6	51	710	1	23.0	25.0	6	48%
'Croissan'wich' w/sausage and cheese	1 sandwich	450	13	21	940	1	35.0	45.0	12	70%
'Croissan'wich' w/sausage, egg, and cheese	1 sandwich	530	18	23	1120	1	41.0	185.0	13	69%
French toast sticks	5 sticks	440	7	51	490	3	23.0	2.0	5	47%
ham	1 serving	35	6	0	770	na	1.0	15.0	0	27%
hash brown rounds, large	1 serving	410	3	42	750	4	26.0	0.0	10	57%
hash brown rounds, small	1 serving	240	2	25	440	2	15.0	0.0	6	56%
BUN										
hamburger	1 serving	130	5	24	250	na	2.0	0.0	0	13%
'Whopper'	1 serving	220	8	39	370	na	4.0	0.0	1	16%
CHEESE, American, processed	2 slices	90	6	0	420	na	8.0	25.0	5	75%
CHEESEBURGER										
bacon double	1 serving	620	41	28	1230	1	38.0	125.0	18	55%
bacon	1 serving	400	24	27	940	1	22.0	70.0	10	49%
double patty	1 serving	580	38	27	1060	1	36.0	120.0	17	55%

Food Name	Serving Size	Calories	Prot. gms	Carbs gms	Sod. mgs	Fiber gms	Fat gms	Sat. Fat gms	Chol. mgs	% Fat Cal.
regular	1 serving	360	21	27	760	1	19.0	60.0	9	47%
'Double Whopper'	1 serving	1010	55	47	1460	3	67.0	180.0	26	60%
'Double Whopper' w/o mayo	1 serving	850	55	47	1460	3	50.0	180.0	26	52%
'Whopper'	1 serving	760	35	47	1380	3	48.0	110.0	17	57%
'Whopper' w/o mayo	1 serving	600	35	47	1380	3	31.0	110.0	17	46%
'Whopper Jr.'	1 serving	450	22	28	770	2	28.0	65.0	10	56%
'Whopper Jr.' w/o mayo	1 serving	370	22	28	770	2	19.0	65.0	10	46%
CHICKEN BREAST PATTY, 'BK Broiler'	1 serving	140	21	4	570	na	4.0	90.0	1	26%
CHICKEN TENDERS										
	5 pieces	230	14	11	590	0	14.0	40.0	4	56%
	4 pieces	180	11	9	470	0	11.0	30.0	3	55%
CONDIMENTS										
barbecue sauce, 'Bull's Eye'	1/2 oz	20	0	5	140	na	0.0	0.0	0	0%
butter, whipped, 'Land O' Lakes Classic Blend'	1 serving	65	0	0	75	na	7.0	0.0	1	100%
catsup	1/2 oz	15	0	4	180	na	0.0	0.0	0	0%
dip, 'A.M. Express'	1 serving	80	0	21	20	na	0.0	0.0	0	0%
dipping sauce	1 serving	170	0	2	200	na	17.0	0.0	3	95%
dipping sauce, barbecue	1 serving	35	0	9	400	na	0.0	0.0	0	0%
dipping sauce, honey flavored	1 serving	90	0	23	10	na	0.0	0.0	0	0%
dipping sauce, honey mustard	1 serving	90	0	10	150	na	6.0	10.0	1	57%
dipping sauce, sweet and sour	1 serving	45	0	11	50	na	0.0	0.0	0	0%
jam, grape, 'A.M. Express'	1 serving	30	0	7	0	na	0.0	0.0	0	0%
jam, strawberry, 'A.M. Express'	1 serving	30	0	8	0	na	0.0	0.0	0	0%
'King Sauce'	1/2 oz	70	0	2	70	na	7.0	4.0	1	89%
mustard	1/9 oz	0	0	0	40	na	0.0	0.0	0	0%
tartar sauce	1.5 oz	260	0	0	330	na	29.0	20.0	4	100%
DESSERT, Dutch apple pie	1 serving	300	3	39	230	2	15.0	0.0	3	45%
HAMBURGER										
'Big King'	1 burger	640	38	28	980	1	42.0	125.0	18	59%
'Double Whopper' w/o mayo	1 serving	760	49	47	980	3	42.0	155.0	21	50%
'Double Whopper'	1 serving	920	49	47	980	3	59.0	155.0	21	58%
regular	1 serving	320	19	27	520	1	15.0	50.0	6	42%
'Whopper'	1 serving	660	29	47	900	3	40.0	85.0	12	54%
'Whopper Jr.' w/o mayo	1 serving	320	19	28	530	2	15.0	55.0	8	42%
'Whopper Jr.'	1 serving	400	19	28	530	2	24.0	55.0	8	53%
'Whopper' w/o mayo	1 serving	510	29	47	900	3	23.0	85.0	12	41%
HAMBURGER PATTY										
regular	1 serving	170	14	0	55	na	13.0	50.0	6	68%
'Whopper'	1 serving	250	20	0	85	na	19.0	70.0	9	68%
LETTUCE	3/4 oz	0	0	0	0	na	0.0	0.0	0	0%
ONION	1/2 oz	5	0	1	0	na	0.0	0.0	0	0%
PICKLE	4 slices	0	0	0	140	na	0.0	0.0	0	0%
SANDWICH										
'Chick 'N Crisp'	1 sandwich	460	16	37	890	3	27.0	35.0	6	53%
'Chick 'N Crisp' w/o mayo	1 sandwich	360	16	37	890	3	16.0	35.0	6	40%
chicken	1 sandwich	710	26	54	1400	2	43.0	60.0	9	55%
chicken, w/o mayo	1 sandwich	500	26	54	1400	2	20.0	60.0	9	36%
chicken, 'BK Broiler'	1 sandwich	530	29	45	1060	2	26.0	105.0	5	44%
chicken, 'BK Broiler' w/o mayo	1 sandwich	370	29	45	1060	2	9.0	105.0	5	21%
fish, 'BK Big'	1 sandwich	720	23	59	1180	3	43.0	80.0	9	54%
SIDE DISH										
French fries, king size, salted	1 serving	590	5	74	1110	5	30.0	0.0	12	46%
French fries, medium, salted	1 serving	400	3	50	820	4	21.0	0.0	8	47%
French fries, medium, unsalted	1 serving	400	3	50	760	4	21.0	0.0	8	47%
French fries, small, salted	1 serving	250	2	32	550	2	13.0	0.0	5	46%

Food Name	Serving Size	Calories	Prot. gms	Carbs gms	Sod. mgs	Fiber gms	Fat gms	Sat. Fat gms	Chol. mgs	% Fat Cal.
French fries, small, unsalted	1 serving	250	2	32	480	2	13.0	0.0	5	46%
onion rings, king size, salted	1 serving	600	8	74	880	6	30.0	4.0	7	45%
onion rings, medium	1 serving	380	5	46	550	4	19.0	2.0	4	46%
TOMATO	2 slices	5	0	1	0	na	0.0	0.0	0	0%

CAPTAIN D'S
CONDIMENTS
salad dressing, Italian, nonfat, low-calorie	2 tbsp	9	0	2	568	0	0.0	0.0	0	0%
sweet and sour sauce	2 tbsp	52	0	13	5	0	0.0	0.0	0	0%

ENTRÉE
chicken, w/rice, green beans, breadstick, salad	1 serving	414	30	55	2615	0	8.0	71.0	0	17%
fish, baked, w/rice, green beans, breadstick, coleslaw	1 serving	659	36	62	1767	0	30.0	54.0	0	41%
orange roughy, w/rice, green beans, breadstick, salad	1 serving	537	35	56	2156	0	19.0	39.0	0	32%
shrimp, w/rice, green beans, breadstick, salad	1 serving	457	56	34	2194	0	10.0	191.0	0	20%

SIDE DISH
breadstick, plain	1 stick	91	3	17	210	0	1.0	0.0	0	10%
green beans, seasoned	1 serving	46	2	5	752	0	2.0	4.0	0	39%
rice serving	124	3	28	9	0.0	0.0	0	0%		
salad, dinner, no dressing	1 salad	27	1	3	67	0	1.0	1.0	0	36%
white bean	1 serving	126	8	22	99	0	1.0	2.0	0	7%

CARL'S JR.
BACON	2 strips	50	3	0	140	0	4.0	10.0	2	75%

BEVERAGE
chocolate shake	13.5 fl oz	390	9	74	280	0	7.0	30.0	5	16%
'Coca-Cola Classic' regular	16 fl oz	200	0	54	25	0	0.0	0.0	0	0%
coffee	12 fl oz	5	1	1	5	0	0.0	0.0	0	0%
'Diet Coke,' regular	16 fl oz	0	0	0	40	0	0.0	0.0	0	0%
'Diet 7-Up,' regular	16 fl oz	0	0	0	80	0	0.0	0.0	0	0%
'Dr. Pepper,' regular	16 fl oz	200	0	52	70	0	0.0	0.0	0	0%
hot chocolate	12 fl oz	110	2	22	80	1	2.0	0.0	2	16%
iced tea, regular	16 fl oz	5	0	0	55	0	0.0	0.0	0	0%
lemonade, 'Minute Maid' original style, regular	16 fl oz	190	0	52	95	0	0.0	0.0	0	0%
milk, 1%	10 fl oz	150	14	18	180	0	3.0	15.0	2	17%
'Nestea,' raspberry, regular	16 fl oz	160	0	42	40	0	0.0	0.0	0	0%
orange juice	10 fl oz	140	2	33	30	0	0.0	0.0	0	0%
orange soda, 'Minute Maid' regular	16 fl oz	210	0	58	20	0	0.0	0.0	0	0%
root beer, 'Barq's,' regular	16 fl oz	220	0	60	70	0	0.0	0.0	0	0%
'Sprite,' regular	16 fl oz	190	0	54	65	0	0.0	0.0	0	0%
strawberry shake	13.5 fl oz	400	9	77	240	0	7.0	30.0	5	15%
vanilla shake	13.5 fl oz	330	11	54	250	0	8.0	35.0	5	22%
BREADSTICK	1 stick	35	1	7	60	1	0.5	0.0	0	12%

BREAKFAST
burrito	1 burrito	480	27	26	750	2	30.0	465.0	13	56%
cheese Danish	1 serving	400	5	49	390	1	22.0	15.0	5	48%
English muffin, w/margarine	1 muffin	210	5	27	300	2	9.0	0.0	1	39%
French toast dips, w/o syrup	1 serving	370	6	42	430	1	20.0	0.0	3	48%
hash brown nuggets	1 serving	330	3	32	470	3	21.0	0.0	5	57%
quesadilla	1 quesadilla	310	14	27	670	2	16.0	230.0	6	47%
scrambled egg	1 egg	160	13	1	125	0	11.0	425.0	4	64%
'Sunrise Sandwich' no bacon or sausage	1 sandwich	360	14	28	700	2	21.0	225.0	5	53%

CHEESE
American	1 slice	60	3	0	280	0	5.0	15.0	3	79%
Swiss	1 slice	50	4	0	250	0	3.5	10.0	3	66%

Food Name	Serving Size	Calories	Prot. gms	Carbs gms	Sod. mgs	Fiber gms	Fat gms	Sat. Fat gms	Chol. mgs	% Fat Cal.
CHEESEBURGER										
double Western bacon	1 burger	900	51	64	1770	2	49.0	155.0	21	49%
Western bacon	1 burger	650	32	63	1430	2	30.0	80.0	12	42%
CHICKEN STARS	1 serving	280	12	15	330	0	19.0	40.0	5	61%
CONDIMENTS. See also Salad Dressing.										
barbecue sauce	1 pkt	50	1	11	270	0	0.0	0.0	0	0%
croutons, salad bar item	1 crouton	35	0	5	65	0	1.0	0.0	0	31%
honey sauce	1 pkt	90	0	22	0	0	0.0	0.0	0	0%
jam, strawberry	1 pkt	35	0	9	0	0	0.0	0.0	0	0%
jelly, grape	1 pkt	35	0	9	0	0	0.0	0.0	0	0%
mustard sauce	1 serving	50	0	11	210	0	0.0	0.0	0	0%
salsa	1 serving	10	0	2	160	0	0.0	0.0	0	0%
sweet and sour sauce	1 serving	50	0	12	80	0	0.0	0.0	0	0%
syrup, table	1 serving	90	0	21	0	0	0.0	0.0	0	0%
DESSERT										
chocolate cake	1 cake	300	3	49	260	4	10.0	23.0	3	30%
chocolate chip cookie	1 cookie	370	3	49	350	1	19.0	25.0	8	45%
strawberry swirl cheesecake	1 serving	290	6	30	230	0	17.0	55.0	9	52%
HAMBURGER										
'Famous Star'	1 burger	580	25	49	910	2	32.0	70.0	9	49%
'Jr.'	1 burger	330	18	34	480	1	13.0	45.0	5	36%
'Super Star'	1 burger	790	42	50	970	2	46.0	130.0	14	53%
SALAD										
'Salad-To-Go,' charbroiled chicken	1 salad	200	25	12	440	3	7.0	75.0	4	30%
'Salad-To-Go,' gardeb	1 salad	50	3	4	60	2	2.5	10.0	2	45%
SALAD DRESSING										
blue cheese	1 pkt	320	2	1	370	0	35.0	25.0	6	96%
French, nonfat	1 pkt	60	0	16	660	0	0.0	0.0	0	0%
house	1 pkt	220	1	3	440	0	22.0	20.0	4	93%
Italian, nonfat	1 pkt	15	0	4	770	0	0.0	0.0	0	0%
Thousand Island	1 pkt	230	1	5	420	0	23.0	20.0	4	90%
SANDWICH										
bacon Swiss crispy chicken	1 sandwich	690	31	60	1560	4	36.0	75.0	9	47%
barbecue chicken	1 sandwich	280	25	37	830	2	3.0	60.0	1	10%
chicken club	1 sandwich	460	32	33	1110	2	22.0	90.0	7	43%
fish, 'Carl's Catch'	1 sandwich	510	18	50	1030	1	27.0	80.0	7	47%
ranch crispy chicken	1 sandwich	590	24	59	1170	4	29.0	50.0	6	44%
Santa Fe chicken	1 sandwich	510	28	32	1240	2	31.0	95.0	7	54%
SAUSAGE PATTY	1 patty	200	8	2	480	1	19.0	30.0	17	81%
SIDE DISH										
baked potato, w/bacon and cheese	1 serving	630	20	76	1700	6	29.0	35.0	7	40%
baked potato, w/broccoli and cheese	1 serving	530	11	74	950	7	21.0	15.0	5	36%
baked potato, plain	1 serving	290	6	68	20	6	0.0	0.0	0	0%
baked potato, w/sour cream and chives	1 serving	430	7	70	135	6	14.0	10.0	3	29%
French fries	1 serving	290	5	37	170	3	14.0	0.0	3	43%
French fries, criss cut	1 serving	410	5	43	950	4	24.0	0.0	5	53%
onion rings	1 serving	430	7	53	700	3	21.0	0.0	5	44%
zucchini	1 serving	340	5	37	860	2	19.0	0.0	5	50%
CARVEL										
ICE CREAM										
'Caravella'	1 serving	164	4	16	92	0	8.0	61.0	0	47%
'Thinny-Thin'	1 serving	92	4	16	80	0	0.0	4.0	0	0%
ICE CREAM CONE										
plain	1 cone	25	1	5	25	0	0.0	0.0	0	0%

Food Name	Serving Size	Calories	Prot. gms	Carbs gms	Sod. mgs	Fiber gms	Fat gms	Sat. Fat gms	Chol. mgs	% Fat Cal.
sugar	1 cone	45	1	10	30	0	1.0	0.0	0	17%
YOGURT, FROZEN										
'Lo-Yo'	1 serving	124	4	20	76	0	4.0	16.0	0	27%
sugarless, low-fat	1 serving	104	4	20	80	0	4.0	8.0	0	27%
CHICK-FIL-A										
BEVERAGE										
'Coca-Cola Classic' small	1 serving	110	0	28	10	0	0.0	0.0	0	0%
'Diet Coke' small	1 serving	0	0	0	10	0	0.0	0.0	0	0%
iced tea, sweetened, small	1 serving	150	0	38	50	0	0.0	0.0	0	0%
iced tea, unsweetened, small	1 serving	0	0	0	50	0	0.0	0.0	0	0%
lemonade, small	1 serving	90	0	23	4	0	0.0	0.0	0	0%
lemonade, diet, small	1 serving	5	0	2	4	0	0.0	0.0	0	0%
CHICKEN PIECES										
'Chick-N-Strips' 4 per serving	1 strip	230	29	10	380	0	8.0	20.0	2	32%
nuggets, fried, 8 per serving	1 serving	290	28	12	770	0	14.0	60.0	3	44%
DESSERT										
brownie, fudge nut	1 brownie	350	10	41	650	0	16.0	30.0	3	41%
cheesecake	1 slice	300	6	23	200	0	21.0	115.0	13	62%
'Ice Dream Cone' small	1 serving	140	11	16	240	0	4.0	40.0	1	25%
lemon pie	1 slice	280	1	19	550	0	22.0	5.0	6	71%
SALAD										
chargrilled chicken garden	1 salad	190	26	12	800	4	5.0	83.0	4	23%
'Chick-N-Strips'	1 salad	370	32	21	724	4	17.0	113.0	6	42%
chicken Caesar	1 salad	230	31	5	940	2	10.0	85.0	6	38%
side	1 salad	70	5	13	0	1	0.0	0.0	0	0%
SANDWICH										
chicken	1 sandwich	290	24	29	870	1	9.0	50.0	2	28%
chicken, chargrilled	1 sandwich	280	27	36	640	1	3.0	40.0	1	10%
chicken club	1 sandwich	390	33	38	980	2	12.0	70.0	5	28%
chicken salad	1 sandwich	320	25	42	810	1	5.0	10.0	2	14%
SIDE DISH										
carrot and raisin salad	1 cup	150	5	28	650	2	2.0	6.0	0	12%
coleslaw	1 cup	130	6	11	430	1	6.0	15.0	1	44%
French fries, potato waffle, small	1 serving	290	1	49	960	0	10.0	5.0	4	31%
SOUP, breast of chicken, hearty	1 cup	110	16	10	760	1	1.0	45.0	0	8%
CHURCH'S FRIED CHICKEN										
CHICKEN										
breast, fried	4.3 oz serving	278	21	9	560	0	17.0	0.0	0	56%
breast, fried	3.5 oz	228	17	7	459	0	13.9	0.0	0	56%
breast, w/o bone	3.5 oz	252	24	5	642	0	15.6	81.9	0	54%
breast, w/o bone	2.8 oz	200	19	4	510	0	12.4	65.0	0	54%
breast fillet	1 serving	608	27	46	725	0	34.0	0.0	0	51%
breast fillet, w/cheese	1 serving	661	30	47	921	0	38.0	0.0	0	53%
leg	3.5 oz	179	16	6	348	0	10.9	0.0	0	53%
leg	2.9-oz serving	147	13	5	286	0	9.0	0.0	0	53%
leg, w/o bone	3.5 oz	247	22	4	282	0	16.1	79.4	0	58%
leg, w/o bone	2 oz	140	13	2	160	0	9.1	45.0	0	58%
thigh	4.2-oz serving	306	19	9	448	0	22.0	0.0	0	64%
thigh	3.5 oz	257	16	8	376	0	18.5	0.0	0	64%
thigh, w/o bone	3.5 oz	290	20	7	655	0	20.4	100.8	0	63%
thigh, w/o bone	2.8 oz	230	16	5	520	0	16.2	80.0	0	63%
wing, fried	4.8-oz serving	303	22	9	583	0	20.0	0.0	0	59%
wing, fried	3.5 oz	223	16	7	428	0	14.7	0.0	0	59%
wing, w/o bone	3.5 oz	284	21	9	614	0	18.3	68.3	0	58%

Food Name	Serving Size	Calories	Prot. gms	Carbs gms	Sod. mgs	Fiber gms	Fat gms	Sat. Fat gms	Chol. mgs	% Fat Cal.
wing, w/o bone	3.1 oz	250	19	8	540	0	16.1	60.0	0	58%
DESSERT										
apple pie	3.1 oz	280	2	41	340	1	12.3	5.0	0	39%
frozen dessert	1 serving	180	4	27	65	0	6.0	0.0	0	30%
FISH										
fillet	1 serving	430	20	45	675	0	18.0	0.0	0	38%
fillet, w/cheese	1 serving	483	23	46	870	0	22.0	0.0	0	42%
HOT DOG										
super	1 serving	520	17	44	1365	0	27.0	0.0	0	50%
w/cheese	1 serving	330	15	21	990	0	21.0	0.0	0	57%
w/cheese, super	1 serving	580	22	45	1605	0	34.0	0.0	0	53%
w/chili	1 serving	320	13	23	985	0	20.0	0.0	0	56%
w/chili, super	1 serving	570	21	47	1595	0	32.0	0.0	0	51%
SIDE DISH										
biscuit	2.1 oz	250	2	26	640	1	16.4	5.0	0	57%
Cajun rice	3.5 oz	148	1	18	296	1	8.0	5.7	0	48%
Cajun rice	3.1 oz	130	1	16	260	1	7.0	5.0	0	48%
coleslaw	3 oz	92	4	8	230	2	5.5	0.0	0	50%
corn on the cob	5.7 oz	190	8	32	15	4	5.4	0.0	0	23%
corn on the cob, w/butter oil	1 med ear	237	4	33	20	0	9.0	0.0	0	35%
French fries	2.7 oz	210	3	29	60	2	10.5	0.0	0	43%
French fries, large	1 serving	320	3	40	185	0	16.0	0.0	0	46%
hushpuppy	2 pieces	156	3	23	110	0	6.0	0.0	0	34%
mashed potatoes, w/gravy	3.7 oz	90	1	14	520	1	3.3	0.0	0	33%
mashed potatoes, w/gravy	3.5 oz	86	1	13	496	1	3.1	0.0	0	33%
okra	2.8 oz	210	3	19	520	4	16.1	0.0	0	62%
onion rings	1 serving	280	4	31	140	0	16.0	0.0	0	51%
COLOMBO										
YOGURT, FROZEN										
French vanilla	8 oz	215	8	30	140	0	7.0	0.0	0	29%
'Gourmet'										
Bavarian chocolate chunk	3 oz	120	3	18	40	0	4.0	10.0	0	30%
caramel pecan chunk	3 oz	120	4	19	150	0	3.0	10.0	0	23%
dream	3 oz	90	3	16	45	0	2.0	10.0	0	19%
'Heath Bar Crunch'	3 oz	130	3	19	75	0	5.0	15.0	0	34%
mocha Swiss almond	3 oz	120	3	17	45	0	5.0	10.0	0	36%
peanut butter cup	3 oz	140	4	16	90	0	7.0	5.0	0	44%
'Strawberry Passion'	3 oz	100	1	18	40	0	2.0	5.0	0	19%
wild raspberry cheesecake	3 oz	100	2	18	40	0	2.0	5.0	0	18%
low-fat	4 oz	99	3	18	35	0	2.0	10.0	0	18%
nonfat	4 oz	95	4	21	70	0	0.0	0.0	0	0%
'Sundae Style'										
banana split, 'Sundae Style'	3 oz	100	2	20	50	0	1.0	5.0	0	9%
caramel fudge sundae, low-fat, 'Sundae Style'	3 oz	100	3	21	60	0	1.0	5.0	0	9%
chocolate peanut butter twist, 'Sundae Style'	3 oz	110	3	18	65	0	3.0	5.0	0	24%
COUSIN'S SUBS										
BACON	3 strips	50	3	1	145	na	4.0	8.0	2	69%
BREAD										
Italian	1 oz	85	4	12	410	0	2.0	1.0	1	22%
wheat, 2 3/4 oz per half sub	1 oz	85	5	11	450	0	2.0	1.0	1	22%
CONDIMENT, tzatziki sauce	1 serving	50	1	1	110	na	4.0	20.0	2	82%
DESSERT										
chocolate chip cookie	1 cookie	210	2	25	190	na	11.0	20.0	na	48%
cranberry walnut cookie	1 cookie	187	2	24	66	na	8.4	na	2	42%

Food Name	Serving Size	Calories	Prot. gms	Carbs gms	Sod. mgs	Fiber gms	Fat gms	Sat. Fat gms	Chol. mgs	% Fat Cal.
PEPPERONI.	6 slices	70	5	0	180	na	6.0	25.0	3	73%
SALAD										
chef, low-fat.	1 salad	194	25	6	998	na	7.9	109.0	4	37%
garden, low-fat.	1 salad	136	15	6	383	na	5.9	65.0	3	39%
Italian.	1 salad	288	26	6	1063	na	17.9	106.0	7	56%
seafood, low-fat.	1 salad	176	21	12	1043	na	5.9	65.0	3	29%
side, low-fat.	1 salad	71	8	0	198	na	4.2	39.0	2	53%
tuna.	1 salad	306	26	6	483	na	19.9	85.0	4	59%
SANDWICH										
Cold										
bacon, lettuce, and tomato sub.	1/2 sub	593	20	34	1418	na	39.8	48.0	14	63%
bacon, lettuce, and tomatoy sub, w/o mayo	1/2 sub	337	20	34	1418	na	13.5	18.0	5	36%
cheese sub.	1/2 sub	664	31	30	1636	na	46.3	87.0	23	63%
cheese sub, mini	1/2 sub	354	17	16	872	na	24.7	46.0	12	63%
cheese sub, mini, w/o mayo	1/2 sub	228	17	16	872	na	10.7	30.0	8	42%
cheese sub, w/o mayo.	1/2 sub	427	31	30	1636	na	20.1	57.0	14	42%
club sub.	1/2 sub	730	50	30	2828	na	45.4	173.0	18	56%
club sub, w/o mayo	1/2 sub	494	50	30	2828	na	19.2	143.0	9	35%
'Cousins Special' sub, mini	1/2 sub	290	13	25	680	na	14.0	6.0	5	45%
ham and cheese sub.	1/2 sub	622	35	30	1748	na	40.1	107.0	15	58%
ham and cheese sub, mini	1/2 sub	332	19	16	932	na	21.4	57.0	8	58%
ham and cheese sub, mini, w/o mayo.	1/2 sub	206	19	16	932	na	7.4	41.0	3	32%
ham and cheese sub, w/o mayo	1/2 sub	386	35	30	1748	na	13.8	77.0	6	32%
ham sub	1/2 sub	547	29	30	1441	na	34.3	85.0	12	56%
ham sub, low-fat, mini, w/o mayo	1/2 sub	167	16	16	768	na	4.3	29.0	2	23%
ham sub, low-fat, w/o mayo.	1/2 sub	311	29	30	1441	na	8.0	55.0	3	23%
ham sub, mini	1/2 sub	292	16	16	768	na	18.3	45.0	6	56%
Italian cappacolla and cheese sub	1/2 sub	567	35	30	1850	na	33.9	73.0	11	54%
Italian cappacolla and Genoa sub.	1/2 sub	567	32	30	1771	na	35.5	58.0	9	56%
Italian Cousins Special sub.	1/2 sub	731	43	30	2490	na	48.6	111.0	15	60%
Italian Genoa and cheese sub	1/2 sub	668	37	30	2023	na	44.5	75.0	15	60%
Italian sub, regular.	1/2 sub	622	35	30	2008	na	40.0	79.0	12	58%
meatball and cheese sub, mini	1/2 sub	365	23	16	1927	na	23.1	55.0	10	57%
roast beef sub.	1/2 sub	598	41	30	1571	na	34.8	54.0	12	52%
roast beef sub, w/o mayo	1/2 sub	361	41	30	1571	na	8.5	24.0	3	21%
seafood w/crab sub.	1/2 sub	555	25	38	1747	na	33.6	35.0	11	54%
seafood w/crab sub, mini.	1/2 sub	296	13	20	932	na	17.9	19.0	6	54%
tuna sub	1/2 sub	756	30	32	1450	na	54.3	95.0	16	66%
tuna sub, made w/o added mayo on bread.	1/2 sub	500	30	32	1450	na	28.0	65.0	7	50%
tuna sub, mini	1/2 sub	495	14	22	670	na	37.0	56.0	10	70%
tuna sub, mini, made w/o added mayo on bread	1/2 sub	290	14	22	670	na	16.0	32.0	3	50%
turkey sub.	1/2 sub	561	32	30	2021	na	34.8	102.0	12	56%
turkey sub, low-fat, mini, w/o mayo	1/2 sub	172	17	16	1078	na	4.4	38.0	2	23%
turkey sub, low-fat, w/o mayo	1/2 sub	325	32	30	2021	na	8.5	72.0	3	24%
turkey sub, mini.	1/2 sub	299	17	16	1078	na	18.5	54.0	6	56%
veggie sub.	1/2 sub	360	26	33	1590	na	14.3	35.0	7	35%
Hot										
cheese steak sub	1/2 sub	470	33	46	540	na	17.0	40.0	11	33%
chicken breast sub	1/2 sub	556	37	30	1391	na	31.8	33.0	11	51%
chicken breast sub, w/o mayo	1/2 sub	320	37	30	1391	na	5.5	3.0	2	15%
double cheese steak sub	1/2 sub	550	44	35	640	na	26.0	61.0	16	43%
gyro sub	1/2 sub	550	28	57	650	na	23.0	36.0	8	38%
Italian sausage sub.	1/2 sub	816	44	30	5204	na	57.5	35.0	19	63%
meatball and cheese sub	1/2 sub	685	44	30	3613	na	43.3	104.0	18	57%

Food Name	Serving Size	Calories	Prot. gms	Carbs gms	Sod. mgs	Fiber gms	Fat gms	Sat. Fat gms	Chol. mgs	% Fat Cal.
pepperoni melt sub	1/2 sub	702	41	30	1908	na	46.1	131.0	18	59%
pepperoni melt sub, w/o mayo	1/2 sub	466	41	30	1908	na	19.8	101.0	9	38%
Philly cheese steak sub	1/2 sub	510	32	43	430	na	23.0	45.0	15	41%
steak sub	1/2 sub	425	28	51	360	na	12.0	40.0	8	25%
veggie sub	1/2 sub	380	21	48	320	na	11.0	0.0	0	26%
SIDE DISH										
French fries, large	1 serving	525	7	72	464	na	24.5	21.0	11	41%
French fries, medium	1 serving	400	5	55	353	na	18.7	16.0	8	41%
French fries, small	1 serving	275	4	38	243	na	12.8	11.0	6	41%
SOUP										
cheese, large	1 serving	330	11	23	1760	na	22.0	28.0	8	59%
cheese, regular	1 serving	210	7	15	1120	na	14.0	18.0	5	59%
cheese broccoli, large	1 serving	261	8	22	1224	na	16.5	21.0	6	55%
cheese broccoli, regular	1 serving	166	5	14	779	na	10.5	13.0	4	55%
chicken noodle, low-fat, large	1 serving	165	10	21	1444	na	4.1	28.0	1	23%
chicken noodle, low-fat, regular	1 serving	105	6	13	919	na	2.6	18.0	1	23%
chicken w/wild rice, large	1 serving	289	11	23	1691	na	16.5	28.0	3	52%
chicken w/wild rice, regular	1 serving	184	7	15	1076	na	10.5	18.0	2	52%
chili, large	1 serving	344	25	32	1485	na	13.8	62.0	6	36%
chili, low-fat, regular	1 serving	219	16	20	945	na	8.8	39.0	4	36%
clam chowder, low-fat, large	1 serving	248	12	30	1004	na	8.3	21.0	3	30%
clam chowder, low-fat, regular	1 serving	158	8	19	639	na	5.3	13.0	2	30%
potato, cream of, large	1 serving	261	7	30	1031	na	12.4	7.0	4	43%
potato, cream of, low-fat, regular	1 serving	166	4	19	656	na	7.9	4.0	3	43%
red rice and beans, low-fat, large	1 serving	179	7	36	1059	na	2.1	0.0	0	10%
red rice and beans, low-fat, regular	1 serving	114	4	23	674	na	1.3	0.0	0	10%
tomato basil, low-fat, large	1 serving	138	4	21	949	na	4.1	7.0	2	27%
tomato basil, low-fat, regular	1 serving	88	3	13	604	na	2.6	4.0	1	27%
vegetable beef, low-fat, large	1 serving	110	7	19	1403	na	2.1	14.0	0	15%
vegetable beef, low-fat, regular	1 serving	70	4	12	893	na	1.3	9.0	0	15%
DAIRY QUEEN/BRAZIER										
BEVERAGE										
chocolate milkshake, large	1 serving	990	19	168	360	0	26.0	70.0	0	24%
chocolate milkshake, regular	14 fl oz	540	12	94	290	0	14.0	45.0	8	23%
malted, 'Queen' large	21 fl oz	889	16	157	304	0	21.0	60.0	0	21%
milkshake, 'Queen' large	21 fl oz	831	16	140	304	0	22.0	60.0	0	24%
vanilla malt	14.7 fl oz	610	13	106	230	0	14.0	45.0	8	21%
vanilla malt milkshake	14.7 fl oz	610	13	106	230	0	14.0	45.0	8	21%
vanilla milkshake, large	16.3 fl oz	600	13	101	260	0	16.0	50.0	10	24%
vanilla milkshake, regular	14 fl oz	520	12	88	230	0	14.0	45.0	8	24%
DESSERT										
Banana split	1 serving	510	8	96	180	3	12.0	30.0	8	21%
'Blizzard'										
Heath	14.3 oz	820	16	114	410	0	36.0	60.0	17	38%
Heath	10.3 oz	560	11	79	280	0	23.0	40.0	11	37%
Heath	3.5 oz	202	4	28	101	0	8.9	14.8	4	38%
strawberry	13.5 oz	740	13	92	230	0	16.0	50.0	11	26%
strawberry	9.4 oz	500	9	64	160	0	12.0	35.0	8	27%
strawberry	3.5 oz	193	3	24	60	0	4.2	13.1	3	26%
'Brownie Delight'										
hot fudge	10.8-oz serving	710	11	102	340	0	29.0	35.0	14	37%
hot fudge	3.5 oz	232	4	33	111	0	9.5	11.4	5	37%
'Breeze'										
Heath	13.4 oz	680	15	113	360	0	21.0	15.0	6	27%

Food Name	Serving Size	Calories	Prot. gms	Carbs gms	Sod. mgs	Fiber gms	Fat gms	Sat. Fat gms	Chol. mgs	% Fat Cal.
Heath...	9.6 oz	450	11	78	230	0	12.0	10.0	3	23%
Heath...	3.5 oz	179	4	30	95	0	5.5	4.0	2	27%
strawberry.....................................	12.5 oz	590	12	90	170	0	1.0	5.0	1	2%
strawberry.....................................	8.7 oz	400	9	63	115	0	1.0	5.0	1	3%
strawberry.....................................	3.5 oz	166	3	25	48	0	0.3	1.4	0	2%
'Buster Bar'										
....	3.5 oz	299	7	27	146	0	19.3	10.0	6	56%
....	5.3 oz	450	11	40	220	0	29.0	15.0	9	56%
'Chipper Sandwich'............................	1 serving	318	5	56	170	0	7.0	13.0	0	21%
'Dilly Bar'										
....	3.5 oz	247	4	25	59	0	15.3	11.8	7	55%
....	3 oz	210	3	21	50	0	13.0	10.0	6	55%
'Double Delight'...............................	1 serving	490	9	69	150	0	20.0	25.0	0	37%
'DQ Frozen Cake'										
undecorated..................................	3.5 oz	231	4	30	128	0	10.9	12.2	5	42%
undecorated..................................	5.8 oz	380	6	50	210	0	18.0	20.0	8	42%
'DQ Sandwich'.................................	1 serving	140	3	24	40	0	4.0	5.0	0	25%
'Fudge Nut Bar'...............................	1 serving	406	8	40	167	0	25.0	10.0	0	54%
Ice cream cone										
chocolate.....................................	3.5 oz	162	4	25	81	0	4.9	14.1	4	27%
chocolate.....................................	5 oz	230	6	36	115	0	7.0	20.0	5	27%
chocolate.....................................	7.5 oz	350	8	54	170	0	11.0	30.0	8	29%
chocolate, chocolate dipped	1 serving	525	9	61	145	0	24.0	30.0	12	44%
chocolate, chocolate dipped	5.5 oz	330	6	40	100	0	16.0	20.0	8	44%
chocolate, 'Queen's Choice'	1 serving	326	5	40	84	0	16.0	52.0	0	44%
vanilla	3 oz	140	4	22	60	0	4.0	15.0	3	26%
vanilla	3.5 oz	162	4	25	67	0	4.9	14.1	4	27%
vanilla	5 oz	230	6	36	95	0	7.0	20.0	5	27%
vanilla	7.5 oz	340	9	53	140	0	10.0	30.0	7	27%
vanilla, 'Queen's Choice'	1 serving	322	4	40	71	0	16.0	52.0	0	45%
'Mr. Misty Float'..............................	1 serving	390	5	74	95	0	7.0	20.0	0	17%
'Mr. Misty Freeze'............................	1 serving	500	9	91	140	0	12.0	30.0	0	21%
'Mr. Misty'										
large	1 serving	340	0	84	10	0	0.0	0.0	0	0%
regular.......................................	11.6 oz serving	250	0	63	10	0	0.0	0.0	0	0%
'Nutty Double Fudge'										
....	3.5 oz	211	4	31	62	0	8.0	12.7	4	34%
....	9.7 oz	580	10	85	170	0	22.0	35.0	10	34%
'Peanut Buster Parfait'										
....	10.8 oz	710	16	94	410	0	32.0	30.0	10	40%
....	3.5 oz	232	5	31	134	0	10.4	9.8	3	40%
'QC Big Scoop'										
chocolate.....................................	4.5 oz	310	5	40	100	0	14.0	35.0	10	41%
chocolate.....................................	3.5 oz	243	4	31	78	0	11.0	27.4	8	41%
vanilla	4.5 oz	300	5	39	100	0	14.0	35.0	9	42%
vanilla	3.5 oz	235	4	31	78	0	11.0	27.4	7	42%
Strawberry shortcake..........................	1 serving	540	10	100	215	0	11.0	25.0	0	18%
Sundae										
chocolate.....................................	6.2 oz	300	6	54	100	0	7.0	20.0	5	21%
chocolate.....................................	3.5 oz	171	3	31	57	0	4.0	11.4	3	21%
chocolate, large...............................	1 serving	440	8	78	165	0	10.0	30.0	0	21%
strawberry, waffle cone	3.5 oz	202	5	32	127	0	6.9	11.6	3	30%
strawberry, waffle cone	6.1 oz	350	8	56	220	0	12.0	20.0	5	30%
Yogurt, frozen										
....	7 oz	230	8	49	100	0	1.0	5.0	1	4%

Food Name	Serving Size	Calories	Prot. gms	Carbs gms	Sod. mgs	Fiber gms	Fat gms	Sat. Fat gms	Chol. mgs	% Fat Cal.
cone, large	7.5 oz	260	9	56	115	0	1.0	5.0	1	3%
cone, regular	5 oz	180	6	38	80	0	1.0	5.0	1	5%
cup, regular	5 oz	170	6	35	70	0	1.0	5.0	1	5%
strawberry sundae	12.5 oz	200	6	43	80	0	1.0	5.0	1	4%
CHEESEBURGER										
double patty	3.5 oz	251	16	14	472	0	15.0	52.9	8	53%
double patty	8 oz	570	37	31	1070	0	34.0	120.0	18	53%
regular	3.5 oz	234	13	19	513	0	11.5	38.5	6	45%
regular	5.5 oz	365	20	30	800	0	18.0	60.0	9	45%
triple patty	1 serving	820	58	34	1010	0	50.0	140.0	0	55%
CHICKEN NUGGETS, all white meat	1 serving	276	16	13	505	0	18.0	39.0	0	58%
HAMBURGER										
double patty	3.5 oz	232	16	15	317	0	12.6	47.9	6	48%
double patty	7 oz	460	31	29	630	0	25.0	95.0	12	48%
'Homestar Ultimate'	3.5 oz	255	16	11	404	0	17.1	50.9	8	59%
'Homestar Ultimate'	9.7 oz	700	43	30	1110	0	47.0	140.0	21	59%
regular	3.5 oz	219	12	20	409	0	9.2	31.8	4	39%
regular	5 oz	310	17	29	580	0	13.0	45.0	6	39%
triple patty	1 serving	710	51	33	690	0	45.0	135.0	0	55%
HOT DOG										
'DQ Hounder' w/cheese	1 serving	533	19	22	1995	0	40.0	89.0	0	69%
'DQ Hounder' w/chili	1 serving	575	22	25	1900	0	41.0	89.0	0	66%
'DQ Hounder'	1 serving	480	16	21	1800	0	36.0	80.0	0	69%
'Super Dog' w/cheese	1 serving	580	22	45	1605	0	34.0	100.0	0	53%
'Super Dog' w/chili	1 serving	570	21	47	1595	0	32.0	100.0	0	51%
'Super Dog'	3.5 oz	297	10	21	685	0	19.1	30.2	8	58%
'Super Dog'	7 oz	590	20	41	1360	0	38.0	60.0	16	58%
SALAD										
garden, w/o dressing	10 oz	200	13	7	240	0	13.0	185.0	7	59%
side, w/o dressing	4.8 oz	25	1	4	15	0	0.0	0.0	0	0%
SALAD DRESSING										
French, diet	2 oz	90	1	11	450	0	5.0	0.0	1	48%
Thousand Island	2 oz	225	1	10	570	0	21.0	25.0	3	81%
SANDWICH										
barbecue beef	3.5 oz	176	9	27	549	0	3.1	15.7	1	16%
barbecue beef	4.5 oz	225	12	34	700	0	4.0	20.0	1	16%
chicken fillet, breaded	3.5 oz	226	13	19	400	0	10.5	29.0	2	42%
chicken fillet, breaded	6.7 oz	430	24	37	760	0	20.0	55.0	4	42%
chicken fillet, breaded, w/cheese	3.5 oz	235	13	19	480	0	12.3	34.3	3	46%
chicken fillet, breaded, w/cheese	7.2 oz	480	27	38	980	0	25.0	70.0	7	46%
chicken fillet, grilled	6.5 oz	300	25	33	800	0	8.0	50.0	2	24%
chicken fillet, grilled	3.5 oz	163	14	18	434	0	4.3	27.1	1	24%
fish fillet	3.5 oz	218	9	23	370	0	9.4	26.5	2	40%
fish fillet	6 oz	370	16	39	630	0	16.0	45.0	3	40%
fish fillet, w/cheese	3.5 oz	228	10	22	461	0	11.4	32.6	3	44%
fish fillet, w/cheese	6.5 oz	420	19	40	850	0	21.0	60.0	6	44%
SIDE DISH										
French fries	3.5 oz	300	4	40	160	0	14.0	0.0	3	42%
French fries, large	4.5 oz	390	5	52	200	0	18.0	0.0	4	42%
onion rings	3 oz	240	4	29	135	0	12.0	0.0	3	45%
DEL TACO										
BURRITO										
beef, deluxe	1 serving	440	23	43	878	0	20.0	63.0	0	41%
'Big Del'	1 serving	453	22	49	1047	0	20.0	59.0	0	39%
breakfast	1 burrito	256	9	30	409	0	11.0	90.0	0	39%

Food Name	Serving Size	Calories	Prot. gms	Carbs gms	Sod. mgs	Fiber gms	Fat gms	Sat. Fat gms	Chol. mgs	% Fat Cal.
chicken	1 serving	264	13	32	771	0	10.0	36.0	0	33%
chicken, spicy	1 serving	480	23	65	1620	8	16.0	40.0	10	29%
chicken fajita, 'Deluxe'	1 serving	435	22	41	944	0	22.0	84.0	0	44%
combination	1 serving	413	21	46	1035	0	17.0	49.0	0	36%
combo	1 serving	490	26	53	1380	8	21.0	55.0	13	37%
combo, deluxe	1 serving	530	27	56	1390	9	25.0	60.0	15	40%
'Del Beef'	1 serving	590	32	45	1110	4	33.0	95.0	19	49%
'Del Beef' deluxe	1 serving	550	31	42	1090	3	30.0	90.0	17	48%
green	1 serving	229	9	32	714	0	8.0	15.0	0	31%
green, large	1 serving	330	14	46	1149	0	11.0	22.0	0	29%
red	1 serving	235	10	32	656	0	8.0	17.0	0	30%
red, large	1 serving	342	14	46	1149	0	11.0	22.0	0	29%
'The Works'	1 serving	480	18	69	1500	9	18.0	25.0	11	32%
CHEESEBURGER	1 serving	284	14	26	852	0	13.0	42.0	0	42%
CONDIMENTS										
guacamole	2 tbsp	60	1	2	130	0	6.0	0.0	0	82%
hot sauce	1 tbsp	2	0	1	38	0	0.0	0.0	0	0%
salsa	4 tbsp	14	1	3	308	0	0.0	1.0	0	0%
HAMBURGER	1 serving	231	11	26	649	0	8.0	29.0	0	33%
QUESADILLA										
cheese	1 serving	260	10	24	530	1	12.0	30.0	9	44%
chicken	1 serving	580	33	41	1240	2	31.0	104.0	21	49%
SALAD										
chicken, deluxe	1 serving	710	31	75	2130	14	32.0	65.0	13	40%
taco, deluxe	1 salad	760	31	76	2010	14	37.0	70.0	17	44%
SIDE DISH										
French fries	1 serving	242	3	32	136	0	11.0	0.0	0	41%
refried beans, w/cheese	1 serving	122	7	17	890	0	7.0	9.0	0	40%
TACO										
	1 serving	160	7	11	150	1	10.0	20.0	4	56%
beef	1 serving	210	11	11	240	1	13.0	35.0	6	57%
beef, double, deluxe	1 serving	240	11	13	250	1	16.0	40.0	8	60%
beef, double, soft, deluxe	1 serving	250	12	18	440	1	14.0	40.0	7	51%
beef, soft	1 serving	210	12	16	430	1	11.0	35.0	6	47%
chicken fajita, deluxe	1 serving	211	11	18	492	0	10.0	53.0	0	44%
chicken fajita, soft, deluxe	1 serving	210	11	16	520	1	12.0	30.0	4	50%
regular	1 serving	211	9	19	320	0	10.0	32.0	0	45%
soft	1 serving	146	5	17	223	0	6.0	16.0	0	38%
TOSTADA	1 serving	210	9	24	640	6	9.0	15.0	5	38%

DENNY'S

Food Name	Serving Size	Calories	Prot. gms	Carbs gms	Sod. mgs	Fiber gms	Fat gms	Sat. Fat gms	Chol. mgs	% Fat Cal.
APPETIZER										
'Kids Heads N' Tails Cracker'	0.5 oz	70	2	9	165	0	3.0	0.0	1	38%
mozzarella sticks, 8 sticks	8 oz	710	36	49	5220	6	41.0	48.0	24	52%
sampler	17 oz	1405	47	124	5305	4	80.0	75.0	24	51%
BEVERAGE										
'Blender Blaster' Butterfinger	13 oz	768	13	97	345	0	38.0	106.0	23	44%
'Blender Blaster' kids jr.	7 oz	370	7	46	175	0	18.0	49.0	11	43%
apple juice	10 fl oz	125	0	33	24	0	0.0	0.0	0	0%
coffee, French vanilla flavored	8 fl oz	76	0	16	4	0	1.0	2.0	1	12%
coffee, hazelnut flavored	8 fl oz	66	0	14	4	0	1.0	2.0	1	14%
coffee, Irish cream flavored	8 fl oz	73	0	16	4	0	1.0	2.0	1	12%
cola float	12 oz	280	3	47	109	0	10.0	39.0	6	31%
grapefruit juice	10 fl oz	115	1	29	0	0	0.0	0.0	0	0%
hot chocolate	8 fl oz	90	4	18	155	0	2.0	0.0	0	17%

Food Name	Serving Size	Calories	Prot. gms	Carbs gms	Sod. mgs	Fiber gms	Fat gms	Sat. Fat gms	Chol. mgs	% Fat Cal.
iced tea, raspberry flavored	16 fl oz	78	0	21	0	0	0.0	0.0	0	0%
lemonade, w/ice	16 fl oz	150	0	35	38	0	0.0	0.0	0	0%
milk, chocolate, whole milk	10 fl oz	235	9	30	189	0	9.0	37.0	6	34%
milk, 2%										
	5 fl oz	90	5	7	70	0	5.0	19.0	3	48%
milkshake, malted, vanilla, or chocolate	12 oz	583	12	82	278	0	26.0	100.0	16	38%
milkshake, vanilla or chocolate	12 oz	560	11	76	272	0	26.0	100.0	16	40%
orange juice	10 fl oz	125	2	31	31	0	0.0	0.0	0	0%
orange-strawberry-banana juice drink, 10% juice	10 fl oz	137	0	38	0	0	0.0	0.0	0	0%
root beer float	12 oz	280	3	47	109	0	10.0	39.0	6	31%
tomato juice	10 fl oz	55	2	11	921	2	0.0	0.0	0	0%
BREAKFAST MEAL. See also individual listings.										
'All American Slam' w/o bread, choice of potato or grits	13 oz	712	38	9	1281	1	62.0	686.0	20	75%
'Cinnamon Swirl Slam'	13 oz	1105	38	68	1374	2	78.0	635.0	26	62%
'Country Slam'	18 oz	1000	41	61	2727	1	66.0	467.0	21	59%
'Farmer's Slam'	19 oz	1200	51	82	3204	3	80.0	704.0	24	58%
'French Slam'	14 oz	1029	44	58	1428	2	71.0	777.0	20	61%
'Kids Frenchtastic Slam' w/o bread, potato, or meat	6 oz	452	19	22	664	1	33.0	311.0	9	64%
'Kids Junior Grand Slam' w/o bread, potato, or meat	5 oz	397	17	33	1118	1	25.0	230.0	7	53%
'Moons Over My Hammy' w/o bread, choice of potato										
or grits	12 oz	807	44	46	2247	2	48.0	430.0	8	55%
'Original Grand Slam'	10 oz	795	34	65	2237	2	50.0	460.0	14	53%
'Play It Again Slam'	15 oz	1192	51	98	3555	3	75.0	690.0	21	53%
'Sausage Lover's Slam'	17 oz	960	31	33	1934	9	68.0	480.0	22	71%
'Scram Slam'	18 oz	740	39	14	1293	3	62.0	686.0	20	72%
'Senior Belgian Waffle Slam' w/o syrup, margarine	6 oz	399	16	12	612	0	33.0	302.0	8	73%
'Senior Triple Play' w/o bread, potato, or meat	8 oz	537	20	64	1445	2	25.0	409.0	6	40%
sirloin steak and eggs, w/o bread, choice of potato										
or grits	9 oz	622	43	1	632	1	49.0	572.0	18	71%
'Slim Slam' w/o topping	12 oz	495	34	98	1746	1	12.0	34.0	3	17%
'Southern Slam'	13 oz	1065	37	47	2449	0	84.0	484.0	23	69%
T-bone steak and eggs, w/o bread, choice of potato										
or grits	14 oz	991	73	1	1003	1	77.0	657.0	31	70%
BREAD AND ROLLS. See also French Toast.										
bagel, w/o added condiments	3 oz	235	9	46	495	0	1.0	0.0	0	4%
biscuit, w/butter	3 oz	272	5	39	790	0	11.0	0.0	4	36%
English muffin, 1 muffin, w/o added condiments	4 oz	125	5	24	198	1	1.0	0.0	0	7%
toast, dry, 1 slice	1 oz	90	3	17	166	1	1.0	0.0	0	10%
toast, herb	2 oz	170	2	15	325	1	11.0	1.0	2	59%
BUFFALO CHICKEN BURGER										
burger only, w/o added condiments	13 oz	803	37	67	2143	5	45.0	77.0	9	49%
BUFFALO WINGS, 12 wings	15 oz	940	80	3	2126	2	68.0	460.0	17	65%
CEREAL, ready to eat, 'Kellogg's' average dry	1 oz	100	2	23	276	1	0.0	0.0	0	0%
CHEESE	8 oz	293	6	13	895	4	23.0	19.0	13	73%
CHEESEBURGER										
classic, burger only, w/o added condiments	13 oz	836	47	43	1595	3	53.0	137.0	19	57%
'Kids The Big Cheese' w/o fries or substitute	3 oz	334	9	28	828	2	20.0	24.0	2	55%
w/bacon, burger only, w/o added condiments	14 oz	875	53	58	1672	5	52.0	163.0	19	51%
CHICKEN DINNER										
breast, grilled, w/o salad dressing, bread	4 oz	130	24	0	560	0	4.0	67.0	1	27%
Charleston, w/o choice of side dishes	6 oz	327	25	16	993	1	18.0	65.0	4	50%
'Senior Grilled Chicken Breast Dinner' w/o bread, soup,										
salad, fruit, vegetable	6 oz	200	25	15	824	1	5.0	67.0	1	22%

Food Name	Serving Size	Calories	Prot. gms	Carbs gms	Sod. mgs	Fiber gms	Fat gms	Sat. Fat gms	Chol. mgs	% Fat Cal.
CHICKEN NUGGETS										
'Kids Dennysaur' w/o fries or substitute	2 oz	190	9	9	340	0	13.0	30.0	4	62%
CHICKEN STRIPS DINNER										
5 strips, w/o choice of side dishes	10 oz	720	7	56	1666	0	33.0	95.0	4	54%
Buffalo, 5 strips, w/o choice of side dishes	10 oz	734	48	43	1673	0	42.0	96.0	4	51%
CHILI, with cheese topping	11 oz	401	26	21	1039	7	19.0	57.0	8	48%
CONDIMENTS										
bacon, 4 strips	1 oz	162	12	1	640	0	18.0	36.0	5	76%
bacon, peppered, 4 strips	1 oz	175	12	2	930	0	13.0	38.0	5	68%
barbecue sauce	1.5 oz	47	0	11	595	0	1.0	0.0	0	17%
cream cheese	1 oz	100	2	1	90	0	10.0	31.0	6	88%
guacamole	1.5 oz	74	1	4	264	1	6.0	0.0	2	73%
honey	0.5 oz	40	0	12	1	0	0.0	0.0	0	0%
margarine, whipped	0.5 oz	87	0	0	117	0	10.0	0.0	2	100%
marinara sauce	1.5 oz	48	1	7	206	1	2.0	0.0	1	36%
mushroom, grilled	2 oz	14	2	2	0	1	0.0	0.0	0	0%
raisins	0.75 oz	65	1	17	3	1	0.0	0.0	0	0%
salsa	1.5 oz	14	0	1	241	0	0.0	0.0	0	0%
sour cream	1.5 oz	91	1	2	23	0	9.0	19.0	6	87%
sugar, brown	1 oz	110	0	30	10	0	0.0	0.0	0	0%
syrup, blueberry flavored	1.5 oz	102	0	26	15	0	0.0	0.0	0	0%
syrup, maple favored, 3 tbsp	1.5 oz	143	0	36	26	0	0.0	0.0	0	0%
syrup, maple favored, sugar free	1.5 oz	23	0	9	71	0	0.0	0.0	0	0%
syrup, strawberry flavored	1.5 oz	91	0	23	36	0	0.0	0.0	0	0%
tartar sauce	1.5 oz	230	0	5	185	0	24.0	17.0	3	92%
tomato, sliced, 3 slices	2 oz	13	1	3	6	1	0.0	0.0	0	0%
DESSERT										
apple pie, 1/6 pie	7 oz	470	3	64	470	1	24.0	0.0	6	45%
banana royale	10 oz	548	6	80	184	6	25.0	64.0	15	40%
banana split	19 oz	894	15	121	177	6	43.0	78.0	19	42%
'Butterfinger Hot Fudge Sundae'	9 oz	780	9	106	333	1	38.0	71.0	25	43%
cheescake, w/o topping	4 oz	470	6	48	280	0	27.0	90.0	13	53%
cherry pie, 1/6 pie	7 oz	630	3	101	550	2	25.0	0.0	6	35%
chocolate layer cake	3 oz	275	4	42	62	0	12.0	26.0	3	37%
chocolate peanut butter pie, 1/6 pie	6 oz	653	15	64	319	3	39.0	27.0	19	53%
chocolate silk pie, 1/6 pie	6 oz	650	10	60	220	2	43.0	165.0	26	58%
Dutch apple pie, 1/6 pie	7 oz	440	10	65	290	1	19.0	0.0	5	36%
hot fudge cake	7 oz	620	7	73	170	1	35.0	60.0	17	50%
key lime pie, 1/6 pie	6 oz	600	6	79	300	0	27.0	35.0	15	42%
'Kids Jr. Butterfinger Hot Fudge Sundae'	4 oz	341	3	46	141	0	17.0	25.0	11	44%
Oreo cookies and creme pie, 1/6 pie	6 oz	590	10	73	390	3	30.0	20.0	17	45%
rainbow sherbet	4 oz	120	1	25	30	0	1.5	5.0	1	11%
sundae, double scoop, w/o topping	6 oz	375	6	29	86	0	27.0	74.0	12	63%
sundae, single scoop, w/o topping, 'Delicious Dip'	3 oz	188	3	14	43	0	14.0	37.0	6	65%
yogurt, frozen, chocolate chocolate chip, low-fat	4 oz	110	4	19	60	1	2.0	5.0	1	16%
EGGS BENEDICT, w/o choice of potato or grits	15 oz	695	34	34	1718	1	46.0	515.0	11	60%
FISH DINNER										
	9 oz	732	30	48	1335	3	47.0	105.0	7	58%
'Senior Fish Dinner' w/o bread, soup, salad, fruit, vegetable	5 oz	465	15	25	743	1	34.0	68.0	5	66%
FRENCH TOAST										
plain, w/o choice of meat, fruit topping or syrup, margarine	2 pieces	507	16	54	594	3	24.0	219.0	6	44%

Food Name	Serving Size	Calories	Prot. gms	Carbs gms	Sod. mgs	Fiber gms	Fat gms	Sat. Fat gms	Chol. mgs	% Fat Cal.
cinnamon swirl, w/o choice of meat, fruit topping or syrup, margarine	12 oz	1030	23	124	675	4	49.0	280.0	21	43%
GARDEN BURGER, burger only, w/o added condiments	11 oz	665	18	75	1051	8	33.0	36.0	8	44%
GRAVY										
biscuit and sausage	7 oz	398	8	45	1267	0	21.0	12.0	6	47%
brown	1 oz	13	0	2	184	0	0.0	0.0	0	0%
chicken	1 oz	14	0	2	139	0	0.5	2.0	0	36%
country	1 oz	17	0	2	93	0	1.0	0.0	0	53%
sausage	4 oz	126	3	6	477	0	10.0	12.0	2	71%
HAM, grilled, grilled slice	3 oz	94	15	2	761	0	3.0	23.0	1	28%
HAMBURGER										
'Big Texas Barbecue' burger only, w/o added condiments	14 oz	929	53	53	2271	3	58.0	163.0	24	55%
'Classic' burger only, w/o added condiments	11 oz	673	37	42	1142	3	40.0	106.0	15	53%
'Double Decker' burger only, w/o added condiments	15 oz	1247	55	82	2200	4	80.0	125.0	13	57%
'Garlic Mushroom Swiss' burger only, w/o added condiments	15 oz	872	48	58	1529	5	51.0	116.0	14	52%
'Kid's Burgerlicious' w/cheese, w/o fries or substitute	4 oz	341	15	24	580	1	20.0	40.0	6	54%
'Kid's Burgerlicious' w/o fries or substitute	4 oz	296	13	24	368	1	17.0	28.0	6	51%
HOT DOG MEAL, 'Kids Pig in a Blanket'	5 oz	479	16	63	1684	2	21.0	32.0	7	37%
HOTCAKES										
buttermilk, w/o choice of meat, fruit topping or syrup, margarine	3 hotcakes	491	12	95	1818	3	7.0	0.0	1	13%
'Kids Smiley-Face Hotcakes' w/meat, w/o syrup, margarine	6 oz	463	14	63	1410	2	22.0	38.0	7	39%
'Kids Smiley-Face Hotcakes' w/omeat, w/o syrup, margarine	4 oz	344	7	62	1014	2	9.0	13.0	3	23%
OATMEAL										
'Quaker'	4 oz	100	5	18	175	3	2.0	0.0	0	16%
and fixings, w/o juice, bread	20 oz	535	13	115	95	7	6.0	12.0	3	10%
OMELET										
farmer's, w/o bread, choice of potato or grits	14 oz	650	29	17	1158	1	51.0	655.0	15	71%
ham and cheddar, w/o bread, choice of potato or grits	10 oz	581	37	4	1180	0	45.0	672.0	8	71%
'Senior Omelette' w/o bread, potato, or meat	9 oz	429	25	8	755	2	20.0	515.0	12	58%
'Ultimate' w/o bread, choice of potato or grits	13 oz	564	30	9	939	2	47.0	639.0	12	73%
'Veggie-Cheese' w/o bread, choice of potato or grits	12 oz	480	26	9	535	2	39.0	644.0	13	71%
PIZZA MEAL, 'Kids Pizza Party'	6 oz	400	18	47	1090	7	15.0	10.0	3	34%
POT ROAST DINNER										
w/gravy	7 oz	292	42	5	927	0	11.0	87.0	5	34%
'Senior Pot Roast Dinner' w/o bread, soup, salad, fruit, vegetable	4 oz	160	25	3	512	0	6.0	48.0	3	33%
POTATO PANCAKE, w/o meat, w/o choice of fruit topping or syrup, margarine	13 oz	530	14	59	1125	6	27.0	253.0	8	45%
SALAD										
Buffalo chicken, w/o dressing, bread	16 oz	516	33	26	1197	4	35.0	79.0	8	57%
Caesar, side, w/dressing, w/o bread	6 oz	362	11	20	913	3	26.0	23.0	7	65%
California grilled chicken, w/o dressing, bread	13 oz	277	33	10	720	4	12.0	89.0	6	39%
fried chicken, w/o dressing, bread	15 oz	438	33	26	1030	4	26.0	78.0	6	50%
garden, side, w/o dressing, bread	7 oz	113	3	16	147	3	4.0	0.0	1	32%
'Garden Chicken Delight' w/o dressing, bread	16 oz	277	30	30	785	6	5.0	67.0	1	16%
grilled chicken Caesar, w/dressing, w/o bread	13 oz	600	37	19	1792	4	41.0	101.0	10	62%
SALAD DRESSING										
blue cheese	1 oz	163	1	1	205	0	18.0	20.0	3	95%
Caesar	1 oz	133	1	1	380	0	14.0	2.0	2	94%
French	1 oz	106	0	3	274	0	10.0	7.0	2	88%

Food Name	Serving Size	Calories	Prot. gms	Carbs gms	Sod. mgs	Fiber gms	Fat gms	Sat. Fat gms	Chol. mgs	% Fat Cal.
honey mustard, nonfat.	1 oz	38	0	9	121	0	0.0	0.0	0	0%
Italian, lower calorie, reduced calorie	1 oz	15	0	3	385	0	0.5	0.0	0	27%
ranch.	1 oz	101	1	1	215	0	11.0	8.0	2	93%
Thousand Island	1 oz	118	0	5	170	0	11.0	15.0	2	83%
SALMON DINNER										
Alaskan salmon, grilled, w/o salad dressing, bread	6 oz	210	43	1	103	0	4.0	101.0	1	17%
SANDWICH										
bacon, lettuce and tomato, sandwich only, w/o added condiments.	6 oz	634	18	37	1116	2	46.0	54.0	8	65%
Charleston chicken, sandwich only, w/o added condiments.	11 oz	632	35	53	1967	4	32.0	81.0	7	45%
club, sandwich only, w/o added condiments	11 oz	718	32	62	1666	3	38.0	75.0	7	48%
grilled cheese, sandwich only	7 oz	510	19	40	1360	3	30.0	54.0	14	53%
grilled chicken, fit-fare, sandwich only.	14 oz	434	35	56	1705	4	9.0	82.0	3	18%
grilled chicken, sandwich only, w/o added condiments	11 oz	520	35	64	1613	3	14.0	77.0	3	24%
ham and swiss, on rye, sandwich only, w/o added condiments.	9 oz	533	23	40	1638	5	31.0	36.0	4	53%
ham and swiss, sandwich only, w/o added condiments . . .	9 oz	497	22	34	1537	4	30.0	36.0	4	55%
Reuben, sandwich only, w/o added condiments	9 oz	580	27	37	2726	5	35.0	69.0	6	55%
'Super Bird' sandwich only, w/o added condiments.	9 oz	620	35	48	1880	2	32.0	60.0	5	46%
turkey breast, on multigrain bread, sandwich only, w/o added condiments	9 oz	476	23	39	1107	5	26.0	57.0	5	49%
turkey sub, sandwich only	9 oz	476	23	39	1107	5	26.0	57.0	3	49%
SHRIMP DINNER										
'Kids Shrimpsational Basket' w/o fries or substitute	5 oz	291	10	27	774	2	16.0	68.0	3	49%
fried.	8 oz	558	19	49	1114	3	32.0	135.0	6	51%
SIDE DISH										
applesauce, 'Musselmans'	3 oz	60	0	15	13	1	0.0	0.0	0	0%
banana, slices	4 oz	100	1	27	0	3	0.0	0.0	0	0%
banana, whole.	4 oz	110	1	29	0	4	0.0	0.0	0	0%
baked potato, plain, w/skin	7 oz	220	5	51	16	5	0.0	0.0	0	0%
broccoli, w/butter	4 oz	65	3	7	280	3	3.0	5.0	2	40%
carrots, w/honey glaze	4 oz	80	1	12	220	3	3.0	0.0	1	34%
corn, w/butter	4 oz	120	3	19	260	5	4.0	5.0	2	29%
cottage cheese	3 oz	72	9	2	281	0	3.0	10.0	2	38%
country fried potato	6 oz	515	3	23	805	9	35.0	8.0	8	75%
French fries, chili cheese.	12 oz	816	29	77	917	3	44.0	74.0	17	48%
French fries, unsalted	4 oz	323	5	44	130	0	14.0	0.0	3	39%
fries, seasoned	4 oz	261	5	35	556	0	12.0	0.0	3	40%
fries, smothered cheese	9 oz	767	27	69	875	0	48.0	78.0	17	53%
fruit mix	3 oz	36	1	9	16	1	0.0	0.0	0	0%
grapefruit, 1/2 grapefruit	5 oz	60	1	16	0	6	0.0	0.0	0	0%
grapes	3 oz	55	1	15	0	1	1.0	0.0	0	12%
green beans, w/bacon.	4 oz	60	1	6	390	3	4.0	5.0	2	56%
green peas, w/butter	4 oz	100	5	14	360	4	3.0	5.0	2	26%
grits	4 oz	80	2	18	520	0	0.0	0.0	0	0%
hash browns	4 oz	218	2	20	424	2	14.0	0.0	2	59%
hash browns, covered	6 oz	318	9	21	604	2	23.0	30.0	7	63%
hash browns, covered and smothered	8 oz	359	9	26	790	2	26.0	30.0	7	63%
hash browns, doubled, covered, smothered	13 oz	460	12	48	1213	5	26.0	30.0	7	49%
mashed potato, plain.	6 oz	105	3	21	378	2	1.0	0.0	0	9%
melon, cantaloupe, 1/4 melon.	3 oz	32	1	8	16	1	0.0	0.0	0	0%
melon, honeydew, 1/4 melon.	3 oz	31	1	8	22	1	0.0	0.0	0	0%
onion rings.	4 oz	381	5	38	1003	1	23.0	6.0	6	55%

Food Name	Serving Size	Calories	Prot. gms	Carbs gms	Sod. mgs	Fiber gms	Fat gms	Sat. Fat gms	Chol. mgs	% Fat Cal.
sausage link, 1 link	3 oz	354	16	0	944	0	32.0	64.0	12	82%
sausage patty, 2 patties	3 oz	300	10	1	466	0	28.0	56.0	10	85%
strawberry-banana medley	4 oz	108	1	27	6	2	1.0	0.0	0	7%
stuffing, bread, plain	3 oz	100	3	19	405	1	1.0	0.0	0	9%
vegetable rice pilaf	3 oz	85	2	16	325	1	1.0	0.0	0	11%
SKILLET MEAL										
'Big Texas Chicken Fajita' w/o bread	17 oz	1217	49	25	1817	8	70.0	518.0	19	68%
'Meat Lover's' w/o bread	15 oz	1147	41	24	2507	7	93.0	460.0	26	76%
'Sausage Supreme' w/o bread	16 oz	1054	17	30	1740	8	83.0	430.0	23	80%
SOUP										
broccoli, cream of	8 oz	193	4	15	818	2	12.0	0.0	9	59%
chicken noodle	8 oz	60	2	8	640	0	2.0	10.0	0	31%
clam chowder	8 oz	214	5	22	903	1	11.0	5.0	9	48%
potato, cream of	8 oz	222	4	23	761	2	12.0	0.0	9	50%
split pea	8 oz	146	8	18	819	2	6.0	5.0	2	34%
vegetable beef	8 oz	79	6	11	820	2	1.0	5.0	1	12%
STEAK MEAL										
chicken-fried steak and eggs, w/o choice of bread, potato or grits	8 oz	430	22	9	861	4	36.0	440.0	12	72%
'Senior Chicken-Fried Steak Dinner' w/o bread, soup, salad, fruit, or vegetable	8 oz	341	16	29	943	2	18.0	27.0	8	47%
sirloin	6 oz	271	22	0	273	0	21.0	62.0	9	68%
T-bone	12 oz	642	45	1	719	0	50.0	170.0	21	71%
chicken-fried steak	7 oz	495	29	24	1150	1	32.0	53.0	15	58%
steak and shrimp dinner	9 oz	645	36	31	1143	2	42.0	150.0	14	59%
STIR-FRY										
grilled chicken, w/o bread	18 oz	524	34	72	1886	11	11.0	43.0	3	19%
vegetable, w/o bread	20 oz	470	13	90	1780	16	6.0	0.0	1	12%
TOPPING										
blueberry	3 oz	106	0	26	15	0	0.0	0.0	0	0%
blueberry	2 oz	71	0	17	10	0	0.0	0.0	0	0%
cherry	3 oz	86	0	21	5	0	0.0	0.0	0	0%
cherry	2 oz	57	0	14	3	0	0.0	0.0	0	0%
chocolate	2 oz	317	2	27	83	0	25.0	0.0	0	66%
fudge	2 oz	201	1	30	96	1	10.0	3.0	7	42%
nut, 1 tsp	0.3 oz	42	1	1	0	0	4.0	0.0	0	82%
strawberry	3 oz	115	1	26	12	1	1.0	0.0	0	8%
strawberry	2 oz	77	1	17	8	1	1.0	0.0	0	11%
whipped cream, 2 tbsp	0.3 oz	23	0	2	3	0	2.0	7.0	0	69%
TURKEY DINNER										
roast turkey and stuffing, w/gravy, w/o salad dressing, bread	14 oz	388	46	38	2467	2	3.0	116.0	1	7%
'Senior Turkey and Stuffing Dinner' w/o bread, soup, salad, fruit, vegetable	8 oz	220	25	25	1378	1	2.0	60.0	0	8%
WAFFLE										
'Kids Wacky Waffles' w/o syrup or margarine	5 oz	215	4	23	102	0	12.0	78.0	3	50%
w/o choice of meat, fruit topping or syrup, and margarine	1 waffle	304	7	23	200	0	21.0	146.0	3	61%
D'LITES OF AMERICA										
CHEESE, light	1 slice	53	5	2	0	0	3.0	0.0	0	49%
CHEESEBURGER										
w/bacon, on multigrain bun	1 serving	370	32	20	0	0	18.0	0.0	0	44%
w/bacon, on sesame seed bun	1 serving	370	32	20	0	0	18.0	0.0	0	44%

Food Name	Serving Size	Calories	Prot. gms	Carbs gms	Sod. mgs	Fiber gms	Fat gms	Sat. Fat gms	Chol. mgs	% Fat Cal.
CONDIMENTS										
salad dressing, lower calorie	1 tbsp	40	0	1	0	0	4.0	0.0	0	90%
salad dressing, mayonnaise type										
mayonnaise, light	1 tbsp	40	0	1	0	0	4.0	0.0	0	90%
tartar sauce, light	1 tbsp	60	0	2	0	0	6.0	0.0	0	87%
DESSERT										
frozen, 'Chocolate D'Lite'	1 serving	203	6	36	0	0	4.0	0.0	0	18%
HAMBURGER										
'Double D'Lite' on multigrain bun	1 serving	450	44	19	0	0	22.0	0.0	0	44%
'Double D'Lite' on sesame seed bun	1 serving	450	44	19	0	0	22.0	0.0	0	44%
'Junior D'Lite' on multigrain bun	1 serving	200	15	19	0	0	7.0	0.0	0	32%
'Junior D'Lite' on sesame seed bun	1 serving	200	15	19	0	0	7.0	0.0	0	32%
'Quarter Pound D'Lite' on multigrain bun	1 serving	280	25	19	0	0	12.0	0.0	0	38%
'Quarter Pound D'Lite' on sesame seed bun	1 serving	280	25	19	0	0	12.0	0.0	0	38%
SANDWICH										
chicken fillet, on multigrain bun	1 sandwich	280	23	24	0	0	11.0	0.0	0	34%
chicken fillet, on sesame seed bun	1 sandwich	280	23	24	0	0	11.0	0.0	0	34%
fish fillet, on multigrain bun	1 sandwich	390	22	29	0	0	21.0	0.0	0	48%
fish fillet, on sesame bun	1 sandwich	390	22	29	0	0	21.0	0.0	0	48%
ham and cheese, on multigrain bun	1 sandwich	280	27	26	0	0	8.0	0.0	0	25%
ham and cheese, on sesame seed bun	1 sandwich	280	27	26	0	0	8.0	0.0	0	25%
vegetarian, 'Vegetarian D'Lite'	1 sandwich	270	16	20	0	0	14.0	0.0	0	47%
SIDE DISH										
baked potato	10-oz serving	230	6	50	0	0	1.0	0.0	0	4%
baked potato	3.5 oz	81	2	18	0	0	0.3	0.0	0	4%
baked potato, 'Mexican'	1 serving	510	27	61	0	0	18.0	0.0	0	32%
baked potato, w/bacon and cheddar	1 serving	490	25	52	0	0	20.0	0.0	0	37%
baked potato, w/broccoli and cheddar	1 serving	410	15	51	0	0	16.0	0.0	0	35%
French fries, large	1 serving	320	4	42	0	0	15.0	0.0	0	42%
French fries, regular	1 serving	260	3	34	0	0	12.0	0.0	0	42%
potato skin, 'Mexi-Skins'	1 piece	99	4	6	0	0	7.0	0.0	0	61%
salad bar platter	1 salad	130	10	9	0	0	6.0	0.0	0	42%
SOUP										
broccoli, cream of	1 serving	180	8	21	0	0	7.0	0.0	0	35%
'D'Lite'	1 serving	130	14	10	0	0	4.0	0.0	0	27%
DOMINO'S										
BREADSTICK	1 piece	116	3	18	152	1	4.0	0.0	1	30%
BUFFALO WINGS										
barbecue	1 piece	50	6	2	175	0	2.0	26.0	1	36%
hot	1 piece	45	5	1	354	0	2.0	26.0	1	43%
CHEESY BREAD	1 piece	142	4	18	183	1	6.0	6.0	2	38%
PIZZA										
Deep-dish										
cheese, individual, 6-inch	1 serving	598	23	68	1341	4	28.0	36.0	10	41%
cheese, large, 14-inch diam	2 slices	677	26	80	1575	5	30.0	41.0	11	39%
cheese, medium, 12-inch diam	2 slices	482	19	56	1123	3	22.0	30.0	8	40%
ham, individual, 6-inch diam	1 serving	615	25	69	1497	4	28.0	43.0	10	40%
ham, large, 14-inch diam	2 slices	708	31	81	1868	5	31.0	53.0	11	38%
ham, medium, 12-inch diam	2 slices	505	22	57	1338	3	23.0	39.0	8	40%
pepperoni, individual, 6-inch diam	1 serving	647	25	69	1524	4	32.0	47.0	12	43%
pepperoni, large, 14-inch diam	2 slices	775	31	81	1940	5	38.0	61.0	14	43%
pepperoni, medium, 12-inch diam	2 slices	556	22	56	1397	3	28.0	45.0	11	45%
sausage, individual, 6-inch diam	1 serving	642	25	70	1478	4	31.0	45.0	11	42%
sausage, large, 14-inch diam	2 slices	787	31	83	1917	5	38.0	64.0	14	43%

Food Name	Serving Size	Calories	Prot. gms	Carbs gms	Sod. mgs	Fiber gms	Fat gms	Sat. Fat gms	Chol. mgs	% Fat Cal.
sausage, medium, 12-inch diam	2 slices	559	22	58	1362	4	28.0	45.0	10	44%
vegetable, w/mushrooms, green peppers, onions, olives, individual, 6-inch diam	1 serving	616	23	70	1399	5	29.0	36.0	10	41%
vegetable, w/mushrooms, green peppers, onions, olives, large, 14-inch diam	2 slices	697	27	83	1636	5	31.0	41.0	11	39%
vegetable, w/mushrooms, green peppers, onions, olives, medium, 12-inch diam	2 slices	498	19	58	1172	4	23.0	30.0	8	40%
Hand-tossed										
cheese, medium, 12-inch diam	2 slices	375	15	55	776	3	11.0	23.0	5	26%
cheese, large, 14-inch diam	2 slices	516	21	75	1080	4	15.0	32.0	7	26%
ham, medium, 12-inch diam	2 slices	398	19	55	990	3	12.0	32.0	5	27%
ham, large, 14-inch diam	2 slices	547	26	76	1372	4	17.0	44.0	7	27%
pepperoni, medium, 12-inch diam	2 slices	448	19	55	1049	3	17.0	38.0	7	34%
pepperoni, large, 14-inch diam	2 slices	614	26	75	1444	4	24.0	52.0	10	35%
sausage, medium, 12-inch diam	2 slices	452	19	57	1015	3	17.0	39.0	7	33%
sausage, large, 14-inch diam	2 slices	626	26	78	1422	5	24.0	54.0	10	34%
vegetable, w/mushrooms, green peppers, onions, olives, medium, 12-inch diam	2 slices	391	16	57	824	4	12.0	23.0	5	27%
vegetable, w/mushrooms, green peppers, onions, olives, large, 14-inch diam	2 slices	536	22	77	1141	5	17.0	32.0	7	28%
Thin crust										
cheese, medium, 12-inch diam	1/4 of pizza	273	12	31	835	2	12.0	23.0	5	39%
cheese, large, 14-inch diam	1/4 of pizza	382	17	43	1172	2	17.0	32.0	7	39%
ham, medium, 12-inch diam	1/4 of pizza	296	15	31	1050	2	13.0	32.0	5	39%
ham, large, 14-inch diam	1/4 of pizza	414	21	44	1464	2	18.0	44.0	7	38%
pepperoni, medium, 12-inch diam	1/4 of pizza	347	15	31	1109	2	18.0	38.0	7	47%
pepperoni, large, 14-inch diam	1/4 of pizza	481	21	44	1536	2	25.0	52.0	10	46%
sausage, medium, 12-inch diam	1/4 of pizza	350	15	33	1074	2	18.0	39.0	7	46%
sausage, large, 14-inch diam	1/4 of pizza	492	22	47	1513	3	25.0	54.0	10	45%
vegetable, w/mushrooms, green peppers, onions, olives, medium, 12-inch diam	1/4 of pizza	289	12	33	884	2	13.0	23.0	5	39%
vegetable, w/mushrooms, green peppers, onions, olives, large, 14-inch diam	1/4 of pizza	402	17	46	1232	3	18.0	32.0	7	39%
DRUTHER'S										
BISCUITS AND GRAVY	8.1-oz serving	331	6	42	1233	1	14.7	3.0	0	41%
BREAKFAST MEAL										
bacon and fried egg platter	1 serving	721	25	62	1224	2	41.9	500.0	0	52%
bacon and scrambled egg platter	1 serving	742	26	64	1243	2	43.0	501.0	0	52%
biscuit, bacon, and egg	3.1-oz serving	258	12	15	653	1	16.3	253.0	0	58%
biscuit, ham, and egg	3.5-oz serving	217	13	15	796	1	11.2	256.0	0	47%
ham and fried egg platter	1 serving	681	29	62	1622	2	35.3	511.0	0	46%
ham and scrambled egg platter	1 serving	762	27	64	1408	2	44.6	515.0	0	52%
sausage and biscuit platter, two of each	3.4-oz serving	358	12	26	894	1	22.3	34.0	0	57%
sausage and egg biscuit	3.3-oz serving	246	11	15	674	1	15.1	257.0	0	56%
sausage and fried egg platter	1 serving	741	26	63	1390	2	43.4	515.0	0	52%
sausage and scrambled egg platter	1 serving	742	26	64	1243	2	43.0	501.0	0	52%
CHEESEBURGER										
'Deluxe Quarter'	8.7 oz	660	33	46	768	1	37.6	127.0	0	52%
double patty	6.4 oz	500	29	35	618	0	26.1	105.0	0	48%
regular	4.7 oz	380	19	35	585	0	17.8	69.0	0	43%
CHICKEN										
12 pieces	3.9 lbs	5496	319	637	12904	16	171.2	902.0	0	29%
8 pieces	2.6 lbs	3664	213	425	8558	11	114.1	601.0	0	29%
breast, w/wing, dinner or snack	2 pieces	595	48	28	1607	1	30.7	154.0	0	48%

Food Name	Serving Size	Calories	Prot. gms	Carbs gms	Sod. mgs	Fiber gms	Fat gms	Sat. Fat gms	Chol. mgs	% Fat Cal.
leg, w/thigh, dinner or snack	2 pieces	549	38	29	1205	1	29.8	152.0	0	50%
thigh and leg, dinner or snack	3 pieces	1281	78	90	2566	2	66.9	273.0	0	47%
thigh and wing, dinner or snack	3 pieces	1309	80	87	2465	2	70.3	271.0	0	49%
CHICKEN ENTRÉE										
breast and wing, w/potatoes and coleslaw	2 pieces	970	54	76	1899	2	49.9	159.0	0	46%
leg and thigh, w/potatoes and coleslaw	2 pieces	925	44	77	1530	2	49.0	157.0	0	48%
FISH ENTRÉE										
	13.3-oz entrée	770	43	79	1306	4	31.3	117.0	0	37%
fried, w/fries	11.2 oz	729	42	71	1292	4	29.8	112.0	0	37%
FISH SANDWICH	4.8 oz	349	22	33	821	2	14.4	56.0	0	37%
HAMBURGER	4.4 oz	327	16	35	382	0	13.4	55.0	0	37%

DUNKIN' DONUTS

BAGEL

Food Name	Serving Size	Calories	Prot. gms	Carbs gms	Sod. mgs	Fiber gms	Fat gms	Sat. Fat gms	Chol. mgs	% Fat Cal.
blueberry	1 bagel	340	10	75	670	0	1.0	0.0	0	3%
cinnamon raisin	1 bagel	340	10	74	480	1	1.0	0.0	0	3%
egg	1 bagel	350	11	72	610	0	1.5	25.0	0	4%
everything	1 bagel	360	11	74	710	0	2.0	0.0	0	5%
garlic	1 bagel	360	11	76	720	0	1.0	0.0	0	3%
onion	1 bagel	330	10	70	660	0	1.0	0.0	0	3%
plain	1 bagel	340	10	73	710	0	1.0	0.0	0	3%
poppyseed	1 bagel	360	11	74	710	0	2.5	0.0	0	6%
pumpernickel	1 bagel	350	11	75	560	2	1.5	0.0	0	4%
salt	1 bagel	340	10	73	3030	0	1.0	0.0	0	3%
sesame	1 bagel	380	12	74	720	0	4.5	0.0	1	11%
wheat	1 bagel	330	12	73	670	4	1.5	0.0	0	4%

BEVERAGE

Food Name	Serving Size	Calories	Prot. gms	Carbs gms	Sod. mgs	Fiber gms	Fat gms	Sat. Fat gms	Chol. mgs	% Fat Cal.
'Coolatta' coffee w/cream	16 fl oz	410	3	51	65	0	22.0	75.0	14	48%
'Coolatta' coffee w/milk	16 fl oz	260	4	52	75	0	4.0	15.0	3	14%
'Coolatta' coffee w/skim milk	16 fl oz	230	4	52	80	0	0.0	0.0	0	0%
'Coolatta' coffee w/2% milk	16 fl oz	240	4	52	80	0	2.0	10.0	2	7%
'Coolatta' orange mango fruit	16 fl oz	290	0	71	30	0	0.0	0.0	0	0%
'Coolatta' pink lemonade	16 fl oz	350	0	88	30	0	0.0	0.0	0	0%
'Coolatta' raspberry lemonade	16 fl oz	280	0	68	35	0	0.0	0.0	0	0%
'Coolatta' strawberry fruit	16 fl oz	280	0	70	30	1	0.0	0.0	0	0%
'Coolatta' vanilla	16 fl oz	450	1	94	170	0	7.0	0.0	4	14%
'Dunkaccino'	18.75 fl oz	480	4	67	470	1	22.0	20.0	7	41%
'Dunkaccino'	10 fl oz	250	2	34	240	0	11.0	10.0	4	41%
'Dunkaccino'	14 fl oz	360	3	51	360	1	17.0	15.0	5	41%
'Dunkaccino'	20 fl oz	510	4	71	500	1	23.0	20.0	7	41%
hot cocoa	18.75 fl oz	440	4	75	610	3	15.0	0.0	4	30%
hot cocoa	10 fl oz	230	2	38	310	2	8.0	0.0	2	31%
hot cocoa	14 fl oz	330	3	57	460	2	11.0	0.0	3	29%
hot cocoa	20 fl oz	470	5	79	640	3	16.0	0.0	4	30%

BREAKFAST SANDWICH

Food Name	Serving Size	Calories	Prot. gms	Carbs gms	Sod. mgs	Fiber gms	Fat gms	Sat. Fat gms	Chol. mgs	% Fat Cal.
'Omwich' bagel, w/bacon and cheddar	1 sandwich	600	26	79	1630	0	21.0	295.0	8	31%
'Omwich' bagel, Spanish, cheese	1 sandwich	570	24	79	1370	0	18.0	280.0	6	28%
'Omwich' bagel, three cheese	1 sandwich	610	25	78	1630	0	22.0	305.0	9	32%
'Omwich' croissant, w/bacon and cheddar	1 sandwich	560	21	33	1190	1	38.0	295.0	13	61%
'Omwich' croissant, Spanish, cheese	1 sandwich	530	19	33	930	1	36.0	285.0	11	61%
'Omwich' croissant, three cheese	1 sandwich	560	20	33	1200	1	39.0	305.0	15	62%
'Omwich' English muffin, w/bacon and cheddar	1 sandwich	400	21	33	1440	2	21.0	295.0	8	47%
'Omwich' English muffin, Spanish, cheese	1 sandwich	370	18	34	1180	2	18.0	280.0	6	44%
'Omwich' English muffin, three cheese	1 sandwich	400	19	33	1450	2	22.0	305.0	9	49%
'Omwich' ham, egg, cheese	1 sandwich	320	22	31	1340	2	12.0	195.0	6	34%

Food Name	Serving Size	Calories	Prot. gms	Carbs gms	Sod. mgs	Fiber gms	Fat gms	Sat. Fat gms	Chol. mgs	% Fat Cal.
CINNAMON BUN	1 bun	510	8	85	420	0	15.0	10.0	4	27%
COOKIE										
chocolate chocolate chunk	1 cookie	210	3	26	110	2	11.0	35.0	7	46%
chocolate chunk	1 cookie	220	3	28	105	1	11.0	35.0	7	44%
chocolate chunk w/nuts	1 cookie	230	3	27	110	1	12.0	35.0	6	47%
chocolate-white chocolate chunk	1 cookie	230	3	28	120	1	12.0	35.0	7	47%
oatmeal raisin pecan	1 cookie	220	3	29	110	1	10.0	30.0	5	41%
peanut butter chocolate chunk w/nuts	1 cookie	240	4	24	125	2	14.0	25.0	6	53%
peanut butter w/nuts	1 cookie	240	5	24	150	1	14.0	30.0	6	52%
CREAM CHEESE										
chive	1 packet	190	3	3	220	0	19.0	55.0	13	88%
garden vegetable	1 packet	180	3	3	310	0	17.0	45.0	11	86%
lite	1 packet	130	5	3	250	0	11.0	30.0	7	76%
plain	1 packet	200	4	3	230	0	19.0	60.0	13	86%
salmon	1 packet	180	5	2	150	0	17.0	50.0	11	85%
CROISSANT										
almond	1 croissant	350	6	34	270	2	22.0	5.0	5	55%
chocolate	1 croissant	400	5	37	240	2	25.0	5.0	9	57%
plain	1 croissant	290	5	26	270	0	18.0	5.0	6	57%
DOUGHNUT										
apple crumb	1 donut	230	3	34	270	0	10.0	0.0	3	38%
apple fritter	1 donut	300	4	41	360	1	14.0	0.0	3	41%
apple n' spice	1 donut	200	3	29	270	0	8.0	0.0	2	36%
Bavarian kreme	1 donut	210	3	30	270	0	9.0	0.0	2	38%
bismark, chocolate-iced	1 donut	340	3	50	290	0	15.0	0.0	4	39%
black raspberry	1 donut	210	3	32	280	0	8.0	0.0	2	34%
blueberry cake	1 donut	290	3	35	400	0	16.0	10.0	4	49%
blueberry crumb	1 donut	240	3	36	260	0	10.0	0.0	3	37%
Boston kreme	1 donut	240	3	36	280	0	9.0	0.0	2	34%
bow tie	1 donut	300	4	34	340	0	17.0	0.0	4	50%
butternut cake ring	1 donut	300	3	36	360	0	16.0	0.0	5	48%
cake, glazed	1 donut	270	3	33	360	0	15.0	0.0	3	48%
chcolate cake glazed	1 donut	290	3	33	370	1	16.0	0.0	4	50%
chocolate coconut cake	1 donut	300	4	31	370	1	19.0	0.0	6	55%
chocolate cruller, glazed	1 donut	280	3	35	360	1	15.0	0.0	3	47%
chocolate kreme filled	1 donut	270	3	35	260	0	13.0	0.0	3	43%
chocolate-frosted cake	1 donut	300	3	38	370	0	16.0	0.0	3	47%
chocolate-frosted	1 donut	200	3	29	260	0	9.0	0.0	2	39%
cinnamon cake	1 donut	270	3	31	360	0	15.0	0.0	3	50%
coconut cake	1 donut	290	3	33	360	0	17.0	0.0	5	52%
coffee roll	1 donut	270	4	33	340	1	14.0	0.0	3	46%
coffee roll, chocolate-frosted	1 donut	290	4	36	340	1	15.0	0.0	3	46%
coffee roll, maple frosted	1 donut	290	4	36	340	1	14.0	0.0	3	44%
cruller, glazed	1 donut	290	3	37	350	0	15.0	0.0	3	46%
double chocolate cake	1 donut	310	3	37	370	2	17.0	0.0	4	49%
dunkin'	1 donut	240	3	25	340	0	15.0	0.0	3	55%
éclair	1 donut	270	3	39	290	0	11.0	0.0	3	37%
fritter, glazed	1 donut	260	4	31	330	1	14.0	0.0	3	47%
glazed	1 donut	180	3	25	250	0	8.0	0.0	2	39%
jelly stick	1 donut	290	3	44	390	0	12.0	0.0	3	36%
jelly-filled	1 donut	210	3	32	280	0	8.0	0.0	2	34%
lemon	1 donut	200	3	28	270	0	9.0	0.0	2	40%
maple frosted	1 donut	210	3	30	260	0	9.0	0.0	2	38%
marble frosted	1 donut	200	3	29	260	0	9.0	0.0	2	39%

Food Name	Serving Size	Calories	Prot. gms	Carbs gms	Sod. mgs	Fiber gms	Fat gms	Sat. Fat gms	Chol. mgs	% Fat Cal.
old fashioned cake	1 donut	250	3	26	360	0	15.0	0.0	3	54%
plain cruller	1 donut	240	3	25	340	0	15.0	0.0	3	55%
powdered cake	1 donut	270	3	32	350	0	15.0	0.0	3	49%
powdered cruller	1 donut	270	3	30	340	0	15.0	0.0	3	51%
strawberry	1 donut	210	3	32	260	0	8.0	0.0	2	34%
strawberry-frosted	1 donut	210	3	30	260	0	9.0	0.0	2	38%
sugar cruller	1 donut	250	3	27	340	0	15.0	0.0	3	53%
sugar raised	1 donut	170	3	22	250	0	8.0	0.0	2	42%
sugared cake	1 donut	250	3	27	350	0	15.0	0.0	3	53%
toasted coconut cake	1 donut	300	3	35	370	0	17.0	0.0	5	50%
vanilla kreme filled	1 donut	270	3	36	250	0	13.0	0.0	3	43%
vanilla-frosted	1 donut	210	3	30	260	0	9.0	0.0	2	38%
whole wheat glazed cake	1 donut	310	4	32	380	2	19.0	0.0	4	54%
DOUGHNUT HOLE										
'Munchkin' cake butternut	3 munchkins	200	2	25	240	0	11.0	0.0	3	48%
'Munchkin' cake chocolate glazed	3 munchkins	200	2	26	250	0	10.0	0.0	2	45%
'Munchkin' cake cinnamon	4 munchkins	250	3	30	330	0	14.0	0.0	3	49%
'Munchkin' cake coconut	3 munchkins	200	2	23	240	0	12.0	0.0	4	52%
'Munchkin' cake glazed	3 munchkins	200	2	27	250	0	10.0	0.0	2	44%
'Munchkin' cake plain	4 munchkins	220	2	22	310	0	14.0	0.0	3	57%
'Munchkin' cake powdered	4 munchkins	250	2	29	310	0	14.0	0.0	3	50%
'Munchkin' cake sugared	4 munchkins	240	2	28	310	0	14.0	0.0	3	51%
'Munchkin' cake toasted coconut	3 munchkins	200	2	24	250	0	11.0	0.0	3	49%
'Munchkin' yeast glazed	5 munchkins	200	3	27	220	0	9.0	0.0	2	40%
'Munchkin' yeast jelly filled	5 munchkins	210	3	30	240	0	9.0	0.0	2	38%
'Munchkin' yeast lemon filled	4 munchkins	170	2	23	190	0	8.0	0.0	2	42%
'Munchkin' yeast sugar raised	7 munchkins	220	4	26	290	0	12.0	0.0	3	47%
MUFFIN										
apple and spice, low-fat	1 muffin	240	4	54	460	0	1.5	0.0	0	6%
apple cinnamon pecan	1 muffin	510	8	74	590	1	21.0	70.0	6	37%
apple n' spice	1 muffin	350	5	57	390	2	12.0	35.0	3	30%
banana nut	1 muffin	360	7	52	490	3	15.0	35.0	3	36%
banana, low-fat	1 muffin	250	4	57	430	0	1.5	0.0	0	5%
blueberry, 4-oz muffin	1 muffin	320	6	49	480	3	12.0	35.0	3	33%
blueberry, 6-oz muffin	1 muffin	490	8	76	610	2	17.0	75.0	6	31%
blueberry, lower fat	1 muffin	450	8	77	590	2	12.0	65.0	9	24%
blueberry, low-fat	1 muffin	250	4	55	430	1	1.5	0.0	0	5%
bran	1 muffin	390	11	60	620	3	12.0	20.0	2	28%
bran, low-fat	1 muffin	240	4	57	430	4	1.0	0.0	0	4%
cherry	1 muffin	340	6	53	510	2	12.0	40.0	3	31%
cherry, low-fat	1 muffin	250	4	56	430	0	1.5	0.0	0	5%
chocolate chip, 4 oz muffin	1 muffin	400	6	58	440	4	17.0	35.0	6	37%
chocolate chip, 6 oz muffin	1 muffin	590	9	88	560	3	24.0	75.0	10	36%
chocolate hazelnut chunk	1 muffin	610	10	87	610	3	26.0	70.0	8	38%
chocolate, low-fat	1 muffin	250	4	53	470	2	2.5	0.0	1	9%
corn, 4 oz muffin	1 muffin	390	8	57	590	2	15.0	55.0	3	34%
corn, 6 oz muffin	1 muffin	500	10	78	920	1	16.0	80.0	5	29%
corn, low-fat	1 muffin	240	3	52	480	0	2.5	45.0	1	9%
corn, reduced fat	1 muffin	460	10	79	900	1	11.0	75.0	7	22%
cranberry orange	1 muffin	470	8	76	600	2	15.0	75.0	5	29%
cranberry orange nut	1 muffin	350	6	52	500	3	15.0	35.0	3	37%
cranberry orange, low-fat	1 muffin	240	4	55	430	1	1.5	0.0	0	5%
honey bran raisin	1 muffin	490	7	84	880	5	16.0	30.0	4	28%

Food Name	Serving Size	Calories	Prot. gms	Carbs gms	Sod. mgs	Fiber gms	Fat gms	Sat. Fat gms	Chol. mgs	% Fat Cal.
lemon poppyseed	1 muffin	360	5	56	530	1	13.0	35.0	3	32%
oat bran	1 muffin	370	11	55	620	3	13.0	20.0	2	31%

EL POLLO LOCO

BEANS

Food Name	Serving Size	Calories	Prot. gms	Carbs gms	Sod. mgs	Fiber gms	Fat gms	Sat. Fat gms	Chol. mgs	% Fat Cal.
pinto	6 oz	185	11	29	744	8	4.0	0.0	0	18%
black, smoky	5 oz	255	6	29	609	4	13.0	11.0	5	46%
black, smoky, bowl	16 oz	604	29	75	1955	6	23.0	54.0	7	33%

BEVERAGE

Food Name	Serving Size	Calories	Prot. gms	Carbs gms	Sod. mgs	Fiber gms	Fat gms	Sat. Fat gms	Chol. mgs	% Fat Cal.
smoothie, kiwi strawberry	9.5 oz	357	5	66	141	2	7.0	23.0	3	18%
smoothie, 'Minute Maid' orange	20 oz	526	9	99	198	0	4.0	44.0	7	8%
smoothie, 'Minute Maid' orange	16 oz	457	8	84	176	0	4.0	41.0	6	9%
smoothie, strawberry banana	11 oz	367	3	68	136	2	7.0	23.0	3	18%

BURRITO

Food Name	Serving Size	Calories	Prot. gms	Carbs gms	Sod. mgs	Fiber gms	Fat gms	Sat. Fat gms	Chol. mgs	% Fat Cal.
black bean, smoky	8 oz	515	15	71	1197	9	20.0	21.0	7	34%
'BRC'	7 oz	440	15	64	1105	9	14.0	15.0	5	29%
chicken, classic	11 oz	580	31	66	1595	9	22.0	108.0	7	34%
chicken, Southwest	12 oz	627	30	69	1795	5	27.0	60.0	4	38%
chicken Caesar, Mexican	11 oz	734	36	65	1214	2	35.0	79.0	8	44%
'Chicken Grande'	14 oz	648	33	72	1705	10	26.0	120.0	7	36%
'Chicken Lovers'	9 oz	476	29	47	1373	8	19.0	143.0	6	36%
'Ultimate Chicken'	12.8 oz	633	92	66	1237	5	23.0	89.0	8	25%

CHICKEN

Food Name	Serving Size	Calories	Prot. gms	Carbs gms	Sod. mgs	Fiber gms	Fat gms	Sat. Fat gms	Chol. mgs	% Fat Cal.
breast, flame-broiled, w/o bone	3 oz	160	26	0	390	0	6.0	110.0	2	34%
leg, flame-broiled, w/o bone	1.75 oz	90	11	0	150	0	5.0	75.0	2	51%
thigh, flame-broiled, w/o bone	2 oz	180	16	0	230	0	12.0	130.0	4	63%
wing, flame-broiled, w/o bone	1.5 oz	110	12	0	220	0	6.0	80.0	2	53%
CHICKEN NUGGETS, 'Dinosaur Chicken Bites' 4 oz	4 pieces	185	12	11	345	2	10.4	64.0	2	50%
CHURROS	1.75 oz	179	3	18	221	1	11.0	5.0	3	54%

CONDIMENTS. See also Salad Dressing.

Food Name	Serving Size	Calories	Prot. gms	Carbs gms	Sod. mgs	Fiber gms	Fat gms	Sat. Fat gms	Chol. mgs	% Fat Cal.
gravy	1 oz	14	0	2	139	0	0.0	2.0	0	0%
guacamole	1.75 oz	52	0	5	280	0	3.0	0.0	0	57%
jalapeño hot sauce, 0.5 oz	1 pkt	5	0	1	110	0	0.0	0.0	0	0%
salsa, avocado	1 oz	12	0	1	204	0	1.0	0.0	0	69%
salsa, house	1 oz	6	0	1	96	0	0.0	0.0	0	0%
salsa, pico de gallo	1 oz	11	0	2	131	0	0.5	0.0	0	43%
salsa, spicy chipotle	1 oz	7	0	1	179	0	0.0	0.0	0	0%
sour cream, light	1 oz	45	2	2	25	0	3.0	12.0	0	63%

DESSERT

Food Name	Serving Size	Calories	Prot. gms	Carbs gms	Sod. mgs	Fiber gms	Fat gms	Sat. Fat gms	Chol. mgs	% Fat Cal.
banana split	15 oz	717	12	107	310	3	28.0	56.0	11	35%
cheesecake	3.5 oz	310	8	30	228	0	18.0	58.0	9	52%
'Foster's Freeze' w/o topping	4.6 oz	180	4	30	100	0	5.0	20.0	3	25%

SALAD

Food Name	Serving Size	Calories	Prot. gms	Carbs gms	Sod. mgs	Fiber gms	Fat gms	Sat. Fat gms	Chol. mgs	% Fat Cal.
'Pollo Bowl'	17 oz	469	30	66	1868	8	11.0	42.0	2	21%
bowl, flame-broiled chicken	12 oz	357	25	39	1079	4	13.0	42.0	2	31%
bowl, Mexican Caesar chicken	11 oz	491	25	32	1170	2	30.0	55.0	6	54%
bowl, Southwest chicken	13 oz	529	25	40	1332	4	31.0	52.0	5	52%
garden, large	14 oz	225	14	17	214	4	13.0	30.0	6	49%
garden, regular	4 oz	105	5	7	99	1	7.0	15.0	3	57%
tostada, w/o shell and sour cream	14 oz	304	29	28	1175	4	11.0	57.0	3	30%

SALAD DRESSING

Food Name	Serving Size	Calories	Prot. gms	Carbs gms	Sod. mgs	Fiber gms	Fat gms	Sat. Fat gms	Chol. mgs	% Fat Cal.
blue cheese	2 oz	300	2	2	590	0	32.0	50.0	6	95%
cilantry, creamy	1.75 oz	266	1	1	306	0	29.0	13.0	4	97%
Italian, light	2 oz	25	0	3	990	0	1.0	0.0	1	43%
ranch	2 oz	350	1	2	500	0	39.0	5.0	6	97%

Food Name	Serving Size	Calories	Prot. gms	Carbs gms	Sod. mgs	Fiber gms	Fat gms	Sat. Fat gms	Chol. mgs	% Fat Cal.
Southwest	1.75 oz	301	0	2	443	0	32.0	18.0	4	97%
Thousand Island	2 oz	270	1	9	460	0	27.0	30.0	4	86%
SIDE DISH. See also Beans.										
coleslaw	5 oz	206	2	12	358	2	16.0	11.0	3	72%
corn cobbette	3 oz	80	3	18	10	1	1.0	0.0	0	10%
French fries	5.5 oz	444	6	61	605	0	19.0	0.0	5	39%
macaroni and cheese	1 serving	330	14	32	1290	4	16.0	30.0	6	44%
mashed potato	5 oz	97	3	21	369	2	1.0	0.0	0	9%
potato salad	6 oz	256	3	30	527	3	14.0	15.0	2	49%
Spanish rice	4 oz	130	2	24	397	1	3.0	0.0	1	21%
vegetables, fresh	4 oz	57	2	8	79	3	2.0	0.0	1	31%
TACO										
'Al Carbon'	3 oz	164	13	14	21	1	6.0	68.0	2	33%
chicken, soft	4.5 oz	237	17	15	629	0	12.0	74.0	4	46%
taquito, chicken	5 oz	370	15	43	690	3	17.0	25.0	4	40%
TORTILLA										
corn, 6-inch diam	1 oz	70	1	14	35	1	1.0	0.0	0	13%
corn, 4.5-inch diam	0.5 oz	32	1	6	21	0	0.5	0.0	0	14%
flour, 11-inch diam	3 oz	260	7	42	583	6	7.0	0.0	2	24%
flour, 6-inch diam	1 oz	90	3	13	224	0	3.0	0.0	0	30%
spicy tomato	3 oz	254	7	42	577	2	6.0	0.0	1	22%
TORTILLA CHIPS, no salt	5 oz	760	9	86	22	7	42.0	0.0	10	50%
TOSTADA SHELL	5.6 oz	440	7	42	610	0	27.0	0.0	4	55%
EVERYTHING YOGURT										
YOGURT, FROZEN										
low-fat	1 serving	95	3	18	30	0	1.0	5.0	0	10%
nonfat	1 serving	80	3	17	40	0	0.0	0.0	0	0%
GODFATHER'S PIZZA										
PIZZA										
Cheese										
golden crust, large	1/10 pizza	261	8	31	314	0	11.0	23.0	0	39%
golden crust, medium	1/8 pizza	229	8	28	272	0	9.0	19.0	0	36%
golden crust, small	1/6 pizza	213	8	27	258	0	8.0	19.0	0	34%
original crust, large	1/10 pizza	271	12	37	329	0	8.0	28.0	0	27%
original crust, medium	1/8 pizza	242	10	35	285	0	7.0	22.0	0	26%
original crust, mini	1/4 pizza	138	6	20	159	0	4.0	13.0	0	26%
original crust, small	1/6 pizza	239	10	32	289	0	7.0	25.0	0	27%
thin crust, large	1/10 pizza	228	11	28	464	0	7.0	16.0	0	29%
thin crust, medium	1/8 pizza	210	10	26	410	0	7.0	14.0	0	30%
thin crust, small	1/6 pizza	180	9	21	370	0	6.0	0.0	0	31%
Combo										
golden crust, large	1/10 pizza	322	14	33	602	0	15.0	34.0	0	42%
golden crust, medium	1/8 pizza	283	13	30	526	0	13.0	29.0	0	40%
golden crust, small	1/6 pizza	273	13	29	542	0	12.0	31.0	0	39%
original crust, large	1/10 pizza	332	16	39	617	0	12.0	39.0	0	33%
original crust, medium	1/8 pizza	318	16	37	569	0	12.0	38.0	0	34%
original crust, mini	1/4 pizza	164	8	21	287	0	5.0	17.0	0	28%
original crust, small	1/6 pizza	299	15	34	573	0	11.0	37.0	0	34%
thin crust, large	1/10 pizza	336	17	31	870	0	16.0	27.0	0	43%
thin crust, medium	1/8 pizza	310	15	29	790	0	14.0	25.0	0	42%
thin crust, small	1/6 pizza	270	13	23	710	0	13.0	25.0	0	45%
STUFFED PIZZA										
cheese, large	1/10 pizza	381	16	44	677	0	16.0	32.0	0	38%
cheese, medium	1/8 pizza	350	14	42	610	0	13.0	25.0	0	34%

Food Name	Serving Size	Calories	Prot. gms	Carbs gms	Sod. mgs	Fiber gms	Fat gms	Sat. Fat gms	Chol. mgs	% Fat Cal.
cheese, small	1/6 pizza	310	13	38	560	0	11.0	25.0	0	33%
combo, large	1/10 pizza	521	23	47	1204	0	26.0	48.0	0	46%
combo, medium	1/8 pizza	480	21	45	1105	0	23.0	43.0	0	44%
combo, small	1/6 pizza	430	19	41	1000	0	20.0	40.0	0	43%

GOLDEN CORRAL

Food Name	Serving Size	Calories	Prot. gms	Carbs gms	Sod. mgs	Fiber gms	Fat gms	Sat. Fat gms	Chol. mgs	% Fat Cal.
BREAD, 'Texas Toast'	1 serving	170	5	26	230	0	6.0	0.0	0	30%
CHICKEN										
fillet, 'Golden Fried'	1 serving	370	37	14	570	0	19.0	85.0	0	46%
fillet, 'Golden Grilled'	1 serving	170	32	0	520	0	5.0	100.0	0	26%
POTATO, baked	1 serving	220	5	46	60	0	2.0	0.0	0	8%
RIBEYE STEAK, regular	1 serving	450	34	0	220	0	35.0	120.0	0	70%
SHRIMP, 'Golden Fried'	1 serving	250	12	24	470	0	12.0	90.0	0	43%
SIRLOIN STEAK										
	5-oz serving	230	27	0	270	0	14.0	85.0	0	54%
chopped	4-oz serving	320	28	0	160	0	23.0	100.0	0	65%
tips, w/onions and pepper	8.2-oz serving	290	30	8	260	0	13.0	120.0	0	43%

HARDEE'S

Food Name	Serving Size	Calories	Prot. gms	Carbs gms	Sod. mgs	Fiber gms	Fat gms	Sat. Fat gms	Chol. mgs	% Fat Cal.
BEVERAGE										
chocolate shake	12.3 fl oz	370	13	67	270	na	5.0	30.0	3	12%
orange juice	10 fl oz	140	2	34	5	na	0.0	0.0	0	0%
vanilla shake	12.3 fl oz	350	12	65	300	na	5.0	20.0	3	13%
BISCUIT										
and gravy	1 serving	530	10	56	1550	na	30.0	15.0	9	51%
apple cinnamon n' raisin	1 serving	250	2	42	350	na	8.0	0.0	2	29%
jelly	1 serving	440	6	57	1000	na	21.0	0.0	6	43%
chicken	1 sandwich	590	24	62	1820	na	27.0	45.0	7	41%
country ham	1 sandwich	440	14	44	1710	na	22.0	30.0	7	46%
egg and cheese	1 sandwich	520	17	45	1420	na	30.0	210.0	11	52%
ham	1 sandwich	410	13	45	1200	na	20.0	25.0	6	44%
'Made From Scratch'	1 serving	390	6	44	1000	na	21.0	0.0	6	49%
omelet	1 sandwich	550	20	45	1350	na	32.0	225.0	12	53%
plain or buttermilk	1 biscuit	353	6	47	1020	1	16.0	2.4	1	40%
sausage and egg	1 sandwich	620	19	45	1370	na	41.0	225.0	13	59%
sausage biscuit	1 sandwich	550	12	44	1310	na	36.0	25.0	11	59%
steak	1 sandwich	580	15	56	1580	na	32.0	30.0	10	50%
CHICKEN										
breast, w/o bone	1 serving	370	29	29	1190	na	15.0	75.0	4	37%
leg, w/o bone	1 serving	170	13	15	570	na	7.0	45.0	2	36%
thigh, w/o bone	1 serving	330	19	30	1000	na	15.0	60.0	4	41%
wing, w/o bone	1 serving	200	10	23	740	na	8.0	30.0	2	35%
DESSERT										
apple turnover	1 serving	270	4	38	250	na	12.0	0.0	4	39%
cone, twist	1 serving	180	4	34	120	na	2.0	10.0	1	11%
peach cobbler	1 serving	310	2	60	360	na	7.0	0.0	1	20%
GRAVY	1 serving	20	0	3	260	na	0.0	0.0	0	0%
HAMBURGER										
'All-Star'	1 burger	660	29	41	1260	na	43.0	100.0	14	58%
'Famous Star'	1 burger	570	24	41	860	na	35.0	80.0	10	55%
'Frisco Burger'	1 burger	720	31	37	1180	na	49.0	95.0	15	62%
'Monster Burger'	1 burger	1060	49	37	1860	na	79.0	185.0	29	67%
regular	1 burger	270	13	29	550	na	11.0	35.0	4	37%
'Super Star'	1 burger	790	40	41	970	na	53.0	145.0	17	60%
HOT DOG, w/condiments	1 serving	450	15	25	1240	na	32.0	55.0	12	64%

Food Name	Serving Size	Calories	Prot. gms	Carbs gms	Sod. mgs	Fiber gms	Fat gms	Sat. Fat gms	Chol. mgs	% Fat Cal.
SANDWICH										
bacon Swiss crispy chicken	1 sandwich	670	24	45	1600	na	44.0	55.0	9	59%
chicken fillet	1 sandwich	480	24	44	1190	na	23.0	55.0	4	43%
chicken, grilled	1 sandwich	350	23	28	860	na	16.0	65.0	3	41%
'Fisherman's Fillet'	1 sandwich	530	25	45	1280	na	28.0	75.0	7	47%
'Frisco Ham'	1 sandwich	450	22	42	1290	na	22.0	225.0	8	44%
ham and cheese, hot	1 sandwich	300	16	34	1390	na	12.0	50.0	6	35%
roast beef, big	1 sandwich	410	24	26	1140	na	24.0	40.0	9	52%
roast beef, monster	1 sandwich	610	35	26	1940	na	39.0	105.0	18	59%
roast beef, regular	1 sandwich	310	17	26	800	na	16.0	40.0	6	46%
SIDE DISH										
coleslaw	1 serving	240	2	13	340	na	20.0	10.0	3	75%
crispy curl potatoes, large	1 serving	520	7	62	1450	na	28.0	0.0	5	48%
crispy curl potatoes, medium	1 serving	340	5	41	950	na	18.0	0.0	4	47%
crispy curl potatoes, monster	1 serving	590	8	70	1640	na	31.0	0.0	6	47%
French fries, large	1 serving	440	5	59	520	na	21.0	0.0	3	42%
French fries, monster	1 serving	510	6	67	590	na	24.0	0.0	3	43%
French fries, regular	1 serving	340	4	45	390	na	16.0	0.0	2	42%
hash rounds, regular	1 serving	230	3	24	560	na	14.0	0.0	3	54%
mashed potato, small	1 serving	70	2	14	330	na	0.0	0.0	0	0%
HARVEY'S FOODS										
BREAKFAST										
pancake	1 serving	89	2	17	0	0	1.0	8.0	0	11%
sausage	1 serving	167	9	3	0	0	14.0	12.0	0	72%
toast, plain	1 serving	250	8	48	0	0	3.0	0.0	0	11%
CHEESEBURGER	1 serving	415	22	41	0	0	18.0	30.0	0	39%
CHICKEN FINGERS	1 serving	240	15	18	0	0	12.0	57.0	0	45%
DESSERT, apple turnover	1 serving	179	1	28	0	0	7.0	7.0	0	35%
HAMBURGER										
double	1 burger	530	31	44	0	0	26.0	34.0	0	44%
regular	1 burger	355	18	40	0	0	14.0	17.0	0	35%
super	1 burger	477	37	38	0	0	19.0	112.0	0	36%
HOT DOG	1 serving	332	12	32	0	0	15.0	50.0	0	43%
MUFFIN										
blueberry	1 muffin	254	4	45	0	0	6.0	0.0	0	22%
bran	1 muffin	301	5	42	0	0	13.0	0.0	0	38%
SANDWICH										
chicken	1 sandwich	419	19	46	0	0	16.0	110.0	0	36%
'Western'	1 sandwich	347	15	58	0	0	10.0	265.0	0	24%
SIDE DISH										
French fries	1 serving	478	10	56	0	0	24.0	5.0	0	45%
hash browns	1 serving	146	2	15	0	0	9.0	2.0	0	54%
onion rings	1 serving	288	4	36	0	0	14.0	5.0	0	44%
HUNGRY HUNTER										
CHICKEN, breast, teriyaki, boneless, charbroiled	1 serving	413	71	9	237	0	8.0	193.0	0	18%
CRAB										
Alaskan king, w/1 tbsp butter	1 serving	432	73	0	3436	0	13.0	194.0	0	29%
Alaskan king, w/o butter	1 serving	332	73	0	3319	0	2.0	163.0	0	6%
STEAK										
filet mignon	8 oz	539	69	0	150	0	27.0	203.0	0	47%
filet mignon, choice	3.5 oz	238	30	0	66	0	11.9	89.5	0	47%
LOBSTER										
cooked, w/o butter	1 serving	139	29	2	539	0	1.0	102.0	0	7%
cooked, w/ 1 tbsp. butter	1 serving	241	29	2	657	0	12.0	133.0	0	47%

Food Name	Serving Size	Calories	Prot. gms	Carbs gms	Sod. mgs	Fiber gms	Fat gms	Sat. Fat gms	Chol. mgs	% Fat Cal.
SIDE DISH										
baked potato	1 serving	185	4	43	13	4	0.0	0.0	0	0%
rice pilaf	1 serving	142	4	26	223	1	2.0	0.0	0	13%
SNAPPER, RED, fresh, cooked in 1/2 oz. butter	1 serving	329	47	0	262	0	15.0	114.0	0	42%
IN-N-OUT										
BEVERAGE										
chocolate shake	15 fl oz	690	9	83	350	0	36.0	95.0	24	47%
'Coca-Cola Classic'	16 fl oz	198	0	54	12	0	0.0	0.0	0	0%
coffee	10 fl oz	5	0	1	3	0	0.0	0.0	0	0%
'Diet Coke'	16 fl oz	0	0	0	20	0	0.0	0.0	0	0%
'Dr. Pepper'	16 fl oz	200	0	52	0	0	0.0	0.0	0	0%
iced tea	16 fl oz	0	0	0	0	0	0.0	0.0	0	0%
lemonade	16 fl oz	180	0	40	20	0	0.0	0.0	0	0%
milk	10 fl oz	180	12	18	190	0	6.0	30.0	4	31%
root beer	16 fl oz	222	0	60	48	0	0.0	0.0	0	0%
'Seven-Up'	16 fl oz	220	0	52	40	0	0.0	0.0	0	0%
strawberry shake	15 fl oz	690	8	91	280	2	33.0	85.0	22	43%
vanilla shake	15 fl oz	680	9	78	390	2	37.0	90.0	25	49%
CHEESEBURGER										
'Protein Style' w/lettuce leaves, w/o bun	1 serving	330	18	11	720	2	25.0	60.0	9	66%
regular	1 serving	480	22	39	1000	3	27.0	60.0	10	50%
w/o spread, w/mustard and ketchup	1 serving	400	22	41	1080	3	18.0	55.0	9	39%
HAMBURGER										
'Double Double'	1 serving	670	37	40	1430	3	41.0	120.0	18	55%
'Double Double' protein style, w/lettuce leaves, w/o bun	1 serving	520	33	11	1160	2	39.0	120.0	17	67%
'Double Double' w/o spread, w/mustard and ketchup	1 serving	590	37	42	1510	3	32.0	115.0	17	48%
regular	1 serving	390	16	39	640	3	19.0	40.0	5	44%
regular, protein style, w/lettuce leaves, w/o bun	1 serving	240	12	10	370	2	17.0	40.0	5	63%
regular, w/o spread, w/mustard and ketchup	1 serving	310	16	41	720	3	10.0	35.0	4	28%
SIDE DISH, French fries	1 serving	400	7	54	245	2	18.0	0.0	5	40%
JACK IN THE BOX										
BEVERAGE										
cappuccino ice cream shake, regular	16 fl oz	630	11	80	320	0	29.0	90.0	17	42%
chocolate ice cream shake, regular	16 fl oz	630	11	85	330	0	27.0	85.0	16	39%
'Coca Cola Classic' regular	20 fl oz	170	0	46	8	0	0.0	0.0	0	0%
coffee, regular	12 fl oz	5	0	1	5	0	0.0	0.0	0	0%
'Diet Coke' regular	20 fl oz	0	0	0	15	0	0.0	0.0	0	0%
'Dr. Pepper' regular	20 fl oz	190	0	49	25	0	0.0	0.0	0	0%
iced tea, regular	20 fl oz	0	0	0	0	0	0.0	0.0	0	0%
lemonade, 'Minute Maid' regular	20 fl oz	190	0	65	100	0	0.0	0.0	0	0%
milk, 2%	8 fl oz	130	9	14	85	0	5.0	25.0	3	33%
orange juice	10 fl oz	150	2	34	20	1	0.0	0.0	0	0%
Oreo cookie ice cream shake, regular	16 fl oz	740	13	91	490	2	36.0	95.0	19	44%
root beer, 'Barq's' regular	20 fl oz	180	0	50	40	0	0.0	0.0	0	0%
'Sprite' regular	20 fl oz	160	0	41	40	0	0.0	0.0	0	0%
BREAKFAST										
'Breakfast Jack'	1 sandwich	280	17	28	750	1	12.0	190.0	5	38%
French toast sticks, w/bacon	1 serving	470	12	53	700	2	23.0	30.0	4	44%
pancake, w/bacon	1 serving	370	12	59	1020	3	9.0	30.0	2	22%
sausage croissant	1 sandwich	700	21	38	1000	0	51.0	240.0	20	66%
'Supreme Croissant'	1 sandwich	530	22	37	960	0	32.0	225.0	13	55%
'Ultimate Breakfast Sandwich'	1 sandwich	600	34	39	1470	2	34.0	400.0	10	51%

Food Name	Serving Size	Calories	Prot. gms	Carbs gms	Sod. mgs	Fiber gms	Fat gms	Sat. Fat gms	Chol. mgs	% Fat Cal.
CHEESE										
American	1 slice	45	2	1	230	0	4.0	10.0	2	75%
Swiss style	1 slice	40	2	1	210	0	4.0	10.0	2	75%
CHEESEBURGER										
'Bacon Ultimate'	1 burger	1020	58	37	1740	1	71.0	210.0	26	63%
double patty	1 burger	460	24	32	1090	2	27.0	80.0	12	52%
'Jumbo Jack'	1 burger	680	31	39	1130	2	45.0	115.0	16	59%
regular	1 burger	320	14	30	720	2	16.0	40.0	6	45%
'Ultimate'	1 burger	950	52	37	1370	1	66.0	195.0	26	63%
CHICKEN, breast pieces	5 pieces	360	27	24	970	1	17.0	80.0	3	43%
CHICKEN MEAL										
chicken teriyaki bowl	1 serving	670	26	128	1730	3	4.0	15.0	1	6%
4 chicken pieces, w/French fries	1 serving	730	26	79	1690	5	34.0	65.0	7	42%
CONDIMENTS. See also Salad Dressing.										
barbecue dipping sauce	1 serving	45	1	11	310	0	0.0	0.0	0	0%
buttermilk dipping house sauce	1 serving	130	1	3	240	1	13.0	10.0	5	88%
catsup	1 serving	10	0	2	105	0	0.0	0.0	0	0%
croutons, salad bar item	1 serving	50	1	8	105	0	2.0	0.0	1	33%
jelly, grape	1 serving	40	0	10	5	0	0.0	0.0	0	0%
margarine-like spread, 'Country Crock'	1 serving	25	0	0	45	0	2.5	0.0	1	100%
salsa	1 serving	10	0	2	200	0	0.0	0.0	0	0%
sour cream	1 serving	60	1	1	30	0	6.0	20.0	4	87%
soy sauce	1 serving	5	1	1	480	0	0.0	0.0	0	0%
sweet and sour sauce	1 serving	45	1	11	160	0	0.0	0.0	0	0%
syrup	1 serving	130	0	30	5	0	0.0	0.0	0	0%
tartar sauce	1 serving	210	1	2	340	0	22.0	30.0	3	94%
DESSERT										
apple turnover, hot	1 serving	340	4	41	510	2	18.0	0.0	4	47%
carrot cake	1 serving	370	3	54	340	2	16.0	40.0	3	39%
double fudge cake	1 serving	300	3	50	320	1	10.0	50.0	2	30%
cheesecake	1 serving	320	7	32	220	1	18.0	65.0	10	51%
strawberry ice cream, regular	16 fl oz	640	10	85	300	0	28.0	85.0	15	40%
vanilla ice cream, regular	16 fl oz	610	12	73	320	0	31.0	95.0	18	45%
FISH AND CHIPS	1 serving	780	19	86	1740	6	39.0	45.0	9	46%
HAMBURGER										
'Jumbo Jack'	1 burger	590	27	39	670	2	37.0	90.0	11	56%
regular	1 burger	280	12	30	490	2	12.0	30.0	4	39%
'Sourdough Jack'	1 burger	690	34	37	1180	2	45.0	105.0	15	59%
SALAD										
chicken garden	1 salad	200	23	8	420	3	9.0	65.0	4	40%
side	1 salad	50	2	3	75	1	3.0	10.0	2	57%
SALAD DRESSING										
blue cheese	1 serving	210	1	11	750	0	15.0	25.0	3	74%
house, buttermilk	1 serving	290	1	6	560	0	30.0	20.0	11	91%
Italian, low-calorie	1 serving	25	0	2	670	0	1.5	0.0	0	63%
Thousand Island	1 serving	250	1	10	570	0	24.0	35.0	4	83%
SANDWICH										
chicken	1 sandwich	420	16	39	950	2	23.0	40.0	4	48%
chicken, 'Jack's Spicy'	1 sandwich	570	24	52	1020	2	29.0	50.0	3	46%
'Chicken Fajita Pita'	1 sandwich	280	24	25	840	3	9.0	75.0	4	29%
chicken fillet, grilled	1 sandwich	480	27	39	1110	4	24.0	65.0	6	45%
'Chicken Supreme'	1 sandwich	830	33	67	2130	3	48.0	75.0	7	52%
'Philly Cheesesteak'	1 sandwich	580	33	56	1860	1	16.0	80.0	8	29%
'Sourdough Breakfast'	1 sandwich	450	21	36	1040	2	24.0	205.0	8	49%

Food Name	Serving Size	Calories	Prot. gms	Carbs gms	Sod. mgs	Fiber gms	Fat gms	Sat. Fat gms	Chol. mgs	% Fat Cal.
SIDE DISH										
eggroll	3 egg rolls	440	15	40	1020	4	24.0	35.0	6	50%
French fries, curly, chili cheese	1 serving	650	14	60	1760	4	41.0	25.0	12	55%
French fries, curly, seasoned	1 serving	410	6	45	1010	4	23.0	0.0	5	50%
French fries, jumbo	1 serving	430	4	58	890	4	20.0	0.0	5	42%
French fries, regular	1 serving	350	4	46	710	3	16.0	0.0	4	42%
French fries, super scoop	1 serving	610	6	82	1250	5	28.0	0.0	6	42%
hash browns	1 serving	170	1	14	250	1	12.0	0.0	2	64%
jalapeños, stuffed	7 jalapeños	530	14	46	1730	3	31.0	60.0	12	54%
onion rings	1 serving	410	6	45	1010	4	23.0	0.0	5	50%
potato, bacon cheddar wedges	1 serving	800	20	49	1470	4	58.0	55.0	16	65%
TACO										
monster	1 serving	270	12	19	670	4	17.0	30.0	6	55%
regular	1 serving	170	7	12	460	2	10.0	20.0	4	54%
KENTUCKY FRIED CHICKEN										
BISCUIT	1 biscuit	180	4	20	560	0	10.0	0.0	3	48%
CHICKEN										
breast, extra crispy, w/o bone, 5.9 oz	1 breast	470	39	17	874	1	28.0	160.0	8	53%
breast, hot and spicy, w/o bone, 6.5 oz	1 breast	505	38	23	1170	1	29.0	162.0	8	52%
breast, original recipe, w/o bone, 5.4 oz	1 breast	400	29	16	1116	1	24.0	135.0	6	55%
drumstick, extra crispy, w/o bone, 2.4 oz	1 drumstick	195	15	7	375	1	12.0	77.0	3	55%
drumstick, hot and spicy, w/o bone, 2.3 oz	1 drumstick	175	13	9	360	1	10.0	77.0	3	51%
drumstick, original recipe, w/o bone, 2.2 oz	1 drumstick	140	13	4	422	0	9.0	75.0	2	54%
popcorn, large	6.0 oz	620	30	36	1046	0	40.0	73.0	10	58%
popcorn, small	3.5 oz	362	17	21	610	0	23.0	43.0	6	58%
thigh, extra crispy, w/o bone, 4.2 oz	1 thigh	380	21	14	625	1	27.0	118.0	7	63%
thigh, hot and spicy, w/o bone, 3.8 oz	1 thigh	355	19	13	630	1	26.0	126.0	7	65%
thigh, original recipe, w/o bone, 3.2 oz	1 thigh	250	16	6	747	1	18.0	95.0	5	65%
wing, honey barbecue	6 pieces	607	33	33	1145	1	38.0	193.0	10	56%
wing, hot	6 pieces	471	27	18	1230	2	33.0	150.0	8	62%
wing, whole, extra crispy, w/o bone, 1.9 oz	1 wing	220	10	10	415	1	15.0	55.0	4	63%
wing, whole, hot and spicy, w/o bone, 1.9 oz	1 wing	210	10	9	360	1	15.0	55.0	4	64%
wing, whole, original recipe, w/o bone, 1.6 oz	1 wing	140	9	5	414	0	10.0	55.0	3	62%
CHICKEN POT PIE, chunky	13 oz	770	29	69	2160	5	42.0	70.0	13	49%
CHICKEN SANDWICH										
honey barbecue, w/sauce, 5.3 oz	1 sandwich	310	28	37	560	2	6.0	125.0	2	17%
original recipe, w/o sauce, 6.6 oz	1 sandwich	360	28	3	890	1	13.0	60.0	4	49%
original recipe, w/sauce, 7.3 oz	1 sandwich	450	29	33	940	2	22.0	70.0	5	44%
'Tender Roast' w/o sauce, 6.2 oz	1 sandwich	270	31	26	690	1	5.0	65.0	2	16%
'Tender Roast' w/sauce, 7.4 oz	1 sandwich	350	32	23	880	1	15.0	75.0	3	38%
'Triple Crunch Zinger' w/o sauce, 6.2 oz	1 sandwich	390	25	39	650	2	15.0	50.0	5	35%
'Triple Crunch Zinger' w/sauce, 7.4 oz	1 sandwich	550	28	36	830	2	32.0	85.0	7	53%
'Triple Crunch' w/o sauce, 6.2 oz	1 sandwich	390	25	39	650	2	15.0	50.0	5	35%
'Triple Crunch' w/o sauce, 6.6 oz	1 sandwich	490	28	29	710	2	29.0	70.0	6	53%
CHICKEN STRIPS										
crispy	3 strips	300	26	18	1165	1	16.0	56.0	4	45%
crispy, spicy	3 strips	335	25	23	1140	1	15.0	70.0	4	41%
DESSERT										
apple pie, 4.0 oz	1 slice	310	2	44	280	0	14.0	0.0	3	41%
double chocolate chip, 2.7 oz	1 serving	320	4	41	230	1	16.0	55.0	4	44%
'Little Bucket Parfait' chocolate creme, 4.0 oz	1 serving	290	3	37	330	2	15.0	15.0	11	46%
'Little Bucket Parfait' fudge brownie, 3.5 oz	1 serving	280	3	44	190	1	10.0	145.0	4	32%
'Little Bucket Parfait' lemon creme, 4.5 oz	1 serving	410	7	62	290	4	14.0	20.0	8	31%
'Little Bucket Parfait' strawberry shortcake, 3.5 oz	1 serving	200	1	33	220	1	7.0	10.0	6	32%

Food Name	Serving Size	Calories	Prot. gms	Carbs gms	Sod. mgs	Fiber gms	Fat gms	Sat. Fat gms	Chol. mgs	% Fat Cal.
pecan pie, 4.0 oz	1 slice	490	5	66	510	2	23.0	65.0	5	42%
strawberry creme pie, 2.7 oz	1 slice	280	4	32	130	2	15.0	15.0	8	48%
SIDE DISH										
barbecue baked beans	5.5 oz	190	6	33	760	6	3.0	5.0	1	15%
coleslaw	5 oz	232	2	26	284	3	13.5	8.0	2	52%
corn on the cob	5.7 oz	150	5	35	20	2	1.5	0.0	0	8%
macaroni and cheese	5.4 oz	180	7	21	860	2	8.0	10.0	3	39%
mashed potato, w/gravy	4.8 oz	120	1	17	440	2	6.0	1.0	1	43%
potato salad	5.6 oz	230	4	23	540	3	14.0	15.0	2	54%
potato wedges	4.8 oz	280	5	28	750	5	13.0	5.0	4	47%
KRYSTAL										
BREAKFAST										
bacon biscuit	3.6 oz	355	9	36	1055	0	20.0	14.0	5	50%
egg biscuit	4.8 oz	372	10	36	813	0	21.0	133.0	5	51%
gravy biscuit	8.2 oz	445	9	43	1306	0	26.0	13.0	5	53%
plain biscuit	3.2 oz	289	5	35	777	0	14.0	1.0	3	44%
sausage biscuit	4.3 oz	429	10	37	987	0	27.0	29.0	7	56%
'Sunriser'	3.6 oz	264	13	17	551	0	17.0	157.0	6	56%
CHEESEBURGER										
regular	1 serving	189	11	16	456	0	10.0	30.0	4	45%
w/bacon	6.4 oz	583	36	34	935	0	35.0	114.0	14	53%
'Burger Plus'	7 oz	545	33	37	962	0	31.0	105.0	12	50%
double patty	1 serving	214	11	22	674	0	8.0	16.0	2	35%
CHILI										
large	12-oz serving	322	17	33	1012	0	11.0	25.0	0	33%
regular	8-oz serving	214	11	22	674	0	8.0	16.0	0	35%
CORN DOG, 'Corn Pup'	2.3 oz	214	6	17	566	0	14.0	24.0	6	58%
DESSERT										
apple pie	4.5 oz	320	3	45	420	0	14.0	0.0	4	40%
lemon meringue pie	4 oz	340	7	60	130	0	9.0	45.0	3	23%
pecan pie	4 oz	450	5	61	290	0	24.0	55.0	6	45%
DOUGHNUT										
plain	1.3 oz	100	1	17	130	0	9.0	6.0	2	53%
w/chocolate icing	1.8 oz	162	1	27	149	0	11.0	6.0	3	47%
w/vanilla icing	1.8 oz	148	1	29	130	0	9.0	6.0	2	40%
HAMBURGER										
'Big K'	7.3 oz	608	40	35	1281	0	36.0	125.0	14	52%
'Burger Plus'	6.4 oz	488	30	36	709	0	27.0	90.0	9	48%
double patty	4 oz serving	276	18	24	532	0	14.0	43.0	5	43%
small	2.2 oz serving	158	9	15	339	0	7.0	21.0	0	40%
HOT DOG										
'Chili Cheese Pup'	2.6 oz	203	8	15	623	0	13.0	24.0	5	56%
'Chili Pup'	2.5 oz	184	7	14	593	0	12.0	19.0	4	56%
plain	1.9 oz	164	6	14	469	0	10.0	15.0	4	53%
MILKSHAKE, chocolate	12.8 fl oz	271	8	41	175	0	10.0	32.0	5	31%
SANDWICH										
chicken, 6.4 oz	1 sandwich	392	21	44	707	0	16.0	33.0	0	36%
country ham, 4.5 oz	1 sandwich	379	15	36	1488	0	19.0	23.0	5	46%
SIDE DISH										
French fries, crisscut, 'Krys Kross'	2.6 oz	242	3	33	589	0	11.0	10.0	5	41%
French fries, crisscut, 'Krys Kross' w/cheese	3.6 oz	292	4	35	789	0	15.0	11.0	6	46%
French fries, regular, large	5 oz serving	615	5	111	191	0	17.0	15.0	8	25%
French fries, regular, medium	3.9 oz serving	474	4	86	147	0	13.0	12.0	6	25%
French fries, regular, small	2.8 oz serving	338	3	61	105	0	9.0	8.0	0	24%

Food Name	Serving Size	Calories	Prot. gms	Carbs gms	Sod. mgs	Fiber gms	Fat gms	Sat. Fat gms	Chol. mgs	% Fat Cal.
LITTLE CAESARS										
BREAD, 'Crazy Bread'	1 serving	98	4	18	119	0	1.0	2.0	0	9%
CONDIMENTS, 'Crazy Sauce'	1 serving	63	3	11	360	0	1.0	0.0	0	14%
PIZZA										
'Baby Pan! Pan!'	1 serving	525	28	53	1180	0	22.0	60.0	0	38%
cheese, single slice, 2.2 oz	1 slice	170	9	20	285	0	6.0	10.0	0	32%
pepperoni combination, single slice	1 serving	190	10	20	340	1	7.0	15.0	0	34%
'Pizza! Pizza!' large	1 serving	169	11	18	240	0	6.0	15.0	0	32%
'Pizza! Pizza!' medium	1 serving	154	10	16	220	0	5.0	15.0	0	30%
'Pizza! Pizza!' small	1 serving	138	9	14	200	0	5.0	15.0	0	33%
'Pizza! Pizza!' square, large	1 serving	188	10	22	380	0	6.0	20.0	0	30%
'Pizza! Pizza!' square, medium	1 serving	185	10	22	370	0	6.0	20.0	0	30%
PIZZA MEAL										
cheese pizza, hand-tossed, w/individual tossed salad	1 serving	600	30	73	1605	3	21.0	35.0	0	31%
vegetable pizza, w/individual tossed salad	1 serving	640	34	76	1715	4	22.0	40.0	0	31%
SALAD										
antipasto, w/low-calorie dressing	12 oz serving	170	10	12	1145	0	9.0	40.0	0	48%
Greek, w/low-calorie dressing	11 oz serving	140	8	8	1075	0	8.0	25.0	0	53%
tossed, small	1 serving	37	2	7	85	0	1.0	0.0	0	20%
tossed, w/low-calorie dressing	11 oz serving	80	4	11	745	0	2.0	0.0	0	23%
SANDWICH										
ham and cheese	1 sandwich	520	28	55	1045	1	21.0	45.0	0	36%
submarine, Italian	1 sandwich	590	29	55	1230	2	28.0	60.0	0	43%
tuna melt	1 sandwich	700	34	58	825	1	37.0	65.0	0	48%
turkey	1 sandwich	450	24	49	1590	0	17.0	45.0	0	34%
vegetarian	1 sandwich	620	30	58	1000	1	30.0	55.0	0	43%
LONG JOHN SILVER'S										
CHICKEN										
batter-dipped, 2 oz	1 piece	120	8	11	400	3	6.0	15.0	2	42%
'FlavorBaked'	2.6 oz	110	19	1	600	1	3.0	55.0	1	25%
CLAMS, batter-dipped	3 oz	300	11	31	670	5	17.0	40.0	4	48%
CONDIMENTS. See also Salad Dressing.										
catsup	0.32 oz	10	0	2	110	0	0.0	0.0	0	0%
honey mustard sauce	0.42 oz	20	0	5	60	na	0.0	0.0	0	0%
malt vinegar	0.28 oz	0	0	0	15	na	0.0	0.0	0	0%
margarine	0.18 oz	35	0	0	35	na	4.0	0.0	1	100%
shrimp sauce	0.42 oz	15	0	3	180	na	0.0	0.0	0	0%
sour cream	1 oz	60	1	1	15	na	6.0	15.0	4	87%
sweet and sour sauce	0.42 oz	20	0	5	45	na	0.0	0.0	0	0%
tartar sauce	0.42 oz	35	0	5	35	na	1.5	0.0	na	40%
FISH										
batter-dipped, 2.98 oz	1 piece	170	11	12	470	5	11.0	30.0	3	52%
'Flavorbaked' 2.3 oz	1 piece	90	14	1	320	0	2.5	35.0	1	27%
SALAD										
garden	1 salad	45	3	9	25	4	0.0	0.0	0	0%
grilled chicken	1 salad	140	20	10	260	4	2.5	45.0	1	16%
ocean chef	1 salad	130	14	15	540	4	2.0	60.0	0	13%
side	4.3 oz	25	1	4	15	1	0.0	0.0	0	0%
SALAD DRESSING										
French, fat-free	1.5 oz	50	0	14	360	na	0.0	0.0	0	0%
Italian	1 oz	130	0	2	280	na	14.0	0.0	2	94%
ranch	1 oz	170	0	1	260	na	18.0	5.0	3	98%
ranch, nonfat	1.5 oz	50	2	13	380	na	0.0	0.0	0	0%
Thousand Island	1 oz	110	0	5	280	na	10.0	15.0	2	82%

Food Name	Serving Size	Calories	Prot. gms	Carbs gms	Sod. mgs	Fiber gms	Fat gms	Sat. Fat gms	Chol. mgs	% Fat Cal.
SANDWICH										
chicken, 'Flavorbaked'	5.8 oz	290	24	27	970	2	10.0	60.0	2	31%
fish, batter-dipped, no sauce	5.4 oz	320	17	40	800	6	13.0	20.0	4	34%
fish, 'Ultimate'	6.4 oz	430	18	44	1340	3	21.0	35.0	7	43%
fish, 'Flavorbaked'	6 oz	320	23	28	930	2	14.0	55.0	7	38%
SHRIMP, batter-dipped, 0.4 oz	1 piece	35	1	2	95	0	2.5	10.0	1	65%
SIDE DISH										
baked potato	8 oz	210	4	49	10	3	0.0	0.0	0	0%
cheese sticks	1.6 oz	160	6	12	360	1	9.0	10.0	4	53%
coleslaw	3.4 oz	140	1	20	260	3	6.0	0.0	na	39%
corn cobbette, w/butter	3.3 oz	140	3	19	0	0	8.0	0.0	2	45%
corn cobbette w/o butter	3.05 oz	80	3	19	0	0	0.5	0.0	0	5%
French fries	3 oz	250	3	28	500	3	15.0	0.0	3	52%
green beans	3.5 oz	30	2	5	310	2	0.5	5.0	0	14%
hushpuppy, 0.8 oz	1 piece	60	1	9	25	0	2.5	0.0	0	36%
rice pilaf	3 oz	140	3	26	210	1	3.0	0.0	1	19%
MAZZIO'S										
CHICKEN PARMESAN, noodles chicken Parmesan	17.5 oz	590	39	68	1600	0	19.0	50.0	3	29%
FETTUCCINE ALFREDO, small	1 serving	440	14	34	680	0	28.0	55.0	16	57%
GARLIC BREAD, w/cheese	2 slices	700	21	74	1280	0	35.0	15.0	7	45%
LASAGNA, meat, small	1 serving	460	24	26	1370	0	25.0	95.0	10	53%
NACHOS, meat	4.5 oz	500	21	21	1200	0	37.0	75.0	17	66%
PIZZA										
cheese, deep pan	1 serving	350	17	42	620	0	8.0	15.0	0	23%
cheese, original, medium	2 slices	260	14	33	450	0	8.0	10.0	0	28%
cheese, thick crust	1 serving	220	13	22	440	0	9.0	15.0	0	37%
combination, deep pan, medium	1 slice	410	19	42	930	0	18.0	20.0	6	40%
combination, original, medium	1 slice	320	17	34	780	0	13.0	25.0	6	36%
'Light' medium	1 slice	240	10	30	460	0	8.0	20.0	4	31%
pepperoni, deep pan, medium	1 slice	380	18	38	740	0	17.0	25.0	6	41%
pepperoni, original, medium	1 slice	280	16	30	600	0	11.0	30.0	5	35%
sausage, deep pan, medium	1 slice	430	21	41	1040	0	21.0	25.0	8	43%
sausage, original, medium	1 slice	350	18	34	890	0	16.0	20.0	7	41%
SANDWICH										
barbecue beef and cheddar	1 sandwich	580	39	53	1260	0	24.0	95.0	11	37%
chicken and cheddar	1 sandwich	570	33	56	1350	0	24.0	70.0	8	38%
ham and cheese sandwich	1 sandwich	790	40	71	1900	0	39.0	85.0	13	44%
SPAGHETTI ENTRÉE, small	1 serving	290	11	39	800	0	10.0	5.0	0	31%
MCDONALD'S										
BEVERAGE										
apple bran muffin, low-fat	1 serving	300	6	61	380	3	3.0	0.0	1	9%
chocolate shake, small	1 small	360	11	60	250	1	9.0	40.0	6	22%
'Coca Cola Classic' medium	21 fl oz	310	0	58	20	0	0.0	0.0	0	0%
'Diet Coke' medium	21 fl oz	0	0	0	40	0	0.0	0.0	0	0%
English muffin	1 serving	140	4	25	210	1	2.0	0.0	0	13%
orange drink, 'Hi-C' medium	21 fl oz	240	0	64	40	0	0.0	0.0	0	0%
milk, 1%										
	8 fl oz	100	8	13	115	0	2.5	10.0	2	21%
orange juice	6 fl oz	80	0	20	20	0	0.0	0.0	0	0%
'Sprite' medium	21 fl oz	210	0	56	80	0	0.0	0.0	0	0%
strawberry shake, small	1 serving	360	11	60	180	0	9.0	40.0	6	22%
vanilla shake, small	1 serving	360	11	59	250	0	9.0	40.0	6	22%
BREAKFAST										
apple Danish	1 serving	340	5	47	340	2	15.0	20.0	3	39%

Food Name	Serving Size	Calories	Prot. gms	Carbs gms	Sod. mgs	Fiber gms	Fat gms	Sat. Fat gms	Chol. mgs	% Fat Cal.
biscuit, plain or buttermilk	1 serving	262	4	35	757	1	11.9	1.8	1	40%
bacon, egg, and cheese biscuit	1 sandwich	540	21	36	1550	1	34.0	250.0	10	57%
cheese Danish	1 serving	400	7	45	400	2	21.0	40.0	5	48%
cinnamon roll	1 serving	390	6	50	310	2	18.0	65.0	5	42%
hash browns	1 serving	130	1	14	330	1	8.0	0.0	2	55%
hotcakes, plain	1 serving	340	9	58	630	3	8.0	20.0	2	21%
hotcakes, w/margarine and syrup	1 serving	600	9	104	770	3	17.0	20.0	3	25%
sausage biscuit	1 sandwich	470	11	35	1080	1	31.0	35.0	9	60%
sausage and egg biscuit	1 sandwich	550	18	35	1160	1	37.0	245.0	10	61%
breakfast burrito	1 serving	320	13	21	660	1	20.0	195.0	7	57%
'Egg McMuffin'	1 sandwich	290	17	27	790	1	12.0	235.0	5	38%
ham, egg, and cheese bagel	1 sandwich	550	26	58	1490	9	23.0	255.0	8	38%
sausage	1 serving	170	6	0	290	0	16.0	35.0	5	86%
'Sausage McMuffin'	1 sandwich	360	13	26	740	1	23.0	45.0	8	57%
'Sausage w/Egg McMuffin'	1 sandwich	440	19	27	890	1	28.0	255.0	10	58%
scrambled eggs	2 eggs	160	13	1	170	0	11.0	425.0	4	64%
Spanish omelette bagel	1 sandwich	690	27	59	1560	10	38.0	275.0	14	50%
steak egg and cheese bagel	1 sandwich	660	36	57	1300	9	31.0	285.0	11	43%
CHEESEBURGER										
'Big Xtra!'	1 burger	810	29	52	1870	4	55.0	120.0	19	60%
'Quarter Pounder with Cheese'	1 burger	530	28	38	1310	2	30.0	95.0	13	51%
regular	1 burger	320	16	35	830	2	13.0	40.0	6	36%
CHICKEN NUGGETS										
'Chicken McNuggets'	4 pieces	190	10	13	360	1	11.0	35.0	3	52%
'Chicken McNuggets'	6 piece	290	15	20	540	2	17.0	55.0	4	52%
'Chicken McNuggets'	9 piece	430	23	29	810	2	25.0	80.0	5	52%
CONDIMENTS. See also Salad Dressing.										
barbecue sauce	1 pkg	45	0	10	250	0	0.0	0.0	0	0%
croutons, salad bar item	1 pkg	50	1	9	105	1	1.0	0.0	0	18%
honey	1 pkg	45	0	12	0	0	0.0	0.0	0	0%
honey mustard sauce	1 pkg	50	0	3	85	0	4.5	10.0	1	77%
hot mustard sauce	1 pkg	60	1	7	240	0	3.5	5.0	0	50%
mayonnaise, light	1 pkg	40	0	0	80	0	4.0	5.0	1	100%
sweet and sour sauce	1 pkg	50	0	11	140	0	0.0	0.0	0	0%
DESSERT										
apple pie, baked	1 serving	260	3	34	200	0	13.0	0.0	4	44%
chocolate chip cookie	1 serving	170	2	22	120	1	10.0	20.0	6	48%
ice cream cone, vanilla, reduced fat	1 serving	150	4	23	75	0	4.5	20.0	3	27%
'McDonaldland'	1 pkg	180	3	32	190	1	5.0	0.0	1	24%
'McFlurry' Butterfinger	1 serving	620	16	90	260	0	22.0	70.0	14	32%
'McFlurry' M&M	1 serving	630	16	90	210	1	23.0	75.0	15	33%
'McFlurry' Nestle Crunch	1 serving	630	16	89	230	0	24.0	75.0	16	34%
'McFlurry' Oreo	1 serving	570	15	82	280	0	20.0	70.0	12	32%
nut topping, for sundae	1 serving	40	2	2	55	0	3.5	0.0	0	66%
sundae, hot caramel	1 serving	360	7	61	180	0	10.0	35.0	6	25%
sundae, hot fudge	1 serving	340	8	52	170	1	12.0	30.0	9	31%
sundae, strawberry	1 serving	290	7	50	95	0	7.0	30.0	5	22%
HAMBURGER										
'Big Mac'	1 burger	570	26	45	1100	3	32.0	85.0	10	50%
'Big Xtra!'	1 burger	710	24	51	1400	4	46.0	95.0	15	58%
'Quarter Pounder'	1 burger	430	23	37	840	2	21.0	70.0	8	44%
regular	1 burger	270	13	35	600	2	8.0	30.0	4	27%
SALAD										
shaker, chef	1 salad	150	17	5	740	2	8.0	95.0	4	45%

Food Name	Serving Size	Calories	Prot. gms	Carbs gms	Sod. mgs	Fiber gms	Fat gms	Sat. Fat gms	Chol. mgs	% Fat Cal.
shaker, garden	1 salad	100	7	4	120	2	6.0	75.0	3	55%
shaker, grilled chicken Caesar	1 salad	100	17	3	240	2	2.5	40.0	2	22%
SALAD DRESSING										
Caesar	1 pkg	150	2	5	390	0	13.0	15.0	3	81%
herb vinaigrette, nonfat	1 pkg	30	0	7	220	0	0.0	0.0	0	0%
honey mustard	1 pkg	150	1	13	290	0	11.0	15.0	2	64%
ranch	1 pkg	170	0	2	480	0	18.0	10.0	3	95%
red ranch, reduced calorie	1 pkg	130	0	18	370	0	6.0	0.0	1	43%
Thousand Island	1 pkg	130	0	11	360	0	9.0	15.0	2	65%
SANDWICH										
chicken, crispy	1 sandwich	550	23	54	1180	2	27.0	50.0	5	44%
'Chicken McGrill'	1 sandwich	450	26	46	970	2	18.0	60.0	3	36%
'Chicken McGrill' w/o mayo	1 sandwich	340	26	45	890	2	7.0	50.0	2	18%
'Fillet-O-Fish'	1 sandwich	470	15	45	890	1	26.0	50.0	5	49%
SIDE DISH										
French fries, large	1 serving	540	8	68	350	6	26.0	0.0	5	43%
French fries, medium	1 serving	450	6	57	290	5	22.0	0.0	4	44%
French fries, small	1 serving	210	3	26	135	2	10.0	0.0	2	44%
French fries, super size	1 serving	610	9	77	390	7	29.0	0.0	5	43%

MRS. WINNER

Food Name	Serving Size	Calories	Prot. gms	Carbs gms	Sod. mgs	Fiber gms	Fat gms	Sat. Fat gms	Chol. mgs	% Fat Cal.
BISCUIT	1 serving	245	4	45	503	0	5.0	0.0	0	19%
CHICKEN										
breast, fried, no skin	4 oz	280	23	14	480	0	15.0	115.0	0	48%
fillet, baked	1 serving	120	10	0	360	0	2.0	33.0	0	31%
leg, fried, no skin	1.7 oz	110	10	5	115	0	6.0	50.0	0	47%
HAM, country	1 serving	60	4	0	565	0	1.0	14.0	0	36%
ROLL, honey yeast	1 roll	200	8	35	290	0	4.0	7.0	0	17%
SALAD										
chicken	1 salad	583	9	39	875	0	8.0	3.0	0	27%
seafood	1 salad	553	5	41	756	0	9.0	4.0	0	31%
tossed	1 salad	6	1	1	439	0	0.0	1.0	0	0%
SANDWICH										
chicken, breaded	1 sandwich	203	19	12	1000	0	10.0	37.0	0	42%
chicken fillet	1 sandwich	379	12	45	541	0	7.0	28.0	0	22%
chicken salad	1 sandwich	313	10	33	599	0	6.0	1.0	0	24%
steak	1 sandwich	429	11	43	644	0	11.0	21.0	0	31%
SAUSAGE, patty	1 serving	200	6	0	400	0	10.0	8.0	0	79%
SIDE DISH										
coleslaw	1 serving	188	1	9	549	0	16.0	1.0	0	78%
French fries	1 serving	225	6	27	214	0	9.0	1.0	0	38%
mashed potato, w/gravy	1 serving	148	3	22	823	0	3.0	2.0	0	21%
potato wedges, oven roasted	1 serving	139	4	31	132	0	1.0	1.0	0	6%
STEAK ENTRÉE, country fried	1 serving	220	12	0	205	0	14.0	7.0	0	72%

PERKINS

Food Name	Serving Size	Calories	Prot. gms	Carbs gms	Sod. mgs	Fiber gms	Fat gms	Sat. Fat gms	Chol. mgs	% Fat Cal.
BROCCOLI, raw	4 oz	31	3	6	31	0	0.4	0.0	0	9%
CHICKEN ENTRÉE										
lemon pepper, w/rice pilaf, broccoli, salad	1 serving	620	59	60	1364	0	12.5	136.0	0	19%
FRUIT CUP, w/cantaloupe, honeydew, blueberries	4.5 oz serving	48	1	12	12	0	0.3	0.0	0	5%
HASH BROWNS	3 oz	101	2	17	28	0	2.6	0.0	0	24%
MUFFIN										
apple	1 muffin	543	9	76	728	0	24.0	95.0	0	39%
banana nut	1 muffin	586	9	75	702	0	29.0	92.0	0	44%
blueberry	1 muffin	506	7	71	671	0	23.0	88.0	0	40%

Food Name	Serving Size	Calories	Prot. gms	Carbs gms	Sod. mgs	Fiber gms	Fat gms	Sat. Fat gms	Chol. mgs	% Fat Cal.
bran	1 muffin	478	9	83	572	0	17.0	0.0	0	29%
carrot	1 muffin	560	7	88	780	0	23.0	81.0	0	35%
chocolate chocolate chip	1 muffin	546	10	73	629	0	26.0	83.0	0	41%
corn	1 muffin	683	12	121	1550	0	17.0	33.0	0	22%
cranberry nut	1 muffin	558	9	71	671	0	28.0	88.0	0	44%
oat bran	1 muffin	513	10	87	588	0	16.0	0.0	0	27%
plain	1 muffin	586	9	81	797	0	26.0	104.0	0	39%
plain, low-fat	1 muffin	495	12	111	802	0	1.2	5.0	0	2%
OMELET										
'Country Club'	1 serving	932	47	6	1134	1	79.1	1154.0	0	77%
'Country Club' w/3 oz hash browns	1 serving	1033	49	23	1162	1	81.7	1154.0	0	72%
'Deli Ham and Lotsa Cheese'	1 serving	962	53	8	1832	1	79.1	864.0	0	74%
'Deli Ham and Lotsa Cheese' w/3 oz hash browns	1 serving	1063	55	25	1860	1	81.7	864.0	0	70%
'Denver' w/fruit cup	1 serving	235	23	22	795	0	6.5	154.0	0	24%
'Everything'	1 serving	697	45	9	870	0	53.4	814.0	0	69%
'Everything' w/3 oz hash browns	1 serving	798	46	25	898	2	56.0	814.0	0	64%
'Granny's Country'	1 serving	941	43	7	786	1	81.5	810.0	0	79%
'Granny's Country' w/9 oz hash browns	1 serving	1245	48	57	869	1	89.2	810.0	0	66%
ham and cheese	1 serving	644	41	3	832	0	51.3	743.0	0	73%
ham and cheese, w/3 oz hash browns	1 serving	745	42	19	860	0	53.9	743.0	0	66%
mushroom and cheese	1 serving	687	32	5	925	1	59.9	744.0	0	79%
mushroom and cheese, w/3 oz hash browns	1 serving	788	34	22	953	1	62.5	744.0	0	72%
seafood, w/fruit cup	1 serving	271	29	28	595	0	5.7	197.0	0	19%
ORANGE ROUGHY ENTRÉE,										
w/rice pilaf, broccoli, salad	1 serving	467	33	60	1387	0	7.0	133.0	0	14%
PANCAKE										
buttermilk	3 pancakes	442	13	70	988	0	12.0	24.0	0	25%
'Harvest Grain' w/1.5 oz low-cal syrup	5 pancakes	473	11	93	1640	0	3.4	0.0	0	7%
'Short Stack Harvest Grain'	3 pancakes	268	7	56	1020	0	2.0	0.0	0	7%
PIE										
apple	1 slice	521	3	72	457	0	26.0	0.0	0	44%
apple, w/Equal sugar substitute	1 slice	420	3	55	371	0	24.0	0.0	0	48%
cherry	1 slice	571	4	84	702	0	26.0	0.0	0	40%
cherry, w/Equal sugar substitute	1 slice	425	4	55	513	0	24.0	0.0	0	48%
coconut cream	1 slice	437	6	56	488	0	33.0	5.0	0	55%
French silk	1 slice	551	4	59	478	0	37.0	53.0	0	57%
lemon meringue	1 slice	395	2	63	528	0	16.0	0.0	0	36%
peanut butter brownie	1 slice	455	9	44	436	0	35.0	29.0	0	60%
pecan	1 slice	669	7	106	670	0	26.0	17.0	0	34%
SALAD										
chef, mini	1 salad	214	23	7	643	0	11.0	55.0	0	45%
dinner, 'Lite and Healthy'	1 salad	103	3	15	496	0	2.1	0.0	0	21%
SYRUP, low-calorie	1.5 oz	26	0	7	0	0	0.0	0.0	0	0%
TOAST, w/.5 oz margarine, grape jelly	0.75-oz slice	219	2	28	224	1	12.2	8.0	0	48%
VEGETABLE STIR-FRY, w/mixed vegetables	6 oz	49	3	10	23	0	0.4	0.0	0	6%
VEGETABLE SANDWICH										
stir-fry, on pita	1 sandwich	308	44	41	752	0	9.2	26.0	0	20%
stir-fry, on pita, w/coleslaw	1 sandwich	441	45	54	877	0	17.8	36.0	0	29%
stir-fry, on pita, w/coleslaw and pasta salad	1 sandwich	626	49	63	1395	0	32.5	37.0	0	40%
stir-fry, on pita, w/pasta salad	1 sandwich	493	48	50	1270	0	23.9	27.0	0	35%

PETER PIPER PIZZA

PIZZA

Beef

Food Name	Serving Size	Calories	Prot. gms	Carbs gms	Sod. mgs	Fiber gms	Fat gms	Sat. Fat gms	Chol. mgs	% Fat Cal.
extra large	1 slice	280	15	36	446	0	8.0	20.0	0	26%

Food Name	Serving Size	Calories	Prot. gms	Carbs gms	Sod. mgs	Fiber gms	Fat gms	Sat. Fat gms	Chol. mgs	% Fat Cal.
large	1 slice	296	15	39	482	0	8.0	20.0	0	25%
express lunch	1 slice	165	9	21	257	0	5.0	13.0	0	27%
medium	1 slice	222	12	29	359	0	6.0	15.0	0	25%
small	1 slice	194	10	25	319	0	5.0	14.0	0	24%
Cheese										
express lunch pizza	1 pizza	608	32	83	609	0	16.0	47.0	0	24%
express lunch pizza	1 slice	152	8	21	152	0	4.0	12.0	0	24%
extra large	1 pizza	3078	160	437	3113	0	73.0	211.0	0	22%
extra large	1 slice	257	13	36	260	0	6.1	18.0	0	22%
large	1 pizza	2159	112	311	2176	0	49.4	140.0	0	21%
large	1 slice	270	14	39	271	0	6.2	18.0	0	21%
medium	1 pizza	1622	84	235	1614	0	37.0	105.0	0	21%
medium	1 slice	203	11	29	201	0	5.0	13.0	0	22%
small	1 pizza	1059	60	152	1073	0	25.0	70.0	0	21%
small	1 slice	177	9	25	179	0	4.0	12.0	0	21%
w/black olive, large	1 slice	259	24	22	407	0	8.0	12.0	0	28%
w/black olive, medium	1 slice	193	18	17	303	0	6.0	9.0	0	28%
w/black olive, small	1 slice	171	16	15	276	0	6.0	8.0	0	30%
w/green pepper, large	1 slice	245	24	22	339	0	7.0	12.0	0	26%
w/green pepper, medium	1 slice	183	18	17	256	0	5.0	9.0	0	24%
w/green pepper, small	1 slice	163	16	15	283	0	4.0	8.0	0	23%
w/ham, large	1 slice	258	26	22	473	0	7.0	17.0	0	25%
w/ham, medium	1 slice	194	19	16	356	0	6.0	13.0	0	28%
w/ham, small	1 slice	172	17	15	317	0	5.0	11.0	0	26%
w/jalapeño, large	1 slice	244	24	22	424	0	7.0	12.0	0	26%
w/jalapeño, medium	1 slice	183	18	17	319	0	5.0	9.0	0	24%
w/jalapeño, small	1 slice	163	16	15	283	0	4.0	8.0	0	23%
w/mushroom, large	1 slice	245	24	22	379	0	7.0	12.0	0	26%
w/mushroom, medium	1 slice	183	18	17	283	0	5.0	9.0	0	24%
w/mushroom, small	1 slice	162	16	15	245	0	4.0	8.0	0	23%
w/onion, large	1 slice	243	24	22	341	0	7.0	12.0	0	26%
w/onion, medium	1 slice	183	18	17	257	0	5.0	9.0	0	24%
w/onion, small	1 slice	162	16	15	228	0	4.0	8.0	0	23%
w/pineapple, large	1 slice	246	23	23	341	0	7.0	12.0	0	26%
w/pineapple, medium	1 slice	185	18	17	256	0	5.0	8.0	0	24%
w/pineapple, small	1 slice	164	16	15	228	0	4.0	8.0	0	23%
Salami										
express lunch	1 slice	164	9	21	199	0	5.0	15.0	0	27%
extra large	1 slice	273	14	37	322	0	7.5	22.0	0	25%
large	1 slice	288	15	39	342	0	8.0	23.0	0	25%
medium	1 slice	216	11	29	254	0	6.0	17.0	0	25%
small	1 slice	189	8	25	223	0	5.0	15.0	0	25%
PIZZA HUT										
BREADSTICK	1 serving	130	3	20	170	1	4.0	0.0	1	28%
BREADSTICK DIPPING SAUCE	1 serving	30	1	5	170	1	0.5	0.0	0	16%
CHICKEN										
Buffalo wings, hot	4 pieces	210	22	4	900	0	12.0	130.0	3	51%
Buffalo wings, mild	5 pieces	200	23	1	510	0	12.0	150.0	4	53%
GARLIC BREAD	1 slice	150	3	16	240	1	8.0	0.0	2	49%
PASTA										
'Cavatini Supreme'	1 serving	560	24	73	1400	10	19.0	10.0	8	31%
cavatini	1 serving	480	21	66	1170	9	14.0	8.0	6	27%
spaghetti, w/marinara sauce	1 serving	490	18	91	730	8	6.0	0.0	1	11%
spaghetti, w/meat sauce	1 serving	600	23	98	910	9	13.0	8.0	5	19%

Food Name	Serving Size	Calories	Prot. gms	Carbs gms	Sod. mgs	Fiber gms	Fat gms	Sat. Fat gms	Chol. mgs	% Fat Cal.
spaghetti, w/meatballs.	1 serving	850	37	120	1120	10	24.0	17.0	10	26%
PIZZA										
Apple, dessert	1 slice	250	3	48	230	2	4.5	0.0	1	17%
Beef										
hand-tossed, medium	1 slice	347	16	44	943	4	12.0	21.0	6	31%
pan, medium	1 slice	399	15	45	773	4	18.0	20.0	7	40%
Sicilian, medium	1 slice	282	13	31	824	3	12.0	19.0	7	38%
stuffed crust, medium	1 slice	466	23	46	1137	3	22.0	30.0	10	42%
thin and crispy, medium.	1 slice	305	14	28	814	3	15.0	24.0	7	45%
Cheese										
'Big New Yorker'	1 slice	393	20	42	1099	3	16.6	18.5	8	38%
hand-tossed, medium	1 slice	309	14	43	848	3	9.0	11.0	5	26%
pan, medium	1 slice	361	13	44	678	3	15.0	11.0	6	37%
pan, personal	1 pizza	813	31	110	1581	8	27.0	24.0	12	30%
Sicilian, medium	1 slice	295	12	32	815	3	13.0	11.0	7	40%
stuffed crust, medium	1 slice	445	22	46	1090	3	19.0	24.0	10	39%
thin and crispy, medium.	1 slice	243	11	27	653	2	10.0	11.0	5	37%
Cherry, dessert	1 slice	250	3	47	220	3	4.5	0.0	1	17%
'Chicken Supreme'										
hand-tossed, medium	1 slice	291	15	44	841	4	6.0	17.0	3	19%
pan, medium	1 slice	343	15	45	671	3	12.0	16.0	4	31%
Sicilian, medium	1 slice	269	13	32	732	3	10.0	15.0	5	33%
stuffed crust, medium	1 slice	432	24	47	1111	3	17.0	32.0	8	35%
'The New Edge' medium	1 slice	90	7	9	290	1	3.5	15.0	2	33%
thin and crispy, medium.	1 slice	232	13	29	681	3	7.0	19.0	3	27%
Ham										
hand-tossed, medium	1 slice	279	13	43	857	3	6.0	15.0	3	19%
pan, medium	1 slice	331	12	44	687	3	12.0	15.0	4	33%
Sicilian, medium	1 slice	257	11	30	745	3	10.0	14.0	5	35%
stuffed crust, medium	1 slice	404	24	45	1190	2	22.0	39.0	12	42%
thin and crispy, medium.	1 slice	212	10	27	662	2	7.0	15.0	3	30%
Italian sausage										
hand-tossed, medium	1 slice	363	16	44	975	4	14.0	26.0	6	34%
pan, medium	1 slice	415	15	45	805	3	20.0	26.0	7	43%
Sicilian, medium	1 slice	333	13	31	855	3	18.0	24.0	7	48%
stuffed crust, medium	1 slice	478	22	46	1164	3	23.0	35.0	10	43%
thin and crispy, medium.	1 slice	325	14	28	865	3	18.0	32.0	7	49%
'Meat Lover's'										
hand-tossed, medium	1 slice	376	17	44	1077	4	15.0	30.0	6	36%
pan, medium	1 slice	428	16	45	607	3	21.0	29.0	7	44%
Sicilian, medium	1 slice	344	14	31	948	3	18.0	27.0	8	47%
stuffed crust, medium	1 slice	543	26	46	1427	3	29.0	48.0	13	48%
'The New Edge' medium	1 slice	160	7	8	440	1	11.0	20.0	5	62%
thin and crispy, medium.	1 slice	339	15	28	970	3	19.0	35.0	8	50%
Pepperoni										
'Big New Yorker'	1 slice	380	18	42	1116	3	16.0	22.4	7	38%
hand-tossed, medium	1 slice	301	13	43	867	3	8.0	15.0	4	24%
pan, medium	1 slice	353	12	44	697	3	14.0	14.0	5	36%
pan, personal	1 pizza	810	30	111	1661	8	28.0	32.0	11	31%
Sicilian, medium	1 slice	227	11	31	754	3	113.0	13.0	5	86%
stuffed crust, medium	1 slice	438	21	45	1116	2	19.0	27.0	9	39%
thin and crispy, medium.	1 slice	235	10	27	672	2	10.0	14.0	4	38%
'Pepperoni Lover's'										
hand-tossed, medium	1 slice	372	17	43	1123	3	14.0	26.0	7	34%

Food Name	Serving Size	Calories	Prot. gms	Carbs gms	Sod. mgs	Fiber gms	Fat gms	Sat. Fat gms	Chol. mgs	% Fat Cal.
pan, medium	1 slice	370	13	44	767	3	16.0	18.0	5	39%
Sicilian, medium	1 slice	321	13	31	899	3	16.0	19.0	8	45%
stuffed crust, medium	1 slice	525	26	46	1413	3	26.0	40.0	13	45%
thin and crispy, medium	1 slice	289	13	28	859	2	14.0	22.0	6	43%
Pork										
hand-tossed, medium	1 slice	342	16	44	990	4	12.0	20.0	5	31%
pan, medium	1 slice	394	15	45	820	4	18.0	20.0	6	40%
Sicilian, medium	1 slice	314	13	31	868	3	16.0	18.0	7	45%
stuffed crust, medium	1 slice	461	22	46	1176	3	21.0	29.0	10	41%
thin and crispy, medium	1 slice	298	14	28	875	3	15.0	23.0	6	45%
'Super Supreme'										
hand-tossed, medium	1 slice	359	16	45	1024	4	12.0	23.0	5	31%
pan, medium	1 slice	401	15	46	854	4	18.0	22.0	6	40%
Sicilian, medium	1 slice	323	13	32	911	3	16.0	21.0	7	44%
stuffed crust, medium	1 slice	505	25	46	1371	3	25.0	44.0	11	44%
thin and crispy, medium	1 slice	304	14	29	902	3	15.0	26.0	6	44%
'Supreme'										
'Big New Yorker'	1 slice	459	10	44	1310	4	22.3	33.2	9	48%
hand-tossed, medium	1 slice	333	15	44	927	4	11.0	18.0	5	30%
pan, medium	1 slice	385	14	45	757	4	17.0	18.0	6	39%
pan, personal	1 pizza	808	30	111	1579	8	27.0	28.0	10	30%
Sicilian, medium	1 slice	307	13	32	815	3	15.0	17.0	7	43%
stuffed crust, medium	1 slice	487	24	47	1227	3	23.0	33.0	11	42%
thin and crispy, medium	1 slice	284	13	29	784	3	13.0	20.0	6	41%
Taco										
beef, hand-tossed, medium	1 slice	270	13	35	870	3	8.0	15.0	4	27%
beef, pan, medium	1 slice	300	12	36	770	3	12.0	15.0	5	36%
beef, thin and crispy, medium	1 slice	260	13	29	850	2	10.0	20.0	5	35%
chicken, hand-tossed, medium	1 slice	290	12	35	940	3	11.0	15.0	5	34%
chicken, pan, medium	1 slice	320	12	36	830	3	15.0	15.0	5	41%
chicken, thin and crispy, medium	1 slice	260	11	26	850	2	12.0	20.0	5	42%
hand-tossed, medium	1 slice	280	12	34	870	3	11.0	15.0	5	35%
meatless, hand-tossed, medium	1 slice	250	11	35	790	3	8.0	10.0	4	28%
meatless, pan, medium	1 slice	290	10	36	680	3	12.0	10.0	4	37%
meatless, thin and crispy, medium	1 slice	230	9	27	700	2	8.0	10.0	4	33%
pan, medium	1 slice	310	12	36	800	3	13.0	15.0	5	38%
pan, personal	1 pizza	780	27	90	1900	7	35.0	30.0	10	40%
thin and crispy, medium	1 slice	260	12	27	860	2	11.0	20.0	5	39%
'The Works' 'The New Edge' medium	1 slice	110	5	9	270	1	6.0	10.0	3	49%
'Veggie Lover's'										
hand-tossed, medium	1 slice	281	12	45	771	4	6.0	7.0	3	19%
pan, medium	1 slice	333	11	46	601	4	12.0	7.0	4	32%
Sicilian, medium	1 slice	252	10	32	627	3	10.0	7.0	5	35%
stuffed crust, medium	1 slice	421	20	48	1039	3	17.0	19.0	8	36%
'The New Edge' medium	1 slice	70	4	9	180	1	3.0	5.0	2	34%
thin and crispy, medium	1 slice	222	9	30	621	3	8.0	7.0	3	32%
SANDWICH										
ham and cheese	1 sandwich	550	33	57	2150	4	21.0	22.0	7	34%
'Supreme'	1 sandwich	640	34	62	2150	4	28.0	28.0	10	40%

PONDEROSA
CHICKEN ENTRÉE

Food Name	Serving Size	Calories	Prot. gms	Carbs gms	Sod. mgs	Fiber gms	Fat gms	Sat. Fat gms	Chol. mgs	% Fat Cal.
breast	5.5 oz	98	20	1	400	0	2.1	54.0	0	19%
wing	2 pieces	213	11	11	610	0	9.0	75.0	0	49%

Food Name	Serving Size	Calories	Prot. gms	Carbs gms	Sod. mgs	Fiber gms	Fat gms	Sat. Fat gms	Chol. mgs	% Fat Cal.
CONDIMENTS. See also Salad Bar Items; Salad Dressing.										
cheese sauce	2 oz	52	1	6	355	0	2.0	4.0	0	37%
cheese topping, herb and garlic	1 tbsp	100	0	0	120	0	10.0	0.0	0	100%
gravy, brown	2 oz	25	1	4	167	0	1.0	0.0	0	33%
gravy, turkey	2 oz	25	1	5	228	0	0.2	0.0	0	7%
margarine, liquid	1 tbsp	100	0	0	110	0	11.0	0.0	0	100%
margarine, whipped	1 tbsp	34	0	0	65	0	1.2	0.0	0	100%
tartar sauce	1 oz	85	0	11	477	0	10.9	9.0	0	69%
DESSERT										
dougnut, winter mix	3.5 oz	25	2	4	371	0	0.0	0.0	0	0%
gelatin dessert, plain, nonfat	4 oz	71	1	17	73	0	0.0	0.0	0	0%
ice milk, chocolate	3.5 oz	152	4	30	70	0	3.0	22.0	0	17%
ice milk, vanilla	3.5 oz	150	4	30	58	0	3.0	20.0	0	17%
mousse, chocolate	4 oz	312	0	28	72	0	18.0	0.0	0	59%
mousse, chocolate	1 oz	78	0	7	18	0	4.4	0.0	0	59%
mousse, strawberry	4 oz	297	0	25	68	0	18.0	0.0	0	62%
mousse, strawberry	1 oz	74	0	6	17	0	4.6	0.0	0	62%
pudding, banana	4 oz	207	1	27	114	0	10.0	0.0	0	45%
vanilla wafer cookie, peanut butter	2 wafers	35	0	6	25	0	1.0	5.0	0	27%
DESSERT TOPPING										
caramel	1 oz	100	0	26	72	0	0.7	2.0	0	6%
chocolate	1 oz	89	1	24	37	0	0.3	0.0	0	3%
peanut, granulated	.2 oz	30	1	1	0	0	2.3	0.0	0	69%
strawberry	1 oz	71	0	24	29	0	0.2	0.0	0	2%
strawberry glaze	1 oz	37	0	10	4	0	0.0	0.0	0	0%
whipped	1 oz	80	0	5	16	0	7.0	0.0	0	76%
FISH. See also individual listings.										
nuggets	1 piece	31	2	2	52	0	1.7	8.0	0	52%
baked, 'Bake 'R Broil' baked	5.2 oz	230	19	10	330	0	13.0	50.0	0	50%
fried	3.2 oz	190	9	17	170	0	9.0	15.0	0	44%
HALIBUT, broiled	6 oz	170	35	0	68	0	2.4	0.0	0	13%
HOT DOG	1.6 oz	144	5	1	460	0	13.0	27.0	0	83%
MEATBALLS	2 pieces	115	5	2	16	0	4.0	21.0	0	56%
ORANGE ROUGHY, broiled	5 oz	139	0	21	88	0	5.0	28.0	0	35%
ROLL										
dinner	1 piece	184	5	33	311	0	3.0	0.0	0	15%
sourdough	1 piece	110	4	22	230	0	1.0	0.0	0	8%
SALAD BAR ITEMS										
banana	1 medium	87	1	23	1	0	0.2	0.0	0	2%
banana chips	.2 oz	25	0	3	0	0	1.3	0.0	0	46%
breadstick, Italian	1 stick	100	4	19	200	0	1.0	0.0	0	9%
breadstick, sesame	2 sticks	35	1	6	60	0	0.0	0.0	0	0%
broccoli, raw	1 oz	9	1	2	4	0	0.9	0.0	0	43%
cabbage, green	1 oz	9	1	2	7	0	0.0	0.0	0	0%
cheese, imitation, shredded	1 oz	90	6	1	420	0	7.0	5.0	0	69%
chicken macaroni salad	3.5 oz	335	8	49	431	0	12.0	9.0	0	32%
chicken salad	3.5 oz	212	11	8	334	0	15.0	42.0	0	64%
chow mein noodles	.2 oz	25	1	3	42	0	1.2	0.0	0	43%
coconut, shredded	.2 oz	25	0	2	14	0	1.9	0.0	0	66%
croutons	1 oz	115	4	18	351	0	4.0	0.0	0	29%
fruit cocktail	4 oz	97	1	25	7	0	0.2	0.0	0	2%
granola	.2 oz	24	1	3	0	0	1.0	0.0	0	38%
grapes	10 grapes	34	0	9	2	0	0.2	0.0	0	5%
ham, diced	2 oz	120	9	1	780	0	10.0	76.0	0	69%

Food Name	Serving Size	Calories	Prot. gms	Carbs gms	Sod. mgs	Fiber gms	Fat gms	Sat. Fat gms	Chol. mgs	% Fat Cal.
lemon	1 wedge	3	0	1	0	0	0.1	0.0	0	20%
macaroni salad	3.5 oz	335	8	49	431	0	11.7	9.0	0	32%
onion, green	1 piece	7	0	2	1	0	0.1	0.0	0	11%
onion, yellow	1 oz	11	0	3	3	0	0.0	0.0	0	0%
orange	1 piece	45	1	11	1	0	0.1	0.0	0	2%
pasta salad	3.5 oz	268	6	34	441	0	12.0	0.0	0	40%
pickle chips, sweet	.14 oz	4	0	1	1	0	0.0	0.0	0	0%
pickle spear, dill	.14 oz	1	0	0	54	0	0.0	0.0	0	0%
potato salad	3.5 oz	126	2	16	300	0	6.0	7.0	0	43%
turkey ham salad	3.5 oz	186	8	10	654	0	13.0	12.0	0	62%
turkey, julienne	1 oz	29	5	1	192	0	1.0	15.0	0	27%
yogurt, frozen, fruit flavor	4 oz	115	5	23	70	0	1.0	5.0	0	7%
yogurt, frozen, vanilla	4 oz	110	5	18	75	0	2.0	6.0	0	16%
SALAD DRESSING										
blue cheese	1 oz	130	1	1	266	0	14.0	27.0	0	94%
coleslaw	1 oz	150	0	6	284	0	14.0	31.0	0	84%
creamy Italian	1 oz	103	0	3	373	0	10.0	0.0	0	88%
cucumber, lower calorie	1 oz	69	0	3	315	0	6.0	0.0	0	82%
Italian, lower calorie	1 oz	31	0	1	371	0	3.0	0.0	0	87%
oil	1 tbsp	120	0	0	0	0	14.0	0.0	0	100%
Parmesan pepper	1 oz	150	1	2	281	0	15.0	9.0	0	92%
ranch	1 oz	147	0	1	297	0	15.0	3.0	0	97%
sweet-n-tangy	1 oz	122	0	8	347	0	10.0	1.0	0	74%
Thousand Island	1 oz	113	0	8	405	0	10.0	9.0	0	74%
SALMON, broiled	6 oz	192	37	3	72	0	3.0	60.0	0	14%
SCROD, baked	7 oz	120	27	0	80	0	1.0	65.0	0	8%
SHRIMP										
fried	7 pieces	230	22	31	612	0	1.0	105.0	0	4%
mini	6 pieces	47	5	6	125	0	1.0	22.0	0	17%
SIDE DISH										
baked beans	4 oz	170	6	21	330	0	6.0	0.0	0	33%
baked potato	7.2 oz	145	4	33	6	0	0.0	0.0	0	0%
corn	3.5 oz	90	3	21	5	0	0.4	0.0	0	4%
French fries	3 oz	120	2	17	39	0	4.0	3.0	0	32%
green beans	3.5 oz	20	1	3	391	0	0.0	0.0	0	0%
macaroni and cheese	1 oz	17	1	4	80	0	0.5	1.0	0	18%
macaroni salad	3.5 oz	335	8	49	431	0	11.7	9.0	0	32%
mashed potato	4 oz	62	2	13	191	0	0.0	20.0	0	0%
okra, breaded	4 oz	124	3	23	483	0	1.0	1.0	0	8%
onion rings, breaded	4 oz	213	3	30	620	0	9.0	2.0	0	38%
pasta/noodles	2 oz	78	2	16	1	0	0.3	0.0	0	4%
potato wedges	3.5 oz	130	3	16	170	0	6.0	0.0	0	42%
rice pilaf	4 oz	160	4	26	450	0	4.0	22.0	0	23%
spinach	1 oz	7	1	1	20	0	0.1	0.0	0	10%
stuffing	4 oz	230	6	27	800	0	11.0	22.0	0	43%
SPAGHETTI, w/sauce	6 oz	188	5	33	520	0	5.0	0.0	0	23%
STEAK										
chopped	4 oz	225	19	1	150	0	16.0	80.0	0	64%
kabobs, meat only	3 oz	153	26	2	280	0	5.0	67.0	0	29%
Kansas City strip	5 oz	138	21	1	850	0	5.7	76.0	0	37%
New York strip, choice	8 oz	314	45	1	570	0	10.5	50.0	0	34%
Porterhouse, choice	16 oz	640	57	3	1130	0	30.9	82.0	0	54%
Porterhouse, non-graded	13 oz	440	43	1	1844	0	30.0	67.0	0	61%
ribeye, choice	6 oz	282	29	1	570	0	14.0	60.0	0	51%

Food Name	Serving Size	Calories	Prot. gms	Carbs gms	Sod. mgs	Fiber gms	Fat gms	Sat. Fat gms	Chol. mgs	% Fat Cal.
ribeye, non-graded	5 oz	219	25	1	1130	0	13.0	75.0	0	53%
sirloin, choice	7 oz	241	35	1	570	0	11.0	63.0	0	41%
sirloin tips, choice	5 oz	197	29	1	280	0	8.0	71.0	0	38%
T-bone, choice	10 oz	444	44	2	850	0	18.0	80.0	0	47%
T-bone, non-graded	8 oz	178	25	2	850	0	8.5	71.0	0	42%
teriyaki	5 oz	174	32	5	1420	0	3.0	64.0	0	15%
STEAK SANDWICH	4 oz	208	20	2	850	0	11.0	62.0	0	53%
SWORDFISH, broiled	5.9 oz	271	44	0	0	0	10.0	84.0	0	34%
TROUT	5 oz	228	30	1	51	0	4.0	110.0	0	23%

POPEYES

Food Name	Serving Size	Calories	Prot. gms	Carbs gms	Sod. mgs	Fiber gms	Fat gms	Sat. Fat gms	Chol. mgs	% Fat Cal.
BISCUIT, plain or buttermilk	1 biscuit	233	4	31	673	1	10.6	1.6	1	40%
CHICKEN										
breast, mild, w/o bone	3.7 oz	270	23	9	660	2	15.9	60.0	0	53%
breast, spicy, w/o bone	3.7 oz	270	23	9	590	2	15.9	60.0	0	53%
leg, mild, w/o bone	1.7 oz	120	10	4	240	0	7.3	40.0	0	53%
leg, spicy, w/o bone	1.7 oz	120	10	4	240	0	7.3	40.0	0	53%
nuggets, fried	4.2 oz	410	17	18	660	3	31.9	55.0	0	67%
thigh, mild, w/o bone	3.1 oz	300	15	9	620	1	22.7	70.0	0	68%
thigh, spicy, w/o bone	3.1 oz	300	15	9	450	1	22.7	70.0	0	68%
wing, mild, w/o bone	1.6 oz	160	9	7	290	0	10.7	40.0	0	60%
wing, spicy, w/o bone	1.6 oz	160	9	7	290	0	10.7	40.0	0	60%
DESSERT										
apple pie	3.1 oz	290	3	37	820	2	15.8	10.0	0	48%
SHRIMP	2.8 oz	250	16	13	650	3	16.4	110.0	0	56%
SIDE DISH										
Cajun rice	3.9 oz	150	10	17	1260	3	5.4	25.0	0	31%
coleslaw	4 oz	149	1	14	271	3	11.2	3.0	0	63%
corn on the cob	5.2 oz	90	4	21	20	9	2.9	0.0	0	20%
French fries	3 oz	240	4	31	610	3	12.2	10.0	0	44%
mashed potato, w/gravy	3.8 oz	100	5	11	460	3	6.0	5.0	0	47%
onion rings	3.1 oz	310	5	31	210	2	19.3	25.0	0	55%
red beans and rice	5.9 oz	270	8	30	680	7	16.9	10.0	0	51%

QUINCY'S

Food Name	Serving Size	Calories	Prot. gms	Carbs gms	Sod. mgs	Fiber gms	Fat gms	Sat. Fat gms	Chol. mgs	% Fat Cal.
CATFISH, fillet, 2 pieces	6.9-oz serving	309	26	19	101	0	12.0	0.0	0	38%
CHEESEBURGER, 1/4 lb precooked	1 serving	451	28	32	432	0	23.0	0.0	0	46%
CHICKEN										
breast, grilled	5-oz serving	145	35	0	140	0	0.4	72.0	0	3%
strips, 4 pieces	4.5 oz	318	39	4	0	0	15.0	0.0	0	44%
CHILI, w/beans	9.2-oz serving	346	20	32	1380	0	16.0	0.0	0	41%
CORNBREAD	1.9-oz serving	178	4	28	263	0	6.0	0.0	0	30%
HAMBURGER, 1/4 lb precooked	1 serving	403	25	32	284	0	19.0	0.0	0	43%
MUSHROOM SAUCE	3-oz serving	27	1	5	366	0	1.0	0.0	0	27%
SHRIMP, 7 pieces	3.9-oz serving	248	22	11	205	0	12.0	0.0	0	45%
SIDE DISH										
baked potato, w/o butter	8.8-oz serving	181	5	41	8	0	1.0	0.0	0	5%
coleslaw	2.1-oz serving	60	1	4	75	0	5.0	0.0	0	69%
green beans	4.3-oz serving	40	2	7	500	0	1.0	0.0	0	20%
peppers and onions	4-oz serving	80	1	8	11	0	5.0	0.0	0	56%
steak fries	5.5-oz serving	426	7	56	90	0	21.0	0.0	0	43%
SOUP										
broccoli, cream of	9.2-oz serving	193	3	13	1045	0	14.0	0.0	0	66%
clam chowder	9.2-oz serving	198	6	15	1185	0	14.0	0.0	0	60%
vegetable beef soup	8.6-oz serving	78	5	10	1045	0	2.0	0.0	0	23%

Food Name	Serving Size	Calories	Prot. gms	Carbs gms	Sod. mgs	Fiber gms	Fat gms	Sat. Fat gms	Chol. mgs	% Fat Cal.
STEAK										
chopped, luncheon	4-oz serving	350	30	0	72	0	25.0	0.0	0	65%
country style, w/mushroom sauce	6-oz serving	288	18	17	315	0	19.0	0.0	0	55%
fillet	5.6-oz serving	331	51	0	159	0	12.0	0.0	0	35%
ribeye	7.3-oz serving	665	31	0	205	0	60.0	0.0	0	81%
sirloin club	4.8-oz serving	283	44	0	160	0	10.0	0.0	0	34%
sirloin tips	4-oz serving	236	37	0	113	0	9.0	0.0	0	35%
sirloin	5.9-oz serving	649	38	0	206	0	54.0	0.0	0	76%
sirloin, large	7.7-oz serving	852	50	0	241	0	70.0	0.0	0	76%
sirloin, petite	4-oz serving	446	26	0	118	0	37.0	0.0	0	76%
T-bone	7.8-oz serving	1045	43	0	222	0	95.0	0.0	0	83%
RALLY'S										
CHEESEBURGER										
'Rallyburger w/Cheese'	1 burger	486	24	33	1185	0	29.4	79.0	0	53%
'Bacon Cheeseburger'	1 burger	622	33	35	1629	0	40.3	99.0	0	57%
'Double Cheeseburger'	1 burger	733	42	34	1473	0	49.1	92.0	0	59%
CHEESEBURGER MEAL										
'Large Combo' w/soft drink	1 meal	1018	29	129	1645	0	45.0	89.0	0	39%
'Small Combo' w/soft drink	1 meal	764	33	85	1416	0	37.2	84.0	0	42%
CHICKEN SANDWICH	1 sandwich	531	18	40	364	0	30.8	18.0	0	55%
CHILI	8 oz	340	22	21	1199	0	19.0	67.0	0	50%
FRENCH FRIES										
large	1 serving	317	5	39	439	0	15.6	10.0	0	44%
regular	1 serving	158	3	20	219	0	7.8	5.0	0	44%
HAMBURGER 'Rallyburger'	1 burger	436	21	33	955	0	24.9	67.0	0	51%
HAMBURGER MEAL										
'Large Combo' w/soft drink	1 meal	968	26	129	1415	0	40.5	76.0	0	37%
'Small Combo' w/soft drink	1 meal	714	24	84	1186	0	32.7	71.0	0	41%
SAUSAGE										
'Smokin' Sausage'	1 serving	724	28	31	1998	0	55.0	40.0	0	68%
'Smokin' Sausage' w/chili	1 serving	830	35	35	2163	0	62.0	67.0	0	67%
TACO, soft	1 taco	223	12	17	377	0	9.9	36.0	0	43%
RAX										
BEEF, roast beef	2.8 oz	140	14	1	524	0	9.0	36.0	0	57%
BREADSTICK, sesame, salad bar item	1 oz	150	3	13	405	0	10.0	0.0	0	58%
CHEESE, American, processed, slices	0.5 oz	60	3	1	180	0	5.0	15.0	0	74%
CONDIMENTS. See also SALAD DRESSING.										
Alfredo sauce, pasta bar item	3.5 oz	80	2	12	70	0	3.0	10.0	0	33%
banana pepper, Mexican bar item	1 tbsp	2	1	1	20	0	1.0	0.0	0	53%
barbecue meat topping	3.25 oz	140	13	13	898	0	4.0	24.0	0	26%
celery, salad bar item	1 tbsp	1	1	1	10	0	1.0	0.0	0	53%
cheese sauce, regular, Mexican bar item	3.5 oz	420	10	58	365	0	17.0	11.0	0	36%
chili topping	3 oz	80	8	8	221	0	2.0	18.0	0	22%
chow mein noodles, salad bar item	1 oz	140	4	17	242	0	6.0	1.0	0	39%
coconut, salad bar item	1 oz	160	1	15	1	0	11.0	0.0	0	61%
croutons, salad bar item	0.5 oz	40	2	8	155	0	1.0	1.0	0	18%
green onion, Mexican bar item	1/4 cup	10	1	2	1	0	1.0	0.0	0	43%
margarine, liquid	1 tbsp	100	1	1	100	0	11.0	0.0	0	93%
mushroom sauce	1 oz	16	1	1	113	0	1.0	0.0	0	53%
nacho cheese sauce, Mexican bar item	3.5 oz	470	10	57	190	0	22.0	11.0	0	42%
onion, diced	0.5 oz	10	1	1	1	0	1.0	0.0	0	53%
pickle	1 spear	8	1	2	928	0	1.0	0.0	0	43%
sour topping	3.5 oz	130	3	5	79	0	11.0	1.0	0	76%

Food Name	Serving Size	Calories	Prot. gms	Carbs gms	Sod. mgs	Fiber gms	Fat gms	Sat. Fat gms	Chol. mgs	% Fat Cal.
spaghetti sauce, pasta bar item	3.5 oz	80	1	19	635	0	1.0	1.0	0	10%
spaghetti sauce, w/meat, pasta bar item	3.5 oz	150	7	12	419	0	8.0	1.0	0	49%
spicy meat sauce, Mexican bar item	3.5 oz	80	5	6	751	0	4.0	12.0	0	45%
sunflower seeds and raisins, salad bar item	1 oz	130	5	6	5	0	10.0	0.0	0	67%
taco sauce, Mexican bar item	3.5 oz	30	1	6	806	0	1.0	0.0	0	24%
taco shell, Mexican bar item	1 shell	40	1	6	53	0	2.0	0.0	0	39%
turkey bits, salad bar item	2 oz	70	10	1	686	0	3.0	49.0	0	38%
DESSERT										
butterscotch pudding, salad bar item	3.5 oz	141	2	20	151	0	6.0	2.0	0	38%
chocolate chip cookie	1 cookie	130	1	17	65	0	6.0	1.0	0	43%
chocolate pudding, salad bar item	3.5 oz	141	2	20	121	0	6.0	2.0	0	38%
lime gelatin, salad bar item	1/2 cup	90	2	20	90	0	1.0	0.0	0	9%
strawberry gelatin, salad bar item	1/2 cup	90	2	20	90	0	1.0	0.0	0	9%
vanilla pudding, salad bar item	3.5 oz	141	2	20	121	0	6.0	2.0	0	38%
DESSERT TOPPING, whipped	1 dollop	50	1	4	6	0	4.0	2.0	0	64%
PASTA										
rainbow rotini, pasta bar item	3.5 oz	180	6	30	9	0	4.0	2.0	0	20%
shells, pasta bar item	3.5 oz	170	7	27	2	0	4.0	0.0	0	21%
spaghetti, pasta bar item	3.5 oz	140	3	23	1	0	4.0	0.0	0	26%
vegetable, pasta bar item	3.5 oz	100	4	12	11	0	4.0	0.0	0	36%
SALAD										
chef, w/o dressing	12.5-oz serving	230	22	4	1048	0	14.0	322.0	0	55%
garden, gourmet, 'Lighterside'	1 serving	134	7	13	350	0	6.0	2.0	0	40%
garden, w/o dressing	10.5-oz serving	160	12	4	362	0	11.0	273.0	0	61%
SALAD DRESSING										
blue cheese	1 tbsp	50	1	1	110	0	5.0	8.0	0	85%
blue cheese, 'Lite'	1 tbsp	35	1	2	240	0	3.0	3.0	0	69%
French	1 tbsp	60	1	6	140	0	4.0	0.0	0	56%
Italian	1 tbsp	50	1	3	159	0	4.0	0.0	0	69%
Italian, 'Lite'	1 tbsp	30	1	1	152	0	3.0	0.0	0	77%
oil	1 tbsp	130	1	1	1	0	14.0	0.0	0	94%
poppyseed	1 tbsp	60	1	5	107	0	4.0	6.0	0	60%
ranch	1 tbsp	45	1	1	103	0	5.0	5.0	0	85%
Thousand Island	1 tbsp	70	1	6	110	0	6.0	8.0	0	66%
Thousand Island, 'Lite'	1 tbsp	40	1	3	143	0	3.0	5.0	0	63%
vinegar	1 tbsp	2	1	1	5	0	1.0	0.0	0	53%
SANDWICH										
barbecue	5.7-oz serving	420	21	53	1343	0	14.0	24.0	0	30%
beef, bacon, and chicken, 'BBC'	8-oz serving	720	30	40	1873	0	49.0	137.0	0	61%
fish	7-oz serving	460	14	58	935	0	17.0	1.0	0	35%
ham and Swiss	7.9-oz serving	430	23	42	1737	0	23.0	37.0	0	44%
Philly beef and cheese	8.25-oz serving	480	25	44	1346	0	22.0	49.0	0	42%
roast beef, large	8-oz serving	570	22	41	1169	0	35.0	36.0	0	56%
roast beef, regular	5.25-oz serving	320	20	33	969	0	11.0	36.0	0	32%
roast beef, 'Uncle Al' small	3.1-oz serving	260	12	21	562	0	14.0	19.0	0	49%
turkey bacon club	9-oz serving	670	29	41	1878	0	43.0	87.0	0	58%
SIDE DISH										
baked potato, barbecue, w/2 oz cheese	1 serving	730	24	104	1071	0	24.0	18.0	0	30%
baked potato, cheese and bacon	3-oz serving	780	22	110	910	0	28.0	23.0	0	32%
baked potato, cheese and broccoli	3-oz serving	760	19	112	489	0	26.0	11.0	0	31%
baked potato, chili, w/2 oz cheese	1 serving	700	22	101	599	0	23.0	25.0	0	30%
baked potato, plain	8.8-oz serving	270	8	60	70	0	1.0	0.0	0	3%
baked potato, w/margarine	9.3-oz serving	370	8	60	170	0	11.0	0.0	0	27%

Food Name	Serving Size	Calories	Prot. gms	Carbs gms	Sod. mgs	Fiber gms	Fat gms	Sat. Fat gms	Chol. mgs	% Fat Cal.
baked potato, w/sour cream topping	1 serving	400	11	65	149	0	11.0	0.0	0	25%
broccoli, salad bar item	1/2 cup	16	2	2	7	0	1.0	0.0	0	36%
coleslaw, salad bar item	3.5 oz	70	1	8	187	0	4.0	1.0	0	50%
French fries, large, salted	4.5-oz serving	390	3	50	104	0	20.0	16.0	0	46%
French fries, large, unsalted	4.5-oz serving	390	3	50	66	0	20.0	16.0	0	46%
French fries, regular, salted	3-oz serving	260	2	33	69	0	13.0	10.0	0	46%
French fries, regular, unsalted	3-oz serving	260	2	33	44	0	13.0	10.0	0	46%
grapefruit sections, salad bar item	1 cup	80	2	18	10	0	1.0	0.0	0	10%
grapes, salad bar item	1 cup	100	1	25	5	0	1.0	0.0	0	8%
kale, salad bar item	1 oz	16	2	2	21	0	1.0	0.0	0	36%
kidney beans, salad bar item	1 cup	220	14	40	8	0	1.0	0.0	0	4%
macaroni salad, salad bar item	3.5 oz	160	2	21	216	0	7.0	1.0	0	41%
pasta salad, salad bar item	3.5 oz	80	2	16	322	0	1.0	1.0	0	11%
potato salad, salad bar item	1 cup	260	7	41	0	0	7.0	7.0	0	25%
refried beans, Mexican bar item	3 oz	120	6	16	375	0	4.0	2.0	0	29%
Spanish rice, Mexican bar item	3.5 oz	90	3	20	442	0	1.0	0.0	0	9%
three-bean salad	1/2 cup	100	3	23	450	0	1.0	0.0	0	8%
SOUP										
broccoli, cream of	3.5 oz	50	1	6	219	0	2.0	1.0	0	39%
chicken soup w/noodles, pasta bar item	3.5 oz	40	2	8	1040	0	1.0	10.0	0	18%
RED LOBSTER										
CALAMARI										
breaded, fried, dinner portion	10 oz	720	26	60	2300	0	42.0	280.0	12	52%
breaded, fried, lunch portion	5 oz	360	13	30	1150	0	21.0	140.0	6	52%
CATFISH										
dinner portion	10 oz	340	40	0	100	0	20.0	170.0	6	53%
lunch portion	5 oz	170	20	0	50	0	10.0	85.0	3	53%
CHICKEN, breast	4-oz serving	120	24	0	60	0	3.0	65.0	1	22%
CLAMS										
cherrystone, dinner portion	10 oz	260	36	22	1080	0	4.0	160.0	0	13%
cherrystone, lunch portion	5 oz	130	18	11	540	0	2.0	80.0	0	13%
COD										
Atlantic, fillet, dinner portion	10 oz	200	46	0	400	0	2.0	140.0	0	9%
Atlantic, fillet, lunch portion	5 oz	100	23	0	200	0	1.0	70.0	0	9%
CRAB										
king, legs, 1 lb.	1 serving	170	32	6	900	0	2.0	100.0	0	11%
snow, legs, 1 lb.	1 serving	150	33	1	1630	0	2.0	130.0	1	12%
FLOUNDER										
dinner portion	10 oz	200	42	2	190	0	2.0	140.0	0	9%
lunch portion	5 oz	100	21	1	95	0	1.0	70.0	0	9%
GROUPER										
dinner portion	10 oz	220	52	0	140	0	2.0	130.0	0	8%
lunch portion	5 oz	110	26	0	70	0	1.0	65.0	0	8%
HADDOCK										
dinner portion	10 oz	220	48	4	360	0	2.0	170.0	0	8%
lunch portion	5 oz	110	24	2	180	0	1.0	85.0	0	8%
HALIBUT										
dinner portion	10 oz	220	50	2	210	0	2.0	120.0	0	8%
lunch portion	5 oz	110	25	1	105	0	1.0	60.0	0	8%
HAMBURGER, 1/3 lb before cooked	1 serving	320	27	0	70	0	23.0	105.0	11	66%
LANGOSTINO										
dinner portion	10 oz	240	52	4	820	0	2.0	420.0	0	7%
lunch portion	5 oz	120	26	2	410	0	1.0	210.0	0	7%

Food Name	Serving Size	Calories	Prot. gms	Carbs gms	Sod. mgs	Fiber gms	Fat gms	Sat. Fat gms	Chol. mgs	% Fat Cal.
LOBSTER										
Maine, cooked, 1 1/4 lb	1 serving	240	36	5	550	0	8.0	310.0	2	31%
rock, tail, cooked	1 serving	230	49	2	1090	0	3.0	200.0	1	12%
MACKEREL										
dinner portion	10 oz	380	2	40	500	0	24.0	200.0	8	56%
raw weight	5 oz	190	1	20	250	0	12.0	100.0	4	56%
MONKFISH										
dinner portion	10 oz	220	0	48	190	0	2.0	160.0	0	9%
lunch portion	5 oz	110	0	24	95	0	1.0	80.0	0	9%
MUSSELS	3-oz serving	70	9	3	150	0	2.0	50.0	0	27%
OCEAN PERCH										
Atlantic, dinner portion	10 oz	260	48	2	380	0	8.0	150.0	2	26%
Atlantic, lunch portion	5 oz	130	24	1	190	0	4.0	75.0	1	26%
OYSTERS, on half shell	6 oysters	110	8	11	90	0	4.0	60.0	2	32%
POLLACK										
dinner portion	10 oz	240	56	2	180	0	2.0	180.0	0	7%
lunch portion	5 oz	120	28	1	90	0	1.0	90.0	0	7%
RED ROCKFISH										
dinner portion	10 oz	180	42	0	190	0	2.0	170.0	0	10%
lunch portion	5 oz	90	21	0	95	0	1.0	85.0	0	10%
RED SNAPPER										
dinner portion	10 oz	220	50	0	280	0	2.0	140.0	0	8%
lunch portion	5 oz	110	25	0	140	0	1.0	70.0	0	8%
SALMON										
Norwegian, dinner portion	10 oz	460	54	6	120	0	24.0	160.0	6	47%
Norwegian, lunch portion	5 oz	230	27	3	60	0	12.0	80.0	3	47%
sockeye, dinner portion	10 oz	320	56	6	120	0	8.0	100.0	2	23%
sockeye, lunch portion	5 oz	160	28	3	60	0	4.0	50.0	1	23%
SCALLOPS										
calico, dinner portion	10 oz	360	64	16	320	0	4.0	230.0	0	10%
calico, lunch portion	5 oz	180	32	8	260	0	2.0	115.0	0	10%
deep sea, dinner portion	10 oz	260	52	4	520	0	4.0	100.0	0	14%
deep sea, lunch portion	5 oz	130	26	2	260	0	2.0	50.0	0	14%
SHARK										
blacktip, dinner portion	10 oz	300	70	0	180	0	2.0	120.0	0	6%
blacktip, lunch portion	5 oz	150	35	0	90	0	1.0	60.0	0	6%
mako, dinner portion	10 oz	280	68	0	120	0	2.0	200.0	0	6%
mako, lunch portion	5 oz	140	34	0	60	0	1.0	100.0	0	6%
SHRIMP, 8–12 pieces	1 serving	120	25	0	110	0	2.0	230.0	0	15%
SOLE										
w/lemon, dinner portion	10 oz	240	54	2	180	0	2.0	130.0	0	7%
w/lemon, lunch portion	5 oz	120	27	1	90	0	1.0	65.0	0	7%
STEAK, strip	7 oz	690	29	0	70	0	64.0	140.0	27	83%
SWORDFISH										
dinner portion	10 oz	200	34	0	280	0	8.0	200.0	2	35%
lunch portion	5 oz	100	17	0	140	0	4.0	100.0	1	35%
TILEFISH										
dinner portion	10 oz	200	40	0	120	0	4.0	160.0	2	18%
lunch portion	5 oz	100	20	0	60	0	2.0	80.0	1	18%
TROUT										
rainbow, dinner portion	10 oz	340	46	0	180	0	18.0	180.0	6	47%
rainbow, lunch portion	5 oz	170	23	0	90	0	9.0	90.0	3	47%
TUNA										
yellowfin, dinner portion	10 oz	360	64	0	140	0	12.0	140.0	4	30%
yellowfin, lunch portion	5 oz	180	32	0	70	0	6.0	70.0	2	30%

Food Name	Serving Size	Calories	Prot. gms	Carbs gms	Sod. mgs	Fiber gms	Fat gms	Sat. Fat gms	Chol. mgs	% Fat Cal.
ROUND TABLE										
PIZZA										
'Alfredo Contempo'										
pan crust	1 slice	220	12	27	240	1	7.4	25.0	4	30%
thin crust	1 slice	170	9	17	210	1	6.5	25.0	4	36%
'Bacon Super Deli'										
pan crust	1 slice	260	12	26	380	0	13.5	25.0	5	44%
thin crust	1 slice	200	9	16	360	0	12.6	25.0	5	53%
Cheese										
pan	1 slice	210	10	26	250	1	7.2	20.0	5	31%
thin crust	1 slice	170	8	17	330	1	5.6	25.0	4	34%
Chicken and garlic										
pan, gourmet	1 slice	230	11	27	310	1	8.1	25.0	4	32%
thin crust, gourmet	1 slice	170	9	17	280	0	7.2	25.0	4	38%
'Classic Pesto'										
pan	1 slice	230	9	27	240	1	8.8	15.0	4	35%
thin crust	1 slice	170	7	18	210	1	7.9	15.0	4	42%
'Garden Delight'										
pan crust	1 slice	200	9	27	250	1	6.2	15.0	4	28%
thin crust	1 slice	150	7	18	250	1	5.6	15.0	3	34%
'Garden Pesto'										
pan crust	1 slice	230	9	28	230	1	8.6	15.0	4	34%
thin crust	1 slice	170	7	18	200	1	7.7	15.0	4	41%
'Gourmet Veggie'										
pan crust	1 slice	220	9	28	230	1	7.4	20.0	4	31%
thin crust	1 slice	160	7	18	200	1	6.5	15.0	3	37%
Italian Garlic Supreme'										
pan crust	1 slice	250	10	27	240	1	10.5	25.0	4	39%
thin crust	1 slice	200	8	17	220	0	10.4	25.0	4	48%
'King Arthur's Supreme'										
pan crust	1 slice	240	10	27	320	1	9.8	25.0	4	37%
thin crust	1 slice	200	9	18	340	1	10.1	25.0	4	46%
Pepperoni										
pan crust	1 slice	220	9	26	240	1	8.1	20.0	4	34%
thin crust	1 slice	170	8	17	240	0	8.0	20.0	3	42%
'Salute Chicken Cashew'										
pan crust	1 slice	200	9	31	260	1	4.5	15.0	2	20%
thin crust	1 slice	150	7	21	240	1	4.1	15.0	2	25%
'Salute Chicken and Garlic'										
pan crust	1 slice	200	9	28	270	1	5.8	20.0	3	26%
thin crust	1 slice	150	8	18	250	1	5.4	20.0	3	32%
'Salute Veggie'										
pan crust	1 slice	190	8	28	190	1	5.1	10.0	3	24%
thin crust	1 slice	140	6	19	170	1	4.7	10.0	2	30%
'Santa Fe Chicken'										
pan crust	1 slice	240	11	27	360	1	9.2	30.0	5	35%
thin crust	1 slice	180	9	17	310	1	7.8	25.0	4	40%
ROY ROGERS										
BISCUIT	1 serving	231	4	26	575	0	12.0	5.0	0	47%
BREAKFAST										
crescent, regular	1 serving	408	13	28	820	0	27.0	207.0	0	60%
crescent, w/bacon	1 serving	446	15	28	982	0	30.0	212.0	0	61%
crescent, w/ham	1 serving	456	20	29	1243	0	29.0	227.0	0	57%

Food Name	Serving Size	Calories	Prot. gms	Carbs gms	Sod. mgs	Fiber gms	Fat gms	Sat. Fat gms	Chol. mgs	% Fat Cal.
crescent, w/sausage	1 serving	564	19	28	1145	0	42.0	248.0	0	67%
apple swirl Danish	1 serving	328	5	62	279	0	7.0	0.0	0	19%
cheese swirl Danish	1 serving	383	8	54	369	0	15.0	0.0	0	35%
cinnamon rod pastry,	1 serving	376	5	55	339	0	15.0	0.0	0	36%
egg platter, w/bacon and biscuit	1 serving	607	21	44	1236	0	39.0	424.0	0	57%
egg platter, w/biscuit, regular	1 serving	557	18	44	1020	0	34.0	417.0	0	55%
egg platter, w/ham and biscuit,	1 serving	605	25	44	1442	0	36.0	437.0	0	54%
egg platter, w/sausage and biscuit	1 serving	713	25	44	1345	0	49.0	458.0	0	62%
pancake platter, regular, w/syrup and butter, regular	1 serving	386	5	63	547	0	13.0	51.0	0	30%
pancake platter, w/bacon, w/syrup and butter	1 serving	436	8	63	763	0	17.0	58.0	0	35%
pancake platter, w/ham, w/syrup and butter	1 serving	434	11	64	969	0	15.0	71.0	0	31%
pancake platter, w/sausage, w/syrup and butter	1 serving	542	11	63	872	0	28.0	92.0	0	46%
CHEESEBURGER										
'Express'	1 serving	613	30	42	1122	0	37.0	82.0	0	54%
'Express' w/bacon	1 serving	641	33	36	1317	0	41.0	89.0	0	57%
regular	1 serving	525	29	37	830	0	29.0	76.0	0	50%
regular, w/bacon	1 sandwich	520	24	32	1620	na	33.0	72.0	18	57%
small	1 serving	275	15	24	558	0	13.0	36.0	0	43%
CHICKEN										
breast, fried	1 serving	412	33	17	609	0	24.0	118.0	0	52%
breast and wing, fried	1 serving	604	44	25	894	0	37.0	165.0	0	55%
breast and wing, w/o skin, 'Roy's Roaster'	1 serving	190	32	2	0	0	6.0	0.0	0	28%
dark meat, 1/4 'Roy's Roaster'	1 serving	490	43	2	1120	0	34.0	225.0	10	63%
dark meat, w/o skin, 1/4 'Roy's Roaster'	1 serving	190	24	1	400	0	10.0	110.0	3	47%
leg, fried	1 serving	140	12	6	190	0	8.0	40.0	0	50%
leg and thigh, fried	1 serving	436	30	17	596	0	28.0	125.0	0	57%
nuggets, fried, 9 pieces	9 pieces	435	18	30	915	na	27.0	22.5	6	56%
nuggets, fried, 6 pieces	6 pieces	290	12	20	610	na	18.0	15.0	4	56%
thigh, fried	1 serving	296	18	12	406	0	20.0	85.0	0	60%
white meat, 1/4 'Roy's Roaster'	1 serving	500	56	3	1450	0	29.0	240.0	9	53%
white meat, w/o skin, '1/4 Roy's Roaster'	1 serving	190	32	2	700	0	6.0	100.0	2	28%
wing, fried	1 serving	192	11	9	285	0	13.0	47.0	0	59%
CONDIMENTS. See also Salad Dressing.										
Chinese noodles, salad bar item	1/4 cup	55	2	7	113	0	3.0	1.0	0	43%
croutons, salad bar item	2 tbsp	14	1	3	50	0	0.0	0.0	0	0%
granola, salad bar item	1/4 cup	65	2	9	8	0	3.0	0.0	0	38%
grapes, salad bar item	5 grapes	20	0	5	1	0	0.0	0.0	0	0%
onion, chopped, salad bar item	2 tbsp	7	0	2	0	0	0.0	0.0	0	0%
DESSERT										
caramel sundae	1 serving	293	7	52	193	0	9.0	23.0	0	26%
chocolate sundae	1 serving	358	8	61	290	0	10.0	37.0	0	25%
gelatin parfait, salad bar item	1/4 cup	50	1	10	23	0	2.0	0.0	0	29%
hot fudge sundae	1 serving	337	7	53	186	0	13.0	23.0	0	33%
strawberry shortcake	1 serving	440	8	39	420	na	19.0	15.0	5	48%
strawberry sundae	1 serving	216	6	33	99	0	7.0	23.0	0	29%
vanilla sundae	1 serving	306	8	45	282	0	11.0	40.0	0	32%
HAMBURGER										
'Express'	1 serving	561	27	42	899	0	32.0	70.0	0	51%
regular	1 serving	472	26	37	607	0	25.0	64.0	0	47%
'Roy Rogers Bar'	1 serving	573	36	38	1252	0	31.0	96.0	0	49%
small	1 serving	222	12	23	336	0	9.0	26.0	0	37%
ROLL, crescent	1 serving	287	5	27	547	0	18.0	5.0	0	56%
SALAD, grilled chicken	1 salad	120	18	2	520	0	4.0	60.0	0	31%

Food Name	Serving Size	Calories	Prot. gms	Carbs gms	Sod. mgs	Fiber gms	Fat gms	Sat. Fat gms	Chol. mgs	% Fat Cal.
SALAD DRESSING										
bacon and tomato	2 tbsp	136	0	6	150	0	12.0	0.0	0	82%
blue cheese	2 tbsp	150	2	2	153	0	16.0	0.0	0	90%
Italian, low-calorie	2 tbsp	70	0	2	100	0	6.0	0.0	0	87%
ranch	2 tbsp	155	0	4	100	0	14.0	0.0	0	89%
Thousand Island	2 tbsp	160	0	4	150	0	16.0	0.0	0	90%
SANDWICH										
chicken, 'Gold Rush'	1 sandwich	558	22	51	1326	na	30.0	35.0	9	48%
fish	1 sandwich	514	18	58	857	0	24.0	62.0	0	42%
roast beef	1 sandwich	329	31	29	875	na	10.0	62.0	3	27%
roast beef, large	1 sandwich	373	35	31	840	0	12.0	82.0	0	29%
roast beef, w/cheese	1 sandwich	403	29	37	954	0	15.0	70.0	0	34%
roast beef, w/cheese, large	1 sandwich	427	38	31	1062	0	17.0	94.0	0	36%
SIDE DISH										
baked potato, plain, 'Hot Topped'	1 serving	211	6	48	65	0	0.0	0.0	0	0%
broccoli, salad bar item	1/4 cup	6	1	1	6	0	0.0	0.0	0	0%
coleslaw	1 serving	110	1	11	261	0	7.0	5.0	0	57%
French fries, large	5.5 oz serving	440	6	54	225	0	22.0	19.0	0	45%
French fries, regular	4 oz serving	320	4	39	164	0	16.0	13.0	0	46%
French fries, small	3 oz serving	238	3	29	122	0	12.0	10.0	0	46%
fruit cocktail, salad bar item	1/4 cup	46	0	12	1	0	0.0	0.0	0	0%
Greek noodles, salad bar item	1/4 cup	159	3	19	328	0	9.0	0.0	0	48%
lettuce, Romaine, salad bar item	1 cup	9	1	1	5	0	0.0	0.0	0	0%
macaroni salad, salad bar item	1/4 cup	93	2	10	301	0	5.0	0.0	0	48%
potato salad, salad bar item	1/4 cup	54	1	5	348	0	3.0	0.0	0	53%
SCHLOTZSKY'S DELI										
BEVERAGE										
'Coca-Cola' regular	20 fl oz	248	na	68	15	na	0.0	na	na	0%
'Diet Coke' regular	20 fl oz	0	na	0	25	na	0.0	na	na	0%
iced tea, regular	20 fl oz	na	na	na	na	na	na	na	na	0%
lemonade, 'All Natural' regular	20 fl oz	183	na	43	14	0	0.0	0.0	0	0%
'Mr. Pibb' regular	20 fl oz	243	na	65	35	na	0.0	na	na	0%
orange, 'Minute Maid' regular	20 fl oz	265	na	73	0	na	0.0	na	na	0%
root beer, 'Barq's' regular	20 fl oz	278	na	75	60	na	0.0	na	na	0%
'Sprite' regular	20 fl oz	243	na	65	55	na	na	na	na	0%
CHILI, 'Timberline'	8 oz cup	210	14	24	814	7	7.0	32.0	3	29%
CONDIMENTS. See also Salad Dressing.										
croutons, garlic cheese, salad bar item	1 crouton	46	1	5	142	0	2.0	0.0	0	43%
chow mein noodles	1 serving	74	2	9	111	1	4.0	0.0	1	45%
DESSERT										
fudge brownie cake	1 serving	410	5	46	135	3	25.0	35.0	11	52%
cookies and creme cheesecake	1 serving	330	6	36	320	1	18.0	35.0	9	49%
New York style cheesecake	1 serving	310	7	31	230	0	18.0	60.0	10	52%
strawberry swirl cheesecake	1 serving	300	6	30	230	0	17.0	55.0	9	52%
chocolate chip cookie	1 cookie	160	2	23	150	0	7.0	10.0	3	39%
chocolate chunk cookie	1 cookie	160	2	23	150	1	7.0	10.0	2	39%
chocolate pecan chunk cookie	1 cookie	170	2	23	140	1	8.0	10.0	2	42%
fudge chocolate chunk cookie	1 cookie	170	2	22	170	1	8.0	10.0	3	43%
oatmeal raisin cookie	1 cookie	150	2	1	na	na	1.0	200.0	10	43%
peanut butter cookie	1 cookie	170	2	21	190	1	8.0	10.0	2	44%
peanut butter chocolate cookie	1 cookie	170	2	21	160	1	8.0	10.0	3	44%
sugar cookie	1 cookie	160	2	23	180	0	6.0	15.0	1	35%
white chocolate macadamia cookie	1 cookie	170	2	22	140	0	8.0	10.0	3	43%

Food Name	Serving Size	Calories	Prot. gms	Carbs gms	Sod. mgs	Fiber gms	Fat gms	Sat. Fat gms	Chol. mgs	% Fat Cal.
PIZZA										
bacon, tomato, and mushroom, sourdough crust, 8-inch	1 pizza	635	27	78	1891	4	24.0	38.0	10	34%
barbecue chicken, sourdough crust, 8-inch	1 pizza	653	38	78	2103	3	20.0	74.0	9	28%
chicken and pesto, sourdough crust, 8-inch	1 pizza	649	40	78	2187	4	19.0	74.0	9	27%
double cheese and pepperoni, sourdough crust, 8-inch	1 pizza	744	32	77	2206	4	34.0	62.0	16	41%
double cheese, sourdough crust, 8-inch	1 pizza	603	26	77	1772	4	21.0	34.0	10	31%
fresh tomato and pesto, sourdough crust, 8-inch	1 pizza	539	23	76	1670	4	16.0	27.0	8	27%
Mediterranean, sourdough crust, 8-inch	1 pizza	564	24	84	1787	3	19.0	36.0	10	28%
New Orleans, sourdough crust, 8-inch	1 pizza	666	40	79	2493	4	20.0	74.0	9	27%
original combination, sourdough crust, 8-inch	1 pizza	648	26	79	1994	5	25.0	41.0	10	35%
smoked turkey and jalapeno, sourdough crust, 8-inch	1 pizza	647	38	81	2591	4	19.0	62.0	8	26%
Southwestern, sourdough crust, 8-inch	1 pizza	635	38	76	2015	4	19.0	71.0	8	27%
Thai chicken, sourdough crust, 8-inch	1 pizza	681	40	88	2303	5	19.0	72.0	9	25%
vegetarian special, sourdough crust, 8-inch	1 pizza	551	24	76	1757	4	17.0	27.0	8	28%
SALAD										
Caesar, w/o dressing, croutons, chow mein noodles	1 salad	152	11	11	505	4	8.0	15.0	4	45%
chef's, ham and turkey, dressing, croutons, chow mein noodles	1 salad	248	23	15	1442	3	11.0	51.0	5	39%
chef's, smoked turkey, w/o dressing, croutons, chow mein noodles	1 salad	243	24	15	1275	3	10.0	53.0	5	37%
chicken Caesar, w/o dressing, croutons, chow mein noodles	1 salad	254	28	13	935	4	10.0	63.0	5	35%
chicken, Chinese, w/o dressing, croutons, chow mein noodles	1 salad	150	20	11	448	3	3.0	47.0	1	18%
garden, small, w/o dressing, croutons, chow mein noodles	1 salad	25	1	3	55	1	1.0	0.0	0	36%
garden, w/o dressing, croutons, chow mein noodles	1 salad	61	3	8	119	3	1.0	0.0	0	17%
Greek, w/o dressing, croutons, chow mein noodles	1 salad	220	13	25	563	4	12.0	27.0	8	42%
SALAD DRESSING										
Caesar, 'Olde World'	1 pkt	260	2	1	250	0	27.0	25.0	5	95%
Greek balsamic vinaigrette	1 pkt	170	0	2	330	0	17.0	0.0	3	95%
Italian, light	1 pkt	90	0	3	690	0	8.0	0.0	2	86%
ranch, spicy	1 pkt	230	1	2	310	0	25.0	15.0	4	95%
ranch, spicy, light	1 pkt	140	1	9	350	0	11.0	15.0	3	71%
ranch, traditional	1 pkt	270	0	1	370	0	29.0	5.0	5	98%
sesame ginger vinaigrette	1 pkt	170	1	8	370	0	15.0	0.0	3	79%
Thousand Island	1 pkt	220	0	6	360	0	21.0	30.0	3	89%
SANDWICH										
Bacon, lettuce and tomato										
large, on sourdough bun	1 sandwich	1141	41	140	3066	6	46.0	80.0	14	36%
regular, on sourdough bun	1 sandwich	578	21	70	1548	3	24.0	41.0	7	37%
small, on sourdough bun	1 sandwich	379	13	47	1010	2	15.0	26.0	5	36%
Cheese										
large, on sourdough bun	1 sandwich	1857	87	159	4365	8	98.0	180.0	56	47%
regular, on sourdough bun	1 sandwich	854	38	79	2107	4	44.0	72.0	23	46%
small, on sourdough bun	1 sandwich	596	27	53	1432	3	31.0	54.0	17	47%
Chicken										
breast, large, on sourdough bun	1 sandwich	1008	72	158	4522	6	15.0	155.0	4	13%
breast, regular, on sourdough bun	1 sandwich	535	37	81	2365	3	10.0	85.0	3	16%
breast, small, on sourdough bun	1 sandwich	363	25	55	1596	2	7.0	58.0	2	16%
Chicken club										
large, on sourdough bun	1 sandwich	1351	88	149	4678	8	45.0	209.0	17	30%
medium on sourdough bun	1 sandwich	686	44	75	2403	4	23.0	106.0	9	30%
small, on sourdough bun	1 sandwich	458	29	50	1591	3	15.0	71.0	6	30%

Food Name	Serving Size	Calories	Prot. gms	Carbs gms	Sod. mgs	Fiber gms	Fat gms	Sat. Fat gms	Chol. mgs	% Fat Cal.
Corned beef										
large, on sourdough bun	1 sandwich	1134	81	139	4751	6	25.0	167.0	5	20%
regular, on dark rye bun	1 sandwich	587	40	70	2488	4	15.0	84.0	3	23%
small, on dark rye bun	1 sandwich	388	27	47	1625	3	10.0	56.0	2	23%
'Deluxe Original'										
large, on sourdough bun	1 sandwich	2638	143	173	10762	8	152.0	451.0	62	52%
regular, on sourdough bun	1 sandwich	1296	69	87	5405	4	75.0	217.0	29	52%
small, on sourdough bun	1 sandwich	1044	55	60	4275	3	65.0	192.0	26	56%
Dijon chicken										
large, on sourdough bun	1 sandwich	972	74	150	3981	8	10.0	137.0	2	9%
regular, on wheat bun	1 sandwich	497	38	74	2091	6	6.0	68.0	1	11%
small, on wheat bun	1 sandwich	330	25	50	1373	4	4.0	46.0	1	11%
Ham and cheese										
original, large, on sourdough bun	1 sandwich	1625	93	163	6807	8	67.0	183.0	29	37%
original, regular, on sourdough bun	1 sandwich	789	44	82	3428	4	32.0	83.0	12	36%
original, small, on sourdough bun	1 sandwich	537	30	55	2298	3	22.0	58.0	9	37%
'Original'										
large, on sourdough bun	1 sandwich	1917	90	161	6155	8	102.0	246.0	46	48%
regular, on sourdough bun	1 sandwich	941	42	81	3166	4	50.0	122.0	22	48%
small, on sourdough bun	1 sandwich	713	32	55	2327	3	41.0	100.0	17	51%
Pastrami and Swiss										
large, on sourdough bun	1 sandwich	1681	114	148	7211	6	69.0	304.0	32	37%
regular, on dark rye bun	1 sandwich	861	57	74	3718	4	37.0	152.0	17	39%
small, on dark rye bun	1 sandwich	570	38	49	2445	3	24.0	101.0	11	38%
Pesto chicken										
large, on sourdough bun	1 sandwich	999	73	145	3799	7	15.0	141.0	3	13%
regular, on sourdough bun	1 sandwich	512	37	73	1927	4	9.0	71.0	2	16%
small, on sourdough bun	1 sandwich	346	25	49	1297	2	6.0	48.0	1	15%
Philly										
large, on sourdough bun	1 sandwich	1709	121	157	4477	7	66.0	244.0	32	35%
regular, on sourdough bun	1 sandwich	824	57	78	2189	4	32.0	113.0	14	35%
small, on sourdough bun	1 sandwich	559	39	52	1467	2	22.0	78.0	10	35%
Reuben										
corned beef, large, on sourdough bun	1 sandwich	1594	102	147	6944	7	62.0	262.0	25	36%
corned beef, regular, on dark rye bun	1 sandwich	833	51	74	3514	4	35.0	132.0	13	39%
corned beef, small, on dark rye bun	1 sandwich	528	32	50	2269	3	21.0	80.0	7	37%
pastrami, large, on sourdough bun	1 sandwich	1777	113	152	7765	7	77.0	308.0	34	40%
pastrami, regular, on dark rye bun	1 sandwich	924	56	77	3924	4	43.0	155.0	18	42%
pastrami, small, on dark rye bun	1 sandwich	619	38	51	2679	3	29.0	103.0	12	42%
turkey, large, on sourdough bun	1 sandwich	1656	101	159	7704	7	69.0	247.0	31	37%
turkey, regular, on dark rye bun	1 sandwich	863	50	80	3893	4	39.0	124.0	16	40%
turkey, small, on dark rye bun	1 sandwich	579	33	54	2659	3	26.0	83.0	11	40%
Roast beef										
large, on sourdough bun	1 sandwich	1185	87	145	3362	6	28.0	164.0	6	21%
regular, on sourdough bun	1 sandwich	617	43	73	1733	3	17.0	83.0	3	25%
small, on sourdough bun	1 sandwich	413	29	49	1162	2	11.0	55.0	2	24%
Roast beef and cheese										
large, on sourdough bun	1 sandwich	1749	120	163	4987	8	70.0	255.0	33	36%
regular, on sourdough bun	1 sandwich	848	57	82	2451	4	34.0	119.0	14	36%
small, on sourdough bun	1 sandwich	580	39	55	1666	3	24.0	83.0	10	36%
Santa Fe chicken										
large, on sourdough bun	1 sandwich	1182	82	155	4232	9	29.0	185.0	14	22%
regular, on jalapeño cheese bun	1 sandwich	642	43	77	2302	4	19.0	106.0	9	26%
small, on jalapeño cheese bun	1 sandwich	431	29	52	1547	3	13.0	72.0	6	27%

Food Name	Serving Size	Calories	Prot. gms	Carbs gms	Sod. mgs	Fiber gms	Fat gms	Sat. Fat gms	Chol. mgs	% Fat Cal.
'Texas Schlotzsky's'										
large, on sourdough bun	1 sandwich	1544	84	155	6446	6	65.0	184.0	27	38%
regular, on jalapeno cheese bun	1 sandwich	816	43	76	3357	3	37.0	98.0	16	41%
small, on jalapeno cheese bun	1 sandwich	561	30	51	2263	2	26.0	69.0	12	42%
Tuna										
albacore, large, on sourdough bun	1 sandwich	1000	59	147	3099	6	26.0	122.0	6	22%
albacore, regular, on wheat bun	1 sandwich	533	31	74	1655	4	16.0	69.0	4	26%
albacore, small, on wheat bun	1 sandwich	361	21	50	1122	3	11.0	47.0	3	26%
Tuna melt										
albacore, large, on sourdough bun	1 sandwich	1631	93	158	4474	7	77.0	214.0	34	41%
albacore, regular, on wheat bun	1 sandwich	818	45	79	2293	5	40.0	106.0	16	42%
albacore, small, on wheat bun	1 sandwich	562	31	53	1552	3	28.0	74.0	12	43%
Turkey										
breast, smoked, large, on sourdough bun	1 sandwich	988	68	150	4229	6	13.0	118.0	2	12%
breast, smoked, regular, on sourdough bun	1 sandwich	498	34	75	2123	3	7.0	60.0	1	13%
breast, smoked, small, on sourdough bun	1 sandwich	335	23	50	1426	2	5.0	40.0	1	13%
original, large, on sourdough bun	1 sandwich	2083	123	166	7535	8	104.0	324.0	45	45%
original, regular, on sourdough bun	1 sandwich	1017	58	83	3744	4	51.0	154.0	20	45%
original, small, on sourdough bun	1 sandwich	763	43	56	2789	3	41.0	125.0	17	48%
Turkey bacon club										
large, on sourdough bun	1 sandwich	1790	108	161	6086	7	80.0	240.0	35	40%
regular, on wheat bun	1 sandwich	874	52	79	3009	5	40.0	113.0	15	41%
small, on wheat bun	1 sandwich	596	35	53	2012	3	27.0	78.0	11	41%
Turkey guacamole										
large, on sourdough bun	1 sandwich	1317	73	166	5255	6	42.0	118.0	6	28%
regular, on sourdough bun	1 sandwich	683	36	84	2680	3	24.0	60.0	3	31%
small, on sourdough bun	1 sandwich	448	24	56	1764	2	15.0	40.0	2	30%
Vegetable club										
large, on sourdough bun	1 sandwich	1112	39	151	2716	9	41.0	46.0	13	33%
regular, on sourdough bun	1 sandwich	584	19	76	1435	5	24.0	24.0	7	36%
small, on sourdough bun	1 sandwich	393	13	50	962	3	16.0	17.0	5	36%
Vegetarian										
large, on sourdough bun	1 sandwich	966	34	150	2398	8	26.0	48.0	12	24%
regular, on wheat bun	1 sandwich	519	18	75	1329	5	17.0	32.0	7	29%
small, on wheat bun	1 sandwich	351	12	51	889	4	11.0	22.0	5	28%
Western, large, on sourdough bun	1 sandwich	1261	35	150	2235	8	61.0	125.0	28	43%
Western, regular, on sourdough bun	1 sandwich	651	18	75	1161	4	33.0	62.0	14	44%
Western, small, on sourdough bun	1 sandwich	449	12	51	790	3	23.0	47.0	10	45%
SIDE DISH										
coleslaw, country style	5 oz	225	1	16	288	1	16.0	5.0	3	68%
coleslaw, shredded	5 oz	225	1	16	388	1	16.0	19.0	3	68%
macaroni salad	5 oz	338	4	23	619	1	23.0	9.0	4	66%
potato salad, 'Choice'	5 oz	253	2	18	525	1	18.0	9.0	3	67%
potato salad, diced, w/egg	5 oz	216	3	18	600	1	13.0	38.0	2	58%
potato salad, mustard/egg	5 oz	225	2	17	534	1	15.0	5.0	2	64%
seven bean medley	8 oz cup	145	7	24	1260	8	2.0	0.0	1	13%
SOUP										
Boston clam chowder	8 oz cup	233	5	24	1062	1	15.0	10.0	1	54%
broccoli cheese	8 oz cup	252	7	23	1104	1	17.0	17.0	4	56%
broccoli, cream of	8 oz cup	206	4	25	1152	1	13.0	15.0	3	50%
cauliflower cheese	8 oz cup	252	3	24	993	1	19.0	11.0	4	61%
chicken gumbo	8 oz cup	110	4	13	1114	2	5.0	20.0	1	40%
chicken noodle, old-fashioned	8 oz cup	122	8	18	1104	1	2.0	39.0	1	15%
chicken tortilla	8 oz cup	167	10	24	1026	3	3.0	22.0	1	17%

Food Name	Serving Size	Calories	Prot. gms	Carbs gms	Sod. mgs	Fiber gms	Fat gms	Sat. Fat gms	Chol. mgs	% Fat Cal.
chicken, w/wild rice	8 oz cup	378	10	24	1201	1	28.0	78.0	12	65%
corn chowder	8 oz cup	284	2	38	1010	1	17.0	6.0	3	49%
creamy turkey vegetable	8 oz cup	218	7	21	871	1	14.0	22.0	2	53%
French onion	8 oz cup	78	3	9	1716	0	3.0	0.0	1	36%
minestrone	8 oz cup	89	3	17	1048	3	1.0	0.0	0	10%
potato, cream of, w/bacon	8 oz cup	226	2	31	1209	2	13.0	5.0	1	47%
ravioli tomato	8 oz cup	111	6	21	1115	1	2.0	17.0	0	14%
red beans and rice	8 oz cup	167	8	32	934	4	1.0	0.0	0	5%
tomato Florentine	8 oz cup	100	3	19	1182	1	1.0	0.0	0	9%
vegetable beef barley	8 oz cup	100	6	12	1160	2	3.0	11.0	1	27%
vegetable cheese	8 oz cup	289	6	24	1338	2	19.0	28.0	6	59%
vegetable, lumberjack	8 oz cup	133	3	19	1482	6	6.0	6.0	2	38%
vegetable, vegetarian	8 oz cup	138	3	20	1536	6	6.0	6.0	2	37%
Wisconsin cheese	8 oz cup	319	4	26	1104	1	25.0	22.0	7	65%

SHAKEY'S PIZZA
CHICKEN ENTRÉE

Food Name	Serving Size	Calories	Prot. gms	Carbs gms	Sod. mgs	Fiber gms	Fat gms	Sat. Fat gms	Chol. mgs	% Fat Cal.
fried, w/potatoes	3 pieces	947	57	51	2293	0	56.0	0.0	0	54%
fried, w/potatoes	5 pieces	1700	97	130	5327	0	90.0	0.0	0	47%

PIZZA
Cheese

Food Name	Serving Size	Calories	Prot. gms	Carbs gms	Sod. mgs	Fiber gms	Fat gms	Sat. Fat gms	Chol. mgs	% Fat Cal.
homestyle pan crust, 12-inch pie	1/10 pie	303	14	31	591	0	13.7	21.0	0	41%
thick crust, 'Shakey's Special' 12-inch pie	1/10 pie	208	13	22	423	0	8.3	18.0	0	35%
thick crust, regular, 12-inch pie	1/10 pie	170	9	22	421	0	4.8	13.0	0	26%
thin crust, 'Shakey's Special' 12-inch pie	1/10 pie	171	13	14	475	0	8.7	16.0	0	42%
thin crust, regular, 12-inch pie	1/10 pie	133	8	13	323	0	5.2	14.0	0	35%
Ham and cheese, 'Hot Ham and Cheese'	1 serving	550	36	56	2135	0	21.0	0.0	0	34%

Pepperoni

Food Name	Serving Size	Calories	Prot. gms	Carbs gms	Sod. mgs	Fiber gms	Fat gms	Sat. Fat gms	Chol. mgs	% Fat Cal.
homestyle pan crust 12-inch pie	1/10 pie	343	16	31	740	0	15.4	27.0	0	42%
thick crust, 12-inch pie	1/10 pie	185	10	22	422	0	6.4	17.0	0	31%
thin crust, 12-inch pie	1/10 pie	148	8	13	403	0	6.9	14.0	0	42%

Sausage and mushroom

Food Name	Serving Size	Calories	Prot. gms	Carbs gms	Sod. mgs	Fiber gms	Fat gms	Sat. Fat gms	Chol. mgs	% Fat Cal.
homestyle pan crust, 12-inch pie	1/10 pie	343	16	31	677	0	16.9	24.0	0	44%
thick crust, 12-inch pie	1/10 pie	179	10	22	420	0	5.6	15.0	0	28%
thin crust, 12-inch pie	1/10 pie	141	9	13	336	0	6.0	13.0	0	38%

Sausage and pepperoni

Food Name	Serving Size	Calories	Prot. gms	Carbs gms	Sod. mgs	Fiber gms	Fat gms	Sat. Fat gms	Chol. mgs	% Fat Cal.
homestyle pan crust, 12-inch pie	1/10 pie	374	17	31	676	0	19.9	24.0	0	48%
thick crust, 12-inch pie	1/10 pie	177	11	22	424	0	8.0	19.0	0	35%
thin crust, 12-inch pie	1/10 pie	166	9	13	397	0	8.4	17.0	0	46%

'Sausage Supreme'

Food Name	Serving Size	Calories	Prot. gms	Carbs gms	Sod. mgs	Fiber gms	Fat gms	Sat. Fat gms	Chol. mgs	% Fat Cal.
homestyle pan crust, vegetable, 12-inch pie	1/10 pie	320	15	32	652	0	14.7	21.0	0	41%
'Special' homestyle pan crust, 12-inch pie	1/10 pie	384	18	32	878	0	20.7	29.0	0	48%
'Thai Chicken' thick crust, 12-inch pie	1/10 pie	162	9	22	418	0	4.1	13.0	0	23%
POTATO, wedges	15 pieces	950	17	120	3703	0	36.0	0.0	0	37%

SANDWICH

Food Name	Serving Size	Calories	Prot. gms	Carbs gms	Sod. mgs	Fiber gms	Fat gms	Sat. Fat gms	Chol. mgs	% Fat Cal.
'Hot Ham and Cheese'	1 sandwich	550	36	56	2135	0	21.0	0.0	0	34%
'Super Hot Hero'	1 sandwich	810	36	67	2688	0	44.0	0.0	0	49%
SPAGHETTI ENTRÉE, w/meat sauce and garlic bread	1 serving	940	26	134	1904	0	33.0	0.0	0	32%

SHONEY'S

Food Name	Serving Size	Calories	Prot. gms	Carbs gms	Sod. mgs	Fiber gms	Fat gms	Sat. Fat gms	Chol. mgs	% Fat Cal.
BISCUIT	1 serving	170	3	22	364	0	8.1	0.0	0	43%
BREAD, Grecian	1 serving	80	2	13	94	0	2.2	0.0	0	25%
BREAKFAST										
bacon	3 strips	109	6	0	303	0	9.4	16.0	0	78%

Food Name	Serving Size	Calories	Prot. gms	Carbs gms	Sod. mgs	Fiber gms	Fat gms	Sat. Fat gms	Chol. mgs	% Fat Cal.
croissant, plain	1 serving	260	5	22	260	0	16.0	2.0	0	57%
egg, fried	1 egg	159	6	1	69	0	14.7	274.0	0	83%
ham	2 slices	59	7	1	526	0	2.1	28.0	0	38%
honey bun	1 bun	265	4	32	33	0	14.0	3.0	0	47%
pancake, 6-inch	1 cake	91	2	20	522	0	0.2	0.0	0	2%
sausage	1 patty	103	4	0	161	0	9.6	17.0	0	85%
syrup, low calorie	2.2 oz	98	0	24	0	0	0.0	0.0	0	0%
toast, w/butter	2 slices	163	4	25	296	1	5.2	0.0	0	29%
CHEESEBURGER, 'Mushroom/Swiss Burger'	1 burger	616	32	29	1135	1	41.7	106.0	0	61%
CHICKEN ENTRÉE										
charbroiled, 'LightSide'	1 serving	239	39	1	592	0	7.0	85.0	0	28%
tenders, 'America's Favorites'	1 serving	388	35	17	239	0	20.4	64.0	0	47%
COMBINATION ENTRÉE										
'Fish N' Shrimp'	1 serving	487	28	37	644	0	25.5	127.0	0	47%
'Italian Feast'	1 serving	500	38	44	369	1	19.6	74.0	0	35%
ribeye steak and chicken, charbroiled	1 serving	605	35	0	211	0	50.5	141.0	0	76%
sirloin and chicken, charbroiled	1 serving	357	32	0	160	0	24.5	99.0	0	63%
steak and chicken, charbroiled	8-oz serving	435	31	0	280	0	34.4	123.0	0	71%
'Steak N' Shrimp' charbroiled shrimp	1 serving	361	37	1	198	0	22.6	141.0	0	58%
'Steak N' Shrimp' fried shrimp	1 serving	507	37	15	249	0	32.7	150.0	0	59%
CONDIMENTS. See also Salad dressing.										
gravy, country	3 oz	114	1	6	358	0	9.8	2.0	0	76%
onion, sauteed	2.5-oz serving	37	1	4	221	1	2.1	0.0	0	48%
sweet and sour sauce, souffle cup	1 cup	58	0	15	5	0	0.0	0.0	0	0%
tartar sauce, souffle cup	1 cup	84	0	4	177	0	7.7	11.0	0	82%
DESSERT										
apple pie, à la mode	1 serving	492	6	67	574	0	23.0	35.0	0	41%
brownie, walnut, à la mode	1 serving	576	10	61	435	0	33.7	35.0	0	52%
carrot cake	1 serving	500	9	56	476	0	26.0	37.0	0	47%
hot fudge cake	1 serving	522	7	82	485	0	19.7	27.0	0	33%
hot fudge sundae	1 serving	451	7	60	226	0	22.0	60.0	0	42%
strawberry pie	1 serving	332	2	45	247	2	16.7	0.0	0	45%
strawberry sundae	1 serving	380	6	48	145	0	19.0	69.0	0	44%
FISH										
baked, 'LightSide'	1 serving	170	35	2	1641	0	1.0	83.0	0	6%
fried, 'Light'	1 serving	297	20	22	536	0	14.4	65.0	0	44%
FISH ENTRÉE, fried, w/fries	1 serving	639	32	50	873	3	34.8	103.0	0	49%
HAMBURGER										
'All-American'	1 burger	501	25	27	597	1	32.6	86.0	0	59%
'Old Fashioned'	1 burger	470	25	26	681	1	28.2	82.0	0	56%
'Shoney Burger'	1 burger	498	23	22	782	0	35.7	79.0	0	64%
w/bacon	1 burger	591	29	29	801	1	40.0	86.0	0	61%
HAMBURGER PATTY, beef, light	1 serving	289	21	0	187	0	22.9	82.0	0	71%
LASAGNA ENTRÉE										
'America's Favorites'	1 serving	297	8	45	870	3	9.8	26.0	0	29%
light, 'LightSide'	1 serving	297	8	45	870	0	10.0	26.0	0	30%
LIVER ENTRÉE, w/onions, 'America's Favorites'	1 serving	411	35	15	321	1	22.9	529.0	0	51%
SALAD DRESSING										
Biscayne, low-calorie	2 tbsp	62	6	1	334	0	1.0	0.0	0	24%
blue cheese	2 tbsp	113	0	0	109	0	13.0	15.0	0	100%
French	2 tbsp	124	2	2	204	0	12.0	12.0	0	87%
French rue	2 tbsp	122	5	2	364	0	10.0	0.0	0	76%
honey mustard	2 tbsp	165	2	2	5	0	17.0	18.0	0	89%
Italian, creamy	2 tbsp	135	0	1	454	0	15.0	0.0	0	97%
Italian, golden	2 tbsp	141	0	1	302	0	15.0	0.0	0	97%

Food Name	Serving Size	Calories	Prot. gms	Carbs gms	Sod. mgs	Fiber gms	Fat gms	Sat. Fat gms	Chol. mgs	% Fat Cal.
Italian, nonfat.	2 tbsp	10	0	2	615	0	0.0	0.0	0	0%
Ranch	2 tbsp	95	0	0	10	0	10.0	15.0	0	100%
Thousand Island	2 tbsp	130	1	2	179	0	13.0	12.0	0	91%
SANDWICH										
cheese and bacon, grilled	1 sandwich	440	18	28	1200	1	28.2	36.0	0	58%
cheese, grilled	1 sandwich	454	17	29	1519	0	29.0	0.0	0	59%
chicken fillet	1 sandwich	464	30	39	585	1	21.2	51.0	0	41%
chicken, charbroiled	1 sandwich	451	43	28	1002	1	17.0	90.0	0	35%
fish	1 sandwich	323	12	41	740	0	12.7	21.0	0	35%
ham club, on whole wheat	1 sandwich	642	37	45	2105	11	35.5	78.0	0	49%
ham, baked	1 sandwich	290	19	28	1263	2	10.3	42.0	0	33%
patty melt	1 sandwich	640	39	30	826	7	41.7	121.0	0	58%
Philly steak	1 sandwich	673	32	37	1242	0	44.0	103.0	0	59%
Reuben	1 sandwich	596	33	32	3873	6	34.7	138.0	0	55%
'Slim Jim'	1 sandwich	484	27	40	1620	1	23.9	57.0	0	44%
steak, country fried	1 sandwich	588	25	67	1501	1	25.8	29.0	0	39%
turkey club, on whole wheat	1 sandwich	635	44	44	1289	10	32.7	100.0	0	46%
SEAFOOD PLATTER ENTRÉE	1 serving	566	33	46	893	0	28.0	127.0	0	45%
SHRIMP										
bite-sized	1 serving	387	16	25	1266	0	24.7	140.0	0	57%
charbroiled	1 serving	138	25	3	170	0	3.0	162.0	0	20%
SHRIMP ENTRÉE										
boiled	1 serving	93	20	0	210	0	1.0	182.0	0	10%
sampler	1 serving	412	26	26	783	0	22.7	217.0	0	50%
'Shrimper's Feast' regular	1 serving	383	17	30	216	0	22.2	125.0	0	52%
'Shrimper's Feast' large	1 serving	575	25	45	324	0	33.3	188.0	0	52%
SIDE DISH										
ambrosia salad	1/4 cup	75	1	12	167	1	3.3	0.0	0	38%
apple grape surprise salad	1/4 cup	19	0	5	2	0	0.0	0.0	0	0%
baked potato	10-oz serving	264	6	61	16	7	0.3	0.0	0	1%
beet-onion salad	1/4 cup	25	1	3	167	1	1.3	0.0	0	45%
broccoli-cauliflower-ranch salad	1/4 cup	65	1	2	12	1	6.4	9.0	0	85%
carrot-apple salad	1/4 cup	99	1	4	10	1	9.1	8.0	0	81%
coleslaw	1/4 cup	69	1	5	106	1	5.1	7.0	0	65%
cucumber salad, lite	1/4 cup	12	0	3	344	0	0.1	0.0	0	7%
'Don's Pasta Salad'	1/4 cup	82	2	9	223	0	4.6	0.0	0	50%
French fries	3-oz serving	189	3	29	273	3	7.5	0.0	0	35%
French fries	4-oz serving	252	4	39	364	4	9.9	0.0	0	34%
'Fruit Delight Salad'	1/4 cup	54	1	10	2	1	1.6	0.0	0	25%
grits	3 oz	57	1	6	62	0	3.2	0.0	0	51%
grits, instant	100 grams	67	1	7	73	0	3.8	0.0	0	51%
hash browns	3 oz	90	2	14	50	0	3.1	0.0	0	31%
home fries	3 oz	115	2	19	53	0	3.7	0.0	0	29%
Italian vegetable salad	1/4 cup	11	0	3	110	1	0.1	0.0	0	7%
kidney bean salad	1/4 cup	55	3	7	154	2	2.1	2.0	0	33%
macaroni salad	1/4 cup	207	4	17	382	0	13.9	14.0	0	60%
mixed squash salad	1/4 cup	49	1	2	230	0	4.1	0.0	0	73%
mushroom, sauteed	3-oz serving	75	2	4	968	1	6.5	0.0	0	71%
onion rings	1 ring	52	1	5	102	0	3.1	2.0	0	54%
Oriental salad	1/4 cup	79	1	13	31	1	2.7	1.0	0	30%
pea salad	1/4 cup	73	3	4	89	2	5.5	42.0	0	67%
rice	3.5-oz serving	137	2	23	765	0	3.7	1.0	0	25%
rotelli pasta	1/4 cup	78	1	9	82	0	4.0	0.0	0	47%
seigan salad	1/4 cup	72	2	8	122	1	3.6	5.0	0	44%
snow salad	1/4 cup	72	1	9	18	0	4.1	0.0	0	49%

Food Name	Serving Size	Calories	Prot. gms	Carbs gms	Sod. mgs	Fiber gms	Fat gms	Sat. Fat gms.	Chol. mgs	% Fat Cal.
spaghetti salad	1/4 cup	81	2	9	20	0	4.6	0.0	0	50%
spring salad	1/4 cup	38	1	2	162	1	2.9	0.0	0	67%
summer salad	1/4 cup	114	1	2	233	1	11.6	0.0	0	89%
three-bean salad	1/4 cup	96	1	12	189	1	5.1	0.0	0	46%
Waldorf salad	1/4 cup	81	1	9	68	1	5.2	2.0	0	55%
SOUP										
bean	6 oz	63	4	10	479	1	1.1	4.0	0	15%
beef, w/cabbage	6 oz	86	6	9	503	2	3.0	13.0	0	30%
broccoli, cream of	6 oz	75	2	11	415	0	4.6	1.0	0	46%
cauliflower	6 oz	124	4	12	560	1	9.2	12.0	0	57%
Cheddar chowder	6 oz	91	3	14	948	0	2.3	0.0	0	23%
cheese Florentine, w/ham	6 oz	110	4	12	890	1	7.8	11.0	0	53%
chicken, cream of	6 oz	136	5	14	1164	0	8.9	11.0	0	53%
chicken gumbo	6 oz	60	4	7	1050	0	2.0	0.0	0	29%
chicken noodle	6 oz	62	3	9	127	0	1.4	14.0	0	20%
chicken vegetable, cream of	6 oz	79	4	13	714	0	1.3	0.0	0	15%
chicken w/rice	6 oz	72	3	13	117	1	0.5	6.0	0	6%
clam chowder	6 oz	94	2	10	66	0	5.4	0.0	0	52%
corn chowder	6 oz	148	4	22	510	0	4.7	0.0	0	29%
onion	6 oz	29	1	2	88	0	2.0	1.0	0	63%
potato	6 oz	102	1	17	335	2	3.4	0.0	0	30%
tomato, w/vegetable	6 oz	46	2	10	314	0	0.3	0.0	0	5%
tomato Florentine	6 oz	63	2	11	683	0	1.1	0.0	0	16%
vegetable beef	6 oz	82	4	14	1254	0	1.5	5.0	0	16%
SPAGHETTI ENTRÉE										
'America's Favorites'	1 serving	496	24	63	387	2	16.3	55.0	0	30%
SPAGHETTI ENTRÉE, LIGHT										
light, 'LightSide'	1 serving	248	12	32	194	0	8.0	28.0	0	29%
STEAK, sirloin, charbroiled	6 oz	357	32	0	160	0	24.5	99.0	0	63%
STEAK ENTRÉE, country fried steak 'America's Favorites'	1 serving	449	19	34	1177	1	27.2	27.0	0	53%
SIZZLER										
BEEF										
roast beef, sliced	2/3 oz	17	3	0	276	0	0.3	8.0	0	16%
steak, New York strip	12 oz	600	70	5	200	0	35.0	180.0	0	51%
steak, sirloin	6.25 oz	447	55	0	245	0	34.0	120.0	12	58%
BEEF PATTY	8 oz	530	42	0	150	0	38.0	156.0	15	67%
BREAD, focaccia	2 pieces	108	2	9	134	0	7.0	1.0	1	59%
BREADSTICK, garlic, soft	1 oz	75	2	15	112	0	0.5	0.0	0	6%
CHICKEN										
breast, lemon herb	5 oz	151	27	27	0	0	4.0	0.0	0	14%
wing	1 oz	73	4	4	136	0	4.0	20.0	1	53%
wing, Cajun	3 oz	201	16	2	435	0	14.4	111.0	0	65%
wing, Southern	1 oz	73	5	4	135	0	6.0	20.0	1	62%
wing, whole, Southern	1 oz	74	4	4	285	0	4.8	18.0	2	59%
CHICKEN ENTRÉE, w/noodles	6 oz	164	13	20	524	0	4.0	40.0	1	21%
CHICKEN PATTY, 'Malibu'	1 patty	368	27	12	0	0	25.0	0.0	0	59%
CHILI, 'Grande' w/beans	6 oz	100	5	18	1190	0	1.0	0.0	0	9%
CONDIMENTS										
buttery dipping sauce	1.5 oz	330	0	0	0	0	37.0	0.0	7	100%
guacamole	1 oz	42	0	2	425	0	4.0	0.0	1	82%
guacamole, extra chunky	3.5 oz serving	285	3	7	0	0	18.4	0.0	0	80%
hibachi sauce	1.5 oz	57	0	11	707	0	0.0	0.0	0	0%
Malibu sauce	1.5 oz	283	0	0	354	0	31.0	28.0	6	100%
margarine, whipped	1.5 tbsp	105	0	0	146	0	12.0	0.0	2	100%

Food Name	Serving Size	Calories	Prot. gms	Carbs gms	Sod. mgs	Fiber gms	Fat gms	Sat. Fat gms	Chol. mgs	% Fat Cal.
marinade	1 oz	13	0	3	90	0	0.0	0.0	0	0%
nacho cheese sauce	2 oz	120	5	3	600	0	10.0	30.0	5	74%
pepper, bell, salad bar item	2 oz	8	1	2	1	1	0.0	0.0	0	0%
salsa	1 oz	7	0	2	156	0	0.0	0.0	0	0%
tartar sauce	1.5 oz	170	0	6	453	0	17.0	14.0	3	86%
turkey ham, salad bar item	1 oz	62	4	0	376	0	5.0	19.0	2	74%
CORNED BEEF, sliced	1 oz	45	8	0	55	0	1.5	0.0	0	30%
CRAB, snow, legs and claws,	3.5 oz	91	21	0	539	0	1.1	55.0	0	11%
CRAB, IMITATION, shredded	3.5 oz serving	104	12	14	864	0	1.0	22.0	0	8%
CROISSANT, mini	1 croissant	120	2	12	95	0	8.0	4.0	3	56%
DESSERT										
'Parfait Salad'	3.5 oz serving	84	2	17	66	0	1.7	0.0	2	18%
yogurt, frozen, chocolate, soft-serve	4 oz	136	1	24	100	0	4.0	0.0	4	26%
yogurt, frozen, vanilla, soft-serve	4 oz	136	1	24	100	0	4.0	0.0	4	26%
DESSERT TOPPING										
chocolate syrup	1 oz	90	0	21	15	0	0.0	0.0	0	0%
strawberry, nonfat	1 oz	70	0	18	5	0	0.0	0.0	0	0%
whipped	1 tbsp	12	0	1	0	0	1.0	0.0	1	69%
FISH NUGGETS	1 oz	40	4	5	100	0	0.0	10.0	0	0%
HALIBUT, steak	6 oz	180	36	0	103	0	2.0	86.0	1	11%
HAMBURGER, w/lettuce and tomato	1 serving	626	45	36	335	1	33.0	142.0	12	48%
LASAGNA										
w/meat	8 oz	327	21	23	657	0	13.0	37.0	6	40%
vegetable	8 oz	245	15	29	553	0	8.0	19.0	5	29%
MACARONI AND CHEESE	6 oz	214	10	22	590	0	9.0	26.0	5	39%
MEATBALL	4 meatballs	157	9	5	461	1	11.0	30.0	5	64%
PASTA										
fettuccine	2 oz	80	3	15	5	0	1.0	5.0	0	11%
fettuccine, whole egg, dry	2 oz	210	9	40	8	0	1.0	0.0	1	4%
ravioli, cheese	4 oz	260	10	47	270	0	4.0	20.0	2	14%
spaghetti	2 oz	80	3	16	1	1	0.0	0.0	0	0%
POLLACK, breaded	4 oz	140	14	18	280	0	1.0	35.0	0	7%
SALAD DRESSING										
bacon, hot	1 tbsp	40	0	58	90	0	20.0	0.0	0	44%
blue cheese	1 oz	111	1	1	168	0	12.0	8.0	4	93%
honey mustard	1 oz	160	0	4	110	0	16.0	10.0	2	90%
Italian, lite	1 oz	14	0	2	350	0	0.0	0.0	0	0%
Italian, Parmesan	1 oz	100	0	2	450	0	10.0	0.0	2	92%
Japanese rice vinegar, nonfat	1 oz	10	0	2	172	0	0.0	0.0	0	0%
Malibu	1 tbsp	100	0	0	125	0	11.0	10.0	2	100%
ranch	1 oz	120	0	2	240	0	12.0	10.0	2	93%
ranch, lower calorie	1 oz	90	0	4	270	0	8.0	10.0	2	82%
sour	1.5 oz	89	0	0	44	0	9.0	0.0	8	100%
sour	2 tbsp	60	0	0	30	0	6.0	0.0	5	100%
Thousand Island	1 oz	143	0	3	125	0	15.0	11.0	2	92%
SALMON	8 oz	247	32	0	232	0	12.0	41.0	2	46%
SCALLOP, breaded, approx 30-40	4 oz	160	14	24	393	0	1.0	18.0	0	6%
SHRIMP										
broiled	5 oz	150	23	0	377	0	6.0	218.0	1	37%
butterfly, breaded, approx 16–20	3.5 oz	220	10	16	440	0	13.0	50.0	0	53%
butterfly, breaded, approx 10–12	3.5 oz	145	10	14	280	0	0.1	0.0	0	1%
butterfly, Cajun, breaded, approx 16–20	3.5 oz	145	10	24	280	0	0.1	0.0	0	1%
butterfly, lemon pepper, breaded, approx 21–25	2 oz	190	5	38	211	0	1.0	5.0	0	5%
Cajun, breaded, approx 80–90	3.5 oz	140	10	22	198	0	0.9	0.0	0	6%

Food Name	Serving Size	Calories	Prot. gms	Carbs gms	Sod. mgs	Fiber gms	Fat gms	Sat. Fat gms	Chol. mgs	% Fat Cal.
mini, breaded, approx 50–60	3.5 oz	140	10	22	198	0	0.9	0.0	0	6%
mini, Cajun, breaded, approx 40–50	3.5 oz	141	10	22	200	0	0.9	0.0	0	6%
scampi	5 oz	143	27	0	386	0	3.0	150.0	1	20%
tempura-battered, approx 21–25	3 oz	155	10	13	442	0	8.0	74.0	3	44%
SIDE DISH										
avocado, salad bar item	1/2 avocado	153	2	6	11	3	15.0	0.0	2	81%
broccoli, salad bar item	1/2 cup	12	1	2	12	1	0.0	0.0	0	0%
carrot-raisin salad	2 oz	130	1	10	104	1	10.0	10.0	2	67%
cauliflower, battered, not fried	3.5 oz serving	184	3	21	49	0	10.3	1.0	0	49%
cheese toast	1 piece	273	6	16	494	1	21.0	5.0	5	68%
Chinese chicken salad	2 oz	54	4	6	119	1	2.0	10.0	0	31%
corn nuggets	3 oz	117	3	22	325	0	8.4	0.0	0	44%
cottage cheese, low-fat	1/2 cup	100	14	4	390	0	2.0	8.0	1	20%
four-bean salad	3.5 oz serving	104	3	19	226	0	2.5	0.0	0	21%
french fries	4 oz	358	5	45	245	4	12.0	0.0	6	35%
grapes, salad bar item	1/2 cup	29	0	8	1	1	0.0	0.0	0	0%
jicama, salad bar item	2 oz	13	1	3	1	0	0.0	0.0	0	0%
jicama salad, spicy	2 oz	16	0	4	28	0	0.0	0.0	0	0%
kidney beans, salad bar item	1/4 cup	52	3	10	222	4	0.0	0.0	0	0%
kiwifruit, salad bar item	2 oz	35	1	8	3	2	0.0	0.0	0	0%
lettuce, Romaine, salad bar item	1 cup	9	1	1	4	1	0.0	0.0	0	0%
macaroni and cheddar salad	3.5 oz serving	185	3	16	476	0	12.5	14.0	4	60%
Mediterranean Minted fruit salad	2 oz	29	1	7	11	0	0.0	0.0	0	0%
'Mexican Fiesta Salad'	2 oz	54	2	10	99	1	1.0	0.0	0	16%
okra, breaded, not fried	3.5 oz serving	105	3	24	503	0	0.5	1.0	0	4%
onion rings, steak cut, breaded, not fried	.5 oz serving	395	5	39	558	0	24.4	0.0	0	56%
'Oriental Pasta Salad'	3.5 oz serving	114	4	23	781	0	1.6	1.0	0	12%
potato and egg salad	3.5 oz serving	140	2	16	340	0	7.8	28.0	1	50%
potato, baked, flesh only	4 oz	105	2	24	6	2	0.0	0.0	0	0%
potato salad, 'Old Fashioned'	2 oz	84	1	10	231	1	5.0	8.0	1	51%
potato salad, 'Old Fashioned'	3.5 oz serving	150	2	17	416	0	8.7	23.0	1	51%
potato salad, red, herb	2 oz	121	1	9	271	1	9.0	9.0	1	67%
potato salad, red, herb	3.5 oz serving	213	2	15	437	0	16.2	15.0	2	68%
potato skin	2 oz	160	2	22	463	3	8.0	0.0	1	43%
refried beans	3 oz	120	5	16	320	0	4.0	2.0	2	30%
rice pilaf	6 oz	256	4	47	866	1	5.0	0.0	1	18%
'Seafood Louis' pasta salad	2 oz	64	3	9	139	1	2.0	17.0	0	27%
seafood salad	2 oz	56	3	4	255	0	3.0	7.0	1	49%
shell pasta salad	3.5 oz serving	112	3	19	591	0	2.7	1.0	1	21%
spinach, salad bar item	1/2 cup	6	1	1	22	1	0.0	0.0	0	0%
teriyaki beef salad	2 oz	49	4	5	136	1	2.0	7.0	1	33%
tuna pasta salad	2 oz	133	6	6	188	0	10.0	10.0	1	65%
tuna salad	3.5 oz serving	353	8	7	296	0	32.9	44.0	5	83%
SOUP										
broccoli cheese soup	4 oz	139	3	10	355	0	9.0	8.0	2	61%
chicken w/noodle	4 oz	31	2	4	495	0	1.0	7.0	0	27%
clam chowder	4 oz	118	3	11	511	0	6.0	6.0	0	49%
minestrone, nonfat	4 oz	36	1	7	443	2	0.0	1.0	0	0%
vegetable, vegetarian	6 oz	50	2	6	630	0	1.0	0.0	0	22%
vegetable sirloin soup	4 oz	60	6	6	364	0	2.0	10.0	1	27%
SWORDFISH	8 oz	315	45	0	331	0	14.0	89.0	3	41%
TACO SHELL	1 shell	50	1	7	20	1	2.0	0.0	0	36%
TUNA, yellowfin	3.5 oz serving	125	15	0	50	0	4.0	65.0	1	38%

Food Name	Serving Size	Calories	Prot. gms	Carbs gms	Sod. mgs	Fiber gms	Fat gms	Sat. Fat gms	Chol. mgs	% Fat Cal.
SKIPPER'S										
CHICKEN ENTRÉE										
'Lite Catch' 3 pieces, w/small green salad	1 serving	305	26	17	673	0	15.0	58.0	0	44%
tenderloin strips, 5 pieces, w/fries	1 serving	793	44	69	798	0	38.0	77.0	0	43%
CHICKEN STRIPS, 'Create A Catch'	1 serving	82	8	4	150	0	4.0	15.0	0	43%
CLAM ENTRÉE, 'Basket' strips w/fries	1 serving	1003	22	90	569	0	70.0	14.0	0	58%
COD ENTRÉE										
3 pieces, thick cut, w/fries	1 serving	665	27	68	1054	0	32.0	38.0	0	43%
4 pieces, thick cut w/fries	1 serving	759	34	74	1388	0	36.0	50.0	0	43%
5 pieces, thick cut, w/fries	1 serving	853	42	80	1723	0	41.0	62.0	0	43%
COMBINATION ENTRÉE										
'Combos' clam strips, 1 piece fish, fries	1 serving	868	25	81	667	0	54.0	61.0	0	53%
'Combos' jumbo shrimp, 1 piece fish, fries	1 serving	720	24	75	1268	0	36.0	91.0	0	45%
'Combos' original shrimp, 1 piece fish, fries	1 serving	728	24	77	943	0	37.0	105.0	0	45%
'Combos' oysters, 1 piece fish, fries	1 serving	885	25	95	809	0	44.0	80.0	0	45%
'Lite Catch' 1 piece fish, 2 pieces chicken, small green salad	1 serving	399	29	24	880	0	21.0	96.0	0	47%
3-piece, chicken strip, fish, fries	1 serving	805	80	72	858	0	40.0	100.0	0	37%
3-piece, chicken strip, shrimp, fries	1 serving	800	36	77	1036	0	39.0	97.0	0	44%
DESSERT										
gelatin, nonfat, 'Jell-O' 'Create A Catch'	1 serving	55	1	12	35	0	0.0	0.0	0	0%
root beer float	1 serving	302	3	33	66	0	10.0	10.0	0	38%
FISH										
fillet, 'Create A Catch'	1 serving	175	11	11	357	0	10.0	53.0	0	51%
FISH ENTRÉE										
1 fish fillet, w/fries	1 serving	558	17	51	408	0	28.0	55.0	0	48%
2 fish fillets, w/fries	1 serving	733	28	71	765	0	38.0	108.0	0	46%
3 fish fillets, w/fries	1 serving	908	39	82	1122	0	48.0	160.0	0	47%
'Lite Catch' 2 pieces, w/small green salad	1 serving	409	25	27	937	0	23.0	119.0	0	50%
FISH SANDWICH										
'Create A Catch'	1 sandwich	524	19	43	1191	0	33.0	86.0	0	55%
'Create A Catch' double	1 sandwich	698	30	54	1548	0	73.0	139.0	0	66%
SIDE DISH										
baked potato	1 serving	145	4	32	6	0	0.0	0.0	0	0%
coleslaw	.5 oz serving	289	2	10	329	0	27.0	50.0	0	84%
French fries, 'Create A Catch'	1 serving	383	6	50	51	0	18.0	2.0	0	42%
SOUP										
clam chowder, 'Create A Catch' cup	1 serving	100	3	14	525	0	3.5	12.0	0	32%
clam chowder, 'Create A Catch' pint	1 serving	200	5	19	1050	0	7.0	24.0	0	40%
salmon chowder, 'Alder Smoked Salmon'	6 oz	166	13	14	73	0	7.0	0.0	0	37%
OYSTER ENTRÉE, w/fries 'Basket'	1 serving	1038	28	118	853	0	51.0	52.0	0	44%
SALAD										
green, small, 'Lite Catch'	1 salad	59	3	6	223	0	3.0	13.0	0	43%
shrimp and seafood	1 salad	167	23	15	657	0	3.0	80.0	0	15%
side	1 salad	24	0	4	8	0	0.0	0.0	0	0%
SALAD DRESSING										
salad dressing, blue cheese, premium	1 pouch	222	1	4	240	0	23.0	8.0	0	91%
salad dressing, Italian, gourmet	1 pouch	140	0	2	200	0	15.0	0.0	0	94%
salad dressing, Italian, low-calorie	1 pouch	17	0	2	680	0	1.0	0.0	0	53%
salad dressing, ranch house	1 pouch	188	1	2	302	0	20.0	0.0	0	94%
salad dressing, Thousand Island	1 pouch	160	0	8	415	0	14.0	6.0	0	80%
tartar sauce	1 tbsp	65	0	0	102	0	7.0	4.0	0	100%
SALMON, baked	4.4 oz	270	39	1	504	0	11.0	70.0	0	38%
SEAFOOD ENTRÉE, w/fries 'Skipper's Platter Basket'	1 serving	1038	32	97	1202	0	63.0	111.0	0	52%

Food Name	Serving Size	Calories	Prot. gms	Carbs gms	Sod. mgs	Fiber gms	Fat gms	Sat. Fat gms	Chol. mgs	% Fat Cal.
SHRIMP ENTRÉE										
w/fries, 'Basket'	1 serving	723	20	82	1121	0	36.0	102.0	0	44%
w/fries, jumbo, 'Basket'	1 serving	707	20	79	911	0	35.0	73.0	0	44%
w/seafood salad, 'Lite Catch'	1 serving	167	23	15	657	0	3.0	80.0	0	15%
SONIC										
CHEESEBURGER										
#1	1 serving	70	4	0	267	0	5.8	18.0	0	75%
#2	1 serving	70	4	0	267	0	5.8	18.0	0	74%
w/bacon	1 serving	548	28	23	839	0	38.6	87.0	0	63%
jalapeño, double meat and cheese	1 serving	638	44	22	1358	0	40.6	136.0	0	58%
mini	1 serving	281	17	20	644	0	14.4	45.0	0	47%
CHILI PIE	1 serving	327	12	20	313	0	22.6	28.0	0	62%
CORN DOG	1 sandwich	280	7	30	700	0	15.0	35.0	0	48%
HAMBURGER										
#1	1 serving	409	20	23	444	0	26.6	58.0	0	58%
#2	1 serving	323	20	23	549	0	15.7	50.0	0	45%
hickory	1 serving	314	20	23	459	0	15.7	50.0	0	45%
mini	1 serving	246	14	20	510	0	11.5	36.0	0	43%
'Super Sonic' double meat and cheese, w/mayo	1 serving	730	44	24	1023	0	51.5	144.0	0	63%
'Super Sonic' double meat and cheese, w/mustard	1 serving	644	44	24	1128	0	40.7	136.0	0	57%
HOT DOG										
'Cheese Coney' extra long	1 serving	635	24	45	632	0	39.0	65.0	0	56%
'Cheese Coney' w/onions, extra long	1 serving	640	25	47	632	0	39.2	65.0	0	55%
'Cheese Coney' regular	1 serving	358	14	23	341	0	23.3	40.0	0	59%
regular	1 serving	258	8	21	241	0	15.3	23.0	0	54%
'Cheese Coney' regular, w/onions	1 serving	361	14	24	341	0	23.3	40.0	0	58%
SANDWICH										
bacon, lettuce, tomato	1 sandwich	327	8	27	600	0	19.3	9.0	0	56%
cheese, grilled	1 sandwich	288	12	25	841	0	17.0	36.0	0	51%
chicken	1 sandwich	319	21	41	890	0	9.0	47.0	0	25%
chicken, breaded	1 sandwich	455	23	36	755	0	24.7	42.0	0	48%
chicken, grilled, no dressing	1 sandwich	215	21	23	716	0	4.3	63.0	0	18%
fish	1 sandwich	277	17	38	655	0	7.0	6.0	0	22%
steak	1 sandwich	631	19	46	1047	0	41.6	50.0	0	59%
SIDE DISH										
French fries, large	1 serving	315	5	50	67	0	11.2	11.0	0	32%
French fries, regular	1 serving	233	3	37	50	0	8.0	8.0	0	31%
French fries, w/cheese, large	1 serving	420	11	51	468	0	20.2	38.0	0	43%
onion rings, large	1 serving	577	8	54	532	0	37.8	0.0	0	58%
onion rings, regular	1 serving	404	5	38	372	0	26.5	0.0	0	58%
potato pieces, 'Tater Tots'	1 serving	150	2	19	330	0	7.0	10.0	0	43%
potato pieces, 'Tater Tots' w/cheese	1 serving	220	6	19	569	0	13.0	28.0	0	54%
SPAGHETTI WAREHOUSE										
MARINADE, dinner serving	1 serving	403	13	75	303	5	5.0	0.0	0	11%
MINESTRONE SOUP	1 serving	56	3	8	155	2	1.0	3.0	0	17%
TOMATO SAUCE, dinner serving	1 serving	410	13	76	454	6	5.0	0.0	0	11%
STEAK 'N SHAKE										
CHEESEBURGER										
'Steakburger'	1 serving	353	23	33	658	0	13.0	0.0	0	34%
'Steakburger' super	1 serving	451	35	33	680	0	18.0	0.0	0	37%
'Steakburger' triple patty	1 serving	626	52	34	934	0	30.0	0.0	0	44%

Food Name	Serving Size	Calories	Prot. gms	Carbs gms	Sod. mgs	Fiber gms	Fat gms	Sat. Fat gms	Chol. mgs	% Fat Cal.
CHILI										
'Chili Mac' w/4 saltines	1 serving	310	15	34	1301	0	12.0	0.0	0	36%
'Chili 3 Ways' w/4 saltines	1 serving	411	19	45	1734	0	16.0	0.0	0	36%
w/oyster crackers	1 serving	337	16	37	1157	0	14.0	0.0	0	37%
DESSERT										
apple Danish	1 piece	391	6	35	352	0	24.0	0.0	0	57%
apple pie à la mode	1 serving	549	4	76	525	0	25.0	0.0	0	41%
brownie	1 brownie	258	3	39	165	0	12.0	0.0	0	39%
cheesecake	1 serving	368	7	61	294	0	11.0	0.0	0	27%
cheesecake, w/strawberries	1 serving	386	7	65	294	0	11.0	0.0	0	26%
cherry pie à la mode'	1 serving	476	6	63	314	0	22.0	0.0	0	42%
'Coca-Cola Float'	1 serving	514	16	76	230	0	17.0	0.0	0	29%
fudge brownie sundae	1 serving	645	7	81	262	0	35.0	0.0	0	47%
hot fudge nut sundae	1 serving	530	5	51	121	0	34.0	0.0	0	58%
'Lemon Float'	1 serving	555	18	82	248	0	19.0	0.0	0	30%
'Lemon Freeze'	1 serving	548	15	69	213	0	25.0	0.0	0	40%
'Orange Float'	1 serving	502	16	74	224	0	17.0	0.0	0	30%
'Orange Freeze'	1 serving	516	14	63	198	0	24.0	0.0	0	41%
'Root Beer Float'	1 serving	529	17	78	237	0	17.0	0.0	0	29%
strawberry sundae	1 serving	330	2	29	81	0	22.0	0.0	0	61%
HAMBURGER										
'Steakburger'	1 serving	277	18	33	425	0	7.0	0.0	0	24%
'Steakburger' super	1 serving	375	30	33	447	0	12.0	0.0	0	30%
'Steakburger' triple patty	1 serving	474	43	33	468	0	17.0	0.0	0	33%
SALAD										
chef	1 salad	313	41	6	1582	0	18.0	0.0	0	46%
lettuce and tomato, w/1 oz Thousand Island dressing	1 salad	168	1	7	223	0	15.0	0.0	0	81%
SANDWICH										
cheese, toasted	1 sandwich	250	9	24	606	0	13.0	0.0	0	47%
egg	1 sandwich	275	12	33	490	0	10.0	0.0	0	33%
ham, baked	1 sandwich	451	29	37	1858	0	22.0	0.0	0	43%
ham and egg	1 sandwich	434	36	33	1850	0	17.0	0.0	0	36%
SIDE DISH										
baked beans	1 serving	173	9	27	656	0	4.0	0.0	0	20%
French fries	1 serving	211	3	28	297	0	10.0	0.0	0	42%
STEAK PLATTER, low calorie	1 serving	293	37	3	242	0	14.0	0.0	0	44%
SUBWAY										
BEVERAGE										
'Berry'Lishus Fruizle Smoothie'	12 oz	154	1	40	9	3	0.3	0.0	0	2%
'Berry Blitz Fruizle Smoothie'	12 oz	129	1	37	7	7	0.0	0.0	0	0%
'Berry Breeze Fruizle Smoothie'	12 oz	120	0	32	7	2	0.1	0.0	0	1%
'Island Berry Fruizle Smoothie'	12 oz	120	0	32	7	2	0.1	0.0	0	1%
'Island Fever Fruizle Smoothie'	12 oz	137	0	36	7	1	0.2	0.0	0	1%
'Peach Paradise Fruizle Smoothie'	12 oz	119	0	32	7	1	0.1	0.0	0	1%
'Peach Pizazz Fruizle Smoothie'	12 oz	126	0	33	10	1	0.0	0.0	0	0%
'Pineapple Delite Fruizle Smoothie'	12 oz	142	1	38	6	1	0.3	0.0	0	2%
'Pineapple Passion Fruizle Smoothie'	12 oz	140	1	38	6	1	0.2	0.0	0	1%
'Sunrise Energizer Fruizle Smoothie'	12 oz	160	1	42	8	2	0.3	0.0	0	2%
'Tropical Trio Fruizle Smoothie'	12 oz	138	0	36	7	1	0.2	0.0	0	1%
'Wild Berries Fruizle Smoothie'	12 oz	130	1	36	8	5	0.1	0.0	0	1%
BREAD										
Italian, 12-inch	1 large	380	14	76	840	0	2.0	0.0	2	5%
Italian, 6-inch	1 small	190	7	38	420	0	1.0	0.0	1	5%
wheat, 12-inch	1 serving	420	16	78	860	6	5.0	0.0	2	11%

Food Name	Serving Size	Calories	Prot. gms	Carbs gms	Sod. mgs	Fiber gms	Fat gms	Sat. Fat gms	Chol. mgs	% Fat Cal.
wheat, 6-inch	1 serving	210	8	39	430	3	3.0	0.0	1	13%
wrap, 10.5-inch	1 wrap	200	0	45	720	1	2.0	0.0	1	9%
CONDIMENTS										
bacon, 'Optional Fixin's'	2 slices	42	3	0	160	0	3.0	9.0	1	69%
cheese	2 triangles	41	2	0	204	0	3.0	10.0	2	77%
lettuce, deli style, 'Standard Fixin's'	1 serving	2	0	0	1	0	0.0	0.0	0	0%
lettuce, 'Standard Fixin's'	1 serving	4	0	1	3	0	0.0	0.0	0	0%
mayonnaise, regular, 'Optional Fixin's'	1 tsp	37	0	0	27	0	4.0	3.0	1	100%
mayonnaise, light, 'Optional Fixin's'	1 tsp	18	0	0	33	0	2.0	2.0	0	100%
mustard, 'Optional Fixin's'	2 tsp	7	0	1	115	0	0.0	0.0	0	0%
oil, 'Optional Fixin's'	1 tsp	45	0	0	0	0	5.0	0.0	1	100%
olives, deli style, 'Standard Fixin's'	2 rings	2	0	0	6	0	0.0	0.0	0	0%
olives, 'Standard Fixin's'	2 rings	2	0	0	6	0	0.0	0.0	0	0%
onion, deli style, 'Standard Fixin's'	1 serving	2	0	1	0	0	0.0	0.0	0	0%
onion 'Standard Fixin's'	1 serving	5	0	1	0	0	0.0	0.0	0	0%
peppers, deli style 'Standard Fixin's'	2 strips	1	0	0	0	na	0.0	0.0	0	0%
peppers, 'Standard Fixin's'	2 strips	1	0	0	0	0	0.0	0.0	0	0%
pickle, deli style, 'Standard Fixin's'	2 chips	1	0	0	92	0	0.0	0.0	0	0%
pickle, 'Standard Fixin's'	3 chips	2	0	0	139	0	0.0	0.0	0	0%
tomato, deli style, 'Standard Fixin's'	2 slices	8	0	2	4	0	0.0	0.0	0	0%
tomato, 'Standard Fixin's'	2 slices	6	0	1	2	0	0.0	0.0	0	0%
vinegar, 'Optional Fixin's'	1 tsp	1	0	0	0	0	0.0	0.0	0	0%
COOKIE										
Brazil nut	1 cookie	215	2	29	153	1	10.0	14.0	3	42%
chocolate chip, 'M&M's'	1 cookie	212	2	29	144	1	10.0	13.0	3	42%
chocolate chip	1 cookie	214	3	29	144	1	10.0	12.0	3	41%
chocolate chunk	1 cookie	215	2	29	144	1	10.0	13.0	3	42%
macadamia nut	1 cookie	222	2	28	144	1	11.0	12.0	2	45%
oatmeal raisin	1 cookie	199	3	29	159	1	8.0	14.0	2	36%
oatmeal raisin, low-fat	1 cookie	168	3	33	171	2	3.0	15.0	1	16%
peanut butter	1 cookie	223	3	27	214	1	12.0	0.0	2	47%
sugar	1 cookie	225	2	28	180	0	12.0	18.0	3	47%
ROLL, deli style	1 serving	170	6	31	350	1	2.0	0.0	1	11%
SALAD										
chicken breast, roasted, w/o dressing, cheese, condiments	1 salad	162	20	13	693	1	4.0	48.0	1	21%
'Classic Italian BMT, w/o dressing, cheese, condiments	1 salad	269	14	11	1305	1	19.0	52.0	7	63%
'Cold Cut Trio' w/o dressing, cheese, condiments	1 salad	193	12	12	1162	1	12.0	47.0	4	53%
ham, w/o dressing, cheese, condiments	1 salad	112	12	11	1068	1	3.0	25.0	1	23%
meatball, w/o dressing, cheese, condiments	1 salad	232	13	17	751	3	13.0	35.0	5	49%
roast beef, w/o dressing, cheese, condiments	1 salad	115	12	11	654	1	3.0	20.0	1	23%
seafood and crab, w/light mayo, w/o dressing	1 salad	157	7	17	761	2	7.0	14.0	1	40%
steak and cheese, w/o dressing	1 salad	182	17	13	887	2	8.0	37.0	4	38%
'Subway Club' w/o dressing, cheese, condiments	1 salad	123	14	12	965	1	3.0	26.0	1	21%
'Subway Melt' w/o dressing	1 salad	190	16	12	1346	1	9.0	41.0	4	42%
tuna, made w/light mayo, w/o dressing, cheese, condiments	1 salad	198	11	11	669	1	12.0	32.0	2	55%
turkey and ham, w/o dressing, cheese, condiments	1 salad	107	11	11	982	1	2.0	23.0	1	17%
turkey breast, w/o dressing, cheese, condiments	1 salad	101	11	12	896	1	2.0	20.0	0	16%
'Veggie Delite' w/o dressing, cheese, condiments	1 salad	51	2	10	308	1	1.0	0.0	0	16%
SANDWICH										
Bacon and egg										
deli style sub	1 sandwich	323	14	33	569	1	14.0	185.0	4	40%
6-inch sub	1 sandwich	363	16	41	649	3	15.0	185.0	4	37%

Food Name	Serving Size	Calories	Prot. gms	Carbs gms	Sod. mgs	Fiber gms	Fat gms	Sat. Fat gms	Chol. mgs	% Fat Cal.
wrap	1 sandwich	353	8	47	939	1	14.0	185.0	4	36%
Bologna, deli style sub, w/o cheese, condiments	1 sandwich	283	11	37	785	1	10.0	19.0	3	32%
Cheese and egg										
deli style sub	1 sandwich	323	14	33	613	1	14.0	187.0	5	40%
6-inch sub	1 sandwich	363	16	41	693	3	15.0	187.0	5	37%
wrap	1 sandwich	353	8	47	983	1	14.0	187.0	5	36%
Chicken breast										
roasted, 6-inch hot sub, w/o cheese, condiments	1 sandwich	342	26	46	966	3	6.0	48.0	2	16%
roasted, super, 6-inch hot sub, w/o cheese, condiments	1 sandwich	453	44	49	1351	4	9.0	96.0	3	18%
Chicken Parmesan wrap	1 sandwich	333	17	56	1393	2	5.0	45.0	2	13%
'Classic Italian BMT'										
6-inch sub, w/o cheese, condiments	1 sandwich	450	21	45	1579	3	21.0	52.0	8	42%
super, 6-inch sub, w/o cheese, condiments	1 sandwich	668	33	47	2576	3	39.0	104.0	354	52%
'Cold Cut Trio'										
6-inch sub, w/o cheese, condiments	1 sandwich	374	19	45	1435	3	14.0	47.0	5	33%
super, 6-inch sub, w/o cheese, condiments	1 sandwich	517	29	47	2289	3	24.0	93.0	220	42%
Ham and egg										
deli style sub	1 sandwich	312	16	33	789	1	12.0	189.0	3	36%
6-inch sub	1 sandwich	352	18	41	869	3	13.0	189.0	3	33%
wrap	1 sandwich	342	10	47	1159	1	12.0	189.0	3	32%
Ham										
deli style sub, w/o cheese, condiments	1 sandwich	224	12	37	827	1	3.0	12.0	0	12%
6-inch sub, w/o cheese, condiments	1 sandwich	293	18	45	1342	3	5.0	25.0	2	15%
super, 6-inch sub, w/o cheese, condiments	1 sandwich	354	27	47	2101	3	7.0	50.0	60	18%
Meatball										
6-inch hot sub, w/o cheese, condiments	1 sandwich	413	19	50	1025	5	15.0	35.0	6	33%
super, 6-inch hot sub, w/o cheese, condiments	1 sandwich	594	30	58	1468	7	27.0	70.0	11	41%
Roast beef										
deli style sub, w/o cheese, condiments	1 sandwich	236	14	37	678	1	4.0	13.0	0	15%
6-inch sub, w/o cheese, condiments	1 sandwich	296	19	45	928	3	5.0	20.0	2	15%
super, 6-inch sub, w/o cheese, condiments	1 sandwich	360	29	47	1273	3	7.0	40.0	61	17%
Seafood and crab										
super, w/light mayo, 6-inch sub	1 sandwich	444	18	58	1486	5	15.0	27.0	137	31%
w/light mayo, 6-inch sub	1 sandwich	338	14	51	1034	4	9.0	14.0	2	24%
Steak and cheese										
6-inch hot sub	1 sandwich	363	24	47	1160	4	10.0	37.0	4	24%
super, 6-inch sub	1 sandwich	495	39	50	1739	5	17.0	75.0	8	30%
wrap	1 sandwich	353	16	53	1450	2	9.0	37.0	4	23%
'Subway Club'										
6-inch sub, w/o cheese, condiments	1 sandwich	304	21	46	1239	3	5.0	26.0	2	14%
super, 6-inch sub, w/o cheese, condiments	1 sandwich	377	32	48	1895	3	7.0	52.0	59	16%
'Subway Melt'										
6-inch hot sub	1 sandwich	370	23	46	1619	3	11.0	41.0	5	26%
super, 6-inch hot sub	1 sandwich	509	36	48	2657	3	19.0	83.0	9	34%
Tuna										
w/light mayo, deli style sub, w/o cheese, condiments	1 sandwich	267	12	37	627	1	8.0	16.0	1	27%
w/light mayo, 6-inch sub, w/o cheese, condiments	1 sandwich	378	18	45	942	3	14.0	32.0	3	33%
w/light mayo, super, 6-inch sub, w/o cheese, condiments	1 sandwich	525	27	46	1303	3	26.0	64.0	5	44%
Turkey and ham										
6-inch sub, w/o cheese, condiments	1 sandwich	288	18	45	1256	3	4.0	23.0	2	13%
super, 6-inch sub, w/o cheese, condiments	1 sandwich	343	27	47	1929	3	6.0	45.0	50	15%
Turkey bacon wrap, deluxe	1 sandwich	355	14	52	1823	1	10.0	39.0	4	25%
Turkey breast										
deli style sub, w/o cheese, condiments	1 sandwich	227	13	37	678	1	4.0	13.0	0	15%

Food Name	Serving Size	Calories	Prot. gms	Carbs gms	Sod. mgs	Fiber gms	Fat gms	Sat. Fat gms	Chol. mgs	% Fat Cal.
6-inch sub, w/o cheese, condiments	1 sandwich	282	17	45	1170	3	4.0	20.0	1	13%
super, 6-inch sub, w/o cheese, condiments	1 sandwich	333	26	47	1758	3	4.0	40.0	40	11%
'Veggie Delite' 6-inch sub, w/o cheese, condiments	1 sandwich	232	9	43	582	3	3.0	0.0	1	11%
Western egg										
deli style sub	1 sandwich	311	14	36	603	2	12.0	182.0	3	35%
6-inch sub	1 sandwich	351	16	44	683	4	12.0	182.0	3	31%
wrap	1 sandwich	341	8	50	973	2	12.0	182.0	3	32%
SWENSEN'S										
ICE CREAM										
'Almond Praline Delight' low-fat	1/2 cup	130	3	25	85	0	2.0	5.0	1	14%
caramel apple crisp, low-fat	1/2 cup	130	3	26	75	0	1.0	5.0	1	7%
caramel turtle fudge, light	1 serving	120	3	18	50	0	4.0	10.0	0	30%
caramel turtle fudge, low-fat	1/2 cup	140	3	26	70	0	2.5	5.0	1	16%
chocolate chocolate chip cheesecake, low-fat	1/2 cup	130	3	26	80	0	2.5	5.0	1	16%
chocolate fudge brownie, low-fat	1/2 cup	120	3	24	70	0	2.5	5.0	1	17%
cookies and cream, light	1 serving	130	3	20	60	0	4.0	10.0	0	28%
ice cream, cookies and cream, low-fat	1/2 cup	130	3	25	80	0	2.5	5.0	1	17%
vanilla, light	1 serving	110	3	15	50	0	4.0	10.0	0	33%
YOGURT, FROZEN										
Black Forest cake	1 serving	95	3	21	130	0	1.0	5.0	0	9%
Black Forest cake, low-fat	1/2 cup	110	4	22	55	1	1.5	0.0	1	11%
blueberry and cream, gourmet, sugar-free	1 serving	110	3	17	90	0	4.0	10.0	0	31%
butter pecan, low-fat	1/2 cup	120	4	20	55	0	3.0	5.0	1	22%
cherry, nonfat	1/2 cup	90	3	20	45	0	0.0	0.0	0	0%
chocolate raspberry truffle, gourmet, sugar-free	1 serving	130	3	18	80	0	5.0	8.0	0	35%
coconut pineapple	1 serving	120	4	26	65	0	1.0	5.0	0	7%
hazelnut amaretto, low-fat	1/2 cup	120	4	20	50	0	3.0	0.0	0	22%
mocha chip, low-fat	1/2 cup	110	4	22	50	0	1.5	0.0	1	11%
strawberry banana and cream, nonfat	1/2 cup	90	3	20	45	0	0.0	0.0	0	0%
triple chocolate, low-fat	1/2 cup	120	4	24	50	1	1.5	0.0	1	11%
triple chocolate, nonfat	1 serving	100	4	21	65	0	0.0	0.0	0	0%
vanilla Swiss almond, gourmet, sugar-free	1 serving	140	4	15	100	0	7.0	10.0	0	45%
vanilla, nonfat	1/2 cup	90	3	20	60	0	0.0	0.0	0	0%
SWISS CHALET										
CHICKEN	1/2 chicken	634	72	1	0	0	38.0	0.0	0	54%
DESSERT										
apple pie	1 serving	394	3	45	0	0	23.0	0.0	0	52%
Black Forest cake	1 piece	278	3	36	0	0	14.0	0.0	0	45%
chocolate éclair	1 serving	205	2	27	0	0	10.0	0.0	0	44%
coconut pie	1 serving	292	2	40	0	0	14.0	0.0	0	43%
fudge nut cake	1 piece	346	4	48	0	0	16.0	0.0	0	41%
vanilla ice cream	1 serving	195	3	16	0	0	14.0	0.0	0	62%
GRAVY, sandwich	1 serving	35	1	5	0	0	1.0	0.0	0	27%
ROLL	1 roll	116	3	24	0	0	1.0	0.0	0	8%
SALAD, chicken	1 salad	500	42	23	0	0	42.0	0.0	0	59%
SANDWICH										
chicken	1 sandwich	360	33	42	0	0	5.0	0.0	0	13%
chicken, hot	1 sandwich	310	30	30	0	0	6.0	0.0	0	18%
SIDE DISH										
baked potato	1 serving	227	8	52	0	0	0.0	0.0	0	0%
coleslaw, 'Chalet'	1 serving	56	2	10	0	0	1.0	0.0	0	16%
French fries	1 serving	478	10	57	0	0	24.0	0.0	0	45%
SOUP, chicken, 'Chalet'	1 serving	97	9	11	0	0	2.0	0.0	0	18%

Food Name	Serving Size	Calories	Prot. gms	Carbs gms	Sod. mgs	Fiber gms	Fat gms	Sat. Fat gms	Chol. mgs	% Fat Cal.
TCBY										
YOGURT, FROZEN										
nonfat, giant	31.6 oz	869	32	182	356	0	0.0	0.0	0	0%
nonfat, kiddie	3.2 oz	88	3	18	36	0	0.0	0.0	0	0%
nonfat, large	10.5 oz	289	10	60	118	0	0.0	0.0	0	0%
nonfat, medium	8.2 oz	226	8	47	92	0	0.0	0.0	0	0%
nonfat, small	5.9 oz	162	6	34	66	0	0.0	0.0	0	0%
nonfat, super	15.2 oz	418	15	87	171	0	0.0	0.0	0	0%
regular, giant	31.6 oz	1027	32	182	474	0	24.0	79.0	16	20%
regular, kiddie	3.2 oz	104	3	18	48	0	2.0	8.0	2	18%
regular, large	10.5 oz	342	10	60	156	0	8.0	26.0	5	20%
regular, medium	8.2 oz	267	8	47	126	0	6.0	20.0	4	20%
regular, small	5.9 oz	192	6	34	90	0	4.0	15.0	3	18%
regular, super	15.2 oz	494	15	87	228	0	11.0	38.0	8	20%
strawberry	8 oz	220	9	43	150	0	2.0	0.0	0	8%
sugarless, nonfat, giant	31.6 oz	632	32	142	316	0	0.0	0.0	0	0%
sugarless, nonfat, kiddie	3.2 oz	64	3	14	32	0	0.0	0.0	0	0%
sugarless, nonfat, large	10.5 oz	210	10	47	105	0	0.0	0.0	0	0%
sugarless, nonfat, medium	8.2 oz	164	8	37	82	0	0.0	0.0	0	0%
sugarless, nonfat, small	5.9 oz	118	6	27	59	0	0.0	0.0	0	0%
sugarless, nonfat, super	15.2 oz	304	15	68	152	0	0.0	0.0	0	0%
TACO BELL										
BURRITO										
bacon and egg, double, 6.25 oz	1 serving	480	18	39	1240	2	27.0	400.0	9	52%
bean, 7 oz	1 serving	370	13	54	1080	12	12.0	10.0	4	29%
'Big Beef Supreme' 10.5 oz	1 serving	510	23	52	1500	11	23.0	60.0	9	41%
'Big Beef' 7 oz	1 serving	400	19	43	1320	6	17.0	50.0	6	38%
'Big Chicken Supreme' 9 oz	1 serving	460	27	50	1200	3	17.0	70.0	6	33%
chicken, grilled, 7 oz	1 serving	390	19	49	1240	3	13.0	40.0	4	30%
chili cheese, 5 oz	1 serving	330	13	40	900	4	13.0	25.0	5	36%
'Country Breakfast' 4 oz	1 serving	270	8	26	690	2	14.0	195.0	5	48%
'Fiesta Breakfast' 3.5 oz	1 serving	280	9	25	580	2	16.0	25.0	6	51%
'Grande Breakfast' 6.25 oz	1 serving	420	13	43	1050	3	22.0	205.0	7	47%
7-layer, 10 oz	1 serving	520	16	65	1270	13	22.0	25.0	7	38%
'Supreme' 9 oz	1 serving	430	17	50	1210	9	18.0	40.0	7	38%
CHALUPA										
'Baja Beef' 5.5 oz	1 serving	420	14	30	760	3	27.0	35.0	7	58%
'Baja Chicken' 5.5 oz	1 serving	400	17	28	660	2	24.0	40.0	5	55%
'Baja Steak' 5.5 oz	1 serving	400	17	27	680	2	24.0	30.0	6	55%
beef, supreme, 5.5 oz	1 serving	380	14	29	580	3	23.0	40.0	8	55%
chicken, supreme, 5.5 oz	1 serving	360	17	28	490	2	20.0	45.0	7	50%
'Santa Fe Beef' 5.5 oz	1 serving	440	14	31	660	4	29.0	35.0	7	59%
'Santa Fe Chicken' 5.5 oz	1 serving	420	17	30	560	2	26.0	40.0	6	55%
'Santa Fe Steak' 5.5 oz	1 serving	430	18	29	580	2	27.0	35.0	6	56%
steak, supreme, 5.5 oz	1 serving	360	17	27	500	2	20.0	35.0	7	51%
CINNAMON TWIST, 1 oz	1 serving	180	1	25	290	1	8.0	0.0	2	41%
DESSERT, chaco taco ice cream, 4 oz	1 serving	310	3	37	100	1	17.0	20.0	10	49%
GORDITA										
'Baja Beef' 5.5 oz	1 serving	360	13	29	810	4	21.0	35.0	5	53%
'Baja Chicken' 5.5 oz	1 serving	340	16	28	710	3	18.0	40.0	4	48%
'Baja Steak' 5.5 oz	1 serving	340	17	27	730	3	18.0	30.0	4	48%
beef, supreme, 5.5 oz	1 serving	300	17	27	550	3	14.0	35.0	5	42%
chicken, supreme, 5.5 oz	1 serving	300	16	28	530	3	13.0	45.0	5	40%
'Santa Fe Beef' 5.5 oz	1 serving	380	14	31	700	5	23.0	35.0	5	53%

Food Name	Serving Size	Calories	Prot. gms	Carbs gms	Sod. mgs	Fiber gms	Fat gms	Sat. Fat gms	Chol. mgs	% Fat Cal.
'Santa Fe Chicken' 5.5 oz	1 serving	370	17	30	610	3	20.0	40.0	4	49%
'Santa Fe Steak' 5.5 oz	1 serving	370	17	29	620	3	20.0	35.0	5	49%
steak, supreme, 5.5 oz	1 serving	300	17	27	550	3	14.0	35.0	5	42%
MEXIMELT, big beef, 4.75 oz	1 serving	290	15	22	830	4	15.0	45.0	7	48%
NACHOS										
'Bellegrande' 11 oz	1 serving	760	20	83	1300	17	39.0	35.0	11	46%
'Big Beef Supreme' 7 oz	1 serving	440	14	44	800	9	24.0	35.0	7	48%
chicken, 'Bellegrande' 11 oz	1 serving	740	23	82	1200	15	36.0	40.0	9	44%
regular, 3.5 oz	1 serving	320	5	34	560	3	18.0	5.0	4	51%
steak, 'Bellegrande' 11 oz	1 serving	740	24	81	1220	15	37.0	35.0	9	44%
PIZZA										
Mexican, 7.75 oz	1 serving	540	20	42	1030	7	35.0	45.0	10	56%
Mexican beef, 7.75 oz	1 serving	530	24	39	950	6	33.0	45.0	9	54%
Mexican chicken, 7.75 oz	1 serving	520	23	41	940	6	32.0	50.0	8	53%
QUESADILLA										
cheese, 4.25 oz	1 serving	350	16	31	860	3	18.0	50.0	9	46%
cheese, breakfast, 5.5 oz	1 serving	380	15	33	1010	1	21.0	280.0	9	50%
chicken, 6 oz	1 serving	400	25	33	1050	3	19.0	75.0	9	42%
w/bacon, breakfast, 6 oz	1 serving	450	19	33	1200	2	27.0	290.0	11	54%
w/sausage, breakfast, 6 oz	1 serving	430	17	33	1090	1	25.0	285.0	10	53%
SALAD										
taco, w/salsa, 19 oz	1 salad	850	30	69	2250	16	52.0	70.0	14	54%
taco, w/salsa, w/o shell, 16.5 oz	1 salad	430	25	36	1990	15	22.0	70.0	10	45%
SIDE DISH										
hash brown nuggets, 3.5 oz	1 serving	280	2	29	570	1	18.0	0.0	5	57%
Mexican rice, 4.75 oz	1 serving	190	5	23	750	1	9.0	15.0	4	42%
pintos and cheese, 4.5 oz	1 serving	180	9	18	640	10	8.0	15.0	4	40%
TACO										
'Double Decker' 5.75 oz	1 serving	330	14	37	740	9	15.0	30.0	5	40%
'Double Decker Supreme' 7 oz	1 serving	380	15	39	760	9	18.0	40.0	7	43%
'Supreme' 4 oz	1 serving	210	9	14	350	3	14.0	40.0	6	58%
grilled chicken, soft, 4.5 oz	1 serving	200	14	20	530	2	7.0	35.0	3	32%
grilled steak, soft, 4.5 oz	1 serving	200	14	19	570	2	7.0	25.0	3	32%
grilled steak, soft, 'Supreme' 5.75 oz	1 serving	240	15	21	580	2	11.0	35.0	5	41%
regular, 2.75 oz	1 serving	170	9	12	340	3	10.0	30.0	4	52%
soft, 'Supreme' 5 oz	1 serving	260	11	22	590	3	13.0	40.0	6	47%
soft, 3.5 oz	1 serving	210	11	20	570	3	10.0	30.0	4	42%
TOSTADA, 6.25 oz	1 serving	250	10	27	640	11	12.0	15.0	5	42%

TACO JOHN'S

Food Name	Serving Size	Calories	Prot. gms	Carbs gms	Sod. mgs	Fiber gms	Fat gms	Sat. Fat gms	Chol. mgs	% Fat Cal.
BURRITO										
bean	5 oz	249	10	36	636	0	6.0	0.0	0	23%
beef	5 oz	355	16	25	666	0	18.0	0.0	0	50%
chicken, super, w/o sour cream, cheese	1 serving	366	30	40	844	0	14.0	0.0	0	31%
chicken, w/o sour cream, cheese	1 serving	227	27	19	639	0	10.0	0.0	0	33%
combination	5 oz	302	11	30	651	0	12.0	0.0	0	40%
super	8.3 oz	434	17	66	1022	0	11.0	0.0	0	23%
super, w/o sour cream, cheese	1 serving	389	18	51	856	0	16.0	0.0	0	34%
Texas chili	12.3 oz	518	23	48	746	0	24.0	0.0	0	43%
w/green chili	12.3 oz	405	18	38	995	0	24.0	0.0	0	49%
w/green chili, w/o sour cream, cheese	1 serving	367	20	40	998	0	18.0	0.0	0	40%
CHILI, Texas	9.5 oz	430	23	35	1580	0	22.0	0.0	0	46%
CHIMICHANGA	12 oz	487	16	54	1226	0	19.0	0.0	0	38%
ENCHILADA	7 oz	379	19	33	431	0	18.0	0.0	0	44%

Food Name	Serving Size	Calories	Prot. gms	Carbs gms	Sod. mgs	Fiber gms	Fat gms	Sat. Fat gms	Chol. mgs	% Fat Cal.
NACHOS										
regular	4 oz	407	11	42	307	0	19.0	0.0	0	45%
super	11.25 oz	657	23	57	857	0	34.0	0.0	0	49%
PASTRY										
'Apple Grande' Danish	3 oz	257	5	44	231	0	8.0	0.0	0	27%
churro	1.2 oz	122	2	12	153	0	7.0	0.0	0	53%
SALAD										
chicken taco, super, w/o dressing, sour cream	1 salad	377	26	56	882	0	15.0	0.0	0	29%
taco, w/o shell, dressing, sour cream, cheese	1 salad	228	13	30	440	0	13.0	0.0	0	40%
taco, super	12.3 oz	450	16	48	880	0	18.0	0.0	0	39%
SANDWICH, chicken fillet, 'Sierra'	8.5 oz	500	31	46	1493	23	21.0	41.0	0	38%
SIDE DISH										
'Potato Ole' large	6 oz	414	6	96	1595	0	6.0	0.0	0	12%
refried beans	9.5 oz	331	19	79	1195	0	6.0	0.0	0	12%
Mexican rice	1 serving	340	7	59	1280	0	8.0	0.0	0	21%
TACO										
'Taco Bravo' w/o sour cream	1 serving	319	16	42	658	0	14.0	0.0	0	35%
'Taco Bravo' super	8 oz	485	18	51	1006	0	20.0	0.0	0	39%
chicken, soft shell	1 serving	180	18	20	490	0	8.0	0.0	0	32%
regular	4.3 oz	228	11	15	347	0	13.0	0.0	0	53%
soft	5 oz	276	13	23	505	0	13.0	0.0	0	45%
TACOBURGER	6 oz	332	14	31	660	0	14.0	0.0	0	41%
TOSTADA	4.3 oz	228	11	15	347	0	13.0	0.0	0	53%
TACO TIME										
BEEF, shredded	2.5 oz	70	1	1	31	0	0.0	0.0	0	0%
BURRITO										
bean, crisp	5.25 oz	427	15	53	453	9	18.0	12.0	5	37%
bean, soft, double	9.5 oz	506	23	77	860	19	12.0	22.0	6	21%
bean, soft, single, 'Value'	6.75 oz	380	16	58	715	13	10.0	15.0	4	23%
chicken, crisp	4.75 oz	422	17	32	795	2	25.0	54.0	8	53%
combination, soft, double	9.5 oz	617	39	66	1343	18	23.0	63.0	10	33%
meat, 'Casita'	12 oz	647	40	54	1233	16	31.0	89.0	15	43%
meat, crisp	5.25 oz	552	34	39	1000	7	30.0	58.0	10	48%
meat, soft, double	9.5 oz	726	57	55	1809	17	33.0	99.0	14	40%
meat, soft, single, 'Value'	6.75 oz	491	31	48	1197	12	21.0	56.0	8	37%
veggie	11 oz	491	21	70	643	10	16.0	24.0	6	28%
CHEESE, Cheddar	0.75 oz	86	5	0	132	0	7.0	22.0	4	76%
CHEESEBURGER, taco, meat	7.5 oz	633	31	48	1291	7	36.0	66.0	10	51%
CHICKEN	2.5 oz	109	11	2	402	0	6.0	33.0	2	51%
CHIPS	2 oz	266	4	35	461	3	12.0	0.0	3	41%
CRUSTOS	3.5 oz	373	9	47	86	na	15.0	0.0	na	38%
CONDIMENTS										
enchilada sauce	1 oz	12	0	3	133	1	0.0	0.0	0	0%
guacamole	1 oz	29	0	2	94	1	2.0	0.0	0	69%
hot sauce	1 oz	10	0	2	120	0	0.0	0.0	0	0%
salad dressing, sour cream	1.5 oz	137	1	2	207	0	14.0	8.0	5	91%
salad dressing, Thousand Island	1 oz	160	0	4	220	0	16.0	10.0	2	90%
salsa, ranchero	2 oz	21	1	3	192	1	1.0	0.0	0	36%
sour cream	1 oz	55	1	1	11	0	5.0	19.0	3	85%
EMPANADA, cherry	4 oz	250	5	37	46	na	9.0	0.0	na	33%
LETTUCE	0.5 oz	2	0	0	1	0	0.0	0.0	0	0%
NACHOS										
deluxe	15.25 oz	1048	46	91	2252	17	57.0	109.0	23	48%
regular	10.5 oz	680	26	61	1250	11	38.0	78.0	19	50%

Food Name	Serving Size	Calories	Prot. gms	Carbs gms	Sod. mgs	Fiber gms	Fat gms	Sat. Fat gms	Chol. mgs	% Fat Cal.
QUESADILLA, cheese	3.25 oz	205	11	17	255	1	11.0	30.0	6	47%
SALAD										
chicken taco, w/o dressing	9 oz	370	19	27	861	3	21.0	48.0	7	51%
taco, regular, w/o dressing	7.5 oz	479	30	30	895	7	28.0	63.0	11	51%
'Tostada Delight' w/meat	9.75 oz	628	36	48	1004	13	33.0	82.0	14	47%
SIDE DISH										
French fries, 'Mexi'	8 oz	532	6	54	1598	na	34.0	0.0	na	56%
French fries, 'Mexi' regular	4 oz	266	3	27	799	na	17.0	0.0	na	56%
Refritos	7 oz	326	18	44	525	13	10.0	22.0	5	27%
Mexican rice	4 oz	159	3	30	530	1	2.0	0.0	1	12%
TACO										
chicken, soft	7 oz	387	21	41	933	7	16.0	48.0	6	37%
crisp	4 oz	295	22	16	609	5	17.0	48.0	7	50%
flour, soft, rolled	7 oz	512	33	46	1111	12	23.0	63.0	10	40%
meat	2.5 oz	208	22	7	576	5	11.0	38.0	4	46%
meat, natural, 'Super'	11.25 oz	627	41	60	915	14	27.0	82.0	13	38%
shredded beef, soft, 'Super'	8 oz	368	12	38	556	7	11.0	22.0	6	33%
soft, 'Value'	5.25 oz	316	24	23	599	5	15.0	48.0	7	42%
TACO SHELL, 6-inch	1.25 oz	110	2	14	48	2	6.0	0.0	1	46%
TOMATO	0.5 oz	3	0	1	1	0	0.0	0.0	0	0%
TORTILLA										
flour, 10-inch	2.75 oz	213	6	31	393	6	4.0	0.0	1	20%
flour, 8-inch	1.25 oz	107	5	16	33	2	3.0	0.0	1	24%
flour, 7-inch	1.75 oz	88	4	16	42	1	1.0	0.0	0	10%
flour, fried, 10-inch	2.75 oz	318	6	37	315	2	16.0	0.0	4	46%
flour, fried, 8-inch	1.3 oz	205	4	24	203	1	11.0	0.0	2	47%
wheat, 11-inch	3.5 oz	175	8	33	84	2	3.0	0.0	1	14%
WENDY'S										
BACON	1 slice	20	2	0	65	0	1.5	5.0	0	63%
BEVERAGE										
coffee	6 fl oz	0	0	1	0	0	0.0	0.0	0	0%
coffee, decaffeinated	6 fl oz	0	0	1	0	0	0.0	0.0	0	0%
cola, diet, small	8 fl oz	0	0	0	20	0	0.0	0.0	0	0%
cola, small	8 fl oz	90	0	24	10	0	0.0	0.0	0	0%
'Frosty' large	20 oz	540	14	91	320	0	14.0	60.0	9	23%
'Frosty' medium	16 oz	440	11	73	260	0	11.0	50.0	7	23%
'Frosty' small	12 oz	330	8	56	200	0	8.0	35.0	5	22%
hot chocolate	6 fl oz	80	1	15	135	0	3.0	0.0	0	30%
lemonade, small	8 fl oz	90	0	24	5	0	0.0	0.0	0	0%
lemon-lime soft drink	8 fl oz	90	0	24	25	0	0.0	0.0	0	0%
milk, 2%	8 fl oz	110	8	11	115	0	4.0	15.0	3	32%
tea, hot or iced	6 fl oz	0	0	0	0	0	0.0	0.0	0	0%
BREAD, pita, 'Classic Greek'	1 pita	440	15	50	1050	4	20.0	35.0	8	41%
BREADSTICK, soft	1 stick	130	4	23	250	1	3.0	5.0	1	20%
BUN										
Kaiser	1 bun	190	6	36	340	2	3.0	0.0	1	14%
sandwich	1 bun	160	5	29	280	2	2.5	0.0	1	14%
CHEESE										
American	1 slice	70	3	1	320	0	5.0	15.0	4	74%
American, junior	1 slice	45	2	0	220	0	3.5	10.0	3	80%
Cheddar, shredded	2 tbsp	70	4	1	110	0	6.0	15.0	4	73%
imitation, shredded, salad bar item	2 tbsp	50	3	1	260	0	4.0	0.0	1	69%

Food Name	Serving Size	Calories	Prot. gms	Carbs gms	Sod. mgs	Fiber gms	Fat gms	Sat. Fat gms	Chol. mgs	% Fat Cal.
CHEESEBURGER										
junior	1 burger	320	17	34	830	2	13.0	45.0	6	36%
bacon, junior	1 burger	380	20	34	850	2	19.0	60.0	7	44%
deluxe, junior	1 burger	360	18	36	890	3	17.0	50.0	6	41%
kid's meal	1 burger	320	17	33	830	2	13.0	45.0	6	37%
CHICKEN										
fillet, breaded	1 piece	230	22	10	490	0	12.0	55.0	3	46%
fillet, grilled	1 fillet	110	22	0	450	0	3.0	60.0	1	23%
fillet, spicy	1 piece	210	22	10	920	0	9.0	60.0	2	39%
nuggets, fried	5 pieces	210	14	7	460	0	14.0	45.0	3	60%
nuggets, fried	4 pieces	170	11	5	370	0	11.0	35.0	3	61%
CHILI										
large	12 oz	310	23	32	1190	7	10.0	45.0	4	29%
small	8 oz	210	15	21	800	5	7.0	30.0	3	30%
CONDIMENTS. See also Salad Dressing.										
bacon bits, salad bar item	2 tbsp	45	6	0	550	0	2.5	10.0	1	48%
barbecue sauce	1 packet	45	1	10	160	0	0.0	0.0	0	0%
buffalo wing sauce, spicy	1 packet	25	0	4	210	0	1.0	0.0	0	36%
catsup	1 tsp	10	0	2	75	0	0.0	0.0	0	0%
croutons, salad bar item	2 tbsp	14	1	4	65	0	1.0	0.0	0	31%
honey mustard sauce	1 packet	130	0	6	220	0	12.0	10.0	2	82%
honey mustard, lower calorie	1 tsp	25	0	2	45	0	1.5	0.0	0	63%
lettuce	1 leaf	0	0	0	0	0	0.0	0.0	0	0%
lettuce, iceberg/Romaine, salad bar item	1 cup	10	0	2	5	1	0.0	0.0	0	0%
margarine, whipped	1 packet	60	0	0	115	0	7.0	0.0	2	100%
mayonnaise	1 tsp	30	0	1	60	0	3.0	5.0	0	87%
mustard	1 tsp	0	0	0	50	0	0.0	0.0	0	0%
onion, red, sliced, salad bar item	3 rings	0	0	1	0	0	0.0	0.0	0	0%
onion, sliced	4 rings	5	0	1	0	0	0.0	0.0	0	0%
Parmesan blend, grated, salad bar item	2 tbsp	70	4	5	290	0	4.0	10.0	2	50%
pepperoni, sliced, salad bar item	6 slices	30	1	0	70	0	3.0	5.0	1	87%
pickle	4 slices	0	0	0	140	0	0.0	0.0	0	0%
salad oil	1 tbsp	120	0	0	0	0	14.0	0.0	2	100%
sour cream	1 packet	60	1	1	15	0	6.0	10.0	4	87%
sunflower seeds and raisins, salad bar item	2 tbsp	80	0	5	0	1	5.0	0.0	1	69%
sweet and sour sauce	1 packet	50	0	12	120	0	0.0	0.0	0	0%
tomato, sliced	1 slice	5	0	1	0	0	0.0	0.0	0	0%
tomato, wedges, salad bar item	1 piece	5	0	1	0	0	0.0	0.0	0	0%
turkey ham, diced, salad bar item	2 tbsp	50	3	0	280	0	4.0	25.0	1	75%
COOKIE, chocolate chip	1 cookie	270	3	36	120	1	13.0	30.0	6	43%
CRACKERS, saltine	2 crackers	25	1	4	80	0	0.5	0.0	0	18%
HAMBURGER										
'Big Bacon Classic'	1 burger	580	34	46	1460	3	30.0	100.0	12	46%
junior	1 burger	270	15	34	610	2	10.0	30.0	4	31%
kid's meal	1 burger	270	15	33	610	2	10.0	30.0	4	32%
single, plain	1 burger	360	24	31	580	2	16.0	65.0	6	40%
w/everything	1 burger	420	25	37	920	3	20.0	70.0	7	42%
HAMBURGER PATTY										
regular	2 oz	100	9	0	150	0	7.0	30.0	3	64%
quarter-pound	0.25 lb	200	19	0	290	0	14.0	65.0	6	62%
SALAD										
Caesar, side	1 salad	100	8	8	620	1	4.0	10.0	2	36%
chicken Caesar	1 salad	260	26	17	1170	2	9.0	60.0	3	32%
chicken, grilled	1 salad	200	25	9	720	3	8.0	50.0	2	35%

Food Name	Serving Size	Calories	Prot. gms	Carbs gms	Sod. mgs	Fiber gms	Fat gms	Sat. Fat gms	Chol. mgs	% Fat Cal.
garden, deluxe	1 salad	110	7	9	350	3	6.0	0.0	1	46%
side	1 salad	60	4	5	180	2	3.0	0.0	0	43%
taco	1 salad	380	26	28	1040	7	19.0	65.0	10	44%
SALAD DRESSING										
blue cheese	2 tbsp	180	1	0	180	0	19.0	15.0	4	98%
Caesar vinaigrette, pita dressing	1 tbsp	70	0	1	170	0	7.0	0.0	1	94%
French	2 tbsp	120	0	6	330	0	10.0	0.0	2	79%
French, nonfat	2 tbsp	35	0	8	150	0	0.0	0.0	0	0%
garden ranch, pita dressing	1 tbsp	50	0	1	125	0	4.5	10.0	1	91%
Italian Caesar	2 tbsp	150	1	1	240	0	16.0	20.0	3	95%
Italian, reduced fat	2 tbsp	40	0	2	340	0	3.0	0.0	0	77%
ranch, 'Hidden Valley'	2 tbsp	100	1	1	220	0	10.0	10.0	2	92%
ranch, reduced fat, 'Hidden Valley'	2 tbsp	60	1	2	240	0	5.0	10.0	1	79%
Thousand Island	2 tbsp	90	0	2	125	0	8.0	10.0	2	90%
wine vinegar	1 tbsp	0	0	0	0	0	0.0	0.0	0	0%
SANDWICH										
chicken, breaded	1 sandwich	440	28	44	840	2	18.0	60.0	4	36%
chicken, grilled	1 sandwich	310	27	35	790	2	8.0	65.0	2	23%
chicken, spicy	1 sandwich	410	28	43	1280	2	15.0	65.0	3	32%
chicken Caesar pita	1 pita	490	34	48	1320	4	18.0	65.0	5	33%
chicken club	1 sandwich	470	31	44	970	2	20.0	70.0	4	38%
'Garden Ranch Chicken Pita'	1 pita	480	30	51	1180	5	18.0	70.0	4	33%
'Garden Veggie Pita'	1 pita	400	11	52	760	5	17.0	20.0	4	38%
SIDE DISH										
applesauce, salad bar item	2 tbsp	30	0	7	0	0	0.0	0.0	0	0%
baked potato, plain	10 oz	310	7	71	25	7	0.0	0.0	0	0%
baked potato, w/bacon and cheese	1 serving	530	17	78	1390	7	18.0	20.0	4	30%
baked potato, w/broccoli and cheese	1 serving	470	9	80	470	9	14.0	5.0	3	26%
baked potato, w/cheese	1 serving	570	14	78	640	7	23.0	30.0	8	36%
baked potato, w/chili and cheese	1 serving	630	20	83	770	9	24.0	40.0	9	34%
baked potato, w/sour cream and chives	1 serving	380	8	74	40	8	6.0	15.0	4	14%
cantaloupe, sliced, salad bar item	1 piece	15	0	4	0	0	0.0	0.0	0	0%
chicken salad, salad bar item	2 tbsp	70	4	2	135	0	5.0	0.0	1	65%
cottage cheese, salad bar item	2 tbsp	30	4	1	125	0	1.5	5.0	1	40%
cucumbers, salad bar item	2 slices	0	0	0	0	0	0.0	0.0	0	0%
egg, hard cooked, salad bar item	2 tbsp	40	3	0	30	0	3.0	110.0	1	69%
French fries, 'Biggie'	5.6 oz	470	6	61	150	6	23.0	0.0	4	44%
French fries, 'Great Biggie'	6.7 oz	570	8	73	180	7	27.0	0.0	4	43%
French fries, small	3.2 oz	270	4	35	85	3	13.0	0.0	2	43%
green peas, salad bar item	2 tbsp	15	1	3	25	1	0.0	0.0	0	0%
green peppers, salad bar item	2 pieces	0	0	1	0	0	0.0	0.0	0	0%
orange, sliced, salad bar item	2 slices	15	0	4	0	1	0.0	0.0	0	0%
pasta salad, salad bar item	2 tbsp	35	1	4	180	1	1.5	0.0	0	40%
peaches, sliced, salad bar item	1 piece	15	0	4	0	0	0.0	0.0	0	0%
potato salad, salad bar item	2 tbsp	80	0	5	180	0	7.0	5.0	3	76%
watermelon, wedges, salad bar item	1 piece	20	0	4	0	0	0.0	0.0	0	0%
TACO CHIPS	15 chips	210	3	24	180	2	11.0	0.0	2	48%
WHATABURGER										
BACON	1 slice	38	2	0	106	na	3.3	6.0	na	79%
BEVERAGE										
'Cherry Coke' medium	1 serving	227	0	60	11	na	0.0	0.0	na	0%
chocolate shake, junior	1 serving	364	9	61	172	na	9.3	36.0	na	23%
'Coca Cola Classic' medium	1 serving	211	0	56	19	na	0.0	0.0	na	0%
coffee, small	1 serving	5	0	1	5	na	0.0	0.0	na	0%

Food Name	Serving Size	Calories	Prot. gms	Carbs gms	Sod. mgs	Fiber gms	Fat gms	Sat. Fat gms	Chol. mgs	% Fat Cal.
'Diet Coke' medium	1 serving	2	0	1	26	na	0.0	0.0	na	0%
'Dr. Pepper' medium	1 serving	207	0	52	51	na	0.0	0.0	na	0%
iced tea, 'Lipton" medium	1 serving	5	0	2	15	na	0.0	0.0	na	0%
orange juice, 'Tropicana'	10 fl oz	140	2	33	0	na	0.0	0.0	na	0%
milk, 2%	1 serving	113	8	11	113	na	4.3	18.0	na	34%
'Sprite' medium	1 serving	211	0	48	45	na	0.0	0.0	na	0%
strawberry shake, junior	1 serving	352	9	60	168	na	8.9	35.0	na	23%
root beer, medium	1 serving	237	0	63	25	na	0.0	0.0	na	0%
vanilla shake, junior	1 serving	325	9	51	172	na	9.5	37.0	na	26%
BISCUIT, plain	1 serving	280	5	37	509	na	13.4	3.0	na	42%
BREAKFAST										
bacon biscuit	1 sandwich	359	10	37	730	na	20.2	15.0	na	50%
bacon, egg, and cheese biscuit	1 sandwich	511	18	38	1010	na	32.9	213.0	na	57%
'Breakfast on a Bun' w/bacon biscuit	1 sandwich	365	18	29	815	na	19.4	210.0	na	48%
'Breakfast on a Bun' w/sausage biscuit	1 sandwich	455	20	30	886	na	28.1	232.0	na	56%
cinnamon roll	1 serving	320	4	39	190	na	16.0	10.0	na	46%
egg and cheese biscuit	1 sandwich	434	14	38	797	na	26.3	202.0	na	54%
egg omelet sandwich	1 sandwich	288	13	29	602	na	12.8	198.0	na	40%
pancake	3 pancakes	259	11	40	842	na	5.8	0.0	na	21%
pancake, 3 pancakes w/2 slices bacon	1 serving	335	15	40	1074	na	12.4	12.0	na	34%
pancake, 3 pancakes w/1 sausage patty	1 serving	426	18	40	1127	na	21.1	34.0	na	45%
platter, w/bacon, scrambled eggs, biscuit, hash browns	1 serving	695	22	54	1162	na	44.0	389.0	na	57%
platter, w/sausage, scrambled eggs, biscuit, hash browns	1 serving	785	25	54	1234	na	52.7	412.0	na	60%
sausage and gravy biscuit	1 sandwich	479	9	48	1253	na	27.4	20.0	na	52%
sausage biscuit	1 sandwich	446	12	37	794	na	28.7	37.0	na	57%
sausage, egg, and cheese biscuit	1 sandwich	601	21	38	1081	na	41.6	236.0	na	62%
toast, Texas	1 slice	147	4	22	250	na	4.5	0.0	na	28%
CHEESE, large slice	1 slice	89	5	0	338	na	7.4	22.0	na	75%
CHICKEN STRIPS	2 strips	300	16	15	630	na	20.0	35.0	na	59%
COOKIE										
chocolate chunk	1 serving	247	4	28	75	na	16.0	36.0	na	53%
white chocolate macadamia nut	1 serving	269	3	31	80	na	16.0	34.0	na	51%
FAJITA										
beef	1 serving	326	22	34	670	na	11.9	28.0	na	33%
chicken, grilled	1 serving	272	18	35	691	na	6.7	33.0	na	22%
GRAVY, peppered	3 oz	75	0	8	375	na	4.5	0.0	na	57%
HAMBURGER										
'Justaburger'	1 burger	298	15	30	598	na	13.0	42.0	na	39%
'Whataburger'	1 burger	598	30	61	1096	na	26.0	84.0	na	39%
'Whataburger' double meat	1 burger	823	49	62	1298	na	42.4	168.0	na	46%
'Whataburger' on small bun, w/o oil	1 burger	407	25	34	839	na	18.8	84.0	na	42%
'Whataburger Jr.'	1 burger	322	16	35	603	na	13.3	42.0	na	37%
MUFFIN, blueberry	1 serving	239	6	36	538	na	7.9	0.0	na	30%
SALAD										
garden	1 salad	56	3	11	32	na	0.6	0.0	na	9%
chicken, grilled	1 salad	150	23	14	434	na	1.2	49.0	na	7%
SANDWICH										
chicken, grilled	1 sandwich	442	34	48	1103	na	14.2	66.0	na	28%
chicken, grilled, on small white bun, w/mustard, w/o oil, dressing	1 sandwich	300	33	35	994	na	3.2	66.0	na	10%
chicken, grilled, w/o dressing	1 sandwich	385	34	46	989	na	8.5	66.0	na	19%
chicken, grilled, w/o dressing, oil	1 sandwich	358	34	46	989	na	5.5	66.0	na	13%
fish, 'Whatacatch'	1 sandwich	467	18	43	636	na	25.0	33.0	na	48%

Food Name	Serving Size	Calories	Prot. gms	Carbs gms	Sod. mgs	Fiber gms	Fat gms	Sat. Fat gms	Chol. mgs	% Fat Cal.
SIDE DISH										
French fries, junior	1 serving	221	4	25	139	na	12.1	0.0	na	49%
French fries, large	1 serving	442	7	49	227	na	24.2	0.0	na	49%
French fries, regular	1 serving	332	5	37	208	na	18.1	0.0	na	49%
onion rings, large	1 serving	498	8	51	893	na	28.7	0.0	na	52%
onion rings, regular	1 serving	329	5	34	596	na	19.1	0.0	na	52%
TAQUITO										
bacon and egg	1 serving	335	15	32	761	na	16.1	286.0	na	44%
potato and egg	1 serving	446	14	48	883	na	21.8	281.0	na	44%
sausage and egg	1 serving	443	20	32	790	na	25.9	315.0	na	53%
TURNOVER, apple, fried	1 serving	215	2	27	241	na	10.8	0.0	na	45%
WHITE CASTLE										
BEVERAGE										
chocolate shake	14 fl oz	220	8	32	140	0	7.0	25.0	1	28%
'Coca Cola Classic'	14 fl oz	120	0	32	12	0	0.0	0.0	0	0%
coffee, black, small	1 serving	6	0	1	5	0	0.0	0.0	0	0%
'Diet Coke'	14 fl oz	1	0	0	13	0	0.0	0.0	0	0%
tea, iced	14 fl oz	45	0	12	15	0	0.0	0.0	0	0%
vanilla shake	14 fl oz	230	8	35	150	0	7.0	25.0	1	27%
BREAKFAST, egg, sausage, cheese on bun	1 sandwich	340	14	17	900	0	25.0	130.0	10	64%
CHEESEBURGER										
double patty	1 sandwich	285	14	16	430	5	18.0	30.0	8	57%
regular	1 sandwich	160	7	11	250	2	9.0	15.0	4	53%
w/bacon	1 sandwich	200	10	12	400	3	13.0	25.0	6	57%
CHICKEN RINGS	6 rings	310	16	14	620	0	21.0	70.0	4	61%
CHILI	12 oz	375	30	45	1635	0	15.0	0.0	0	31%
HAMBURGER										
double	1 burger	235	11	16	200	4	14.0	20.0	6	54%
regular	1 burger	135	6	11	135	2	7.0	10.0	3	48%
SANDWICH										
chicken	1 sandwich	190	8	21	360	0	8.0	20.0	2	38%
fish	1 sandwich	160	8	18	220	0	6.0	15.0	1	34%
SIDE DISH										
cheese sticks	3 sticks	290	15	19	730	0	17.0	0.0	5	53%
French fries, small	1 serving	115	0	15	15	2	6.0	0.0	1	47%
onion rings	8 rings	540	8	69	1300	0	26.0	0.0	0	43%